Drug compatibility chart (Y-site / syringe compatibility). Column headers (left to right): insulin (regular); isoproterenol; lactated Ringer's; lidocaine; methylprednisolone sodium succinate; mezlocillin; midazolam; morphine sulfate; nafcillin; norepinephrine; normal saline solution; ondansetron; oxacillin; oxytocin; penicillin G potassium; phenylephrine; phenytoin; phytonadione; piperacillin; potassium chloride; procainamide; ranitidine; sodium; ticarcil; tobran; vanco; verap.

Drug (row)	insulin (regular)	isoproterenol	lactated Ringer's	lidocaine	methylprednisolone sod. succ.	mezlocillin	midazolam	morphine sulfate	nafcillin	norepinephrine	normal saline sol.	ondansetron	oxacillin	oxytocin	penicillin G potassium	phenylephrine	phenytoin	phytonadione	piperacillin	potassium chloride	procainamide	ranitidine	sodium	ticarcil	tobran	vanco	verap
acyclovir			4		4			4	4				4		4			4	4			4	4	4	4		
albumin																											
amikacin			24			24	4		24	24	4	8		8				24		4		24	24			24	24
aminophylline			24	24	?			24		24									4		24	24					
amiodarone	24	24		24			24	24		24	24					4	24			24	24				4	4	24
ampicillin	2						4		8								3	4	?	?			?				?
calcium gluconate			24	24			24			24									4					1		48	
cefazolin	2		24				24	4		24	4							?					?		?	24	
cefoxitin	24		24					4		24	4									24		24				24	
ceftazidime							4		24	4							?	6								24	
cimetidine	24	24		24	24		24			48	4			24			24		24						24	24	
ciprofloxacin		48	24		24													24	24		24			24		24	
clindamycin			24		24		24	4		24	4			24				48	24	?	24		48			24	
dexamethasone sodium phosphate							4			4									4	24	4					24	
dextrose 5% in water (D5W)		24		24	?	24			24	24			48	6	6	24		24	24	24	48	24	24	24	24	24	24
D5W in lactated Ringer's		24		24						24			24		24				24							24	
D5W in normal saline solution		24		24	?			24			48	?		24			24	24		24		48				24	
diazepam																						?					24
diphenhydramine							4	¼			4			24					4	1							24
dobutamine		24	24	24			4	4		24	24					24			?	24	48					24	
dopamine		48	24	18			4	4			48		24						24	48						24	
epinephrine		24					4	4		4	24					3		4	24							24	
erythromycin lactobionate		18					24	4		22								24	24	24						24	24
esmolol		24				24	8	24	24	4				24	24		24	24	24					24	24	24	24
gentamicin	2		24				24	1		24	4				1					24							24
heparin sodium	2	24		24	?		24	1			4	4	4	?		4	6	24	4	24	24	6					24
hydrocortisone sodium succinate	4	4	24		?		4			24	4	4				4	24		4	24	3	2	2	2			48
insulin (regular)			24				24	1			4				2					4		24	3	2			24
isoproterenol			24													24					24						24
lactated Ringer's		24		24	?	72		24				24		24			24	24				24	24				24
lidocaine	24		24				4	48		24					24					24	24	24					48
methylprednisolone sodium succinate		?			24	4		?				24						?	48	2							24
mezlocillin		72						48																			24
midazolam	24			24		24		24							24	24								24	24		24
morphine sulfate	1		4	4		24		4	4		4		4	1	4			4	4		1	3	4	1		4	24
nafcillin		24	48				4	24			24								24		24						24
norepinephrine			24				24	4		24								4			24						24
normal saline solution		24		24	?	48		24	24			48	24		24				24	24	24	48	24	24	48	24	24
ondansetron				24	4					48									4	4			4		4		24
oxacillin		24					4			4																	24
oxytocin	2							1											4		24						24
penicillin G potassium		24		24			4			24									24		24						24
phenylephrine																			24		24						48
phenytoin																			24		24						48
phytonadione																			4		24						24
piperacillin		24		24	4		24											24		4							24
potassium chloride	4		24		?		24	4		24	4		4		4		24		4		24	4	48	24			24
procainamide			24							24											4		24				48
ranitidine	24	24		24	48			1		4	48	4					24				4	48	24		24	24	24
sodium bicarbonate	3		24	2			3	24			24			24		24	24	24									
ticarcillin	2		24								24	4											24				24
tobramycin	2		24				24	1			48											24					24
vancomycin	2							24	4			24	4									24					24
verapamil	48	24	24	48	24			24			24	24					24	24		48		24	24	24	24	24	

Springhouse
Nurse's
Drug Guide
2007

EIGHTH EDITION

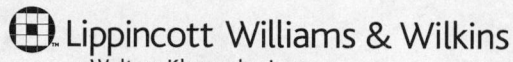

Lippincott Williams & Wilkins
a Wolters Kluwer business
Philadelphia · Baltimore · New York · London
Buenos Aires · Hong Kong · Sydney · Tokyo

Staff

Executive Publisher
Judith A. Schilling McCann, RN, MSN

Editorial Director
William J. Kelly

Clinical Director
Joan M. Robinson, RN, MSN

Senior Art Director
Arlene Putterman

Art Director
Elaine Kasmer

Clinical Manager
Eileen Cassin Gallen, RN, BSN

Electronic Project Manager
John Macalino

Editorial Project Manager
Christiane L. Brownell, ELS

Clinical Project Manager
Carol A. Saunderson, RN, BA, BS

Editors
Toby Brener, Rita Doyle, Catherine E. Harold,
Patricia Nale

Clinical Editors
Lisa Morris Bonsall, RN, MSN, CRNP;
Christine M. Damico, RN, MSN, CPNP;
Shari A. Regina-Cammon, RN, MSN, CCRN;
Kimberly Zalewski, RN, MSN

Copy Editor
Jenifer F. Walker

Digital Composition Services
Diane Paluba (manager), Joyce Rossi Biletz,
Donald G. Knauss

Manufacturing
Beth J. Welsh

Editorial Assistants
Megan Aldinger, Karen Kirk, Linda Ruhf

Indexer
Deborah Tourtlotte

Visit our Web site at eDrugInfo.com

SNDG07010606
ISBN 1-58255-932-5
ISSN 1088-8063

Contents

Contributors and consultants

At the time of publication, the contributors and consultants held the following positions.

Elizabeth A. Archer, EdD, RN
Associate Professor
Baptist College of Health Sciences
Memphis, Tenn.

Dana Bartlett, RN, MSN, MA
Poison Information Specialist
Philadelphia Poison Control Center

Tricia Berry, PharmD, BCPS
Associate Professor of Pharmacy Practice
St. Louis College of Pharmacy

Jennalie Blackwood, PharmD
Clinical Infusion Pharmacist
Interlock Pharmacy
Florissant, Mo.

Lawrence Carey, PharmD
Assistant Professor, Academic Coordinator
Philadelphia University

Janice W. Chapman, RN, BSN, MSN
Health Careers Coordinator & Instructor
Reid State College
Atmore, Ala.

Victor Cohen, BS, PharmD, BCPS
Clinical Manager of Emergency Medicine
Director, Maimonides Medical Center
   Pharmacy Practice Residency Program
Assistant Professor of Pharmacy Practice
Arnold & Marie Schwartz College of Pharmacy
   & Health Sciences
Brooklyn, N.Y.

Jason C. Cooper, PharmD
Clinical Pharmacist
Medical University of South Carolina
Charleston

Melissa Devlin, PharmD
Clinical Pharmacist
Excellerx, Inc.
Philadelphia, Penn.

Jennifer Faulkner, PharmD, BCPP
Clinical Pharmacy Specialist
Central Texas Veterans Health Care System
Temple

Dawn Feltner, RPh, PharmD
Pharmacist
Acme Pharmacy
Burlington, N.J.

Margaret Gingrich, RN, MSN
Associate Professor
Harrisburg (Penn.) Area Community College

Tatyana Gurvich, PharmD
Clinical Pharmacologist
Glendale (Calif.) Adventist Family Practice
   Residency Program

AnhThu Hoang, PharmD
Pharmacist
Drug Information & Research Centre
Don Mills, Ontario

Samantha P. Jellinek, PharmD, BCPS
Manager of Medication Reconciliation
Clinical Coordinator, Pharmacy Practice
   Residency Program
Maimonides Medical Center
Dept. of Pharmaceutical Services
Brooklyn, N.Y.

Julia N. Kleckner, PharmD
Clinical Coordinator
Mercy Fitzgerald Hospital
Darby, Penn.

Christopher Miller, PharmD
Assistant Professor, Pharmacy Practice
Albany (N.Y.) College of Pharmacy

Mary Miller-Bell, PharmD
Clinical Pharmacist, Neonatology
Associate Clinical Professor
Duke University Medical Center
Durham, N.C.

William O'Hara, RPh, BS, PharmD
Clinical Team Leader
Thomas Jefferson Hospital
Philadelphia, Penn.

Priti Patel, PharmD, BCPS
Assistant Clinical Professor
St. John's University
Queens, N.Y.

Jeffrey B. Purcell, PharmD
Clinical Lead Pharmacist
Clinical Associate Professor
Harborview Medical Center, University of
    Washington
Seattle

Dana Reeves, RN, MSN
Assistant Professor
University of Arkansas at Fort Smith

Kendra S. Seiler, RN, BSN, MSN
Nursing Instructor
Rio Hondo Community College
Whittier, Calif.

Joseph F. Steiner, PharmD, RPh
Dean and Professor of Pharmacy Practice
College of Pharmacy
Idaho State University
Pocatello

Maria Sulli, PharmD
Assistant Clinical Professor
St. John's University
Jamaica, N.Y.

Maria Summa, PharmD, BS, BCPS
Assistant Director for Clinical Programs,
    Pharmacy
St. Francis Hospital & Medical Center
Hartford, Conn.

Sheryl Thomas, MSN, RN
Nursing Instructor
Wayne County Community College
Detroit, Mich.

Laurie A. Willhite, PharmD, CSPI
Clinical Assistant Professor
University of Minnesota College of Pharmacy
Minneapolis

Foreword

As a nurse practitioner and nursing professor teaching pharmacology, I understand the daunting task of delivering safe, effective care to patients receiving drug therapy. Drug administration doesn't stop with handing a patient a pill or hanging an I.V. piggyback correctly. Every nurse has an ongoing responsibility to assess drug effects, help patients understand and manage their drug therapy, and identify possible adverse effects as quickly and accurately as possible.

It's impossible to remember all the drug information you need to know to deliver world class nursing care. That's why you need a great drug reference, a reference that's reliable, concise, comprehensive, nursing-focused--and easy to use and understand. I believe *Springhouse Nurse's Drug Guide 2007* is just such a reference. Whether you're a student nurse, a new graduate, or an experienced practicing nurse, this book will help you deliver safe, effective nursing care to patients receiving drug therapy.

New in this 2007 edition, you'll find more than 30 new monographs, an incompatibilities section for every I.V. drug, more pediatric dosages and off-label uses, and helpful new appendices covering combination drug products, toxic drug–drug interactions, and dangerous abbreviations.

The book starts with a section of helpful hints for making the most of this book's special features. Next is a list of the abbreviations used throughout the book. And then you'll find a set of four chapters that concisely review drug therapy and the nursing process, essential dosage calculations, routes of administration, and safety tips to help you avoid medication errors.

The next section describes 40 classes of drugs with examples, a prototype for each class, and administration information that applies to the entire class.

Individual drug monographs are listed alphabetically by generic name. Each monograph describes the drug's indications and dosages; I.V. administration and incompatibilities, if applicable; contraindications and cautions; lifespan considerations; adverse reactions; interactions with drugs, herbs, foods, and lifestyle; effects on lab test results; pharmacokinetics; onset, peak, and duration; the drug's chemical and therapeutic action; and its available forms. In addition, each monograph uses the nursing process to review assessment, nursing diagnoses, planning and implementation, patient teaching, and evaluation. Make sure to look for the handy color logos that highlight dosage adjustment, lifespan, and incompatibility information. An "alert" logo calls attention to especially important nursing practice information.

The photoguide to tablets and capsules provides pictures of common drugs in their actual size and color. In my experience, many patients remember the name of their medication but not the dose. Using this convenient photoguide can help you identify a drug with certainty.

The excellent section on herbal medicines offers key information to help you counsel patients about the risks and effects of these products. It includes reported uses, preparations and amounts, cautions, potential adverse reactions, action and components, common forms, nursing considerations, and patient teaching.

The appendices offer an abundance of useful information. The section includes a glossary, pregnancy risk categories, controlled substance schedules, and appendices reviewing combination drug products, toxic drug–drug interactions, dangerous abbreviations, dialyzable drugs, herb–drug interactions, equivalents and conversions, drugs that shouldn't be crushed, normal laboratory test values, adverse reactions misinterpreted as age-related changes, and an English-to-Spanish drug phrase translator.

In addition to this great text, *Springhouse Nurse's Drug Guide 2007* includes a mini-CD that contains review questions for an NCLEX-style test. I'm sure you can see for yourself why this book is the perfect tool whether you're novice or expert.

Samantha Venable, RN, MS, FNP

How to use Springhouse Nurse's Drug Guide 2007

Springhouse Nurse's Drug Guide 2007 is the premier drug reference for all nursing students—beginning to advanced. Tightly organized entries offer consistent, practical drug information for more than 750 common generic drugs, presented in a clear writing style that beginning students can understand. The book is also a must-have for advanced students: it includes comprehensive pharmacokinetic and pharmacodynamic information and route-onset-peak-duration tables that give a clear understanding of drug actions. Because each entry also follows the nursing process, the book even helps students formulate accurate care plans. Students of all levels will find that *Springhouse Nurse's Drug Guide 2007* offers a comprehensive and convenient resource.

The book begins with introductory material crucial to safe, accurate drug administration. Chapter 1 discusses drug therapy as it relates to the nursing process. Chapter 2 explains how to calculate dosages and provides examples for each step in the calculations. Chapter 3 discusses how to give drugs by common routes and includes illustrations to guide students through the steps of each procedure. Chapter 4 focuses on common medication errors and explains how to avoid them.

Drug classifications

Springhouse Nurse's Drug Guide 2007 provides complete overviews of 40 pharmacologic and therapeutic drug classifications, from alkylating drugs to xanthine derivatives. After each class name is an alphabetical list of drugs in that class; the drug highlighted in color represents the prototype drug for the class. Each class entry has specific information on indications, actions, adverse reactions, contraindications, and precautions. Look for the special Lifespan logo (🝆) for contraindications and cautions for specific populations, such as children, pregnant and breast-feeding women, and elderly patients.

Alphabetical listing of drugs

Drug entries appear alphabetically by generic name for quick reference. The generic name is followed by a pronunciation guide and an alphabetical list of brand (trade) names. Brands that don't need a prescription are designated with a dagger (†); those available only in Canada with a closed diamond (♦); those available only in Australia with an open diamond (◊); and those that contain alcohol with an asterisk (*). A trade name may also have a capsule (✐), meaning that the drug appears in the full-color photoguide. The mention of a brand name in no way implies endorsement of that product or guarantees its legality.

Each entry then identifies the drug's pharmacologic (chemical category) and therapeutic (main use) classes. Seeing both classes helps you grasp the multiple, varying, and sometimes overlapping uses of drugs within a single pharmacologic class and among different classes. Each entry then lists the drug's pregnancy risk category and, if appropriate, its controlled substance schedule.

Indications and dosages

The next section lists the drug's indications and provides dosage information for adults, children, and elderly patients. Off-label indications (uses not approved by the FDA) are designated with a double dagger (‡). Because the double dagger now appears in color, off-label indications are easier than ever to find. Dosage instructions reflect current trends in therapeutics but can't be considered absolute or universal. For your patient, dosage instructions must be considered in light of his condition.

When giving a drug to a patient who needs special dosage considerations, look for the

Adjust-a-Dose label and logo (⊠) at the end of the indication.

I.V. administration

This section, only found in drugs that can be given I.V., addresses preparation, administration, and storage information, as well as cautions and other information about the safe use of I.V. drugs. A special section highlighted with a logo (⊗) lists incompatibilities in I.V. administration.

Contraindications and cautions

This section specifies situations in which the drug shouldn't be used and details recommendations for cautious use. The Lifespan logo (🜨) draws your attention to contraindications and cautions for special populations, such as children, pregnant or breast-feeding women, and elderly patients.

Adverse reactions

This section lists adverse reactions by body system. The most common adverse reactions (those experienced by at least 10% of people taking the drug in clinical trials) are in *italic* type; less common reactions are in roman type; life-threatening reactions are in ***bold italic*** type; and reactions that are common *and* life-threatening are in BOLD CAPITAL letters.

Interactions

This section lists confirmed, significant interactions with other drugs (added, increased, or decreased effects), herbs, foods, and lifestyle behaviors (such as alcohol use and smoking).

Drug interactions are listed under the drug that is adversely affected. For example, antacids that contain magnesium may decrease absorption of tetracycline so this interaction is listed under tetracycline. To determine the possible effects of using two or more drugs simultaneously, check the interactions section for each of the drugs in question.

Drugs that cause interactions that arise quickly and require immediate attention, called rapid-onset interactions, are shown in color.

Effects on lab test results

This section lists increased and decreased levels, counts, false results, and other laboratory test results that may be affected by the drug.

Pharmacokinetics

This section describes absorption, distribution, metabolism, and excretion, along with the drug's half-life. It also provides a quick reference table highlighting onset, peak, and duration for each route of administration. Values for half-life, onset, peak, and duration are for patients with normal renal function, unless specified otherwise.

Action

This section explains the drug's chemical and therapeutic actions. For example, although all antihypertensives lower blood pressure, they don't all do so in the same way.

Available forms

This section lists all available preparations for each drug (for example, tablets, capsules, solutions for injection) and all available dosage forms and strengths. As with the brand names discussed above, over-the-counter dosage forms and strengths are marked with a dagger (†); those available only in Canada with a closed diamond (♦); those available only in Australia with an open diamond (◊); and those that contain alcohol with an asterisk (*).

Nursing process

This section uses the nursing process as its organizational framework. It also contains an Alert logo (🜨) to call your attention to vital, need-to-know information or to warn you about a common drug error.

• *Assessment* focuses on observation and monitoring of key patient data, such as vital signs, weight, intake and output, and laboratory values.

• *Nursing diagnoses* represent those most commonly applied to drug therapy. In actual use, nursing diagnoses must be relevant to an individual patient so they may not include the listed examples and may include others not listed.

• *Planning and implementation* offers detailed recommendations for drug administration, including full coverage of P.O., I.M., subcutaneous, and other routes.

• *Patient teaching* focuses on explaining the drug's purpose, promoting compliance, and ensuring proper use and storage of the drug. It also includes instructions for preventing or minimizing adverse reactions.

• *Evaluation* identifies the expected patient outcomes for the listed nursing diagnoses.

Because nursing considerations in this text emphasize drug-specific recommendations, they don't include standard recommendations that apply to all drugs, such as "assess the six rights of drug therapy before administration" or "teach the patient the name, dose, frequency, route, and strength of the prescribed drug."

Photoguide to tablets and capsules

To make drug identification easier and to enhance patient safety, *Springhouse Nurse's Drug Guide 2007* offers a full-color photoguide to the most commonly prescribed tablets and capsules. Shown in their actual sizes, the drugs are arranged alphabetically by generic names. Trade names and most common dosage strengths are included. Page references appear under each drug name so you can turn quickly to information about the drug.

Herbal medicines

Herbal medicine entries appear alphabetically by name, followed by a phonetic spelling.

Reported uses

This section lists reported uses of herbal medicines. Some of these uses are based on anecdotal claims; other uses have been studied. A listing in this section should not be considered a recommendation; herbal medicines aren't regulated by the FDA.

Preparations and amounts

This section lists the preparation and amounts for each form of the herb according to its reported use. This information has been gathered from the herbal literature, anecdotal reports, and available clinical data. Not all uses have specific information; often, no consensus exists. Amounts shown reflect current trends and shouldn't be considered as recommendations by the publisher.

Cautions

This section lists any condition, especially a disease, in which use of the herbal remedy is undesirable. It also provides recommendations for cautious use, as appropriate.

Adverse reactions

This section lists undesirable effects that may follow use of an herbal supplement. Some of these effects haven't been reported but are theoretically possible, given the chemical composition or action of the herb.

Interactions

This section lists each herb's clinically significant interactions, actual or potential, with other herbs, drugs, foods, and lifestyle choices. Each statement describes the effect of the interaction and then offers a specific suggestion for avoiding the interaction. As with adverse reactions, some interactions have not been proven but are theoretically possible.

Actions and components

This section describes the herb's chemical and therapeutic actions and active components.

Common forms

This section lists the available preparations for each herbal medicine as well as forms and strengths.

Nursing considerations

This section offers helpful information, such as monitoring techniques and methods for the prevention and treatment of adverse reactions. Patient teaching tips that focus on educating the patient about the herb's purpose, preparation, administration, and storage are also included, as are suggestions for promoting patient compliance with the therapeutic regimen and steps the patient can take to prevent or minimize the risk or severity of adverse reactions.

Appendices and index

The appendices include a list of combination drug products with dosage forms and strengths, indications, and dosages; a list of dangerous abbreviations that you should avoid; a list of toxic drug–drug interactions; a list of dialyzable drugs; a glossary explaining unfamiliar medical words and phrases; a list of drugs that shouldn't be crushed; a table of equivalents and conversions; an English-to-Spanish translator of common drug-related phrases; a list of normal laboratory test values; and a table of adverse reactions that can be misinterpreted as normal changes of aging.

The comprehensive index lists drug classifications, generic drugs, brand names, indications, and herbal medicines included in this book. Drugs that appear in the photoguide are listed in the index with the photoguide page number in **bold**.

PharmDisk 2007

New to *PharmDisk 2007,* is a pharmacology self-test with NCLEX®-style questions, including alternate-format. *PharmDisk 2007* also provides a link to eDrugInfo.com.

eDrugInfo.com

This Web site keeps *Springhouse Nurse's Drug Guide 2007* current by providing the following features:

● updates on new drugs, indications, and warnings
● patient teaching aids on new drugs
● news summaries of pertinent drug information.

The Web site also gives you:

● two QuikTools, *Construct-a-card,* which lets you create custom drug information cards, and *Construct-a-calendar,* which lets you create individualized drug regimen calendars for your patients.
● information on herbs
● links to pharmaceutical companies, government agencies, and other drug information sites
● a bookstore full of nursing books, PDAs, software, and more.

Plus, registering with eDrugInfo.com entitles you to e-mail notifications when new drug updates are posted.

Guide to abbreviations

ACE	angiotensin-converting enzyme	ECG	electrocardiogram
ACT	activated clotting time	EEG	electroencephalogram
ADH	antidiuretic hormone	EENT	eyes, ears, nose, throat
AIDS	acquired immunodeficiency syndrome	F	Fahrenheit
		FDA	Food and Drug Administration
ALT	alanine transaminase	g	gram
APTT	activated partial thromboplastin time	G	gauge
AST	aspartate transaminase	GABA	gamma-aminobutyric acid
AV	atrioventricular	GFR	glomerular filtration rate
b.i.d.	twice daily	GGT	gamma-glutamyltransferase
BPH	benign prostatic hyperplasia	GI	gastrointestinal
BUN	blood urea nitrogen	gtt	drops
C	celsius	GU	genitourinary
cAMP	cyclic adenosine monophosphate	G6PD	glucose-6-phosphate dehydrogenase
CBC	complete blood count	H_1, H_2	histamine$_1$, histamine$_2$
CK	creatine kinase	HDL	high-density lipoprotein
CMV	cytomegalovirus	HIV	human immunodeficiency virus
CNS	central nervous system	HMG-CoA	3-hydroxy-3-methylglutaryl coenzyme A
COMT	catechol-O-methyltransferase	hr	hour
COPD	chronic obstructive pulmonary disease	h.s.	at bedtime
CPK	creatine phosphokinase	ICU	intensive care unit
CSF	cerebrospinal fluid	I.D.	intradermal
CV	cardiovascular	I.M.	intramuscular
CVA	cerebrovascular accident	INR	international normalized ratio
CYP	cytochrome P450	IPPB	intermittent positive-pressure breathing
DIC	disseminated intravascular coagulation	IU	international unit
D_5W	dextrose 5% in water	I.V.	intravenous
dl	deciliter	kg	kilogram
DNA	deoxyribonucleic acid	L	liter

lb	pound	RSV	respiratory syncytial virus
LDH	lactate dehydrogenase	SA	sinoatrial
LDL	low-density lipoprotein	S.C.	subcutaneous
M	molar, moles	SIADH	syndrome of inappropriate antidiuretic hormone
m^2	square meter		
MAO	monoamine oxidase	S.L.	sublingual
mcg	microgram	SSRI	selective serotonin reuptake inhibitor
mEq	milliequivalent	T_3	triiodothyronine
mg	milligram	T_4	thyroxine
MI	myocardial infarction	tbs	tablespoon
min	minute	t.i.d.	three times daily
ml	milliliter	tsp	teaspoon
mm^3	cubic millimeter	USP	United States Pharmacopeia
Na	sodium	UTI	urinary tract infection
NG	nasogastric	WBC	white blood cell
NSAID	nonsteroidal anti-inflammatory drug	wk	week
OTC	over-the-counter		
oz	ounce		
PABA	para-aminobenzoic acid		
$Paco_2$	partial carbon dioxide pressure		
Pao_2	partial oxygen pressure		
PCA	patient-controlled analgesia		
P.O.	by mouth		
P.R.	by rectum		
p.r.n.	as needed		
PT	prothrombin time		
PTT	partial thromboplastin time		
PVC	premature ventricular contraction		
q	every		
q.i.d.	four times daily		
RBC	red blood cell		
RDA	recommended daily allowance		
REM	rapid eye movement		
RNA	ribonucleic acid		

Drug therapy and the nursing process

Springhouse Nurse's Drug Guide 2007 uses the nursing process as its organizing principle for good reason. The nursing process guides the way that nurses give drugs, ensuring patient safety and medical and legal standards. The process has four parts:
- assessment
- nursing diagnoses
- planning and implementation
- evaluation.

Assessment

Assessment begins with the patient history. After taking the patient's history, perform a thorough physical examination. Also, assess the patient's knowledge and understanding of the drug therapy he's about to receive.

History

When taking a history, investigate the patient's allergies, use of drugs and herbs, medical history, lifestyle and beliefs, and socioeconomic status.

Allergies

Specify drugs and foods to which the patient is allergic. Describe the reaction he has; its situation, time, and setting; and other contributing causes, such as a significant change in eating habits or the use of stimulants, tobacco, alcohol, or illegal drugs. Don't forget to place an allergy label conspicuously on the front of the patient's chart and place an allergy band on the patient.

Drugs and herbs

Take a complete drug history that includes both prescription and over-the-counter drugs. Also find out which herbs the patient takes. Ask the patient why he uses this drug or herb and how much he knows about its purpose. Explore the patient's thoughts and attitudes about drug use to find out if he may have trouble complying with his drug therapy. Note any special procedures the patient will need to perform himself,

such as monitoring glucose level or checking heart rate; make sure he can perform them correctly.

After the patient starts taking the drug, discuss with him the effects of therapy to determine whether new symptoms or adverse drug reactions have developed. Also talk about measures the patient has taken to recognize, minimize, or avoid adverse drug reactions or accidental overdose. Ask the patient where medication is stored and what system he uses to help remember to take it as prescribed.

Medical history

Note any chronic disorders the patient has, and record the date of diagnosis, the prescribed treatment, and the name of the prescriber. Careful attention during this part of the history can uncover one of the most important problems with drug therapy: incompatible drug regimens.

Lifestyle and beliefs

Ask about the patient's support systems, marital and childbearing circumstances, attitudes toward health and health care, and daily patterns of activity. These influences all affect patient compliance and, consequently, the patient's care plan.

Also ask about the patient's diet. Certain foods can influence the effectiveness of many drugs. Don't forget to inquire about the patient's use of alcohol, tobacco, caffeine, and illegal drugs, such as marijuana, cocaine, and heroin. Note any substance used and the amount and frequency of use.

Socioeconomic status

Note the patient's age, educational level, occupation, and insurance coverage. These characteristics help determine the plan of care, the likelihood of compliance, and the possible need for financial assistance, counseling, or other social services.

Physical examination

Examine the patient closely for expected drug effects and for adverse reactions. Every drug has a desired effect on one body system, but it also may have one or more undesired effects on that or another body system. For example, chemotherapeutic drugs destroy cancer cells but also affect normal cells. These drugs typically cause hair loss, diarrhea, and nausea. Besides looking for adverse drug effects, investigate whether the patient has any sensory impairments or changes in mental state.

Sensory impairment

Assess the patient for sensory impairments that could influence his care plan. For example, impaired vision or paralysis can hinder the patient's ability to give a subcutaneous injection, break a scored tablet, or open a drug vial. Impaired hearing can prevent a patient from finding out from you all that he needs to know about the drug.

Mental state

Note whether the patient is alert, oriented, and able to interact appropriately. Assess whether he can think clearly and talk properly. Check the patient's short-term and long-term memory, which are both needed to follow the prescribed regimen correctly. Also, determine whether the patient can read and, if he can, at what level.

Understanding drug therapy

A patient is more likely to comply if he understands the reason for drug therapy. During your assessment, evaluate your patient's understanding of the therapy and the reason for it. Pay particular attention to his emotional acceptance of the need for drug therapy. For instance, a young patient being prescribed an antihypertensive may need more education than an older patient to ensure compliance.

Nursing diagnosis

Using the information you gathered during assessment, define drug-related problems by formulating each problem into a relevant nursing diagnosis. The most common problem statements related to drug therapy are "Deficient knowledge," "Ineffective health maintenance," and "Noncompliance." Nursing diagnoses provide the framework for planning interventions and outcome criteria, also known as patient goals.

Planning and implementation

Make sure that your patient goals state the desired patient behaviors or responses that should result from nursing care. Such criteria should be:
- measurable
- objective
- concise
- realistic for the patient
- attainable by nursing interventions.

Express patient behavior in terms of expectations, and specify a time frame. An example of a good outcome statement is "Before discharge, the patient verbalizes major adverse effects related to his chemotherapy."

After developing outcome criteria, determine the interventions needed to help the patient reach the desired goals. Appropriate interventions may include administration procedures and techniques, legal and ethical concerns, patient teaching, and special actions for pregnant, breast-feeding, pediatric, or geriatric patients. Interventions also may be independent nursing actions, such as turning a bedridden patient every 2 hours.

Evaluation

The final piece of the nursing process is a formal and systematic determination of your nursing care's effectiveness. This evaluation lets you determine whether outcome criteria were met so you can make informed decisions about subsequent interventions. If you stated the outcome criteria in measurable terms, you can easily evaluate whether the criteria were met.

For example, if a patient experiences relief from headache pain within 1 hour after receiving an analgesic, the outcome criterion was met. If the headache was the same or worse, the outcome criterion wasn't met. In that case, you need to reassess the patient, which may produce new data that might go against the original nursing diagnosis, new nursing interventions that are more specific or more appropriate for the patient, or a new care plan. This reassessment could lead to a higher dosage, a different analgesic, or the discovery of the underlying cause of the headache pain.

2

Essentials of dosage calculations

Because nurses frequently perform drug and intravenous (I.V.) fluid calculations, it's important to understand how drugs are weighed and measured, how to convert between systems and measures, how to compute drug dosages, and how to make adjustments for children.

Systems of drug weights and measures

Several systems of measurement can be used to determine the proper drug dosage. They include the metric, household, apothecary, and avoirdupois systems.

The metric and household systems are so widely used that most brands of medication cups for liquid measurements are standardized in both systems. The apothecary system isn't widely used but is still encountered in practice. A fourth system, the avoirdupois system, is rarely used. This system uses solid units of measure, such as the ounce and the pound. Also, some special systems of measurement — such as units, international units, and milliequivalents — have been developed by international scientists for standardization and only pertain to particular drugs or biological agents.

Metric system

The metric system is the international system of measurement, the most widely used system, and the system used by the U.S. Pharmacopoeia. This system has units for both liquid and solid measures. Among its many advantages, the metric system enables accuracy in calculating small drug dosages. The metric system uses Arabic numerals, which are commonly used by health care professionals worldwide. And most manufacturers standardize newly developed drugs in the metric system.

Liquid measures

In the metric system, one liter (L) is equal to about 1 quart in the apothecary system. Liters are often used when ordering and administering I.V. solutions. Milliliters are frequently used for parenteral and some oral drugs. One milliliter (ml) equals $\frac{1}{1,000}$ of a liter.

Solid measures

The gram (g) is the basis for solid measures or units of weight in the metric system. One milligram (mg) equals $\frac{1}{1,000}$ of a gram. Drugs are frequently ordered in grams, milligrams, or an even smaller unit, the microgram (mcg), depending on the drug. One microgram equals $\frac{1}{1,000}$ of a milligram. Body weight is usually recorded in kilograms (kg). One kilogram equals 1,000 g.

The following are examples of drug orders using the metric system:
- 30 ml Milk of Magnesia P.O. at bedtime
- 1 g Ancef I.V. q 6 hours
- 0.125 mg Lanoxin P.O. daily.

Household system

Most foods, recipes, over-the-counter drugs, and home remedies use the household system. Health care professionals seldom use this system for drug administration; however, knowledge of household measures may be useful in some home care and patient teaching situations.

Liquid measures

Liquid measurements in the household system include teaspoons (tsp) and tablespoons (tbs). For medical use, these measurements have been standardized to 5 milliliters and 15 milliliters, respectively. Using these standardized amounts, 3 teaspoons equal 1 tablespoon, 6 teaspoons equal 1 ounce, and so forth. Patients who need to measure doses by teaspoon or tablespoon should do so using standardized medical devices to make sure they receive exactly the prescribed amount. Advise patients not to use an ordinary spoon to measure a teaspoonful of a drug because the amount will most likely be inaccurate. Teaspoon sizes vary from 4 to 6 milliliters or more.

The following are examples of drug orders using the household system:
- 2 tsp Bactrim P.O. twice daily

• 2 tbs Riopan P.O. 1 hour before meals and at bedtime.

Apothecary system

Two unique features distinguish the apothecary system from other systems: the use of Roman numerals and the placement of the unit of measurement before the Roman numeral. For example, a measurement of 5 grains would be written as *grains V.*

In the apothecary system, equivalents among the various units of measure are close approximations of one another. By contrast, equivalents in the metric system are exact. When using apothecary equivalents for calculations and conversions, the calculations won't be precise but still must fall within acceptable standards. (See *Imprecision of dosage computations,* page 9.)

The apothecary system is the only system of measurement that uses both symbols and abbreviations to represent units of measure. Although the apothecary system isn't used frequently in health care today, you must still be able to read dosages that have been written in the apothecary system and convert them to the metric system.

Liquid measures

The smallest unit of liquid measurement in the apothecary system is the minim (℞), which is about the size of a drop of water; 15 to 16 minims equal about 1 ml.

Solid measures

The grain (gr) is the smallest solid measure or unit of weight in the apothecary system. It equals about 60 milligrams; 1 dram equals about 60 grains.

The following are examples of drug orders using the apothecary system:
• Robitussin fȝ (fluidrams) IV P.O. every 6 hours
• Mylanta fȝ (fluidounce) I P.O. 1 hour after meals
• Tylenol gr X P.O. every 4 hours as needed for headache.

Units, international units, and milliequivalents

For some drugs, you'll need to use a measuring system developed by drug companies. Three of the most common special systems of measurement are units, international units, and milliequivalents.

Units

Insulin is one of the drugs measured in units. Although many types of insulin exist, all are measured in units. The international standard of U-100 insulin means that 1 ml of insulin solution contains 100 units of insulin, regardless of type. Heparin, an anticoagulant, is also measured in units, as are several antibiotics available in liquid, solid, and powder forms for oral or parenteral use. Each drug company provides specific information about the measurement of its drugs that are measured in units.

The following are examples of drug orders using units:
• Inject 14 units NPH insulin subcutaneously this a.m.
• Heparin 5,000 units subcutaneously q 12 hours
• Nystatin 200,000 units P.O. q 12 hours.
The unit is not a standard measure. Different drugs, although all measured in units, may have no relationship to one another in quality or activity.

Units should never be abbreviated as "U" because of the potential for confusing a "U" with a "0."

International units

International units are used to measure biologicals, such as vitamins, enzymes, and hormones. For instance, the activity of calcitonin, a synthetic hormone used in calcium regulation, is expressed in international units.

The following are examples of drug orders using international units:
• 100 international units calcitonin (salmon) subcutaneously daily
• 8 international units somatropin subcutaneously three times a week.

Milliequivalents

Electrolytes may be measured in milliequivalents (mEq). Drug companies provide information about the number of metric units needed to provide a prescribed number of milliequivalents. Potassium chloride (KCl), for example, is usually ordered in milliequivalents.

The following are examples of drug orders using milliequivalents:
• 30 mEq KCl P.O. b.i.d.
• 1 L dextrose 5% in normal saline solution with 40 mEq KCl to be run at 125 ml/hour.

Conversions between measurement systems

You may need to convert from one measurement system to another, particularly when a drug is ordered in one system but only available in another. To perform conversion calculations, you need to know the equivalent measurements for the different systems. One of the most commonly used methods for converting drug measurements is the fraction method.

Fraction method

The fraction method for converting between measurement systems involves an equation consisting of two fractions. Set up the first fraction by placing the ordered dosage over an unknown number of units of the available dosage.

For example, say a prescriber orders 7.5 ml of acetaminophen elixir to be given by mouth. To find the equivalent in teaspoons, first set up a fraction in which the top of the fraction (numerator) represents the ordered dosage in milliliters and the bottom of the fraction (denominator) represents the unknown (x) number of teaspoons:

$$\frac{7.5 \text{ ml}}{x \text{ tsp}}$$

Then, set up the second fraction, which appears on the right side of the equation. This fraction consists of the standard equivalents between the ordered (ml) and the available (tsp) measures. Because milliliters must be converted to teaspoons, the right side of the equation appears as follows:

$$\frac{5 \text{ ml}}{1 \text{ tsp}}$$

The same unit of measure should appear in the numerator of both fractions. Likewise, the same unit of measure should appear in both denominators. The entire equation should appear as:

$$\frac{7.5 \text{ ml}}{x \text{ tsp}} = \frac{5 \text{ ml}}{1 \text{ tsp}}$$

To solve for x, cross multiply:

$$x \text{ tsp} \times 5 \text{ ml} = 7.5 \text{ ml} \times 1 \text{ tsp}$$

$$x \text{ tsp} = \frac{7 \text{ ml} \times 1 \text{ tsp}}{5 \text{ ml}}$$

$$x \text{ tsp} = \frac{7.5 \times 1 \text{ tsp}}{5}$$

$$x \text{ tsp} = 1.5 \text{ tsp}$$

The patient should receive 1.5 teaspoons of acetaminophen elixir.

Computing drug dosages

Computing drug dosages is a two-step process that you complete after verifying the drug order. Determine whether the ordered drug is available in units in the same system of measurement in which the order was written. If not, convert the measurement for the ordered drug to the system used for the available drug.

If the ordered units of measurement are available, calculate how much of the available dosage form should be given. For example, if the prescribed dose is 250 mg, determine the quantity of tablets, powder, or liquid that would equal 250 mg. To determine that quantity, use one of the methods described below.

Fraction method

When using the fraction method to compute a drug dosage, write an equation consisting of two fractions. First, set up a fraction showing the number of units to be given over x, which represents the quantity of the dosage form you are trying to find. In this case, this dosage form is tablets (tab).

For example, if the number of units to be administered equals 250 mg, the first fraction in the equation would appear as:

$$\frac{250 \text{ mg}}{x \text{ tab}}$$

On the other side of the equation, set up a fraction showing the number of units of the drug in its dosage form over the quantity of dosage forms that supply that number of units. The number of units and the quantity of dosage forms are specific for each drug. In most cases, the stated quantity equals 1. You can find all of the information for the second fraction on the drug label.

The drug label states that each tablet contains 125 mg, so the second fraction would appear as:

$$\frac{125 \text{ mg}}{1 \text{ tab}}$$

Note that in the two equations, the numerator units are the same (mg) and the denominator units are the same (tab).

The entire equation would appear as:

$$\frac{250 \text{ mg}}{x \text{ tab}} = \frac{125 \text{ mg}}{1 \text{ tab}}$$

Solving for x by cross-multiplying determines the quantity of the dosage form — 2 tablets, in this example.

Ratio method

To use the ratio method, write the amount of the drug to be given and the x quantity of the dosage form as a ratio. Using the example above, you would write:

$$250 \text{ mg} : x \text{ tab}$$

Next, complete the equation by forming a second ratio from the number of units in each tablet. The drug label provides this information. The entire equation is:

$$250 \text{ mg} : x \text{ tab} :: 125 \text{ mg} : 1 \text{ tab}$$

Solve for x by multiplying the inner portions (means) and outer portions (extremes) of the equation. The patient should receive 2 tablets.

Desired-available method

You can also use the desired-available method, also known as the dose-over-on hand (D/H) method. This method converts ordered units into available units and computes the drug dosage all in one step. The desired-available equation appears as:

$$\begin{array}{c} x \\ \text{quantity} \\ \text{to give} \end{array} = \frac{\begin{array}{c}\text{ordered} \\ \text{units}\end{array}}{1} \times \frac{\text{conversion}}{\text{fraction}} \times \frac{\begin{array}{c}\text{quantity} \\ \text{of dosage} \\ \text{form}\end{array}}{\begin{array}{c}\text{stated} \\ \text{quantity of} \\ \text{drug within} \\ \text{each dosage} \\ \text{form}\end{array}}$$

For example, say you receive an order for grains (gr) X of a drug. The drug is available only in 300-mg tablets. To determine what number of tablets to give the patient, substitute gr X (the ordered number of units) for the first element of the equation. Then use the conversion fraction as the second portion of the formula. The conversion factor is:

$$\frac{60 \text{ mg}}{\text{gr I}}$$

The measure in the denominator must be the same as the measure in the ordered units. In this case, the order specified gr X. As a result, grains will appear in the denominator of the conversion fraction.

The third element of the equation shows the dosage form over the stated drug quantity for that dosage form. Because the drug is available in 300-mg tablets, the fraction appears as:

$$\frac{1 \text{ tab}}{300 \text{ mg}}$$

The dosage form should always appear in the numerator, and the quantity of drug in each dosage form should always appear in the denominator. The completed equation is:

$$x \text{ tab} = \text{gr X} \times \frac{60 \text{ mg}}{\text{gr I}} \times \frac{1 \text{ tab}}{300 \text{ mg}}$$

Solving for x shows that the patient should receive 2 tablets.

The desired-available method has the advantage of using only one equation. However, you need to memorize an equation more elaborate than the one used in the fraction method or the ratio method. Relying on your memorization of a more complicated equation may increase the chance of error.

Dimensional analysis

A variation of the ratio method, dimensional analysis (also known as factor analysis or factor labeling) eliminates the need to memorize formulas and requires only one equation. To compare the two methods at a glance, read the following problem and solutions, and then read the paragraphs that follow for a detailed explanation.

Say the prescriber orders 0.25 g of streptomycin sulfate I.M. The vial reads 2 ml = 1 g. How many milliliters should you give?

Dimensional analysis

$$\frac{0.25 \text{ g}}{1} \times \frac{2 \text{ ml}}{1 \text{ g}} = 0.5 \text{ ml}$$

Ratio method

$$1 \text{ g} : 2 \text{ ml} :: 0.25 \text{ g} : x \text{ ml}$$

$$x = 2 \times 0.25$$

$$x = 0.5 \text{ ml}$$

Explanation

When using dimensional analysis you arrange a series of ratios, called factors, in a single (although sometimes lengthy) fractional equation. Each factor, written as a fraction, consists of two quantities and their related units of measurement. For instance, if 1,000 ml of a drug should be given over 8 hours, the relationship between the dose and time is expressed by the fraction:

$$\frac{1,000 \text{ ml}}{8 \text{ hr}}$$

When a problem includes a quantity or a unit of measurement that doesn't have an equivalent in the problem, these numbers appear in the numerator of the fraction, and 1 becomes the denominator. In the problem and solutions above, 0.25 g is such a number.

Some mathematical problems contain all the information you need to identify the factors, set up the equation, and find the solution. Other problems require you to use a conversion factor. Conversion factors are equivalents (for example, 1 g = 1,000 mg) that you can memorize or get from a conversion chart. Because the two quantities and units of measurement are equivalent, they can serve as the numerator or the denominator; thus, the conversion factor 1 g = 1,000 mg can be written in fraction form as:

$$\frac{1,000 \text{ mg}}{1 \text{ g}} \quad \text{or} \quad \frac{1 \text{ g}}{1,000 \text{ mg}}$$

The factors given in the problem, plus any conversion factors needed to solve the problem, are called *knowns*. The quantity of the answer, of course, is the *unknown*. When setting up an equation in dimensional analysis, work backward, beginning with the unit of measurement of the answer. After plotting all the knowns, find the solution by following this sequence:
• Cancel similar quantities and units of measurement.
• Multiply the numerators.
• Multiply the denominators.
• Divide the numerator by the denominator.

Mastering dimensional analysis can take practice, but it will be well worth it. To understand more fully how dimensional analysis works, review the following problem and the steps taken to solve it.

A prescriber orders grains X of a drug. The pharmacy supplies the drug in 300-mg tablets (tab). How many tablets should you administer?
• Write down the unit of measurement of the answer, followed by an "equal to" symbol:

$$\text{tab} =$$

• Search the problem for the quantity with the same unit of measurement (if one doesn't exist, use a conversion factor); place this in the numerator and its related quantity and unit of measurement in the denominator:

$$\text{tab} = \frac{1 \text{ tab}}{300 \text{ mg}}$$

• Separate the first factor from the next with a multiplication symbol:

$$\text{tab} = \frac{1 \text{ tab}}{300 \text{ mg}} \times$$

• Place the unit of measurement of the first factor's denominator in the second factor's numerator. Then search the problem for the quantity with the same unit of measurement (if one doesn't exist, as in this example, use a conversion factor); place this in the numerator and its related quantity and unit of measurement in the denominator, and follow the fraction with a multiplication symbol. Repeat this step until all known factors are included in the equation:

$$\text{tab} = \frac{1 \text{ tab}}{300 \text{ mg}} \times \frac{60 \text{ mg}}{\text{gr I}} \times \frac{\text{gr X}}{1}$$

• Treat the equation as a large fraction. First, cancel similar units of measurement in the numerator and the denominator. What remains should be what you began with: the unit of measurement of the answer. If not, check your equation to find and correct the error. Next, multiply the numerators and then the denominators. Finally, divide the numerator by the denominator:

$$\text{tab} = \frac{1 \text{ tab}}{300 \text{ mg}} \times \frac{60 \text{ mg}}{\text{gr I}} \times \frac{\text{gr X}}{1}$$

$$= \frac{60 \times 10 \text{ tab}}{300}$$

$$= \frac{600 \text{ tab}}{300}$$

$$= 2 \text{ tab}$$

For more practice, study the following examples, which use dimensional analysis to solve various mathematical problems common to dosage calculations and drug administration.

1. A patient weighs 140 lb. What is his weight in kilograms (kg)?

$$\text{1st factor (conversion factor): } \frac{1 \text{ kg}}{2.2 \text{ lb}}$$

$$\text{2nd factor: } \frac{140 \text{ lb}}{1}$$

$$\text{kg} = \frac{1 \text{ kg}}{2.2 \text{ lb}} \times 140 \text{ lb}$$

$$= \frac{140}{2.2}$$

$$= 63.6 \text{ kg}$$

2. A physician prescribes 75 mg of a drug. The pharmacy stocks a multidose vial containing 100 mg/ml. How many milliliters should you give?

$$\text{1st factor: } \frac{1 \text{ ml}}{100 \text{ mg}}$$

$$\text{2nd factor: } \frac{75 \text{ mg}}{1}$$

$$\text{ml} = \frac{1 \text{ ml}}{100 \text{ mg}} \times \frac{75 \text{ mg}}{1}$$

$$= 0.75 \text{ ml}$$

3. A nurse practitioner prescribes 1 tsp of a cough elixir. The pharmacist sends up a bottle whose label reads 1 ml = 50 mg. How many milligrams should you give?

$$\text{1st factor: } \frac{50 \text{ mg}}{1 \text{ ml}}$$

$$\text{2nd factor (conversion factor): } \frac{5 \text{ ml}}{1 \text{ tsp}}$$

$$\text{3rd factor: } \frac{1 \text{ tsp}}{1}$$

$$\text{mg} = \frac{50 \text{ mg}}{1 \text{ ml}} \times \frac{5 \text{ ml}}{1 \text{ tsp}} \times \frac{1 \text{ tsp}}{1}$$

$$= 50 \text{ mg} \times 5$$

$$= 250 \text{ mg}$$

4. A physician prescribes 1,000 ml of an I.V. solution to be given over 8 hours. The I.V. tub-ing delivers 15 drops (gtt)/ml/minute. What is the infusion rate in gtt/minute?

$$\text{1st factor: } \frac{15 \text{ gtt}}{1 \text{ ml}}$$

$$\text{2nd factor: } \frac{1,000 \text{ ml}}{8 \text{ hr}}$$

$$\text{3rd factor (conversion factor): } \frac{1 \text{ hr}}{60 \text{ min}}$$

$$\text{gtt/minute} = \frac{15 \text{ gtt}}{1 \text{ ml}} \times \frac{1,000 \text{ ml}}{8 \text{ hr}} \times \frac{1 \text{ hr}}{60 \text{ min}}$$

$$= \frac{15 \text{ gtt} \times 1,000 \times 1}{8 \times 60 \text{ min}}$$

$$= \frac{15,000 \text{ gtt}}{480 \text{ min}}$$

$$= 31.3 \text{ or } 31 \text{ gtt/min}$$

5. A physician prescribes 10,000 units of hepa-rin added to 500 ml of 5% dextrose and water at 1,200 units/hour. How many drops per minute should you give if the I.V. tubing deliv-ers 10 gtt/ml?

$$\text{1st factor: } \frac{10 \text{ gtt}}{1 \text{ ml}}$$

$$\text{2nd factor: } \frac{500 \text{ ml}}{10,000 \text{ units}}$$

$$\text{3rd factor: } \frac{1,200 \text{ units}}{1 \text{ hr}}$$

$$\text{4th factor (conversion factor): } \frac{1 \text{ hr}}{60 \text{ min}}$$

$$\frac{\text{gtt}}{\text{minute}} = \frac{10 \text{ gtt}}{1 \text{ ml}} \times \frac{500 \text{ ml}}{10,000 \text{ units}} \times \frac{1,200 \text{ units}}{1 \text{ hr}} \times \frac{1 \text{ hr}}{60 \text{ min}}$$

$$= \frac{10 \times 500 \times 1,200 \text{ gtt}}{10,000 \times 60 \text{ min}}$$

$$= \frac{6,000,000 \text{ gtt}}{600,000 \text{ min}}$$

$$= 10 \text{ gtt/min}$$

Special computations

The fraction, ratio, and desired-available meth-ods, as well as dimensional analysis, can be used to compute drug dosages when the ordered drug and the available form of the drug occur in the same units of measure. These methods can also be used when the availability of a particular dosage form differs from the units in which the dosage form is given.

For example, if a patient is to receive 1,000 mg of a drug available in liquid form and measured in milligrams, with 100 mg contained in 6 ml, how many milliliters should the patient receive? Because the ordered and the available dosages are in milligrams, no initial conversions are needed. The fraction method would be used to determine the number of milliliters the patient should receive, in this case, 60 ml.

Because the drug will be given in ounces (oz), the number of ounces should be determined using a conversion method. For the fraction method of conversion, the equation would appear as:

$$\frac{60 \text{ ml}}{x \text{ oz}} = \frac{30 \text{ ml}}{1 \text{ oz}}$$

Solving for x shows that the patient should receive 2 oz of the drug.

To use the desired-available method, change the order of the elements in the equation to correspond with the situation. The revised equation should appear as:

$$\frac{x}{\text{quantity}} = \frac{\text{ordered}}{1} \times \frac{\text{quantity of dosage form}}{\text{stated quantity of drug within each dosage form}} \times \frac{\text{conversion fraction}}{}$$

Placing the given information into the equation results in:

$$x \text{ oz} = \frac{1,000 \text{ mg}}{1} \times \frac{6 \text{ ml}}{100 \text{ mg}} \times \frac{1 \text{ oz}}{30 \text{ ml}}$$

Solving for x shows that the patient should receive 2 oz of the drug.

Imprecision of dosage computations

Converting drug measurements from one system to another and then determining the amount of a dosage to give can easily produce inexact dosages. A rounding error made during computation or discrepancies in the dosage may occur, depending on the conversion standard used in calculation. Or, you may determine a precise amount to be given, only to find that

giving that amount is impossible. For example, precise computations may indicate that a patient should receive 0.97 tablets. Giving such an amount is impossible.

The following rule helps avoid calculation errors and discrepancies between theoretical and real dosages: No more than a 10% variation should exist between the dosage ordered and the dosage to be given. For example, if you determine that a patient should receive 0.97 tablets, you can safely give 1 tablet. If your calculations don't give you a clear answer, notify the prescriber and request an equivalent dosage in the form you have available.

Computing parenteral dosages

The methods for computing drug dosages can be used not just for oral but also for parenteral routes. The following example shows how to determine a parenteral drug dosage. Say a prescriber orders 75 mg of Demerol. The package label reads: meperidine (Demerol), 100 mg/ml. By using the fraction method to determine the number of milliliters the patient should receive, your equation should look like this:

$$\frac{75 \text{ mg}}{x \text{ ml}} = \frac{100 \text{ mg}}{1 \text{ ml}}$$

To solve for x, cross multiply:

$$x \text{ ml} \times 100 \text{ mg} = 75 \text{ mg} \times 1 \text{ ml}$$

$$x \text{ ml} = \frac{75 \cancel{\text{ mg}} \times 1 \text{ ml}}{100 \cancel{\text{ mg}}}$$

$$x \text{ ml} = \frac{75 \text{ ml}}{100}$$

$$x \text{ ml} = 0.75 \text{ ml}$$

The patient should receive 0.75 ml.

Reconstituting powders for injection

Although a pharmacist usually reconstitutes powders for parenteral use, nurses sometimes perform this function by following the directions on the drug label. The label gives the total quantity of drug in the vial or ampule, the amount and type of diluent to be added to the powder, and the strength and expiration date of the resulting solution.

When you add diluent to a powder, the powder increases the fluid volume. That's why the label calls for less diluent than the total volume of the prepared solution. For example, a label may tell you to add 1.7 ml of diluent to a vial of powdered drug to obtain a 2-ml total volume of prepared solution.

To determine the amount of solution to give, use the manufacturer's information about the concentration of the solution. For example, if you want to give 500 mg of a drug and the concentration of the prepared solution is 1 g (1,000 mg)/10 ml, use the following equation:

$$\frac{500 \text{ mg}}{x \text{ ml}} = \frac{1,000 \text{ mg}}{10 \text{ ml}}$$

The patient would receive 5 ml of the prepared solution.

Intravenous drip rates and flow rates

Make sure you know the difference between I.V. drip and flow rates and also how to calculate each rate. I.V. drip rate refers to the number of drops of solution to be infused per minute. Flow rate refers to the number of milliliters of fluid to be infused over 1 hour.

To calculate an I.V. drip rate, first set up a fraction showing the volume of solution to be delivered over the number of minutes in which that volume should be infused. For example, if a patient should receive 100 ml of solution in 1 hour, the fraction would be written as:

$$\frac{100 \text{ ml}}{60 \text{ min}}$$

Multiply the fraction by the drip factor (the number of drops contained in 1 ml) to determine the number of drops per minute to be infused, or the drip rate. The drip factor varies among different I.V. sets and should appear on the package that contains the I.V. tubing administration set.

Following the manufacturer's directions for drip factor is a crucial step. Standard administration sets have drip factors of 10, 15, or 20 gtt/ml. A microdrip, or minidrip, set has a drip factor of 60 gtt/ml.

Use the following equation to determine the drip rate of an I.V. solution:

$$\text{gtt/min} = \frac{\text{total no. of ml}}{\text{total no. of min}} \times \frac{\text{drip}}{\text{factor}}$$

The equation applies to I.V. solutions that infuse over many hours or to small-volume infusions such as those used for antibiotics usually given in less than an hour. For example, if an order requires 1,000 ml of 5% dextrose in nor-

mal saline solution to infuse over 12 hours and the administration set delivers 15 gtt/ml, what should the drip rate be?

$$x \text{ gtt/min} = \frac{1,000 \text{ ml}}{720 \text{ min}} \times 15 \text{ gtt/ml}$$

$$x \text{ gtt/min} = 20.83 \text{ gtt/min}$$

The drip rate would be rounded to 21 gtt per minute.

You'll use flow-rate calculations when working with I.V. infusion pumps to set the number of milliliters to be delivered in an hour. To perform this calculation, you should know the total volume in milliliters to be infused and the amount of time for the infusion. Use the following equation:

$$\text{flow rate} = \frac{\text{total volume ordered}}{\text{number of hours}}$$

Quick methods for calculating drip rates

To give an I.V. solution through a microdrip set, adjust the flow rate (number of milliliters per hour) to equal the drip rate (gtt per minute).

Using this method, the flow rate is divided by 60 minutes and then multiplied by the drip factor, also 60. Because the flow rate and the drip factor are equal, the two arithmetic operations cancel each other out. For example, if 125 ml/hour represented the ordered flow rate, the equation is:

$$\text{drip rate (125)} = \frac{125 \text{ ml}}{60 \text{ min}} \times 60$$

Rather than spending time calculating the equation, you can use the number assigned to the flow rate as the drip rate.

For I.V. administration sets that deliver 15 gtt/ml, the flow rate divided by 4 equals the drip rate. For sets with a drip factor of 10, the flow rate divided by 6 equals the drip rate.

Critical care calculations

Many drugs given on the critical care unit are used to treat life-threatening disorders. You must be able to perform calculations swiftly and accurately, prepare the drug for infusion, give the drug, and then observe the patient closely to evaluate the drug's effectiveness.

Three calculations must be performed before giving critical care drugs:
• Calculate the concentration of the drug in the I.V. solution.

- Figure the flow rate needed to deliver the desired dose.
- Determine the needed dosage.

Calculating concentration

To calculate the drug's concentration, use the following formula:

concentration in mg/ml = mg of drug/ml of fluid

To express the concentration in mcg/ml, multiply the answer by 1,000.

Figuring flow rate

To determine the I.V. flow rate per minute, use the following formula:

$$\frac{\text{dose/min}}{x \text{ ml/min}} = \frac{\text{concentration of solution}}{1 \text{ ml of fluid}}$$

To calculate the hourly flow rate, first multiply the ordered dose, given in milligrams or micrograms per minute, by 60 minutes to determine the hourly dose. Then use the following equation to compute the hourly flow rate:

$$\frac{\text{hourly dose}}{x \text{ ml/hr}} = \frac{\text{concentration of solution}}{1 \text{ ml of fluid}}$$

Determining dosage

To determine the dosage in mg/kg of body weight/minute, first determine the concentration of the solution in milligrams per milliliter. (If a drug is ordered in micrograms, convert milligrams to micrograms by multiplying by 1,000.) To determine the dose in milligrams per hour, multiply the hourly flow rate by the concentration using the following formula:

$$\frac{\text{dose in}}{\text{mg/hr}} = \frac{\text{hourly}}{\text{flow rate}} \times \text{concentration}$$

Then calculate the dose in milligrams per minute. Divide the hourly dose by 60 minutes.

$$\text{dose in mg/min} = \frac{\text{dose in mg/hr}}{60 \text{ min}}$$

Divide the dose per minute by the patient's weight, using the following formula:

$$\text{mg/kg/min} = \frac{\text{mg/min}}{\text{patient's weight in kg}}$$

Finally, make sure that the drug is being given within a safe and therapeutic range. Compare the amount in milligrams per kilogram per minute to the safe range shown in this book.

The following examples show how to calculate an I.V. flow rate using the different formulas.

Example 1

A patient has frequent runs of ventricular tachycardia that subside after 10 to 12 beats. The prescriber orders 2 g (2,000 mg) of lidocaine in 500 ml of D_5W to infuse at 2 mg/minute. What's the rate in milliliters per minute? Milliliters per hour?

First, find the concentration of the solution by setting up a proportion with the unknown concentration in one fraction and the ordered dose in the other fraction:

$$\frac{x \text{ mg}}{1 \text{ ml}} = \frac{2,000 \text{ mg}}{500 \text{ ml}}$$

Cross multiply the fractions:

$$x \text{ mg} \times 500 \text{ ml} = 2,000 \text{ mg} \times 1 \text{ ml}$$

Solve for x by dividing each side of the equation by 500 ml and canceling units that appear in both the numerator and denominator:

$$\frac{x \text{ mg} \times \cancel{500 \text{ ml}}}{\cancel{500 \text{ ml}}} = \frac{2,000 \text{ mg} \times 1 \cancel{\text{ml}}}{500 \cancel{\text{ml}}}$$

$$x = \frac{2,000 \text{ mg}}{500}$$

$$x = 4 \text{ mg}$$

The concentration of the solution is 4 mg/ml. Next, calculate the flow rate per minute needed to deliver the ordered dose of 2 mg/minute. To do this, set up a proportion with the unknown flow rate per minute in one fraction and the concentration of the solution in the other fraction:

$$\frac{2 \text{ mg}}{x \text{ ml}} = \frac{4 \text{ mg}}{1 \text{ ml}}$$

Cross multiply the fractions:

$$x \text{ ml} \times 4 \text{ mg} = 1 \text{ ml} \times 2 \text{ mg}$$

Solve for x by dividing each side of the equation by 4 mg and canceling units that appear in both the numerator and denominator:

$$\frac{x \text{ ml} \times \cancel{4 \text{ mg}}}{\cancel{4 \text{ mg}}} = \frac{1 \text{ ml} \times 2 \cancel{\text{mg}}}{4 \cancel{\text{mg}}}$$

$$x = \frac{2 \text{ ml}}{4}$$

$$x = 0.5 \text{ ml}$$

The patient should receive 0.5 ml/minute of lidocaine. Because lidocaine must be given with an infusion pump, compute the hourly flow rate. Set up a proportion with the unknown flow rate per hour in one fraction and the drip rate per minute in the other fraction:

$$\frac{x \text{ ml}}{60 \text{ min}} = \frac{0.5 \text{ ml}}{1 \text{ min}}$$

Cross multiply the fractions:

$$x \text{ ml} \times 1 \text{ min} = 0.5 \text{ ml} \times 60 \text{ min}$$

Solve for x by dividing each side of the equation by 1 minute and canceling units that appear in both the numerator and denominator:

$$\frac{x \text{ ml} \times 1 \text{ min}}{1 \text{ min}} = \frac{0.5 \text{ ml} \times 60 \text{ min}}{1 \text{ min}}$$

$$x = 30 \text{ ml}$$

Set the infusion pump to deliver 30 ml/hour.

Example 2

A 200-lb patient is scheduled to receive an I.V. infusion of dobutamine at 10 mcg/kg/minute. The package insert says to dilute 250 mg of the drug in 50 ml of dextrose 5% in water (D_5W). Because the drug vial contains 20 ml of solution, the total to be infused is 70 ml (50 ml of D_5W plus 20 ml of solution). How many micrograms of the drug should the patient receive each minute? Each hour?

First, compute the patient's weight in kilograms. To do this, set up a proportion with the weight in pounds and the unknown weight in kilograms in one fraction and the number of pounds per kilogram in the other fraction:

$$\frac{200 \text{ lb}}{x \text{ kg}} = \frac{2.2 \text{ lb}}{1 \text{ kg}}$$

Cross multiply the fractions:

$$x \text{ kg} \times 2.2 \text{ lb} = 1 \text{ kg} \times 200 \text{ lb}$$

Solve for x by dividing each side of the equation by 2.2 lb and canceling units that appear in both the numerator and denominator:

$$\frac{x \text{ kg} \times 2.2 \text{ lb}}{2.2 \text{ lb}} = \frac{1 \text{ kg} \times 200 \text{ lb}}{2.2 \text{ lb}}$$

$$x = \frac{200 \text{ kg}}{2.2}$$

$$x = 90.9 \text{ kg}$$

The patient weighs 90.9 kg. Next, determine the dose in micrograms per minute by setting up a proportion with the patient's weight in kilograms and the unknown dose in micrograms per minute in one fraction and the known dose in micrograms per kilogram per minute in the other fraction:

$$\frac{90.9 \text{ kg}}{x \text{ mcg/min}} = \frac{1 \text{ kg}}{10 \text{ mcg/min}}$$

Cross multiply the fractions:

$$x \text{ mcg/min} \times 1 \text{ kg} = 10 \text{ mcg/min} \times 90.9 \text{ kg}$$

Solve for x by dividing each side of the equation by 1 kg and canceling units that appear in both the numerator and denominator:

$$\frac{x \text{ mcg/min} \times 1 \text{ kg}}{1 \text{ kg}} = \frac{10 \text{ mcg/min} \times 90.9 \text{ kg}}{1 \text{ kg}}$$

$$x = 909 \text{ mcg/min}$$

The patient should receive 909 mcg of dobutamine every minute. Finally, determine the hourly dose by multiplying the dose per minute by 60:

$$909 \text{ mcg/min} \times 60 \text{ min/hr} = 54,540 \text{ mcg/hr}$$

The patient should receive 54,540 mcg of dobutamine every hour.

Pediatric dosages

To determine the correct pediatric dosage of a drug, prescribers, pharmacists, and nurses use one of two computational methods. One is based on a child's weight in kilograms; the other is based on the child's body surface area. Other methods are less accurate and not recommended.

Dose range per kilogram of body weight

Many drug companies provide information on the safe dosage ranges for drugs given to children. The companies usually provide the dose ranges in milligrams per kilogram of body weight and, in many cases, give similar information for adult dose ranges. The following example and explanation show how to calculate the safe pediatric dosage range for a drug, using the company's suggested safe dose range provided in milligrams per kilogram.

For a child, a prescriber orders a drug with a suggested dosage range of 10 to 12 mg/kg of body weight/day. The child weighs 12 kg. What is the safe daily dose range for the child?

You must calculate the lower and upper limits of the dose range provided by the manufacturer. First, calculate the dose based on 10 mg/kg of body weight. Then, calculate the dose based on 12 mg/kg of body weight. The answers represent the lower and upper limits of the daily dose range, expressed in mg/kg of the child's weight.

Body surface area

A second method for calculating safe pediatric doses uses the child's body surface area. This method may provide a more accurate calculation because the child's body surface area is thought to parallel the child's organ growth and maturation and metabolic rate.

You can determine the body surface area of a child by using a three-column chart called a nomogram. Mark the child's height in the first column and weight in the third column. Then draw a line between the two marks. The point at which the line intersects the vertical scale in the second column is the child's estimated body surface area in square meters. To calculate the child's approximate dose, use the body surface area measurement in the following equation:

$$\frac{\text{body surface area of child}}{\text{average adult body surface area} \ (1.73 \ m^2)} \times \frac{\text{average}}{\text{adult dose}} = \frac{\text{child's}}{\text{dose}}$$

The following example illustrates the use of the equation. The nomogram shows that a 25-lb (11.3-kg) child who is 33 inches (84-cm) tall has a body surface area of 0.52 m². To determine the child's dose of a drug with an average adult dose of 100 mg, the equation would appear as:

$$\frac{0.52 \ m^2}{1.73 \ m^2} \times 100 \ mg = \frac{30.06 \ mg}{\text{(child's dose)}}$$

The child should receive 30 mg of the drug. Many facilities have guidelines that determine acceptable calculation methods for pediatric doses. If you work with children, familiarize yourself with your facility's policies about pediatric doses.

3

Drug administration routes

You will give drugs by many routes, including oral (P.O.), intravenous (I.V.), intramuscular (I.M.), subcutaneous, topical, ophthalmic, rectal (P.R.), buccal and sublingual (S.L.), inhalation, nasogastric (NG), otic, and vaginal. No matter which route you use, you need to follow the established procedure to make sure you give the right drug, in the right dose, to the right patient, at the right time, and by the right route. Immediately after giving the drug, you need to provide the right documentation. This procedure includes:

• checking the order, medication record, and label
• confirming the patient's identity
• following standard drug safety procedures
• addressing all of the patient's questions
• correctly documenting the drug administration in the patient's medical record.

Check the order

Make sure you have a written order for every drug given. Use verbal orders only in emergencies; write them out and get the prescriber to sign them within the time period specified by your facility.

If your facility has a computerized order system, it may allow prescribers to order drugs electronically from the pharmacy. The computer may indicate whether the pharmacy has the drug and trigger the pharmacy staff to fill the prescription. A computerized order also may generate a patient record, either paper or electronic, on which you can document medication administration.

Computer systems offer several advantages over paper systems. Drugs often arrive on the unit or floor more quickly. Documentation is quicker and easier. Prescribers can see at a glance which drugs have been given. Errors can't result from poor handwriting (although typing mistakes may occur). Finally, computerized records are easier to store than paper records.

Check the medication record

Check the order on the patient's medication record against the prescriber's order.

Check the label

Before giving a drug, check its label three times to make sure you're giving the prescribed drug and the prescribed dose. First, check the label when you take the container from the shelf or drawer. Next, check the label right before pouring the drug into the medication cup or drawing it into the syringe. Finally, check the label again before returning the container to the shelf or drawer. If you're giving a unit-dose drug, open the container at the patient's bedside. Check the label for the third time immediately after pouring the drug and again before discarding the wrapper.

Don't give a drug from a poorly labeled or unlabeled container. Also, don't attempt to label a drug or to reinforce a label that is falling off or improperly placed. Instead, return the drug to the pharmacist for verification and proper relabeling.

Confirm the patient's identity

Before giving the drug, ask the patient his full name and confirm his identity by checking the name and medical record number on his patient-identification wristband against the medication administration record. Don't rely on information that can vary during a hospital stay, such as a room or bed number. In nonacute settings, identify the patient by picture or other specific information.

Check again that you have the correct drug, and make sure the patient isn't allergic to it. If the patient has any drug allergies, check to make sure the chart and medication administration record are labeled accordingly and that the patient is wearing an allergy wristband that identifies the allergen.

Follow safety procedures

Whenever you give a drug, follow these safety procedures:
- Never give a drug poured or prepared by someone else.
- Never allow the medication cart or tray out of your sight once you've prepared a dose.
- Never leave a drug at a patient's bedside.
- Always observe the patient during drug administration; make sure he swallows oral drugs or uses an inhaler appropriately. If the patient is giving the drug to himself, make sure his technique is correct.
- Never return unwrapped or prepared drugs to stock containers; instead, dispose of them and notify the pharmacy.
- Keep the medication cart locked at all times.
- Follow your facility's standard precautions.

Respond to questions

If the patient questions you about his drug or dosage, check his medication record again. If the drug you're giving is correct, reassure the patient and explain the reason for the drug. Explain any changes to his drug regimen or drug dosage. Instruct him, as appropriate, about possible adverse reactions, and ask him to report anything that he feels may be an adverse reaction.

Oral administration

Because oral drug administration is usually the safest, most convenient, and least expensive method, most drugs are given this way. Drugs for oral administration are available in many forms: tablets, enteric-coated tablets, capsules, syrups, elixirs, oils, liquids, suspensions, powders, and granules. Some require special preparation before administration, such as mixing with juice to make them more palatable.

Oral drugs are sometimes prescribed in higher dosages than their parenteral equivalents because after the drugs are absorbed through the gastrointestinal (GI) system, the liver breaks them down before they reach the systemic circulation.

Equipment and preparation
- Check the chart and the medication administration record.
- Gather the drug and medication cup.

- If the patient is a child or an elderly person, you may need to gather a mortar and pestle for crushing pills and an appropriate buffer, such as jelly or applesauce for crushed pills or juice, water, or milk for liquid drugs.

Implementation
- Wash your hands.
- Confirm the patient's identity by asking his full name and checking the name and medical record number on his wristband.
- Make sure the patient isn't allergic to the drug or any of its components.
- Assess the patient's condition, including level of consciousness and vital signs. Changes in the patient's condition may call for withholding the drug.
- Give the patient the drug. If needed and verified safe, crush the drug to facilitate swallowing or mix it with a soft food or liquid to aid swallowing, minimize adverse effects, or promote absorption.
- Stay with the patient until he has swallowed the drug. If he seems confused or disoriented, check his mouth to make sure he has indeed swallowed the drug. Return and reassess the patient's response within one hour of giving the drug.

Nursing considerations
- To avoid damaging or staining the patient's teeth, give acid or iron preparations through a straw. An unpleasant-tasting liquid usually can be made more palatable if taken through a straw because the liquid contacts fewer taste buds.
- If the patient can't swallow a whole tablet or capsule, ask the pharmacist if the drug is available in liquid form or if it can be given by another route. If not, ask the pharmacist if the tablet can be crushed or if capsules can be opened and mixed with food.
- Don't crush sustained-action, buccal, S.L., or enteric-coated drugs because this may counteract the safety or effectiveness of these drugs.

Intravenous bolus administration

In this method, rapid I.V. administration allows the drug level to quickly peak in the bloodstream. This method also may be used for drugs that can't be given I.M. because they're toxic or because the patient can't absorb them well. It may also be used for drugs that can't be diluted. Bolus doses may be injected directly into a vein or through an existing I.V. line.

Equipment and preparation
● Check the chart and the medication administration record. Gather the prescribed drug, 20G needle and syringe, diluent (if needed), tourniquet, alcohol sponge, sterile 2″ × 2″ gauze pad, gloves, adhesive bandage, and tape. Other materials may include a winged device primed with normal saline solution and a second syringe (and needle) filled with normal saline solution.
● Draw the drug into the syringe and dilute if needed.

Implementation
● Confirm the patient's identity by asking his full name and checking the name and medical record number on his wristband.
● Make sure the patient isn't allergic to the drug or any of its components.

To give a direct injection
● Wash your hands and put on gloves.
● Select the largest vein suitable to dilute the drug and minimize irritation.
● Apply a tourniquet above the site to distend the vein, and clean the site with an alcohol sponge, working outward in a circle.
● If you're using the needle of the drug syringe, insert it at a 30-degree angle with the bevel up. The bevel should reach ¼″ (0.6 cm) into the vein. Insert a winged device bevel-up at a 10- to 25-degree angle. Lower the angle once you enter the vein. Advance the needle into the vein. Tape the wings in place when you see blood return, and attach the syringe containing the drug.
● Check for blood backflow.
● Remove the tourniquet, and inject the drug at the ordered rate.
● Check for blood backflow to ensure that the needle remained in place and the entire amount of injected drug entered the vein.
● For a winged device, flush the line with normal saline solution from the second syringe to ensure complete delivery.
● Withdraw the needle and discard it in a biohazard container. Apply pressure to the site with the sterile gauze pad for at least 3 minutes to prevent hematoma.
● Apply an adhesive bandage when the bleeding stops.

● Remove and discard your gloves in a designated biohazard container. Wash your hands.

To inject through an existing line
● Wash your hands and put on gloves.
● Check the drug's compatibility with the IV solution.
● If the drug isn't compatible with the I.V. solution, flush the line with normal saline solution before and after the injection.
● Close the flow clamp, wipe the injection port with an alcohol sponge, and inject the drug as you would a direct injection.
● Open the flow clamp and readjust the flow rate.
● Remove and discard your gloves in a designated biohazard container. Wash your hands.

Nursing considerations
● If the existing I.V. line is capped, making it an intermittent infusion device, verify patency and placement of the device before injecting the drug. Then flush the device with normal saline solution, give the drug, and follow with the appropriate flush.
● Immediately report signs of acute allergic reaction or anaphylaxis. If extravasation occurs, stop the injection, estimate the amount of infiltration, and notify the prescriber.
● When giving diazepam or chlordiazepoxide hydrochloride through a steel needle winged device or an I.V. line, flush device with bacteriostatic water before and after use to prevent precipitation.

Intravenous administration through a secondary line

A secondary I.V. line is a complete I.V. set connected to the lower Y-port (secondary port) of a primary line instead of to the I.V. catheter or needle. It features an I.V. container, long tubing, and either a microdrip or a macrodrip system, and this line can be used for continuous or intermittent drug infusion. When used continuously, it permits drug infusion and titration while the primary line maintains a constant total infusion rate.

A secondary I.V. line used only for intermittent drug administration is called a piggyback set. In this case, the primary line maintains venous access between drug doses. A piggyback set includes a small I.V. container, short tubing, and usually a macrodrip system, and it connects to the primary line's upper Y-port (piggyback port).

Equipment and preparation

• Check the chart and the medication administration record.
• Make sure the patient isn't allergic to the drug or any of its components.
• Gather the prescribed I.V. drug, diluent (if needed), prescribed I.V. solution, administration set with secondary injection port, 22G 1″ needle or a needleless system, gloves, alcohol sponges, 1″ (2.5 cm) adhesive tape, time tape, labels, infusion pump, extension hook, and solution for intermittent piggyback infusion.
• Wash your hands and put on gloves.
• Inspect the I.V. container for cracks, leaks, or contamination.
• Check the expiration date.
• Check compatibility with the primary solution.
• Determine whether the primary line has a secondary injection port.
• If needed, add the drug to the secondary I.V. solution (usually 50- to 100-ml of normal saline solution or D_5W). To do so, remove the seals from the secondary container and wipe the main port with an alcohol sponge.
• Inject the prescribed drug and agitate the solution to mix the drug.
• Label the I.V. mixture.
• Insert the administration set spike, and attach the needle or needleless system.
• Open the flow clamp and prime the line. Then close the flow clamp.
• Some drugs come in vials that can hang directly on the I.V. pole. In this case, inject diluent directly into the drug vial. Then spike the vial, prime the tubing, and hang the set.

Implementation

• If the drug is incompatible with the primary I.V. solution, replace the primary solution with a fluid that's compatible with both solutions, and flush the line before starting the drug infusion.
• Hang the container of the secondary set and wipe the injection port of the primary line with an alcohol sponge.

• Insert the needle or needleless system from the secondary line into the injection port, and tape it securely to the primary line.
• To run the container of the secondary set by itself, lower the primary set's container with an extension hook. To run both containers simultaneously, place them at the same height.
• Open the clamp and adjust the drip rate.
• For continuous infusion, set the secondary solution to the desired drip rate; then adjust the primary solution to the desired total infusion rate.
• For intermittent infusion, wait until the secondary solution has completely infused; then adjust the primary drip rate, as needed.
• If the secondary solution tubing is being reused, close the clamp on the tubing and follow your facility's policy: Remove the needle or needleless system and replace it with a new one, or leave it taped to the injection port, and label it with the time it was first used.
• Leave the empty container in place until you replace it with a new dose of drug at the prescribed time. If the tubing won't be reused, discard it appropriately with the I.V. container.

Nursing considerations

• If institutional policy allows, use a pump for drug infusion. Place a time tape on the secondary container to help prevent an inaccurate administration rate.
• When reusing secondary tubing, change it when your facility's policy requires, usually every two or three days. Inspect the injection port for leakage with each use; change it more often, if needed.
• Except for lipids, don't piggyback a secondary I.V. line to a total parenteral nutrition line because this risks contamination.

Intramuscular administration

You'll use intramuscular (I.M.) injections to deposit up to 5 ml of drug deep into well-vascularized muscle for rapid systemic action and absorption.

Equipment and preparation

• Check the chart and the medication administration record.
• Make sure the patient isn't allergic to the drug or any of its components.

• Gather the prescribed drug, diluent, or filter needle (if needed), 3- to 5-ml syringe, 20G to 25G 1″ to 3″ needle, gloves, alcohol sponges, and a nonsterile cotton ball or 2″ × 2″ gauze pad.

• The prescribed drug must be sterile. The needle may be packaged separately or already attached to the syringe. Needles used for I.M. injections are longer than those used for subcutaneous injections because they must reach deep into the muscle. Needle length also depends on the injection site, the patient's size, and the amount of subcutaneous fat covering the muscle. A larger needle gauge can accommodate viscous solutions and suspensions.

• Check the drug for abnormal changes in color and clarity. If in doubt, ask the pharmacist.

• Wipe the stopper that tops the drug vial with alcohol, and draw up the prescribed amount of drug.

• Provide privacy and explain the procedure to the patient.

• Position the patient and drape him appropriately, making sure that the site is well lit and exposed.

Implementation

• Wash your hands.

• Confirm the patient's identity by asking his full name and checking the name and medical record number on his wristband.

• Make sure the patient isn't allergic to the drug or any of its components.

• Select an appropriate injection site. Avoid any site that looks inflamed, edematous, or irritated. Also, avoid using injection sites that contain moles, birthmarks, scar tissue, or other lesions. The dorsogluteal and ventrogluteal muscles are used most commonly for I.M. injections.

Dorsogluteal muscle

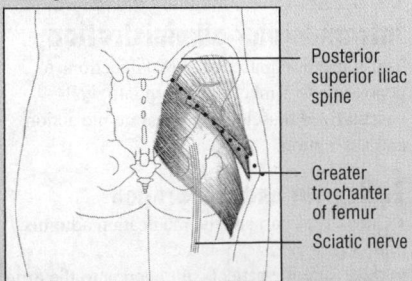

Ventrogluteal muscle

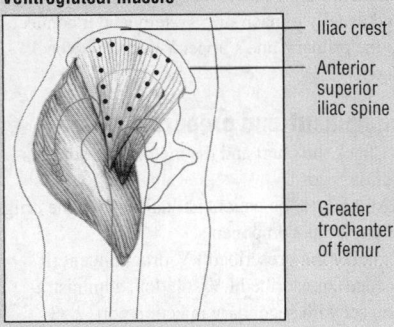

• The deltoid muscle may be used for injections of 2 ml or less.

Deltoid muscle

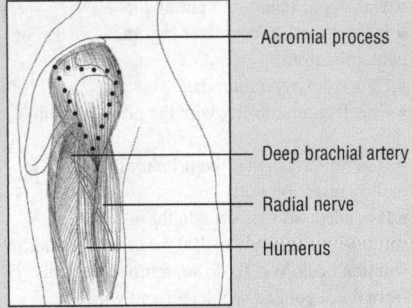

• The vastus lateralis muscle is used most often in children; the rectus femoris may be used in infants.

Vastus lateralis and rectus femoris muscles

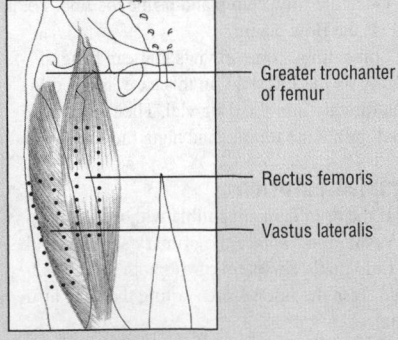

• Loosen, but don't remove, the needle sheath.

• Gently tap the site to stimulate nerve endings and minimize pain.

- Clean the site with an alcohol sponge, starting at the site and moving outward in expanding circles to about 2" (5 cm). Allow the skin to dry because wet alcohol stings in the puncture.
- Put on gloves.
- With the thumb and index finger of your non-dominant hand, gently stretch the skin.
- With the syringe in your dominant hand, remove the needle sheath with the free fingers of the other hand.
- Position the syringe perpendicular to the skin surface and a couple of inches from the skin. Tell the patient that he'll feel a prick. Then quickly and firmly thrust the needle into the muscle.
- Pull back slightly on the plunger to aspirate for blood. If blood appears, the needle is in a blood vessel. Withdraw the needle, prepare a fresh syringe, and inject another site. If no blood appears, inject the drug slowly and steadily to let the muscle distend gradually. You should feel little or no resistance. Gently but quickly remove the needle at a 90-degree angle.
- Using a gloved hand, apply gentle pressure to the site with the cotton ball or 2" × 2" gauze. Massage the relaxed muscle, unless contraindicated, to distribute the drug and promote absorption.
- Inspect the site for bleeding or bruising. Apply pressure as needed.
- Discard all equipment properly. Don't recap needles; put them in an appropriate biohazard container to avoid needle-stick injuries.
- Remove and discard your gloves in a biohazard container. Wash your hands.

Nursing considerations

- To slow absorption, some drugs are dissolved in oil. Mix them well before use.
- ⑤ ALERT: If you must inject more than 5 ml, divide the solution and inject it at two different sites.
- Rotate injection sites for patients who need repeated injections.
- Urge the patient to relax the muscle to reduce pain and bleeding.
- ⑤ ALERT: Never inject into the gluteal muscles of a child who has been walking for less than one year.
- Keep in mind that I.M. injections can damage local muscle cells and elevate CK levels, which can be confused with elevated levels caused by MI. Diagnostic tests can be used to differentiate between them.

Subcutaneous administration

A subcutaneous injection allows slower, more sustained administration than an I.M. injection. Drugs and solutions delivered subcutaneously are injected through a relatively short needle using sterile technique.

Equipment and preparation

- Check the chart and the medication administration record.
- Make sure the patient isn't allergic to the drug or any of its components.
- Gather drug, needle of appropriate gauge and length, 1- to 3-ml syringe, gloves, alcohol sponges, and nonsterile cotton ball or 2" × 2" gauze pad. Other materials may include antiseptic cleanser, filter needle, insulin syringe, and insulin pump.
- Inspect the drug to make sure it's the right color and consistency and is free of precipitates.
- Wash your hands.

For single-dose ampules

- Wrap the neck of the ampule in an alcohol sponge and snap off the top, directing it away from you.
- If desired, attach a filter needle to the needle, slightly tip the ampule, and withdraw the desired amount of the drug.
- Tap the syringe to disperse air bubbles.
- Cover the needle with the attached safety sheath by placing the needle sheath on the counter or medication cart and sliding the needle into the sheath.
- Before discarding the ampule, check the label against the patient's medication record.
- Discard the filter needle and the ampule in a biohazard container.
- Attach the appropriate-sized needle to the syringe.

For single-dose and multidose vials

- Reconstitute powdered drugs according to the instructions on the label.
- Clean the rubber stopper on the vial with an alcohol sponge for at least 15 seconds.
- Pull the syringe plunger back until the volume of air in the syringe equals the volume of drug to be withdrawn from the vial.
- Insert the needle into the vial.

• Inject the air, invert the vial, and keep the bevel tip of the needle below the level of the solution as you withdraw the prescribed amount of drug.
• Tap the syringe to disperse air bubbles.
• Cover the needle with the attached safety sheath by placing the needle sheath on the counter or medication cart and sliding the needle into the sheath.
• Check the drug label against the patient's medication record before returning the multi-dose vial to the shelf or drawer or before discarding the single-dose vial.
• Attach the appropriate-sized needle to the syringe.

Implementation

• Confirm the patient's identity by asking his full name and checking his identity by wristband, picture, or other specific data.
• Make sure the patient isn't allergic to the drug or any of its components.
• Select the injection site from those shown, and tell the patient where you'll be giving the injection.

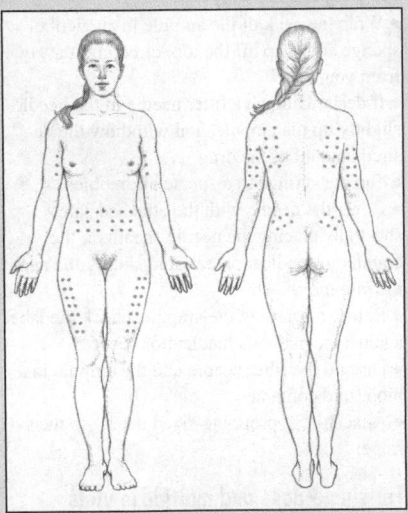

• Wash your hands and put on gloves. Position and drape the patient.
• Clean the injection site with an alcohol sponge. Loosen the protective needle sheath.
• With your nondominant hand, pinch the skin around the injection site firmly to elevate the

subcutaneous tissue, forming a 1″ (2.5 cm) fat fold, as shown.

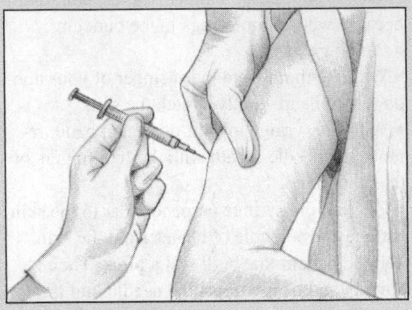

• Holding the syringe in your dominant hand, grip the needle sheath between the fourth and fifth fingers of your nondominant hand while continuing to pinch the skin around the injection site with the index finger and thumb of your nondominant hand. Pull the sheath back to uncover the needle. Don't touch the needle.
• Position the needle with its bevel up.
• Tell the patient he'll feel a prick as you insert the needle. Do so quickly, in one motion, at a 45-degree or 90-degree angle, as shown below. The needle length and the angle you use depend on the amount of subcutaneous tissue at the site. Some drugs, such as heparin, should always be injected at a 90-degree angle.

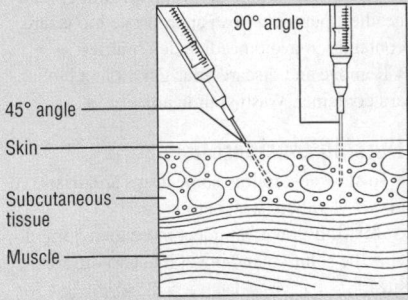

• Release the skin to avoid injecting the drug into compressed tissue and irritating the nerves. Except for insulin and heparin, pull the plunger back slightly to check for blood return. If blood appears, withdraw the needle, prepare another syringe, and repeat the procedure. If no blood appears, slowly inject the drug.
• After injection, remove the needle at the same angle you used to insert it. Using a gloved hand, apply gentle pressure to the site with the

cotton ball or 2″ × 2″ gauze pad. Massage the site gently, unless contraindicated, to distribute the drug and promote absorption.
• Inspect the injection site for bleeding or bruising.
• Discard all equipment properly. Don't recap needles; put them in a biohazard container to avoid needle-stick injuries.
• Remove and discard your gloves in a biohazard container. Wash your hands.

Nursing considerations
✪ **ALERT:** Don't aspirate for blood return when giving insulin or heparin. It isn't necessary with insulin and may cause a hematoma with heparin.
• Don't massage the site after giving heparin.
✪ **ALERT:** Repeated injections in the same site can cause lipodystrophy, a natural immune response. Rotating injection sites can minimize this complication.

Topical administration
Topical drugs, such as patches, lotions, and ointments, are applied directly to the skin. They're commonly used for local rather than systemic effects. Certain types of topical drugs—known as transdermal drugs—are meant to enter the patient's bloodstream and to have a systemic effect after you apply them.

Equipment and preparation
• Check the chart and the drug administration record.
• Make sure the patient isn't allergic to the drug or any of its components.
• Gather the prescribed drug, sterile tongue blades, gloves, sterile gloves for open lesions, sterile 4″ × 4″ gauze pads, transparent semipermeable dressing, adhesive tape, normal saline solution, cotton-tipped applicators, gloves, and linen savers, if needed.

Implementation
• Confirm the patient's identity by asking his full name and checking his identity by wristband, picture, or other specific data.
• Make sure the patient isn't allergic to the drug or any of its components.
• Explain the procedure to the patient because, after discharge, he may have to apply the drug himself.

• If the procedure is uncomfortable, premedicate the patient with an analgesic. Give it time to take effect.
• Wash your hands to reduce the risk of cross-contamination, and glove your dominant hand.
• Help the patient to a comfortable position, and expose the area to be treated. Make sure the skin or mucous membrane is intact (unless the drug is for a skin lesion). Applying the drug to broken or abraded skin may cause unwanted systemic absorption and further irritation.
• If needed, clean debris from the skin. You may have to change your gloves if they become soiled.

To apply paste, cream, or ointment
• Open the container. Place the cap upside down to avoid contaminating its inner surface.
• Remove a tongue blade from its sterile wrapper, and cover one end of the blade with drug from the tube or jar. Then transfer the drug from the blade to your gloved hand.
• Apply the drug to the affected area with long, smooth strokes that follow the direction of hair growth. This technique avoids forcing the drug into hair follicles, which can cause irritation and folliculitis. Don't press too hard because it could abrade the skin and cause discomfort.
• When applying a drug to the patient's face, use cotton-tipped applicators for small areas, such as under the eyes. For larger areas, use a sterile gauze pad.
• To avoid contaminating the drug, use a new sterile tongue blade each time you remove the drug from its container.
• Remove and discard your gloves and wash your hands.

To apply transdermal ointment
• Choose the application site—usually a dry, hairless spot on the patient's chest or upper arm.
• To help absorption, wash the site with soap and warm water and dry thoroughly.
• Wash your hands and put on gloves.
• If the patient has a previously applied medication strip at another site, remove it and swab or wash this area to clear away the drug residue.
• If the area you choose is hairy, clip excess hair rather than shaving it. Shaving causes irritation, which the drug may worsen.
• Squeeze the prescribed amount of ointment onto the application strip or measuring paper. Don't get the ointment on your skin.

• Apply the strip, drug side down, directly to the patient's skin.
• Maneuver the strip slightly to spread a thin layer of the ointment over a 3″ (8-cm) area, but don't rub the ointment into the skin.
• Secure the application strip to the patient's skin by covering it with a semipermeable dressing or plastic wrap.
• Tape the covering securely in place.
• Label the strip with the date, time, and your initials, if required by your facility.
• Remove your gloves and wash your hands.

To apply a transdermal patch

• Remove the old patch and swab or wash the site to remove any residual drug or adhesive.
• Choose a dry, hairless application site.
• Clip (don't shave) hair from the chosen site. Wash the area with warm water and soap, and dry it thoroughly.
• Wash your hands and put on gloves.
• Without touching the adhesive surface, remove the clear plastic backing.
• Apply the patch to the site without touching the adhesive.
• If required by your facility's policy, label the patch with the date, time, and your initials.
• Remove your gloves and wash your hands.

To remove ointment

• Wash your hands and put on gloves.
• Gently swab ointment from the patient's skin using a sterile 4″ × 4″ gauze pad saturated with normal saline solution.
• Don't wipe too hard because you could irritate the skin.
• Remove and discard your gloves and wash your hands.

Nursing considerations

• To prevent skin irritation, always remove previous drug applications by swabbing or washing; then select a new site.
• Always wear gloves to protect your skin.
• Never apply ointment to the eyelids or ear canal. The ointment may congeal and occlude the tear duct or ear canal.
• Inspect the treated area frequently for allergic or other adverse reactions.
• Don't apply a topical drug to scarred or callused skin because this may slow absorption.
• Don't place a defibrillator paddle on a transdermal patch. The aluminum on the patch can cause electrical arcing during defibrillation, re-

sulting in smoke and thermal burns. If a patient has a patch on a standard paddle site, remove the patch and swab the skin quickly before applying the paddle, or use another site, if possible.

Ophthalmic administration

Ophthalmic drugs—drops or ointments—serve both diagnostic and therapeutic purposes. During an ophthalmic examination, drugs can be used to anesthetize the eye, dilate the pupil, and stain the cornea to identify anomalies. Therapeutic uses include eye lubrication and treatment of glaucoma and infections.

Equipment and preparation

• Check the chart and the medication administration record.
• Make sure the patient isn't allergic to the drug or any of its components.
• Gather the prescribed ophthalmic drug, sterile cotton balls, gloves, warm water or normal saline solution, sterile gauze pads, and facial tissue. An ocular dressing also may be used.
• Make sure the drug is labeled for ophthalmic use. Check the expiration date. Remember to date the container after first use. If in doubt, consult the pharmacist.
• Inspect ocular solutions for cloudiness, discoloration, and precipitation, keeping in mind that some drugs are suspensions that normally appear cloudy.

Implementation

• Make sure you know which eye you are treating because different drugs or doses may be ordered for each eye.
• Confirm the patient's identity by asking his full name and checking his identity by wristband, picture, or other specific data.
• Make sure the patient isn't allergic to the drug or any of its components.
• Wash your hands and put on gloves.
• If the patient has an eye dressing, remove it by pulling it down and away from his forehead, being careful not to contaminate your hands. (If you do, remove the contaminated gloves, wash your hands, and put on new gloves.) Don't apply pressure to the area around the eyes.
• To remove exudates or meibomian gland secretions, clean around the eye with sterile cot-

ton balls or sterile gauze pads that have been moistened with warm water or normal saline solution. Have the patient close his eyes; then gently wipe the eyelids from the inner to the outer canthus. Use a fresh cotton ball or gauze pad for each stroke, and use a different cotton ball or pad for each eye.
• Have the patient sit or lie on his back. Tell him to tilt his head back and toward his affected eye so that any excess drug can flow away from the tear duct, minimizing systemic absorption through the nasal mucosa.
• Remove the dropper cap from the drug container, and draw the drug into the dropper. Or, if the bottle has a dropper tip, remove the cap and hold or place it upside down to prevent contamination.
• Before instilling eyedrops, tell the patient to look up and away. This moves the cornea away from the lower lid and minimizes the risk of touching the lid with the dropper.

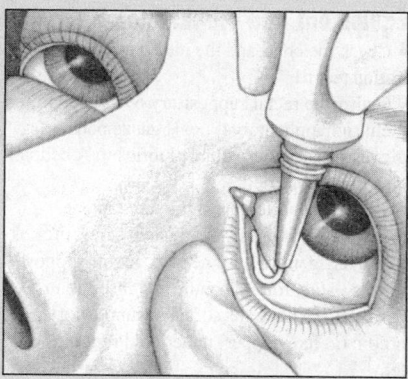

To instill eyedrops
• Steady the hand that's holding the dropper by resting it gently against the patient's forehead. With your other hand, gently pull down the lower lid of the affected eye, and instill the drops in the conjunctival sac. Never instill eyedrops directly onto the eyeball.
• After instilling the eyedrops, tell the patient to close his eyes gently without squeezing the lids shut and not to blink.
• Instruct the patient to place a finger in the corner of the eye between the bridge of the nose and the eyelid and to apply gentle pressure for 2 to 3 minutes to prevent systemic absorption of drops through the lacrimal sac. Then have the patient wipe away any excess drops or tears with a clean tissue before opening the eyes. Use a fresh tissue for each eye.
• Remove and discard your gloves and wash your hands.
• An elderly patient may have difficulty feeling the drops in his eye. When teaching an elderly patient how to instill drops himself, suggest that he chill the drug slightly in the refrigerator because cold drops are easier to feel.

To apply eye ointment
• Squeeze a small ribbon of drug on the edge of the conjunctival sac from the inner to the outer canthus. Cut off the ribbon by turning the tube. Don't touch the eye with the tip of the tube.

• After applying ointment, tell the patient to close his eye gently without squeezing the lid shut and to roll his eye behind a closed lid to help distribute the drug over the eyeball. Have the patient sit with the eye closed for 2 to 3 minutes to facilitate absorption and avoid "clouding" of the vision from the ointment.
• Use a tissue to remove any excess drug that leaks from the eye. Use a fresh tissue for each eye to prevent cross-contamination.
• Apply a new eye dressing, if needed.
• Remove and discard your gloves and wash your hands.

Nursing considerations
• Urge the patient not to rub his eye or blink immediately after eyedrops.
• To maintain the drug container's sterility, don't put the cap down after opening the container, and never touch the eye area with the tip of the dropper or bottle. Discard any solution remaining in the dropper before returning it to the bottle. If the dropper or bottle tip is contaminated, discard it and use another sterile dropper. Never share eyedrops between patients.

Rectal administration
A rectal suppository is a small, solid drug mass, usually cone shaped, with a cocoa butter or glycerin base. It may be inserted to stimulate peristalsis and defecation or to relieve pain, vomiting, and local irritation. An ointment is a semisolid drug used to produce local effects. It may be applied externally to the anus or internally to the rectum.

Equipment and preparation

• Check the chart and the medication administration record.

• Gather the rectal suppository or tube of ointment and applicator, $4'' \times 4''$ gauze pads, gloves, and a water-soluble lubricant. A bedpan also may be needed.

• To prevent softening of the drug and decreased effectiveness, store rectal suppositories in the refrigerator until needed. A soft suppository is also harder to handle and insert than a hard one. To harden a softened suppository, hold it (in its wrapper) under cold running water.

Implementation

• Confirm the patient's identity by asking his full name and checking the name and medical record number on his wristband.

• Make sure the patient isn't allergic to the drug or any of its components.

• Wash your hands.

To insert a rectal suppository

• Place the patient on his left side in Sims' position. Drape him with the bedcovers, exposing only his buttocks.

• Put on gloves. Unwrap the suppository and lubricate it with water-soluble lubricant.

• Lift the patient's right buttock with your nondominant hand to expose the anus.

• Instruct the patient to take several deep breaths through his mouth to relax the anal sphincter and to reduce anxiety and discomfort during drug insertion.

• Using the index finger of your dominant hand, insert the suppository—tapered end first—about $3''$ (8 cm) until you feel it pass the internal anal sphincter, as shown.

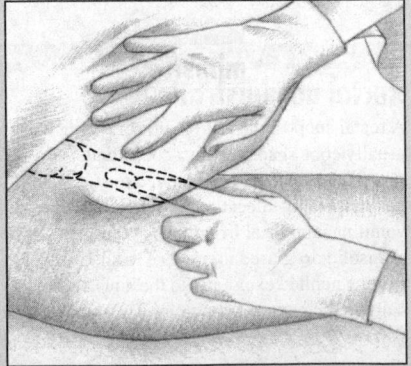

• Direct the tapered end of the suppository toward the side of the rectum so the drug contacts the membranes.

• Encourage the patient to lie quietly and, if possible, to contract his anal sphincter and buttocks together to retain the suppository for the correct length of time. Press on the patient's anus with a gauze pad, if needed, until the urge to defecate passes.

• Discard the used equipment and gloves. Wash your hands thoroughly.

To apply an ointment

• For external application, put on gloves and use a gauze pad to spread the drug over the anal area. For internal application, attach the end of the applicator to the tube of ointment, and coat the applicator with water-soluble lubricant.

• Use about $1''$ (2.5 cm) of ointment. To gauge how much pressure to use during application, try squeezing a small amount from the tube before you attach the applicator.

• Place the patient on his left side in Sims' position. Drape him with the bedcovers, exposing only his buttocks.

• Lift the patient's right buttock with your nondominant hand to expose the anus.

• Tell the patient to take several deep breaths through his mouth to relax the anal sphincter and reduce anxiety and discomfort during insertion. Gently insert the applicator, directing it toward the umbilicus.

• Squeeze the tube to eject drug.

• Remove the applicator and place a folded $4'' \times 4''$ gauze pad between the patient's buttocks to absorb excess ointment.

• Disassemble the tube and applicator and recap the tube. Clean the applicator with soap and warm water and store or discard it. Remove and discard your gloves, and wash your hands thoroughly.

Nursing considerations

• Because eating and drinking stimulates peristalsis, a suppository for relieving constipation should be inserted about 30 minutes before mealtime to help soften the stool and facilitate defecation. A medicated retention suppository should be inserted between meals.

• Tell the patient to try to retain the suppository. If this is difficult, place the patient on a bedpan.

• Make sure that the patient's call button is handy, and watch for his signal because he may be unable to suppress the urge to defecate.
• Inform the patient that the suppository may discolor his next bowel movement.

Buccal and sublingual administration

Certain drugs are given buccally (between the cheek and teeth) or S.L. (under the tongue) to bypass the digestive tract and speed absorption into the bloodstream. When using either method, observe the patient carefully to make sure he doesn't swallow the drug or develop mucosal irritation.

Equipment and preparation
• Check the chart and the medication administration record.
• Gather the prescribed drug, medication cup, and gloves.

Implementation
• Wash your hands. If you'll be placing the drug into the patient's mouth, put on gloves.
• Confirm the patient's identity by asking his full name and checking the name and medical record number on his wristband.
• Make sure the patient isn't allergic to the drug or any of its components.
• For buccal administration, place the tablet in the patient's buccal pouch, between the cheek and teeth, as shown below.

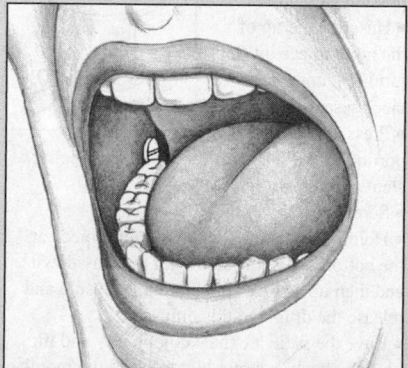

• For S.L. administration, place the tablet under the patient's tongue, as shown below.

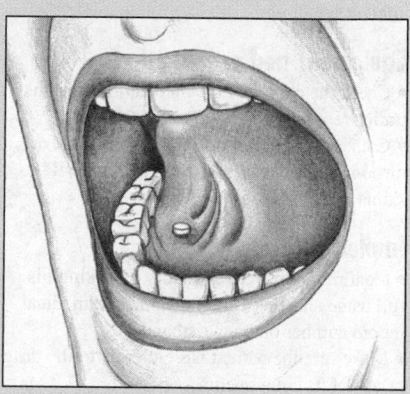

• Remove and discard gloves and wash your hands.
• Instruct the patient to keep the drug in place until it dissolves completely to ensure absorption. Caution the patient against chewing the tablet or touching it with his tongue to prevent accidental swallowing.
• Tell the patient not to smoke before the drug has dissolved because nicotine constricts blood vessels and slows drug absorption.

Nursing considerations
• Don't give liquids until a buccal tablet is absorbed; in some cases, this make take up to an hour.
• If the patient has angina, tell him to wet the nitroglycerin tablet with saliva and keep it under his tongue until it's fully absorbed.
• Make sure a patient with angina knows how to take nitroglycerin, how many doses to take, and when to call for emergency help.

Inhalation administration

Hand-held oropharyngeal inhalers include the metered-dose inhaler, dry-powder multidose inhaler, nasal inhaler, and turbo-inhaler. These devices deliver topical drugs to the respiratory tract, producing local and systemic effects. The mucosal lining of the respiratory tract absorbs the inhalant almost immediately. Examples of oral inhalants are bronchodilators, which improve airway patency and facilitate mucous drainage, and mucolytics, which liquefy tenacious bronchial secretions. Examples of nasal inhalants include corticosteroids, which reduce allergic symptoms.

Equipment and preparation

• Check the chart and the medication administration record.
• Gather the metered-dose inhaler, diskus, or turbo-inhaler, prescribed drug, and normal saline solution.

Implementation

• Confirm the patient's identity by asking his full name and checking the name and medical record number on his wristband.
• Make sure the patient isn't allergic to the drug or any of its components.
• Wash your hands. Apply gloves if there is a risk of aerosol or secretion exposure.

To use a metered-dose inhaler

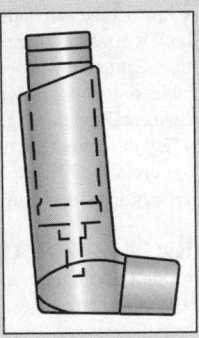

• Shake the inhaler bottle. Remove the cap and insert the stem into the small hole on the flattened portion of the mouthpiece, as shown.
• Place the inhaler about 1" (2.5 cm) in front of the patient's open mouth.
• Tell the patient to exhale.
• If using a spacer, which can make the inhaler more effective, tell the patient to place the spacer mouthpiece in his mouth and to press his lips firmly around the mouthpiece.
• As you push the bottle down against the mouthpiece, tell the patient to inhale slowly through his mouth and to continue inhaling until his lungs feel full. Compress the bottle against the mouthpiece only once.
• Remove the inhaler and tell the patient to hold his breath for several seconds. Then instruct him to exhale slowly through pursed lips to keep distal bronchioles open and allow increased absorption and diffusion of the drug.
• Have the patient gargle with normal saline solution or water to remove the drug from his mouth and the back of his throat and to help prevent oral fungal infections. Warn the patient not to swallow after gargling, but rather to spit out the liquid.

To use a dry-powder multidose inhaler

• Hold the dry-powder multidose inhaler in one hand and put the thumb of your other hand on the thumbgrip. Push your thumb away from you as far as it will go, until the mouthpiece appears and snaps into position.
• Hold the dry-powder multidose inhaler level horizontally with the mouthpiece toward the patient. Slide the lever away from the patient as far as it will go until it clicks.
• Instruct the patient to exhale fully (not into the mouthpiece of the dry-powder multidose inhaler).
• Instruct the patient to breathe in quickly and deeply through the dry-powder multidose inhaler's mouthpiece, then hold the breath for 10 or more seconds. Then have the patient breathe out slowly.
• Wipe off the mouthpiece with a clean tissue, if needed, and close. (It will automatically reset for the next dose.)
• Tell the patient to rinse his mouth with water, without swallowing, after each dose.
• Never take a dry-powder multidose inhaler apart or wash any part of it. Check counter on top of dry-powder multidose inhaler to be sure dose is available and reorder five inhalations from end.

To use a turbo-inhaler

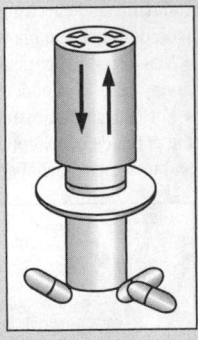

• Hold the mouthpiece in one hand. With the other hand, slide the sleeve away from the mouthpiece as far as possible, as shown.
• Unscrew the tip of the mouthpiece by turning it counter-clockwise.
• Press the colored portion of the drug capsule into the propeller stem of the mouthpiece.
• Screw the inhaler together again.
• Holding the inhaler with the mouthpiece at the bottom, slide the sleeve all the way down and then up again to puncture the capsule and release the drug. Do this only once.
• Have the patient exhale completely and tilt his head back. Instruct him to place the mouthpiece in his mouth, close his lips around it, and inhale once. Tell him to hold his breath for several seconds.

- Remove the inhaler from the patient's mouth, and tell him to exhale as much air as possible.
- Repeat the procedure until the entire amount of drug in the device is inhaled.
- Have the patient gargle and spit with normal saline solution or water, if desired, to remove the drug from his mouth and the back of his throat.

To use a nasal inhaler

- Instruct patient to clear his nasal passages before administration.
- Shake the container to ensure even distribution of contents.
- Wipe the tip of the container with a clean tissue if needed.
- Tell patient to place a finger against the nostril not being treated to block air entrance. Instruct the patient to exhale fully through the mouth.
- Place tip of nasal container into appropriate nostril without directing it onto nasal mucosa. Instruct patient to inhale quickly and deeply through this nostril, with mouth closed, while squeezing the nasal inhaler to release spray along with inhalation.
- Remove the inhaler and have the patient gently press close the medicated nostril, breathing through his mouth for several seconds. Treat the opposite nostril, if indicated, or apply two inhalations to each nostril, if indicated, spaced 3 to 5 seconds apart.

Nursing considerations

- Teach the patient how to use the inhaler so he can continue treatments after discharge, if needed. Explain that overdose can cause the drug to lose its effectiveness. Tell him to record the date and time of each inhalation and his response.
- Some inhalants may cause restlessness, palpitations, nervousness, and other systemic effects. They also may cause hypersensitivity reactions, such as a rash, urticaria, rhinitis, nasal bleeding, or bronchospasms.
- Give oral inhalants cautiously to patients with heart disease because these drugs may lead to coronary insufficiency, cardiac arrhythmias, or hypertension. If paradoxical bronchospasm occurs, stop the drug and use a different drug.
- If the patient is prescribed a bronchodilator and a corticosteroid, give the bronchodilator

first so the air passages can open fully before the patient uses the corticosteroid.
- Instruct the patient to keep an extra inhaler handy.
- Instruct the patient to discard the inhaler after taking the prescribed number of doses and to start a new inhaler.
- Urge the patient to notify his prescriber if he notices an increased use of or need for an inhaler, or if symptoms are not relieved with the prescribed regimen.

Nasogastric administration

Besides providing another way to feed patients who can't eat normally, an NG tube allows for the instillation of drugs directly into the GI system.

Equipment and preparation

- Check the chart and the medication administration record.
- Gather equipment for use at the bedside, including prescribed drug, towel or linen-saver pad, 50- or 60-ml piston-type catheter-tip syringe, feeding tubing, two 4″ × 4″ gauze pads, stethoscope, gloves, diluent (juice, water, or a nutritional supplement), cup for mixing drug and fluid, spoon, 50-ml cup of water, and rubber band. You may also need pill-crushing equipment and a clamp, if it's not already attached to the tube.
- Make sure that liquids are at room temperature to avoid abdominal cramping and that the cup, syringe, spoon, and gauze are clean.

Implementation

- Wash your hands and put on gloves.
- Confirm the patient's identity by asking his full name and checking the name and medical record number on his wristband.
- Make sure the patient isn't allergic to the drug or any of its components.
- Unpin the tube from the patient's gown. To avoid soiling the sheets during the procedure, fold back the bed linens and drape the patient's chest with a towel or linen-saver pad.
- Help the patient into Fowler's position, if possible.
- After unclamping the tube, auscultate the patient's abdomen about 3″ (8 cm) below the sternum as you gently insert 10 ml of air into the

tube with the 50- or 60-ml syringe. You should hear the air bubble entering the stomach. Gently draw back on the piston of the syringe. The appearance of gastric contents indicates that the tube is patent and is properly placed in the stomach.
• If no gastric contents appear or if you meet resistance, the tube may be lying against the gastric mucosa. Withdraw the tube slightly or turn the patient to free it.
• Clamp the tube, detach the syringe, and lay the end of the tube on the 4″ × 4″ gauze pad.
• If the drug is a tablet, crush it before mixing it with the diluent. Make sure the particles are small enough to pass through the eyes at the distal end of the tube. Some drugs (extended release, enteric-coated, or S.L. drugs, for example) shouldn't be crushed. If you aren't sure, ask the pharmacist. Also, check to see if the drug comes as a liquid form or if a capsule may be opened and the contents poured into a diluent. Pour liquid drugs into the diluent and stir well.
• Reattach the syringe, without the piston, to the end of the tube. Holding the tube upright at a level slightly above the patient's nose, open the clamp and pour the drug in slowly and steadily, as shown below.

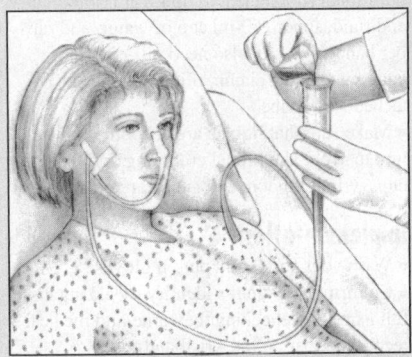

• To keep air from entering the patient's stomach, hold the tube at a slight angle and add more drug before the syringe empties. If the drug flows smoothly, slowly give the entire dose. If it doesn't flow, it may be too thick. If so, dilute it with water. If you suspect that tube placement is inhibiting flow, stop the procedure and reevaluate the placement.
• Watch the patient's reaction. If you see signs of discomfort, stop immediately.

• As the last of the drug flows out of the syringe, start to irrigate the tube by adding 30 to 50 ml of water (15 to 30 ml for a child). Irrigating clears drug from the tube and reduces the risk of clogging.
• When the water stops flowing, clamp the tube. Detach the syringe, and discard it properly.
• Fasten the tube to the patient's gown, and make the patient comfortable.
• Leave the patient in Fowler's position or on his right side with his head partially elevated for at least 30 minutes to ease flow and prevent esophageal reflux.
• Remove and discard your gloves and wash your hands.

Nursing considerations
• If you must give a tube feeding and a drug, give the drug first to make sure the patient receives the entire drug.
• Certain drugs—such as phenytoin (Dilantin)—bind with tube feedings, decreasing the availability of the drug. Stop the tube feeding for 2 hours before and after the dose, according to your facility's policy.
• If residual stomach contents exceed 150 ml, withhold the drug and feeding, and notify the prescriber. Excessive stomach contents may indicate intestinal obstruction or paralytic ileus.
• Never crush enteric-coated, buccal, S.L., or sustained-release drugs.
• If suction is on, turn it off for 20 to 30 minutes after giving a drug.

Otic administration
Eardrops may be instilled to treat infection and inflammation, to soften cerumen for removal, to produce local anesthesia, or to remove an insect trapped in the ear.

Equipment and preparation
• Check the chart and the medication administration record.
• Gather the eardrops, gloves, a light, and facial tissue or cotton-tipped applicators. Cotton balls and a bowl of warm water may be needed.
• First, warm the drug to body temperature in the bowl of warm water, or carry the drug in your pocket for 30 minutes before giving. Test the temperature of the drug by placing a drop

on your wrist. If the drug is too hot, it may burn the patient's eardrum.
• To avoid injuring the ear canal, check the dropper before use to make sure it's not chipped or cracked.

Implementation
• Wash your hands and put on gloves.
• Confirm the patient's identity by asking his full name and checking the name and medical record number on his wristband.
• Make sure the patient isn't allergic to the drug or any of its components.
• Have the patient lie on the side opposite the affected ear.

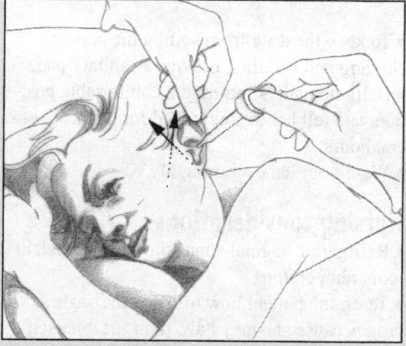

• Straighten the patient's ear canal. For an adult, pull the auricle up and back. For a child younger than age 3, gently pull the auricle down and back because the ear canal is straighter at this age.

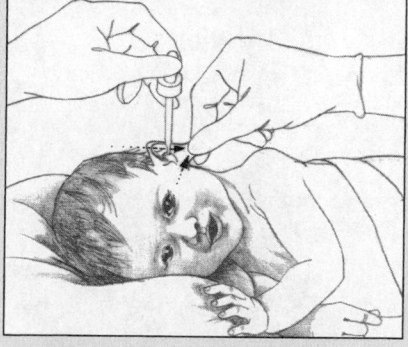

• Using a light, examine the ear canal for drainage. If you see drainage, gently clean the canal with the tissue or cotton-tipped applica-

tors because drainage can reduce the effectiveness of the drug. Never insert an applicator past the point where you can see it.
• Compare the label on the eardrops to the order on the patient's medication record. Check the label again while drawing the drug into the dropper. Check the label for the final time before giving the eardrops.
• Straighten the patient's ear canal once again, and instill the proper number of drops. For the patient's comfort, aim the dropper so that the drops fall against the sides of the ear canal, not on the eardrum. Hold the ear canal in position until you see the drug disappear down the canal. Then release the ear.
• To avoid damaging the ear canal with the dropper, especially with a struggling child, it may be necessary to gently rest the hand that is holding the dropper against the patient's head to secure a safe position before giving the drug.
• Instruct the patient to remain on his side for 5 to 10 minutes to allow the drug to run down into the ear canal.
• Tuck a cotton ball with a small amount of petroleum jelly on it loosely into the opening of the ear canal to prevent the drug from leaking out. Don't insert the cotton too deeply into the canal because this may prevent secretions from draining and may increase pressure on the eardrum.
• Clean and dry the outer ear.
• If needed, repeat the procedure in the other ear after 5 to 10 minutes.
• Help the patient into a comfortable position.
• Remove your gloves and wash your hands.

Nursing considerations
• Some conditions make the normally tender ear canal even more sensitive, so be especially gentle.
• To prevent injury to the eardrum, never insert a cotton-tipped applicator into the ear canal past the point where you can see the tip.
• After instilling eardrops to soften cerumen, irrigate the ear to remove.
• If the patient has vertigo, keep the side rails of his bed up and assist him as needed during the procedure. Also, move slowly to avoid worsening his vertigo.
• Teach the patient to instill the eardrops himself so that he can continue treatment at home. Have the patient try it himself while you observe.

Vaginal administration

Vaginal drugs can be inserted as topical treatment for infection, particularly *Trichomonas vaginalis* and vaginal candidiasis or inflammation. Suppositories melt when they contact the vaginal mucosa, and the drug diffuses topically.

Vaginal drugs usually come with a disposable applicator that enables placement of drug in the anterior and posterior fornices. Vaginal administration is most effective when the patient can remain lying down afterward to retain the drug.

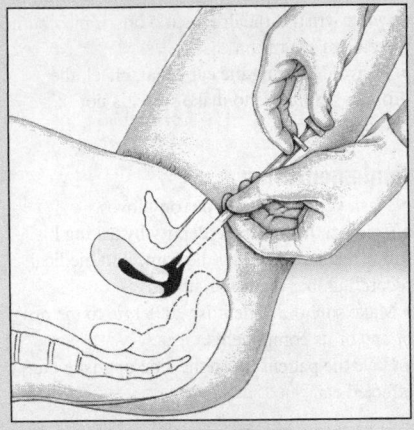

Equipment and preparation
• Check the chart and the medication administration record.
• Gather the prescribed drug and applicator, gloves, water-soluble lubricant, and a small sanitary pad.

Implementation
• If possible, give vaginal drugs at bedtime when the patient is lying down.
• Confirm the patient's identity by asking her full name and checking the name and medical record number on her wristband.
• Make sure the patient isn't allergic to the drug or any of its components.
• Wash your hands, explain the procedure to the patient, and provide privacy.
• Ask the patient to void.
• Ask the patient if she would prefer to insert the drug herself and give instruction.
• Help the patient into the lithotomy position. Drape her, exposing only the perineum.
• Remove the suppository from the wrapper and lubricate it with water-soluble lubricant.
• Put on gloves and expose the vagina by spreading the labia. If you see discharge, wash the area with several cotton balls soaked in warm, soapy water. Clean each side of the perineum and then the center, using a fresh cotton ball for each stroke. Rinse well with clean, warm water. While the labia are still separated, insert the suppository or vaginal applicator about 3″ to 4″ (7.6 to 10 cm) into the vagina.
• After insertion, wash the applicator with soap and warm water, and store or discard it. Label it so it will be used only for this patient.
• Remove and discard gloves.

• To keep the drug from soiling the patient's clothing and bedding, provide a sanitary pad.
• Help the patient return to a comfortable position, and tell her to stay in bed for the next several hours.
• Wash your hands thoroughly.

Nursing considerations
• Refrigerate vaginal suppositories that melt at room temperature.
• Teach the patient how to insert the vaginal drug because she may have to insert it herself after she is discharged. Give her instructions in writing, if possible.
• Instruct the patient not to insert a tampon after inserting a vaginal drug because the tampon will absorb the drug and decrease its effectiveness.

4

Drug administration safety

In the state where you practice nursing, many different health care professionals may be legally permitted to prescribe, dispense, and give drugs, such as doctors, nurse practitioners, dentists, podiatrists, and optometrists. Most often, doctors prescribe drugs, pharmacists dispense them, and nurses give them to patients.

That means that nurses are usually on the front line when it comes to patients and their drugs. It also means that nurses bear a major share of the responsibility for avoiding medication errors. Besides faithfully following their facilities' drug administration policies, nurses can help prevent medication errors by studying and avoiding the common slip ups that allow them to happen. This chapter outlines some common causes of medication errors.

Name game

Drugs with similar-sounding names can be easily confused. Even different-sounding names can look similar when written rapidly by hand on a prescription form. An example is Soriatane and Loxitane, which are both capsules. If the patient's drug order doesn't seem right for his diagnosis, call the prescriber to clarify the order.

🅢 **ALERT:** Many nurses have confused an order for morphine with one for hydromorphone (Dilaudid). Both drugs come in 4-mg prefilled syringes. If you give morphine when the prescriber really ordered hydromorphone, the patient could develop respiratory depression or even arrest. In the place where opioids are kept, consider posting a prominent notice that warns the staff about this common mix-up. Or try attaching a fluorescent sticker printed with NOT MORPHINE to each hydromorphone syringe.

Drug names aren't the only words you can confuse. Patient names can cause problems if you fail to verify the individual's identity before giving a drug. This problem can be especially troublesome if two patients have the same first name.

Consider this clinical scenario: Robert Brewer, age 5, was hospitalized for measles. Robert Brinson, also age 5, was admitted after a severe asthma attack. The boys were assigned to adjacent rooms on a small pediatric unit. Each had a nonproductive cough. When Robert Brewer's nurse came to give him an expectorant, the child's mother told her that Robert had already inhaled a medication through a mask.

The nurse quickly figured out that another nurse, new to the unit, had given Robert Brinson's medication (acetylcysteine, a mucolytic) to Robert Brewer in error. Fortunately, no harmful adverse effects occurred. Had the nurse checked her patient's identity more carefully, however, she wouldn't have made the error.

Always check each patient's full name. Also, teach each patient (or parent) to offer an identification bracelet for inspection and to state his full name when anyone enters the room with the intention of giving a medication. (See *Reducing medication errors through patient teaching,* page 32.) Also, urge patients to tell you if an identification bracelet falls off, is removed, or gets lost. Replace it right away.

Allergy alert

Once you've verified your patient's full name, check to see if he is wearing an allergy bracelet. If he is, the allergy bracelet should conspicuously display the name of the allergen. The allergy information also should be labeled on the front of the patient's chart and on his medication record. Whether the patient is wearing an allergy bracelet or not, take the time to double-check and ask the patient whether he has any drug allergies — even if he's in distress. Consider the following real-life example.

A doctor issued a stat order for chlorpromazine (Thorazine) for a distressed patient. By the time the nurse arrived with the drug, the patient had grown more distressed and was demanding relief. Unnerved by the patient's behavior, the nurse gave the drug without checking the patient's medication administration record or documenting the order, and the patient had an allergic reaction to it.

Any time you're in a tense situation with a patient who needs or wants medication fast, resist the temptation to act first and verify later.

Reducing medication errors through patient teaching

You aren't the only one at risk for making medication errors. Patients taking drugs at home are at an even higher risk because they know so much less about drugs than you do. Clearly, patient teaching is a crucial aspect of your nursing responsibility in minimizing medication errors and their consequences—especially with more patients receiving outpatient instead of inpatient care.

To help minimize medication errors, teach your patient about his diagnosis and the purpose of his drug therapy. Make sure he knows the name of each drug in his regimen, the purpose of each drug, the amount he's supposed to take, and the timing and method by which he's supposed to take it. Use an interpreter if he doesn't speak English. Ideally, the patient should go home with his printed, or at least clearly and legibly written, drug information. Explaining the drug therapy to the patient's family and others closely involved with his care also helps to reduce drug errors.

Remember that some types of drug therapy can be quite confusing for patients. One patient who went home with a warfarin prescription took the 2.5 and 5 mg tablets at the same time rather than 2.5 and 5 mg on alternating days. He eventually was hospitalized with GI bleeding—a problem that might have been avoided had he better understood his dosage regimen. Likewise, any regimen that requires a patient to take more than one drug greatly increases the complexity of the therapy and the chance of confusion and drug errors. The patient may need special help to establish a dosing schedule.

Also, ask if your patient takes OTC drugs at home in addition to his prescribed drugs. Make a special point of asking about herbal remedies and other nutritional supplements. Some herbal remedies have druglike effects and can cause or contribute to a drug-related problem. And, because these preparations aren't regulated like drugs are, government assurance standards don't apply to their labeling or manufacturing, and their ingredients can be misrepresented, substituted, or contaminated.

Finally, tell your patient which kinds of drug-related problems require a call to his prescriber. Encourage him to report anything about his drug therapy that concerns or worries him.

Skipping that crucial assessment step could easily lead to a medication error.

⊛ **ALERT:** A patient who is severely allergic to peanuts could have an anaphylactic reaction to ipratropium bromide (Atrovent) aerosol given by metered-dose inhaler. Ask your patient or his parents whether he's allergic to peanuts before you give this drug. If you find that he is allergic, you'll need to use the nasal spray and inhalation solution form of the drug. Because it doesn't contain soy lecithin, it's safe for patients allergic to peanuts.

Compound errors

Many medication errors occur because of a compound problem — a mistake or group of mistakes that could have been caught at any of several steps along the way. For a drug to be given correctly, each member of the health care team must fill the appropriate role:

• The prescriber must write the order correctly and legibly.
• The pharmacist must evaluate whether the order is appropriate and fill it correctly.
• The nurse must evaluate whether the order is appropriate and give it correctly.

A breakdown anywhere along this chain of events can lead to a medication error. That's why it's so important for members of the health care team to act as a real team so that they can check each other and catch any problems that might arise before those problems affect the patient's health. Encourage an environment in which professionals double-check each other.

For instance, the pharmacist can help clarify the number of times a drug should be given each day. He can help nurses label drugs in the most appropriate way. He can remind nurses to always return unused or discontinued medications to the pharmacy.

Nurses can, in fact they must, clarify any order that doesn't seem clear or correct. They also must correctly handle and store any multidose vials obtained from the pharmacist. Nurses should only give drugs that they've prepared personally and should never give a drug that has an ambiguous label or no label at all. Here's an example of what could happen.

A nurse placed an unlabeled cup of phenol (used in neurolytic procedures) next to a cup of guanethidine (a postganglionic-blocking drug). The doctor accidentally injected the phenol instead of the guanethidine, causing severe tissue damage to a patient's arm. The patient needed emergency surgery and later developed neurologic complications as a result of receiving an unlabeled (and incorrect) injection.

Obviously this was a compound problem. The nurse should have labeled each cup clearly, and the doctor shouldn't have given an unlabeled drug to a patient.

Here's another example of a compound problem: In the neonatal intensive care unit, a nurse prepared and gave a dose of aminophylline to an infant. She didn't have anyone else check her work. After receiving the drug, the infant developed tachycardia and other signs of theophylline toxicity and died. The nurse thought the order read 7.4 ml of aminophylline; instead, it read 7.4 mg.

This tragedy might have been avoided if the doctor had written a clearer order, if the nurse had clarified the order, if a pharmacist had prepared and dispensed the drug, or if another nurse had checked the dose calculation. To help prevent such problems, many facilities require that a pharmacist prepare and dispense nonemergency parenteral doses whenever commercial unit doses aren't available.

Here's another example: A container of 5% acetic acid, used to clean tracheostomy tubing, was left near nebulization equipment in the room of a 10-month-old infant. A respiratory therapist mistook the liquid for normal saline solution and used it to dilute albuterol for the child's nebulizer treatment. During treatment, the child experienced bronchospasm, hypercapnic dyspnea, tachypnea, and tachycardia.

Leaving dangerous chemicals near patients is extremely risky, especially when the container labels don't warn of toxicity. To prevent such problems, read the label on every drug you prepare, and never give any drug that isn't labeled or that is labeled poorly.

Route trouble

Many drug errors happen, at least in part, from problems related to the route of administration. The risk of error increases when a patient has several lines running for different purposes. Consider the following example.

A nurse prepared a dose of digoxin elixir for a patient who had both a central intravenous (I.V.) line and a jejunostomy tube. She mistakenly gave the drug into the central I.V. line. Fortunately, the patient had no adverse reaction.

To help prevent such mix-ups in route of administration, prepare all oral medications in a syringe that has a tip small enough to fit an abdominal tube but too big to fit a central line.

Here's another error that could have been avoided: To clear air bubbles from a 9-year-old patient's insulin infusion, a nurse disconnected the tubing and raised the pump rate to 200 ml/hour to flush the bubbles through quickly. She then reconnected the tubing and restarted the infusion, but she forgot to reset the drip rate back to 2 units/hour. The child received 50 units of insulin before the error was detected. To prevent this kind of error, never increase a drip rate to clear bubbles from a line. Instead, remove the tubing from the pump, disconnect it from the patient, and use the flow-control clamp to establish gravity flow.

Risky abbreviations

Abbreviating drug names is risky. Cancer patients with anemia may receive epoetin alfa, commonly abbreviated EPO, to stimulate red blood cell production. In one case, when a cancer patient was admitted to a hospital, the doctor wrote, "May take own supply of EPO." However, the patient wasn't anemic. Sensing that something was wrong, the pharmacist interviewed the patient, who confirmed that he was taking "EPO," or evening primrose oil, to lower his cholesterol level. Ask all prescribers to spell out drug names.

Unclear orders

A patient was supposed to receive one dose of the antineoplastic lomustine to treat brain cancer. (Lomustine typically is given as a single oral dose once every 6 weeks.) The doctor's order read, "Administer h.s." Because a nurse misinterpreted the order to mean every night, the patient received nine daily doses, developed severe thrombocytopenia and leukopenia, and died.

If you're unfamiliar with a drug, check a drug book before giving it. If a prescriber uses "h.s." but doesn't specify the frequency of administration, ask him to clarify the order. When documenting orders, note "h.s. nightly" or "h.s. one dose today."

Color changes

In two reports, alert nurses noticed that antineoplastics prepared in the pharmacy didn't look the way they should. The first error involved a

6-year-old child who was to receive 12 mg of methotrexate intrathecally. In the pharmacy, a 1-g vial was mistakenly selected instead of a 20-mg vial, and the drug was reconstituted with 10 ml of normal saline. The vial containing 100 mg/ml was incorrectly labeled as containing 2 mg/ml, and 6 ml of the solution was drawn into a syringe. Although the syringe label indicated 12 mg of drug, the syringe actually contained 600 mg of drug.

When the nurse received the syringe and noted that the drug's color didn't appear right, she returned it to the pharmacy for verification. The pharmacist retrieved the vial used to prepare the dose and drew the remaining solution into another syringe. The solutions in both syringes matched, and no one noticed the vial's 1-g label. The pharmacist concluded that a manufacturing change caused the color difference.

The child received the 600-mg dose and experienced seizures 45 minutes later. A pharmacist responding to the emergency detected the error. The child received an antidote and recovered.

A similar case involved a 20-year-old patient with leukemia who received mitomycin instead of mitoxantrone. The nurse had questioned the drug's unusual bluish tint, but the pharmacist assured her that the color difference was due to a change in manufacturer. Fortunately, the patient didn't suffer any harm.

If a familiar drug seems to have an unfamiliar appearance, investigate the cause. If the pharmacist cites a manufacturing change, ask him to double-check whether he has received verification from the manufacturer. Always document the appearance discrepancy, your actions, and the pharmacist's response in the patient record.

Stress levels

A nurse-anesthetist gave the sedative midazolam (Versed) to the wrong patient. When she discovered the error, she reached for what she thought was a vial of the antidote flumazenil (Romazicon), withdrew 2.5 ml of the drug, and gave it. When the patient didn't respond, she realized she'd reached for a vial of ondansetron (Zofran), an antiemetic, instead. Another practitioner assisted with proper I.V. administration of flumazenil, and the patient recovered without harm.

Committing a serious error can cause enormous stress and cloud your judgment. If you're involved in a drug error, ask another professional to give the antidote.

Clearly, you carry a great deal of responsibility for making sure that the right patient gets the right drug, in the right dose, at the right time, and by the right route. By staying aware of potential trouble spots, you can minimize your risk of making medication errors and maximize the therapeutic effects of your patients' drug regimens.

Drug
Classifications

Alkylating drugs

altretamine
busulfan
carboplatin
carmustine
chlorambucil
cisplatin
cyclophosphamide
dacarbazine
ifosfamide
lomustine
mechlorethamine hydrochloride
melphalan
procarbazine hydrochloride
thiotepa

Indications

▶ Various tumors, especially those with large volume and slow cell-turnover rate.

Contraindications and cautions

• Contraindicated in patients hypersensitive to these drugs.
• Use cautiously in patients receiving other cell-destroying drugs or radiation therapy.
⚠ **Lifespan:** In pregnant women, use only when potential benefits to the patient outweigh the known possible risks to the fetus. Breast-feeding women should stop breast-feeding during therapy because drugs are found in breast milk. In children, safety and effectiveness of many alkylating drugs haven't been established. Elderly patients have an increased risk of adverse reactions; monitor these patients closely.

Adverse reactions

The most common adverse reactions are anxiety, bone marrow depression, chills, diarrhea, fever, flank pain, hair loss, leukopenia, nausea, redness or pain at the injection site, sore throat, swelling of the feet or lower legs, thrombocytopenia, and vomiting.

Action

Alkylating drugs appear to act independently of a specific cell-cycle phase. They are polyfunctional compounds that can be divided chemically into five groups: nitrogen mustards, ethyleneimines, alkyl sulfonates, triazines, and nitrosoureas. These drugs are highly reactive;

they primarily target nucleic acids and form links with the nuclei of different molecules. This allows the drugs to cross-link double-stranded DNA and to prevent strands from separating for replication, which may contribute to these drugs' ability to destroy cells.

NURSING PROCESS

℞ Assessment

• Perform a complete assessment before therapy begins.
• Monitor patient for adverse reactions throughout therapy.
• Monitor platelet and total and differential leukocyte counts, hematocrit, and BUN, ALT, AST, LDH, bilirubin, creatinine, uric acid, and other levels as needed.
• Monitor vital signs and patency of catheter or I.V. line throughout administration.

🔑 Key nursing diagnoses

• Ineffective protection related to thrombocytopenia
• Risk for infection related to immunosuppression
• Risk for deficient fluid volume related to adverse GI effects

▶ Planning and implementation

• Give under the supervision of a physician experienced in the use of antineoplastics.
• Follow established procedures for safe and proper handling, administration, and disposal of chemotherapeutic drugs.
• Treat extravasation promptly.
• While giving carboplatin or cisplatin, keep epinephrine, corticosteroids, and antihistamines available. Anaphylactoid reactions may occur.
• Give ifosfamide with mesna to prevent hemorrhagic cystitis.
• Give lomustine 2 to 4 hours after meals. Nausea and vomiting usually last less than 24 hours, although loss of appetite may last for several days.
• Maintain adequate hydration before and for 24 hours after cisplatin treatment.
• Be aware that allopurinol may be prescribed to prevent drug-induced hyperuricemia.

Patient teaching

• Tell patient to avoid people with bacterial or viral infections because chemotherapy can in-

Prototype drug

crease susceptibility. Urge him to report signs of infection promptly.
• Review proper oral hygiene, including cautious use of toothbrush, dental floss, and tooth-picks.
• Advise patient to complete dental work before therapy begins or to delay it until blood counts are normal.
• Warn patient that he may bruise easily because of drug's effect on blood count.

✓ Evaluation
• Patient develops no serious bleeding complications.
• Patient remains free from infection.
• Patient maintains adequate hydration.

Alpha blockers (peripherally acting)
alfuzosin hydrochloride (selective)
doxazosin mesylate (nonselective)
prazosin hydrochloride (nonselective)
tamsulosin hydrochloride (selective)
terazosin hydrochloride (nonselective)

Indications

► Hypertension, or mild to moderate urinary obstruction in men with BPH.

Contraindications and cautions

• Contraindicated in patients with MI, coronary insufficiency, or angina or with hypersensitivity to these drugs or any of their components. Also contraindicated in combination therapy with phosphodiesterase type 5 inhibitors (vardenafil, sildenafil, tadalafil), although tadalafil may be used with tamsulosin 0.4 mg daily.
✸ **Lifespan:** In pregnant or breast-feeding women, use cautiously. In children, the safety and effectiveness of many alpha blockers haven't been established; use cautiously. In elderly patients, hypotensive effects may be more pronounced.

Adverse reactions

Especially with the first few doses, alpha blockers may cause severe orthostatic hypotension and syncope, often called the "first-dose effect." The most common adverse effects of alpha$_1$

blockade are dizziness, headache, drowsiness, somnolence, and malaise. These drugs also may cause tachycardia, palpitations, fluid retention (from excess renin secretion), nasal and ocular congestion, and aggravation of respiratory tract infection.

Action

Selective alpha blockers have readily observable effects. They decrease vascular resistance and increase vein capacity, thereby lowering blood pressure and causing nasal and sclero-conjunctival congestion, ptosis, orthostatic and exercise hypotension, mild to moderate miosis, interference with ejaculation, and pink, warm skin. They also relax nonvascular smooth muscle, especially in the prostate capsule, which reduces urinary problems in men with BPH. Because alpha$_1$ blockers don't block alpha$_2$ receptors, they don't cause transmitter overflow.

Nonselective alpha blockers antagonize both alpha$_1$ and alpha$_2$ receptors. Generally, alpha blockade results in tachycardia, palpitations, and increased renin secretion because of abnormally large amounts of norepinephrine (because of transmitter overflow) released from adrenergic nerve endings as a result of the blockade of alpha$_1$ and alpha$_2$ receptors. Norepinephrine's effects are counterproductive to the major uses of nonselective alpha blockers.

NURSING PROCESS

⚒ Assessment
• Monitor vital signs, especially blood pressure.
• Monitor patient closely for adverse reactions.

⊕ Key nursing diagnoses
• Decreased cardiac output related to hypotension
• Acute pain related to headache
• Excessive fluid volume related to fluid retention

▶ Planning and implementation
• Give at bedtime to minimize dizziness or light-headedness.
• Begin therapy with a small dose to avoid first-dose syncope.

Patient teaching
• Warn patient not to rise suddenly from a lying or sitting position.

• Urge patient to avoid hazardous tasks that require mental alertness until the drug's full effects are known.

• Advise patient that alcohol, excessive exercise, prolonged standing, and heat exposure will intensify adverse effects.

• Tell patient to report promptly dizziness or irregular heartbeat.

• Caution patient to speak to his prescriber before taking a drug for erectile dysfunction.

☑ **Evaluation**

• Patient maintains adequate cardiac output.

• Patient's headache is relieved.

• Patient has no edema.

Aminoglycosides

amikacin sulfate
gentamicin sulfate
neomycin sulfate
streptomycin sulfate
tobramycin sulfate

Indications

▶ Septicemia; postoperative, pulmonary, intra-abdominal, and urinary tract infections; skin, soft tissue, bone, and joint infections; aerobic gram-negative bacillary meningitis not susceptible to other antibiotics; serious staphylococcal, *Pseudomonas aeruginosa,* and *Klebsiella* infections; enterococcal infections; nosocomial pneumonia; anaerobic infections involving *Bacteroides fragilis;* tuberculosis; initial empiric therapy in febrile, leukopenic patients.

Contraindications and cautions

• Contraindicated in patients hypersensitive to these drugs.

• Use cautiously in patients with a neuromuscular disorder and in those taking neuromuscular blockades.

• Use at lower dosages in patients with renal impairment.

☀ **Lifespan:** In pregnant women, use cautiously. In breast-feeding women, safety hasn't been established. In neonates and premature infants, the half-life of aminoglycosides is prolonged because of immature renal systems. In infants and children, dosage adjustment may be

needed. Elderly patients have an increased risk of nephrotoxicity and commonly need a lower dose and longer dosing intervals; they're also susceptible to ototoxicity and superinfection.

Adverse reactions

Ototoxicity and nephrotoxicity are the most serious complications. Neuromuscular blockade also may occur. Oral forms most commonly cause diarrhea, nausea, and vomiting. Parenteral drugs may cause vein irritation, phlebitis, and sterile abscess.

Action

Aminoglycosides are bactericidal. They bind directly and irreversibly to 30S ribosomal subunits, inhibiting bacterial protein synthesis. They're active against many aerobic gram-negative and some aerobic gram-positive organisms.

NURSING PROCESS

☙ **Assessment**

• Obtain patient's history of allergies.

• Monitor patient for adverse reactions.

• Obtain results of culture and sensitivity tests before first dose, and check tests periodically to assess drug effectiveness.

• Monitor vital signs and electrolyte levels. Conduct hearing ability and renal function studies before and during therapy.

• Draw blood for peak level 1 hour after I.M. injection and 30 minutes to 1 hour after I.V. infusion; for trough level, draw sample just before next dose. Time and date all blood samples. Don't use heparinized tube to collect blood samples because it interferes with results.

🔲 **Key nursing diagnoses**

• Risk for injury related to nephrotoxicity and ototoxicity

• Risk for infection related to drug-induced superinfection

• Risk for deficient fluid volume related to adverse GI reactions

▶ **Planning and implementation**

• Keep patient hydrated to minimize chemical irritation of renal tubules.

• Don't add or mix other drugs with I.V. infusions, particularly penicillins, which inactivate

aminoglycosides. If other drugs must be given I.V., temporarily stop infusion of primary drug.
• Follow manufacturer's instructions for reconstitution, dilution, and storage of drugs; check expiration dates.
• Shake oral suspensions well before giving.
• Give I.M. dose deep into the gluteal muscle mass or midlateral thigh; rotate injection sites to minimize tissue injury. Apply ice to injection site to relieve pain.
• Giving I.V. dose too rapidly may cause neuromuscular blockade. Infuse I.V. dose continuously or intermittently over 30 to 60 minutes for adults, 1 to 2 hours for infants; dilution volume for children is determined individually.

Patient teaching
• Teach signs and symptoms of hypersensitivity and other adverse reactions. Urge patient to report unusual effects promptly.
• Emphasize importance of adequate fluid intake.

▓ Evaluation
• Patient maintains pretreatment renal and hearing functions.
• Patient is free from infection.
• Patient maintains adequate hydration.

Angiotensin-converting enzyme inhibitors

benazepril hydrochloride
captopril
enalapril maleate
enalaprilat
fosinopril sodium
lisinopril
moexipril hydrochloride
perindopril erbumine
quinapril hydrochloride
ramipril
trandolapril

Indications

▶ Hypertension, heart failure, left ventricular dysfunction (LVD), MI (with ramipril and lisinopril), and diabetic nephropathy (with captopril).

Contraindications and cautions

• Contraindicated in patients hypersensitive to these drugs.
• Use cautiously in patients with impaired renal function or serious autoimmune disease and in those taking other drugs known to decrease WBC count or immune response.
≈ Lifespan: Women of childbearing age taking ACE inhibitors should report suspected pregnancy immediately to prescriber. High risks of fetal morbidity and mortality are linked to ACE inhibitors, especially in the second and third trimesters. Some ACE inhibitors appear in breast milk. To avoid adverse effects in infants, instruct patient to stop breast-feeding during therapy. In children, safety and effectiveness haven't been established; give drug only if potential benefits outweighs risks. Elderly patients may need lower doses because of impaired drug clearance.

Adverse reactions

The most common adverse effects of therapeutic doses are angioedema of the face and limbs, dry cough, dysgeusia, fatigue, headache, hyperkalemia, hypotension, proteinuria, rash, and tachycardia. Severe hypotension may occur at toxic drug levels.

Action

ACE inhibitors prevent conversion of angiotensin I to angiotensin II, a potent vasoconstrictor. Besides decreasing vasoconstriction and thus reducing peripheral arterial resistance, inhibiting angiotensin II decreases adrenocortical secretion of aldosterone. This reduces sodium and water retention and extracellular fluid volume. ACE inhibition also causes increased levels of bradykinin, which results in vasodilation. This decreases heart rate and systemic vascular resistance.

NURSING PROCESS

▓ Assessment
• Observe patient for adverse reactions.
• Monitor vital signs regularly, and monitor WBC count and electrolyte level periodically.

▓ Key nursing diagnoses
• Risk for trauma related to orthostatic hypotension

• Ineffective protection related to hyperkalemia
• Acute pain related to headache

▶ **Planning and implementation**
• To reduce risk of hypotension, stop diuretic 2 to 3 days before starting ACE inhibitor. If drug doesn't adequately control blood pressure, diuretics may be restarted.
• If patient has impaired renal function, give a reduced dosage.
• Give potassium supplements and potassium-sparing diuretics cautiously because ACE inhibitors may cause potassium retention.
• If patient becomes pregnant, stop ACE inhibitors. These drugs can cause birth defects or fetal death in the second and third trimesters.
• Give captopril and moexipril 1 hour before meals.

Patient teaching
• Tell patient that drugs may cause a dry, persistent, tickling cough that stops when therapy stops.
• Urge patient to report light-headedness, especially in the first few days of therapy so that the dosage can be adjusted. Tell him to report signs of infection, such as sore throat and fever, because these drugs may decrease WBC count; facial swelling or difficulty breathing, because these drugs may cause angioedema; and loss of taste, for which therapy may stop.
• Advise patient to avoid sudden position changes to minimize orthostatic hypotension.
• Warn patient to seek medical approval before taking self-prescribed cold preparations.
• Tell women to report pregnancy at once.
• Warn patient to use salt substitutes containing potassium cautiously because ACE inhibitors may cause potassium retention.

☑ **Evaluation**
• Patient sustains no injury from orthostatic hypotension.
• Patient's WBC count remains normal throughout therapy.
• Patient's headache is relieved by mild analgesic.

Antacids

aluminum hydroxide
calcium carbonate
magaldrate
magnesium hydroxide
magnesium oxide
sodium bicarbonate

Indications

▶ Hyperacidity; hyperphosphatemia (aluminum hydroxide); hypomagnesemia (magnesium oxide); postmenopausal hypocalcemia (calcium carbonate).

Contraindications and cautions

• Calcium carbonate, magaldrate, and magnesium oxide are contraindicated in patients with severe renal disease. Sodium bicarbonate is contraindicated in patients with hypertension, renal disease, or edema; in patients who are vomiting; in patients receiving diuretics or continuous GI suction; and in patients on sodium-restricted diets.
• In patients with mild renal impairment, give magnesium oxide cautiously.
• Give aluminum preparations, calcium carbonate, and magaldrate cautiously in elderly patients; in those receiving antidiarrheals, antispasmodics, or anticholinergics; and in those with dehydration, fluid restriction, chronic renal disease, or suspected intestinal absorption problems.
• ⚖ **Lifespan:** Pregnant women should consult their prescriber before using antacids. Breast-feeding women may take antacids. In infants, serious adverse effects are more likely from changes in fluid and electrolyte balance; monitor them closely. Elderly patients have an increased risk of adverse reactions; monitor them closely; also, give these patients aluminum preparations, calcium carbonate, magaldrate, and magnesium oxide cautiously.

Adverse reactions

Antacids containing aluminum may cause aluminum intoxication, constipation, hypophosphatemia, intestinal obstruction, and osteomalacia. Antacids containing magnesium may cause diarrhea or hypermagnesemia (in renal failure). Calcium carbonate, magaldrate, magnesium oxide, and sodium bicarbonate may cause constipation, milk-alkali syndrome, or rebound hyperacidity.

Action

Antacids reduce the total acid load in the GI tract and elevate gastric pH to reduce pepsin activity. They also strengthen the gastric mucosal barrier and increase esophageal sphincter tone.

NURSING PROCESS

⏰ Assessment
• Assess patient's condition before therapy and regularly thereafter.
• Record number and consistency of stools.
• Observe patient for adverse reactions.
• Monitor patient receiving long-term, high-dose aluminum carbonate and hydroxide for fluid and electrolyte imbalance, especially if patient is on a sodium-restricted diet.
• Monitor phosphate level in a patient taking aluminum carbonate or hydroxide.
• Watch for signs of hypercalcemia in a patient taking calcium carbonate.
• Monitor magnesium level in a patient with mild renal impairment who takes magaldrate.

⊞ Key nursing diagnoses
• Constipation related to adverse effects of aluminum-containing antacid
• Diarrhea related to adverse effects of magnesium-containing antacid
• Ineffective protection related to drug-induced electrolyte imbalance

▶ Planning and implementation
• Manage constipation with laxatives or stool softeners, or switch patient to a magnesium preparation.
• If patient suffers from diarrhea, give an antidiarrheal, and switch patient to an antacid containing aluminum.
• Shake container well, and give with small amount of water or juice to facilitate passage. When giving through an NG tube, make sure the tube is patent and placed correctly. After instilling the drug, flush the tube with water to ensure passage to the stomach and to clear the tube.

Patient teaching
• Warn patient not to take antacids randomly or to switch antacids without prescriber's consent.
• Tell patient not to take calcium carbonate with milk or other foods high in vitamin D.
• Warn patient not to take sodium bicarbonate with milk because doing so could cause hypercalcemia.

☑ Evaluation
• Patient regains normal bowel pattern.
• Patient states that diarrhea is relieved.
• Patient maintains normal electrolyte balance.

Antianginals

Beta blockers
acebutolol
atenolol
bisoprolol fumarate
esmolol hydrochloride
metoprolol
nadolol
propranolol hydrochloride
Calcium channel blockers
amlodipine besylate
diltiazem hydrochloride
nicardipine hydrochloride
nifedipine
verapamil hydrochloride
Nitrates
isosorbide dinitrate
isosorbide mononitrate
nitroglycerin

Indications

▶ Moderate to severe angina (beta blockers); classic, effort-induced angina and Prinzmetal's angina (calcium channel blockers); recurrent angina (long-acting nitrates and topical, transdermal, transmucosal, and oral extended-release nitroglycerin); acute angina (S.L. nitroglycerin and S.L. or chewable isosorbide dinitrate); unstable angina (I.V. nitroglycerin).

Contraindications and cautions

• Beta blockers are contraindicated in patients hypersensitive to them and in patients with cardiogenic shock, sinus bradycardia, heart block greater than first degree, or bronchial asthma.

Calcium channel blockers are contraindicated in patients with severe hypotension or heart block greater than first degree (except with functioning pacemaker). Nitrates are contraindicated in patients with severe anemia, cerebral hemorrhage, head trauma, glaucoma, or hyperthyroidism or in patients using phosphodiesterase type 5 inhibitors (tadalafil, vardenafil, sildenafil).

• Use beta blockers cautiously in patients with nonallergic bronchospastic disorders, diabetes mellitus, or impaired hepatic or renal function. Use calcium channel blockers cautiously in patients with hepatic or renal impairment, bradycardia, heart failure, or cardiogenic shock. Use nitrates cautiously in patients with hypotension or recent MI.

⚖ Lifespan: In pregnant women, use beta blockers cautiously. Recommendations for breast-feeding vary by drug; use beta blockers and calcium channel blockers cautiously. In children, safety and effectiveness haven't been established. Check with prescriber before giving these drugs to children. Elderly patients have an increased risk of adverse reactions; use cautiously.

Adverse reactions

Beta blockers may cause bradycardia, cough, diarrhea, disturbing dreams, dizziness, dyspnea, fatigue, fever, heart failure, hypotension, lethargy, nausea, peripheral edema, and wheezing. Calcium channel blockers may cause bradycardia, confusion, constipation, depression, diarrhea, dizziness, dyspepsia, edema, elevated liver enzyme levels (transient), fatigue, flushing, headache, hypotension, insomnia, nervousness, and rash. Nitrates may cause alcohol intoxication (from I.V. preparations containing alcohol), flushing, headache, orthostatic hypotension, reflex tachycardia, rash, syncope, and vomiting.

Action

Beta blockers decrease catecholamine-induced increases in heart rate, blood pressure, and myocardial contraction. Calcium channel blockers inhibit the flow of calcium through muscle cells, which dilates coronary arteries and decreases systemic vascular resistance, known as afterload. Nitrates decrease afterload and left ventricular end-diastolic pressure, or preload, and increase blood flow through collateral coronary vessels.

NURSING PROCESS

🕮 Assessment
• Monitor vital signs. With I.V. nitroglycerin, monitor blood pressure and pulse rate every 5 to 15 minutes while adjusting dosage and every hour thereafter.
• Monitor the drug's effectiveness.
• Observe patient for adverse reactions.

🔢 Key nursing diagnoses
• Risk for injury related to adverse reactions
• Excessive fluid volume related to adverse CV effects of beta blockers or calcium channel blockers
• Acute pain related to headache

❯ Planning and implementation
• Have patient sit or lie down when receiving the first nitrate dose; take his pulse and blood pressure before giving dose and when drug action starts.
• Don't give a beta blocker or calcium channel blocker to relieve acute angina.
• Withhold the dose and notify prescriber if patient's heart rate is slower than 60 beats/minute or systolic blood pressure is lower than 90 mm Hg.

Patient teaching
• Warn patient not to stop drug abruptly without prescriber's approval.
• Teach patient to take his pulse before taking a beta blocker or calcium channel blocker. Tell him to withhold the dose and alert the prescriber if his pulse rate is slower than 60 beats/minute.
• Instruct patient taking nitroglycerin S.L. to go to the emergency department if 3 tablets taken 5 minutes apart don't relieve angina.
• Caution patient about the dangers of using nitrates with certain erectile dysfunction drugs.
• Tell patient to report serious or persistent adverse reactions.

✓ Evaluation
• Patient sustains no injury from adverse reactions.
• Patient maintains normal fluid balance.
• Patient's headache is relieved with mild analgesic.

Antiarrhythmics

adenosine
Class IA
disopyramide
moricizine hydrochloride
procainamide hydrochloride
quinidine bisulfate
quinidine gluconate
quinidine sulfate
Class IB
lidocaine hydrochloride
mexiletine hydrochloride
phenytoin sodium
tocainide hydrochloride
Class IC
flecainide acetate
propafenone hydrochloride
Class II (beta blockers)
acebutolol hydrochloride
esmolol hydrochloride
propranolol hydrochloride
Class III
amiodarone hydrochloride
bretylium tosylate
dofetilide
ibutilide fumarate
sotalol hydrochloride
Class IV (calcium channel blocker)
verapamil hydrochloride

Indications

▶ Atrial and ventricular arrhythmias.

Contraindications and cautions

• Contraindicated in patients hypersensitive to these drugs.
• Many antiarrhythmics are contraindicated or require cautious use in patients with cardiogenic shock, digitalis toxicity, and second- or third-degree heart block (unless patient has a pacemaker).
⚞ Lifespan: In pregnant women, use only if the potential benefits to the mother outweigh the risks to the fetus. In breast-feeding women, use cautiously; many antiarrhythmics appear in breast milk. In children, monitor closely because they have an increased risk of adverse reactions. In elderly patients, use these drugs cau-

tiously because these patients may exhibit physiologic alterations in CV system.

Adverse reactions

Most antiarrhythmics can aggravate existing arrhythmias or cause new ones. They also may produce CNS disturbances, such as dizziness or fatigue, GI problems, such as nausea, vomiting, or altered bowel elimination; hypersensitivity reactions; and hypotension. Some antiarrhythmics may worsen heart failure. Class II drugs may cause bronchoconstriction.

Action

Class I drugs reduce the inward current carried by sodium ions, which stabilizes neuronal cardiac membranes. Class IA drugs depress phase 0, prolong the action potential, and stabilize cardiac membranes. Class IB drugs depress phase 0, shorten the action potential, and stabilize cardiac membranes. Class IC drugs block the transport of sodium ions, which decreases conduction velocity but not repolarization rate. Moricizine is a class I drug that possesses characteristics of the IA, B, and C classes. Class II drugs decrease the heart rate, myocardial contractility, blood pressure, and AV node conduction. Class III drugs prolong the action potential and refractory period. Class IV drugs decrease myocardial contractility and oxygen demand by inhibiting calcium ion influx; they also dilate coronary arteries and arterioles.

NURSING PROCESS

⚙ **Assessment**
• Monitor ECG continuously when therapy starts and when dosage is adjusted.
• Monitor patient's vital signs frequently and assess for signs of toxicity and adverse reactions.
• Measure apical pulse rate before giving drug.
• Monitor drug level as indicated.

⊞ **Key nursing diagnoses**
• Decreased cardiac output related to arrhythmias or myocardial depression
• Ineffective protection related to adverse reactions
• Noncompliance related to long-term therapy

▷ **Planning and implementation**
• Don't crush sustained-release tablets.

• Take safety precautions if adverse CNS reactions occur.
• Notify prescriber about adverse reactions.

Patient teaching
• Stress the importance of taking drug exactly as prescribed.
• Teach patient to take his pulse before each dose. Tell him to notify prescriber if his pulse is irregular or slower than 60 beats/minute.
• Instruct patient to avoid hazardous activities that require mental alertness if adverse CNS reactions occur.
• Tell patient to limit fluid and salt intake if his prescribed drug causes fluid retention.

☑ Evaluation
• Patient maintains adequate cardiac output, as evidenced by normal vital signs and adequate tissue perfusion.
• Patient has no serious adverse reactions.
• Patient states importance of compliance with therapy.

Antibiotic antineoplastics

bleomycin sulfate
daunorubicin hydrochloride
doxorubicin hydrochloride
epirubicin hydrochloride
idarubicin hydrochloride
mitomycin
mitoxantrone hydrochloride

Indications

▶ Various tumors.

Contraindications and cautions

• Contraindicated in patients hypersensitive to these drugs.
⚘ **Lifespan:** In pregnant women, avoid antineoplastics. Breast-feeding during therapy isn't recommended. In children, safety and effectiveness of some drugs haven't been established; use cautiously. In elderly patients, use cautiously because of their increased risk of adverse reactions.

Adverse reactions

The most common adverse reactions include anxiety, bone marrow depression, chills, confusion, diarrhea, fever, flank or joint pain, hair loss, leukopenia, nausea, redness or pain at the injection site, sore throat, swelling of the feet or lower legs, and vomiting.

Action

Although classified as antibiotics, these drugs destroy cells, thus ruling out their use as antimicrobials alone. They interfere with proliferation of malignant cells in several ways. Their action may be cell–cycle-phase nonspecific, cell–cycle-phase specific, or both. Some of these drugs act like alkylating drugs or antimetabolites. By binding to or creating complexes with DNA, antibiotic antineoplastics directly or indirectly inhibit DNA, RNA, and protein synthesis.

NURSING PROCESS

⬛ Assessment
• Perform a complete assessment before therapy begins.
• Monitor patient for adverse reactions.
• Monitor vital signs and patency of catheter or I.V. line.
• Monitor platelet and total and differential leukocyte counts, and monitor ALT, AST, LDH, bilirubin, creatinine, uric acid, BUN, and hemoglobin levels and hematocrit.
• Monitor pulmonary function tests in a patient receiving bleomycin. Assess lung function regularly.
• Monitor ECG before and during treatment with daunorubicin and doxorubicin.

⬛ Key nursing diagnoses
• Ineffective protection related to thrombocytopenia
• Risk for infection related to immunosuppression
• Risk for deficient fluid volume related to adverse GI effects

⬛ Planning and implementation
• Follow established procedures for safe and proper handling, administration, and disposal of chemotherapeutic drugs.
• Try to ease anxiety in patient and family before treatment.

• Keep epinephrine, corticosteroids, and anti-histamines available during bleomycin therapy. Anaphylactoid reaction may occur.
• Treat extravasation promptly.
• Ensure adequate hydration during idarubicin therapy.
• Stop procarbazine and notify prescriber if patient becomes confused or neuropathies develop.

Patient teaching
• Advise patient to avoid exposure to people with bacterial or viral infections because chemotherapy increases susceptibility. Urge him to report signs of infection immediately.
• Review proper oral hygiene, including cautious use of toothbrush, dental floss, and toothpicks. Chemotherapy can increase the risk of microbial infection, delayed healing, and bleeding gums.
• Urge patient to complete dental work before therapy begins or to delay it until blood counts are normal.
• Warn patient that he may bruise easily.
• Tell patient to report redness, pain, or swelling at injection site immediately. Local tissue injury and scarring may result if I.V. infiltration occurs.
• Advise patient taking daunorubicin, doxorubicin, or idarubicin that his urine may turn orange or red for 1 to 2 days after therapy begins.

☑ Evaluation
• No serious bleeding complications develop.
• Patient remains free from infection.
• Patient maintains adequate hydration.

Anticholinergics

atropine sulfate
benztropine mesylate
dicyclomine hydrochloride
scopolamine
scopolamine butylbromide
scopolamine hydrobromide

Indications

▶ Prevention of motion sickness, preoperative reduction of secretions and blockage of cardiac reflexes, adjunct treatment of peptic ulcers and other GI disorders, blockage of cholinomimetic effects of cholinesterase inhibitors or other drugs, and (for benztropine) various spastic conditions, including acute dystonic reactions, muscle rigidity, parkinsonism, and extrapyramidal disorders.

Contraindications and cautions

• Contraindicated in patients hypersensitive to these drugs and in those with angle-closure glaucoma, renal or GI obstructive disease, reflux esophagitis, or myasthenia gravis.
• Use cautiously in patients with heart disease, GI infection, open-angle glaucoma, prostatic hypertrophy, hypertension, hyperthyroidism, ulcerative colitis, autonomic neuropathy, or hiatal hernia with reflux esophagitis.
⚘ Lifespan: In pregnant women, safe use hasn't been established. In breast-feeding women, avoid anticholinergics because they may decrease milk production; some may appear in breast milk and cause infant toxicity. In children, safety and effectiveness haven't been established. Patients older than age 40 may be more sensitive to these drugs. In elderly patients, use cautiously and give a reduced dosage, as indicated.

Adverse reactions

Therapeutic doses commonly cause blurred vision, constipation, cycloplegia, decreased sweating or anhidrosis, dry mouth, headache, mydriasis, palpitations, tachycardia, and urinary hesitancy and retention. These reactions usually disappear when therapy stops. Toxicity can cause signs and symptoms resembling psychosis (disorientation, confusion, hallucinations, delusions, anxiety, agitation, and restlessness); dilated, nonreactive pupils; blurred vision; hot, dry, flushed skin; dry mucous membranes; dysphagia; decreased or absent bowel sounds; urine retention; hyperthermia; tachycardia; hypertension; and increased respirations.

Action

Anticholinergics competitively antagonize the actions of acetylcholine and other cholinergic agonists at muscarinic receptors.

NURSING PROCESS

🗒 Assessment
• Monitor patient regularly for adverse reactions.
• Check vital signs at least every 4 hours.
• Measure urine output; check for urine retention.
• Assess patient for changes in vision and for signs of impending toxicity.

⊞ Key nursing diagnoses
• Urine retention related to adverse effect on bladder
• Constipation related to adverse effect on GI tract
• Acute pain related to headache

▷ Planning and implementation
• Provide ice chips, cool drinks, or hard candy to relieve dry mouth.
• Relieve constipation with stool softeners or bulk laxatives.
• Give a mild analgesic for headache.
• Notify prescriber of urine retention, and be prepared for catheterization.

Patient teaching
• Teach patient how and when to take the drug and caution him not to take other drugs unless prescribed.
• Warn patient to avoid hazardous tasks if he experiences dizziness, drowsiness, or blurred vision. Inform him that the drug may increase his sensitivity to or intolerance of high temperatures, resulting in dizziness.
• Advise patient to avoid alcohol because it may cause additive CNS effects.
• Urge patient to drink plenty of fluids and to eat a high-fiber diet to prevent constipation.
• Tell patient to notify prescriber promptly if he experiences confusion, rapid or pounding heartbeat, dry mouth, blurred vision, rash, eye pain, significant change in urine volume, or pain or difficulty on urination.
• Advise women to report planned or known pregnancy.

☑ Evaluation
• Patient maintains normal voiding pattern.
• Patient regains normal bowel patterns.
• Patient is free from pain.

Anticoagulants
Coumarin derivative
warfarin sodium
Heparin derivative
heparin sodium
Low–molecular-weight heparins
dalteparin sodium
enoxaparin sodium
tinzaparin sodium
Selective factor Xa inhibitor
fondaparinux sodium
Thrombin inhibitors
argatroban
bivalirudin

Indications
▶ Pulmonary emboli, deep vein thrombosis, thrombus, blood clotting, DIC, unstable angina, MI, atrial fibrillation.

Contraindications and cautions
• Contraindicated in patients hypersensitive to these drugs or any of their components; in patients with aneurysm, active bleeding, CV hemorrhage, hemorrhagic blood dyscrasias, hemophilia, severe hypertension, pericardial effusions, or pericarditis; and in patients undergoing major surgery, neurosurgery, or ophthalmic surgery.
• Use cautiously in patients with severe diabetes, renal impairment, severe trauma, ulcerations, or vasculitis.
❋ **Lifespan:** Most anticoagulants (except warfarin) may only be used in pregnancy if clearly necessary. In pregnant women and those who have just had a threatened or complete spontaneous abortion, warfarin is contraindicated. Women should avoid breast-feeding during therapy. Infants, especially neonates, may be more susceptible to anticoagulants because of vitamin K deficiency. Elderly patients are at greater risk for hemorrhage because of altered hemostatic mechanisms or age-related deterioration of hepatic and renal functions.

Adverse reactions
Anticoagulants commonly cause bleeding and may cause hypersensitivity reactions. Warfarin may cause agranulocytosis, alopecia (long-term use), anorexia, dermatitis, fever, nausea, tissue

necrosis or gangrene, urticaria, and vomiting. Heparin derivatives may cause thrombocytopenia and may increase liver enzyme levels. Nonhemorrhagic adverse reactions associated with thrombin inhibitors may include back pain, bradycardia, and hypotension.

Action

Heparin derivatives accelerate formation of an antithrombin III-thrombin complex. It inactivates thrombin and prevents conversion of fibrinogen to fibrin. The coumarin derivative warfarin inhibits vitamin K-dependent activation of clotting factors II, VII, IX, and X, which are formed in the liver. Thrombin inhibitors directly bind to thrombin and inhibit its action. Selective factor Xa inhibitors bind to antithrombin III, which in turn initiates the neutralization of factor Xa.

NURSING PROCESS

⚰ Assessment
• Monitor patient closely for bleeding and other adverse reactions.
• Check PT, INR, PTT, or APTT.
• Monitor vital signs, hemoglobin, and hematocrit.
• Assess patient's urine, stools, and emesis for blood.

⊕ Key nursing diagnoses
• Ineffective protection related to drug's effects on body's normal clotting and bleeding mechanisms
• Risk for deficient fluid volume related to bleeding
• Noncompliance related to long-term warfarin therapy

▶ Planning and implementation
• Don't give heparin I.M., and avoid I.M. injections of any anticoagulant if possible.
• Keep protamine sulfate available to treat severe bleeding caused by heparin. Keep vitamin K available to treat frank bleeding caused by warfarin.
• Notify prescriber about serious or persistent adverse reactions.
• Maintain bleeding precautions throughout therapy.

Patient teaching
• Urge patient to take drug exactly as prescribed. If he's taking warfarin, tell him to take it at night and to have blood drawn for PT or INR in the morning for accurate results.
• Advise patient to consult his prescriber before taking any other drug, including OTC medications and herbal remedies.
• Review bleeding-prevention precautions to take in everyday living. Urge patient to remove safety hazards and make home repairs to reduce risk of injury.
• Advise patient not to increase his intake of green, leafy vegetables because vitamin K may antagonize anticoagulant effects.
• Instruct patient to report bleeding or other adverse reactions promptly.
• Encourage patient to keep appointments for blood tests and follow-up examinations.
• Advise woman to report planned or known pregnancy.

☑ Evaluation
• Patient has no adverse change in health status.
• Patient has no evidence of bleeding or hemorrhaging.
• Patient demonstrates compliance with therapy, as evidenced by normal bleeding and clotting values.

Anticonvulsants
acetazolamide sodium
carbamazepine
clonazepam
clorazepate dipotassium
diazepam
divalproex sodium
fosphenytoin sodium
gabapentin
lamotrigine
levetiracetam
magnesium sulfate
oxcarbazepine
phenobarbital
phenobarbital sodium
phenytoin sodium
phenytoin sodium (extended)
primidone
tiagabine hydrochloride

topiramate
valproate sodium
valproic acid
zonisamide

Indications

▶ Seizure disorders; acute, isolated seizures not caused by seizure disorders; status epilepticus; prevention of seizures after trauma or craniotomy; neuropathic pain.

Contraindications and cautions

• Contraindicated in patients hypersensitive to these drugs.
• Carbamazepine is contraindicated within 14 days of MAO inhibitor use.
• Use cautiously in patients with blood dyscrasias. Also, use barbiturates cautiously in patients with suicidal ideation.
※ **Lifespan:** In pregnant women, therapy usually continues despite the fetal risks caused by some anticonvulsants (barbiturates, phenytoin). In breast-feeding women, the safety of many anticonvulsants hasn't been established. Children, especially young ones, are sensitive to the CNS depression of some anticonvulsants; use cautiously. Elderly patients are sensitive to CNS effects and may require lower doses. Also, some anticonvulsants may take longer to be eliminated because of decreased renal function, and parenteral use is more likely to cause apnea, hypotension, bradycardia, and cardiac arrest.

Adverse reactions

Anticonvulsants can cause adverse CNS effects, such as ataxia, confusion, somnolence, and tremor. Many anticonvulsants also cause CV disorders, such as arrhythmias and hypotension; GI effects, such as vomiting; and hematologic disorders, such as agranulocytosis, bone marrow depression, leukopenia, and thrombocytopenia. Stevens-Johnson syndrome, other severe rashes, and abnormal liver function test results may occur with certain anticonvulsants.

Action

Anticonvulsants include six classes of drugs: selected hydantoin derivatives, barbiturates, benzodiazepines, succinimides, iminostilbene derivatives (carbamazepine), and carboxylic acid derivatives. Two miscellaneous anticonvulsants are acetazolamide and magnesium sulfate.

Some hydantoin derivatives and carbamazepine inhibit the spread of seizure activity in the motor cortex. Some barbiturates and succinimides limit seizure activity by increasing the threshold for motor cortex stimuli. Selected benzodiazepines and carboxylic acid derivatives may increase inhibition of GABA in brain neurons. Acetazolamide inhibits carbonic anhydrase. Magnesium sulfate interferes with the release of acetylcholine at the myoneural junction.

NURSING PROCESS

❊ Assessment
• Monitor drug level and patient's response as indicated.
• Monitor patient for adverse reactions.
• Assess patient's compliance with therapy at each follow-up visit.

🔁 Key nursing diagnoses
• Risk for trauma related to adverse reactions
• Impaired physical mobility related to sedation
• Noncompliance related to long-term therapy

❯ Planning and implementation
• Give oral forms with food to reduce GI irritation.
• Phenytoin binds with tube feedings, thus decreasing absorption of drug. Turn off tube feedings for 2 hours before and after giving phenytoin, according to your facility's policy.
• Adjust dosage according to patient's response.
• Take safety precautions if patient has adverse CNS reactions.

Patient teaching
• Instruct patient to take drug exactly as prescribed and not to stop drug without medical supervision.
• Urge patient to avoid hazardous activities that require mental alertness if adverse CNS reactions occur.
• Advise patient to wear or carry medical identification at all times.

☑ Evaluation
• Patient sustains no trauma from adverse reactions.
• Patient maintains physical mobility.
• Patient complies with therapy and has no seizures.

Antidepressants, tricyclic

amitriptyline hydrochloride
amitriptyline pamoate
amoxapine
clomipramine hydrochloride
desipramine hydrochloride
doxepin hydrochloride
imipramine hydrochloride
imipramine pamoate
nortriptyline hydrochloride

Indications

▶ Depression, anxiety (doxepin hydrochloride), obsessive-compulsive disorder (clomipramine), enuresis in children older than age 6 (imipramine).

Contraindications and cautions

• Contraindicated in patients hypersensitive to these drugs and in patients with urine retention or angle-closure glaucoma.
• Tricyclic antidepressants are contraindicated within 2 weeks of MAO inhibitor therapy.
• Use cautiously in patients with suicidal tendencies, schizophrenia, paranoia, seizure disorders, CV disease, or impaired hepatic function.
❋ Lifespan: In pregnant and breast-feeding women, safety hasn't been established; use cautiously. In children younger than age 12, tricyclic antidepressants aren't recommended. Elderly patients are more sensitive to therapeutic and adverse effects; they need lower dosages.

Adverse reactions

Adverse reactions include anticholinergic effects, orthostatic hypotension, and sedation. The tertiary amines (amitriptyline, doxepin, and imipramine) exert the strongest sedative effects; tolerance usually develops in a few weeks. Amoxapine is most likely to cause seizures, especially with overdose. Tricyclic antidepressants may cause cardiovascular effects such as T-wave abnormalities, conduction disturbances, and arrhythmias.

Action

Tricyclic antidepressants may inhibit reuptake of norepinephrine and serotonin in CNS nerve terminals (presynaptic neurons), thus enhancing the concentration and activity of neurotransmitters in the synaptic cleft. Tricyclic antidepressants also exert antihistaminic, sedative, anticholinergic, vasodilatory, and quinidine-like effects.

NURSING PROCESS

Assessment

• Observe patient for mood changes to monitor drug effectiveness; benefits may not appear for 3 to 6 weeks.
• Check vital signs regularly for tachycardia or decreased blood pressure; observe patient carefully for other adverse reactions and report changes. Check ECG in patients older than age 40 before starting therapy.
• Monitor patient for anticholinergic adverse reactions, such as urine retention or constipation, which may require dosage reduction.

Key nursing diagnoses

• Disturbed thought processes related to adverse effects
• Risk for injury related to sedation and orthostatic hypotension
• Noncompliance related to long-term therapy

Planning and implementation

• Make sure patient swallows each dose; a depressed patient may hoard pills for suicide attempt, especially when symptoms begin to improve.
• Don't withdraw drug abruptly; instead, gradually reduce dosage over several weeks to avoid rebound effect or other adverse reactions.

Patient teaching

• Explain to patient the rationale for therapy and its anticipated risks and benefits. Inform patient that full therapeutic effect may not occur for several weeks.
• Teach patient how and when to take the drug. Warn him not to increase dosage, stop taking the drug, or take any other drug, including OTC medicines and herbal remedies, without medical approval.
• Because overdose with tricyclic antidepressants is commonly fatal, entrust a reliable family member with the drug, and warn him to store drug safely away from children.
• Advise patient not to take drug with milk or food to minimize GI distress. Suggest taking

full dose at bedtime if daytime sedation is a problem.
- Tell patient to avoid alcohol.
- Advise patient to avoid hazardous tasks that require mental alertness until full effects of drug are known.
- Warn patient that excessive exposure to sunlight, heat lamps, or tanning beds may cause burns and abnormal hyperpigmentation.
- Urge diabetic patient to monitor his glucose level carefully because drug may alter it.
- Recommend sugarless gum or hard candy, artificial saliva, or ice chips to relieve dry mouth.
- Advise patient to report adverse reactions promptly.

☑ **Evaluation**
- Patient regains normal thought processes.
- Patient sustains no injury from adverse reactions.
- Patient complies with therapy, and his depression is alleviated.

Antidiabetics
acarbose
glimepiride
glipizide
glyburide
metformin hydrochloride
miglitol
nateglinide
pioglitazone hydrochloride
repaglinide
rosiglitazone maleate

Indications
▶ Mild to moderately severe, stable, nonketotic, type 2 (non–insulin-dependent) diabetes mellitus that can't be controlled by diet alone.

Contraindications and cautions
- Contraindicated in patients hypersensitive to these drugs and in patients with diabetic ketoacidosis with or without coma. Metformin is also contraindicated in patients with renal disease or metabolic acidosis and generally should be avoided in patients with hepatic disease.
- Use sulfonylureas cautiously in patients with renal or hepatic disease. Use metformin cau-

tiously in patients with adrenal or pituitary insufficiency and in debilitated and malnourished patients. Alpha-glucosidase inhibitors should be used cautiously in patients with mild to moderate renal insufficiency. Thiazolidinediones aren't recommended in patients with edema, heart failure, or liver disease.
⚘ **Lifespan:** In pregnant or breast-feeding women, use is contraindicated. Oral hypoglycemics appear in small amounts in breast milk and may cause hypoglycemia in the infant. In children, oral hypoglycemics aren't effective in type 1 diabetes mellitus. Elderly patients may be more sensitive to these drugs, usually need lower dosages, and are more likely to develop neurologic symptoms of hypoglycemia; monitor these patients closely. In elderly patients, avoid chlorpropamide use because of its long duration of action.

Adverse reactions
Sulfonylureas cause dose-related reactions that usually respond to decreased dosage: anorexia, headache, heartburn, nausea, paresthesia, vomiting, and weakness. Hypoglycemia may follow excessive dosage, increased exercise, decreased food intake, or alcohol use.
    The most serious adverse reaction linked to metformin is lactic acidosis. It's rare and most likely to occur in patients with renal dysfunction. Other reactions to metformin include dermatitis, GI upset, megaloblastic anemia, rash, and unpleasant or metallic taste.
    Thiazolidinediones may cause fluid retention leading to or exacerbating heart failure. Alpha-glucosidase inhibitors can cause abdominal pain, diarrhea, and flatulence.

Action
Oral hypoglycemics come in several types. Sulfonylureas are sulfonamide derivatives that aren't antibacterial. They lower glucose levels by stimulating insulin release from the pancreas. These drugs work only in the presence of functioning beta cells in the islet tissue of the pancreas. After prolonged administration, they produce hypoglycemia by acting outside of the pancreas, including reduced glucose production by the liver and enhanced peripheral sensitivity to insulin. The latter may result from an increased number of insulin receptors or from changes after insulin binding. Sulfonylureas are divided into first-generation drugs, such as

chlorpropamide, and second-generation drugs, such as glyburide, glimepiride, and glipizide. Although their mechanisms of action are similar, the second-generation drugs carry a more lipophilic side chain, are more potent, and cause fewer adverse reactions. Their most important difference is their duration of action.

Meglitinides, such as nateglinide and repaglinide, are nonsulfonylurea hypoglycemics that stimulate the release of insulin from the pancreas.

Metformin decreases hepatic glucose production, reduces intestinal glucose absorption, and improves insulin sensitivity by increasing peripheral glucose uptake and utilization. With metformin therapy, insulin secretion remains unchanged, and fasting insulin levels and all-day insulin response may decrease.

Alpha-glucosidase inhibitors, such as acarbose and miglitol, delay digestion of carbohydrates, resulting in a smaller rise in glucose levels.

Rosiglitazone and pioglitazone are thiazolidinediones, which lower glucose levels by improving insulin sensitivity. These drugs are potent and highly selective agonists for receptors found in insulin-sensitive tissues, such as adipose, skeletal muscle, and liver.

NURSING PROCESS

⚖ Assessment
• Monitor patient's glucose level regularly. Increase monitoring during periods of increased stress, such as infection, fever, surgery, or trauma.
• Monitor patient for adverse reactions.
• Assess patient's compliance with drug therapy and other aspects of diabetic treatment.

🔑 Key nursing diagnoses
• Risk for injury related to hypoglycemia
• Risk for deficient fluid volume related to adverse GI effects
• Noncompliance related to long-term therapy

▶ Planning and implementation
• Give sulfonylurea 30 minutes before morning meal for once-daily dosing or 30 minutes before morning and evening meals for twice-daily dosing. Give metformin with morning and evening meals. Alpha-glucosidase inhibitors

should be taken with the first bite of each main meal three times daily.
• Patients who take a thiazolidinedione should have liver enzyme levels measured at the start of therapy, every 2 months for the first year of therapy, and periodically thereafter.
• Keep in mind that a patient transferring from one oral hypoglycemic to another (except chlorpropamide) usually needs no transition period.
• Anticipate patient's need for insulin during periods of increased stress.

Patient teaching
• Emphasize importance of following the prescribed regimen. Urge patient to adhere to diet, weight reduction, exercise, and personal hygiene recommendations.
• Explain that therapy relieves symptoms but doesn't cure the disease.
• Teach patient how to recognize and treat hypoglycemia.

☑ Evaluation
• Patient sustains no injury.
• Patient maintains adequate hydration.
• Patient complies with therapy, as evidenced by normal or near-normal glucose level.

Antidiarrheals
bismuth subgallate
bismuth subsalicylate
calcium polycarbophil
diphenoxylate hydrochloride and atropine sulfate
kaolin and pectin mixtures
loperamide hydrochloride
octreotide acetate
opium tincture
opium tincture, camphorated

Indications
▶ Mild, acute, or chronic diarrhea. Octreotide acetate is only indicated for diarrhea caused by tumors.

Contraindications and cautions
• Contraindicated in patients hypersensitive to these drugs.

≋ Lifespan: Some antidiarrheals may appear in breast milk; check individual drugs for specific recommendations. For infants younger than age 2, don't give kaolin and pectin mixtures. For children or teenagers recovering from flu or chickenpox, consult prescriber before giving bismuth subsalicylate. For elderly patients, use caution when giving antidiarrheal drugs, especially opium preparations.

Adverse reactions

Bismuth preparations may cause salicylism (with high doses) or temporary darkening of tongue and stools. Kaolin and pectin mixtures may cause constipation and fecal impaction or ulceration. Opium preparations may cause dizziness, light-headedness, nausea, physical dependence (with long-term use), and vomiting.

Action

Bismuth preparations may have a mild water-binding capacity, may absorb toxins, and provide a protective coating for the intestinal mucosa. Kaolin and pectin mixtures decrease fluid in the stool by absorbing bacteria and toxins that cause diarrhea. Opium preparations increase smooth muscle tone in the GI tract, inhibit motility and propulsion, and decrease digestive secretions.

NURSING PROCESS

⏏ Assessment
- Assess patient's condition before therapy and regularly thereafter.
- Monitor fluid and electrolyte balance.
- Observe patient for adverse reactions.

⊞ Key nursing diagnoses
- Constipation related to adverse effect of bismuth preparations on GI tract
- Risk for injury related to adverse CNS reactions
- Risk for deficient fluid volume related to GI upset

▷ Planning and implementation
- Take safety precautions if patient experiences adverse CNS reactions.
- Don't substitute opium tincture for paregoric.
- Notify prescriber about serious or persistent adverse reactions.

Patient teaching
- Instruct patient to take drug exactly as prescribed; warn him that excessive use of opium preparations can lead to dependence.
- Instruct patient to notify prescriber if diarrhea lasts for more than 2 days and to report adverse reactions.
- Warn patient to avoid hazardous activities that require alertness if CNS depression occurs.

☑ Evaluation
- Patient doesn't develop constipation.
- Patient isn't injured during therapy.
- Patient maintains adequate hydration.

Antihistamines

azelastine hydrochloride
brompheniramine maleate
cyproheptadine hydrochloride
desloratadine
diphenhydramine hydrochloride
fexofenadine hydrochloride
hydroxyzine embonate
hydroxyzine hydrochloride
hydroxyzine pamoate
loratadine
meclizine hydrochloride
promethazine hydrochloride

Indications

▶ Allergic rhinitis, urticaria, pruritus, vertigo, motion sickness, nausea and vomiting, sedation, dyskinesia, parkinsonism.

Contraindications and cautions

- Contraindicated in patients hypersensitive to these drugs and in those with angle-closure glaucoma, stenosing peptic ulcer, pyloroduodenal obstruction, or bladder neck obstruction. Also contraindicated in those taking MAO inhibitors.

≋ Lifespan: In pregnant women, safe use hasn't been established. During breast-feeding, antihistamines shouldn't be used because many of these drugs appear in breast milk and may cause unusual excitability in the infant. Neonates, especially premature infants, may experience seizures. Children, especially those younger than age 6, may experience paradoxical hyperexcitability with restlessness, insomnia, nervousness, euphoria, tremors, and seizures; give cautiously. Elderly patients usually are more sensitive to the adverse effects of antihistamines, especially dizziness, sedation, hypotension, and urine retention; use cautiously and monitor these patients closely.

Adverse reactions

Most antihistamines cause drowsiness and impaired motor function early in therapy. They also can cause blurred vision, constipation, and dry mouth and throat. Some antihistamines, such as promethazine, may cause cholestatic jaundice, which may be a hypersensitivity reaction, and may predispose patients to photosensitivity. Promethazine may also cause extrapyramidal reactions with high doses.

Action

Antihistamines are structurally related chemicals that compete with histamine for histamine H_1-receptor sites on smooth muscle of bronchi, GI tract, and large blood vessels, binding to cellular receptors and preventing access to and subsequent activity of histamine. They don't directly alter histamine or prevent its release.

NURSING PROCESS

Assessment
• Monitor patient for adverse reactions.
• Monitor blood counts during long-term therapy; watch for signs of blood dyscrasia.

Key nursing diagnoses
• Risk for injury related to sedation
• Impaired oral mucous membrane related to dry mouth
• Constipation related to anticholinergic effect of antihistamines

Planning and implementation
• Reduce GI distress by giving antihistamines with food.
• Provide sugarless gum, hard candy, or ice chips to relieve dry mouth.
• Increase fluid intake or humidify air to decrease adverse effect of thickened secretions.

Patient teaching
• Advise patient to take drug with meals or snacks to prevent GI upset.

• Suggest that patient use warm water rinses, artificial saliva, ice chips, or sugarless gum or candy to relieve dry mouth. Tell him to avoid overusing mouthwash, which may worsen dryness and destroy normal flora.
• Warn patient to avoid hazardous activities until full CNS effects of drug are known.
• Tell patient to seek medical approval before using alcohol, tranquilizers, sedatives, pain relievers, or sleeping medications.
• For accurate diagnostic skin test results, advise patient to stop taking antihistamines 4 days before test.

Evaluation
• Patient sustains no injury from sedation.
• Patient maintains normal mucous membranes by using preventive measures throughout therapy.
• Patient maintains normal bowel function.

Antihypertensives
Angiotensin-converting enzyme (ACE) inhibitors
benazepril hydrochloride
captopril
enalapril maleate
enalaprilat
fosinopril sodium
lisinopril
moexipril hydrochloride
perindopril erbumine
quinapril hydrochloride
ramipril
trandolapril
Angiotensin II receptor blockers
candesartan cilexetil
eprosartan mesylate
irbesartan
losartan potassium
olmesartan medoxomil
telmisartan
valsartan
Beta blockers
acebutolol hydrochloride
atenolol
bisoprolol fumarate
carvedilol
labetalol hydrochloride
metoprolol tartrate

nadolol
pindolol
propranolol hydrochloride
timolol maleate
Calcium channel blockers
amlodipine besylate
diltiazem hydrochloride
felodipine
nicardipine hydrochloride
nifedipine
nisoldipine
verapamil hydrochloride
Centrally acting alpha blockers (sympatholytics)
clonidine hydrochloride
guanfacine hydrochloride
methyldopa
Peripherally acting alpha blockers
doxazosin mesylate
prazosin hydrochloride
terazosin hydrochloride
Vasodilators
diazoxide
hydralazine hydrochloride
minoxidil
nitroprusside sodium

Indications

▶ Essential and secondary hypertension.

Contraindications and cautions

• Contraindicated in patients hypersensitive to these drugs and in those with hypotension.
• Use cautiously in patients with hepatic or renal dysfunction.
⚖ **Lifespan:** In pregnant women, use cautiously when potential benefits to the patient outweigh risks to the fetus. Check each drug because some are safe only in the first trimester. In breast-feeding women, use cautiously; some antihypertensives appear in breast milk. In children, safety and effectiveness of many antihypertensives haven't been established; give these drugs cautiously and monitor children closely. Elderly patients are more susceptible to adverse reactions and may need lower maintenance doses; monitor these patients closely.

Adverse reactions

Antihypertensives commonly cause orthostatic changes in heart rate, headache, hypotension, nausea, and vomiting. Other reactions vary greatly among different drug types. Centrally acting sympatholytics may cause constipation, depression, dizziness, drowsiness, dry mouth, headache, palpitations, severe rebound hypertension, and sexual dysfunction; methyldopa also may cause aplastic anemia and thrombocytopenia. Rauwolfia alkaloids may cause anxiety, depression, drowsiness, dry mouth, hyperacidity, impotence, nasal stuffiness, and weight gain. Vasodilators may cause ECG changes, diarrhea, dizziness, heart failure, palpitations, pruritus, and rash.

Action

Antihypertensives reduce blood pressure through various mechanisms. For information on the action of ACE inhibitors, alpha blockers, angiotensin II receptor blockers, beta blockers, calcium channel blockers, and diuretics, see their individual drug class entries. Centrally acting sympatholytics stimulate central alpha-adrenergic receptors, reducing cerebral sympathetic outflow, thereby decreasing peripheral vascular resistance and blood pressure. Rauwolfia alkaloids bind to and gradually destroy the norepinephrine-containing storage vesicles in central and peripheral adrenergic neurons. Vasodilators act directly on smooth muscle to reduce blood pressure.

NURSING PROCESS

🕎 **Assessment**
• Obtain baseline blood pressure and pulse rate and rhythm; recheck regularly.
• Monitor patient for adverse reactions.
• Monitor patient's weight and fluid and electrolyte status.
• Monitor patient's compliance with treatment.

🔑 **Key nursing diagnoses**
• Risk for trauma related to orthostatic hypotension
• Risk for deficient fluid volume related to GI upset
• Noncompliance related to long-term therapy or adverse reactions

▷ **Planning and implementation**
• Give drug with food or h.s., as indicated.
• When mixing and giving parenteral drugs, follow manufacturer's guidelines.

• Take steps to prevent or minimize orthostatic hypotension.
• Maintain patient's nondrug therapy, such as sodium restriction, calorie reduction, stress management, and exercise program.

Patient teaching
• Instruct patient to take drug exactly as prescribed. Warn against stopping drug abruptly.
• Review adverse reactions caused by drug, and urge patient to notify prescriber of serious or persistent reactions.
• To prevent dizziness, light-headedness, or fainting, advise patient to avoid sudden changes in position.
• Warn patient to avoid hazardous activities until full effects of drug are known. Also, warn patient to avoid physical exertion, especially in hot weather.
• Advise patient to consult prescriber before taking any OTC medications or herbal remedies; serious drug interactions can occur.
• Encourage patient to comply with therapy.

☑ **Evaluation**
• Patient doesn't experience trauma from orthostatic hypotension.
• Patient maintains adequate hydration.
• Patient complies with therapy, as evidenced by normal blood pressure.

Antilipemics
atorvastatin calcium
cholestyramine
colesevelam hydrochloride
ezetimibe
fenofibrate
fluvastatin sodium
gemfibrozil
lovastatin
pravastatin sodium
rosuvastatin calcium
simvastatin

Indications

▶ Hyperlipidemia, hypercholesterolemia.

Contraindications and cautions

• Contraindicated in patients hypersensitive to these drugs. Also, bile-sequestering drugs are contraindicated in patients with complete biliary obstruction. Fibric acid derivatives are contraindicated in patients with primary biliary cirrhosis or significant hepatic or renal dysfunction. HMG-CoA reductase inhibitors and cholesterol absorption inhibitors are contraindicated in patients with active liver disease or persistently elevated transaminase levels.
• Use bile-sequestering drugs cautiously in constipated patients. Use fibric acid derivatives cautiously in patients with peptic ulcer. Use HMG-CoA inhibitors cautiously in patients who consume large amounts of alcohol or who have a history of liver or renal disease.
☙ **Lifespan:** In pregnant women, use bile-sequestering drugs and fibric acid derivatives cautiously and avoid using HMG-CoA inhibitors. In breast-feeding women, avoid using fibric acid derivatives and HMG-CoA inhibitors; give bile-sequestering drugs cautiously. In children ages 10 to 17, certain antilipemics have been approved to treat heterozygous familial hypercholesterolemia. Elderly patients have an increased risk of severe constipation; use bile-sequestering drugs cautiously and monitor patients closely.

Adverse reactions

Antilipemics commonly cause GI upset. Bile-sequestering drugs may cause bloating, cholelithiasis, constipation, and steatorrhea. Fibric acid derivatives may cause cholelithiasis and have other GI or CNS effects. Use of gemfibrozil with lovastatin may cause myopathy. HMG-CoA reductase inhibitors may affect liver function or cause rash, pruritus, increased CK levels, rhabdomyolysis, and myopathy.

Action

Antilipemics lower elevated lipid levels. Bile-sequestering drugs (cholestyramine and colesevelam) lower LDL level by forming insoluble complexes with bile salts, thus triggering cholesterol to leave the bloodstream and other storage areas to make new bile acids. Fibric acid derivatives (gemfibrozil) reduce cholesterol formation, increase sterol excretion, and decrease lipoprotein and triglyceride synthesis. HMG-CoA reductase inhibitors (atorvastatin, fluvastatin, lovastatin, pravastatin, rosuvastatin, simvastatin) interfere with the activity of enzymes that generate cholesterol in the liver. Selective cholesterol absorption inhibitors (ezetimibe) inhibit the absorption of cholesterol by the small intestine, reducing hepatic cholesterol stores and increasing cholesterol clearance from the blood.

NURSING PROCESS

⬛ Assessment
• Monitor cholesterol and lipid levels before and periodically during therapy.
• Monitor CK level when therapy begins and every 6 months thereafter. Also, check CK level in a patient who complains of muscle pain.
• Monitor patient for adverse reactions.

⬛ Key nursing diagnoses
• Risk for deficient fluid volume related to adverse GI reactions
• Constipation related to adverse effect on bowel
• Noncompliance related to long-term therapy

⬛ Planning and implementation
• Mix powder form of bile-sequestering drugs with 120 to 180 ml of liquid. Never give dry powder alone because patient may inhale it accidentally.
• Give lovastatin with evening meal, simvastatin in the evening, and fluvastatin and pravastatin at bedtime.

Patient teaching
• Instruct patient to take drug exactly as prescribed. If he takes a bile-sequestering drug, warn him never to take the dry form.
• Stress importance of diet in controlling lipid levels.
• Advise patient to drink 2 to 3 L of fluid daily and to report persistent or severe constipation.

⬛ Evaluation
• Patient maintains adequate fluid volume.
• Patient doesn't experience severe or persistent constipation.
• Patient complies with therapy, as evidenced by normal lipid and cholesterol levels.

Antimetabolite antineoplastics
capecitabine
cytarabine
cytarabine liposomal
fludarabine phosphate
fluorouracil
hydroxyurea
mercaptopurine
methotrexate
pentostatin
thioguanine

Indications
▶ Various tumors.

Contraindications and cautions
• Contraindicated in patients hypersensitive to these drugs.
⬛ **Lifespan:** Pregnant women should be informed of the risks to the fetus. Breast-feeding isn't recommended for women taking these drugs. In children, safety and effectiveness of some drugs haven't been established; use cautiously. Elderly patients have an increased risk of adverse reactions; monitor them closely.

Adverse reactions
The most common adverse effects include anemia, anxiety, bone marrow depression, chills, diarrhea, fever, flank or joint pain, hair loss, leukopenia, nausea, redness or pain at injection site, thrombocytopenia, swelling of the feet or lower legs, and vomiting.

Action
Antimetabolites are structurally similar to naturally occurring metabolites and can be divided into three subcategories: purine, pyrimidine, and folinic acid analogues. Most of these drugs interrupt cell reproduction at a specific phase of the cell cycle. Purine analogues are incorporated into DNA and RNA, interfering with nucleic acid synthesis (by miscoding) and replication. They also may inhibit synthesis of purine bases through pseudofeedback mechanisms. Pyrimidine analogues inhibit enzymes in metabolic pathways that interfere with biosynthesis of uridine and thymine. Folic acid antagonists prevent conversion of folic acid to tetrahydrofolate

by inhibiting the enzyme dihydrofolic acid reductase.

NURSING PROCESS

🖎 Assessment
• Perform a complete assessment before therapy begins.
• Monitor patient for adverse reactions.
• Monitor vital signs and patency of catheter or I.V. line throughout administration.
• Monitor platelet and total and differential leukocyte counts, hematocrit, and ALT, AST, LDH, bilirubin, creatinine, uric acid, and BUN levels.

🖎 Key nursing diagnoses
• Ineffective protection related to thrombocytopenia
• Risk for infection related to immunosuppression
• Risk for deficient fluid volume related to adverse GI effects

🖎 Planning and implementation
• Follow established procedures for safe and proper handling, administration, and disposal of drugs.
• Try to ease patient's and family's anxiety before treatment.
• Give an antiemetic to reduce nausea before giving drug.
• Give cytarabine with allopurinol to decrease the risk of hyperuricemia. Encourage patient to drink a lot of fluids.
• Provide diligent mouth care to prevent stomatitis with cytarabine, fluorouracil, or methotrexate therapy.
• Anticipate the need for leucovorin rescue with high-dose methotrexate therapy.
• Treat extravasation promptly.
• Anticipate diarrhea, possibly severe, with prolonged fluorouracil therapy.

Patient teaching
• Teach patient proper oral hygiene, including cautious use of toothbrush, dental floss, and toothpicks. Chemotherapy can increase the incidence of microbial infection, delayed healing, and bleeding gums.
• Advise patient to complete dental work before therapy begins or to delay it until blood counts are normal.

• Tell patient to defer immunizations if possible until hematologic stability is confirmed.
• Warn patient that he may bruise easily because of drug's effect on platelets.
• Advise patient to avoid close contact with people who have taken oral poliovirus vaccine or who have been exposed to people with bacterial or viral infection because chemotherapy may increase susceptibility. Urge patient to notify prescriber promptly if he develops signs or symptoms of infection.
• Instruct patient to report redness, pain, or swelling at injection site. Local tissue injury and scarring may result from tissue infiltration at infusion site.

🖎 Evaluation
• Patient doesn't have serious bleeding complications.
• Patient doesn't have an infection.
• Patient maintains adequate hydration.

Antiparkinsonians
amantadine hydrochloride
apomorphine hydrochloride
benztropine mesylate
bromocriptine mesylate
diphenhydramine hydrochloride
entacapone
levodopa
levodopa and carbidopa
levodopa, carbidopa, and entacapone
pergolide mesylate
pramipexole dihydrochloride
ropinirole hydrochloride
selegiline hydrochloride
tolcapone
trihexyphenidyl hydrochloride

Indications
▶ Signs and symptoms of Parkinson's and drug-induced extrapyramidal reactions.

Contraindications and cautions
• Contraindicated in patients hypersensitive to these drugs.
• Use cautiously in patients with prostatic hyperplasia or tardive dyskinesia and in debilitated patients.

• Neuroleptic malignant-like syndrome involving muscle rigidity, increased body temperature, and mental status changes may occur with abrupt withdrawal of antiparkinsonians.
☀ **Lifespan:** In pregnant women, safe use hasn't been established. Antiparkinsonians may appear in breast milk; a decision should be made to stop the drug or stop breast-feeding, taking into account the importance of the drug to the mother. In children, safety and effectiveness haven't been established. Elderly patients have an increased risk for adverse reactions; monitor them closely.

Adverse reactions

Anticholinergics may cause blurred vision, cycloplegia, constipation, decreased sweating or anhidrosis, dry mouth, headache, mydriasis, palpitations, tachycardia, and urinary hesitancy and urine retention. Dopaminergics may cause arrhythmias, confusion, disturbing dreams, dystonias, hallucinations, headache, muscle cramps, nausea, orthostatic hypotension, and vomiting. Amantadine also causes irritability, insomnia, and livedo reticularis (with prolonged use).

Action

Antiparkinsonians include synthetic anticholinergics, dopaminergics, and the antiviral amantadine. Anticholinergics probably prolong the action of dopamine by blocking its reuptake into presynaptic neurons and by suppressing central cholinergic activity. Dopaminergics act in the brain by increasing dopamine availability, thus improving motor function. Entacapone is a reversible inhibitor of peripheral cathechol-*O*-methyltransferase (commonly known as COMT), which is responsible for elimination of various catecholamines, including dopamine. Blocking this pathway when giving levodopa and carbidopa should result in higher levels of levodopa, thereby allowing greater dopaminergic stimulation in the CNS and leading to a greater effect in treating parkinsonian symptoms. Amantadine is thought to increase dopamine release in the substantia nigra.

NURSING PROCESS

🗒 **Assessment**
• Obtain baseline assessment of patient's impairment, and reassess regularly to monitor the drug's effectiveness.

• Monitor patient for adverse reactions.
• Monitor vital signs, especially during dosage adjustments.

🔑 **Key nursing diagnoses**
• Risk for injury related to adverse CNS effects
• Urine retention related to anticholinergic effect on bladder
• Disturbed sleep pattern related to amantadine-induced insomnia

▶ **Planning and implementation**
• Give drug with food to prevent GI irritation.
• Adjust dosage according to patient's response and tolerance.
• Never withdraw drug abruptly.
• Institute safety precautions.
• Provide ice chips, drinks, or sugarless hard candy or gum to relieve dry mouth. Increase fluid and fiber intake to prevent constipation, as appropriate.
• Notify prescriber about urine retention, and be prepared to catheterize patient, if necessary.

Patient teaching
• Instruct patient to take drug exactly as prescribed, and warn him not to suddenly stop taking the drug.
• Advise patient to take drug with food to prevent GI upset.
• Teach patient how to manage anticholinergic effects.
• Instruct patient to avoid hazardous tasks if adverse CNS effects occur. Tell him to avoid alcohol during therapy.
• Encourage patient to report severe or persistent adverse reactions.

☑ **Evaluation**
• Patient remains free from injury.
• Patient's voiding pattern doesn't change.
• Patient's sleep pattern isn't altered by amantadine.

Antivirals

abacavir sulfate
acyclovir sodium
adefovir dipivoxil
amantadine hydrochloride
amprenavir
atazanavir sulfate
cidofovir
delavirdine mesylate
didanosine
efavirenz
emtricitabine
enfuvirtide
famciclovir
fosamprenavir calcium
foscarnet sodium
ganciclovir
indinavir sulfate
lamivudine
lamivudine and zidovudine
lopinavir and ritonavir
nelfinavir mesylate
nevirapine
oseltamivir phosphate
ribavirin
rimantadine hydrochloride
ritonavir
saquinavir mesylate
stavudine
tenofovir disoproxil fumarate
valacyclovir hydrochloride
valganciclovir hydrochloride
zalcitabine
zanamivir
zidovudine

Indications

▶ Viral infections.

Contraindications and cautions

• Contraindicated in patients hypersensitive to these drugs.
• Use cautiously in patients with suicidal thoughts.
🕮 Lifespan: Some antivirals are contraindicated in pregnancy; see individual drug monographs. In breast-feeding women, some antivirals are contraindicated, while others require cautious use. For infants and children, recom-

mendations vary with the antiviral prescribed. Elderly patients have an increased risk of adverse reactions; monitor them closely.

Adverse reactions

Antivirals may cause anorexia, blood dyscrasias, chills, confusion, depression, diarrhea, dry mouth, edema, fatigue, hallucinations, headache, nausea, and vomiting.

Action

Acyclovir, cidofovir, didanosine, famciclovir, ganciclovir, valacyclovir, valganciclovir, and zalcitabine interfere with DNA synthesis and replication. Amantadine prevents the release of infectious viral nucleic acid into the host cell and possibly prevents viruses from penetrating cells. Foscarnet blocks the pyrophosphate-binding site. Rimantadine prevents viral uncoating. Abacavir, amprenavir, emtricitabine, fosamprenavir, indinavir, ritonavir, saquinavir, and stavudine inhibit the activity of HIV protease. Delavirdine, efavirenz, lamivudine, nevirapine, and zidovudine inhibit reverse transcriptase. Enfuvirtide interferes with entry of HIV-1 into cells by inhibiting fusion of HIV-1 to cell membranes.

NURSING PROCESS

🕮 Assessment
• Obtain baseline assessment of patient's viral infection, and reassess regularly to monitor the drug's effectiveness.
• Monitor renal and hepatic function, CBC, and platelet count regularly. Monitor electrolytes, such as calcium, phosphate, magnesium, potassium, in patients receiving foscarnet.
• Inspect patient's I.V. site regularly for signs of irritation, phlebitis, inflammation, or extravasation.
• If patient has a history of heart failure, watch closely for worsening or recurrence during amantadine therapy.
• Monitor patient's cardiac status during ribavirin therapy.

🕮 Key nursing diagnoses
• Ineffective protection related to adverse hematologic reactions
• Risk for deficient fluid volume related to GI upset
• Noncompliance related to long-term therapy

⏩ Planning and implementation

• Adjust dosage of selected antiviral for patient with decreased renal function, especially during parenteral therapy.
• Obtain an order for an antiemetic or antidiarrheal, if needed.
• If patient has adverse CNS reactions, take safety precautions. For example, place bed in low position, raise bed rails, and supervise ambulation and other activities.
• Notify prescriber about serious or persistent adverse reactions.

Patient teaching
• Instruct patient to take drug exactly as prescribed, even if he feels better.
• Inform patient with HIV that drug doesn't cure HIV infection, that opportunistic infections and other complications of HIV infection may continue to occur, and that transmission of HIV to others through sexual contact or blood contamination is still possible.
• Urge patient to notify prescriber promptly about severe or persistent adverse reactions.
• Encourage patient to keep appointments for follow-up care.

🖪 Evaluation

• Patient doesn't have any serious adverse hematologic effects.
• Patient maintains adequate hydration.
• Patient complies with therapy, and viral infection is eradicated.

Barbiturates

amobarbital sodium
pentobarbital sodium
phenobarbital
phenobarbital sodium
primidone
secobarbital sodium

Indications

▶ Sedation, preanesthetic, short-term treatment of insomnia, seizure disorders.

Contraindications and cautions

• Contraindicated in patients hypersensitive to these drugs and in those with bronchopneumo-

nia, other severe pulmonary insufficiency, or liver dysfunction.
• Use cautiously in patients with blood pressure alterations, pulmonary disease, and CV dysfunction. Use cautiously, if at all, in patients who are depressed or have suicidal tendencies.
⚖ **Lifespan:** Barbiturates can cause fetal abnormalities; avoid use in pregnant women. Barbiturates appear in breast milk and may result in infant CNS depression; use cautiously. Premature infants are more susceptible to depressant effects of barbiturates because of their immature hepatic metabolism. Children may experience hyperactivity, excitement, or hyperalgesia; use cautiously and closely monitor. Elderly patients may experience hyperactivity, excitement, or hyperalgesia; use cautiously.

Adverse reactions

CNS depression, drowsiness, headache, lethargy, and vertigo are common with barbiturates. After hypnotic doses, a hangover effect, subtle distortion of mood, and impaired judgment and motor skills may continue for many hours. After dosage reduction or discontinuation, rebound insomnia or increased dreaming or nightmares may occur. Barbiturates cause hyperalgesia in subhypnotic doses. They can also cause paradoxical excitement at low doses, confusion in elderly patients, and hyperactivity in children. High fever, severe headache, stomatitis, conjunctivitis, or rhinitis may precede potentially fatal skin eruptions. Withdrawal symptoms may occur after as little as 2 weeks of uninterrupted therapy.

Action

Barbiturates act throughout the CNS, especially in the mesencephalic reticular activating system, which controls the CNS arousal mechanism. The main anticonvulsant actions are reduced nerve transmission and decreased excitability of the nerve cell. Barbiturates decrease presynaptic and postsynaptic membrane excitability by promoting the actions of GABA. They also depress respiration and GI motility and raise the seizure threshold.

NURSING PROCESS

⏰ Assessment

• To evaluate the drug's effectiveness, assess patient's level of consciousness and sleeping

patterns before and during therapy. Monitor neurologic status for alteration or deterioration.
• Assess vital signs often, especially during I.V. use.
• Monitor seizure character, frequency, and duration for changes.
• Observe patient to prevent hoarding or self-dosing, especially if patient is depressed, suicidal, or drug dependent.

⬚ Key nursing diagnoses
• Risk for injury related to sedation
• Disturbed thought processes related to confusion
• Impaired adjustment related to drug dependence

⬚ Planning and implementation
• When giving parenteral drug, inject I.V. or deep I.M., to avoid extravasation, which may cause local tissue damage and tissue necrosis. To avoid tissue damage, don't exceed 5 ml for any I.M. injection site.
• Keep resuscitative measures available. Giving I.V. drug too rapidly may cause respiratory depression, apnea, laryngospasm, or hypotension.
• Take seizure precautions as needed.
• Institute safety measures to prevent falls and injury. Raise side rails, assist patient out of bed, and keep call light within easy reach.
• Stop drug slowly. Stopping drug abruptly may cause withdrawal symptoms.

Patient teaching
• Explain that barbiturates can cause physical or psychological dependence.
• Instruct patient to take drug exactly as prescribed. Warn him not to change the dosage or take other drugs, including OTC medications or herbal remedies, without prescriber's approval.
• Reassure patient that a morning hangover is common after therapeutic use of barbiturates.
• Advise patient to avoid hazardous tasks, driving a motor vehicle, or operating machinery while taking the drug, and to review other safety measures to prevent injury.
• Instruct patient to report skin eruptions or other significant adverse effects.

⬚ Evaluation
• Patient sustains no injury from sedation.
• Patient maintains normal thought processes.

• Patient doesn't develop physical or psychological dependence.

Beta blockers

Beta₁ blockers
acebutolol hydrochloride
atenolol
bisoprolol fumarate
esmolol hydrochloride
metoprolol tartrate

Beta₁ and beta₂ blockers
carvedilol
labetalol hydrochloride
nadolol
pindolol
propranolol hydrochloride
sotalol hydrochloride
timolol maleate

Indications

▶ Hypertension (most drugs), angina pectoris (atenolol, metoprolol, nadolol, and propranolol), arrhythmias (acebutolol hydrochloride, esmolol, propranolol, and sotalol), glaucoma (betaxolol and timolol), prevention of MI (atenolol, metoprolol, propranolol, and timolol), prevention of recurrent migraine and other vascular headaches (propranolol and timolol), pheochromocytomas or essential tremors (selected drugs), heart failure (atenolol, bisoprolol, carvedilol, metoprolol).

Contraindications and cautions

• Contraindicated in patients hypersensitive to these drugs and in patients with cardiogenic shock, sinus bradycardia, heart block greater than first degree, bronchial asthma, and heart failure unless failure is caused by tachyarrhythmia treatable with propranolol.
• Use cautiously in patients with nonallergic bronchospastic disorders, diabetes mellitus, or impaired hepatic or renal function.
⚖ Lifespan: In pregnant women, use cautiously. Drugs appear in breast milk. In children, safety and effectiveness haven't been established; use only if the benefits outweigh the risks. Elderly patients may need reduced maintenance doses because of increased bioavail-

ability or delayed metabolism and may also have increased adverse effects; use cautiously.

Adverse reactions

Therapeutic dose may cause bradycardia, dizziness, and fatigue; some may cause other CNS disturbances, such as depression, hallucinations, memory loss, and nightmares. Toxic dose can produce severe hypotension, bradycardia, heart failure, or bronchospasm.

Action

Beta blockers compete with beta agonists for available beta receptors; individual drugs differ in their ability to affect beta receptors. Some drugs are nonselective: they block beta$_1$ receptors in cardiac muscle and beta$_2$ receptors in bronchial and vascular smooth muscle. Several drugs are cardioselective and, in lower doses, inhibit mainly beta$_1$ receptors. Some beta blockers have intrinsic sympathomimetic activity and stimulate and block beta receptors, thereby decreasing cardiac output. Others stabilize cardiac membranes, which affects cardiac-action potential.

NURSING PROCESS

Assessment

• Check apical pulse rate daily; alert prescriber about extremes, such as a pulse rate lower than 60 beats/minute.
• Monitor blood pressure, ECG, and heart rate and rhythm frequently; be alert for progression of AV block or bradycardia.
• If patient has heart failure, weigh him regularly; watch for weight gain of more than 2.25 kg (5 lb) per week.
• Observe diabetic patients for sweating, fatigue, and hunger. Signs of hypoglycemic shock may be masked.

Key nursing diagnoses

• Risk for injury related to adverse CNS effects
• Excessive fluid volume related to edema
• Decreased cardiac output related to bradycardia or hypotension

Planning and implementation

• Stop beta blockers before surgery for pheochromocytoma. Before any surgical procedure, notify anesthesiologist that patient is taking a beta blocker.

• Keep glucagon nearby to reverse beta blocker overdose.

Patient teaching

• Teach patient to take drug exactly as prescribed, even when he feels better.
• Warn patient not to stop taking the drug suddenly. Stopping suddenly can worsen angina or precipitate MI.
• Tell patient not to take OTC medications or herbal remedies without prescriber's approval.
• Explain potential adverse reactions, and stress importance of reporting unusual effects.

Evaluation

• Patient remains free from injury.
• Patient has no signs of edema.
• Patient maintains normal blood pressure and heart rate.

Calcium channel blockers

amlodipine besylate
diltiazem hydrochloride
felodipine
nicardipine hydrochloride
nifedipine
nisoldipine
verapamil hydrochloride

Indications

▶ Prinzmetal's variant angina, chronic stable angina, unstable angina, mild-to-moderate hypertension, arrhythmias.

Contraindications and cautions

• Contraindicated in patients hypersensitive to these drugs and in those with second- or third-degree heart block (except those with a pacemaker) and cardiogenic shock. Use diltiazem and verapamil cautiously in patients with heart failure.
⚠ Lifespan: In pregnant women, use cautiously. Calcium channel blockers may appear in breast milk; instruct patient to stop breastfeeding during therapy. In neonates and infants, adverse hemodynamic effects of parenteral verapamil are possible, but safety and effectiveness of other calcium channel blockers haven't been established; avoid use, if possible. In elderly

patients, the half-life of calcium channel blockers may be increased as a result of decreased clearance; use cautiously.

Adverse reactions

Adverse reactions vary among the drugs. Verapamil may cause bradycardia, hypotension, various degrees of heart block, and worsening of heart failure after rapid I.V. delivery. Prolonged oral verapamil therapy may cause constipation. Nifedipine may cause flushing, headache, heartburn, hypotension, light-headedness, and peripheral edema. The most common adverse reactions with diltiazem are anorexia and nausea; it also may induce bradycardia, heart failure, peripheral edema, and various degrees of heart block.

Action

The main physiologic action of calcium channel blockers is to inhibit calcium influx across the slow channels of myocardial and vascular smooth muscle cells. By inhibiting calcium flow into these cells, calcium channel blockers reduce intracellular calcium concentrations. This, in turn, dilates coronary arteries, peripheral arteries, and arterioles and slows cardiac conduction.

When used to treat Prinzmetal's variant angina, calcium channel blockers inhibit coronary spasm, which then increases oxygen delivery to the heart. Peripheral artery dilation decreases total peripheral resistance, which reduces afterload. This, in turn, decreases the amount of oxygen used by the myocardium. Inhibiting calcium flow into the specialized cardiac conduction cells (specifically, those in the SA and AV nodes) slows conduction through the heart. Of the calcium channel blockers, verapamil and diltiazem have the greatest effect on the AV node, which slows the ventricular rate in atrial fibrillation or flutter and converts supraventricular tachycardia to a normal sinus rhythm.

NURSING PROCESS

Assessment
- Monitor cardiac rate and rhythm and blood pressure carefully when therapy starts or dosage increases.
- Monitor fluids and electrolytes.
- Monitor patient for adverse reactions.

Key nursing diagnoses
- Decreased cardiac output related to adverse CV reactions
- Constipation related to oral verapamil therapy
- Noncompliance related to long-term therapy

Planning and implementation
- Don't give calcium supplements while patient is taking a calcium channel blocker; they may decrease the drug's effectiveness.
- Expect to decrease dosage gradually; don't stop calcium channel blockers abruptly.

Patient teaching
- Teach patient to take drug exactly as prescribed, even if he feels better.
- Instruct patient to take a missed dose as soon as possible, unless it's almost time for his next dose. Warn him never to take a double dose.
- Warn patient not to stop drug suddenly; abrupt discontinuation can produce serious adverse effects.
- Urge patient to report irregular heartbeat, shortness of breath, swelling of hands and feet, pronounced dizziness, constipation, nausea, or hypotension.

Evaluation
- Patient maintains adequate cardiac output throughout therapy, as evidenced by normal blood pressure and pulse rate.
- Patient regains normal bowel pattern.
- Patient complies with therapy, as evidenced by absence of symptoms related to disorder.

Cephalosporins
First generation
cefadroxil monohydrate
cefazolin sodium
cephalexin monohydrate
Second generation
cefaclor
cefotetan disodium
cefoxitin sodium
cefprozil
cefuroxime axetil
cefuroxime sodium
loracarbef

Third generation
cefdinir
cefditoren pivoxil
cefixime
cefoperazone sodium
cefotaxime sodium
cefpodoxime proxetil
ceftazidime
ceftibuten
ceftizoxime sodium
ceftriaxone sodium

Indications

▶ Infections of the lungs, skin, soft tissue, bones, joints, urinary and respiratory tracts, blood, abdomen, and heart; CNS infections caused by susceptible strains of *Neisseria meningitidis, Haemophilus influenzae,* and *Streptococcus pneumoniae;* meningitis caused by *Escherichia coli* or *Klebsiella;* infections that develop after surgical procedures classified as contaminated or potentially contaminated; penicillinase-producing *N. gonorrhoeae;* otitis media and ampicillin-resistant middle ear infection caused by *H. influenzae.*

Contraindications and cautions

• Contraindicated in patients hypersensitive to these drugs.
• Use cautiously in patients with renal or hepatic impairment, history of GI disease, or allergy to penicillins.
⚹ **Lifespan:** In pregnant women, use cautiously; safety hasn't been definitively established. In breast-feeding women, use cautiously because drugs appear in breast milk. In neonates and infants, half-life is prolonged; use cautiously. Elderly patients are susceptible to superinfection and coagulopathies, commonly have renal impairment, and may need a lower dosage; use cautiously.

Adverse reactions

Many cephalosporins have similar adverse effects. Hypersensitivity reactions range from mild rashes, fever, and eosinophilia to fatal anaphylaxis and are more common in patients with penicillin allergy. Adverse GI reactions include abdominal pain, diarrhea, dyspepsia, glossitis, nausea, tenesmus, and vomiting. Hematologic reactions include positive direct and indirect antiglobulin in Coombs' test, thrombocytopenia

or thrombocythemia, transient neutropenia, and reversible leukopenia. Minimal elevation of liver function test results occurs occasionally. Adverse renal effects may occur with any cephalosporin; they are most common in older patients, those with decreased renal function, and those taking other nephrotoxic drugs.

Local venous pain and irritation are common after I.M. injection; these reactions occur more often with higher doses and long-term therapy. Disulfiram-type reactions occur when cefoperazone or cefotetan are given within 3 days of alcohol use. Bacterial and fungal superinfections may result from suppression of normal flora.

Action

Cephalosporins are chemically and pharmacologically similar to penicillin; they act by inhibiting bacterial cell wall synthesis, causing rapid cell destruction. Their sites of action are enzymes known as penicillin-binding proteins. The affinity of certain cephalosporins for these proteins in various microorganisms helps explain the differing actions of these drugs. They are bactericidal: they act against many aerobic gram-positive and gram-negative bacteria and some anaerobic bacteria but don't kill fungi or viruses.

First-generation cephalosporins act against many gram-positive cocci, including penicillinase-producing *Staphylococcus aureus* and *Staphylococcus epidermidis, S. pneumoniae,* group B streptococci, and group A beta-hemolytic streptococci. Susceptible gram-negative organisms include *Klebsiella pneumoniae, E. coli, Proteus mirabilis,* and *Shigella.*

Second-generation cephalosporins are effective against all organisms attacked by first-generation drugs and have additional activity against *Moraxella catarrhalis, H. influenzae, Enterobacter, Citrobacter, Providencia, Acinetobacter, Serratia,* and *Neisseria. Bacteroides fragilis* is susceptible to cefotetan and cefoxitin.

Third-generation cephalosporins are less active than first- and second-generation drugs against gram-positive bacteria but are more active against gram-negative organisms, including those resistant to first- and second-generation drugs. They have the greatest stability against beta-lactamases produced by gram-negative bacteria. Susceptible gram-negative organisms include *E. coli, Klebsiella, Enterobacter, Provi-*

Prototype drug

dencia, Acinetobacter, Serratia, Proteus, Morganella, and *Neisseria.* Some third-generation drugs are active against *B. fragilis* and *Pseudomonas.*

NURSING PROCESS

⛭ Assessment
• Review patient's history of allergies. Try to determine whether any previous reactions were true hypersensitivity reactions or adverse effects (such as GI distress) that patient interpreted as allergy.
• Monitor patient continuously for possible hypersensitivity reactions or other adverse effects.
• Obtain culture and sensitivity specimen before giving first dose; check test results periodically to assess drug's effectiveness.
• Monitor renal function study; dosage of certain cephalosporins must be lowered in a patient with severe renal impairment. In patient with decreased renal function, monitor BUN and creatinine levels and urine output for significant changes.
• Monitor PT and platelet count, and assess patient for signs of hypoprothrombinemia, which may occur, with or without bleeding, during therapy with cefoperazone, cefotetan, or ceftriaxone. It usually occurs in elderly, debilitated, malnourished, or immunocompromised patients and in patients with renal impairment or impaired vitamin K synthesis.
• Monitor patient receiving long-term therapy for possible bacterial and fungal superinfection; this is especially problematic in elderly or debilitated patients and in those receiving immunosuppressants or radiation therapy.
• Monitor at-risk patients for fluid retention while they are taking sodium salts of cephalosporins.

⛭ Key nursing diagnoses
• Ineffective protection related to hypersensitivity
• Risk for infection related to superinfection
• Risk for deficient fluid volume related to adverse GI reactions

⛭ Planning and implementation
• Give these drugs at least 1 hour before bacteriostatic antibiotics, such as tetracyclines, erythromycin, and chloramphenicol; the antibiotics keep bacteria from growing by decreasing cephalosporin uptake by bacterial cell walls.
• Refrigerate oral suspensions, which are stable for 14 days; to ensure correct dosage, shake well before giving.
• Give I.M. dose deep into gluteal muscle mass or midlateral thigh; rotate injection sites to minimize tissue injury.
• Don't add or mix other drugs with I.V. infusions, particularly aminoglycosides, which will be inactivated if mixed with cephalosporins. If other drugs must be given I.V., temporarily stop infusion of primary drug.
• Ensure adequate dilution of I.V. infusion and rotate site every 48 hours to help minimize local vein irritation; using a small-gauge needle in a larger available vein may be helpful.

Patient teaching
• Make sure patient understands how and when to take drug. Urge him to comply with instructions for around-the-clock dosage and to complete the prescribed regimen.
• Advise patient to take oral drug with food if GI irritation occurs.
• Review proper storage and disposal of drug, and remind him to check expiration date.
• Teach signs and symptoms of hypersensitivity and other adverse reactions, and emphasize importance of reporting unusual effects.
• Teach signs and symptoms of bacterial and fungal superinfection, especially if patient is elderly or debilitated or has low resistance from immunosuppressants or irradiation. Emphasize importance of promptly reporting signs or symptoms.
• Warn patient not to ingest alcohol in any form within 3 days of treatment with cefoperazone or cefotetan.
• Advise patient to add yogurt or buttermilk to diet to prevent intestinal superinfection resulting from suppression of normal intestinal flora.
• Advise diabetic patient to monitor glucose level with Diastix, not Clinitest.
• Urge patient to keep follow-up appointments.

⛭ Evaluation
• Patient has no evidence of hypersensitivity.
• Patient is free from infection.
• Patient maintains adequate hydration.

Corticosteroids

betamethasone
betamethasone sodium phosphate
cortisone acetate
dexamethasone
dexamethasone acetate
dexamethasone sodium phosphate
fludrocortisone acetate
hydrocortisone
hydrocortisone acetate
hydrocortisone cypionate
hydrocortisone sodium phosphate
hydrocortisone sodium succinate
methylprednisolone
methylprednisolone acetate
methylprednisolone sodium succinate
prednisolone
prednisolone acetate
prednisolone sodium phosphate
prednisolone tebutate
prednisone
triamcinolone

Indications

► Hypersensitivity; inflammation, particularly of eye, nose, and respiratory tract; to initiate immunosuppression; replacement therapy in adrenocortical insufficiency, dermatologic diseases, respiratory disorders, rheumatic disorders.

Contraindications and cautions

● Contraindicated in patients hypersensitive to these drugs or any of their components and in those with systemic fungal infection.
● Use cautiously in patients with GI ulceration, renal disease, hypertension, osteoporosis, varicella, vaccinia, exanthema, diabetes mellitus, hypothyroidism, thromboembolic disorder, seizures, myasthenia gravis, heart failure, tuberculosis, ocular herpes simplex, hypoalbuminemia, emotional instability, or psychosis.
⚖ Lifespan: In pregnant women, avoid use, if possible, because of risk to the fetus. Women should stop breast-feeding because these drugs appear in breast milk and could cause serious adverse effects in infants. In children, long-term use should be avoided whenever possible because stunted growth may result. Elderly pa-

tients may have an increased risk of adverse reactions; monitor them closely.

Adverse reactions

Systemic corticosteroid therapy may suppress the hypothalamic-pituitary-adrenal (HPA) axis. Excessive use may cause cushingoid symptoms and various systemic disorders, such as diabetes and osteoporosis. Other effects may include dermatologic disorders, edema, euphoria, fluid and electrolyte imbalances, hypertension, immunosuppression, increased appetite, insomnia, peptic ulcer, psychosis, and weight gain.

Action

Corticosteroids suppress cell-mediated and humoral immunity in three ways: by reducing levels of leukocytes, monocytes, and eosinophils; by decreasing immunoglobulin binding to cell-surface receptors; and by inhibiting interleukin synthesis. They reduce inflammation by preventing hydrolytic enzyme release into the cells, preventing plasma exudation, suppressing polymorphonuclear leukocyte migration, and disrupting other inflammatory processes.

NURSING PROCESS

⚗ Assessment
● Establish baseline blood pressure, fluid and electrolyte status, and weight; reassess regularly.
● Monitor patient closely for adverse reactions.
● Evaluate drug effectiveness at regular intervals.

▦ Key nursing diagnoses
● Ineffective protection related to suppression of HPA axis with long-term therapy
● Risk for injury related to severe adverse reactions
● Risk for infection related to immunosuppression

▷ Planning and implementation
● Give drug early in the day to mimic circadian rhythm.
● Give drug with food to prevent GI irritation.
● Take precautions to avoid exposing patient to infection.
● Don't stop drug abruptly.
● Notify prescriber of severe or persistent adverse reactions.

Prototype drug

• Avoid prolonged use of corticosteroids, especially in children.

Patient teaching
• Teach patient to take drug exactly as prescribed, and warn him never to stop it abruptly.
• Tell patient to notify prescriber if stress level increases; dosage may need to be temporarily increased.
• Instruct patient to take oral drug with food.
• Urge patient to report black tarry stools, bleeding, bruising, blurred vision, emotional changes, or other unusual effects.
• Encourage patient to wear or carry medical identification at all times.

✓ Evaluation
• Patient has no evidence of adrenal insufficiency.
• Patient remains free from injury.
• Patient is free from infection.

Diuretics, loop

bumetanide
ethacrynate sodium
ethacrynic acid
furosemide
torsemide

Indications

▶ Edema from heart failure, hepatic cirrhosis, or nephrotic syndrome; mild-to-moderate hypertension; adjunct treatment in acute pulmonary edema or hypertensive crisis.

Contraindications and cautions

• Contraindicated in patients hypersensitive to these drugs and in patients with anuria, hepatic coma, or severe electrolyte depletion.
• Use cautiously in patients with severe renal disease.
• Use cautiously in patients with severe hypersensitivity to sulfonamides because allergic reaction may occur.
⚠ Lifespan: In pregnant women, use cautiously. In breast-feeding women, don't use. In neonates, use cautiously; the usual pediatric dose can be used, but dosage intervals should be extended. Elderly patients are more sus-

ceptible to drug-induced diuresis, and a lower dose may be indicated; monitor these patients closely.

Adverse reactions

Therapeutic dose commonly causes metabolic and electrolyte disturbances, particularly potassium depletion. It also may cause hyperglycemia, hyperuricemia, hypochloremic alkalosis, and hypomagnesemia. Rapid parenteral administration may cause hearing loss (including deafness) and tinnitus. High doses can produce profound diuresis, leading to hypovolemia and CV collapse. Photosensitivity also may occur.

Action

Loop diuretics inhibit sodium and chloride reabsorption in the ascending loop of Henle, thus increasing excretion of sodium, chloride, and water. Like thiazide diuretics, loop diuretics increase excretion of potassium. Loop diuretics produce more diuresis and electrolyte loss than thiazide diuretics.

NURSING PROCESS

🔲 Assessment
• Monitor blood pressure and pulse rate, especially during rapid diuresis. Establish baseline values before therapy begins and watch for significant changes.
• Establish baseline CBC (including WBC count), liver function test results, and electrolyte, carbon dioxide, magnesium, BUN, and creatinine levels. Review periodically.
• Assess patient for evidence of excessive diuresis: hypotension, tachycardia, poor skin turgor, excessive thirst, or dry and cracked mucous membranes.
• Monitor patient for edema and ascites. Observe the legs of ambulatory patients and the sacral area of patients on bed rest.
• Weigh patient each morning immediately after he voids and before breakfast, in the same type of clothing, and on the same scale. Weight provides a reliable indicator of patient's response to diuretic therapy.
• Monitor and record patient's intake and output daily.

🔲 Key nursing diagnoses
• Risk for deficient fluid volume related to excessive diuresis

• Impaired urine elimination related to change in diuresis pattern
• Ineffective protection related to electrolyte imbalance

⬥ Planning and implementation
• Give diuretics in morning to ensure that major diuresis occurs before bedtime. To prevent nocturia, give diuretics before 6 p.m.
• Reduce dosage for patient with hepatic dysfunction, and increase dosage for patient with renal impairment, oliguria, or decreased diuresis. Inadequate urine output may result in circulatory overload, which causes water intoxication, pulmonary edema, and heart failure. Increase dosage of insulin or oral hypoglycemic in diabetic patient, and reduce dosage of other antihypertensives.
• Take safety measures for all ambulatory patients until response to diuretic is known.
• Consult dietitian about need for potassium supplements.
• Keep urinal or commode readily available to patient.

Patient teaching
• Explain rationale for therapy and importance of following prescribed regimen.
• Review adverse effects, and urge patient to report symptoms promptly, especially chest, back, or leg pain; shortness of breath; dyspnea; increased edema or weight; and excess diuresis evidenced by weight loss of more than 0.9 kg (2 lb) daily.
• Advise patient to eat potassium-rich foods and to avoid high-sodium foods, such as lunch meat, smoked meats, and processed cheeses. Instruct him not to add table salt to foods.
• Encourage patient to keep follow-up appointments to monitor effectiveness of therapy.

☑ Evaluation
• Patient maintains adequate hydration.
• Patient states importance of taking diuretic early in the day to prevent nocturia.
• Patient complies with therapy, as evidenced by improvement in underlying condition.

Diuretics, thiazide and thiazide-like
Thiazide
chlorothiazide
hydrochlorothiazide
Thiazide-like
indapamide
metolazone

Indications

▶ Edema from right-sided heart failure, mild-to-moderate left-sided heart failure, or nephrotic syndrome; edema and ascites caused by hepatic cirrhosis; hypertension; diabetes insipidus, particularly nephrogenic diabetes insipidus.

Contraindications and cautions

• Contraindicated in patients hypersensitive to these drugs and in those with anuria.
• Use cautiously in patients with severe renal disease, impaired hepatic function, or progressive liver disease.
⚕ **Lifespan:** In pregnant women, use cautiously. In breast-feeding women, thiazides are contraindicated because they appear in breast milk. In children, safety and effectiveness haven't been established. Elderly patients are more susceptible to drug-induced diuresis, and reduced dosages may be needed; monitor patient closely.

Adverse reactions

Therapeutic dose causes electrolyte and metabolic disturbances, most commonly potassium depletion. Other abnormalities include elevated cholesterol levels, hypercalcemia, hyperglycemia, hyperuricemia, hypochloremic alkalosis, hypomagnesemia, and hyponatremia. Photosensitivity also may occur.

Action

Thiazide and thiazide-like diuretics interfere with sodium transport across the tubules of the cortical diluting segment in the nephron, thereby increasing renal excretion of sodium, chloride, water, potassium, and calcium.
    Thiazide diuretics also exert an antihypertensive effect. Although the exact mechanism is unknown, direct arteriolar dilation may be par-

tially responsible. In diabetes insipidus, thiazides cause a paradoxical decrease in urine volume and an increase in renal concentration of urine, possibly because of sodium depletion and decreased plasma volume. This increases water and sodium reabsorption in the kidneys.

NURSING PROCESS

🜂 Assessment
• Monitor patient's intake, output, and electrolyte level regularly.
• Weigh patient each morning immediately after he voids and before breakfast, in the same type of clothing, and on the same scale. Weight provides a reliable indicator of patient's response to diuretic therapy.
• Monitor diabetic patient's glucose level. Diuretics may cause hyperglycemia.
• Monitor creatinine and BUN levels regularly. Drug isn't as effective if these levels are more than twice normal. Also, monitor uric acid level.

🜂 Key nursing diagnoses
• Risk for deficient fluid volume related to excessive diuresis
• Impaired urine elimination related to change in diuresis pattern
• Ineffective protection related to electrolyte imbalance

❯ Planning and implementation
• Give drug in the morning to prevent nocturia.
• Provide a high-potassium diet.
• Give potassium supplements to maintain acceptable potassium level.
• Keep urinal or commode readily available to patient.

Patient teaching
• Explain the rationale for therapy and the importance of following the prescribed regimen.
• Tell patient to take drug at the same time each day to prevent nocturia. Suggest taking drug with food to minimize GI irritation.
• Urge patient to seek prescriber's approval before taking any other drug, including OTC medications and herbal remedies.
• Advise patient to record his weight each morning after voiding and before breakfast, in the same type of clothing, and on the same scale.

• Review adverse effects, and urge the patient to promptly report symptoms, especially chest, back, or leg pain; shortness of breath; dyspnea; increased edema or weight; or excess diuresis evidenced by weight loss of more than 0.9 kg (2 lb) daily. Warn him about photosensitivity reactions that usually occur 10 to 14 days after initial sun exposure.
• Advise patient to eat potassium-rich foods and to avoid high-sodium foods, such as lunch meat, smoked meats, processed cheeses. Instruct him not to add table salt to foods.
• Encourage patient to keep follow-up appointments to monitor effectiveness of therapy.

🗹 Evaluation
• Patient maintains adequate hydration.
• Patient states importance of taking diuretic early in the day to prevent nocturia.
• Patient complies with therapy, as evidenced by improvement in underlying condition.

Estrogens
esterified estrogens
estradiol
estradiol cypionate
estradiol valerate
estrogenic substances, conjugated
estrone
estropipate

Indications

▶ Prevention of moderate to severe vasomotor symptoms linked to menopause, such as hot flushes and dizziness; stimulation of vaginal tissue development, cornification, and secretory activity; inhibition of hormone-sensitive cancer growth; female hypogonadism; female castration; primary ovulation failure; ovulation control; prevention of conception.

Contraindications and cautions

• Contraindicated in women with thrombophlebitis or thromboembolic disorders, unexplained abnormal genital bleeding, or estrogen-dependent neoplasia.
• Use cautiously in patients with hypertension; metabolic bone disease; migraines; seizures; asthma; cardiac, renal, or hepatic impairment;

blood dyscrasia; diabetes; family history of breast cancer; or fibrocystic disease.
⚖ **Lifespan:** In pregnant or breast-feeding women, use is contraindicated. In adolescents whose bone growth isn't complete, use cautiously because of effects on epiphyseal closure. Postmenopausal women with a history of long-term estrogen use have an increased risk of endometrial cancer and stroke. Postmenopausal women also have increased risk for breast cancer, MI, stroke, and blood clots with long-term use of estrogen plus progestin.

Adverse reactions

Acute adverse reactions include abdominal cramps; bloating caused by fluid and electrolyte retention; breast swelling and tenderness; changes in menstrual bleeding patterns, such as spotting and prolongation or absence of bleeding; headache; loss of appetite; loss of libido; nausea; photosensitivity; swollen feet or ankles; and weight gain.

Long-term effects include benign hepatomas, cholestatic jaundice, elevated blood pressure (sometimes into the hypertensive range), endometrial carcinoma (rare), and thromboembolic disease (risk increases greatly with cigarette smoking, especially in women older than age 35).

Action

Estrogens promote the development and maintenance of the female reproductive system and secondary sexual characteristics. They inhibit the release of pituitary gonadotropins and have various metabolic effects, including retention of fluid and electrolytes, retention and deposition in bone of calcium and phosphorus, and mild anabolic activity. Of the six naturally occurring estrogens in humans, estradiol, estrone, and estriol are present in significant quantities.

Estrogens and estrogenic substances given as drugs have effects related to endogenous estrogen's mechanism of action. They can mimic the action of endogenous estrogen when used as replacement therapy and can inhibit ovulation or the growth of certain hormone-sensitive cancers. Conjugated estrogens and estrogenic substances are normally obtained from the urine of pregnant mares. Other estrogens are manufactured synthetically.

NURSING PROCESS

🔣 Assessment
• Monitor patient regularly to detect improvement or worsening of symptoms; observe patient for adverse reactions.
• If patient has diabetes mellitus, watch closely for loss of diabetes control.
• Monitor PT of patient receiving warfarin-type anticoagulant. Adjust anticoagulant dosage.

🔣 Key nursing diagnoses
• Excessive fluid volume related to drug-induced fluid retention
• Risk of injury related to adverse effects
• Noncompliance related to long-term therapy

🔣 Planning and implementation
• Notify pathologist of patient's estrogen therapy when sending specimens for evaluation.
• Give drug once daily for 3 weeks, followed by 1 week without drugs; repeat as needed.

Patient teaching
• Urge patient to read the package insert describing adverse reactions. Follow this with a verbal explanation. Tell patient to keep the package insert for later reference.
• Advise patient to take drug with meals or at bedtime to relieve nausea. Reassure patient that nausea usually disappears with continued therapy.
• Teach patient how to apply estrogen ointments or transdermal estrogen. Review symptoms that accompany a systemic reaction to ointments.
• Teach patient how to insert intravaginal estrogen suppository. Advise her to use sanitary pads instead of tampons when using suppository.
• Teach patient how to perform routine monthly breast self-examination.
• Tell patient to stop taking drug immediately if she becomes pregnant because estrogens can harm fetus.
• Remind patient not to breast-feed during estrogen therapy.
• If patient is receiving cyclic therapy for postmenopausal symptoms, explain that withdrawal bleeding may occur during the week off, but that fertility hasn't been restored and ovulation won't occur.
• Explain that medical supervision is essential during prolonged therapy.

• Tell man on long-term therapy about possible temporary gynecomastia and impotence, which will disappear when therapy ends.
• Instruct patient to notify prescriber immediately if patient experiences abdominal pain; pain, numbness, or stiffness in legs or buttocks; pressure or pain in chest; shortness of breath; severe headaches; visual disturbances, such as blind spots, flashing lights, or blurriness; vaginal bleeding or discharge; breast lumps; swelling of hands or feet; yellow skin and sclera; dark urine; or light-colored stools.
• Urge diabetic patient to report symptoms of hyperglycemia or glycosuria.

☑ Evaluation
• Patient experiences only minimal fluid retention.
• Patient doesn't develop serious complications of estrogen therapy.
• Patient complies with therapy, as evidenced by improvement in condition or absence of pregnancy.

Hematinics, oral
ferrous fumarate
ferrous gluconate
ferrous sulfate

Indications
▶ Prevention and treatment of iron-deficiency anemia.

Contraindications and cautions
• Contraindicated in patients with hemochromatosis, hemolytic anemia, or hemosiderosis.
• Use cautiously in patients with peptic ulcer disease, Crohn's disease, ulcerative colitis, or sensitivity to sulfites or tartrazine.
❀ Lifespan: In pregnant women and breast-feeding women, iron supplements are commonly recommended; no adverse effects are known. With children, caution parents about possible lethal effects of iron overdose. In elderly patients, iron-induced constipation is common; stress proper diet high in fiber to minimize this effect. Elderly patients also may need higher doses because reduced gastric secretions and

achlorhydria may lower their capacity for iron absorption.

Adverse reactions
Because iron is corrosive, GI intolerance occurs in 5% to 20% of patients. Symptoms of intolerance include anorexia, constipation, dark stools, nausea, and vomiting. Liquid forms may stain teeth.

Action
Iron is an essential component of hemoglobin. It's needed in adequate amounts for erythropoiesis and for efficient oxygen transport in the blood. After absorption into the blood, iron is immediately bound to transferrin, a plasma protein that transports iron to bone marrow, where it's used during hemoglobin synthesis. Some iron is also used during synthesis of myoglobin and other nonhemoglobin heme units.

NURSING PROCESS

🔖 Assessment
• Monitor patient for adverse reactions, especially those related to bowel function.
• Monitor hemoglobin and reticulocyte count during therapy.

🔷 Key nursing diagnoses
• Risk for deficient fluid volume related to GI upset
• Constipation related to adverse effect on bowel function
• Noncompliance related to adverse effects or long-term use

▶ Planning and implementation
• Dilute liquid forms in juice (preferably orange juice, which promotes iron absorption) or water, but not in milk or antacids. To avoid staining teeth, give liquid preparations through a straw. Don't give antacids within 1 hour before or 2 hours after an iron product, if possible, to prevent interference with absorption.
• Don't crush tablets or capsules. If patient has trouble swallowing, use a liquid form.

Patient teaching
• Explain rationale for therapy, and urge patient to follow the prescribed regimen.

• Tell patient to continue his regular dosage schedule if he misses a dose; warn him not to take a double dose.

• Advise patient to dilute liquid form in juice (preferably orange juice) or water. Suggest that he use a straw to avoid staining his teeth.

• Review possible adverse effects. Tell patient that oral iron may turn stools black, and reassure him that this is harmless. Teach dietary measures to help prevent constipation.

• Explain the toxicity of iron, and emphasize the importance of keeping iron away from children to prevent poisoning. As few as 3 or 4 tablets can cause serious iron poisoning.

• Urge patient to report diarrhea or constipation because prescriber may want to adjust dosage, modify diet, or order further tests.

• Explain that iron therapy may be required for 4 to 6 months after anemia resolves. Encourage compliance.

☑ Evaluation
• Patient maintains adequate hydration.
• Patient regains normal bowel pattern.
• Patient complies with therapy, as evidenced by return of normal hemoglobin and resolution of iron deficiency anemia.

Histamine₂-receptor antagonists
cimetidine
famotidine
nizatidine
ranitidine hydrochloride

Indications
▶ Acute duodenal or gastric ulcer, Zollinger-Ellison syndrome, gastroesophageal reflux.

Contraindications and cautions
• Contraindicated in patients hypersensitive to these drugs.
• Use cautiously in patients with impaired renal or hepatic function.
⚖ Lifespan: In pregnant women, use cautiously. In breast-feeding women, histamine₂ (H₂)-receptor antagonists are contraindicated because they may appear in breast milk. In children, safety and effectiveness haven't been established. Elderly patients have increased risk

of adverse reactions, particularly those affecting the CNS; use cautiously.

Adverse reactions
H₂-receptor antagonists rarely cause adverse reactions. Cardiac arrhythmias, dizziness, fatigue, gynecomastia, headache, mild and transient diarrhea, and thrombocytopenia are possible.

Action
All H₂-receptor antagonists inhibit the action of H₂-receptors in gastric parietal cells, reducing gastric acid output and concentration, regardless of stimulants, such as histamine, food, insulin, and caffeine, or basal conditions.

NURSING PROCESS

☜ Assessment
• Monitor patient for adverse reactions, especially hypotension and arrhythmias.
• Periodically monitor laboratory tests, such as CBC and renal and hepatic studies.

⊞ Key nursing diagnoses
• Risk for infection related to drug-induced neutropenia
• Decreased cardiac output related to adverse CV effects (cimetidine)
• Fatigue related to drug's CNS effects

▷ Planning and implementation
• Give once-daily dose h.s., twice-daily doses in morning and evening, and multiple doses with meals and h.s. A once-daily dose h.s. promotes compliance.
• Don't exceed recommended infusion rates when giving drugs I.V.; doing so increases risk of adverse CV effects. Continuous I.V. infusion may suppress acid secretion more effectively.
• Give antacids at least 1 hour before or after H₂-receptor antagonists. Antacids can decrease drug absorption.
• Adjust dosage for patient with renal disease.
• Don't abruptly stop the drug.

Patient teaching
• Teach patient how and when to take drug, and warn him not to abruptly stop taking it.
• Review possible adverse reactions, and urge patient to report unusual effects.

• Caution patient to avoid smoking during therapy; smoking stimulates gastric acid secretion and worsens the disease.

☑ Evaluation
• Patient is free from infection.
• Patient maintains a normal heart rhythm.
• Patient states appropriate management plan for combating fatigue.

Laxatives
Bulk-forming
calcium polycarbophil
methylcellulose
psyllium
Emollient
docusate calcium
docusate potassium
docusate sodium
Hyperosmolar
glycerin
lactulose
magnesium citrate
magnesium hydroxide
magnesium sulfate
sodium phosphates
Stimulant
bisacodyl
senna

Indications

▶ Constipation, irritable bowel syndrome, diverticulosis.

Contraindications and cautions

• Contraindicated in patients with GI obstruction or perforation, toxic colitis, megacolon, nausea and vomiting, or acute surgical abdomen.
• Use cautiously in patients with rectal or anal conditions such as rectal bleeding or large hemorrhoids.
※ **Lifespan:** For pregnant women and breastfeeding women, recommendations vary for individual drugs. Infants and children have an increased risk of fluid and electrolyte disturbances; use cautiously. In elderly patients, dependence is more likely to develop because of age-related changes in GI function. Monitor these patients closely.

Adverse reactions

All laxatives may cause flatulence, diarrhea, abdominal discomfort, weakness, and dependence. Bulk-forming laxatives may cause intestinal obstruction, impaction, or (rarely) esophageal obstruction. Emollient laxatives may cause a bitter taste or throat irritation. Hyperosmolar laxatives may cause fluid and electrolyte imbalances. Stimulant laxatives may cause urine discoloration, malabsorption, and weight loss.

Action

Laxatives promote movement of intestinal contents through the colon and rectum in several ways: bulk-forming, emollient, hyperosmolar, and stimulant.

NURSING PROCESS

✷ Assessment
• Obtain baseline assessment of patient's bowel patterns and GI history before giving.
• Monitor patient for adverse reactions.
• Monitor bowel pattern throughout therapy. Assess bowel sounds and color and consistency of stools.
• Monitor patient's fluid and electrolyte status during administration.

⊞ Key nursing diagnoses
• Diarrhea related to adverse GI effects
• Acute pain related to abdominal discomfort
• Impaired health maintenance related to laxative dependence

▶ Planning and implementation
• Don't crush enteric-coated tablets.
• Time administration so that bowel evacuation doesn't interfere with sleep.
• Make sure patient has easy access to bedpan or bathroom.
• Institute measures to prevent constipation.

Patient teaching
• Advise patient that therapy should be short-term. Point out that abuse or prolonged use can cause nutritional imbalances.

Prototype drug

• Tell patient that stool softeners and bulk-forming laxatives may take several days to achieve results.
• Encourage patient to remain active and to drink plenty of fluids if he's taking a bulk-forming laxative.
• Explain that stimulant laxatives may cause harmless urine discoloration.
• Teach patient about including foods high in fiber into diet.

Evaluation
• Patient regains normal bowel pattern.
• Patient states that pain is relieved with stool evacuation.
• Patient discusses dangers of laxative abuse and importance of limiting laxative use.

Nonsteroidal anti-inflammatory drugs

celecoxib
diclofenac potassium
diclofenac sodium
diflunisal
etodolac
ibuprofen
indomethacin
indomethacin sodium trihydrate
ketoprofen
ketorolac tromethamine
meloxicam
nabumetone
naproxen
naproxen sodium
oxaprozin
piroxicam
sulindac

Indications

▶ Mild to moderate pain, inflammation, stiffness, swelling, or tenderness caused by headache, arthralgia, myalgia, neuralgia, dysmenorrhea, rheumatoid arthritis, juvenile arthritis, osteoarthritis, or dental or surgical procedures.

Contraindications and cautions

• Contraindicated in patients with GI lesions or GI bleeding and in patients hypersensitive to these drugs.
• Use cautiously in patients with cardiac decompensation, hypertension, risk of MI, fluid retention, or coagulation defects.
Lifespan: In pregnant women, use cautiously in the first and second trimesters; don't use in the third trimester. For breast-feeding women, NSAIDs aren't recommended. In children younger than age 14, safety of long-term therapy hasn't been established. Patients older than age 60 may be more susceptible to toxic effects of NSAIDs because of decreased renal function.

Adverse reactions

Adverse reactions chiefly involve the GI tract, particularly erosion of the gastric mucosa. The most common symptoms are abdominal pain, dyspepsia, epigastric distress, heartburn, and nausea. CNS and skin reactions also may occur. Flank pain with other evidence of nephrotoxicity occurs occasionally. Fluid retention may aggravate hypertension or heart failure.

Action

The analgesic effect of NSAIDs may result from interference with the prostaglandins involved in pain. Prostaglandins appear to sensitize pain receptors to mechanical stimulation or to other chemical mediators. NSAIDs inhibit synthesis of prostaglandins peripherally and possibly centrally.

Like salicylates, NSAIDs exert an anti-inflammatory effect that may result in part from inhibition of prostaglandin synthesis and release during inflammation. The exact mechanism isn't clear.

NURSING PROCESS

Assessment
• Assess patient's level of pain and inflammation before therapy begins, and evaluate drug effectiveness.
• Monitor patient for evidence of bleeding. If patient needs surgery, assess bleeding time.
• Monitor ophthalmic and auditory function before and periodically during therapy to detect toxicity.

Prototype drug

• Monitor CBC, platelet count, PT, and hepatic and renal function studies periodically to detect abnormalities.
• Watch for bronchospasm in patients with aspirin hypersensitivity, rhinitis or nasal polyps, and asthma.

▣ Key nursing diagnoses
• Risk for injury related to adverse reactions
• Excessive fluid volume related to fluid retention
• Disturbed sensory perception (visual and auditory) related to toxicity

▷ Planning and implementation
• Give oral NSAIDs with 8 oz (240 ml) of water to ensure adequate passage into the stomach. Have patient sit up for 15 to 30 minutes after taking drug to prevent it from lodging in esophagus.
• Crush tablets or mix with food or fluid to aid swallowing. Give with antacids to minimize GI upset.

Patient teaching
• Encourage patient to take drug as directed to achieve desired effect. Explain that he may not notice benefits of drug for 2 to 4 weeks.
• Review methods to prevent or minimize GI upset.
• Work with patient on long-term therapy to arrange for monitoring of laboratory values, especially BUN and creatinine levels, liver function test results, and CBC.
• Instruct patient to notify prescriber about severe or persistent adverse reactions.

☑ Evaluation
• Patient remains free from injury.
• Patient shows no signs of edema.
• Patient maintains normal visual and auditory function.

Opioids
alfentanil hydrochloride
codeine phosphate
codeine sulfate
difenoxin hydrochloride
diphenoxylate hydrochloride
fentanyl citrate
hydrocodone bitartrate
hydromorphone hydrochloride
meperidine hydrochloride
methadone hydrochloride
morphine sulfate
oxycodone hydrochloride
oxymorphone hydrochloride
propoxyphene hydrochloride
propoxyphene napsylate
sufentanil citrate

Indications
▶ Moderate to severe pain from acute and some chronic disorders; diarrhea; dry, nonproductive cough; management of opiate dependence; anesthesia support; sedation.

Contraindications and cautions
• Contraindicated in patients hypersensitive to these drugs and in those who have recently taken an MAO inhibitor. Also contraindicated in those with acute or severe bronchial asthma or respiratory depression.
• Use cautiously in patients with head injury, increased intracranial or intraocular pressure, and hepatic or renal dysfunction.
• Use cautiously in patients with mental illnesses and emotional disturbances, and in patients exhibiting drug-seeking behaviors.
⚛ Lifespan: In pregnant or breast-feeding women, use cautiously; codeine, meperidine, methadone, morphine, and propoxyphene appear in breast milk. Breast-feeding infants of women taking methadone may develop physical dependence. In children, safety and effectiveness of some opioids haven't been established; use cautiously. Elderly patients may be more sensitive to opioids, and lower doses are usually given.

Adverse reactions

Respiratory and circulatory depression (including orthostatic hypotension) are the major hazards of opioids. Other adverse CNS effects include agitation, coma, depression, dizziness, dysphoria, euphoria, faintness, mental clouding, nervousness, restlessness, sedation, seizures, and visual disturbances, and weakness. Adverse GI effects include biliary colic, constipation, nausea, and vomiting. Urine retention or hypersensitivity also may occur. Tolerance to the drug and psychological or physical dependence may follow prolonged therapy.

Action

Opioids act as agonists at specific opiate-receptor binding sites in the CNS and other tissues, altering the patient's perception of and emotional response to pain.

NURSING PROCESS

■ Assessment
• Obtain baseline assessment of patient's pain, and reassess frequently to determine the drug's effectiveness.
• Evaluate patient's respiratory status before each dose; watch for respiratory rate below patient's baseline level and for restlessness, which may be compensatory signs of hypoxia. Respiratory depression may last longer than the analgesic effect.
• Monitor patient for other adverse reactions.
• Monitor patient for tolerance and dependence. The first sign of tolerance to opioids is usually a shortened duration of effect.

■ Key nursing diagnoses
• Ineffective breathing pattern related to respiratory depression
• Risk for injury related to orthostatic hypotension
• Ineffective individual coping related to drug dependence

■ Planning and implementation
• Keep resuscitative equipment and an opioid antagonist, such as naloxone, available.
• Give I.V. drug by slow injection, preferably in diluted solution. Rapid I.V. injection increases the risk of adverse effects.
• Give drug I.M. or subcutaneously, cautiously, to a patient with decreased platelet count and to a patient who is chilled, hypovolemic, or in shock; decreased perfusion may lead to drug accumulation and toxicity. Rotate injection sites to avoid induration.
• Carefully note the strength of solution when measuring a dose. Oral solutions of varying concentrations are available.
• For maximum effectiveness, give on a regular dosage schedule rather than p.r.n.
• Institute safety precautions.
• Encourage postoperative patient to turn, cough, and breathe deeply every 2 hours to avoid atelectasis.
• Give oral forms with food if GI irritation occurs.
• Withdrawal symptoms—including tremors, agitation, nausea, and vomiting—may occur if drug is stopped abruptly. Monitor patient with these symptoms carefully and provide supportive therapy.

Patient teaching
• Teach patient to take drug exactly as prescribed. Urge him to call prescriber if he isn't experiencing desired effect or is experiencing significant adverse reactions.
• Warn patient to avoid hazardous activities until drug's effects are known.
• Advise patient to avoid alcohol while taking opioid; alcohol will cause additive CNS depression.
• Suggest measures to prevent constipation, such as increasing fiber in diet and using a stool softener.
• Instruct patient to breathe deeply, cough, and change position every 2 hours to avoid respiratory complications.

■ Evaluation
• Patient maintains adequate ventilation, as evidenced by normal respiratory rate and rhythm and pink color.
• Patient remains free from injury.
• Patient doesn't become tolerant to drug.

Penicillins

Natural penicillins
penicillin G benzathine
penicillin G potassium
penicillin G procaine
penicillin G sodium
penicillin V potassium
Aminopenicillins
amoxicillin and clavulanate potassium
amoxicillin trihydrate
ampicillin
ampicillin sodium and sulbactam sodium
ampicillin trihydrate
Penicillinase-resistant penicillins
dicloxacillin sodium
nafcillin sodium
oxacillin sodium
Extended-spectrum penicillins
carbenicillin indanyl sodium
piperacillin sodium and tazobactam sodium
ticarcillin disodium
ticarcillin disodium and clavulanate
potassium

Indications

▶ Streptococcal pneumonia; enterococcal and nonenterococcal group D endocarditis; diphtheria; anthrax; meningitis; tetanus; botulism; actinomycosis; syphilis; relapsing fever; Lyme disease; pneumococcal infections; rheumatic fever; bacterial endocarditis; neonatal group B streptococcal disease; septicemia; gynecologic infections; infections of urinary, respiratory, and GI tracts; infections of skin, soft tissue, bones, and joints.

Contraindications and cautions

• Contraindicated in patients hypersensitive to these drugs.
• Use cautiously in patients with history of asthma or drug allergy, mononucleosis, renal impairment, CV diseases, hemorrhagic condition, or electrolyte imbalance.
🕭 **Lifespan:** In pregnant women, use cautiously. For breast-feeding patients, recommendations vary depending on the drug. For children, dosage recommendations have been established for most penicillins. Elderly patients are susceptible to superinfection and re-

nal impairment, which decreases excretion of penicillins; use cautiously and at a lower dosage.

Adverse reactions

With all penicillins, hypersensitivity reactions range from mild rash, fever, and eosinophilia to fatal anaphylaxis. Hematologic reactions include hemolytic anemia, leukopenia, thrombocytopenia, and transient neutropenia.

Certain adverse reactions are more common with specific classes. For example, bleeding episodes are usually seen with high doses of extended-spectrum penicillins, whereas GI adverse effects are most common with ampicillin. In patients with renal disease, high doses, especially of penicillin G, irritate the CNS by causing confusion, twitching, lethargy, dysphagia, seizures, and coma. Hepatotoxicity may occur with penicillinase-resistant penicillins, and hyperkalemia and hypernatremia have been reported with extended-spectrum penicillins.

Local irritation from parenteral therapy may be severe enough to warrant administration by subclavian or centrally placed catheter or stopping therapy.

Action

Penicillins are generally bactericidal. They inhibit synthesis of the bacterial cell wall, causing rapid cell destruction. They're most effective against fast-growing susceptible bacteria. Their sites of action are enzymes known as penicillin-binding proteins (PBPs). The affinity of certain penicillins for PBPs in various microorganisms helps explain the different activities of these drugs.

Susceptible aerobic gram-positive cocci include *Staphylococcus aureus;* nonenterococcal group D streptococci; groups A, B, D, G, H, K, L, and M streptococci; *Streptococcus viridans;* and *Enterococcus* (usually with an aminoglycoside). Susceptible aerobic gram-negative cocci include *Neisseria meningitidis* and non–penicillinase-producing *N. gonorrhoeae.* Susceptible aerobic gram-positive bacilli include *Corynebacterium, Listeria,* and *Bacillus anthracis.* Susceptible anaerobes include *Peptococcus, Peptostreptococcus, Actinomyces, Clostridium, Fusobacterium, Veillonella,* and non–beta-lactamase–producing strains of *Streptococcus pneumoniae.* Susceptible spirochetes include *Treponema pallidum, T. pertenue, Lep-*

tospira, Borrelia recurrentis, and, possibly, *B. burgdorferi.*

Aminopenicillins have uses against more organisms, including many gram-negative organisms. Like natural penicillins, aminopenicillins are vulnerable to inactivation by penicillinase. Susceptible organisms include *Escherichia coli, Proteus mirabilis, Shigella, Salmonella, S. pneumoniae, N. gonorrhoeae, Haemophilus influenzae, S. aureus, S. epidermidis* (non–penicillinase-producing *Staphylococcus*), and *Listeria monocytogenes.*

Penicillinase-resistant penicillins are semisynthetic penicillins designed to remain stable against hydrolysis by most staphylococcal penicillinases and thus are the drugs of choice against susceptible penicillinase-producing staphylococci. They also act against most organisms susceptible to natural penicillins.

Extended-spectrum penicillins offer a wider range of bactericidal action than the other three classes and usually are given in combination with aminoglycosides. Susceptible strains include *Enterobacter, Klebsiella, Citrobacter, Serratia, Bacteroides fragilis, Pseudomonas aeruginosa, Proteus vulgaris, Providencia rettgeri,* and *Morganella morganii.* These penicillins are also vulnerable to beta-lactamase and penicillinases.

NURSING PROCESS

🔏 Assessment
● Assess patient's history of allergies. Try to find out whether any previous reactions were true hypersensitivity reactions or adverse reactions (such as GI distress) that patient interpreted as allergy.
● Keep in mind that a patient who has never had a penicillin hypersensitivity reaction may still have future allergic reactions; monitor patient continuously for possible allergic reactions or other adverse effects.
● Obtain culture and sensitivity tests before giving first dose; repeat tests periodically to assess drug's effectiveness.
● Monitor vital signs, electrolytes, and renal function studies.
● Assess patient's consciousness and neurologic status when giving high doses; CNS toxicity can occur.
● Coagulation abnormalities, even frank bleeding, can follow high doses, especially of

extended-spectrum penicillins. Monitor PT, INR, and platelet counts. Assess patient for signs of occult or frank bleeding.
● Monitor patients, especially elderly patients, debilitated patients, and patients receiving immunosuppressants or radiation, receiving long-term therapy for possible superinfection.

🔲 Key nursing diagnoses
● Ineffective protection related to hypersensitivity
● Risk for infection related to superinfection
● Risk for deficient fluid volume related to adverse GI reactions

⊳ Planning and implementation
● Give penicillin at least 1 hour before bacteriostatic antibiotics, such as tetracyclines, erythromycin, and chloramphenicol; these drugs inhibit bacterial cell growth and decrease rate of penicillin uptake by bacterial cell walls.
● To enhance GI absorption, give oral penicillin at least 1 hour before or 2 hours after meals.
● Refrigerate oral suspensions, which will be stable for 14 days; to ensure correct dosage, shake suspension well before giving it.
● To minimize tissue injury, give I.M. dose deep into gluteal muscle mass or midlateral thigh, and rotate injection sites. To relieve pain, apply ice to injection site. Don't inject more than 2 g of drug per injection site.
● With I.V. infusions, don't add or mix another drug, especially an aminoglycoside, which will become inactive if mixed with a penicillin. If other drugs must be given I.V., temporarily stop infusion of primary drug.
● Infuse I.V. drug continuously or intermittently over 30 minutes. Rotate infusion site every 48 hours. Intermittent I.V. infusion may be diluted in 50 to 100 ml sterile water, normal saline solution, D_5W, D_5W and half-normal saline solution, or lactated Ringer's solution.

Patient teaching
● Make sure patient understands how and when to take drug. Urge him to complete the prescribed regimen, comply with instructions for around-the-clock scheduling, and keep follow-up appointments.
● Teach patient signs and symptoms of hypersensitivity and other adverse reactions. Urge him to report unusual reactions.

• Tell patient to check drug's expiration date and to discard unused drug. Warn him not to share drug with family or friends.

☑ Evaluation
• Patient shows no signs of hypersensitivity.
• Patient is free from infection.
• Patient maintains adequate hydration.

Phenothiazines

chlorpromazine hydrochloride
fluphenazine
mesoridazine besylate
perphenazine
prochlorperazine
promazine hydrochloride
promethazine
thioridazine hydrochloride
thiothixene
trifluoperazine hydrochloride

Indications

▶ Agitated psychotic states, hallucinations, manic-depressive illness, excessive motor and autonomic activity, nausea and vomiting, moderate anxiety, behavioral problems caused by chronic organic mental syndrome, tetanus, acute intermittent porphyria, intractable hiccups, itching, symptomatic rhinitis.

Contraindications and cautions

• Contraindicated in patients with CNS depression, bone marrow suppression, heart failure, circulatory collapse, coronary artery or cerebrovascular disorders, subcortical damage, or coma. Also contraindicated in patients receiving spinal and epidural anesthetics and adrenergic blockers.
• Use cautiously in debilitated patients and in those with hepatic, renal, or CV disease; respiratory disorders; hypocalcemia; seizure disorders; suspected brain tumor or intestinal obstruction; glaucoma; and prostatic hyperplasia.
⚖ Lifespan: In pregnant women, use only if clearly necessary; safety hasn't been established. Women shouldn't breast-feed during therapy because most phenothiazines appear in breast milk and directly affect prolactin levels. For children younger than age 12, phenoth-

iazines aren't recommended unless otherwise specified; use cautiously for nausea and vomiting. Acutely ill children, such as those with chickenpox, measles, CNS infections, or dehydration have a greatly increased risk of dystonic reactions. Elderly patients are more sensitive to therapeutic and adverse effects, especially cardiac toxicity, tardive dyskinesia, and other extrapyramidal effects; use cautiously and give reduced doses, adjusting dosage to patient response.

Adverse reactions

Phenothiazines may produce extrapyramidal symptoms, such as dystonic movements, torticollis, oculogyric crises, and parkinsonian symptoms ranging from akathisia during early treatment to tardive dyskinesia after long-term use. A neuroleptic malignant syndrome resembling severe parkinsonism may occur, most often in young men taking fluphenazine. The progression of elevated liver enzyme levels to obstructive jaundice usually indicates an allergic reaction.

Other adverse reactions include abdominal pain, agitation, anorexia, arrhythmias, confusion, constipation, dizziness, dry mouth, endocrine effects, fainting, hallucinations, hematologic disorders, local gastric irritation, nausea, orthostatic hypotension with reflex tachycardia, photosensitivity, seizures, skin eruptions, urine retention, visual disturbances, and vomiting.

Action

Phenothiazines are believed to function as dopamine antagonists by blocking postsynaptic dopamine receptors in various parts of the CNS. Their antiemetic effects result from blockage of the chemoreceptor trigger zone. They also produce varying degrees of anticholinergic effects and alpha–adrenergic-receptor blocking.

NURSING PROCESS

☷ Assessment
• Check vital signs regularly for decreased blood pressure, especially before and after parenteral therapy, or tachycardia; observe patient carefully for other adverse reactions.

• Check intake and output for urine retention or constipation, which may require dosage reduction.
• Monitor bilirubin level weekly for the first 4 weeks. Establish baseline CBC, ECG (for quinidine-like effects), liver and renal function test results, electrolyte level (especially potassium), and eye examination findings. Monitor these findings periodically thereafter, especially in patients receiving long-term therapy.
• Observe patient for mood changes and monitor progress.
• Monitor patient for involuntary movements. Check patient receiving prolonged treatment at least once every 6 months.

Key nursing diagnoses
• Risk for injury related to adverse reactions
• Impaired mobility related to extrapyramidal symptoms
• Noncompliance related to long-term therapy

Planning and implementation
• Don't stop drug abruptly. Although physical dependence doesn't occur with antipsychotic drugs, rebound worsening of psychotic symptoms may occur, and many drug effects may persist.
• Follow manufacturer's guidelines for reconstitution, dilution, administration, and storage of drugs. Slightly discolored liquids may or may not be acceptable for use. Check with pharmacist.

Patient teaching
• Teach patient how and when to take drug. Tell him not to increase the dosage or stop taking the drug without prescriber's approval. Suggest taking the full dose at bedtime if daytime sedation occurs.
• Explain that full therapeutic effect may not occur for several weeks.
• Teach signs and symptoms of adverse reactions, and urge patient to report unusual effects, especially involuntary movements.
• Instruct patient to avoid beverages and drugs containing alcohol, and warn him not to take other drugs, including OTC or herbal products, without prescriber's approval.
• Advise patient to avoid hazardous tasks until full effects of drug are established. Explain that sedative effects will lessen after several weeks.

• Inform patient that excessive exposure to sunlight, heat lamps, or tanning beds may cause photosensitivity reactions. Advise him to avoid exposure to extreme heat or cold.
• Explain that phenothiazines may cause pink or brown discoloration of urine.

☑ Evaluation
• Patient remains free from injury.
• Patient doesn't develop extrapyramidal symptoms.
• Patient complies with therapy, as evidenced by improved thought processes.

Skeletal muscle relaxants
baclofen
carisoprodol
chlorzoxazone
cyclobenzaprine hydrochloride
methocarbamol

Indications
▶ Painful musculoskeletal disorders, spasticity caused by multiple sclerosis.

Contraindications and cautions
• Contraindicated in patients hypersensitive to these drugs.
• Use cautiously in patients with impaired renal or hepatic function.
⚜ **Lifespan:** In pregnant women and breast-feeding women, use only when potential benefits to the patient outweigh the risks to the fetus or infant. In children, recommendations vary for use. Elderly patients have an increased risk of adverse reactions; monitor them carefully.

Adverse reactions
Skeletal muscle relaxants may cause ataxia, confusion, depressed mood, dizziness, drowsiness, dry mouth, hallucinations, headache, hypotension, nervousness, tachycardia, tremor, and vertigo. Baclofen also may cause seizures.

Action
All skeletal muscle relaxants, except baclofen, reduce impulse transmission from the spinal cord to skeletal muscle. Baclofen's mechanism of action is unclear.

Assessment

• Monitor patient for hypersensitivity reactions.
• Assess degree of relief obtained to determine when dosage can be reduced.
• Watch for increased seizures in epileptic patient receiving baclofen.
• Monitor CBC results closely.
• In patient receiving cyclobenzaprine, monitor platelet counts.
• In patient receiving methocarbamol, watch for orthostatic hypotension.
• In patient receiving long-term baclofen or chlorzoxazone therapy, monitor hepatic function and urinalysis results.
• In patient receiving long-term therapy, assess compliance.

Key nursing diagnoses

• Risk for trauma related to baclofen-induced seizures
• Disturbed thought processes related to confusion
• Noncompliance related to long-term therapy

Planning and implementation

• Avoid withdrawal symptoms, such as insomnia, headache, nausea, and abdominal pain, by not abruptly stopping baclofen or carisoprodol after long-term therapy, unless patient has severe adverse reactions.
• Institute safety precautions as needed.
• Prevent GI distress by giving oral forms of drug with meals or milk.
• Obtain an order for a mild analgesic to relieve drug-induced headache.

Patient teaching

• Tell patient to take drug exactly as prescribed. Teach him to avoid withdrawal symptoms by not stopping baclofen or carisoprodol abruptly after long-term therapy.
• Instruct patient to avoid hazardous activities that require mental alertness until CNS effects of drug are known.
• Advise patient to avoid alcohol use during therapy.
• Advise patient to follow prescriber's advice regarding rest and physical therapy.
• Instruct patient receiving cyclobenzaprine or baclofen to report urinary hesitancy.

• Inform patient taking methocarbamol or chlorzoxazone that urine may be discolored.

Evaluation

• Patient remains free from seizures.
• Patient exhibits normal thought processes.
• Patient complies with therapy, as evidenced by pain relief or improvement of spasticity.

Sulfonamides

co-trimoxazole (trimethoprim and sulfamethoxazole)
sulfasalazine

Indications

▶ Bacterial infections, nocardiosis, toxoplasmosis, chloroquine-resistant *Plasmodium falciparum* malaria.

Contraindications and cautions

• Contraindicated in patients hypersensitive to these drugs.
• Use cautiously in patients with renal or hepatic impairment, bronchial asthma, severe allergy, or G6PD deficiency.
• **Lifespan:** In pregnant women at term and in breast-feeding women, use is contraindicated; sulfonamides appear in breast milk. In infants younger than age 2 months, sulfonamides are contraindicated unless there is no therapeutic alternative. In children with fragile X chromosome and mental retardation, use cautiously. Elderly patients are susceptible to bacterial and fungal superinfection and have an increased risk of folate deficiency anemia and adverse renal and hematologic effects.

Adverse reactions

Many adverse reactions stem from hypersensitivity, including bronchospasm, conjunctivitis, erythema multiforme, erythema nodosum, exfoliative dermatitis, fever, joint pain, pruritus, leukopenia, Lyell's syndrome, photosensitivity, rash, Stevens-Johnson syndrome, and toxic epidermal necrolysis. GI reactions include anorexia, diarrhea, folic acid malabsorption, nausea, pancreatitis, stomatitis, and vomiting. Hematologic reactions include agranulocytosis, granulocytopenia, hypoprothrombinemia thrombocytopenia, and, in G6PD deficiency, hemolytic anemia. Renal effects usually result from crystalluria caused by precipitation of sulfonamide in renal system.

Action

Sulfonamides are bacteriostatic. They inhibit biosynthesis of tetrahydrofolic acid, which is needed for bacterial cell growth. They're active against some strains of staphylococci, streptococci, *Nocardia asteroides* and *N. brasiliensis, Clostridium tetani* and *C. perfringens, Bacillus anthracis, Escherichia coli,* and *Neisseria gonorrhoeae* and *N. meningitidis.* Sulfonamides are also active against organisms that cause UTIs, such as *E. coli, Proteus mirabilis* and *P. vulgaris, Klebsiella, Enterobacter,* and *Staphylococcus aureus,* and genital lesions caused by *Haemophilus ducreyi* (chancroid).

NURSING PROCESS

Assessment
• Assess patient's history of allergies, especially to sulfonamides or to any drug containing sulfur, such as thiazides, furosemide, and oral sulfonylureas.
• Monitor patient for adverse reactions; patients with AIDS have a much higher risk of adverse reactions.
• Obtain culture and sensitivity tests before first dose; check test results periodically to assess the drug's effectiveness.
• Monitor urine cultures, CBC, and urinalysis before and during therapy.
• During long-term therapy, monitor patient for possible superinfection.

Key nursing diagnoses
• Ineffective protection related to hypersensitivity
• Risk for infection related to superinfection
• Risk for deficient fluid volume related to adverse GI reactions

Planning and implementation
• Give oral dose with 8 oz (240 ml) of water. Give 3 to 4 L of fluids daily, depending on drug; patient's urine output should be at least 1,500 ml daily.
• Follow manufacturer's directions for reconstituting, diluting, and storing drugs; check expiration dates.

• Shake oral suspensions well before giving to ensure correct dosage.

Patient teaching
• Urge patient to take drug exactly as prescribed, to complete the prescribed regimen, and to keep follow-up appointments.
• Advise patient to take oral drug with full glass of water and to drink plenty of fluids; explain that tablet may be crushed and swallowed with water to ensure maximal absorption.
• Teach signs and symptoms of hypersensitivity and other adverse reactions. Urge patient to report bloody urine, difficulty breathing, rash, fever, chills, or severe fatigue.
• Advise patient to avoid direct sun exposure and to use a sunscreen to help prevent photosensitivity reactions.
• Tell diabetic patient that sulfonamides may increase effects of oral hypoglycemics. Tell him not to use Clinitest to monitor glucose level.
• Inform patient taking sulfasalazine that it may cause an orange-yellow discoloration of urine or skin and may permanently stain soft contact lenses yellow.

Evaluation
• Patient exhibits no signs of hypersensitivity.
• Patient is free from infection.
• Patient maintains adequate hydration.

Tetracyclines

doxycycline
doxycycline hyclate
minocycline hydrochloride
oxytetracycline hydrochloride
tetracycline hydrochloride

Indications

▶ Bacterial, protozoal, rickettsial, and fungal infections.

Contraindications and cautions

• Contraindicated in patients hypersensitive to these drugs.
• Use cautiously in patients with renal or hepatic impairment.
Lifespan: In pregnant or breast-feeding women, use is contraindicated; tetracyclines ap-

pear in breast milk. Children younger than age 8 shouldn't take tetracyclines; these drugs can cause permanent tooth discoloration, enamel hypoplasia, and a reversible decrease in bone calcification. Elderly patients may have decreased esophageal motility; use these drugs cautiously and monitor patients for local irritation from slow passage of oral forms. Elderly patients also are more susceptible to superinfection.

Adverse reactions

The most common adverse effects involve the GI tract and are dose related; they include abdominal discomfort; anorexia; bulky, loose stools; epigastric burning; flatulence; nausea; and vomiting. Superinfections also are common. Photosensitivity reactions may be severe. Renal failure may be caused by Fanconi's syndrome after use of outdated tetracycline. Permanent discoloration of teeth occurs if drug is given during tooth formation in children younger than age 8.

Action

Tetracyclines are bacteriostatic but may be bactericidal against certain organisms. They bind reversibly to 30S and 50S ribosomal subunits, which inhibits bacterial protein synthesis.

Susceptible gram-positive organisms include *Bacillus anthracis, Actinomyces israelii, Clostridium perfringens, C. tetani, Listeria monocytogenes,* and *Nocardia.*

Susceptible gram-negative organisms include *Neisseria meningitidis, Pasteurella multocida, Legionella pneumophila, Brucella, Vibrio cholerae, Yersinia enterocolitica, Y. pestis, Bordetella pertussis, Haemophilus influenzae, H. ducreyi, Campylobacter fetus, Shigella,* and many other common pathogens.

Other susceptible organisms include *Rickettsia akari, R. typhi, R. prowazekii, R. tsutsugamushi, Coxiella burnetii, Chlamydia trachomatis, C. psittaci, Mycoplasma pneumoniae, M. hominis, Leptospira, Treponema pallidum, T. pertenue,* and *Borrelia recurrentis.*

NURSING PROCESS

☷ Assessment
• Assess patient's allergic history.
• Monitor patient for adverse reactions.

• Obtain culture and sensitivity tests before first dose; check cultures periodically to assess drug effectiveness.
• Check expiration dates before giving. Outdated tetracyclines may cause nephrotoxicity.
• Monitor patient for bacterial and fungal superinfection, especially if patient is elderly, debilitated, or receiving immunosuppressants or radiation therapy; watch especially for oral candidiasis.

⊞ Key nursing diagnoses
• Ineffective protection related to hypersensitivity
• Risk for infection related to superinfection
• Risk for deficient fluid volume related to adverse GI reactions

⟩ Planning and implementation
• For maximum absorption, give all oral tetracyclines except doxycycline and minocycline 1 hour before or 2 hours after meals. Don't give drug with food, milk or other dairy products, sodium bicarbonate, iron compounds, or antacids, which may impair absorption.
• Give water with and after oral drug to help it pass to the stomach because incomplete swallowing can cause severe esophageal irritation. To prevent esophageal reflux, don't give drug within 1 hour of bedtime.
• Monitor I.V. injection sites and rotate routinely to minimize local irritation. I.V. administration may cause severe phlebitis.

Patient teaching
• Urge patient to take drug exactly as prescribed, to complete the prescribed regimen, and to keep follow-up appointments.
• Warn patient not to take drug with food, milk or other dairy products, sodium bicarbonate, or iron compounds because they may interfere with absorption. Advise him to wait 3 hours after taking tetracycline before taking an antacid.
• Instruct patient to check expiration dates and to discard any expired drug.
• Teach signs and symptoms of adverse reactions, and urge patient to report them promptly.
• Advise patient to avoid direct exposure to sunlight and to use a sunscreen to help prevent photosensitivity reactions.

☑ Evaluation
• Patient shows no signs of hypersensitivity.

- Patient is free from infection.
- Patient maintains adequate hydration.

Thyroid hormones
levothyroxine sodium
liothyronine sodium
thyroid, desiccated

Indications

▶ Hypothyroidism, simple goiter, goitrogenesis.

Contraindications and cautions

- Contraindicated in patients with MI, thyrotoxicosis, or uncorrected adrenal insufficiency.
- Use cautiously in patients with angina pectoris, hypertension, or other CV disorders; renal insufficiency; endocrine disorders; ischemia; or myxedema.

⚞ **Lifespan:** During pregnancy, women may continue thyroid replacement. Minimal amounts of exogenous thyroid hormones appear in breast milk, but problems haven't been reported in breast-feeding infants. Children may have partial hair loss during first few months of therapy; reassure child and parents that this is temporary. In patients older than age 60, initial hormone replacement dose should be 25% less than the usual recommended starting dosage.

Adverse reactions

Adverse reactions include fever, hair gain, hair loss, headache, insomnia, nausea, nervousness, palpitations, sweating, tachycardia, tremor, and weight loss.

Action

Thyroid hormones have catabolic and anabolic effects and influence normal metabolism, growth, and development. These hormones affect every organ system and are vital to normal CNS function. Thyroid-stimulating hormone increases iodine uptake by the thyroid and increases formation and release of thyroid hormone. Thyroid hormones are produced either from bovine anterior pituitary glands (natural hormone) or synthetically. Differing brands and types of thyroid hormone aren't dose compara-

ble, so patients are advised to stay with the original product ordered.

NURSING PROCESS

⚚ Assessment
- Assess patient's thyroid function test results regularly.
- Monitor pulse rate and blood pressure.
- Monitor patient for signs of thyrotoxicosis or inadequate dosage, including diarrhea, fever, irritability, listlessness, rapid heartbeat, vomiting, and weakness.
- Monitor PT and INR in patients taking anticoagulants.

⚇ Key nursing diagnoses
- Risk for injury related to adverse CV reactions
- Disturbed sleep pattern related to insomnia
- Noncompliance related to long-term therapy

▷ Planning and implementation
- Thyroid hormone dosage varies widely. Begin treatment at lowest level, adjusting to higher doses according to patient's symptoms and laboratory data, until euthyroid state is reached.
- Give thyroid hormones at same time each day, preferably in the morning to prevent insomnia.
- Thyroid medications may be supplied either in micrograms (mcg) or in milligrams (mg). Don't confuse these dose measurements.

Patient teaching
- Instruct patient to take drug exactly as prescribed. Suggest taking dose in morning to prevent insomnia.
- Advise patient to report signs and symptoms of overdose (chest pain, palpitations, sweating, nervousness) or aggravated CV disease (chest pain, dyspnea, tachycardia).
- Tell patient who has achieved a stable response not to change brands.
- Inform parents that child may lose hair during first months of therapy, and reassure them that this is temporary.
- Urge patient to keep follow-up appointments and have regular laboratory testing of thyroid levels.

Prototype drug

☑ Evaluation
● Patient sustains no injury from adverse reactions.
● Patient gets adequate sleep during the night.
● Patient complies with therapy, as evidenced by normal thyroid hormone levels and resolution of underlying disorder.

Xanthine derivatives
aminophylline
theophylline

Indications
▶ Asthma and bronchospasm from emphysema and chronic bronchitis.

Contraindications and cautions
● Contraindicated in patients hypersensitive to these drugs.
● Use cautiously in patients with arrhythmias, cardiac or circulatory impairment, cor pulmonale, hepatic or renal disease, active peptic ulcers, hyperthyroidism, or diabetes mellitus.
⚘ **Lifespan:** In pregnant women, use cautiously. In breast-feeding women, avoid these drugs because they appear in breast milk, and infants may have serious adverse reactions. Small children may have excessive CNS stimulation; monitor them closely. In elderly patients, use cautiously.

Adverse reactions
Adverse effects, except for hypersensitivity, are dose related and can be controlled by dosage adjustment. Common reactions include arrhythmias, headache, hypotension, irritability, nausea, palpitations, restlessness, urine retention, and vomiting.

Action
Xanthine derivatives are structurally related; they directly relax smooth muscle, stimulate the CNS, induce diuresis, increase gastric acid secretion, inhibit uterine contractions, and exert weak inotropic and chronotropic effects on the heart. Of these drugs, theophylline exerts the greatest effect on smooth muscle.
    The action of xanthine derivatives isn't completely caused by inhibition of phosphodi-

esterase. Current data suggest that inhibition of adenosine receptors or unidentified mechanisms may be responsible for therapeutic effects. By relaxing smooth muscle of the respiratory tract, they increase airflow and vital capacity. They also slow onset of diaphragmatic fatigue and stimulate the respiratory center in the CNS.

NURSING PROCESS

⚒ Assessment
● Monitor theophylline level closely because therapeutic level ranges from 10 to 20 mcg/ml.
● Monitor patient closely for adverse reactions, especially toxicity.
● Monitor vital signs.

⊞ Key nursing diagnoses
● Disturbed sleep pattern related to CNS effects
● Urine retention related to adverse effects on bladder
● Noncompliance related to long-term therapy

▷ Planning and implementation
● Don't crush or allow patient to chew timed-release preparations.
● Calculate dosage from lean body weight because theophylline doesn't distribute into fatty tissue.
● Adjust daily dosage in elderly patients and in those with heart failure or hepatic disease.
● Provide patient with nondrug sleep aids, such as a back rub or milk-based beverage.

Patient teaching
● Tell patient to take drug exactly as prescribed.
● Advise patient to check with prescriber before using any other drug, including OTC medications or herbal remedies, or before switching brands.
● If patient smokes, tell him that doing so may decrease theophylline level. Urge him to notify prescriber if he quits smoking because the dosage will need adjustment to avoid toxicity.

☑ Evaluation
● Patient sleeps usual number of hours without interruption.
● Patient's voiding pattern doesn't change.
● Patient complies with therapy, as evidenced by maintenance of therapeutic level.

Alphabetical
Listing of Drugs

A

abacavir sulfate
(uh-BACK-uh-veer SUL-fayt)
Ziagen

Pharmacologic class: nucleoside analogue reverse transcriptase inhibitor (NRTI)
Therapeutic class: antiretroviral
Pregnancy risk category: C

Indications and dosages

▶ **HIV-1 infection.** *Adults:* 300 mg P.O. b.i.d. with other antiretrovirals.
Children ages 3 months to 16 years: 8 mg/kg (up to 300 mg) P.O. b.i.d. with other antiretrovirals.
☒ Adjust-a-dose: For patients with mild hepatic impairment, reduce dosage to 200 mg P.O. b.i.d.

Contraindications and cautions

• Contraindicated in patients hypersensitive to the drug or any of its components, and in patients with moderate to severe hepatic impairment.
• Use cautiously in patients at high risk for liver disease. Lactic acidosis and severe hepatomegaly with steatosis may occur, most commonly in women, obese patients, or those with prolonged NRTI exposure.
☀ Lifespan: In pregnant women, use only if potential benefits outweigh risks to the fetus. In elderly patients, use cautiously as they may have decreased renal or hepatic function.

Adverse reactions

CNS: insomnia, sleep disorders, headache, fever.
GI: *nausea, vomiting,* diarrhea, loss of appetite, anorexia.
Hepatic: *hepatotoxicity.*
Metabolic: *lactic acidosis.*
Skin: rash.
Other: *fatal hypersensitivity reaction.*

Interactions

Drug-drug. *Methadone:* Clearance of drug may be increased. Increased methadone dosage may be needed.
Drug-lifestyle. *Alcohol use:* May decrease elimination of drug, increasing overall exposure. Discourage use together.

Effects on lab test results

• May increase GGT, glucose, and triglyceride levels.

Pharmacokinetics

Absorption: Rapid and extensive; oral solution and tablet forms may be used interchangeably.
Distribution: In extravascular space; about 50% bound to plasma proteins.
Metabolism: In the liver, alcohol dehydrogenase and glucuronyl transferase metabolize the drug to form two inactive metabolites.
Excretion: Mainly in urine; about 16% in feces.
Half-life: 1 to 2 hours.

Route	Onset	Peak	Duration
P.O.	Unknown	Unknown	Unknown

Action

Chemical effect: Inhibits the activity of HIV-1 reverse transcriptase, stopping viral DNA growth.
Therapeutic effect: Reduces the symptoms of HIV-1 infection.

Available forms

Oral solution: 20 mg/ml
Tablets: 300 mg

NURSING PROCESS

☒ Assessment
• Assess patient's condition before therapy and regularly thereafter.
• Watch for hypersensitivity reaction.
• Monitor glucose level during therapy.
• Assess patient for risk factors of liver disease. Lactic acidosis and severe hepatomegaly with steatosis may occur, especially in women or patients who are obese or have prolonged exposure to nucleosides. If patient has symptoms of lactic acidosis or pronounced hepatotoxicity, stop treatment. Symptoms may include hepatomegaly and steatosis, even without elevated transaminase levels.

• Assess patient's and family's knowledge of drug therapy.

Nursing diagnoses
• Risk for infection secondary to presence of HIV
• Ineffective individual coping related to HIV infection
• Deficient knowledge related to drug therapy

Planning and implementation
• Drug should always be given with other antiretrovirals, never alone.
• Register pregnant woman with the Antiretroviral Pregnancy Registry at 1-800-258-4263.
ALERT: Drug may cause fatal hypersensitivity reactions. If a patient develops fever, rash, fatigue, nausea, vomiting, diarrhea, or abdominal pain, stop the drug and immediately notify the prescriber.
• Don't restart drug after a hypersensitivity reaction because more severe signs and symptoms, including life-threatening hypotension, may recur within hours. To report hypersensitivity reactions, register patient with the Abacavir Hypersensitivity Registry at 1-800-270-0425.
ALERT: Don't use triple antiretroviral therapy (abacavir, lamivudine, and tenofovir) as a new treatment because of the high rate of early viral resistance. Monitor patients taking this combination; they may need a different therapy.

Patient teaching
• Give written information about drug with each new prescription and refill. Patient also should receive, and be instructed to carry, a warning card summarizing drug's hypersensitivity reaction.
• Tell patient to take drug exactly as prescribed.
• Inform patient that drug can be taken with or without food.
• Inform patient that drug can cause a life-threatening hypersensitivity reaction. Tell patient to stop drug and immediately seek medical attention if he develops symptoms of hypersensitivity, such as fever, rash, severe fatigue, achiness, nausea, vomiting, diarrhea, stomach pain, or a generally ill feeling.
• Explain that the drug neither cures HIV nor reduces the risk of transmitting HIV to others and that its long-term effects are unknown.

Evaluation
• Patient has reduced signs and symptoms of infection.
• Patient demonstrates adequate coping mechanisms.
• Patient and family state understanding of drug therapy.

abacavir sulfate, lamivudine, and zidovudine
uh-BACK-uh-veer SULL-fayt, lah-MIH-vyoo-deen, and zye-DOE-vyoo-deen
Trizivir

Pharmacologic classification: nucleoside analogue reverse transcriptase inhibitor
Therapeutic classification: antiretroviral
Pregnancy risk category: C

Indications and dosages
▶ **HIV-1 infection, given alone or with other antiretrovirals.** *Adults and adolescents who weigh 40 kg (88 lb) or more:* 1 tablet P.O. b.i.d.

Contraindications and cautions
Contraindicated in patients with hepatic impairment and those who have had an allergic reaction to abacavir or any of Trizivir's components. Avoid drug if patient's creatinine clearance is less than 50 ml/minute, if patient weighs less than 40 kg (88 lb), or if patient needs a dosage adjustment.

Use cautiously in patients with anemia, hepatitis B, hepatomegaly, immune reconstitution syndrome, infection that's resistant to nucleoside reverse transcriptase inhibitors, lactic acidosis, myopathy, neutropenia, or signs of fat redistribution. Also use cautiously if patient has risk factors for liver disease, or if patient's granulocyte count is less than 1,000 cells/mm^3 or hemoglobin level is less than 9.5 g/dl.

Lifespan: In pregnant women, give drug only if benefit to mother outweighs risk to fetus. Patients exposed to Trizivir may be registered at 1-800-258-4263 to monitor maternal-fetal outcome. HIV-infected mothers shouldn't breastfeed. Lamivudine and zidovudine appear in breast milk. Don't use drug in children or adolescents who weigh less than 40 kg. In the elderly, use cautiously because of the increased risks of drug interactions, concurrent disease, and decreased hepatic, renal, and cardiac function.

Adverse reactions

CNS: anxiety, depression, *fatigue,* fever, *headache, malaise.*
EENT: ear, nose, or throat infection.
GI: diarrhea, nausea, *pancreatitis,* vomiting.
Hematologic: anemia, *aplastic anemia, neutropenia, thrombocytopenia.*
Hepatic: *hepatic steatosis, lactic acidosis.*
Musculoskeletal: muscle pain, muscle weakness.
Respiratory: viral infection.
Skin: *erythema multiforme,* rash, *Stevens-Johnson syndrome, toxic epidermal necrolysis.*
Other: chills, *hypersensitivity reaction.*

Interactions

Drug-drug. *Atovaquone, fluconazole, methadone, probenecid, valproic acid:* May increase zidovudine level. Dosage adjustment of these drugs may not be needed.
Doxorubicin, ribavirin, stavudine: May antagonize zidovudine. Avoid use together.
Ganciclovir, interferon-alfa, other bone marrow suppressant or cytotoxic drugs: May increase zidovudine toxicity. Monitor patient closely.
Methadone: May increase methadone clearance (abacavir). If needed, increase methadone dose.
Nelfinavir: May increase lamivudine level. Dosage adjustment of these drugs may not be needed.
Nelfinavir, ritonavir: May decrease zidovudine level. Dosage adjustment of these drugs may not be needed.
Other HIV fixed-dose combination drugs or drugs that contain one or more of the active ingredients of Trizivir (Combivir, Emtriva, Epzicom, Epivir, Epivir-HBV, Retrovir, Truvada, Ziagen): May disrupt fixed-dose regimen. Avoid use together.
Trimethoprim and sulfamethoxazole (TMP-SMZ): May increase lamivudine level. Monitor patient closely.
Zalcitabine: May inhibit phosphorylation of both lamivudine and zalcitabine. Avoid use together.
Drug-lifestyle. *Alcohol:* May decrease abacavir elimination. Discourage use together.

Effects on lab test results

● May increase AST, ALT, bilirubin, serum creatinine, BUN, CK, triglyceride, amylase, glucose, and hemoglobin levels and hematocrit.
● May decrease WBC, neutrophil, RBC, and platelet counts.

Pharmacokinetics

Absorption: Rapid.
Distribution: Extensive, with low plasma protein binding.
Metabolism: Significant hepatic for abacavir and zidovudine. Minor for lamivudine.
Excretion: Mainly hepatic for abacavir and zidovudine. About 70% of lamivudine appears in urine unchanged. *Half-life:* 1½ hours for abacavir, 5 to 7 hours for lamivudine, and ½ to 3 hours for zidovudine.

Route	Onset	Peak	Duration
P.O.	Unknown	Unknown	Unknown

Action

Chemical effect: Inhibits HIV-1 reverse transcriptase, stopping viral DNA growth. Also weakly inhibits cellular DNA alpha, beta, and gamma polymerases.
Therapeutic effect: Reduces the symptoms of HIV-1 infection.

Available forms

Tablets (film coated): 300 mg abacavir sulfate, 150 mg lamivudine, 300 mg zidovudine.

NURSING PROCESS

🖹 Assessment

● Assess patient's condition before starting therapy and regularly thereafter to monitor the drug's effectiveness.
🚱 **ALERT:** Monitor patient carefully for hypersensitivity reactions, which may be fatal.
● Monitor patient's weight.
● Monitor patient's renal and hepatic function regularly.
● Monitor blood counts often for evidence of hematologic toxicity, including neutropenia and severe anemia.
● Monitor patient for muscle pain or weakness and increased CK level; long-term use of zidovudine may cause myopathy and myositis.
● Monitor patient for central obesity, dorsocervical fat enlargement (buffalo hump), peripheral

and facial wasting, breast enlargement, and a cushingoid appearance. Patients taking antiretroviral drugs may have redistribution and accumulation of body fat.
• Assess patient's and family's knowledge of drug therapy.

🔷 Nursing diagnoses
• Noncompliance related to long-term therapeutic regimen
• Ineffective protection related to drug-induced adverse hematologic reactions
• Deficient knowledge related to drug therapy

❱ Planning and implementation
• Safety and effectiveness of lamivudine haven't been established in patients infected with both HIV and hepatitis B virus (HBV). Resistant HBV can occur in HIV patients treated with lamivudine. Also, HBV may worsen after lamivudine treatment, possibly increasing patient's risk of death. Monitor patient for increased ALT level and return of HBV DNA.
• Don't give drug if creatinine clearance is less than 50 ml/minute or patient develops hepatic impairment.
• Don't give drug if patient weighs less than 40 kg.
⚠ ALERT: Hypersensitivity to abacavir usually causes two or more of the following reactions: fever; rash; nausea, vomiting, diarrhea, or abdominal pain; malaise, fatigue, or achiness; and dyspnea, cough, or pharyngitis.
• Stop Trizivir immediately if patient may be having an allergic reaction, and never restart any therapy that contains abacavir.
• Call the abacavir Hypersensitivity Registry at 1-800-270-0425 to report allergic reactions.
• Combination antiretroviral therapy may cause an inflammatory response to other opportunistic infections and the need for further treatment.
• All three components of Trizivir may cause lactic acidosis and severe hepatomegaly with steatosis. These may be more likely in patients who are obese, female, or exposed to nucleosides long-term. Watch for evidence of lactic acidosis and hepatotoxicity.
• In the case of overdose, abacavir has no known antidote. Experience with lamivudine overdose is limited. It may cause no signs or symptoms and no changes in blood tests. Zidovudine overdose may cause confusion, dizzi-

ness, drowsiness, headache, lethargy, nausea, vomiting, and transient hematologic changes.
Patient teaching
• Tell patient to take drug exactly as prescribed, with or without food.
• To minimize drug interactions, urge patient to tell prescriber about all other drugs and supplements he takes.
⚠ ALERT: Warn patient to avoid this drug if he has ever had an allergic reaction to any of its components. Tell him to stop drug and seek medical attention immediately if he develops hives, a rash, swelling of the face or throat, or trouble breathing. Describe other allergy-related problems, including fever, rash, nausea, vomiting, diarrhea, stomach pain, extreme fatigue, achiness, cough, and sore throat, and explain that they may worsen or become life threatening if he doesn't stop drug immediately.
• Urge patient to read the medication guide and warning card that accompany drug, and tell him always to carry the warning card.
• Explain that drug may cause blood irregularities, liver damage, and liver enlargement.
• Tell patient to report a history of hepatitis B.
• Advise patient to report any unusual side effects, such as excessive nausea, vomiting, fatigue, abdominal pain, fever, muscle aches and pains, any unusual skin reactions, or worsening of previous infections.
• Tell patient that body appearance may change, and he may develop buffalo hump, fat deposits around the waist, breast enlargement, and wasting of face, arms, and legs.
• Explain that blood counts may be done often to check for adverse effects.
• Tell patient that Trizivir doesn't reduce the risk of transmitting HIV to others.

☑ Evaluation
• Patient is compliant with therapeutic regimen.
• Patient doesn't develop complications from drug therapy.
• Patient and family state understanding of drug therapy.

abciximab
(ab-SICKS-ih-mahb)
ReoPro

Pharmacologic class: glycoprotein IIb/IIIa receptor blocker
Therapeutic class: platelet-aggregation inhibitor
Pregnancy risk category: C

Indications and dosages

▶ **Adjunct for percutaneous coronary intervention (PCI) to prevent acute cardiac ischemic complications in patients at high risk for abrupt closure of treated coronary vessel.** *Adults:* 0.25 mg/kg as I.V. bolus 10 to 60 minutes before PCI, followed by continuous I.V. infusion of 0.125 mcg/kg/minute (maximum, 10 mcg/minute) for 12 hours.
▶ **Patients with unstable angina not responding to conventional medical therapy who are to undergo PCI within 24 hours.** *Adults:* 0.25 mg/kg as I.V. bolus; then an 18- to 24-hour infusion of 10 mcg/minute, concluding 1 hour after PCI.

▼ I.V. administration

• Intended for use with heparin and aspirin.
• Anticipate hypersensitivity reactions. Have epinephrine, dopamine, theophylline, antihistamine, and corticosteroid available for immediate use.
• If solution contains opaque particles, discard it and obtain a new vial.
• For I.V. bolus, withdraw drug into syringe; then inject through a sterile 0.2- or 0.22-micron filter.
• For I.V. infusion, inject drug into normal saline solution or D₅W, and infuse via continuous infusion pump equipped with 0.2- or 0.22-micron in-line filter.
• If hypersensitivity or bleeding occurs, stop infusion immediately and start treatment.
• Discard any unused portion of vials or mixed drug.
⊗ **Incompatibilities**
• Give drug in separate I.V. line; don't add another drug to infusion solution.

Contraindications and cautions

• Contraindicated in patients hypersensitive to a drug component or to murine proteins and in patients with active internal bleeding; bleeding diathesis; platelet count less than 100,000/mm³; intracranial neoplasm, arteriovenous malformation, or aneurysm; severe uncontrolled hypertension; a history of stroke within 2 years or with significant residual neurologic deficit; or a history of vasculitis. Also contraindicated within 6 weeks of major surgery, trauma, or GI or GU bleeding; when oral anticoagulants have been given within 7 days unless PT is less than or equal to 1.2 times control; and when I.V. dextran is used before or during PCI.
• Use cautiously in patients who weigh less than 75 kg (165 lb), have a history of GI disease, or are receiving thrombolytics because these patients are at increased risk for bleeding. Conditions that increase risk of bleeding include PCI within 12 hours of onset of symptoms of acute MI, PCI lasting longer than 70 minutes, failed PCI, and use of heparin.
⚯ **Lifespan:** In pregnant or breast-feeding women, use cautiously. In children, safety and effectiveness of drug haven't been established. In patients older than age 65, use cautiously.

Adverse reactions

CNS: hypoesthesia, confusion, headache, pain.
CV: hypotension, chest pain, *bradycardia,* peripheral edema.
EENT: abnormal vision.
GI: nausea, vomiting, abdominal pain.
Hematologic: *bleeding, thrombocytopenia,* anemia, leukocytosis.
Musculoskeletal: *back pain.*
Respiratory: pleural effusion, pleurisy, pneumonia.

Interactions

Drug-drug. *Antiplatelets, heparin, NSAIDs, other anticoagulants, thrombolytics:* May increase risk of bleeding. Monitor patient closely.

Effects on lab test results

• May decrease hemoglobin level and hematocrit.
• May decrease platelet counts. May increase WBC count.

Pharmacokinetics

Absorption: Given I.V.

Distribution: Rapidly binds to platelet receptors.
Metabolism: Unknown.
Excretion: Unknown. *Half-life:* Initially, less than 10 minutes; second phase, about 30 minutes.

Route	Onset	Peak	Duration
I.V.	Immediate	Immediate	24 hr

Action

Chemical effect: Prevents binding of fibrinogen, von Willebrand factor, and other adhesive molecules to receptor sites on activated platelets.
Therapeutic effect: Inhibits platelet aggregation.

Available forms

Injection: 2 mg/ml

NURSING PROCESS

Assessment
● Note patient history. Patients at risk for abrupt closure include those undergoing PCI with unstable angina, non–Q wave MI, acute Q wave MI within 12 hours of onset of symptoms, two type B lesions in artery to be dilated, one type B lesion in artery to be dilated in a woman older than age 65 or a patient with diabetes, one type C lesion in artery to be dilated, or angioplasty of infarct-related lesion within 7 days of MI.
● Assess vital signs and evaluate bleeding studies before therapy.
● Monitor patient closely for bleeding. Bleeding caused by therapy falls into two categories: that observed at arterial access site used for cardiac catheterization, and internal bleeding involving GI or GU tract or retroperitoneal sites.
● Look for adverse reactions and drug interactions.
● Assess patient's and family's knowledge of drug therapy.

Nursing diagnoses
● Ineffective cerebral or cardiopulmonary tissue perfusion related to patient's underlying condition
● Risk for deficient fluid volume related to drug-induced bleeding
● Deficient knowledge related to drug therapy

Planning and implementation
● Institute bleeding precautions. Keep patient on bed rest for 6 to 8 hours after removing sheath or stopping infusion, whichever is later.
● Drug is intended for use with aspirin and heparin.
⊛ **ALERT:** Keep epinephrine, dopamine, theophylline, antihistamines, and corticosteroids available in case of anaphylaxis.
Patient teaching
● Teach patient about his disease and therapy.
● Stress the importance of reporting adverse reactions.

Evaluation
● Patient maintains adequate tissue perfusion.
● Patient maintains adequate hydration.
● Patient and family state understanding of drug therapy.

acamprosate calcium
(ay-CAM-proh-sate KAL-see-um)
Campral◈

Pharmacologic class: synthetic amino acid neurotransmitter analog
Therapeutic class: alcohol deterrent
Pregnancy risk category: C

Indications and dosages

▶ **Maintenance of alcohol abstinence as part of a comprehensive treatment program.**
Adults: 666 mg P.O. t.i.d.
❒ **Adjust-a-dose:** If patient's creatinine clearance is 30 to 50 ml/min, give 333 mg t.i.d.

Contraindications and cautions

● Contraindicated in patients allergic to drug or its components and in those whose creatinine clearance is 30 ml/minute or less.
● Use cautiously in patients with moderate renal impairment, and patients with a history of depression and suicidal thoughts or attempts.
⚘ **Lifespan:** Use cautiously in women who are pregnant or breast-feeding and in elderly patients. Safety and effectiveness haven't been evaluated in children. Plasma levels are likely to be increased in elderly patients because renal function is commonly decreased in these patients. Consider a reduced dosage and renal function monitoring.

Adverse reactions

CNS: abnormal thinking, amnesia, anxiety, asthenia, depression, dizziness, headache, insomnia, paresthesia, somnolence, *suicidal ideation,* syncope, tremor.
CV: hypertension, palpitations, peripheral edema, vasodilation.
EENT: abnormal vision, pharyngitis, rhinitis.
GI: abdominal pain, anorexia, constipation, *diarrhea,* dry mouth, dyspepsia, flatulence, increased appetite, nausea, taste disturbance, vomiting.
GU: impotence.
Metabolic: weight gain.
Musculoskeletal: arthralgia, back pain, chest pain, myalgia.
Respiratory: bronchitis, dyspnea, increased cough.
Skin: increased sweating, pruritus, rash.
Other: accidental injury, chills, decreased libido, flulike symptoms, infection, pain.

Interactions

None significant.

Effects on lab test results

• May increase ALT, AST, bilirubin, blood glucose, and uric acid levels. May decrease hemoglobin level and hematocrit.
• May decrease platelet count.

Pharmacokinetics

Absorption: Absolute bioavailability is about 11%.
Distribution: Into plasma with negligible protein binding.
Metabolism: Not metabolized.
Excretion: By the kidneys as unchanged drug.
Half-life: 20 to 33 hours.

Route	Onset	Peak	Duration
P.O.	Unknown	3–8 hr	Unknown

Action

Chemical effect: Drug restores the balance of neuronal excitation and inhibition, probably by interacting with glutamate and gamma aminobutyric acid neurotransmitter systems, thus reducing alcohol dependence.
Therapeutic effect: Maintenance of alcohol abstinence.

Available forms

Tablets (delayed-release): 333 mg

NURSING PROCESS

⏲ Assessment
• Obtain a history of patient's alcohol use before therapy.
• Assess patient's support system and his involvement in a comprehensive treatment program.
• Monitor patient for adverse reactions to drug therapy.
• Monitor patient for development of depression or suicidal thoughts.
• Assess patient's and family's knowledge of drug therapy.

⊕ Nursing diagnoses
• Ineffective health maintenance related to alcoholism.
• Risk for injury related to alcoholism and drug-induced adverse CNS effects.
• Deficient knowledge related to drug therapy.

▶ Planning and implementation
• Use drug only after the patient has successfully achieved abstinence.
• Drug doesn't eliminate or reduce withdrawal symptoms.
• Drug doesn't cause alcohol aversion or a disulfiram-like reaction if used with alcohol.
Patient teaching
• Tell patient to continue the alcohol abstinence program, including counseling and support.
• Advise patient to notify his prescriber if he develops depression, anxiety, thoughts of suicide, or severe diarrhea.
• Caution patient's family or caregiver to watch for signs of depression or suicidal ideation.
• Tell patient that drug may be taken without regard to meals, but that taking it with meals may help him remember to take it.
• Tell patient not to crush, break, or chew the tablets but to swallow them whole.
• Advise women to use effective contraception while taking this drug. Tell patient to contact her prescriber if she becomes pregnant or plans to become pregnant.
• Explain that this drug may impair judgment, thinking, or motor skills. Urge patient to use caution when driving or performing hazardous activities until drug's effects are known.

Rapid onset   *Liquid form contains alcohol.   ♦ Canada   ◊ Australia   †OTC   ⌀Photoguide   ‡Off-label use

• Tell patient to continue taking acamprosate and to contact his prescriber if he resumes drinking.

☑ Evaluation
• Patient abstains from alcohol consumption.
• Patient abstains from alcohol and doesn't experience injury.
• Patient and family state understanding of drug therapy.

acarbose
(ay-KAR-bohs)
Precose

Pharmacologic class: alpha-glucosidase inhibitor
Therapeutic class: antidiabetic
Pregnancy risk category: B

Indications and dosages

▶ **Adjunct to diet and exercise to lower glucose level in patients with type 2 (non–insulin-dependent) diabetes mellitus, or in combination with a sulfonylurea, metformin, or insulin.** *Adults:* Initially, 25 mg P.O. t.i.d. with the first bite of each main meal. Dosage adjustments are made q 4 to 8 weeks, based on glucose level and tolerance 1 hour after a meal. Maximum dosage for patients weighing 60 kg (132 lb) or less is 50 mg P.O. t.i.d.; for patients weighing more than 60 kg, maximum dosage is 100 mg P.O. t.i.d.

Contraindications and cautions

• Contraindicated in patients hypersensitive to drug and in patients with diabetic ketoacidosis, cirrhosis, inflammatory bowel disease, colonic ulceration, partial intestinal obstruction, predisposition to intestinal obstruction, chronic intestinal disease with disorder of digestion or absorption, and conditions that may deteriorate because of increased intestinal gas formation.
• Drug isn't recommended in patients with severe renal impairment.
• Use cautiously in patients receiving insulin or a sulfonylurea. Drug may increase the hypoglycemic potential of a sulfonylurea.
☙ **Lifespan:** In pregnant or breast-feeding women, drug isn't recommended. In children,

safety and effectiveness haven't been established.

Adverse reactions
GI: abdominal pain, diarrhea, flatulence.

Interactions
Drug-drug. *Calcium channel blockers, corticosteroids, estrogens, hormonal contraceptives, isoniazid, nicotinic acid, phenothiazines, phenytoin, sympathomimetics, thiazides and other diuretics, thyroid products:* May cause hyperglycemia and loss of glucose control during use or hypoglycemia when withdrawn. Monitor glucose level.
Digestive enzyme preparations containing carbohydrate-splitting enzymes (such as amylase, Beano enzyme, pancreatin), intestinal adsorbents (such as activated charcoal): May reduce effect of acarbose. Don't give together.
Digoxin: May decrease digoxin level. Monitor digoxin level.
Drug-herb. *Aloe, bilberry leaf, bitter melon, burdock, dandelion, fenugreek, garlic, ginseng:* May improve glucose control and allow reduced antidiabetic dosage. Urge patient to discuss herbal products with prescriber before use.

Effects on lab test results
• May increase ALT and AST levels. May decrease calcium, vitamin B_6, and hemoglobin levels and hematocrit.

Pharmacokinetics
Absorption: Minimal.
Distribution: Acts locally in GI tract.
Metabolism: Exclusively in the GI tract, mainly by intestinal bacteria and partly by digestive enzymes.
Excretion: Almost completely excreted by the kidneys. *Half-life:* 2 hours.

Route	Onset	Peak	Duration
P.O.	Unknown	1 hr	2–4 hr

Action
Chemical effect: Delays carbohydrate digestion and glucose absorption.
Therapeutic effect: Lessens postprandial hyperglycemia.

Available forms
Tablets: 25 mg, 50 mg, 100 mg

NURSING PROCESS

⚕ Assessment
• Monitor glucose level 1 hour after a meal to determine effectiveness and to identify appropriate dose. Report hypoglycemia or hyperglycemia to prescriber.
• Monitor glycosylated hemoglobin level every 3 months.
• In a patient receiving 50 mg t.i.d. or more, monitor transaminase level every 3 months in first year of therapy and periodically thereafter. Report abnormalities to prescriber.
• Obtain baseline creatinine level. Drug isn't recommended in patient with a creatinine level greater than 2 mg/dl.
• Assess patient's and family's knowledge of drug therapy.

⊕ Nursing diagnoses
• Risk for imbalanced fluid volume related to adverse GI effect
• Imbalanced nutrition: less than body requirements related to patient's underlying condition
• Deficient knowledge related to drug therapy

⊇ Planning and implementation
• If dosage exceeds 50 mg t.i.d., watch for high transaminase and bilirubin levels and low calcium and vitamin B_6 levels.
• Drug may increase hypoglycemic potential of sulfonylureas. Closely monitor any patient receiving both drugs. If hypoglycemia occurs, treat with dextrose, I.V. glucose infusion, or glucagon. Report hypoglycemia to prescriber.
• Insulin may be needed during increased stress, such as infection, fever, surgery, or trauma.

Patient teaching
• Tell patient to take drug daily with first bite of each of three main meals.
• Explain that therapy relieves symptoms but doesn't cure the disease.
• Stress importance of adhering to specific diet, weight reduction, exercise, and hygiene programs. Show patient how to monitor glucose level and how to recognize and treat hyperglycemia.
• Teach patient to recognize hypoglycemia and to treat symptoms with a form of dextrose rather than with a product containing table sugar.
• Instruct patient to check with the prescriber before using any OTC natural or herbal products such as Beano.

• Urge patient to wear or carry medical identification at all times.

☑ Evaluation
• Patient maintains adequate fluid volume balance.
• Patient doesn't experience hypoglycemia.
• Patient and family state understanding of drug therapy.

acebutolol
(as-ih-BYOO-tuh-lol)
Sectral

Pharmacologic class: beta blocker
Therapeutic class: antihypertensive, antiarrhythmic
Pregnancy risk category: B

Indications and dosages
▶ **Hypertension.** *Adults:* 400 mg P.O. as single daily dosage or in divided doses b.i.d. Maximum, 1,200 mg daily.
▶ **Suppression of PVCs.** *Adults:* 400 mg P.O. in divided doses b.i.d. Increase dosage to provide adequate clinical response. Usual dosage is 600 to 1,200 mg daily.
▶ **Stable angina‡.** *Adults:* Initially, 200 mg P.O. b.i.d. Increase dosage up to 800 mg daily until angina is controlled. Patients with severe stable angina may require higher doses.
⧉ Adjust-a-dose: For patients with renal impairment, if creatinine clearance is less than 50 ml/minute, decrease dosage by 50%; if creatinine clearance is less than 25 ml/minute, decrease dosage by 75%. In elderly patients, don't exceed 800 mg daily.

Contraindications and cautions
• Contraindicated in patients with persistently severe bradycardia, second- or third-degree heart block, overt heart failure, or cardiogenic shock.
• Use cautiously in patients with heart failure, peripheral vascular disease, bronchospastic disease, diabetes, or hepatic impairment.
⚶ Lifespan: In pregnant women, use cautiously. In breast-feeding women, use is contraindicated. In children, safety of drug hasn't been established. In elderly patients, use cautiously and at a reduced dose.

Adverse reactions

CNS: *fatigue,* headache, dizziness, fever, insomnia, depression, abnormal dreams.
CV: chest pain, edema, *bradycardia, heart failure,* hypotension.
EENT: rhinitis, abnormal vision, dry eye, eye pain.
GI: nausea, constipation, diarrhea, dyspepsia, flatulence, vomiting, *mesenteric arterial thrombosis.*
GU: impotence.
Metabolic: *hypoglycemia,* hyperglycemia, unstable diabetes mellitus.
Musculoskeletal: arthralgia, myalgia.
Respiratory: dyspnea, cough, *bronchospasm.*
Skin: rash.

Interactions

Drug-drug. *Alpha-adrenergic stimulants:* May increase hypertensive response. Use together cautiously.
Digoxin, diltiazem: May cause excessive bradycardia and increase depression of the myocardium. Use together cautiously.
Insulin, oral antidiabetics: May alter dosage requirements in previously stabilized patient with diabetes. Observe patient carefully.
NSAIDs: May decrease antihypertensive effect. Monitor blood pressure and adjust dosage.
Prazosin: May increase the risk of orthostatic hypotension in the early phases of use together. Assist patient to stand slowly until effects are known.
Reserpine: May have an additive effect. Monitor patient closely.
Verapamil: May increase the effects of both drugs. Monitor cardiac function closely and decrease dosages as necessary.

Effects on lab test results

• May increase AST and ALT levels.
• May cause false-positive antinuclear antibody test result. May cause false results with glucose or insulin tolerance tests.

Pharmacokinetics

Absorption: Well absorbed after oral use.
Distribution: About 25% protein bound; minimal quantities detected in CSF.
Metabolism: Undergoes extensive first-pass metabolism in liver.

Excretion: 30% to 40% of dose is excreted in urine, the rest in feces and bile. *Half-life:* 3 to 4 hours.

Route	Onset	Peak	Duration
P.O.	1–1½ hr	2½ hr	< 24 hr

Action

Chemical effect: May reduce cardiac output and inhibit renin release. May decrease myocardial contractility and heart rate.
Therapeutic effect: Lowers blood pressure and heart rate and restores normal sinus rhythm.

Available forms

Capsules: 200 mg, 400 mg

NURSING PROCESS

⚗ Assessment

• Assess blood pressure and heart rate and rhythm before and during therapy.
• Monitor energy level.
• Be alert for adverse reactions and drug interactions.
• Assess patient's and family's knowledge of drug therapy.

🔲 Nursing diagnoses

• Risk for injury related to patient's underlying condition
• Fatigue related to drug-induced CNS adverse reactions
• Deficient knowledge related to drug therapy

▶ Planning and implementation

• Drug may be removed by hemodialysis.
• Check apical pulse before giving drug; if it's slower than 60 beats/minute, withhold drug and call prescriber.
Ⓢ **ALERT:** Don't stop drug abruptly. Doing so may worsen angina or cause an MI or rebound hypertension.
• Before surgery, notify anesthesiologist about patient's drug therapy.
Ⓢ **ALERT:** Don't confuse Sectral with Factrel or Septra.
Patient teaching
• Teach patient how to take his pulse, and instruct him to withhold dose and notify prescriber if pulse rate is slower than 60 beats/minute.

• Warn patient that drug may cause dizziness. Instruct him to avoid sudden position changes and to sit down immediately if he feels dizzy.
• Explain the importance of taking drug as prescribed, even when feeling well.
• Tell diabetic patient to monitor glucose level closely because this drug may mask the symptoms of hypoglycemia.

☑ Evaluation
• Patient's blood pressure and heart rate and rhythm are normal.
• Patient effectively combats fatigue.
• Patient and family state understanding of drug therapy.

acetaminophen
(APAP, paracetamol)
(as-ee-tuh-MIH-nuh-fin)
Abenol ◆ †, Acephen†, Aceta†, Aceta Elixir*†, Acetaminophen Uniserts†, Anacin†, Anacin Maximum Strength Aspirin Free†, Apacet†, Apo-Acetaminophen ◆ †, Arthritis Pain Formula Aspirin Free†, Atasol Caplets ◆ †, Atasol Drops ◆ †, Atasol Elixir*†, Atasol Tablets ◆ †, Dymadon ◇ †, FeverAll Infants†, FeverAll Junior Strength†, FeverAll Children's†, Genapap†, Genapap Children's Chewable Tablets†, Genapap Children's Elixir†, Genapap Extra Strength†, Genapap Infants' Drops†, Genebs†, Genebs Extra Strength†, Liquiprin Infants' Drops†, Mapap†, Meda-Cap†, Meda Tab†, Neopap†, Oraphen-PD†, Panadol†, Panadol Children's†, Redutemp†, Silapap Children's, Silapap Infants' Drops, St. Joseph Aspirin-Free Fever Reducer for Children†, Tapanol Extra Strength†, Tempra†, Tempra Infants'†, Tylenol†, Tylenol Arthritis Pain Extended Relief, Tylenol Children's Chewable Tablets†, Tylenol Children's Elixir†, Tylenol Concentrated Infant's' Drops†, Tylenol Extended Relief†, Tylenol Extra Strength†, Tylenol Infants' Drops†, Tylenol Junior Strength†

Pharmacologic class: para-aminophenol derivative
Therapeutic class: nonopioid analgesic, antipyretic

Pregnancy risk category: B

Indications and dosages
▶ Mild pain or fever. Adults and children older than age 12: 325 to 650 mg P.O. or P.R. q 4 hours, p.r.n.; or 1 g P.O. t.i.d. or q.i.d., p.r.n. Alternatively, 2 extended-release caplets P.O. q 8 hours. Maximum, 4 g daily. Dosage for long-term therapy shouldn't exceed 2.6 g daily unless monitored by prescriber. Maximum dosage for chronic alcoholics is 2 g daily.
Children ages 11 to 12: 480 mg P.O. or P.R. q 4 to 6 hours p.r.n.
Children ages 9 to 10: 400 mg P.O. or P.R. q 4 to 6 hours p.r.n.
Children ages 6 to 8: 320 mg P.O. or P.R. q 4 to 6 hours p.r.n.
Children ages 4 to 5: 240 mg P.O. or P.R. q 4 to 6 hours p.r.n.
Children ages 2 to 3: 160 mg P.O. or P.R. q 4 to 6 hours p.r.n.
Children ages 12 to 23 months: 120 mg P.O. q 4 to 6 hours p.r.n.
Infants ages 4 to 11 months: 80 mg P.O. q 4 to 6 hours p.r.n.
Infants age 3 months or younger: 40 mg P.O. q 4 to 6 hours p.r.n.
▶ Osteoarthritis. Adults: Up to 1 g P.O. q.i.d.

Contraindications and cautions
• Contraindicated in patients hypersensitive to drug.
• Use cautiously in patients with history of chronic alcohol abuse because hepatotoxicity may occur after therapeutic doses.
⚜ Lifespan: In pregnant or breast-feeding women, use cautiously.

Adverse reactions
Hematologic: hemolytic anemia, neutropenia, leukopenia, pancytopenia, thrombocytopenia.
Hepatic: liver damage (with toxic doses), jaundice.
Metabolic: hypoglycemia.
Skin: rash, urticaria.

Interactions
Drug-drug. Barbiturates, carbamazepine, hydantoins, isoniazid, rifampin, sulfinpyrazone: With high doses or long-term use of these drugs, may reduce therapeutic effects and enhance hepatotoxic effects of acetaminophen. Avoid use together.

Lamotrigine: May decrease lamotrigine level and effect. Monitor patient closely.
Warfarin: With long-term use at high doses of acetaminophen, may increase hypoprothrombinemic effect. Monitor PT and INR closely.
Zidovudine: May increase risk of bone marrow suppression because of impaired zidovudine metabolism. Monitor patient closely.
Drug-food. *Caffeine:* May enhance analgesic effects. Monitor patient for effect.
Drug-lifestyle. *Alcohol use:* May increase risk of liver damage. Discourage use together.

Effects on lab test results

• May decrease hemoglobin level and hematocrit.
• May decrease neutrophil, WBC, RBC, and platelet counts.
• May produce false-positive decrease in glucose level. May alter laboratory tests for urinary 5-hydroxyindoleacetic acid.

Pharmacokinetics

Absorption: Rapid and complete.
Distribution: 25% protein-bound. Level isn't connected strongly with analgesic effect but is with toxicity.
Metabolism: 90% to 95% metabolized in liver.
Excretion: In urine. *Half-life:* 1 to 4 hours.

Route	Onset	Peak	Duration
P.O., P.R.	Unknown	1–3 hr	1–3 hr

Action

Chemical effect: May produce analgesic effect by blocking pain impulses, by inhibiting prostaglandin or pain receptor sensitizers. May relieve fever by acting in hypothalamic heat-regulating center.
Therapeutic effect: Relieves pain and reduces fever.

Available forms

Caplets: 165 mg†, 500 mg†, 650 mg†
Capsules: 500 mg†
Elixir: 80 mg/2.5 ml†, 80 mg/5 ml†,120 mg/5 ml†,160 mg/5 ml*†
Gelcaps: 500 mg†
Infant drops: 80 mg/0.8 ml†, 100 mg/ml†
Liquid: 160 mg/5 ml†, 500 mg/15 ml†
Solution: 80 mg/1.66 ml†, 100 mg/ml†
Sprinkles: 80 mg/capsule†, 160 mg/capsule†

Suppositories: 80 mg†,120 mg†, 125 mg†, 300 mg†, 325 mg†, 650 mg†
Tablets: 160 mg†, 325 mg†, 500 mg†, 650 mg†
Tablets (chewable): 80 mg†, 160 mg†

NURSING PROCESS

⚖ Assessment

• Assess patient's pain or temperature before and during therapy.
• Assess patient's drug history. Many OTC products and combination prescription pain products contain acetaminophen. Calculate total daily dosage accordingly.
• Be alert for adverse reactions and drug interactions.
• Assess patient's and family's knowledge of drug therapy.

🔲 Nursing diagnoses

• Acute pain related to patient's underlying condition
• Risk for injury related to drug-induced liver damage with toxic doses
• Deficient knowledge related to drug therapy

▶ Planning and implementation

• Give liquid form to children and other patients who have trouble swallowing.
• ⓈALERT: When giving oral form, calculate dosage based on level of drug because drops and elixir have different concentrations.
• Use P.R. in young children or other patients for whom oral forms aren't practical.
Patient teaching
• ⓈALERT: Tell patient that drug is for short-term use only. Prescriber should be consulted if child takes drug for longer than 5 days or, for adults, longer than 10 days.
• ⓈALERT: Tell patient not to use drug for fever that's above 103.1° F (39.5° C), lasts longer than 3 days, or recurs.
• Warn patient that high doses or unsupervised long-term use can cause liver damage. Excessive alcohol use may increase risk of hepatotoxicity.
• Tell patient to keep track of daily acetaminophen intake, including OTC and prescription medications. Warn patient not to exceed total recommended dose of acetaminophen per day because of risk of hepatotoxicity.
• Tell breast-feeding woman that drug appears in breast milk in levels less than 1% of dose.

Reactions may be *common*, uncommon, *life-threatening*, or COMMON AND LIFE-THREATENING.

She may use the recommended dose safely for short-term therapy.

☑ **Evaluation**
• Patient reports pain relief with drug.
• Patient's liver function test results remain normal.
• Patient and family state understanding of drug therapy.

acetazolamide
(ah-see-tuh-ZOH-luh-mighd)
Acetazolam, Apo-Acetazolamide, Diamox, Diamox Sequels

acetazolamide sodium
Diamox

Pharmacologic class: carbonic anhydrase inhibitor
Therapeutic class: anticonvulsant, diuretic
Pregnancy risk category: C

Indications and dosages

▶ **Secondary glaucoma and preoperative management of acute angle-closure glaucoma.** *Adults:* 250 mg P.O. q 4 hours, or 250 mg P.O. or I.V. b.i.d. for short-term therapy. For some acute glaucomas, 500 mg P.O.; then 125 mg to 250 mg P.O. q 4 hours.
▶ **Edema in heart failure.** *Adults:* 250 to 375 mg (5 mg/kg) P.O. daily in a.m.
▶ **Chronic open-angle glaucoma.** *Adults:* 250 mg to 1 g P.O. daily in divided doses q.i.d., or 500 mg extended-release P.O. b.i.d.
▶ **Prevention or amelioration of acute mountain sickness.** *Adults:* 500 mg to 1 g P.O. daily in divided doses q 8 to 12 hours, or 500 mg extended-release P.O. q 12 hours. Therapy should start 24 to 48 hours before ascent and continue for 48 hours while at high altitude.
▶ **Adjunct treatment of myoclonic, refractory generalized tonic-clonic, absence, or mixed seizures.** *Adults and children:* 8 to 30 mg/kg P.O. daily in divided doses. Optimum dosage, 375 mg to 1 g daily. When given with other anticonvulsants, the initial dose is 250 mg daily.
▶ **Drug-induced edema.** *Adults:* 250 to 375 mg (5 mg/kg) P.O. as a single dose for 1 or 2 days alternating with one drug-free day.

▶ **Periodic paralysis.** *Adults:* 250 mg P.O. b.i.d. or t.i.d., not to exceed 1.5 g daily.

▽ **I.V. administration**
• Reconstitute 500-mg vial with at least 5 ml of sterile water for injection.
• Inject 100 to 500 mg/minute into large vein, using 21G or 23G needle.
• Intermittent or continuous infusion isn't recommended.
• Use within 24 hours.
⊗ **Incompatibilities**
Multivitamins.

Contraindications and cautions

• Contraindicated in patients hypersensitive to drug, patients undergoing long-term therapy for chronic noncongestive angle-closure glaucoma, and patients with hyponatremia, hypokalemia, renal or hepatic impairment, adrenal gland failure, and hyperchloremic acidosis.
• Use cautiously in patients with respiratory acidosis, emphysema, or COPD, and in patients receiving other diuretics.
⚘ **Lifespan:** In pregnant women, use cautiously. In breast-feeding women, drug is contraindicated. In children, safety and effectiveness of drug haven't been established, and cases of growth retardation have been reported.

Adverse reactions

CNS: drowsiness, paresthesia, confusion.
EENT: transient myopia.
GI: nausea, vomiting, anorexia, altered taste.
GU: crystalluria, renal calculi, hematuria.
Hematologic: *aplastic anemia,* hemolytic anemia, *leukopenia.*
Metabolic: *hyperchloremic acidosis,* asymptomatic hyperuricemia, hypokalemia.
Skin: rash.
Other: *pain at injection site,* sterile abscesses.

Interactions

Drug-drug. *Amphetamines, anticholinergics, mecamylamine, procainamide, quinidine, tricyclic antidepressants:* May decrease renal clearance of these drugs, increasing toxicity. Monitor patient closely.
Cyclosporine: May increase cyclosporine level, causing toxicity. Use cautiously together.
Lithium: May increase lithium secretion. Monitor patient.

Methenamine: May reduce effectiveness of acetazolamide. Avoid using together.
Salicylates: May cause accumulation and toxicity of acetazolamide, including CNS depression and metabolic acidosis. Monitor patient closely.
Phenytoin: May increase occurrence of osteomalacia with long-term use together. Use cautiously together.
Primidone: May decrease absorption of primidone, reducing anticonvulsant effects. Use cautiously together.

Effects on lab test results

• May increase uric acid level. May decrease potassium and hemoglobin levels and hematocrit. May increase or decrease glucose and theophylline levels.
• May decrease WBC count and thyroid iodine uptake.
• May cause false-positive urine protein test results.

Pharmacokinetics

Absorption: Well absorbed from GI tract.
Distribution: Throughout body tissues.
Metabolism: None.
Excretion: Mainly in urine. *Half-life:* 10 to 15 hours.

Route	Onset	Peak	Duration
P.O.			
capsules	2 hr	8–12 hr	18–24 hr
tablets	1–1½ hr	2–4 hr	8–12 hr
I.V.	2 min	15 min	4–5 hr

Action

Chemical effect: Blocks action of carbonic anhydrase, promoting urine excretion of sodium, potassium, bicarbonate, and water. Decreases secretion of aqueous humor in eye. May decrease abnormal paroxysmal or excessive neuronal discharge. Produces respiratory and metabolic acidosis that may encourage ventilation, increase cerebral blood flow, and help release oxygen from hemoglobin.
Therapeutic effect: Lowers intraocular pressure (IOP), controls seizure activity, and may improve respiratory function.

Available forms

Capsules (extended-release): 500 mg
Injection: 500 mg/vial
Tablets: 125 mg, 250 mg

NURSING PROCESS

✍ Assessment

• In patients with glaucoma, assess eye discomfort and IOP before and during therapy; in those with heart failure, assess edema, and in those with seizures, assess neurologic condition.
• Closely monitor intake and output.
• Be alert for adverse reactions and drug interactions.
• Assess patient's and family's knowledge of drug therapy.

✛ Nursing diagnoses

• Excessive fluid volume related to patient's underlying condition
• Impaired urine elimination related to diuretic action of drug
• Deficient knowledge related to drug therapy

▷ Planning and implementation

• Give oral preparation early in the morning to avoid nocturia. Give second dose early in the afternoon.
• If patient can't swallow oral form, ask pharmacist to make a suspension using crushed tablets in flavored syrup. Although concentrations up to 500 mg/5 ml are possible, concentrations of 250 mg/5 ml are more palatable. Refrigeration improves palatability but doesn't improve stability. Suspensions are stable for 1 week.
• Diuretic effect decreases with acidosis but is re-established by stopping drug for several days and then restarting it, or by using intermittent administration.
⊗ ALERT: Don't confuse acetazolamide with acetohexamide. Also don't confuse acetazolamide sodium (Diamox) with acyclovir sodium (Zovirax). These vials may appear similar.
• If hypersensitivity or adverse reactions occur, withhold drug and notify prescriber.
Patient teaching
• Advise patient to take drug early in the day to avoid sleep interruption caused by nocturia.
• Teach patient to monitor fluid volume by measuring weight, intake, and output daily.
• Encourage patient to avoid high-sodium foods and to choose high-potassium foods.
• Teach patient to recognize and report signs and symptoms of fluid and electrolyte imbalance.

Reactions may be *common,* uncommon, *life-threatening,* or COMMON AND LIFE-THREATENING.

☑ Evaluation
• Patient is free from edema.
• Patient adjusts lifestyle to accommodate altered patterns of urine elimination.
• Patient and family state understanding of drug therapy.

acetylcysteine
(as-ee-til-SIS-teen)
Acetadote, Mucosil-10, Mucosil-20, Mucomyst, Mucomyst-10

Pharmacologic class: amino acid (L-cysteine) derivative
Therapeutic class: mucolytic, antidote for acetaminophen overdose
Pregnancy risk category: B

Indications and dosages

▶ **Pneumonia, bronchitis, tuberculosis, cystic fibrosis, emphysema, atelectasis (adjunct), complications of thoracic and CV surgery.**
Adults and children: 1 to 2 ml of 10% or 20% solution by direct instillation into trachea as often as hourly; or 3 to 5 ml of 20% solution or 6 to 10 ml of 10% solution by nebulization q 2 to 3 hours p.r.n.
▶ **Acetaminophen toxicity.** *Adults and children:* Initially, 140 mg/kg P.O., followed by 70 mg/kg P.O. q 4 hours for 17 doses; or if using I.V. formulation, give 150 mg/kg loading dose in 200 ml of D₅W, infused I.V. over 15 minutes. Then begin maintenance doses of 50 mg/kg in 500 ml of D₅W, infused I.V. over 4 hours, followed by 100 mg/kg in 1 L of D₅W, infused I.V. over 16 hours.
▶ **To prevent acute renal failure related to radiographic contrast media‡.** *Adults:* 600 mg P.O. b.i.d. given the day before and on the day of contrast media administration for a total of four doses. Or, if for hydration, give with half-normal saline solution I.V. infusion at 1 ml/kg/hour for 12 hours before and 12 hours after contrast media administration.

▼ I.V. administration
• Dilute initial dose of 150 mg/kg in 200 ml of D₅W, and infuse over 15 minutes.
• Dilute second dose of 50 mg/kg in 500 ml of D₅W, and infuse over 4 hours.

• Dilute final dose of 100 mg/kg in 1 L of D₅W, and infuse over 16 hours.
• Store unopened vials at controlled room temperature, 68° to 77° F (20° to 25° C). Reconstituted solution is stable for 24 hours.
⊗ **Incompatibilities**
Rubber and metals, particularly iron, copper, and nickel.

Contraindications and cautions
• Contraindicated in patients hypersensitive to drug.
• Use cautiously in debilitated patients with severe respiratory insufficiency. In patients with asthma or a history of bronchospasm, use I.V. formulation cautiously.
Lifespan: In pregnant and breast-feeding women and in elderly patients with severe respiratory insufficiency, use cautiously.

Adverse reactions
EENT: rhinorrhea, hemoptysis.
GI: stomatitis, nausea, vomiting.
Respiratory: BRONCHOSPASM.

Interactions
Drug-drug. *Activated charcoal:* May limit acetylcysteine's effectiveness. Avoid using together in treating drug toxicity.

Effects on lab test results
None reported.

Pharmacokinetics
Absorption: Most inhaled acetylcysteine acts directly on mucus in lungs; remainder is absorbed by pulmonary epithelium. After oral administration, drug is absorbed from GI tract.
Distribution: Protein bound (50%).
Metabolism: In liver.
Excretion: The mean elimination terminal half-life is longer in newborns (11 hours) than in adults (5½ hours). *Half-life:* 6¼ hours.

Route	Onset	Peak	Duration
P.O., I.V., inhalation	Unknown	Unknown	Unknown

Action
Chemical effect: Increases respiratory tract fluids to help liquefy tenacious secretions. Restores glutathione in liver to treat acetaminophen toxicity.

Therapeutic effect: Thins respiratory secretions and reverses toxic effects of acetaminophen.

Available forms

I.V. injection: 20% in 30 ml vials
Oral or inhalation solution: 10%, 20%

NURSING PROCESS

℞ Assessment
• Assess patient's respiratory secretions before and frequently during therapy.
• Be alert for adverse reactions and drug interactions.
• Assess patient's and family's knowledge of drug therapy.

⊕ Nursing diagnoses
• Ineffective airway clearance related to patient's underlying condition
• Impaired oral mucous membrane related to drug-induced stomatitis
• Deficient knowledge related to drug therapy

⧁ Planning and implementation
• Dilute oral doses with cola, fruit juice, or water before giving to treat acetaminophen overdose. Dilute 20% solution to a concentration of 5% by adding 3 ml of diluent to each ml of acetylcysteine. If patient vomits within 1 hour of initial or maintenance dose, repeat dose.
⊛ ALERT: If the time of ingestion is unknown or the acetaminophen level isn't available or can't be interpreted within 8 hours of ingestion, immediately give drug I.V.
⊛ ALERT: Don't confuse acetylcysteine with acetylcholine.
• Use plastic, glass, stainless steel, or another nonreactive metal when giving by nebulization. Drug isn't compatible with rubber or metals, especially iron, copper, and nickel.
• Hand-bulb nebulizers aren't recommended because output is too small and particle size is too large.
• Before aerosol administration, have patient clear airway by coughing.
⊛ ALERT: Drug is incompatible with tetracyclines, erythromycin lactobionate, amphotericin B, and ampicillin sodium. If given by aerosol inhalation, these drugs should be nebulized separately. Iodized oil, trypsin, and hydrogen peroxide are incompatible with drug. Don't add these drugs to nebulizer.

• Have suction equipment available in case patient can't effectively clear his air passages.
• Alert prescriber if patient's respiratory secretions thicken or become purulent or if bronchospasm occurs.
• After opening, store in refrigerator, and use within 4 days.

Patient teaching
• Instruct patient to follow directions on drug label exactly. Explain importance of using drug as directed.
• If patient's condition doesn't improve within 10 days, tell him to notify prescriber. Drug shouldn't be used for prolonged period without direct medical supervision.
• Teach patient how to use and clean nebulizer.
• Inform patient that drug may have foul taste or smell.
• Instruct patient to clear his airway by coughing before aerosol administration to achieve maximum effect.
• Instruct patient to rinse mouth with water after nebulizer treatment because it may leave sticky coating.

☑ Evaluation
• Patient has clear lung sounds, decreased respiratory secretions, and reduced frequency and severity of cough.
• Patient's oral mucous membranes remain unchanged.
• Patient and family state understanding of drug therapy.

activated charcoal
(AK-tih-vay-ted CHAR-kohl)
Actidose†, Actidose-Aqua†, CharcoAid†, CharcoCaps†, Insta-Char Pediatric†, Liqui-Char†, SuperChar†

Pharmacologic class: adsorbent
Therapeutic class: antidote
Pregnancy risk category: C

Indications and dosages

▶ **Poisoning.** *Adults:* Initially, 1 g/kg (30 to 100 g) P.O. or 5 to 10 times amount of poison ingested as suspension in 180 to 240 ml of water.
Children: Five to 10 times estimated weight of poison ingested, with minimum dose being 30 g

P.O. in 240 ml of water to make a slurry, preferably within 30 minutes of poisoning. Larger dose is necessary if food is in stomach.

▶ **Flatulence, dyspepsia.** *Adults:* 600 mg to 5 g P.O. t.i.d. after meals.

Contraindications and cautions

None reported.

Adverse reactions

GI: black stool, nausea, constipation.

Interactions

Drug-drug. *Acetylcysteine, ipecac:* May render charcoal ineffective. Don't use together and don't perform gastric lavage until all charcoal is removed.

Drug-food. *Milk, ice cream, sherbet:* May decrease effectiveness of activated charcoal.

Effects on lab test results

None reported.

Pharmacokinetics

Absorption: None.
Distribution: None.
Metabolism: None.
Excretion: In feces.

Route	Onset	Peak	Duration
P.O.	Immediate	Unknown	Unknown

Action

Chemical effect: Adheres to many drugs and chemicals, inhibiting their absorption.
Therapeutic effect: Used as antidote for selected poisons and overdoses.

Available forms

Liquid: 208 mg/ml
Oral suspension: 0.625 g/5 ml†, 1 g/5 m♦ †
Powder: 15 g†, 30 g†, 40 g†, 50 g†, 120 g†, 240 g†
Tablets: 200 mg ◇ † 300 mg ◇ †

NURSING PROCESS

Assessment

- Find out what substance was ingested and when it was ingested. Drug isn't effective for all drugs and toxic substances.
- Be alert for adverse reactions and drug interactions.
- Assess patient's and family's knowledge of drug therapy.

Nursing diagnoses

- Risk for injury related to ingestion of toxic substance or overdose
- Risk for deficient fluid volume related to drug-induced vomiting
- Deficient knowledge related to drug therapy

Planning and implementation

- Commonly used for treating poisoning or overdose of acetaminophen, aspirin, atropine, barbiturates, cardiac glycosides, poisonous mushrooms, oxalic acid, parathion, phenol, phenytoin, propantheline, propoxyphene, strychnine, or tricyclic antidepressants. Check with poison control center for use in other types of poisonings or overdoses.
- Give after emesis because drug absorbs and inactivates syrup of ipecac.

ALERT: Don't give to a semiconscious or unconscious patient unless airway is protected and NG tube is in place for instillation.

- Mix powder form (most effective) with tap water to form consistency of thick syrup. Add small amount of fruit juice or flavoring to make mix more palatable.
- Give by NG tube after lavage, if needed.
- Don't give in ice cream, milk, or sherbet, which may reduce absorption.
- If patient vomits shortly after administration, repeat dose.
- Keep airway, oxygen, and suction equipment nearby.
- Follow treatment with stool softener or laxative to prevent constipation.

ALERT: Don't confuse Actidose with Actos.

Patient teaching

- Warn patient that feces will be black.
- Instruct patient to report respiratory difficulty immediately.

Evaluation

- Patient doesn't experience injury from ingesting toxic substance or from overdose.
- Patient exhibits no signs of deficient fluid volume.
- Patient and family state understanding of drug therapy.

acyclovir sodium

(ay-SIGH-kloh-veer SOH-dee-um)

Aciclovir ◊, Acihexal ◊, Avirax ♦, Zovirax†

Pharmacologic class: synthetic purine nucleoside
Therapeutic class: antiviral
Pregnancy risk category: B

Indications and dosages

▶ **Chickenpox.** *Adults and children weighing more than 40 kg (88 lb):* 800 mg P.O. q.i.d. for 5 days.
Children age 2 and older weighing less than 40 kg: 20 mg/kg P.O. q.i.d. for 5 days.
▶ **Acute herpes zoster.** *Adults:* 800 mg P.O. q 4 hours, five times daily for 7 to 10 days. Give within 48 hours of rash onset.
▶ **Initial genital herpes.** *Adults:* 200 mg P.O. q 4 hours during waking hours (total of 5 capsules daily) for 10 days.
▶ **Intermittent therapy for recurrent genital herpes.** *Adults:* 200 mg P.O. q 4 hours during waking hours (total of 5 capsules daily) for 5 days. Start therapy at first sign of recurrence.
▶ **Long-term suppressive therapy for recurrent genital herpes.** *Adults:* 400 mg P.O. b.i.d. for up to 12 months.
Adjust-a-dose: For patients with renal impairment, if usual dosage is 800 mg five times daily and creatinine clearance is 10 to 25 ml/minute, decrease dosage to 800 mg q 8 hours. If creatinine clearance is 10 ml/minute or less, decrease the 200 to 400 mg dosage to 200 mg q 12 hours, or the 800 mg dosage to 800 mg q 12 hours.
▶ **Initial and recurrent episodes of mucocutaneous herpes simplex virus (HSV-1 and HSV-2) infections in immunocompromised patients; severe initial episodes of herpes genitalis in immunocompetent patients.** *Adults and children age 12 and older:* 5 mg/kg I.V. at constant rate over 1 hour q 8 hours for 7 days (5 days for herpes genitalis).
Children younger than age 12: 10 mg/kg I.V. at constant rate over 1 hour q 8 hours for 7 days (5 days for herpes genitalis).
▶ **Herpes simplex encephalitis.** *Adults:* 10 mg/kg I.V. infused at a constant rate over 1 hour, q 8 hours for 10 days.

Children ages 3 months to 12 years: 20 mg/kg I.V. at a constant rate over at least 1 hour, q 8 hours for 10 days.
▶ **Neonatal herpes simplex virus infections.** *Children from birth to age 3 months:* 10 mg/kg I.V. at a constant rate for over 1 hour, every 8 hours for 10 days.
▶ **Varicella zoster in immunocompromised patients.** *Adults and children age 12 and older:* 10 mg/kg I.V. infused at a constant rate over 1 hour, q 8 hours for 7 days. Obese patients should be given 10 mg/kg (ideal body weight). Don't exceed maximum dose equivalent to 500 mg/m² q 8 hours.
Children younger than age 12: 20 mg/kg I.V. q 8 hours for 7 days, or 500 mg/m² at a constant rate over at least 1 hour, q 8 hours for 7 days.
Adjust-a-dose: In patients with renal failure, if creatinine clearance exceeds 50 ml/minute, give 100% of the I.V. dose q 8 hours; if creatinine clearance is between 25 and 50 ml/minute, 100% of the dose q 12 hours; if the creatinine clearance is between 10 to 25 ml/minute, 100% of the dose q 24 hours; and if it's below 10 ml/minute, 50% of the dose q 24 hours.
▶ **Recurrent herpes labialis (cold sores).** *Adults and children age 12 and older:* Apply cream five times daily for 4 days. Start therapy as early as possible following onset of signs and symptoms.
▶ **Genital herpes in immunocompromised patients‡.** *Adults:* 400 mg P.O. three to five times daily.
▶ **Long-term suppressive or maintenance therapy for recurrent HSV infections in patients with HIV‡.** *Adults and children older than age 12:* 200 mg P.O. t.i.d. or 400 mg P.O. b.i.d.
Children age 12 and younger: 600 to 1,000 mg P.O. daily in three to five divided doses.
▶ **Acute herpes zoster ophthalmicus‡.** *Adults:* 600 mg P.O. q 4 hours five times daily for 10 days, preferably within 3 days of rash onset, but no longer than 7 days.
▶ **Rectal herpes infection‡.** *Adults:* 400 mg P.O. five times daily for 10 days or until resolved; Or, give 800 mg P.O. q 8 hours for 7 to 10 days.
▶ **Disseminated herpes zoster‡.** *Adults:* 5 to 10 mg/kg I.V. q 8 hours for 7 to 10 days. Infuse over at least 1 hour.

⊠ Adjust-a-dose: Follow oral and I.V. guidelines under Adjust-a-dose for varicella zoster in immunocompromised patients.

▼ I.V. administration

• Dissolve the contents of a 500-mg vial in 10 ml of sterile water for injection, or a 1,000-mg vial in 20 ml sterile water for injection, to yield 50 mg/ml. Then dilute further in appropriate I.V. solution so that final concentration is 7 mg/ml or less. Concentrated solutions (10 mg/ml or more) increase the risk of phlebitis.
• Don't use bacteriostatic water containing benzyl alcohol or parabens.
• Give I.V. infusion over at least 1 hour to prevent renal tubular damage. Don't give by bolus injection.
• Don't exceed a maximum dose equivalent of 20 mg/kg every 8 hours for any patient.
• Make sure I.V. infusion is accompanied by adequate hydration. Monitor intake and output closely during administration.
⊗ **Incompatibilities**
Biological or colloidal solutions, idarubicin hydrochloride, parabens.

Contraindications and cautions

• Contraindicated in patients hypersensitive to drug.
• Use cautiously in patients with underlying neurologic problems, renal disease, or dehydration and in those receiving other nephrotoxic drugs.
⚕ **Lifespan:** In pregnant or breast-feeding women, use cautiously. In children younger than age 2, safety and effectiveness of drug haven't been established.

Adverse reactions

CNS: *encephalopathic changes* (including lethargy, obtundation, tremor, confusion, hallucinations, agitation, *seizures, coma,* headache [with I.V. dosage]), ataxia, aggressive behavior, fatigue, fever, pain.
CV: peripheral edema, hypotension.
GI: nausea, vomiting, diarrhea, abdominal pain.
GU: hematuria.
Hematologic: *DIC, hemolysis, leukopenia.*
Hepatic: *hepatitis,* hyperbilirubinemia, jaundice.
Musculoskeletal: myalgia.
Skin: rash, itching, *vesicular eruptions.*

Other: inflammation, phlebitis at injection site, *anaphylaxis, angioedema.*

Interactions

Drug-drug. *Phenytoin, valproic acid:* May decrease levels of these drugs. Monitor patient closely.
Probenecid: May increase acyclovir level. Monitor patient for possible toxicity.
Zidovudine: May cause drowsiness or lethargy. Use together cautiously.

Effects on lab test results

• May increase BUN, creatinine, liver enzyme, and bilirubin levels. May decrease hemoglobin level and hematocrit.
• May increase or decrease platelet, neutrophil, and WBC counts.

Pharmacokinetics

Absorption: Slow and only 15% to 30% is absorbed. Not affected by food.
Distribution: Widely to organ tissues and body fluids. CSF levels equal about 50% of serum levels, and 9% to 33% binds to plasma proteins.
Metabolism: Primarily inside viral cell to its active form.
Excretion: Up to 92% of systemically absorbed acyclovir is excreted unchanged by kidneys.
Half-life: 2 to 3½ hours with normal renal function; up to 19 hours with renal impairment.

Route	Onset	Peak	Duration
P.O.	Unknown	Unknown	Unknown
I.V.	Immediate	Immediate	Unknown

Action

Chemical effect: Becomes incorporated into viral DNA and inhibits viral multiplication.
Therapeutic effect: Kills susceptible viruses.

Available forms

Injection: 500 mg/vial, 1 g/vial
Suspension: 200 mg/5 ml
Tablets: 400 mg, 800 mg

NURSING PROCESS

⚗ Assessment
• Assess infection before and regularly during therapy.

Rapid onset *Liquid form contains alcohol. ◆ Canada ◇ Australia †OTC ✐Photoguide ‡Off-label use

• Monitor patient for renal toxicity. Dehydration, renal disease, and use of other nephrotoxic drugs increase risk.
• Monitor patient's mental condition when giving drug I.V. Encephalopathic changes are more likely in patients with neurologic disorders or in those who have had neurologic reactions to cytotoxic drugs.
• If adverse GI reactions occur with oral administration, monitor patient's hydration.
• Assess patient's and family's knowledge of drug therapy.

🔁 **Nursing diagnoses**
• Infection related to presence of virus
• Risk for deficient fluid volume related to adverse GI reactions to oral drug
• Deficient knowledge related to drug therapy

▶ **Planning and implementation**
⊛ **ALERT:** Don't give I.M., subcutaneously, or by bolus injection.
⊛ **ALERT:** Don't confuse Zovirax with Zyvox.
⊛ **ALERT:** Don't confuse acyclovir sodium with acetazolamide sodium. The vials may look alike.
Patient teaching
• Explain that drug effectively manages herpes infection but doesn't eliminate or cure it.
• Warn patient that drug won't prevent spread of infection to others.
• Help patient to recognize early symptoms of herpes infection (tingling, itching, pain) so he can take drug before infection fully develops.
• Tell patient to alert nurse if he has pain or discomfort at I.V. injection site.

☑ **Evaluation**
• Patient's infection is eradicated.
• Patient maintains adequate hydration.
• Patient and family state understanding of drug therapy.

adalimumab
(ay-da-LIM-yoo-mab)
Humira

Pharmacologic class: tumor necrosis factor (TNF)-alpha blocker
Therapeutic class: antirheumatic
Pregnancy risk category: B

Indications and dosages
▶ **To reduce signs and symptoms and structural damage and improve physical function in patients with moderate to severe active rheumatoid arthritis that hasn't responded well to disease-modifying antirheumatics.** *Adults:* 40 mg subcutaneously q other week. May increase to 40 mg q week if patient isn't taking methotrexate.
▶ **To reduce signs and symptoms of active psoriatic arthritis.** *Adults:* 40 mg subcutaneously q other week.

Contraindications and cautions
• Contraindicated in patients hypersensitive to drug or any of its components. Don't start drug if patient is immunosuppressed or has a chronic or localized active infection.
• Use cautiously in patients with a history of recurrent infection, those with underlying conditions that predispose them to infections, and those who have lived in areas where tuberculosis and histoplasmosis are common. Use cautiously in patients with CNS-demyelinating disorders.
☀ **Lifespan:** In pregnant women, give only if benefits outweigh risks to the fetus because no well-controlled studies exist. Breast-feeding women should stop nursing or stop using the drug because of the risk for serious adverse reactions. It's unknown whether drug appears in breast milk or would be absorbed by a breast-feeding infant. In children, safety and effectiveness of drug haven't been established. In elderly patients, use cautiously because serious infections and malignancies are more common in these patients.

Adverse reactions
CNS: headache.
CV: hypertension.
EENT: sinusitis.
GI: nausea, abdominal pain.
GU: UTI, hematuria.
Hematologic: *pancytopenia, thrombocytopenia, leukopenia.*
Metabolic: hypercholesterolemia, hyperlipidemia.
Musculoskeletal: back pain.
Respiratory: upper respiratory tract infection, bronchitis.
Skin: rash.

Reactions may be *common*, uncommon, *life-threatening*, or COMMON AND LIFE-THREATENING.

Other: *malignancy, serious infections, sepsis,* flu syndrome, *accidental injury,* allergic reactions, injection site reactions (erythema, itching, hemorrhage, pain, swelling), *anaphylaxis.*

Interactions

Drug-drug. *Anakinra:* May cause serious infections. Avoid use together.
Live-virus vaccines: May cause immunosuppression and susceptibility to disease. Avoid using together.

Effects on lab test results

• May increase cholesterol level.

Pharmacokinetics

Absorption: Average absolute bioavailability is 64%.
Distribution: Levels in synovial fluid are 31% to 96% of those in serum.
Metabolism: Clearance may be higher if anti-adalimumab antibodies are present and lower in patients age 40 and older.
Excretion: Unknown. *Half-life:* Ranges from 10 to 20 days.

Route	Onset	Peak	Duration
SubQ	Variable	Variable	Unknown

Action

Chemical effect: Blocks human TNF-alpha that aids normal inflammatory and immune responses and the inflammation and joint destruction of rheumatoid arthritis.
Therapeutic effect: Reduces signs and symptoms of rheumatoid arthritis.

Available forms

Injection: 40 mg/0.8 ml

NURSING PROCESS

⚗ Assessment

• Assess patient for immunosuppression or active infection before therapy and regularly thereafter.
• Monitor patient for hypersensitivity reaction.

⊞ Nursing diagnoses

• Alteration in mobility status related to rheumatoid arthritis
• Deficient knowledge related to signs and symptoms of immunosuppression or infection

• Deficient knowledge related to drug therapy

⊠ Planning and implementation

• Drug can be given alone or with methotrexate or other disease-modifying antirheumatics.
• Give first dose under supervision of experienced health care provider.
• Evaluate patient for latent tuberculosis and, if present, start treatment before giving drug.
• Serious infections and sepsis, including tuberculosis and invasive opportunistic fungal infections, may occur. If patient develops new infection during treatment, monitor him closely.
Ⓢ **ALERT:** The needle cover contains latex and shouldn't be handled by those with latex sensitivity.
• Stop drug if patient develops a severe infection, anaphylaxis, other serious allergic reaction, or evidence of a lupuslike syndrome.
Patient teaching
• Tell patient to report evidence of tuberculosis.
• If appropriate, teach patient or caregiver how to give drug.
• Tell patient to rotate injection sites and to avoid tender, bruised, red, or hard skin.
• Teach patient to dispose of used vials, needles, and syringes safely.
• Tell patient to refrigerate drug in its original container before use.
Ⓢ **ALERT:** Warn patient to seek immediate medical attention for symptoms of blood dyscrasias or infection, including fever, bruising, bleeding, and pallor.

▨ Evaluation

• Patient experiences reduced signs and symptoms of rheumatoid arthritis.
• Patient remains free from infection during therapy.
• Patient and family state understanding of drug therapy.

adefovir dipivoxil
(uh-DEPH-uh-veer dih-pih-VOCKS-ul)
Hepsera

Pharmacologic class: acyclic nucleotide analogue
Therapeutic class: antiviral
Pregnancy risk category: C

Indications and dosages

▶ **Chronic hepatitis B infection.** *Adults:*
10 mg P.O. daily.
☒ **Adjust-a-dose:** For patients with renal impairment, if creatinine clearance is 20 to 49 ml/minute, give 10 mg P.O. q 2 days. If creatinine clearance is 10 to 19 ml/minute, give 10 mg P.O. q 3 days. In patients receiving hemodialysis, give 10 mg P.O. q 7 days, after dialysis session.

Contraindications and cautions

• Contraindicated in patients hypersensitive to drug or any of its components.
• Use cautiously and at a reduced dose in patients with renal impairment and in those receiving nephrotoxic drugs.
⚠ **Lifespan:** In pregnant women, use drug only if benefits outweigh risks. Women should avoid breast-feeding. It's unknown if drug appears in breast milk. In children, safety and effectiveness of drug haven't been established. In elderly patients, use cautiously because of increased risk of renal or CV dysfunction.

Adverse reactions

CNS: *asthenia,* headache, fever.
EENT: pharyngitis, sinusitis.
GI: abdominal pain, diarrhea, dyspepsia, flatulence, nausea, vomiting.
GU: *renal failure,* renal insufficiency, hematuria, glycosuria.
Hepatic: *hepatomegaly with steatosis, hepatic failure.*
Metabolic: *lactic acidosis.*
Respiratory: cough.
Skin: pruritus, rash.

Interactions

Drug-drug. *Ibuprofen:* May increase adefovir bioavailability. Monitor patient closely.
Nephrotoxic drugs, such as aminoglycosides, cyclosporine, NSAIDs, tacrolimus, vancomycin: May increase risk of nephrotoxicity. Use together cautiously.

Effects on lab test results

• May increase ALT, amylase, AST, CK, creatinine, and lactic acid levels.

Pharmacokinetics

Absorption: Readily from the GI tract with a bioavailability of 59%.

Distribution: Up to 4% bound to plasma and serum proteins.
Metabolism: Rapidly converted to adefovir diphosphate, an active metabolite.
Excretion: Undergoes renal elimination. *Half-life:* Unknown.

Route	Onset	Peak	Duration
P.O.	Unknown	1–4 hr	Unknown

Action

Chemical effect: Inhibits hepatitis B virus reverse transcriptase, which breaks the viral DNA chain.
Therapeutic effect: Reduces symptoms of hepatitis B.

Available forms

Tablets: 10 mg

NURSING PROCESS

⚕ Assessment
• Assess patient's condition before therapy and regularly thereafter.
• Watch for hypersensitivity reaction.
• Monitor renal function, especially in patients with renal dysfunction and in those taking nephrotoxic drugs.
• Monitor hepatic function.

⊕ Nursing diagnoses
• Risk for lactic acidosis, hepatomegaly, and steatosis secondary to liver disease.
• Deficient knowledge related to drug therapy.

⊠ Planning and implementation
• The ideal length of treatment hasn't been established.
• Patients should be offered HIV antibody testing because drug may promote resistance to antiretrovirals in patients with unrecognized or untreated HIV infection.
• Monitor hepatic function. If patient develops signs or symptoms of lactic acidosis and severe hepatomegaly with steatosis, notify prescriber to stop drug.
• Severe exacerbations of hepatitis may result from stopping drug. Monitor hepatic function closely in patients who stop taking drug.
⊛ **ALERT:** Patients may develop lactic acidosis and severe hepatomegaly with steatosis during

---

treatment. Risk is higher in women, obese patients, and those taking other antiretrovirals.

• Overdose causes GI adverse effects. Treating overdose includes monitoring for evidence of toxicity and giving supportive therapy. Dialysis may be helpful.

• Pregnant women exposed to drug may call the Antiretroviral Pregnancy Registry at 1-800-258-4263, to monitor fetal outcome.

Patient teaching

• Inform patient that drug may be taken with or without food.

• Tell patient to immediately report weakness, muscle pain, trouble breathing, stomach pain with nausea and vomiting, dizziness, lightheadedness, fast or irregular heartbeat, or feeling cold in the arms and legs.

• Warn patient not to stop taking drug unless directed because it could cause hepatitis to become worse.

• Instruct women to tell their prescriber if they become pregnant or are breast-feeding. Advise breast-feeding women to either stop breast-feeding or stop taking the drug.

☑ Evaluation

• Patient remains free from lactic acidosis, hepatomegaly, and steatosis during therapy.

• Patient and family state understanding of drug therapy.

adenosine
(uh-DEN-oh-seen)
Adenocard

Pharmacologic class: nucleoside
Therapeutic class: antiarrhythmic
Pregnancy risk category: C

Indications and dosages

▶ **To convert paroxysmal supraventricular tachycardia (PSVT) to sinus rhythm.** *Adults:* 6 mg I.V. by rapid bolus injection over 1 to 2 seconds. If PSVT isn't eliminated in 1 to 2 minutes, give 12 mg by rapid I.V. bolus and repeat, if needed.

▼ I.V. administration

• Check solution for crystals that may form if solution is cold. If crystals are visible, gently warm solution to room temperature. Don't use cloudy solutions.

• Give by rapid I.V. injection over 1 to 2 seconds. Give directly into vein if possible. If I.V. line is used, inject drug into most proximal port.

• Drug has a very short half-life. Follow with rapid saline flush to ensure that drug reaches systemic circulation quickly.

• Don't give single dose that exceeds 12 mg.

• Discard unused drug. It doesn't contain preservatives.

⊗ **Incompatibilities**
Other I.V. drugs.

Contraindications and cautions

• Contraindicated in patients hypersensitive to drug and in those with second- or third-degree heart block or sick-sinus syndrome unless artificial pacemaker is present. Don't repeat dose in patients who develop significant heart block from drug.

• Use cautiously in patients with asthma because bronchoconstriction may occur.

⚕ **Lifespan:** In pregnant and breast-feeding women and in children, safety of drug hasn't been established.

Adverse reactions

CNS: apprehension, burning sensation, *dizziness, headache,* heaviness in arms, *lightheadedness,* numbness, tingling in arms.
CV: *chest pressure, chest pain, facial flushing,* hypotension, palpitations, *ventricular tachycardia, ventricular fibrillation, atrial fibrillation.*
EENT: metallic taste, blurred vision, tightness in throat.
GI: nausea.
Musculoskeletal: back pain, neck pain.
Respiratory: *dyspnea,* shortness of breath, hyperventilation.
Skin: diaphoresis.

Interactions

Drug-drug. *Carbamazepine:* May cause higher degree of heart block. Monitor patient.
Digoxin, verapamil: In rare cases, may cause ventricular fibrillation. Use together cautiously.
Dipyridamole: May potentiate adenosine's effects. A smaller dose may be needed.
Methylxanthines: May antagonize adenosine's effects. A patient receiving theophylline or caffeine may require a higher dose or may not respond to therapy.

Rapid onset   *Liquid form contains alcohol.   ◆ Canada   ◇ Australia   †OTC   ✐Photoguide   ‡Off-label use

Drug-herb. *Guarana:* May decrease therapeutic response. Discourage using together.
Drug-food. *Caffeine:* May antagonize adenosine's effects. Give higher dose.

Effects on lab test results

None reported.

Pharmacokinetics

Absorption: Given I.V.
Distribution: Rapidly taken up by erythrocytes and vascular endothelial cells.
Metabolism: Within tissues to inosine and adenosine monophosphate.
Excretion: Unknown. *Half-life:* Less than 10 seconds.

Route	Onset	Peak	Duration
I.V.	Immediate	Immediate	Seconds

Action

Chemical effect: Acts on AV node to slow conduction and inhibit reentry pathways.
Therapeutic effect: Restores normal sinus rhythm.

Available forms

Injection: 3 mg/ml

NURSING PROCESS

⚕ Assessment
● Monitor patient's heart rate and rhythm before and during therapy.
● Be alert for adverse reactions and drug interactions.
● Assess patient's and family's knowledge of drug therapy.

⊕ Nursing diagnoses
● Decreased cardiac output related to arrhythmias
● Ineffective protection related to drug-induced proarrhythmias
● Deficient knowledge related to drug therapy

▷ Planning and implementation
● If ECG disturbances occur, withhold drug, obtain rhythm strip, and notify prescriber immediately.
⊛ ALERT: Have emergency equipment and drugs on hand to treat new arrhythmias.

Patient teaching
● Teach patient and family about his disease and therapy.
● Stress importance of alerting health care provider if chest pain or dyspnea occurs.
● Advise patient to avoid caffeine.

☑ Evaluation
● Patient's arrhythmias are corrected and his heart maintains normal sinus rhythm.
● Patient doesn't experience proarrhythmias.
● Patient and family state understanding of drug therapy.

albumin 5%
(al-BYOO-min)
Albuminar-5, Albutein 5%, Plasbumin-5

albumin 25%
Albuminar-25, Albutein 25%, Plasbumin-25

Pharmacologic class: blood derivative
Therapeutic class: plasma volume expander
Pregnancy risk category: C

Indications and dosages

▶ **Hypovolemic shock.** *Adults:* Initially, 500 ml 5% solution by I.V. infusion; repeat, p.r.n. Dosage varies with patient's condition and response. Maximum, 250 g in 48 hours.
Children: 10 to 20 ml/kg 5% solution by I.V. infusion, repeated in 15 to 30 minutes if response isn't adequate. Or, 2.5 to 5 ml/kg 25% solution I.V.; repeat after 10 to 30 minutes, if needed.
▶ **Hypoproteinemia.** *Adults:* 1,000 to 1,500 ml 5% solution by I.V. infusion daily, with maximum rate of 5 to 10 ml/minute; or 200 to 300 ml 25% solution by I.V. infusion daily, with maximum rate of 3 ml/minute. Dosage varies with patient's condition and response.
▶ **Hyperbilirubinemia.** *Infants:* 1 g albumin (4 ml 25%)/kg I.V. 1 to 2 hours before transfusion.

▼ I.V. administration

● Don't waste drug when preparing and giving. This drug is expensive, and random shortages are common.
● Dilute with normal saline solution or D_5W. Use solution promptly and discard any unused solution because it doesn't contain preserva-

tives. Don't use cloudy solutions or those containing sediment. Solution should be clear amber.
• Avoid infusing 10 ml/minute or faster. Infusion rate is individualized according to patient's age, condition, and diagnosis. Albumin 5% is infused undiluted; albumin 25% may be undiluted or diluted with normal saline or D_5W injection.
• Follow storage instructions on bottle. Freezing may cause bottle to break.
• Don't give more than 250 g in 48 hours.
⊗ **Incompatibilities**
Verapamil hydrochloride.

Contraindications and cautions

• Contraindicated in patients hypersensitive to drug.
• Use cautiously in patients with hypertension, cardiac disease, severe pulmonary infection, severe chronic anemia, or hypoalbuminemia with peripheral edema.
⚖ **Lifespan:** In pregnant women, use cautiously.

Adverse reactions

CNS: fever.
CV: *vascular overload,* hypotension, altered pulse rate.
GI: increased salivation, nausea, vomiting.
Respiratory: altered respiration.
Skin: urticaria, rash.
Other: chills.

Interactions

None significant.

Effects on lab test results

• May increase albumin level.

Pharmacokinetics

Absorption: Given I.V.
Distribution: Albumin accounts for about 50% of plasma proteins. Ito intravascular space and extravascular sites, including skin, muscle, and lungs.
Metabolism: Unknown.
Excretion: Unknown. *Half-life:* 15 to 20 days.

Route	Onset	Peak	Duration
I.V.	Immediate	15 min	Up to several hr

Action

Chemical effect: Albumin 5% supplies colloid to blood and increases plasma volume. Albumin 25% causes fluid to shift from interstitial spaces to circulation, slightly increasing protein level and providing hemodilution.
Therapeutic effect: Relieves shock by increasing plasma volume and corrects plasma protein deficiency.

Available forms

albumin 5% injection: 50-ml, 250-ml, 500-ml, 1,000-ml vials
albumin 25% injection: 20-ml, 50-ml, 100-ml vials

NURSING PROCESS

Assessment
• Assess patient's underlying condition.
• Be alert for adverse reactions.
• Monitor fluid intake and output; protein, electrolyte, and hemoglobin levels; and hematocrit.
• Monitor patient's blood pressure often during therapy.
• Assess patient's and family's knowledge of drug therapy.

Nursing diagnoses
• Deficient fluid volume related to patient's underlying condition
• Excessive fluid volume related to adverse effects of drug
• Deficient knowledge related to drug therapy

Planning and implementation
• One volume of albumin 25% is equivalent to five volumes of albumin 5% in producing hemodilution and relative anemia.
• Withhold fluids in patient with cerebral edema for 8 hours after infusion to avoid fluid overload.
• If hypotension occurs, slow or stop infusion. Use vasopressor, if needed.
Patient teaching
• Explain how and why albumin is given.
• Tell patient to report chills, fever, dyspnea, nausea, or rash immediately.

Evaluation
• Patient's deficient fluid volume is resolved.
• Patient doesn't experience fluid overload.

• Patient and family state understanding of drug therapy.

albuterol sulfate (salbutamol sulfate)

(al-BYOO-ter-oll SUHL-fayt)
AccuNeb, Airomir ◇, Asmol CFC-free ◇, Proventil, Proventil HFA, Proventil Repetabs, Ventolin, Ventolin CFC-free ◇, Ventolin HFA, Ventolin Rotacaps ◇, Volmax, VoSpire ER

Pharmacologic class: adrenergic
Therapeutic class: bronchodilator
Pregnancy risk category: C

Indications and dosages

▶ **To prevent exercise-induced broncho-spasm.** *Adults and children age 4 and older:* Two aerosol inhalations 15 to 30 minutes before exercise.
▶ **To prevent or treat bronchospasm in patients with reversible obstructive airway disease.** *Aerosol. Adults and children age 4 and older:* One or two inhalations q 4 to 6 hours. More frequent administration and more inhalations aren't recommended. Proventil brand isn't indicated for use in children younger than age 12.
Solution for inhalation. Adults and children age 12 and older: 2.5 mg solution for inhalation by nebulizer t.i.d. or q.i.d. To prepare solution, use 0.5 ml of 0.5% solution diluted with 2.5 ml normal saline solution. Or, use 3 ml of 0.083% solution.
Children ages 2 to 11: Initially, 0.1 to 0.15 mg/kg solution for inhalation by nebulizer, with subsequent dosing adjusted to response. Don't exceed 2.5 mg t.i.d. or q.i.d. by nebulization.
Tablets. Adults and children older than age 12: 2- to 4-mg tablets P.O. t.i.d. or q.i.d. Maximum, 8 mg q.i.d.
Children ages 6 to 12: 2-mg tablets P.O. t.i.d. or q.i.d. Maximum, 6 mg q.i.d. Or, 4- to 8-mg extended-release tablets P.O. q 12 hours. Maximum, 12 to 16 mg b.i.d.
Syrup. Adults and children age 15 and older: 2 to 4 mg (5 to 10 ml) syrup P.O. t.i.d. or q.i.d. Maximum, 8 mg P.O. q.i.d.

Children ages 6 to 14: 2 mg (5 ml) syrup P.O. t.i.d. or q.i.d. Maximum, 24 mg daily in divided doses.
Children ages 2 to 5: Initially, 0.1 mg/kg syrup P.O. t.i.d. Starting dose shouldn't exceed 2 mg (5 ml) t.i.d. Maximum, 4 mg (10 ml) t.i.d.
🔃 **Adjust-a-dose:** For elderly patients and patients sensitive to beta stimulators, 2-mg tablets P.O. t.i.d. or q.i.d. tablets or syrup. Maximum, 8 mg t.i.d. or q.i.d.

Contraindications and cautions

• Contraindicated in patients hypersensitive to drug or its components.
• Use cautiously in patients with CV disorders (including coronary insufficiency and hypertension), hyperthyroidism, or diabetes mellitus and in those unusually responsive to adrenergics.
• Use extended-release tablets cautiously in patients with GI narrowing.
🔅 **Lifespan:** With pregnant women, use cautiously. Breast-feeding women shouldn't take drug. In children, safety of drug hasn't been established in those younger than age 6 for tablets and Repetabs, younger than age 4 for aerosol and capsules for inhalation, and younger than age 2 for inhalation solution and syrup. In elderly patients, use cautiously.

Adverse reactions

CNS: *tremor, nervousness,* dizziness, insomnia, headache.
CV: tachycardia, palpitations, hypertension.
EENT: drying and irritation of nose and throat.
GI: heartburn, nausea, vomiting.
Metabolic: hypokalemia, weight loss.
Musculoskeletal: muscle cramps.
Respiratory: *bronchospasm.*

Interactions

Drug-drug. *CNS stimulants:* May increase CNS stimulation. Avoid using together.
Levodopa: May increase risk of arrhythmias. Monitor patient closely.
MAO inhibitors, tricyclic antidepressants: May increase adverse CV effects. Monitor patient closely.
Propranolol, other beta blockers: May antagonize each other. Monitor patient carefully.
Drug-herb. *Herbs containing caffeine:* May have additive adverse effects. Discourage using together.

Reactions may be *common*, uncommon, *life-threatening*, or COMMON AND LIFE-THREATENING.

Drug-food. *Caffeine:* May increase CNS stimulation. Discourage using together.

Effects on lab test results

• May decrease potassium level.

Pharmacokinetics

Absorption: After inhalation, most of dose is swallowed and absorbed through GI tract.
Distribution: Doesn't cross blood–brain barrier.
Metabolism: Extensively in liver to inactive compounds.
Excretion: Rapidly in urine and feces. *Half-life:* About 4 hours.

Route	Onset	Peak	Duration
P.O.	15–30 min	2–3 hr	6–12 hr
Inhalation	5–15 min	1–1½ hr	3–6 hr

Action

Chemical effect: Relaxes bronchial and uterine smooth muscle by acting on beta$_2$-adrenergic receptors.
Therapeutic effect: Improves ventilation.

Available forms

Aerosol inhaler: 90 mcg/metered spray, 100 mcg/metered spray
Capsules: 200 mcg ◊
Solution for inhalation: 0.083%, 0.5%, 0.63 mg/3 ml, 1.25 mg/3 ml
Syrup: 2 mg/5 ml
Tablets: 2 mg, 4 mg
Tablets (extended-release): 4 mg, 8 mg

NURSING PROCESS

Assessment
• Obtain baseline assessment of patient's respiratory status, and assess patient often during therapy.
• Be alert for adverse reactions and drug interactions.
• Assess patient's and family's knowledge of drug therapy.

Nursing diagnoses
• Impaired gas exchange related to underlying respiratory condition
• Risk for injury related to drug-induced adverse reactions
• Deficient knowledge related to drug therapy

Planning and implementation
• Pleasant-tasting syrup may be taken by children as young as age 2. Syrup contains no alcohol or sugar.
• If more than one dose is ordered, wait at least 2 minutes between nebulized doses. If corticosteroid inhaler also is used, first have patient use bronchodilator, wait 5 minutes, and then have patient use corticosteroid inhaler. This permits bronchodilator to open air passages for maximum effectiveness.
• Aerosol form may be prescribed for use 15 minutes before exercise to prevent exercise-induced bronchospasm.
• Patients may use tablets and aerosol together.
• **ALERT:** Don't confuse albuterol with atenolol or Albutein.

Patient teaching
• Warn patient to stop drug immediately if paradoxical bronchospasm occurs.
• Give these instructions for using metered-dose inhaler: Clear nasal passages and throat. Breathe out, expelling as much air from lungs as possible. Place mouthpiece well into mouth and inhale deeply as dose is released. Hold breath for several seconds, remove mouthpiece, and exhale slowly.
• Advise patient to wait at least 2 minutes before repeating procedure if more than one inhalation is ordered.
• Warn patient to avoid accidentally spraying inhalant into eyes, which may cause temporary blurred vision.
• Tell patient to reduce intake of foods and herbs containing caffeine, such as coffee, cola, and chocolate, when using a bronchodilator.
• Show patient how to take his pulse. Instruct him to check pulse before and after using bronchodilator and to call prescriber if pulse rate increases more than 20 to 30 beats/minute.

Evaluation
• Patient's respiratory signs and symptoms improve.
• Patient has no injury from adverse drug reactions.
• Patient and family state understanding of drug therapy.

alefacept
(ALE-fuh-sept)
Amevive

Pharmacologic class: immunosuppressive
Therapeutic class: antipsoriatic
Pregnancy risk category: B

Indications and dosages

▶ **Moderate to severe chronic plaque psoriasis in candidates for systemic therapy or phototherapy.** *Adults:* 15 mg I.M. once weekly for 12 weeks. Another 12-week course may be given if CD4+ T lymphocyte count is normal and at least 12 weeks have passed since the previous treatment.
▷ **Adjust-a-dose:** If CD4+ T lymphocyte count is below 250 cells/mm³, withhold dose. Stop drug if CD4+ count remains below 250 cells/mm³ for 1 month.

Contraindications and cautions

• Contraindicated in patients hypersensitive to drug or its components, in patients with a history of systemic malignancy or clinically important infection, and in patients with HIV infection.
• Use cautiously in patients at high risk for malignancy and in those with chronic or recurrent infections.
✴ **Lifespan:** In pregnant women, use only if clearly needed because effects on fetus aren't known. Breast-feeding women should stop nursing or using the drug because it's not known whether drug appears in breast milk. In children, safety and effectiveness of drug haven't been established. In elderly patients, give drug cautiously because of their increased rate of infection and malignancies.

Adverse reactions

CNS: dizziness.
CV: *coronary artery disorder, MI.*
EENT: pharyngitis.
GI: nausea.
Hematologic: *lymphopenia.*
Musculoskeletal: myalgia.
Respiratory: cough.
Skin: pruritus.
Other: infection; chills; *malignancy;* hypersensitivity reaction; antibody formation; *injection site pain, inflammation,* bleeding, edema, or mass.

Interactions

Drug-drug. *Immunosuppressants, phototherapy:* May increase risk of excessive immunosuppression. Avoid using together.

Effects on lab test results

• May decrease CD4+ and CD8+ T lymphocyte counts.

Pharmacokinetics

Absorption: Unknown.
Distribution: 63% bioavailable after I.M. injection.
Metabolism: Unknown.
Excretion: Unknown.

Route	Onset	Peak	Duration
I.M.	Unknown	Unknown	Unknown

Action

Chemical effect: Interferes with lymphocyte activation and reduces CD4+ and CD8+ T lymphocyte counts.
Therapeutic effect: Reduces symptoms of psoriasis.

Available forms

Powder for injection: 15-mg single-dose vial

NURSING PROCESS

✍ Assessment
• Monitor CD4+ T lymphocyte count weekly for the 12-week course. Ensure that patient has normal CD4+ T lymphocyte count before starting therapy.
• Monitor patient carefully for evidence of infection or malignancy, and stop drug if it appears.

✎ Nursing diagnoses
• Impaired skin integrity related to psoriasis
• Risk for infection related to immunosuppressive drug therapy
• Deficient knowledge related to drug therapy

▷ Planning and implementation
⚠ **ALERT:** Rotate I.M. injection sites so that the new injection is given at least 1 inch away from

the old site and not in an area that is bruised, tender, or hard.

• Overdose may cause chills, headache, arthralgia, and sinusitis. Provide supportive care and closely monitor total lymphocyte and CD4+ T lymphocyte counts.

• Enroll pregnant women receiving drug into the Biogen Pregnancy Registry by phoning 1-866-263-8483 so that drug effects can be studied.

Patient teaching

• Warn patient about potential adverse reactions.

• Urge patient to report evidence of infection immediately.

• Inform patient that blood tests will be done regularly to monitor WBC count.

• Tell patient to notify prescriber if she is or could be pregnant within 8 weeks of receiving drug.

☑ Evaluation

• Patient's psoriasis improves.

• Patient remains free from infection.

• Patient and family state understanding of drug therapy.

alemtuzumab

(ah-lem-TOO-zeh-mab)
Campath

Pharmacologic class: monoclonal antibody
Therapeutic class: antineoplastic
Pregnancy risk category: C

Indications and dosages

▶ **B-cell chronic lymphocytic leukemia in patients treated with alkylating drugs, and for whom fludarabine therapy has failed.** *Adults:* Initially, 3 mg I.V. infusion over 2 hours daily; if tolerated, increase dose to 10 mg daily; then increase to 30 mg daily. Escalation to 30 mg usually can be accomplished in 3 to 7 days. As maintenance, give 30 mg I.V. three times weekly on nonconsecutive days (such as Monday, Wednesday, Friday) for up to 12 weeks. Don't give a single dose greater than 30 mg or a weekly dose greater than 90 mg.

🅐 Adjust-a-dose: At the first occurrence of absolute neutrophil count (ANC) of 250/mm³ or less or platelet count of 25,000/mm³ or less, stop therapy; resume at same dose when there is ANC of 500/mm³ or more or platelet count of

50,000/mm³ or more. If delay between doses is 7 days or longer, start therapy at 3 mg; increase to 10 mg, then 30 mg as tolerated. At the second occurrence of ANC of 250/mm³ or less or platelet count of 25,000/mm³ or less, stop therapy; when ANC returns to 500/mm³ or more or platelet count to 50,000/mm³ or more, resume at 10 mg; if delay between doses is 7 days or longer, start therapy at 3 mg; increase to 10 mg only. At the third occurrence of ANC of 250/mm³ or less or platelet count of 25,000/mm³ or less, stop therapy. For a decrease in ANC or platelet count that's 50% or less of the baseline value in patients starting therapy with a baseline ANC of 500/mm³ or less or a baseline platelet count 25,000/mm³ or less, stop therapy; when ANC or platelet count returns to baseline, resume therapy. If delay between doses is 7 days or longer, start therapy at 3 mg and increase to 10 mg, then 30 mg, as tolerated.

▼ I.V. administration

• Don't use solution if it's discolored or contains precipitate. Don't shake ampule before use. Filter with a sterile, low–protein-binding, 5-micron filter before dilution. Add to 100 ml normal saline solution or D₅W. Gently invert bag to mix solution.

• Premedicate with 50 mg diphenhydramine and 650 mg acetaminophen 30 minutes before initial infusion and before each dose increase. May give 200 mg hydrocortisone to decrease severe infusion-related adverse events. Give anti-infective prophylaxis, such as TMP-sulfa DS b.i.d. three times weekly and 250 mg famciclovir (or equivalent) b.i.d. Prophylaxis should continue for 2 months, or until CD4+ count is 200/mm³ or more, whichever occurs later.

• Don't give as I.V. push or bolus.

• Infuse over 2 hours.

• Protect solution from light.

• Use within 8 hours of dilution.

⊗ Incompatibilities
Other I.V. drugs.

Contraindications and cautions

• Contraindicated in patients with active systemic infections, underlying immunodeficiency (such as HIV), or type I hypersensitivity or anaphylactic reactions to drug or any of its components.

⚖ Lifespan: In pregnant women, benefits of drug should be weighed against risks to the fetus. Breast-feeding women should stop breast-feeding during treatment and for at least 3 months after taking last dose of drug. In children, safety and effectiveness of drug haven't been established.

Adverse reactions

CNS: fever, insomnia, depression, somnolence, asthenia, headache, dysthenias, dizziness, fatigue, malaise, tremor, syncope.
CV: edema, peripheral edema, hypotension, hypertension, tachycardia, SUPRAVENTRICULAR TACHYCARDIA.
EENT: epistaxis, rhinitis, *pharyngitis*.
GI: anorexia, nausea, vomiting, diarrhea, stomatitis, ulcerative stomatitis, mucositis, abdominal pain, dyspepsia, constipation.
Hematologic: NEUTROPENIA, *anemia*, *pancytopenia*, THROMBOCYTOPENIA, purpura.
Musculoskeletal: pain, skeletal pain, back pain, myalgias.
Respiratory: dyspnea, cough, bronchitis, *pneumonia*, pneumonitis, *bronchospasm*.
Skin: rash, urticaria, pruritus, increased sweating.
Other: SEPSIS, infection, herpes simplex, rigors, chills, candidiasis.

Interactions

None reported.

Effects on lab test results

• May decrease hemoglobin level and hematocrit.
• May decrease CD4+, lymphocyte, neutrophil, WBC, RBC, and platelet counts.
• May interfere with diagnostic tests that use antibodies.

Pharmacokinetics

Absorption: Given I.V.
Distribution: Binds to various tissues.
Metabolism: Unknown.
Excretion: Unknown. *Half-life:* 12 days.

Route	Onset	Peak	Duration
I.V.	Unknown	Unknown	Unknown

Action

Chemical effect: Binds to CD52 and causes antibody-dependent destruction of leukemic cells following cell-surface binding.
Therapeutic effect: Destroys leukemic cells.

Available forms

Ampules: 10 mg/ml, in 3-ml ampules

NURSING PROCESS

Assessment
• Assess patient before therapy for signs or symptoms of active infection or compromised immune function.
• Obtain baseline CBC and platelet count before starting therapy.
• Monitor blood pressure and be alert for hypotensive symptoms during drug administration.
⚑ **ALERT:** Monitor hematologic studies during therapy. Even with normal dosages, patients may experience signs and symptoms of hematologic toxicity, including myelosuppression, bone marrow dysplasia, and thrombocytopenia. Initial doses greater than 3 mg aren't well tolerated. Extremely high doses can be fatal or cause acute bronchospasm, cough, shortness of breath, and anuria. If these occur, stop drug and provide supportive treatment.
• Monitor CBC and platelet counts weekly during therapy and more frequently if anemia, neutropenia, or thrombocytopenia worsens.
• After treatment, monitor CD4+ count until it reaches 200 cells/mm³.

Nursing diagnoses
• Risk for infection related to immunocompromised state
• Fatigue caused by drug therapy
• Deficient knowledge related to alemtuzumab therapy

Planning and implementation
• Irradiate blood if transfusions are needed to protect against graft-versus-host disease.
• Don't immunize with live viral vaccines.
• If therapy is stopped for longer than 7 days, restart with gradual dose increase.
⚑ **ALERT:** Don't confuse alemtuzumab with trastuzumab.
Patient teaching
• Tell patient to immediately report any infusion reaction, such as rigors, chills, fever, nausea, or vomiting.
• Advise patient to report signs or symptoms of infection immediately.
• Inform patient that blood tests will be done frequently during therapy to observe for adverse effects.

Reactions may be *common*, uncommon, *life-threatening*, or COMMON AND LIFE-THREATENING.

• Tell women of childbearing age and men to use effective contraceptive methods during therapy and for at least 6 months after completion of therapy.

🔲 **Evaluation**
• Patient remains free from infection.
• Patient doesn't suffer any harmful drug-induced adverse reactions.
• Patient and family state understanding of drug therapy.

alendronate sodium
(ah-LEN-droh-nayt SOH-dee-um)
Fosamax◊, Fosamax Plus D

Pharmacologic class: inhibitor of osteoclast-mediated bone resorption
Therapeutic class: antiosteoporotic
Pregnancy risk category: C

Indications and dosages

▶ **Osteoporosis in postmenopausal women; to increase bone mass in men with osteoporosis.** *Adults:* 10 mg P.O. daily or 70-mg tablet, one bottle of 70-mg oral solution, or one 70 mg/2,800 international units vitamin D_3 tablet, P.O. once weekly with water at least 30 minutes before first food, beverage, or medication of the day.
▶ **Prevention of osteoporosis in postmenopausal women.** *Women:* 5 mg P.O. daily or 35-mg tablet P.O. once weekly taken with water at least 30 minutes before first food, beverage, or medication of the day.
▶ **Corticosteroid-induced osteoporosis, given with calcium and vitamin D supplements.** *Adults:* 5 mg P.O. daily.
Postmenopausal women not receiving estrogen replacement therapy: 10 mg P.O. daily.
▶ **Paget's disease of bone.** *Adults:* 40 mg P.O. daily for 6 months taken with water at least 30 minutes before first food, beverage, or drug of the day.

Contraindications and cautions

• Contraindicated in patients with hypocalcemia, severe renal insufficiency, inability to stand or sit upright for at least 30 minutes, abnormalities of the esophagus that delay esophageal emptying, such as stricture or achalasia, patients

with increased risk of aspiration (oral solution), or hypersensitivity to drug or its components.
• Use cautiously in patients with dysphagia, esophageal diseases, gastritis, duodenitis, ulcers, or mild to moderate renal insufficiency.
⚠ **Lifespan:** In pregnant women, use only if benefits outweigh the risks to the fetus. In breast-feeding women and in children, safety of drug hasn't been established.

Adverse reactions

CNS: headache.
GI: abdominal pain, nausea, dyspepsia, constipation, diarrhea, flatulence, acid regurgitation, esophageal ulcer, vomiting, dysphagia, abdominal distention, gastritis, taste perversion.
Musculoskeletal: musculoskeletal pain.

Interactions

Drug-drug. *Antacids, calcium supplements, and many other oral medications:* May interfere with alendronate absorption. Give 30 minutes after alendronate dose.
Aspirin, NSAIDs: May increase risk of upper GI reactions with alendronate doses greater than 10 mg daily. Monitor patient closely.
Drug-food. *Any food:* May decrease absorption of drug. Don't give drug with food.

Effects on lab test results

• May mildly decrease calcium and phosphate levels.

Pharmacokinetics

Absorption: Food or beverages can significantly decrease bioavailability.
Distribution: Initially to soft tissues, but rapidly redistributed to bone or excreted in urine; about 78% protein-bound.
Metabolism: None.
Excretion: In urine. *Half-life:* More than 10 years.

Route	Onset	Peak	Duration
P.O.	1 mo	3–6 mo	3 wk after therapy

Action

Chemical effect: Suppresses osteoclast activity on newly formed resorption surfaces, reducing bone turnover.
Therapeutic effect: Increases bone mass.

Available forms

Oral solution: 70 mg/75 ml
Tablets: 5 mg, 10 mg, 35 mg, 40 mg, 70 mg,
70 mg tablet also containing 2,800 international
units vitamin D_3

NURSING PROCESS

🏥 Assessment
• Obtain history of patient's underlying disorder
before therapy.
• Monitor calcium and phosphate levels
throughout therapy.
• Be alert for adverse reactions and drug interactions.
• Assess patient's and family's knowledge of
drug therapy.

🏥 Nursing diagnoses
• Risk for injury related to decreased bone mass
• Risk for deficient fluid volume related to
drug-induced GI upset
• Deficient knowledge related to drug therapy

🏥 Planning and implementation
• Hypocalcemia and other disturbances of mineral metabolism (such as vitamin D deficiency)
should be corrected before therapy begins.
• Give drug in the morning at least 30 minutes
before first meal, fluid, or other oral drug administration.
🏥 **ALERT:** Don't confuse Fosamax with Flomax.
• The recommended daily intake of vitamin D
is 400 to 800 international units. Fosamax Plus
D provides 400 international units daily in the
once-weekly formulation. Patients at risk for
vitamin D deficiency, such as those who are
chronically ill, have a GI malabsorption syndrome, or are older than age 70, may require additional supplementation.
Patient teaching
• Advise patient to take tablets when he awakes,
with 6 to 8 oz of water or oral solution with at
least 2 oz of water.
🏥 **ALERT:** Warn patient not to lie down for at
least 30 minutes after taking drug and until after
the first food of the day to aid passage to stomach and reduce potential for esophageal irritation.
• Tell patient to take calcium and vitamin D
supplements if daily dietary intake is inadequate.

• Show patient how to perform weight-bearing
exercises, which help increase bone mass.
• Urge patient to limit or restrict smoking and
alcohol use, if appropriate.

☑ Evaluation
• Patient remains free from bone fracture.
• Patient maintains adequate hydration.
• Patient and family state understanding of drug
therapy.

alfuzosin hydrochloride
(al-FYOO-zoe-sin)
Uroxatral

Pharmacologic class: selective post-synaptic
alpha$_1$-adrenergic antagonist
Therapeutic class: benign prostatic hypertrophy (BPH) drug
Pregnancy risk category: B

Indications and dosages
▶ **BPH.** *Men:* 10 mg P.O. after the same meal
daily.

Contraindications and cautions
• Contraindicated in patients hypersensitive to
drug or any of its components, in those with
moderate or severe hepatic insufficiency
(Child–Pugh categories B and C), and those also
being treated with potent inhibitors of CYP
3A4.
• Use cautiously in patients with severe renal
insufficiency, congenital or acquired prolonged
QT interval, or symptomatic hypotension and in
those who have hypotension with other drugs.
🏥 **Lifespan:** In women and children, drug is
contraindicated.

Adverse reactions
CNS: dizziness, headache, fatigue, pain.
CV: angina, orthostatic hypotension, tachycar-
dia, chest pain.
EENT: sinusitis, pharyngitis.
GI: abdominal pain, dyspepsia, constipation,
nausea.
GU: impotence, priapism.
Respiratory: upper respiratory tract infection,
bronchitis.
Skin: rash.

Reactions may be *common*, uncommon, *life-threatening*, or COMMON AND LIFE-THREATENING.

Interactions

Drug-drug. *Alpha blockers:* May interact. Don't use together.
Antihypertensives: May cause hypotension. Monitor blood pressure and use together cautiously.
Atenolol: May cause reductions in blood pressure and heart rate. Monitor blood pressure and heart rate.
Cimetidine: May increase alfuzosin level. Use together cautiously.
CYP 3A4 inhibitors (itraconazole, ketoconazole, and ritonavir): May increase alfuzosin level. Don't use together.
Drug-food. *Any food:* May increase absorption by 50%. Give with food.

Effects on lab test results

None significant.

Pharmacokinetics

Absorption: When taken with food, bioavailability is 49% and peak levels are achieved in 8 hours.
Distribution: 82% to 90% bound to plasma proteins.
Metabolism: Extensive, principally by CYP 3A4.
Excretion: 11% unchanged in urine. *Half-life:* 10 hours.

Route	Onset	Peak	Duration
P.O.	Unknown	8 hr	Unknown

Action

Chemical effect: Blocks $alpha_1$-adrenergic receptors in the lower urinary tract, causing smooth muscle in the bladder, neck, and prostate to relax.
Therapeutic effect: Improves urine flow and reduces symptoms of BPH.

Available forms

Tablets (extended-release): 10 mg

NURSING PROCESS

⚗ Assessment
● Assess patient's condition before therapy and regularly thereafter.
● Monitor patient for adverse reactions.
● Assess patient's and family's knowledge of drug therapy.

⊞ Nursing diagnoses
● Risk of injury related to adverse reactions from drug therapy
● Deficient knowledge related to drug therapy

❱ Planning and implementation
● Prostate cancer and BPH may cause similar symptoms. Make sure prostate cancer is ruled out before starting therapy.
● Orthostatic hypotension may occur within a few hours after therapy. Provide safety precautions.
● If angina appears or worsens, stop drug.
⑤ ALERT: If overdose leads to hypotension, provide CV support by restoring blood pressure and heart rate. Have patient lie down and give I.V. fluids and vasopressors, if needed.
⑤ ALERT: Don't use alfuzosin to treat hypertension.
Patient teaching
● Tell patient to take drug with food and with the same meal each day.
● Advise patient to rise slowly to prevent orthostatic hypotension.
● Warn patient that he may be dizzy, and caution him to avoid hazardous tasks until the effects of the drug are known.
● Advise patient not to crush or chew tablets.

☑ Evaluation
● Patient remains free from any adverse effects.
● Patient and family state understanding of drug therapy.

allopurinol
(al-oh-PYOOR-ih-nol)
Allorin◇, Apo-Allopurinol♦, Capurate◇, Zyloprim

allopurinol sodium
Aloprim

Pharmacologic class: xanthine oxidase inhibitor
Therapeutic class: antigout drug
Pregnancy risk category: C

Indications and dosages

▶ **Gout.** *Adults:* Mild gout, 200 to 300 mg P.O. daily; severe gout with large tophi, 400 to 600 mg P.O. daily. Dosage varies with severity of disease and can be given as single dose or in divided doses; doses larger than 300 mg should be divided. Maximum dosage, 800 mg daily.

▶ **To prevent acute gouty attacks.** *Adults:* 100 mg P.O. daily; increase at weekly intervals by 100 mg to a maximum of 800 mg daily, or until uric acid level falls to 6 mg/dl or less.

▶ **Hyperuricemia secondary to malignancies.** *Adults and children older than age 10:* 200 to 400 mg/m^2/day I.V. 1 to 2 days before chemotherapy as a single infusion or in equally divided doses q 6, 8, or 12 hours. Maximum 600 mg daily.

Children age 10 and younger: Initially, 200 mg/ m^2/day I.V. as a single infusion or in equally divided doses q 6, 8, or 12 hours. Then, titrate according to uric acid level. For children ages 6 to 10, give 300 mg P.O. daily or divided t.i.d. For children younger than age 6, give 150 mg P.O. daily.

▶ *To prevent uric acid nephropathy during cancer chemotherapy. Adults:* 600 to 800 mg P.O. daily for 2 to 3 days, with high fluid intake.

▶ **Recurrent calcium oxalate calculi.** *Adults:* 200 to 300 mg P.O. daily in single or divided doses.

⌧ **Adjust-a-dose:** For patients with renal impairment, if creatinine clearance is 10 to 20 ml/ minute, give 200 mg P.O. or I.V. daily; if less than 10 ml/minute, give 100 mg P.O. or I.V. daily; if less than 3 ml/minute, give 100 mg P.O. or I.V. at extended intervals.

▼ **I.V. administration**

• Dissolve contents of vial in 25 ml sterile water for injection. Dilute solution to desired concentration (no greater than 6 mg/ml) with normal saline solution for injection or D$_5$W. Don't use solution that contains sodium bicarbonate.

• Store solution at 68° to 77° F (20° to 25° C) and use within 10 hours. Don't use if solution has particulates or is discolored.

⊗ **Incompatibilities**
Amikacin, amphotericin B, carmustine, cefotaxime, chlorpromazine, cimetidine, clindamycin phosphate, cytarabine, dacarbazine, daunorubicin, diphenhydramine, doxorubicin, doxycycline hyclate, droperidol, floxuridine, gentamicin, haloperidol lactate, hydroxyzine, idarubicin, imipenem and cilastatin sodium, mechlorethamine, meperidine, methylprednisolone sodium succinate, metoclopramide, minocycline, nalbuphine, netilmicin, ondan-

setron, prochlorperazine edisylate, promethazine, sodium bicarbonate, streptozocin, tobramycin sulfate, vinorelbine.

Contraindications and cautions

• Contraindicated in patients hypersensitive to drug and in those with idiopathic hemochromatosis.

⚖ **Lifespan:** In pregnant or breast-feeding women, use cautiously.

Adverse reactions

CNS: drowsiness, headache.
EENT: cataracts, retinopathy.
GI: nausea, vomiting, diarrhea, abdominal pain.
GU: *renal failure,* uremia.
Hematologic: *agranulocytosis,* anemia, *aplastic anemia, thrombocytopenia.*
Hepatic: *hepatitis.*
Skin: rash, usually maculopapular; *exfoliative lesions;* urticarial and purpuric lesions; *erythema multiforme;* ichthyosis; *toxic epidermal necrolysis.*
Other: severe furunculosis of nose.

Interactions

Drug-drug. ACE inhibitors: May increase risk of hypersensitivity reaction. Monitor patient closely.
Amoxicillin, ampicillin, bacampicillin: May increase risk of rash. Avoid using together.
Anticoagulants, dicumarol: May potentiate anticoagulant effect. Adjust dosage, if needed.
Antineoplastics: May increase risk of bone marrow suppression. Monitor patient carefully.
Azathioprine, mercaptopurine: May increase levels of these drugs. Adjust dosage, if needed.
Chlorpropamide: May increase hypoglycemic effect. Avoid using together.
Cyclosporine: May increase cyclosporine levels. Monitor and adjust cyclosporine dose as needed.
Diazoxide, diuretics, mecamylamine, pyrazinamide: May increase uric acid level. Adjust allopurinol dosage, if needed.
Ethacrynic acid, thiazide diuretics: May increase risk of allopurinol toxicity. Reduce allopurinol dosage and closely monitor renal function.
Uricosurics: May have an additive effect. Use to therapeutic advantage.

Urine-acidifying drugs: May increase possibility of kidney stone formation. Monitor patient carefully.
Xanthines: May increase theophylline level. Adjust theophylline dosage.
Drug-lifestyle. *Alcohol use:* May increase uric acid level. Discourage using together.

Effects on lab test results

• May increase alkaline phosphatase, AST, ALT, BUN, and creatinine levels. May decrease hemoglobin level and hematocrit.
• May decrease granulocyte and platelet counts.

Pharmacokinetics

Absorption: 80% to 90%.
Distribution: Widely throughout body except brain, where levels are 50% of those found elsewhere.
Metabolism: To oxypurinol by xanthine oxidase.
Excretion: Primarily in urine; minute amount excreted in feces. *Half-life:* Allopurinol, 1 to 2 hours; oxypurinol, about 15 hours.

Route	Onset	Peak	Duration
P.O.	2–3 days	½–2 hr	1–2 wk
I.V.	Unknown	½ hr	Unknown

Action

Chemical effect: Reduces uric acid production by inhibiting the necessary biochemical reactions.
Therapeutic effect: Alleviates gout symptoms.

Available forms

allopurinol
Capsules: 100 mg ◊, 300 mg ◊
Tablets (scored): 100 mg, 200 mg ◊, 300 mg
allopurinol sodium
Injection: 500 mg/30-ml vial

NURSING PROCESS

⟐ Assessment

• Assess patient's history. Gout may be secondary to diseases such as acute or chronic leukemia, polycythemia vera, multiple myeloma, and psoriasis.
• Assess patient's uric acid level, joint stiffness, and pain before and during therapy. Optimal benefits may require 2 to 6 weeks of therapy.

• Monitor fluid intake and output. Daily urine output of at least 2 L and maintenance of neutral or slightly alkaline urine are desirable.
• Monitor CBC and hepatic and renal function at start of therapy and periodically during therapy.
• Be alert for adverse reactions and drug interactions.
• Assess patient's and family's knowledge of drug therapy.

⟐ Nursing diagnoses

• Acute pain (joint) related to patient's underlying condition
• Risk for infection related to drug-induced agranulocytosis
• Deficient knowledge related to drug therapy

⟐ Planning and implementation

• Give drug with or immediately after meals to minimize adverse GI reactions.
• Have patient drink plenty of fluids while taking drug, unless contraindicated.
• Notify prescriber if renal insufficiency occurs during treatment because this usually warrants dosage reduction.
⟐ **ALERT:** Don't confuse Zyloprim with ZORprin.
• Give colchicine with allopurinol. This combination prophylactically treats acute gout attacks that may occur in first 6 weeks of therapy.
Patient teaching
• Advise patient to refrain from driving or performing hazardous tasks requiring mental alertness until CNS effects of drug are known.
• Advise patient taking allopurinol for recurrent calcium oxalate stones to reduce intake of animal protein, sodium, refined sugars, oxalate-rich foods, and calcium.
• Tell patient to stop drug at first sign of rash, which may precede severe hypersensitivity or other adverse reaction. Rash is more common in patients taking diuretics and in those with renal disorders. Tell patient to report all adverse reactions immediately.
• Advise patient not to use alcohol during drug therapy.

⟐ Evaluation

• Patient expresses relief from joint pain.
• Patient is free from infection.
• Patient and family state understanding of drug therapy.

---

almotriptan malate
(AL-moh-trip-tan MAH-layt)
Axert

Pharmacologic class: serotonin 5-HT$_1$ receptor agonist
Therapeutic class: antimigraine drug
Pregnancy risk category: C

Indications and dosages

▶ **Acute migraine with or without aura.**
Adults: 6.25-mg or 12.5-mg tablet P.O., with one additional dose after 2 hours if headache is unresolved or recurs. Maximum, two doses within 24 hours.
⧉ **Adjust-a-dose:** For patients with hepatic or renal impairment, initially, 6.25 mg P.O. daily, with a maximum daily dosage of 12.5 mg.

Contraindications and cautions

• Contraindicated in patients hypersensitive to drug or its components. Also contraindicated in those with angina pectoris, history of MI, silent ischemia, uncontrolled hypertension, other CV disease, hemiplegic and basilar migraine, and coronary artery vasospasm, such as with Prinzmetal's variant angina.
• Don't give within 24 hours after other serotonin agonists or ergotamine drugs.
• Use cautiously in patients with renal or hepatic impairment and in those with cataracts because of the potential for corneal opacities.
• Also use cautiously in patients with risk factors for coronary artery disease (CAD), such as obesity, diabetes, and family history of CAD.
⚘ **Lifespan:** In pregnant women, use only if the potential benefits outweigh the potential risks to the fetus. In breast-feeding women, use cautiously because it isn't known whether drug appears in breast milk. In children, safety and effectiveness of drug haven't been established.

Adverse reactions

CNS: paresthesia, headache, dizziness, somnolence.
CV: *coronary artery vasospasm, transient myocardial ischemia, MI, ventricular tachycardia, ventricular fibrillation.*
GI: nausea, dry mouth.

Interactions

Drug-drug. *MAO inhibitors, verapamil:* May increase almotriptan level. No dosage adjustment is needed.
CYP 3A4 inhibitors, such as ketoconazole: May increase almotriptan level. Monitor patient for adverse reactions. Reduce dosage, if needed.
Ergot-containing drugs, serotonin 5-HT$_{1B/1D}$ agonists: May cause additive effects. Avoid using within 24 hours of almotriptan.
SSRIs: May cause additive serotonin effects, resulting in weakness, hyperreflexia, or incoordination. Monitor patient closely if given together.

Effects on lab test results

None reported.

Pharmacokinetics

Absorption: Rapid and extensive; reaches peak level in 1 to 3 hours. Food doesn't affect absorption.
Distribution: High, with minimal protein-binding.
Metabolism: Monoamine oxidase-A and CYP 3A4 and 2D6 are mainly responsible.
Excretion: 75% through renal excretion. *Half-life:* 3 to 4 hours.

Route	Onset	Peak	Duration
P.O.	1–3 hr	1–3 hr	3–4 hr

Action

Chemical effect: Binds selectively to various serotonin receptors, mainly serotonin 5-HT$_{1B/1D}$ receptors, resulting in cranial vessel constriction, which inhibits migraine headache.
Therapeutic effect: Blocks neuropeptide release to the pain pathways to prevent migraine headaches.

Available forms

Tablets: 6.25 mg, 12.5 mg

NURSING PROCESS

⧫ Assessment
• Assess patient's condition before and during drug therapy.
• Obtain list of patient's drug intake within 24 hours to prevent drug interactions. Use caution when giving drug to patient who is taking an MAO inhibitor or a CYP 3A4 or 2D6 inhibi-

tor. Don't give drug with other serotonin agonist or ergotamine derivatives.
• Be alert for any adverse reactions.
• Monitor ECG in patients with risk factors for CAD or with symptoms similar to those of CAD, such as chest or throat tightness, pain, and heaviness.
• Assess patient's and family's knowledge of drug therapy.

🔲 **Nursing diagnoses**
• Acute pain related to presence of acute migraine attack
• Risk for injury related to drug-induced interactions
• Deficient knowledge related to almotriptan therapy

▶ **Planning and implementation**
• Give dose as soon as patient complains of migraine symptoms.
• Repeat dose after 2 hours if needed.
• Don't give more than two doses within 24 hours.
Ⓢ **ALERT:** Don't confuse Axert with Antivert.
Patient teaching
• Advise patient to take drug only when he is having a migraine.
• Teach patient to avoid possible migraine triggers, such as cheese, chocolate, citrus fruits, caffeine, and alcohol.
• Tell patient to repeat dose only once within 24 hours and no sooner than 2 hours after initial dose.
• Inform patient that other commonly prescribed migraine medications may interact with this drug.
• Tell patient to immediately report to the prescriber any chest, throat, jaw, or neck tightness, pain, or heaviness, and to stop using the drug.
• Advise patient to use caution while driving or operating machinery.

☑ **Evaluation**
• Patient's symptoms are alleviated and patient is free from pain.
• Serious complications from drug interactions don't develop.
• Patient and family state understanding of drug therapy.

alosetron hydrochloride
(a-LOE-se-tron high-droh-KLOR-ighd)
Lotronex

Pharmacologic class: selective 5-HT$_3$ receptor antagonist
Therapeutic class: GI drug
Pregnancy risk category: B

Indications and dosages
▶ **Irritable bowel syndrome (IBS) in women with severe diarrhea who haven't responded adequately to conventional therapy.** *Women:* Initially, 1 mg P.O. daily for 4 weeks. If response is inadequate, the dose may be increased to 1 mg P.O. b.i.d. If adequate relief isn't achieved at 1 mg b.i.d. after 4 weeks, stop drug.

Contraindications and cautions
• Contraindicated in women hypersensitive to the drug or any of its components, those with Crohn's disease, ulcerative colitis, or diverticulitis or a history of chronic or severe constipation, sequelae from constipation, intestinal obstruction, stricture, toxic megacolon, GI perforation, GI adhesions, ischemic colitis, impaired intestinal circulation, thrombophlebitis, or hypercoagulable state.
• Women shouldn't take drug if they are constipated or if their chief bowel symptom is constipation.
🔥 **Lifespan:** In pregnant women, use only if clearly needed. In breast-feeding women, use cautiously because it's unknown whether drug or its metabolites appear in breast milk. In children, use hasn't been studied and therefore isn't recommended. In elderly women, use cautiously because they may be at greater risk for complications of constipation.

Adverse reactions
CNS: headache, sedation, abnormal dreams, anxiety, sleep and depressive disorders.
CV: *arrhythmias, hypertension.*
EENT: *photophobia, allergic rhinitis, throat and tonsil discomfort and pain, bacterial ear, nose, and throat infections.*
GI: *constipation,* nausea, GI discomfort and pain, abdominal discomfort and pain, abdominal distention, gaseous symptoms, viral GI infections, proctitis, hemorrhoids, dyspeptic symp-

toms, *ileus, perforation, ischemic colitis, small bowel mesenteric ischemia, obstruction,* impaction.
GU: UTI, polyuria, diuresis.
Respiratory: *cough.*
Skin: rash, acne, folliculitis.

Interactions

Drug-drug. *Hydralazine, isoniazid, procainamide:* May slow metabolism and increase level of these drugs because of inhibition of N-acetyltransferase. Monitor patient for toxicity.

Effects on lab test results

• May increase ALT, AST, alkaline phosphatase, and bilirubin levels.

Pharmacokinetics

Absorption: Rapid. Mean absolute bioavailability is 50% to 60%. Food decreases rate by 25%.
Distribution: 82% bound to plasma proteins.
Metabolism: Extensive, by CYP enzymes (2C9, 3A4, 1A2).
Excretion: 7% unchanged in urine. Radiolabeled dose 73% in urine and 24% in feces. *Half-life:* 1½ hour.

Route	Onset	Peak	Duration
P.O.	Unknown	1 hr	Variable

Action

Chemical effect: Selectively inhibits 5-HT$_3$ receptors on enteric neurons in the GI tract. Blocks neuronal depolarization, which decreases visceral pain, colonic transit, and GI secretions.
Therapeutic effect: Relieves pain and decreases frequency of loose stools caused by IBS.

Available forms

Tablets: 0.5 mg, 1 mg

NURSING PROCESS

🔖 Assessment
⑤ ALERT: Effectiveness in men hasn't been established.
• Only physicians enrolled in the prescribing program can prescribe this drug. Call 1-888-825-5249 or visit www.lotronex.com to enroll or report adverse reactions.
• Don't use in patient whose main symptom is constipation.
• Assess patient before and during drug therapy.

⊕ Nursing diagnoses

• Diarrhea related to underlying IBS condition
• Acute pain related to underlying IBS condition
• Deficient knowledge related to drug therapy

⟩ Planning and implementation

• If patient develops constipation, therapy should be suspended and the usual care of laxatives and fiber should be prescribed until the constipation resolves.
⑤ ALERT: Death may occur in patients who develop ischemic colitis and serious complications of constipation. If patient complains of rectal bleeding or sudden worsening of abdominal pain, stop therapy and rule out acute ischemic colitis.
• Acute symptoms of toxicity include labored respiration, ataxia, subdued behavior, tremors, and seizures. No antidote exists for overdose. Treatment for overdose includes supportive care.

Patient teaching
⑤ ALERT: Explain to patient that she must be enrolled in the prescribing program. Counsel patient about the risks and benefits of the drug, give instructions, answer questions, and provide information about the drug. The patient must review and sign a patient–physician agreement. A special program sticker must be affixed to all written prescriptions; no telephone, facsimile, or computerized prescriptions are permitted.
• Instruct patient not to start drug if she is constipated.
⑤ ALERT: Urge patient to look for constipation or signs and symptoms of ischemic colitis, such as rectal bleeding, bloody diarrhea, or worsened abdominal pain or cramping. Tell her to stop drug and consult prescriber immediately if symptoms occur.
• Explain that this drug isn't a cure but may alleviate some of the symptoms of IBS. If the drug doesn't adequately control symptoms after twice-daily therapy, advise patient to stop taking drug and contact prescriber.
• Inform patient that most women notice their symptoms improving after about 1 week of therapy, but some may take up to 4 weeks to experience relief. Symptoms usually return within 1 week of stopping therapy.

Evaluation

- Patient's symptoms related to IBS, including pain and frequency of loose stools, are relieved.
- Patient and family state understanding of drug therapy.

alprazolam

(al-PRAH-zoh-lam)

Apo-Alpraz♦, Novo-Alprazol♦, Niravam, Nu-Alpraz♦, Xanax◇, Xanax XR

Pharmacologic class: benzodiazepine
Therapeutic class: anxiolytic
Pregnancy risk category: D
Controlled substance schedule: IV

Indications and dosages

► **Anxiety.** *Adults:* Usual initial dose, 0.25 to 0.5 mg P.O. t.i.d. Maximum, 4 mg daily in divided doses.
◪ **Adjust-a-dose:** For elderly or debilitated patients or those with advanced liver disease, usual initial dose is 0.25 mg P.O. b.i.d. or t.i.d. Maximum, 4 mg daily in divided doses.
► **Panic disorders.** *Adults:* 0.5 mg P.O. t.i.d., increased q 3 to 4 days in increments of no more than 1 mg. Maximum, 10 mg daily in divided doses. Or initially 0.5 to 1 mg extended-release P.O. daily. Increase dose by no more than 1 mg daily at intervals of 3 to 4 days. Usual dosage is 3 to 6 mg P.O. once daily, preferably in the morning. Individualize dosage as necessary. Maximum dosage is 10 mg daily. If dosage reduction is necessary, decrease by no more than 0.5 mg every 3 days.
► **Social phobias‡.** *Adults:* 2 to 8 mg P.O. daily.

Contraindications and cautions

- Contraindicated in patients hypersensitive to drug or other benzodiazepines and in those with acute angle-closure glaucoma or taking azole antifungals.
- Use cautiously in patients with hepatic, renal, or pulmonary disease. Also use cautiously in patients with cardiac disease because hypotension may occur.
- ⚘ **Lifespan:** In pregnant women, don't use during first trimester. Use cautiously in second and third trimesters because neonates may experience withdrawal symptoms. In breast-feeding

women, drug isn't recommended. In children, safety of drug hasn't been established. In elderly patients, use cautiously because they may be more sensitive to sedation and ataxia.

Adverse reactions

CNS: *drowsiness, light-headedness, sedation, somnolence, difficulty speaking, impaired coordination, memory impairment, fatigue, depression,* mental impairment, ataxia, paresthesia, dyskinesia, emergence of anxiety between doses, hypoesthesia, lethargy, *confusion, anxiety,* vertigo, malaise, *headache, dizziness,* tremor, *irritability, insomnia,* nervousness, restlessness, agitation, nightmare, syncope, akathisia, mania, *suicidal thoughts.*
CV: palpitation, chest pain, hypotension.
EENT: sore throat, allergic rhinitis, blurred vision, nasal congestion.
GI: *dry mouth, constipation,* nausea, increased or decreased appetite, anorexia, *diarrhea,* vomiting, dyspepsia, abdominal pain.
GU: dysmenorrhea, premenstrual syndrome, difficulty urinating.
Metabolic: increased or decreased weight.
Musculoskeletal: arthralgia, myalgia, limb and back pain; muscle rigidity, cramps, or twitch.
Respiratory: upper respiratory tract infection, dyspnea, hyperventilation.
Skin: pruritus, increased sweating, dermatitis.
Other: hot flushes, influenza, injury, decreased or increased libido, sexual dysfunction, dependence.

Interactions

Drug-drug. *Anticonvulsants, antidepressants, antihistamines, barbiturates, benzodiazepines, general anesthetics, opioids, phenothiazines:* May increase CNS depressant effects. Avoid using together.
Carbamazepine, propoxyphene: May decrease alprazolam concentrations. Use together cautiously.
Cimetidine, fluoxetine, fluvoxamine, hormonal contraceptives, nefazodone: May increase alprazolam level. Use together cautiously and consider reducing alprazolam dosage.
Fluconazole, itraconazole, ketoconazole, miconazole: May increase and prolong levels, CNS depression, and psychomotor impairment. Don't use together.
Tricyclic antidepressants: May increase levels of these drugs. Monitor patient closely.

Drug-herb. *Calendula, hops, lemon balm, skullcap, valerian:* May enhance sedative effects. Discourage using together.
Kava: May enhance CNS sedation. Discourage using together.
Drug-food. *Grapefruit:* May increase alprazolam levels. Use cautiously together.
Drug-lifestyle. *Alcohol use:* May cause additive CNS effects. Strongly discourage using together.
Smoking: May decrease effectiveness of drug. Help patient to quit smoking.

Effects on lab test results

• May increase ALT and AST levels.

Pharmacokinetics

Absorption: Well absorbed.
Distribution: Wide; 80% of dose is bound to plasma protein.
Metabolism: In liver by CYP 3A4 pathway equally to alpha-hydroxyalprazolam and inactive metabolites.
Excretion: In urine. *Half-life:* Immediate-release is 12 to 15 hours; extended-release is 11 to 16 hours.

Route	Onset	Peak	Duration
P.O.	Unknown	1–2 hr	Unknown
P.O. extended	Unknown	Unknown	Unknown

Action

Chemical effect: May potentiate effects of GABA, an inhibitory neurotransmitter, and depress CNS at limbic and subcortical levels of brain.
Therapeutic effect: Decreases anxiety.

Available forms

Oral solution: 0.5 mg/5 ml, 1 mg/ml (concentrate)
Tablets: 0.25 mg, 0.5 mg, 1 mg, 2 mg
Tablets (extended-release): 0.5 mg, 1 mg, 2 mg, 3 mg
Tablets (orally disintegrating): 0.25 mg, 0.5 mg, 1 mg

NURSING PROCESS

Assessment

• Assess patient's anxiety before and frequently after therapy.

• In patient receiving repeated or prolonged therapy, monitor liver, renal, and hematopoietic function test results periodically.
• Be alert for adverse reactions and drug interactions.
• Assess patient's and family's knowledge of drug therapy.

Nursing diagnoses

• Anxiety related to patient's underlying condition
• Risk for injury related to drug-induced CNS reactions
• Deficient knowledge related to drug therapy

Planning and implementation

• Drug shouldn't be given for everyday stress or for use longer than 4 months.
• When giving drug, check to see that patient has swallowed tablets before leaving.
ALERT: Paradoxic excitation has occurred. Episodes of hostility, mania, hypomania, and insomnia have been reported.
ALERT: Don't stop drug abruptly after long-term use because withdrawal symptoms may occur. Abuse or addiction is possible.
ALERT: Don't confuse alprazolam with alprostadil; also don't confuse Xanax with Zantac or Tenex.
• To switch patient from immediate-release to extended-release tablets, calculate the total daily dose of immediate-release tablets and give the same dose of extended-release tablets once daily.
• Withdrawal symptoms include seizures, status epilepticus, impaired concentration, muscle cramps or twitch, diarrhea, blurred vision, decreased appetite, and weight loss.
Patient teaching
• Warn patient to avoid hazardous activities that require alertness and psychomotor coordination until CNS effects of drug are known.
• Tell patient to avoid alcohol use and smoking while taking drug.
• Advise patient to take drug as prescribed and not to stop without prescriber's approval. Inform him of potential for dependence if taken longer than directed.
• Instruct patient to swallow extended-release tablets whole; don't chew or crush them.
• Tell patient using orally disintegrating tablets to remove tablet from bottle using dry hands and immediately place on top of his tongue

where the tablet will dissolve and can be swallowed with saliva.

• Tell patient using half of a scored orally disintegrating tablet to destroy the unused portion.

• Advise patient to discard any cotton from the bottle of orally disintegrating tablets and keep tightly sealed to prevent moisture from entering the bottle and dissolving the tablets.

• Teach patient how to manage or avoid adverse reactions, such as constipation and drowsiness.

☑ **Evaluation**

• Patient is less anxious.

• Patient doesn't experience injury from adverse CNS reactions.

• Patient and family state understanding of drug therapy.

alprostadil
(al-PROS-tuh-dil)
Prostin VR Pediatric

Pharmacologic class: prostaglandin
Therapeutic class: ductus arteriosus patency adjunct
Pregnancy risk category: NR

Indications and dosages

▶ **Temporary maintenance of patent ductus arteriosus until surgery can be performed.**
Infants: 0.05 to 0.1 mcg/kg per minute by I.V. infusion. When therapeutic response is achieved, reduce infusion rate to lowest effective dosage. Maximum dosage is 0.4 mcg/kg/minute. Alternatively, drug can be given through umbilical artery catheter placed at ductal opening.

▼ I.V. administration

• Keep respiratory and emergency equipment available.

• Before giving, dilute 500 mcg of drug with sodium chloride or dextrose injection. Dilute to appropriate volume for pump delivery system.

• Drug isn't recommended for direct injection or intermittent infusion. Give by continuous infusion using constant-rate pump. Infuse through large peripheral or central vein or through umbilical artery catheter placed at level of ductus arteriosus. If flushing occurs as a result of peripheral vasodilation, reposition catheter.

• If fever or significant hypotension develops in an infant, reduce the infusion rate.

• If apnea and bradycardia develop, stop infusion immediately. This may be a sign of drug overdose.

• In prolonged infusions, infant may develop gastric outlet obstruction, morphologic changes in pulmonary arteries, and proliferation of long bones.

• Discard solution after 24 hours.

⊗ **Incompatibilities**
Diluents that contain benzyl alcohol; fatal toxic syndrome may occur.

Contraindications and cautions

⚖ **Lifespan:** In neonates with bleeding tendencies, use cautiously because drug inhibits platelet aggregation. In neonates with respiratory distress syndrome or in premature infants with a patent ductus arteriosus, drug is contraindicated. Infants on long-term infusions may experience cortical growth of long bones.

Adverse reactions

CNS: fever, *seizures.*
CV: flushing, *bradycardia, cardiac arrest,* hypotension, tachycardia.
GI: diarrhea.
Hematologic: *DIC.*
Respiratory: APNEA.
Other: *sepsis.*

Interactions

None significant.

Effects on lab test results

• May decrease potassium level.

Pharmacokinetics

Absorption: Given I.V.
Distribution: Rapid.
Metabolism: About 68% of dose is metabolized in one pass through lung, mainly by oxidation; 100% is metabolized within 24 hours.
Excretion: All metabolites are excreted in urine within 24 hours. *Half-life:* About 5 to 10 minutes.

Route	Onset	Peak	Duration
I.V.	5–10 min	20 min	1–3 hr

Action

Chemical effect: Relaxes smooth muscle of ductus arteriosus.
Therapeutic effect: Improves cardiac circulation.

Available forms

Injection: 500 mcg/ml

NURSING PROCESS

⚚ Assessment
• Obtain baseline assessment of infant's cardiopulmonary status before therapy.
• Measure drug's effectiveness by monitoring blood oxygenation of infants with restricted pulmonary blood flow and by systemic blood pressure and blood pH of infants with restricted systemic blood flow.
• Be alert for adverse reactions throughout therapy.
• Evaluate parent's knowledge of drug therapy.

⚙ Nursing diagnoses
• Ineffective cardiopulmonary tissue perfusion related to underlying condition
• Risk for injury related to drug-induced adverse reactions
• Deficient knowledge related to drug therapy

▶ Planning and implementation
• A differential diagnosis should be made between respiratory distress syndrome and cyanotic heart disease before drug is given. Don't use drug in neonates with respiratory distress syndrome.
ⓈALERT: Don't confuse alprostadil with alprazolam.
Patient teaching
• Keep parents informed of infant's status.
• Explain that parents will be allowed as much time and physical contact with infant as possible.

☑ Evaluation
• Patient is stable with a working cardiopulmonary system.
• Patient isn't injured by adverse drug reactions.
• Parents state understanding of drug therapy.

alteplase (tissue plasminogen activator, recombinant; t-PA)
(AL-teh-plays)
Actilyse ◇, Activase, Cathflo Activase

Pharmacologic class: enzyme
Therapeutic class: thrombolytic enzyme
Pregnancy risk category: C

Indications and dosages

▶ **Lysis of thrombi obstructing coronary arteries in acute MI.** *Adults:* 100 mg I.V. infusion over 3 hours as follows: 60 mg in first hour, with 6 to 10 mg given as bolus over first 1 to 2 minutes. Then, 20 mg/hour infusion for 2 hours. Adults weighing less than 65 kg (143 lb) should receive 1.25 mg/kg using the same method (60% in first hour with 10% as bolus, then 20% of total dose per hour for 2 hours). Don't exceed 100-mg dose. Higher doses may increase risk of intracranial bleeding.
▶ **To manage acute massive pulmonary embolism.** *Adults:* 100 mg I.V. infusion over 2 hours. Heparin begun at end of infusion when APTT or PT returns to twice normal or less. Don't exceed 100-mg dose. Higher doses may increase risk of intracranial bleeding. Also,‡ may infuse 30 or 50 mg via intrapulmonary artery over 1½ or 2 hours, respectively, with heparin therapy.
▶ **To manage acute ischemic stroke.** *Adults:* 0.9 mg/kg (maximum 90 mg) I.V. over 60 minutes with 10% of the total dose given as initial bolus over 1 minute.
▶ **To restore function to central venous access devices as assessed by the ability to withdraw blood.** *Adults and children older than age 2:* For patients weighing 30 kg (66 lb) or more, instill 2 mg Cathflo Activase in 2 ml sterile water into catheter. For patients weighing 10 kg (22 lb) to 30 kg (66 lb), instill 110% of the internal lumen volume of the catheter, not to exceed 2 mg. After 30 minutes of dwell time, assess catheter function by aspirating blood. If function is restored, aspirate 4 to 5 ml of blood to remove Cathflo Activase and residual clot, and gently irrigate the catheter with normal saline solution. If catheter function isn't restored after 120 minutes, instill a second dose.
▶ **To prevent reocclusion after thrombolysis for acute MI‡.** *Adults:* 3.3 mcg/kg/minute by

I.V. infusion for 4 hours with heparin therapy immediately following initial thrombolytic infusion.
▶ **Lysis of arterial occlusion in a peripheral vessel or bypass graft.** *Adults:* 0.05 to 0.1 mg/kg/hour infused via the intrapulmonary artery for 1 to 8 hours.

▼ I.V. administration

• Reconstitute drug with sterile water (without preservatives) for injection only. Check manufacturer's label for specific information. Don't use vial if vacuum seal isn't present. Reconstitute with large-bore (18G) needle, directing stream of sterile water at lyophilized cake. Don't shake, but make sure that drug is dissolved completely. Slight foaming is common, and solution should be clear or pale yellow.
• Drug may be given as reconstituted (1 mg/ml) or diluted with equal volume of normal saline solution or D_5W to make 0.5 mg/ml solution.
• Reconstitute alteplase solution immediately before use, and give within 8 hours because it contains no preservatives. Drug may be stored temporarily at 35° to 86° F (2° to 30° C), but it's stable for only 8 hours at room temperature. Discard unused solution.
To restore function of a central venous catheter
• Reconstitute Cathflo Activase with 2.2 ml sterile water, dissolve completely into a colorless to pale yellow solution that yields a concentration of 1 mg/ml. Solutions are stable for up to 8 hours at room temperature.
• Assess the cause of catheter dysfunction before using Cathflo Activase. Some conditions that may occlude a catheter include incorrect catheter position, mechanical failure, constriction by a suture, and lipid deposits or drug precipitates within the catheter lumen. Don't attempt to suction because of the risk of damage to the vascular wall or collapse of soft-walled catheters.
• Don't use excessive pressure while instilling Cathflo Activase into the catheter because it could cause catheter rupture or expulsion of the clot into the circulation.
⊗ **Incompatibilities**
None reported, but don't mix with other drugs.

Contraindications and cautions

• Contraindicated in patients with active internal bleeding, intracranial neoplasm, arteriove-

nous malformation, aneurysm, severe uncontrolled hypertension, history of stroke, known bleeding diathesis, or intraspinal or intracranial trauma or surgery within past 2 months.
• Use cautiously in patients who had major surgery within past 10 days; in those receiving anticoagulants; and in those with organ biopsy, trauma (including cardiopulmonary resuscitation), GI or GU bleeding, cerebrovascular disease, hypertension, acute pericarditis or subacute bacterial endocarditis, septic thrombophlebitis, or diabetic hemorrhagic retinopathy; or in those with mitral stenosis, atrial fibrillation, or other conditions that may lead to left-sided heart thrombus.
⚖ **Lifespan:** During pregnancy, the first 10 days postpartum, and lactation, use cautiously. In children, safety of drug hasn't been established. In patients age 75 and older, use cautiously.

Adverse reactions

CNS: *cerebral hemorrhage,* fever.
CV: hypotension, *arrhythmias,* edema.
GI: nausea, vomiting, *GI bleed.*
GU: genitourinary bleed.
Hematologic: *severe, spontaneous bleeding.*
Musculoskeletal: arthralgia.
Skin: urticaria.
Other: bleeding at puncture sites, hypersensitivity reactions, *angioedema, anaphylaxis.*

Interactions

Drug-drug. *Abciximab, aspirin, coumarin anticoagulants, dipyridamole, heparin:* May increase risk of bleeding. Monitor patient carefully.
ACE inhibitors: May increase the risk of angioedema. Monitor patient closely during and for several hours after infusion.
Nitroglycerin: May decrease tPA antigen concentrations. Avoid using together. If use together is unavoidable, use the lowest effective dose of nitroglycerin.
Drug-herb. *Dong quai, garlic, ginkgo:* May increase risk of bleeding. Discourage using together.

Effects on lab test results

None reported.

Pharmacokinetics

Absorption: Given I.V.

Distribution: Rapidly cleared from plasma by liver (about 80% cleared within 10 minutes after infusion stops).
Metabolism: Primarily hepatic.
Excretion: Over 85% excreted in urine, 5% in feces. *Half-life:* Less than 10 minutes.

Route	Onset	Peak	Duration
I.V.	Immediate	45 min	4 hr

Action

Chemical effect: Binds to fibrin in thrombus and locally converts plasminogen to plasmin, which initiates local fibrinolysis.
Therapeutic effect: Dissolves blood clots in coronary arteries and lungs.

Available forms

Injection: 50-mg (29 million international units), 100-mg (58 million international units) vials
Lyophilized powder for intracatheter instillation: 2-mg single-patient vials
Solution for intracatheter clearance: 2-mg single-use vials

NURSING PROCESS

Assessment

- Assess patient's cardiopulmonary status (including ECG, vital signs, and coagulation studies) before and during therapy.
- Be alert for adverse reactions and drug interactions.
- Monitor patient for internal bleeding, and check puncture site frequently.
- Assess patient's and family's knowledge of drug therapy.

Nursing diagnoses

- Ineffective cardiopulmonary tissue perfusion related to patient's underlying condition
- Risk for injury related to adverse effects of drug therapy
- Deficient knowledge related to drug therapy

Planning and implementation

- Recanalization of occluded coronary arteries and improvement of heart function require starting drug as soon as possible after onset of symptoms.
- Heparin is frequently started after treatment with alteplase to reduce risk of rethrombosis.
- For arterial puncture, select site on arm and apply pressure for 30 minutes afterward. Also use pressure dressings, sand bags, or ice packs on recent puncture sites to prevent bleeding.
- Notify prescriber if severe bleeding occurs and doesn't stop with intervention; alteplase and heparin infusions will need to be stopped.

ALERT: Have antiarrhythmics available. Coronary thrombolysis is linked to arrhythmias induced by reperfusion of ischemic myocardium.

- Avoid invasive procedures during thrombolytic therapy.

Patient teaching

- Tell patient to immediately report chest pain, dyspnea, changes in heart rate or rhythm, nausea, and bleeding.

Evaluation

- Patient's cardiopulmonary assessment findings demonstrate improved perfusion.
- Patient has no serious adverse drug reactions.
- Patient and family state understanding of drug therapy.

aluminum hydroxide

(uh-LOO-mih-num high-DROKS-ighd)
AlternaGEL†, Alu-Cap†, Alu-Tab†, Amphojel†, Dialume†

Pharmacologic class: aluminum salt
Therapeutic class: antacid
Pregnancy risk category: C

Indications and dosages

▶ **Antacid; relief from peptic ulcer or gastric symptoms; hyperphosphatemia.** *Adults:* 500- to 1,500-mg tablet or capsule P.O. 1 hour after meals and h.s.; or 5- to 30-ml suspension, p.r.n. 1 hour after meals and h.s.

Contraindications and cautions

- Use cautiously in patients with chronic renal disease.

Lifespan: In pregnant women, consult prescriber before giving.

Adverse reactions

GI: anorexia, constipation, intestinal obstruction.
Metabolic: hypophosphatemia.

Interactions

Drug-drug. *Allopurinol, antibiotics (including tetracyclines), corticosteroids, diflunisal, digoxin, ethambutol, H_2-receptor antagonists, iron, isoniazid, penicillamine, phenothiazines, thyroid hormones:* May decrease pharmacologic effect because of possible impaired absorption. Give aluminum hydroxide separately.
Ciprofloxacin, gatifloxacin, levofloxacin, lomefloxacin, moxifloxacin, norfloxacin, ofloxacin: May decrease effects of quinolone. Give antacid at least 6 hours before or 2 hours after the quinolone.
Enteric-coated drugs: May release prematurely in stomach. Separate doses by at least 1 hour.

Effects on lab test results

• May increase gastrin level. May decrease phosphate level.

Pharmacokinetics

Absorption: Small amounts absorbed.
Distribution: None.
Metabolism: None.
Excretion: In feces. *Half-life:* Unknown.

Route	Onset	Peak	Duration
P.O.	Liquids more rapid than tablets or capsules	Unknown	20–60 min if fasting; 3 hr if taken 1 hr after meal

Action

Chemical effect: Reduces total acid load in GI tract, elevates gastric pH to reduce pepsin activity, strengthens gastric mucosal barrier, and increases esophageal sphincter tone.
Therapeutic effect: Relieves GI discomfort.

Available forms

Capsules: 400 mg†, 500 mg†
Liquid: 600 mg/5 ml†
Suspension: 450 mg/5 ml†, 675 mg/5 ml†, 320-mg/5 ml†
Tablets: 300 mg†, 500 mg†, 600 mg†

NURSING PROCESS

Assessment
• Assess patient's discomfort before therapy and regularly thereafter.
• In patient with restricted sodium intake, monitor long-term, high-dose use. Each tablet, cap-

sule, or 5 ml of suspension contains 2 to 3 mg of sodium.
• Be alert for adverse reactions and drug interactions.
• Assess patient's and family's knowledge of drug therapy.

Nursing diagnoses
• Acute pain related to gastric hyperacidity
• Constipation related to drug's adverse effects
• Deficient knowledge related to drug therapy

Planning and implementation
• Shake suspension well; give with small amount of milk or water to ease passage.
• When giving through NG tube, make sure tube is patent and placed correctly; after instilling, flush tube with water to ensure passage to stomach and to clear tube.
• Don't give other oral drug within 2 hours of antacid administration. This may cause premature release of enteric-coated drugs in stomach.
Patient teaching
• Advise patient not to take aluminum hydroxide indiscriminately or to switch antacids without prescriber's advice.
• Instruct patient to shake suspension well and to follow with sips of water or juice.
• Warn patient that drug may color stool white or cause white streaks.
• Teach patient how to prevent constipation.

Evaluation
• Patient's pain is relieved.
• Patient maintains normal bowel function.
• Patient and family state understanding of drug therapy.

amantadine hydrochloride
(uh-MAN-tah-deen high-droh-KLOR-ighd)
Symmetrel

Pharmacologic class: synthetic cyclic primary amine
Therapeutic class: antiviral, antiparkinsonian
Pregnancy risk category: C

Indications and dosages
▶ **Prophylactic or symptomatic treatment of influenza type A virus; respiratory tract ill-**

nesses in elderly or debilitated patients.
Adults age 65 and older: 100 mg P.O. once daily. Treatment should continue for 24 to 48 hours after symptoms disappear. Prophylaxis should start as soon as possible after initial exposure and continue for at least 10 days. When inactivated influenza A vaccine is unavailable, may continue prophylactic treatment for the duration of known influenza A in the community because of repeated or suspected exposures. If used with influenza vaccine, dose is continued for 2 to 4 weeks until protection develops from vaccine.
Adults age 65 and younger and children age 13 and older: 200 mg P.O. daily in single dose or divided b.i.d.
Children ages 9 to 12: 100 mg P.O. b.i.d.
Children ages 1 to 8: 4.4 to 8.8 mg/kg P.O. daily in single dose or divided b.i.d. Maximum, 150 mg daily.

▶ **Drug-induced extrapyramidal reactions.**
Adults: 100 mg P.O. b.i.d. Occasionally, patients whose responses aren't optimal may benefit from an increase to 300 mg P.O. daily in divided doses.

▶ **Idiopathic parkinsonism, parkinsonian syndrome.** *Adults:* 100 mg P.O. b.i.d.; in patients who are seriously ill or receiving other antiparkinsonians, 100 mg daily for at least 1 week, then 100 mg b.i.d., p.r.n.

☒ Adjust-a-dose: For patients with creatinine clearance of 30 to 50 ml/minute, give 200 mg the first day, and 100 mg daily thereafter; for clearance of 15 to 29 ml/minute, give 200 mg the first day then 100 mg every other day; for clearance of less than 15 ml/minute, give 200 mg once weekly.

Contraindications and cautions

• Contraindicated in patients hypersensitive to drug.
• Use cautiously in patients with seizure disorders, heart failure, peripheral edema, hepatic disease, mental illness, eczematoid rash, renal impairment, orthostatic hypotension, or CV disease. Adjust dosage in patients with renal impairment.
🎋 Lifespan: In pregnant and breast-feeding women, use cautiously. In children younger than age 1, safety of drug hasn't been established. In elderly patients, use cautiously.

Adverse reactions

CNS: depression, fatigue, confusion, dizziness, psychosis, hallucinations, anxiety, irritability, ataxia, insomnia, weakness, headache, lightheadedness, difficulty concentrating, *neuroleptic malignant syndrome.*
CV: peripheral edema, orthostatic hypotension, *heart failure.*
GI: anorexia, nausea, constipation, vomiting, dry mouth, diarrhea.
GU: urine retention.
Skin: livedo reticularis.

Interactions

Drug-drug. *Anticholinergics:* May increase adverse anticholinergic effects. Use together cautiously.
CNS stimulants: May cause additive CNS stimulation. Use together cautiously.
Hydrochlorothiazide, sulfamethoxazole, triamterene, trimethoprim: May increase amantadine levels. Use together cautiously.
Quinidine, quinine: May reduce renal clearance of amantadine. Use together cautiously.
Thioridazine: May worsen tremor in elderly patients. Monitor these patients closely.
Drug-herb. *Jimsonweed:* May adversely affect CV function. Discourage using together.

Effects on lab test results

None reported.

Pharmacokinetics

Absorption: Well absorbed from the GI tract.
Distribution: Widely throughout the body; crosses the blood–brain barrier.
Metabolism: About 10% of drug is metabolized.
Excretion: About 90% unchanged in urine, primarily by tubular secretion. Portion of drug may be excreted in breast milk. Excretion rate depends on urine pH. *Half-life:* About 24 hours; with renal dysfunction, may be prolonged to 10 days.

Route	Onset	Peak	Duration
P.O.	Unknown	2–4 hr	Unknown

Action

Chemical effect: May interfere with influenza A virus penetration into susceptible cells. In parkinsonism, action is unknown.

Reactions may be *common,* uncommon, *life-threatening*, or COMMON AND LIFE-THREATENING.

Therapeutic effect: Protects against and reduces symptoms of influenza A viral infection and extrapyramidal symptoms.

Available forms

Capsules: 100 mg
Syrup: 50 mg/5 ml
Tablets: 100 mg

NURSING PROCESS

☑ Assessment
• Obtain baseline assessment of patient's exposure to influenza A virus or history of Parkinson's disease.
• Watch for adverse reactions and drug interactions.
• Monitor patient's hydration status if adverse GI reactions occur.
• Assess patient's and family's knowledge of drug therapy.

⊞ Nursing diagnoses
• Ineffective health maintenance related to patient's underlying condition
• Risk for deficient fluid volume related to adverse GI reactions
• Deficient knowledge related to drug therapy

▷ Planning and implementation
• Elderly patients are more susceptible to neurologic adverse effects. Giving drug in two daily doses rather than as single dose may reduce these effects.
• Give drug after meals for best absorption.
• **ALERT:** Don't confuse amantadine with rimantadine.
Patient teaching
• To prevent insomnia, advise patient to take drug several hours before bedtime.
• To prevent orthostatic hypotension, advise patient not to stand or change positions too quickly.
• Instruct patient to report adverse reactions, especially dizziness, depression, anxiety, nausea, and urine retention.
• Warn patient with parkinsonism not to stop drug abruptly because doing so could cause a parkinsonian crisis.

☑ Evaluation
• Patient exhibits improved health.
• Patient maintains adequate hydration.

• Patient and family state understanding of drug therapy.

amikacin sulfate
(am-eh-KAY-sin SUL-fayt)
Amikin

Pharmacologic class: aminoglycoside
Therapeutic class: antibiotic
Pregnancy risk category: D

Indications and dosages

▶ **Serious infections caused by sensitive strains of** *Pseudomonas aeruginosa, Escherichia coli, Proteus, Klebsiella, Serratia, Enterobacter, Acinetobacter, Providencia, Citrobacter, Staphylococcus;* **meningitis.** *Adults and children:* 15 mg/kg daily divided q 8 to 12 hours I.M. or I.V. infusion.
Neonates: Initially, loading dose of 10 mg/kg I.V., followed by 7.5 mg/kg q 12 hours.
§ **Adjust-a-dose:** For patients with renal impairment, initially, 7.5 mg/kg I.M. or I.V. Subsequent doses and frequency determined by drug level and renal function test results.
▶ **Uncomplicated UTI.** *Adults:* 250 mg I.M. or I.V. b.i.d.
▶ *Mycobacterium avium* **complex, with other drugs‡.** *Adults:* 15 mg/kg I.V. daily, in divided doses q 8 to 12 hours.
§ **Adjust-a-dose:** For patients with renal impairment, initially, 7.5 mg/kg I.M or I.V. Subsequent doses and frequency determined by drug level. Keep peak level between 15 and 35 mcg/ml. Trough level shouldn't exceed 10 mcg/ml.

▼ I.V. administration
• For adults, dilute in 100 to 200 ml of D₅W or normal saline solution. Volume for children depends on dose.
• For adults, infuse over 30 to 60 minutes. Infants should receive a 1- to 2-hour infusion.
• After I.V. infusion, flush line with normal saline solution or D₅W.
⊗ **Incompatibilities**
Amphotericin B, bacitracin, cephapirin, cisplatin, heparin sodium, other I.V. drugs, phenytoin, thiopental, vancomycin, vitamin B complex with C.

Rapid onset   *Liquid form contains alcohol.   ◆ Canada   ◇ Australia   †OTC   ✐Photoguide   ‡Off-label use

Contraindications and cautions

• Contraindicated in patients hypersensitive to drug or other aminoglycosides.
• Use cautiously in patients with impaired renal function or neuromuscular disorders.
⚠ **Lifespan:** In pregnant women, use cautiously and only if benefit outweighs risk to the fetus. In breast-feeding women, don't give drug. In neonates and infants, use cautiously. In elderly patients, use cautiously because they are more likely to have ototoxicity.

Adverse reactions

CNS: headache, lethargy, *neuromuscular block-ade.*
EENT: ototoxicity.
GU: nephrotoxicity.
Hepatic: *hepatic necrosis.*
Other: hypersensitivity reactions, *anaphylaxis.*

Interactions

Drug-drug. *Acyclovir, amphotericin B, cephalothin, cisplatin, methoxyflurane, other aminoglycosides, vancomycin:* May increase nephrotoxicity. Use together cautiously.
Atracurium, doxacurium, mivacurium, pancuronium, rocuronium, tubocurarine, vecuronium: May increase the effects of nondepolarizing neuromuscular blockade, including prolonged respiratory depression. Use together only when necessary. Dose of nondepolarizing muscle relaxant may need to be reduced.
Dimenhydrinate: May mask symptoms of ototoxicity. Use cautiously.
Indomethacin: May increase trough and peak levels of amikacin. Monitor amikacin level closely.
I.V. loop diuretics (such as furosemide): May increase ototoxicity. Use together cautiously.
Parenteral penicillins (such as ticarcillin): May cause amikacin inactivation in vitro. Don't mix.

Effects on lab test results

• May increase BUN, creatinine, nonprotein nitrogen, and urine urea levels.

Pharmacokinetics

Absorption: Rapidly after I.M. administration.
Distribution: Widely; protein-binding is minimal; drug crosses placenta.
Metabolism: None.

Excretion: Primarily in urine by glomerular filtration. *Half-life:* 2 to 3 hours (adults); 30 to 86 hours (patients with severe renal damage).

Route	Onset	Peak	Duration
I.V.	Immediate	Immediate	8–12 hr
I.M.	Unknown	1 hr	8–12 hr

Action

Chemical effect: Inhibits protein synthesis by binding directly to 30S ribosomal subunit. Generally bactericidal.
Therapeutic effect: Kills susceptible bacteria and many aerobic gram-negative organisms (including most strains of *P. aeruginosa*) and some aerobic gram-positive organisms. Ineffective against anaerobes.

Available forms

Injection: 50 mg/ml, 250 mg/ml

NURSING PROCESS

⚙ Assessment

• Assess patient's infection, hearing, weight, and renal function test values before therapy and regularly thereafter.
• Watch for signs of ototoxicity, including tinnitus, vertigo, and hearing loss.
• Monitor amikacin level. Obtain blood for peak amikacin level 1 hour after I.M. injection and 30 minutes to 1 hour after infusion ends; for trough level, draw blood just before next dose. Don't collect blood in heparinized tube because heparin is incompatible with aminoglycosides. Peak level higher than 35 mcg/ml and trough level higher than 10 mcg/ml may raise the risk of toxicity.
• Be alert for signs of nephrotoxicity, including cells or casts in urine, oliguria, proteinuria, decreased creatinine clearance, and increased BUN and creatinine levels.
• Assess patient's and family's knowledge of drug therapy.

⚙ Nursing diagnoses

• Risk for infection related to bacteria
• Impaired urine elimination related to amikacin-induced nephrotoxicity
• Deficient knowledge related to drug therapy

Planning and implementation

• Obtain specimen for culture and sensitivity tests before first dose. Therapy may begin before receiving results.
• Therapy usually lasts 7 to 10 days.
• Drug potency isn't affected if solution turns light yellow.
• Patient should be well hydrated while taking drug to minimize renal tubule irritation.
• If no response occurs after 5 days, therapy may be stopped and new specimens obtained for culture and sensitivity testing.

ALERT: Don't confuse Amikin with Amicar or amikacin with anakinra.

Patient teaching

• Tell patient to immediately report changes in hearing or in urine appearance or elimination pattern. Teach patient how to measure intake and output.
• Emphasize importance of drinking 2 L of fluid daily, unless contraindicated.
• Teach patient to watch for and promptly report signs of superinfection, such as continued fever and other signs of new infections, especially of upper respiratory tract.

Evaluation

• Patient's infection is eradicated.
• Patient's renal function test values remain unchanged.
• Patient and family state understanding of drug therapy.

aminophylline (theophylline and ethylenediamine)

(am-mih-NOF-il-in)

Pharmacologic class: xanthine derivative
Therapeutic class: bronchodilator
Pregnancy risk category: C

Indications and dosages

▶ **Symptomatic relief of bronchospasm.** *Patients receiving theophylline products who require rapid relief of symptoms:* Loading dose is 6 mg/kg (equivalent to 4.7 mg/kg anhydrous theophylline) I.V. infusion at a rate of 25 mg/minute or less; then maintenance infusion.
Adults (nonsmokers): 0.7 mg/kg/hour I.V. for 12 hours; then 0.5 mg/kg/hour.
Otherwise healthy adult smokers: 1 mg/kg/hour I.V. for 12 hours; then 0.8 mg/kg/hour.
Older patients and adults with cor pulmonale: 0.6 mg/kg/hour I.V. for 12 hours; then 0.3 mg/kg/hour.
Adults with heart failure or liver disease: 0.5 mg/kg/hour I.V. for 12 hours; then 0.1 to 0.2 mg/kg/hour.
Children ages 9 to 16: 1 mg/kg/hour I.V. for 12 hours; then 0.8 mg/kg/hour.
Children ages 6 months to 8 years: 1.2 mg/kg/hour for 12 hours; then 1 mg/kg/hour.
Patients receiving theophylline products: Aminophylline infusion of 0.63 mg/kg (0.5 mg/kg anhydrous theophylline) increases level of theophylline by 1 mcg/ml. Some clinicians recommend a dose of 3.1 mg/kg (2.5 mg/kg anhydrous theophylline) with no obvious signs of theophylline toxicity.

▶ **Chronic bronchial asthma.** Dosage is highly individualized. Rectal dosage is same as oral dosage.
Adults: 600 to 1,600 mg P.O. daily in divided doses t.i.d. or q.i.d.
Children: 12 mg/kg P.O. daily in divided doses t.i.d. or q.i.d.

▶ **Periodic apnea related to Cheyne-Stokes respirations, promote diuresis, paroxysmal nocturnal dyspnea‡.** *Adults:* 200 to 400 mg I.V. bolus.

▶ **Reduce severe bronchospasm in infants with cystic fibrosis‡.** *Infants:* 10 to 12 mg/kg I.V. daily.

I.V. administration

• Because I.V. drug can burn, dilute with compatible I.V. solution.
• Exceeding recommended I.V. infusion rates increases the risk of adverse reactions. Inject at no more than 25 mg/minute.
• Theophylline concentration should range from 10 to 20 mcg/ml; toxicity may occur with level above 20 mcg/ml.
• Aminophylline is a soluble salt of theophylline. Dosage is adjusted by monitoring response, tolerance, pulmonary function, and theophylline level.

⊗ Incompatibilities

Amikacin, amiodarone, ascorbic acid, bleomycin, cephapirin, chlorpromazine, ciprofloxacin, clindamycin phosphate, codeine phosphate, corticotropin, dimenhydrinate, dobutamine, doxapram, doxorubicin, epinephrine hydrochloride, fat emulsion 10%, fructose 10% in normal saline, hydralazine, hydroxyzine hydrochloride, invert sugar 10% in normal saline injection, invert sugar 10% in water, levorphanol, meperidine, methadone, methylprednisolone sodium succinate, morphine, nafcillin, norepinephrine, ondansetron, papaverine, penicillin G potassium, pentazocine lactate, phenobarbital sodium, phenytoin sodium, procaine, prochlorperazine edisylate, promazine, promethazine hydrochloride, regular insulin, vancomycin, verapamil hydrochloride, vitamin B complex with C.

Contraindications and cautions

• Contraindicated in patients with active peptic ulcer disease, seizure disorders (unless anticonvulsants are given), and hypersensitivity to xanthine compounds (caffeine, theobromine) or ethylenediamine.
• Use cautiously in patients with heart failure or other cardiac or circulatory impairment, COPD, cor pulmonale, renal or hepatic disease, hyperthyroidism, diabetes mellitus, peptic ulcer, severe hypoxemia, or hypertension.
⚖ **Lifespan:** In pregnant or breast-feeding women, young children, and elderly patients, use cautiously.

Adverse reactions

CNS: nervousness, restlessness, dizziness, headache, insomnia, light-headedness, *seizures, muscle twitching.*
CV: palpitations, tachycardia, extrasystole, flushing, hypotension, *arrhythmias.*
GI: nausea, vomiting, anorexia, dyspepsia, heavy feeling in stomach, diarrhea, bitter aftertaste.
Respiratory: increased respiratory rate, *respiratory arrest.*
Skin: urticaria, local irritation with rectal suppositories.

Interactions

Drug-drug. *Adenosine:* May decrease antiarrhythmic effectiveness. Higher doses of adenosine may be needed.
Alkali-sensitive drugs: May reduce drug's activity. Don't add to I.V. fluids containing aminophylline.
Allopurinol (high doses), cimetidine, influenza virus vaccine, macrolide antibiotics (such as erythromycin), hormonal contraceptives, quinolone antibiotics (such as ciprofloxacin):

May decrease hepatic clearance of theophylline and increase theophylline level. Monitor patient for toxicity.
Amiodarone, ticlopidine, verapamil: May increase theophylline level. Use together cautiously.
Barbiturates, carbamazepine, nicotine, phenytoin, rifampin: May enhance metabolism and decrease theophylline level. Monitor patient for decreased aminophylline effect.
Carteolol, pindolol, propranolol, timolol: May act antagonistically, reducing the effects of one or both drugs. Monitor patient closely.
Ephedrine, other sympathomimetics: Theophylline may exhibit synergistic toxicity with these drugs, predisposing patient to arrhythmias. Monitor patient closely.
Isoniazid, ketoconazole: May decrease theophylline absorption.
Lithium: Theophylline may increase lithium level. Monitor patient closely.
Drug-herb. *Caffeine-containing herbs (such as guarana):* May increase adverse effects. Discourage using together.
St. John's wort: May decrease level and effectiveness of drug. Monitor patient for lack of therapeutic effect. Discourage using together.
Drug-food. *Caffeinated foods, colas:* May increase CNS adverse effects. Advise patient to monitor caffeine intake.
Drug-lifestyle. *Smoking:* May increase clearance and decrease half-life of theophylline. Higher doses may be needed to achieve desired effect.

Effects on lab test results

• May increase glucose and free fatty acid levels.

Pharmacokinetics

Absorption: Well absorbed except for suppository form, which is unreliable and slow. Food may alter rate but not extent of absorption of oral doses.
Distribution: In all tissues and extracellular fluids except fatty tissue.
Metabolism: Converted to theophylline, then metabolized to inactive compounds.
Excretion: 10% in urine as theophylline. *Half-life:* Depends on many variables, including smoking status, illness, age, and formulation used.

Reactions may be *common,* uncommon, *life-threatening,* or COMMON AND LIFE-THREATENING.

Route	Onset	Peak	Duration
P.O.			
tablets	15–60 min	2 hr	Varies
solution	15–60 min	1 hr	Varies
I.V.	15 min	Immediate	Varies
P.R.	Varies	Varies	Varies

Action

Chemical effect: Inhibits phosphodiesterase, the enzyme that degrades cAMP, thereby relaxing smooth muscle of bronchial airways and pulmonary blood vessels. **Therapeutic effect:** Eases breathing.

Available forms

Injection: 25 mg/ml
Oral liquid: 105 mg/5 ml
Rectal suppositories: 250 mg, 500 mg
Tablets: 100 mg, 200 mg

NURSING PROCESS

🔁 Assessment
• Monitor drug's effectiveness by regularly auscultating lungs and by noting respiratory rate and results of laboratory studies, such as arterial blood gas analysis.
• Monitor patient's hydration status if adverse GI reactions occur.
• Be alert for adverse reactions and drug interactions.
• Assess patient's and family's knowledge of drug therapy.

🔷 Nursing diagnoses
• Impaired gas exchange related to bronchospasm
• Risk for deficient fluid volume related to drug-induced adverse GI reactions
• Deficient knowledge related to drug therapy

🔷 Planning and implementation
• Make sure that patient hasn't had recent theophylline therapy before giving loading dose.
• Give drug with full glass of water at meals. Food in stomach delays absorption. Enteric-coated tablets may delay and impair absorption.
• Give suppository only if patient can't take drug orally. Schedule after bowel evacuation, if possible. Suppository may be retained better if given before meal. Have patient remain recumbent for 15 to 20 minutes after insertion.

⊗ ALERT: Don't confuse aminophylline with amitriptyline or ampicillin.

Patient teaching
• Supply instructions for home care and dosage schedule. Some patients may need an around-the-clock schedule.
• Warn elderly patients that dizziness is common at start of therapy.
• Warn patient to check with prescriber or pharmacist before combining aminophylline with other prescription drugs, OTC products, or herbal remedies that may contain ephedrine. Excessive CNS stimulation may result.
• Advise patient to avoid switching brands without consulting prescriber.
• Tell patient to notify prescriber if he quits smoking. Dosage may need to be reduced.
• Advise patient to notify prescriber if he experiences signs of toxicity, including anxiety, insomnia, irritability, or diarrhea.

☑ Evaluation
• Patient's appearance, vital signs, and laboratory test results demonstrate improved gas exchange.
• Patient remains hydrated throughout therapy.
• Patient and family state understanding of drug therapy.

amiodarone hydrochloride
(am-ee-OH-dah-rohn high-droh-KLOR-ighd)
Cordarone, Pacerone

Pharmacologic class: benzofuran derivative
Therapeutic class: ventricular antiarrhythmic
Pregnancy risk category: D

Indications and dosages

▶ **Recurrent ventricular fibrillation, unstable ventricular tachycardia, atrial fibrillation‡, angina‡, and hypertrophic cardiomyopathy‡.** *Adults:* loading dose of 800 to 1,600 mg P.O. daily for 1 to 3 weeks until initial therapeutic response occurs, then 650 to 800 mg P.O. daily for 1 month, then 200 to 600 mg P.O. daily as maintenance dosage. Or, for first 24 hours, 150 mg I.V. over 10 minutes (mix in 100 ml D_5W); then 360 mg I.V. over 6 hours (mix 900 mg in 500 ml D_5W); then maintenance dose of 540 mg I.V. over 18 hours at 0.50 mg/minute. After first 24 hours, continue a

maintenance infusion of 0.5 mg/minute in a concentration of 1 to 6 mg/ml. For infusions longer than 1 hour, concentrations shouldn't exceed 2 mg/ml unless you use a central venous catheter. Don't use for longer than 3 weeks.
▶ **Conversion from I.V. to P.O. route.** *Adults:* After daily dose of 720 mg I.V. (assuming rate of 0.5 mg/minute) for less than 1 week, start 800 to 1,600 mg P.O. daily; for 1 to 3 weeks, give 600 to 800 mg P.O. daily; and for longer than 3 weeks, give 400 mg P.O. daily.
▶ **Supraventricular arrhythmias‡.** *Adults:* 600 to 800 mg P.O. for 1 to 4 weeks or until supraventricular tachycardia is controlled. Maintenance dose is 100 to 400 mg P.O. daily.

▼ I.V. administration

• Drug may be given I.V. in facilities in which close monitoring of cardiac function and resuscitation is available. Initial dosage of 5 mg/kg should be mixed in 250 ml of D_5W.
• Repeat doses should be given through central venous catheter. Patient should receive maximum of 1.2 g in up to 500 ml D_5W daily.
• Maintain ECG monitoring during start and any change of dosage. Notify prescriber of significant change in ECG.
• Because of significant risk of life-threatening adverse reactions, drug is endline therapy used when other antiarrhythmics have been ineffective.
⊗ **Incompatibilities**
Aminophylline, cefazolin sodium, heparin sodium, sodium bicarbonate.

Contraindications and cautions

• Contraindicated in patients hypersensitive to drug and in those with severe sinus node disease, bradycardia, second- or third-degree AV block (unless artificial pacemaker is present), and bradycardia-induced syncope.
• Use cautiously in patients receiving other antiarrhythmics and in patients with pulmonary or thyroid disease because use may result in fatal toxicity.
⑤ **ALERT:** Some I.V. Cordarone preparations contain benzyl alcohol, which has caused "gasping syndrome" in neonates younger than age 1 month. Monitor patient for symptoms of sudden onset of gasping respiration, hypotension, bradycardia, and CV collapse.
❧ **Lifespan:** In pregnant women, use only when benefits outweigh risks to patient and fe-

tus. In breast-feeding women, drug is contraindicated. In children, safety of drug hasn't been established. I.V. Cordarone leaches plasticizers from administration tubing, which can adversely affect male reproductive tract development in the fetus, infants, and toddlers.

Adverse reactions

CNS: peripheral neuropathy, extrapyramidal symptoms, abnormal gait, ataxia, dizziness, paresthesias, headache, malaise, fatigue.
CV: *bradycardia, hypotension, arrhythmias, heart failure, heart block, sinus arrest.*
EENT: *corneal microdeposits,* vision disturbances.
GI: *nausea, vomiting,* constipation, anorexia.
Hepatic: *hepatic dysfunction.*
Metabolic: hypothyroidism, hyperthyroidism.
Musculoskeletal: muscle weakness.
Respiratory: SEVERE PULMONARY TOXICITY (PNEUMONITIS, ALVEOLITIS).
Skin: *photosensitivity,* blue-gray skin.
Other: gynecomastia.

Interactions

Drug-drug. *Antiarrhythmics:* Amiodarone may reduce hepatic or renal clearance of certain antiarrhythmics (especially flecainide and procainamide), and use of amiodarone with other antiarrhythmics (especially disopyramide, mexiletine, procainamide, and propafenone) may induce torsades de pointes. Monitor ECG closely.
Antihypertensives: May increase hypotensive effect. Use together cautiously.
Beta blockers, calcium channel blockers: May increase cardiac depressant effects and potentiate slowing of sinus node and AV conduction. Use together cautiously.
Digoxin: May increase digoxin level by an average of 70% to 100%. Monitor digoxin level closely.
Cholestyramine, rifampin: May decrease amiodarone level. Use together cautiously.
Cimetidine, protease inhibitors: May increase amiodarone level. Avoid using together.
Cyclosporine: May increase cyclosporine level. Monitor patient for cyclosporine toxicity.
Phenytoin: May decrease phenytoin metabolism. Monitor phenytoin level.
Quinidine: May increase quinidine concentrations producing potentially fatal cardiac arrhythmias. Monitor quinidine concentrations closely

---

if combination cannot be avoided. Adjust quinidine as needed.
Theophylline: May increase theophylline level and lead to toxicity. Monitor theophylline level.
Warfarin: May increase INR by an average of 100% within 1 to 4 weeks of therapy. Warfarin dosage should be decreased 33% to 50% when amiodarone is started. Monitor patient closely.
Drug-herb. *Pennyroyal:* May change the rate at which toxic metabolites of pennyroyal form. Discourage using together.
St. John's Wort: May decrease amiodarone levels. Discourage using together.
Drug-food. *Grapefruit juice:* May increase amiodarone levels. Discourage using together.
Drug-lifestyle. *Sun exposure:* May cause photosensitivity reaction. Advise against prolonged or unprotected sun exposure.

Effects on lab test results
● May increase ALT, AST, alkaline phosphatase, and GGT levels.
● May increase PT and INR.
● May alter thyroid function test results.

Pharmacokinetics
Absorption: Slow and variable.
Distribution: Wide, accumulating in adipose tissue and in organs with marked perfusion, such as lungs, liver, and spleen. Drug is 96% protein-bound.
Metabolism: Extensive in liver to active metabolite, desethyl amiodarone.
Excretion: Mainly hepatic through biliary tree.
Half-life: 25 to 110 days (usually 40 to 50 days).

Route	Onset	Peak	Duration
P.O.	2–21 days	3–7 hr	Varies
I.V.	Unknown	Unknown	Unknown

Action
Chemical effect: Unknown; thought to prolong refractory period and duration of action potential and decrease repolarization.
Therapeutic effect: Abolishes ventricular arrhythmia.

Available forms
Injection: 50 mg/ml
Tablets: 100 mg, 200 mg, 400 mg

NURSING PROCESS

⚖ Assessment
● Assess CV status before therapy.
● Review pulmonary, liver, and thyroid function test results before and regularly during therapy.
● Continuously monitor cardiac status of patient receiving I.V. amiodarone to evaluate its effectiveness.
● Watch for adverse reactions and drug interactions.
● Monitor patient carefully for pulmonary toxicity, which can be fatal. Risk increases in patients receiving more than 400 mg daily.
● Monitor electrolytes, particularly potassium and magnesium levels, and PT and INR if on warfarin.
● Assess patient's and family's knowledge of drug therapy.

⊞ Nursing diagnoses
● Decreased cardiac output related to ventricular arrhythmia
● Risk for injury related to drug-induced adverse reactions
● Deficient knowledge related to drug therapy

▶ Planning and implementation
● Adverse reactions commonly limit drug's use.
③ **ALERT:** Drug may pose life-threatening risks for patients already at risk for sudden death. Drug may cause fatal toxicities, including hepatic and pulmonary toxicity. Drug should be used only in patients with life-threatening, recurrent ventricular arrhythmias unresponsive to other antiarrhythmics or when alternative drugs can't be tolerated. Drug may also be used to treat atrial fibrillation, atrial flutter, paroxysmal supraventricular tachycardia, and, at low doses, heart failure.
● Divide oral loading dose into three equal doses and give with meals to decrease GI intolerance. Maintenance dosage may be given once daily or divided into two doses taken with meals if GI intolerance occurs.
● Instillation of methylcellulose ophthalmic solution during amiodarone therapy is recommended to minimize corneal microdeposits.
③ **ALERT:** Don't confuse amiodarone with amiloride.
Patient teaching
● Stress importance of taking drug exactly as prescribed.

Rapid onset   *Liquid form contains alcohol.   ◆ Canada   ◇ Australia   †OTC   ✐Photoguide   ‡Off-label use

• Emphasize importance of close follow-up and regular diagnostic studies to monitor drug action and assess for adverse reactions.
• Warn patient that drug may cause blue-gray skin pigmentation.
• Advise patient to use sunscreen to prevent photosensitivity reaction (burning or tingling skin followed by erythema and possible blistering).
• Inform patient that adverse effects are more prevalent at high doses but are generally reversible when therapy stops. Resolution of adverse reactions may take up to 4 months.

☑ **Evaluation**

• Patient's arrhythmia is corrected.
• Patient has no injury from adverse reactions.
• Patient and family state understanding of drug therapy.

amitriptyline hydrochloride

(am-ih-TRIP-tuh-leen high-droh-KLOR-ighd)
Apo-Amitriptyline ♦ , Elavil, Endep ◇ ,
Tryptanol ◇

Pharmacologic class: tricyclic antidepressant
Therapeutic class: antidepressant
Pregnancy risk category: C

Indications and dosages

▶ **Depression.** *Adults:* 50 to 100 mg P.O. h.s., gradually increasing to 150 mg daily; maximum dosage is 300 mg daily, if needed.
Elderly patients and adolescents: 10 mg P.O. t.i.d. and 20 mg h.s. daily.
▶ **Anorexia or bulimia related to depression or as adjunctive therapy for neurogenic pain‡.** *Adults:* If outpatient, initially 75 to 100 mg P.O. in divided doses daily. If inpatient, 100 to 300 mg P.O. in divided doses daily. After maximum effect is achieved, gradually lower dose to maintenance dose of 50 to 100 mg or less P.O. daily for a minimum of 3 months.

Contraindications and cautions

• Contraindicated during acute recovery phase of MI, in patients hypersensitive to drug, and within 14 days of MAO inhibitor therapy.
• Use cautiously in patients with history of seizures, urine retention, prostatic hypertrophy, angle-closure glaucoma, or increased intraocu-

lar pressure; in those with hyperthyroidism, CV disease, diabetes, or impaired liver function; and in those receiving thyroid medications.
⚘ **Lifespan:** In pregnant women, use cautiously. In breast-feeding women, drug is contraindicated. In children younger than age 12, don't use drug. In elderly patients, who may experience increased falls and increased anticholinergic effects while taking this drug, use cautiously.

Adverse reactions

CNS: *drowsiness,* dizziness, excitation, tremors, weakness, confusion, headache, *stroke,* nervousness, EEG alterations, *seizures,* extrapyramidal reactions.
CV: *orthostatic hypotension,* tachycardia, ECG changes, hypertension, *MI, arrhythmias.*
EENT: blurred vision, tinnitus, mydriasis.
GI: *dry mouth, constipation,* nausea, vomiting, anorexia, paralytic ileus.
GU: *urine retention.*
Hematologic: *agranulocytosis, thrombocytopenia.*
Skin: diaphoresis, rash, urticaria, photosensitivity reaction.
Other: hypersensitivity reactions.

Interactions

Drug-drug. *Barbiturates, CNS depressants:* May enhance CNS depression. Avoid using together.
Cimetidine, methylphenidate: May increase tricyclic antidepressant level. Monitor patient for enhanced antidepressant effect.
Clonidine: May cause loss of blood pressure control with potentially life threatening elevations in blood pressure. Don't use together.
Epinephrine, norepinephrine: May increase hypertensive effect. Use together cautiously.
Guanethidine: May antagonize antihypertensive action of guanethidine. Monitor patient.
MAO inhibitors: Especially at high dosage, may cause severe excitation, hyperpyrexia, or seizures. Avoid using within 14 days of each other.
Drug-herb. *St. John's wort, SAMe, yohimbe:* May cause serotonin level to become too high. Discourage using together.
Drug-lifestyle. *Alcohol use:* May enhance CNS depression. Discourage using together.
Smoking: May lower drug level. Monitor patient for lack of effect.

Sun exposure: May increase risk of photosensitivity reactions. Advise against prolonged or unprotected sun exposure.

Effects on lab test results

• May increase or decrease glucose level.
• May increase eosinophil count. May decrease granulocyte, platelet, and WBC counts.
• May increase liver function test values.

Pharmacokinetics

Absorption: Rapid.
Distribution: Widely into body, including CNS and breast milk. Drug is 96% protein-bound.
Metabolism: By liver to active metabolite nortriptyline; significant first-pass effect may account for variable levels in different patients taking same dosage.
Excretion: Primarily in urine. *Half-life:* Not established, wide interpatient variations.

Route	Onset	Peak	Duration
P.O., I.M.	Unknown	2–12 hr	Unknown

Action

Chemical effect: Unknown, but tricyclic antidepressant increases norepinephrine, serotonin, or both in CNS by blocking their reuptake by presynaptic neurons.
Therapeutic effect: Relieves depression.

Available forms

Syrup: 10 mg/5 ml
Tablets: 10 mg, 25 mg, 50 mg, 75 mg, 100 mg, 150 mg

NURSING PROCESS

Assessment

• Assess patient's depression before therapy.
• Be alert for adverse reactions and drug interactions.
• Assess patient's and family's knowledge of drug therapy.

Nursing diagnoses

• Ineffective individual coping related to depression
• Risk for injury related to adverse CNS reactions
• Deficient knowledge related to drug therapy

Planning and implementation

• Oral therapy should replace injection as soon as possible.
• Give full dose h.s. when possible.
• Don't withdraw drug abruptly.
• If signs of psychosis occur or increase, reduce dosage. Allow patient only minimum supply of drug.
• Because hypertensive episodes may occur during surgery in patients receiving tricyclic antidepressants, drug should be gradually stopped several days before surgery.
ⓈALERT: Don't confuse amitriptyline with nortriptyline or aminophylline, Elavil with Equanil or Mellaril, or Endep with Depen.
Patient teaching
• Advise patient to take full dose at bedtime, but warn him of possible morning orthostatic hypotension.
• Tell patient to avoid using alcohol and smoking while taking drug.
• Warn patient to avoid hazardous activities until full CNS effects of drug are known. Drowsiness and dizziness usually subside after a few weeks.
• Advise patient to consult prescriber before taking other prescription drugs, OTC medications, or herbal remedies.
• Teach patient to relieve dry mouth with sugarless hard candy or gum. Saliva substitutes may be needed.
• Advise patient to use sunblock, wear protective clothing, and avoid prolonged exposure to strong sunlight.
• Warn patient not to stop drug therapy abruptly. After abrupt withdrawal of long-term therapy, patient may experience nausea, headache, and malaise. These symptoms don't indicate addiction.
• Tell patient to watch for urine retention and constipation. Instruct him to increase fluids and suggest stool softener or high-fiber diet, as needed.
• Advise patient that effects of drug may not be apparent for 2 to 3 weeks.

Evaluation

• Patient's behavior and communication indicate improvement of depression.
• Patient doesn't experience injury from CNS adverse reactions.
• Patient and family state understanding of drug therapy.

amlodipine besylate
(am-LOW-dih-peen BEH-sih-layt)
Norvasc◊

Pharmacologic class: calcium channel blocker
Therapeutic class: antianginal, antihypertensive
Pregnancy risk category: C

Indications and dosages

▶ **Chronic stable angina; vasospastic angina (Prinzmetal's [variant] angina).** *Adults:* Initially, 10 mg P.O. daily.
Ⓝ Adjust-a-dose: For small, frail, or elderly patients or patients with hepatic insufficiency, begin therapy at 5 mg daily. Most patients need 10 mg daily for adequate results.
▶ **Hypertension.** *Adults:* Initially, 5 mg P.O. daily.
Ⓝ Adjust-a-dose: For small, frail, or elderly patients, patients receiving other antihypertensives, and patients with hepatic insufficiency, begin therapy at 2.5 mg daily. Dosage adjusted based on patient response and tolerance. Maximum, 10 mg daily.

Contraindications and cautions

• Contraindicated in patients hypersensitive to drug.
• Use cautiously in patients receiving other peripheral vasodilators (especially those with severe aortic stenosis) and in those with heart failure.
• In patients with severe hepatic disease, use cautiously and in reduced dosage because drug is metabolized by liver.
⚘ **Lifespan:** In pregnant women, use cautiously. In breast-feeding women, drug is contraindicated. In children, safety of drug hasn't been established.

Adverse reactions

CNS: headache, fatigue, somnolence.
CV: *edema,* dizziness, flushing, palpitations.
GI: nausea, abdominal pain, dyspepsia.

Interactions

Drug-food. *Grapefruit juice:* May increase drug level and adverse effects. Tell patient not to take drug with grapefruit juice. However, if he has been stabilized on the drug while routinely drinking grapefruit juice, caution him not to abruptly stop doing so.

Effects on lab test results
None reported.

Pharmacokinetics

Absorption: Absolute bioavailability from 64% to 90%.
Distribution: About 93% of circulating drug is bound to plasma proteins.
Metabolism: About 90% of drug is converted to inactive metabolites in liver.
Excretion: Primarily in urine. *Half-life:* 30 to 50 hours.

Route	Onset	Peak	Duration
P.O.	Unknown	6–9 hr	24 hr

Action

Chemical effect: Inhibits calcium ion influx across cardiac and smooth-muscle cells, thus decreasing myocardial contractility and oxygen demand. Also dilates coronary arteries and arterioles.
Therapeutic effect: Reduces blood pressure and prevents angina.

Available forms

Tablets: 2.5 mg, 5 mg, 10 mg

NURSING PROCESS

⚘ Assessment
• Assess patient's blood pressure or angina before therapy and regularly thereafter.
• Monitor patient carefully for pain. In some patients, especially those with severe obstructive coronary artery disease, increased frequency, duration, or severity of angina or even acute MI has developed after start of calcium channel blocker therapy or at time of dosage increase.
• Be alert for adverse reactions.
• Assess patient's and family's knowledge of drug therapy.

⚙ Nursing diagnoses
• Acute pain related to increased oxygen demand in cardiac tissue
• Risk for injury related to hypertension
• Deficient knowledge related to drug therapy

A

⊠ Planning and implementation
- Adjust dosage based on patient response and tolerance.
- Give S.L. nitroglycerin as needed for acute angina.
- ⊛ **ALERT:** Don't confuse amlodipine with amiloride.

Patient teaching
- Tell patient that S.L. nitroglycerin may be taken as needed for acute angina. If patient continues nitrate therapy during adjustment of amlodipine dosage, urge continued compliance.
- Advise patient to continue taking drug even when feeling better.

☑ Evaluation
- Patient's blood pressure is normal.
- Patient states anginal pain occurs with less frequency and severity.
- Patient and family state understanding of drug therapy.

amlodipine besylate and atorvastatin calcium
(am-LOW-dih-peen BEH-sih-layt AND ah-tore-vah-STAT-in CAL-see-um)
Caduet

Pharmacologic class: calcium channel blocker; HMG-CoA reductase inhibitor
Therapeutic class: Antianginal, antihypertensive; antilipemic
Pregnancy risk category: X

Indications and dosages
▶ **Patients who need amlodipine for hypertension, chronic stable angina, or vasospastic angina and atorvastatin for heterozygous familial or nonfamilial hypercholesterolemia, mixed dyslipidemia, elevated serum triglyceride levels, primary dysbetalipoproteinemia, or homozygous familial hypercholesterolemia.** *Adults:* 5 to 10 mg amlodipine with 10 to 80 mg atorvastatin P.O. once daily. Determine the most effective dose for each component, and then select the most appropriate combination product.
▶ **Hypertension and heterozygous familial hypercholesterolemia in children.** *Postpubertal boys and postmenarchal girls age 10 and*

older: 5 mg amlodipine with 10 to 20 mg atorvastatin P.O. once daily. Determine the most effective dose for each component, and then select the most appropriate combination product. If patient needs less than 5 mg of amlodipine, don't use the combination product.

Contraindications and cautions
- Contraindicated in patients hypersensitive to the drug or any of its components and in patients with active liver disease or an unexplained persistently elevated serum transaminase level.
- Use cautiously in patients who consume large amounts of alcohol or have a history of liver disease. Also use cautiously in patients who take a peripheral vasodilator or have severe aortic stenosis or heart failure.
- ⚘ **Lifespan:** In pregnant women, breastfeeding women, and women of childbearing age, use is contraindicated. In prepubertal patients, safety isn't known for combination product. In elderly patients, consider initiating with lower amlodipine doses.

Adverse reactions
CNS: asthenia, dizziness, fatigue, *headache,* insomnia, somnolence, vertigo.
CV: chest pain, *edema,* flushing, palpitations.
EENT: pharyngitis, rhinitis, sinusitis.
GI: abdominal pain, constipation, diarrhea, dyspepsia, flatulence, nausea.
GU: urinary tract infection.
Musculoskeletal: arthralgia, arthritis, back pain, myalgia.
Respiratory: bronchitis, dyspnea.
Skin: pruritus, rash.
Other: accidental injury, *allergic reaction, anaphylaxis,* flulike syndrome, *infection.*

Interactions
Drug-drug. *Azole antifungals, cyclosporine, erythromycin, fibric acid derivatives, niacin:* May increase risk of rhabdomyolysis with acute renal failure. Assess patient for muscle pain, tenderness, or weakness.
Digoxin: May increase digoxin level. Monitor serum digoxin levels.
Erythromycin: May increase atorvastatin level. Monitor patient.
Hormonal contraceptives: May increase hormone levels and adverse effects of hormonal contraceptive. Monitor patient.

Effects on lab test results

• May elevate liver function test results.

Pharmacokinetics

Absorption: Absolute availability for amlodipine is 64% to 90% and 14% for atorvastatin.
Distribution: In hypertensive patients, about 93% of amlodipine and 98% of atorvastatin are bound to plasma proteins. Atorvastatin penetrates RBCs poorly. Both drugs probably appear in breast milk.
Metabolism: Amlodipine undergoes extensive hepatic metabolism, with 90% converted to inactive metabolites. Atorvastatin is extensively metabolized, with about 70% of HMG-CoA reductase inhibition from active metabolites.
Excretion: Amlodipine is excreted mainly in urine. Half-life is 30 to 50 hours. Atorvastatin is excreted mainly in bile, but it doesn't seem to undergo enterohepatic recirculation. Mean plasma elimination half-life is about 14 hours, but the half-life for HMG-CoA reductase inhibition is 20 to 30 hours. Less than 2% of a dose is recovered in urine.

Route	Onset	Peak	Duration
P.O.			
amlodipine	Unknown	6–12 hr	24 hr
atorvastatin	Unknown	1–2 hr	Unknown

Action

Chemical effect: A peripheral arterial vasodilator, amlodipine inhibits calcium ion influx across cell membranes. It acts directly on vascular smooth muscle to reduce peripheral vascular resistance and blood pressure. Antianginal effects probably result from reduced afterload and myocardial oxygen demand. In vasospastic angina, amlodipine blocks constriction and restores blood flow in coronary arteries and arterioles. Atorvastatin inhibits HMG-CoA reductase, which reduces cholesterol synthesis.
Therapeutic effect: Reduces blood pressure, prevents angina, and lowers serum cholesterol levels.

Available forms

Tablets: 5 mg amlodipine with 10, 20, 40, or 80 mg atorvastatin; 10 mg amlodipine with 10, 20, 40, or 80 mg atorvastatin

NURSING PROCESS

✐ Assessment

• Assess patient's blood pressure, anginal pain, and lipid levels before therapy and regularly thereafter.
• Monitor liver function test results before therapy starts, after 12 weeks, whenever the dosage increases, and periodically during therapy.
• Assess the patient for myalgias, muscle tenderness or weakness, and marked elevation in CK level. Stop drug if it exceeds 10 times the upper limit of normal (ULN) or if myopathy is diagnosed or suspected.
• Assess patient's and family's knowledge of drug therapy.

✪ Nursing diagnoses

• Risk for deficient fluid volume related to adverse GI reactions
• Noncompliance related to long-term therapy or adverse reactions
• Deficient knowledge related to drug therapy

⧉ Planning and implementation

• Adjust dose based on patient response and tolerance.
• Reduce dose or stop drug if AST or ALT level increases to more than three times the ULN and stays elevated.
• Stop drug if patient has evidence of myopathy or has a condition that increases the risk of renal failure secondary to rhabdomyolysis, such as a severe acute infection, hypotension, major surgery, trauma, uncontrolled seizures, or severe metabolic, endocrine, or electrolyte disorders.
Patient teaching
• Advise patient to promptly report unexplained muscle pain, tenderness, or weakness, especially if accompanied by malaise or fever.
• Urge patient to continue appropriate diet, exercise, and weight loss regimens.

✔ Evaluation

• Patient maintains adequate fluid volume.
• Patient complies with therapy as evidenced by controlled blood pressure or angina and decreased lipid levels.
• Patient and family state understanding of drug therapy.

Reactions may be *common*, uncommon, *life-threatening*, or COMMON AND LIFE-THREATENING.

amoxicillin and clavulanate potassium

(uh-moks-uh-SIL-in and
KLAV-yoo-lan-ayt poh-TAH-see-um)
Augmentin, Augmentin ES-600,
Augmentin XR, Clavulin◆

Pharmacologic class: aminopenicillin, beta-lactamase inhibitor
Therapeutic class: antibiotic
Pregnancy risk category: B

Indications and dosages

▶ **Lower respiratory tract infections, otitis media, sinusitis, skin and skin-structure infections, and UTI caused by susceptible strains of gram-positive and gram-negative organisms.** *Adults:* 250 mg (based on amoxicillin component) P.O. q 8 hours. For more severe infections, 500 mg q 8 hours, or 875 mg P.O. q 12 hours.
Children: 20 to 40 mg/kg (based on amoxicillin component) P.O. daily in divided doses q 8 hours.
Neonates and infants younger than age 12 weeks: 30 mg/kg (based on amoxicillin component) P.O. daily in divided doses q 12 hours.
▶ **Recurrent or persistent acute otitis media caused by** *Streptococcus pneumoniae, Haemophilus influenzae,* **or** *Moraxella catarrhalis,* **in children with antibiotic exposure within the previous 3 months and who either are age 2 or younger or attend daycare.** *Infants and children age 3 months and older:* 90 mg/kg daily Augmentin ES-600 (based on amoxicillin component) P.O. q 12 hours for 10 days. Experience with this drug in patients weighing 40 kg (88 lb) or more is unavailable.
▶ **Community-acquired pneumonia or acute bacterial sinusitis from confirmed, or suspected beta-lactamase–producing pathogens** (*H. influenzae, M. catarrhalis, H. parainfluenzae, K. pneumoniae,* **or methicillin-susceptible** *S. aureus*) **and** *S. pneumoniae* **with reduced susceptibility to penicillin.** *Adults and children age 16 and older:* 2,000 mg/125 mg Augmentin XR q 12 hours for 7 to 10 days for pneumonia, or 10 days for sinusitis. Take with meals.

Contraindications and cautions

• Contraindicated in patients hypersensitive to drug or other penicillins and in those with a history of amoxicillin-related cholestatic jaundice or hepatic dysfunction.
• Augmentin XR is contraindicated in hemodialysis patients and in patients with renal impairment and a creatinine clearance less than 30 ml/minute. Augmentin XR is also contraindicated for infections from *S. pneumoniae* with penicillin minimal inhibitory concentrations (commonly known as MICs) of 4 mcg/ml or more.
• Use cautiously in patients with other drug allergies, especially to cephalosporins (possible cross-sensitivity), and in those with mononucleosis (high risk of maculopapular rash) or hepatic impairment.
 Lifespan: In pregnant and breast-feeding women, use cautiously. In children younger than age 16, safety and effectiveness of Augmentin XR haven't been established.

Adverse reactions

CNS: agitation, anxiety, insomnia, confusion, behavioral changes, dizziness.
GI: nausea, vomiting, *diarrhea,* indigestion, gastritis, stomatitis, glossitis, mucocutaneous candidiasis, abdominal pain, black "hairy" tongue, enterocolitis, *pseudomembranous colitis.*
GU: vaginitis, vaginal candidiasis.
Hematologic: anemia, *thrombocytopenia, thrombocytopenic purpura,* eosinophilia, *leukopenia, agranulocytosis.*
Other: hypersensitivity reactions (*rash,* urticaria, pruritus, *angioedema, anaphylaxis*), overgrowth of nonsusceptible organisms, serum sickness-like reactions (urticaria or skin rash accompanied by arthritis, arthralgia, myalgia, and frequently fever).

Interactions

Drug-drug. *Allopurinol:* May cause rash. Monitor patient.
Probenecid: May increase level of amoxicillin and other penicillins. Probenecid may be used for this purpose.

Effects on lab test results

• May decrease hemoglobin level and hematocrit.

Rapid onset   *Liquid form contains alcohol.   ◆Canada   ◇ Australia   †OTC   ⌀Photoguide   ‡Off-label use

• May increase eosinophil count. May decrease granulocyte, platelet, and WBC counts.
• May cause false-positive urine glucose determinations with copper sulfate tests, such as Benedict's solution and Clinitest.

Pharmacokinetics

Absorption: Well absorbed.
Distribution: Both drugs are distributed into pleural fluid, lungs, and peritoneal fluid, with high urine levels. Amoxicillin also is distributed into synovial fluid, liver, prostate, muscle, and gallbladder and penetrates into middle ear effusions, maxillary sinus secretions, tonsils, sputum, and bronchial secretions. Both drugs have minimal protein-binding.
Metabolism: Amoxicillin is metabolized only partially; clavulanate potassium, extensively.
Excretion: Amoxicillin is excreted mainly in urine; clavulanate potassium by glomerular filtration. *Half-life:* 1 to 1½ hours (in severe renal impairment, 7½ hours for amoxicillin and 4½ hours for clavulanate).

Route	Onset	Peak	Duration
P.O.			
Augmentin	Unknown	1–2½ hr	6–8 hr
Augmentin ES-600	Unknown	1–4 hr	Unknown
Augmentin XR	Unknown	1–6 hr	Unknown

Action

Chemical effect: Prevents bacterial cell-wall synthesis during replication. Clavulanic acid increases amoxicillin's effectiveness by inactivating beta lactamases, which destroy amoxicillin.
Therapeutic effect: Kills susceptible bacteria.

Available forms

Oral suspension: 125 mg amoxicillin trihydrate and 31.25 mg clavulanic acid/5 ml (after reconstitution); 200 mg amoxicillin trihydrate and 28.5 mg clavulanic acid/5 ml (after reconstitution); 250 mg amoxicillin trihydrate and 62.5 mg clavulanic acid/5 ml (after reconstitution); 400 mg amoxicillin trihydrate and 57 mg clavulanic acid/5 ml (after reconstitution); 600 mg amoxicillin trihydrate and 42.9 mg clavulanic acid/5 ml (after reconstitution)
Tablets: 875 mg amoxicillin trihydrate, 125 mg clavulanic acid
Tablets (chewable): 125 mg amoxicillin trihydrate, 31.25 mg clavulanic acid; 200 mg amoxicillin trihydrate, 28.5 mg clavulanic acid; 250 mg amoxicillin trihydrate, 62.5 mg clavulanic acid; 400 mg amoxicillin trihydrate, 57 mg clavulanic acid
Tablets (extended-release): 1,000 mg amoxicillin trihydrate, 62.5 mg clavulanic acid
Tablets (film-coated): 250 mg amoxicillin trihydrate, 125 mg clavulanic acid; 500 mg amoxicillin trihydrate, 125 mg clavulanic acid

NURSING PROCESS

🔍 Assessment

• Before therapy begins, assess patient's infection, ask him about past allergic reactions to penicillin (although negative history is no guarantee against allergic reaction), and obtain specimen for culture and sensitivity tests. Therapy may begin pending results.
• Be alert for adverse reactions and drug interactions.
• Monitor hydration status if adverse GI reactions occur.
• Assess patient's and family's knowledge of drug therapy.

🔷 Nursing diagnoses

• Infection related to susceptible bacteria
• Risk for deficient fluid volume related to drug-induced adverse GI reactions
• Deficient knowledge related to drug therapy

▶ Planning and implementation

• Give drug with food to prevent GI distress. Adverse effects for this combination drug, especially diarrhea, are more common than with plain amoxicillin.
• Give drug at least 1 hour before bacteriostatic antibiotics.
🔆 **ALERT:** Both 250-mg and 500-mg film-coated tablets contain 125 mg of clavulanic acid. Therefore, two 250-mg film-coated tablets don't equal one 500-mg film-coated tablet. Also, don't interchange the oral suspensions because of clavulanic acid content.
🔆 **ALERT:** Augmentin ES-600 is intended for children only.
• This drug combination is particularly useful with amoxicillin-resistant organisms.
• After reconstitution, refrigerate oral suspension and discard after 10 days.
🔆 **ALERT:** Don't confuse amoxicillin with amoxapine.

Reactions may be *common,* uncommon, *life-threatening,* or COMMON AND LIFE-THREATENING.

ALERT: Augmentin (250 mg or 500 mg amoxicillin) and Augmentin XR extended-release tablets aren't interchangeable because of the different amounts of clavulanic acid in each and the fact that Augmentin XR is an extended-release formulation. Don't give two Augmentin 500 mg tablets to replace one Augmentin XR 1,000 mg tablet.

Patient teaching

- Tell patient to take entire quantity of drug exactly as prescribed, even after he feels better.
- Tell patient to call prescriber if rash develops (sign of allergic reaction).
- Instruct patient to take drug with food to prevent GI distress.

Evaluation

- Patient is free from infection.
- Patient maintains adequate hydration.
- Patient and family state understanding of drug therapy.

amoxicillin trihydrate (amoxycillin trihydrate ◇)

(uh-moks-uh-SIL-in trigh-HIGH-drayt)

Alphamox ◇, Amoxil, Apo-Amoxil, Cilamox ◇, DisperMox, Maxamox ◇, Moxacin ◇, Novamoxin ♦, Nu-Amoxi ♦, Trimox

Pharmacologic class: aminopenicillin
Therapeutic class: antibiotic
Pregnancy risk category: B

Indications and dosages

▶ **Mild to moderate infections of the ear, nose and throat, skin and skin structure, or genitourinary tracts.** *Adults and children who weigh 40 kg (88 lb) or more:* 500 mg P.O. q 12 hours or 250 mg P.O. q 8 hours.
Children older than 3 months who weigh less than 40 kg: 25 mg/kg/day P.O. divided q 12 hours or 20 mg/kg/day P.O. divided q 8 hours.
Neonates and infants up to age 3 months: Up to 30 mg/kg/day P.O. divided q 12 hours.

▶ **Mild to severe infections of the lower respiratory tract and severe infections of the ear, nose and throat, skin and skin structure, or genitourinary tracts.** *Adults and children weighing 40 kg or more:* 875 mg P.O. q 12 hours or 500 mg P.O. q 8 hours.
Children older than 3 months who weigh less than 40 kg: 45 mg/kg/day P.O. divided q 12 hours or 40 mg/kg/day P.O. divided q 8 hours.

▶ **Uncomplicated gonorrhea.** *Adults:* 3 g P.O. as a single dose.
Children older than age 2: 50 mg/kg with 25 mg/kg probenecid as a single dose.

▶ **Chlamydial and mycoplasmal infections during pregnancy.** *Adults:* 500 mg P.O. t.i.d. for 7 to 10 days.

Adjust-a-dose: Patients with renal failure who need repeated doses may need adjustment of dosing interval. If creatinine clearance is 10 to 30 ml/minute, increase interval to q 12 hours; if it's less than 10 ml/minute, give drug q 24 hours. Supplemental doses may be needed after hemodialysis. Don't give 875-mg tablet if creatinine clearance is less than 30 ml/minute.

▶ **Oral prophylaxis of bacterial endocarditis.** Consult current American Heart Association recommendations before giving drug. *Adults:* 2 g 1 hour before procedure.
Children: 50 mg/kg (maximum, 2 g) 1 hour before procedure.

▶ **Postexposure prophylaxis for penicillin-susceptible anthrax.** *Adults and children age 9 and older:* 500 mg P.O. t.i.d. for 60 days.
Children younger than age 9: 80 mg/kg/day P.O., divided t.i.d. for 60 days.

▶ **Lyme disease‡.** *Adults:* 250 to 500 mg P.O. t.i.d. or q.i.d. for 10 to 30 days.
Children: 25 to 50 mg/kg daily (maximum, 1 to 2 g daily) P.O. in three divided doses for 10 to 30 days.

▶ **Acute complicated UTI in nonpregnant women‡.** *Adults:* 3 g P.O. as a single dose.

Contraindications and cautions

- Contraindicated in patients hypersensitive to drug or other penicillins.
- Use cautiously in patients with other drug allergies, especially to cephalosporins (possible cross-sensitivity), and in those with mononucleosis (high risk of maculopapular rash).

Lifespan: In pregnant or breast-feeding women, use cautiously.

Adverse reactions

CNS: *seizures.*
GI: nausea, vomiting, diarrhea.

Hematologic: anemia, *thrombocytopenia, thrombocytopenic purpura,* eosinophilia, *leukopenia, agranulocytosis.*
Other: hypersensitivity reactions (erythematous maculopapular rash, urticaria, *anaphylaxis*), overgrowth of nonsusceptible organisms.

Interactions

Drug-drug. *Allopurinol:* May increase risk of rash. Monitor patient.
Probenecid: May increase level of amoxicillin and other penicillins. Probenecid may be used for this purpose.

Effects on lab test results

• May decrease hemoglobin level and hematocrit.
• May increase eosinophil count. May decrease granulocyte, platelet, and WBC counts.
• May cause false-positive urine glucose determinations with copper sulfate tests (such as Benedict's solution and Clinitest).

Pharmacokinetics

Absorption: About 80%.
Distribution: Into pleural, peritoneal, and synovial fluids; lungs; prostate; muscle; liver; and gallbladder. Also penetrates middle ear, maxillary sinus and bronchial secretions, tonsils, and sputum. Amoxicillin readily crosses placenta and is 17% to 20% protein-bound.
Metabolism: Only partially.
Excretion: Principally in urine by renal tubular secretion and glomerular filtration; also excreted in breast milk. *Half-life:* 1 to 1½ hours (7½ hours in severe renal impairment).

Route	Onset	Peak	Duration
P.O.	Unknown	1–2 hr	6–8 hr

Action

Chemical effect: Inhibits cell-wall synthesis during bacterial multiplication.
Therapeutic effect: Kills susceptible bacteria.

Available forms

Capsules: 250 mg, 500 mg
Suspension: 50 mg/ml (pediatric drops) 125 mg/5 ml, 200 mg/5 ml, 250 mg/5 ml, 400 mg/5 ml
Tablets (chewable): 200 mg, 400 mg
Tablets (film-coated): 500 mg, 875 mg

Tablets (for oral suspension): 200 mg, 400 mg, 600 mg

NURSING PROCESS

⚕ Assessment

• Before therapy, assess patient's infection, ask him about allergic reactions to drug or other forms of penicillin (although negative history doesn't guarantee against future reaction), and obtain specimen for culture and sensitivity tests. Therapy may begin pending test results.
• Be alert for adverse reactions and drug interactions.
• Monitor patient's hydration status if adverse GI reactions occur.
• Assess patient's and family's knowledge of drug therapy.

🔟 Nursing diagnoses

• Infection related to susceptible bacteria
• Risk for deficient fluid volume related to drug-induced adverse GI reactions
• Deficient knowledge related to drug therapy

▶ Planning and implementation

• Give amoxicillin at least 1 hour before bacteriostatic antibiotics.
• May be taken with or without food.
• Trimox oral suspension may be stored at room temperature for up to 2 weeks. Check individual product labels for storage information.
• For DisperMox, mix 1 tablet in 10 ml of water and have patient drink mixture. Rinse container with a small amount of water to make sure the entire tablet is taken. Don't let the patient chew, swallow, or allow tablet to dissolve in mouth.
⊛ ALERT: Don't confuse amoxicillin with amoxapine.
Patient teaching
• If drug allergy develops, advise patient to wear or carry medical identification stating penicillin allergy.
• Tell patient to take entire quantity of drug exactly as prescribed, even after he feels better.
• Tell patient to call prescriber if rash (most common), fever, or chills develop.
• Inform patient drug may be taken with or without food.
• Warn patient never to use leftover amoxicillin for a new illness or to share it with others.
• Tell patient to mix DisperMox tablet in 10 ml of water and drink. Rinse container with small

---

Reactions may be *common,* uncommon, *life-threatening,* or **COMMON AND LIFE-THREATENING.**

amount of water and drink to get entire dosage. Only mix tablet with water. Don't chew or swallow tablets or let dissolve in mouth.

☑ Evaluation
• Patient is free from infection.
• Patient maintains adequate hydration.
• Patient and family state understanding of drug therapy.

amphotericin B desoxycholate
(am-foh-TER-ah-sin bee)
Amphocin, Fungizone

Pharmacologic class: polyene macrolide
Therapeutic class: antifungal
Pregnancy risk category: B

Indications and dosages

► **Systemic (potentially fatal) fungal infections caused by susceptible organisms, fungal endocarditis, fungal septicemia.** *Adults and children:* Some clinicians recommend an initial dose of 1 mg I.V. in 20 ml D₅W infused over 20 minutes. If test dose is tolerated, then give daily doses of 0.25 to 0.3 mg/kg, gradually increasing by 5 to 10 mg daily until dose is 1 mg/kg daily or 1.5 mg/kg q alternate day. Duration of therapy depends on the severity and nature of infection.
► **Sporotrichosis.** *Adults and children:* 0.4 to 0.5 mg/kg daily I.V. for up to 9 months. Total I.V. dosage of 2.5 g over 9 months.
► **Aspergillosis.** *Adults and children:* 0.5 to 1.5 mg/kg daily initially and a total I.V. dosage of 1.5 to 4 g over 11 months.
► **Disseminated or invasive candidal infections.** *Adults and children:* 0.4 to 0.6 mg/kg I.V. daily. Higher doses of up to 1.5 mg/kg have been used in rapidly progressing or potentially fatal infections. Therapy may last 7 to 14 days to more than 6 weeks depending on severity.
► **Coccidioidomycosis.** *Adults:* 0.5 to 1 mg/kg I.V. daily. Therapy usually lasts 4 to 12 weeks.
► **Cryptococcosis.** *Adults:* 0.3 to 1 mg/kg I.V. daily. Therapy may last 2 weeks to several months. Drug may be given with flucytosine P.O.
► **Cryptococcal meningitis in HIV-infected patients.** *Adults:* 0.7 mg/kg I.V. daily for 4

weeks followed by 0.7 mg/kg I.V. every other day for another 4 weeks.
► **Mucocutaneous leishmaniasis.** *Adults and children:* 0.25 to 0.5 mg/kg/day I.V., increased gradually to 0.5 to 1 mg/kg/day. Then give on alternate days. Treat for 3 to 12 weeks.
► **Visceral leishmaniasis.** *Adults and children:* 0.5 to 1 mg/kg/day I.V. on alternate days for 14 to 20 doses.
► **Paracoccidioidomycosis‡.** *Adults:* 0.4 to 0.5 mg/kg I.V. daily for 4 to 12 weeks.
► **Empiric therapy of presumed fungal infections in febrile, neutropenic patients, including cancer and bone marrow transplant patients ‡.** *Adults:* 0.1 mg/kg daily.

▼ I.V. administration

• Reconstitute only with 10 ml sterile water. To avoid precipitation, don't mix with solutions containing sodium chloride, other electrolytes, or bacteriostatic drugs (such as benzyl alcohol).
• Don't use if solution contains precipitate or foreign matter.
• Amphotericin B appears to be compatible with limited amounts of heparin sodium, hydrocortisone sodium succinate, and methylprednisolone sodium succinate.
• Give drug parenterally only in hospitalized patients, under close supervision, after diagnosis of potentially fatal fungal infection is confirmed.
• Be prepared to give an initial test dose, for which 1 mg is added to 20 ml of D₅W and infused over 20 to 30 minutes.
• Use an infusion pump and in-line filter with a mean pore diameter larger than 1 micron. Infuse over 2 to 6 hours because rapid infusion may cause CV collapse.
• Use I.V. sites in distal veins. If thrombosis occurs, alternate sites.
• If patient has severe adverse infusion reactions to first dose, stop infusion, notify prescriber, and give antipyretics, antihistamines, antiemetics, or small doses of corticosteroids. To prevent reactions during subsequent infusions, premedicate with these drugs or give amphotericin B on an alternate-day schedule.
• Reconstituted solution is stable for 1 week in refrigerator, 24 hours at room temperature, and 8 hours in room light.
• Store dry form at 36° to 46° F (2° to 8° C). Protect from light.

⊗ Incompatibilities

Amikacin, calcium chloride, chlorpromazine, cimetidine, diphenhydramine, edetate calcium disodium, gentamicin, kanamycin, lactated Ringer's injection, melphalan, methyldopate, normal saline solution, paclitaxel, penicillin G potassium, penicillin G sodium, polymyxin B, potassium chloride, prochlorperazine mesylate, streptomycin, verapamil. Give antibiotics separately; don't mix or piggyback with amphotericin B.

Contraindications and cautions

• Contraindicated in patients hypersensitive to drug or its components.
• Use cautiously in patients with impaired renal function.
☆ **Lifespan:** In pregnant women, use cautiously. Breast-feeding women must stop breast-feeding or stop the drug. In children, safety and dosage haven't been fully established, but therapy may be successful.

Adverse reactions

CNS: fever, malaise, headache, peripheral neuropathy, encephalopathy, *seizures,* peripheral nerve pain, paresthesia (with I.V. use).
CV: hypotension, hypertension, *arrhythmias, asystole,* phlebitis, thrombophlebitis.
EENT: tinnitus, vertigo, hearing loss, visual impairment.
GI: anorexia, weight loss, nausea, vomiting, dyspepsia, diarrhea, epigastric cramps, *hemorrhagic gastroenteritis.*
GU: abnormal renal function with hypokalemia, azotemia, hyposthenuria, hypomagnesemia, renal tubular acidosis, nephrocalcinosis, *permanent renal impairment,* anuria, oliguria.
Hematologic: normochromic normocytic anemia, eosinophilia, *thrombocytopenia, agranulocytosis.*
Hepatic: *hepatitis, acute liver failure.*
Metabolic: hypokalemia, hypomagnesemia.
Musculoskeletal: arthralgia, myalgia.
Respiratory: pulmonary edema, hypersensitivity pneumonitis, dyspnea.
Skin: burning, stinging, irritation, tissue damage with extravasation, pain at injection site, rash, pruritus.
Other: chills, generalized pain; *anaphylactoid reactions.*

Interactions

Drug-drug. *Corticosteroids:* May cause potassium depletion. Monitor potassium level.
Digoxin: May increase risk of digitalis toxicity in potassium-depleted patients. Monitor patient closely.
Flucytosine: May increase flucytosine toxicity. Monitor patient closely.
Other nephrotoxic drugs (such as antibiotics, antineoplastics): May increase risk of nephrotoxicity. Use together cautiously.
Skeletal muscle relaxants: May increase effects of muscle relaxants. Monitor patient for increased effects.
Thiazide diuretics: May increase potassium loss. Monitor patient for signs of hypokalemia; monitor potassium level.

Effects on lab test results

• May increase urine urea, uric acid, BUN, creatinine, alkaline phosphatase, ALT, AST, GGT, LDH, and bilirubin levels. May decrease phosphate, magnesium, and hemoglobin levels and hematocrit. May increase or decrease glucose, potassium, and calcium levels.
• May decrease platelet and granulocyte counts. May increase or decrease WBC and eosinophil counts.

Pharmacokinetics

Absorption: Poor.
Distribution: Well into pleural cavities and joints; less so into aqueous humor, bronchial secretions, pancreas, bone, muscle, and parotid gland. Drug is 90% to 95% bound to plasma proteins.
Metabolism: Not well defined.
Excretion: Up to 5% unchanged in urine. *Half-life:* Adults and children older than age 9, 24 hours; children age 9 and younger, 18 hours.

Route	Onset	Peak	Duration
I.V.	Immediate	Immediate	Unknown

Action

Chemical effect: May bind to sterol in fungal cell membrane and alter cell permeability, allowing leakage of intracellular components.
Therapeutic effect: Decreases activity of or kills susceptible fungi.

Available forms

Powder for injection: 50-mg lyophilized cake

NURSING PROCESS

⚕ Assessment
• Obtain history of fungal infection and samples for culture and sensitivity tests before first dose. Reevaluate condition during therapy.
• Be alert for adverse reactions and drug interactions.
• Monitor patient's pulse, respiratory rate, temperature, and blood pressure every 30 minutes for at least 4 hours after giving drug I.V.; fever, shaking chills, anorexia, nausea, vomiting, headache, tachypnea, and hypotension may appear 1 to 3 hours after start of I.V. infusion. Symptoms are usually more severe with initial dose.
• Monitor BUN, creatinine or creatinine clearance, and electrolyte levels; CBC; and liver function test results at least weekly.
• Drug is linked to rhinocerebral phycomycosis, especially in patients with uncontrolled diabetes. Leukoencephalopathy also may occur. Monitor pulmonary function. Acute reactions are characterized by dyspnea, hypoxemia, and infiltrates.
• Assess patient's and family's knowledge of drug therapy.

⊕ Nursing diagnoses
• Infection related to presence of susceptible fungal species
• Risk for injury related to drug-induced adverse reactions
• Deficient knowledge related to drug therapy

▶ Planning and implementation
🚫 **ALERT:** Different amphotericin B preparations aren't interchangeable, and dosages vary.
• If BUN level exceeds 40 mg/dl, or if creatinine level exceeds 3 mg/dl, prescriber may reduce or stop drug until renal function improves. Drug may be stopped if alkaline phosphatase or bilirubin level increases.
Patient teaching
• Teach patient signs and symptoms of hypersensitivity, and stress importance of reporting them immediately.
• Warn patient that therapy may take several months; teach personal hygiene and other measures to prevent spread and recurrence of lesions.

• Urge patient to comply with prescribed regimen and recommended follow-up.
• Warn patient that discomfort at injection site and adverse reactions may occur during therapy, which may last several months.

☑ Evaluation
• Patient is free from fungal infection.
• Patient doesn't experience injury as a result of drug-induced adverse reactions.
• Patient and family state understanding of drug therapy.

amphotericin B lipid complex
(am-foe-TER-ah-sin bee LIP-id KOM-pleks)
Abelcet

Pharmacologic class: polyene antibiotic
Therapeutic class: antifungal
Pregnancy risk category: B

Indications and dosages
▶ **Invasive fungal infections, including those caused by** *Aspergillus fumigatus, Candida albicans, C. guilliermondii, C. stellatoidea,* **and** *C. tropicalis, Coccidioidomycosis* **sp.,** *Cryptococcus* **sp.,** *Histoplasma* **sp., and** *Blastomyces* **sp. in patients refractory to or intolerant of conventional amphotericin B therapy.** *Adults and children:* 5 mg/kg daily as a single I.V. infusion. Give by continuous I.V. infusion at 2.5 mg/kg/hour.

▼ I.V. administration
• To prepare, shake the vial gently until you see no yellow sediment. Using aseptic technique, draw the calculated dose into one or more 20-ml syringes, using an 18G needle. You'll need more than one vial.
• Attach a 5-micron filter needle to the syringe and inject the dose into an I.V. bag of D_5W. One filter needle can be used for up to four vials of drug. The volume of D_5W should be sufficient to yield a final concentration of 1 mg/ml.
• For children and patients with CV disease, the recommended final concentration is 2 mg/ml.
• Shake the bag and check the contents for foreign matter.
• Don't use an in-line filter.
• If infusing through an existing I.V. line, flush first with D_5W.

Rapid onset   *Liquid form contains alcohol.   ◆ Canada   ◇ Australia   †OTC   ⵠPhotoguide   ‡Off-label use

• Solutions are stable for up to 48 hours when refrigerated at 36° to 46° F (2° to 8° C) and for up to 6 hours at room temperature.
• Refrigerate and protect from light. Don't freeze.
• Discard unused drug; it contains no preservatives.
• Slowing the infusion rate also may decrease the risk of infusion-related reactions.
• For infusions lasting longer than 2 hours, shake the I.V. bag every 2 hours to ensure an even suspension.

⊗ **Incompatibilities**
Electrolytes, other I.V. drugs, saline solutions.

Contraindications and cautions

• Contraindicated in patients hypersensitive to amphotericin B or its components.
• Use cautiously in patients with renal impairment.
☲ **Lifespan:** In pregnant women, safety hasn't been established. Use only if benefits outweigh risks to the fetus. Breast-feeding women must stop breast-feeding or stop drug. In infants younger than 1 month, safety and effectiveness haven't been established.

Adverse reactions

CNS: fever, headache, pain.
CV: chest pain, *cardiac arrest,* hypertension, hypotension.
GI: abdominal pain, diarrhea, nausea, vomiting, *GI hemorrhage.*
GU: *renal failure.*
Hematologic: anemia, *leukopenia, thrombocytopenia.*
Hepatic: bilirubinemia.
Metabolic: hypokalemia.
Respiratory: dyspnea, respiratory disorder, *respiratory failure.*
Skin: rash.
Other: chills, infection, MULTIPLE ORGAN FAILURE, *sepsis.*

Interactions

Drug-drug. *Antineoplastics:* May increase risk of renal toxicity, bronchospasm, and hypotension. Use cautiously.
Digoxin: May increase risk of digoxin toxicity and induce hypokalemia. Monitor potassium level closely.
Corticosteroids, corticotropin: May enhance hypokalemia, which may lead to cardiac dys-

function. Monitor electrolytes and cardiac function.
Cyclosporin A: May increase renal toxicity. Monitor patient closely.
Flucytosine: May increase risk of flucytosine toxicity due to increased cellular uptake or impaired renal excretion. Use together cautiously.
Imidazoles (clotrimazole, fluconazole, itraconazole, ketoconazole, miconazole): May decrease effectiveness of amphotericin B because of inhibition of ergosterol synthesis. Clinical significance is unknown.
Leukocyte transfusions: May cause acute pulmonary toxicity. Avoid using together.
Nephrotoxic drugs (aminoglycosides, pentamidine): May increase risk of renal toxicity. Use together cautiously. Monitor renal function closely.
Skeletal muscle relaxants: May enhance effects of skeletal muscle relaxants because of drug-induced hypokalemia. Monitor potassium level closely.
Zidovudine: May increase myelotoxicity and nephrotoxicity. Monitor renal and hematologic function.

Effects on lab test results

• May increase BUN, creatinine, alkaline phosphatase, ALT, AST, bilirubin, GGT, and LDH levels. May decrease potassium and hemoglobin levels and hematocrit.
• May decrease WBC and platelet counts.

Pharmacokinetics

Absorption: Given I.V.
Distribution: Well distributed. Volume increases with dose. Amphotericin B lipid complex yields measurable amphotericin B levels in spleen, lung, liver, lymph nodes, kidney, heart, and brain.
Metabolism: Unknown.
Excretion: Rapidly cleared from blood. *Terminal half-life:* About a week, probably because of slow elimination from tissues.

Route	Onset	Peak	Duration
I.V.	Unknown	Unknown	Unknown

Action

Chemical effect: Amphotericin B binds to sterols in fungal cell membranes, resulting in enhanced cellular permeability and cell damage.

Reactions may be *common,* uncommon, *life-threatening,* or COMMON AND LIFE-THREATENING.

It has fungistatic or fungicidal effects, depending on fungal susceptibility.
Therapeutic effect: Decreases activity of or kills susceptible fungi.

Available forms

Suspension for injection: 50 mg/10-ml vial; 100 mg/20-ml vial

NURSING PROCESS

≈ Assessment

• Obtain history of fungal infection and samples for culture and sensitivity tests before therapy. Reevaluate condition during therapy.
• Be alert for adverse reactions and drug interactions.
• Assess renal function before therapy starts.
• Monitor liver function, creatinine, and electrolyte levels (especially magnesium and potassium), and CBC during therapy.
• Assess patient's and family's knowledge of drug therapy.

✤ Nursing diagnoses

• Risk for infection related to presence of susceptible fungal infection
• Risk for injury related to drug-induced adverse reactions
• Deficient knowledge related to drug therapy

❯ Planning and implementation

• If severe respiratory distress develops, stop the infusion, provide supportive therapy for anaphylaxis, and notify prescriber. Don't resume the infusion.
⑤ **ALERT:** Different amphotericin B preparations aren't interchangeable, and dosages vary.
• Premedicate patient with acetaminophen, antihistamines, and corticosteroids to prevent or lessen the severity of infusion-related reactions, such as fever, chills, nausea, and vomiting, which occur 1 to 2 hours after the start of infusion.
Patient teaching
• Inform patient that fever, chills, nausea, and vomiting may occur during the infusion and that these reactions usually subside with subsequent doses.
• Instruct patient to report any redness or pain at the infusion site.

• Teach patient to recognize and report any symptoms of acute hypersensitivity, such as respiratory distress.
• Tell patient to expect frequent laboratory testing to monitor kidney and liver function.

✓ Evaluation

• Patient is free from fungal infection.
• Patient has no injury from adverse drug reactions.
• Patient and family state understanding of drug therapy.

amphotericin B liposomal
(am-foh-TER-ah-sin bee lye-poh-SOW-mul)
AmBisome

Pharmacologic class: polyene antibiotic
Therapeutic class: antifungal
Pregnancy risk category: B

Indications and dosages

❯ **Empirical therapy for presumed fungal infection in febrile, neutropenic patients.** *Adults and children:* 3 mg/kg I.V. infusion daily.
❯ **Systemic fungal infections caused by** *Aspergillus* sp., *Candida* sp., or *Cryptococcus* sp. **refractory to amphotericin B deoxycholate or in patients with renal impairment or unacceptable toxicity that precludes the use of amphotericin B deoxycholate.** *Adults and children:* 3 to 5 mg/kg I.V. infusion daily.
❯ **Visceral leishmaniasis in immunocompetent patients.** *Adults and children:* 3 mg/kg I.V. infusion daily on days 1 to 5, 14, and 21. A repeat course of therapy may be beneficial if initial treatment fails to achieve parasitic clearance.
❯ **Visceral leishmaniasis in immunocompromised patients.** *Adults and children:* 4 mg/kg I.V. infusion daily on days 1 to 5, 10, 17, 24, 31, and 38. Expert advice regarding further treatment is recommended if initial therapy fails or relapse occurs.
❯ **Cryptococcal meningitis in HIV-infected patients.** *Adults and children:* 6 mg/kg daily I.V. infusion over 2 hours. Infusion time may be reduced to 1 hour if well tolerated or increased if discomfort occurs.

▽ I.V. administration

• Reconstitute each 50-mg vial of amphotericin B liposomal with 12 ml of sterile water for injection to yield a solution of 4 mg amphotericin B per milliliter.

• After reconstitution, shake vial vigorously for 30 seconds or until particulate matter disappears. Withdraw calculated amount of reconstituted solution into a sterile syringe and inject through a 5-micron filter into the appropriate amount of D_5W to a final concentration of 1 to 2 mg/ml. Lower concentrations (0.2 to 0.5 mg/ml) may be appropriate for children to provide sufficient volume for infusion.

• Flush existing I.V. line with D_5W before infusing drug. If this isn't feasible, give drug through a separate line.

• Use a controlled infusion device and an in-line filter with a mean pore diameter larger than 1 micron. Initially, infuse drug over at least 2 hours. Infusion time may be reduced to 1 hour if the treatment is well tolerated. If the patient has discomfort during infusion, the duration of infusion may be increased.

• Observe patient closely for adverse reactions during infusion. If anaphylaxis occurs, stop the infusion immediately, provide supportive therapy, and notify the prescriber.

• Refrigerate unopened drug at 36° to 46° F (2° to 8° C). Once reconstituted, the product may be stored for up to 24 hours at 36° to 46° F. Don't freeze.

⊗ **Incompatibilities**
Other I.V. drugs, saline solutions, bacteriostatic water for injection and bacteriostatic drugs.

Contraindications and cautions

• Contraindicated in patients hypersensitive to drug or any of its components.

• Use cautiously in patients with renal impairment.

❋ **Lifespan:** In pregnant women, safety hasn't been established. Use only if benefits outweigh risks to the fetus. Breast-feeding women must stop breast-feeding or stop drug. In infants younger than 1 month, safety and effectiveness haven't been established.

Adverse reactions

CNS: anxiety, confusion, fever, headache, insomnia, asthenia, pain.

CV: chest pain, hypotension, tachycardia, hypertension, edema, vasodilation, phlebitis.
EENT: *epistaxis,* rhinitis.
GI: *GI hemorrhage,* nausea, vomiting, anorexia, abdominal pain, diarrhea.
GU: hematuria.
Hepatic: hepatomegaly.
Metabolic: hyperglycemia, hypernatremia, hypocalcemia, hypokalemia, hypomagnesemia.
Musculoskeletal: back pain.
Respiratory: cough, dyspnea, hypoxia, pleural effusion, lung disorder, hyperventilation.
Skin: *pruritus, rash,* sweating.
Other: chills, infection, *anaphylaxis, sepsis, blood product infusion reaction.*

Interactions

Drug-drug. *Antineoplastics:* May enhance potential for renal toxicity, bronchospasm, and hypotension. Use cautiously.
Corticosteroids, corticotropin: May potentiate hypokalemia, which could result in cardiac dysfunction. Monitor potassium level and cardiac function.
Digoxin: May increase risk of digoxin toxicity in potassium-depleted patients. Monitor potassium level closely.
Flucytosine: May increase flucytosine toxicity by increasing cellular uptake or impairing renal excretion of flucytosine. Monitor renal function closely.
Imidazole antifungals (clotrimazole, ketoconazole, miconazole): May induce fungal resistance to amphotericin B. Use together cautiously
Leukocyte transfusions: May increase risk of acute pulmonary toxicity. Avoid using together.
Other nephrotoxic drugs (antibiotics, antineoplastics): May increase risk of nephrotoxicity. Use together cautiously. Monitor renal function closely.
Skeletal muscle relaxants: May enhance effects of skeletal muscle relaxants because of amphotericin-induced hypokalemia. Monitor potassium level.

Effects on lab test results

• May increase BUN, creatinine, glucose, sodium, alkaline phosphatase, ALT, AST, bilirubin, GGT, and LDH levels. May decrease potassium, calcium, and magnesium levels.

Pharmacokinetics

Absorption: Given I.V.

Reactions may be *common,* uncommon, *life-threatening,* or COMMON AND LIFE-THREATENING.

A

Distribution: Unknown.
Metabolism: Unknown.
Excretion: Unknown. *Initial half-life:* 7 to
10 hours with 24-hour dosing; *Terminal elimination half-life:* About 4 to 6 days.

Route	Onset	Peak	Duration
I.V.	Unknown	Unknown	Unknown

Action

Chemical effect: Binds to the sterol component of a fungal cell membrane, leading to alterations in cell permeability and cell death.
Therapeutic effect: Decreases activity of or kills susceptible fungi. Treats visceral protozoal infections.

Available forms

Injection: 50-mg vial

NURSING PROCESS

Assessment
• Obtain history of fungal infection and samples for culture and sensitivity tests before therapy. Reevaluate condition during therapy.
• Carefully assess patients who are also receiving chemotherapy or bone marrow transplantation because they are at greater risk for additional adverse reactions, including seizures, arrhythmias, thrombocytopenia, and respiratory failure.
• Monitor CBC, liver function test results, and creatinine, BUN, and CBC and electrolyte levels, particularly magnesium and potassium.
• Monitor patient for signs of hypokalemia, such as ECG changes, muscle weakness, cramping, and drowsiness.
• Watch for adverse reactions. Patients who receive drug may have fewer chills, decreased BUN level, a lower risk of hypokalemia, and less vomiting than patients who receive regular amphotericin B.
• Assess patient's and family's knowledge of drug therapy.

Nursing diagnoses
• Risk for infection related to presence of susceptible fungal or parasite infections
• Risk for injury related to drug-induced adverse reactions
• Deficient knowledge related to drug therapy

Planning and implementation
⊛ **ALERT:** Different amphotericin B preparations aren't interchangeable, and dosages vary.
• To lessen the risk or severity of adverse reactions, premedicate patient with antipyretics, antihistamines, antiemetics, or corticosteroids.
• Therapy may take several weeks to months.
Patient teaching
• Teach patient signs and symptoms of hypersensitivity, and stress importance of reporting them immediately.
• Warn patient that therapy may take several months; teach personal hygiene and other measures to prevent spread and recurrence of lesions.
• Instruct patient to report adverse reactions.
• Instruct patient to watch for and report signs of hypokalemia, such as muscle weakness, cramping, and drowsiness.
• Advise patient that frequent laboratory testing will be performed.

Evaluation
• Patient is free from fungal or parasitic infection.
• Patient doesn't experience injury as a result of drug-induced adverse reactions.
• Patient and family state understanding of drug therapy.

ampicillin
(am-pih-SIL-in)
Apo-Ampi ♦ , Novo-Ampicillin ♦ ,
Nu-Ampi ♦ , Principen

ampicillin sodium
Ampicin ♦ , Ampicyn Injection ◇ ,
Penbritin ♦

ampicillin trihydrate
Ampicyn Oral ◇ , D-Amp, Penbritin ◇ ,
Totacillin

Pharmacologic class: aminopenicillin
Therapeutic class: antibiotic
Pregnancy risk category: B

Indications and dosages

▶ **Respiratory tract or skin and skin-structure infection.** *Adults and children weighing 40 kg (88 lb) or more:* 250 to 500 mg P.O. q 6 hours.

Rapid onset   *Liquid form contains alcohol.   ♦ Canada   ◇ Australia   †OTC   ⌀Photoguide   ‡Off-label use

Children weighing less than 40 kg: 25 to 50 mg/kg/day P.O. in equally divided doses q 6 hours. Pediatric dosages shouldn't exceed recommended adult dosages.

▶ **GI infection, UTI.** *Adults and children weighing 40 kg (88 lb) or more:* 500 mg P.O. q 6 hours. For severe infections, larger doses may be needed.

Children weighing less than 40 kg: 50 to 100 mg/kg/day P.O. in equally divided doses q 6 hours.

▶ **Bacterial meningitis or septicemia.** *Adults:* 150 to 200 mg/kg/day I.V. in divided doses q 3 to 4 hours. May be given I.M. after 3 days of I.V. therapy. Maximum recommended daily dose is 14 g.

Children: 100 to 200 mg/kg I.V. daily in divided doses q 3 to 4 hours. Give I.V. for 3 days; then give I.M.

▶ **Uncomplicated gonorrhea.** *Adults and children weighing more than 45 kg (99 lb):* 3.5 g P.O. with 1 g probenecid given as a single dose.

▶ **To prevent endocarditis in patients having dental procedures.** *Adults:* 2 g I.M. or I.V. within 30 minutes before procedure.

Children: 50 mg/kg I.M. or I.V. within 30 minutes before procedure.

⚲ **Adjust-a-dose:** In patients who have severe renal impairment, increase drug interval to 12 hours. Use same dose.

▽ I.V. administration

● Don't give I.V. unless infection is severe or patient can't take oral dose.

● For direct injection, reconstitute with bacteriostatic water for injection. Use 5 ml for 125-mg, 250-mg, or 500-mg vials; 7.4 ml for 1-g vials; and 14.8 ml for 2-g vials. Use initial dilution within 1 hour.

● Give direct I.V. injections over 3 to 5 minutes for doses of 500 mg or less; over 10 to 15 minutes for larger doses. Don't exceed 100 mg/minute.

● For an intermittent infusion, dilute in 50 to 100 ml of normal saline solution and give over 15 to 30 minutes. Follow manufacturer's directions for stability data when ampicillin is further diluted for I.V. infusion.

● Give intermittently to prevent vein irritation. Change site every 48 hours.

⊗ **Incompatibilities**
Amikacin, amino acid solutions, chlorpromazine, dextran solutions, dopamine, erythromycin lactobionate, 10% fat emulsions, fructose, gentamicin, heparin sodium, hetastarch, hydrocortisone sodium succinate, hydromorphone, kanamycin, lidocaine, lincomycin, polymyxin B, prochlorperazine edisylate, sodium bicarbonate, streptomycin, tobramycin.

Contraindications and cautions

● Contraindicated in patients hypersensitive to drug or other penicillins.

● Use cautiously in patients with other drug allergies, especially to cephalosporins (possible cross-sensitivity), and in those with mononucleosis (high risk of maculopapular rash).

※ **Lifespan:** In pregnant or breast-feeding women, use cautiously.

Adverse reactions

CNS: *seizures.*
CV: vein irritation, thrombophlebitis.
GI: nausea, vomiting, diarrhea, glossitis, stomatitis.
Hematologic: anemia, *thrombocytopenia, thrombocytopenic purpura,* eosinophilia, *leukopenia, agranulocytosis.*
Other: hypersensitivity reactions (maculopapular rash, urticaria, *anaphylaxis*), overgrowth of nonsusceptible organisms, pain at injection site.

Interactions

Drug-drug. *Allopurinol:* May increase risk of rash. Monitor patient.
Probenecid: May increase level of ampicillin and other penicillins. Probenecid may be used for this purpose.

Effects on lab test results

● May decrease hemoglobin level and hematocrit.

● May increase eosinophil count. May decrease platelet, WBC, and granulocyte counts.

● May cause false-positive urine glucose determinations with copper sulfate tests (Clinitest).

Pharmacokinetics

Absorption: About 42% after P.O. use; unknown after I.M. use.
Distribution: Into pleural, peritoneal, and synovial fluids; lungs; prostate; liver; and gallbladder. Also penetrates middle ear effusions, maxillary sinus and bronchial secretions, tonsils, and sputum. Ampicillin is minimally protein-bound at 15% to 25%.

Reactions may be *common,* uncommon, *life-threatening*, or COMMON AND LIFE-THREATENING.

Metabolism: Only partial.
Excretion: In urine by renal tubular secretion and glomerular filtration. *Half-life:* About 1 to 1½ hours (10 to 24 hours in severe renal impairment).

Route	Onset	Peak	Duration
P.O.	Unknown	2 hr	6–8 hr
I.V.	Immediate	Immediate	Unknown
I.M.	Unknown	1 hr	Unknown

Action

Chemical effect: Inhibits cell-wall synthesis during microorganism multiplication.
Therapeutic effect: Kills susceptible bacteria, including non-penicillinase–producing gram-positive bacteria and many gram-negative organisms.

Available forms

Capsules: 250 mg, 500 mg
Infusion: 500 mg, 1 g, 2 g
Injection: 125 mg, 250 mg, 500 mg, 1 g, 2 g
Oral suspension: 125 mg/5 ml, 250 mg/5 ml (after reconstitution)

NURSING PROCESS

☒ Assessment

• Obtain history of patient's infection before therapy and observe throughout therapy to assess improvement.
• Ask patient about previous allergic reaction to penicillin. A negative history of penicillin allergy doesn't rule out future reaction.
• Obtain specimen for culture and sensitivity tests before giving first dose.
• Be alert for adverse reactions and drug interactions.
• Monitor patient's hydration status if adverse GI reactions occur.
• Assess patient's and family's knowledge of drug therapy.

⊞ Nursing diagnoses

• Risk for infection related to presence of susceptible bacterial infection
• Risk for deficient fluid volume related to drug-induced adverse GI reactions
• Deficient knowledge related to drug therapy

▷ Planning and implementation

• Give orally either 1 hour before or 2 hours after meals. Food may interfere with absorption.
• Don't give I.M. unless infection is severe or patient can't take oral dose.
• Give at least 1 hour before bacteriostatic antibiotics.
• In children with meningitis, give with parenteral chloramphenicol for 24 hours pending culture results.
• Stop drug immediately if anaphylaxis occurs. Notify prescriber and prepare to give immediate treatment, such as epinephrine, corticosteroids, antihistamines, and other resuscitative measures.
Patient teaching
• Tell patient to take entire quantity of drug exactly as prescribed, even after he feels better.
• Tell patient to call prescriber if a rash (most common), fever, or chills develop.
• Warn patient never to use leftover ampicillin for a new illness or to share it with others.
• Advise patient to take oral ampicillin 1 hour before or 2 hours after meals for best absorption.

☑ Evaluation

• Patient is free from infection.
• Patient maintains adequate hydration.
• Patient and family state understanding of drug therapy.

ampicillin sodium and sulbactam sodium
(am-pih-SIL-in SOH-dee-um and sul-BAC-tam SOH-dee-um)
Unasyn

Pharmacologic class: aminopenicillin and beta-lactamase inhibitor
Therapeutic class: antibiotic
Pregnancy risk category: B

Indications and dosages

▶ Intra-abdominal, gynecologic, and skin and skin-structure infections caused by susceptible gram-positive, gram-negative, and beta-lactamase–producing strains. *Adults:* Dosage expressed as total drug (each 1.5-g vial contains 1 g ampicillin sodium and 0.5 g sulbactam sodium). 1.5 to 3 g I.M. or I.V. q 6 hours. Maximum daily dosage is 4 g sulbactam (12 g of combined drugs).

▶ **Skin and skin-structure infections caused by susceptible organisms.** *Children older than age 1*: 300 mg/kg I.V. daily in equally divided doses q 6 hours. Children should receive a maximum of 14 days of therapy. Children weighing 40 kg (88 lb) or more may receive the usual adult dosage shown above.

▶ **Pelvic inflammatory disease.** *Adults and children:* 3 g (2 g ampicillin and 1 g sulbactam) I.V. or I.M. q 6 hours, given with doxycycline 100 mg P.O. q 12 hours. Continue parenteral therapy for 24 hours after clinical improvement. Continue with oral doxycycline 100 mg P.O. b.i.d. to complete the 14-day cycle.

▼ I.V. administration

• When preparing injection, reconstitute powder with any of the following diluents: normal saline solution, D_5W, lactated Ringer's solution, 1/6 M sodium lactate, dextrose 5% in half-normal saline solution for injection, or 10% inert sugar. Stability varies with diluent, temperature, and concentration of solution.

• After reconstitution, allow vials to stand for a few minutes to allow foam to dissipate to permit visual inspection of contents for particles.

• Give dose by injection over 10 to 15 minutes, or dilute in 50 to 100 ml of a compatible diluent and infuse over 15 to 30 minutes. If permitted, give intermittently to prevent vein irritation. Change site every 48 hours.

⊗ **Incompatibilities**
Amikacin, amino acid solutions, chlorpromazine, dextran solutions, dopamine, erythromycin lactobionate, 10% fat emulsions, fructose, gentamicin, heparin sodium, hetastarch, hydrocortisone sodium succinate, kanamycin, lidocaine, lincomycin, netilmicin, polymyxin B, prochlorperazine edisylate, sodium bicarbonate, streptomycin, tobramycin. Don't add or mix with other drugs because they might be physically or chemically incompatible.

Contraindications and cautions

• Contraindicated in patients hypersensitive to drug or other penicillins.

• Use cautiously in patients with other drug allergies, especially to cephalosporins (possible cross-sensitivity), and in those with mononucleosis (high risk of maculopapular rash).

🜲 **Lifespan:** In pregnant and breast-feeding women, use cautiously. In children younger than age 1, safety of drug hasn't been established. In children age 1 and older, drug can be used I.V. for skin and skin-structure infections. Children shouldn't receive the drug I.M.

Adverse reactions

CV: vein irritation, thrombophlebitis.
GI: nausea, vomiting, *diarrhea,* glossitis, stomatitis.
Hematologic: anemia, *thrombocytopenia, thrombocytopenic purpura,* eosinophilia, *leukopenia, agranulocytosis.*
Other: hypersensitivity reactions (erythematous maculopapular rash, urticaria, *anaphylaxis*), overgrowth of nonsusceptible organisms, pain at injection site.

Interactions

Drug-drug. *Allopurinol:* May increase risk of rash. Monitor patient.
Hormonal contraceptives: May decrease effectiveness of hormonal contraceptives. Advise patient to use barrier contraception until therapy is complete.
Probenecid: May increase ampicillin level. Probenecid may be used for this purpose.

Effects on lab test results

• May increase BUN, creatinine, ALT, AST, alkaline phosphatase, bilirubin, LDH, CK, and GGT levels. May decrease hemoglobin level and hematocrit.

• May increase eosinophil count. May decrease platelet, WBC, and granulocyte counts.

• May cause false-positive urine glucose determinations with copper sulfate tests (Clinitest).

Pharmacokinetics

Absorption: Given I.V.
Distribution: Both drugs into pleural, peritoneal, and synovial fluids; lungs; prostate; liver; and gallbladder. They also penetrate middle ear effusions, maxillary sinus and bronchial secretions, tonsils, and sputum. Ampicillin is minimally protein-bound at 15% to 25%; sulbactam is about 38% protein-bound.
Metabolism: Both drugs only partially.
Excretion: Both drugs in urine by renal tubular secretion and glomerular filtration. *Half-life:* 1

to 1½ hours (10 to 24 hours in severe renal impairment).

Route	Onset	Peak	Duration
I.V.	Immediate	Immediate	Unknown
I.M.	Unknown	Unknown	Unknown

Action

Chemical effect: Ampicillin inhibits cell-wall synthesis during microorganism multiplication; sulbactam inactivates bacterial beta-lactamase, the enzyme that inactivates ampicillin and provides bacterial resistance to it.
Therapeutic effect: Kills susceptible bacteria.

Available forms

Injection: Vials and piggyback vials containing 1.5 g (1 g ampicillin sodium with 0.5 g sulbactam sodium); 3 g (2 g ampicillin sodium with 1 g sulbactam sodium)

NURSING PROCESS

🔧 Assessment
● Obtain history of patient's infection before therapy and observe throughout therapy to determine improvement.
● Ask patient about previous allergic reaction to penicillin. A negative history of penicillin allergy doesn't rule out future reaction.
● Obtain specimen for culture and sensitivity tests before giving first dose.
● Be alert for adverse reactions and drug interactions.
● Monitor patient's hydration status if adverse GI reactions occur.
● Assess patient's and family's knowledge of drug therapy.

🔧 Nursing diagnoses
● Risk for infection related to presence of susceptible bacterial infection
● Risk for deficient fluid volume related to drug-induced adverse GI reactions
● Deficient knowledge related to drug therapy

🔧 Planning and implementation
● When giving drug I.M., reconstitute with sterile water for injection or with 0.5% or 2% lidocaine hydrochloride. Add 3.2 ml to a 1.5-g vial (or 6.4 ml to a 3-g vial) to yield a concentration of 375 mg/ml. Give deep into muscle.

● Dosage should be altered in patients with renal impairment.
● Give drug at least 1 hour before bacteriostatic antibiotics.
● Stop drug immediately if anaphylaxis occurs. Notify prescriber and prepare to give immediate treatment, such as epinephrine, corticosteroids, antihistamines; and other resuscitative measures.

Patient teaching
● Tell patient to call prescriber if rash (most common), fever, or chills develop.
● Advise women taking hormonal contraceptives to use a barrier form of contraception during drug therapy.

✅ Evaluation
● Patient is free from infection.
● Patient maintains adequate hydration.
● Patient and family state understanding of drug therapy.

amprenavir
(am-PREH-nah-veer)
Agenerase

Pharmacologic class: protease inhibitor
Therapeutic class: antiretroviral
Pregnancy risk category: C

Indications and dosages

▶ **HIV-1 infection, with other antiretrovirals.**
Adults and children ages 13 to 16 weighing 50 kg (110 lb) or more: 1,200 mg (eight 150-mg capsules) P.O. b.i.d. with other antiretrovirals.
Children ages 4 to 12 or 13 to 16 weighing less than 50 kg (110 lb): Give 20 mg/kg P.O. capsules b.i.d. or 15 mg/kg P.O. t.i.d. (maximum, 2,400 mg daily) with other antiretrovirals. Or, give 22.5 mg/kg (1.5 ml/kg) oral solution P.O. b.i.d. or 17 mg/kg (1.1 ml/kg) P.O. t.i.d. (maximum, 2,800 mg daily) with other antiretrovirals.
🔲 **Adjust-a-dose:** For patients with hepatic impairment and a Child-Pugh score of 5 to 8, reduce dosage to 450-mg capsules P.O. b.i.d.

For patients with hepatic impairment and a Child-Pugh score of 9 to 12, reduce dosage to 300-mg capsules P.O. b.i.d.

Contraindications and cautions

- Contraindicated in patients hypersensitive to drug or its components. Coadministration with drugs dependent on the CYP 3A4 enzyme pathway is contraindicated.
- Use cautiously in patients with moderate or severe hepatic impairment, diabetes mellitus, sulfonamide allergy, or hemophilia A or B.
- Drug can cause severe or life-threatening rash, including Stevens-Johnson syndrome. Therapy should be stopped if patient develops a severe or life-threatening rash or a moderate rash with systemic signs and symptoms.
- ⚜ **Lifespan:** In pregnant women, use only if potential benefits outweigh risks; no adequate studies exist. In children age 4 and younger, drug is contraindicated because of risk of toxicity.

Adverse reactions

CNS: *paresthesia*, headache, depressive or mood disorders.
GI: nausea, vomiting, diarrhea or loose stools, taste disorders.
Hepatic: hypertriglyceridemia, hypercholesterolemia.
Metabolic: hyperglycemia.
Skin: rash, *Stevens-Johnson syndrome.*

Interactions

Drug-drug. *Antacids:* Interferes with absorption. Separate administration by at least 1 hour.
Antiarrhythmics, such as amiodarone; lidocaine (systemic); quinidine; anticoagulants, such as warfarin; tricyclic antidepressants, cyclosporine, tacrolimus: Levels of these drugs may be affected. Monitor patient closely.
Calcium channel blockers, dihydroergotamine, midazolam, rifampin, triazolam: May cause serious and life-threatening interactions. Avoid using together.
Cimetidine, indinavir, nelfinavir, ritonavir: May increase amprenavir level. Monitor patient closely for increased adverse effects.
Efavirenz: May decrease exposure of amprenavir to the body. Increase dose accordingly.
Ethinyl estradiol and norethindrone: Loss of virologic response and possible resistance to amprenavir. Tell patient to use alternative method of birth control.
HMG-CoA reductase inhibitors, such as atorvastatin, lovastatin, and simvastatin: May increase levels of these drugs and increase risk of

myopathy, including rhabdomyolysis. Avoid using together.
Indinavir, nelfinavir, ritonavir: May increase plasma levels of amprenavir. Monitor patient closely.
Ketoconazole, itraconazole: May increase levels of both drugs. Monitor patient closely for adverse reactions.
Macrolides: May increase amprenavir level. No adjustment necessary.
Methadone: May decrease amprenavir level. Alternative antiretroviral or pain therapy should be considered. Dosage of methadone may need to be increased.
Psychotherapeutic drugs: May increase CNS effects. Monitor patient closely.
Rifabutin: May decrease exposure of amprenavir to the body and increase rifabutin level by 200%. Decrease rifabutin dose to 150 mg daily or 300 mg two to three times weekly.
Saquinavir: May decrease exposure of amprenavir to the body. Monitor patient closely.
Sildenafil, tadalafil, vardenafil: May increase levels of these drugs, increasing risk of adverse effects, including hypotension and priapism. Don't exceed recommended dose restrictions.
Drug-herb. *St. John's wort:* May decrease amprenavir level. Avoid using together.
Drug-food. *Grapefruit juice:* May affect blood levels of amprenavir. Monitor patient closely.
High-fat meals: May reduce drug absorption. Discourage taking drug with a high-fat meal.

Effects on lab test results

- May increase glucose, triglyceride, AST, ALT, and cholesterol levels.

Pharmacokinetics

Absorption: Rapid.
Distribution: Apparent volume of distribution is about 430 L. In vitro, about 90% of drug binds to plasma proteins.
Metabolism: By CYP 3A4 enzymes in the liver.
Excretion: Minimal, in urine and feces. *Elimination half-life:* 7 to 10½ hours.

Route	Onset	Peak	Duration
P.O.	Unknown	1–2 hr	Unknown

Action
Chemical effect: Inhibits HIV-1 protease by binding to the active site of HIV-1 protease, which causes immature noninfectious viral particles to form.
Therapeutic effect: Reduces symptoms of HIV-1 infection.

Available forms
Capsules: 50 mg, 150 mg
Oral solution: 15 mg/ml

NURSING PROCESS

⚗ Assessment
• Assess patient for appropriateness of drug therapy.
• Because drug may interact with other drugs, obtain patient's complete drug history.
• Patients with moderate or severe hepatic impairment, diabetes mellitus, known sulfonamide allergy, or hemophilia A or B must be monitored very closely while taking this drug.
• Determine whether patient is pregnant or plans to become pregnant.
• Assess patient's and family's knowledge about drug therapy.

⊕ Nursing diagnoses
• Risk for infection secondary to presence of HIV
• Ineffective individual coping related to HIV infection
• Deficient knowledge related to drug therapy

▷ Planning and implementation
• Don't give patient high-fat foods because they may decrease absorption of oral drug.
• **ⓢ ALERT:** Amprenavir capsules aren't interchangeable with amprenavir oral solution on a milligram-per-milligram basis.
• Monitor coagulation studies. Drug provides high daily doses of vitamin E.
• Protease inhibitors cause spontaneous bleeding in some patients with hemophilia A or B. In some patients, additional factor VIII may be required. Treatment with protease inhibitors can then continue.
Patient teaching
• Inform patient that drug doesn't cure HIV infection and that opportunistic infections and other complications may develop. Also explain

that drug doesn't reduce the risk of transmitting HIV to others.
• Tell patient that drug can be taken with or without food, but that he shouldn't take it with a high-fat meal because doing so may decrease drug absorption.
• Urge patient to report adverse reactions, especially rash.
• Warn patient that he may experience a redistribution of body fat, including central obesity, dorsocervical fat enlargement (buffalo hump), peripheral wasting, breast enlargement, and cushingoid appearance.
• Advise patient to take drug every day as prescribed, always with other antiretrovirals. Warn against changing the dosage or stopping the drug without prescriber's approval.
• If patient takes an antacid or didanosine, tell him to do so 1 hour before or after amprenavir to avoid interfering with amprenavir absorption.
• If patient misses a dose by more than 4 hours, tell him to wait and take the next dose at the regularly scheduled time. If he misses a dose by less than 4 hours, tell him to take the dose as soon as possible and then take the next dose at the regularly scheduled time. Caution against doubling the dose.
• Advise patient not to take supplemental vitamin E because high levels of this vitamin may worsen the blood coagulation defect of vitamin K deficiency caused by anticoagulant therapy or malabsorption.
• If patient uses a hormonal contraceptive, warn her to use another contraceptive during amprenavir therapy.
• Urge patient to notify prescriber about planned, suspected, or known pregnancy during therapy.
• Advise patients taking sildenafil, tadalafil, and vardenafil of the increased risk of adverse affects, including hypotension, visual changes, and priapism. These patients should promptly report symptoms to their prescribers and shouldn't exceed 25 mg of sildenafil in a 48-hour period.

☑ Evaluation
• Patient exhibits reduced signs and symptoms of infection.
• Patient demonstrates adequate coping mechanisms.
• Patient and family state understanding of drug therapy.

anakinra
(ann-uh-KIN-ruh)
Kineret

Pharmacologic class: recombinant human interleukin-1 receptor antagonist
Therapeutic class: disease-modifying antirheumatic drug (DMARD)
Pregnancy risk category: B

Indications and dosages

▶ **Reduction in signs and symptoms and slowing the progression of structural damage in moderate-to-severe active rheumatoid arthritis (RA) after one failure with DMARDs, used alone or combined with DMARDs other than tumor necrosis factor (TNF) blockers.** *Adults:* 100 mg subcutaneously daily.

Contraindications and cautions

• Contraindicated in patients hypersensitive to *Escherichia coli*–derived proteins or components of the product. Don't use in immunosuppressed patients or in those with chronic or active infection.
• Use caution with TNF blockers because of the increased risk of neutropenia.
⚠ **Lifespan:** In pregnant women, use only if necessary because no adequate, well-controlled studies exist. In breast-feeding women, use cautiously because it's unknown whether drug appears in breast milk. In patients with juvenile RA, safety and effectiveness of drug haven't been established. In elderly patients, use drug cautiously because they have a greater risk of infection and are more likely to have renal impairment.

Adverse reactions

CNS: headache.
EENT: sinusitis.
GI: abdominal pain, diarrhea, nausea.
Hematologic: *neutropenia.*
Respiratory: upper respiratory tract infection.
Other: infection (cellulitis, pneumonia, bone and joint), flulike symptoms, injection site reactions (erythema, ecchymosis, inflammation, pain).

Interactions

Drug-drug. *Etanercept, other TNF blockers:* May increase risk of severe infection. Use together cautiously.
Vaccines: May decrease effectiveness of vaccines or increase risk of secondary transmission of infection with live vaccines. Avoid using together.

Effects on lab test results

• May increase differential percentage of eosinophils. May decrease neutrophil, WBC, and platelet counts.

Pharmacokinetics

Absorption: Absolute bioavailability is 95% after a 70-mg subcutaneous injection.
Distribution: In plasma.
Metabolism: Unknown.
Excretion: Renal. Clearance increases with increasing creatinine clearance and body weight. Mean plasma clearance decreases 70% to 75% in patients with creatinine clearance less than 30 ml/minute. *Half-life:* 4 to 6 hours.

Route	Onset	Peak	Duration
SubQ	Unknown	3–7 hr	Unknown

Action

Chemical effect: A recombinant, nonglycosylated form of the human interleukin-1 receptor antagonist (IL-1Ra). The level of naturally occurring IL-1Ra in synovium and synovial fluid from patients with RA isn't enough to compete with the elevated level of locally produced IL-1. Drug blocks the activity of IL-1 by competitively inhibiting IL-1 from binding to the interleukin-1–type receptors.
Therapeutic effect: Decreases inflammation and cartilage degradation.

Available forms

Injection: 100 mg/ml in prefilled glass syringe

NURSING PROCESS

⚕ Assessment
• Assess patient before therapy for signs and symptoms of chronic or active infection. If patient has active infection, don't start treatment.
• Obtain neutrophil count before treatment, monthly for the first 3 months of treatment, and then quarterly for up to 1 year.

• Monitor patient for infections and injection site reactions.

🔢 Nursing diagnoses
• Risk of infection related to anakinra therapy
• Risk of pain from underlying rheumatoid arthritis
• Risk of impaired skin integrity from injection site reaction

❯ Planning and implementation
• Inject the entire contents of the prefilled syringe subcutaneously.
• Stop drug if patient develops a serious infection.
③ ALERT: Don't confuse anakinra with amikacin.
Patient teaching
• Tell patient to store drug in refrigerator and not to freeze or expose to excessive heat. Tell patient to allow drug to come to room temperature before injecting.
• Teach patient proper technique for administration and disposal of syringes in a puncture-resistant container. Also, warn patient not to reuse needles.
• Urge patient to rotate injection sites.
• Review with patient the signs and symptoms of allergic and other adverse reactions and the symptoms of infection. Urge patient to contact prescriber immediately if they arise. Inform patient that injection site reactions are common, are usually mild, and typically last 14 to 28 days.
• Tell patient to avoid live-virus vaccines while taking anakinra.

☑ Evaluation
• Patient is free from infection or adverse reactions during drug therapy.
• Patient's symptoms of RA are relieved.
• Patient and family state understanding of drug therapy and give drug properly.

anastrozole
(uh-NASS-truh-zohl)
Arimidex⊘

Pharmacologic class: nonsteroidal aromatase inhibitor
Therapeutic class: antineoplastic
Pregnancy risk category: D

Indications and dosages
▶ **First-line therapy for hormone-receptor–positive or hormone-receptor–unknown locally advanced or metastatic breast cancer; advanced breast cancer with disease progression following tamoxifen; adjuvant therapy for hormone-receptor–positive early breast cancer.** *Postmenopausal women:* 1 mg P.O. daily.

Contraindications and cautions
• Contraindicated in patients hypersensitive to the drug or any of its components.
• Use cautiously in patients with hepatic impairment.
⚞ Lifespan: In pregnant women, drug isn't recommended because it may cause fetal harm. In breast-feeding women, use cautiously. In children, safety of drug hasn't been established.

Adverse reactions
CNS: pain, asthenia, headache, dizziness, depression, insomnia, anxiety, paresthesia.
CV: chest pain, hypertension, edema, ***thromboembolic disease,*** peripheral edema, *vasodilation.*
EENT: cataracts, pharyngitis.
GI: nausea, vomiting, diarrhea, constipation, dry mouth, abdominal pain, anorexia.
GU: pelvic pain, ***vaginal hemorrhage,*** vaginal dryness.
Metabolic: weight gain, increased appetite.
Musculoskeletal: back pain, bone pain, arthralgia.
Respiratory: dyspnea, increased cough.
Skin: rash, sweating.
Other: *hot flushes.*

Interactions
Drug-drug. *Estrogen-containing therapies, tamoxifen:* May decrease anastrozole's effect. Avoid using together.

Effects on lab test results
• May increase liver enzyme and cholesterol levels.

Pharmacokinetics
Absorption: Food doesn't affect extent of absorption.
Distribution: 40% bound to plasma proteins.

Metabolism: In liver.
Excretion: In urine. *Half-life:* About 50 hours.

Route	Onset	Peak	Duration
P.O.	Unknown	Unknown	Unknown

Action

Chemical effect: Lowers estradiol level.
Therapeutic effect: Hinders cancer cell growth.

Available forms

Tablets: 1 mg

NURSING PROCESS

🔍 Assessment

• Obtain history of patient's neoplastic disease before therapy.
• Be alert for adverse reactions.
• Assess patient's and family's knowledge of drug therapy.

🔷 Nursing diagnoses

• Ineffective health maintenance related to neoplastic disease
• Risk for deficient fluid volume related to drug-induced adverse GI reactions
• Deficient knowledge related to drug therapy

🔳 Planning and implementation

• Rule out pregnancy before treatment begins.
• Give drug under supervision of a prescriber experienced in using antineoplastics.
• Patients with hormone-receptor–negative disease and those who didn't respond to previous tamoxifen therapy, rarely respond to anastrozole.
• Patients with advanced breast cancer should continue therapy until tumor progression is evident.

Patient teaching

• Instruct patient to report adverse reactions.
• Stress importance of follow-up care.

🔲 Evaluation

• Patient has positive response to therapy.
• Patient maintains adequate hydration.
• Patient and family state understanding of drug therapy.

apomorphine hydrochloride
(ah-poe-MORE-feen high-droh-KLOR-ide)
Apokyn

Pharmacologic class: dopamine agonist
Therapeutic class: antiparkinsonian drug
Pregnancy risk category: C

Indications and dosages

▶ **Intermittent hypomobility, "off" episodes caused by advanced Parkinson's disease (with an antiemetic).** *Adults:* Initially, give a 0.2-ml test dose subcutaneously. Measure supine and standing blood pressure q 20 minutes for the first hour. If patient tolerates and responds to drug, start with 0.2 ml subcutaneously p.r.n. (outpatient). Doses must be separated by at least 2 hours. Increase by 0.1 ml every few days, as needed.

If initial 0.2-ml dose is ineffective but tolerated, give 0.4 ml at next "off" period, measuring supine and standing blood pressure q 20 minutes for the first hour. If drug is tolerated, start with 0.3 ml (outpatient). If needed, increase by 0.1 ml every few days

If patient doesn't tolerate 0.4-ml dose, give 0.3 ml as a test dose at the next "off" period, measuring supine and standing blood pressure as before. If drug is tolerated, give 0.2 ml (outpatient). Increase by 0.1 ml every few days, p.r.n., but doses higher than 0.4 ml usually aren't tolerated if 0.2 ml is the starting dose.

Maximum recommended dose is usually 0.6 ml p.r.n. Most patients take drug about three times daily. Experience is limited at more than five times daily or more than 2 ml daily.
🔲 **Adjust-a-dose:** In patients with mild to moderate renal impairment, the test and starting doses should be 0.1 ml, given subcutaneously.

Contraindications and cautions

• Contraindicated in patients allergic to apomorphine or its ingredients, including sulfites, and in patients who take 5-HT_3 antagonists.
• Use cautiously in patients at risk for prolonged QTc interval, such as those with hypokalemia, hypomagnesemia, bradycardia, or genetic predisposition. Also use cautiously in patients with cardiovascular or cerebrovascular disease and in those with renal or hepatic impairment.

Reactions may be *common*, uncommon, *life-threatening*, or COMMON AND LIFE-THREATENING.

⚡ **Lifespan:** Drug effects are unknown in pregnant and breast-feeding women. Give drug only if clearly needed. In children, safety and effectiveness haven't been established.

Adverse reactions

CNS: aggravated Parkinson's disease, anxiety, *confusion,* depression, *dizziness, drowsiness,* fatigue, *hallucinations,* headache, insomnia, *somnolence,* syncope, weakness.
CV: *angina,* **cardiac arrest,** *chest pain, chest pressure, edema, flushing,* **heart failure,** *hypotension, orthostatic hypotension, MI.*
EENT: *rhinorrhea.*
GI: constipation, diarrhea, *nausea, vomiting.*
GU: UTI.
Metabolic: dehydration.
Musculoskeletal: arthralgia, back pain, *dyskinesias,* limb pain.
Respiratory: dyspnea, pneumonia.
Skin: bruising, injection site reaction, pallor, sweating.
Other: *falls, yawning.*

Interactions

Drug-drug. *Antihypertensives, vasodilators:* May increase risk of hypotension, MI, pneumonia, falls, and joint injury. Use together cautiously.
Dopamine antagonists, metoclopramide: May reduce apomorphine effectiveness. Use together cautiously.
Drugs that prolong the QTc interval: May prolong the QTc interval. Give cautiously with other drugs that prolong QTc interval.
5-HT3 antagonists (ondansetron, granisetron, dolasetron, palonosetron, alosetron): May cause serious hypotension and loss of consciousness. Don't use together.
Drug-lifestyle. *Alcohol use:* May increase risk of sedation and hypotension. Discourage use together.

Effects on lab test results

None known.

Pharmacokinetics

Absorption: Rapid. Patients with hepatic or renal impairment may have higher serum level.
Distribution: Large, but CSF penetration is poor.
Metabolism: Unknown.

Excretion: Unknown. *Elimination half-life* is about 30 to 60 minutes in patients with normal or impaired renal function.

Route	Onset	Peak	Duration
SubQ	20 min	10–60 min	2 hr

Action

Chemical effect: Apomorphine is thought to improve motor function by stimulating dopamine D2 receptors in the caudate-putamen area of the brain.
Therapeutic effect: Relieves signs and symptoms of parkinsonism.

Available forms

Solution for injection: 10 mg/ml (contains benzyl alcohol)

NURSING PROCESS

🔎 Assessment
• Monitor supine and standing blood pressure every 20 minutes for the first hour after therapy starts or dosage changes.
⑤ ALERT: Monitor patient for drowsiness or sleepiness, which may occur well after treatment starts. Stop drug if patient develops significant daytime sleepiness that interferes with activities of daily living.
• Watch for evidence of coronary or cerebral ischemia, and stop drug if they occur.
• Assess elderly patients carefully because adverse effects are more likely in elderly patients, particularly hallucinations, falls, CV events, respiratory problems, and GI effects.
• Assess patient's and family's knowledge of drug therapy.

⊕ Nursing diagnoses
• Impaired physical mobility related to presence of parkinsonism
• Risk for deficient fluid volume related to drug-induced nausea and vomiting
• Deficient knowledge related to drug therapy

▷ Planning and implementation
⑤ ALERT: Drug is for subcutaneous injection only. Avoid I.V. use.
• Give with an antiemetic to avoid severe nausea and vomiting. Start with trimethobenzamide 300 mg P.O. t.i.d. 3 days before starting apo-

morphine, and continue antiemetic at least 2 months.

❸ **ALERT:** The prescribed dose should always be specified in milliliters rather than milligrams to avoid confusion. The dosing pen is marked in milliliters.

• When programming the dosing pen, it's possible to select the appropriate dose even though insufficient drug remains in the pen. To avoid insufficient dosing, track the amount of drug received at each dose and change the cartridge before drug runs out.

• Give test dose in a medically supervised setting to determine tolerability and effect.

Patient teaching

• Tell patient to avoid sudden position changes, especially rising too quickly from lying down. A sudden drop in blood pressure, dizziness, or fainting can occur.

• Urge patient to keep taking the prescribed antiemetic because nausea and vomiting are likely.

• Instruct patient or caregiver to document each dose to make sure enough drug remains in the cartridge to provide a full next dose.

• Tell patient or caregiver to wait at least 2 hours between doses.

• Show patient or caregiver how to read the dosing pen, and make sure he understands that it's marked in milliliters and not milligrams.

• Tell patient or caregiver to rotate injection sites and to wash hands before each injection. Applying ice to the site before and after the injection may reduce soreness, redness, pain, itching, swelling, or bruising at the site.

• Explain that hallucinations (either visual or auditory) may occur, and urge patient or caregiver to report them immediately.

• Explain that headaches may occur and urge patient or caregiver to notify the prescriber if they become severe or don't go away.

• Advise patient to avoid hazardous activities that require alertness until drug effects are known.

• Caution patient to avoid consuming alcohol.

☑ **Evaluation**

• Patient has improved physical mobility.

• Patient doesn't experience nausea and vomiting.

• Patient and family state understanding of drug therapy.

aprepitant
(uh-pre-PIH-tant)
Emend

Pharmacologic class: substance P and neurokinin-1 receptor antagonist
Therapeutic class: centrally acting antiemetic
Pregnancy risk category: B

Indications and dosages

▶ **To prevent nausea and vomiting after moderately or highly emetogenic chemotherapy (including cisplatin); given with a 5-HT$_3$ antagonist and a corticosteroid.**
Adults: 125 mg P.O. on day 1 of treatment (1 hour before chemotherapy); then 80 mg P.O. q a.m. on days 2 and 3. Single doses up to 600 mg of aprepitant have been well tolerated.

Contraindications and cautions

• Contraindicated in patients hypersensitive to drug or any of its components, and in those also receiving pimozide because drug may increase pimozide level, causing life-threatening reactions such as ventricular arrhythmias.

• Administration beyond 3 days per cycle of chemotherapy isn't recommended because of the potential for CYP 3A4- and 2C9-related drug interactions.

⚠ **Lifespan:** In pregnant women, use with caution; drug hasn't been well studied in pregnant women. In breast-feeding women, use cautiously because it's unknown whether drug appears in breast milk. In children, safety and effectiveness haven't been established.

Adverse reactions

CNS: dizziness, *fatigue,* headache, insomnia.
EENT: tinnitus.
GI: abdominal pain, *anorexia, constipation, diarrhea,* gastritis, *nausea,* vomiting.
GU: proteinuria.
Hematologic: *neutropenia, febrile neutropenia.*
Respiratory: *hiccups.*
Skin: drug-induced rash with urticaria, *Stevens-Johnson syndrome.*
Other: *angioedema.*

Interactions

Drug-drug. *Benzodiazepines, such as alprazolam and midazolam:* May increase levels of

---

these drugs. Monitor patient for increased sedation and other CNS effects. Decrease the dose of benzodiazepines by 50% if use together is necessary.

Chemotherapy metabolized by CYP 3A4, such as etoposide, ifosfamide, irinotecan, taxanes, and vinca alkaloids: May increase levels of these drugs, leading to increased toxicity. Avoid using together if possible.

Corticosteroids: May increase levels of these drugs, leading to increased toxicity. Decrease the dose of corticosteroids by 50% if use together is necessary.

CYP 3A4 inducers (carbamazepine, phenytoin, rifampin): May decrease aprepitant level and decrease antiemetic effect. Avoid using together if possible.

CYP 3A4 inhibitors (azole antifungals, diltiazem, erythromycin, nelfinavir, ritonavir): May increase aprepitant level, leading to increased toxicity. Avoid using together if possible.

Diltiazem: May increase diltiazem level. Monitor heart rate and blood pressure. Avoid using together if possible.

Hormonal contraceptives: May decrease the effectiveness of these drugs. Women should be advised to use an additional form of birth control if use together is necessary.

Phenytoin: May decrease phenytoin level. Monitor phenytoin levels carefully. An increased dose may be needed when used together. Avoid using together if possible.

SSRIs: May decrease the effectiveness of these drugs. Avoid using together if possible.

Tolbutamide: May decrease the effectiveness of tolbutamide. Only use together if necessary, and monitor glucose level carefully.

Warfarin: May decrease the effectiveness of warfarin. Monitor INR levels carefully in the 2 weeks after each treatment, especially days 7 to 10. Avoid using together whenever possible.

Drug-herb. *St. John's wort:* May decrease the drug's antiemetic effects. Discourage using together.

Drug-food. *Grapefruit juice:* May increase drug level, leading to increased toxicity. Discourage using together.

Effects on lab test results

- May increase creatinine, AST, and ALT levels.
- May decrease neutrophil counts.

Pharmacokinetics

Absorption: Well absorbed, with an average bioavailability of 60% to 65%. Food doesn't appear to have an effect. Peak level occurs approximately 4 hours after each dose.
Distribution: 95% protein-bound. May cross the placenta and blood–brain barrier.
Metabolism: Extensively in the liver by CYP 3A4 and to a lesser degree by CYP 1A2 and 2C19.
Excretion: In the urine and in the feces. *Half-life:* 9 to 13 hours.

Route	Onset	Peak	Duration
P.O.	Unknown	4 hr	9–13 hr

Action

Chemical effect: Selectively antagonizes substance P and neurokinin-1 receptors in the brain.
Therapeutic effect: Inhibits emesis caused by cytotoxic chemotherapy.

Available forms

Capsules: 80 mg, 125 mg

NURSING PROCESS

✍ Assessment
- Monitor patients thoroughly for potential drug and herbal interactions before giving.
- Assess patient's condition before administration and regularly thereafter.
- Watch for hypersensitivity reactions.
- Monitor therapy with other drugs for potential interactions, particularly drugs metabolized by the liver.

✛ Nursing diagnoses
- Imbalanced nutrition: less than body requirements related to chemotherapy-induced nausea and vomiting
- Ineffective individual coping related to effects of chemotherapy
- Deficient knowledge related to drug therapy

❯ Planning and implementation
- Give the first dose of drug 1 hour before chemotherapy.
- Give drug with other antiemetics, usually a 5-HT$_3$ antagonist and a corticosteroid.
- Don't give for longer than 3 days per chemotherapy cycle.

• Don't give to treat established nausea and vomiting. Make sure patient has other antiemetics to treat breakthrough emesis.

• Higher doses may lead to drowsiness and headache. Provide supportive treatment for overdose; because of the drug's mechanism of action, antiemetics may not be effective. Don't attempt to remove by hemodialysis because removal doesn't occur.

• Monitor CBC, liver function tests, and creatinine periodically during drug therapy.

Patient teaching

• Advise patient that drug is given with other antiemetics and shouldn't be taken alone in an attempt to prevent chemotherapy-induced nausea and vomiting.

• Tell patient that you will give the first dose 1 hour before each chemotherapy cycle, and that he should take the second and third doses of the drug in the morning on days 2 and 3 of the treatment cycle. It may be taken with or without food.

• Instruct patient to treat breakthrough emesis with other antiemetics.

• Advise patient to tell his oncologist if he starts or stops any other drugs or herbal supplements during therapy because of the drug's many drug and herb interactions.

• Advise women of childbearing age who are taking hormonal contraceptives to use an additional form of birth control during therapy.

☑ Evaluation

• Patient doesn't experience chemotherapy-induced nausea or vomiting.

• Patient maintains adequate nutrition and hydration during chemotherapy treatments.

• Patient and family state understanding of drug therapy.

argatroban
(ahr-GAH-troh-ban)
Argatroban

Pharmacologic class: direct thrombin inhibitor
Therapeutic class: anticoagulant
Pregnancy risk category: B

Indications and dosages

▶ **Prevention or treatment of thrombosis in patients with heparin-induced thrombocytopenia.** *Adults:* 2 mcg/kg/minute, given as a continuous I.V. infusion; adjust dose until steady state APTT is 1½ to 3 times the initial baseline value, not to exceed 100 seconds; maximum dose is 10 mcg/kg/minute.

The standard infusion rates for 2 mcg/kg/minute are shown below.

Body weight (kg)	Infusion rate (ml/hour)
50	6
60	7
70	8
80	10
90	11
100	12
110	13
120	14
130	16
140	17

⊠ Adjust-a-dose: For patients with moderate hepatic impairment, initial dose should be reduced to 0.5 mcg/kg/minute, given as a continuous infusion. Monitor APTT closely and adjust dosage as needed.

▶ **Anticoagulation in patients with or at risk for heparin-induced thrombocytopenia during percutaneous coronary interventions (PCI).** *Adults:* 350 mcg/kg I.V. bolus over 3 to 5 minutes. Start a continuous I.V. infusion at 25 mcg/kg/minute. Activated clotting time (ACT) should be checked 5 to 10 minutes after the bolus dose is given and every 5 to 10 minutes during the infusion until it stabilizes at 300 seconds or longer.
⊠ Adjust-a-dose: See table below.

Activated clotting time	Additional I.V. bolus	Continuous I.V. infusion
< 300 sec	150 mcg/kg	30 mcg/kg/min***
300–450 sec	None needed	25 mcg/kg/min
> 450 sec	None needed	15 mcg/kg/min***

***Check ACT again after 5 to 10 minutes

In case of dissection, impending abrupt closure, thrombus formation during the procedure, or inability to achieve or maintain an ACT longer than 300 seconds, give an additional bolus of 150 mcg/kg and increase infusion rate to 40 mcg/kg/minute. Check ACT again after 5 to 10 minutes.
⑧ ALERT: ACT should be checked every 20 to 30 minutes during a prolonged PCI.

▼ I.V. administration

• Dilute in normal saline solution, D_5W, or lactated Ringer's injection to a final concentration of 1 mg/ml.
• Each 2.5-ml vial should be diluted 1:100 by mixing it with 250 ml of diluent.
• Mix the constituted solution by repeatedly turning over the diluent bag for 1 minute.
• Prepared solutions are stable for up to 24 hours at 77° F (25° C).
⊗ **Incompatibilities**
Other I.V. drugs.

Contraindications and cautions

• Contraindicated in patients hypersensitive to the drug or any of its components, and in patients with active bleeding.
• Use cautiously in patients with hepatic disease; disease states that create an increased risk of hemorrhage, such as severe hypertension; very recent lumbar puncture, spinal anesthesia, or major surgery, especially involving the brain, spinal cord, or eye; and hematologic conditions linked to increased bleeding tendencies, such as congenital or acquired bleeding disorders and GI lesions and ulcerations.
⚜ **Lifespan:** In pregnant women, use only if clearly needed. Breast-feeding women should either stop the drug or stop breast feeding, taking into account the importance of the drug to the mother. In children, safety and effectiveness haven't been established.

Interactions

Drug-drug. *Oral anticoagulants, antiplatelet drugs:* May prolong PT and INR and increase risk of bleeding. Avoid using together.
Thrombolytics: May increase risk of intracranial bleeding. Avoid using together.

Adverse reactions

CNS: fever, pain.
CV: atrial fibrillation, *cardiac arrest, cerebrovascular disorder, hemorrhage,* hypotension, *ventricular tachycardia,* vasodilation.
GI: abdominal pain, diarrhea, *GI bleeding,* hemoptysis, nausea, vomiting.
GU: abnormal renal function, groin bleeding, *hematuria,* UTI.
Hematologic: anemia.
Respiratory: cough, dyspnea, pneumonia.
Skin: rash, bullous eruptions.

Other: brachial bleeding, infection, *sepsis, allergic reactions (in patients also receiving thrombolytic therapy for acute MI).*

Effects on lab test results

• May decrease hemoglobin level and hematocrit.
• May increase WBC and platelet counts, APTT, ACT, and INR.

Pharmacokinetics

Absorption: Given I.V.
Distribution: Mainly in the extracellular fluid. Drug is 54% protein-bound, of which 34% is bound to a_1-acid glycoprotein and 20% to albumin.
Metabolism: Mainly in the liver by hydroxylation. The formation of four metabolites is catalyzed in the liver by CYP 3A4 and 5. The primary metabolite is 20% weaker than that of the parent drug. The other metabolites are detected in low levels in urine.
Excretion: Primarily in the feces, presumably through the biliary tract. *Half-life:* 39 to 51 minutes.

Route	Onset	Peak	Duration
I.V.	Rapid	1–3 hr	Until infusion stops

Action

Chemical effect: Reversibly binds to the thrombin active site and inhibits reactions catalyzed or induced by thrombin, including fibrin formation, activation of coagulation factors V, VIII, and XIII and protein C, and platelet aggregation. Inhibits the action of both free and clot-related thrombin.
Therapeutic effect: Prevents clot formation.

Available forms

Injection: 100 mg/ml

NURSING PROCESS

📝 Assessment
• Assess patient for increased risk of bleeding or overt bleeding before starting drug therapy.
• Obtain baseline coagulation tests, platelet counts, hemoglobin level, and hematocrit before therapy. Check APTT and ACT. Note abnormalities and notify prescriber.

• Stop all parenteral anticoagulants before giving drug.
• Assess patient's and family's knowledge of drug therapy.

Nursing diagnoses
• Ineffective tissue perfusion due to blood clots
• Increased risk for injury related to increased APTT and increased risk of bleeding from drug therapy
• Deficient knowledge related to argatroban therapy and anticoagulant safety precautions

Planning and implementation
• If an unexplained drop in hematocrit or blood pressure or another unexplained symptom occurs, suspect a hemorrhage and notify prescriber.
⚠ ALERT: Excessive anticoagulation, with or without bleeding, may occur with overdose. Symptoms of acute toxicity include loss of reflex, tremors, clonic seizures, limb paralysis, and coma. No specific antidote is available. Stop drug immediately and monitor APTT and other coagulation tests. Provide symptomatic and supportive therapy.
• To convert to oral anticoagulant therapy, give warfarin with argatroban at doses of up to 2 mcg/kg/minute until INR is higher than 4. After stopping argatroban, repeat INR in 4 to 6 hours. If the repeat INR is below the desired therapeutic range, resume argatroban. Repeat the procedure daily until the desired therapeutic range is reached on warfarin alone.
⚠ ALERT: Don't confuse argatroban with Aggrastat.
Patient teaching
• Advise patient that drug can cause bleeding, and urge him to immediately report any unusual bruising, bleeding (nosebleeds, bleeding gums, ecchymosis, or hematuria), or tarry or bloody stools.
• Advise patient to avoid activities that carry a risk of injury or cuts, and instruct him to use a soft toothbrush and electric razor while taking argatroban.
• Tell patient to notify prescriber if she is pregnant, breast-feeding, or recently had a baby.
• Tell patient to notify prescriber if he has stomach ulcers or liver disease; if he's had recent surgery, radiation treatments, falls, or other injury; or if wheezing, difficulty breathing, or rash occurs.

☑ Evaluation
• Patient doesn't have any unnecessary bruising or bleeding.
• Patient doesn't develop blood clots while on drug.
• Patient and family state understanding of drug therapy.

---

aripiprazole
(air-uh-PIP-rah-zol)
Abilify⬦

Pharmacologic class: psychotropic
Therapeutic class: atypical antipsychotic
Pregnancy risk category: C

Indications and dosages
▶ **Schizophrenia.** *Adults:* Initially, 10 to 15 mg P.O. daily, increasing to a maximum daily dose of 30 mg if needed, after at least 2 weeks. Maintenance doses of 15 mg P.O. daily may be effective.
▶ **Manic and mixed episodes associated with bipolar disorder.** *Adults:* Initially, 30 mg P.O. once daily. May decrease to 15 mg daily based on patient response.
⬦ Adjust-a-dose: Give half the dose when giving with CYP 3A4 or CYP 2D6 inhibitors, particularly ketoconazole, quinidine, fluoxetine, or paroxetine. Double the dose when giving with CYP 3A4 inducers, such as carbamazepine. Give original dose once other drugs are stopped.

Contraindications and cautions
• Contraindicated in patients hypersensitive to drug.
• Use cautiously in patients with CV disease, cerebrovascular disease, or conditions that could predispose the patient to hypotension, such as dehydration or hypovolemia. Also use cautiously in patients with history of seizures or with conditions that lower the seizure threshold and in those at risk for aspiration pneumonia, such as those with Alzheimer's disease. Use caution in patients who engage in strenuous exercise, are exposed to extreme heat, take anticholinergic medications, or are susceptible to dehydration.
※ Lifespan: In pregnant women, use only if the benefits outweigh the risks. In breast-feeding women, use cautiously because it's unknown whether drug appears in breast milk.

In children, safety and effectiveness of drug haven't been established. In elderly patients, use cautiously because they may experience greater sensitivity to drug.

Adverse reactions

CNS: *headache, anxiety, insomnia, lightheadedness, somnolence, akathisia,* tremor, asthenia, depression, nervousness, hostility, *suicidal thoughts,* manic behavior, confusion, abnormal gait, cogwheel rigidity, *seizures,* fever, tardive dyskinesia, cognitive and motor impairment, *neuroleptic malignant syndrome.*
CV: peripheral edema, chest pain, hypertension, tachycardia, orthostatic hypotension, *bradycardia.*
EENT: rhinitis, blurred vision, increased salivation, conjunctivitis, ear pain.
GI: *nausea, vomiting, constipation,* anorexia, diarrhea, abdominal pain, esophageal dysmotility.
GU: urinary incontinence.
Hematologic: anemia.
Metabolic: weight gain, weight loss, *hyperglycemia.*
Musculoskeletal: neck pain, neck stiffness, muscle cramps.
Respiratory: dyspnea, pneumonia, cough.
Skin: rash, dry skin, ecchymosis, pruritus, sweating, ulcer.
Other: flulike syndrome, inability to regulate body temperature.

Interactions

Drug-drug. *Antihypertensives:* May enhance antihypertensive and orthostatic hypotensive effects. Monitor blood pressure.
Carbamazepine and other CYP 3A4 inducers: May decrease level and effectiveness of aripiprazole. Double the usual dose of aripiprazole and monitor the patient closely.
Ketoconazole and other CYP 3A4 inhibitors; quinidine, fluoxetine, paroxetine, and other CYP 2D6 inhibitors: May increase level and toxicity of aripiprazole. Halve the usual dose of aripiprazole and monitor patient closely.
Drug-food. *Grapefruit juice:* May increase drug level. Advise patient to avoid grapefruit juice during treatment.
Drug-lifestyle. *Alcohol use:* May increase CNS effects. Discourage using together.

Effects on lab test results
● May increase glucose and CK levels.

Pharmacokinetics
Absorption: Good. Absolute bioavailability is 87% and isn't affected by food.
Distribution: Extensive. Protein-binding, mainly to albumin, is 99% for drug and major metabolites.
Metabolism: Extensively through the CYP 3A4 and CYP 2D6 systems, with one active metabolite.
Excretion: In urine and feces. *Elimination half-life:* About 75 hours in patients with normal metabolism and about 146 hours in those unable to metabolize the drug through CYP 2D6.

Route	Onset	Peak	Duration
P.O.	Unknown	3–5 hr	Unknown

Action
Chemical effect: May exhibit its antipsychotic effects through partial agonist activity at D2 and serotonin 5-HT$_{1A}$ receptors and antagonist activity at serotonin 5-HT$_{2A}$ receptors.
Therapeutic effect: Decreases psychotic behaviors.

Available forms
Tablets: 5 mg, 10 mg, 15 mg, 20 mg, 30 mg
Oral solution: 1 mg/ml

NURSING PROCESS

Assessment
● Assess patient's condition before and after therapy.
● Assess for potential compliance issues with drug regimen.
● Be alert for adverse reactions and drug interactions.
● Assess patient and family's knowledge of drug therapy.

Nursing diagnoses
● Risk for recurrence of signs and symptoms of schizophrenia if not compliant with medication regimen
● Potential noncompliance with medication regimen related to underlying mental illness
● Deficient knowledge related to drug therapy

▷ Planning and implementation

⚄ **ALERT:** Neuroleptic malignant syndrome may occur. Monitor patient for hyperpyrexia, muscle rigidity, altered mental status, irregular pulse or blood pressure, tachycardia, diaphoresis, and cardiac arrhythmias. If signs and symptoms of neuroleptic malignant syndrome occur, stop drug immediately.

• Monitor patient for signs and symptoms of tardive dyskinesia. Elderly patients, especially elderly women, are at higher risk of developing this adverse effect. If it occurs, stop drug.

⚄ **ALERT:** Hyperglycemia may occur in patients taking this drug. Monitor patients with diabetes regularly. Patients with risk factors for diabetes should undergo fasting blood glucose testing at baseline and periodically. Monitor patient for symptoms of hyperglycemia, including polydipsia, polyuria, polyphagia, and weakness. If symptoms develop, have patient undergo fasting blood glucose testing. In some cases, hyperglycemia is reversible by stopping use of the drug.

• Give the smallest dose for the shortest time. Periodically reassess need for treatment.

• To reduce risk of overdose, make sure only a small quantity of tablets is available at any time.

• The oral solution can be substituted on a mg-per-mg basis in place of the 5-, 10-, 15-, or 20-mg tablets up to 25 mg. Patients taking 30-mg tablets should receive 25 mg of solution.

• Overdose may cause somnolence and vomiting. Give activated charcoal within the first hours of overdose because 50% of a 15-mg dose is absorbed within the first hour. Dialysis isn't helpful because drug is highly protein-bound.

Patient teaching

• Tell patient to use caution when driving or operating hazardous machinery because psychoactive drugs may impair judgment, thinking, or motor skills.

• Tell patient that drug may be taken without regard to meals.

• Advise patient to avoid taking drug with grapefruit juice.

• Inform patient that gradual improvement in symptoms should occur over several weeks rather than immediately.

• Explain to patient that periodic blood work will be required.

• Tell patient to avoid alcohol use while taking drug.

• Advise patient to limit strenuous activity while taking drug to avoid dehydration and becoming overheated.

• Tell patient to store oral solution in refrigerator and that it can be used up to 6 months after opening.

☑ Evaluation

• Patient demonstrates reduced signs and symptoms of schizophrenia.

• Patient is compliant with drug regimen.

• Patient and family state understanding of drug therapy.

arsenic trioxide
(AR-sen-ik try-OX-ide)
Trisenox

Pharmacologic class: antineoplastic
Therapeutic class: antileukemia drug
Pregnancy risk category: D

Indications and dosages

▶ **Acute promyelocytic leukemia (APL) in patients who have relapsed from or are refractory to retinoid and anthracycline chemotherapy.** *Adults and children age 5 and older:* During induction phase, 0.15 mg/kg I.V. daily until bone marrow remission. Maximum 60 doses. During consolidation phase, 0.15 mg/kg I.V. daily for 25 doses over a period of up to 5 weeks, starting 3 to 6 weeks after completion of induction therapy.

▼ I.V. administration

• Follow facility policy for preparing and handling antineoplastics because the active ingredient is a carcinogen.

• Dilute with 100 to 250 ml of D_5W or normal saline solution. After dilution, drug is stable for 24 hours at room temperature and for 48 hours if refrigerated.

• Give over 1 to 2 hours. If vasomotor reactions occur, extend to 4 hours.

⊗ **Incompatibilities**
Other I.V. drugs.

Contraindications and cautions

• Contraindicated in patients hypersensitive to arsenic.

• Use cautiously in patients with heart failure or a history of torsades de pointes, prolonged QT interval, or conditions that result in hypokalemia or hypomagnesemia.

☀ **Lifespan:** Women of childbearing age should avoid becoming pregnant during therapy. In breast-feeding women, avoid use because arsenic appears in breast milk and may cause fetal harm. In children younger than age 5, safety and effectiveness haven't been established.

Adverse reactions

CNS: *fever;* headache, insomnia, paresthesia, dizziness, *pain,* tremor, *seizures,* somnolence, *coma,* anxiety, depression, agitation, confusion, fatigue, weakness.
CV: *hemorrhage,* tachycardia, PROLONGED QT INTERVAL, COMPLETE AV BLOCK, *palpitations, edema, chest pain,* ECG abnormalities, *hypotension, flushing, facial edema, hypertension.*
EENT: *eye irritation, epistaxis, blurred vision,* dry eye, earache, tinnitus, *sore throat, postnasal drip,* facial and eyelid edema, *sinusitis,* nasopharyngitis, painful red eye.
GI: *nausea, vomiting, diarrhea, anorexia, abdominal pain, constipation, loose stools, dyspepsia,* oral blistering, fecal incontinence, *GI hemorrhage,* dry mouth, abdominal tenderness or distension, bloody diarrhea, oral candidiasis.
GU: *renal failure,* renal impairment, oliguria, incontinence, *vaginal hemorrhage,* intermenstrual bleeding.
Hematologic: *leukocytosis, anemia,* THROMBOCYTOPENIA, NEUTROPENIA, DIC, lymphadenopathy.
Metabolic: hypokalemia, hypomagnesemia, hyperglycemia, hypocalcemia, *hypoglycemia,* acidosis, weight gain, weight loss, HYPERKALEMIA.
Musculoskeletal: arthralgia, myalgia, bone pain, back pain, neck pain, limb pain.
Respiratory: cough, dyspnea, hypoxia, pleural effusion, wheezing, decreased breath sounds, crepitations, rales, hemoptysis, tachypnea, rhonchi, upper respiratory tract infection.
Skin: *dermatitis, pruritus, dry skin, erythema, increased sweating,* night sweats, petechiae, hyperpigmentation, urticaria, skin lesions, local exfoliation, *pallor,* ecchymosis.
Other: drug hypersensitivity, *erythema or edema at injection site, rigors, herpes simplex infection,* bacterial infection, herpes zoster, *sepsis.*

Interactions

Drug-drug. *Drugs that can lead to electrolyte abnormalities (diuretics or amphotericin B):* May increase risk of electrolyte abnormalities. Use together cautiously.
Drugs that can prolong QT interval (antiarrhythmics or thioridazine): May further prolong QT interval. Use together cautiously and monitor ECG closely.

Effects on lab test results

• May increase AST, ALT, BUN, magnesium, calcium, and creatinine levels. May decrease sodium and hemoglobin levels and hematocrit. May increase or decrease glucose and potassium levels.
• May decrease RBC, WBC, neutrophil, and platelet counts.

Pharmacokinetics

Absorption: Given I.V.
Distribution: Stored mainly in the liver, kidneys, heart, lungs, hair, and nails.
Metabolism: In the liver.
Excretion: In urine in the methylated form. *Half-life:* Not established.

Route	Onset	Peak	Duration
I.V.	Unknown	Unknown	Unknown

Action

Chemical effect: Causes morphologic changes and DNA fragmentation resulting in death of promyelocytic leukemic cells.
Therapeutic effect: Destroys promyelocytic leukemic cells.

Available forms

Injection: 1 mg/ml

NURSING PROCESS

✍ Assessment
Ⓢ **ALERT:** May cause fatal arrhythmias and complete AV block.
• Monitor patient closely for altered blood pressure.
• Perform ECG; obtain potassium, calcium, magnesium, and creatinine levels; and correct electrolyte abnormalities before starting therapy.
• Monitor electrolyte levels and hematologic and coagulation profiles at least twice weekly during treatment. Keep potassium levels above

4 mEq/dl and magnesium levels above 1.8 mg/dl.

• Monitor patient for syncope and rapid or irregular heart rate. If these occur, stop drug, hospitalize patient, and monitor electrolyte levels and QT interval. Drug may be restarted when electrolyte abnormalities are corrected and QTc interval falls below 460 msec.

• Monitor ECG at least weekly during therapy. QT interval commonly is prolonged between 1 and 5 weeks after infusion and returns to baseline about 8 weeks after infusion. If QTc interval is longer than 500 msec at any time during therapy, assess patient carefully and stop drug.

• Assess patient's and family's knowledge of drug therapy.

✪ Nursing diagnoses
• Risk of decreased cardiac output due to drug-induced toxicity
• Risk for infection related to drug-induced thrombocytopenia or neutropenia
• Deficient knowledge related to arsenic trioxide therapy

⦥ Planning and implementation
• Monitor patient carefully for adverse reactions or drug toxicity. Symptoms of acute arsenic toxicity include confusion, muscle weakness, and seizures. If overdose occurs, stop drug immediately. Give 3 mg/kg dimercaprol I.M. q 4 hours until life-threatening toxicity subsides; then give 250 mg penicillamine P.O. up to q.i.d.

⦿ **ALERT:** May cause fatal APL differentiation syndrome, characterized by fever, dyspnea, weight gain, pulmonary infiltrates, and pleural or pericardial effusions with or without leukocytosis. If this occurs, give high-dose steroids.

Patient teaching
• Tell patient to immediately report any fever, shortness of breath, bloody stools, or weight gain.
• Instruct patient to tell prescriber about all drugs currently being taken and to check with prescriber before starting any new drug.
• Inform patient with diabetes that drug may cause hyperglycemia or hypoglycemia, and instruct him to monitor glucose level closely.
• Caution women of childbearing age to avoid becoming pregnant during therapy.

☑ Evaluation
• Patient tolerates therapy and responds positively to drug therapy.
• Patient doesn't have infection or life-threatening adverse events.
• Patient and family state understanding of drug therapy.

asparaginase (L-asparaginase)
(as-PAR-ah-jin-ays)
Elspar, Kidrolase ♦

Pharmacologic class: enzyme
Therapeutic class: antineoplastic
Pregnancy risk category: C

Indications and dosages
▶ **Acute lymphocytic leukemia (ALL) (with other drugs).** *Adults and children:* For ALL Regimen I treatment period, on day 22 of treatment, give 1,000 international units/kg I.V. daily for 10 days, injected over at least 30 minutes, or for ALL Regimen II treatment protocol, give 6,000 international units/m² I.M. at intervals specified in protocol.
▶ **Sole induction drug for remission of ALL.** *Adults and children:* 200 international units/kg I.V. daily for 28 days.

▽ I.V. administration
• Follow facility policy to reduce risks. Preparing and giving parenteral form may carry carcinogenic, mutagenic, and teratogenic risks.
• Reconstitute with 5 ml of either sterile water or normal saline solution for injection. Don't shake vial. Don't use cloudy solutions.
• Filtration through a 5-micron filter during administration will remove particles without decreasing potency.
• Give injection over no less than 30 minutes through a running infusion of normal saline solution for injection or D₅W injection.
• If drug contacts skin or mucous membranes, wash with copious amounts of water for at least 15 minutes.
• Keep epinephrine, diphenhydramine, and I.V. corticosteroids available to treat anaphylaxis.
• Refrigerate unopened dry powder. Reconstituted solution is stable for 8 hours if refrigerated.

⊗ **Incompatibilities**
None reported.

Contraindications and cautions

• Contraindicated in patients with pancreatitis or a history of pancreatitis and in patients with previous hypersensitivity unless desensitized.
• Use cautiously in patients with hepatic dysfunction.
🔥 **Lifespan:** In pregnant women, use cautiously. In breast-feeding women, drug shouldn't be used.

Adverse reactions

CNS: fever, chills, coma, confusion, drowsiness, depression, hallucinations, headache, nervousness, lethargy, somnolence.
GI: *vomiting, anorexia, nausea,* cramps, weight loss, HEMORRHAGIC PANCREATITIS.
GU: azotemia, *renal impairment,* uric acid nephropathy, glycosuria, polyuria, *increased blood ammonia level.*
Hematologic: *anemia, hypofibrinogenemia, thrombocytopenia, leukopenia.*
Hepatic: *hepatotoxicity.*
Metabolic: *hyperuricemia, hyperglycemia.*
Skin: rash, urticaria.
Other: ANAPHYLAXIS, *fatal hyperthermia.*

Interactions

Drug-drug. *Methotrexate:* May decrease methotrexate's effectiveness when given immediately before or with methotrexate. Monitor levels of methotrexate. Watch patient for signs of decreased effect.
Prednisone, vincristine: May increase toxicity. Monitor patient closely.

Effects on lab test results

• May increase BUN, AST, ALT, bilirubin, glucose, uric acid, and ammonia levels. May decrease calcium, fibrinogen, albumin, other clotting factor, and hemoglobin levels and hematocrit. May increase or decrease total lipid level.
• May decrease WBC and platelet counts.
• May decrease thyroid function test values.

Pharmacokinetics

Absorption: Unknown.
Distribution: Primarily within intravascular space, with detectable levels in thoracic and cervical lymph. Minimal amount crosses blood–brain barrier.

Metabolism: Hepatic sequestration by reticuloendothelial system may occur.
Excretion: Unknown. *Half-life:* 8 to 30 hours.

Route	Onset	Peak	Duration
I.V.	Immediate	Immediate	23–33 days after stopping drug
I.M.	Immediate	4–24 hr after stopping drug	23–33 days

Action

Chemical effect: Destroys amino acid asparagine, which is needed for protein synthesis in acute lymphocytic leukemia.
Therapeutic effect: Kills leukemia cells.

Available forms

Injection: 10,000–international unit vial

NURSING PROCESS

🩺 **Assessment**
• Obtain history of patient's leukemia.
• Monitor effectiveness by evaluating CBC and bone marrow function test results. Bone marrow regeneration may take 5 to 6 weeks.
• Be alert for adverse reactions and drug interactions.
• Assess patient's and family's knowledge of drug therapy.

Nursing diagnoses
• Ineffective health maintenance related to leukemic condition
• Ineffective protection related to drug-induced adverse reactions
• Deficient knowledge related to drug therapy

Planning and implementation
• Give drug in a hospital under close supervision with emergency resuscitation equipment readily available.
• Drug shouldn't be used alone to induce remission unless combination therapy is inappropriate. Not recommended for maintenance therapy.
• Increase patient's fluid intake to prevent tumor lysis, which can result in uric acid nephropathy. Start allopurinol before therapy begins.
🔵 **ALERT:** Repeated doses increase the risk of hypersensitivity reactions. Perform an I.D. skin test before initial dose and repeat after an interval of a week or more, between doses. To per-

form skin test, give 2 international units of drug I.D. Observe site for at least 1 hour for erythema or a wheal, which indicates a positive response. An allergic reaction to the drug may still develop in a patient with a negative skin test.
• Give 1 international unit I.V. as a desensitizing dose. Dose is doubled every 10 minutes if no reaction occurs, until total amount given equals patient's total dose for that day.
• Limit I.M. dose at single injection site to 2 ml.
• Because patient may vomit, give parenteral fluids for 24 hours or until patient can tolerate oral fluids.

Patient teaching
• Tell patient to watch for signs of infection (fever, sore throat, fatigue) and bleeding (easy bruising, nosebleeds, bleeding gums, tarry or bloody stools). Instruct patient to take temperature daily.
• Encourage patient to maintain an adequate fluid intake to increase urine output and facilitate excretion of uric acid.
• Tell patient that drowsiness may occur during therapy or for several weeks after treatment ends. Warn patient to avoid hazardous activities requiring mental alertness.

⚕ Evaluation
• Patient is free from leukemia.
• Patient doesn't experience injury as a result of drug-induced adverse reactions.
• Patient and family state understanding of drug therapy.

aspirin (acetylsalicylic acid)
(AS-prin)
Ancasal ♦ †, Arthrinol ♦ †, Artria S.R.†, ASA†, ASA Enseals†, Aspergum†, Aspro Preparations ◇, Astrin ♦ †, Bayer Aspirin†, Bex Powders ◇, Coryphen ♦ †, Easprin†, Ecotrin†, Empirin†, Entrophen ♦ †, Halfprin, Measurin ♦ †, Norwich Extra Strength†, Novasen†, Riphen-10 ♦ †, Sal-Adult ♦ †, Sal-Infant ♦ †, Solprin ◇, Supasa ♦ †, Triaphen-10 ♦ †, Vincent's Powders ◇, ZORprin†

Pharmacologic class: salicylate
Therapeutic class: nonopioid analgesic, antipyretic, anti-inflammatory, antiplatelet drug

Pregnancy risk category: C (D in third trimester)

Indications and dosages
▶ **Arthritis.** *Adults:* Initially, 2.4 to 3.6 g P.O. daily in divided doses. Maintenance dosage is 3.6 to 5.4 g P.O. daily in divided doses. *Children:* 60 to 130 mg/kg P.O. daily in divided doses.
▶ **Mild pain or fever.** *Adults:* 325 to 650 mg P.O. or P.R. q 4 hours, p.r.n. *Children:* For mild pain only, 65 mg/kg P.O. or P.R. daily in four to six divided doses.
▶ **Prevention of thrombosis.** *Adults:* 1.3 g P.O. daily in two to four divided doses.
▶ **Reduction of risk of MI in patients with previous MI or unstable angina.** *Adults:* 160 to 325 mg P.O. daily.
▶ **Kawasaki syndrome (mucocutaneous lymph node syndrome).** *Adults:* 80 to 100 mg/kg P.O. daily in four divided doses during febrile phase. Some patients may need up to 120 mg/kg. When fever subsides, decrease dosage to 3 to 8 mg/kg once daily, adjusted according to salicylate level.
▶ **Prophylaxis for transient ischemic attack (TIA).** *Adults:* 50 to 325 mg P.O. daily.
▶ **TIA.** *Adults:* 160 to 325 mg P.O. immediately within 48 hours of onset of stroke.
▶ **Prevention of reocclusion in coronary revascularization procedures.** *Adults:* 325 mg P.O. q 6 hours after surgery and for 1 year.
▶ **Rheumatic fever‡.** *Adults:* 4.9 to 7.8 g P.O. daily in divided doses q 4 to 6 hours for 1 to 2 weeks. Decrease to 60 to 70 mg/kg daily for 1 to 6 weeks, then gradually withdraw over 1 to 2 weeks. *Children:* 90 to 130 mg/kg P.O. daily in divided doses q 4 to 6 hours.
▶ **Pericarditis after acute MI‡.** *Adults:* 160 to 325 mg P.O. daily.
▶ **Stent implantation‡.** *Adults:* 80 to 325 mg P.O. 2 hours before stent placement and 160 to 325 mg P.O. daily thereafter.

Contraindications and cautions
• Contraindicated in patients hypersensitive to drug and those with G6PD deficiency; bleeding disorders such as hemophilia, von Willebrand's disease, and telangiectasia; and NSAID-induced sensitivity reactions.
• Use cautiously in patients with GI lesions, impaired renal function, hypoprothrombinemia, vitamin K deficiency, thrombocytopenia, throm-

botic thrombocytopenic purpura, or severe hepatic impairment.

≋ Lifespan: In pregnant women, use cautiously. In breast-feeding women, safety hasn't been established.

⊛ ALERT: Because of the risk of Reye's syndrome, the Centers for Disease Control and Prevention recommends not giving salicylates to children or teenagers who have or are recovering from chickenpox or flulike illness or who have acute febrile illnesses. In elderly patients, use cautiously because GI and renal adverse effects may be exacerbated.

Adverse reactions

EENT: *tinnitus, hearing loss.*
GI: *nausea, vomiting, GI distress, occult bleeding,* dyspepsia, *GI bleeding.*
GU: transient renal insufficiency.
Hematologic: *prolonged bleeding time, thrombocytopenia.*
Hepatic: *hepatitis.*
Skin: *rash,* bruising, urticaria.
Other: *angioedema,* hypersensitivity reactions (*anaphylaxis,* asthma), *Reye's syndrome.*

Interactions

Drug-drug. *Ammonium chloride, other urine acidifiers:* May increase levels of aspirin products. Watch for aspirin toxicity.
Antacids in high doses (and other urine alkalinizers): May decrease levels of aspirin products. Watch for decreased aspirin effect.
Beta blockers: May decrease antihypertensive effect. Avoid long-term aspirin use if patient is taking antihypertensives.
Corticosteroids: May enhance salicylate elimination. Watch for decreased salicylate effect.
Heparin: May increase risk of bleeding. Monitor patient and coagulation studies closely if used together.
Methotrexate: May increase risk of methotrexate toxicity. Monitor patient closely.
NSAIDs: May alter pharmacokinetics of these drugs, leading to lower levels and decreased effectiveness. Avoid using together. May also increase risk of GI bleeding. Monitor patient closely.
Oral anticoagulants: May increase risk of bleeding. Monitor patient for signs of bleeding.
Oral antidiabetics: May increase hypoglycemic effect. Monitor patient closely.

Probenecid, sulfinpyrazone: May decrease uricosuric effect. Avoid aspirin during therapy with these drugs.
Steroids: May increase risk of GI bleeding. Monitor patient closely.
Drug-herb. *Dong quai, feverfew, garlic, ginger, horse chestnut, red clover:* May increase risk of bleeding. Monitor patient for increased effects, and discourage using together.
Drug-food. *Caffeine:* May increase the absorption of aspirin. Monitor patient for increased effects.
Drug-lifestyle. *Alcohol use:* May increase risk of GI bleeding. Discourage using together.

Effects on lab test results

• May increase liver enzyme levels.
• May decrease WBC and platelet counts.

Pharmacokinetics

Absorption: Rapid and complete.
Distribution: Wide. Protein-binding to albumin is concentration-dependent. It ranges from 75% to 90% and decreases as level increases.
Metabolism: Hydrolyzed partially in GI tract to salicylic acid, but almost completely in liver.
Excretion: In urine as salicylate and its metabolites. *Half-life:* 15 to 20 minutes.

Route	Onset	Peak	Duration
P.O.			
buffered	5–30 min	1–2 hr	1–4 hr
enteric-coated	5–30 min	4–8 hr	1–4 hr
extended-release	5–30 min	1–2 hr	4–8 hr
regular	5–30 min	25–40 min	1–4 hr
solution	5–30 min	15–60 min	1–4 hr
P.R.	5–30 min	3–4 hr	1–4 hr

Action

Chemical effect: Produces analgesia by blocking prostaglandin synthesis (peripheral action). Drug and other salicylates may prevent lowering of pain threshold that occurs when prostaglandins sensitize pain receptors to stimulation. Exerts its anti-inflammatory effect by inhibiting prostaglandin synthesis; also may inhibit synthesis or action of other mediators of inflammatory response. Relieves fever by acting on hypothalamic heat-regulating center to cause peripheral vasodilation, which increases peripheral blood supply and promotes sweating, which leads to heat loss and to cooling by evaporation. In low doses, aspirin also appears to impede clotting by blocking prostaglandin synthesis, which prevents formation of platelet-aggregating substance thromboxane A2.

Therapeutic effect: Relieves pain, reduces fever and inflammation, and decreases risk of transient ischemic attacks and MI.

Available forms

Capsules: 325 mg†, 500 mg†
Chewing gum: 227.5 mg†
Suppositories: 60 mg†, 65 mg†, 120 mg†, 125 mg†, 130 mg†, 195 mg†, 200 mg†, 300 mg†, 325 mg†, 600 mg†, 650 mg†
Tablets†: 325 mg, 500 mg, 600 mg, 650 mg
Tablets (chewable): 81 mg†
Tablets (enteric-coated): 81 mg†, 165 mg, 325 mg†, 500 mg†, 650 mg†, 975 mg
Tablets (extended-release): 800 mg
Tablets (timed-release): 650 mg†

NURSING PROCESS

Assessment
• Obtain history of patient's pain or fever before therapy, and monitor patient throughout therapy.
• Be alert for adverse reactions and drug interactions.
• During long-term therapy, monitor salicylate level. Therapeutic level in arthritis is 10 to 30 mg/dl. With long-term therapy, mild toxicity may occur at levels of 20 mg/dl. Tinnitus may occur at levels of 30 mg/dl and above but doesn't reliably indicate toxicity, especially in very young patients and those older than age 60.
• Assess patient's and family's knowledge of drug therapy.

Nursing diagnoses
• Acute pain related to underlying condition
• Risk for injury related to drug-induced adverse GI reactions
• Deficient knowledge related to drug therapy

Planning and implementation
• Give aspirin with food, milk, antacid, or large glass of water to reduce adverse GI reactions.
• If patient has trouble swallowing, crush aspirin, combine it with soft food, or dissolve it in liquid. Give immediately after mixing with liquid because drug doesn't stay in solution. Don't crush enteric-coated aspirin.

• Enteric-coated products are slowly absorbed and not suitable for acute effects. These products cause less GI bleeding and may be more suited for long-term therapy, such as for arthritis.
• Give P.R. after a bowel movement or at night to maximize absorption.
• Hold dose and notify prescriber if bleeding, salicylism (tinnitus, hearing loss), or adverse GI reactions develop.
• Stop aspirin 5 to 7 days before elective surgery.
⊛ **ALERT:** Don't confuse aspirin with Asendin or Afrin.

Patient teaching
• Encourage patient to retain suppository for as long as possible, preferably at least 10 hours to maximize absorption.
• Advise patient receiving high-dose prolonged treatment to watch for petechiae, bleeding gums, and signs of GI bleeding and to maintain adequate fluid intake. Encourage use of a soft toothbrush.
• Because of many possible drug interactions involving aspirin, warn patient who takes prescription form to check with prescriber or pharmacist before taking herbal preparations or OTC combinations containing aspirin.
• Explain that various OTC preparations contain aspirin. Warn patient to read labels carefully to avoid overdose.
• Advise patient to avoid alcohol use during drug therapy.
• Advise patient to restrict intake of caffeine during drug therapy.
• Instruct patient to take aspirin with food or milk.
• Instruct patient not to chew enteric-coated products.
• Aspirin is a leading cause of poisoning in children. Emphasize safe storage of drugs in the home. Teach patient to keep aspirin and other drugs out of children's reach. Encourage use of child-resistant containers, even if children only visit occasionally.

Evaluation
• Patient states that aspirin has relieved pain.
• Patient remains free from adverse GI effects throughout drug therapy.
• Patient and family state understanding of drug therapy.

Reactions may be *common*, uncommon, *life-threatening*, or COMMON AND LIFE-THREATENING.

atazanavir sulfate

(att-uh-za-NUH-veer sul-FAYT)
Reyataz

Pharmacologic class: protease inhibitor
Therapeutic class: antiretroviral
Pregnancy risk category: B

Indications and dosages

▶ **HIV-1 infection, with other antiretrovirals.**
Adults: In antiretroviral-experienced patients,
give 300 mg (as two 150-mg capsules) once
daily plus 100 mg ritonavir once daily taken
with food. For antiretroviral-naive patients,
400 mg (as two 200-mg capsules) P.O. once
daily with food. When giving with efavirenz in
antiretroviral-naive patients, give 300 mg
atazanavir and 100 mg ritonavir with 600 mg
efavirenz, all as a single daily dose with food.
Dosing recommendations for efavirenz and
atazanavir in treatment-experienced patients
haven't been established.
◙ **Adjust-a-dose:** For patients with Child-Pugh
class B hepatic insufficiency, reduce dosage to
300 mg P.O. once daily.

Contraindications and cautions

• Contraindicated in patients hypersensitive to
drug or any of its components. Also contraindicated with drugs, such as midazolam, triazolam,
dihydroergotamine, ergotamine, ergonovine,
methylergonovine, cisapride, pimozide, that are
highly dependent on CYP 3A4 for clearance
and for which elevated levels are linked to life-
threatening effects.
• Use cautiously in patients with preexisting
conduction system disease or hepatic impairment.
▲ **Lifespan:** In pregnant women, drug should
be used only if potential benefits outweigh risk.
To help monitor maternal-fetal outcomes of
pregnant women, register pregnant women in
the Antiretroviral Pregnancy Registry (1-800-
258-4263). In breast-feeding women, use cautiously because it's unknown whether drug appears in breast milk. In children, an optimal
dosing regimen hasn't been established. In children younger than age 3, the drug shouldn't be
used because of a risk for kernicterus. In elderly
patients, use cautiously because they may retain
more of the drug.

Adverse reactions

CNS: *headache,* fever, pain, fatigue, depression,
insomnia, dizziness, peripheral neurology
symptoms.
CV: first degree heart block.
GI: *nausea, abdominal pain,* vomiting, diar-
rhea.
Hepatic: *hepatitis,* jaundice or scleral icterus.
Metabolic: lipodystrophy, *lactic acidosis,* lipo-
hypertrophy.
Musculoskeletal: back pain, arthralgia.
Respiratory: increased cough.
Skin: *rash.*

Interactions

Drug-drug. *Antacids and buffered medications:*
May decrease atazanavir levels. Give atazanavir
2 hours before or 1 hour after these medications.
Amiodarone, lidocaine (systemic), quinidine:
May increase levels of these drugs. Monitor levels.
Atorvastatin, lovastatin, simvastatin: May increase statin level and the risk of myopathy and
rhabdomyolysis. Use atorvastatin cautiously,
don't use lovastatin or simvastatin.
Clarithromycin: May increase clarithromycin
and atazanavir levels and decrease 14-OH clarithromycin levels. Reduce clarithromycin dose
by 50% when giving with atazanavir. Because
levels of the active metabolite 14-OH clarithromycin are significantly reduced, consider alternative therapy for indications other than infections caused by *Mycobacterium avium* complex.
Cyclosporine, sirolimus, tacrolimus: May increase immunosuppressant levels. Monitor immunosuppressant levels.
Didanosine buffered formulations: May decrease atazanavir level. Give atazanavir 2 hours
before or 1 hour after didanosine buffered formulations.
*Dihydroergotamine, ergonovine, ergotamine,
methylergonovine:* May cause life-threatening
reactions, such as acute ergot toxicity characterized by peripheral vasospasm and ischemia of
the limbs and other tissues. Don't use together.
Diltiazem: May increase diltiazem and
desacetyl-diltiazem levels. Use cautiously. Reduce dose of diltiazem by 50%. Monitor ECG.
Efavirenz: May decrease atazanavir levels. If
used together, give 300 mg atazanavir with
100 mg ritonavir with 600 mg efavirenz all as a
single daily dose with food because this combination results in atazanavir exposure that

approximates the exposure to 400 mg of atazanavir alone. Atazanavir shouldn't be given with efavirenz without ritonavir.

Ethinyl estradiol and norethindrone: May increase ethinyl estradiol and norethindrone. Use cautiously. The lowest effective dose of each hormonal contraceptive component should be used.

Felodipine, nicardipine, nifedipine, verapamil: May increase calcium channel blocker levels. Use cautiously. Adjust dose of the calcium channel blocker. Monitor ECG.

Fluticasone: Significantly increases fluticasone exposure, causing decreased serum cortisol levels, leading to systemic corticosteroid effects (including Cushing syndrome). Don't use together, if possible.

H_2-receptor antagonists: May decrease atazanavir levels. Give 12 hours apart.

Indinavir: May increase risk of hyperbilirubinemia. Use together isn't recommended.

Irinotecan: May interfere with the metabolism of irinotecan, resulting in increased irinotecan toxicities. Don't use together.

Itraconazole, ketoconazole: May interact with ritonavir-boosted atazanavir. Use together cautiously.

Midazolam, triazolam: May cause life-threatening reactions, such as prolonged or increased sedation or respiratory depression. Don't use together.

Nevirapine: May decrease atazanavir levels. Use together isn't recommended.

Pimozide: May cause life-threatening reactions such as cardiac arrhythmias. Don't use together.

Proton pump inhibitors: May substantially decrease atazanavir levels and reduce its therapeutic effect. Use together isn't recommended.

Rifabutin: May increase rifabutin levels. Reduce rifabutin dose by up to 75%.

Rifampin: May decrease level of most protease inhibitors, resulting in loss of therapeutic effect and development of resistance. Don't use together.

Ritonavir: May increase atazanavir levels. Give 300 mg atazanavir once daily with 100 mg ritonavir once daily, with food.

Saquinavir (soft gelatin capsules): May increase saquinavir level. Appropriate dose for this combination hasn't been established.

Sildenafil, tadalafil, vardenafil: May increase sildenafil, tadalafil, and vardenafil levels. Use together may result in increased sildenafil-

associated adverse events, including hypotension, visual changes, and priapism. Use sildenafil with caution at a reduced dose of 25 mg every 48 hours; use tadalafil with caution at reduced dosages of 10 mg every 72 hours, and use vardenafil with caution at reduced dosages of 2.5 mg every 72 hours. Monitor patient for adverse events.

Tenofovir: May decrease atazanavir level, causing resistance. Give both drugs with ritonavir.

Trazadone: May increase trazadone level causing nausea, dizziness, hypotension, and syncope. Avoid using together, or use cautiously with a lower dose of trazadone.

Tricyclic antidepressants: May increase levels of tricyclic antidepressants. Monitor levels.

Voriconazole: May interact. Monitor for toxicities. Avoid use with ritonavir-boosted atazanavir.

Warfarin: May increase warfarin levels. Monitor INR.

Drug-herb. *St. John's wort:* May reduce atazanavir level, resulting in loss of therapeutic effect and development of resistance. Discourage using together.

Effects on lab test results

● May increase AST, ALT, total bilirubin, amylase, and lipase levels. May decrease hemoglobin level and hematocrit.

● May decrease neutrophil count.

Pharmacokinetics

Absorption: Rapid. Peak level occurs in approximately 2½ hours. Food enhances bioavailability.

Distribution: 86% protein-bound and binds to $alpha_1$-acid glycoprotein and albumin to a similar extent.

Metabolism: Extensively, primarily by the liver.

Excretion: In urine and feces. About 7% excreted unchanged in urine. *Elimination half-life:* About 7 hours.

Route	Onset	Peak	Duration
P.O.	Unknown	2 hr	Unknown

Action

Chemical effect: Prevents the formation of mature virions within HIV-1 infected cells.

Therapeutic effect: Treats symptoms of HIV infection.

Available forms

Capsules: 100 mg, 150 mg, 200 mg

NURSING PROCESS

⚖ Assessment
• Monitor cardiac status during therapy.
• Test women for pregnancy before starting therapy.
• Monitor liver function tests periodically during therapy.
• Assess patient's and family's knowledge of drug therapy.

🔲 Nursing diagnoses
• Infection related to underlying HIV infection
• Risk of injury related to adverse reactions
• Deficient knowledge related to drug therapy

⧉ Planning and implementation
• Drug may prolong PR interval.
• Most patients experience asymptomatic elevations in indirect bilirubin, which may be accompanied by yellowing of the skin or whites of the eyes. Hyperbilirubinemia is reversible when drug is stopped.
• Various degrees of cross-resistance among protease inhibitors may occur. Resistance to this drug doesn't preclude the subsequent use of other protease inhibitors. Give drug with other antiretrovirals.
• Patients should remain under the care of a physician while taking drug.
• At high doses, jaundice is caused by indirect (unconjugated) hyperbilirubinemia (without associated liver function test changes), or prolonged PR interval may occur.
• Treat overdose with general supportive measures, including monitoring of vital signs and ECG, and observations of the patient's clinical status. Induce vomiting or use gastric lavage to eliminate unabsorbed drug. Also give activated charcoal to aid removal of unabsorbed drug. Because drug is highly metabolized by the liver and is highly protein-bound, dialysis is unlikely to be beneficial.
Patient teaching
• Tell patient that sustained decreases in HIV RNA have been linked to a reduced risk of progression to AIDS and death.
• Tell patient he should remain under the care of a physician while taking drug.

• Advise patient to take drug with food every day, and to take other antiretrovirals as prescribed.
• Inform patient that drug isn't a cure for HIV and that he may develop opportunistic infections and other complications of HIV disease. Also explain that the drug doesn't reduce the risk of transmitting HIV to others.
• Tell patient not to alter dose or stop therapy without consulting his prescriber.
• If a dose is missed, advise patient to take the dose as soon as possible and then return to his normal schedule. However, if he skips a dose, tell him not to double the next dose.
• Tell patient to consult prescriber if he experiences dizziness or light-headedness.
• Tell patient that elevations in indirect bilirubin may occur and to report yellowing of the skin or the whites of the eyes.
• Inform patient that redistribution or accumulation of body fat may occur.
• Recommend that HIV-infected mothers avoid breast-feeding to prevent postnatal transmission of HIV.

☑ Evaluation
• Patient remains free from infection.
• Patient doesn't suffer injury from adverse reactions.
• Patient and family state understanding of drug therapy.

atenolol
(uh-TEN-uh-lol)
Apo-Atenol ♦ , Noten ◇ , Nu-Atenol ♦ , Tenormin⌀

Pharmacologic class: beta blocker
Therapeutic class: antihypertensive, antianginal
Pregnancy risk category: D

Indications and dosages
▶ **Hypertension.** *Adults:* Initially, 50 mg P.O. daily as a single dose. Increase dosage to 100 mg once daily after 7 to 14 days. Doses higher than 100 mg are unlikely to produce further benefit.
🔲 **Adjust-a-dose:** *Elderly patients:* Initially, 25 mg P.O. daily and increase slowly until desired response. Also reduce dosage in patients

with creatinine clearance less than 35 ml/ minute.

▶ **Angina pectoris.** *Adults:* 50 mg P.O. once daily. Increase p.r.n. to 100 mg daily after 7 days for optimal effect. Maximum dosage is 200 mg daily.

▶ **To reduce CV mortality rate and risk of reinfarction in patients with acute MI.** *Adults:* 5 mg I.V. over 5 minutes, followed by another 5 mg 10 minutes later. After another 10 minutes, 50 mg P.O., followed by 50 mg P.O. in 12 hours. Thereafter, 100 mg P.O. daily (as a single dose or 50 mg b.i.d.) for at least 7 days.

▶ **To slow rapid ventricular response to atrial tachyarrhythmias after acute MI without left ventricular dysfunction and AV block‡.** *Adults:* 2.5 to 5 mg I.V. over 2 to 5 minutes, p.r.n. to control rate. Maximum, 10 mg over a 10- to 15-minute period.

▼ I.V. administration

• Mix doses with D_5W, normal saline solution, or dextrose and sodium chloride solutions.
• Give by slow injection, not to exceed 1 mg/ minute.
• Solution is stable for 48 hours after mixing.
⊗ **Incompatibilities**
Other I.V. drugs.

Contraindications and cautions

• Contraindicated in patients with sinus bradycardia, greater than first-degree heart block, overt cardiac failure, or cardiogenic shock.
• Use cautiously in patients at risk for heart failure and in those with bronchospastic disease, diabetes, and hyperthyroidism.
⚘ **Lifespan:** In pregnant women, don't use unless absolutely necessary because fetal harm can occur. In breast-feeding women, use cautiously. In children, safety of drug hasn't been established.

Adverse reactions

CNS: fever, fatigue, hallucinations, headache, lethargy.
CV: BRADYCARDIA, PROFOUND HYPOTENSION, intermittent claudication, *second- or third-degree AV block.*
EENT: visual disturbances
GI: nausea, vomiting, diarrhea, dry mouth.
GU: impotence, Peyronie's disease
Respiratory: dyspnea, *bronchospasm.*
Skin: rash, reversible alopecia.

Interactions

Drug-drug. *Antihypertensives:* May enhance hypotensive effect. Use together cautiously.
Digoxin, diltiazem: May cause excessive bradycardia and may increase depressant effect on myocardium. Use together cautiously.
Insulin, oral antidiabetics: May alter dosage requirements in previously stabilized patient with diabetes. Observe patient carefully.
I.V. lidocaine: May reduce hepatic metabolism of lidocaine, increasing the risk of toxicity. Give bolus doses of lidocaine at a slower rate and monitor lidocaine levels closely.
Prazosin: May increase the risk of orthostatic hypotension in the early phases of use together. Assist patient to stand slowly until effects are known.
Reserpine: May cause hypotension. Use together cautiously.
Verapamil: May increase the effects of both drugs. Monitor cardiac function closely and decrease dosages as necessary.

Effects on lab test results

• May increase BUN, creatinine, potassium, uric acid, transaminase, alkaline phosphatase, triglyceride, and LDH levels. May increase or decrease glucose level.
• May increase platelet count.

Pharmacokinetics

Absorption: About 50% to 60%.
Distribution: Into most tissues and fluids except brain and CSF. About 5% to 15% protein-bound.
Metabolism: Minimal.
Excretion: From 40% to 50% of dose is excreted unchanged in urine; remainder is excreted as unchanged drug and metabolites in feces. *Half-life:* 6 to 7 hours.

Route	Onset	Peak	Duration
P.O.	1 hr	2–4 hr	24 hr
I.V.	5 min	5 min	12 hr

Action

Chemical effect: Selectively blocks $beta_1$ receptors; decreases cardiac output, peripheral resistance, and cardiac oxygen consumption; and depresses renin secretion.
Therapeutic effect: Decreases blood pressure, relieves angina, and reduces CV mortality rate and risk of reinfarction after acute MI.

Reactions may be *common,* uncommon, *life-threatening,* or COMMON AND LIFE-THREATENING.

Available forms

Injection: 5 mg/10 ml
Tablets: 25 mg, 50 mg, 100 mg

NURSING PROCESS

Assessment

• Obtain history of patient's underlying condition.
• If prescribed for hypertension, monitor drug's effectiveness by frequently checking patient's blood pressure. Full antihypertensive effect may not occur for 1 to 2 weeks after therapy starts. For angina pectoris, monitor frequency and severity of anginal pain. For reducing CV mortality rate and risk of reinfarction after acute MI, monitor signs of reinfarction.
• Be alert for adverse reactions and drug interactions.
• Assess patient's and family's knowledge of drug therapy.

Nursing diagnoses

• Risk for injury related to underlying condition
• Decreased cardiac output related to drug-induced adverse CV reactions
• Deficient knowledge related to drug therapy

Planning and implementation

• Adjust dosage in patients with renal insufficiency and those receiving hemodialysis.
• Check patient's apical pulse before giving drug; if slower than 60 beats/minute, withhold drug and call prescriber.
• Give as a single daily dose.
• Be prepared to treat shock or hypoglycemia because this drug masks common signs of these conditions.
• Notify prescriber immediately if patient shows signs of decreased cardiac output.
ⓈALERT: Withdraw drug gradually over 1 to 2 weeks to avoid serious adverse reactions.
ⓈALERT: Don't confuse atenolol with timolol or albuterol.
Patient teaching
• Warn patient that stopping drug abruptly can worsen angina and MI. Drug should be withdrawn gradually over a 2-week period.
• Counsel patient to take drug at same time every day.
• Tell woman to notify prescriber if she becomes pregnant because drug must be stopped.

• Teach patient how to take his pulse. Tell patient not to take the drug and to call his prescriber if pulse rate is slower than 60 beats/minute.
• Tell patient to notify prescriber of excessive fatigue.

Evaluation

• Patient's underlying condition improves with drug therapy.
• Patient's cardiac output remains unchanged throughout drug therapy.
• Patient and family state understanding of drug therapy.

atomoxetine hydrochloride
(ATT-oh-mocks-uh-teen high-droh-KLOR-ighd)
Strattera◆

Pharmacologic class: selective norepinephrine reuptake inhibitor
Therapeutic class: attention deficit hyperactivity disorder (ADHD) drug
Pregnancy risk category: C

Indications and dosages

▶ **Adjunct therapy for ADHD.** *Adults and children weighing more than 70 kg (154 lb):* Initially, 40 mg P.O. daily; increase after a minimum of 3 days to a target total daily dose of 80 mg P.O. as a single dose in the morning or two evenly divided doses in the morning and late afternoon or early evening. After 2 to 4 weeks, increase total dosage to a maximum of 100 mg, if needed.
Children weighing 70 kg or less: Initially, 0.5 mg/kg P.O. daily; increase after a minimum of 3 days to a target total daily dose of 1.2 mg/kg P.O. as a single dose in the morning or two evenly divided doses in the morning and late afternoon or early evening. Don't exceed 1.4 mg/kg or 100 mg daily, whichever is less.
ⓈAdjust-a-dose: For patients with moderate hepatic impairment, reduce to 50% of the normal dose; in those with severe hepatic impairment, reduce to 25% of the normal dose.

Contraindications and cautions

• Contraindicated in patients hypersensitive to the drug or any of its components, in those who have used an MAO inhibitor within the past

14 days, those who have jaundice or laboratory evidence of liver injury, and in those with narrow-angle glaucoma.
• Use cautiously in patients with hypertension, tachycardia, moderate to severe hepatic insufficiency, or CV or cerebrovascular disease.
Lifespan: In pregnant and breast-feeding women, use cautiously. In children younger than age 6, safety and effectiveness of drug haven't been established. In the elderly, safety and effectiveness haven't been established.

Adverse reactions

CNS: dizziness, *headache,* somnolence, crying, irritability, mood swings, pyrexia, fatigue, *insomnia,* sedation, depression, tremor, early morning awakening, paresthesia, abnormal dreams, sleep disorder, ***suicidal thoughts.***
CV: orthostatic hypotension, tachycardia, hypertension, palpitations.
EENT: ear infection, rhinorrhea, sore throat, nasal congestion, nasopharyngitis, sinus congestion, mydriasis, sinusitis.
GI: abdominal pain, constipation, dyspepsia, nausea, vomiting, decreased appetite, gastroenteritis, dry mouth, flatulence.
GU: urinary retention, urinary hesitation, ejaculatory problems, difficulty in micturition, dysmenorrhea, erectile disturbance, impotence, delayed menses, menstrual disorder, prostatitis.
Metabolic: weight loss.
Musculoskeletal: arthralgia, myalgia.
Respiratory: *cough,* upper respiratory tract infection.
Skin: dermatitis, pruritus, increased sweating.
Other: decreased libido, influenza, rigors, hot flashes.

Interactions

Drug-drug. *Albuterol:* May increase CV effects. Use together cautiously.
MAO inhibitors: May cause hyperthermia, rigidity, myoclonus, autonomic instability with possible rapid fluctuations of vital signs, and mental status changes. Don't combine with an MAO inhibitor, and separate atomoxetine and MAO inhibitor doses by 14 days.
Pressor agents: May increase blood pressure. Use together cautiously.
Strong CYP 2D6 inhibitors (fluoxetine, paroxetine, quinidine): May increase atomoxetine level. In children weighing less than 70 kg (154 lb), adjust dosage to 0.5 mg/kg daily and increase only to 1.2 mg/kg daily if symptoms don't improve after 4 weeks. In children and adults weighing more than 70 kg, start at 40 mg daily and increase only to 80 mg daily if symptoms don't improve after 4 weeks.

Effects on lab test results

• May increase liver enzyme levels.

Pharmacokinetics

Absorption: Rapid.
Distribution: Primarily into total body water. It's 98% bound to plasma proteins, primarily albumin.
Metabolism: Primarily through CYP 2D6. Absolute bioavailability is about 63% in patients with extensive metabolism and 94% in those with poor metabolism.
Excretion: More than 80% of the dose in urine, and less than 17% of the dose via feces. *Half-life:* 21½ hours.

Route	Onset	Peak	Duration
P.O.	Rapid	1–2 hr	Unknown

Action

Chemical effect: Unknown. May relate to selective inhibition of the presynaptic norepinephrine transporter.
Therapeutic effect: Decreases symptoms of ADHD.

Available forms

Capsules: 10 mg, 18 mg, 25 mg, 40 mg, 60 mg, 80 mg, 100 mg

NURSING PROCESS

Assessment

• Assess patient's condition before therapy and regularly thereafter.
• Watch for hypersensitivity reaction, or signs of liver injury (nausea, anorexia, pruritus, jaundice, right upper quadrant pain, flulike symptoms).
• Assess patient's and family's knowledge related to disease and drug therapy.

Nursing diagnoses

• Alteration in patient's comprehension and concentration related to underlying disease

• Risk for imbalanced nutrition: less than the body requires, related to side effect of medication
• Deficient knowledge related to drug therapy

▶ Planning and implementation

• Use drug as part of a total treatment program for ADHD, with psychological, educational, and social intervention.
• Periodically reevaluate patients taking drug for extended periods to determine drug's usefulness.
⊛ **ALERT:** Monitor children and adolescents closely for agitation, irritability, and suicidal thinking or behaviors.
• Monitor growth during treatment. If growth or weight gain is unsatisfactory, consider stopping therapy.
• Monitor blood pressure and pulse at baseline, after each dose increase, and periodically during treatment.
• Monitor patient for urinary hesitancy or retention, and sexual dysfunction.
⊛ **ALERT:** If patient becomes jaundiced or has abnormal liver function test results, stop drug.
• Stop drug without tapering.
• In case of overdose, monitor patient closely and provide supportive care. Perform gastric lavage and give activated charcoal to prevent absorption.

Patient teaching

• Advise parents to call prescriber immediately if their child develops unusual behaviors or suicidal thoughts.
• Tell pregnant women, women planning to become pregnant, and breast-feeding women to consult prescriber before taking drug.
• Tell patient to use caution when operating a vehicle or machinery until drug effects are known.
• Tell patient to report itching, yellow skin, yellow sclera, nausea or decreased appetite, abdominal pain, or flulike symptoms to prescriber immediately.

☑ Evaluation

• Patient has reduced signs and symptoms of underlying disease.
• Patient maintains adequate nutritional status.
• Patient and family state understanding of drug therapy.

atorvastatin calcium
(uh-TOR-vah-stah-tin KAL-see-um)
Lipitor◊

Pharmacologic class: HMG-CoA reductase inhibitor
Therapeutic class: antilipemic
Pregnancy risk category: X

Indications and dosages

▶ **Adjunct to diet to reduce elevated LDL, total cholesterol, apo B, and triglyceride levels and to increase HDL level in patients with primary hypercholesterolemia (heterozygous familial and nonfamilial) and mixed dyslipidemia (Fredrickson Types IIa and IIb).**
Adults: Initially, 10 or 20 mg P.O. once daily. Start dosage at 40 mg once daily for patients who require a reduction in LDL cholesterol level of more than 45%. Increase dose, p.r.n., to maximum of 80 mg daily as single dose. Base dosage on lipid levels drawn within 2 to 4 weeks after starting therapy.
▶ **Alone or as an adjunct to lipid-lowering treatments such as LDL apheresis to reduce total cholesterol and LDL levels in patients with homozygous familial hypercholesterolemia.** *Adults:* 10 to 80 mg P.O. daily.
▶ **Heterozygous familial hypercholesterolemia.** *Children ages 10 to 17:* 10 mg P.O. once daily. Adjust dosage after 4 weeks to 20 mg daily.
▶ **To reduce the risk of MI, stroke, angina, and revascularization procedures in patients with no evidence of CAD but with multiple risk factors.** *Adults:* 10 mg P.O. daily.

Contraindications and cautions

• Contraindicated in patients hypersensitive to drug and in those with active liver disease or conditions linked with unexplained persistent increases in transaminase levels. Also contraindicated in patients with serious, acute conditions that suggest myopathy and in those at risk for renal failure caused by rhabdomyolysis from trauma; major surgery; severe metabolic, endocrine, and electrolyte disorders; severe acute infection; hypotension; or uncontrolled seizures.
• Adolescent girls must be at least 1 year postmenarche.

☙ **Lifespan:** In pregnant or breast-feeding women and in women who may become pregnant, drug is contraindicated.

Adverse reactions

CNS: *headache,* asthenia, fever, malaise.
CV: chest pain.
EENT: sinusitis, pharyngitis.
GI: abdominal pain, constipation, diarrhea, dyspepsia, flatulence.
Musculoskeletal: back pain, arthralgia, *rhabdomyolysis,* myalgia.
Skin: rash, *erythema multiforme, Stevens-Johnson syndrome, toxic epidermal necrolysis.*
Other: infection, accidental injury, flulike syndrome, hypersensitivity reaction, *anaphylaxis, angioedema.*

Interactions

Drug-drug. *Antacids:* May decrease bioavailability. Give separately.
Azole antifungals, cyclosporine, erythromycin, fibric acid derivatives, niacin: May increase risk of myopathy. Avoid using together.
Colestipol and other bile-acid sequestrants: May decrease atorvastatin level; however, these drugs may be used together for therapeutic effect. Monitor patient.
Digoxin: May increase digoxin level. Monitor digoxin level.
Erythromycin: May increase drug level. Monitor patient.
Fluconazole, itraconazole, ketoconazole: May increase level and adverse effects of atorvastatin. Avoid this combination. If they must be given together, reduce dose of atorvastatin.
Hormonal contraceptives: May increase hormone levels. Consider when selecting a hormonal contraceptive.
Warfarin: May increase anticoagulant effect. Monitor INR and patient for bleeding.

Effects on lab test results

● May increase ALT and AST levels.

Pharmacokinetics

Absorption: Rapid.
Distribution: 98% bound to plasma proteins.
Metabolism: By liver.
Excretion: In bile. *Half life:* 14 hours

Route	Onset	Peak	Duration
P.O.	Unknown	1–2 hr	20–30 hr

Action

Chemical effect: Selectively inhibits HMG-CoA reductase, which converts HMG-CoA to mevalonate, a precursor of sterols.
Therapeutic effect: Lowers cholesterol and lipoprotein levels.

Available forms

Tablets: 10 mg, 20 mg, 40 mg, 80 mg

NURSING PROCESS

⚗ Assessment

● Monitor patient's lipid and liver function levels at baseline and periodically thereafter.
● Monitor patient for signs of rhabdomyolysis especially if taking more than one class of lipid-lowering drugs.
● Assess patient's and family's knowledge of drug therapy.

⊕ Nursing diagnoses

● Risk for injury related to elevated cholesterol levels
● Deficient knowledge related to drug therapy

▷ Planning and implementation

● Use drug only after diet and other nonpharmacologic treatments prove ineffective. Patient should follow a standard low-cholesterol diet before and during therapy.
● Drug can be given as a single dose at any time of the day, with or without food.
● After starting drug and upon adjustment, monitor lipid levels within 4 weeks and adjust dosage accordingly.
● Before starting treatment, perform a baseline lipid profile to exclude secondary causes of hypercholesterolemia. Liver function test results and lipid levels should be obtained before therapy, after 6 and 12 weeks, or following a dosage increase and periodically thereafter.
● Check CK level if patient complains of muscle pain, tenderness, or weakness.
⊛ **ALERT:** Don't confuse Lipitor with Levatol.
Patient teaching
● Teach patient about proper dietary management, weight control, and exercise, and explain their role in controlling elevated lipid levels.
● Warn patient to avoid alcohol.
● Tell patient to inform prescriber of adverse reactions, such as muscle pain, tenderness, or

weakness, especially if accompanied by fever or malaise.
• Urge woman to notify prescriber immediately if pregnancy is suspected.

☑ **Evaluation**
• Patient's cholesterol level is within normal limits.
• Patient and family state understanding of drug therapy.

atovaquone
(uh-TOH-vuh-kwohn)
Mepron

Pharmacologic class: ubiquinone analogue
Therapeutic class: antiprotozoal
Pregnancy risk category: C

Indications and dosages

▶ **Prevention of *Pneumocystis jiroveci* (carinii) pneumonia in patients who are intolerant to co-trimoxazole, including HIV-infected individuals.** *Adults and children age 13 and older:* 1,500 mg (10 ml) P.O. daily with food.
Infants ages 1 to 3 months and children older than 24 months‡: 30 mg/kg P.O. once daily.
Infants ages 4 to 24 months‡: 45 mg/kg P.O. daily.
▶ **Mild to moderate *P. jiroveci* (carinii) pneumonia in patients who can't tolerate co-trimoxazole.** *Adults and children age 13 and older:* 750 mg P.O. b.i.d. for 21 days.
▶ **Prevention of toxoplasmosis in HIV-infected patients‡.** *Adults and children age 13 and older:* 1,500 mg P.O. daily.

Contraindications and cautions

• Contraindicated in patients hypersensitive to drug.
• Use cautiously with other highly protein-bound drugs because drug is more than 99.9% protein-bound. Also use cautiously in those with liver disease.
※ **Lifespan:** In pregnant and breast-feeding women, use cautiously. In children, safety of drug hasn't been established. In elderly patients, use cautiously.

Adverse reactions

CNS: fever, asthenia, dizziness, depression, *headache,* dreams, insomnia.
EENT: visual difficulties.
GI: *abdominal pain,* diarrhea, anorexia, *nausea, vomiting,* dyspepsia, gastritis, oral ulcers.
Musculoskeletal: myalgia.
Respiratory: cough, rhinitis, sinusitis.
Skin: pruritus, rash, sweating.
Other: flulike syndrome.

Interactions

Drug-drug. *Highly protein-bound drugs:* May compete for receptor sites affecting drug levels. Use together cautiously.
Rifabutin, rifampin: May decrease atovaquone's steady-state levels. Avoid using together.

Effects on lab test results

• May increase alkaline phosphatase, ALT, and AST levels. May decrease hemoglobin level and hematocrit.
• May decrease WBC count.

Pharmacokinetics

Absorption: Limited. Bioavailability is increased twofold when given with meals. Fat enhances absorption significantly.
Distribution: 99.9% bound to plasma proteins.
Metabolism: Not metabolized.
Excretion: Undergoes enterohepatic cycling and is primarily excreted in feces. *Half-life:* 2 to 3 days.

Route	Onset	Peak	Duration
P.O.	Unknown	1–8 hr	Unknown

Action

Chemical effect: Unknown; may interfere with electron transport in protozoal mitochondria, inhibiting enzymes needed for synthesis of nucleic acids and adenosine triphosphate.
Therapeutic effect: Kills *Pneumocystis jiroveci (carinii)* protozoa.

Available forms

Suspension: 750 mg/5 ml
Tablet: 250 mg

NURSING PROCESS

🖉 Assessment
- Obtain history of patient's protozoal respiratory infection and reassess regularly.
- Be alert for adverse reactions.
- Monitor patient's hydration if adverse GI reactions occur.
- Assess patient's and family's knowledge of drug therapy.

⊕ Nursing diagnoses
- Infection related to presence of susceptible protozoal organisms
- Risk for deficient fluid volume related to drug-induced adverse GI reactions
- Deficient knowledge related to drug therapy

▶ Planning and implementation
- Give drug with food to improve bioavailability.

Patient teaching
- Instruct patient to take drug with meals because food significantly enhances absorption.
- Warn patient not to perform hazardous activities if dizziness occurs.
- Emphasize importance of taking drug as prescribed, even if patient is feeling better.
- Tell patient to notify prescriber if serious adverse reactions occur.

☑ Evaluation
- Patient's infection is eradicated.
- Patient remains adequately hydrated throughout therapy.
- Patient and family state understanding of drug therapy.

atovaquone and proguanil hydrochloride
(uh-TOH-vuh-kwohn and pro-GWAN-ill high-droh-KLOR-ighd)
Malarone, Malarone Pediatric

Pharmacologic class: pyrimidine biosynthesis inhibitors
Therapeutic class: antimalarial
Pregnancy risk category: C

Indications and dosages

▶ **Prevention of *Plasmodium falciparum* malaria in areas where chloroquine resistance has been reported.** *Adults and children weighing more than 40 kg (88 lb):* 1 adult-strength tablet (250 mg atovaquone and 100 mg proguanil) P.O. once daily with food or milk. Begin 1 or 2 days before entering a malaria-endemic area. Continue prophylactic treatment during stay and for 7 days after return.
Children weighing 31 to 40 kg (68 to 88 lb): 3 pediatric-strength tablets P.O. once daily with food or milk, beginning 1 or 2 days before entering endemic area. Total daily dose is 187.5 mg atovaquone and 75 mg proguanil. Treatment should continue during stay and for 7 days after return.
Children weighing 21 to 30 kg (46 to 66 lb): 2 pediatric-strength tablets P.O. once daily with food or milk, beginning 1 or 2 days before entering endemic area. Total daily dose is 125 mg atovaquone and 50 mg proguanil. Treatment should continue during stay and for 7 days after return.
Children weighing 11 to 20 kg (24 to 44 lb): 1 pediatric-strength tablet P.O. daily with food or milk, beginning 1 or 2 days before entering endemic area. Continue treatment during stay and for 7 days after return.
▶ **Acute, uncomplicated *P. falciparum* malaria.** *Adults and children weighing more than 40 kg:* 4 adult-strength tablets with food or milk, P.O. once daily for 3 consecutive days. Total daily dose is 1 g atovaquone and 400 mg proguanil.
Children weighing 31 to 40 kg: 3 adult-strength tablets P.O. once daily with food or milk, for 3 consecutive days. Total daily dose is 750 mg atovaquone and 300 mg proguanil.
Children weighing 21 to 30 kg: 2 adult-strength tablets P.O. once daily with food or milk, for 3 consecutive days. Total daily dose is 500 mg atovaquone and 200 mg proguanil.
Children weighing 11 to 20 kg: 1 adult-strength tablet P.O. once daily with food or milk, for 3 consecutive days.
Children weighing 9 to 10 kg: 3 pediatric-strength tablets P.O. daily with food or milk, for 3 consecutive days.
Children weighing 5 to 8 kg: 2 pediatric-strength tablets P.O. daily, with food or milk, for 3 consecutive days.

Contraindications and cautions

• Contraindicated in patients hypersensitive to atovaquone, proguanil, or any component of the formulation. Not intended for patients with severe malaria or for those with a fresh breakout of *P. falciparum* infection after treatment with Malarone or failure of preventative treatment with Malarone.

• Use cautiously in patients with severe renal impairment because proguanil is renally eliminated. Use cautiously in vomiting patients.

⚜ **Lifespan:** In pregnant women, drug shouldn't be used as prophylaxis but may be used for treatment of chloroquine-resistant disease when other options are unavailable or not tolerated and if the potential benefits outweigh the risks. In breast-feeding women, use cautiously because drug appears in breast milk in small amounts. In children weighing less than 5 kg, safety and effectiveness of drug haven't been established. In elderly patients, use cautiously because they are more likely to have decreased renal function.

Adverse reactions

CNS: asthenia, dizziness, dreams, hallucinations, *headache.*
EENT: visual difficulties.
GI: *abdominal pain,* diarrhea, anorexia, dyspepsia, oral ulcers, gastritis, *nausea, vomiting.*
Respiratory: cough.
Skin: pruritus.
Other: *anaphylaxis,* flulike syndrome.

Interactions

Drug-drug. *Drugs containing proguanil:* Proguanil is eliminated renally and a high level may cause renal impairment. Avoid using together.
Metoclopramide: May decrease atovaquone bioavailability. Consider alternative antiemetics.
Rifabutin: May reduce atovaquone level by about 34%. Avoid using together.
Rifampin: May reduce atovaquone level by about 50%. Avoid using together.
Tetracycline: May reduce atovaquone level by about 40%. Monitor patient closely for signs and symptoms of parasitemia.

Effects on lab test results

• May increase alkaline phosphatase, ALT, AST, and creatinine levels. May decrease hemoglobin level and hematocrit.

• May decrease WBC count.

Pharmacokinetics

Absorption: Bioavailability of atovaquone is 23% when tablets are taken with food. Atovaquone bioavailability varies considerably. Dietary fat increases the rate and extent of atovaquone absorption compared with fasting. Proguanil is well absorbed without regard to food. Absorption of both drugs is decreased in patients with diarrhea and vomiting.
Distribution: Atovaquone is more than 99% protein-bound; proguanil, 75%.
Metabolism: Atovaquone undergoes virtually no metabolism. Proguanil is metabolized in the liver to cycloguanil (primarily by CYP 2C19) and 4-chlorophenylbiguanide.
Excretion: More than 94% of atovaquone is eliminated unchanged in the feces over 21 days. The kidneys eliminate 40% to 60% of proguanil and its metabolites. *Half-life* in children is decreased. *Atovaquone half-life:* 2 to 3 days in adults. *Proguanil half-life:* 12 to 21 hours in adults and children.

Route	Onset	Peak	Duration
P.O.	Unknown	Unknown	Unknown

Action

Chemical effect: May interfere with nucleic acid replication in the malarial parasite by inhibiting biosynthesis of pyrimidine compounds in two different pathways. Atovaquone selectively inhibits parasitic mitochondrial electron transport. Proguanil disrupts deoxythymidylate synthesis through inhibition of dihydrofolate reductase.
Therapeutic effect: Prevents and treats symptoms of malaria.

Available forms

Tablets: 250 mg atovaquone and 100 mg proguanil (adult-strength); 62.5 mg atovaquone and 25 mg proguanil (pediatric-strength)

NURSING PROCESS

⚏ **Assessment**
• Assess patient for signs and symptoms of malaria.
• Assess patient and travel plans for need for antimalarial prophylaxis.
• Be alert for adverse reactions.

• Monitor patient's liver and renal function during drug therapy.

🔷 **Nursing diagnoses**
• Risk of infection related to exposure to *P. falciparum* in malaria-endemic areas
• Deficient knowledge related to drug therapy

▧ **Planning and implementation**
• Atovaquone absorption may be decreased by persistent diarrhea or vomiting. Consider another antimalarial for a patient with persistent diarrhea or vomiting and give antiemetics.
• If treatment or prophylaxis fails, give another antimalarial.
• Give drug at the same time each day with food or milk.
• Store tablets at controlled room temperature 59° to 86° F (15° to 30° C).
Patient teaching
• Tell patient to take dose at the same time each day with food or milk.
• Tell patient that if he vomits within 1 hour after taking a dose, he should repeat it.
• Advise patient to contact prescriber if he can't complete the course of therapy as prescribed.
• Instruct patient that in addition to drug therapy, malaria prophylaxis should include the use of protective clothing, bed nets, and insect repellents.

✅ **Evaluation**
• Patient doesn't have malaria.
• Patient and family state understanding of antimalarial drug therapy.

atracurium besylate
(at-truh-KYOO-ree-um BES-eh-layt)
Tracrium

Pharmacologic class: nondepolarizing neuromuscular blocker
Therapeutic class: skeletal muscle relaxant
Pregnancy risk category: C

Indications and dosages

▶ **Adjunct to general anesthesia, to facilitate endotracheal intubation and cause skeletal muscle relaxation during surgery or mechanical ventilation.** *Adults and children older than age 2:* 0.4 to 0.5 mg/kg by I.V. bolus. Mainte-

nance dosage of 0.08 to 0.1 mg/kg within 20 to 45 minutes of initial dose should be given during prolonged surgical procedures. Maintenance dosages may be given q 15 to 25 minutes in patients receiving balanced anesthesia. For prolonged surgical procedures, a constant infusion of 5 to 9 mcg/kg/minute may be used after initial bolus.
Children ages 1 month to 2 years: Initial dose, 0.3 to 0.4 mg/kg. Frequent maintenance doses may be needed.

▽ **I.V. administration**
• In lactated Ringer's solution for injection, atracurium is stable for 8 hours at a concentration of 0.5 mg/ml. Because of increased drug degradation in this solution, it isn't recommended.
• Drug usually is given by rapid I.V. bolus injection but may be given by intermittent or continuous infusion. At 0.2 to 0.5 mg/ml, drug is compatible for 24 hours in D_5W, normal saline solution injection, or dextrose 5% in normal saline solution injection.
⊗ **Incompatibilities**
Acidic and alkaline solutions, lactated Ringer's solution.

Contraindications and cautions

• Contraindicated in patients hypersensitive to drug.
• Use cautiously in patients with CV disease; severe electrolyte disorders; bronchogenic carcinoma; hepatic, renal, or pulmonary impairment; neuromuscular diseases; or myasthenia gravis; and in debilitated patients.
⚘ **Lifespan:** In pregnant women, breastfeeding women, and elderly patients, use cautiously.

Adverse reactions

CV: *flushing,* increased heart rate, **bradycardia,** hypotension.
Respiratory: *prolonged dose-related apnea,* wheezing, increased bronchial secretions.
Skin: erythema, pruritus, urticaria.
Other: *anaphylaxis.*

Interactions

Drug-drug. *Amikacin, gentamicin, neomycin, streptomycin, tobramycin:* May increase the effects of nondepolarizing muscle relaxant, including prolonged respiratory depression. Use together only when necessary, and reduce dose of nondepolarizing muscle relaxant.

Carbamazepine, phenytoin: May decrease the effects of atracurium, causing it to be less effective. Increase dose of atracurium.

Kanamycin; polymyxin antibiotics (colistin, polymyxin B sulfate); clindamycin; general anesthetics (such as enflurane, halothane, isoflurane); quinidine: May potentiate neuromuscular blockade, leading to increased skeletal muscle relaxation and prolongation of effect. Use cautiously during surgical and postoperative periods.

Lithium, magnesium salts, opioid analgesics: May potentiate neuromuscular blockade, which may lead to increased skeletal muscle relaxation and, possibly, respiratory paralysis. Reduce dose of atracurium.

Effects on lab test results

None reported.

Pharmacokinetics

Absorption: Given I.V.
Distribution: Into extracellular space. About 82% protein-bound.
Metabolism: Rapidly by Hofmann elimination and by nonspecific enzymatic ester hydrolysis. The liver doesn't appear to play a major role.
Excretion: Drug and its metabolites are excreted in urine and feces. *Half-life:* 20 minutes.

Route	Onset	Peak	Duration
I.V.	2 min	3–5 min	35–70 min

Action

Chemical effect: Prevents acetylcholine from binding to receptors on muscle end plate, thus blocking depolarization and resulting in skeletal muscle paralysis.
Therapeutic effect: Relaxes skeletal muscles.

Available forms

Injection: 10 mg/ml

NURSING PROCESS

🏥 Assessment
• Obtain history of patient's neuromuscular status before therapy and reassess regularly.
• Be alert for adverse reactions and interactions.
• Monitor respirations closely until patient fully recovers from neuromuscular blockade, as evi-

denced by tests of muscle strength (hand grip, head lift, and ability to cough).
• A nerve stimulator and train-of-four monitoring are recommended to confirm antagonism of neuromuscular blockade and recovery of muscle strength. Before attempting pharmacologic reversal with neostigmine, some evidence of spontaneous recovery should be seen.
• Assess patient's and family's knowledge of drug therapy.

💬 Nursing diagnoses
• Risk for injury related to underlying condition
• Impaired spontaneous ventilation related to drug-induced respiratory paralysis
• Deficient knowledge related to drug therapy

⟫ Planning and implementation
• Give sedatives or general anesthetics before neuromuscular blockers. Neuromuscular blockers don't decrease consciousness or alter pain threshold.
⊛ **ALERT:** Use this drug only under direct medical supervision by personnel skilled in use of neuromuscular blockers and techniques for maintaining a patent airway. Don't use unless facilities and equipment for mechanical ventilation, oxygen therapy, and intubation as well as an antagonist are immediately available.
• Don't give by I.M. injection.
• Prior use of succinylcholine doesn't prolong duration of action but quickens onset and may deepen neuromuscular blockade.
• Explain all events to patient because he can still hear.
• Give analgesics for pain. Patient may have pain but be unable to express it.
• Keep airway clear. Have emergency equipment and drugs available.
• After spontaneous recovery starts, reverse atracurium-induced neuromuscular blockade with an anticholinesterase (such as neostigmine or edrophonium). These drugs usually are given with an anticholinergic (such as atropine).
Patient teaching
• Instruct patient and family about drug therapy.
• Reassure patient and family that patient will be monitored at all times and that respiratory life support will be used during paralysis.
• Reassure patient that pain medication will be given as needed.

☑ **Evaluation**
• Patient's underlying condition is resolved without causing injury.
• Patient sustains spontaneous ventilation after effects of atracurium besylate wear off.
• Patient and family state understanding of drug therapy.

atropine sulfate
(AT-truh-peen SUL-fayt)
AtroPen Auto-Injector, Sal-Tropine

Pharmacologic class: anticholinergic, belladonna alkaloid
Therapeutic class: antiarrhythmic, vagolytic
Pregnancy risk category: C

Indications and dosages

▶ **Symptomatic bradycardia, bradyarrhythmia (junctional or escape rhythm).** *Adults:* Usually 0.5 to 1 mg I.V. push; repeat q 3 to 5 minutes to maximum of 2 mg, p.r.n. Lower doses (less than 0.5 mg) can cause bradycardia. *Children:* 0.02 mg/kg I.V. to a maximum of 1 mg; or 0.3 mg/m²; may repeat q 5 minutes.
▶ **Anticholinesterase insecticide poisoning.** *Adults and children:* 1 to 2 mg I.M. or I.V. repeated q 20 to 30 minutes until muscarinic symptoms disappear or signs of atropine toxicity appear. Patient with severe poisoning may require up to 6 mg q hour.
▶ **Preoperatively for decreasing secretions and blocking cardiac vagal reflexes.** *Adults and children weighing 20 kg (44 lb) or more:* 0.4 mg I.M. or subcutaneously 30 to 60 minutes before anesthesia.
Children weighing less than 20 kg: 0.1 mg I.M. for 3 kg, 0.2 mg I.M. for 4 to 9 kg, 0.3 mg I.M. for 10 to 20 kg, given 30 to 60 minutes before anesthesia.
▶ **Adjunct in peptic ulcer disease; functional GI disorders such as irritable bowel syndrome.** *Adults:* 0.4 to 0.6 mg P.O. q 4 to 6 hours.
Children: 0.01 mg/kg or 0.3 mg/m² (not to exceed 0.4 mg) q 4 to 6 hours.

▼I.V. administration

• Give by direct injection into a large vein or I.V. tubing over 1 to 2 minutes.

⊗ **Incompatibilities**
Alkalies, bromides, iodides, isoproterenol, methohexital, norepinephrine, pentobarbital sodium, sodium bicarbonate.

Contraindications and cautions

• Contraindicated in patients hypersensitive to drug and those with acute angle-closure glaucoma, obstructive uropathy, obstructive disease of GI tract, paralytic ileus, toxic megacolon, intestinal atony, unstable CV status in acute hemorrhage, asthma, or myasthenia gravis.
• Use cautiously in patients with Down syndrome.
⚜ **Lifespan:** In pregnant women, use cautiously. Use in breast-feeding women isn't recommended. In children and elderly patients, use cautiously because they may have increased adverse effects.

Adverse reactions

CNS: *headache, restlessness,* ataxia, disorientation, hallucinations, delirium, *coma, insomnia, dizziness,* excitement, agitation, confusion.
CV: *tachycardia, palpitations, angina, arrhythmias,* flushing.
EENT: photophobia, *blurred vision, mydriasis.*
GI: *dry mouth,* thirst, *constipation,* nausea, vomiting.
GU: urine retention.
Hematologic: leukocytosis.
Other: *anaphylaxis.*

Interactions

Drug-drug. *Antacids:* May decrease absorption of anticholinergics. Give at least 1 hour apart.
Anticholinergics, drugs with anticholinergic effects (such as amantadine, antiarrhythmics, antiparkinsonians, glutethimide, meperidine, phenothiazines, tricyclic antidepressants): May cause additive anticholinergic effects. Use together cautiously.
Ketoconazole, levodopa: May decrease absorption. Avoid using together.
Methotrimeprazine: May produce extrapyramidal symptoms. Monitor patient carefully.
Potassium chloride wax matrix tablets: May increase risk of mucosal lesions. Use together cautiously.

Effects on lab test results

• May increase WBC count.

Reactions may be *common,* uncommon, *life-threatening*, or COMMON AND LIFE-THREATENING.

Pharmacokinetics

Absorption: Well absorbed after P.O. and I.M. use; unknown for subcutaneous use.
Distribution: Throughout the body, including CNS. Only 18% binds with plasma protein.
Metabolism: In liver to several metabolites.
Excretion: Mainly through kidneys; small amount in feces and expired air. *Half-life:* Initial, 2 hours; second phase, 12½ hr.

Route	Onset	Peak	Duration
P.O.	½ hr	2 hr	4 hr
I.V.	Immediate	2–4 min	4 hr
I.M.	30 min	1–1½ hr	4 hr
SubQ	Unknown	Unknown	4 hr

Action

Chemical effect: Inhibits acetylcholine at parasympathetic neuroeffector junction, blocking vagal effects on SA node. This enhances conduction through AV node and speeds heart rate.
Therapeutic effect: Increases heart rate, decreases secretions, and slows GI motility. Antidote for anticholinesterase insecticide poisoning.

Available forms

Injection: 0.05 mg/ml, 0.1 mg/ml, 0.3 mg/ml, 0.4 mg/ml, 0.5 mg/ml, 0.6 mg/ml, 0.8 mg/ml, 1 mg/ml, 1.2 mg/ml
Tablets: 0.4 mg, 0.6 mg

NURSING PROCESS

Assessment
● Obtain history of patient's underlying condition and reassess regularly.
● Be alert for adverse reactions and drug interactions.
● Monitor patients, especially those receiving doses of 0.4 to 0.6 mg, for paradoxical initial bradycardia, which is caused by a drug effect in CNS and usually disappears within 2 minutes.
● **ALERT:** Watch for tachycardia in cardiac patients because it may cause ventricular fibrillation.
● Assess patient's and family's knowledge of drug therapy.

Nursing diagnoses
● Ineffective health maintenance related to underlying condition

● Risk for injury related to drug-induced adverse reactions
● Deficient knowledge related to drug therapy

Planning and implementation
● Give with or without food.
● If ECG disturbances occur, withhold drug, obtain a rhythm strip, and notify prescriber immediately.
● Have emergency equipment and drugs on hand to treat new arrhythmias. Other anticholinergics may increase vagal blockage.
● Use physostigmine salicylate as antidote for atropine overdose.
Patient teaching
● Teach patient about atropine sulfate therapy.
● Instruct patient to ask for assistance with activities if adverse CNS reactions occur.
● Teach patient how to handle distressing anticholinergic effects.

Evaluation
● Patient's underlying condition improves.
● Patient has no injury as a result of therapy.
● Patient and family state understanding of drug therapy.

azacitidine
(az-uh-SIT-uh-deen)
Vidaza

Pharmacologic class: pyrimidine nucleoside analog
Therapeutic class: antineoplastic
Pregnancy risk category: D

Indications and dosages

▶ **Myelodysplastic syndrome, including refractory anemia, refractory anemia with ringed sideroblasts (if patient has neutropenia or thrombocytopenia or needs transfusions), refractory anemia with excess blasts, refractory anemia with excess blasts in transformation, or chronic myelomonocytic leukemia.** *Adults:* Initially, 75 mg/m² subcutaneously daily for 7 days, repeating cycle q 4 weeks. May increase to 100 mg/m² if no response after two treatment cycles and nausea and vomiting are the only toxic reactions. At least four treatment cycles are recommended.

⊠ Adjust-a-dose: If bicarbonate level is less than 20 mEq/L, reduce next dose by 50%. If BUN or creatinine levels rise during treatment, delay the next cycle until they are normal, and then give 50% of previous dose.

Make further adjustments during therapy based on hematologic and renal toxicities.

Contraindications and cautions

• Contraindicated in patients hypersensitive to azacitidine or mannitol and in patients with advanced malignant hepatic tumors.
• Use cautiously in patients with hepatic and renal disease.
⚐ **Lifespan:** In pregnant patients, avoid use. In breast-feeding women, avoid use because drug may cause cancer in fetus. In children, safety and effectiveness haven't been established.

Adverse reactions

CNS: *anxiety, depression, dizziness, fatigue, headache,* hypoesthesia, *insomnia,* lethargy, *malaise,* pain, syncope, *weakness.*
CV: *cardiac murmur, chest pain, edema,* hypotension, peripheral swelling, tachycardia.
EENT: *epistaxis,* nasal congestion, *nasopharyngitis, pharyngitis,* postnasal drip, *rhinorrhea,* sinusitis.
GI: abdominal distension, *abdominal pain and tenderness,* anorexia, constipation, *decreased appetite, diarrhea,* dyspepsia, dysphagia, gingival bleeding, hemorrhoids, loose stools, mouth hemorrhage, *nausea,* oral mucosal petechiae, stomatitis, tongue ulceration, *vomiting.*
GU: dysuria, UTI.
Hematologic: *anemia,* FEBRILE NEUTROPENIA, hematoma, LEUKOPENIA, NEUTROPENIA, postprocedural hemorrhage, THROMBOCYTOPENIA.
Metabolic: *weight loss.*
Musculoskeletal: *arthralgia, back pain, limb pain,* muscle cramps, *myalgia.*
Respiratory: *atelectasis,* cough, *crackles, dyspnea,* pleural effusion, *rales, rhonchi, pneumonia, upper respiratory tract infection,* wheezing.
Skin: *bruising,* dry skin, granuloma, *pain,* pigmentation, pruritus, or swelling at injection site; cellulitis; *contusion; ecchymosis; erythema; increased sweating; injection site reaction;* night sweats; *pallor; petechiae; pitting edema; rash; skin lesion;* skin nodules; urticaria.
Other: *rigors, pyrexia,* lymphadenopathy, herpes simplex.

Interactions

None reported.

Effects on lab test results

• May increase creatinine and BUN levels. May decrease bicarbonate, potassium, and hemoglobin levels and hematocrit.
• May decrease WBC, neutrophil, and platelet counts.

Pharmacokinetics

Absorption: Rapid.
Distribution: Mean volume isn't known.
Metabolism: By the liver.
Excretion: Mainly in urine, with less than 1% excreted in feces. *Half-life:* About 40 minutes.

Route	Onset	Peak	Duration
SubQ	Unknown	30 min	Unknown

Action

Chemical effect: Causes hypomethylation of DNA and is toxic to abnormal hematopoietic cells in bone marrow. Hypomethylation may restore normal function to genes needed for proliferation and differentiation. Drug has little effect on nonproliferating cells.
Therapeutic effect: Restores normal bone marrow function.

Available forms

Powder for injection: 100-mg vials

NURSING PROCESS

⁂ Assessment
• Assess patient's condition before therapy and regularly thereafter.
• Check liver function test results and creatinine levels before therapy starts.
• Obtain CBC before each cycle or more often.
• If patient has renal impairment, monitor him closely.
• Assess patient's and family's knowledge of drug therapy.

⊞ Nursing diagnoses
• Ineffective health maintenance related to presence of underlying disease
• Ineffective protection related to both underlying disease and drug-induced adverse hematologic reactions
• Deficient knowledge related to drug therapy

Reactions may be *common,* uncommon, *life-threatening,* or COMMON AND LIFE-THREATENING.

> **Planning and implementation**
• Give antiemetic before therapy.
• Dilute using aseptic and hazardous substances techniques. Reconstitute with 4 ml sterile water for injection. Invert vial two to three times and gently rotate until a uniform suspension forms. The resulting cloudy suspension will be 25 mg/ml. Draw up suspension into syringes for injection (no more than 4 ml per syringe).
• Just before giving drug, resuspend drug by inverting the syringe two to three times and gently rolling between palms for 30 seconds. Divide doses greater than 4 ml into two syringes and inject into two separate sites. Give new injections at least 1" from previous site, and never into tender, bruised, red, or hardened skin.
• Store unreconstituted vials at room temperature (59° to 86° F [15° to 30° C]).
• Reconstituted drug is stable 1 hour at room temperature and 8 hours refrigerated (36° to 46° F [2° to 8° C]). After refrigeration, suspension may be allowed to equilibrate for 30 minutes at room temperature.
⑤ **ALERT:** Don't confuse azacitidine with gemcitabine.
Patient teaching
• Inform patient about potential decrease in blood counts with febrile neutropenia, thrombocytopenia, and anemia.
• Advise men and women to use birth control during azacitidine therapy.

☑ **Evaluation**
• Patient responds well to the drug.
• Patient doesn't develop serious complications from adverse hematologic reactions.
• Patient and family state understanding of drug therapy.

azathioprine
(ay-zuh-THIGH-oh-preen)
Azasan, Imuran, Thioprine ◊

Pharmacologic class: purine antagonist
Therapeutic class: immunosuppressant
Pregnancy risk category: D

Indications and dosages

> **Immunosuppression in kidney transplantation.** *Adults and children:* Initially, 3 to 5 mg/kg P.O. or I.V. daily, usually beginning on

day of transplantation. Maintain at 1 to 3 mg/kg daily depending on patient response.
> **Severe, refractory rheumatoid arthritis.**
Adults: Initially, 1 mg/kg (about 50 mg to 100 mg) P.O. daily as single dose or as two doses. If patient response isn't satisfactory after 6 to 8 weeks, increase dosage by 0.5 mg/kg daily (up to maximum of 2.5 mg/kg daily) at 4-week intervals.

▽ I.V. administration

• Reconstitute 100-mg vial with 10 ml of sterile water for injection. Inspect for particles before giving.
• Drug may be given by direct I.V. injection or further diluted in normal saline solution or D_5W and infused over 30 to 60 minutes.
• Use only for patient who can't tolerate P.O. drugs.
⊗ **Incompatibilities**
None reported.

Contraindications and cautions

• Contraindicated in patients hypersensitive to drug.
• Use cautiously in patients with hepatic or renal dysfunction.
☀ **Lifespan:** In pregnant women, don't use for rheumatoid arthritis. In breast-feeding women, drug isn't recommended.

Adverse reactions

GI: nausea, vomiting, esophagitis, anorexia, *pancreatitis,* steatorrhea, mouth ulceration.
Hematologic: LEUKOPENIA, *bone marrow suppression,* anemia, *pancytopenia,* THROMBOCYTOPENIA.
Hepatic: *hepatotoxicity,* jaundice.
Musculoskeletal: arthralgia, muscle wasting.
Skin: rash, alopecia, pruritus.
Other: *immunosuppression,* infections, *neoplasia.*

Interactions

Drug-drug. *ACE inhibitors:* May cause severe leukopenia. Monitor patient closely.
Allopurinol: May impair inactivation of azathioprine. Decrease azathioprine dose to one-fourth or one-third normal dose.
Co-trimoxazole and other drugs that interfere with myelopoiesis: Severe leukopenia, especially in renal transplant patients. Use together cautiously.

Cyclosporine: May decrease cyclosporine level. Monitor level.

Methotrexate: May increase 6-MP metabolite level. Monitor patient for increased adverse effects.

Nondepolarizing neuromuscular blockers: May decrease or reverse effects of these agents. Monitor patient for clinical effects.

Vaccines: May decrease immune response. Postpone routine immunization.

Warfarin: May inhibit anticoagulant effect of warfarin. Monitor PT and INR.

Effects on lab test results

• May increase AST, ALT, alkaline phosphatase, and bilirubin levels. May decrease uric acid and hemoglobin levels and hematocrit.

• May decrease WBC, RBC, and platelet counts.

Pharmacokinetics

Absorption: Good.

Distribution: Throughout body; I.V. and P.O. forms are 30% protein-bound.

Metabolism: Primarily to mercaptopurine; tissue levels of thiopurine nucleotide produce clinical effects.

Excretion: Small amounts of azathioprine and mercaptopurine intact in urine; most of given dose is excreted in urine as secondary metabolites. *Half-life:* about 5 hours.

Route	Onset	Peak	Duration
P.O., I.V.	Unknown	1–2 hr	Unknown

Action

Chemical effect: Unknown.

Therapeutic effect: Suppresses immune system activity.

Available forms

Injection: 100 mg
Tablets: 25 mg, 50 mg, 75 mg, 100 mg

NURSING PROCESS

Assessment

• Obtain history of patient's immune status before therapy.

• Monitor effectiveness by observing patient for signs of organ rejection. Therapeutic response usually occurs within 8 weeks.

• Be alert for adverse reactions and drug interactions.

• Monitor hemoglobin level, hematocrit, and WBC and platelet counts at least once monthly—more often at beginning of treatment.

• Assess patient's and family's knowledge of drug therapy.

Nursing diagnoses

• Ineffective protection related to threat of organ rejection

• Risk for infection related to drug-induced immunosuppression

• Deficient knowledge related to drug therapy

Planning and implementation

• Give in divided doses or after meals to minimize adverse GI effects.

• Benefits must be weighed against risks with systemic viral infections, such as chickenpox and herpes zoster.

• Patients with rheumatoid arthritis previously treated with alkylating drugs, such as cyclophosphamide, chlorambucil, and melphalan, may have prohibitive risk of neoplasia if treated with azathioprine.

• To prevent irreversible bone marrow suppression, stop drug immediately when WBC count is less than 3,000/mm^3. Notify prescriber.

• To prevent bleeding, avoid I.M. injections when platelet count is below 100,000/mm^3.

⚠ ALERT: Don't confuse azathioprine with azidothymidine, Azulfidine, or azatadine. Don't confuse Imuran with Inderal.

Patient teaching

• Warn patient to report even mild infections (colds, fever, sore throat, and malaise) because drug is a potent immunosuppressant.

• Instruct woman to avoid conception during therapy and for 4 months after stopping therapy.

• Warn patient that thinning of hair is possible.

• Tell patient taking this drug for refractory rheumatoid arthritis that it may take up to 12 weeks to be effective.

Evaluation

• Patient exhibits no signs of organ rejection.

• Patient demonstrates no signs and symptoms of infection.

• Patient and family state understanding of drug therapy.

A

azelastine hydrochloride

(ah-zuh-LAST-een high-droh-KLOR-ighd)
Astelin, Optivar

Pharmacologic class: H_1-receptor antagonist
Therapeutic class: antihistamine
Pregnancy risk category: C

Indications and dosages

▶ **Seasonal allergic rhinitis, such as rhinorrhea, sneezing, and nasal pruritus.** *Adults and children age 12 and older:* 2 sprays (274 mcg/2 sprays) per nostril b.i.d.
Children ages 5 to 11 years: 1 spray (137 mcg/spray) per nostril b.i.d.

▶ **Vasomotor rhinitis, such as rhinorrhea, nasal congestion, and postnasal drip.** *Adults and children age 12 and older:* 2 sprays (274 mcg/2 sprays) per nostril b.i.d.

▶ **Allergic conjunctivitis.** *Adults and children older than age 3:* Give 1 drop into affected eye b.i.d.

Contraindications and cautions

- Contraindicated in patients hypersensitive to drug.
- Use cautiously in patients with pulmonary conditions because it can cause thickened secretions.

Lifespan: In pregnant women, drug should be used only if benefit justifies risk to fetus. Breast-feeding women shouldn't take drug. In children younger than age 5, safety and effectiveness of drug haven't been established for treatment of seasonal allergic rhinitis. In children younger than age 12, don't use drug for vasomotor rhinitis.

Adverse reactions

CNS: fatigue, *headaches, somnolence,* dysesthesia, dizziness.
EENT: transient eye burning, stinging, nasal burning, conjunctivitis, eye pain, pharyngitis, rhinitis, paroxysmal sneezing, temporary eye blurring, epistaxis, sinusitis.
GI: *bitter taste,* dry mouth, nausea.
Metabolic: weight increase.
Respiratory: ***asthma,*** dyspnea.
Skin: pruritus.
Other: flulike symptoms.

Interactions

Drug-drug. *Cimetidine:* May increase azelastine level. Avoid using together.
CNS depressants: May reduce alertness and impair CNS performance. Avoid using together.
Drug-lifestyle. *Alcohol use:* May reduce alertness and cause CNS impairment if using the nasal spray. Discourage using together.

Effects on lab test results

None reported.

Pharmacokinetics

Absorption: Ophthalmic solution has low absorption.
Distribution: Systemic bioavailability is 40%.
Metabolism: After dosing to a steady state, level ranges from 20% to 50%.
Excretion: Oral drug is 75% excreted in feces. Less than 10% remains unchanged. *Half-life:* 22 hours.

Route	Onset	Peak	Duration
Nasal	Unknown	2–3 hr	12 hr
Ophthalmic	3 min	Unknown	8 hr

Action

Chemical effect: Exhibits histamine H_1-receptor antagonist activity.
Therapeutic effect: Relieves seasonal allergic rhinitis and conjunctivitis.

Available forms

Nasal solution: 1 mg/ml (137 mcg/spray)
Ophthalmic solution: 0.05%

NURSING PROCESS

Assessment

- Obtain history of patient's allergy condition before therapy begins, and reassess regularly thereafter.
- Be alert for adverse reactions and drug interactions.
- Assess patient's and family's knowledge of drug therapy.

Nursing diagnoses

- Ineffective health maintenance related to underlying allergic condition
- Deficient knowledge related to drug therapy

⬗ Planning and implementation
• Don't contaminate eye dropper tip or solution.
• Make sure patient removes contact lenses before giving eyedrops. Tell patient to wait at least 10 minutes before reinserting them.
• When using nasal spray, avoid spraying into patient's eyes.

Patient teaching
• Warn patient not to drive or perform hazardous activities if somnolence occurs.
• Advise patient not to use alcohol, CNS depressants, or other antihistamines while taking drug.
• Teach patient proper use of nasal spray. Instruct patient to replace child-resistant screw top on bottle with pump unit. Prime delivery system with four sprays or until a fine mist appears. If 3 or more days have elapsed since last use, reprime system with 2 sprays or until a fine mist appears. Store bottle upright at room temperature with pump closed tightly. Keep unit away from children.
• Tell patient to avoid getting nasal spray in eyes.

⬗ Evaluation
• Patient's allergic symptoms are relieved with drug therapy.
• Patient and family state understanding of drug therapy.

azithromycin
(uh-zith-roh-MIGH-sin)
Zithromax✦

Pharmacologic class: azalide macrolide
Therapeutic class: antibiotic
Pregnancy risk category: B

Indications and dosages

▶ **Acute bacterial exacerbations of chronic obstructive pulmonary disease caused by** *Haemophilus influenzae, Moraxella catarrhalis,* **or** *Streptococcus pneumoniae;* **uncomplicated skin and skin-structure infections caused by** *Staphylococcus aureus, Streptococcus pyogenes,* **or** *Streptococcus agalactiae;* **and second-line therapy for pharyngitis or tonsillitis caused by** *S. pyogenes. Adults and children age 16 and older:* Initially, 500 mg P.O. as a single dose on day 1, followed by 250 mg daily on days 2 through 5. Total cumu-

lative dose is 1.5 g. Or for COPD exacerbations, 500 mg P.O. daily for 3 days.
▶ **Community-acquired pneumonia caused by** *Chlamydia pneumoniae, H. influenzae, Mycoplasma pneumoniae, S. pneumoniae;* **I.V. form is also used for** *Legionella pneumophila, M. catarrhalis,* **and** *S. aureus. Adults and children age 16 and older:* 500 mg P.O. as a single dose on day 1, followed by 250 mg P.O. daily on days 2 through 5. Total dosage is 1.5 g. For patients requiring initial I.V. therapy, 500 mg I.V. as a single daily dose for 2 days, followed by 500 mg P.O. as a single daily dose to complete a 7- to 10-day course of therapy. Switch from I.V. to P.O. therapy should be done at prescriber's discretion and based on patient's clinical response.
Children age 6 months and older: 10 mg/kg (max 500 mg) P.O. as a single dose on day 1, followed by 5 mg/kg (max 250 mg) daily on days 2 through 5.
▶ **Nongonococcal urethritis or cervicitis caused by** *Chlamydia trachomatis. Adults and children age 16 and older:* 1 g P.O. as a single dose.
▶ **Prevention of disseminated** *Mycobacterium avium* **complex (MAC) disease in patients with advanced HIV infection.** *Adults:* 1,200 mg P.O. once weekly, as indicated. *Infants and children‡:* 20 mg/kg P.O. (maximum dosage of 1.2 g) weekly or 5 mg/kg (maximum dosage of 250 mg) can be given P.O. daily. Children 6 years and older may also receive rifabutin 300 mg P.O. daily.
▶ **Disseminated MAC in patients with advanced HIV infection.** *Adults:* 600 mg P.O. daily with ethambutol 15 mg/kg daily.
▶ **Urethritis and cervicitis caused by** *Neisseria gonorrhoeae. Adults:* 2 g P.O. as a single dose.
▶ **Pelvic inflammatory disease caused by** *C. trachomatis, N. gonorrhoeae,* **or** *Mycoplasma hominis* **in patients who require initial I.V. therapy.** *Adults and adolescents age 16 and older:* 500 mg I.V. as a single daily dose for 1 to 2 days, followed by 250 mg P.O. daily to complete a 7-day course of therapy. Switch from I.V. to P.O. therapy should be done at prescriber's discretion and based on patient's clinical response.
▶ **Genital ulcer disease caused by** *Haemophilus ducreyi* **(chancroid) in men, women‡, and children‡.** *Adults:* 1 g P.O. as a single dose.

Children and infants‡: 20 mg/kg (maximum, 1 g) P.O. as a single dose.
► **Acute otitis media.** *Children older than age 6 months:* 30 mg/kg P.O. as a single dose. Or, 10 mg/kg P.O. once daily for 3 days. Or 10 mg/kg P.O. on day 1; then 5 mg/kg once daily on days 2 to 5.
► **Pharyngitis, tonsillitis caused by *S. pyogenes.*** *Children age 2 and older:* 12 mg/kg (maximum, 500 mg) P.O. daily for 5 days.
► **Prophylaxis for sexual assault victims‡.** *Adults:* 1 g P.O. as a single dose with metronidazole and ceftriaxone.
► **Prophylaxis of bacterial endocarditis in penicillin-allergic patients at moderate-to-high risk‡.** *Adults:* 500 mg P.O. 1 hour before the procedure.
Children: 15 mg/kg P.O. 1 hour before the procedure. Don't exceed adult dose.
► *Chlamydial ophthalmia* **neonatorum** ◊. *Infants:* 20 mg/kg once daily P.O. for 3 days.

▼ I.V. administration

• Reconstitute drug by adding 4.8 ml sterile water for injection to 500-mg vial and shake until all the drug is dissolved. Further dilute in 250 to 500 ml D₅W, normal saline solution, or other compatible solution.
• Infuse over 1 to 3 hours.
• Reconstituted solution is stable for 7 days if stored in refrigerator (41° F [5° C]).
• Don't give by I.V. injection or bolus.
⊗ **Incompatibilities**
Amikacin, aztreonam, cefotaxime, ceftazidime, ceftriaxone, cefuroxime, ciprofloxacin, clindamycin, famotidine, fentanyl, furosemide, gentamicin, imipenem and cilastin, ketorolac, levofloxacin, morphine, ondansetron, piperacillin and tazobactam sodium potassium chloride, ticarcillin disodium and clavulanate potassium, tobramycin.

Contraindications and cautions

• Contraindicated in patients hypersensitive to erythromycin or other macrolides.
• Use cautiously in patients with impaired hepatic function.
⚘ **Lifespan:** In pregnant or breast-feeding women, use cautiously.

Adverse reactions

CNS: dizziness, vertigo, headache, fatigue, somnolence, aggressive reaction, anxiety, *seizure.*

CV: palpitations, chest pain, *QT prolongation, torsade de pointes.*
EENT: hearing loss, tinnitus, taste perversion.
GI: *nausea, vomiting, diarrhea, abdominal pain,* dyspepsia, flatulence, melena, cholestatic jaundice, *pseudomembranous colitis.*
GU: candidiasis, vaginitis, nephritis.
Hematologic: *thombocytopenia,* mild neutropenia.
Hepatic: hepatitis, cholestatic jaundice, *hepatic necrosis, hepatic failure.*
Skin: rash, photosensitivity, *Stevens-Johnson syndrome, toxic epidermal necrolysis,* urticaria.
Other: *angioedema, anaphylaxis.*

Interactions

Drug-drug. *Antacids containing aluminum and magnesium:* May lower peak azithromycin level. Separate administration times by at least 2 hours.
Digoxin: May elevate digoxin level. Monitor patient closely.
Dihydroergotamine, ergotamine: May cause acute ergot toxicity. Avoid using together.
Drugs metabolized by CYP system: May elevate carbamazepine, cyclosporine, hexobarbital, and phenytoin levels. Monitor patient closely.
Theophylline: May increase theophylline level with other macrolides; effect of azithromycin is unknown. Monitor theophylline level carefully.
Triazolam: May increase pharmacologic effect of triazolam. Use together cautiously.
Warfarin: May increase PT with other macrolides; effect of azithromycin is unknown. Monitor PT and INR carefully.
Drug-food. *Any food:* May decrease rate of absorption, but not effectiveness of drug.
Drug-lifestyle. *Sun exposure:* May cause photosensitivity reactions. Advise against prolonged or unprotected sun exposure.

Effects on lab test results

None reported.

Pharmacokinetics

Absorption: Rapid. Food decreases both maximum level and amount of drug absorbed.
Distribution: Rapid throughout body and readily penetrates cells; drug doesn't readily enter CNS. Drug concentrates in fibroblasts and phagocytes. Significantly higher levels are reached in tissues compared with plasma.
Metabolism: None.

Rapid onset   *Liquid form contains alcohol.   ♦ Canada   ◊ Australia   †OTC   ✐Photoguide   ‡Off-label use

Excretion: Mostly in feces after excretion into bile. Less than 10% in urine. *Terminal elimination half-life:* 68 hours.

Route	Onset	Peak	Duration
P.O.	Unknown	2½–4½ hr	Unknown
I.V.	Unknown	Unknown	Unknown

Action

Chemical effect: Binds to 50S subunit of bacterial ribosomes, blocking protein synthesis; bacteriostatic or bactericidal, depending on concentration.
Therapeutic effect: Hinders or kills susceptible bacteria, including many gram-positive and gram-negative aerobic and anaerobic bacteria.

Available forms

Injection: 500 mg
Powder for oral suspension: 100 mg/5 ml, 200 mg/5 ml; 1,000 mg/packet
Tablets: 250 mg, 500 mg, 600 mg

NURSING PROCESS

Assessment
• Obtain history of patient's infection before therapy and reassess regularly thereafter.
• Obtain specimen for culture and sensitivity tests before first dose. Therapy may begin pending test results.
• Be alert for adverse reactions and drug interactions.
• Assess patient's and family's knowledge of drug therapy.

Nursing diagnoses
• Infection related to presence of susceptible bacteria
• Ineffective protection related to drug-induced superinfection
• Deficient knowledge related to drug therapy

Planning and implementation
ALERT: Don't give drug I.M. or by I.V. bolus injection.
• Don't give with antacids.
Patient teaching
• Tell patient that tablets or oral suspension may be taken with or without food, but that taking with food may decrease risk of nausea.
• Tell patient to take all medication as prescribed, even after he feels better.

• Instruct patient to use sunblock and avoid prolonged exposure to the sun to decrease risk of photosensitivity reactions.

Evaluation
• Patient's infection is eliminated.
• Patient doesn't experience superinfection during therapy.
• Patient and family state understanding of drug therapy.

aztreonam
(az-TREE-oh-nam)
Azactam

Pharmacologic class: monobactam
Therapeutic class: antibiotic
Pregnancy risk category: B

Indications and dosages

▶ **UTI, lower respiratory tract infections, septicemia, skin and skin-structure infections, intra-abdominal infections, surgical infections, gynecologic infections caused by various aerobic organisms; or as adjunct therapy to pelvic inflammatory disease‡ or gonorrhea‡.** *Adults:* 500 mg to 2 g I.V. or I.M. q 8 to 12 hours. For severe systemic or life-threatening infection, 2 g q 6 to 8 hours. Maximum dosage is 8 g daily.
▶ **Infections of the respiratory or GU tract, bone, skin, and soft tissues caused by susceptible organisms‡.** *Neonates ages 1 to 4 weeks weighing more than 2 kg:* 30 mg/kg I.V. q 6 hours.
Neonates ages 1 to 4 weeks weighing 2 kg or less: 30 mg/kg I.V. q 8 hours.
Neonates younger than 7 days weighing more than 2 kg (4.4 lb): 30 mg/kg I.V. q 8 hours.
Neonates younger than 7 days weighing 2 kg or less: 30 mg/kg I.V. q 12 hours

I.V. administration
• Inject bolus dose drug over 3 to 5 minutes directly into vein or I.V. tubing.
• Give infusion over 20 minutes to 1 hour.
⊗ **Incompatibilities**
Acyclovir, amphotericin B, ampicillin sodium, azithromycin, cephradine, chlorpromazine, daunorubicin, ganciclovir, lorazepam, metronidazole, mitomycin, mitoxantrone, nafcillin,

other I.V. drugs, prochlorperazine, streptozocin, vancomycin.

Contraindications and cautions

• Contraindicated in patients hypersensitive to drug.
• Use cautiously in patients with impaired renal function. Dosage adjustment may be needed.
⚠ **Lifespan:** In breast-feeding women, drug isn't recommended. In children, safety of drug hasn't been established. In elderly patients, use cautiously because dosage adjustment may be needed.

Adverse reactions

CNS: *seizures,* headache, insomnia, confusion.
CV: hypotension.
EENT: halitosis, altered taste.
GI: diarrhea, nausea, vomiting.
Hematologic: *neutropenia,* anemia, *thrombo-cytopenia, pancytopenia.*
Other: hypersensitivity reactions (rash, *ana-phylaxis*); rash, thrombophlebitis at I.V. site; discomfort, swelling at I.M. injection site.

Interactions

Drug-drug. *Aminoglycosides, beta-lactam antibiotics, other anti-infectives:* May have synergistic effect and increase risk of ototoxicity, nephrotoxicity. Monitor patient closely.
Cefoxitin, imipenem: May have antagonistic effect. Avoid using together.
Furosemide, probenecid: May increase aztreonam level. Avoid using together.

Effects on lab test results

• May increase BUN, creatinine, ALT, AST, and LDH levels. May decrease hemoglobin level and hematocrit.
• May increase PT, APTT, and INR. May decrease neutrophil and RBC counts. May increase or decrease WBC and platelet counts.

Pharmacokinetics

Absorption: Rapid and complete.
Distribution: Rapid and wide to all body fluids and tissues, including bile, breast milk, and CSF.
Metabolism: From 6% to 16% metabolized to inactive metabolites by nonspecific hydrolysis of beta-lactam ring; 56% to 60% protein-bound, less if renal impairment is present.

Excretion: Primarily unchanged in urine by glomerular filtration and tubular secretion; 1.5% to 3.5% excreted unchanged in feces. *Half-life:* Average 2 hours.

Route	Onset	Peak	Duration
I.V.	Immediate	Immediate	Unknown
I.M.	Unknown	½–1¼ hr	Unknown

Action

Chemical effect: Inhibits bacterial cell-wall synthesis, ultimately causing cell-wall destruction.
Therapeutic effect: Kills susceptible bacteria.

Available forms

Injection: 500-mg, 1-g, 2-g vials

NURSING PROCESS

✏ Assessment
• Obtain history of patient's infection before therapy and reassess regularly thereafter.
• Obtain urine specimen for culture and sensitivity tests before giving first dose. Therapy may begin pending test results.
• Be aware of adverse reactions and drug interactions.
• Patients who are allergic to penicillins or cephalosporins may not be allergic to this drug. However, closely monitor patients who have had an immediate hypersensitivity reaction to these antibiotics.
• Assess patient's and family's knowledge of drug therapy.

⊞ Nursing diagnoses
• Infection related to presence of susceptible bacteria
• Ineffective protection related to drug-induced superinfection
• Deficient knowledge related to drug therapy

▷ Planning and implementation
• Give I.M. injection deep into large muscle mass, such as the upper outer quadrant of gluteus maximus or the outer thigh. Give doses larger than 1 g by I.V. route.
• Report diarrhea to the prescriber. Pseudomembranous colitis may need to be ruled out.
• Monitor renal and hepatic function.

Patient teaching

• Tell patient to report pain or discomfort at I.V. site.
• Warn patient receiving drug I.M. that pain and swelling may develop at injection site.
• Instruct patient to report signs or symptoms that suggest superinfection.

☑ Evaluation

• Patient is free from infection.
• Patient doesn't develop superinfection as a result of therapy.
• Patient and family state understanding of drug therapy.

baclofen
(BAH-kloh-fen)
Clofen◇, Kemstro, Lioresal, Lioresal Intrathecal

Pharmacologic class: chlorophenyl derivative (GABA derivative)
Therapeutic class: skeletal muscle relaxant
Pregnancy risk category: C

Indications and dosages

▶ **Spasticity in multiple sclerosis, spinal cord injury.** *Adults:* Initially, 5 mg P.O. t.i.d. for 3 days. Increase dosage based on response at 3-day intervals by 15 mg (5 mg/dose) daily up to maximum of 80 mg daily (20 mg q.i.d.).
▶ **Management of severe spasticity in patients who don't respond to or can't tolerate oral baclofen therapy.** *Adults (screening phase):* After test dose, give drug by an implantable infusion pump. The test dose is 50 mcg in 1-ml dilution given into intrathecal space by barbotage over 1 minute or longer. Significantly decreased severity or frequency of muscle spasm or reduced muscle tone should be evident in 4 to 8 hours. If response is inadequate, give a second test dose of 75 mcg/1.5 ml 24 hours after the first. If response is still inadequate, give a final test dose of 100 mcg/2 ml 24 hours later. Patients unresponsive to 100-mcg

dose shouldn't be considered candidates for implantable pump.
Adults (maintenance therapy): Adjust initial dose based on screening dose that elicits an adequate response. This effective dose is doubled and given over 24 hours. If screening-dose effectiveness is maintained for 8 hours or longer, dosage isn't doubled. After first 24 hours, increase dose slowly, as needed and tolerated, by 10% to 30% daily until desired effects occur. Dose may be decreased by 10% to 20% if intolerable adverse effects occur.
Children younger than age 12: Testing dose is the same as for adults (50 mcg); but for very small children, an initial dose of 25 mcg may be given.

Contraindications and cautions

• Contraindicated in patients hypersensitive to drug. Orally disintegrating tablets are contraindicated in patients hypersensitive to aspartame.
• Use cautiously in patients with impaired renal function or seizure disorder or when spasticity is used to maintain motor function.
⚕ **Lifespan:** In pregnant or breast-feeding women, use cautiously. In children younger than age 12, safety of oral dosage form hasn't been established. In children younger than age 4, safety of intrathecal dosage form hasn't been established.

Adverse reactions

CNS: *high fever,* drowsiness, dizziness, *headache,* weakness, fatigue, *hypotonia, confusion,* somnolence, paresthesias, SEIZURES.
CV: ankle edema, hypotension.
EENT: nasal congestion, blurred vision.
GI: nausea, constipation, vomiting.
GU: sexual dysfunction, impotence, urinary frequency, urinary incontinence.
Metabolic: hyperglycemia, weight gain.
Musculoskeletal: *muscle rigidity or spasticity,* dysarthria, *rhabdomyolysis.*
Respiratory: dyspnea.
Skin: rash, pruritus, excessive perspiration.
Other: *multiple organ-system failure.*

Interactions

Drug-drug. *CNS depressants:* May increase CNS depression. Avoid using together.
MAO inhibitors, tricyclic antidepressants: CNS and respiratory depression and hypotension may occur. Avoid using together.

Drug-lifestyle. *Alcohol use:* May increase CNS depression. Discourage using together.

Effects on lab test results

• May increase AST, alkaline phosphatase, and glucose levels.

Pharmacokinetics

Absorption: Rapid and extensive with P.O. administration; may vary.
Distribution: Widely distributed throughout body, with small amounts crossing blood–brain barrier. About 30% protein-bound.
Metabolism: About 15% metabolized in liver by deamination.
Excretion: 70% to 80% in urine unchanged or as metabolites; remainder in feces. *Half-life:* 2½ to 4 hours.

Route	Onset	Peak	Duration
P.O.	Rapid	2–3 hr	8 hr
P.O. orally disintegrating	Rapid	1½ hr	8 hr
Intrathecal	½–1 hr	4 hr	4–8 hr

Action

Chemical effect: Unknown; appears to reduce transmission of impulses from spinal cord to skeletal muscle.
Therapeutic effect: Relieves muscle spasms.

Available forms

Intrathecal injection: 500 mcg/ml, 2,000 mcg/ml, 5,000 mcg/ml
Orally disintegrating tablets: 10 mg, 20 mg
Tablets: 10 mg, 20 mg, 25 mg

NURSING PROCESS

Assessment

• Obtain history of patient's pain and muscle spasms from underlying condition before therapy, and reassess regularly thereafter.
• Be alert for adverse reactions and drug interactions.
• Watch for increased seizures in patients with seizure disorder. Seizures have been reported during overdose and withdrawal of intrathecal baclofen, as well as in patients maintained on therapeutic doses. Monitor patient carefully, and institute seizure precautions.

• Assess patient's and family's understanding of drug therapy.

Nursing diagnoses

• Acute pain related to spasticity
• Risk for injury related to drug-induced adverse CNS reactions
• Deficient knowledge related to drug therapy

Planning and implementation

• Give with meals or milk to prevent GI distress.
• Don't give orally to treat muscle spasm caused by rheumatic disorders, cerebral palsy, Parkinson's disease, or stroke because effectiveness hasn't been established.
• Treatment for oral overdose is supportive; don't induce emesis or use respiratory stimulant in an unconscious patient.
• Implantable pump or catheter failure can result in sudden loss of effectiveness of intrathecal baclofen.
ALERT: Don't give intrathecal injection by I.V., I.M., subcutaneous, or epidural route.
• The amount of relief determines whether dose (and drowsiness) can be reduced.
• Don't stop intrathecal baclofen abruptly. Early symptoms of baclofen withdrawal may include return of baseline spasticity, pruritus, hypotension, and paresthesias. Symptoms that have occurred include high fever, altered mental status, exaggerated rebound spasticity, and muscle rigidity that in rare cases has advanced to rhabdomyolysis, multiple organ-system failure, and death. Treat intrathecal baclofen withdrawal by restoring intrathecal baclofen at or near the same dosage as before therapy was stopped. However, if delayed, treat with P.O. or enteral baclofen, or P.O., enteral, or I.V. benzodiazepines to prevent potentially fatal sequelae. P.O. or enteral baclofen alone shouldn't be relied upon to halt the progression of intrathecal baclofen withdrawal.
• About 10% of patients may develop tolerance to drug. In some cases, this may be treated by hospitalizing patient and by slowly withdrawing drug over a 2-week period.
Patient teaching
• Tell patient to avoid activities that require alertness until drug's CNS effects are known. Drowsiness usually is transient.
• Inform patient with phenylketonuria that orally disintegrating tablets contain phenylalanine (3.9 mg/10-mg tablet and 7.9 mg/20-mg tablet).

• Instruct patient to remove orally disintegrating tablet from blister pack and immediately place on tongue to dissolve, then swallow with or without water.
• Tell patient to avoid alcohol while taking drug.
• Advise patient to follow prescriber's orders about rest and physical therapy.
• Advise patient to take drug with food or milk to prevent GI distress.

☑ **Evaluation**

• Patient reports that pain and muscle spasms have ceased with drug therapy.
• Patient doesn't experience injury as a result of drug-induced drowsiness.
• Patient and family state understanding of drug therapy.

balsalazide disodium
(bal-SAL-uh-zide digh-SOH-dee-um)
Colazal

Pharmacologic class: GI drug
Therapeutic class: anti-inflammatory
Pregnancy risk category: B

Indications and dosages

▶ **Ulcerative colitis.** *Adults:* 2.25 g (three 750-mg capsules) P.O. t.i.d. for a total of 6.75 g daily for 8 to 12 weeks.

Contraindications and cautions

• Contraindicated in patients hypersensitive to salicylates or to any component of balsalazide metabolites.
• Use cautiously in patients with history of renal disease or renal dysfunction.
• Use judiciously in patients with pyloric stenosis because of prolonged retention of drug. Safety and effectiveness beyond 12 weeks of treatment haven't been established.
⚘ **Lifespan:** In breast-feeding women, use cautiously because it's unknown whether drug appears in breast milk. In children, safety and effectiveness haven't been established.

Adverse reactions

CNS: fever, dizziness, fatigue, headache, insomnia.
EENT: pharyngitis, rhinitis, sinusitis.

GI: abdominal pain, anorexia, constipation, cramps, diarrhea, dyspepsia, flatulence, frequent stools, nausea, rectal bleeding, vomiting, dry mouth.
GU: UTI.
Hepatic: *hepatotoxicity.*
Musculoskeletal: arthralgia, back pain, myalgia.
Respiratory: cough, respiratory infection.
Other: flulike symptoms.

Interactions

Drug-drug. *Azathioprine and 6-mercaptopurine:* Balsalazide may interfere with the metabolism of these drugs. Use with caution.
Oral antibiotics and anti-infectives: May interfere with release of mesalamine in the colon. Monitor patient for worsening of symptoms.

Effects on lab test results

• May increase AST, ALT, LDH, alkaline phosphatase, and bilirubin levels.

Pharmacokinetics

Absorption: Very low and variable in healthy patients; 60 times greater in patients with ulcerative colitis.
Distribution: 99% or more protein-bound.
Metabolism: Metabolized to mesalamine (5-aminosalicylic acid), the active component of the drug.
Excretion: By the kidneys. Less than 1% recovered in urine. *Half-life:* Unknown.

Route	Onset	Peak	Duration
P.O.	Unknown	Unknown	Unknown

Action

Chemical effect: Balsalazide is converted in the colon to mesalamine, which is then converted to 5-aminosalicylic acid. The mechanism of action is unknown, but it appears to be local rather than systemic. In patients with chronic inflammatory bowel disease, the production of arachidonic acid metabolites is increased. Balsalazide likely blocks the production of arachidonic acid metabolites in the colon.
Therapeutic effect: Decreases inflammation in the colon.

Available forms

Capsules: 750 mg

Reactions may be *common*, uncommon, *life-threatening*, or COMMON AND LIFE-THREATENING.

B

NURSING PROCESS

☞ Assessment
• Assess patient's underlying condition and note frequency of bowel movements before starting drug therapy.
• Hepatotoxicity, including elevated liver function test results, jaundice, cirrhosis, liver necrosis, and liver failure, has occurred with other products containing or metabolized to mesalamine. Although no signs of hepatotoxicity have been reported with balsalazide disodium, monitor patient closely for evidence of hepatic dysfunction.
• Assess patient's and family's knowledge of drug therapy and ulcerative colitis.

⊕ Nursing diagnoses
• Diarrhea related to underlying disease process
• Risk of imbalanced nutrition: less than body requirements related to frequent bowel movements due to ulcerative colitis
• Deficient knowledge related to balsalazide disodium therapy

▶ Planning and implementation
• Notify prescriber if drug has been given for 8 to 12 weeks or longer.
Patient teaching
• Advise patient not to take drug if he is allergic to aspirin or salicylate derivatives.
• Advise patient to promptly report adverse reactions to prescriber.

☑ Evaluation
• Patient states that diarrhea has improved.
• Because of decreasing symptoms of ulcerative colitis, patient is able to tolerate and absorb a balanced diet.
• Patient and family state understanding of balsalazide disodium therapy.

basiliximab
(ba-sil-IK-si-mab)
Simulect

Pharmacologic class: recombinant chimeric human monoclonal antibody IgG$_{1k}$
Therapeutic class: immunosuppressant
Pregnancy risk category: B

Indications and dosages.
▶ **To prevent acute organ rejection in renal transplant patients when used as part of immunosuppressive regimen including cyclosporine and corticosteroids.** *Adults and children weighing 35 kg (77 lb) or more:* 20 mg I.V. given within 2 hours before transplant surgery and 20 mg I.V. given 4 days after transplantation.
Children weighing less than 35 kg: 10 mg I.V. given within 2 hours before transplant and 10 mg I.V. given 4 days post-transplantation.

▽ I.V. administration
• Reconstitute with 5 ml sterile water for injection. Shake vial gently to dissolve powder. Dilute reconstituted solution to volume of 50 ml with normal saline solution or D$_5$W for infusion. When mixing solution, gently invert bag to avoid foaming. Don't shake.
• Infuse over 20 to 30 minutes by a central or peripheral vein.
• Use reconstituted solution immediately, or it may be refrigerated between 36° and 46° F (2° and 8° C) for up to 24 hours or kept at room temperature for 4 hours.
⊗ **Incompatibilities**
Other I.V. drugs.

Contraindications and cautions
• Contraindicated in patients hypersensitive to drug or any of its components.
⚘ **Lifespan:** In pregnant women, use only if potential benefits outweigh risks to the fetus. Breast-feeding women should stop nursing or stop taking the drug because of potential for adverse effects. It's unknown whether drug appears in breast milk. In elderly patients, use cautiously.

Adverse reactions
CNS: *fever,* agitation, anxiety, asthenia, depression, *dizziness, headache,* hypoesthesia, *insomnia,* neuropathy, paresthesia, *tremor,* fatigue.
CV: *hemorrhage,* angina pectoris, *arrhythmias,* atrial fibrillation, *heart failure,* chest pain, abnormal heart sounds, *aggravated hypertension, hypertension, leg or peripheral edema,* general edema, hypotension, tachycardia.
EENT: abnormal vision, cataract, conjunctivitis, *rhinitis,* sinusitis, *pharyngitis.*
GI: *abdominal pain, candidiasis, constipation, diarrhea, dyspepsia,* esophagitis, enlarged ab-

domen, flatulence, gastroenteritis, GI disorder, *GI hemorrhage,* gum hyperplasia, melena, *nausea,* ulcerative stomatitis, *vomiting.*
GU: abnormal renal function, albuminuria, bladder disorder, *dysuria,* frequent micturition, genital edema, hematuria, *increased nonprotein nitrogen,* oliguria, *renal tubular necrosis,* ureteral disorder, *UTI,* urine retention, impotence.
Hematologic: *anemia,* hematoma, *polycythemia, purpura, thrombocytopenia, thrombosis.*
Metabolic: *acidosis,* dehydration, *diabetes mellitus,* fluid overload, hypercalcemia, *hypercholesterolemia, hyperglycemia,* HYPERKALEMIA, hyperlipemia, *hyperuricemia, hypocalcemia, hypokalemia,* hypomagnesemia, hypophosphatemia, hypoproteinemia, *weight gain.*
Musculoskeletal: arthralgia, arthropathy, *back pain,* bone fracture, cramps, hernia, *leg pain,* myalgia.
Respiratory: abnormal chest sounds, bronchitis, *bronchospasm, cough, dyspnea,* pneumonia, pulmonary disorder, *pulmonary edema, upper respiratory tract infection.*
Skin: *acne,* cyst, herpes simplex, herpes zoster, hypertrichosis, pruritus, rash, skin disorder or ulceration.
Other: accidental trauma, *viral infection,* infection, *sepsis, surgical wound complications.*

Interactions

None significant.

Effects on lab test results

• May increase calcium, cholesterol, glucose, lipid, and uric acid levels. May decrease magnesium, phosphorus, protein, and hemoglobin levels and hematocrit. May increase or decrease potassium level.
• May increase RBC count. May decrease platelet count.

Pharmacokinetics

Absorption: Given I.V.
Distribution: Unknown.
Metabolism: Unknown.
Excretion: Unknown. *Half-life:* About 7¼ days in adults, 9½ days in children, 9 days in adolescents.

Route	Onset	Peak	Duration
I.V.	Unknown	Immediate	Unknown

Action

Chemical effect: Binds specifically to and blocks the interleukin (IL)-2 receptor alpha chain on the surface of activated T lymphocytes, inhibiting IL-2–mediated activation of lymphocytes, a critical pathway in the cellular immune response involved in allograft rejection.
Therapeutic effect: Prevents organ rejection.

Available forms

Injection: 20-mg vials

NURSING PROCESS

℞ Assessment
• Monitor patient for anaphylactoid reactions. Be sure that drugs for treating severe hypersensitivity reactions are available for immediate use.
• Check for electrolyte imbalances and acidosis.
• Monitor patient's intake and output, vital signs, hemoglobin level, and hematocrit.
• Be alert for signs and symptoms of opportunistic infections.
• Assess patient's and family's knowledge of drug therapy.

Nursing diagnoses
• Risk for injury related to potential for organ rejection
• Ineffective protection related to drug-induced immunosuppression
• Deficient knowledge related to drug therapy

Planning and implementation
• Use drug only under supervision of prescriber experienced in this type of therapy and management of organ transplantation.
• Patients who have a severe hypersensitivity reaction shouldn't receive the drug again.
Patient teaching
• Inform patient of potential benefits and risks of therapy, including decreased risk of graft loss or acute rejection. Advise patient that therapy increases risks of developing lymphoproliferative disorders and opportunistic infections. Tell him to report signs and symptoms of infection immediately.
• Tell women of childbearing age to use effective contraception before therapy starts and for 4 months after therapy ends.
• Instruct patient to immediately report adverse effects to prescriber.

Reactions may be *common,* uncommon, *life-threatening*, or COMMON AND LIFE-THREATENING.

• Explain that drug is used with cyclosporine and corticosteroids.

☑ Evaluation
• Patient doesn't experience organ rejection while taking this drug.
• Patient is free from infection and serious bleeding episodes throughout drug therapy.
• Patient and family state understanding of drug therapy.

beclomethasone dipropionate
(bek-loh-METH-eh-sohn digh-proh-PIGH-uh-nayt)
QVAR

Pharmacologic class: synthetic corticosteroid
Therapeutic class: antiasthmatic
Pregnancy risk category: C

Indications and dosages
▶ **Chronic asthma.** *Adults and children age 12 and older:* Starting dose, 40 to 80 mcg b.i.d. by aerosol inhalation when used with bronchodilators alone, or 40 to 160 mcg b.i.d. when used with other inhaled corticosteroids. Maximum, 320 mcg b.i.d.
Children ages 5 to 11: 40 mcg b.i.d., up to 80 mcg b.i.d. by aerosol inhalation when used with bronchodilators alone or with inhaled corticosteroids.

Contraindications and cautions
• Contraindicated in patients hypersensitive to drug or any of its components, and in those with status asthmaticus, nonasthmatic bronchial diseases, or asthma controlled by bronchodilators or other noncorticosteroids alone.
• Use with extreme caution, if at all, in patients with tuberculosis, fungal or bacterial infections, ocular herpes simplex, or systemic viral infections.
• Use with caution in patients receiving systemic corticosteroid therapy.
≋ **Lifespan:** In pregnant or breast-feeding women, use cautiously. In children younger than age 5, safety and effectiveness haven't been established.

Adverse reactions
EENT: *hoarseness, fungal infection of throat, throat irritation.*

GI: dry mouth, *fungal infection of mouth.*
Metabolic: *suppression of hypothalamic-pituitary-adrenal function,* adrenal insufficiency.
Respiratory: *bronchospasm,* wheezing, cough.
Other: *angioedema,* hypersensitivity reactions, facial edema.

Interactions
None significant.

Effects on lab test results
None reported.

Pharmacokinetics
Absorption: Rapid from lungs and GI tract.
Distribution: No evidence of tissue storage of beclomethasone or its metabolites.
Metabolism: Mostly in liver.
Excretion: Unknown, although when drug is given systemically, its metabolites are excreted mainly in feces and, to a lesser extent, in urine. *Half-life:* 15 hours.

Route	Onset	Peak	Duration
Inhalation	1–4 wk	Unknown	Unknown

Action
Chemical effect: Decreases inflammation, mainly by stabilizing leukocyte lysosomal membranes.
Therapeutic effect: Helps alleviate asthma symptoms.

Available forms
Oral inhalation aerosol: 40 mcg/metered spray, 80 mcg/metered spray

NURSING PROCESS

⚖ Assessment
• Obtain history of patient's asthma before therapy and reassess regularly thereafter.
• Be alert for adverse reactions.
• Monitor patient closely during times of stress (trauma, surgery, or infection) because systemic corticosteroids may be needed to prevent adrenal insufficiency in previously steroid-dependent patients.
• Periodic measurement of growth and development may be necessary during high-dose or prolonged therapy in children.

• Assess patient's and family's understanding of drug therapy.

🔁 Nursing diagnoses
• Impaired gas exchange related to asthma
• Impaired oral mucous membranes related to drug-induced fungal infections
• Deficient knowledge related to drug therapy

▧ Planning and implementation
⊛ **ALERT:** Never give drug to relieve an emergency asthma attack because onset of action is too slow.
• Give prescribed bronchodilators several minutes before beclomethasone.
• Have patient hold breath for a few seconds after each puff and rest 1 minute between puffs to enhance drug action.
• Use of a spacer device isn't necessary.
⊛ **ALERT:** Taper oral corticosteroid therapy slowly. Acute adrenal insufficiency and death have occurred in patients with asthma who changed abruptly from oral corticosteroids to beclomethasone.
• Notify prescriber if decreased response is noted after giving drug.
• Have patient gargle and rinse mouth with water after inhalations to help prevent oral fungal infections.
Patient teaching
• Tell patient to prime the inhaler before first use, or after 10 days of not using it, by depressing canister twice into the air.
• Inform patient that drug doesn't relieve acute asthma attacks.
• Tell patient who needs a bronchodilator to use it several minutes before beclomethasone.
• Instruct patient to carry or wear medical identification indicating his need for supplemental systemic corticosteroids during stress.
• Advise patient to allow 1 minute to elapse between inhalations of drug and to hold his breath for a few seconds to enhance drug action.
• Tell patient it may take up to 4 weeks to feel the full benefit of the drug.
• Tell patient to keep inhaler clean by wiping it weekly with a dry tissue or cloth; don't get it wet.
• Advise patient to prevent oral fungal infections by gargling or rinsing his mouth with water after each use. Caution him not to swallow the water.

• Tell patient to report evidence of corticosteroid withdrawal, including fatigue, weakness, arthralgia, orthostatic hypotension, and dyspnea.
• Instruct patient to store drug at 77° F (25° C) and advise patient to give at room temperature.

☑ Evaluation
• Patient's lungs are clear, and breathing and skin color are normal.
• Patient doesn't exhibit an oral fungal infection during therapy.
• Patient and family state understanding of drug therapy.

beclomethasone dipropionate monohydrate
(bek-loh-METH-eh-sohn digh-proh-PIGH-uh-nayt mon-oh-HIGH-drayt)
Beconase AQ

Pharmacologic class: corticosteroid
Therapeutic class: anti-inflammatory
Pregnancy risk category: C

Indications and dosages

▶ **Symptoms of allergic rhinitis; prevention of recurrence of nasal polyps after surgical removal.** *Adults and children age 12 and older:* 1 to 2 inhalations or sprays in each nostril, b.i.d. Maximum dosage, 256 mcg daily, given in each nostril as 128 mcg (4 sprays) once daily.
Children ages 6 to 11: 1 inhalation or spray in each nostril b.i.d. Those with more severe symptoms may need 2 inhalations in each nostril twice daily.

Contraindications and cautions

• Contraindicated in patients hypersensitive to drug and in those experiencing status asthmaticus or other acute episodes of asthma.
• Use cautiously, if at all, in patients with active or quiescent respiratory tract tubercular infections, or untreated fungal, bacterial, systemic viral, or ocular herpes simplex infections. Also use cautiously in patients who've recently had nasal septal ulcers, nasal surgery, or trauma.
� **Lifespan:** In pregnant or breast-feeding women, use cautiously. In children younger than age 6, safety and effectiveness of drug haven't been established.

Reactions may be *common,* uncommon, *life-threatening,* or COMMON AND LIFE-THREATENING.

Adverse reactions

CNS: headache.
EENT: *mild, transient nasal burning* and stinging; nasal congestion; sneezing; epistaxis; watery eyes; nasopharyngeal fungal infections; irritation of nasal mucosa.
GI: nausea, vomiting.

Interactions

None significant.

Effects on lab test results

None reported.

Pharmacokinetics

Absorption: Primarily through nasal mucosa with minimal systemic absorption.
Distribution: Unknown.
Metabolism: Most of drug in liver.
Excretion: Unknown. *Half-life:* 15 hours.

Route	Onset	Peak	Duration
Inhalation	5–7 days	≤ 3 wk	Unknown

Action

Chemical effect: Decreases nasal inflammation, mainly by stabilizing leukocyte lysosomal membranes.
Therapeutic effect: Helps relieve nasal allergy symptoms.

Available forms

Nasal aerosol: 42 mcg/metered spray
Nasal spray: 42 mcg/metered spray

NURSING PROCESS

⚕ Assessment

• Obtain history of patient's allergy symptoms and nasal congestion before therapy, and reassess regularly thereafter.
• Be alert for adverse reactions.
• Monitor patient's hydration status if adverse GI reactions occur.
• Check for irritation of nasal mucosa.
• Assess patient's and family's understanding of drug therapy.

⊕ Nursing diagnoses

• Ineffective health maintenance related to allergy-induced nasal congestion

• Risk for deficient fluid volume related to drug-induced adverse GI reactions
• Deficient knowledge related to drug therapy

▷ Planning and implementation

• Drug isn't effective for acute rhinitis. Decongestants or antihistamines may be needed.
• Shake container and invert. Have patient clear his nasal passages and then tilt his head backward. Insert nozzle (pointed away from septum) into nostril, holding other nostril closed. Deliver spray while patient inhales. Shake container and repeat in other nostril.
• Notify prescriber if relief isn't obtained or signs of infection appear.
Patient teaching
• Teach patient how to give himself nasal spray.
• Advise patient to pump new nasal spray three or four times before first use and once or twice before first use each day thereafter. Also tell patient to clean cap and nosepiece of activator in warm water every day and air-dry them.
• Advise patient to use drug regularly, as prescribed, because its effectiveness depends on regular use.
• Explain that drug's therapeutic effects, unlike those of decongestants, aren't immediate. Most patients achieve benefit within a few days, but some may require 2 to 3 weeks.
• Warn patient not to exceed recommended doses because of risk of hypothalamic-pituitary-adrenal function suppression.
• Tell patient to notify prescriber if symptoms don't improve within 3 weeks or if nasal irritation persists.
• Teach patient good nasal and oral hygiene.

☑ Evaluation

• Patient's nasal congestion subsides with therapy.
• Patient maintains adequate hydration throughout therapy.
• Patient and family state understanding of drug therapy.

benazepril hydrochloride

(ben-AY-zuh-pril high-droh-KLOR-ighd)
Lotensin

Pharmacologic class: ACE inhibitor
Therapeutic class: antihypertensive
Pregnancy risk category: C (D in second and third trimesters)

Indications and dosages

▶ **Hypertension.** *Adults not taking diuretics:* Initially, 10 mg P.O. daily. Dosage adjusted, as needed and tolerated; usually, 20 to 40 mg daily, equally divided into one or two doses. Maximum, 80 mg daily.
Adults taking diuretics: Stop diuretic 2 to 3 days before starting benazepril hydrochloride to minimize hypotension. If unable to stop diuretic, start dose at 5 mg daily.
Adjust-a-dose: For adults with renal impairment, if creatinine clearance is less than 30 ml/minute, start dose at 5 mg daily. Don't exceed 40 mg P.O. daily.
Children age 6 and older with creatinine clearance greater than 30 ml/minute: 0.2 mg/kg P.O. daily. Doses exceeding 0.6 mg/kg (or in excess of 40 mg/day) haven't been studied.

Contraindications and cautions

- Contraindicated in patients hypersensitive to ACE inhibitors.
- Use cautiously in patients with impaired hepatic or renal function.

Lifespan: In pregnant women, stop drug as soon as possible; it can cause injury and death to the fetus during the second and third trimesters. With breast-feeding women, use cautiously. In children younger than age 6 years or those with a glomerular filtration rate less than 30 ml/minute, safety of drug hasn't been established.

Adverse reactions

CNS: asthenia, headache, dizziness, lightheadedness, anxiety, amnesia, depression, insomnia, nervousness, neuralgia, neuropathy, paresthesia, somnolence, syncope.
CV: ***symptomatic hypotension,*** angina, ***arrhythmias,*** palpitations, edema.
GI: nausea, vomiting, abdominal pain, constipation, dyspepsia, gastritis, dysphagia, increased salivation.
GU: impotence.
Metabolic: ***hyperkalemia,*** weight gain.
Musculoskeletal: arthralgia, arthritis, myalgia.
Respiratory: dry, persistent, tickling, nonproductive cough; dyspnea.
Skin: rash, dermatitis, increased diaphoresis, pruritus, photosensitivity, purpura.
Other: ***angioedema,*** hypersensitivity reactions.

Interactions

Drug-drug. *ACE inhibitors, diuretics, other antihypertensives:* May cause excessive hypotension. Stop diuretic or lower dose of benazepril, if needed.
Digoxin: May increase digoxin level. Monitor patient for toxicity.
Indomethacin, aspirin: May reduce hypotensive effects. Monitor blood pressure.
Lithium: May increase lithium level and lithium toxicity. Avoid using together.
Potassium-sparing diuretics, potassium supplements: May cause hyperkalemia. Monitor patient closely.
Drug-herb. *Capsicum:* May aggravate or cause ACE-induced cough. Discourage using together.
Licorice: May cause sodium retention, thus decreasing ACE effects. Discourage using together.
Sodium substitutes containing potassium: May cause hyperkalemia. Monitor patient closely.

Effects on lab test results

- May increase BUN, creatinine, uric acid, glucose, bilirubin, liver enzymes, and potassium levels.

Pharmacokinetics

Absorption: At least 37%.
Distribution: Highly protein-bound.
Metabolism: Almost completely in liver to benazeprilat, which has much greater ACE inhibitory activity than benazepril.
Excretion: Primarily in urine. *Half-life:* Benazepril, 0.6 hours; benazeprilat, 10 to 12 hours.

Route	Onset	Peak	Duration
P.O.	≤ 1 hr	2–6 hr	24 hr

Action

Chemical effect: Inhibits ACE, preventing conversion of angiotensin I to angiotensin II, a potent vasoconstrictor. Reduced formation of angiotensin II decreases peripheral arterial resistance, thus decreasing aldosterone secretion. This reduces sodium and water retention and lowers blood pressure. Benazepril also has antihypertensive activity in patients with low-renin hypertension.

Therapeutic effect: Lowers blood pressure.

Available forms

Tablets: 5 mg, 10 mg, 20 mg, 40 mg

NURSING PROCESS

Assessment
• Obtain history of patient's blood pressure before therapy and reassess regularly thereafter. Measure blood pressure when drug levels are at peak (2 to 6 hours after dose) and at trough (just before dose) to verify adequate blood pressure control.
• Be alert for adverse reactions and drug interactions.
• Monitor patient's ECG.
• Monitor renal and hepatic function periodically. Also monitor potassium levels.
• Monitor patient's CBC with differential every 2 weeks for first 3 months of therapy and periodically thereafter. Other ACE inhibitors have been linked to agranulocytosis and neutropenia.
• Assess patient's and family's understanding of drug therapy.

Nursing diagnoses
• Risk for injury related to hypertension
• Decreased cardiac output related to drug-induced arrhythmias
• Deficient knowledge related to drug therapy

Planning and implementation
• If patient is taking a diuretic, dose should be lower than if patient isn't taking a diuretic; excessive hypotension can occur when drug is given with diuretics.
• For children who can't swallow pills, an oral suspension can be made from the tablet.
• Give drug at about the same time every day to maintain consistent effect on blood pressure.
• Give drug when patient's stomach is empty.

Patient teaching
• Instruct patient to take drug on an empty stomach; meals, particularly those high in fat, can impair absorption.
• Tell patient to avoid sodium substitutes because such products may contain potassium,

which can cause hyperkalemia in patients taking drug.
• Tell patient to rise slowly to minimize risk of dizziness, which may occur during first few weeks of therapy. Advise patient to stop taking drug and call prescriber immediately if dizziness occurs.
• Tell patient to use caution in hot weather and during exercise. Inadequate fluid intake, vomiting, diarrhea, and excessive perspiration can lead to light-headedness and syncope.
• Urge patient to report signs of infection, such as fever and sore throat. Also tell him to call prescriber if any of the following signs or symptoms occur: easy bruising or bleeding; swelling of tongue, lips, face, eyes, mucous membranes, or limbs; difficulty swallowing or breathing; or hoarseness.
• Tell woman to notify prescriber if pregnancy occurs. Drug will need to be stopped.

Evaluation
• Patient's blood pressure is normal.
• Patient maintains adequate cardiac output during drug therapy.
• Patient and family state understanding of drug therapy.

benztropine mesylate
(BENZ-troh-peen MES-ih-layt)
Apo-Benztropine ♦, Cogentin

Pharmacologic class: anticholinergic
Therapeutic class: antiparkinsonian
Pregnancy risk category: C

Indications and dosages

► **Drug-induced extrapyramidal disorders (except tardive dyskinesia).** *Adults:* 1 to 4 mg P.O. or I.M. once or twice daily.
► **Acute dystonic reaction.** *Adults:* 1 to 2 mg I.V. or I.M., followed by 1 to 2 mg P.O. b.i.d. to prevent recurrence.
► **Parkinsonism.** *Adults:* 0.5 to 6 mg P.O. daily. Initial dose is 0.5 to 1 mg. I.M. or P.O. Because of cumulative action, initiate at a low dose and increase by 0.5 mg q 5 to 6 days. Adjust dosage to meet individual requirements. Maximum daily dose is 6 mg.

▼ I.V. administration

• Drug is seldom used I.V. because of small difference in onset compared with I.M. route.

⊗ **Incompatibilities**

None reported.

Contraindications and cautions

• Contraindicated in patients hypersensitive to drug or any of its components, and in those with acute angle-closure glaucoma.

• Use cautiously in patients exposed to hot weather; those with mental disorders; and those with prostatic hyperplasia, arrhythmias, seizure disorder, obstructive disease of the GI or GU tract, or tendency of urinary retention.

Lifespan: In pregnant women, use cautiously. In breast-feeding women and children younger than age 3, drug is contraindicated. In children age 3 and older and patients older than age 60, use cautiously.

Adverse reactions

CNS: disorientation, restlessness, irritability, incoherence, hallucinations, headache, sedation, depression, nervousness, confusion.

CV: palpitations, tachycardia, ***paradoxical bradycardia,*** flushing.

EENT: dilated pupils, blurred vision, photophobia, difficulty swallowing.

GI: dry mouth, *constipation,* nausea, vomiting, epigastric distress.

GU: urinary hesitancy, urine retention.

Musculoskeletal: muscle weakness.

Interactions

Drug-drug. *Amantadine, phenothiazines, tricyclic antidepressants:* May cause additive anticholinergic adverse reactions, such as hyperthermia or heat intolerance. Notify prescriber immediately if adverse GI effects, fever, or heat intolerance occurs.

Anticholinergics and other antiparkinsonians: May increase anticholinergic effects and may be fatal. Use cautiously.

Cholinesterase inhibitors: May decrease effectiveness of cholinesterase inhibitors.

Effects on lab test results

None reported.

Pharmacokinetics

Absorption: Unknown.

Distribution: Largely unknown; however, drug crosses blood–brain barrier.

Metabolism: Unknown.

Excretion: In urine as unchanged drug and metabolites. *Half-life:* Unknown.

Route	Onset	Peak	Duration
P.O.	1–2 hr	Unknown	24 hr
I.V., I.M.	≤ 15 min	Unknown	24 hr

Action

Chemical effect: Unknown; thought to block central cholinergic receptors, helping to balance cholinergic activity in basal ganglia.

Therapeutic effect: Improves capability for voluntary movement.

Available forms

Injection: 1 mg/ml in 2-ml ampules

Tablets: 0.5 mg, 1 mg, 2 mg

NURSING PROCESS

Assessment

• Obtain history of patient's dyskinetic movements and underlying condition before therapy.

• Monitor effectiveness by regularly checking body movements for signs of improvement. Full effect of drug may take 2 to 3 days.

• Be alert for adverse reactions and drug interactions. Some adverse reactions may result from atropine-like toxicity and are dose related.

• Assess patient's and family's understanding of drug therapy.

Nursing diagnoses

• Impaired physical mobility related to dyskinetic movements

• Risk for injury related to drug-induced adverse CNS reactions

• Deficient knowledge related to drug therapy

Planning and implementation

ALERT: Never stop drug abruptly. Reduce dose gradually.

• Give drug after meals to help prevent GI distress.

• The I.M. route is preferred for parenteral administration.

• Give drug h.s. if patient is to receive single daily dose.

Patient teaching
• Warn patient to avoid activities requiring alertness until CNS effects of drug are known.
• If patient will receive single daily dose, tell him to take it at bedtime.
• If patient will receive drug orally, tell him to take it after meals.
• Advise patient to report signs of urinary hesitancy or urine retention.
• Tell patient to relieve dry mouth with cool drinks, ice chips, sugarless gum, or hard candy.
• Advise patient to limit activities during hot weather because drug-induced anhidrosis may result in hyperthermia.

☑ Evaluation
• Patient exhibits improved mobility with reduction in muscle rigidity, akinesia, and tremors.
• Patient doesn't experience injury as a result of drug-induced adverse CNS reactions.
• Patient and family state understanding of drug therapy.

bethanechol chloride
(beh-THAN-eh-kol KLOR-ighd)
Duvoid ◆ , Urecholine

Pharmacologic class: cholinergic agonist
Therapeutic class: urinary tract stimulant
Pregnancy risk category: C

Indications and dosages
▶ **Acute postoperative and postpartum nonobstructive (functional) urinary retention, neurogenic atony of urinary bladder with urinary retention.** *Adults:* 10 to 50 mg P.O. t.i.d. to q.i.d. When used for urine retention, some patients may need 50 to 100 mg P.O. per dose. Use such doses with extreme caution. All doses must be adjusted individually.
▶ **Bladder dysfunction caused by phenothiazines‡.** *Adults:* 50 to 100 mg P.O. q.i.d.
▶ **Chronic gastroesophageal reflux‡.** *Adults:* 25 mg P.O. q.i.d.
Infants and children: 3 mg/m² P.O. t.i.d.

Contraindications and cautions
• Contraindicated when increased muscle activity of GI or urinary tract is harmful. Also contraindicated in patients hypersensitive to the drug or any of its components and in those with hyperthyroidism, peptic ulceration, latent or active bronchial asthma, pronounced bradycardia or hypotension, vasomotor instability, cardiac or coronary artery disease, seizure disorder, Parkinson's disease, spastic GI disturbances, acute inflammatory lesions of GI tract, peritonitis, mechanical obstruction of GI or urinary tract, marked vagotonia, or uncertain strength or integrity of bladder wall.
🕮 **Lifespan:** In pregnant women, use cautiously. In breast-feeding women, use should be avoided. In children, safety of drug for labeled uses hasn't been established.

Adverse reactions
CNS: headache, malaise.
CV: *bradycardia,* hypotension, flushing, reflex tachycardia.
EENT: lacrimation, miosis.
GI: *abdominal cramps, diarrhea,* excessive salivation, nausea, vomiting, belching, borborygmi, esophageal spasms.
GU: urinary urgency.
Respiratory: *bronchoconstriction,* increased bronchial secretions.
Skin: sweating.

Interactions
Drug-drug. *Anticholinergics, atropine, procainamide, quinidine:* May reverse cholinergic effects. Watch for lack of drug effect.
Anticholinesterases, cholinergic agonists: May cause additive effects or increase toxicity. Avoid using together.
Ganglionic blockers: May cause severe abdominal pain followed by a critical drop in blood pressure. Avoid using together.

Effects on lab test results
• May increase liver enzyme, amylase, and lipase levels.

Pharmacokinetics
Absorption: Poor.
Distribution: Unknown.
Metabolism: Unknown.
Excretion: Unknown. *Half life:* Unknown

Route	Onset	Peak	Duration
P.O.	30–90 min	1 hr	1–6 hr

Action

Chemical effect: Directly stimulates cholinergic receptors, mimicking action of acetylcholine.
Therapeutic effect: Relieves urine retention.

Available forms

Tablets: 5 mg, 10 mg, 25 mg, 50 mg

NURSING PROCESS

⚗ Assessment

• Obtain history of patient's bladder condition before therapy and reassess regularly throughout therapy.
• Be alert for adverse reactions and drug interactions.
• Assess patient's and family's understanding of drug therapy.

⊞ Nursing diagnoses

• Impaired urinary elimination related to underlying bladder condition
• Ineffective breathing pattern related to drug-induced bronchoconstriction
• Deficient knowledge related to drug therapy

▷ Planning and implementation

• Give P.O. drug on empty stomach to prevent nausea and vomiting.
• **ALERT:** When inpatient, always have atropine injection readily available and be prepared to give 0.5 mg subcutaneously or by slow I.V. push. Provide respiratory support, p.r.n.
Patient teaching
• Advise patient to take oral dose on an empty stomach.
• Tell patient to report breathing difficulty immediately.

☑ Evaluation

• Patient is able to void without urine retention.
• Patient's respiratory function remains normal during therapy.
• Patient and family state understanding of drug therapy.

bevacizumab
(bev-a-SIZ-u-mab)
Avastin

Pharmacologic class: monoclonal antibody
Therapeutic class: antineoplastic
Pregnancy risk category: C

Indications and dosages

▶ **First-line use with fluorouracil-based therapy for metastatic colon or rectal cancer.**
Adults: 5 mg/kg I.V. every 14 days until disease progression is detected.

▼ I.V. administration

• Dilute using aseptic technique. Don't freeze or shake the vials. Withdraw proper dose and mix into I.V. bag in a total volume of 100 ml normal saline solution.
• Give the first infusion over 90 minutes and, if tolerated, the second infusion over 60 minutes. Later infusions can be given over 30 minutes if patient tolerated previous infusions.
• Don't give by I.V. push or bolus.
• Drug is stable for 8 hours if refrigerated at 36° to 46° F (2° to 8° C) and protected from light.
⊗ **Incompatibilities**
Dextrose solutions.

Contraindications and cautions

• Contraindicated in patients with recent hemoptysis or within 28 days after major surgery.
• Use with extreme caution if patient has significant cardiovascular disease or history of arterial thromboembolism.
• Use cautiously in patients hypersensitive to drug or any of its components. Also use cautiously in patients who need surgery.
⚘ **Lifespan:** In pregnant women, use during pregnancy only if potential benefits to the mother outweigh risks to the fetus. In breast-feeding women, stop nursing during therapy and for 60 days after therapy stops because of the drug's long half-life. In children, safety and effectiveness haven't been established. In patients age 65 or older, increased risk of serious to fatal arterial thromboembolic events.

Adverse reactions

CNS: abnormal gait, *asthenia*, confusion, *dizziness, headache,* pain, syncope.

CV: deep vein thrombosis, heart failure, *hypertension,* hypotension, INTRA-ABDOMINAL THROMBOSIS, *thromboembolism.*
EENT: *epistaxis,* excess lacrimation, gum bleeding, taste disorder, voice alteration.
GI: abdominal pain, *anorexia,* colitis, *constipation, diarrhea,* dry mouth, *dyspepsia, flatulence, GI hemorrhage,* nausea, *stomatitis, vomiting.*
GU: proteinuria, urinary urgency, *vaginal hemorrhage.*
Hematologic: *leukopenia, neutropenia, thrombocytopenia.*
Metabolic: bilirubinemia, *hypokalemia, weight loss.*
Musculoskeletal: *myalgia.*
Respiratory: *dyspnea,* HEMOPTYSIS, *upper respiratory tract infection.*
Skin: *alopecia, dermatitis, discoloration, dry skin, exfoliative dermatitis,* nail disorder, skin ulcer.
Other: decreased wound healing, hypersensitivity.

Interactions

Drug-drug. *Irinotecan:* May increase levels of irinotecan metabolite (SN-38). Monitor patient.

Effects on lab test results

• May increase bilirubin and urine protein levels. May decrease potassium level.
• May decrease WBC, neutrophil, and platelet counts.

Pharmacokinetics

Absorption: Given I.V.
Distribution: Unknown.
Metabolism: Degraded to basic peptides via phagocytosis by the reticuloendothelial system.
Excretion: Via the reticuloendothelial system. *Half-life:* 11 to 50 days.

Route	Onset	Peak	Duration
I.V.	Unknown	Unknown	Unknown

Action

Chemical effect: Inhibits actions between proteins and cell surface receptors that would normally allow proliferation of endothelial cells and new blood vessel growth.
Therapeutic effect: Inhibits metastatic colon or rectal tumor growth.

Available forms

Solution: 25 mg/ml in 4-ml and 16-ml vials

NURSING PROCESS

✒ Assessment

• Assess patient's condition before therapy and regularly thereafter.
• Monitor CBC, platelet count, and serum electrolytes before and during therapy.
• Monitor patient for hypersensitivity reactions, which can occur during infusions.
• Monitor urinalysis for presence of worsening of proteinuria. Patients with 2+ or greater urine dipstick test should undergo 24-hour urine collection.
• Monitor patient's blood pressure every 2 to 3 weeks.
• Assess patient's and family's knowledge of drug therapy.

Nursing diagnoses

• Ineffective health maintenance related to presence of neoplastic disease
• Delayed surgical recovery related to decreased wound healing effects of drug
• Deficient knowledge related to bevacizumab therapy

▶ Planning and implementation

• Monitor patient for serious adverse effects during therapy. Stop drug if patient develops nephrotic syndrome, severe hypertension, hypertensive crisis, serious hemorrhage, GI perforation, or wound dehiscence that needs intervention.
• Stop drug before elective surgery, taking into account drug's half-life of about 20 days. Don't resume therapy until surgical incision is fully healed.
• ⚠ ALERT: Increased risk of serious to fatal arterial thromboembolic events, including MI, transient ischemic attacks, stroke, and angina have been reported in patients age 65 or older. Patients age 65 or older, those with a history of arterial thromboembolism, and those previously treated with bevacizumab are at the highest risk. Patients who experience any type of arterial thrombotic event should permanently stop the drug.
• Treat symptoms and provide supportive care if overdose occurs. Large doses may cause head-

ache, and the maximum tolerated dose is un-
known.
Patient teaching
• Inform patient about potential adverse reactions.
• Tell patient to immediately report adverse reactions, especially abdominal pain, constipation, or vomiting.
• Advise patient that blood pressure and urinalysis will be monitored during treatment.
• Caution women of childbearing age to avoid pregnancy during treatment.
• Urge patient to alert other health care providers about treatment and to avoid elective surgery during treatment.

☑ **Evaluation**
• Patient responds to drug therapy.
• Drug is stopped prior to surgery. Drug therapy isn't started until surgical incision is fully healed.
• Patient and family state understanding of drug therapy.

bexarotene

(bex-AHR-oh-teen)
Targretin

Pharmacologic class: retinoid (selective retinoid X receptor activator)
Therapeutic class: tumor cell growth inhibitor
Pregnancy risk category: X

Indications and dosages

▶ **Cutaneous effects of cutaneous T-cell lymphoma in patients refractory to at least one previous systemic therapy.** *Adults:* 300 mg/m² P.O. daily as a single dose with a meal. If no response after 8 weeks, increase to 400 mg/m² daily. Adjust dosage to 200 mg/m² daily, and then to 100 mg/m² daily if toxicity occurs, or drug may be temporarily suspended. When toxicity is controlled, dosage may be carefully readjusted upward. Or, for topical application, apply a sufficient amount of 1% gel and rub into the affected areas once every other day, for the first week. Allow gel to dry before applying a dressing. Then increase at weekly intervals to b.i.d., t.i.d., and q.i.d., according to the individual skin response.

⊠ **Adjust-a-dose:** For patients with hepatic insufficiency, lower doses may be needed. If toxicity occurs, dosage may be adjusted to 200 mg/m² daily, then to 100 mg/m² daily, or drug may be temporarily suspended. When toxicity is controlled, adjust upward carefully.

Contraindications and cautions

• Contraindicated in patients hypersensitive to the drug or any of its components.
• Drug isn't recommended for patients taking drugs that increase triglyceride levels or cause pancreatic toxicity or those who have risk factors for pancreatitis, such as prior pancreatitis, uncontrolled hyperlipidemia, excessive alcohol consumption, uncontrolled diabetes mellitus, or biliary tract disease.
• Use cautiously in patients with hepatic insufficiency and in patients hypersensitive to retinoids.
⚘ **Lifespan:** In pregnant women, drug is contraindicated. In women of childbearing age, use cautiously. In breast-feeding women, stop the drug or breast-feeding, taking into account the importance of the drug to the mother. In children younger than 18 years, safety and effectiveness haven't been established.

Adverse reactions

CNS: fever, *headache,* insomnia, *asthenia,* fatigue, syncope, depression, agitation, ataxia, **stroke,** confusion, dizziness, hyperesthesia, hypoesthesia, neuropathy.
CV: *peripheral edema,* chest pain, **hemorrhage,** hypertension, angina, **heart failure,** tachycardia.
EENT: cataracts, pharyngitis, rhinitis, dry eyes, conjunctivitis, ear pain, blepharitis, corneal lesion, keratitis, otitis externa, visual field defect.
GI: *nausea,* diarrhea, vomiting, anorexia, **pancreatitis,** *abdominal pain,* constipation, dry mouth, flatulence, colitis, dyspepsia, cheilitis, gastroenteritis, gingivitis, melena.
GU: albuminuria, hematuria, incontinence, UTI, urinary urgency, dysuria, abnormal kidney function.
Hematologic: *leukopenia,* anemia, eosinophilia, *thrombocythemia,* lymphocytosis, ***thrombocytopenia.***
Hepatic: bilirubinemia, *liver failure.*
Metabolic: *hyperlipemia, hypercholesteremia, hypothyroidism,* hyperglycemia, hypoproteine-

---

Reactions may be *common,* uncommon, *life-threatening,* or COMMON AND LIFE-THREATENING.

mia, hypocalcemia, hyponatremia, weight change.

Musculoskeletal: arthralgia, myalgia, back pain, bone pain, myasthenia, arthrosis.

Respiratory: pneumonia, dyspnea, hemoptysis, pleural effusion, bronchitis, cough, *lung edema, hypoxia.*

Skin: (P.O.) rash, dry skin, exfoliative dermatitis, alopecia, photosensitivity, pruritus, cellulitis, acne, skin ulcer, skin nodule; **(Topical)** *contact dermatitis, pain, skin disorders, pruritus, rash.*

Other: breast pain, *infection,* chills, flulike syndrome, *sepsis.*

Interactions

Drug-drug. *Diethyltoluamide (DEET):* May increase DEET toxicity with gel form. Avoid using together.

Erythromycin, gemfibrozil, itraconazole, ketoconazole, other inhibitors of CYP 3A4: May increase level of bexarotene. Avoid using together.

Hormonal contraceptives: May decrease plasma concentration of contraceptive. Use alternative method of birth control.

Insulin, sulfonylureas: May enhance hypoglycemic action of these drugs, resulting in hypoglycemia in patients with diabetes mellitus. Use together cautiously.

Phenobarbital, phenytoin, rifampin, other inducers of CYP 3A4: May decrease level of bexarotene. Avoid using together.

Vitamin A preparations: May increase potential for vitamin A toxicity. Avoid vitamin A supplements.

Drug-food. *Any food:* Enhances drug absorption. Give with food.

Grapefruit juice: May inhibit CYP 3A4. Don't give together.

Drug-lifestyle. *Sun exposure:* Retinoids may cause photosensitivity. Advise patient to minimize exposure to sunlight and artificial ultraviolet light.

Effects on lab test results

• May increase creatinine, LDH, AST, ALT, bilirubin, amylase, lipid, cholesterol, glucose, and thyroid-stimulating hormone (TSH) levels. May decrease protein, calcium, sodium, and hemoglobin levels and hematocrit.

• May increase eosinophil count. May decrease WBC and lymphocyte counts. May alter platelet count.

• May increase CA 125 assay values in patients with ovarian cancer.

Pharmacokinetics

Absorption: Increased if given P.O. with a meal that contains fat. Unknown for topical use.

Distribution: More than 99% protein-bound. Low level with topical use.

Metabolism: Metabolized through oxidative pathways, primarily by the cytochrome P450 3A4 system, to four metabolites. These may maintain retinoid receptor activity.

Excretion: Thought to be eliminated primarily through the hepatobiliary system. *Terminal half-life:* 7 hours.

Route	Onset	Peak	Duration
P.O., topical	Unknown	Unknown	Unknown

Action

Chemical effect: Selectively binds and activates retinoid X receptor subtypes. Once activated, these receptors regulate the expression of genes that control cellular differentiation and proliferation.

Therapeutic effect: Inhibits tumor growth in cutaneous T-cell lymphoma.

Available forms

Capsules: 75 mg
Topical gel: 1%

NURSING PROCESS

☞ Assessment

• Assess women of childbearing age carefully. A negative pregnancy test should be obtained within 1 week before therapy starts and monthly during therapy.

• Men with sexual partners who are pregnant, who could be pregnant, or who could become pregnant must use a condom during sexual intercourse during therapy and for at least 1 month after therapy ends.

• Obtain total cholesterol, HDL, and triglyceride levels when therapy starts, weekly until the lipid response is established (2 to 4 weeks) and at 8-week intervals thereafter. Elevated triglycerides during treatment should be treated with antilipemic therapy and the dose of bexarotene reduced or suspended, p.r.n.

• Obtain baseline thyroid function tests, and monitor results during treatment.
• Monitor WBC with differential at baseline and periodically during treatment.
• Monitor liver function test results at baseline and after 1, 2, and 4 weeks of treatment. If patient is stable, monitor test results every 8 weeks during treatment. The prescriber may consider suspending treatment if results are three times the upper limit of normal.
• Monitor TSH levels and patient for signs and symptoms of hypothyroidism.
• Obtain ophthalmologic evaluation for cataracts in patients who experience visual difficulties.
• Assess patient's and family's knowledge of drug therapy.

Nursing diagnoses
• Ineffective health maintenance related to underlying condition
• Risk for injury related to drug-induced adverse reactions
• Deficient knowledge related to drug therapy

Planning and implementation
• Lower doses may be needed for patients with hepatic insufficiency.
• Give drug with food for better absorption, although not with grapefruit or grapefruit juice.
• Start therapy on the second or third day of a normal menstrual period.
• No more than a 1-month supply of bexarotene should be given to a patient who could become pregnant so the results of pregnancy testing can be assessed regularly and the patient can be reminded to avoid pregnancy.
Patient teaching
• Advise patient to minimize unprotected or prolonged exposure to sunlight or artificial ultraviolet light.
• Teach patient that it may take several capsules to make the necessary dose and that these capsules should all be taken at the same time and with a meal.
• Teach women of childbearing age the dangers of becoming pregnant while taking bexarotene and the need for monthly pregnancy tests.
• Explain the need for obtaining baseline laboratory tests and for periodic monitoring of these tests.
• Tell patient to report any visual changes.

• Advise patient to wait at least 20 minutes after bathing before applying the gel and to avoid the use of occlusive dressings.
• Tell patient to avoid gel contact with healthy skin or mucous membranes.
• Tell patient to allow the gel to dry for 5 to 10 minutes before covering area with clothing.
• Tell patient to use effective contraception at least 1 month before therapy starts, during therapy, and for at least 1 month after therapy stops.
• Tell patient to use two reliable forms of contraception simultaneously during therapy unless abstinence is the chosen method.

✓ Evaluation
• Patient exhibits positive response to therapy.
• Patient has no injury as a result of drug-induced adverse reactions.
• Patient and family state understanding of drug therapy.

bimatoprost
(by-MAT-oh-prost)
Lumigan

Pharmacologic class: prostaglandin analogue
Therapeutic class: antiglaucoma drug, ocular antihypertensive
Pregnancy risk category: C

Indications and dosages
▶ **To reduce elevated intraocular pressure (IOP) in patients with open-angle glaucoma or ocular hypertension who are intolerant of or unresponsive to other IOP-lowering drugs.**
Adults: Instill 1 drop in the conjunctival sac of the affected eye or eyes once daily in the evening.

Contraindications and cautions
• Contraindicated in patients hypersensitive to bimatoprost, benzalkonium chloride, or any of the drug's components. Also contraindicated in patients with angle-closure glaucoma, inflammatory glaucoma, or neovascular glaucoma.
• Use cautiously in patients with renal or hepatic impairment, active intraocular inflammation (iritis or uveitis), aphakic patients, pseudophakic patients with a torn posterior lens capsule, or patients at risk for macular edema.

🌢 Lifespan: In pregnant women, drug isn't recommended. In breast-feeding women, use cautiously because it's unknown whether drug appears in breast milk. In children, safety and effectiveness of drug haven't been established.

Adverse reactions

CNS: headache, asthenia.
EENT: *conjunctival hyperemia, growth of eyelashes, ocular pruritus,* ocular dryness, visual disturbance, ocular burning, foreign body sensation, eye pain, pigmentation of the periocular skin, blepharitis, cataract, superficial punctate keratitis, eyelid erythema, ocular irritation, eyelash darkening, eye discharge, tearing, photophobia, allergic conjunctivitis, asthenopia, increased iris pigmentation, conjunctival edema, gradual change in eye color.
Respiratory: *upper respiratory tract infection.*
Skin: hirsutism.
Other: *infection.*

Interactions

None significant.

Effects on lab test results

• May cause abnormal liver function test values.

Pharmacokinetics

Absorption: Through the cornea.
Distribution: Moderately into tissues. About 12% remains unbound.
Metabolism: Mainly by oxidation.
Excretion: Metabolites are 67% eliminated in urine; 25% are eliminated in feces. *Half life:* 45 minutes.

Route	Onset	Peak	Duration
Ophthalmic	4 hr	10 min	1½ hr

Action

Chemical effect: May increase the outflow of aqueous humor through the trabecular meshwork and uveoscleral routes.
Therapeutic effect: Reduces IOP.

Available forms

Ophthalmic solution: 0.03%

NURSING PROCESS

🗊 Assessment
⊕ ALERT: Obtain complete medication history. If more than one ophthalmic drug is being used, give drugs at least 5 minutes apart.
• Assess patient's underlying condition and eyes before giving eyedrops.
• Monitor patient for excessive ocular irritation and evaluate the success of treatment.
• Assess patient's and family's knowledge of drug therapy and administration.

⊕ Nursing diagnoses
• Risk for injury to the eye related to improper administration of drug
• Impaired visual perception related to underlying condition
• Deficient knowledge related to bimatoprost therapy

▶ Planning and implementation
⊕ ALERT: Contact lenses must be removed before using solution. Lenses may be reinserted 15 minutes after administration.
• Don't touch the tip of the dropper to the eye. Avoid contamination to the dropper.
• Apply light pressure on lacrimal sac for 1 minute after instillation to minimize systemic absorption of the drug.
• Store drug in original container at 59° to 77° F (15° to 25° C).
• Be aware that an increase in pigmentation of the iris, eyelid, and eyelashes may occur, as well as growth of the eyelashes.
Patient teaching
• Explain to patients receiving treatment in only one eye the possibility for increased brown pigmentation of iris, eyelid skin darkening, and increased length, thickness, pigmentation, or number of lashes in the treated eye.
• Teach patient to instill drops properly, and advise him to wash hands before and after instilling solution. Warn him not to touch tip of dropper to eye or surrounding tissue.
• If eye trauma or infection occurs or if eye surgery is needed, tell patient to seek immediate medical advice before continuing to use multidose container.
• Urge patient to immediately report conjunctivitis or lid reactions to prescriber.

B

☑ Evaluation

● Patient demonstrates proper administration of the drug, and no injury occurs.
● Patient's underlying eye condition responds positively to drug.
● Patient and family state understanding of drug therapy.

bisacodyl
(bigh-suh-KOH-dil)
Bisac-Evac†, **Bisacodyl Uniserts**†, **Bisacolax** ♦ †, **Bisalax** ◊, **Bisco-Lax**†, **Carter's Little Pills**†, **Correctol**†, **Dacodyl**†, **Deficol**†, **Dulcolax**†, **Durolax** ◊, **Feen-a-Mint**†, **Fleet Bisacodyl**†, **Fleet Laxative**†, **Fleet Prep Kit**†, **Laxit** ♦ †, **Modane**†, **Theralax**†

Pharmacologic class: diphenylmethane derivative
Therapeutic class: stimulant laxative
Pregnancy risk category: NR

Indications and dosages

▶ **Chronic constipation; preparation for childbirth, surgery, or rectal or bowel examination.** *Adults and children age 12 and older:* 10 to 15 mg P.O. in evening or before breakfast; maximum 30 mg P.O. For evacuation before examination or surgery, 10 mg P.R.
Children ages 6 to 12: 5 mg P.O. or P.R. h.s. or before breakfast.

Contraindications and cautions

● Contraindicated in patients hypersensitive to drug and in those with rectal bleeding, gastroenteritis, intestinal obstruction, or symptoms of appendicitis or acute surgical abdomen, such as abdominal pain, nausea, or vomiting.
⚕ **Lifespan:** In pregnant women and children younger than age 10, safety hasn't been established.

Adverse reactions

GI: *nausea, vomiting, abdominal cramps,* diarrhea (with high doses), *burning sensation in rectum* (with suppositories), protein-losing enteropathy (with excessive use), laxative dependence (with long-term or excessive use).
Metabolic: *alkalosis,* hypokalemia, fluid and electrolyte imbalance.

Musculoskeletal: muscle weakness (with excessive use), tetany.

Interactions

Drug-drug. *Antacids:* May cause gastric irritation or dyspepsia from premature dissolution of enteric coating. Avoid using together.
Drug-food. *Milk:* May cause gastric irritation or dyspepsia from premature dissolution of enteric coating. Avoid using together.

Effects on lab test results

● May increase phosphate and sodium levels. May decrease calcium, magnesium, and potassium levels.

Pharmacokinetics

Absorption: Minimal.
Distribution: Locally.
Metabolism: Up to 15% of P.O. dose may enter enterohepatic circulation.
Excretion: Primarily in feces; some excreted in urine. *Half-life:* unknown.

Route	Onset	Peak	Duration
P.O.	6–12 hr	Variable	Variable
P.R.	15–60 min	Variable	Variable

Action

Chemical effect: Increases peristalsis, probably by acting directly on smooth muscle of intestine. May irritate musculature, stimulate colonic intramural plexus, and promote fluid accumulation in colon and small intestine.
Therapeutic effect: Relieves constipation.

Available forms

Enema: 0.33 mg/dl†, 10 mg/5 ml (microenema) ◊, 10 mg/30 ml
Powder for rectal solution (*bisacodyl tannex*): 1.5 mg bisacodyl and 2.5 g tannic acid
Suppositories: 10 mg†
Tablets (enteric-coated): 5 mg†

NURSING PROCESS

☒ Assessment

● Obtain history of bowel disorder, GI status, fluid intake, nutritional status, exercise habits, and normal patterns of elimination.
● Monitor effectiveness by checking frequency and characteristics of stools.

Reactions may be *common,* uncommon, *life-threatening*, or COMMON AND LIFE-THREATENING.

- Be alert for adverse reactions and drug interactions.
- Auscultate bowel sounds at least once per shift. Check for pain and cramping.
- Assess patient's and family's understanding of drug therapy.

🔷 Nursing diagnoses
- Constipation related to interruption of normal pattern of elimination
- Acute pain related to drug-induced abdominal cramps
- Deficient knowledge related to drug therapy

❯ Planning and implementation
- Don't give tablets within 60 minutes of milk or antacid.
- Insert suppository as high as possible into rectum, and try to position suppository against rectal wall. Avoid embedding within fecal material because this may delay onset of action.
- Time administration of drug so as not to interfere with scheduled activities or sleep. Soft, formed stool usually is produced 15 to 60 minutes after P.R. administration.
- Tablets and suppositories are used together to clean colon before and after surgery and before barium enema.
- Store tablets and suppositories below 86° F (30° C).

Patient teaching
- Advise patient to swallow enteric-coated tablet whole to avoid GI irritation. Tell him not to take tablet within 1 hour of milk or antacid.
- Advise patient to report adverse effects to prescriber.
- Teach patient about dietary sources of fiber, including bran and other cereals, fresh fruit, and vegetables.
- Warn patient against excessive use of drug.

☑ Evaluation
- Patient reports return of normal bowel pattern of elimination.
- Patient is free from abdominal pain and cramping.
- Patient and family state understanding of drug therapy.

bismuth subgallate
(BIS-muth sub-GAL-ayt)
Devrom

bismuth subsalicylate
Children's Kaopectate†, Extra Strength Kaopectate†, Kaopectate (Regular)†, Maximum Strength Pepto-Bismol†, Pepto-Bismol†

Pharmacologic class: adsorbent
Therapeutic class: antidiarrheal
Pregnancy risk category: NR

Indications and dosages

▶ **To control fecal odors in colostomy, ileostomy, or incontinence.** *Adults:* 1 to 2 tablets subgallate P.O. t.i.d. with meals. Tablet can be chewed or swallowed whole.

▶ **Mild, nonspecific diarrhea.** *Adults and children age 12 and older:* 30 ml or 2 tablets subsalicylate P.O. q 30 minutes to 1 hour up to a maximum of eight doses in 24 hours and for no longer than 2 days.
Children ages 9 to 12: 15 ml or 1 tablet subsalicylate P.O. q 30 minutes to 1 hour up to a maximum of eight doses in 24 hours and for no longer than 2 days.
Children ages 6 to 9: 10 ml or ⅔ tablet subsalicylate P.O. q 30 minutes to 1 hour up to a maximum of eight doses in 24 hours and for no longer than 2 days.
Children ages 3 to 6: 5 ml or ½ tablet subsalicylate P.O. q 30 minutes to 1 hour up to a maximum of eight doses in 24 hours and for no longer than 2 days.

Contraindications and cautions

- Contraindicated in patients hypersensitive to salicylates.
- Use cautiously in patients already taking aspirin.
- ⚠ **Lifespan:** In pregnant or breast-feeding women, use cautiously.

Adverse reactions

GI: temporary darkening of tongue and stools.
Other: salicylism (with high doses).

Interactions

Drug-drug. *Aspirin, other salicylates:* May increase risk of salicylate toxicity. Monitor patient closely.
Oral anticoagulants, oral antidiabetics: Theoretical risk of increased effects of these drugs after high doses of bismuth subsalicylate. Monitor patient closely.
Probenecid: May decrease uricosuric effects after high doses of bismuth subsalicylate. Monitor patient closely.
Tetracycline: May decrease tetracycline absorption. Give drugs at least 2 hours apart.

Effects on lab test results

● May increase lipid levels.

Pharmacokinetics

Absorption: Poor; significant salicylate absorption may occur after using bismuth subsalicylate.
Distribution: Locally in gut.
Metabolism: Minimal.
Excretion: Bismuth subsalicylate is excreted in urine. *Half life:* Unknown.

Route	Onset	Peak	Duration
P.O.	1 hr	Unknown	Unknown

Action

Chemical effect: May adsorb toxins and provide protective coating for mucosa.
Therapeutic effect: Relieves diarrhea.

Available forms

bismuth subgallate
Tablets (chewable): 200 mg†
bismuth subsalicylate
Caplet: 262 mg
Liquid (Children's): 87 mg/5 ml
Liquid (Extra Strength): 175 mg/5 ml
Liquid (Regular): 87.3 mg/ml
Oral suspension: 130 mg/15 ml, 262.5 mg/15 ml†, 525 mg/15 ml†
Tablets (chewable): 262.5 mg†

NURSING PROCESS

Assessment
● Obtain history of patient's bowel disorder, GI status, and frequency of loose stools.
● Monitor drug's effectiveness by checking frequency and characteristics of stools.

● Be alert for adverse reactions and drug interactions.
● Check patient's hearing if he takes drug in large doses.
● Assess patient's and family's understanding of drug therapy.

Nursing diagnoses
● Diarrhea related to underlying GI condition
● Disturbed sensory perception (auditory) related to drug-induced salicylism
● Deficient knowledge related to drug therapy

Planning and implementation
● Avoid use before GI radiologic procedures because bismuth is radiopaque and may interfere with X-rays.
● Read label carefully because dosage varies with form of drug.
● If tinnitus occurs, stop drug and notify prescriber.
Patient teaching
⑤ ALERT: Oral nonprescription drug products containing bismuth subsalicylate or kaolin are the only ones generally recognized as safe and effective for use as antidiarrheal agents. (This doesn't affect the availability of loperamide products.)
● Advise patient that drug contains large amount of salicylate. Each tablet contains 102 mg; regular-strength liquid contains 130 mg/15 ml, and extra-strength liquid contains 230 mg/15 ml.
● Instruct patient to chew tablets well or to shake liquid before measuring dose.
● Tell patient to report diarrhea that persists for longer than 2 days or is accompanied by high fever.
● Tell patient to consult with prescriber before giving bismuth subsalicylate to children or teenagers who have or are recovering from flu or chickenpox.
● Inform patient that both liquid and tablet forms of Pepto-Bismol are effective against traveler's diarrhea. Tablets may be more convenient to carry.
● Tell patient that any darkening of stool or the tongue is temporary.

Evaluation
● Patient reports decrease or absence of loose stools.

Reactions may be *common*, uncommon, *life-threatening*, or COMMON AND LIFE-THREATENING.

- Patient remains free from signs and symptoms of salicylism.
- Patient and family state understanding of drug therapy.

bisoprolol fumarate
(bis-OP-roh-lol FYOO-muh-rayt)
Zebeta

Pharmacologic class: beta blocker
Therapeutic class: antihypertensive
Pregnancy risk category: C

Indications and dosages

▶ **Hypertension.** *Adults:* Initially, 5 mg P.O. once daily. If response is inadequate, increase to 10 mg or 20 mg P.O. daily; 20 mg is maximum recommended dosage.

⧄ **Adjust-a-dose:** For patients with renal impairment, a creatinine clearance of less than 40 ml/minute, hepatic dysfunction, cirrhosis, or hepatitis, start with 2.5 mg P.O. daily. Adjust dose cautiously.

▶ **Heart failure‡.** *Adults:* 1.25 mg P.O. daily for 2 to 4 weeks. This low-dose strength isn't available in the United States. If dose is tolerated, increase dose to 2.5 mg daily for 2 to 4 weeks. Subsequent doses can be doubled q 2 to 4 weeks, if tolerated.

Contraindications and cautions

- Contraindicated in patients hypersensitive to drug and in those with cardiogenic shock, overt cardiac failure, marked sinus bradycardia, or second- or third-degree AV block.
- Use cautiously in patients with bronchospastic disease. These patients should avoid beta blockers because blockade of beta₁ receptors isn't absolute and blockage of pulmonary beta₂ receptors may result in worsening of symptoms. If avoiding beta blockers is impossible, have a bronchodilator available. Also use cautiously in patients with diabetes, peripheral vascular disease, or thyroid disease, and in those with history of heart failure.
- ✵ **Lifespan:** In pregnant or breast-feeding women, use cautiously. In children, safety and effectiveness of drug haven't been established.

Adverse reactions

CNS: asthenia, fatigue, dizziness, headache, hypoesthesia, vivid dreams, depression, insomnia.
CV: *bradycardia,* peripheral edema, chest pain, *heart failure.*
EENT: pharyngitis, rhinitis, sinusitis.
GI: nausea, vomiting, diarrhea, dry mouth.
Musculoskeletal: arthralgia
Respiratory: cough, dyspnea.
Skin: sweating.

Interactions

Drug-drug. *Beta blockers:* May cause extreme hypotension. Don't use together.
Calcium channel blockers: May cause myocardial depression and AV conductive inhibition. Monitor ECG closely.
Guanethidine, reserpine: Can cause hypotension. Monitor patient closely.
NSAIDs: May decrease antihypertensive effect. Monitor blood pressure and adjust dosage.
Rifampin: May increase metabolic clearance of bisoprolol. Monitor patient.

Effects on lab test results

None reported.

Pharmacokinetics

Absorption: Bioavailability after 10-mg dose is about 80%.
Distribution: About 30% protein-bound.
Metabolism: First-pass metabolism of drug is about 20%.
Excretion: Equally by renal and nonrenal pathways, with about 50% of dose appearing unchanged in urine and remainder appearing as inactive metabolites. Less than 2% of dose is excreted in feces. *Half-life:* 9 to 12 hours.

Route	Onset	Peak	Duration
P.O.	Unknown	2–4 hr	24 hr

Action

Chemical effect: May decrease myocardial contractility, heart rate, and cardiac output; lowers blood pressure; and reduces myocardial oxygen consumption.
Therapeutic effect: Decreases blood pressure.

Available forms

Tablets: 5 mg, 10 mg

NURSING PROCESS

⚕ Assessment
• Obtain history of patient's hypertensive status before therapy, and check blood pressure regularly throughout therapy.
• Be alert for adverse reactions and drug interactions.
• Monitor patient's hydration status if adverse GI reactions occur.
• Closely monitor glucose level in patient with diabetes. Beta blockers may mask some evidence of hypoglycemia, such as tachycardia.
• Assess patient's and family's understanding of drug therapy.

⊕ Nursing diagnoses
• Risk for injury related to presence of hypertension
• Risk for deficient fluid volume related to drug-induced adverse GI reactions
• Deficient knowledge related to drug therapy

▷ Planning and implementation
• Have a beta$_2$ agonist (bronchodilator) available for patients with bronchospastic disease.
⧗ ALERT: Don't stop drug abruptly; angina may occur in patients with unrecognized coronary artery disease.
⧗ ALERT: Don't confuse Zebeta with Zestril, Zetia, or Zyrtec.
Patient teaching
• Tell patient to take drug as prescribed, even when he's feeling better. Warn him that abruptly discontinuing drug can worsen angina and precipitate MI. Explain that drug must be withdrawn gradually over 1 to 2 weeks.
• Instruct patient to call prescriber if adverse reactions occur.
• Tell patient with diabetes to closely monitor glucose levels.
• Tell patient to check with prescriber or pharmacist before taking OTC medications or herbal remedies.

✓ Evaluation
• Patient's blood pressure is normal.
• Patient maintains adequate fluid balance throughout therapy.
• Patient and family state understanding of drug therapy.

bivalirudin
(bye-VAL-ih-roo-din)
Angiomax

Pharmacologic class: direct thrombin inhibitor
Therapeutic class: anticoagulant
Pregnancy risk category: B

Indications and dosages

▶ **Anticoagulation in patients with unstable angina undergoing percutaneous transluminal coronary angioplasty (PTCA); anticoagulation in patients with unstable angina undergoing percutaneous coronary intervention (PCI), with provisional use of a glycoprotein IIb/IIIa platelet inhibitor (GPI).** *Adults:* Give 0.75 mg/kg I.V. bolus followed by a continuous infusion of 1.75 mg/kg/hour for the duration of the procedure. Check activated clotting time 5 minutes after bolus dose is given. May give additional 0.3 mg/kg bolus dose if needed. Infusion may continue for up to 4 hours after procedure. After 4-hour infusion, may give an additional infusion of 0.2 mg/kg/hour for up to 20 hours, if needed. Use with 300 to 325 mg aspirin.
▨ **Adjust-a-dose:** For patients with creatinine clearance of 30 ml/minute or less, decrease infusion rate to 1 mg/kg/hour. For patients on hemodialysis, reduce infusion rate to 0.25 mg/kg/hour. No reduction of bolus dose is needed.
▶ **Patients with or at risk for heparin-induced thrombocytopenia (HIT) or heparin-induced thrombocytopenia and thrombosis syndrome (HITTS) undergoing PCI.** *Adults:* 0.75 mg/kg I.V. bolus followed by continuous infusion of 1.75 mg/kg/hour for the duration of the procedure. The prescriber may continue the infusion after PCI.

▼ I.V. administration

• Reconstitute each 250-mg vial with 5 ml of sterile water for injection. Further dilute each reconstituted vial in 50 ml D$_5$W or normal saline solution to yield a final concentration of 5 mg/ml.
• To prepare low-rate infusion, further dilute each reconstituted vial in 500 ml D$_5$W or normal saline solution to yield a final concentration of 0.5 mg/ml.

• The prepared solution is stable and may be stored for up to 24 hours at 36° to 46° F (2° to 8° C).

⊗ **Incompatibilities**
Alteplase, amiodarone, amphotericin B, chlorpromazine, diazepam, prochlorperazine edisylate, reteplase, streptokinase, vancomycin, all I.V. drugs.

Contraindications and cautions

• Contraindicated in patients hypersensitive to the drug or any of its components, and in patients with active major bleeding. Don't use drug in patients with unstable angina who aren't undergoing PTCA or PCI, in patients with other acute coronary conditions, or in patients who aren't taking aspirin.
• Use cautiously in patients with HIT or HITTS, and in patients with an increased risk of bleeding.
⚖ **Lifespan:** In pregnant women, use only if clearly needed due to the risk of maternal bleeding. In breast-feeding women, use cautiously because it isn't known whether drug appears in breast milk. In children, safety and effectiveness of drug haven't been established. In elderly patients, use with caution because they are more likely to have puncture site hemorrhage and catheterization site hematoma.

Adverse reactions

CNS: *cerebral ischemia,* anxiety, *headache,* insomnia, nervousness, fever, *pain,* confusion.
CV: *bradycardia,* hypertension, hypotension, syncope, *ventricular fibrillation,* vascular anomaly.
GI: abdominal pain, dyspepsia, *nausea,* vomiting.
GU: urine retention, *renal failure,* oliguria.
Hematologic: *severe, spontaneous bleeding (cerebral, retroperitoneal, GU, GI), arterial site hemorrhage.*
Musculoskeletal: *back pain,* pelvic pain, facial paralysis.
Respiratory: *pulmonary edema.*
Other: pain at injection site, infection, *sepsis.*

Interactions

Drug-drug. *GPI inhibitors:* Safety and effectiveness haven't been established. Avoid using together.
Heparin, warfarin, other oral anticoagulants: May increase risk of bleeding. Use together cau-

tiously. If using low–molecular-weight heparin, stop it at least 8 hours before giving bivalirudin.

Effects on lab test results

• May increase activated clotting time, APTT, thrombin time, and PT.

Pharmacokinetics

Absorption: Given I.V.
Distribution: Binds rapidly to thrombin and has a rapid onset of action.
Metabolism: Rapidly cleared by a combination of renal mechanisms and proteolytic cleavage.
Excretion: Renal. Total body clearance is similar in patients with normal renal function and mild renal impairment. Clearance is reduced about 20% in patients with moderate and severe renal impairment and is reduced about 80% in dialysis-dependent patients. Bivalirudin is hemodialyzable. *Half-life:* 25 minutes in patients with normal renal function.

Route	Onset	Peak	Duration
I.V.	Rapid	Immediate	Duration of infusion

Action

Chemical effect: Directly inhibits both clot-bound and circulating thrombin, preventing generation of fibrin and further activation of the clotting cascade. Inhibits thrombin-induced platelet activation, granule release, and aggregation.
Therapeutic effect: Prevents blood clots.

Available forms

Injection: 250-mg vial

NURSING PROCESS

⚕ Assessment
• Obtain and monitor baseline coagulation tests, and hemoglobin level and hematocrit, before and throughout therapy.
• Monitor effectiveness by measuring APTT, PT, and thrombin time values regularly.
• Monitor venipuncture sites for bleeding, hematoma, or inflammation.
• Be alert for adverse reactions.
⊛ ALERT: If the patient has an unexplained drop in hematocrit, blood pressure, or other unexplained symptom, consider the possibility of hemorrhage.

• Assess access site regularly for bleeding.
• Assess patient's and family's knowledge of drug therapy.

⊕ **Nursing diagnoses**
• Risk for injury related to potential acute ischemic event caused by impaired CV status
• Ineffective protection related to increased risk of bleeding from anticoagulant therapy
• Deficient knowledge related to drug therapy

❯ **Planning and implementation**
• Patients with renal failure require reduced dosage.
• Don't give I.M.
Patient teaching
• Advise patient that drug can cause bleeding. Urge patient to report immediately to prescriber any unusual bruising or bleeding (nosebleeds, bleeding gums, petechiae, and hematuria), or tarry or bloody stools.
• Warn patient to avoid other aspirin-containing drugs and drugs used to treat swelling or pain (such as Motrin, Naprosyn, Aleve).
• Advise patient to avoid activities that carry a risk of injury, and instruct patient to use a soft toothbrush and electric razor while taking drug.

◪ **Evaluation**
• Patient doesn't suffer acute ischemic event after PTCA or PCI.
• Patient doesn't suffer drug-induced adverse reactions or bleeding.
• Patient and family state understanding of drug therapy.

bleomycin sulfate
(blee-oh-MIGH-sin SUL-fayt)
Blenoxane

Pharmacologic class: antibiotic
Therapeutic class: antineoplastic
Pregnancy risk category: D

Indications and dosages

▶ **Hodgkin's lymphoma, squamous cell carcinoma, non-Hodgkin's lymphoma, testicular cancer.** *Adults:* 10 to 20 units/m² (0.25 to 0.5 units/kg) I.V., I.M., or subcutaneously once or twice weekly. After 50% response in patients with Hodgkin's disease, maintenance dosage is

1 unit I.V. or I.M. daily or 5 units I.V. or I.M. weekly.
▶ **Malignant pleural effusion, prevention of recurrent pleural effusions or to manage pneumothorax related to AIDS or *Pneumocystis jiroveci (carinii)* pneumonia.** *Adults:* Give 60 units as a single-dose bolus in 50 to 100 ml of normal saline solution by intrapleural injection through a thoracostomy tube. Leave in for 4 hours, then drain and resume suction. Maximum dose is 1 unit/kg.
Elderly patients receiving intrapleural injection: Don't exceed 40 units/m².
▶ **AIDS-related Kaposi's sarcoma‡.** *Adults:* 20 units/m² daily I.V. continuously over 72 hours q 3 weeks.

▼ **I.V. administration**
• Follow institutional policy for giving drug to reduce risks. Preparation and administration of parenteral form of this drug carries carcinogenic, mutagenic, and teratogenic risks for personnel.
• Reconstitute drug with 5 ml or more of normal saline solution for injection.
• For I.V. infusion, further dilute with 50 to 100 ml of normal saline solution for injection. Infuse slowly over 10 minutes.
• Drug may adsorb to plastic I.V. bags. For prolonged stability, use glass containers.
⊗ **Incompatibilities**
Amino acids; aminophylline; ascorbic acid injection; cefazolin; diazepam; drugs containing sulfhydryl groups; fluids containing dextrose; furosemide; hydrocortisone; methotrexate; mitomycin; nafcillin; penicillin G; riboflavin; solutions containing divalent and trivalent cations, especially calcium salts and copper; terbutaline sulfate.

Contraindications and cautions
• Contraindicated in patients hypersensitive to drug.
• Use cautiously in patients with renal or pulmonary impairment.
⚠ **Lifespan:** In pregnant or breast-feeding women and in children, safety of drug hasn't been established.

Adverse reactions
CNS: hyperesthesia of scalp and fingers, headache, fever.

GI: *stomatitis, prolonged anorexia,* nausea, vomiting, diarrhea.
Hematologic: leukocytosis.
Musculoskeletal: swelling of interphalangeal joints.
Respiratory: PNEUMONITIS, *pulmonary fibrosis, fine crackles, dyspnea, nonproductive cough.*
Skin: *reversible alopecia; erythema; vesiculation; hardening and discoloration of palmar and plantar skin;* desquamation of hands, feet, and pressure areas; *hyperpigmentation; acne.*
Other: *hypersensitivity reactions (fever up to 106° F [41.1° C] with chills after injection), anaphylaxis.*

Interactions

Drug-drug. *Digoxin:* May decrease digoxin level. Monitor patient closely for loss of therapeutic effect.
Oxygen: Give supplemental oxygen, if ordered after treatment, at a fraction of inspired oxygen no higher than 25% to avoid potential lung damage.
Phenytoin: May decrease phenytoin level. Monitor patient closely.

Effects on lab test results

• May increase uric acid level.
• May increase WBC count.

Pharmacokinetics

Absorption: I.M. administration results in lower levels than those produced by equivalent I.V. doses.
Distribution: Widely into total body water, mainly in skin, lungs, kidneys, peritoneum, and lymphatic tissue.
Metabolism: Unknown; however, extensive tissue inactivation occurs in liver and kidneys, with much less in skin and lungs.
Excretion: Drug and its metabolites excreted primarily in urine. *Half-life:* 2 hours.

Route	Onset	Peak	Duration
I.V., I.M., SubQ, intrapleural	Unknown	Unknown	Unknown

Action

Chemical effect: May inhibit DNA synthesis and cause scission of single- and double-stranded DNA.

Therapeutic effect: Kills selected types of cancer cells.

Available forms

Injection: 15- and 30-unit vials (1 unit = 1 mg)

NURSING PROCESS

Assessment
• Obtain history of patient's overall physical status (especially respiratory status, CBC, and pulmonary and renal function tests) before therapy and reassess regularly thereafter.
• Be alert for adverse reactions and drug interactions. Adverse pulmonary reactions are common in patients older than age 70. Fatal pulmonary fibrosis occurs in 1% of patients, especially when cumulative dose exceeds 400 units.
• Monitor patient for bleomycin-induced fever, which is common and usually occurs within 3 to 6 hours after giving drug.
• Watch for hypersensitivity reactions, which may be delayed for several hours, especially in patients with lymphoma.
• Assess patient for development of fine crackles and dyspnea.
• Assess patient's and family's understanding of drug therapy.

Nursing diagnoses
• Risk for injury related to underlying neoplastic condition
• Impaired gas exchange related to drug-induced adverse pulmonary reactions
• Deficient knowledge related to drug therapy

Planning and implementation
• Follow institutional policy for giving drug to reduce risks. Preparation and administration of parenteral form of this drug carries carcinogenic, mutagenic, and teratogenic risks for personnel.
• Dilute drug for I.M. or subcutaneous administration in 1 to 5 ml of sterile water for injection, bacteriostatic water for injection, or normal saline solution for injection.
• Follow manufacturer's guidelines for giving bleomycin subcutaneously.
• For intrapleural use, dissolve drug in 50 to 100 ml normal saline solution for injection. Give through a thoracotomy tube after excess intrapleural fluid has been drained and complete lung expansion has been confirmed.

• Refrigerate unopened vials containing dry powder.

• Refrigerated, reconstituted solution for injection is stable for 4 weeks; at room temperature, it's stable for 2 weeks.

• Stop drug if pulmonary function test shows a marked decline.

• Don't use adhesive dressings on skin. This helps prevent linear streaking from drug concentrating in keratin of squamous epithelium.

• Give acetaminophen before treatment and for 24 hours after treatment in patients susceptible to post-treatment fever.

Patient teaching
• Explain the risks of drug therapy, especially the danger of serious pulmonary reactions in high-risk patients.

• Explain the need for monitoring and the type of monitoring to be done.

• Tell patient that alopecia may occur, but that it's usually reversible.

☑ **Evaluation**
• Patient exhibits positive response to therapy, as evidenced by follow-up diagnostic test results.

• Patient's gas exchange remains normal throughout therapy.

• Patient and family state understanding of drug therapy.

bortezomib
(bore-TEHZ-uh-mihb)
Velcade

Pharmacologic class: proteosome inhibitor
Therapeutic class: antineoplastic
Pregnancy risk category: D

Indications and dosages

▶ **Multiple myeloma that's progressing after at least one previous therapy.** *Adults:* 1.3 mg/m^2 by I.V. bolus twice weekly for 2 weeks (days 1, 4, 8, and 11) followed by a 10-day rest period (days 12 to 21). This 3-week period is a treatment cycle. For extended therapy of longer than 8 weeks, may adjust dosage schedule to once weekly for 4 weeks (days 1, 8, 15, and 22) followed by a 13-day rest period (days 23 to 35). Separate consecutive doses of drug by at least 72 hours.

⧄ **Adjust-a-dose:** If patient develops a grade 3 nonhematologic or a grade 4 hematologic toxicity (excluding neuropathy), withhold drug. When toxicity resolves, restart at a 25% reduced dose. If patient has neuropathic pain, peripheral neuropathy, or both, use the following table.

Severity of neuropathy	Dosage adjustment
Grade 1 (paresthesias, loss of reflexes, or both) without pain or loss of function	No change.
Grade 1 with pain or grade 2 (function altered but not activities of daily living)	Reduce to 1 mg/m^2.
Grade 2 with pain or grade 3 (interference with activities of daily living)	Hold drug until toxicity resolves; then start at 0.7 mg/m^2 once weekly.
Grade 4 (permanent sensory loss that interferes with function)	Stop drug.

▽ **I.V. administration**
• Reconstitute with 3.5 ml of normal saline solution. Use caution and aseptic technique when preparing and handling drug. Wear gloves and protective clothing to prevent skin contact.

• Give by I.V. bolus within 8 hours of reconstitution.

• Drug may be stored up to 3 hours in a syringe, but total storage time for reconstituted solution mustn't exceed 8 hours when exposed to normal indoor lighting.

• Store unopened vials at a controlled room temperature, in original packaging, and protect from light.

⊗ **Incompatibilities**
None reported.

Contraindications and cautions

• Contraindicated in patients hypersensitive to bortezomib, boron, or mannitol.

• Use cautiously if patient is dehydrated, is receiving other drugs known to cause hypotension, or has a history of syncope. Use cautiously, and only after careful assessment of risks and benefits, in patients with severe neuropathy.

⚕ **Lifespan:** In pregnant or breast-feeding women, avoid use. Women should avoid breast-feeding or becoming pregnant during drug therapy. In children, safety and effectiveness of drug haven't been established.

B

Adverse reactions

CNS: anxiety, *asthenia,* dizziness, dysesthesia, *fever,* headache, insomnia, paresthesia, *peripheral neuropathy,* rigors.
CV: edema, orthostatic and postural hypotension.
EENT: blurred vision.
GI: abdominal pain, *constipation, decreased appetite, diarrhea,* dysgeusia, dyspepsia, *nausea, vomiting.*
GU: dehydration.
Hematologic: *anemia,* NEUTROPENIA, THROMBOCYTOPENIA.
Musculoskeletal: arthralgia, back pain, bone pain, limb pain, muscle cramps, myalgia.
Respiratory: cough, dyspnea, pneumonia, upper respiratory tract infection.
Skin: rash, pruritus.
Other: herpes zoster.

Interactions

Drug-drug. *Antihypertensives:* May cause hypotension. Monitor patient's blood pressure closely.
Drugs linked to peripheral neuropathy, such as amiodarone, antivirals, isoniazid, nitrofurantoin, statins: May worsen neuropathy. Use together cautiously.
Inhibitors or inducers of CYP 3A4: Monitor patient closely for either toxicity or reduced effects.
Oral antidiabetics: May cause hypoglycemia or hyperglycemia. Monitor glucose levels closely.

Effects on lab test results

• May decrease hemoglobin level and hematocrit.
• May decrease neutrophil and platelet counts.

Pharmacokinetics

Absorption: Given I.V.
Distribution: 83% is protein-bound.
Metabolism: Mainly in the liver by CYP enzymes.
Excretion: Unknown. *Half-life:* 9 to 15 hours.

Route	Onset	Peak	Duration
I.V.	Unknown	Unknown	Unknown

Action

Chemical effect: Disrupts intracellular homeostatic mechanisms by inhibiting the 26S proteosome, which regulates intracellular levels of certain proteins and causes cells to die.
Therapeutic effect: Destroys cancer cells.

Available forms

Injection: 3.5 mg

NURSING PROCESS

✐ Assessment

• Assess patient's condition before therapy and regularly thereafter.
• Assess patient's nutrition and hydration status before and during therapy.
• Assess patient's and family's knowledge of drug therapy.

⊞ Nursing diagnoses

• Risk for injury related to potential neuropathy as an adverse effect
• Risk for hypotension related to dehydration
• Risk for imbalanced nutrition: less than body requires related to underlying disease and drug adverse effects

⊳ Planning and implementation

• Monitor patient's reaction. An antiemetic, an antidiarrheal, or both may be needed because drug may cause nausea, vomiting, diarrhea, or constipation.
• Adjust antihypertensive dosage, maintain hydration status, and give mineralocorticoids to manage orthostatic hypotension.
• Watch for evidence of neuropathy, such as a burning sensation, hyperesthesia, hypoesthesia, paresthesia, discomfort, or neuropathic pain.
• Change dose and schedule if patient develops new or worsening peripheral neuropathy.
Patient teaching
• Tell patient to notify prescriber about new or worsening peripheral neuropathy.
• Urge women to use effective contraception during treatment.
• Teach patient how to avoid dehydration, and stress the need to tell prescriber about dizziness, light-headedness, or fainting spells.
• Tell patient to use caution when driving or performing potentially hazardous activities because drug may cause fatigue, dizziness, faintness, light-headedness, and double or blurred vision.

☑ Evaluation

• Patient has no serious drug reactions.
• Patient maintains adequate nutritional status.
• Patient maintains adequate hydration status.
• Patient and family state understanding of drug therapy.

bosentan
(bow-SEN-tan)
Tracleer

Pharmacologic class: endothelin receptor antagonist
Therapeutic class: vasodilator
Pregnancy risk category: X

Indications and dosages

▶ **Pulmonary arterial hypertension in patients with World Health Organization class III or IV symptoms to improve exercise ability and decrease clinical worsening.** *Adults:* 62.5 mg P.O. b.i.d. for 4 weeks. Increase to maintenance dose of 125 mg P.O. b.i.d. In patients older than 12 years who weigh less than 40 kg (88 lb), the initial and maintenance dose is 62.5 mg b.i.d. Adjust dose based on ALT and AST levels.

Contraindications and cautions

• Contraindicated in patients hypersensitive to drug. Don't use in patients with moderate-to-severe liver impairment or in those with aminotransferase (ALT/AST) levels more than three times upper limit of normal.
• Use cautiously in patients with mild liver impairment.
⚠ **Lifespan:** In pregnant women, drug is contraindicated. In breast-feeding women, drug isn't recommended because it's unknown whether drug appears in breast milk. In children 12 years old or younger, safety and effectiveness of drug haven't been established. In elderly patients, select dose cautiously because of greater likelihood of decreased organ function.

Adverse reactions

CNS: *headache,* fatigue.
CV: hypotension, palpitations, flushing, edema, lower leg edema.
EENT: *nasopharyngitis.*
GI: dyspepsia.

Hematologic: anemia.
Hepatic: *liver failure.*
Skin: pruritus.

Interactions

Drug-drug. *Cyclosporin A:* May increase concentrations of bosentan and decrease levels of cyclosporine. Avoid using together.
Glyburide: May increase risk of elevated liver enzyme levels and decrease levels of both drugs. Avoid using together.
Hormonal contraceptives: May cause contraceptive failure. Advise use of a barrier method of birth control.
Ketoconazole: May increase bosentan level. Monitor patient for increased effects of bosentan.
Simvastatin, other statins: May decrease levels of these drugs. Monitor cholesterol levels to assess need for statin dosage adjustment.

Effects on lab test results

• May increase liver aminotransferase (such as AST, ALT, and bilirubin) levels. May decrease hemoglobin level and hematocrit.

Pharmacokinetics

Absorption: 50% bioavailability after oral use.
Distribution: More than 98% protein-bound, mainly albumin.
Metabolism: Hepatically into three metabolites. Bosentan induces CYP 2C9 and CYP 3A4, and possibly CYP 2C19.
Excretion: By biliary excretion. Less than 3% of oral dose is recovered in urine. *Half life:* About 5 hours.

Route	Onset	Peak	Duration
P.O.	Unknown	3–5 hr	Unknown

Action

Chemical effect: Antagonizes endothelin-1 (ET-1). ET-1 levels are elevated in patients with pulmonary arterial hypertension.
Therapeutic effect: Increases exercise capacity and cardiac index. Decreases blood pressure, pulmonary arterial pressure, vascular resistance, and mean right arterial pressure.

Available forms

Tablets: 62.5 mg, 125 mg

Reactions may be *common,* uncommon, *life-threatening*, or COMMON AND LIFE-THREATENING.

B

NURSING PROCESS

🔧 Assessment
• Assess patient's underlying condition before therapy and reassess regularly thereafter.
• Make sure patient isn't pregnant. Obtain monthly pregnancy tests.
• Serious liver injury may occur. Measure aminotransferase levels before treatment and monthly thereafter, and adjust dosage accordingly.
• This drug may cause hematologic changes. Monitor hemoglobin level after 1 and 3 months of therapy and then every 3 months thereafter.
• Be alert for adverse events.
• Assess patient's and family's knowledge of drug therapy.

🔄 Nursing diagnoses
• Risk of injury related to drug-induced liver enzyme elevations
• Ineffective tissue perfusion (cardiopulmonary) related to underlying condition
• Deficient knowledge related to drug therapy

▶ Planning and implementation
• To decrease the possibility of potential serious liver injury and to limit the chance for fetal exposure, Tracleer may be prescribed only through the Tracleer access program at 1-866-228-3546. Adverse effects also may be reported through this number.
• For patients who develop aminotransferase abnormalities, the dosage may need to be decreased or therapy stopped until aminotransferase levels return to normal. If liver function abnormalities are accompanied by symptoms of liver injury, such as nausea, vomiting, fever, abdominal pain, jaundice, or unusual lethargy or fatigue, or if bilirubin level is greater than or equal to two times upper limit of normal, stop treatment and don't restart.
• Overdose may cause headache, nausea and vomiting, mildly decreased blood pressure, and increased heart rate. Massive overdose may cause severe hypotension requiring CV support. Treat symptoms, and provide supportive care.
• To avoid the potential for deterioration, gradually reduce the dosage when stopping drug.
Patient teaching
• Advise patient to take drug only as prescribed.
• Warn patient to avoid becoming pregnant while taking this drug. Major birth defects may result with fetal exposure. Reliable contraception must be used and a monthly pregnancy test performed.
• Advise patient to have liver tests and blood counts performed regularly.
• Tell patient not to use hormonal contraceptives, including oral, implantable, and injectable, as her only means of contraception because failure may occur.

☑ Evaluation
• Patient doesn't suffer from adverse reactions or liver damage from drug therapy.
• Patient's pulmonary artery pressure decreases, and patient reaches pulmonary hemodynamic stability.
• Patient and family state understanding of drug therapy.

bromfenac ophthalmic solution
BROM-fehn-ack
Xibrom

Pharmacologic classification: nonsteroidal anti-inflammatory drug
Therapeutic classification: anti-inflammatory, ophthalmic
Pregnancy risk category: C

Indications and dosages

▶ **Postoperative inflammation following cataract surgery.** *Adults:* 1 drop in affected eye twice daily starting 24 hours after surgery and continuing for 2 weeks.

Contraindications and cautions

Contraindicated in patients hypersensitive to any ingredient in the product. Bromfenac ophthalmic solution contains sulfite, which may cause allergic-type reactions, including anaphylaxis and life-threatening or less severe asthmatic episodes in patients sensitive to sulfites.

Use cautiously in patients with bleeding tendencies, patients taking anticoagulants, and patients sensitive to acetylsalicylic acid, phenylacetic acid derivatives, and other NSAIDs because of the risk of cross-sensitivity reactions. Also use cautiously in patients with complicated ocular surgeries, corneal denervation, corneal epithelial defects, diabetes mellitus, ocular surface diseases (such as dry eye syndrome), rheumatoid arthritis, or recent repeat ocular surgeries because the risk of corneal adverse effects, which may be sight-threatening, is increased.

⚘ **Lifespan:** Use during pregnancy only if potential benefit justifies the risk. Avoid giving drug late in pregnancy because NSAIDs may cause premature closure of the ductus arteriosus, a necessary structure of fetal circulation. Use cautiously in breast-feeding women. Safety and effectiveness haven't been established in patients younger than age 18.

Adverse reactions

CNS: headache.
EENT: abnormal sensation in the eye, burning, conjunctival hyperemia, eye irritation, eye pain, eye pruritus, eye redness, iritis, keratitis, stinging.
Other: *anaphylaxis,* hypersensitivity reactions.

Interactions

Drug-drug: *Drugs that affect coagulation:* May further increase bleeding tendency or prolong bleeding time. Avoid use together, if possible, or monitor bleeding closely.
Topical corticosteroids: May disrupt healing. Avoid use together, if possible, or monitor healing closely.

Effects on lab test results

None reported.

Pharmacokinetics

Absorption: Unknown.
Distribution: Intraocular.
Metabolism: Unknown.
Excretion: Unknown. *Half-life:* Unknown.

Route	Onset	Peak	Duration
Ophthalmic	Unknown	Unknown	Unknown

Action

Chemical effect: Blocks prostaglandin synthesis by inhibiting cyclooxygenase 1 and 2.
Therapeutic effect: Reduces postoperative inflammation after cataract surgery.

Available forms

Ophthalmic solution: 0.09%

⚗ Assessment

• Assess patient's risk for allergic reaction; ask patient before treatment if he is sensitive to sulfites, aspirin, or other NSAIDs.
• If patient takes an anticoagulant, watch closely for increased bleeding.
• Monitor PT and INR if appropriate.
• Assess patient's and family's knowledge of drug therapy.

⊕ Nursing diagnoses

• Disturbed visual sensory perception related to cataract surgery and potential adverse effects of medication.
• Risk for activity intolerance related to decreased visual acuity.
• Deficient knowledge related to drug therapy.

⟩ Planning and implementation

• Be aware that sulfite sensitivity is more common in patients with asthma than without.
• Begin treatment at least 24 hours after surgery and continue for 2 weeks.
• Giving drug less than 24 hours after surgery or more than 14 days after surgery increases risk for ocular adverse effects.
• If overdose or significant ocular adverse effect occurs, stop drug and monitor ocular health closely.

Patient teaching

• Advise patient not to use drops while wearing contact lenses.
• Teach patient how to instill the drops.
• Instruct patient to start using drops 24 hours after surgery and to continue for 14 days.
• Tell him not to use drops for longer than 2 weeks after surgery or to save unused drops for other conditions.
• Review the signs and symptoms of adverse effects. If bothersome or serious adverse effects occur, inform the patient to stop the drops and contact his prescriber.
• Tell patient to store drops at room temperature.

☑ Evaluation

• Patient doesn't experience adverse effects.
• Patient's activity level improves.
• Patient and family state understanding of drug therapy.

Reactions may be *common,* uncommon, *life-threatening,* or COMMON AND LIFE-THREATENING.

bromocriptine mesylate
(broh-moh-KRIP-teen MES-ih-layt)
Parlodel, Parlodel SnapTabs

Pharmacologic class: dopamine receptor agonist
Therapeutic class: antiparkinsonian, inhibitor of prolactin and growth hormone release
Pregnancy risk category: B

Indications and dosages

▶ **Parkinson's disease.** *Adults:* 1.25 to 2.5 mg P.O. b.i.d. with meals. Increase dosage q 14 to 28 days, up to 100 mg daily, p.r.n. Usual dosage, 10 to 40 mg daily.

▶ **Acromegaly.** *Adults:* 1.25 to 2.5 mg P.O. h.s. with snack for 3 days. An additional 1.25 to 2.5 mg may be added q 3 to 7 days until patient receives therapeutic benefit. Usual therapeutic dose is 20 to 30 mg daily. Maximum dosage, 100 mg daily.

▶ **Amenorrhea and galactorrhea related to hyperprolactinemia; infertility or hypogonadism in women.** *Adults:* 1.25 to 2.5 mg P.O. daily. Increase by 2.5 mg daily at 3- to 7-day intervals until desired effect is achieved. Maintenance dosage is usually 5 to 7.5 mg daily, but may be 2.5 to 15 mg daily.

▶ **Premenstrual syndrome‡.** *Adults:* 2.5 to 7.5 mg P.O. b.i.d. from day 10 of menstrual cycle until onset of menstruation.

▶ **Cushing's syndrome‡.** *Adults:* 1.25 to 2.5 mg P.O. b.i.d. to q.i.d.

▶ **Hepatic encephalopathy‡.** *Adults:* 1.25 mg P.O. daily, increase by 1.25 mg q 3 days until 15 mg is reached.

▶ **Neuroleptic malignant syndrome related to neuroleptic drug therapy‡.** *Adults:* 2.5 to 5 mg P.O. 2 to 6 times daily.

Contraindications and cautions

• Contraindicated in patients hypersensitive to ergot derivatives and in those with uncontrolled hypertension, severe ischemic heart disease or peripheral vascular disease, or toxemia of pregnancy.
• Use cautiously in patients with renal or hepatic impairment or history of MI with residual arrhythmias.
☀ **Lifespan:** In pregnant women, use only if benefits outweigh risks to fetus. In breast-feeding women, avoid use because it inhibits lactation. In children younger than age 15, safety and effectiveness of drug haven't been established.

Adverse reactions

CNS: confusion, hallucinations, uncontrolled body movements, *dizziness, headache,* fatigue, mania, delusions, nervousness, insomnia, depression, *seizures, stroke, syncope.*
CV: *hypotension,* orthostatic hypotension, hypertension, *acute MI.*
EENT: nasal congestion, tinnitus, blurred vision.
GI: *nausea,* vomiting, *abdominal cramps,* constipation, diarrhea.
GU: urine retention, urinary frequency.
Skin: coolness and pallor of fingers and toes.

Interactions

Drug-drug. *Antihypertensives:* May increase hypotensive effects. Dosage adjustment of antihypertensive may be needed.
Ergot alkaloids, estrogens, hormonal contraceptives, progestins: May interfere with effects of bromocriptine. Don't use together.
Erythromycin: May increase bromocriptine levels. Adjustment of bromocriptine may be needed.
Haloperidol, loxapine, MAO inhibitors, methyldopa, metoclopramide, phenothiazines, reserpine: May interfere with effects of bromocriptine. Increase of bromocriptine dosage may be needed.
Levodopa: May have additive effects. Adjustment of levodopa dosage may be needed.
Drug-lifestyle. *Alcohol use:* May cause disulfiram-like reaction. Discourage use together.

Effects on lab test results

• May increase BUN, alkaline phosphatase, uric acid, AST, ALT, and CK levels.

Pharmacokinetics

Absorption: 28% absorbed.
Distribution: 90% to 96% bound to albumin.
Metabolism: First-pass metabolism occurs with more than 90% of absorbed dose. Drug is metabolized completely in liver.

Excretion: Major route of excretion is through bile. Only 2.5% to 5.5% of dose excreted in urine. *Half-life:* 15 hours.

Route	Onset	Peak	Duration
P.O.	½–2 hr	1–3 hr	12–24 hr

Action

Chemical effect: Inhibits secretion of prolactin and acts as a dopamine-receptor agonist by activating postsynaptic dopamine receptors.
Therapeutic effect: Reverses amenorrhea and galactorrhea caused by hyperprolactinemia, increases fertility in women, improves voluntary movement, and inhibits prolactin and growth hormone release.

Available forms

Capsules: 5 mg
Tablets: 2.5 mg

NURSING PROCESS

Assessment

• Obtain history of patient's underlying condition before therapy and reassess regularly thereafter.
• Before treatment, assess patient for evidence of dementia. Monitor patient for mental changes during therapy.
• Perform baseline and periodic evaluations of cardiac, hepatic, renal, and hematopoietic functions during prolonged therapy.
• Be alert for adverse reactions and drug interactions. Risk of adverse reactions is high, particularly at start of therapy and with doses greater than 20 mg. Adverse reactions are more frequent when drug is used for Parkinson's disease.
• Assess patient's and family's knowledge of drug therapy.

Nursing diagnoses

• Ineffective health maintenance related to underlying condition
• Risk for injury related to drug-induced adverse CNS or CV reactions
• Deficient knowledge related to drug therapy

Planning and implementation

• Patients with impaired renal function may require dosage adjustments.
• Give drug with meals.

• Gradually adjust dose to effective level to minimize adverse reactions.
• For Parkinson's disease, bromocriptine is usually given with either levodopa or levodopa-carbidopa.

Patient teaching

• Advise patient to use methods other than hormonal contraceptives during treatment.
• Advise patient to rise slowly to an upright position and avoid sudden position changes to avoid dizziness and fainting.
• Advise patient that resumption of menses and suppression of galactorrhea may take 6 weeks or longer.
• Warn patient to avoid hazardous activities that require alertness until CNS and CV effects of drug are known.
• Tell patient to take drug with meals to minimize GI distress.

✓ Evaluation

• Patient exhibits improvement in underlying condition.
• Patient doesn't experience injury as a result of drug-induced adverse reactions.
• Patient and family state understanding of drug therapy.

budesonide (inhalation)

(byoo-DES-oh-nighd)
Pulmicort Respules, Pulmicort Turbuhaler, Rhinocort Aqua

Pharmacologic class: glucocorticoid
Therapeutic class: anti-inflammatory
Pregnancy risk category: B

Indications and dosages

▶ **Symptoms of seasonal or perennial allergic rhinitis and nonallergic perennial rhinitis.**
Adults and children age 6 and older: 1 spray in each nostril once daily. In adults and children age 12 and older, may increase to 4 sprays in each nostril once daily; in children younger than age 12, may increase to 2 sprays in each nostril once daily. Maintenance dosage is fewest number of sprays needed to control symptoms.
▶ **Chronic asthma.** *Adults:* 200 to 400 mcg oral inhalation via Turbuhaler b.i.d. when patient previously used bronchodilators alone or inhaled corticosteroids; 400 to 800 mcg oral in-

halation b.i.d. when patient previously used oral corticosteroids. Maximum dosage 800 mcg b.i.d.
Children age 6 and older: Initially, 200 mcg oral inhalation via Turbuhaler b.i.d. Maximum dosage is 400 mcg b.i.d.
Children ages 1 to 8: 0.25 mg Pulmicort Respules by jet nebulizer with compressor once daily. Increase to 0.5 mg once daily or 0.25 mg b.i.d. in child not receiving systemic or inhaled corticosteroids or 1 mg daily or 0.5 mg b.i.d. if child is receiving oral corticosteroids.

Contraindications and cautions

• Contraindicated in patients hypersensitive to the drug or any of its components, and in those who have had recent septal ulcers, nasal surgery, or nasal trauma, until total healing has occurred. Pulmicort Turbuhaler and Pulmicort Respules are contraindicated in the primary treatment of status asthmaticus.
• Use cautiously in patients with tuberculous infections, ocular herpes simplex, or untreated fungal, bacterial, or systemic viral infections.
⚘ **Lifespan:** In pregnant or breast-feeding women, use cautiously. In children younger than age 1, don't use Pulmicort Respules via jet nebulizer. In children younger than age 6, safety of oral inhalation via Turbuhaler hasn't been established.

Adverse reactions

CNS: nervousness, *headache.*
CV: facial edema.
EENT: nasal irritation, epistaxis, pharyngitis, sinusitis, reduced sense of smell, nasal pain, hoarseness.
GI: bad taste, dry mouth, dyspepsia, nausea, vomiting.
Metabolic: weight gain.
Musculoskeletal: myalgia.
Respiratory: cough, candidiasis, wheezing, dyspnea.
Skin: rash, pruritus, contact dermatitis.
Other: hypersensitivity reactions.

Interactions

Drug-drug. *Alternate-day prednisone therapy, inhaled corticosteroids:* May increase risk of hypothalamic-pituitary-adrenal suppression. Monitor patient closely.
Ketoconazole: May increase budesonide level. Use together cautiously.

Effects on lab test results

None reported.

Pharmacokinetics

Absorption: Amount of intranasal dose that reaches systemic circulation is typically about 20%.
Distribution: 88% protein-bound.
Metabolism: Rapidly and extensively in liver.
Excretion: About 67% in urine and about 33% in feces. *Half-life:* About 2 hours.

Route	Onset	Peak	Duration
Nasal inhalation	Unknown	45 min	8–10 hr
Oral inhalation	5–15 min	30 min	Unknown

Action

Chemical effect: Decreases nasal and pulmonary inflammation, mainly by inhibiting activities of specific cells and mediators involved in allergic response.
Therapeutic effect: Decreases nasal and pulmonary congestion.

Available forms

Inhalation suspension: 0.25 mg/2 ml, 0.5 mg/2 ml
Nasal spray: 32 mcg/metered spray (7-g canister)
Oral inhalation powder: 200 mcg/dose

NURSING PROCESS

📝 **Assessment**
• Obtain history of patient's condition before therapy and reassess regularly thereafter.
• Be alert for adverse reactions.
• Assess patient's and family's knowledge of drug therapy.

⊕ **Nursing diagnoses**
• Ineffective health maintenance related to allergy-induced nasal congestion
• Impaired gas exchange related to drug-induced wheezing
• Deficient knowledge related to drug therapy

▶ **Planning and implementation**
• Before using nasal inhaler, shake container. Have patient clear his nasal passages. Insert nozzle (pointed away from septum) into nostril,

holding other nostril closed. Have patient tilt head slightly forward so spray is directed up nasal passage. Deliver spray while patient inhales. Have patient tilt head back for a few seconds. Repeat in other nostril. Wipe off tip of inhaler before capping.
• Notify prescriber if relief isn't obtained or signs of infection appear.
• Obtain specimen for culture if signs of nasal infection occur.

Patient teaching
• Teach patient how to use nasal inhaler himself, as above.
• Instruct patient to hold the inhaler upright while orally inhaling the dose. When loading Pulmicort Turbuhaler, tell him not to blow or exhale into the inhaler and not to shake it while loaded. Tell him to place the mouthpiece between his lips and inhale forcefully and deeply. Have him rinse mouth after use to decrease risk of fungal growth.
• Pulmicort Respules can be given only by jet nebulizer connected to an air compressor with minimum airflow of 5.5 L/minute. System should be equipped with a mouthpiece or face mask. Have patient rinse mouth after administration. When using face mask, teach him to wash face after use to decrease risk of contact dermatitis or rash.
• Inform patient that use of an oral inhaler results in improvement in asthma control in 10 to 24 hours, with maximum benefit at 1 to 2 weeks, or possibly longer.
• Advise parent that antihistamines can cause paradoxical excitement in small children.
⊕ **ALERT:** Advise patient that Pulmicort Turbuhaler and Pulmicort Respules aren't indicated for relief of acute asthma attacks.
• Tell patient that product should be used by only one person to prevent spread of infection.
• Advise patient not to break or incinerate canister or store it in extreme heat. Contents are under pressure.
• Warn patient not to exceed prescribed dose or use for long periods because of risk of hypothalamic-pituitary-adrenal axis suppression.
• Tell patient to report worsened condition or symptoms that don't improve in 3 weeks.
• Teach patient good nasal and oral hygiene.

☑ **Evaluation**
• Patient's nasal congestion subsides.

• Patient has adequate gas exchange.
• Patient and family state understanding of drug therapy.

budesonide (oral)
(byoo-DES-oh-nighd)
Entocort EC

Pharmacologic class: corticosteroid
Therapeutic class: anti-inflammatory
Pregnancy risk category: B

Indications and dosages

▶ **Mild to moderate active Crohn's disease involving the ileum or the ascending colon.**
Adults: 9 mg P.O. once daily in the morning for up to 8 weeks. For recurrent episodes of active Crohn's disease, a repeat 8-week course may be given.
▶ **To maintain remission of mild to moderate Crohn's disease involving the ileum or ascending colon.** *Adults:* 6 mg P.O. daily for up to 3 months. If symptom control maintained at 3 months, taper drug to complete stop. Maintenance treatment beyond 3 months doesn't provide additional benefit.

Contraindications and cautions

• Contraindicated in patients hypersensitive to drug.
• Use cautiously in patients with tuberculosis, hypertension, diabetes mellitus, osteoporosis, peptic ulcer disease, glaucoma, or cataracts. Also use cautiously in patients with a family history of diabetes or glaucoma and those with any other condition in which glucocorticosteroids may have unwanted effects.
⚘ **Lifespan:** In pregnant women, use only if potential benefit justifies risks. In breast-feeding women, the decision to breast-feed should be based on importance of drug to the mother; glucocorticoids appear in breast milk and infants may have adverse reactions. In children, safety and effectiveness of drug haven't been established. In elderly patients, give drug cautiously, starting at the lower end of the dosage range.

Adverse reactions

CNS: *headache,* dizziness, asthenia, hyperkinesia, paresthesia, syncope, tremor, vertigo, fatigue, malaise, agitation, confusion, insomnia,

nervousness, somnolence, migraine, fever, pain, sleep disorder.
CV: chest pain, dependent edema, facial edema, hypertension, palpitations, tachycardia, flushing.
EENT: *pharyngitis,* ear infection, eye abnormality, abnormal vision, sinusitis, voice alteration, neck pain.
GI: *nausea,* dyspepsia, abdominal pain, flatulence, vomiting, anus disorder, aggravated Crohn's disease, gastroenteritis, epigastric pain, fistula, glossitis, hemorrhoids, intestinal obstruction, tongue edema, dry mouth, tooth disorder, taste perversion, increased appetite, oral candidiasis, *diarrhea.*
GU: dysuria, micturition frequency, nocturia, intermenstrual bleeding, menstrual disorder.
Hematologic: leukocytosis, anemia.
Metabolic: *hypercorticism,* hypokalemia, weight gain, ADRENAL INSUFFICIENCY.
Musculoskeletal: back pain, aggravated arthritis, cramps, myalgia, arthralgia, hypotonia.
Respiratory: *respiratory tract infection,* bronchitis, dyspnea, cough.
Skin: acne, alopecia, dermatitis, eczema, skin disorder, increased sweating, ecchymosis.
Other: flulike syndrome, infection, viral infection.

Interactions

Drug-drug. *CYP 3A4 inhibitors (erythromycin, ketoconazole, indinavir, itraconazole, ritonavir, saquinavir):* May increase the effects of budesonide. If drugs must be given together, monitor patient for signs of hypercorticism and consider reducing budesonide dosage.
Drug-food. *Grapefruit or grapefruit juice:* May increase drug effects. Discourage using together.

Effects on lab test results

• May increase alkaline phosphatase and C-reactive protein levels. May decrease hemoglobin level and hematocrit. May increase or decrease potassium level.
• May increase erythrocyte sedimentation rate and atypical neutrophil and WBC counts.

Pharmacokinetics

Absorption: Complete.
Distribution: 85% to 90% protein-bound.
Metabolism: Extensive first-pass metabolism and rapidly and extensively biotransformed by CYP 3A4 to two major metabolites that have very little glucocorticoid activity.

Excretion: In urine and feces as metabolites, which primarily are excreted renally. *Half-life:* Unknown.

Route	Onset	Peak	Duration
P.O.	Unknown	½–10 hr	Unknown

Action

Chemical effect: Has high affinity for glucocorticoid receptors.
Therapeutic effect: Alleviates symptoms of Crohn's disease.

Available forms

Capsules: 3 mg

NURSING PROCESS

Assessment
• Assess patient's underlying condition before starting therapy and reassess regularly thereafter.
• Monitor patient's laboratory values regularly. Monitor patient for adverse effects.
• Be alert for signs and symptoms of hypercorticism.
• Assess patient's and family's knowledge of drug therapy.

Nursing diagnoses
• Diarrhea caused by underlying Crohn's disease
• Imbalanced nutrition: less than body requirements related to underlying Crohn's disease
• Deficient knowledge related to drug therapy

Planning and implementation
• Patients undergoing surgery or another stressful situation may need systemic glucocorticoid supplementation in addition to budesonide therapy.
• When a patient is transferred from systemic glucocorticoid therapy to budesonide, monitor him carefully for signs and symptoms of steroid withdrawal. Taper glucocorticoid therapy when budesonide treatment starts.
• Watch for immunosuppression, especially in a patient who hasn't had diseases such as chickenpox or measles because these diseases can be fatal in a patient who is immunosuppressed or receiving glucocorticoids. Monitor adrenocortical function carefully and reduce dosage cautiously.

• Prevent patient exposure to chickenpox or measles. If patient is exposed to measles, consider therapy with pooled intravenous immunoglobulin. If patient develops chickenpox, antiviral treatment and varicella zoster immune globulin may be considered.
• Acute toxicity after overdose is rare.
• Prolonged use of drug may cause hypercorticism (symptoms include swelling of the face and neck, acne, bruising, hirsutism, buffalo hump, and skin striae) and adrenal suppression. Treat with immediate gastric lavage or emesis, followed by treatment of symptoms and supportive therapy. For chronic overdose in serious disease requiring continuous steroid therapy, dosage may be reduced temporarily. Dosage may need to be reduced in patients with moderate to severe liver disease if they have increased signs or symptoms of hypercorticism.

Patient teaching
• Tell patient to swallow capsules whole and not to chew or break them.
• Advise patient not to drink grapefruit juice while taking drug.
• Tell patient to notify prescriber immediately if exposed to chickenpox or measles.

☑ Evaluation
• Patient's symptoms of Crohn's disease, including diarrhea and abdominal pain, are relieved.
• Patient's nutrition improves as symptoms improve.
• Patient and family state understanding of drug therapy.

bumetanide
(byoo-MEH-tuh-nighd)
Bumex, Burinex ◇

Pharmacologic class: loop diuretic
Therapeutic class: diuretic
Pregnancy risk category: C

Indications and dosages
▶ **Hypertension.** *Adults:* 0.5 mg P.O. daily. Oral maintenance dosage is 1 to 4 mg daily, not to exceed 5 mg P.O. daily.
▶ **Heart failure.** *Children:* 0.015 mg/kg every other day to 0.1 mg/kg daily. Use with extreme caution in neonates.
▶ **Heart failure, hepatic or renal disease, postoperative edema‡, premenstrual syndrome‡, disseminated cancer‡.** *Adults:* 0.5 to 2 mg P.O. once daily. If diuretic response isn't adequate, give second or third dose at 4- to 5-hour intervals. Maximum dosage is 10 mg daily. Give parenterally if P.O. use isn't feasible. Usual initial dose is 0.5 to 1 mg given I.V. over 1 to 2 minutes or I.M. If response isn't adequate, give second or third dose at 2- to 3-hour intervals. Maximum dosage is 10 mg daily.
Adjust-a-dose: For patients with severe chronic renal insufficiency, a continuous infusion of 12 mg over 12 hours may be more effective and less toxic than intermittent bolus therapy.

I.V. administration
• For direct injection, use 21G or 23G needle and give drug over 1 to 2 minutes.
• For intermittent infusion, give diluted drug through an intermittent infusion device or piggyback into an I.V. line containing free-flowing compatible solution. Infuse at ordered rate.
• Continuous infusion not recommended.
⊗ Incompatibilities
Dobutamine, midazolam.

Contraindications and cautions
• Contraindicated in patients hypersensitive to drug or sulfonamides (possible cross-sensitivity), in those with anuria or hepatic coma, and in those with severe electrolyte depletion.
• Use cautiously in patients with depressed renal function or hepatic cirrhosis or ascites.
Lifespan: In pregnant women, use cautiously. In breast-feeding women, drug is contraindicated. In children, safety and effectiveness of drug haven't been established.

Adverse reactions
CNS: dizziness, headache.
CV: volume depletion and dehydration, orthostatic hypotension, ECG changes.
EENT: transient deafness.
GI: nausea.
GU: ***renal failure,*** nocturia, polyuria, azotemia, frequent urination, oliguria.
Hematologic: ***thrombocytopenia.***
Metabolic: hypokalemia; hypochloremic alkalosis; asymptomatic hyperuricemia; fluid and electrolyte imbalances, including dilutional hy-

ponatremia, hypocalcemia, and hypomagnesemia; hyperglycemia; impaired glucose tolerance.
Musculoskeletal: muscle pain and tenderness.
Skin: rash.

Interactions

Drug-drug. *Aminoglycoside antibiotics:* May potentiate ototoxicity. Use together cautiously.
Antihypertensives: May increase risk of hypotension. Use together cautiously.
Chlorothiazide, chlorthalidone, hydrochlorothiazide, indapamide, metolazone: May cause excessive diuretic response, resulting in serious electrolyte abnormalities or dehydration. Adjust dosages carefully while monitoring the patient for excessive diuretic responses.
Digoxin: May increase risk of digitalis toxicity from bumetanide-induced hypokalemia. Monitor potassium and digoxin levels.
Indomethacin, NSAIDs, probenecid: May inhibit diuretic response. Use together cautiously.
Lithium: May decrease lithium clearance, increasing risk of lithium toxicity. Monitor lithium level.
Other potassium-wasting drugs: May increase risk of hypokalemia. Use together cautiously.
Drug-herb. *Licorice:* May contribute to excessive potassium loss. Discourage use together.

Effects on lab test results

• May increase creatinine, urine urea, glucose, and cholesterol levels. May decrease potassium, magnesium, sodium, and calcium levels.
• May decrease platelet count.

Pharmacokinetics

Absorption: After P.O. administration, 85% to 95%; food delays absorption. Complete after I.M. administration.
Distribution: About 92% to 96% protein-bound; unknown whether drug enters CSF.
Metabolism: By liver to at least five metabolites.
Excretion: In urine (80%) and feces (10% to 20%). *Half-life:* 1 to 1½ hours.

Route	Onset	Peak	Duration
P.O.	30–60 min	1–2 hr	4–6 hr
I.V.	3 min	15–30 min	3½–4 hr
I.M.	40 min	Unknown	Unknown

Action

Chemical effect: Inhibits sodium and chloride reabsorption at ascending portion of loop of Henle.
Therapeutic effect: Promotes sodium and water excretion.

Available forms

Injection: 0.25 mg/ml
Tablets: 0.5 mg, 1 mg, 2 mg

NURSING PROCESS

⚡ Assessment
• Obtain history of patient's urine output, vital signs, electrolyte levels, breath sounds, peripheral edema, and weight before therapy, and reassess regularly thereafter.
• Be alert for adverse reactions and drug interactions.
• Assess patient's and family's knowledge of drug therapy.

Nursing diagnoses
• Excess fluid volume related to underlying condition
• Impaired urinary elimination related to therapeutic effect of drug therapy
• Deficient knowledge related to drug therapy

Planning and implementation
• Give P.O. dose with food to prevent GI upset.
• To prevent nocturia, give in morning. If second dose is needed, give in early afternoon.
• The safest and most effective dosage schedule for control of edema is intermittent dosage either given on alternate days or given for 3 to 4 days with 1- or 2-day rest periods.
• Drug can be used safely in patients allergic to furosemide: 1 mg of bumetanide equals 40 mg of furosemide. Bumetanide may be less ototoxic than furosemide.
• If oliguria or azotemia develops or increases, anticipate that prescriber may stop drug.
• Notify prescriber if drug-related hearing changes occur.
⚠ ALERT: Don't confuse bumetanide with budesonide.

Patient teaching
• Advise patient to stand up slowly to prevent dizziness; also tell him to limit alcohol intake and strenuous exercise in hot weather to avoid exacerbating orthostatic hypotension.

• Teach patient to monitor fluid volume by measuring weight daily.
• Advise patient to take drug early in day to avoid sleep interruption caused by nocturia.
• Tell patient with diabetes to monitor glucose levels closely.

☑ **Evaluation**
• Patient is free from edema.
• Patient demonstrates adjustment of lifestyle to deal with altered patterns of urinary elimination.
• Patient and family state understanding of drug therapy.

buprenorphine hydrochloride
(byoo-preh-NOR-feen high-droh-KLOR-ighd)
Buprenex, Subutex

buprenorphine hydrochloride and naloxone hydrochloride dihydrate
Suboxone

Pharmacologic class: opioid agonist-antagonist, opioid partial agonist
Therapeutic class: analgesic
Pregnancy risk category: C
Controlled substance schedule: III

Indications and dosages

▶ **Moderate to severe pain.** *Adults and children age 13 and older:* 0.3 mg I.M. or slow I.V. q 6 hours, p.r.n., or around-the-clock. May repeat 0.3 mg or increase to 0.6 mg, if needed, 30 to 60 minutes after initial dose.
Children ages 2 to 12: 2 to 6 mcg/kg I.V. or I.M. q 4 to 6 hours.
▶ **Opioid dependence.** *Adults:* 12 to 16 mg Suboxone or Subutex S.L. daily. Maintenance therapy with Suboxone is preferred; target dose is 16 mg/day. Increase or decrease in increments of 2 mg or 4 mg according to withdrawal effects, usual range is 4 to 24 mg.
▶ **Postoperative pain‡.** *Adults:* 25 to 250 mcg/hour I.V. infusion over 48 hours.
▶ **Pain‡.** *Adults:* 60 to 80 mcg epidural injection.
▶ **Circumcision‡.** *Children ages 9 months to 9 years:* 3 mcg/kg I.M. with surgical anesthesia.

▼ I.V. administration

• Give by direct I.V. injection into vein or through tubing of free-flowing compatible I.V. solution over at least 2 minutes.
⊗ **Incompatibilities**
Diazepam, furosemide, lorazepam.

Contraindications and cautions

• Contraindicated in patients hypersensitive to drug.
• Use cautiously in debilitated patients and patients with head injury, intracranial lesions, increased intracranial pressure, or severe respiratory, liver, or kidney impairment. Also use cautiously in patients with CNS depression or coma, thyroid irregularities, adrenal insufficiency, prostatic hyperplasia, urethral stricture, acute alcoholism, alcohol withdrawal syndrome, or kyphoscoliosis.
⚠ **Lifespan:** In pregnant and breast-feeding women and in elderly patients, use cautiously.

Adverse reactions

CNS: *dizziness, sedation,* headache, confusion, nervousness, euphoria, *vertigo,* **increased intracranial pressure,** fatigue, weakness, depression, dreaming, psychosis, slurred speech, paresthesia.
CV: *hypotension,* **bradycardia,** tachycardia, hypertension, Wenckebach block, **cyanosis,** flushing.
EENT: *miosis,* blurred vision, diplopia, visual abnormalities, tinnitus, conjunctivitis.
GI: *nausea,* vomiting, constipation, dry mouth.
GU: urine retention.
Respiratory: **respiratory depression,** hypoventilation, dyspnea.
Skin: *pruritus, diaphoresis.*
Other: *injection site reactions,* chills, withdrawal syndrome.

Interactions

Drug-drug. *CNS depressants, MAO inhibitors:* May have additive effects. Monitor patient.
Opioid analgesics: Possible decreased analgesic effect. Avoid using together.
Drug-lifestyle. *Alcohol use:* May have additive effects. Discourage using together.

Effects on lab test results

• May decrease alkaline phosphatase and hemoglobin levels and hematocrit.

• May decrease erythrocyte count and sedimentation rate.

Pharmacokinetics

Absorption: Rapid.
Distribution: About 96% protein-bound.
Metabolism: In liver.
Excretion: Primarily in feces. *Half-life:* 1 to 7 hours. *Combination drug half-life:* Buprenorphine, 37 hours; naloxone, 1 hour.

Route	Onset	Peak	Duration
I.V., I.M.	15 min	1 hr	6 hr
S.L.	Unknown	Unknown	2–8 hr

Action

Chemical effect: Binds with opiate receptors in CNS, altering perception of and emotional response to pain.
Therapeutic effect: Relieves pain.

Available forms

Injection: 0.324 mg (0.3 mg base/ml)
Sublingual: 2 mg, 8 mg
Sublingual (combination): 2 mg buprenorphine and 0.5 mg naloxone, 8 mg buprenorphine and 2 mg naloxone

NURSING PROCESS

Assessment
• Obtain history of patient's pain.
• Monitor respiratory status frequently for at least 1 hour after administration. Notify prescriber if respiratory depression occurs.
• Cytolytic hepatitis and hepatitis with jaundice can occur in an opioid-dependent patient. Monitor closely.
• Assess patient's and family's knowledge of drug therapy.

Nursing diagnoses
• Acute pain related to underlying condition
• Ineffective breathing pattern related to drug-induced respiratory depression
• Deficient knowledge related to drug therapy

Planning and implementation
• Data are insufficient to give single I.M. doses greater than 0.6 mg for long-term use.
• Analgesic potency of 0.3 mg buprenorphine is equal to that of 10 mg morphine and 75 mg

meperidine, but buprenorphine has a longer duration of action.
• Notify prescriber if pain isn't relieved.
• If patient's respiratory rate falls below 8 breaths per minute, withhold dose, rouse patient to stimulate breathing, and notify prescriber.
• Naloxone won't completely reverse respiratory depression caused by buprenorphine overdose; mechanical ventilation may be necessary. Doxapram and larger-than-usual doses of naloxone also may be ordered.
• Drug may precipitate withdrawal syndrome in opioid-dependent patients.
• If dependence occurs, withdrawal symptoms may appear up to 14 days after drug is stopped.

Patient teaching
• Warn ambulatory patient about getting out of bed slowly or walking cautiously because of risk of dizziness or hypotension.
• When drug is used postoperatively, encourage patient to turn, cough, and deep-breathe to prevent atelectasis.
• Teach patient to avoid activities that require full alertness until CNS effects are known.
• Instruct patient to avoid alcohol and other CNS depressants.

Evaluation
• Patient reports pain relief.
• Patient's respiratory status is within normal limits.
• Patient and family state understanding of drug therapy.

bupropion hydrochloride
(byoo-PROH-pee-on high-droh-KLOR-ighd)
Wellbutrin, Wellbutrin SR✐, Wellbutrin XL, Zyban

Pharmacologic class: aminoketone
Therapeutic class: antidepressant, aid to smoking cessation
Pregnancy risk category: B

Indications and dosages

▶ **Depression.** *Adults:* 100 mg immediate-release Wellbutrin P.O. b.i.d. initially, increased after 3 days to 100 mg P.O. t.i.d., if needed. If no response occurs after several weeks of therapy, increase to 150 mg t.i.d. Don't exceed 150 mg for a single dose. Allow at least 6 hours between successive doses. Maximum, 450 mg daily. Or, initially, 150 mg sustained-release Wellbutrin P.O. q morning; increase to target dose of 150 mg P.O. b.i.d. as tolerated as early as day 4 of dosing. Allow at least 8 hours between successive doses. Maximum, 400 mg daily. Or, initially, 150 mg extended-release Wellbutrin P.O. q morning; increase to target dose of 300 mg P.O. daily as tolerated as early as day 4 of dosing. Allow at least 24 hours between successive doses. Maximum, 450 mg daily.

S Adjust-a-dose: For patients with mild to moderate hepatic cirrhosis or renal impairment, reduce dosage. For patients with severe hepatic cirrhosis, don't exceed 75 mg immediate-release P.O. daily; 100 mg sustained-release P.O. daily; 150 mg sustained release P.O. q other day; or 150 mg extended-release P.O. q other day.

▶ **Aid to smoking cessation.** *Adults:* 150 mg Zyban P.O. daily for 3 days; increase to maximum dosage of 150 mg P.O. b.i.d. at least 8 hours apart. Start therapy 1 to 2 weeks before patient stops smoking.

▶ **Attention deficit hyperactivity disorder‡.** *Adults:* 150 mg Wellbutrin P.O. daily with regular-release tablets. Adjust dosage to a maximum of 450 mg P.O. daily.

Contraindications and cautions

• Contraindicated in patients hypersensitive to drug, in those who have taken MAO inhibitors during the previous 14 days, and in those with seizure disorders, a history of bulimia, or anorexia nervosa because of a higher risk of seizures. Also contraindicated in patients undergoing abrupt stoppage of alcohol or sedatives (including benzodiazepines). Don't use Wellbutrin with Zyban or other drugs containing bupropion that are used for smoking cessation.

• Use cautiously in patients with renal or hepatic impairment and in patients with recent MI or unstable heart disease.

• Adults and children with major depressive disorders may experience a worsening of depression and the emergence of suicidal ideation and behavior even while taking an antidepressant. Health care professionals are reminded that these drugs haven't been approved for use in children and are advised to carefully monitor patients for worsening depression or suicidal ideation, especially at the beginning of therapy and during dosage changes.

⚖ Lifespan: In pregnant women, use cautiously. If drug must be given to breast-feeding woman, breast-feeding should be stopped. In children, safety and effectiveness of drug haven't been established.

Adverse reactions

CNS: fever, *headache,* akathisia, *seizures, agitation,* anxiety, *confusion,* delusions, euphoria, hostility, impaired sleep quality, insomnia, sedation, sensory disturbance, syncope, tremor.
CV: *arrhythmias,* hypertension, hypotension, palpitations, tachycardia.
EENT: auditory disturbance, blurred vision.
GI: dry mouth, taste disturbance, increased appetite, constipation, dyspepsia, nausea, vomiting, anorexia.
GU: impotence, menstrual complaints, urinary frequency.
Metabolic: hyperglycemia, weight gain or loss.
Musculoskeletal: arthritis.
Skin: pruritus, rash, cutaneous temperature disturbance, diaphoresis.
Other: chills, decreased libido.

Interactions

Drug-drug. *Amantadine, levodopa, MAO inhibitors, phenothiazines, tricyclic antidepressants; recent and rapid withdrawal of benzodiazepines:* May increase risk of adverse reactions, including seizures. Monitor patient closely.
Antipsychotics, beta blockers, SSRIs, type 1C antiarrhythmics: May inhibit CYP 2D6 used to metabolize the listed drugs. If used together, consider reducing dosage of listed drugs.
Carbamazepine: May decrease bupropion levels. Monitor patient for loss of therapeutic effect.
Nicotine replacement drugs: May cause hypertension. Monitor blood pressure.
Ritonavir: May increase bupropion levels, increasing toxicity risk. Monitor patient closely.
Warfarin: May alter PT and INR. Monitor patient for bleeding or clotting when drugs are used together.
Drug-lifestyle. *Alcohol use:* May alter seizure threshold. Discourage using together.
Sun exposure: Photosensitivity reactions may occur. Advise patient to wear protective clothing and sunblock and to avoid sun exposure.

Reactions may be *common,* uncommon, *life-threatening*, or COMMON AND LIFE-THREATENING.

B

Effects on lab test results

- May decrease hemoglobin level and hematocrit. May increase or decrease glucose level.
- May decrease platelet count. May increase or decrease WBC count, PT, and INR.

Pharmacokinetics

Absorption: Unknown.
Distribution: About 80% protein-bound.
Metabolism: Probably in liver; several active metabolites have been identified.
Excretion: Mainly in urine. *Half-life:* 8 to 24 hours.

Route	Onset	Peak	Duration
P.O.	1–3 wk	2 hr	Unknown
Wellbutrin SR	Unknown	3 hr	Unknown
Wellbutrin XL	Unknown	5 hr	Unknown

Action

Chemical effect: Unknown. May work through noradrenergic, dopaminergic, or both mechanisms.
Therapeutic effect: Relieves depression; smoking deterrent.

Available forms

Tablets (extended-release): 150 mg, 300 mg
Tablets (immediate-release): 75 mg, 100 mg
Tablets (sustained-release): 100 mg, 150 mg, 200 mg

NURSING PROCESS

Assessment

- Obtain history of patient's condition before therapy and reassess regularly thereafter.
- Be alert for adverse reactions and drug interactions.
- Closely monitor a patient with history of bipolar disorder. Antidepressants can cause manic episodes during depressed phase of bipolar disorder.
- Assess patient's and family's knowledge of drug therapy.

Nursing diagnoses

- Ineffective individual coping related to underlying condition
- Risk for injury related to drug-induced adverse CNS reactions
- Deficient knowledge related to drug therapy

Planning and implementation

ALERT: Risk of seizure may be minimized by not exceeding 450 mg/day (immediate-release) and by giving drug daily in three equally divided doses. Increases in doses shouldn't exceed 100 mg/day in a 3-day period. For sustained-release formulations, don't exceed 400 mg/day and give drug daily in two equally divided doses. Increases in doses shouldn't exceed 200 mg/day in a 3-day period. Patients who experience seizures often have predisposing factors, including history of head trauma, prior seizures, or CNS tumors, or they may be taking a drug that lowers seizure threshold.

ALERT: Don't confuse bupropion with buspirone.

- Make sure patient has swallowed dose.
- Patient may experience period of increased restlessness, agitation, insomnia, and anxiety, especially at beginning of therapy.
- Reassess patient on warfarin regularly for changes in PT and INR, risk for bleeding, and clotting.
- For smoking cessation, begin therapy while patient is still smoking because about 1 week is needed to achieve steady state levels of drug. Course of treatment is usually 7 to 12 weeks.

Patient teaching

- Advise patient to take drug as scheduled and to take each day's dose in three divided doses (immediate-release) or two divided doses (sustained-release) to minimize risk of seizures.
- Tell patient to avoid alcohol while taking drug because alcohol may contribute to development of seizures.
- Advise patient to avoid hazardous activities that require alertness and good psychomotor coordination until CNS effects of drug are known.

ALERT: Advise patient not to take Wellbutrin with Zyban and to seek medical advice before taking other prescription drugs, OTC medications, or herbal remedies.

- Tell patient not to crush, chew, or divide sustained-release tablets.

Evaluation

- Patient's behavior and communication indicate improvement of depression.
- Patient doesn't experience injury from drug-induced adverse CNS reactions.
- Patient and family state understanding of drug therapy.

buspirone hydrochloride
(byoo-SPEER-ohn high-droh-KLOR-ighd)
BuSpar

Pharmacologic class: azaspirodecanedione derivative
Therapeutic class: anxiolytic
Pregnancy risk category: B

Indications and dosages

▶ **Anxiety disorders, short-term relief of anxiety.** *Adults:* Initially, 10 to 15 mg P.O. daily, usually in two or three divided doses. Increase dosage at 2- to 4-day intervals in 5-mg/day increments. Usual maintenance dosage is 15 to 30 mg daily in two or three divided doses. Don't exceed 60 mg daily.
⊠ Adjust-a-dose: When given with a CYP 3A4 inhibitor, lower initial dosage to 2.5 mg P.O. b.i.d. Subsequent dosage adjustment of either drug also may be needed.

Contraindications and cautions

• Contraindicated in patients hypersensitive to drug and in those who have taken an MAO inhibitor within 14 days.
• Use cautiously in patients with hepatic or renal failure.
� **Lifespan:** In pregnant women, use cautiously. In breast-feeding women, don't use. In children, safety and effectiveness of drug haven't been established.

Adverse reactions

CNS: *dizziness, drowsiness,* nervousness, excitement, insomnia, headache, fatigue.
GI: dry mouth, nausea, diarrhea.

Interactions

Drug-drug. *CNS depressants:* May increase CNS depression. Avoid using together.
Erythromycin: May increase buspirone concentrations. Consider initial dose of 2.5 mg b.i.d.
Itraconazole: May increase buspirone concentrations. Consider initial dose of 2.5 mg once daily.
MAO inhibitors: May elevate blood pressure. Avoid using together.
Drug-food. *Grapefruit juice:* May increase buspirone level. Don't use together.
Drug-lifestyle. *Alcohol use:* May increase CNS depression. Discourage using together.

Effects on lab test results

• May increase aminotransferase level.
• May decrease WBC and platelet counts.

Pharmacokinetics

Absorption: Rapidly and completely, but extensive first-pass metabolism limits absolute bioavailability to between 1% and 13% of P.O. dose. Food slows absorption but increases amount of unchanged drug in systemic circulation.
Distribution: 95% protein-bound; doesn't displace other highly protein-bound medications.
Metabolism: In liver.
Excretion: 29% to 63% in urine in 24 hours, primarily as metabolites; 18% to 38% in feces.
Half-life: 2 to 3 hours.

Route	Onset	Peak	Duration
P.O.	Unknown	40–90 min	Unknown

Action

Chemical effect: May inhibit neuronal firing and reduce serotonin turnover in cortical, amygdaloid, and septohippocampal tissue.
Therapeutic effect: Relieves anxiety.

Available forms

Tablets: 5 mg, 10 mg, 15 mg

NURSING PROCESS

⚗ Assessment
• Obtain history of patient's anxiety before therapy and reassess regularly thereafter.
• Signs of improvement usually appear within 7 to 10 days; optimal results occur after 3 to 4 weeks of therapy.
• Be alert for adverse reactions and drug interactions.
• Assess patient's and family's knowledge of drug therapy.

🔲 Nursing diagnoses
• Anxiety related to underlying condition
• Fatigue related to drug-induced adverse reactions
• Deficient knowledge related to drug therapy

▷ Planning and implementation
• Although drug has shown no potential for abuse and hasn't been classified as a controlled substance, it isn't recommended for relief from everyday stress.

Reactions may be *common*, uncommon, *life-threatening*, or COMMON AND LIFE-THREATENING.

B

• Before starting therapy in patient already being treated with a benzodiazepine, make sure he doesn't stop benzodiazepine abruptly because withdrawal reaction may occur.
• Give drug with food or milk but not grapefruit juice.
• Dosage may be increased in 2- to 4-day intervals.

Patient teaching
• Tell patient to take drug with food but avoid grapefruit juice.
• Warn patient to avoid hazardous activities that require alertness and psychomotor coordination until the drug's CNS effects are known.
• Review energy-saving measures with patient and family.
• If patient is already being treated with a benzodiazepine, warn him not to abruptly stop it because withdrawal reaction can occur. Teach him how and when benzodiazepine can be withdrawn safely.

☑ Evaluation
• Patient's anxiety is reduced.
• Patient states that energy-saving measures help combat fatigue caused by therapy.
• Patient and family state understanding of drug therapy.

busulfan
(byoo-SUL-fan)
Busulfex, Myleran

Pharmacologic class: alkylating drug
Therapeutic class: antineoplastic
Pregnancy risk category: D

Indications and dosages

▶ **Palliative treatment of chronic myelocytic (granulocytic) leukemia (CML).** *Adults:* For remission induction, 4 to 8 mg P.O. daily (0.06 mg/kg or 1.8 mg/m²). For maintenance therapy, 1 to 3 mg P.O. daily. Dosages may vary. *Children:* 0.06 mg/kg or 1.8 mg/m² P.O. daily. Dosages may vary.
▶ **With cyclophosphamide as a conditioning regimen before allogeneic hematopoietic progenitor cell transplantation for CML.** *Adults:* 0.8 mg/kg of ideal body weight or actual body weight (whichever is lower) I.V. by central venous catheter as a 2-hour infusion q 6 hours for

4 consecutive days for a total of 16 doses. Give phenytoin for seizure prophylaxis. Dosages may vary.
▶ **Myelofibrosis‡.** *Adults:* Initially, give 2 to 4 mg P.O. daily, then followed by the same dose two to three times weekly. Dosages may vary.

▼ I.V. administration

• Use aseptic technique when preparing and handling drug. Wear gloves and other protective clothing to prevent skin contact.
• Dilute with normal saline solution or D_5W, to a final concentration of at least 0.5 mg/ml.
• Flush catheter with diluent before and after infusion.
• Give by infusion pump over 2 hours.
• If solution is kept at room temperature, use within 8 hours of preparing; if refrigerated, within 12 hours.
• Refrigerate unopened ampules.
⊗ **Incompatibilities**
Other I.V. drugs.

Contraindications and cautions

• Contraindicated in patients with drug-resistant CML.
• Use cautiously in patients recently given other myelosuppressive drugs or radiation therapy and in those with depressed neutrophil or platelet count. Because high-dose therapy has been linked to seizures, use such therapy cautiously in patients with history of head trauma or seizures and in patients receiving other drugs that lower seizure threshold.
⚖ **Lifespan:** In pregnant women, use cautiously, if at all. In breast-feeding women, drug is contraindicated.

Adverse reactions

CNS: *fever, headache, asthenia, pain, insomnia, anxiety, dizziness, depression,* delirium, agitation, *encephalopathy,* confusion, hallucination, lethargy, somnolence, *seizures.*
CV: *edema, chest pain, tachycardia, hypertension, hypotension, thrombosis, vasodilation, heart rhythm abnormalities,* cardiomegaly, *ECG abnormalities, heart failure, pericardial effusion.*
EENT: *rhinitis, epistaxis, pharyngitis,* sinusitis, ear disorder, cataracts.
GI: *cheilosis (P.O.); nausea, stomatitis, mucositis, vomiting, anorexia, diarrhea, abdominal*

pain and enlargement, dyspepsia, constipation, dry mouth, rectal disorder, pancreatitis.
GU: dysuria, *oliguria,* hematuria, hemorrhagic cystitis.
Hematologic: *granulocytopenia, thrombocytopenia, leukopenia,* anemia.
Hepatic: *jaundice,* **hepatic necrosis,** hepatomegaly.
Metabolic: *hypomagnesemia, hyperglycemia, hypokalemia, hypocalcemia, hypervolemia, weight gain, hypophosphatemia,* hyponatremia.
Musculoskeletal: *back pain, myalgia, arthralgia.*
Respiratory: *lung disorder, cough, dyspnea, **irreversible pulmonary fibrosis, alveolar hemorrhage, asthma,*** atelectasis, pleural effusion, hypoxia, hemoptysis.
Skin: *rash, pruritus, alopecia,* exfoliative dermatitis, erythema nodosum, acne, skin discoloration, *hyperpigmentation,* anhidrosis.
Other: inflammation at injection site, Addison-like wasting syndrome, gynecomastia (P.O.); *chills, allergic reaction, **graft-versus-host disease, infection,*** hiccup.

Interactions

Drug-drug. *Acetaminophen within 72 hours:* May decrease busulfan clearance. Use together cautiously.
Anticoagulants, aspirin: May increase risk of bleeding. Avoid using together.
Cyclophosphamide: May increase risk of cardiac tamponade in patients with thalassemia. Monitor patient.
Itraconazole: May decrease busulfan clearance. Use together cautiously.
Myelosuppressives: May increase myelosuppression. Monitor patient.
Other cytotoxic drugs that cause pulmonary injury: May cause additive pulmonary toxicity. Avoid using together.
Phenytoin: May decrease busulfan level. Monitor busulfan levels.
Thioguanine: May cause hepatotoxicity, esophageal varices, or portal hypertension. Use together cautiously.

Effects on lab test results

• May increase serum glucose, ALT, bilirubin, alkaline phosphatase, uric acid, creatinine, and BUN levels. May decrease magnesium, calcium, potassium, phosphorus, sodium, and hemoglobin levels and hematocrit.

• May decrease WBC, and platelet counts.

Pharmacokinetics

Absorption: Well absorbed from GI tract.
Distribution: Unknown.
Metabolism: In liver.
Excretion: Cleared rapidly and excreted in urine. *Half-life:* About 2½ hours.

Route	Onset	Peak	Duration
P.O.	1–2 wk	Unknown	Unknown
I.V.	Unknown	Unknown	Unknown

Action

Chemical effect: Unknown; thought to cross-link strands of cellular DNA and interfere with RNA transcription, causing an imbalance of growth that leads to cell death.
Therapeutic effect: Kills selected type of cancer cell.

Available forms

Injection: 6 mg/ml
Tablets: 2 mg

NURSING PROCESS

Assessment
• Obtain history of patient's underlying neoplastic disease.
• Monitor WBC and platelet counts weekly while patient is receiving drug. WBC count falls about 10 days after the start of therapy and continues to fall for 2 weeks after stopping drug.
• Monitor uric acid, liver and kidney function, and glucose levels.
⊛ ALERT: Be alert for adverse reactions and drug interactions. Pulmonary fibrosis may occur as late as 4 to 6 months after treatment.
• Assess patient's and family's knowledge of drug therapy.

Nursing diagnoses
• Ineffective health maintenance related to presence of neoplastic disease
• Risk for infection related to drug-induced immunosuppression
• Deficient knowledge related to drug therapy

Planning and implementation
• Premedicate patient with phenytoin to decrease risk of seizures that can occur with I.V. infusion.

B

• Follow facility policy regarding preparation and handling of drug. Label as hazardous drug.
• Give drug at same time each day.
• Make sure patient is adequately hydrated.
• Adjust dosage based on patient's weekly WBC counts and temporarily stop drug therapy if severe leukocytopenia develops. Therapeutic effects are often accompanied by toxicity.
• Give with allopurinol in addition to adequate hydration to prevent hyperuricemia with resulting uric acid nephropathy.

Patient teaching

• Warn patient to watch for signs of infection, such as fever, sore throat, and fatigue, and for symptoms of bleeding, such as easy bruising, nosebleeds, bleeding gums, and melena. Advise patient to take his temperature daily.
⊛ **ALERT:** Instruct patient to report symptoms of toxicity so that dosage adjustments can be made. Symptoms include persistent cough and progressive dyspnea with alveolar exudate, suggestive of pneumonia.
• Instruct patient to avoid OTC products that contain aspirin.
• Advise woman of childbearing age to avoid becoming pregnant during therapy. Recommend that patient consult with prescriber before becoming pregnant.
• Advise breast-feeding woman to stop breast-feeding because of possible risk of toxicity in infant.

☑ **Evaluation**

• Patient exhibits positive response to drug therapy.
• Patient remains free from infection.
• Patient and family state understanding of drug therapy.

butorphanol tartrate

(byoo-TOR-fah-nohl TAR-trayt)
Stadol, Stadol NS

Pharmacologic class: opioid agonist-antagonist
Therapeutic class: analgesic, adjunct to anesthesia
Pregnancy risk category: C

Indications and dosages

▶ **Moderate to severe pain.** *Adults:* 0.5 to 2 mg I.V. q 3 to 4 hours, p.r.n., or around the clock. Or 1 to 4 mg I.M. q 3 to 4 hours, p.r.n. or around-the-clock. Maximum 4 mg per dose. Alternatively, 1 mg by nasal spray q 3 to 4 hours (1 spray in one nostril); repeat in 60 to 90 minutes if pain relief is inadequate.
▶ **Labor for pregnant women at full term and in early labor.** *Adults:* 1 to 2 mg I.V. or I.M., repeated after 4 hours, p.r.n.
▶ **Preoperative anesthesia or preanesthesia.** *Adults:* 2 mg I.M. 60 to 90 minutes before surgery.
▶ **Adjunct to balanced anesthesia.** *Adults:* 2 mg I.V. shortly before induction or 0.5 to 1 mg I.V. in increments during anesthesia.
◪ **Adjust-a-dose:** For patients with hepatic or renal impairment and elderly patients, reduce dosage to 50% of the usual parenteral adult dose at 6-hour intervals p.r.n. For nasal spray, the initial dose (1 spray in one nostril) is the same, but repeat dose is in 90 to 120 minutes, if needed. Repeat doses thereafter q 6 hours, p.r.n.

▼ I.V. administration

• Give drug by direct I.V. injection into vein or into I.V. line containing free-flowing compatible solution.
⊗ **Incompatibilities**
Dimenhydrinate, pentobarbital sodium.

Contraindications and cautions

• Contraindicated in patients with opioid addiction; may precipitate withdrawal syndrome. Also contraindicated in patients hypersensitive to drug or to preservative (benzethonium chloride).
• Use cautiously in patients with head injury, increased intracranial pressure, acute MI, ventricular dysfunction, coronary insufficiency, respiratory disease or depression, or renal or hepatic dysfunction. Also use cautiously in patients who have recently received repeated doses of an opioid analgesic.
⚖ **Lifespan:** In pregnant women, use only when benefits outweigh risks to the fetus. In breast-feeding women, drug is contraindicated. In children, safety and effectiveness haven't been established. In the elderly, mean half life of the drug is extended; use cautiously due to possible increased adverse reactions.

Adverse reactions

CNS: *sedation, headache, vertigo, floating sensation*, lethargy, *confusion*, nervousness, unusu-

al dreams, agitation, euphoria, hallucinations, flushing, *increased intracranial pressure.*
CV: palpitations, fluctuation in blood pressure.
EENT: diplopia, blurred vision, *nasal congestion* (with nasal spray).
GI: nausea, vomiting, constipation, *dry mouth.*
Respiratory: *respiratory depression.*
Skin: rash, urticaria, clamminess, excessive sweating.

Interactions

Drug-drug. *CNS depressants:* May have additive effects. Use together cautiously.
Opioid analgesics: Possible decreased analgesic effect. Avoid using together.
Drug-lifestyle. *Alcohol use:* May have additive depressant effects. Discourage using together.

Effects on lab test results

None reported.

Pharmacokinetics

Absorption: Good after I.M. use.
Distribution: 80% protein-bound. Drug rapidly crosses placenta, and neonatal levels are 0.4 to 1.4 times maternal levels.
Metabolism: Extensive, in liver to inactive metabolites.
Excretion: In inactive form, mainly by kidneys. About 11% to 14% of parenteral dose excreted in feces. *Half-life:* About 2 to 9¼ hours.

Route	Onset	Peak	Duration
I.V.	2–3 min	½–1 hr	2–4 hr
I.M.	10–30 min	½–1 hr	3–4 hr
Intranasal	≤ 15 min	1–2 hr	4–5 hr

Action

Chemical effect: Binds with opiate receptors in CNS, altering both perception of and emotional response to pain through unknown mechanism.
Therapeutic effect: Relieves pain and enhances anesthesia.

Available forms

Injection: 1 mg/ml, 2 mg/ml
Nasal spray: 10 mg/ml

NURSING PROCESS

▧ Assessment
• Obtain history of patient's pain before therapy, and reassess during therapy.

• Be alert for adverse reactions and drug interactions.
• Periodically monitor postoperative vital signs and bladder function. Drug decreases both rate and depth of respirations, and monitoring arterial oxygen saturation may aid in assessing respiratory depression.
• Assess patient's and family's knowledge of drug therapy.

⊞ Nursing diagnoses
• Acute pain related to underlying condition
• Risk for injury related to drug-induced adverse CNS reactions
• Deficient knowledge related to drug therapy

≫ Planning and implementation
• For intranasal use, have patient clear nasal passages before giving drug. Shake container. Tilt patient's head slightly backward; insert nozzle into nostril, pointing away from septum. Have patient hold other nostril closed, and spray while patient inhales gently.
• Subcutaneous route isn't recommended.
• Monitor patient for psychological and physical addiction, which may occur.
• Notify prescriber and discuss increasing dose or frequency if pain persists.
• Keep opioid antagonist (naloxone) and resuscitative equipment available.
Patient teaching
• Caution ambulatory patient to get out of bed slowly and walk carefully until CNS effects are known.
• Warn outpatient to refrain from driving and performing other activities that require mental alertness until drug's CNS effects are known.
• Warn patient that drug can cause physical and psychological dependence. Tell him to use drug only as directed and that abrupt withdrawal after prolonged use produces intense withdrawal symptoms.

☑ Evaluation
• Patient reports relief from pain.
• Patient doesn't experience injury as a result of therapy.
• Patient and family state understanding of drug therapy.

Reactions may be *common*, uncommon, *life-threatening*, or COMMON AND LIFE-THREATENING.

C

calcitonin (salmon)
(kal-sih-TOH-nin)
Calcimar, Miacalcin

Pharmacologic class: thyroid hormone, calcium and bone metabolism regulator
Therapeutic class: hypocalcemic, bone resorption inhibitor
Pregnancy risk category: C

Indications and dosages

▶ **Osteoporosis.** *Postmenopausal women:* 100 international units daily I.M. or subcutaneously. Or, 200 international units (one activation) daily intranasally, alternating nostrils daily.
▶ **Paget's disease of bone (osteitis deformans).** *Adults:* Initially, 100 international units daily I.M. or subcutaneously; maintenance dosage is 50 to 100 international units daily or q other day.
▶ **Hypercalcemia.** *Adults:* 4 international units/kg q 12 hours I.M. or subcutaneously. If response is inadequate after 1 or 2 days, increase dosage to 8 international units/kg I.M. q 12 hours. If response remains unsatisfactory after 2 more days, increase dosage to maximum of 8 international units/kg q 6 hours.
▶ **Osteogenesis imperfecta‡.** *Adults:* 2 international units/kg subcutaneously or I.M. three times weekly with daily calcium supplementation.

Contraindications and cautions

● Contraindicated in patients hypersensitive to drug.
⚜ **Lifespan:** In pregnant women, use cautiously. In breast-feeding women, don't use because drug may inhibit lactation. In children, safety and effectiveness haven't been established.

Adverse reactions

CNS: dizziness, headache, paresthesia, weakness.
CV: facial flushing, hypertension.
EENT: nasal symptoms (irritation, redness, sores) with intranasal use, *rhinitis,* epistaxis.
GI: anorexia, diarrhea, *nausea,* unusual taste, *vomiting.*
GU: nocturia, urinary frequency.
Metabolic: goiter, hyperglycemia, hyperthyroidism, hypocalcemia.
Musculoskeletal: arthralgia, back pain.
Skin: facial and hand flushing, rash.
Other: *anaphylaxis;* hand swelling, tingling, and tenderness; hypersensitivity reactions; *inflammation at injection site.*

Interactions

None significant.

Effects on lab test results

● May increase glucose, T_3, and T_4 levels. May decrease serum calcium and thyroid-stimulating hormone levels.

Pharmacokinetics

Absorption: Rapid with intranasal use.
Distribution: Unknown; however, calcitonin doesn't cross the placenta.
Metabolism: Rapidly in kidneys; additional activity in blood and peripheral tissues.
Excretion: In urine as inactive metabolites.
Half-life: Calcitonin human, 60 minutes; calcitonin salmon, 43 to 60 minutes.

Route	Onset	Peak	Duration
I.M., SubQ	≤ 15 min	≤ 4 hr	8–24 hr
Intranasal	Rapid	30 min	1 hr

Action

Chemical effect: Decreases osteoclastic activity by inhibiting osteocytic lysis; decreases mineral release and matrix or collagen breakdown in bone.
Therapeutic effect: Prohibits bone and kidney (tubular) resorption of calcium.

Available forms

Injection: 200 international units/ml, 2-ml ampules
Nasal spray: 200 international units/activation in 2-ml bottle (0.09 ml/dose)

NURSING PROCESS

📝 **Assessment**
⑤ **ALERT:** Assess postmenopausal woman's history. Drug is given only if patient can't take es-

trogen. Patient requires continued vitamin D and calcium supplements in addition to drug.
• Assess patient's calcium level before therapy and regularly thereafter.
• If using nasal spray, assess nasal passages before therapy and periodically thereafter.
• For Paget's disease, monitor alkaline phosphatase and 24-hour urine hydroxyproline levels to evaluate the drug's effectiveness.
• Monitor glucose level and thyroid studies before treatment and periodically during treatment. Repeat DEXA bone scan to assess effectiveness of therapy at least yearly.
• Examine urine sediment periodically for casts, particularly in immobilized patients.
• Look for adverse reactions.
• Assess patient's and family's knowledge of drug therapy.

NURSING DIAGNOSES

• Risk for injury related to patient's underlying bone condition
• Ineffective protection related to potential for drug-induced anaphylaxis
• Deficient knowledge related to drug therapy

▷ Planning and implementation
• Perform skin test before therapy.
• Give drug h.s. to minimize nausea and vomiting; remind patient that these symptoms usually resolve after 1 to 2 months of treatment.
• If dose is larger than 2 ml, give it I.M.
• Alternate nostrils daily when using nasal spray.
• Keep parenteral calcium available during first doses in case hypocalcemic tetany occurs.
• Refrigerate calcitonin salmon at 36° to 46° F (2° to 8° C). Store open nasal spray at room temperature.
• In patient who relapses after a positive initial response, evaluate for antibody response to hormone protein.
• Systemic allergic reactions may occur because hormone is a protein; keep epinephrine handy.
• If symptoms have been relieved after 6 months, stop drug until symptoms or radiologic signs recur.
⊛ ALERT: Don't confuse calcitonin with calciferol or calcitriol.
Patient teaching
• For outpatient therapy for Paget's disease, teach patient how to give drug subcutaneously.

• Teach patient to activate nasal spray before first use by holding bottle upright and depressing side arms six times until a faint mist appears. This signifies that the pump is primed and ready for use. Patient doesn't need to reprime the pump before each use.
• Instruct patient to report signs of nasal irritation from spray.
• Tell patient to handle missed doses as follows: With daily use, take as soon as possible, but don't double the dose. With alternate-day use, take missed dose as soon as possible, and then resume alternate-day schedule from that point.
• Remind patient with postmenopausal osteoporosis to take adequate calcium and vitamin D supplements.

☑ Evaluation
• Patient's calcium level is normal.
• Patient doesn't experience anaphylaxis.
• Patient and family state understanding of drug therapy.

calcitriol
(1,25-dihydroxycholecalciferol)
(kal-SIH-try-ohl)
Calcijex, Rocaltrol

Pharmacologic class: vitamin D analogue
Therapeutic class: antihypocalcemic
Pregnancy risk category: C

Indications and dosages
▶ **Hypocalcemia in patients undergoing long-term dialysis.** *Adults:* Initially, 0.25 mcg P.O. daily. Increase by 0.25 mcg daily at 4- to 8-week intervals. Maintenance dosage is 0.25 mcg q other day up to 1.25 mcg daily or 1 to 2 mcg I.V. three times weekly. Dosages from 0.5 to 4 mcg three times weekly may be used initially. If response to initial dose is inadequate, increase by 0.5 to 1 mcg at 2- to 4-week intervals. Maintenance dosage is 0.5 to 3 mcg I.V. three times weekly.
▶ **Hypoparathyroidism and pseudohypoparathyroidism.** *Adults and children age 6 and older:* Initially, 0.25 mcg P.O. daily. Increase dosage at 2- to 4-week intervals. Maintenance dosage is 0.25 to 2 mcg daily.

C

▶ **Hypoparathyroidism.** *Children and infants ages 1 to 5:* 0.25 to 0.75 mcg P.O. daily.
▶ **To manage secondary hyperparathyroidism and resulting metabolic bone disease in predialysis patients (moderate-to-severe chronic renal impairment with creatinine clearance of 15 to 55 ml/minute).** *Adults and children age 3 and older:* Initially, 0.25 mcg P.O. daily. Increase dosage to 0.5 mcg daily, if needed.
Children younger than age 3: Initially, 0.01 to 0.015 mcg/kg P.O. daily.

▼ I.V. administration

• For hypocalcemic patients with chronic renal impairment who are undergoing hemodialysis, give I.V. dose by rapid injection via dialysis catheter after treatment.
• Discard unused portions because drug contains no preservatives.
• Store injection at room temperature; avoid excessive heat or freezing. Protect from light.
⊗ **Incompatibilities**
None reported.

Contraindications and cautions

• Contraindicated in patients with hypercalcemia or vitamin D toxicity.
🜲 **Lifespan:** In pregnant or breast-feeding women, use cautiously.

Adverse reactions

CNS: headache, somnolence.
EENT: conjunctivitis, photophobia, rhinorrhea.
GI: anorexia, constipation, dry mouth, metallic taste, nausea, vomiting.
GU: polyuria.
Musculoskeletal: bone and muscle pain, weakness.

Interactions

Drug-drug. *Antacids containing magnesium:* May induce hypermagnesemia, especially in patients with chronic renal impairment. Avoid using together.
Cholestyramine, colestipol, excessive use of mineral oil: May decrease absorption of orally given vitamin D analogues. Avoid using together.
Corticosteroids: Counteracts vitamin D analogue effects. Avoid using together.
Digoxin: May increase occurrence of arrhythmias. Avoid using together.

Ketoconazole: May decrease endogenous calcitriol level. Monitor patient.
Phenytoin, phenobarbital: May reduce calcitriol level. Higher doses of calcitriol may be needed.
Thiazides: May induce hypercalcemia. Monitor calcium level and patient closely.
Verapamil: May cause atrial fibrillation because of increased risk of hypercalcemia. Monitor calcium level and patient closely.

Effects on lab test results

• May increase BUN, ALT, AST, albumin, and cholesterol levels.

Pharmacokinetics

Absorption: Readily.
Distribution: Wide; protein-bound.
Metabolism: In liver and kidneys.
Excretion: Mainly in feces. *Half-life:* 3 to 6 hours.

Route	Onset	Peak	Duration
P.O.	2–6 hr	3–6 hr	3–5 days
I.V.	Immediate	Unknown	3–5 days

Action

Chemical effect: Stimulates calcium absorption from GI tract; promotes calcium secretion from bone to blood.
Therapeutic effect: Raises calcium level.

Available forms

Capsules: 0.25 mcg, 0.5 mcg
Injection: 1 mcg/ml, 2 mcg/ml
Oral solution: 1 mcg/ml

NURSING PROCESS

🔲 **Assessment**

• Assess patient's calcium and phosphate levels before therapy and regularly thereafter to monitor the drug's effectiveness; make sure that calcium level times phosphate level isn't more than 70. During dosage adjustment, determine calcium level twice weekly.
• Monitor patient for vitamin D intoxication, which may cause headache, somnolence, weakness, irritability, hypertension, arrhythmias, conjunctivitis, photophobia, rhinorrhea, nausea, vomiting, constipation, polydipsia, pancreatitis, metallic taste, dry mouth, anorexia, nephrocalcinosis, polyuria, nocturia, weight loss, bone and

muscle pain, pruritus, hyperthermia, and decreased libido.
• Look for adverse reactions and drug interactions.
• Assess patient's and family's knowledge of drug therapy.

🔄 **Nursing diagnoses**
• Risk for injury related to patient's underlying condition
• Ineffective protection related to potential for drug-induced vitamin D intoxication
• Deficient knowledge related to drug therapy

▷ **Planning and implementation**
• Keep drug away from heat, light, and moisture.
• Give drug at same time each day.
• If hypercalcemia occurs, stop drug and notify prescriber; resume drug after calcium level returns to normal. Make sure that patient receives adequate daily calcium intake.
🔆 **ALERT:** Don't confuse calcitriol with calciferol or calcitonin.
Patient teaching
• Tell patient to immediately report early symptoms of vitamin D intoxication, such as weakness, nausea, vomiting, dry mouth, constipation, muscle or bone pain, or metallic taste.
• Instruct patient to adhere to diet and calcium supplements and to avoid OTC drugs and antacids containing magnesium.
• Warn patient that drug is the most potent form of vitamin D available and that severe toxicity can occur if ingested by anyone for whom it isn't prescribed.
• Tell patient to protect drug from light, moisture, and heat.

☑ **Evaluation**
• Patient's calcium level is normal.
• Patient doesn't experience injury from drug-induced vitamin D toxicity.
• Patient and family state understanding of drug therapy.

calcium acetate
(KAL-see-um AS-ih-tayt)
Phos-Lo

calcium carbonate
Apo-Cal ◆ †, Cal-Carb-HD†, Calci-Chew†, Calciday 667†, Calci-Mix†, Calcite 500 ◆ †, Calcium 600†, Cal-Plus†, Calsan ◆ †, Caltrate†, Caltrate 600 ◆ †, Chooz†, Fem Cal†, Florical†, Gencalc 600†, Mallamint†, Nephro-Calci, Nu-Cal† ◆, Os-Cal†, Os-Cal 500 ◆, Os-Cal Chewable† ◆, Oysco†, Oysco 500 Chewable†, Oyst-Cal 500†, Oystercal 500†, Oyster Shell Calcium-500†, Rolaids Calcium Rich†, Super Calcium 1200†, Titralac†, Tums†, Tums 500†, Tums E-X†

calcium chloride†
Calciject ◆

calcium citrate†
Citracal†, Citracal Liquitabs ◆ †

calcium glubionate†
Calcium-Sandoz ◆, Neo-Calglucon

calcium gluconate

calcium lactate†

calcium phosphate, dibasic†

calcium phosphate, tribasic
Posture†

Pharmacologic class: mineral, electrolyte
Therapeutic class: calcium supplement, antiarrhythmic
Pregnancy risk category: C

Indications and dosages

▶ **Hypocalcemic emergency.** *Adults:* 7 to 14 mEq calcium I.V. May be given as 10% calcium gluconate solution or 2% to 10% calcium chloride solution.
Children: 1 to 7 mEq calcium I.V.
Infants: Up to 1 mEq calcium I.V.
▶ **Hypocalcemic tetany.** *Adults:* 4.5 to 16 mEq calcium I.V. Repeat until tetany is controlled.

Children: 0.5 to 0.7 mEq/kg calcium I.V. t.i.d. or q.i.d. until tetany is controlled.
Neonates: 2.4 mEq/kg I.V. daily in divided doses.
▶ **Adjunct in cardiac arrest.** *Adults:* 500 mg to 1 g calcium chloride I.V.; rate not to exceed 1 ml/min. Determine calcium level before giving further doses.
▶ **Adjunct in magnesium intoxication.** *Adults:* Initially, 7 mEq I.V. Base subsequent doses on patient's response.
▶ **During exchange transfusions.** *Adults:* 1.35 mEq I.V. with each 100 ml citrated blood. *Neonates:* 0.45 mEq I.V. with each 100 ml citrated blood.
▶ **Hyperphosphatemia in end-stage renal failure.** *Adults:* 2 to 4 tablets calcium acetate P.O. with each meal.
▶ **Dietary supplement.** *Adults:* 800 mg to 1.2 g P.O. daily.

▼ I.V. administration

• Calcium salts aren't interchangeable. Verify preparation before use.
• Give calcium chloride and calcium gluconate I.V only.
• When adding calcium chloride to parenteral solutions that contain other additives (especially phosphorus or phosphate), observe solution closely for precipitate. Use in-line filter.
• Monitor ECG when giving calcium I.V. If patient complains of discomfort, stop and notify prescriber. After injection, make sure patient remains recumbent for 15 minutes.
• Severe necrosis and tissue sloughing can occur after extravasation. Calcium gluconate is less irritating to veins and tissues than calcium chloride.
Direct injection
• Warm solution to body temperature before giving it.
• Give direct injection slowly through small needle into large vein or through I.V. line containing free-flowing, compatible solution at no more than 1 ml/minute (1.5 mEq/minute) for calcium chloride or 0.5 to 2 ml/minute for calcium gluconate. Don't use scalp veins in children.
• Rapid injection may cause syncope, vasodilation, bradycardia, arrhythmias, or cardiac arrest.
Intermittent infusion
• When giving intermittent infusion, infuse diluted solution through I.V. line containing com-

patible solution. Maximum, 200 mg/minute for calcium gluconate.
• Precipitate will form if drug is given I.V. with sodium bicarbonate or other alkaline drugs. Use an in-line filter.
⊗ **Incompatibilities**
Calcium chloride: amphotericin B, chlorpheniramine, dobutamine.
Calcium gluconate: amphotericin B, cefamandole, dobutamine, fluconazole, indomethacin sodium trihydrate, methylprednisolone sodium succinate, prochlorperazine edisylate.

Contraindications and cautions

• Contraindicated in patients with ventricular fibrillation, hypercalcemia, hypophosphatemia, or renal calculi.
• Use all calcium products cautiously in patients taking digitalis and in patients with sarcoidosis and renal or cardiac disease.
• Use calcium chloride cautiously in patients with cor pulmonale, respiratory acidosis, or respiratory impairment.
⚕ **Lifespan:** In children, use I.V. drug cautiously; safety and effectiveness haven't been established.

Adverse reactions

CNS: pain, sense of oppression or heat waves, syncope, tingling.
CV: *arrhythmias, bradycardia, cardiac arrest,* mild decrease in blood pressure, vasodilation.
GI: chalky taste; constipation, *hemorrhage,* or irritation with oral use; nausea; thirst; vomiting.
GU: polyuria, renal calculi.
Metabolic: hypercalcemia.
Skin: burning, cellulitis, necrosis, soft-tissue calcification, and tissue sloughing with I.M. use; irritation with subcutaneous injection.
Other: *vein irritation with I.V. use.*

Interactions

Drug-drug. *Atenolol, fluoroquinolones, tetracyclines:* May decrease bioavailability of these drugs and calcium when oral forms are taken together. Give drugs at different times.
Calcium channel blockers: May decrease calcium effectiveness. Avoid using together.
Ciprofloxacin, gatifloxacin, levofloxacin, lomefloxacin, moxifloxacin, norfloxacin, ofloxacin: May decrease effects of quinolone. Give antacid at least 6 hours before or 2 hours after the quinolone.

Digoxin: May increase digitalis toxicity. Use together cautiously (if at all).

Sodium polystyrene sulfonate: May increase risk of metabolic acidosis in patients with renal disease. Avoid using together in patients with renal disease.

Thiazide diuretics: May increase risk of hypercalcemia. Avoid using together.

Thyroid hormone: May inhibit the absorption of thyroid drugs. Give drugs at least 2 hours apart.

Drug-food. *Foods containing oxalic acid (rhubarb, spinach), phytic acid (bran, whole cereals), or phosphorus (hard cheese, nuts, dried fruits, sardines):* May interfere with calcium absorption. Tell patient to avoid these foods.

Effects on lab test results

• May increase calcium and 11-hydroxycorticosteroid levels.

• May produce false-negative values for serum and urinary magnesium as measured by the Titan yellow method.

Pharmacokinetics

Absorption: Pregnancy and reduced calcium intake may enhance absorption. Vitamin D in active form is required for absorption.

Distribution: Enters extracellular fluid and is incorporated rapidly into skeletal tissue. Bone contains 99% of total calcium; 1% is distributed equally between intracellular and extracellular fluids. Level in CSF is about half that in blood.

Metabolism: Insignificant.

Excretion: Mainly in feces, minimally in urine.

Half-life: Unknown.

Route	Onset	Peak	Duration
P.O.	Unknown	Unknown	Unknown
I.V.	Immediate	Immediate	½–2 hr

Action

Chemical effect: Replaces and maintains calcium.

Therapeutic effect: Raises calcium level.

Available forms

calcium acetate
Contains 253 mg or 12.7 mEq of elemental calcium/g
Injection: 0.5 mEq elemental calcium/ml
Tablets: 250 mg†, 500 mg†, 667 mg, 668 mg†, 1,000 mg†

calcium carbonate
Contains 400 mg or 20 mEq of elemental calcium/g
Capsules: 364 mg†, 1.25 g†
Oral suspension: 1.25 g/5 ml†
Powder packets: 6.5 g (2,400 mg calcium) per packet†
Tablets: 650 mg†, 667 mg†, 750 mg†, 1.25 g†, 1.5 g†
Tablets (chewable): 350 mg†, 420 mg†, 500 mg†, 625 mg†, 750 mg†, 850 mg†, 1.25 g†

calcium chloride
Contains 270 mg or 13.5 mEq of elemental calcium/g
Injection: 10% solution in 10-ml ampules, vials, and syringes

calcium citrate
Contains 211 mg or 10.6 mEq of elemental calcium/g
Effervescent tablets: 2,376 mg†
Tablets: 950 mg†

calcium glubionate
Contains 64 mg or 3.2 mEq of elemental calcium/g
Syrup: 1.8 g/5 ml

calcium gluconate
Contains 90 mg or 4.5 mEq of elemental calcium/g
Injection: 10% solution in 10-ml ampules and vials, 10-ml or 50-ml vials
Tablets: 500 mg†, 650 mg†, 975 mg†, 1 g†

calcium lactate
Contains 130 mg or 6.5 mEq of elemental calcium/g
Tablets: 325 mg, 650 mg

calcium phosphate, dibasic
Contains 230 mg or 11.5 mEq of elemental calcium/g
Tablets: 468 mg†

calcium phosphate, tribasic
Contains 400 mg or 20 mEq of elemental calcium/g
Tablets: 600 mg†

NURSING PROCESS

Assessment

• Assess patient's calcium level before therapy and frequently thereafter to monitor the drug's effectiveness. Hypercalcemia may result after large doses in patients with chronic renal impairment.

Reactions may be *common,* uncommon, *life-threatening,* or COMMON AND LIFE-THREATENING.

• Look for adverse reactions and drug interactions.
• Assess patient's and family's knowledge of drug therapy.

⊞ **Nursing diagnoses**
• Ineffective protection related to calcium deficiency
• Risk for injury related to drug-induced adverse reactions
• Deficient knowledge related to drug therapy

▷ **Planning and implementation**
• If hypercalcemia occurs, stop drug and notify prescriber. Provide emergency supportive care until calcium level returns to normal.
• Signs and symptoms of severe hypercalcemia may include stupor, confusion, delirium, and coma. Signs and symptoms of mild hypercalcemia may include anorexia, nausea, and vomiting.
⊛ ALERT: Make sure prescriber specifies which calcium form to use because code carts usually contain both calcium gluconate and calcium chloride.
Patient teaching
• Tell patient to take oral calcium 1 to 1½ hours after meals if GI upset occurs.
⊛ ALERT: Warn patient to avoid foods containing oxalic acid, phytic acid, and phosphorus because interactions may interfere with calcium absorption.
• Teach patient to recognize and report signs and symptoms of hypercalcemia.
• Stress importance of follow-up care and regular blood samples to monitor calcium level.

☑ **Evaluation**
• Patient's calcium level is normal.
• Patient doesn't experience injury from calcium-induced adverse reactions.
• Patient and family state understanding of drug therapy.

calcium carbonate
(KAL-see-um KAR-buh-nayt)
Alka-Mints†, Amitone†, Cal-Sup◇, Chooz†, Equilet†, Mallamint†, Rolaids Calcium Rich†, Titralac†, Titralac Extra Strength†, Titralac Plus†, Tums†, Tums E-X†, Tums Extra Strength†

Pharmacologic class: mineral, electrolyte
Therapeutic class: antacid, calcium supplement
Pregnancy risk category: NR

Indications and dosages
▶ **Gastric hyperacidity, calcium supplement.**
Adults: 350 mg to 1.25 g P.O. or two pieces of chewing gum 1 hour after meals and h.s. p.r.n.

Contraindications and cautions
• Contraindicated in patients with ventricular fibrillation or hypercalcemia.
• Use cautiously, if at all, in patients receiving digoxin and in those with sarcoidosis, dehydration, electrolyte imbalance, renal impairment, or cardiac disease.
⚹ Lifespan: In pregnant women, consult provider before use.

Adverse reactions
GI: constipation, flatulence, gastric distention, nausea, rebound hyperacidity.

Interactions
Drug-drug. *Antibiotics (including tetracyclines), hydantoins, iron, isoniazid, salicylates, thyroid hormones:* May decrease effects of these drugs because of impaired absorption. Give at different times.
Ciprofloxacin, gatifloxacin, levofloxacin, lomefloxacin, moxifloxacin, norfloxacin, ofloxacin: May decrease effects of quinolone. Give antacid at least 6 hours before or 2 hours after the quinolone.
Enteric-coated drugs: May release prematurely in stomach. Don't give within an hour of each other.
Sodium bicarbonate: May cause milk-alkali syndrome (headache, confusion, nausea, vomiting, hypercalcemia, hypercalciuria, metabolic alkalosis, weakness, and hypophosphatemia). Discourage using together.

Effects on lab test results

• May increase calcium level. May decrease phosphate level.

Pharmacokinetics

Absorption: Pregnancy and reduced calcium intake may enhance absorption. Vitamin D in its active form is required for absorption.
Distribution: Enters extracellular fluid and is incorporated rapidly into skeletal tissue. Bone contains 99% of total calcium; 1% is distributed equally between intracellular and extracellular fluids. Level in CSF is about half that in blood.
Metabolism: Insignificant.
Excretion: Mainly in feces, minimally in urine.
Half-life: Unknown.

Route	Onset	Peak	Duration
P.O.			
fasting	≤ 20 min	Unknown	20–60 min
nonfasting	≤ 20 min	Unknown	3 hr

Action

Chemical effect: Reduces total acid load in GI tract, elevates gastric pH to reduce pepsin activity, strengthens gastric mucosal barrier, and increases esophageal sphincter tone.
Therapeutic effect: Raises calcium level and relieves mild gastric discomfort.

Available forms

Contains 40% calcium; 20 mEq calcium/g
Chewing gum: 500 mg/piece
Oral suspension: 400 mg/5 ml, 1.25 g/5 ml†
Tablets: 500 mg†, 600 mg†, 650 mg†, 1,250 mg†
Tablets (chewable): 350 mg†, 420 mg†, 500 mg†, 750 mg, 850 mg, 1,000 mg, 1,250 mg ◊

NURSING PROCESS

⁂ Assessment
• Assess patient's underlying condition before therapy and regularly thereafter.
• Monitor calcium level, especially in patient with mild renal impairment or dehydration.
• Look for adverse reactions and drug interactions.
• Assess patient's and family's knowledge of drug therapy.

⊕ Nursing diagnoses
• Imbalanced nutrition: less than body requirements related to insufficient calcium intake
• Risk for injury related to calcium-induced hypercalcemia
• Deficient knowledge related to drug therapy

▶ Planning and implementation
• Give 1 hour after meals, p.r.n.
• Make sure patient with calcium deficiency is receiving adequate calcium, fiber, and fluid in diet.
• Divide daily oral calcium supplements into three or four doses.
Patient teaching
• Advise patient not to take drug indiscriminately and not to switch antacids without consulting prescriber.
• Tell patient to take drug 1 hour after meals and at bedtime, p.r.n.
• Tell patient to notify prescriber of continuing symptoms and of tarry stools or "coffee ground" vomitus. Tell him not to use antacids continuously for more than 2 weeks without prescriber consent.

✓ Evaluation
• Patient's symptoms are alleviated.
• Patient's calcium level is normal.
• Patient and family state understanding of drug therapy.

calfactant
(kal-FAK-tant)
Infasurf

Pharmacologic class: surfactant
Therapeutic class: respiratory distress syndrome (RDS) drug
Pregnancy risk category: NR

Indications and dosages

▶ **Confirmed RDS in neonates younger than 72 hours old who need endotracheal intubation.** *Neonates:* 3 ml/kg birth weight, intratracheally, given in 2 aliquots of 1.5 ml/kg. Repeat doses of 3 ml/kg of birth weight, given in 2 aliquots of 1.5 ml/kg, up to a total of three doses given 12 hours apart.
▶ **Prevention of RDS in premature infants younger than 29 weeks' gestational age at**

high risk for RDS. 3 ml/kg birth weight, given intratracheally within 30 minutes of birth, in 2 aliquots of 1.5 ml/kg each.

Contraindications and cautions

None reported.
❋ **Lifespan:** Indicated for premature infants only.

Adverse reactions

CV: BRADYCARDIA, *cyanosis.*
Respiratory: AIRWAY OBSTRUCTION, APNEA, *dislodgment of endotracheal tube, hypoventilation, reflux of drug into endotracheal tube.*

Interactions

None significant.

Effects on lab test results

None reported.

Pharmacokinetics

Absorption: Unknown.
Distribution: Unknown.
Metabolism: Unknown.
Excretion: Unknown. *Half-life:* Unknown.

Route	Onset	Peak	Duration
Intratracheal	24–48 hr	Unknown	Unknown

Action

Chemical effect: Modifies alveolar surface tension, thereby stabilizing the alveoli.
Therapeutic effect: Prevents or treats RDS in premature neonates with specific characteristics.

Available forms

Intratracheal suspension: 35 mg phospholipids and 0.65 mg proteins/ml; 6-ml vial

NURSING PROCESS

☡ Assessment
• Assess patient's underlying condition before therapy and regularly thereafter.
• Monitor patient for reflux of drug into endotracheal tube, cyanosis, bradycardia, or airway obstruction. If these occur, stop the drug and stabilize infant. After infant is stable, give the remainder of the dose, with appropriate monitoring.

• After giving drug, carefully monitor infant so oxygen therapy and ventilation can be adjusted for improved oxygenation and lung compliance.
• Evaluate parents' knowledge of drug therapy.

⊞ Nursing diagnoses
• Risk for injury related to potential for RDS
• Impaired gas exchange related to presence of RDS
• Deficient knowledge related to drug therapy

▶ Planning and implementation
• Give drug under supervision of a prescriber experienced in the acute care of neonates with respiratory impairment who need intubation.
• Drug is intended only for intratracheal use; to prevent RDS, give immediately after birth, preferably within 30 minutes.
• Suspension settles during storage. Gently swirl or agitate the vial to redisperse, but don't shake. Visible flecks in the suspension and foaming at the surface are normal.
• Withdraw dose into a syringe from single-use vial using a 20G or larger needle; avoid excessive foaming.
• Use each single-use vial only once; discard unused material.
• Give through a side-port adapter into the endotracheal tube. Two health care providers should be present. Give dose in 2 aliquots of 1.5 ml/kg each. Continue ventilation over 20 to 30 breaths for each aliquot, with small bursts timed to occur during inspiration. Evaluate respiration and reposition infant between each aliquot.
• Store drug at 36° to 46° F (2° to 8° C). Don't warm drug before use; it's not needed. Unopened, unused vials that have warmed to room temperature can be returned to refrigerated storage within 24 hours for future use. Avoid repeated warming to room temperature.

Patient teaching
• Explain to parents the reason for using drug to prevent or treat RDS.
• Notify parents that although the infant may improve rapidly after therapy, he may still need intubation and mechanical ventilation.
• Notify parents of the adverse effects of drug, including bradycardia, reflux into endotracheal tube, airway obstruction, cyanosis, dislodgment of endotracheal tube, and hypoventilation.
• Reassure parents that infant will be carefully monitored.

☑ **Evaluation**
- Premature infant doesn't develop RDS.
- Patient's gas exchange improves because of oxygenation and increased lung compliance.
- Parents state understanding of drug therapy.

candesartan cilexetil
(kan-dih-SAR-ten se-LEKS-ih-til)
Atacand

Pharmacologic class: angiotensin II receptor antagonist
Therapeutic class: antihypertensive
Pregnancy risk category: C (D in second and third trimesters)

Indications and dosages

▶ **Heart failure.** *Adults:* Initially, 4 mg P.O. once daily. Double the dose approximately every 2 weeks as tolerated, to a target dose of 32 mg once daily.
▶ **Hypertension (alone or with other antihypertensives).** *Adults:* Initially, 16 mg P.O. once daily when used as monotherapy; usual dosage is 8 to 32 mg P.O. daily as single dose or divided b.i.d.
Adjust-a-dose: In patients with volume depletion or moderate hepatic impairment, consider giving lower initial dose.

Contraindications and cautions

- Contraindicated in patients hypersensitive to drug or its components.
- Use cautiously in patients whose renal function depends on the renin-angiotensin-aldosterone system (such as patients with heart failure) because of risk of oliguria and progressive azotemia resulting in acute renal impairment. Also use cautiously in patients who are volume- or salt-depleted because of risk of symptomatic hypotension.

Lifespan: In pregnant women, don't use because drug acts directly on the renin-angiotensin system and may harm the fetus or neonate. If drug is absolutely needed, limit to first trimester. If pregnancy is suspected, stop the drug. In breast-feeding women, use cautiously because the effects on the infant are unknown.

Adverse reactions

CNS: dizziness, fatigue, headache.
CV: chest pain, peripheral edema.
EENT: pharyngitis, rhinitis, sinusitis.
GI: abdominal pain, diarrhea, nausea, vomiting.
GU: albuminuria.
Musculoskeletal: arthralgia, back pain.
Respiratory: bronchitis, cough, upper respiratory tract infection.

Interactions

Drug-drug. *Lithium:* May increase lithium level. Carefully monitor lithium level for toxicity.

Effects on lab test results

- May increase bilirubin, lithium, BUN, creatinine, potassium, and uric acid levels. May decrease hemoglobin level and hematocrit.
- May increase liver function test results.

Pharmacokinetics

Absorption: Absolute bioavailability is about 15%.
Distribution: More than 99% binds to protein and doesn't penetrate RBCs.
Metabolism: Rapid and complete.
Excretion: About 33% is in urine (26% unchanged) and 67% in feces. *Half-life:* 9 hours.

Route	Onset	Peak	Duration
P.O.	Unknown	3–4 hr	24 hr

Action

Chemical effect: Blocks the angiotensin II receptor on the surface of vascular smooth muscle and other tissue cells.
Therapeutic effect: Dilates blood vessels and decreases blood pressure.

Available forms

Tablets: 4 mg, 8 mg, 16 mg, 32 mg

NURSING PROCESS

Assessment
- Monitor patient's electrolytes, and assess patient for volume or salt depletion (as from vigorous diuretic use) before starting therapy.
- Carefully monitor therapeutic response and adverse reactions, especially in elderly patients and patients with renal or moderate liver impairment
- Assess patient's and family's knowledge of drug therapy.

🖅 Nursing diagnoses

• Decreased cardiac output related to risk for symptomatic hypotension in volume- or salt-depleted patients
• Risk for imbalanced fluid volume in patients with impaired renal function related to drug-induced oliguria
• Deficient knowledge related to drug therapy

🖅 Planning and implementation

• Make sure patient is adequately hydrated before starting therapy.
• Observe patient for hypotension. If it occurs after a dose, place patient in supine position and, if needed, give an I.V. infusion of normal saline solution.
• Most of antihypertensive effect occurs within 2 weeks. Maximal antihypertensive effect is obtained within 4 to 6 weeks. If blood pressure isn't controlled by drug alone, add diuretic.
• Drug can't be removed by hemodialysis.

Patient teaching

• Advise woman of childbearing age about risk of second- and third-trimester exposure to drug. If pregnancy is suspected, tell her to notify prescriber immediately.
• Tell patient to report adverse reactions promptly.
• Instruct patient to take drug exactly as directed.
• Tell patient that drug may be taken with or without food.

🖅 Evaluation

• Patient's volume or salt depletion is corrected so that symptomatic hypotension doesn't occur.
• Patient maintains fluid balance.
• Patient and family state understanding of drug therapy.

capecitabine
(kape-SITE-a-been)
Xeloda

Pharmacologic class: fluoropyrimidine carbamate
Therapeutic class: antineoplastic
Pregnancy risk category: D

Indications and dosages

▶ First-line therapy for metastatic colorectal cancer; Dukes C colon cancer after complete resection of primary tumor when treatment with fluoropyrimidine therapy alone is preferred; metastatic breast cancer resistant to combined paclitaxel and anthracycline therapy, or paclitaxel after anthracycline therapy, or with docetaxel after anthracycline failure. *Adults:* 1,250 mg/m^2 P.O. within 30 minutes after morning and evening meals for 2 weeks; followed by a 1-week rest period. Continue as a q-3-week cycle, adjusted for toxicity and individual needs.
🖅 **Adjust-a-dose:** For patients with renal impairment, if creatinine clearance is 30 to 50 ml/minute, reduce initial dose by 75%.

Contraindications and cautions

• Contraindicated in patients hypersensitive to 5-fluorouracil (5-FU).
🖅 **Lifespan:** In pregnant women, use only in life-threatening situations or severe disease for which safer drugs can't be used or are ineffective. Breast-feeding should be stopped during therapy. In children, safety and effectiveness haven't been established. In patients older than age 80, use cautiously because they may have a greater risk of GI adverse effects.

Adverse reactions

CNS: dizziness, *fatigue, headache,* insomnia, mood alteration, *pain, paresthesia, peripheral neuropathy,* tremor.
CV: dysrhythmias, *edema,* venous thrombosis.
EENT: *eye irritation, increased lacrimation,* rhinorrhea, sore throat.
GI: *abdominal pain, anorexia, constipation, diarrhea,* dyspepsia, *nausea, stomatitis,* taste disturbance, *vomiting.*
Hematologic: anemia, *leukopenia, lymphopenia, neutropenia, thrombocytopenia.*
Hepatic: *hyperbilirubinemia.*
Musculoskeletal: *back pain,* limb pain, myalgia.
Respiratory: cough, *dyspnea,* pharyngeal disorder.
Skin: alopecia, *dermatitis, hand-foot syndrome,* nail disorder.
Other: dehydration, *fever.*

Interactions

Drug-drug. *Leucovorin:* May increase 5-FU level and toxicity. Monitor patient carefully.

Phenytoin: May increase phenytoin level. Monitor level carefully. Consider decreased phenytoin dose.

Warfarin: May increase risk of bleeding and death. Avoid this combination, or monitor PT and INR often, and adjust warfarin dose, if needed.

Drug-food. *Any food:* May decrease rate and extent of absorption. Give drug 30 minutes after a meal to decrease GI adverse events, but avoid excessive drug inactivation.

Effects on lab test results
• May increase bilirubin, AST, ALT, alkaline phosphatase, and hemoglobin levels and hematocrit.
• May increase PT and INR. May decrease platelet, lymphocyte, and neutrophil counts.

Pharmacokinetics
Absorption: Good.
Distribution: About 60% is bound to proteins.
Metabolism: Extensively in the liver and tumor cells.
Excretion: 70% in urine. *Half-life:* About 45 minutes.

Route	Onset	Peak	Duration
P.O.	Unknown	1½–2 hr	Unknown

Action
Chemical effect: Interferes with DNA synthesis to inhibit cell division and with RNA processing and protein synthesis.
Therapeutic effect: Inhibits cell growth of selected cancers.

Available forms
Tablets: 150 mg, 500 mg

NURSING PROCESS

Assessment
• Assess patient's underlying condition before therapy and regularly thereafter.
• Assess patient for coronary artery disease, mild-to-moderate hepatic impairment caused by liver metastases, hyperbilirubinemia, and renal insufficiency.
• Monitor PT and INR in patients also taking warfarin because of increased risk of bleeding. Patients older than age 60 are also at risk for coagulopathies, even if they aren't taking warfarin.

• Monitor patient for severe diarrhea; if it occurs, notify prescriber.
• Monitor patient for hand-foot syndrome (numbness, paresthesia, tingling, painless or painful swelling, erythema, desquamation, blistering, and severe pain of hands or feet), hyperbilirubinemia, and severe nausea. If these reactions occur, adjust therapy immediately.
• Assess patient's and family's knowledge of drug therapy.

Nursing diagnoses
• Risk for infection related to adverse effects of drug
• Risk for impaired skin integrity related to potential for hand-foot syndrome
• Deficient knowledge related to drug therapy

Planning and implementation
• If diarrhea occurs and patient becomes dehydrated, give fluid and electrolyte replacement. Stop the drug immediately until diarrhea resolves or decreases in intensity.
• If hyperbilirubinemia occurs, stop the drug.
• Monitor patient for toxicity. To manage toxicity, treat symptoms, stop the drug temporarily, and reduce the dosage.
Patient teaching
• Inform patient and family of expected adverse drug effects, especially nausea, vomiting, diarrhea, and hand-foot syndrome. Explain that dose will be adjusted.
ⓢ ALERT: Instruct patient to stop taking the drug and to contact prescriber immediately if he develops diarrhea (more than four bowel movements daily or diarrhea at night), vomiting (two to five episodes in 24 hours), nausea, appetite loss or decrease in amount of food taken each day, stomatitis (pain, redness, swelling or sores in mouth), hand-foot syndrome, fever of 100.5° F (38° C) or more, or other evidence of infection.
• Tell patient that most adverse effects improve within 2 or 3 days after stopping drug and that if they don't, he should contact prescriber.
• Tell patient how to take drug. Dosage cycle is usually to take drug for 14 days followed by 7-day rest period. Inform him how many cycles he should take.
• Instruct patient to take drug with water within 30 minutes after breakfast and after dinner.

• If a combination of tablets is prescribed, teach patient importance of correctly identifying the tablets.

• For missed doses, instruct patient not to take the missed dose and not to double the next one. Instead, he should continue with regular schedule and check with prescriber.

• Instruct patient to inform prescriber if he's taking folic acid.

☑ **Evaluation**

• Patient doesn't develop infection.

• Patient doesn't develop hand-foot syndrome.

• Patient and family state understanding of drug therapy.

captopril
(KAP-toh-pril)
Capoten◆

Pharmacologic class: ACE inhibitor
Therapeutic class: antihypertensive, adjunct treatment of heart failure and diabetic nephropathy
Pregnancy risk category: C (D in second and third trimesters)

Indications and dosages

▶ **Hypertension.** *Adults:* Initially, 25 mg P.O. b.i.d. or t.i.d. If blood pressure isn't controlled in 1 to 2 weeks, increase dosage to 50 mg b.i.d. or t.i.d. If not controlled after another 1 to 2 weeks, add thiazide diuretic. If blood pressure needs to be reduced further, raise dosage as high as 150 mg t.i.d. while continuing diuretic. Maximum daily dose, 450 mg.

▶ **Heart failure.** *Adults:* 6.25 to 12.5 mg P.O. t.i.d. initially. Gradually increase to 50 to 100 mg t.i.d. p.r.n. Maximum daily dose, 450 mg.

▶ **Diabetic nephropathy.** *Adults:* 25 mg P.O. t.i.d.

▶ **Left ventricular dysfunction after MI.**
Adults: 6.25 mg P.O. as a single dose 3 days after MI; then 12.5 mg t.i.d., increasing dosage to 25 mg t.i.d. Target dosage is 50 mg t.i.d.

Contraindications and cautions

• Contraindicated in patients hypersensitive to drug or other ACE inhibitors.

• Use cautiously in patients with renal impairment or serious autoimmune disease (particularly systemic lupus erythematosus), and in patients exposed to other drugs known to affect WBC counts or immune response.

☀ **Lifespan:** In pregnant women, use cautiously. If patient becomes pregnant, drug usually is stopped. In breast-feeding women, use cautiously. In children, safety and effectiveness haven't been established.

Adverse reactions

CNS: dizziness, fainting, fever.
CV: angina pectoris, *heart failure, hypotension,* pericarditis, tachycardia.
GI: anorexia, dysgeusia.
GU: proteinuria, membranous glomerulopathy, nephrotic syndrome, *renal impairment* (in patients with renal disease or those receiving high dosages), urinary frequency.
Hematologic: *agranulocytosis, leukopenia, pancytopenia, thrombocytopenia.*
Hepatic: cholestatic jaundice, elevated liver enzyme levels.
Metabolic: *hyperkalemia.*
Respiratory: cough.
Skin: maculopapular rash, pruritus, urticaria.
Other: *angioedema.*

Interactions

Drug-drug. *Antacids:* May decrease captopril effect. Separate doses.
Digoxin: May increase digoxin level by 15% to 30%. Monitor patient for digitalis toxicity.
Diuretics, other antihypertensives: May increase risk of excessive hypotension. Stop diuretic or lower captopril dosage.
Insulin, oral antidiabetics: May increase risk of hypoglycemia when captopril therapy starts. Monitor patient closely.
Lithium: May increase lithium level and cause lithium toxicity. Monitor patient closely.
NSAIDs: May reduce antihypertensive effect. Monitor blood pressure.
Potassium supplements, potassium-sparing diuretics: May increase risk of hyperkalemia. Avoid these drugs unless hypokalemic level is confirmed.
Probenecid: May increase captopril level. Avoid using together.
Drug-food. *Any food:* May reduce absorption of drug. Give drug 1 hour before meals.

Drug-herb. *Black catechu:* May have additional hypotensive effects of catechu. Discourage using together.
Capsaicin: May worsen captopril-related cough. Discourage herb use.
Licorice: May cause sodium retention, which counteracts ACE effects. Monitor blood pressure.

Effects on lab test results

• May increase alkaline phosphatase, bilirubin, and potassium levels and may cause a transient increase in hepatic enzyme levels. May decrease hemoglobin level and hematocrit.
• May decrease WBC, granulocyte, RBC, and platelet counts.

Pharmacokinetics

Absorption: Through GI tract; food may reduce absorption by up to 40%.
Distribution: Into most body tissues except CNS; 25% to 30% protein-bound.
Metabolism: About 50% in liver.
Excretion: Mainly in urine, minimally in feces.
Half-life: Less than 2 hours.

Route	Onset	Peak	Duration
P.O.	15–60 min	30–90 min	6–12 hr

Action

Chemical effect: Thought to inhibit ACE, preventing conversion of angiotensin I to angiotensin II. Reduced formation of angiotensin II decreases peripheral arterial resistance, thus decreasing aldosterone secretion.
Therapeutic effect: Reduces sodium and water retention, lowers blood pressure, and helps improve renal function adversely affected by diabetes.

Available forms

Tablets: 12.5 mg, 25 mg, 50 mg, 100 mg

NURSING PROCESS

Assessment

• Assess patient's underlying condition before therapy and regularly thereafter.
• Monitor blood pressure and pulse rate often.
• Monitor WBC and differential counts before therapy, every 2 weeks for first 3 months, and periodically thereafter.

• Monitor potassium level and renal function (BUN and creatinine clearance levels, urinalysis).
• Be alert for adverse reactions and drug interactions.
• Assess patient's and family's knowledge of drug therapy.

Nursing diagnoses

• Risk for injury related to patient's underlying condition
• Ineffective protection related to drug-induced blood disorder
• Deficient knowledge related to drug therapy

Planning and implementation

• If patient has persistent dry, tickling, nonproductive cough, watch closely for adverse reaction and respiratory impairment.
• Because antacids decrease drug's effect, separate doses.
• If patient develops fever, sore throat, leukopenia, hypotension, or tachycardia, withhold dose and notify prescriber.
• Notify prescriber of abnormal laboratory studies.
ALERT: Don't confuse captopril with carvedilol.
Patient teaching
• Instruct patient to take drug 1 hour before meals because food decreases drug absorption.
• Inform patient that light-headedness may occur, especially during the first few days of therapy. Tell patient to rise slowly to minimize this effect and to report symptoms to prescriber. Tell patient who experiences syncope to stop taking drug and call prescriber immediately.
• Tell patient to use caution in hot weather and during exercise. Inadequate fluid intake, vomiting, diarrhea, and excessive perspiration can lead to light-headedness and syncope.
• Advise patient to report signs of infection, such as fever and sore throat.
• Tell woman to notify prescriber if she becomes pregnant because drug will be stopped.
• Tell patient to notify prescriber if cough interferes with sleep or required activities so that drug can be changed.

Evaluation

• Patient's underlying condition improves.
• Patient's WBC and differential counts are normal.

• Patient and family state understanding of drug therapy.

carbamazepine
(kar-buh-MAH-zuh-peen)
Apo-Carbamazepine ♦, Atretol, Carbatrol, Epitol, Equetro, Novo-Carbamaz ♦, Tegretol, Tegretol CR ♦, Tegretol-XR, Teril

Pharmacologic class: iminostilbene derivative
Therapeutic class: anticonvulsant, analgesic
Pregnancy risk category: D

Indications and dosages

► **Generalized tonic-clonic and complex partial seizures, mixed seizure patterns.** *Adults and children older than age 12:* Initially, 200 mg P.O. b.i.d. for tablets or 100 mg of suspension P.O. q.i.d. Increase at weekly intervals by 200 mg P.O. daily, in divided doses at 6- to 8-hour intervals. Adjust to minimum effective level when control is achieved. Maximum daily dosage, 1 g in children ages 12 to 15, or 1.2 g in patients older than age 15.
Children ages 6 to 12: Initially, 100 mg P.O. b.i.d., or 50 mg of suspension P.O. q.i.d. Increase at weekly intervals by 100 mg P.O. daily. Maximum daily dose is 1 g.
Children younger than age 6: 10 to 20 mg/kg P.O. daily in two to three divided doses (tablets) or four divided doses (suspension). Increase weekly to achieve optimal response. Maximum, 35 mg/kg/day.
► **Trigeminal neuralgia.** *Adults:* Initially, 100 mg P.O. b.i.d. or 50 mg of suspension P.O. q.i.d. with meals. Increase by 100 mg q 12 hours for tablets or 50 mg of suspension q.i.d. until pain is relieved. Maintenance dosage, 200 to 1,200 mg P.O. daily. Maximum daily dosage is 1,200 mg. Decrease dose to minimum effective level, or stop drug at least once q 3 months.
► **Restless leg syndrome‡.** *Adults:* 100 to 300 mg P.O. q h.s.
► **Chorea‡.** *Children:* 15 to 25 mg/kg P.O. daily.
► **Acute manic and mixed episodes in bipolar 1 disorder (Equetro).** *Adults:* Initially, 200 mg P.O. b.i.d. Increase by 200 mg daily to achieve therapeutic response. Doses higher than 1,600 mg daily haven't been studied.

Contraindications and cautions

• Contraindicated in patients hypersensitive to drug or tricyclic antidepressants, in patients with previous bone marrow suppression, and within 14 days of MAO inhibitor therapy.
• Use cautiously in patients with mixed seizure disorders because drugs may increase risk of seizures, usually atypical absence or generalized.
⚥ **Lifespan:** In pregnant women, use cautiously. If breast-feeding woman must take drug, breast-feeding should be stopped.

Adverse reactions

CNS: ataxia, dizziness, drowsiness, fatigue, fever, vertigo, *worsening of seizures* (usually in patients with mixed seizure disorders, including atypical absence seizures).
CV: aggravation of coronary artery disease, *heart failure,* hypertension, hypotension.
EENT: blurred vision, conjunctivitis, diplopia, dry mouth and pharynx, nystagmus.
GI: abdominal pain, anorexia, diarrhea, glossitis, nausea, stomatitis, vomiting.
GU: albuminuria, glycosuria, impotence, urinary frequency, urine retention.
Hematologic: *agranulocytosis, aplastic anemia,* eosinophilia, leukocytosis, *thrombocytopenia.*
Hepatic: *hepatitis.*
Respiratory: pulmonary hypersensitivity.
Skin: erythema multiforme, excessive sweating, rash, *Stevens-Johnson syndrome,* urticaria.
Other: chills, *water intoxication.*

Interactions

Drug-drug. *Atracurium, cisatracurium, doxacurium, mivacurium, pancuronium, rocuronium, tubocurarine, vecuronium:* May decrease the effects of nondepolarizing muscle relaxant, causing it to be less effective. May need to increase the dose of the nondepolarizing muscle relaxant.
Charcoal: May decrease GI absorption of carbamazepine. Use only in cases of overdose to promote drug clearance.
Cimetidine, danazol, diltiazem, macrolides, isoniazid, propoxyphene, valproic acid, verapamil: May increase carbamazepine level. Use together cautiously.
Clarithromycin, erythromycin, troleandomycin: May inhibit carbamazepine metabolism, causing

increased level and risk of toxicity. Avoid using together.
Doxycycline, haloperidol, hormonal contraceptives, phenytoin, tiagabine, theophylline, topiramate, valproate, warfarin: May decrease levels of these drugs. Monitor patient for decreased effect.
Lithium: May increase risk of CNS toxicity of lithium. Avoid using together.
MAO inhibitors: May increase depressant and anticholinergic effects. Don't use together.
Phenobarbital, phenytoin, primidone: May decrease carbamazepine level. Monitor patient for decreased effect.
Drug-herb. *Plantains:* Psyllium seeds may inhibit GI absorption. Discourage using together.

Effects on lab test results

• May increase BUN level. May decrease hemoglobin level and hematocrit.
• May increase eosinophil count. May decrease granulocyte, WBC, and platelet counts and thyroid and liver function test values.

Pharmacokinetics

Absorption: Slow.
Distribution: Widely throughout body; about 75% protein-bound.
Metabolism: By liver to active metabolite; may also induce its own metabolism.
Excretion: 70% in urine and 30% in feces.
Half-life: 25 to 65 hours with single dose; 8 to 29 hours with long-term use.

Route	Onset	Peak	Duration
P.O.			
extended-release	Unknown	4–8 hr	Unknown
suspension	1 hr	1½ hr	Unknown
tablets	1 hr	4–12 hr	Unknown

Action

Chemical effect: May stabilize neuronal membranes and limit seizure activity by increasing efflux or decreasing influx of sodium ions across cell membranes in motor cortex during generation of nerve impulses.
Therapeutic effect: Prevents seizure activity; eliminates pain caused by trigeminal neuralgia.

Available forms

Capsules (extended-release): 100 mg, 200 mg, 300 mg

Oral suspension: 100 mg/5 ml
Tablets: 200 mg
Tablets (chewable): 100 mg, 200 mg
Tablets (extended-release): 100 mg, 200 mg, 400 mg

NURSING PROCESS

✐ Assessment

• Assess patient's seizure disorder or trigeminal neuralgia before therapy and regularly thereafter.
• Obtain baseline determinations of urinalysis, BUN level, liver function, CBC, platelet and reticulocyte counts, and iron level. Reassess regularly.
• Monitor drug level and effects closely. Therapeutic level is 4 to 12 mcg/ml.
• Be alert for adverse reactions and drug interactions.
• Assess patient's and family's knowledge of drug therapy.

Nursing diagnoses

• Risk for injury related to seizure disorder
• Acute pain related to trigeminal neuralgia
• Deficient knowledge related to drug therapy

Planning and implementation

⊛ ALERT: Don't confuse Tegretol or Tegretol-XR with Topamax or Toprol-XL.
• Give drug in divided doses to maintain consistent level.
• Give drug with food to minimize GI distress.
• Shake oral suspension well before measuring dose.
• When giving by NG tube, mix dose with equal volume of water, normal saline solution, or D_5W. Flush tube with 100 ml of diluent after giving dose.
⊛ ALERT: When treating seizures or status epilepticus, never abruptly stop giving the drug. If adverse reactions occur, notify prescriber immediately. Increase dosage gradually to minimize adverse reactions.
Patient teaching
• Tell patient to take drug with food to minimize GI distress.
• Tell patient to keep tablets in original container, tightly closed, and away from moisture. Some formulations may harden when exposed to excess moisture, resulting in decreased bioavailability and loss of seizure control.

Reactions may be *common*, uncommon, *life-threatening*, or COMMON AND LIFE-THREATENING.

C

• Inform patient with trigeminal neuralgia that prescriber may attempt to decrease dosage or withdraw drug every 3 months.

⑤ **ALERT:** Tell patient to notify prescriber immediately about fever, sore throat, mouth ulcers, or easy bruising or bleeding.

• Warn patient that drug may cause mild-to-moderate dizziness and drowsiness at first. Advise patient to avoid hazardous activities until effects disappear (usually within 3 to 4 days).

• Advise patient to have periodic eye examinations.

☑ Evaluation

• Patient remains free from seizures.

• Patient reports pain relief.

• Patient and family state understanding of drug therapy.

carboplatin

(KAR-boh-plat-in)
Paraplatin, Paraplatin-AQ ♦

Pharmacologic class: alkylating drug
Therapeutic class: antineoplastic
Pregnancy risk category: D

Indications and dosages

▶ **Palliative therapy for ovarian cancer.**
Adults: 360 mg/m² I.V. on day 1 q 4 weeks; don't repeat dosages until platelet count exceeds 100,000/mm³ and neutrophil count exceeds 2,000/mm³. Base later dosages on blood counts.
◣ **Adjust-a-dose:** For patients with renal impairment, if creatinine clearance is 41 to 59 ml/minute, starting dose is 250 mg/m² I.V. If creatinine clearance is 16 to 40 ml/minute, it's 200 mg/m². Recommended dosage adjustments aren't available for patients with creatinine clearance of 15 ml/minute or less.

▶ **Initial therapy for advanced ovarian cancer, with cyclophosphamide.** *Adults:* Initial dose is 300 mg/m² I.V. on day 1 q 4 weeks for six cycles. Don't repeat cycles until the neutrophil count is greater than or equal to 2,000/mm³ and the platelet count is greater than or equal to 100,000/mm³.

▽ I.V. administration

• Have epinephrine, corticosteroids, and antihistamines available when giving drug because anaphylactoid reactions may occur within minutes of administration.

• Preparing and giving I.V. form is linked to mutagenic, teratogenic, and carcinogenic risks for personnel. Follow facility policy to reduce risks.

• Reconstitute powder for injection with D_5W, normal saline solution, or sterile water for injection to make 10 mg/ml. Add 5 ml of diluent to 50-mg vial, 15 ml of diluent to 150-mg vial, or 45 ml of diluent to 450-mg vial. Then, further dilute reconstituted powder or aqueous solution for injection with normal saline solution or D_5W before infusion. Concentrations as low as 0.5 mg/ml can be prepared.

• Give drug by continuous or intermittent infusion over at least 15 minutes.

• Don't give carboplatin with needles or I.V. administration sets that contain aluminum because drug may precipitate or lose potency.

• Store unopened vials at room temperature. Once reconstituted and diluted, drug is stable at room temperature for 8 hours. Discard unused drug at this time.

⊗ **Incompatibilities**
Amphotericin B cholesteryl sulfate complex, fluorouracil, mesna, sodium bicarbonate.

Contraindications and cautions

• Contraindicated in patients hypersensitive to cisplatin, platinum-containing compounds, or mannitol. Also contraindicated in patients with severe bone marrow suppression or bleeding.

✾ **Lifespan:** In pregnant women, drug is contraindicated. In breast-feeding women and in children, safety and effectiveness haven't been established. In patients older than age 65, use cautiously because of greater risk for neurotoxicity.

Adverse reactions

CNS: CENTRAL NEUROTOXICITY, confusion, dizziness, *peripheral neuropathy, stroke.*
EENT: *ototoxicity.*
CV: *embolism, heart failure.*
GI: constipation, diarrhea, nausea, vomiting.
Hematologic: *anemia,* bone marrow suppression, *leukopenia, neutropenia, thrombocytopenia.*
Hepatic: *hepatotoxicity.*
Skin: alopecia.
Other: hypersensitivity reactions.

Interactions

Drug-drug. *Bone marrow depressants, including radiation therapy:* May increase hematologic toxicity. Monitor hematologic studies.
Nephrotoxic drugs: May enhance nephrotoxicity of carboplatin. Monitor renal function tests.

Effects on lab test results

• May increase BUN, creatinine, bilirubin, AST, and alkaline phosphatase levels. May decrease magnesium, calcium, potassium, sodium, and hemoglobin levels and hematocrit.
• May decrease neutrophil, WBC, RBC, and platelet counts.

Pharmacokinetics

Absorption: Given I.V.
Distribution: Volume distributed is about equal to that of total body water; no significant protein binding occurs.
Metabolism: Hydrolyzed to form hydroxylated and aquated types.
Excretion: 65% by kidneys within 12 hours, 71% within 24 hours. *Half-life:* 5 hours.

Route	Onset	Peak	Duration
I.V.	Unknown	Unknown	Unknown

Action

Chemical effect: Probably produces cross-linking of DNA strands.
Therapeutic effect: Impairs ovarian cancer cell replication.

Available forms

Powder for injection: 50-mg, 150-mg, 450-mg vials
Solution for injection: 50 mg/5 ml, 150 mg/15 ml, 450 mg/45 ml

NURSING PROCESS

⚗ Assessment

• Assess patient's condition before therapy and regularly thereafter.
• Determine electrolyte, creatinine, and BUN levels; creatinine clearance; CBC; and platelet count before first infusion and before each course of therapy. Lowest WBC and platelet counts usually occur by day 21. They usually return to baseline by day 28.
• Be alert for adverse reactions and drug interactions.

• Assess patient's and family's knowledge of drug therapy.

⊕ Nursing diagnoses

• Ineffective health maintenance related to ovarian cancer
• Ineffective protection related to drug-induced adverse reactions
• Deficient knowledge related to drug therapy

▶ Planning and implementation

• Check dose carefully against laboratory test results. Only increase dose once. Don't exceed 125% of starting dose in subsequent doses.
• Bone marrow suppression may be more severe in patients with creatinine clearance below 60 ml/minute. Adjust dosage in these patients.
⑤ **ALERT:** Don't repeat dose unless platelet count exceeds $100,000/mm^3$.
• Provide antiemetic therapy. Carboplatin can produce severe vomiting.
⑤ **ALERT:** Don't confuse carboplatin with cisplatin.
Patient teaching
• Warn patient to watch for signs of infection (fever, sore throat, fatigue) and bleeding (easy bruising, nosebleed, bleeding gums, melena). Tell patient to take his own temperature daily.
• Instruct patient to avoid OTC products that contain aspirin.
• Advise woman of childbearing age to avoid pregnancy during therapy and to consult prescriber before becoming pregnant.
• Advise breast-feeding patient to stop breast-feeding because of risk of toxicity to infant.

☑ Evaluation

• Patient has positive response to carboplatin as evidenced by follow-up diagnostic tests.
• Patient doesn't experience injury from drug therapy.
• Patient and family state understanding of drug therapy.

carisoprodol
(kar-ih-soh-PROH-dol)
Soma

Pharmacologic class: carbamate derivative
Therapeutic class: skeletal muscle relaxant
Pregnancy risk category: NR

Reactions may be *common,* uncommon, *life-threatening,* or COMMON AND LIFE-THREATENING.

Indications and dosages

▶ **Adjunct in acute, painful musculoskeletal conditions.** *Adults:* 350 mg P.O. t.i.d. and h.s.

Contraindications and cautions

• Contraindicated in patients hypersensitive to related compounds (such as meprobamate) and in patients with intermittent porphyria.
• Use cautiously in patients with hepatic or renal impairment. Prolonged use may lead to dependence; use cautiously in addiction-prone patients.
❀ **Lifespan:** In pregnant or breast-feeding women and in children younger than age 12, safety and effectiveness haven't been established.

Adverse reactions

CNS: agitation, ataxia, depressive reactions, *dizziness, drowsiness,* fever, headache, insomnia, irritability, tremor, vertigo.
CV: facial flushing, orthostatic hypotension, tachycardia.
GI: epigastric distress, increased bowel activity, nausea, vomiting.
Hematologic: eosinophilia.
Respiratory: *asthmatic episodes,* hiccups.
Skin: *erythema multiforme,* pruritus, rash.
Other: *anaphylaxis, angioedema.*

Interactions

Drug-drug. *CNS depressants:* May increase CNS depression. Avoid using together.
Drug-lifestyle. *Alcohol use:* May increase CNS depression. Discourage using together.

Effects on lab test results

• May increase eosinophil count.

Pharmacokinetics

Absorption: Unknown.
Distribution: Widely throughout body.
Metabolism: In liver.
Excretion: In urine mainly as metabolites; less than 1% excreted unchanged. *Half-life:* 8 hours.

Route	Onset	Peak	Duration
P.O.	≤ 30 min	≤ 4 hr	4–6 hr

Action

Chemical effect: Appears to modify central perception of pain without modifying pain reflexes. Blocks interneuronal activity in descend-

ing reticular activating system and in spinal cord.
Therapeutic effect: Relieves musculoskeletal pain.

Available forms

Tablets: 350 mg

NURSING PROCESS

📖 Assessment

• Assess patient's pain before and after giving drug.
• Monitor the drug's effectiveness by regularly assessing severity and frequency of muscle spasms.
• Be alert for adverse reactions and drug interactions.
🔵 **ALERT:** Watch for idiosyncratic reactions after first to fourth doses (weakness, ataxia, visual and speech difficulties, fever, skin eruptions, and mental changes) and for severe reactions (bronchospasm, hypotension, and anaphylaxis).
• Assess patient for history of drug addiction. Prolonged use of drug may lead to dependence.
• Assess patient's and family's knowledge of drug therapy.

🔷 Nursing diagnoses

• Acute pain related to patient's underlying condition
• Risk for injury related to drug-induced drowsiness
• Deficient knowledge related to drug therapy

▷ Planning and implementation

• Give drug with meals or milk to prevent GI distress.
• Once pain is adequately relieved, reduce dose.
• Stop giving the drug and notify prescriber immediately if unusual reactions occur.
• Don't stop drug abruptly because mild withdrawal effects, such as insomnia, headache, nausea, and abdominal cramps, may result.
Patient teaching
• Warn patient to avoid activities that require alertness or physical dexterity, such as operating machinery or a motor vehicle, until drug's CNS effects are known.
• Advise patient not to consume alcohol or other CNS depressants.
• Advise patient to follow prescriber's orders about rest and physical therapy.

• Tell patient to take drug with meals or milk to prevent GI distress.

☑ **Evaluation**
• Patient reports pain has ceased.
• Patient doesn't experience injury from drug-induced CNS adverse reactions.
• Patient and family state understanding of drug.

carmustine (BCNU)
(kar-MUHS-teen)
BiCNU, Gliadel

Pharmacologic class: alkylating drug
Therapeutic class: antineoplastic
Pregnancy risk category: D

Indications and dosages

▶ **Hodgkin's disease, non-Hodgkin's lymphoma, and multiple myeloma.** *Adults:* 150 to 200 mg/m^2 I.V. by slow infusion as single dose, repeat q 6 weeks; or 75 to 100 mg/m^2 I.V. by slow infusion daily for 2 days; repeat q 6 weeks. Don't repeat dose until platelet count is above 100,000/mm^3 and WBC count is above 4,000/mm^3.
⬧ **Adjust-a-dose:** Reduce dosage by 30% when WBC count is 2,000 to 3,000/mm^3 and platelet count is 25,000 to 75,000/mm^3. Reduce dosage by 50% when WBC count is below 2,000/mm^3 and platelet count is below 25,000/mm^3.
▶ **Recurrent glioblastoma multiforme (adjunct to surgery); newly diagnosed high-grade malignant glioma patients (adjunct to surgery and radiation).** *Adults:* 8 wafers implanted into resection cavity as size of cavity allows.
▶ **Brain‡, breast‡, GI tract‡, lung‡, and hepatic cancer‡; malignant melanomas‡.** *Adults:* 75 to 100 mg/m^2 I.V. by slow infusion daily for 2 days; repeat q 6 weeks if platelet count is above 100,000/mm^3 and WBC count is above 4,000/mm^3.

▼ I.V. administration

• To reconstitute, dissolve 100 mg of drug in 3 ml of absolute alcohol provided by manufacturer. Dilute solution with 27 ml of sterile water for injection. Resulting solution contains 3.3 mg of drug/ml in 10% alcohol. Dilute in normal saline solution or D$_5$W for I.V. infusion.
• If powder liquefies or appears oily, discard drug because decomposition has occurred.
• Give only in glass containers. Solution is unstable in plastic I.V. bags.
• Give at least 250 ml over 1 to 2 hours. To reduce pain of infusion, dilute further or slow infusion rate.
• Avoid contact with skin because drug will cause brown stain. If drug contacts skin, wash it off thoroughly.
• Store reconstituted solution in refrigerator for 48 hours. May decompose at temperatures above 80° F (27° C).
⊗ **Incompatibilities**
Sodium bicarbonate. Don't mix with other drugs.

Contraindications and cautions

• Contraindicated in patients hypersensitive to drug.
🕮 **Lifespan:** In pregnant or breast-feeding women, use is contraindicated. In children, safety and effectiveness haven't been established.

Adverse reactions

CNS: ataxia, *brain edema,* drowsiness, *seizures.*
CV: facial flushing.
EENT: ocular toxicities.
GI: anorexia, diarrhea, dysphagia, esophagitis, nausea, vomiting.
GU: *nephrotoxicity,* renal impairment.
Hematologic: *acute leukemia or bone marrow dysplasia* (may occur after long-term use), *cumulative bone marrow suppression* (delayed 4 to 6 weeks, lasting 1 to 2 weeks), *leukopenia, thrombocytopenia.*
Hepatic: *hepatotoxicity.*
Metabolic: hyperuricemia (in lymphoma patients when rapid cell lysis occurs).
Respiratory: *pulmonary fibrosis.*
Skin: hyperpigmentation (if drug contacts skin).
Other: *intense pain* (at infusion site from venous spasm).

Interactions

Drug-drug. *Anticoagulants, aspirin, NSAIDs:* May increase risk of bleeding. Avoid using together.
Cimetidine: May increase carmustine's bone marrow toxicity. Avoid using together.

Digoxin, phenytoin: May reduce levels of these drugs. Use together cautiously; monitor levels.
Mitomycin: May increase corneal and conjunctival damage with high doses. Monitor patient.
Myelosuppressives: May increase risk of myelosuppression. Monitor patient's CBC periodically.

Effects on lab test results

• May increase urine urea, AST, bilirubin, and alkaline phosphatase levels. May decrease hemoglobin level and hematocrit.
• May decrease WBC and platelet counts.

Pharmacokinetics

Absorption: Given I.V.
Distribution: Rapidly into CSF.
Metabolism: Extensively in liver.
Excretion: 60% to 70% in urine within 96 hours, 6% to 10% as carbon dioxide by lungs, and 1% in feces. *Half-life:* 15 to 30 minutes.

Route	Onset	Peak	Duration
I.V., wafer	Unknown	Unknown	Unknown

Action

Chemical effect: Inhibits enzymatic reactions involved with DNA synthesis, cross-links strands of cellular DNA, and interferes with RNA transcription, causing growth imbalance that leads to cell death.
Therapeutic effect: Kills selected cancer cells.

Available forms

Injection: 100-mg vial (lyophilized), with 3-ml vial of absolute alcohol supplied as diluent
Wafer: 7.7 mg

NURSING PROCESS

✍ Assessment

• Assess patient's neoplastic disorder before therapy and regularly thereafter.
• Obtain baseline pulmonary function tests before starting therapy because pulmonary toxicity appears to be dose related. Evaluate results of liver, renal, and pulmonary function tests periodically thereafter.
• Monitor CBC and uric acid levels.
• Be alert for adverse reactions and drug interactions.
• Assess patient's and family's knowledge of drug therapy.

⊕ Nursing diagnoses

• Ineffective health maintenance related to neoplastic disease
• Risk for injury related to drug-induced adverse reactions
• Deficient knowledge related to drug therapy

▷ Planning and implementation

• Preparing and giving drug has carcinogenic, mutagenic, and teratogenic risks. Follow facility policy to reduce risks.
• To reduce nausea, give antiemetic before giving drug.
• Unopened foil packs containing wafers are stable at room temperature for 6 hours. Store below –4° F (–20° C).
• If handling wafer in operating room, use double gloves.
• Allopurinol may be used with adequate hydration to prevent hyperuricemia and uric acid nephropathy.
Patient teaching
• Warn patient to watch for signs of infection (fever, sore throat, fatigue) and bleeding (easy bruising, nosebleed, bleeding gums, melena). Tell patient to take temperature daily.
• Instruct patient to avoid OTC products containing aspirin.
• Advise breast-feeding women to stop breast-feeding because of toxicity to infant.
• Advise women of childbearing age to avoid pregnancy during therapy and to consult prescriber before becoming pregnant.

☑ Evaluation

• Patient shows positive response to drug therapy as evidenced by follow-up diagnostic studies.
• Patient doesn't experience injury from drug-induced adverse reactions.
• Patient and family state understanding of drug therapy.

carvedilol

(kar-VAY-deh-lol)
Coreg

Pharmacologic class: alpha$_1$ and beta blocker
Therapeutic class: antihypertensive, adjunct treatment for heart failure
Pregnancy risk category: C

Indications and dosages

▶ **Hypertension.** *Adults:* Dosage highly individualized. Initially, 6.25 mg P.O. b.i.d. with food. Obtain a standing blood pressure 1 hour after initial dose. If tolerated, continue dosage for 7 to 14 days. May increase to 12.5 mg P.O. b.i.d. for 7 to 14 days, monitor blood pressure as above. Maximum dosage, 25 mg P.O. b.i.d. as tolerated.

▶ **Mild to severe heart failure.** *Adults:* Individualize and adjust dosage carefully. Initially, 3.125 mg P.O. b.i.d. with food for 2 weeks; if tolerated, increase to 6.25 mg P.O. b.i.d. Double dose q 2 weeks as tolerated. At start of new dose, observe patient for dizziness or lightheadedness for 1 hour. Maximum dosage for patients weighing less than 85 kg (187 lb) is 25 mg P.O. b.i.d.; for those weighing over 85 kg, maximum dosage is 50 mg P.O. b.i.d.

▶ **Left ventricular dysfunction after MI.** *Adults:* Individualize dosage. Start therapy after patient is hemodynamically stable and fluid retention has been minimized. Initially, 6.25 mg P.O. b.i.d. with food. Increase after 3 to 10 days to 12.5 mg b.i.d., then again to a target dose of 25 mg b.i.d. Or, start with 3.25 mg b.i.d. May adjust dosage more slowly. Monitor blood pressure; observe patient for light-headedness with each dosage change.

⊠ **Adjust-a-dose:** In patients with pulse rate below 55 beats/minute, reduce dosage.

Contraindications and cautions

• Contraindicated in patients hypersensitive to drug and in those with New York Heart Association class IV decompensated heart failure requiring I.V. inotropic therapy, bronchial asthma or related bronchospastic conditions, second- or third-degree AV block, sick sinus syndrome (unless a permanent pacemaker is in place), cardiogenic shock, or severe bradycardia.

• Drug isn't recommended for patients with symptomatic hepatic impairment.

• Use cautiously in hypertensive patients with left ventricular failure, perioperative patients who receive anesthetics that depress myocardial function, patients with diabetes who receive insulin or oral antidiabetics, and patients subject to spontaneous hypoglycemia. Also use cautiously in patients with thyroid disease, pheochromocytoma, Prinzmetal's variant angina, bronchospastic disease, or peripheral vascular disease.

⚱ **Lifespan:** In pregnant women, use only if benefits outweigh risks to the fetus. Women should stop breast-feeding during therapy. In children, safety and effectiveness haven't been established. In elderly patients, drug levels are about 50% higher than in other adults. Monitor these patients closely.

Adverse reactions

CNS: asthenia, depression, *dizziness,* fatigue, fever, headache, hypesthesia, insomnia, pain, paresthesia, somnolence, *stroke,* syncope, vertigo.

CV: angina pectoris, *AV block, bradycardia,* edema, fluid overload, hypertension, *hypotension,* hypovolemia, orthostatic hypotension, palpitations, peripheral edema, peripheral vascular disorder.

EENT: abnormal vision, blurred vision, pharyngitis, rhinitis, sinusitis.

GI: abdominal pain, *diarrhea,* dyspepsia, melena, nausea, periodontitis, vomiting.

GU: abnormal renal function, albuminuria, hematuria, impotence, UTI.

Hematologic: anemia, purpura, *thrombocytopenia.*

Metabolic: diabetes mellitus, glycosuria, gout, hypercholesterolemia, *hyperglycemia, hyperkalemia,* hypertriglyceridemia, hyperuricemia, hypervolemia, *hypoglycemia,* hyponatremia, *weight gain,* weight loss.

Musculoskeletal: arthralgia, arthritis, back pain, hypotonia, muscle cramps.

Respiratory: bronchitis, cough, dyspnea, *lung edema,* rales, *upper respiratory tract infection.*

Other: flulike syndrome, hypersensitivity reactions, infection, injury, viral infection.

Interactions

Drug-drug. *Calcium channel blockers:* May cause isolated conduction disturbances. Monitor patient's heart rhythm and blood pressure.

Catecholamine-depleting drugs (such as MAO inhibitors, reserpine): May cause bradycardia or severe hypotension. Monitor patient closely.

Cimetidine: May increase bioavailability of carvedilol. Monitor vital signs carefully.

Clonidine: May increase blood pressure and heart rate-lowering effects. Monitor vital signs closely.

Digoxin: May increase digoxin level by about 15% during therapy. Monitor digoxin level and vital signs carefully.

Fluoxetine, paroxetine, propafenone, quinidine: May increase level of R (+) enantiomer of carvedilol. Monitor patient for hypotension and dizziness.

Insulin, oral antidiabetics: May enhance hypoglycemic properties. Monitor glucose level.

Rifampin: May reduce level of carvedilol by 70%. Monitor vital signs closely.

Drug-food. *Any food:* Delays carvedilol absorption but doesn't alter extent of bioavailability. Advise patient to take drug with food to minimize orthostatic effects.

Effects on lab test results

• May increase creatinine, BUN, ALT, AST, GGT, cholesterol, triglyceride, alkaline phosphatase, sodium, uric acid, potassium, and nonprotein nitrogen levels. May increase or decrease glucose level.

• May decrease PT, INR, and platelet counts.

Pharmacokinetics

Absorption: Rapidly and extensively with absolute bioavailability of 25% to 35% because of significant first-pass metabolism.

Distribution: Extensively into extravascular tissues; about 98% bound to proteins.

Metabolism: Mainly by aromatic ring oxidation and glucuronidation.

Excretion: Metabolites are excreted mainly via bile in feces. Less than 2% excreted unchanged in urine. *Half-life:* 7 to 10 hours.

Route	Onset	Peak	Duration
P.O.	Unknown	1–2 hr	7–10 hr

Action

Chemical effect: Causes significant reductions in systemic blood pressure, pulmonary arterial pressure, pulmonary capillary wedge pressure, and heart rate.

Therapeutic effect: Lowers blood pressure and heart rate.

Available forms

Tablets: 3.125 mg, 6.25 mg, 12.5 mg, 25 mg

NURSING PROCESS

☡ Assessment

• Monitor patient for decreased PT and increased alkaline phosphatase, BUN, ALT, and AST levels.

• Assess patient with heart failure for worsened condition, renal impairment, or fluid retention; add or increase diuretics p.r.n.

• Monitor patient with diabetes closely because drug may mask signs of hypoglycemia or worsen hyperglycemia.

• Monitor elderly patients carefully because drug level is about 50% higher in elderly patients than in younger patients.

• Observe patient for dizziness or lightheadedness for 1 hour after giving each dose.

• Assess patient's and family's knowledge of drug therapy.

⊕ Nursing diagnoses

• Ineffective health maintenance related to underlying disorder

• Ineffective cerebral tissue perfusion secondary to therapeutic action of drug

• Deficient knowledge related to drug therapy

⧁ Planning and implementation

• Before therapy begins, stabilize dose of digoxin, diuretics, and ACE inhibitors.

⊛ **ALERT:** Patient taking a beta blocker who has a history of anaphylactic reaction to several allergens may be more reactive to repeated challenges (accidental, diagnostic, or therapeutic). Such a patient may be unresponsive to the doses of epinephrine typically used to treat allergic reactions.

• Give drug with food to reduce risk of orthostatic hypotension.

• If pulse drops below 55 beats/minute, notify prescriber and reduce the dose.

⊛ **ALERT:** Don't confuse carvedilol with captopril or carteolol.

Patient teaching

• Tell patient not to interrupt or stop taking the drug without medical approval. Drug should be withdrawn gradually over 1 to 2 weeks.

• Advise patient with heart failure to call prescriber about weight gain or shortness of breath.

• Inform patient that he may develop low blood pressure when standing. If he's dizzy or faint, advise him to sit or lie down.

• Warn patient not to drive or perform hazardous tasks until the drug's CNS effects are known.

• Tell patient to notify prescriber about dizziness or faintness. Dose may need to be adjusted.

• Advise patient with diabetes to promptly report changes in glucose level.

• Inform patient who wears contact lenses that decreased lacrimation may occur.

☑ Evaluation
• Patient responds well to therapy.
• Patient doesn't experience dizziness or light-headedness.
• Patient and family state understanding of drug therapy.

caspofungin acetate
(kas-poh-FUN-jin AS-ih-tayt)
Cancidas

Pharmacologic class: echinocandin
Therapeutic class: antifungal
Pregnancy risk category: C

Indications and dosages

▶ **Invasive aspergillosis in patients refractory to or intolerant of other drugs, such as amphotericin B, lipid formulations of amphotericin B, itraconazole.** *Adults:* A single 70-mg loading dose I.V. on day 1, followed by 50 mg daily. Duration of therapy based on severity of patient's underlying disease, recovery from immunosuppression, and response.
▶ **Candidemia and *Candida* infections including intra-abdominal abscesses, peritonitis, and pleural space infections.** *Adults:* Give a single 70-mg loading dose I.V. on day 1, followed by 50 mg daily thereafter. Duration of therapy is based on response. In general, antifungal therapy should continue for at least 14 days after the last positive culture. Patients with persistent neutropenia may warrant a longer course of therapy while neutropenia resolves.
▶ **Esophageal candidiasis.** *Adults:* 50 mg I.V. daily. Because of the risk of relapse of oropharyngeal candidiasis in patients with HIV infections, suppressive oral therapy could be considered.
▶ **Empirical therapy for presumed fungal infections in febrile, neutropenic patients.** *Adults:* A single 70-mg loading dose I.V. on day 1, followed by 50 mg daily thereafter. Duration of therapy based on response. Empirical therapy should continue until neutropenia resolves. Patients found to have a fungal infection should be treated for a minimum of 14 days; treatment should continue for at least 7 days after both

neutropenia and clinical symptoms are resolved. If the 50-mg dose is well tolerated but doesn't provide an adequate response, increase the daily dose to 70 mg.
◙ **Adjust-a-dose:** For patients with moderate hepatic impairment and a Child-Pugh score of 7 to 9, give 35 mg daily after initial 70-mg loading dose.

▼ I.V. administration
• Allow refrigerated vial to warm to room temperature before diluting.
• Dilute all doses (70 mg, 50 mg, 35 mg) in 250 ml of normal saline solution. In patients with fluid restrictions, dilute the 50-mg and 35-mg doses in 100 ml of normal saline solution.
• Give by slow I.V. infusion over about 1 hour; don't give by I.V. bolus injection.
• Use reconstituted vials within 1 hour or discard.
• Diluted solutions may be stored at 77° F (25° C) for up to 24 hours.
⊗ **Incompatibilities**
Dextrose solutions, other I.V. drugs.

Contraindications and cautions
• Contraindicated in patients hypersensitive to the drug or any of its components.
🌡 **Lifespan:** In pregnant women, use only when potential benefits to the mother outweigh risks to the fetus. In breast-feeding women, use cautiously because it isn't known whether drug appears in breast milk. In children, safety and effectiveness haven't been established.

Adverse reactions
CNS: *chills, fever, headache,* paresthesia.
CV: peripheral edema, *phlebitis,* swelling, *tachycardia, thrombophlebitis.*
GI: abdominal pain, anorexia, diarrhea, nausea, vomiting.
GU: hematuria, proteinuria.
Hematologic: anemia, eosinophilia.
Hepatic: hepatic dysfunction.
Metabolic: hypercalcemia.
Musculoskeletal: myalgia, pain.
Respiratory: *tachypnea.*
Skin: *anaphylaxis,* histamine-mediated symptoms (rash, facial swelling, phlebitis, pruritus, sensation of warmth, erythema, sweating), *infusion site complication.*

C

Interactions

Drug-drug. *Carbamazepine, dexamethasone, efavirenz, nelfinavir, nevirapine, phenytoin, rifampin:* May decrease caspofungin level. Consider increasing caspofungin dosage to 70 mg daily if patient doesn't respond to lower dosage. *Cyclosporine:* May significantly increase AST and ALT levels and bioavailability of caspofungin. Avoid using together unless potential benefit outweighs potential risk.
Tacrolimus: May decrease tacrolimus level. Monitor tacrolimus level, and adjust dosage accordingly.

Effects on lab test results

• May increase ALT, AST, alkaline phosphatase, and urine protein levels. May decrease potassium and hemoglobin levels and hematocrit.
• May increase eosinophil and urine RBC counts.

Pharmacokinetics

Absorption: Rapid into plasma; slower into tissue.
Distribution: Extensively bound to albumin (about 97%).
Metabolism: Slowly in the tissues and liver.
Excretion: 35% of drug and metabolites in feces and 41% in urine. *Half-life:* 9 to 11 hours.

Route	Onset	Peak	Duration
I.V.	Immediate	Unknown	36–48 hr

Action

Chemical effect: Inhibits synthesis of beta (1, 3)-D-glucan, an integral component of the cell walls of susceptible filamentous fungi that isn't found in mammal cells.
Therapeutic effect: Prevents fungi formation.

Available forms

Lyophilized powder for injection: 50-mg, 70-mg single-use vials

NURSING PROCESS

✎ Assessment

• Assess patient's hepatic function before starting drug.
• Observe patient for histamine-mediated reactions (rash, facial swelling, pruritus, sensation of warmth, sweating).
• Monitor I.V. site carefully for phlebitis.

• Monitor patient's liver function test results carefully during therapy.
• Assess patient's and family's knowledge of drug therapy.

⊞ Nursing diagnoses

• Risk for infection and impaired skin integrity related to adverse effects of I.V. drug administration
• Ineffective health maintenance related to underlying disease process and immunocompromised state
• Deficient knowledge related to drug therapy

⟩ Planning and implementation

• An increase in dose to 70 mg daily hasn't been studied but may be well tolerated.
• A long course of therapy hasn't been studied but may be well tolerated.
• Adjust dose in a patient with moderate hepatic insufficiency.
Patient teaching
• Instruct patient to report signs and symptoms of phlebitis.
• Tell patient to report any adverse events during drug therapy.

✓ Evaluation

• Patient has no adverse reactions during drug therapy.
• Patient responds positively to antifungal drug therapy.
• Patient and family state understanding of drug therapy.

cefaclor
(SEH-fuh-klor)
Ceclor, Ceclor CD

Pharmacologic class: second-generation cephalosporin
Therapeutic class: antibiotic
Pregnancy risk category: B

Indications and dosages

▶ **Respiratory, urinary tract, skin, and soft-tissue infections and otitis media caused by** *Haemophilus influenzae, Streptococcus pneumoniae, S. pyogenes, Escherichia coli, Proteus mirabilis, Klebsiella,* **and staphylococci.**
Adults: 250 to 500 mg P.O. q 8 hours. Maxi-

mum total daily dosage, 4 g. For extended-release forms, 500 mg P.O. q 12 hours for 7 days for bronchitis. For pharyngitis, 375 mg P.O. q 12 hours for 10 days. For skin and skin-structure infections, 375 mg P.O. q 12 hours for 7 to 10 days.

Children: 20 mg/kg P.O. daily divided t.i.d., q 8 hours. For pharyngitis or otitis media, b.i.d. q 12 hours. For more serious infections, 40 mg/kg daily are recommended, not to exceed 1 g daily.

▶ **Acute uncomplicated UTI‡.** *Adults:* 2 g P.O. as a single dose.

Contraindications and cautions

• Contraindicated in patients hypersensitive to other cephalosporins.
• Use cautiously in patients with a history of sensitivity to penicillin because of reports of potential allergic reaction. Also use cautiously in patients with renal impairment.
✾ **Lifespan:** In pregnant and breast-feeding women, use cautiously. In children younger than age 1 month, safety and effectiveness of oral suspension haven't been established. In children younger than age 16, safety and effectiveness of extended-release tablets and capsules haven't been established.

Adverse reactions

CNS: dizziness, fever, headache, malaise, somnolence.
GI: abdominal cramps, anorexia, *diarrhea,* dyspepsia, *nausea,* oral candidiasis, ***pseudomembranous colitis,*** vomiting.
GU: red and white cells in urine, vaginal candidiasis, vaginitis.
Hematologic: anemia, eosinophilia, lymphocytosis, ***thrombocytopenia, transient leukopenia.***
Skin: dermatitis, maculopapular rash.
Other: hypersensitivity reactions (serum sickness, *anaphylaxis*).

Interactions

Drug-drug. *Aminoglycosides:* May increase risk of nephrotoxicity. Avoid using together.
Antacids: May decrease absorption of extended-release tablets. Separate doses by at least 1 hour.
Anticoagulants: May increase anticoagulant effects. Monitor coagulation studies.
Chloramphenicol: May have an antagonistic effect. Avoid using together.
Probenecid: May inhibit excretion and increase level of cefaclor. Monitor patient.

Effects on lab test results

• May increase ALT, AST, alkaline phosphatase, bilirubin, GGT, and LDH levels. May decrease hemoglobin level and hematocrit.
• May increase eosinophil count. May decrease WBC and platelet counts.
• May cause false-positive urine glucose determinations with copper sulfate tests (Clinitest).

Pharmacokinetics

Absorption: Well absorbed from GI tract. Food will delay but not prevent complete GI tract absorption.
Distribution: Wide; CSF penetration is poor. Drug is 25% protein-bound.
Metabolism: None.
Excretion: Mainly in urine by renal tubular secretion and glomerular filtration. *Half-life:* ½ to 1 hour.

Route	Onset	Peak	Duration
P.O.	Unknown	½–1 hr	Unknown

Action

Chemical effect: Inhibits cell-wall synthesis, promoting osmotic instability; usually bactericidal.
Therapeutic effect: Hinders or kills susceptible bacteria.

Available forms

Capsules: 250 mg, 500 mg
Oral suspension: 125 mg/5 ml, 187 mg/5 ml, 250 mg/5 ml, 375 mg/5 ml
Tablets: (extended-release): 375 mg, 500 mg

NURSING PROCESS

⚕ Assessment

• Assess patient's infection before therapy and regularly thereafter.
• Before giving first dose, obtain specimen for culture and sensitivity tests. Begin therapy pending test results.
• Before giving first dose, ask patient about previous reactions to cephalosporins or penicillin.
• Be alert for adverse reactions and drug interactions.
• If adverse GI reactions occur, monitor patient's hydration.
• Assess patient's and family's knowledge of drug therapy.

⊕ Nursing diagnoses

- Infection related to bacteria susceptible to drug
- Risk for deficient fluid volume related to drug-induced adverse GI reactions
- Deficient knowledge related to drug therapy

▶ Planning and implementation

- Give drug with food to prevent or minimize GI upset.
- Store reconstituted suspension in refrigerator where it will remain stable for 14 days. Keep tightly closed and shake well before using.

ALERT: Don't confuse with other cephalosporins with similar-sounding names.

Patient teaching

- Tell patient that drug should be taken with food to minimize GI upset.
- Advise patient to take drug exactly as prescribed, even after he feels better.
- Instruct patient to call prescriber if rash develops.
- Teach patient how to store drug.

☑ Evaluation

- Patient is free from infection.
- Patient maintains adequate hydration.
- Patient and family state understanding of drug therapy.

cefadroxil monohydrate

(seh-fuh-DROKS-il MON-oh-HIGH-drayt)

Duricef✎

Pharmacologic class: first-generation cephalosporin
Therapeutic class: antibiotic
Pregnancy risk category: B

Indications and dosages

▶ **UTI caused by *Escherichia coli, Proteus mirabilis,* and *Klebsiella;* skin and soft-tissue infections; and streptococcal pharyngitis.** *Adults:* 1 to 2 g P.O. daily, depending on infection treated, usually as a single dose or in two divided doses.
Children: 30 mg/kg P.O. daily in two divided doses. Course of therapy is usually at least 10 days.

Adjust-a-dose: For adults with renal impairment, give initial dosage of 1 g P.O. daily. Reduce maintenance dosage as follows: If creatinine clearance is 25 to 50 ml/minute, give 500 mg q 12 hours. If creatinine clearance is 10 to 25 ml/minute, give 500 mg q 24 hours. If creatinine clearance is less than 10 ml/minute, give 500 mg q 36 hours.

Contraindications and cautions

- Contraindicated in patients hypersensitive to drug or other cephalosporins.
- Use cautiously in patients with renal impairment or a history of sensitivity to penicillin.

Lifespan: In pregnant or breast-feeding women, use cautiously.

Adverse reactions

CNS: dizziness, headache, malaise, paresthesia, ***seizures.***
GI: abdominal cramps, anal pruritus, anorexia, diarrhea, dyspepsia, glossitis, oral candidiasis, ***pseudomembranous colitis,*** nausea, tenesmus, vomiting.
GU: candidiasis, genital pruritus.
Hematologic: ***agranulocytosis,*** anemia, eosinophilia, ***leukopenia, thrombocytopenia, transient neutropenia.***
Respiratory: dyspnea.
Skin: maculopapular and erythematous rashes.
Other: hypersensitivity reactions (serum sickness, ***anaphylaxis***).

Interactions

Drug-drug. *Probenecid:* May inhibit excretion and increase level of cefadroxil. Monitor patient.

Effects on lab test results

- May increase ALT, AST, alkaline phosphatase, bilirubin, GGT, and LDH levels. May decrease hemoglobin level and hematocrit.
- May increase eosinophil count. May decrease neutrophil, WBC, granulocyte, and platelet counts.
- May cause false-positive urine glucose determinations with copper sulfate tests (Clinitest).

Pharmacokinetics

Absorption: Rapid and complete.
Distribution: Wide; CSF penetration is poor. Drug is 20% protein-bound.
Metabolism: None.

Excretion: Mainly unchanged in urine. *Half-life:* About 1 to 2 hours.

Route	Onset	Peak	Duration
P.O.	Unknown	1–2 hr	6–9 hr

Action

Chemical effect: Inhibits cell-wall synthesis, promoting osmotic instability; usually bactericidal.
Therapeutic effect: Hinders or kills susceptible bacteria.

Available forms

Capsules: 500 mg
Oral suspension: 125 mg/5 ml, 250 mg/5 ml, 500 mg/5 ml
Tablets: 1 g

NURSING PROCESS

🔖 Assessment
• Assess patient's infection before therapy and regularly thereafter.
• Before giving first dose, obtain specimen for culture and sensitivity tests. Begin therapy pending test results.
• Be alert for adverse reactions and drug interactions.
• If adverse GI reactions occur, monitor patient's hydration.
• Assess patient's and family's knowledge of drug therapy.

🔳 Nursing diagnoses
• Infection related to bacteria susceptible to drug
• Risk for deficient fluid volume related to drug-induced adverse GI reactions
• Deficient knowledge related to drug therapy

▷ Planning and implementation
• Drug's half-life permits once- or twice-daily use.
• If creatinine clearance is less than 50 ml/minute, expect prescriber to lengthen dosage interval to prevent drug accumulation.
• Store reconstituted suspension in refrigerator. Keep container tightly closed and shake well before using.
• About 40% to 75% of patients receiving cephalosporins show false-positive direct Coombs' tests.

⚠ ALERT: Don't confuse with other cephalosporins with similar-sounding names.
Patient teaching
• Tell patient to take drug exactly as prescribed, even after he feels better.
• Advise patient to take drug with food or milk to lessen GI discomfort.
• Tell patient to call prescriber if rash develops.
• Inform patient using oral suspension to shake it well before using and to refrigerate mixture in tightly closed container.

✅ Evaluation
• Patient is free from infection.
• Patient maintains adequate hydration.
• Patient and family state understanding of drug therapy.

cefazolin sodium
(sef-EH-zoh-lin SOH-dee-um)
Ancef, Zolicef

Pharmacologic class: first-generation cephalosporin
Therapeutic class: antibiotic
Pregnancy risk category: B

Indications and dosages

▶ **Serious infections of respiratory, biliary, and GU tracts; skin, soft-tissue, bone, and joint infections; septicemia; endocarditis caused by *Escherichia coli*, *Enterobacteriaceae gonococci*, *Haemophilus influenzae*, *Klebsiella*, *Proteus mirabilis*, *Staphylococcus aureus*, *Streptococcus pneumoniae*, and group A beta-hemolytic streptococci.** *Adults:* 250 mg I.V. or I.M. q 8 hours to 1 g q 6 hours. Maximum 12 g daily in life-threatening situations. *Children and infants older than 1 month:* 25 to 100 mg/kg daily I.V. or I.M. in three or four divided doses.
▶ **Perioperative prophylaxis in contaminated surgery.** *Adults:* 1 g I.V. or I.M. 30 to 60 minutes before surgery; then 0.5 to 1 g I.V. or I.M. q 6 to 8 hours for 24 hours. In operations lasting more than 2 hours, another 0.5- to 1-g dose may be given intraoperatively. In cases where infection would be devastating, prophylaxis may continue for 3 to 5 days.
◨ Adjust-a-dose: For patients with renal impairment, after initial dose, adjust dosage as fol-

lows. If creatinine clearance is 35 to 54 ml/ minute, give full dose q 8 hours; if creatinine clearance is 11 to 34 ml/minute, give 50% of usual dose q 12 hours; if creatinine clearance is less than 10 ml/minute, give 50% of usual dose q 18 to 24 hours.

▼ I.V. administration

• Reconstitute with sterile water, bacteriostatic water, or normal saline solution as follows: 2 ml to 500-mg vial to yield 225 mg/ml; or 2.5 ml to 1-g vial to yield 330 mg/ml. Shake well until dissolved.
• For direct injection, further dilute with 5 ml of sterile water. Inject into large vein or into tubing of free-flowing I.V. solution over 3 to 5 minutes. For intermittent infusion, add reconstituted drug to 50 to 100 ml of compatible solution or use premixed solution. Give premixed frozen solutions of drug in D_5W only by intermittent or continuous I.V. infusion.
• If I.V. therapy lasts longer than 3 days, alternate injection sites. Use of small I.V. needles in larger veins may be preferable.
• Reconstituted drug is stable for 24 hours at room temperature and 96 hours if refrigerated.
⊗ **Incompatibilities**
Aminoglycosides, amiodarone, amobarbital, ascorbic acid injection, bleomycin, calcium gluconate, cimetidine, colistimethate, hydrocortisone, idarubicin, lidocaine, norepinephrine, oxytetracycline, pentobarbital sodium, polymyxin B, ranitidine, tetracycline, theophylline, vitamin B complex with C.

Contraindications and cautions

• Contraindicated in patients hypersensitive to other cephalosporins.
• Use cautiously in patients with a history of sensitivity to penicillin because of cross-allergic reaction, and in patients with renal impairment.
⚕ **Lifespan:** In pregnant and breast-feeding women, use cautiously.

Adverse reactions

CNS: dizziness, headache, malaise, paresthesia.
GI: abdominal cramps, anal pruritus, anorexia, *diarrhea,* dyspepsia, glossitis, nausea, oral candidiasis, *pseudomembranous colitis,* vomiting, tenesmus.
GU: genital pruritus and candidiasis, vaginitis.
Hematologic: anemia, eosinophilia, *leukopenia, thrombocytopenia, transient neutropenia.*

Respiratory: dyspnea.
Skin: injection site reactions (pain, induration, abscess, tissue sloughing), *maculopapular and erythematous rashes,* **Stevens-Johnson syndrome,** *urticaria.*
Other: hypersensitivity reactions (serum sickness, *anaphylaxis*).

Interactions

Drug-drug. *Probenecid:* May inhibit excretion and increase level of cefazolin. Monitor patient.

Effects on lab test results

• May increase ALT, AST, alkaline phosphatase, bilirubin, GGT, and LDH levels.
• May increase eosinophil count. May decrease neutrophil, WBC, and platelet counts.
• May cause false-positive urine glucose determinations with copper sulfate tests (Clinitest).

Pharmacokinetics

Absorption: Unknown after I.M. use.
Distribution: Wide; CSF penetration is poor; 74% to 86% protein-bound.
Metabolism: None.
Excretion: Mainly in urine. *Half-life:* About 1 to 2 hours.

Route	Onset	Peak	Duration
I.V.	Immediate	Immediate	Unknown
I.M.	Unknown	1–2 hr	Unknown

Action

Chemical effect: Inhibits cell-wall synthesis, promoting osmotic instability; usually bactericidal.
Therapeutic effect: Hinders or kills susceptible bacteria.

Available forms

Infusion: 500 mg/50-ml or 100-ml vial, 1 g/ 50-ml or 100-ml vial, 500 mg or 1 g RediVials, Faspaks, or ADD-Vantage vials
Injection (parenteral): 250 mg, 500 mg, 1 g

NURSING PROCESS

🏵 **Assessment**
• Assess patient's infection before therapy and regularly thereafter.
• Before giving first dose, obtain specimen for culture and sensitivity tests. Begin therapy pending test results.

- Before giving first dose, ask patient about previous reactions to cephalosporins or penicillin.
- If adverse GI reactions occur, monitor patient's hydration.
- Assess patient's and family's knowledge of drug therapy.

Nursing diagnoses
- Infection related to bacteria susceptible to drug
- Risk for deficient fluid volume related to drug-induced adverse GI reactions
- Deficient knowledge related to drug therapy

Planning and implementation
- Because of long duration of effect, most infections can be treated with q-8-hour use.
- After reconstitution, inject I.M. drug without further dilution (not as painful as other cephalosporins). Inject deep into large muscle mass, such as gluteus maximus or lateral aspect of thigh.
- **ALERT:** Don't confuse with other cephalosporins with similar-sounding names.

Patient teaching
- Tell patient to report adverse reactions.

Evaluation
- Patient is free from infection.
- Patient maintains adequate hydration.
- Patient and family state understanding of drug therapy.

cefdinir
(SEF-dih-neer)
Omnicef

Pharmacologic class: third-generation cephalosporin
Therapeutic class: antibiotic
Pregnancy risk category: B

Indications and dosages
▶ **Mild to moderate infections caused by susceptible strains of microorganisms for conditions of community-acquired pneumonia and uncomplicated skin and skin-structure infections.** *Adults and children older than age 12:* 300 mg P.O. q 12 hours for 10 days.
Children ages 6 months to 12 years: For uncomplicated skin and skin-structure infections,

7 mg/kg P.O. q 12 hours for 10 days; maximum daily dosage, 600 mg.
▶ **Acute exacerbations of chronic bronchitis; acute bacterial otitis media; acute maxillary sinusitis.** *Adults and children older than age 12:* 300 mg P.O. q 12 hours for 10 days or 600 mg P.O. q 24 hours for 10 days.
Children ages 6 months to 12 years: 7 mg/kg P.O. q 12 hours for 10 days or 14 mg/kg P.O. q 24 hours for 10 days, up to a maximum dose of 600 mg daily.
▶ **Pharyngitis, tonsillitis.** *Adults and children older than age 12:* 300 mg P.O. q 12 hours for 5 to 10 days or 600 mg P.O. q 24 hours for 10 days.
Children ages 6 months to 12 years: 7 mg/kg P.O. q 12 hours for 5 to 10 days or 14 mg/kg P.O. q 24 hours for 10 days, up to a maximum dosage of 600 mg daily.
Adjust-a-dose: For patients with renal impairment, if creatinine clearance is less than 30 ml/minute, reduce adult dosage to 300 mg P.O. once daily; for children, reduce to 7 mg/kg up to 300 mg P.O. once daily. In patients receiving long-term hemodialysis, dosage is 300 mg or 7 mg/kg P.O. at end of each dialysis session and subsequently q other day.

Contraindications and cautions
- Contraindicated in patients hypersensitive to cephalosporins.
- Use cautiously in patients hypersensitive to penicillin because of risk of cross-sensitivity with other beta-lactam antibiotics. Also use cautiously in patients with history of colitis or renal impairment.
Lifespan: In breast-feeding women, use cautiously. In children younger than age 6 months, safety and effectiveness haven't been established.

Adverse reactions
CNS: headache.
GI: abdominal pain, *diarrhea,* nausea, vomiting.
GU: vaginal candidiasis, vaginitis.
Skin: rash.

Interactions
Drug-drug. *Antacids containing aluminum or magnesium, iron supplements, multivitamins containing iron:* May decrease cefdinir's ab-

sorption and bioavailability. Give such preparations 2 hours before or after cefdinir dose. *Probenecid:* May inhibit the renal excretion of cefdinir. Monitor patient.

Effects on lab test results

- May increase GGT, alkaline phosphatase, and urine protein levels.
- May increase RBC count.

Pharmacokinetics

Absorption: Bioavailability of drug is about 21% after 300-mg capsule dose, 16% after 600-mg capsule dose, and 25% for suspension.
Distribution: 60% to 70% bound to proteins.
Metabolism: Not appreciably metabolized; activity results mainly from parent drug.
Excretion: Mainly by renal excretion. *Half-life:* 1¾ hours.

Route	Onset	Peak	Duration
P.O.	Unknown	2–4 hr	Unknown

Action

Chemical effect: Kills bacteria by inhibiting cell-wall synthesis.
Therapeutic effect: Is stable in the presence of some beta-lactamase enzymes, causing some microorganisms resistant to penicillins and cephalosporins to be susceptible to this drug.

Available forms

Capsules: 300 mg
Suspension: 125 mg/5 ml

NURSING PROCESS

Assessment

- Before giving first dose, obtain specimen for culture and sensitivity tests. Begin therapy pending test results.
- Before giving first dose, ask patient about previous reactions to cephalosporins or penicillin.
- Monitor patient for symptoms of superinfection.
- Assess patient with diarrhea carefully because pseudomembranous colitis has been reported with drug.
- Assess patient's and family's knowledge of drug therapy.

Nursing diagnoses

- Infection related to susceptible bacteria
- Risk for deficient fluid volume related to drug-induced adverse GI reactions
- Deficient knowledge related to drug therapy

Planning and implementation

- If allergic reaction is suspected, notify prescriber; stop drug and give emergency care.

ALERT: Don't confuse with other cephalosporins with similar-sounding names.

Patient teaching

- If patient is taking antacids or iron supplements, instruct him to take them 2 hours before or after dose of cefdinir.
- Inform patient with diabetes that each teaspoon of suspension contains 2.86 g of sucrose.
- Tell patient that drug may be taken with or without food.
- Advise patient to report severe diarrhea or diarrhea accompanied by abdominal pain.
- Tell patient to promptly report adverse reactions or symptoms of superinfection.

Evaluation

- Patient is free from infection.
- Patient maintains adequate hydration.
- Patient and family state understanding of drug therapy.

cefditoren pivoxil

(sef-da-TOR-en pa-VOX-ill)
Spectracef

Pharmacologic class: semisynthetic third-generation cephalosporin
Therapeutic class: antibiotic
Pregnancy risk category: B

Indications and dosages

▶ **Acute bacterial exacerbation of chronic bronchitis caused by *Haemophilus influenzae, H. parainfluenzae, Streptococcus pneumoniae* (penicillin-susceptible strains only), or *Moraxella catarrhalis.*** *Adults and children age 12 and older:* 400 mg P.O. b.i.d. with meals for 10 days.

▶ **Pharyngitis, tonsillitis, and uncomplicated skin and skin-structure infections caused by *Streptococcus pyogenes.*** *Adults and children age 12 and older:* 200 mg P.O. b.i.d. with meals for 10 days.

⧉ **Adjust-a-dose:** For patients with renal impairment, if creatinine clearance is 30 to 49 ml/minute, don't give more than 200 mg b.i.d. If creatinine clearance is less than 30 ml/minute, give 200 mg daily.

Contraindications and cautions

• Contraindicated in patients hypersensitive to drug, other cephalosporins, and penicillins. Also contraindicated in patients with carnitine deficiency or inborn errors of metabolism that may result in significant carnitine deficiency. Because tablets contain sodium caseinate, a milk protein, don't give them to patients hypersensitive to milk protein (distinct from those with lactose intolerance).
• Use cautiously in patients with renal impairment. Drug is dialyzable.
• Not recommended for prolonged antibiotic therapy.
⚕ **Lifespan:** In breast-feeding women, use cautiously because cephalosporins appear in breast milk. In children younger than age 12, safety and effectiveness haven't been established.

Adverse reactions

CNS: headache.
GI: abdominal pain, *colitis, diarrhea,* dyspepsia, hepatic dysfunction (including cholestasis), nausea, vomiting.
GU: hematuria, *nephrotoxicity,* vaginal candidiasis.
Hematologic: anemia.
Metabolic: hyperglycemia.
Skin: *Stevens-Johnson syndrome, toxic epidermal necrolysis.*
Other: *hypersensitivity reactions* (including serum sickness, rash, fever, *anaphylaxis*).

Interactions

Drug-drug. *Aluminum antacids, H₂-receptor antagonists, magnesium:* May reduce cefditoren absorption. Avoid using together. If used together, separate doses.
Oral anticoagulants: May increase bleeding time. Monitor PT and patient closely for unusual bleeding or bruising.
Probenecid: May increases cefditoren level. Avoid using together.
Drug-food. *Moderate- to high-fat meals:* May increase drug bioavailability. Advise patient to take drug with meals.

Effects on lab test results

• May increase liver enzyme levels. May decrease carnitine and hemoglobin levels and hematocrit.
• May decrease PT.
• May cause a false-positive direct Coombs' test result and false-positive reaction for glucose in urine using copper reduction tests (those involving Benedict's solution, Fehling's solution, or Clinitest tablets).

Pharmacokinetics

Absorption: From the GI tract and hydrolyzed by esterases to cefditoren.
Distribution: Wide based on volume of distribution. CSF penetration is unknown. Drug is about 88% protein-bound.
Metabolism: Not appreciably metabolized.
Excretion: Unchanged mainly in urine by glomerular filtration and tubular secretion. *Half-life:* 1¼ to 2 hours in patients with normal renal function.

Route	Onset	Peak	Duration
P.O.	Unknown	1½–3 hr	Unknown

Action

Chemical effect: Mainly bactericidal. Drug acts by adhering to bacterial penicillin-binding proteins, thereby inhibiting cell-wall synthesis. Active against many gram-positive and gram-negative organisms.
Therapeutic effects: Kills susceptible bacteria.

Available forms

Tablets: 200 mg

NURSING PROCESS

℞ Assessment

• Assess patient's history for hypersensitivity to cefditoren, cephalosporins, penicillins, or other contraindications for drug therapy.
• Monitor patient for overgrowth or recurrence of resistant organisms with prolonged or repeated drug therapy.
• Because cefditoren has been linked to *Clostridium difficile*–related colitis, monitor patient for diarrhea during therapy.
• Monitor patient for hypersensitivity reactions during therapy, as well as for any unusual bleeding or bruising.

Reactions may be *common*, uncommon, *life-threatening*, or COMMON AND LIFE-THREATENING.

• Assess patient's and family's knowledge of drug therapy.

⚙ Nursing diagnoses
• Noncompliance related to completion of 10-day antibiotic regimen
• Risk for infection with nonsusceptible bacteria or fungi related to prolonged or repeated drug therapy
• Deficient knowledge related to cephalosporin therapy

⟩ Planning and implementation
• Give drug with a meal to increase its bioavailability.
• If patient develops diarrhea after receiving cefditoren, keep in mind that this drug may cause pseudomembranous colitis. Notify prescriber immediately because colitis may be fatal.
• Don't use this drug if patient needs prolonged therapy.
• Signs and symptoms of overdose may include nausea, vomiting, epigastric distress, diarrhea, and seizures. Treat symptoms and provide supportive therapy.
• If hypersensitivity or allergic reaction occurs, stop drug and provide emergency care.
⑧ ALERT: Don't confuse with other cephalosporins with similar-sounding names.
Patient teaching
• Instruct patient to take drug with food to increase its absorption.
• Caution patient not to take drug with an H_2 antagonist or an antacid because they may reduce cefditoren absorption. If an H_2 antagonist or antacid must be used, instruct the patient to take them 2 hours before or after drug.
• Explain to patient the importance of taking drug for the prescribed duration, despite feeling better, to prevent any future drug resistance.
• Instruct patient to immediately stop taking drug and call prescriber if any adverse reactions develop, such as rash, hives, difficulty breathing, unusual bleeding or bruising, or diarrhea.
• Encourage patient to contact prescriber if signs and symptoms of infection don't improve after several days of therapy.
• Urge patient not to miss any doses. However, if patient misses a dose, instruct him to take the missed dose immediately after he realizes he has missed a dose and to wait 12 hours before

taking the next dose. Tell him not to double the dose.

☑ Evaluation
• Patient completes prescribed 10-day therapy.
• Patient doesn't experience any adverse reactions during drug therapy.
• Patient and family state understanding of drug therapy and importance of completing entire drug regimen as prescribed.

cefixime
(sef-IKS-eem)
Suprax

Pharmacologic class: third-generation cephalosporin
Therapeutic class: antibiotic
Pregnancy risk category: B

Indications and dosages
▶ **Uncomplicated UTIs caused by** *Escherichia coli* **and** *Proteus mirabilis;* **otitis media caused by** *Haemophilus influenzae* **(beta-lactamase–positive and –negative strains),** *Moraxella catarrhalis,* **and** *Streptococcus pyogenes;* **pharyngitis and tonsillitis caused by** *S. pyogenes;* **acute bronchitis and acute exacerbations of chronic bronchitis caused by** *S. pneumoniae* **and** *H. influenzae* **(beta-lactamase–positive and –negative strains).**
Adults and children older than age 12 who weigh more than 50 kg (110 lb): 400 mg P.O. daily or 200 mg q 12 hours.
Children age 6 months to 12 years: 8 mg/kg P.O. daily in one or two divided doses. For otitis media, use suspension only.
▶ **Uncomplicated gonorrhea caused by** *Neisseria gonorrhoeae.* *Adults:* 400 mg P.O. as single dose.
▶ **Disseminated gonococcal infections.** *Adults:* 400 mg P.O. b.i.d. after initial therapy with I.M. or I.V. antibiotics for a total of 7 days of therapy.

Contraindications and cautions
• Contraindicated in patients hypersensitive to drug, other cephalosporins, or beta-lactam antibiotics.
• Use cautiously in patients with renal dysfunction or history of sensitivity to penicillin. Re-

duce dosage in patients with creatinine clearance less than 60 ml/minute.
※ **Lifespan:** Use cautiously in pregnant or breast-feeding women.

Adverse reactions

CNS: dizziness, fatigue, headache, insomnia, malaise, nervousness, somnolence.
GI: abdominal pain, *diarrhea,* dyspepsia, flatulence, loose stools, nausea, *pseudomembranous colitis,* vomiting.
GU: genital candidiasis, genital pruritus, vaginitis.
Hematologic: eosinophilia, *leukopenia, thrombocytopenia.*
Hepatic: *hepatitis,* jaundice.
Skin: pruritus, rash, *Stevens-Johnson syndrome,* urticaria.
Other: drug fever, *hypersensitivity reactions* (serum sickness, *anaphylaxis*).

Interactions

Drug-drug. *Nifedipine:* May increase cefixime level. Avoid using together.
Probenecid: May inhibit excretion and increase level of cefixime. Monitor patient.
Salicylates: May displace cefixime from protein-binding sites. Significance is unknown.

Effects on lab test results

● May increase BUN, creatinine, ALT, AST, alkaline phosphatase, bilirubin, GGT, and LDH levels.
● May increase eosinophil count. May decrease platelet and WBC counts.
● May cause false-positive results in urine glucose tests that use copper sulfate (Clinitest).

Pharmacokinetics

Absorption: Good.
Distribution: Wide; enters CSF in patients with inflamed meninges; 65% bound to proteins.
Metabolism: 50% of drug.
Excretion: Mainly in urine. *Half-life:* 3 to 4 hours.

Route	Onset	Peak	Duration
P.O.	Unknown	2–6 hr	Unknown

Action

Chemical effect: Inhibits cell-wall synthesis, promoting osmotic instability; usually bactericidal.

Therapeutic effect: Hinders or kills bacteria, including *H. influenzae, M. catarrhalis, S. pyogenes, S. pneumoniae, E. coli,* and *P. mirabilis.*

Available forms

Oral suspension: 100 mg/5 ml (after reconstitution)
Tablets: 200 mg, 400 mg

NURSING PROCESS

⚷ Assessment
● Assess patient's infection before therapy and regularly thereafter.
● Before giving first dose, obtain specimen for culture and sensitivity tests. Begin therapy pending test results.
● Before giving first dose, ask patient about previous reactions to cephalosporins or penicillin.
● Be alert for adverse reactions and drug interactions.
● If adverse GI reactions occur, monitor patient's hydration.
● Assess patient's and family's knowledge of drug therapy.

⊞ Nursing diagnoses
● Infection related to bacteria susceptible to drug
● Risk for deficient fluid volume related to drug-induced adverse GI reactions
● Deficient knowledge related to drug therapy

▶ Planning and implementation
● To prepare oral suspension, add required amount of water to powder in two portions. Shake well after each addition. After mixing, suspension is stable for 14 days (no need to refrigerate). Keep tightly closed. Shake well before using.
⊛ **ALERT:** Don't confuse with other cephalosporins with similar-sounding names.
Patient teaching
● Tell patient to take drug exactly as prescribed, even after he feels better.
● Tell patient to call prescriber if rash develops.
● Teach patient how to store drug.

☑ Evaluation
● Patient is free from infection.
● Patient maintains adequate hydration.
● Patient and family state understanding of drug therapy.

Reactions may be *common,* uncommon, *life-threatening*, or COMMON AND LIFE-THREATENING.

cefoperazone sodium
(sef-oh-PER-ah-zohn SOH-dee-um)
Cefobid

Pharmacologic class: third-generation cephalosporin
Therapeutic class: antibiotic
Pregnancy risk category: B

Indications and dosages

▶ Serious infections of respiratory tract; intra-abdominal, gynecologic, and skin infections; bacteremia; and septicemia caused by susceptible microorganisms including *Streptococcus pneumoniae* and *S. pyogenes; Staphylococcus aureus* (penicillinase– and non-penicillinase–producing) and *Staphylococcus epidermidis;* enterococci; *Escherichia coli; Klebsiella; Haemophilus influenzae; Enterobacter; Citrobacter; Proteus;* some *Pseudomonas,* including *P. aeruginosa;* and *Bacteroides fragilis. Adults:* Usual dosage is 1 to 2 g q 12 hours I.V. or I.M. In severe infections or those caused by less sensitive organisms, increase total daily dosage to 16 g.
🔲 **Adjust-a-dose:** For patients with hepatic or biliary obstruction, give 4 g daily, cautiously. Larger amounts require monitoring of level.
    For patients with hepatic and substantial renal impairment, maximum total dosage is 2 g daily. Because the drug's half-life is slightly reduced during hemodialysis, give dose after a hemodialysis session.

▼ I.V. administration

● Before reconstituting sterile powder, protect it from light and store at 77° F (25° C) or lower. After drug is reconstituted, it need not be protected from light.
● Reconstitute 1- or 2-g vial with at least 2.8 ml of compatible I.V. solution. Manufacturer recommends 5 ml/g.
● Give by direct injection into large vein or into tubing of free-flowing I.V. solution over 3 to 5 minutes.
● When giving by intermittent infusion, add reconstituted drug to 20 to 40 ml of compatible I.V. solution and infuse over 15 to 30 minutes.
⊗ **Incompatibilities**
Amifostine, aminoglycosides, diltiazem, filgrastim, hetastarch, labetalol hydrochloride, meperi-

dine hydrochloride, ondansetron hydrochloride, pentamidine isethionate, perphenazine, promethazine hydrochloride, sargramostim, vinorelbine tartrate.

Contraindications and cautions

● Contraindicated in patients hypersensitive to drug or other cephalosporins.
● Use cautiously in patients with renal impairment and in patients with a history of sensitivity to penicillin.
🧬 **Lifespan:** In pregnant or breast-feeding women, use cautiously. In children younger than age 12, safety and effectiveness haven't been established.

Adverse reactions

CNS: dizziness, headache, malaise, paresthesia.
GI: abdominal cramps, anal pruritus, anorexia, *diarrhea,* dyspepsia, glossitis, oral candidiasis, *pseudomembranous colitis,* nausea, tenesmus, vomiting.
GU: genital pruritus and candidiasis.
Hematologic: bleeding, eosinophilia, hemolytic anemia, *hypoprothrombinemia, transient neutropenia.*
Respiratory: dyspnea.
Skin: maculopapular and erythematous rashes, urticaria.
Other: hypersensitivity reactions (serum sickness, *anaphylaxis*); pain, induration, sterile abscesses, warmth, tissue sloughing at injection site; phlebitis, thrombophlebitis with I.V. injection.

Interactions

Drug-drug. *Aminoglycosides:* May increase risk of nephrotoxicity. Monitor patient's renal condition closely.
Anticoagulants: May increase anticoagulant effects. Use with caution, and monitor patient for bleeding.
Probenecid: May inhibit excretion and increase level of cefoperazone. Monitor patient.
Drug-lifestyle. *Alcohol use:* May cause a disulfiram-like reaction, including flushing, tachycardia, bronchospasm, sweating, nausea, and vomiting. Strongly discourage alcohol use with these drugs. This reaction could also occur after several days.

Effects on lab test results

• May increase BUN, creatinine, ALT, AST, alkaline phosphatase, bilirubin, GGT, and LDH levels. May decrease hemoglobin level and hematocrit.
• May increase INR and eosinophil count. May decrease neutrophil count. May increase or decrease PT.
• May cause false-positive urine glucose determinations with copper sulfate tests (Clinitest).

Pharmacokinetics

Absorption: Unknown after I.M. use.
Distribution: Wide; CSF penetration in patients with inflamed meninges; 82% to 93% protein-bound.
Metabolism: Insignificant.
Excretion: Mainly in urine. *Half-life:* About 1½ to 2½ hours.

Route	Onset	Peak	Duration
I.V.	Immediate	Immediate	Unknown
I.M.	Unknown	1–2 hr	Unknown

Action

Chemical effect: Inhibits cell-wall synthesis, promoting osmotic instability; usually bactericidal.
Therapeutic effect: Hinders or kills susceptible bacteria.

Available forms

Infusion: 1 g, 2 g piggyback
Parenteral: 1 g, 2 g

NURSING PROCESS

Assessment
• Assess patient's infection before therapy and regularly thereafter.
• Before giving first dose, obtain specimen for culture and sensitivity tests. Begin therapy pending test results.
• Before giving first dose, ask patient about previous reactions to cephalosporins or penicillin.
• Be alert for adverse reactions and drug interactions.
• If patient develops adverse GI reactions, monitor hydration. Drug may increase the risk of diarrhea more than other cephalosporins.
• Assess patient's and family's knowledge of drug therapy.

Nursing diagnoses
• Infection related to bacteria susceptible to drug
• Risk for deficient fluid volume related to drug-induced adverse GI reactions
• Deficient knowledge related to drug therapy

Planning and implementation
• To prepare drug for I.M. injection, using 1-g vial, dissolve drug with 2 ml of sterile water for injection; add 0.6 ml of 2% lidocaine hydrochloride for final concentration of 333 mg/ml. Or dissolve drug with 2.8 ml of sterile water for injection; then add 1 ml of 2% lidocaine hydrochloride for final concentration of 250 mg/ml. When using 2-g vial, dissolve drug with 3.8 ml of sterile water for injection; then add 1.2 ml of 2% lidocaine hydrochloride for final concentration of 333 mg/ml. Or dissolve drug with 5.4 ml of sterile water for injection; then add 1.8 ml of 2% lidocaine hydrochloride for final concentration of 250 mg/ml.
• Inject deep into large muscle mass, such as gluteus maximus or lateral aspect of thigh.
ALERT: Don't confuse with other cephalosporins with similar-sounding names.
Patient teaching
• Tell patient to report adverse reactions.

Evaluation
• Patient is free from infection.
• Patient maintains adequate hydration.
• Patient and family state understanding of drug therapy.

cefotaxime sodium
(sef-oh-TAKS-eem SOH-dee-um)
Claforan

Pharmacologic class: third-generation cephalosporin
Therapeutic class: antibiotic
Pregnancy risk category: B

Indications and dosages

▶ **Perioperative prophylaxis in contaminated surgery.** *Adults:* 1 g I.V. or I.M. 30 to 90 minutes before surgery. In patients undergoing cesarean delivery, give dose as soon as umbilical cord is clamped, followed by 1 g I.V. or I.M. 6 and 12 hours later.

▶ Serious infections of lower respiratory and urinary tracts, CNS, skin, bone, and joints; gynecologic and intra-abdominal infections; bacteremia; and septicemia. Susceptible microorganisms include streptococci, including *Streptococcus pneumoniae* and *S. pyogenes; Staphylococcus aureus* (penicillinase– and non-penicillinase–producing) and *S. epidermidis; Escherichia coli; Klebsiella; Haemophilus influenzae; Enterobacter; Proteus;* and *Peptostreptococcus*. Pelvic inflammatory disease‡. *Adults:* Usual dosage is 1 g I.V. or I.M. q 6 to 12 hours. Up to 12 g daily can be given in life-threatening infections.
Children weighing at least 50 kg (110 lb): Usual adult dose but don't exceed 12 g daily.
Children ages 1 month to 12 years weighing less than 50 kg: 50 to 180 mg/kg I.V. or I.M. daily in four to six divided doses.
Neonates ages 1 to 4 weeks: 50 mg/kg I.V. q 8 hours.
Neonates up to age 1 week: 50 mg/kg I.V. q 12 hours.
▶ Disseminated gonococcal infection‡.
Adults: 1 g I.V. q 8 hours.
Neonates and infants: 25 to 50 mg/kg I.V. q 8 to 12 hours for 7 days, or 50 to 100 mg/kg I.M or I.V. q 12 hours for 7 days.
▶ Gonococcal ophthalmia‡. *Adults:* 500 mg I.V. q.i.d.
Neonates: 100 mg I.V. or I.M. for one dose; may continue until ocular cultures are negative at 48 to 72 hours.
▶ Gonorrheal meningitis or arthritis‡.
Neonates and infants: 25 to 50 mg/kg I.V. q 8 to 12 hours for 10 to 14 days. Or 50 to 100 mg/kg I.M. or I.V. q 12 hours for 10 to 14 days.
⊠ **Adjust-a-dose:** For patients with renal impairment, if creatinine clearance is less than 20 ml/minute, give half the usual dose at the usual interval.

▼ I.V. administration

• Reconstitute infusion vials with 50 to 100 ml D₅W or normal saline solution.
• For direct injection, reconstitute 500-mg, 1-g, or 2-g vials with 10-ml sterile water for injection. Solutions containing 1 g/14 ml are isotonic.
• Inject drug into large vein or into tubing of free-flowing I.V. solution over 3 to 5 minutes.
• Infuse drug over 20 to 30 minutes. Interrupt flow of primary I.V. solution during infusion.

⊗ **Incompatibilities**
Allopurinol, aminoglycosides, aminophylline, azithromycin, doxapram, filgrastim, fluconazole, hetastarch, pentamidine isethionate, sodium bicarbonate injection, vancomycin.

Contraindications and cautions

• Contraindicated in patients hypersensitive to drug or other cephalosporins.
• Use cautiously in patients with history of sensitivity to penicillin and in patients with renal impairment.
⚘ **Lifespan:** In pregnant or breast-feeding women, use cautiously.

Adverse reactions

CNS: dizziness, elevated temperature, headache, malaise, paresthesia.
GI: abdominal cramps, anal pruritus, anorexia, *diarrhea,* dyspepsia, glossitis, nausea, oral candidiasis, *pseudomembranous colitis,* tenesmus, vomiting.
GU: genital pruritus and candidiasis.
Hematologic: *agranulocytosis,* eosinophilia, hemolytic anemia, *thrombocytopenia, transient neutropenia.*
Respiratory: dyspnea.
Skin: maculopapular and erythematous rashes, urticaria.
Other: hypersensitivity reactions (serum sickness, *anaphylaxis*); pain, induration, sterile abscesses, warmth, tissue sloughing at injection site; phlebitis, thrombophlebitis with I.V. injection.

Interactions

Drug-drug. *Aminoglycosides:* May increase risk of nephrotoxicity. Monitor renal function closely.
Probenecid: May inhibit excretion and increase level of cefotaxime. Use together cautiously.

Effects on lab test results

• May increase ALT, AST, alkaline phosphatase, bilirubin, GGT, and LDH levels. May decrease hemoglobin level and hematocrit.
• May increase eosinophil count. May decrease neutrophil, platelet, and granulocyte counts.
• May cause false-positive urine glucose determinations with copper sulfate tests (Clinitest).

Pharmacokinetics

Absorption: Unknown after I.M. use.

Distribution: Wide; adequate CSF penetration when meninges are inflamed; 13% to 38% protein-bound.
Metabolism: Partially to active metabolite.
Excretion: Mainly in urine. *Half-life:* 1 to 2 hours.

Route	Onset	Peak	Duration
I.V.	Immediate	Immediate	8–12 hr
I.M.	Unknown	30 min	8–12 hr

Action

Chemical effect: Inhibits cell-wall synthesis, promoting osmotic instability; usually bactericidal.
Therapeutic effect: Hinders or kills susceptible bacteria.

Available forms

Infusion: 1 g, 2 g
Injection: 500 mg, 1 g, 2 g

NURSING PROCESS

🔍 Assessment

• Assess patient's infection before therapy and regularly thereafter.
• Before giving first dose, obtain specimen for culture and sensitivity tests. Begin therapy pending test results.
• Before giving first dose, ask patient about previous reactions to cephalosporins or penicillin.
• Be alert for adverse reactions and drug interactions.
• If adverse GI reactions occur, monitor patient's hydration.
• Assess patient's and family's knowledge of drug therapy.

🔷 Nursing diagnoses

• Infection related to bacteria susceptible to drug
• Risk for deficient fluid volume related to drug-induced adverse GI reactions
• Deficient knowledge related to drug therapy

⋙ Planning and implementation

• For I.M. use, inject deeply into large muscle mass, such as gluteus maximus or lateral aspect of thigh.
• **⚠ ALERT:** Don't confuse with other cephalosporins with similar-sounding names.

Patient teaching
• Tell patient to report adverse reactions.
• Teach patient to report decrease in urinary output. May have to decrease total daily dose.

✔ Evaluation

• Patient is free from infection.
• Patient maintains adequate hydration.
• Patient and family state understanding of drug therapy.

cefoxitin sodium
(sef-OKS-ih-tin SOH-dee-um)
Mefoxin

Pharmacologic class: second-generation cephalosporin
Therapeutic class: antibiotic
Pregnancy risk category: B

Indications and dosages

▶ **Serious infections of respiratory and GU tracts; skin, soft-tissue, bone, and joint infections; bloodstream and intra-abdominal infections caused by susceptible** *Escherichia coli* **and other coliform bacteria,** *Staphylococcus aureus* **(penicillinase– and non-penicillinase–producing),** *S. epidermidis,* **streptococci,** *Klebsiella, Haemophilus influenzae,* **and** *Bacteroides,* **including** *B. fragilis;* **and perioperative prophylaxis.** *Adults:* 1 to 2 g I.V. q 6 to 8 hours for uncomplicated forms of infection. In life-threatening infections, up to 12 g daily.
Children and infants age 3 months and older: 80 to 160 mg/kg I.V. daily in four to six equally divided doses. Maximum daily dose is 12 g.
▶ **Prophylactic use in surgery.** *Adults:* 2 g I.V. 30 to 60 minutes before surgery; then 2 g I.V. q 6 hours for 24 hours. If used in cesarean section give 2 g I.V. as soon as cord is clamped. Or, if a three-dose regimen is used, give 2 g I.V. as soon as cord is clamped, then 2 g I.V. 4 and 8 hours after first dose.
Children older than age 3 months: 30 to 40 mg/kg I.V. 30 to 60 minutes before surgery; then 30 to 40 mg/kg q 6 hours for 24 hours.
⬛ Adjust-a-dose: For patients with renal impairment, if creatinine clearance is 30 to 50 ml/minute, give 1 to 2 g q 8 to 12 hours; if clearance is 10 to 29 ml/minute, give 1 to 2 g q 12 to

24 hours; and if clearance is 5 to 10 ml/minute, give 500 mg to 1 g q 12 to 24 hours. If clearance is less than 5 ml/minute, give 500 mg to 1 g q 24 to 48 hours. For hemodialysis patients, give loading dose of 1 to 2 g after each session, and maintenance dose as indicated above.

▼ I.V. administration

• Reconstitute 1 g with at least 10 ml of sterile water for injection and 2 g with 10 to 20 ml of sterile water for injection. Solutions of D_5W and normal saline solution for injection also can be used.
• For direct injection, inject reconstituted drug into large vein or into tubing of free-flowing I.V. solution over 3 to 5 minutes.
• For intermittent infusion, add reconstituted drug to 50 or 100 ml D_5W, $D_{10}W$, or normal saline solution for injection. Interrupt flow of primary I.V. solution during infusion.
• Assess I.V. site frequently for thrombophlebitis.
⊗ **Incompatibilities**
Aminoglycosides, filgrastim, gatifloxacin, hetastarch, pentamidine isethionate, ranitidine.

Contraindications and cautions

• Contraindicated in patients hypersensitive to drug or other cephalosporins.
• Use cautiously in patients with history of sensitivity to penicillin and in patients with renal impairment.
🌣 **Lifespan:** In pregnant or breast-feeding women, use cautiously.

Adverse reactions

CNS: fever.
CV: hypotension, *phlebitis, thrombophlebitis* with I.V. injection.
GI: *diarrhea, pseudomembranous colitis.*
GU: *acute renal failure.*
Hematologic: eosinophilia, hemolytic anemia, *thrombocytopenia, transient neutropenia.*
Respiratory: dyspnea.
Skin: *maculopapular and erythematous rashes, urticaria.*
Other: hypersensitivity reactions (serum sickness, *anaphylaxis*).

Interactions

Drug-drug. *Nephrotoxic drugs:* May increase risk of nephrotoxicity. Monitor renal function closely.

Probenecid: May inhibit excretion and increase level of cefoxitin. Sometimes used for this effect.

Effects on lab test results

• May increase ALT, AST, alkaline phosphatase, bilirubin, and LDH levels. May decrease hemoglobin level and hematocrit.
• May increase eosinophil count. May decrease neutrophil and platelet counts.
• May cause false-positive urine glucose determinations with copper sulfate tests (Clinitest).

Pharmacokinetics

Absorption: Unknown.
Distribution: Wide; CSF penetration is poor; 50% to 80% protein-bound.
Metabolism: Insignificant (about 2%).
Excretion: Mainly in urine. *Half-life:* About ½ to 1 hour.

Route	Onset	Peak	Duration
I.V.	Immediate	Immediate	Unknown

Action

Chemical effect: Inhibits cell-wall synthesis, promoting osmotic instability; usually bactericidal.
Therapeutic effect: Hinders or kills susceptible bacteria.

Available forms

Infusion: 1 g, 2 g, 10 g
Injection: 1 g, 2 g

NURSING PROCESS

Assessment

• Assess patient's infection before therapy and regularly thereafter.
• Before giving first dose, obtain specimen for culture and sensitivity tests. Begin therapy pending test results.
• Before giving first dose, ask patient about previous reactions to cephalosporins or penicillin.
• Be alert for adverse reactions and drug interactions.
• If adverse GI reactions occur, monitor patient's hydration.
• Assess patient's and family's knowledge of drug therapy.

🔯 Nursing diagnoses

- Infection related to bacteria susceptible to drug
- Risk for deficient fluid volume related to drug-induced adverse GI reactions
- Deficient knowledge related to drug therapy

⊠ Planning and implementation

- Patients with renal impairment require dosage adjustment.
- After reconstitution, drug may be stored for 24 hours at room temperature or refrigerated for 1 week.
- ⚱ **ALERT:** Don't confuse with other cephalosporins with similar-sounding names.

Patient teaching
- Tell patient to report adverse reactions and signs and symptoms of superinfection promptly.
- Instruct patient to notify prescriber if he has loose stools or diarrhea.

☑ Evaluation

- Patient is free from infection.
- Patient maintains adequate hydration.
- Patient and family state understanding of drug therapy.

cefpodoxime proxetil

(sef-poh-DOKS-eem PROKS-eh-til)
Vantin

Pharmacologic class: third-generation cephalosporin
Therapeutic class: antibiotic
Pregnancy risk category: B

Indications and dosages

▶ **Acute, community-acquired pneumonia caused by non–beta-lactamase–producing strains of *Haemophilus influenzae* or *Streptococcus pneumoniae*.** *Adults and children age 12 and older:* 200 mg P.O. q 12 hours for 14 days.
▶ **Acute bacterial exacerbation of chronic bronchitis caused by *S. pneumoniae*, *H. influenzae* (non–beta-lactamase–producing strains), or *Moraxella catarrhalis*.** *Adults and children age 12 and older:* 200 mg P.O. q 12 hours for 10 days.
▶ **Uncomplicated gonorrhea in men and women; rectal gonococcal infections in**
women. *Adults and children age 12 and older:* 200 mg P.O. as single dose. Follow with doxycycline 100 mg P.O. b.i.d. for 7 days.
▶ **Uncomplicated skin and skin-structure infections caused by *Staphylococcus aureus* or *Streptococcus pyogenes*.** *Adults and children age 12 and older:* 400 mg P.O. q 12 hours for 7 to 14 days.
▶ **Acute otitis media caused by *Streptococcus pneumoniae*, *H. influenzae*, or *M. catarrhalis*.** *Children ages 2 months to 12 years:* 5 mg/kg (not to exceed 200 mg) P.O. q 12 hours or 10 mg/kg (not to exceed 400 mg) P.O. daily for 10 days.
▶ **Pharyngitis or tonsillitis caused by *S. pyogenes*.** *Adults and children age 12 and older:* 100 mg P.O. q 12 hours for 5 to 10 days. *Children ages 2 months to 12 years:* 5 mg/kg (not to exceed 100 mg) P.O. q 12 hours for 10 days.
▶ **Uncomplicated UTIs caused by *E. coli*, *Klebsiella pneumoniae*, *Proteus mirabilis*, or *Staphylococcus saprophyticus*.** *Adults and children age 12 and older:* 100 mg P.O. q 12 hours for 7 days.
▶ **Mild to moderate acute maxillary sinusitis caused by *H. influenzae*, *S. pneumoniae*, or *M. catarrhalis*.** *Adults and children age 12 and older:* 200 mg P.O. q 12 hours for 10 days. *Children ages 2 months to 12 years:* 5 mg/kg P.O. q 12 hours for 10 days; maximum dosage is 200 mg.
🔲 **Adjust-a-dose:** For patients with renal impairment, if creatinine clearance is less than 30 ml/minute, increase dosage interval to q 24 hours. For patients undergoing dialysis, give dose three times weekly, after dialysis.

Contraindications and cautions

- Contraindicated in patients hypersensitive to drug or other cephalosporins.
- Use cautiously in patients with history of hypersensitivity to penicillin (risk of cross-sensitivity) and in patients receiving nephrotoxic drugs (other cephalosporins have had nephrotoxic potential).
- ⚹ **Lifespan:** In pregnant or breast-feeding women, use cautiously.

Adverse reactions

CNS: headache.
GI: abdominal pain, *diarrhea,* nausea, vomiting.

GU: vaginal fungal infections.
Skin: rash.
Other: hypersensitivity reactions *(anaphylaxis)*.

Interactions

Drug-drug. *Antacids, H_2-receptor antagonists:* May decrease cefpodoxime absorption. Avoid using together.
Probenecid: May decrease cefpodoxime excretion. Monitor patient for toxicity.
Drug-food. *Any food:* May increase absorption of tablets. Give tablet form with food. Oral suspension isn't affected by food.

Effects on lab test results

• May increase BUN, creatinine, AST, ALT, GGT, alkaline phosphatase, bilirubin, and LDH levels. May decrease albumin, potassium, sodium, and hemoglobin levels and hematocrit. May increase or decrease glucose level.
• May increase eosinophil, WBC, granulocyte, lymphocyte, basophil, and platelet counts. May prolong PT and PTT.
• May cause false-positive urine glucose determinations with copper sulfate tests (Clinitest). May cause positive Coombs' test.

Pharmacokinetics

Absorption: From GI tract.
Distribution: Widely into most body tissues and fluids except CSF.
Metabolism: Drug is de-esterified to its active metabolite, cefpodoxime. **Excretion:** Mainly in urine. *Half-life:* 2 to 3 hours.

Route	Onset	Peak	Duration
P.O.	Unknown	2–3 hr	Unknown

Action

Chemical effect: Inhibits cell-wall synthesis, promoting osmotic instability; usually bactericidal.
Therapeutic effect: Hinders or kills susceptible bacteria.

Available forms

Oral suspension: 50 mg/5 ml, 100 mg/5 ml in 100-ml bottles
Tablets (film-coated): 100 mg, 200 mg

NURSING PROCESS

☲ Assessment

• Assess patient's infection before therapy and regularly thereafter.
• Before giving first dose, obtain specimen for culture and sensitivity tests. Begin therapy pending test results.
• Before giving first dose, ask patient about previous reactions to cephalosporins or penicillin.
• Be alert for adverse reactions and drug interactions.
• If adverse GI reactions occur, monitor patient's hydration.
• Assess patient's and family's knowledge of drug therapy.

⊕ Nursing diagnoses

• Infection related to bacteria susceptible to drug
• Risk for deficient fluid volume related to drug-induced adverse GI reactions
• Deficient knowledge related to drug therapy

▷ Planning and implementation

• Give drug with food to minimize adverse GI reactions. Shake well before using.
• Store suspension in refrigerator (36° to 46° F [2° to 8° C]). Discard unused portion after 14 days.
⚠ **ALERT:** Don't confuse with other cephalosporins with similar-sounding names.
Patient teaching
• Advise patient to take drug with meals to minimize GI adverse effects.
• Tell patient to take drug exactly as prescribed, even after he feels better.
• Instruct patient to notify prescriber if rash develops.
• Teach patient how to store drug.
• Instruct patient to notify prescriber about a reduction in urinary output, especially if patient takes a diuretic.

☑ Evaluation

• Patient is free from infection.
• Patient maintains adequate hydration.
• Patient and family state understanding of drug therapy.

---

cefprozil
(SEF-pruh-zil)
Cefzil

Pharmacologic class: second-generation cephalosporin
Therapeutic class: antibiotic
Pregnancy risk category: B

Indications and dosages

▶ **Pharyngitis or tonsillitis caused by** *Streptococcus pyogenes. Adults and children older than age 12:* 500 mg P.O. daily for 10 days.
Children ages 2 to 12: 7.5 mg/kg P.O. q 12 hours for 10 days.
▶ **Otitis media caused by** *Streptococcus pneumoniae, Haemophilus influenzae,* **or** *Moraxella catarrhalis. Infants and children ages 6 months to 12 years:* 15 mg/kg P.O. q 12 hours for 10 days.
▶ **Secondary bacterial infections of acute bronchitis and acute bacterial exacerbation of chronic bronchitis caused by** *S. pneumoniae, H. influenzae,* **and** *M. catarrhalis. Adults and children older than age 12:* 500 mg P.O. q 12 hours for 10 days.
▶ **Uncomplicated skin and skin-structure infections caused by** *Staphylococcus aureus* **or** *S. pyogenes. Adults and children older than age 12:* 250 mg P.O. b.i.d., or 500 mg daily to b.i.d. for 10 days.
Children ages 2 to 12: 20 mg/kg P.O. q 24 hours for 10 days. Maximum dose is 1 g P.O. daily.
▶ **Acute sinusitis caused by** *S. pneumoniae, H. influenzae,* **and** *M. (Branhamella) catarrhalis. Adults and children older than age 12:* 250 mg or 500 mg P.O. q 12 hours for 10 days.
Children ages 6 months to 12 years: 7.5 mg/kg P.O. q 12 hours or 15 mg/kg P.O. daily for 10 days.
⧄ Adjust-a-dose: For patients with renal impairment, if creatinine clearance is less than 30 ml/minute, give 50% of usual dose.

Contraindications and cautions

• Contraindicated in patients hypersensitive to drug or other cephalosporins.
• Use cautiously in patients with history of sensitivity to penicillin and patients with hepatic or renal impairment.

⚶ Lifespan: In pregnant and breast-feeding women, use cautiously. Don't give children more than the recommended adult dose.

Adverse reactions

CNS: dizziness, headache, hyperactivity, insomnia, nervousness.
GI: abdominal pain, diarrhea, *nausea,* vomiting.
GU: genital pruritus, vaginitis.
Hematologic: eosinophilia.
Skin: rash, urticaria.
Other: *hypersensitivity reactions* (serum sickness, **anaphylaxis**), superinfection.

Interactions

Drug-drug. *Aminoglycosides:* May increase risk of nephrotoxicity. Monitor patient closely.
Probenecid: May inhibit excretion and increase level of cefprozil. Monitor patient.

Effects on lab test results

• May increase BUN, creatinine, ALT, AST, alkaline phosphatase, bilirubin, and LDH levels.
• May increase eosinophil count. May decrease WBC, leukocyte, and platelet counts.
• May cause false-positive results in urine glucose tests that use copper sulfate (Clinitest).

Pharmacokinetics

Absorption: About 95% from GI tract.
Distribution: About 35% protein-bound; distributed into various body tissues and fluids.
Metabolism: Probably by the liver.
Excretion: Mainly in urine. *Half-life:* 1¼ hours in patients with normal renal function; 2 hours in patients with impaired hepatic function; and 5¼ to 6 hours in patients with end-stage renal disease.

Route	Onset	Peak	Duration
P.O.	Unknown	Unknown	Unknown

Action

Chemical effect: Inhibits cell-wall synthesis, promoting osmotic instability; usually bactericidal.
Therapeutic effect: Hinders or kills susceptible bacteria.

Available forms

Oral suspension: 125 mg/5 ml, 250 mg/5 ml
Tablets: 250 mg, 500 mg

Reactions may be *common,* uncommon, *life-threatening*, or COMMON AND LIFE-THREATENING.

C

NURSING PROCESS

⌘ Assessment
• Assess patient's infection before therapy and regularly thereafter.
• Before giving first dose, obtain specimen for culture and sensitivity tests. Begin therapy pending test results.
• Before giving first dose, ask patient about previous reactions to cephalosporins or penicillin.
• Be alert for adverse reactions and drug interactions.
• If adverse GI reactions occur, monitor patient's hydration.
• Monitor patient's renal function.
• Assess patient's and family's knowledge of drug therapy.

⌘ Nursing diagnoses
• Infection related to bacteria susceptible to drug
• Risk for deficient fluid volume related to drug-induced adverse GI reactions
• Deficient knowledge related to drug therapy

⌘ Planning and implementation
• Give drug after hemodialysis is completed because it removes drug.
• Refrigerate reconstituted suspension (stable for 14 days). Keep tightly closed, and shake well before using.
• **ALERT:** Don't confuse with other cephalosporins with similar-sounding names.
Patient teaching
• Tell patient to shake suspension well before measuring dose.
• Advise patient to take drug as prescribed, even after he feels better.
• Inform patient that oral suspensions contain drug in bubble-gum flavor to improve palatability and promote compliance in children. Tell him to refrigerate reconstituted suspension and to discard any unused portion after 14 days.
• Advise elderly patients also receiving diuretic therapy to notify prescriber of decreased urine output.

⌘ Evaluation
• Patient is free from infection.
• Patient maintains adequate hydration.
• Patient and family state understanding of drug therapy.

ceftazidime
(sef-TAZ-ih-deem)
Ceptaz, Fortaz, Tazicef, Tazidime

Pharmacologic class: third-generation cephalosporin
Therapeutic class: antibiotic
Pregnancy risk category: B

Indications and dosages

▶ **Serious infections of lower respiratory and urinary tracts; gynecologic, intra-abdominal, CNS, and skin infections; bacteremia; and septicemia. Among susceptible microorganisms are streptococci, including *Streptococcus pneumoniae* and *S. pyogenes; Staphylococcus aureus; Escherichia coli; Klebsiella; Proteus; Enterobacter; Haemophilus influenzae; Pseudomonas;* and some strains of *Bacteroides.***
Adults and children older than age 12: 1 g I.V. or I.M. q 8 to 12 hours; maximum 6 g daily for life-threatening infections.
Children ages 1 month to 12 years: 25 to 50 mg/kg I.V. q 8 hours. Maximum 6 g daily.
Neonates age 4 weeks or younger: 30 mg/kg I.V. q 12 hours.
▶ **Uncomplicated UTI.** *Adults:* 250 mg I.V. or I.M. q 12 hours.
▶ **Complicated UTI.** *Adults:* 500 mg I.V. or I.M. q 8 to 12 hours.
▶ **Uncomplicated pneumonia or mild skin and skin-structure infection.** *Adults:* 0.5 to 1 g I.V. or I.M. q 8 hours.
▶ **Bone and joint infection.** *Adults:* 2 g I.V. q 12 hours.
▶ **Empiric therapy in febrile neutropenic patients‡.** *Adults:* 100 mg/kg I.V. daily in three divided doses; or 2 g I.V. q 8 hours either alone or with an aminoglycoside, such as amikacin.
▶ **Adjust-a-dose:** For patients with renal impairment, if creatinine clearance is 31 to 50 ml/minute, give 1 g q 12 hours; if clearance is 16 to 30 ml/minute, give 1 g q 24 hours; if clearance is 6 to 15 ml/minute, give 500 mg q 24 hours; if clearance is less than 5 ml/minute, give 500 mg q 48 hours. Drug is removed by hemodialysis; give a supplemental dose of drug after each dialysis session.

▼ I.V. administration

• Reconstitute solutions containing sodium carbonate with sterile water for injection. Add 5 ml to 500-mg vial; 10 ml to 1- or 2-g vial. Shake well to dissolve drug.
• Carbon dioxide is released during dissolution, and positive pressure will develop in vial. Don't add air to the vial when removing dose.
• Reconstitute solutions containing arginine with 10 ml sterile water for injection; this formulation won't release gas bubbles.
• Infuse drug over 15 to 30 minutes.
⊗ Incompatibilities
Aminoglycosides, aminophylline, amiodarone, amphotericin B cholesteryl sulfate complex, azithromycin, clarithromycin, fluconazole, idarubicin, midazolam, pentamidine isethionate, ranitidine hydrochloride, sargramostim, sodium bicarbonate solutions, vancomycin.

Contraindications and cautions

• Contraindicated in patients hypersensitive to drug or other cephalosporins.
• Use cautiously in patients with history of sensitivity to penicillin and in patients with renal impairment.
⚖ Lifespan: In pregnant and breast-feeding women, use cautiously. In children age 12 and younger, safety and effectiveness haven't been established.

Adverse reactions

CNS: dizziness, headache, *seizures.*
GI: abdominal cramps, diarrhea, dysgeusia, nausea, *pseudomembranous colitis,* vomiting.
GU: candidiasis, genital pruritus.
Hematologic: *agranulocytosis,* eosinophilia, *leukopenia,* thrombocytosis.
Respiratory: dyspnea.
Skin: *maculopapular and erythematous rashes, urticaria.*
Other: elevated temperature; hypersensitivity reactions (serum sickness, *anaphylaxis*); *pain, induration, sterile abscesses, tissue sloughing at injection site; phlebitis, thrombophlebitis with I.V. injection.*

Interactions

Drug-drug. *Chloramphenicol:* May have an antagonistic effect. Avoid using together.

Effects on lab test results

• May increase ALT, AST, alkaline phosphatase, bilirubin, and LDH levels. May decrease hemoglobin level and hematocrit.
• May increase eosinophil count. May decrease WBC and granulocyte counts. May increase or decrease platelet count.
• May cause false-positive urine glucose determinations with copper sulfate tests (Clinitest).

Pharmacokinetics

Absorption: Unknown with I.M. use.
Distribution: Wide, including CSF (unlike most other cephalosporins); 5% to 24% protein-bound.
Metabolism: None.
Excretion: Mainly in urine. *Half-life:* About 1½ to 2 hours.

Route	Onset	Peak	Duration
I.V.	Immediate	Immediate	Unknown
I.M.	Unknown	1 hr	Unknown

Action

Chemical effect: Inhibits cell-wall synthesis, promoting osmotic instability; usually bactericidal.
Therapeutic effect: Hinders or kills susceptible bacteria.

Available forms

Infusion: 1 g, 2 g in 50-ml and 100-ml vials (premixed)
Injection (with arginine): 1 g, 2 g, 6 g
Injection (with sodium carbonate): 500 mg, 1 g, 2 g

NURSING PROCESS

⏀ Assessment
• Assess patient's infection before therapy and regularly thereafter.
• Before giving first dose, obtain specimen for culture and sensitivity tests. Begin therapy pending test results.
• Before giving first dose, ask patient about previous reactions to cephalosporins or penicillin.
• Be alert for adverse reactions and drug interactions.
• If adverse GI reactions occur, monitor patient's hydration.
• Assess patient's and family's knowledge of drug therapy.

Nursing diagnoses
• Infection related to bacteria susceptible to drug
• Risk for deficient fluid volume related to drug-induced adverse GI reactions
• Deficient knowledge related to drug therapy

Planning and implementation
• Inject deep into large muscle mass, such as gluteus maximus or lateral aspect of thigh.
ALERT: Commercially available forms contain either sodium carbonate (Fortaz, Tazicef, Tazidime) or arginine (Ceptaz) to facilitate dissolution of drug.
ALERT: Don't confuse with other cephalosporins with similar-sounding names.

Patient teaching
• Tell patient to report adverse reactions.
• Instruct patient to immediately report to prescriber any change in urinary output. Dose may need to be reduced to compensate for decreased excretion.

Evaluation
• Patient is free from infection.
• Patient maintains adequate hydration.
• Patient and family state understanding of drug therapy.

ceftibuten
(sef-tih-BYOO-tin)
Cedax

Pharmacologic class: third-generation cephalosporin
Therapeutic class: antibiotic
Pregnancy risk category: B

Indications and dosages
▶ **Acute bacterial exacerbation of chronic bronchitis caused by *Haemophilus influenzae, Moraxella catarrhalis,* or penicillin-susceptible strains of *Streptococcus pneumoniae.*** *Adults and children age 12 and older:* 400 mg P.O. daily for 10 days.
▶ **Pharyngitis and tonsillitis caused by *Streptococcus pyogenes,* acute bacterial otitis media caused by *H. influenzae, M. catarrhalis,* or *S. pyogenes.*** *Adults and children age 12 and older:* 400 mg capsules P.O. daily for 10 days.
Children younger than age 12: 9 mg/kg capsules P.O. daily for 10 days. Maximum daily dose is 400 mg.
Children weighing more than 45 kg (99 lb): 400 mg oral suspension P.O. daily for 10 days.
Children older than age 6 months and weighing 45 kg or less: 9 mg/kg oral suspension P.O. daily for 10 days. Maximum daily dose is 400 mg.
Adjust-a-dose: For patients with renal impairment, if creatinine clearance is 30 to 49 ml/minute, give 4.5 mg/kg or 200 mg P.O. q 24 hours; if creatinine clearance is 5 to 29 ml/minute, give 2.25 mg/kg or 100 mg P.O. q 24 hours. For patients undergoing hemodialysis, give 400 mg P.O. as a single dose at the end of each dialysis session.

Contraindications and cautions
• Contraindicated in patients hypersensitive to cephalosporins.
• Use cautiously in patients with history of hypersensitivity to penicillin and in patients with GI disease or renal impairment.
Lifespan: In pregnant women, use cautiously. In breast-feeding women, use cautiously; it isn't known whether drug appears in breast milk. In elderly patients, use cautiously. Monitor their renal function, and adjust dosage p.r.n.

Adverse reactions
CNS: aphasia, dizziness, headache, psychosis.
GI: abdominal pain, diarrhea, dyspepsia, loose stools, nausea, ***pseudomembranous colitis,*** vomiting.
GU: renal dysfunction, ***toxic nephropathy.***
Hematologic: ***agranulocytosis, aplastic anemia, hemolytic anemia, hemorrhage, neutropenia, pancytopenia.***
Hepatic: hepatic cholestasis.
Skin: ***Stevens-Johnson syndrome.***
Other: allergic reaction, ***anaphylaxis,*** drug fever.

Interactions
Drug-food. *Any food:* May decrease bioavailability of drug. Give drug 2 hours before or 1 hour after a meal.

Effects on lab test results
• May increase ALT, AST, alkaline phosphatase, bilirubin, and BUN and creatinine levels. May decrease hemoglobin level and hematocrit.

• May increase eosinophil count. May decrease leukocyte count. May increase or decrease platelet count.

Pharmacokinetics

Absorption: Rapid.
Distribution: 65% bound to proteins.
Metabolism: By the kidneys.
Excretion: Mainly in urine. *Half-life:* 2 to 2½ hours.

Route	Onset	Peak	Duration
P.O.	Unknown	2–4 hr	Unknown

Action

Chemical effect: Exerts bacterial action by binding to essential target proteins of the bacterial cell wall, thus inhibiting cell-wall synthesis.
Therapeutic effect: Hinders or kills susceptible bacteria.

Available forms

Capsules: 400 mg
Oral suspension: 90 mg/5 ml, 180 mg/5 ml

NURSING PROCESS

Assessment
• Before giving first dose, obtain specimen for culture and sensitivity tests. Begin therapy pending test results.
• Monitor patient for superinfection.
• Obtain specimen for *Clostridium difficile* in patient who develops diarrhea after therapy.
• Assess patient's and family's knowledge of drug therapy.

Nursing diagnoses
• Infection related to bacteria susceptible to drug
• Deficient knowledge related to drug therapy

Planning and implementation
• To prepare oral suspension, tap bottle to loosen powder. Follow chart supplied by manufacturer for mixing instructions. Suspension is stable for 14 days if refrigerated.
• Shake suspension well before use.
• Stop giving the drug and notify prescriber if allergic reaction occurs.
ALERT: Don't confuse with other cephalosporins with similar-sounding names.

Patient teaching
• Instruct patient to take drug as prescribed, even if he feels better.
• Instruct patient using oral suspension to shake bottle before use and to take it at least 2 hours before or 1 hour after a meal.
• Instruct patient to store oral suspension in the refrigerator, with lid tightly closed, and to discard unused drug after 14 days.
• Warn breast-feeding woman that it's unclear whether drug appears in breast milk.
• Tell patient with diabetes that suspension has 1 g sucrose per teaspoon.

Evaluation
• Patient is free from infection.
• Patient and family state understanding of drug therapy.

ceftizoxime sodium
(sef-tih-ZOKS-eem SOH-dee-um)
Cefizox

Pharmacologic class: third-generation cephalosporin
Therapeutic class: antibiotic
Pregnancy risk category: B

Indications and dosages

▶ **Serious infections of lower respiratory and urinary tracts, gynecologic infections, bacteremia, septicemia, meningitis, intraabdominal infections, bone and joint infections, and skin infections. Among susceptible microorganisms are** *Streptococcus pneumoniae* **and** *Streptococcus pyogenes,* *Staphylococcus aureus* **(penicillinase- and non–penicillinase-producing) and** *Staphylococcus epidermidis, Escherichia coli, Klebsiella, Haemophilus influenzae, Enterobacter, Proteus,* **some** *Pseudomonas,* **and** *Peptostreptococcus. Adults:* 1 to 2 g I.V. or I.M. q 8 to 12 hours. In life-threatening infections, 3 to 4 g I.V. q 8 hours.
Children older than age 6 months: 50 mg/kg I.V. q 6 to 8 hours. For serious infections, up to 200 mg/kg daily in divided doses may be used. Maximum, 12 g daily.
Adjust-a-dose: For patients with renal impairment, if creatinine clearance is 50 to 79 ml/minute, give 500 mg q 8 hours for less severe

C

infections or 750 mg to 1.5 g q 8 hours for life-threatening infections; if clearance is 5 to 49 ml/minute, give 250 to 500 mg q 12 hours for less-severe infections or 500 mg to 1 g q 12 hours for life-threatening infections; if clearance is less than 5 ml/minute or patient undergoes hemodialysis, give 500 mg q 48 hours or 250 q 24 hours for less severe infections or 500 mg to 1 g q 48 hours or 500 mg q 24 hours for life-threatening infections.

▼ I.V. administration

• To reconstitute powder, add 5 ml sterile water to 500-mg vial, 10 ml to 1-g vial, or 20 ml to 2-g vial.
• Reconstitute piggyback vials with 50 to 100 ml of normal saline solution or D₅W. Shake vial well.
• Inject directly into vein over 3 to 5 minutes or slowly into I.V. tubing with free-flowing compatible solution.
• Give intermittent infusion over 15 to 30 minutes.
• After reconstitution or dilution, solutions are stable for 1 day at room temperature and 4 days if refrigerated.
⊗ **Incompatibilities**
Aminoglycosides.

Contraindications and cautions

• Contraindicated in patients hypersensitive to drug or other cephalosporins.
• Use cautiously in patients with history of sensitivity to penicillin and in patients with renal impairment.
⚘ **Lifespan:** In pregnant and breast-feeding women, use cautiously. In infants younger than age 6 months, safety and effectiveness haven't been established.

Adverse reactions

CNS: dizziness, fever, headache, malaise, paresthesia.
GI: abdominal cramps, anal pruritus, anorexia, diarrhea, dyspepsia, glossitis, nausea, *pseudomembranous colitis,* tenesmus, vomiting.
GU: genital pruritus and candidiasis.
Hematologic: eosinophilia, hemolytic anemia, *thrombocytopenia, transient neutropenia.*
Respiratory: dyspnea.
Skin: *maculopapular and erythematous rashes, urticaria.*

Other: hypersensitivity reactions (serum sickness, *anaphylaxis*); induration, sterile abscesses, tissue sloughing at injection site; phlebitis, thrombophlebitis with I.V. injection.

Interactions

Drug-drug. *Probenecid:* May inhibit excretion and increase level of ceftizoxime. Sometimes used for this effect.

Effects on lab test results

• May increase BUN, creatinine, ALT, AST, alkaline phosphatase, bilirubin, GGT, and LDH levels. May decrease albumin, protein, and hemoglobin levels and hematocrit.
• May increase eosinophil count. May decrease PT and RBC, WBC, platelet, granulocyte, and neutrophil counts.
• May cause false-positive urine glucose determinations with copper sulfate tests (Clinitest).

Pharmacokinetics

Absorption: Unknown with I.M. use.
Distribution: Wide; unlike many other cephalosporins, ceftizoxime has good CSF penetration and achieves adequate level in inflamed meninges. Drug is 28% to 31% protein-bound.
Metabolism: None.
Excretion: Mainly in urine. *Half-life:* About 1½ to 2 hours.

Route	Onset	Peak	Duration
I.V.	Immediate	Immediate	Unknown
I.M.	Unknown	½–1½ hr	Unknown

Action

Chemical effect: Inhibits cell-wall synthesis, promoting osmotic instability; usually bactericidal.
Therapeutic effect: Hinders or kills susceptible bacteria.

Available forms

Infusion: 1 g, 2 g in 100-mg vials or in 50 ml of D₅W
Injection: 500 mg, 1 g, 2 g

NURSING PROCESS

▨ **Assessment**
• Assess patient's infection before therapy and regularly thereafter.

• Before giving first dose, obtain specimen for culture and sensitivity tests. Begin therapy pending test results.
• Before giving first dose, ask patient about previous reactions to cephalosporins or penicillin.
• Be alert for adverse reactions and drug interactions.
• If adverse GI reactions occur, monitor patient's hydration.
• Assess patient's and family's knowledge of drug therapy.

⊕ Nursing diagnoses
• Infection related to bacteria susceptible to drug
• Risk for deficient fluid volume related to drug-induced adverse GI reactions
• Deficient knowledge related to drug therapy

⧉ Planning and implementation
• Inject I.M. dose deep into large muscle mass, such as gluteus maximus or lateral aspect of thigh. Divide doses of 2 g or more and give divided doses at two different sites.
⊛ **ALERT:** Don't confuse with other cephalosporins with similar-sounding names.
Patient teaching
• Tell patient to report adverse reactions and signs and symptoms of superinfection promptly.
• Instruct patient to report discomfort at the I.V. site.
• Tell patient to notify prescriber if loose stools or diarrhea occur.

✓ Evaluation
• Patient is free from infection.
• Patient maintains adequate hydration.
• Patient and family state understanding of drug therapy.

ceftriaxone sodium
(sef-trigh-AKS-ohn SOH-dee-um)
Rocephin

Pharmacologic class: third-generation cephalosporin
Therapeutic class: antibiotic
Pregnancy risk category: B

Indications and dosages
▶ **Uncomplicated gonococcal vulvovaginitis.** *Adults and children older than age 12 or weighing more than 45 kg (99 lb):* 125 to 250 mg I.M. as single dose, followed by either 100 mg of doxycycline P.O. q 12 hours for 7 days, or a single oral dose of azithromycin 1 g.
Children younger than age 12 or weighing less than 45 kg: 125 mg I.M. as a single dose.
▶ **Serious infections of lower respiratory and urinary tracts; gynecologic, bone, joint, intra-abdominal, and skin infections; bacteremia; and septicemia caused by susceptible microorganisms such as** *Streptococcus pneumoniae, S. pyogenes, Staphylococcus aureus, S. epidermidis, Escherichia coli, Klebsiella, Haemophilus influenzae, Neisseria meningitides, N. gonorrhoeae, Enterobacter, Proteus, Pseudomonas, Peptostreptococcus,* **and** *Serratia marcescens. Adults and children older than age 12:* 1 to 2 g I.V. or I.M. daily or in equally divided doses; maximum 4 g daily for 4 to 14 days depending on severity of infection.
Children age 12 and younger: 50 to 75 mg/kg, maximum 2 g daily, given in divided doses q 12 hours.
▶ **Meningitis.** *Adults and children:* Initially, 100 mg/kg I.M. or I.V. (maximum 4 g); thereafter, 100 mg/kg I.M. or I.V. given once daily or in divided doses q 12 hours. Maximum, 4 g, for 7 to 14 days.
▶ **Preoperative prophylaxis.** *Adults:* 1 g I.V. as single dose 30 minutes to 2 hours before surgery.
▶ **Acute bacterial otitis media.** *Children:* 50 mg/kg I.M. as a single dose; maximum I.M. dose is 1 g.
▶ **Persisting or relapsing otitis media in children‡.** *Children and infants age 3 months and older:* 50 mg/kg I.M daily for 3 days.
▶ **Sexually transmitted epididymitis, pelvic inflammatory disease‡.** *Adults:* 250 mg I.M. as a single dose; follow up with other antibiotics.
▶ **Anti-infectives for sexual assault victims‡.** *Adults:* 125 mg I.M. as a single dose given with other antibiotics.
▶ **Lyme disease‡.** *Adults:* 1 to 2 g I.M. or I.V. q 12 to 24 hours.

▼ I.V. administration
• Reconstitute with sterile water for injection, normal saline solution for injection, D_5W or $D_{10}W$ injection, or combination of saline solu-

tion and dextrose injection and other compatible solutions.
- Reconstitute by adding 2.4 ml of diluent to 250-mg vial, 4.8 ml to 500-mg vial, 9.6 ml to 1-g vial, and 19.2 ml to 2-g vial. All reconstituted solutions yield concentration that averages 100 mg/ml.
- After reconstitution, dilute further to desired concentration for intermittent infusion.
- Dilutions are stable for 24 hours at room temperature.

⊗ **Incompatibilities**
Aminoglycosides, aminophylline, azithromycin, clindamycin phosphate, filgrastim, fluconazole, labetalol, lidocaine hydrochloride, pentamidine isethionate, theophylline, vancomycin, vinorelbine tartrate.

Contraindications and cautions

- Contraindicated in patients hypersensitive to drug or other cephalosporins.
- Use cautiously in patients with history of sensitivity to penicillin.
- **Lifespan:** In pregnant and breast-feeding women, use cautiously.

Adverse reactions

CNS: dizziness, fever, headache.
GI: diarrhea, dysgeusia, nausea, *pseudomembranous colitis,* vomiting.
GU: genital pruritus and candidiasis.
Hematologic: eosinophilia, *leukopenia,* thrombocytosis.
Skin: phlebitis, *rash.*
Other: hypersensitivity reactions (serum sickness, *anaphylaxis*); pain, induration, and tenderness at injection site.

Interactions

Drug-drug. *Aminoglycosides:* May have additive effect. Monitor drug level and adjust dosage as needed.
Probenecid: May shorten half-life of ceftriaxone in large doses. Avoid using together.
Quinolones: May have synergistic effect against *S. pneumoniae.* Using together against this organism is recommended.
Drug-lifestyle. *Alcohol use:* May cause disulfiram-like reaction. Discourage use together.

Effects on lab test results

- May increase BUN, ALT, AST, alkaline phosphatase, bilirubin, and LDH levels.
- May increase eosinophil and platelet counts. May decrease WBC count.
- May cause false-positive urine glucose determinations with copper sulfate tests (Clinitest).

Pharmacokinetics

Absorption: Unknown.
Distribution: Wide; unlike many other cephalosporins, ceftriaxone has good CSF penetration. Drug is 58% to 96% protein-bound.
Metabolism: Partial.
Excretion: Mainly in urine, minimally in bile.
Half-life: About 5½ to 11 hours.

Route	Onset	Peak	Duration
I.V.	Immediate	Immediate	Unknown
I.M.	Unknown	1½–4 hr	Unknown

Action

Chemical effect: Inhibits cell-wall synthesis, promoting osmotic instability; usually bactericidal.
Therapeutic effect: Hinders or kills susceptible bacteria.

Available forms

Infusion: 1 g, 2 g
Injection: 250 mg, 500 mg, 1 g, 2 g

NURSING PROCESS

Assessment

- Assess patient's infection before therapy and regularly thereafter.
- Before giving first dose, obtain specimen for culture and sensitivity tests. Begin therapy pending test results.
- Before giving first dose, ask patient about previous reactions to cephalosporins or penicillin.
- Be alert for adverse reactions and drug interactions.
- If adverse GI reactions occur, monitor patient's hydration.
- Assess patient's and family's knowledge of drug therapy.

Nursing diagnoses

- Infection related to bacteria susceptible to drug

• Risk for deficient fluid volume related to drug-induced adverse GI reactions
• Deficient knowledge related to drug therapy

⟫ Planning and implementation
• Inject deep into large muscle mass, such as gluteus maximus or lateral aspect of thigh. May use lidocaine 1% without epinephrine to dilute for I.M. use.
⑤ **ALERT:** Don't confuse with other cephalosporins with similar-sounding names.

Patient teaching
• Tell patient to promptly report adverse reactions and signs and symptoms of superinfection.
• Instruct patient to report pain at the I.V. site.
• Tell patient to notify prescriber if loose stools or diarrhea occur.

☑ Evaluation
• Patient is free from infection.
• Patient maintains adequate hydration.
• Patient and family state understanding of drug therapy.

cefuroxime axetil
(sef-yoor-OKS-eem AKS-eh-til)
Ceftin

cefuroxime sodium
Kefurox, Zinacef

Pharmacologic class: second-generation cephalosporin
Therapeutic class: antibiotic
Pregnancy risk category: B

Indications and dosages
▶ **Pharyngitis, tonsillitis, infections of urinary and lower respiratory tracts, and skin and skin-structure infections.** Susceptible organisms are *Streptococcus pneumoniae, S. pyogenes, Haemophilus influenzae, Klebsiella, Staphylococcus aureus, Escherichia coli, Moraxella catarrhalis* (including beta-lactamase-producing strains), *Enterobacter,* and *Neisseria gonorrhoeae. Adults and children age 13 and older:* 250 mg P.O. q 12 hours. For severe infections, increase dose to 500 mg q 12 hours.
▶ **Serious infections of lower respiratory and urinary tracts, skin and skin-structure infec-**

tions, bone and joint infections, septicemia, meningitis, gonorrhea, and perioperative prophylaxis. *Adults and children age 13 and older:* 750 mg to 1.5 g I.V. or I.M. q 8 hours for 5 to 10 days. For life-threatening infections and infections caused by less-susceptible organisms, 1.5 g I.V. or I.M. q 6 hours; for bacterial meningitis, up to 3 g I.V. q 8 hours.
Children age 3 months to 12 years: 50 to 100 mg/kg daily I.V. or I.M. in equally divided doses q 6 to 8 hours. Use higher doses of 100 mg/kg daily (not to exceed adult maximum dosage) for more severe or serious infections. For bacterial meningitis, 200 to 240 mg/kg I.V. in divided doses q 6 to 8 hours.
▶ **Uncomplicated UTIs.** *Adults and children age 13 and older:* 125 to 250 mg P.O. q 12 hours for 7 to 10 days.
▶ **Otitis media.** *Children ages 3 months to 12 years:* 30 mg/kg oral suspension P.O. daily divided in two doses (maximum dose, 1 g) for children who can't swallow tablets, or 250-mg tablet P.O. b.i.d. for 10 days for children who can swallow tablets whole.
▶ **Pharyngitis and tonsillitis.** *Children ages 3 months to 12 years:* 125 mg P.O. q 12 hours for 10 days, in children who can swallow tablets whole. Or 20 mg/kg daily of oral suspension (maximum 500 mg) in two divided doses for 10 days, in children who can't swallow tablets.
▶ **Perioperative prophylaxis.** *Adults:* 1.5 g I.V. 30 to 60 minutes before surgery; in lengthy operations, 750 mg I.V. or I.M. q 8 hours. For open-heart surgery, 1.5 g I.V. at induction of anesthesia and q 12 hours; total dosage, 6 g.
▶ **Acute bacterial maxillary sinusitis caused by *S. pneumoniae* or *H. influenzae* (only strains that don't produce beta-lactamase).** *Adults and children age 13 and older:* 250 mg (tablet) P.O. b.i.d. for 10 days.
Infants and children ages 3 months to 12 years: 30 mg/kg (suspension) by mouth daily in two divided doses for 10 days. Maximum daily suspension dosage is 1,000 mg. For children who can swallow tablets whole, give 250 mg (tablet) by mouth b.i.d. for 10 days.
▶ **Secondary bacterial infection of acute bronchitis.** *Adults and children age 13 and older:* 250 mg to 500 mg P.O. b.i.d. for 5 to 10 days.
▶ **Early Lyme disease as manifested by erythema migrans.** *Adults and children age 13 and older:* 500 mg P.O. b.i.d. for 20 days.

Reactions may be *common,* uncommon, *life-threatening*, or COMMON AND LIFE-THREATENING.

▶ **Gonorrhea.** *Adults and children age 13 and older:* Give a one-time dose of 1.5 g I.M. (I.M. dose to be divided and given at two different sites) with 1 g oral probenecid. Or 1 g P.O. as a single dose.

§ **Adjust-a-dose:** For patients with renal impairment, if creatinine clearance is 10 to 20 ml/minute give 750 mg I.V. or I.M. q 12 hours; if clearance is less than 10 ml/minute, give 750 mg I.V. or I.M q 24 hours.

▼ I.V. administration

• For each 750-mg vial of Zinacef, reconstitute with 8 ml sterile water for injection; for each 1.5-g vial, reconstitute with 16 ml. In each case, withdraw entire contents of vial for dose.

• For direct injection, inject into large vein or into tubing of free-flowing I.V. solution over 3 to 5 minutes.

• For intermittent infusion, add reconstituted drug to 100 ml D_5W, normal saline solution for injection, or other compatible I.V. solution. Infuse over 15 to 60 minutes.

⊗ **Incompatibilities**
Aminoglycosides, ciprofloxacin, clarithromycin, filgrastim, fluconazole, midazolam, ranitidine, sodium bicarbonate injection, vinorelbine tartrate.

Contraindications and cautions

• Contraindicated in patients hypersensitive to drug or other cephalosporins.

• Use cautiously in patients with history of sensitivity to penicillin and in patients with renal impairment.

⚘ **Lifespan:** In pregnant and breast-feeding women, use cautiously. In infants younger than age 3 months, safety and effectiveness haven't been established.

Adverse reactions

CNS: dizziness, headache, malaise, paresthesia.
GI: abdominal cramps, anal pruritus, anorexia, diarrhea, dyspepsia, glossitis, nausea, *pseudomembranous colitis,* tenesmus, vomiting.
GU: genital pruritus and candidiasis.
Hematologic: eosinophilia, hemolytic anemia, *thrombocytopenia, transient neutropenia.*
Respiratory: dyspnea.
Skin: *maculopapular and erythematous rashes, urticaria.*

Other: hypersensitivity reactions (serum sickness, *anaphylaxis*); pain, induration, sterile abscesses, warmth, tissue sloughing at injection site; phlebitis, thrombophlebitis with I.V. injection.

Interactions

Drug-drug. *Diuretics:* May increase risk of adverse renal reactions. Monitor renal function closely.
Probenecid: May inhibit excretion and increase level of cefuroxime. Sometimes used for this effect.
Drug-food. *Any food:* May increase drug absorption and bioavailability of suspension. Give suspension with food. Tablets may be given without regard to food.

Effects on lab test results

• May increase ALT, AST, alkaline phosphatase, bilirubin, and LDH levels. May decrease hemoglobin level and hematocrit.
• May increase eosinophil count, PT, and INR. May decrease neutrophil and platelet counts.
• May cause false-positive urine glucose determinations with copper sulfate tests (Clinitest).

Pharmacokinetics

Absorption: 37% to 52% of oral cefuroxime axetil reaches systemic circulation. Food appears to enhance absorption. Cefuroxime sodium isn't well absorbed from GI tract; absorption after I.M. use is unknown.
Distribution: Wide; CSF penetration is greater than that of most first- and second-generation cephalosporins and achieves adequate therapeutic level in inflamed meninges. 33% to 50% protein-bound.
Metabolism: None.
Excretion: Mainly in urine. *Half-life:* 1 to 2 hours.

Route	Onset	Peak	Duration
P.O.	Unknown	2–3 hr	Unknown
I.V.	Unknown	Immediate	Unknown
I.M.	Unknown	15–60 min	Unknown

Action

Chemical effect: Inhibits cell-wall synthesis, promoting osmotic instability; usually bactericidal.

Therapeutic effect: Hinders or kills susceptible bacteria, including many gram-positive organisms and enteric gram-negative bacilli.

Available forms

cefuroxime axetil
Suspension: 125 mg/5 ml, 250 mg/5 ml
Tablets: 125 mg, 250 mg, 500 mg
cefuroxime sodium
Infusion: 750 mg, 1.5 g premixed, frozen solution
Injection: 750 mg, 1.5 g

NURSING PROCESS

⚡ Assessment
• Assess patient's infection before therapy and regularly thereafter.
• Before giving first dose, obtain specimen for culture and sensitivity tests. Begin therapy pending test results.
• Before giving first dose, ask patient about previous reactions to cephalosporins or penicillin.
• Be alert for adverse reactions and drug interactions.
• If adverse GI reactions occur, monitor patient's hydration.
• Assess patient's and family's knowledge of drug therapy.

⊕ Nursing diagnoses
• Infection related to bacteria susceptible to drug
• Risk for deficient fluid volume related to drug-induced adverse GI reactions
• Deficient knowledge related to drug therapy

⬦ Planning and implementation
• Food enhances absorption of cefuroxime axetil.
• Cefuroxime axetil is available only in tablet form, which may be crushed for patients who can't swallow tablets. Tablets may be dissolved in small amounts of apple, orange, or grape juice or chocolate milk. However, drug has bitter taste that's difficult to mask, even with food.
⚠ **ALERT:** Cefuroxime tablets and oral suspensions aren't bioequivalent and can't be substituted on a milligram-for-milligram basis.
• Inject deep into large muscle mass, such as gluteus maximus or lateral aspect of thigh. Before I.M. injection, aspirate to avoid injection into a blood vessel.

• Cefuroxime isn't considered the drug of choice for meningitis or gonorrhea infections.
⚠ **ALERT:** Don't confuse with other cephalosporins with similar-sounding names.
Patient teaching
• Instruct patient to take drug exactly as prescribed, even after he feels better.
• Advise patient to take oral drug with food to enhance absorption. Explain that tablets may be crushed, but drug has bitter taste that's difficult to mask, even with food.
• Tell patient to report adverse reactions.

✓ Evaluation
• Patient is free from infection.
• Patient maintains adequate hydration.
• Patient and family state understanding of drug therapy.

celecoxib
(sel-eh-COKS-ib)
Celebrex✒

Pharmacologic class: cyclooxygenase-2 (COX-2) inhibitor
Therapeutic class: anti-inflammatory
Pregnancy risk category: C (D in third trimester)

Indications and dosages

▶ **Relief of signs and symptoms of osteoarthritis.** *Adults:* 200 mg P.O. daily as a single dose or divided equally b.i.d.
▶ **Relief of signs and symptoms of rheumatoid arthritis.** *Adults:* 100 to 200 mg P.O. b.i.d.
▶ **Relief of signs and symptoms of ankylosing spondylitis.** *Adults:* 200 mg P.O. once daily or divided b.i.d. If no response after 6 weeks, may increase to 400 mg daily. If no response after 6 more weeks, different treatment should be considered.
▶ **Adjunct to familial adenomatous polyposis to reduce the number of adenomatous colorectal polyps.** *Adults:* 400 mg P.O. b.i.d. with food for up to 6 months.
▶ **Acute pain and primary dysmenorrhea.** *Adults:* Initially, give 400 mg P.O., followed by an additional 200-mg dose on the first day, if needed. On subsequent days, 200 mg P.O. b.i.d. p.r.n.

Reactions may be *common*, uncommon, *life-threatening*, or COMMON AND LIFE-THREATENING.

Adjust-a-dose: For patients with hepatic impairment, reduce dose by 50%. For elderly patients who weigh less than 50 kg (110 lb), use the lowest recommended dose.

Contraindications and cautions

• Contraindicated in patients hypersensitive to drug, sulfonamides, or aspirin or other NSAIDs and in patients with severe hepatic or renal impairment. Also contraindicated for treating perioperative pain after coronary artery bypass graft surgery.
• Use cautiously in patients with known or suspected history of poor CYP 2C9 metabolism and in patients with history of ulcers, GI bleeding, dehydration, anemia, symptomatic liver disease, hypertension, edema, heart failure, or asthma. Also use cautiously in patients who smoke or drink alcohol frequently, take oral corticosteroids or anticoagulants, or are at a high risk for CV complications, such as those who have recently had heart surgery.
Lifespan: In women in the third trimester of pregnancy, avoid use. In children younger than age 18, safety and effectiveness haven't been established. In elderly and debilitated patients, use cautiously because of the increased risk of GI bleeding and acute renal impairment.

Adverse reactions

CNS: dizziness, *headache,* insomnia, ***stroke.***
CV: hypertension, *MI,* peripheral edema.
EENT: pharyngitis, rhinitis, sinusitis.
GI: *abdominal pain,* diarrhea, *dyspepsia,* flatulence, *nausea.*
Metabolic: hyperchloremia, hypophosphatemia.
Musculoskeletal: back pain.
Respiratory: upper respiratory tract infection.
Skin: *erythema multiforme, exfoliative dermatitis,* rash, ***Stevens-Johnson syndrome, toxic epidermal necrolysis.***
Other: accidental injury.

Interactions

Drug-drug. *ACE inhibitors:* May decrease antihypertensive effects. Monitor patient's blood pressure.
Aluminum- and magnesium-containing antacids: May decrease celecoxib level. Separate doses.
Aspirin: May increase risk of ulcers; low aspirin dosages can be used safely to prevent CV events. Monitor patient for evidence of GI bleeding.
Diuretics: May decrease sodium excretion of diuretics, leading to sodium retention. Monitor patient for swelling and increased blood pressure.
Fluconazole: May increase celecoxib level. Reduce dosage of celecoxib to minimal effective level.
Lithium: May increase lithium level. Monitor lithium level.
Warfarin: May increase PT level and bleeding complications. Monitor PT and INR, and check for evidence of bleeding.
Drug-herb. *Dong quai, feverfew, garlic, ginger, ginkgo, horse chestnut, red clover:* May increase the risk of bleeding. Discourage use together.
Drug-lifestyle. *Chronic alcohol use, smoking:* May increase risk of GI irritation or bleeding. Check for evidence of bleeding, and discourage use together.

Effects on lab test results

• May increase BUN, ALT, AST, and chloride levels. May decrease phosphate level.

Pharmacokinetics

Absorption: Level peaks in about 3 hours. If patient receives multiple doses, expect steady-state level within 5 days. Elderly patients have higher level than younger adults.
Distribution: Extensive. Highly protein-bound, mainly to albumin.
Metabolism: By CYP 2C9. No active metabolites have been identified.
Excretion: Mainly through hepatic metabolism, with less than 3% as unchanged drug in urine and feces. *Half-life:* 11 hours.

Route	Onset	Peak	Duration
P.O.	Unknown	3 hr	Unknown

Action

Chemical effect: May selectively inhibit COX-2, decreasing prostaglandin synthesis.
Therapeutic effect: Relieves pain and inflammation in joints and smooth muscle tissue.

Available forms

Capsules: 100 mg, 200 mg, 400 mg

⅍ Assessment

• Assess patient for appropriateness of therapy. Drug must be used cautiously in patients with history of ulcers or GI bleeding, advanced renal disease, dehydration, anemia, symptomatic liver disease, hypertension, edema, heart failure, or asthma.

⊛ **ALERT:** Obtain accurate list of patient's allergies. Patients may be allergic to celecoxib if they're allergic and have had anaphylactic reactions to sulfonamides, aspirin, or other NSAIDs.

• Assess patients for risk factors for GI bleeding, including corticosteroid or anticoagulant therapy, long-term NSAID therapy, smoking, alcoholism, older age, and poor overall health. Patients with a history of ulcers or GI bleeding are at higher risk for GI bleeding while taking NSAIDs such as celecoxib.

• Monitor patient for evidence of overt and occult bleeding.

⊛ **ALERT:** Assess patient's CV status, CV risk factors, and history, particularly for recent heart surgery, MI, or stroke, before starting therapy. NSAIDs may increase the risk of serious thrombotic events; the risk increases with duration of use and may be higher in patients with CV disease or risk factors for it.

• Monitor patient for signs and symptoms of liver toxicity. Celecoxib may be hepatotoxic.

• Assess patient's and family's knowledge of drug therapy.

⊞ Nursing diagnoses

• Acute pain related to underlying condition
• Risk for injury related to drug-induced adverse reactions
• Deficient knowledge related to drug therapy

⊡ Planning and implementation

⊛ **ALERT:** Use cautiously in patients at a high risk for CV complications and in those taking the drug long term because such use may increase risk of MI and stroke.

• In patients weighing less than 50 kg (110 lb), start therapy at lowest recommended dose.

• Although drug can be given with or without food, food may decrease GI upset.

• Before therapy, rehydrate patient.

• Although celecoxib may be used with low-dose aspirin, the combination may increase the risk of GI bleeding.

• NSAIDs such as celecoxib can cause fluid retention. Closely monitor patient who has hypertension, edema, or heart failure while taking this drug.

⊛ **ALERT:** Don't confuse Celebrex with Cerebyx or Celexa.

Patient teaching

• Instruct patient to immediately report to prescriber signs of GI bleeding (such as bloody vomitus, blood in urine or stool, and black, tarry stools).

⊛ **ALERT:** Advise patient to immediately report to prescriber rash, unexplained weight gain, or edema.

• Tell woman to notify prescriber if she becomes pregnant or is planning to become pregnant while taking this drug.

• Instruct patient to take drug with food if stomach upset occurs.

• Advise patient that all NSAIDs, including celecoxib, may adversely affect the liver. Signs and symptoms of liver toxicity include nausea, fatigue, lethargy, itching, jaundice, right upper quadrant tenderness, and flulike syndrome. Advise patient to stop therapy and seek immediate medical advice if he has any of these signs or symptoms.

• Inform patient that it may take several days before he feels consistent pain relief.

⍈ Evaluation

• Patient is free from pain.
• Patient doesn't experience injury as a result of drug-induced adverse reactions.
• Patient and family state understanding of drug therapy.

cephalexin
Apo-Cephalex♦, Biocef, Keflex, Novo-Lexin♦, Nu-Cephalex◇

cephalexin hydrochloride monohydrate
(sef-uh-LEK-sin high-droh-KLOR-ighd)
Keftab

Pharmacologic class: first-generation cephalosporin
Therapeutic class: antibiotic
Pregnancy risk category: B

Reactions may be *common,* uncommon, *life-threatening*, or COMMON AND LIFE-THREATENING.

Indications and dosages

▶ **Respiratory tract, GI tract, skin, soft-tissue, bone, and joint infections and otitis media caused by** *Escherichia coli* **and other coliform bacteria, group A beta-hemolytic streptococci,** *Haemophilus influenzae, Klebsiella, Moraxella catarrhalis, Proteus mirabilis, Streptococcus pneumoniae,* **and staphylococci.** *Adults:* 250 mg to 1 g P.O. q 6 hours or 500 mg q 12 hours; maximum, 4 g daily.

Children: 6 to 12 mg/kg P.O. q 6 hours (monohydrate only); maximum, 25 mg/kg q 6 hours or 4 g daily.

◩ **Adjust-a-dose:** For patients with renal impairment, if creatinine clearance is 11 to 40 ml/minute, give 500 mg q 8 to 12 hours; if clearance is 5 to 10 ml/minute, give 250 mg q 12 hours; if clearance is less than 5 ml/minute, give 250 mg q 12 to 24 hours.

Contraindications and cautions

• Contraindicated in patients hypersensitive to cephalosporins.
• Use cautiously in patients hypersensitive to penicillin and in patients with renal impairment.
⚘ **Lifespan:** In pregnant and breast-feeding women, use cautiously.

Adverse reactions

CNS: dizziness, headache, malaise, paresthesia.
GI: abdominal cramps, anal pruritus, *anorexia, diarrhea,* dyspepsia, glossitis, *nausea,* oral candidiasis, *pseudomembranous colitis,* tenesmus, vomiting.
GU: candidiasis, genital pruritus, vaginitis.
Hematologic: anemia, eosinophilia, *thrombocytopenia, transient neutropenia.*
Respiratory: dyspnea.
Skin: maculopapular and erythematous rashes, urticaria.
Other: hypersensitivity reactions (serum sickness, *anaphylaxis*).

Interactions

Drug-drug. *Probenecid:* May increase cephalosporin level. Sometimes used for this effect.

Effects on lab test results

• May increase ALT, AST, alkaline phosphatase, bilirubin, and LDH levels. May decrease hemoglobin level and hematocrit.

• May increase eosinophil count. May decrease neutrophil and platelet counts.
• May cause false-positive urine glucose determinations with copper sulfate tests (Clinitest).

Pharmacokinetics

Absorption: Rapid and complete. Food delays but doesn't prevent complete absorption.
Distribution: Wide; CSF penetration is poor. Drug is 6% to 15% protein-bound.
Metabolism: None.
Excretion: Mainly unchanged in urine. *Half-life:* 30 minutes to 1 hour.

Route	Onset	Peak	Duration
P.O.	Unknown	≤ 1 hr	Unknown

Action

Chemical effect: Inhibits cell-wall synthesis, promoting osmotic instability; usually bactericidal.
Therapeutic effect: Hinders or kills susceptible bacteria.

Available forms

cephalexin
Capsules: 250 mg, 500 mg
Oral suspension: 125 mg/5 ml, 250 mg/5 ml
Tablets: 250 mg, 500 mg, 1 g
cephalexin hydrochloride monohydrate
Tablets: 500 mg

NURSING PROCESS

⚕ **Assessment**
• Assess patient's infection before therapy and regularly thereafter.
• Before giving first dose, obtain specimen for culture and sensitivity tests. Begin therapy pending test results.
• Before giving first dose, ask patient about previous reactions to cephalosporins or penicillin.
• Be alert for adverse reactions and drug interactions.
• If adverse GI reactions occur, monitor patient's hydration.
• Assess patient's and family's knowledge of drug therapy.

⊕ **Nursing diagnoses**
• Infection related to bacteria susceptible to drug

• Risk for deficient fluid volume related to drug-induced adverse GI reactions
• Deficient knowledge related to drug therapy

⚡ Planning and implementation
• To prepare oral suspension, first add required amount of water to powder in two portions. Shake well after each addition. After mixing, store in refrigerator (stable for 14 days without significant loss of potency). Keep tightly closed, and shake well before using.
• To minimize adverse GI reactions, give drug with food or milk.
• Treat group A beta-hemolytic streptococcal infections for at least 10 days.
• If giving more than 4 g daily, give initial treatment with a parenteral cephalosporin; switch to oral form when patient is stable.
⊕ ALERT: Don't confuse with other cephalosporins with similar-sounding names.
Patient teaching
• Inform patient that drug may be taken with meals.
• Instruct patient to take drug exactly as prescribed, even after he feels better.
• Tell patient to call prescriber if rash develops.
• Teach patient how to store drug.

☑ Evaluation
• Patient is free from infection.
• Patient maintains adequate hydration.
• Patient and family state understanding of drug therapy.

cetuximab
(seh-TUX-eh-mab)
Erbitux

Pharmacologic class: recombinant monoclonal antibody
Therapeutic class: epidermal growth factor receptor (EGFR) antagonist
Pregnancy risk category: C

Indications and dosages
▶ **Epidermal growth factor-expressing metastatic colorectal cancer as monotherapy in patients intolerant of irinotecan-based chemotherapy, or, with irinotecan, in patients refractory to irinotecan therapy alone.**
Adults: Initial loading dose, 400 mg/m² I.V.

over 2 hours (maximum, 5 ml/minute), alone or with irinotecan. Maintenance dosage, 250 mg/m² I.V. weekly over 1 hour (maximum, 5 ml/minute). Premedicate with an H_1 antagonist (such as 50 mg of diphenhydramine I.V.).
⧉ Adjust-a-dose: If patient develops a grade 1 or 2 infusion reaction, permanently reduce infusion rate by 50%. If patient develops a grade 3 or 4 reaction, stop drug immediately and permanently.

▼ I.V. administration
• Solution should be clear and colorless and may contain a small amount of particulates.
• Don't shake or dilute.
• Give by infusion pump or syringe pump. Piggyback into the patient's infusion line.
• Don't give drug by I.V. push or bolus.
• Give drug through a low–protein-binding 0.22-micrometer in-line filter.
• Flush line with normal saline solution at the end of the infusion.
• Monitor patient for 1 hour after the infusion.
• If patient develops a severe acneiform rash, follow these guidelines: The first time, delay infusion 1 to 2 weeks. If the patient improves, continue at 250 mg/m². If the patient doesn't improve, stop the drug. The second time, delay infusion 1 to 2 weeks. If the patient improves, reduce dose to 200 mg/m². If the patient doesn't improve, stop the drug. The third time, delay infusion 1 to 2 weeks. If the patient improves, reduce dose to 150 mg/m². If the patient doesn't improve, stop the drug. The fourth time, stop the drug permanently.
• Store vials at 36° to 46° F (2° to 8° C). Don't freeze. Solution in infusion container is stable up to 12 hours in refrigerator and up to 8 hours at room temperature (68° to 77° F [20° to 25° C]).
⊗ **Incompatibilities**
• Don't dilute cetuximab with other solutions.

Contraindications and cautions
• Use cautiously in patients hypersensitive to drug, its components, or murine proteins.
⚘ Lifespan: It isn't known whether drug can harm fetus, so give drug to a pregnant woman only if potential benefits justify risks to fetus. Before therapy starts, caution mother about risks to fetus. Urge women to stop breast-feeding while receiving drug and for 60 days after the last dose. In children, safety and effectiveness haven't been established.

Adverse reactions

CNS: asthenia, fever, depression, headache, insomnia.
CV: edema.
EENT: conjunctivitis.
GI: abdominal pain, anorexia, constipation, diarrhea, dyspepsia, nausea, stomatitis, vomiting.
GU: *acute renal failure.*
Hematologic: *anemia,* LEUKOPENIA.
Metabolic: dehydration, weight loss.
Musculoskeletal: *back pain.*
Respiratory: *bronchospasm,* cough, dyspnea, hoarseness, *pulmonary embolus,* stridor.
Skin: *acneiform rash,* alopecia, maculopapular rash, nail disorder, pruritus.
Other: infection, infusion reaction, pain, *sepsis.*

Interactions

Drug-lifestyle. *Sun exposure:* May worsen skin reactions. Urge patient to take precautions.

Effects on lab test results

None reported.

Pharmacokinetics

Absorption: Given I.V.
Distribution: Binds to EGFR, which is expressed in many normal epithelial tissues, such as skin and hair follicles, and in many cancers.
Metabolism: Unknown.
Excretion: Unknown. *Half-life:* 5 days.

Route	Onset	Peak	Duration
I.V.	Unknown	Unknown	Unknown

Action

Chemical effect: Binds to the EGFR on normal and tumor cells, keeping epidermal growth factor from binding, which inhibits cell growth, causes cell death, and decreases growth factor production.
Therapeutic effect: Inhibits tumor cells that overexpress EGFR in colorectal cancer patients.

Available forms

Injection: 2 mg/ml in 50-ml vial

NURSING PROCESS

⏳ Assessment
⚠ **ALERT:** Assess patient for signs and symptoms of severe infusion reactions, including acute airway obstruction, urticaria, and hypotension,

usually with the first infusion and despite premedication. If a severe infusion reaction occurs, immediately stop giving the drug and treat symptoms. Treat mild to moderate infusion reactions by cutting infusion rate in half and continuing antihistamines.
• Monitor patient for infusion reactions for 1 hour after the infusion.
• Assess patient for acute onset or worsening of pulmonary symptoms. If interstitial lung disease is confirmed, stop the drug.
• Monitor patient for skin toxicity, which starts most often during the first 2 weeks of therapy. Give topical and oral antibiotics.
• Assess hematologic and renal function studies before therapy and periodically thereafter.
• Assess patient's and family's knowledge of drug therapy.

⊞ Nursing diagnoses
• Risk for injury related to drug infusion reaction
• Impaired skin integrity related to dermatologic toxicity
• Deficient knowledge related to cetuximab therapy

▶ Planning and implementation
• To reduce risk of pulmonary drug reactions, premedicate with 50 mg diphenhydramine I.V.
• Keep epinephrine, corticosteroids, I.V. antihistamines, bronchodilators, and oxygen available to treat severe infusion reactions.
Patient teaching
• Tell patient to promptly report adverse reactions.
• Inform patient that skin reactions may occur, typically during the first 2 weeks.
• Advise patient to avoid prolonged or unprotected sun exposure, which can worsen adverse skin reactions.

☑ Evaluation
• Patient doesn't experience a drug infusion reaction.
• Patient doesn't develop dermatologic toxicity.
• Patient and family state understanding of drug therapy.

chloral hydrate
(KLOR-ul HIGH-drayt)
Aquachloral Supprettes, Somnote

Pharmacologic class: general CNS depressant
Therapeutic class: sedative-hypnotic
Pregnancy risk category: C
Controlled substance schedule: IV

Indications and dosages

▶ **Sedation.** *Adults:* 250 mg P.O. or P.R. t.i.d. after meals.
Children: 8.3 mg/kg P.O. or P.R. t.i.d.; maximum 500 mg per dose daily; doses may be divided.
▶ **Insomnia.** *Adults:* 500 mg to 1 g P.O. or P.R. 15 to 30 minutes before bedtime.
Children: 50 mg/kg P.O. or P.R. 15 to 30 minutes before bedtime; maximum single dose, 1 g.
▶ **Preoperative use.** *Adults:* 500 mg to 1 g P.O. or P.R. 30 minutes before surgery.
▶ **Premedication for EEG.** *Children:* 20 to 25 mg/kg P.O. or P.R.
▶ **Alcohol withdrawal.** *Adults:* 500 mg to 1 g P.O. or P.R.; repeat at 6-hour intervals, p.r.n. Maximum daily dosage is 2 g.

Contraindications and cautions

• Contraindicated in patients hypersensitive to drug and in those with hepatic or renal impairment. Oral administration contraindicated in patients with gastric disorders.
• Use cautiously in patients with severe cardiac disease and in patients with mental depression, suicidal tendencies, or history of drug abuse.
⚜ **Lifespan:** In breast-feeding women, avoid use because small amounts of drug appear in breast milk and may cause drowsiness in infants.

Adverse reactions

CNS: ataxia, dizziness, drowsiness, hangover, nightmares, paradoxical excitement.
GI: diarrhea, flatulence, nausea, vomiting.
Hematologic: eosinophilia, *leukopenia.*
Other: hypersensitivity reactions.

Interactions

Drug-drug. *Alkaline solutions:* May be incompatible with aqueous solutions of chloral hydrate. Don't mix together.

CNS depressants, including opioid analgesics: May cause excessive CNS depression or vasodilation reaction. Use together cautiously.
Furosemide I.V.: May cause sweating, flushing, variable blood pressure, and uneasiness. Use together cautiously or use different hypnotic drug.
Oral anticoagulants: May increase risk of bleeding. Monitor patient closely.
Phenytoin: May decrease phenytoin level. Monitor level closely.
Drug-lifestyle. *Alcohol use:* May react synergistically, increasing CNS depression, or may cause a disulfiram-like reaction (rarely). Strongly discourage alcohol use.

Effects on lab test results

• May increase BUN level.
• May increase eosinophil count. May decrease WBC count.
• May interfere with fluorometric tests for urine catecholamines and Reddy-Jenkins-Thorn test for urine 17-hydroxycorticosteroids. May cause false-positive tests for urine glucose in copper sulfate tests (Clinitest).

Pharmacokinetics

Absorption: Good.
Distribution: Throughout body tissue and fluids; trichloroethanol (the active metabolite) is 35% to 41% protein-bound.
Metabolism: Rapid and nearly complete in liver and erythrocytes to trichloroethanol; then again in liver and kidneys to trichloroacetic acid and other inactive metabolites.
Excretion: Inactive metabolites mainly in urine, minimally in bile. *Half-life:* 8 to 10 hours for trichloroethanol.

Route	Onset	Peak	Duration
P.O.	≤ 30 min	Unknown	4–8 hr
P.R.	Unknown	Unknown	4–8 hr

Action

Chemical effect: Unknown; sedative effects may be caused by trichloroethanol.
Therapeutic effect: Promotes sleep and calmness.

Available forms

Capsules: 500 mg
Suppositories: 324 mg, 500 mg, 648 mg
Syrup: 250 mg/5 ml, 500 mg/5 ml

Reactions may be *common,* uncommon, *life-threatening*, or COMMON AND LIFE-THREATENING.

NURSING PROCESS

⚕ Assessment
• Assess patient's underlying condition.
• Evaluate drug's effectiveness.
• Be alert for adverse reactions and drug interactions.
• Assess patient's and family's knowledge of drug therapy.

⊕ Nursing diagnoses
• Disturbed sleep pattern related to patient's underlying condition
• Risk for trauma related to adverse CNS reactions
• Deficient knowledge related to drug therapy

▶ Planning and implementation
⦿ **ALERT:** Oral liquid form comes in two strengths; double-check dose, especially when giving to children. Fatal overdose may occur.
• To minimize unpleasant taste and stomach irritation, dilute or give drug with liquid and after meals.
• Store rectal suppositories in refrigerator.
• Don't use for long-term therapy because drug loses its effectiveness in promoting sleep after 14 days of continued use. Long-term use may also cause drug dependence, and patient may experience withdrawal symptoms if drug is suddenly stopped.
⦿ **ALERT:** Some products may contain tartrazine, which may cause hypersensitivity reactions in susceptible people.
Patient teaching
• Warn patient about performing activities that require mental alertness or physical coordination. For inpatients, particularly elderly patients, supervise walking and raise bed rails.
• Tell patient to store capsules or syrup in dark container and to store suppositories in refrigerator.
• Explain that drug may cause morning hangover. Encourage patient to report severe hangover or feelings of oversedation so that prescriber can adjust the dose or change drug.

✓ Evaluation
• Patient states drug effectively induced sleep.
• Patient's safety is maintained.
• Patient and family state understanding of drug therapy.

chlorambucil
(klor-AM-byoo-sil)
Leukeran

Pharmacologic class: alkylating drug
Therapeutic class: antineoplastic
Pregnancy risk category: D

Indications and dosages

▶ **Chronic lymphocytic leukemia; malignant lymphomas, including lymphosarcoma, giant follicular lymphoma, non-Hodgkin's lymphoma, Hodgkin's disease, autoimmune hemolytic anemia‡, nephrotic syndrome‡, polycythemia vera‡, and ovarian neoplasms‡.**
Adults: 0.1 to 0.2 mg/kg P.O. daily for 3 to 6 weeks; then adjust for maintenance (usually 4 to 10 mg daily).
Children: 0.1 to 0.2 mg/kg or 3 to 6 mg/m² P.O. as a single daily dose. Reduce initial dose if given within 4 weeks after a full course of radiation therapy or myelosuppressive drugs or if pretreatment leukocyte or platelet counts are depressed from bone marrow disease.
▶ **Macroglobulinemia‡.** *Adults:* 2 to 10 mg P.O. daily. Or 8 mg/m² for 10 days with prednisone 30 mg/m² daily; repeat cycle q 6 to 8 weeks p.r.n.
▶ **Metastatic trophoblastic neoplasia‡.**
Adults: 6 to 10 mg P.O. daily for 5 days; repeat q 1 to 2 weeks.
▶ **Idiopathic uveitis‡.** *Adults:* 6 to 12 mg P.O. daily for 1 year.
▶ **Rheumatoid arthritis‡.** *Adults:* 0.1 to 0.3 mg/kg P.O. daily.

Contraindications and cautions

• Contraindicated in patients hypersensitive or resistant to previous therapy (those hypersensitive to other alkylating drugs also may be hypersensitive to chlorambucil).
• Use cautiously in patients with history of head trauma or seizures and in patients receiving other drugs that lower seizure threshold.
❧ **Lifespan:** In pregnant women, use cautiously, if at all, because drug may harm fetus. In breast-feeding women, drug is contraindicated. In children, safety and effectiveness haven't been established, and potential benefits must be weighed against risks.

Adverse reactions

CNS: *seizures.*
GI: *nausea, stomatitis, vomiting.*
GU: *azoospermia, infertility.*
Hematologic: *anemia, myelosuppression* (usually moderate, gradual, and rapidly reversible), *neutropenia* (delayed up to 3 weeks, lasting up to 10 days after last dose), *thrombocytopenia.*
Hepatic: *hepatotoxicity.*
Metabolic: hyperuricemia.
Respiratory: interstitial pneumonitis, *pulmonary fibrosis.*
Skin: exfoliative dermatitis, rash, *Stevens-Johnson syndrome.*
Other: *allergic febrile reaction.*

Interactions

Drug-drug. *Anticoagulants, aspirin:* May increase risk of bleeding. Avoid using together. If drugs must be used together, monitor patient's coagulation studies.

Effects on lab test results

• May increase AST, ALT, alkaline phosphatase, and blood and urine uric acid levels. May decrease hemoglobin level and hematocrit.
• May decrease neutrophil, platelet, WBC, granulocyte, and RBC counts.

Pharmacokinetics

Absorption: Good.
Distribution: Highly bound to proteins.
Metabolism: Main metabolite, phenylacetic acid mustard, also has cytotoxic activity.
Excretion: In urine. *Half-life:* 2 hours for parent compound; 2½ hours for phenylacetic acid metabolite.

Route	Onset	Peak	Duration
P.O.	3–4 wk	1 hr	Unknown

Action

Chemical effect: Cross-links strands of cellular DNA and interferes with RNA transcription, causing growth imbalance that leads to cell death.
Therapeutic effect: Kills selected cancer cells.

Available forms

Tablets: 2 mg

NURSING PROCESS

✍ Assessment
• Assess patient's underlying neoplastic disorder before and regularly during therapy.
• Monitor CBC and uric acid level.
• Be alert for adverse reactions and drug interactions.
• Assess patient's and family's knowledge of drug therapy.

✣ Nursing diagnoses
• Ineffective health maintenance related to presence of neoplastic disease
• Ineffective protection related to drug-induced hematologic adverse reactions
• Deficient knowledge related to drug therapy

❯ Planning and implementation
• Dosage is based on patient's response.
• Give drug 1 hour before breakfast and at least 2 hours after evening meal.
• Drug-related nausea and vomiting usually can be controlled with antiemetics.
• Allopurinol may be used with adequate hydration to prevent hyperuricemia with resulting uric acid nephropathy.
• Follow institutional policy for infection control in immunocompromised patients if WBC count falls below 2,000/mm^3 or granulocyte count falls below 1,000/mm^3. Severe neutropenia is reversible up to cumulative dosage of 6.5 mg/kg in single course.
Patient teaching
• Warn patient to watch for signs of infection (fever, sore throat, fatigue) and bleeding (easy bruising, nosebleed, bleeding gums, melena). Tell him to take temperature daily.
• Instruct patient to avoid OTC products that contain aspirin.
• Tell patient to take drug 1 hour before breakfast and 2 hours after evening meal if bothered by nausea and vomiting.
• Instruct patient to maintain fluid intake of 2,400 to 3,000 ml daily, if not contraindicated.
• Tell patient to use contraceptive measures while using this drug.

☑ Evaluation
• Patient shows improvement in underlying neoplastic condition on follow-up diagnostic tests.

Reactions may be *common*, uncommon, *life-threatening*, or COMMON AND LIFE-THREATENING.

- Patient remains infection free and doesn't bleed abnormally.
- Patient and family state understanding of drug therapy.

chloramphenicol sodium succinate
(klor-am-FEN-eh-kol SOH-dee-um SUK-seh-nayt)
Chloromycetin, Chloromycetin Sodium Succinate

Pharmacologic class: dichloroacetic acid derivative
Therapeutic class: antibiotic
Pregnancy risk category: C

Indications and dosages

▶ **Haemophilus influenzae meningitis; acute Salmonella typhi infection; meningitis, bacteremia, or other severe infection caused by sensitive Salmonella, Rickettsia, or various sensitive gram-negative organisms; lymphogranuloma; or psittacosis.** *Adults and children:* 50 to 100 mg/kg P.O. or I.V. daily (depending on the severity of infection), divided q 6 hours. Maximum dosage is 100 mg/kg daily.
Full-term infants older than age 2 weeks with normal metabolic processes: Up to 50 mg/kg I.V. daily, divided q 6 hours.
Premature infants, neonates younger than age 2 weeks, and infants and children with immature metabolic processes: 25 mg/kg I.V. once daily. Use I.V. route to treat meningitis.
▶ **Meningitis and other severe infections caused by Streptococcus pneumoniae.** *Children and infants age 1 month and older:* 75 mg to 100 mg/kg/day I.V. in divided doses q 6 hours.

▽ I.V. administration

- Reconstitute 1-g vial of powder for injection with 10 ml sterile water for injection. Concentration will be 100 mg/ml.
- Give I.V. slowly over at least 1 minute. Check injection site daily for phlebitis and irritation.
- Stable for 30 days at room temperature, but refrigeration is recommended. Don't use cloudy solutions.
⊗ **Incompatibilities**
Chlorpromazine, fluconazole, glycopyrrolate, hydroxyzine, metoclopramide, polymyxin B sulfate, prochlorperazine, promethazine, vancomycin.

Contraindications and cautions

- Contraindicated in patients hypersensitive to drug.
- Use cautiously in patients with impaired hepatic or renal function, acute intermittent porphyria, or G6PD deficiency, and in those taking other drugs that cause bone marrow suppression or blood disorders.
- Indicated only for serious infections that can't be treated with other antibiotics.
※ **Lifespan:** In pregnant women, use cautiously. Women shouldn't breast-feed during therapy because drug appears in breast milk.

Adverse reactions

CNS: confusion, delirium, headache, mild depression, peripheral neuropathy (with prolonged therapy).
EENT: decreased visual acuity, glossitis, optic neuritis (in patients with cystic fibrosis).
GI: diarrhea, enterocolitis, nausea, stomatitis, vomiting.
Hepatic: jaundice.
Hematologic: *agranulocytosis, aplastic anemia, granulocytopenia, hypoplastic anemia, thrombocytopenia.*
Other: *gray syndrome* (in neonates), hypersensitivity reactions (fever, rash, urticaria, *anaphylaxis*), infection with nonsusceptible organisms, jaundice.

Interactions

Drug-drug. *Chlorpropamide, dicumarol, phenobarbital, phenytoin, tolbutamide:* May increase drug levels. Monitor patient for toxicity.
Folic acid, iron supplements, vitamin B_{12}: May delay response in patients with anemia. Monitor patient closely.

Effects on lab test results

- May decrease hemoglobin level and hematocrit.
- May decrease RBC, granulocyte, and platelet counts.

Pharmacokinetics

Absorption: Good.
Distribution: Wide. About 50% to 60% bound to protein.

Metabolism: Mainly by hepatic glucuronyl transferase to inactive metabolites.
Excretion: 8% to 12% by kidneys as unchanged drug; remainder as inactive metabolites. *Half-life:* 1½ to 4½ hours.

Route	Onset	Peak	Duration
P.O.	Unknown	1–3 hr	Unknown
I.V.	Immediate	Immediate	Unknown

Action

Chemical effect: Inhibits bacterial protein synthesis by binding to 50S subunit of ribosome; bacteriostatic.
Therapeutic effect: Inhibits growth of susceptible bacteria.

Available forms

Capsules: 250 mg
Injection: 100 mg/ml (as sodium succinate)
Oral suspension: 150 mg/5 ml (as palmitate)

NURSING PROCESS

▓ Assessment
• Assess patient's infection before and regularly during therapy.
• Before giving first dose, obtain specimen for culture and sensitivity tests. Begin therapy pending test results.
• Monitor drug level. Therapeutic drug level is 5 to 20 mcg/ml.
• Monitor CBC, platelets, iron, and reticulocytes before and every 2 days during therapy.
• Be alert for adverse reactions and drug interactions.
⊛ **ALERT:** Signs and symptoms of gray syndrome in neonates include abdominal distention, gray cyanosis, vasomotor collapse, and respiratory distress. Gray syndrome can lead to death within a few hours after onset of symptoms.
• Assess patient's and family's knowledge about drug therapy.

⊕ Nursing diagnoses
• Infection related to presence of bacteria susceptible to drug
• Impaired protection related to drug-induced aplastic anemia
• Deficient knowledge related to drug therapy

▷ Planning and implementation
• Give oral drug 1 hour before or 2 hours after meals. If patient develops adverse GI effects, give with food.
• If anemia, reticulocytopenia, leukopenia, or thrombocytopenia develops, stop drug immediately and notify prescriber.
• If patient's drug level exceeds 25 mcg/ml, take bleeding precautions and infection-control measures because bone marrow suppression can occur.
Patient teaching
• Instruct patient to report adverse reactions to prescriber, especially nausea, vomiting, diarrhea, fever, confusion, sore throat, or mouth sores.
• Stress importance of having frequent blood tests to monitor therapeutic effectiveness and adverse reactions.

☑ Evaluation
• Patient is free from infection.
• Patient's hematologic condition remains unchanged with drug therapy.
• Patient and family state understanding of drug therapy.

chlordiazepoxide hydrochloride
(klor-digh-eh-zuh-POKS-ighd high-droh-KLOR-ighd)
Apo-Chlordiazepoxide ◆ , Librium

Pharmacologic class: benzodiazepine
Therapeutic class: anxiolytic, sedative-hypnotic
Pregnancy risk category: D
Controlled substance schedule: IV

Indications and dosages

▶ **Mild to moderate anxiety.** *Adults:* 5 to 10 mg P.O. t.i.d. or q.i.d.
Children age 6 and older: 5 mg P.O. b.i.d. to q.i.d. Maximum dosage, 10 mg P.O. b.i.d. or t.i.d.
▶ **Severe anxiety.** *Adults:* 20 to 25 mg P.O. t.i.d. or q.i.d. Or 50 to 100 mg I.V. or I.M. initially, followed by 25 to 50 mg I.V. 3 or 4 times daily p.r.n.
Elderly patients: 5 mg P.O. b.i.d. to q.i.d.
▶ **Withdrawal symptoms of acute alcoholism.** *Adults:* 50 to 100 mg P.O., I.V., or I.M.

Repeat in 2 to 4 hours, p.r.n. Maximum dosage is 300 mg daily.
▶ **Preoperative apprehension and anxiety.**
Adults: 5 to 10 mg P.O. t.i.d. or q.i.d. on day preceding surgery. Or 50 to 100 mg I.M. 1 hour before surgery.

▼ I.V. administration

• Make sure equipment and staff needed for emergency airway management are available.
• Don't give packaged diluent I.V. because air bubbles may form.
• Use 5 ml normal saline solution or sterile water for injection as diluent for an ampule containing 100 mg of drug. Give slowly over 1 minute.
• Monitor respirations every 5 to 15 minutes after use and before each repeated dose.
⊗ Incompatibilities
Other I.V. drugs.

Contraindications and cautions

• Contraindicated in patients hypersensitive to drug.
• Use cautiously in patients with mental depression, porphyria, or hepatic or renal disease. In debilitated patients, use cautiously and at a reduced dosage.
⚠ Lifespan: In pregnant women, drug is contraindicated. Breast-feeding women shouldn't use drug because of risk of adverse effects in infant. In children younger than age 6, safety and effectiveness haven't been established. In children younger than age 12, parenteral use isn't recommended. In elderly patients, use smallest effective dose to avoid ataxia and oversedation

Adverse reactions

CNS: confusion, drowsiness, fainting, hangover, lethargy, psychosis, restlessness, *suicidal tendencies.*
CV: *thrombophlebitis,* transient hypotension.
EENT: visual disturbances.
GI: abdominal discomfort, constipation, nausea, vomiting.
GU: incontinence, menstrual irregularities, urine retention.
Hematologic: *agranulocytosis.*
Skin: pain at injection site, swelling.

Interactions

Drug-drug. *Cimetidine:* May increase sedation. Monitor patient carefully.

CNS depressants: May increase CNS depression. Avoid using together.
Digoxin: May increase digoxin level and risk of toxicity. Monitor patient closely; monitor level.
Fluconazole, itraconazole, ketoconazole, miconazole: May increase and prolong levels, CNS depression, and psychomotor impairment. Avoid using together.
Drug-herb. *Kava:* May lead to excessive sedation. Discourage use together.
Drug-lifestyle. *Alcohol use:* May cause additive CNS effects. Strongly discourage alcohol use.
Smoking: May increase clearance of drug. Monitor patient for lack of effectiveness.

Effects on lab test results

• May increase liver function test values. May decrease granulocyte count.
• May cause false-positive reaction in Gravindex pregnancy test. May interfere with certain tests for urine 17-ketosteroids.

Pharmacokinetics

Absorption: Good with P.O. use.
Distribution: Wide. 80% to 90% protein-bound.
Metabolism: In liver to several active metabolites.
Excretion: Most metabolites in urine. *Half-life:* 5 to 30 hours.

Route	Onset	Peak	Duration
P.O., I.V.	Unknown	½–4 hr	Unknown
I.M.	¼–½ hr	½–4 hr	Unknown

Action

Chemical effect: May potentiate the effects of GABA in brain and suppress the spread of seizure activity produced by epileptogenic foci in the cortex, thalamus, and limbic structures.
Therapeutic effect: Relieves anxiety and promotes sleep and calmness.

Available forms

Capsules: 5 mg, 10 mg, 25 mg
Powder for injection: 100 mg/ampule

NURSING PROCESS

▨ **Assessment**
• Assess patient's underlying condition before and regularly during therapy.

- Monitor liver, renal, and hematopoietic function studies periodically in patients receiving repeated or prolonged therapy.
- Monitor patient for abuse and addiction.
- Be alert for adverse reactions and drug interactions.
- Assess patient's and family's knowledge of drug therapy.

⊞ Nursing diagnoses
- Anxiety related to patient's underlying condition
- Risk for injury related to drug-induced CNS reactions
- Deficient knowledge related to drug therapy

⊞ Planning and implementation
- Don't give drug regularly for everyday stress.
- Make sure patient has swallowed tablets before you leave the bedside.
- **⑨ ALERT:** 5 mg and 25 mg unit-dose capsules may appear similar in color when viewed through the package. Verify contents and read label carefully.
- When using I.M., add 2 ml of diluent to powder and agitate gently until clear. Use immediately. I.M. form may be erratically absorbed.
- Recommended for I.M. use only, but may be given I.V.
- Injectable form comes in two types of ampules: as diluent and as powdered drug. Read directions carefully.
- Don't mix injectable form with any other parenteral drug.
- Refrigerate powder and keep away from light; mix just before use and discard remainder.
- Don't stop drug abruptly after long-term use because withdrawal symptoms may occur.

Patient teaching
- Warn patient to avoid hazardous activities that require alertness and good psychomotor coordination until CNS effects of drug are known.
- Tell patient to avoid alcohol while taking drug.
- Warn patient to take this drug only as directed and not to stop taking it without prescriber's approval. Inform patient of drug's potential for dependence if taken longer than directed.

☑ Evaluation
- Patient says he's less anxious.
- Patient's safety is maintained.

- Patient and family state understanding of drug therapy.

chloroquine hydrochloride
(KLOR-oh-qwin high-droh-KLOR-ighd)
Aralen HCl

chloroquine phosphate
Chlorquin ◇, Aralen Phosphate

Pharmacologic class: 4-amino-quinoline
Therapeutic class: antimalarial, amebicide
Pregnancy risk category: C

Indications and dosages

▶ **Acute malarial attacks caused by** *Plasmodium vivax, P. malariae, P. ovale,* **and susceptible strains of** *P. falciparum. Adults:* 1 g (600-mg base) P.O. followed by 500 mg (300-mg base) P.O. after 6 to 8 hours; for next 2 days, a single dose of 500 mg (300-mg base) P.O. Or 4 to 5 ml (160- to 200-mg base) I.M., repeated in 6 hours, if needed, changing to P.O. as soon as possible.
Children: Initially, 10 mg (base)/kg P.O.; then 5 mg (base)/kg at 6, 24, and 48 hours (don't exceed adult dosage). Or, 5 mg (base)/kg I.M. initially; repeated in 6 hours p.r.n. Don't exceed 10 mg (base)/kg/24 hours. Switch to P.O. as soon as possible.
▶ **Malaria prophylaxis.** *Adults:* 500 mg (300-mg base) P.O. on the same day once weekly, beginning 2 weeks before exposure. Continue for 4 weeks after leaving endemic area.
Children: 5 mg (base)/kg P.O. on the same day once weekly (not to exceed adult dosage), beginning 2 weeks before exposure.
▶ **Extraintestinal amebiasis.** *Adults:* 1 g (600-mg base) chloroquine phosphate P.O. daily for 2 days; then 500 mg (300-mg base) daily for at least 2 to 3 weeks. Therapy usually is combined with intestinal amebicide.
▶ **Rheumatoid arthritis‡.** *Adults:* 250 mg P.O. daily (chloroquine phosphate) with evening meal.
▶ **Lupus erythematosus‡.** *Adults:* 250 mg P.O. daily (chloroquine phosphate) with evening meal; reduce dosage gradually over several months when lesions regress.

Contraindications and cautions

• Contraindicated in patients hypersensitive to drug and in patients with retinal changes, visual field changes, or porphyria.
• Use cautiously in patients with severe GI, neurologic, or blood disorders. Also use cautiously in patients with hepatic disease or alcoholism (drug concentrates in liver), and in those with G6PD deficiency or psoriasis (drug may exacerbate these conditions).
☀ **Lifespan:** In pregnant women, don't use except in women who may have been exposed to active malaria because fetal risks of malaria outweigh risks of drug. Warn pregnant women or those planning to become pregnant to avoid exposure to malaria. Breast-feeding women should stop breast-feeding or stop the drug.

Adverse reactions

CNS: dizziness, fatigue, irritability, mild and transient headache, neuromyopathy, nightmares, psychic stimulation, *seizures.*
CV: ECG changes, hypotension.
EENT: ototoxicity (with prolonged high doses), *visual disturbances* (blurred vision; trouble focusing; reversible corneal changes; typically irreversible, sometimes progressive or delayed retinal changes, such as narrowing of arterioles; macular lesions; pallor of optic disk; optic atrophy; patchy retinal pigmentation, typically leading to blindness).
GI: abdominal cramps, anorexia, diarrhea, nausea, stomatitis, vomiting.
Hematologic: *agranulocytosis, aplastic anemia, hemolytic anemia, thrombocytopenia.*
Skin: lichen planus eruptions, pleomorphic skin eruptions, pruritus, skin and mucosal pigment changes.

Interactions

Drug-drug. *Aluminum salts, kaolin, magnesium:* May decrease GI absorption. Separate doses.
Cimetidine: May decrease hepatic metabolism of chloroquine. Monitor patient for toxicity.
Drug-lifestyle. *Sun exposure:* May worsen drug-induced dermatoses. Tell patient to avoid excessive sun exposure and to wear protective clothing and sunblock.

Effects on lab test results

• May decrease hemoglobin level and hematocrit.

• May decrease granulocyte and platelet counts.

Pharmacokinetics

Absorption: Quick and almost complete.
Distribution: In liver, spleen, kidneys, heart, and brain and is strongly bound to melanin-containing cells.
Metabolism: 30%.
Excretion: 70% unchanged in urine; unabsorbed drug in feces. Small amounts of drug may be present in urine for months after drug is stopped. Renal excretion is enhanced by urine acidification. *Half-life:* 1 to 2 months.

Route	Onset	Peak	Duration
P.O.	Unknown	1–3 hr	Unknown
I.M.	Unknown	30 min	Unknown

Action

Chemical effect: May bind to and alter properties of DNA in susceptible parasites.
Therapeutic effect: Prevents or eradicates malarial infections; eradicates amebiasis.

Available forms

chloroquine hydrochloride
Injection: 50 mg/ml (40-mg/ml base)
chloroquine phosphate
Tablets: 250 mg (150-mg base), 500 mg (300mg base)

NURSING PROCESS

⚷ Assessment

• Assess patient's infection before and regularly during therapy.
• Make sure baseline and periodic ophthalmic examinations are performed. After long-term use, check periodically for ocular muscle weakness.
• Assist patient with obtaining audiometric examinations before, during, and after therapy, especially long-term therapy.
• Monitor CBC and liver function studies periodically during long-term therapy.
• Be alert for adverse reactions and drug interactions.
• Assess patient for potential overdose, which can quickly lead to toxic symptoms: headache, drowsiness, visual disturbances, CV collapse, and seizures, followed by cardiopulmonary arrest. Children are highly susceptible to toxicity.

• Assess patient's and family's knowledge of drug therapy.

⊞ Nursing diagnoses
• Infection related to presence of organisms susceptible to drug
• Disturbed sensory perception (visual or auditory) related to adverse reactions to drug
• Deficient knowledge related to drug therapy

⧄ Planning and implementation
• Give drug at same time of same day each week.
⊛ ALERT: Give missed doses as soon as possible. To avoid doubling doses in regimens requiring more than one dose per day, give missed dose within 1 hour of scheduled time or omit dose altogether.
• Replace I.M. with P.O. use as quickly as possible.
• Give drug with milk or meals to minimize GI distress. Tablets may be crushed and mixed with food or chocolate syrup for patients who have trouble swallowing; however, drug has bitter taste and patients may find mixture unpleasant. Crushed tablets may be placed inside empty gelatin capsules, which are easier to swallow.
• Store drug in amber-colored containers to protect from light.
• Begin prophylactic antimalarial therapy 2 weeks before exposure and continue for 4 weeks after patient leaves endemic area.
• Monitor patient's weight for significant changes because dose is based on weight.
• If patient develops severe blood disorder not attributable to disease, notify prescriber and stop drug.
Patient teaching
• Tell patient to take drug with food at same time on same day each week.
• Instruct patient to avoid excessive sun exposure to avoid worsening drug-induced dermatoses.
• Tell patient to report blurred vision, increased sensitivity to light, trouble hearing, ringing in the ears, and muscle weakness.
• Warn patient to avoid alcohol while taking drug.
• Teach patient how to take missed doses.

✓ Evaluation
• Patient is free from infection.

• Patient maintains normal visual and auditory function.
• Patient and family state understanding of drug therapy.

---

chlorothiazide
(klor-oh-THIGH-uh-zighd)
Chlotride ◇ , Diurigen, Diuril

chlorothiazide sodium
Diuril Sodium Intravenous

Pharmacologic class: diuretic
Therapeutic class: thiazide diuretic, antihypertensive
Pregnancy risk category: C

Indications and dosages
▶ **Edema, hypertension.** *Adults:* 500 mg to 1 g P.O. or I.V. daily or in divided doses.
▶ **Diuresis, hypertension.** *Children and infants age 6 months and older:* 10 to 20 mg/kg P.O. daily in divided doses, not to exceed 375 mg daily.
Infants age 6 months and younger: May require 30 mg/kg P.O. daily in two divided doses.

▽ I.V. administration
• Reconstitute 500 mg with 18 ml sterile water for injection.
• Inject reconstituted drug directly into vein; through I.V. line containing free-flowing, compatible solution; or through intermittent infusion device. Compatible solutions include dextrose and saline.
• Monitor the patient for signs and symptoms of I.V. infiltration.
• Avoid simultaneous administration with whole blood and its derivatives.
• If hypersensitivity reactions occur, stop drug and notify prescriber.
• Store reconstituted solutions at room temperature up to 24 hours.
⊗ **Incompatibilities**
Amikacin; chlorpromazine; codeine; hydralazine; insulin (regular); Ionosol B, D, or K and invert sugar 10%; Ionosol B or D-CM and dextrose 5%; Ionosol PSL; levorphanol; methadone; morphine; norepinephrine; Normosol-M (900 calories); Normosol-M in dextrose 5%; Normosol-R in dextrose 5%;

Reactions may be *common,* uncommon, *life-threatening,* or COMMON AND LIFE-THREATENING.

polymyxin B; procaine; prochlorperazine; promazine; promethazine hydrochloride; streptomycin; triflupromazine; vancomycin; vitamin B complex with C; whole blood and its derivatives.

Contraindications and cautions

• Contraindicated in patients hypersensitive to other thiazides or other sulfonamide-derived drugs and in patients with anuria.
• Use cautiously in patients with severe renal disease or impaired hepatic function.
⚹ **Lifespan:** In pregnant or breast-feeding women, safety and effectiveness haven't been established. In children, I.V. use isn't recommended.

Adverse reactions

CV: orthostatic hypotension.
GI: anorexia, nausea, *pancreatitis.*
GU: frequent urination, impotence, nocturia, polyuria, *renal impairment.*
Hematologic: *agranulocytosis, aplastic anemia, leukopenia, thrombocytopenia.*
Hepatic: hepatic encephalopathy.
Metabolic: asymptomatic hyperuricemia; fluid and electrolyte imbalances, including dilutional hyponatremia and hypochloremia, metabolic alkalosis and hyperkalemia; gout; hyperglycemia and impaired glucose tolerance; hypokalemia.
Skin: dermatitis, photosensitivity, rash.
Other: hypersensitivity reaction.

Interactions

Drug-drug. *Barbiturates, opioids:* May increase risk of orthostatic hypotension. Monitor blood pressure closely.
Chlorthalidone, ethacrynic acid, furosemide, hydrochlorothiazide, indapamide, metolazone and bumetanide, torsemide: May cause excessive diuretic response and serious electrolyte abnormalities or dehydration. Adjust doses carefully while monitoring the patient closely.
Cholestyramine, colestipol: May decrease intestinal absorption of thiazides. Separate doses.
Diazoxide: May increase antihypertensive, hyperglycemic, and hyperuricemic effects. Use together cautiously.
Digoxin: May increase risk of digitalis toxicity from chlorothiazide-induced hypokalemia. Monitor potassium and digitalis levels.

Lithium: May decrease lithium clearance, increasing risk of lithium toxicity. Monitor lithium level.
NSAIDs: May increase risk of NSAID-induced renal impairment. Monitor patient for this reaction.
Drug-herb. *Licorice root:* May worsen the potassium depletion caused by thiazides. Avoid using together.
Drug-lifestyle. *Alcohol use:* May increase orthostatic hypotension. Monitor patient closely and place patient on fall precautions.

Effects on lab test results

• May increase uric acid, glucose, and calcium levels. May decrease potassium, sodium, chloride, and hemoglobin levels and hematocrit.
• May decrease granulocyte, WBC, and platelet counts.

Pharmacokinetics

Absorption: Incomplete and variable.
Distribution: Unknown.
Metabolism: None.
Excretion: Unchanged in urine. *Half-life:* 1 to 2 hours.

Route	Onset	Peak	Duration
P.O.	≤ 2 hr	4 hr	6–12 hr
I.V.	≤ 15 min	30 min	6–12 hr

Action

Chemical effect: Increases sodium and water excretion by inhibiting sodium reabsorption in nephron's cortical diluting site.
Therapeutic effect: Promotes sodium and water excretion.

Available forms

Injection: 500-mg vial
Oral suspension: 250 mg/5 ml
Tablets: 250 mg, 500 mg

NURSING PROCESS

Assessment

• Assess patient's underlying condition before therapy and regularly thereafter.
• Monitor the drug's effectiveness by regularly checking blood pressure, fluid intake, urine output, blood pressure, and weight.
• Expect therapeutic response to be delayed several days in patients with hypertension.

Rapid onset   *Liquid form contains alcohol.   ♦ Canada   ◊ Australia   †OTC   ✐Photoguide   ‡Off-label use

- Monitor electrolyte and glucose levels.
- Monitor creatinine and BUN levels regularly. If they're more than twice normal, drug isn't as effective.
- Monitor blood uric acid level, especially in patients with history of gout.
- Be alert for adverse reactions and drug interactions.
- Assess patient's and family's knowledge of drug therapy.

⊞ Nursing diagnoses
- Excessive fluid volume related to patient's underlying condition
- Impaired urinary elimination related to drug therapy
- Deficient knowledge related to drug therapy

▷ Planning and implementation
- To prevent nocturia, give drug in the morning.
- Many patients with edema respond to intermittent therapy. Intermittent use reduces the risk of excessive response and electrolyte imbalances.
- **⊛ ALERT:** Never inject I.M. or subcutaneously.
- Drug may be used with potassium-sparing diuretic to prevent potassium loss.
- Stop thiazides and thiazide-like diuretics before parathyroid function tests are performed.

Patient teaching
- Teach patient and family to identify and report signs of hypersensitivity and hypokalemia.
- Teach patient to monitor fluid intake and output and daily weight.
- Instruct patient to avoid high-sodium foods and to choose high-potassium foods.
- Tell patient to take drug in the morning to avoid nocturia.
- Advise patient to avoid sudden posture changes and to rise slowly to avoid orthostatic hypotension.
- Advise patient to use sunblock in order to prevent photosensitivity reactions.
- Teach patient the importance of periodic laboratory tests to detect electrolyte imbalances.

☑ Evaluation
- Patient is free from edema.
- Patient adjusts lifestyle to cope with altered patterns of urine elimination.
- Patient and family state understanding of drug therapy.

chlorpromazine hydrochloride
(klor-PROH-meh-zeen high-droh-KLOR-ighd)
Chlorpromanyl-20 ◆ , Chlorpromanyl-40 ◆ ,
Largactil ◆ ◇ , Novo-Chlorpromazine ◆ ,
Thorazine

Pharmacologic class: aliphatic phenothiazine
Therapeutic class: antipsychotic, antiemetic
Pregnancy risk category: C

Indications and dosages

▶ **Psychosis.** *Adults:* Initially, 30 to 75 mg P.O. daily in two to four divided doses. Increase dosage by 20 to 50 mg twice weekly until symptoms are controlled. Some patients may need up to 800 mg daily. Or, for prompt control of severe symptoms, 25 mg I.M., followed by 25 to 50 mg I.M. in 1 hour if needed, then gradually increase dosage q 4 to 6 hours to maximum of 400 mg/dose. Switch to P.O. use as soon as symptoms are controlled.
Children age 6 months and older: 0.55 mg/kg P.O. q 4 to 6 hours or I.M. q 6 to 8 hours. Or 1.1 mg/kg P.R. q 6 to 8 hours. Maximum I.M. dose in children younger than age 5 or weighing less than 22.7 kg (50 lb) is 40 mg. Maximum I.M. dose in children ages 5 to 12 or weighing 22.7 to 45.5 kg (100 lb) is 75 mg.
▶ **Nausea and vomiting.** *Adults:* 10 to 25 mg P.O. q 4 to 6 hours, p.r.n. Or 50 to 100 mg P.R. q 6 to 8 hours, p.r.n. Or, 25 mg I.M. If no hypotension occurs, give 25 to 50 mg I.M. q 3 to 4 hours p.r.n. until vomiting stops.
Children and infants age 6 months and older: 0.55 mg/kg P.O. q 4 to 6 hours or I.M. q 6 to 8 hours. Or 1.1 mg/kg P.R. q 6 to 8 hours. Maximum I.M. dose in children younger than age 5 or weighing less than 22.7 kg is 40 mg. Maximum I.M. dose in children ages 5 to 12 or weighing 22.7 to 45.5 kg is 75 mg.
▶ **Intractable hiccups, acute intermittent porphyria.** *Adults:* 25 to 50 mg P.O. t.i.d. or q.i.d. If symptoms persist for 2 to 3 days, 25 to 50 mg I.M. If symptoms still persist, 25 to 50 mg diluted in 500 to 1,000 ml normal saline solution and infused slowly.
▶ **Adjunct treatment of tetanus.** *Adults:* 25 to 50 mg I.V. or I.M. t.i.d. or q.i.d., usually with barbiturates.
Children and infants age 6 months and older: 0.55 mg/kg I.M. or I.V. q 6 to 8 hours. Maxi-

mum parenteral dosage in children weighing less than 22.7 kg is 40 mg daily; in children weighing 22.7 to 45.5 kg, 75 mg daily, except in severe cases.

▶ **To relieve apprehension and nervousness before surgery and to control acute nausea and vomiting during surgery.** *Adults:* Preoperatively, 25 to 50 mg P.O. 2 to 3 hours before surgery or 12.5 to 25 mg I.M. 1 to 2 hours before surgery. To control acute nausea and vomiting during surgery, 12.5 mg I.M.; repeat after 30 minutes if needed or fractional 2-mg doses I.V. at 2-minute intervals; maximum dose, 25 mg. Postoperatively, 10 to 25 mg P.O. q 4 to 6 hours or 12.5 mg to 25 mg I.M.; repeat in 1 hour if needed.

Children and infants age 6 months and older: Preoperatively, 0.55 mg/kg P.O. 2 to 3 hours before surgery or I.M. 1 to 2 hours before surgery. To control acute nausea and vomiting during surgery, 0.275 mg/kg I.M. repeated after 30 minutes, if needed or fractional 1-mg doses I.V. at 2-minute intervals, maximum dose, 0.275 mg/kg. May repeat fractional I.V. regimen in 30 minutes, if needed; postoperatively, 0.55 mg/kg P.O. q 4 to 6 hours or 0.55 mg/kg I.M.; repeat in 1 hour if needed and hypotension doesn't occur.

▽ I.V. administration

• Drug is compatible with most common I.V. solutions, including D_5W, Ringer's injection, lactated Ringer's injection, and normal saline solution for injection.
• For direct injection, drug may be diluted with normal saline solution for injection and injected into large vein or through tubing of free-flowing I.V. solution.
• Don't exceed 1 mg/minute for adults or 0.5 mg/minute for children.
• For I.V. infusion, dilute with 500 or 1,000 ml normal saline solution and infuse slowly.
⊗ **Incompatibilities**
Aminophylline, amphotericin B, ampicillin, chloramphenicol sodium succinate, chlorothiazide, cimetidine, dimenhydrinate, furosemide, heparin sodium, linezolid, melphalan, methohexital, paclitaxel, penicillin, pentobarbital, phenobarbital, solutions having a pH of 4 to 5, thiopental.

Contraindications and cautions

• Contraindicated in patients hypersensitive to drug and in patients with CNS depression, bone marrow suppression, subcortical damage, and coma.
• Use cautiously in debilitated patients and in those with hepatic or renal disease, severe CV disease (may cause sudden drop in blood pressure); exposure to extreme heat or cold (including antipyretic therapy); exposure to organophosphate insecticides, respiratory disorders, hypocalcemia, seizure disorders; severe reactions to insulin or electroconvulsive therapy; glaucoma; or prostatic hyperplasia.
⚖ **Lifespan:** In pregnant or breast-feeding women, drug isn't recommended. In acutely ill or dehydrated children, use cautiously. In elderly patients, use cautiously.

Adverse reactions

CNS: dizziness, extrapyramidal reactions, *neuroleptic malignant syndrome,* pseudoparkinsonism, sedation, *seizures,* tardive dyskinesia.
CV: ECG changes, *orthostatic hypotension,* tachycardia.
EENT: blurred vision, ocular changes.
GI: constipation, dry mouth.
GU: *erectile dysfunction,* inhibited ejaculation, menstrual irregularities, urine retention.
Hematologic: *agranulocytosis,* aplastic anemia, *hyperprolactinemia, thrombocytopenia, transient leukopenia.*
Hepatic: cholestatic jaundice.
Skin: mild photosensitivity.
Other: allergic reactions, gynecomastia, I.M. injection site pain, sterile abscess.

Interactions

Drug-drug. *Antacids:* May inhibit absorption of oral phenothiazines. Separate antacid and phenothiazine doses by at least 2 hours.
Anticholinergics, including antidepressants and antiparkinsonians: May increase anticholinergic activity and aggravate parkinsonian symptoms. Use with caution.
Barbiturates, lithium: May decrease phenothiazine effect. Observe patient.
Centrally acting antihypertensives: May decrease antihypertensive effect. Monitor patient's blood pressure carefully.
CNS depressants: May increase CNS depression. Avoid using together.

Meperidine: May cause excessive sedation and hypotension. Don't use together.

Propranolol: May increase propranolol and chlorpromazine levels. Monitor patient.

Warfarin: May decrease effect of oral anticoagulants. Monitor PT and INR.

Drug-herb. *Dong quai, St. John's wort:* May increase risk of photosensitivity. Advise patient to avoid prolonged or unprotected exposure to sunlight.

Kava: May increase the risk or severity of dystonic reactions. Discourage using together.

Yohimbe: May increase risk of toxicity. Discourage using together.

Drug-lifestyle. *Alcohol use:* May increase CNS depression, particularly psychomotor skills. Strongly discourage alcohol use.

Sun exposure: May increase photosensitivity. Discourage prolonged or unprotected exposure to sun.

Effects on lab test results

• May increase CK, GGT, and prolactin levels. May decrease hemoglobin level and hematocrit.

• May increase eosinophil count. May decrease WBC, granulocyte, and platelet counts.

Pharmacokinetics

Absorption: Erratic and variable with oral use; rapid with I.M. use.

Distribution: Wide; level usually is higher in CNS than plasma. 91% to 99% protein-bound.

Metabolism: Extensive. Forms 10 to 12 metabolites, and some are pharmacologically active.

Excretion: Most of drug as metabolites in urine; some in feces. Drug may undergo enterohepatic circulation. *Half-life:* 20 to 24 hours.

Route	Onset	Peak	Duration
P.O.	30–60 min	1–4 hr	4–6 hr
P.O. controlled-release	30–60 min	1–4 hr	10–12 hr
I.V., I.M.	Unknown	Unknown	Unknown
P.R.	>1 hr	1–4 hr	3–4 hr

Action

Chemical effect: May block postsynaptic dopamine receptors in brain and inhibit medullary chemoreceptor trigger zone.

Therapeutic effect: Relieves nausea and vomiting, hiccups, signs and symptoms of psychosis,

acute intermittent porphyria, and tetanus. Produces calmness and sleep preoperatively.

Available forms

Capsules (controlled-release): 30 mg, 75 mg, 150 mg
Injection: 25 mg/ml
Oral concentrate: 30 mg/ml, 100 mg/ml
Suppositories: 25 mg, 100 mg
Syrup: 10 mg/5 ml
Tablets: 10 mg, 25 mg, 50 mg, 100 mg, 200 mg

NURSING PROCESS

☜ Assessment

• Assess patient's underlying condition before therapy and regularly thereafter.

• Be alert for adverse reactions and drug interactions.

• Monitor blood pressure regularly. Watch for orthostatic hypotension, especially with parenteral use. Monitor blood pressure before and after I.M. use.

• Monitor patient for tardive dyskinesia, which may occur after prolonged use. It may not appear until months or years later and may disappear spontaneously or persist for life despite stopping drug.

• Watch for symptoms of neuroleptic malignant syndrome. It's rare, but commonly fatal. It isn't necessarily related to length of drug use or type of neuroleptic, but more than 60% of affected patients are men.

• Monitor therapy with weekly bilirubin tests during the first month, periodic blood tests (CBC and liver function), and ophthalmic tests (long-term use).

• Assess patient's and family's knowledge of drug therapy.

⊕ Nursing diagnoses

• Ineffective health maintenance related to patient's underlying condition

• Impaired physical mobility related to drug-induced extrapyramidal reactions

• Deficient knowledge related to drug therapy

▷ Planning and implementation

⚠ **ALERT:** Wear gloves when preparing solutions, and prevent contact with skin and clothing. Oral liquid and parenteral forms can cause contact dermatitis.

Reactions may be *common*, uncommon, *life-threatening*, or COMMON AND LIFE-THREATENING.

• Slight yellowing of injection or concentrate is common; potency isn't affected. Discard very discolored solutions.

• Protect liquid concentrate from light.

• Dilute liquid forms with fruit juice, milk, or semisolid food just before giving.

• Don't give chlorpromazine oral solution and carbamazepine oral solutions together. Mixing causes orange, rubbery precipitate with unknown effect on bioavailability of either drug.

• Shake syrup before giving.

• Don't crush controlled-release form.

• Give deep I.M. only in upper outer quadrant of buttocks. Massage slowly afterward to prevent sterile abscess. Injection stings.

• Store suppositories in cool place.

• Keep patient supine for 1 hour after parenteral delivery, and advise him to get up slowly.

• Don't stop drug abruptly unless required by severe adverse reactions. After abruptly stopping long-term therapy, the patient may experience gastritis, nausea, vomiting, dizziness, and tremors.

• Don't give a dose, and notify prescriber, if patient develops jaundice; symptoms of blood dyscrasia (fever, sore throat, infection, cellulitis, weakness); extrapyramidal reactions that last longer than a few hours or any extrapyramidal reaction in pregnant patients or in children.

• Dystonic reactions may often be treated with diphenhydramine or an antiparkinsonian drug.

⊛ **ALERT:** Don't confuse chlorpromazine with chlorpropamide or clomipramine.

Patient teaching

• Warn patient to avoid activities that require alertness or good psychomotor coordination until CNS effects of drug are known. Drowsiness and dizziness usually subside after first few weeks.

• Instruct patient to avoid alcohol while taking drug.

• Tell patient to notify prescriber about urine retention or constipation.

• Urge patient to use sunblock and wear protective clothing to avoid photosensitivity reactions. Chlorpromazine causes higher risk of photosensitivity than other drugs in its class.

• Instruct patient to use sugarless gum or hard candy to relieve dry mouth.

• Caution patient not to stop taking drug suddenly but to take it exactly as prescribed and not to double doses to compensate for missed ones.

• Tell patient which fluids are appropriate for diluting concentrate, and show dropper technique for measuring dose. Warn patient to avoid spilling liquid on skin because it may cause rash and irritation.

• Advise patient that injection stings.

☑ **Evaluation**

• Patient has fewer signs and symptoms.

• Patient maintains physical mobility throughout drug therapy.

• Patient and family state understanding of drug therapy.

cholestyramine
(koh-leh-STIGH-ruh-meen)
LoCHOLEST, Prevalite, Questran, Questran Light, Questran Lite ◇

Pharmacologic class: anion exchange resin
Therapeutic class: antilipemic, bile acid sequestrant
Pregnancy risk category: C

Indications and dosages

▶ **Primary hyperlipidemia or pruritus caused by partial bile obstruction; adjunct for reduction of elevated cholesterol level in patients with primary hypercholesterolemia.** *Adults:* 4 g P.O. t.i.d. before meals. Maintenance dosage is 4 g t.i.d. or q.i.d. before meals or before meals and at bedtime. Maximum daily dosage is 24 g.

Contraindications and cautions

• Contraindicated in patients hypersensitive to bile-acid sequestering resins and in patients with complete biliary obstruction.

• Use cautiously in patients at risk for constipation and those with conditions aggravated by constipation, such as severe, symptomatic coronary artery disease.

⚕ **Lifespan:** In pregnant and breast-feeding women, use cautiously because of interference with fat-soluble vitamin absorption. In children, safety and effectiveness haven't been established.

Adverse reactions

GI: *abdominal discomfort, constipation,* fecal impaction, flatulence, hemorrhoids, *nausea,* steatorrhea, vomiting.
Metabolic: folic acid deficiency; *hyperchloremic acidosis* (with long-term use or very high dosage); vitamin A, D, E, and K deficiency.
Skin: irritation of skin, tongue, and perianal area; rash.

Interactions

Drug-drug. *Acetaminophen, beta blockers, digoxin, corticosteroids, fat-soluble vitamins (A, D, E, and K), iron preparations, thiazide diuretics, thyroid hormones, warfarin and other coumarin derivatives:* May reduce absorption of the drugs listed. Give at least 1 hour before or 4 to 6 hours after cholestyramine.

Effects on lab test results

• May increase alkaline phosphatase and chloride levels. May decrease cholesterol; vitamins A, D, E, and K; folic acid; and hemoglobin levels and hematocrit.

Pharmacokinetics

Absorption: Not absorbed.
Distribution: None.
Metabolism: None.
Excretion: Insoluble drug with bile acid complex in feces. *Half-life:* Unknown.

Route	Onset	Peak	Duration
P.O.	1–2 wk	Unknown	2–4 wk

Action

Chemical effect: Combines with bile acid to form insoluble compound that's excreted. The liver must synthesize new bile acid from cholesterol, which reduces LDL cholesterol levels. Excretion of excess bile acids may decrease pruritus associated with partial cholestasis.
Therapeutic effect: Reduces cholesterol level and pruritus.

Available forms

Powder: 210-, 231-, 239-, 378-g cans; 5-, 5.7-, 9-g single-dose packets. Each scoop of powder or single-dose packet contains 4 g of cholestyramine resin

NURSING PROCESS

✎ Assessment

• Assess patient's cholesterol level and pruritus before therapy.
• Monitor drug effectiveness by checking cholesterol and triglyceride levels in 4 weeks and every 3 to 6 months thereafter; also, ask patient whether pruritus has diminished or abated.
• Be alert for adverse reactions and drug interactions.
• Monitor patient for fat-soluble vitamin deficiency because long-term use may be linked to deficiency of vitamins A, D, E, and K and folic acid.
• Assess patient's and family's knowledge of drug therapy.

Nursing diagnoses

• Risk for injury related to elevated cholesterol level
• Constipation related to drug-induced adverse GI reactions
• Deficient knowledge related to drug therapy

Planning and implementation

• To mix powder, sprinkle on surface of preferred beverage or wet food (soup, applesauce, crushed pineapple). Let stand a few minutes; then stir to obtain uniform suspension. Mixing with carbonated beverages may cause excess foaming. Use large glass, and mix slowly.
• Give drug before meals and at bedtime.
• If therapy is stopped, lower the dose of digoxin to avoid toxicity.
• If severe constipation develops, lower the dose, add stool softener, increase fiber, and give a laxative if needed; or stop drug.
• Give all other drugs at least 1 hour before or 4 to 6 hours after cholestyramine to avoid blocking their absorption.
Patient teaching
• Instruct patient never to take drug in its dry form; esophageal irritation or severe constipation may result. Tell the patient to sprinkle powder on surface of preferred beverage in a large glass; to let mixture stand a few minutes; then to stir thoroughly. The best diluents are water, milk, and juice (especially pulpy fruit juice). Tell him that mixing with carbonated beverages could cause excess foaming. Tell him to swirl small additional amount of liquid in same glass

and then to drink it all to make sure he took the whole dose.

• Advise patient to take all other drugs at least 1 hour before or 4 to 6 hours after cholestyramine to avoid blocking their absorption.

• Teach patient about proper dietary management of serum lipids (restricting total fat and cholesterol intake), as well as measures to control other cardiac disease risk factors.

• When appropriate, recommend weight control, exercise, and smoking-cessation programs.

☑ Evaluation

• Patient's cholesterol level is normal with drug therapy.

• Patient maintains normal bowel patterns throughout drug therapy.

• Patient and family state understanding of drug therapy.

cidofovir
(sigh-doh-FOH-veer)
Vistide

Pharmacologic class: inhibitor of viral DNA synthesis
Therapeutic class: antiviral
Pregnancy risk category: C

Indications and dosages

▶ **CMV retinitis in patients with AIDS.**
Adults: 5 mg/kg I.V. infused over 1 hour once weekly for 2 consecutive weeks, followed by maintenance dosage of 5 mg/kg I.V. infused over 1 hour once q 2 weeks. Probenecid and prehydration with normal saline solution I.V. must be given at the same time and may reduce risk of nephrotoxicity.

◧ Adjust-a-dose: For patients with renal impairment, if creatinine level increases 0.3 to 0.4 mg/dl above baseline, reduce dose to 3 mg/kg at same rate and frequency. If creatinine level increases 0.5 mg/dl or more above baseline, or if patient develops 3+ proteinuria, stop drug.

▽ I.V. administration

• Because of the mutagenic properties of drug, prepare in a class II laminar flow biological safety cabinet. Wear surgical gloves and a closed front surgical gown with knit cuffs.

• If drug contacts skin or membranes, wash and flush thoroughly with water. Place excess drug and all other materials used in the admixture preparation and administration in a leak-proof, puncture-proof container. Dispose of by high-temperature.

• To prepare drug for infusion, remove it from vial using syringe, and transfer dose to an infusion bag containing 100 ml normal saline solution.

• Compatibility with Ringer's solution, lactated Ringer's solution, or bacteriostatic infusion fluids hasn't been evaluated.

• Infuse entire volume I.V. at constant rate over 1 hour. Use a standard infusion pump. Because of the risk of increased nephrotoxicity, don't exceed recommended dose, frequency, or rate of administration.

• Give admixtures for infusion within 24 hours of preparation.

• If admixtures aren't used immediately, they may be refrigerated at 36° to 46° F (2° to 8° C) for longer than 24 hours. Let drug reach room temperature before use.

⊗ **Incompatibilities**
Don't add other drugs or supplements to admixture.

Contraindications and cautions

• Contraindicated in patients hypersensitive to drug and in those with history of severe hypersensitivity to probenecid or other sulfa-containing drugs.

• Use cautiously in patients with renal impairment.

❀ **Lifespan:** In pregnancy, use only if potential benefits to mother outweigh potential risks to fetus. In women who are breast-feeding, use cautiously. It isn't known whether drug appears in breast milk. In children, safety and effectiveness haven't been studied.

Adverse reactions

CNS: abnormal gait, amnesia, anxiety, *asthenia*, confusion, depression, dizziness, *fever*, hallucinations, *headache*, insomnia, malaise, neuropathy, paresthesia, **seizures**, somnolence, syncope.
CV: facial edema, hypotension, orthostatic hypotension, pallor, tachycardia, vasodilation.
EENT: abnormal vision, amblyopia, conjunctivitis, eye disorders, iritis, *ocular hypotony*, pharyngitis, retinal detachment, rhinitis, sinusitis, uveitis.

GI: *abdominal pain, anorexia,* aphthous stomatitis, colitis, constipation, *diarrhea,* dry mouth, dyspepsia, dysphagia, flatulence, gastritis, melena, mouth ulcerations, *nausea,* oral candidiasis, taste disturbance, tongue discoloration, rectal disorders, stomatitis, *vomiting.*
GU: glycosuria, hematuria, ***nephrotoxicity,*** *proteinuria,* urinary incontinence, UTI.
Hematologic: *anemia,* ***neutropenia, thrombocytopenia.***
Hepatic: hepatomegaly.
Metabolic: decreased bicarbonate level, fluid imbalance, hyperglycemia, hyperlipidemia, hyperkalemia, hypocalcemia, hypokalemia, weight loss.
Musculoskeletal: arthralgia; myalgia; myasthenia; pain in back, chest, or neck.
Respiratory: *asthma,* bronchitis, cough, *dyspnea,* hiccups, increased sputum, lung disorders, pneumonia.
Skin: acne, *alopecia,* dry skin, pruritus, *rash,* skin discoloration, sweating, urticaria.
Other: allergic reactions, *chills,* herpes simplex, *infections,* ***sarcoma, sepsis.***

Interactions

Drug-drug. *Nephrotoxic drugs (such as aminoglycosides, amphotericin B, foscarnet, I.V. pentamidine):* May increase nephrotoxicity. Avoid using together.
Probenecid: Interacts with metabolism or renal tubular excretion of many drugs. May be used with drug to decrease nephrotoxicity.

Effects on lab test results

• May increase BUN, creatinine, urine glucose, protein, alkaline phosphatase, ALT, AST, and LDH levels. May decrease calcium, bicarbonate, and hemoglobin levels and hematocrit. May increase or decrease potassium level.
• May decrease neutrophil and platelet counts.

Pharmacokinetics

Absorption: Given I.V.
Distribution: Less than 6% protein-bound.
Metabolism: Mainly by kidneys.
Excretion: By renal tubular secretion. *Half-life:* Unknown.

Route	Onset	Peak	Duration
I.V.	Unknown	Unknown	Unknown

Action

Chemical effect: Selective inhibition of CMV DNA polymerase; inhibits DNA viral synthesis.
Therapeutic effect: Reduces CMV replication.

Available forms

Injection: 75 mg/ml in 5-ml ampule

NURSING PROCESS

⚐ Assessment
• Before each dose, check WBC and neutrophil counts, with differential, and renal function.
• Monitor intraocular pressure, visual acuity, and ocular symptoms periodically.
• Don't use drug in patients with baseline creatinine greater than 1.5 mg/dl or calculated creatinine clearance of 55 ml/minute or less unless potential benefits outweigh risks. Monitor creatinine and urine protein within 48 hours before each dose and adjust dose according to renal function.
• Assess patient's and family's knowledge of drug therapy.

⊕ Nursing diagnoses
• Infection related to presence of virus
• Ineffective protection related to adverse renal reactions
• Deficient knowledge related to drug therapy

▷ Planning and implementation
• Give 1 L normal saline solution, usually over 1- to 2-hour period, immediately before each cidofovir infusion.
• Give probenecid with each cidofovir infusion.
Patient teaching
• Inform patient that drug doesn't cure CMV retinitis and that regular ophthalmologic follow-up examinations are needed.
• Explain that close monitoring of renal function is critical.
• Tell patient to take probenecid with food to reduce drug-related nausea and vomiting.
• Advise men to use barrier contraception during and for 3 months after drug therapy.

✓ Evaluation
• Patient's infection is eradicated.
• Patient doesn't experience serious renal reactions.
• Patient and family state understanding of drug therapy.

Reactions may be *common,* uncommon, *life-threatening,* or COMMON AND LIFE-THREATENING.

cilostazol
(sil-OS-tah-zol)
Pletal

Pharmacologic class: quinolinone phosphodiesterase inhibitor
Therapeutic class: antiplatelet, arterial vasodilator
Pregnancy risk category: C

Indications and dosages

▶ **To reduce symptoms of intermittent claudication.** *Adults:* 100 mg P.O. b.i.d. taken at least 30 minutes before or 2 hours after breakfast and dinner.
⎅ **Adjust-a-dose:** Decrease dosage to 50 mg P.O. b.i.d. during use with CYP 3A4– or CYP 2C19–inhibiting drugs, which may interact to increase cilostazol level.

Contraindications and cautions

• Contraindicated in patients hypersensitive to drug or its components and in those with heart failure.
• Use cautiously in patients with severe underlying heart disease and with other drugs that have antiplatelet activity.
⚠ **Lifespan:** In breast-feeding women, avoid use. In children, safety and effectiveness haven't been established.

Adverse reactions

CNS: *dizziness, headache,* vertigo.
CV: *palpitations,* peripheral edema, tachycardia.
EENT: *pharyngitis, rhinitis.*
GI: abdominal pain, *abnormal stools, diarrhea,* dyspepsia, flatulence, nausea.
Musculoskeletal: back pain, myalgia.
Respiratory: increased cough.
Other: *infection.*

Interactions

Drug-drug. *Diltiazem:* May increase cilostazol level. Reduce cilostazol dosage to 50 mg b.i.d.
Erythromycin, other macrolides: May increase levels of cilostazol and one of the metabolites. Reduce cilostazol dosage to 50 mg b.i.d.
Omeprazole: May increase level of active cilostazol metabolite. Reduce cilostazol dosage to 50 mg b.i.d.

Strong inhibitors of CYP 3A4, such as fluconazole, fluoxetine, fluvoxamine, itraconazole, ketoconazole, miconazole, nefazodone, sertraline: May increase levels of cilostazol and its metabolites. Reduce cilostazol dosage to 50 mg b.i.d.
Drug-food. *Grapefruit juice:* May increase cilostazol level. Tell patient to avoid grapefruit juice during therapy.
Drug-lifestyle. *Smoking:* May decrease cilostazol exposure by about 20%. Monitor patient closely and discourage patient from smoking.

Effects on lab test results

• May increase HDL level. May decrease triglyceride level.

Pharmacokinetics

Absorption: Increases by 90% when given with a high-fat meal. Absolute bioavailability is unknown.
Distribution: Highly protein-bound, mainly to albumin.
Metabolism: Extensive, mainly by CYP 3A4. There are two active metabolites, one of which accounts for at least 50% of activity.
Excretion: 74% through urine. 20% in feces.
Half-life: 11 to 13 hours.

Route	Onset	Peak	Duration
P.O.	Unknown	2–4 hr	Unknown

Action

Chemical effect: Drug is thought to inhibit the enzyme phosphodiesterase III, causing an increase of cAMP in platelets and blood vessels, thus inhibiting platelet aggregation. Drug also has a vasodilating effect that's greatest in the femoral vascular beds.
Therapeutic effect: Reduces symptoms of intermittent claudication.

Available forms

Tablets: 50 mg, 100 mg

NURSING PROCESS

☜ Assessment
• Assess patient's underlying condition and pain level before therapy and regularly thereafter.
• Before therapy starts, make sure patient has a thorough physical examination for signs and symptoms of heart failure.

• Be alert for adverse reactions and drug interactions.
• Assess patient's and family's knowledge of drug therapy.

✤ **Nursing diagnoses**
• Acute pain related to underlying disease
• Ineffective peripheral tissue perfusion secondary to underlying disease
• Deficient knowledge related to drug therapy

❯ **Planning and implementation**
• Beneficial effects may not appear for up to 12 weeks.
• Dose can be reduced or drug stopped without rebound effects, such as platelet hyperaggregability. Notify prescriber of coagulation study results.
• Monitor heart rate and CV condition regularly for evidence of heart failure or tachyarrhythmias.
Patient teaching
• Advise patient to read the patient package insert carefully before starting therapy.
• Instruct patient to take cilostazol on an empty stomach, at least 30 minutes before or 2 hours after breakfast and dinner.
• Tell patient that the beneficial effect of drug on intermittent claudication isn't likely to be noticed for 2 to 4 weeks and that it may take as long as 12 weeks.
• Instruct patient not to drink grapefruit juice while taking drug.
• Inform patient that CV risk is unknown in patients who use the drug on a long-term basis and in patients who have severe underlying heart disease.
• Tell patient that drug may cause dizziness. Warn patient not to drive or perform other activities that require alertness until response to drug is known.

☑ **Evaluation**
• Patient experiences a decrease in pain.
• Patient has adequate tissue perfusion.
• Patient and family state understanding of drug therapy.

cimetidine
(sih-MEH-tih-deen)
Tagamet, Tagamet HB†

Pharmacologic class: H_2-receptor antagonist
Therapeutic class: antiulcerative
Pregnancy risk category: B

Indications and dosages

▶ **Duodenal ulcer (short-term therapy).**
Adults and children age 16 and older: 800 mg P.O. h.s. Or 400 mg P.O. b.i.d. or 300 mg q.i.d. (with meals and h.s.). Therapy continues for 4 to 6 weeks unless endoscopy shows healing. For maintenance therapy, 400 mg h.s.
▶ **Active benign gastric ulceration.** *Adults:* 800 mg P.O. h.s., or 300 mg P.O. q.i.d., with meals and h.s., for up to 8 weeks.
▶ **Pathologic hypersecretory conditions (such as Zollinger-Ellison syndrome, systemic mastocytosis, and multiple endocrine adenomas).** *Adults and children age 16 and older:* 300 mg P.O. q.i.d. with meals and h.s.; adjust to patient's needs. Maximum oral daily dosage is 2,400 mg.
▶ **Gastroesophageal reflux disease.** *Adults:* 800 mg P.O. b.i.d. or 400 mg q.i.d. before meals and h.s. for up to 12 weeks.
▶ **Heartburn.** *Adults:* 200 mg Tagamet HB† P.O. with water as symptoms occur, or as directed, up to b.i.d. Maximum, 400 mg daily. Don't give daily for more than 2 weeks.
▶ **To prevent upper GI bleeding in critically ill patients.** *Adults:* 50 mg/hour by continuous I.V. infusion for up to 7 days.
▧ **Adjust-a-dose:** For patients with renal impairment, if creatinine clearance is less than 30 ml/minute, give 25 mg/hour by continuous I.V. infusion.
▶ **Hospitalized patients with intractable ulcers or hypersecretory conditions or patients who can't take oral drugs.** *Adults:* 300 mg I.M. q 6 to 8 hours. Or 300 mg diluted to 20 ml with normal saline solution or other compatible solution by I.V. push over 5 minutes q 6 to 8 hours. Or 300 mg diluted in 50 ml D_5W or other compatible solution by I.V. infusion over 15 to 20 minutes q 6 to 8 hours. To increase dosage, give 300-mg doses more frequently to maximum daily dosage of 2,400 mg. Or, 37.50 mg/hour (900 mg/day) I.V. continuous

infusion diluted in 100 to 1,000 ml of compatible solution.
► **Active upper GI bleeding, peptic esophagitis, stress ulcers‡.** *Adults:* 1 to 2 g I.V. or P.O. daily in four divided doses.
◙ **Adjust-a-dose:** For patients with creatinine clearance less than 30 ml/minute, decrease dosage to 300 mg P.O. or I.V. q 12 hours. If patient also has liver impairment, may need to further reduce dosage. May increase cautiously to q 8 hours based on patient response.

▼ I.V. administration

• Dilute I.V. solutions with normal saline solution, D_5W, dextrose 10% in water, combinations of them, lactated Ringer's solution, or 5% sodium bicarbonate injection. Don't dilute with sterile water for injection. Cimetidine may be added to total parenteral nutrition solutions with or without fat emulsion.
• Direct injection requires dilution of drug in 20 ml of compatible solution. Give direct injection over at least 5 minutes. Rapid I.V. injection may result in arrhythmias and hypotension.
• Infuse drug over at least 30 minutes to minimize risk of adverse cardiac effects. If giving continuous I.V. infusion, use infusion pump if giving a total volume of 250 ml over 24 hours or less.
• In children younger than age 16, dosages of 20 to 40 mg/kg are seldom used.
⊗ **Incompatibilities**
Allopurinol, amphotericin B, barbiturates, cefepime, chlorpromazine, combination atropine sulfate and pentobarbital sodium, indomethacin sodium trihydrate, pentobarbital sodium, warfarin.

Contraindications and cautions

• Contraindicated in patients hypersensitive to drug.
• Use cautiously in debilitated patients because they may be more susceptible to drug-induced confusion.
≋ **Lifespan:** In pregnant women, use cautiously. In breast-feeding women, drug is contraindicated. In patients younger than age 16, experience with drug is limited, and drug should only be used when anticipated benefits outweigh the potential risks. In elderly patients, use cautiously.

Adverse reactions

CNS: confusion, dizziness, headaches, peripheral neuropathy.
CV: *bradycardia.*
GI: mild and transient diarrhea.
Hematologic: *agranulocytosis, aplastic anemia, neutropenia, thrombocytopenia.*
Hepatic: jaundice.
Musculoskeletal: muscle pain.
Skin: acnelike rash, urticaria.
Other: hypersensitivity reactions, mild gynecomastia (if taken longer than 1 month).

Interactions

Drug-drug. *Antacids:* May interfere with cimetidine absorption. Separate administration by at least 1 hour.
Calcium channel blockers, carbamazepine, labetalol, pentoxifylline, phenytoin, some benzodiazepines, sulfonylureas, tacrine, theophylline, valproic acid, warfarin: May inhibit hepatic microsomal enzyme metabolism of these drugs. Monitor levels of these drugs.
Lidocaine (I.V.): May decrease clearance of lidocaine, increasing the risk of toxicity. Consider using a different H2 antagonist. Monitor lidocaine level closely.
Metoprolol, propranolol, timolol: May increase the pharmacologic effects of beta blocker. Consider using another H_2 antagonist or decrease the dose of beta blocker.
Procainamide: May increase procainamide level. Use cautiously. Monitor procainamide level closely and adjust the dose p.r.n.
Drug-herb. *Pennyroyal:* May change the rate at which toxic metabolites of pennyroyal form. Discourage use together.
Yerba maté: May decrease clearance of yerba maté methylxanthines and cause toxicity. Tell patient to use together cautiously.

Effects on lab test results

• May increase creatinine, alkaline phosphatase, AST, and ALT levels. May decrease hemoglobin level and hematocrit.
• May decrease neutrophil, granulocyte, leukocyte, and platelet counts.

Pharmacokinetics

Absorption: 60% to 75% of oral amount. Rate, but not extent, may be affected by food. Unknown after I.M. use.

Distribution: To many body tissues. 15% to 20% of drug is protein-bound.
Metabolism: 30% to 40%.
Excretion: Mainly in urine (48% of oral dose, 75% of parenteral dose); 10% of oral dose in feces. *Half-life:* 2 hours.

Route	Onset	Peak	Duration
P.O.	Unknown	45–90 min	4–5 hr
I.V.	Unknown	Immediate	Unknown
I.M.	Unknown	Unknown	Unknown

Action

Chemical effect: Competitively inhibits action of H_2 at receptor sites of parietal cells, decreasing gastric acid secretion.
Therapeutic effect: Lessens upper GI irritation caused by increased gastric acid secretion.

Available forms

Injection: 150 mg/ml; 300 mg in 50 ml normal saline solution for injection
Oral liquid: 300 mg/5 ml
Tablets: 200 mg†, 300 mg, 400 mg, 800 mg

NURSING PROCESS

Assessment
• Assess patient's underlying upper GI condition before and regularly throughout therapy.
• Be alert for adverse reactions and drug interactions.
• Identify tablet strength when obtaining drug history.
• Monitor patient's CV condition during I.V. use because drug can cause profound bradycardia and other cardiotoxic effects when given too rapidly.
• Assess patient's and family's knowledge of drug therapy.

Nursing diagnoses
• Impaired tissue integrity related to patient's underlying condition
• Diarrhea related to drug-induced adverse reaction
• Deficient knowledge related to drug therapy

Planning and implementation
• Give tablets with meals to ensure more consistent therapeutic effect.
• I.M. administration may be painful.

• Hemodialysis reduces level of drug. Schedule dose at end of hemodialysis. Lower dose in patients with renal impairment.
• Cimetidine shouldn't be used for self-medication (Tagamet HB†) in children younger than age 12 unless directed by a physician.
⚠ ALERT: Don't confuse cimetidine with simethicone.

Patient teaching
• Remind patient taking drug once daily to take it at bedtime for best results.
• Instruct patient to take drug as directed and to continue taking it even after pain subsides, to allow for adequate healing.
• Remind patient not to take antacid within 1 hour of taking drug.
• Advise patient to tell prescriber if he's taking other drugs.
• Urge patient to avoid cigarette smoking because it may increase gastric acid secretion and worsen disease.
• Instruct patient to immediately report black tarry stools, diarrhea, confusion, or rash.

Evaluation
• Patient experiences decrease in or relief of upper GI symptoms with drug therapy.
• Patient maintains normal bowel habits throughout drug therapy.
• Patient and family state understanding of drug therapy.

cinacalcet hydrochloride
(syn-uh-KAL-seht)
Sensipar

Pharmacologic class: calcimimetic
Therapeutic class: hyperparathyroidism drug
Pregnancy risk category: C

Indications and dosages

▶ **Secondary hyperparathyroidism in patients with chronic kidney disease on dialysis.** *Adults:* Initially, 30 mg P.O. once daily; adjust no more than q 2 to 4 weeks through sequential doses of 60 mg, 90 mg, 120 mg, and 180 mg P.O. once daily, to reach target range of 150 to 300 picograms (pg)/ml of intact parathyroid hormone (iPTH).
▶ **Hypercalcemia in patients with parathyroid carcinoma.** *Adults:* Initially, 30 mg P.O.

b.i.d.; adjust q 2 to 4 weeks through sequential doses of 60 mg, and 90 mg P.O. b.i.d., and 90 mg P.O. t.i.d. or q.i.d. daily p.r.n. to normalize calcium level.

Contraindications and cautions

• Contraindicated in patients hypersensitive to drug or any of its components and in patients with calcium level below 8.4 mg/dl.
• Use cautiously in patients with a history of a seizure disorder and patients with moderate to severe hepatic impairment.
☀ **Lifespan:** In women who are breast-feeding, use cautiously. It's not known if drug appears in breast milk. In children, safety and effectiveness haven't been established.

Adverse reactions

CNS: asthenia, *dizziness.*
CV: chest pain, hypertension.
GI: anorexia, diarrhea, nausea, vomiting.
Musculoskeletal: *myalgia.*
Other: dialysis venous access site infection.

Interactions

Drug-drug. *Drugs metabolized mainly by CYP 2D6 with a narrow therapeutic index (such as flecainide, thioridazine, most tricyclic antidepressants, vinblastine):* May strongly inhibit CYP 2D6. Adjust dosages of these drugs p.r.n. *Drugs that strongly inhibit CYP 3A4 (such as erythromycin, itraconazole, ketoconazole):* May increase cinacalcet level. Monitor parathyroid hormone (PTH) and calcium level closely, and adjust cinacalcet dosage p.r.n. if patient starts or stops therapy with one of these drugs.
Drug-food. *Food:* Improved concentrations of drug. Give with food or shortly after a meal.

Effects on lab test results

• May decrease calcium, phosphorous, and testosterone levels.

Pharmacokinetics

Absorption: Increases when drug is given with meals. Level peaks in about 2 to 6 hours.
Distribution: High volume. Drug reaches steady-state drug level within 7 days; 93 to 97% bound to proteins.
Metabolism: Mainly by CYP 3A4, CYP 2D6, and CYP 1A2.
Excretion: 80% in urine, 15% in feces. *Half-life:* 30 to 40 hours.

Route	Onset	Peak	Duration
P.O.	Unknown	2–6 hr	Unknown

Action

Chemical effect: Increases the sensitivity of calcium-sensing receptor to extracellular calcium.
Therapeutic effect: Decreases both iPTH and calcium level.

Available forms

Tablet: 30 mg, 60 mg, 90 mg

NURSING PROCESS

Assessment
⊛ **ALERT:** Monitor calcium level closely, especially if patient has a history of seizures, because a decreased calcium level lowers the threshold for seizures.
• Measure calcium level within 1 week of starting therapy or adjusting dose. Once the maintenance dosage has been established, measure calcium level monthly in patients with chronic kidney disease on dialysis and every 2 months in patients with parathyroid carcinoma.
• Watch carefully for evidence of hypocalcemia, such as paresthesias, myalgias, cramping, tetany, and seizures.
• Measure iPTH 1 to 4 weeks after therapy starts or dosage is changed. Once the maintenance dosage is established, monitor PTH every 1 to 3 months. Keep level at 150 to 300 pg/ml in patients with chronic kidney disease on dialysis.
• Assess patient's and family's knowledge of drug therapy.

Nursing diagnoses
• Risk for injury related to drug-induced hypocalcemia
• Noncompliance related to GI adverse effects of drug
• Deficient knowledge related to drug therapy

Planning and implementation
• In patient with moderate to severe hepatic impairment, adjust dose based on PTH and calcium level. Monitor patient closely.
• Give drug alone or with vitamin D sterols, phosphate binders, or both.
• If calcium level is 7.5 to 8.4 mg/dl or patient develops symptoms of hypocalcemia, give phosphate binders containing calcium, vitamin D

sterols, or both to raise level. If level is below 7.5 mg/dl or hypocalcemia symptoms persist, and the vitamin D dose has reached the maximum, withhold drug until level reaches 8 mg/dl, hypocalcemia symptoms resolve, or both. Resume with the next lowest dose.
• A dynamic bone disease may develop if iPTH levels are suppressed below 100 pg/ml. If this occurs, reduce the dosage of drug or vitamin D sterols, or stop therapy.
⑤ ALERT: Drug isn't approved for patients with chronic kidney disease who aren't on dialysis because they have an increased risk of hypocalcemia.

Patient teaching
• Tell patient to take tablets whole, with food or shortly after a meal.
• Advise patient to report adverse reactions and signs of hypocalcemia, which include paresthesias, muscle weakness, muscle cramping, and muscle spasm.

🗹 Evaluation
• Patient doesn't develop hypocalcemia.
• Patient doesn't experience GI adverse effects.
• Patient and family state understanding of drug therapy.

ciprofloxacin
(sih-proh-FLOKS-uh-sin)
Cipro◆, Cipro I.V., Ciproxin◇, Cipro XR

Pharmacologic class: fluoroquinolone
Therapeutic class: antibiotic
Pregnancy risk category: C

Indications and dosages
▶ **Mild to moderate UTI.** *Adults:* 250 mg P.O. or 200 mg I.V., q 12 hours.
▶ **Severe or complicated UTI; mild to moderate bone and joint infections; mild to moderate respiratory tract infections; mild to moderate skin and skin-structure infections; infectious diarrhea; intra-abdominal infection.** *Adults:* 500 mg P.O. or 400 mg I.V., q 12 hours.
▶ **Severe or complicated bone or joint infections; severe respiratory tract infections; severe skin and skin-structure infections.** *Adults:* 750 mg P.O. q 12 hours. Or 400 mg I.V. q 8 hours.

▶ **Mild to moderate acute sinusitis caused by** *Haemophilus influenzae, Streptococcus pneumoniae,* **or** *Moraxella catarrhalis;* **mild-to-moderate chronic bacterial prostatitis caused by** *Escherichia coli* **or** *Proteus mirabilis.*
Adults: 500 mg P.O. q 12 hours or 400 mg I.V. infusion q 12 hours.
▶ **Febrile neutropenia.** *Adults:* 400 mg I.V. q 8 hours for 7 to 14 days given in conjunction with piperacillin sodium (50 mg/kg I.V. q 4 hours, not to exceed 24 g daily).
▶ **Inhalation anthrax (postexposure).** *Adults:* 400 mg I.V. q 12 hours initially until susceptibility tests are known, then switch to 500 mg P.O. b.i.d. when patient's condition improves. *Children:* 10 mg/kg I.V. q 12 hours, then switch to 15 mg/kg P.O. q 12 hours when patient's condition improves. Don't exceed 800 mg I.V. daily or 1 g P.O. daily.
For all patients: Also use one or two additional antimicrobials. Treat for a total of 60 days (I.V. and P.O. combined).
▶ **Acute uncomplicated cystitis.** *Women:* 100 or 250 mg P.O. q 12 hours for 3 days.
▶ **Cutaneous anthrax‡.** *Adults:* 500 mg P.O. b.i.d. for 60 days. *Children:* 10 to 15 mg/kg q 12 hours, not to exceed 1 g daily, for 60 days.
▶ **Uncomplicated urethral, endocervical, rectal‡, or pharyngeal‡ gonorrhea.** *Adults:* 500 mg P.O. as a single dose with other anti-infectives if chlamydial infection isn't ruled out.
▶ **Neisseria meningitidis in nasal passages‡.** *Adults:* 500 to 750 mg P.O. as a single dose, or 250 mg P.O. b.i.d. for 2 days, or 500 mg P.O. b.i.d. for 5 days.
◩ Adjust-a-dose: For all indications above, in patients with renal impairment, if creatinine clearance is 30 to 50 ml/minute, give 250 to 500 mg P.O. q 12 hours or the usual I.V. dose; if clearance is 5 to 29 ml/minute, give 250 to 500 mg q 18 hours or 200 to 400 mg I.V. q 18 to 24 hours. If patient is on hemodialysis, give 250 to 500 mg P.O. q 24 hours after dialysis.
▶ **UTI.** *Adults:* If uncomplicated, 500 mg (extended-release) P.O. once daily for 3 days. If complicated, 1 g (extended-release) P.O. once daily for 3 days.
◩ Adjust-a-dose: For patients with renal impairment, if creatinine clearance is less than 30 ml/minute, give 500 mg (extended-release) P.O. daily. For dialysis patients, give dose after dialysis session.

▼ I.V. administration

• Dilute drug using D_5W or normal saline solution for injection to final concentration of 1 to 2 mg/ml. Infuse over 1 hour into large vein.
• If giving drug through a Y-type set, stop the other I.V. solution during infusion.

⊗ **Incompatibilities**
Aminophylline, ampicillin-sulbactam, azithromycin, cefepime, clindamycin phosphate, dexamethasone sodium phosphate, furosemide, heparin sodium, methylprednisolone sodium succinate, phenytoin sodium.

Contraindications and cautions

• Contraindicated in patients hypersensitive to fluoroquinolones.
• Use cautiously in patients with CNS disorders, such as severe cerebral arteriosclerosis or seizure disorders, and in those at increased risk for seizures. May cause CNS stimulation.
• Immunocompromised patients may receive the usual dose and regimen for anthrax.
☀ **Lifespan:** In pregnant women, use cautiously. Pregnant women may receive the usual dose and regimen for anthrax. In breast-feeding women, drug is contraindicated because it appears in breast milk. In children, safety and effectiveness for indications other than anthrax haven't been established. In children younger than age 18, avoid use of Cipro XR because its safety and effectiveness haven't been established.

Adverse reactions

CNS: confusion, hallucinations, headache, light-headedness, paresthesia, restlessness, *seizures,* tremor.
CV: thrombophlebitis.
GI: abdominal pain or discomfort, *diarrhea, nausea,* oral candidiasis, vomiting.
GU: crystalluria, interstitial nephritis.
Hematologic: eosinophilia, *leukopenia, neutropenia, thrombocytopenia.*
Musculoskeletal: achiness, arthralgia, joint inflammation, joint or back pain, joint stiffness, neck or chest pain.
Skin: photosensitivity, rash, *Stevens-Johnson syndrome.*
Other: burning, erythema, pruritus, swelling with I.V. use.

Interactions

Drug-drug. *Aluminum hydroxide, aluminum-magnesium hydroxide, calcium carbonate, magnesium hydroxide:* May decrease effects of ciprofloxacin. Give antacid at least 6 hours before or 2 hours after ciprofloxacin.
Iron salts: May decrease absorption of ciprofloxacin, reducing anti-infective response. Give at least 2 hours apart.
Probenecid: May elevate level of ciprofloxacin. Monitor patient for toxicity.
Sucralfate: May decrease absorption of ciprofloxacin, reducing anti-infective response. Give at least 6 hours apart.
Theophylline: May increase theophylline level and prolong theophylline half-life. Monitor level of theophylline and observe patient for adverse effects.
Tizanidine: May increase plasma level of tizanidine and cause low blood pressure, somnolence, dizziness, and slowed psychomotor skills. Avoid use together.
Warfarin: May enhance anticoagulant effects. Monitor PT closely.
Drug-herb. *Yerba maté:* May decrease clearance of yerba maté methylxanthines and cause toxicity. Discourage using together.
Drug-food. *Orange juice fortified with calcium:* May decrease absorption of drug, reducing effects. Advise patient to avoid taking drug with calcium-fortified orange juice.
Drug-lifestyle. *Caffeine:* May increase effects of caffeine. Monitor patient.

Effects on lab test results

• May increase BUN, creatinine, ALT, AST, alkaline phosphatase, bilirubin, LDH, and GGT levels.
• May increase eosinophil count. May decrease WBC, neutrophil, and platelet counts.

Pharmacokinetics

Absorption: About 70%. Food delays rate but not extent; 35% of Cipro XR is an immediate-release form, whereas 65% is a slow-release matrix.
Distribution: 20% to 40% protein-bound; CSF level is only 10% of this level.
Metabolism: May be hepatic. Four metabolites have been identified; each has less antimicrobial activity than parent compound.

Excretion: Mainly renal. *Half-life:* 4 hours. *Half-life of Cipro XR:* 6 hours in adults with normal renal function.

Route	Onset	Peak	Duration
P.O.	Unknown	1–2 hr	Unknown
P.O. extended-release	Unknown	1–4 hr	Unknown
I.V.	Immediate	Immediate	Unknown

Action

Chemical effect: Unknown. Bactericidal effects may result from inhibition of bacterial DNA gyrase and prevention of replication in susceptible bacteria.
Therapeutic effect: Kills susceptible bacteria.

Available forms

Infusion (premixed): 200 mg in 100 ml D₅W, 400 mg in 200 ml D₅W
Injection: 200 mg, 400 mg
Oral suspension: 250 mg/5 ml; 500 mg/5 ml
Tablets: 100 mg, 250 mg, 500 mg, 750 mg
Tablets (extended-release, film-coated): 500 mg, 1,000 mg

NURSING PROCESS

▨ Assessment
• Assess patient's infection before therapy and regularly throughout.
• Before giving first dose, obtain specimen for culture and sensitivity tests. Begin therapy pending results.
• Be alert for adverse reactions and drug interactions.
• If adverse GI reactions occur, monitor patient's hydration.
• Assess patient's and family's knowledge of drug therapy.

⊕ Nursing diagnoses
• Infection related to presence of bacteria susceptible to drug
• Risk for deficient fluid volume related to drug-induced adverse GI reactions
• Deficient knowledge related to drug therapy

⊳ Planning and implementation
• Give oral form 2 hours after meal or 2 hours before or 6 hours after taking antacids, sucralfate, or products that contain iron (such as vita-

mins with mineral supplements). Food doesn't affect absorption but may delay peak level.
• Reduce dose in patients with renal impairment.
• Have patient drink plenty of fluids to reduce risk of crystalluria.
• Additional antimicrobials for anthrax multidrug regimen can include rifampin, vancomycin, penicillin, ampicillin, chloramphenicol, imipenem, clindamycin, and clarithromycin.
• Steroids may be considered as adjunctive therapy for anthrax patients with severe edema and for meningitis, based on experience with bacterial meningitis of other etiologies.
• Ciprofloxacin and doxycycline are first-line therapy for anthrax. Amoxicillin 500 mg P.O. t.i.d. for adults and 80 mg/kg daily divided q 8 hours for children is an option for completion of therapy after improvement.
• Follow current Centers for Disease Control and Prevention recommendations for anthrax.

Patient teaching
• Tell patient to take drug 2 hours after meal and to take prescribed antacids at least 2 hours after taking drug.
• Advise patient not to crush, split, or chew the extended-release tablets, but to swallow them whole.
• Advise patient to drink plenty of fluids to reduce risk of crystalluria.
• Warn patient to avoid hazardous tasks that require alertness, such as driving, until CNS effects of drug are known.
• Advise patient to avoid caffeine while taking drug because of potential for cumulative caffeine effects.
• Advise patient that hypersensitivity reactions may occur even after first dose. If he notices rash or other allergic reaction, tell him to stop taking the drug and notify prescriber immediately.
• Instruct patient either to stop breast-feeding or request a different drug.

☑ Evaluation
• Patient is free from infection.
• Patient maintains adequate hydration throughout drug therapy.
• Patient and family state understanding of drug therapy.

Reactions may be *common,* uncommon, *life-threatening,* or COMMON AND LIFE-THREATENING.

cisplatin (cis-platinum)

(sis-PLAH-tin)
Platinol-AQ

Pharmacologic class: alkylating drug
Therapeutic class: antineoplastic
Pregnancy risk category: D

Indications and dosages

▶ **Adjunct therapy in metastatic testicular cancer.** *Adults:* 20 mg/m² I.V. daily for 5 days. Repeat q 3 weeks for three cycles or longer.
▶ **Adjunct therapy in metastatic ovarian cancer.** *Adults:* 100 mg/m² I.V.; repeat q 4 weeks. Or 75 to 100 mg/m² I.V. once q 3 to 4 weeks with cyclophosphamide.
▶ **Advanced bladder cancer.** *Adults:* 50 to 70 mg/m² I.V. q 3 to 4 weeks. Give 50 mg/m² q 4 weeks to patients who have received other antineoplastics or radiation therapy.
▶ **Head and neck cancer‡.** *Adults:* 80 to 120 mg/m² I.V. once q 3 weeks.
▶ **Metastatic or recurrent cervical cancer‡.** *Adults:* 50 mg/m² I.V. once q 3 weeks.
▶ **Invasive cervical cancer‡.** *Adults:* 40 to 75 mg/m² I.V. weekly or daily with radiation therapy.
▶ **Non–small-cell lung cancer‡.** *Adults:* 75 to 100 mg/m² I.V. q 3 to 4 weeks with other drugs.
▶ **Brain tumor‡.** *Children:* 60 mg/m² I.V. for 2 days q 3 to 4 weeks.
▶ **Osteogenic sarcoma or neuroblastoma‡.** *Children:* 90 mg/m² I.V. q 3 weeks.
▶ **Advanced esophageal cancer‡.** *Adults:* 50 to 120 mg/m² I.V. q 3 to 4 weeks when used alone, or 75 to 100 mg/m² I.V. q 3 to 4 weeks when used with other chemotherapy.

▽ I.V. administration

● Preparing and giving drug are linked to carcinogenic, mutagenic, and teratogenic risks. Follow facility policy to reduce risks.
● Reconstitute powder using sterile water for injection. Add 10 ml to 10-mg vial or 50 ml to 50-mg vial to make a solution containing 1 mg/ml. Further dilute with D₅W in one-third normal saline solution for injection or dextrose 5% in half-normal saline solution for injection. Solutions are stable for 20 hours at room temperature. Don't refrigerate.

● Infusions are most stable in chloride-containing solutions (such as normal, half-normal, and one-quarter saline solution). Don't use D₅W alone.
● To prevent hypokalemia, potassium chloride (10 to 20 mEq/L) is commonly added to I.V. fluids before and after therapy. Magnesium sulfate may be added to prevent hypomagnesemia.
● Hydrate patient with normal saline solution before giving drug. Maintain urine output of at least 100 ml/hour for 4 consecutive hours before therapy and for 24 hours after therapy. Prehydration and diuresis may reduce renal toxicity and ototoxicity significantly.
● Give mannitol or furosemide boluses or infusions before and with infusion to maintain diureses of 100 to 400 ml/hour during and for 24 hours after therapy. I.V. infusion in 2 L dextrose 5% in half-normal saline solution or dextrose 5% in 0.33% sodium chloride solution with 37.5 g mannitol over 6 to 8 hours is recommended.

⊗ Incompatibilities

Amifostine, cefepime, D₅W, fluorouracil, mesna, 0.1% sodium chloride solution, piperacillin sodium with tazobactam sodium, sodium bicarbonate, sodium bisulfate, sodium thiosulfate, solutions with a chloride content less than 2%, thiotepa. Don't use needles or I.V. administration sets that contain aluminum because it will displace platinum, causing loss of potency and formation of black precipitate.

Contraindications and cautions

● Contraindicated in patients hypersensitive to drug or other platinum-containing compounds. Also contraindicated in patients with severe renal disease, hearing impairment, or myelosuppression.
✻ **Lifespan:** In pregnant women, use cautiously and only when absolutely needed because fetal harm may occur. In breast-feeding women, drug isn't recommended. In children, safety and effectiveness haven't been established.

Adverse reactions

CNS: *peripheral neuritis, seizures.*
EENT: *hearing loss, tinnitus.*
GI: diarrhea, loss of taste, metallic taste, *nausea and vomiting beginning 1 to 4 hours after dose and lasting 24 hours.*
GU: *nephrotoxicity.*

Hematologic: *anemia, leukopenia,* MILD MYELOSUPPRESSION, nadirs in circulating platelet and WBC counts on days 18 to 23 with recovery by day 39, *thrombocytopenia.*
Metabolic: hypocalcemia, hypokalemia, hypomagnesemia.
Other: *anaphylactoid reaction.*

Interactions

Drug-drug. *Aminoglycoside antibiotics:* May cause additive nephrotoxicity. Monitor renal function studies carefully.
Bumetanide, furosemide: May cause additive ototoxicity. Avoid using together.
Phenytoin: May decrease phenytoin level. Monitor level.

Effects on lab test results

• May increase uric acid, liver enzyme, and bilirubin levels. May decrease magnesium, potassium, calcium, sodium, phosphate, and hemoglobin levels and hematocrit.
• May decrease WBC, RBC, and platelet counts.

Pharmacokinetics

Absorption: Given I.V.
Distribution: Wide, with highest level in kidneys, liver, and prostate. Doesn't readily cross blood–brain barrier. Extensively and irreversibly bound to plasma and tissue proteins.
Metabolism: Unknown.
Excretion: Mainly unchanged in urine. *Half-life:* Initial phase, 25 to 79 minutes; terminal phase, 58 to 78 hours.

Route	Onset	Peak	Duration
I.V.	Unknown	Immediate	Several days

Action

Chemical effect: Probably cross-links strands of cellular DNA and interferes with RNA transcription, causing imbalance of growth that leads to cell death.
Therapeutic effect: Kills selected cancer cells.

Available forms

Injection: 1 mg/ml

NURSING PROCESS

☝ Assessment

• Assess patient's underlying neoplastic disease before and regularly throughout therapy.
• Monitor CBC, electrolyte levels (especially potassium and magnesium), platelet count, and renal function studies before initial and subsequent dosages.
• To detect permanent hearing loss, obtain audiometry test results before initial dose and subsequent courses.
• Be alert for adverse reactions and drug interactions.
• Assess patient's and family's knowledge of drug therapy.

Nursing diagnoses

• Ineffective health maintenance related to presence of neoplastic disease
• Ineffective protection related to drug-induced adverse reactions
• Deficient knowledge related to drug therapy

Planning and implementation

• Renal toxicity is cumulative. Renal function must return to normal before next dose can be given.
• Don't repeat dose unless platelet count is over 100,000/mm^3, WBC count is over 4,000/mm^3, creatinine level is under 1.5 mg/dl, or BUN level is under 25 mg/dl.
• I.V. sodium thiosulfate may be used to minimize toxicity. Check current protocol.
• Nausea and vomiting may be severe and protracted (up to 24 hours). Provide I.V. hydration until patient can tolerate adequate oral intake.
• Antiemetics, such as ondansetron, granisetron, and high-dose metoclopramide, may be used to prevent and treat nausea and vomiting. Metoclopramide may be combined with dexamethasone and antihistamines, or ondansetron or granisetron with dexamethasone.
• Delayed-onset vomiting (3 to 5 days after therapy) may occur. Patients may need prolonged antiemetic treatment.
• Immediately give epinephrine, corticosteroids, or antihistamines for anaphylactoid reactions.
⚕ **ALERT:** Don't confuse cisplatin with carboplatin.

Patient teaching

• Warn patient to watch for signs of infection (fever, sore throat, fatigue) and bleeding (easy

---

bruising, nosebleeds, bleeding gums, melena).
Tell him to take his temperature daily.
• Tell patient to immediately report tinnitus.
• Instruct patient to avoid OTC products that
contain aspirin.
• Teach patient to record intake and output on
daily basis and to report edema or decrease in
urine output.
• Encourage patient to notify prescriber if any
concerns arise during therapy.

☑ Evaluation
• Patient has positive response to cisplatin therapy according to follow-up diagnostic studies.
• Patient doesn't have permanent injury from
drug-induced adverse reactions.
• Patient and family state understanding of drug
therapy.

citalopram hydrobromide
(sih-TAL-oh-pram high-droh-BROH-mighd)
Celexa◆

Pharmacologic class: SSRI
Therapeutic class: antidepressant
Pregnancy risk category: C

Indications and dosages
▶ **Depression.** *Adults:* Initially, 20 mg P.O.
once daily, increasing to maximum dosage of
40 mg daily after no less than 1 week.
▶ **Panic disorder‡.** *Adults:* 20 to 30 mg P.O.
once daily.
🔲 **Adjust-a-dose:** For elderly patients and patients with hepatic impairment, give 20 mg P.O.
once daily, increase to 40 mg daily only for patients not responding to therapy.

Contraindications and cautions
• Contraindicated within 14 days of MAO inhibitor therapy. Also contraindicated in patients
hypersensitive to drug, any of its components,
or escitalopram. Contraindicated in patients taking pimozide.
• Use cautiously in patients with history of mania, seizures, suicidal ideation, hepatic impairment, or renal impairment.
⚠ **Lifespan:** In breast-feeding women, avoid
drug because it appears in breast milk and may
cause serious adverse reactions in infants. Drug
isn't approved for pediatric use and shouldn't be

used in children and adolescents younger than
age 18 for major depressive disorder because of
possible increased risk of suicidal behavior. In
elderly patients, reduce dosage.

Adverse reactions
CNS: agitation, amnesia, anxiety, apathy, confusion, depression, dizziness, fatigue, fever, impaired concentration, insomnia, migraine, paresthesia, *somnolence, **suicide attempt,** tremor.
CV: hypotension, orthostatic hypotension,
tachycardia.
EENT: abnormal accommodation, rhinitis, sinusitis.
GI: abdominal pain, anorexia, diarrhea, dry
mouth, dyspepsia, flatulence, increased appetite,
increased saliva, nausea, taste disturbance, vomiting, weight changes.
GU: amenorrhea, dysmenorrhea, ejaculation
disorder, impotence, polyuria.
Musculoskeletal: arthralgia, myalgia.
Respiratory: cough, upper respiratory tract in-
fection.
Skin: increased sweating, pruritus, rash.
Other: decreased libido, yawning.

Interactions
Drug-drug. *Carbamazepine:* May increase
citalopram clearance. Monitor patient for effects.
CNS drugs: May increase CNS effects. Use together cautiously.
*Drugs that inhibit CYP 3A4 (such as flucona-
zole) and CYP 2C19 (such as omeprazole):* May
decrease citalopram clearance. Monitor patient
for toxicity.
Imipramine, other tricyclic antidepressants:
May increase level of imipramine metabolite
desipramine by about 50%. Use together cautiously.
Lithium: May enhance serotonergic effect of
citalopram. Use cautiously and monitor lithium
level.
Phenelzine, selegiline, tranylcypromine: May
cause serotonin syndrome, including CNS irritability, shivering, and altered consciousness.
Don't give together. Wait at least 2 weeks after
stopping an MAO inhibitor before giving any
SSRI.
Sumatriptan: May cause weakness, hyperreflexia, and incoordination. Monitor patient closely.
Warfarin: PT increases by 5%. Monitor patient
carefully; monitor PT and INR.

Drug-herb. *St. John's wort:* May raise serotonin level, causing serotonin syndrome. Discourage using together.
Drug-lifestyle. *Alcohol use:* May increase CNS effects. Discourage use together.

Effects on lab test results

• May increase liver function test values.

Pharmacokinetics

Absorption: Absolute bioavailability is 80%.
Distribution: Wide, about 80% bound to proteins.
Metabolism: Mainly by the liver.
Excretion: 10% is recovered in urine. *Half-life:* 35 hours.

Route	Onset	Peak	Duration
P.O.	Unknown	4 hr	Unknown

Action

Chemical effect: May enhance serotonergic activity in CNS by inhibiting neuronal reuptake of serotonin.
Therapeutic effect: Relieves depression.

Available forms

Oral solution: 10 mg/5 ml
Tablets: 10 mg, 20 mg, 40 mg

NURSING PROCESS

⚕ Assessment
• Assess patient's underlying condition before therapy and regularly thereafter.
• Check vital signs regularly for decreased blood pressure or tachycardia.
• Closely supervise high-risk patients at start of drug therapy.
• Assess patient's and family's knowledge of drug therapy.

⊞ Nursing diagnoses
• Risk for injury related to patient's underlying condition
• Ineffective coping related to patient's underlying condition
• Deficient knowledge related to drug therapy

⚕ Planning and implementation
⑤ **ALERT:** Don't start citalopram therapy within 14 days of MAO inhibitor therapy.

• For patient with hepatic impairment, reduce dosage.
• May increase risk of suicide in adolescents.
• Don't stop drug abruptly.
⑤ **ALERT:** Don't confuse Celexa with Celebrex, Cerebyx, or Concerta.
Patient teaching
• Urge patient to continue therapy as prescribed even if he improves within 1 to 4 weeks.
• Instruct patient to exercise caution when operating hazardous machinery, including automobiles, because psychoactive drugs can impair judgment, thinking, and motor skills.
• Warn patient that drug may cause photosensitivity; advise patient to take protective measures until tolerance is determined.
• Advise patient to consult prescriber before taking other prescription drugs, OTC medicines, or herbal remedies.
⑤ **ALERT:** If patient wishes to switch from an SSRI to St. John's wort, tell him to wait a few weeks for the SSRI to leave his system before he starts the herb. Urge him to ask his prescriber for advice.
• Warn patient not to consume alcohol during therapy.
• Instruct woman of childbearing age to use birth control during therapy and to notify prescriber immediately if she suspects pregnancy.

☑ Evaluation
• Patient's safety is maintained.
• Patient's condition is improved with drug.
• Patient and family state understanding of drug therapy.

clarithromycin

(klah-rith-roh-MIGH-sin)
Biaxin, Biaxin XL

Pharmacologic class: macrolide
Therapeutic class: antibiotic
Pregnancy risk category: C

Indications and dosages

▶ **Pharyngitis or tonsillitis caused by** *Streptococcus pyogenes.* *Adults:* 250 mg P.O. q 12 hours for 10 days.
Children: 7.5 mg/kg, up to 500 mg, P.O., q 12 hours for 10 days.

▶ **Acute maxillary sinusitis caused by** *Streptococcus pneumoniae, Haemophilus influenzae*, **or** *Moraxella catarrhalis. Adults:* 500 mg P.O. q 12 hours for 14 days. Or, two 500-mg extended-release tablets P.O. daily for 14 days. *Children:* 7.5 mg/kg, up to 500 mg, P.O. daily q 12 hours for 10 days.

▶ **Acute exacerbation of chronic bronchitis caused by** *M. catarrhalis, S. pneumoniae, H. influenzae*, **or** *H. parainfluenzae. Adults:* 250 mg P.O. q 12 hours for 7 to 14 days (for *M. catarrhalis* and *S. pneumoniae*), or 500 mg P.O. q 12 hours for 7 days for *H. parainfluenzae* (up to 14 days for *H. influenzae*). Or two 500-mg extended-release tablets P.O. daily for 7 days.

▶ **Uncomplicated skin and skin-structure infections caused by** *Staphylococcus aureus* **or** *S. pyogenes. Adults:* 250 mg P.O. q 12 hours for 7 to 14 days.

▶ **Prophylaxis and treatment of disseminated infection from** *Mycobacterium avium* **complex.** *Adults:* 500 mg P.O. b.i.d. *Children:* 7.5 mg/kg, up to 500 mg, P.O. b.i.d.

▶ **Acute otitis media caused by** *H. influenzae, M. catarrhalis*, **or** *S. pneumoniae. Children:* 7.5 mg/kg, up to 500 mg, P.O. q 12 hours,

▶ *Helicobacter pylori* **eradication to reduce risk of duodenal ulcer recurrence.** *Adults:* For triple therapy, 500 mg clarithromycin with 30 mg lansoprazole and 1 g amoxicillin, all given P.O. q 12 hours for 10 to 14 days; or 500 mg clarithromycin with 20 mg omeprazole and 1 g amoxicillin, all given P.O. q 12 hours for 10 days; or clarithromycin 500 mg with 20 mg rabeprazole and 1 g amoxicillin, all given P.O. q 12 hours for 7 days. For dual therapy, 500 mg clarithromycin q 8 hours and 40 mg omeprazole once daily P.O. for 14 days. *Children:* 7.5 mg/kg P.O., up to 500 mg, q 12 hours for 10 days.

▶ **Community-acquired pneumonia from** *Chlamydia pneumoniae, Mycoplasma pneumoniae, S. pneumoniae, H. influenzae, H. parainfluenzae, M. catarrhalis. Adults:* 250 mg P.O. q 12 hours for 7 to 14 days (for *H. influenzae,* 7 days). Or two 500-mg extended-release tablets P.O. daily for 7 days for all listed organisms. Don't use conventional tablets to treat pneumonia caused by *H. parainfluenzae* or *M. catarrhalis. Children:* 7.5 mg/kg P.O., up to 500 mg, q 12 hours for 10 days (for *C. pneumoniae, M. pneumoniae,* or *S. pneumoniae* only).

▶ **Lyme disease‡.** *Adults:* 500 mg P.O. b.i.d. for 14 to 21 days. *Children:* 7.5 mg/kg P.O., up to 500 mg, b.i.d. for 14 to 21 days

Ṉ Adjust-a-dose: For patients with renal impairment, if creatinine clearance is less than 30 ml/minute, reduce dose by 50% or double frequency interval.

Contraindications and cautions

● Contraindicated in patients hypersensitive to drug and other macrolides. Use with pimozide, cisapride, or other drugs that prolong QT interval or may cause ventricular arrhythmias is contraindicated.

● Use cautiously in patients with hepatic or renal impairment.

▓ **Lifespan:** In pregnant or breast-feeding women, use cautiously. In infants younger than age 6 months, safety and effectiveness haven't been established.

Adverse reactions

CNS: headache.
CV: *ventricular arrhythmias.*
GI: abdominal pain or discomfort, abnormal taste, diarrhea, dyspepsia, nausea, *pseudomembranous colitis,* vomiting (pediatric).
Hematologic: coagulation abnormalities, *leukopenia, neutropenia, thrombocytopenia.*
Skin: rash (pediatric), *Stevens-Johnson syndrome, toxic epidermal necrolysis.*

Interactions

Drug-drug. *Alprazolam, midazolam, triazolam:* May increase adverse CNS effects. Assess patient carefully.
Carbamazepine: May inhibit metabolism of carbamazepine and increase level and risk of toxicity. Avoid using together.
Digoxin, theophylline: May increase levels of these drugs; dosage may be reduced at start of clarithromycin therapy. Monitor patient for toxicity.
Dihydroergotamine, ergotamine: May increase risk of acute ergot toxicity with severe peripheral vasospasm and dysesthesia. Monitor patient closely.
Drugs metabolized by the CYP 3A system (alfentanil, bromocriptine, cilostazol, cyclosporine, disopyramide, hexobarbital, HMG-CoA reductase inhibitors, methylprednisolone, phenytoin, quinidine, rifabutin, rifampin, silde-

nafil, tacrolimus, valproate): May decrease clearance of these drugs, increasing risk of toxicity. Monitor drug levels and effects closely.
Fluconazole: May increase clarithromycin level. Monitor patient.
Ritonavir: May prolong absorption of clarithromycin. Don't adjust dosage in patients with normal renal function; if creatinine clearance is 30 to 60 ml/minute, give 50% of clarithromycin dose; if less than 30 ml/minute, give 25% of clarithromycin dose.
Warfarin: May increase bleeding times. Monitor PT and INR.
Zidovudine: May alter zidovudine level. Monitor patient closely for effectiveness of both drugs.

Effects on lab test results

- May increase AST, ALT, GGT, alkaline phosphatase, LDH, total bilirubin, creatinine, and BUN levels.
- May increase PT and INR. May decrease WBC counts.

Pharmacokinetics

Absorption: Rapid.
Distribution: Wide. Protein binding is 40% to 70%.
Metabolism: Extensive. Major metabolite has significant antimicrobial activity.
Excretion: In urine and feces. *Half-life:* 5 to 6 hours with 250 mg q 12 hours; 7 hours with 500 mg q 12 hours.

Route	Onset	Peak	Duration
P.O.	Unknown	2–3 hr	Unknown
P.O. extended-release	Unknown	5–6 hr	Unknown

Action

Chemical effect: Binds to 50S subunit of bacterial ribosomes, blocking protein synthesis; bacteriostatic or bactericidal, depending on concentration.
Therapeutic effect: Hinders or kills susceptible bacteria.

Available forms

Suspension: 125 mg/5 ml, 250 mg/5 ml
Tablets: 250 mg, 500 mg
Tablets (extended-release): 500 mg

NURSING PROCESS

Assessment

- Assess patient's infection before and regularly throughout therapy.
- Obtain urine specimen for culture and sensitivity tests before giving the first dose. Begin therapy pending results.
- Be alert for adverse reactions and drug interactions.
- If adverse GI reactions occur, monitor patient's hydration.
- Assess patient's and family's knowledge of drug therapy.

Nursing diagnoses

- Infection related to presence of bacteria susceptible to drug
- Risk for deficient fluid volume related to drug-induced adverse GI reactions
- Deficient knowledge related to drug therapy

Planning and implementation

- Give drug with or without food. It may be taken with milk.
- Don't refrigerate oral suspension after reconstitution. Discard unused portion after 14 days.

ALERT: Don't confuse or interchange Biaxin XL (extended-release) with Biaxin (immediate release).

Patient teaching

- Tell patient to complete therapy as prescribed, even after he feels better.
- Urge patient to notify prescriber about all prescription and OTC medications taken, and to immediately report any adverse reactions.
- Instruct patient to report persistent diarrhea to prescriber, even if it occurs a month after antibiotic therapy has ended.
- Tell patient not to chew or crush extended-release tablets.

Evaluation

- Patient is free from infection.
- Patient maintains adequate hydration throughout drug therapy.
- Patient and family state understanding of drug therapy.

clindamycin hydrochloride
(klin-duh-MIGH-sin high-droh-KLOR-ighd)
Cleocin, Dalacin C ◆ ◊

clindamycin palmitate hydrochloride
Cleocin Pediatric

clindamycin phosphate
Clindesse, Cleocin T, Clindagel, ClindaMax, Clindets, ClindaMax Lotion, Evoclin Foam

Pharmacologic class: lincomycin derivative
Therapeutic class: antibiotic
Pregnancy risk category: B

Indications and dosages

▶ **Infections caused by sensitive staphylococci, streptococci, pneumococci, *Bacteroides, Fusobacterium, Clostridium perfringens,* and other sensitive aerobic and anaerobic organisms.** *Adults:* 150 to 450 mg P.O. q 6 hours. Or 600 to 2,700 mg I.M. or I.V. daily divided into two to four doses. Don't exceed 600 mg in one I.M. dose. Don't give more than 1.2 g I.V. in a 1-hour period. Maximum adult I.V. dosage is 4.8 g daily.
Children ages 1 month to 16 years: 8 to 25 mg/kg P.O. daily in three or four equally divided doses. Or 20 to 40 mg/kg I.M. or I.V. daily, in three or four equally divided doses, or 350 to 450 mg/m² daily.
Neonates younger than age 1 month: 15 to 20 mg/kg I.V. daily in three or four equally divided doses.
▶ **Endocarditis prophylaxis for dental procedures in patients allergic to penicillin.** *Adults:* 600 mg P.O. 1 hour before procedure or 600 mg I.V. 30 minutes before procedure.
Children ages 1 month to 16 years: 20 mg/kg P.O. 1 hour before procedure or 20 mg/kg I.V. 30 minutes before procedure (not to exceed adult dosage).
▶ **Acne vulgaris.** *Adults:* Apply a thin film of topical suspension, gel, or lotion to affected areas b.i.d. Or apply foam to skin once daily after washing with mild soap and water. Cover affected areas completely and massage in until foam disappears. Or, 150 mg P.O. b.i.d.‡
▶ **Bacterial vaginosis.** *Adults:* One applicatorful intravaginally h.s. daily for 3 to 7 days per

prescriber instructions. Or, 1 suppository intravaginally h.s. daily for 3 days.
▶ ***Pneumocystis jiroveci (carinii)* pneumonia‡.** *Adults:* 600 mg I.V. q 6 hours. Or 300 to 450 mg P.O. q.i.d. With primaquine, give 30 mg P.O. daily for 21 days.
▶ **Toxoplasmosis (cerebral or ocular) in immunocompromised patients‡.** *Adults:* 300 to 450 mg P.O. q 6 to 8 hours with pyrimethamine (25 to 75 mg once daily) and leucovorin (10 to 25 mg once daily).
Infants and children age 16 and younger: 20 to 30 mg/kg P.O. daily in four divided doses with oral pyrimethamine (1 mg/kg daily) and oral leucovorin (5 mg once q 3 days).

▼ I.V. administration

● For I.V. infusion, dilute each 300 mg in 50 ml solution.
● Give no faster than 30 mg/minute (over 10 to 60 minutes). Never give undiluted as bolus.
● Check I.V. site daily for phlebitis and irritation.
⊗ **Incompatibilities**
Allopurinol; aminophylline; ampicillin; azithromycin; barbiturates; calcium gluconate; ceftriaxone; ciprofloxacin hydrochloride; filgrastim; fluconazole; idarubicin; magnesium sulfate; phenytoin sodium; rubber closures, such as those on I.V. tubing; tobramycin sulfate.

Contraindications and cautions

● Contraindicated in patients hypersensitive to drug or lincomycin.
● Use cautiously in patients with renal or hepatic disease, asthma, history of GI disease, or significant allergies.
🜲 **Lifespan:** Breast-feeding women should stop breast-feeding. In neonates, use cautiously.

Adverse reactions

CNS: *headache.*
CV: thrombophlebitis.
EENT: pharyngitis.
GI: abdominal pain, anorexia, *bloody or tarry stools,* constipation, *diarrhea, dysphagia,* esophagitis, flatulence, *nausea, pseudomembranous colitis,* unpleasant or bitter taste, vomiting.
GU: UTI, vaginal discharge.
Hematologic: eosinophilia, *thrombocytopenia, transient leukopenia.*
Skin: maculopapular rash, urticaria.

Other: *anaphylaxis;* erythema, pain (I.V. use); *induration, pain, sterile abscess* (I.M. use).

Interactions

Drug-drug. *Erythromycin:* May block clindamycin site of action. Avoid using together.
Kaolin: May decrease absorption of oral clindamycin. Separate doses.
Neuromuscular blockers: May potentiate neuromuscular blockade. Monitor patient closely.

Effects on lab test results

• May increase bilirubin, AST, alkaline phosphatase, and CK levels.
• May increase eosinophil count. May decrease WBC and platelet counts.

Pharmacokinetics

Absorption: Rapid and almost complete when given P.O. Good after I.M. administration. Minimal vaginal absorption.
Distribution: Widely to most body tissues and fluids (except CSF). Drug is about 93% bound to proteins.
Metabolism: Partially, to inactive metabolites.
Excretion: 10% unchanged in urine; rest as inactive metabolites. *Half-life:* 2½ to 3 hours; 1½ to 2½ hours for cream.

Route	Onset	Peak	Duration
P.O.	Unknown	45–60 min	Unknown
I.V.	Immediate	Immediate	Unknown
I.M.	Unknown	3 hr	Unknown
Topical	Unknown	Unknown	Unknown
Vaginal	Unknown	10–14 hr	20–24 hr

Action

Chemical effect: Inhibits bacterial protein synthesis by binding to 50S subunit of ribosome.
Therapeutic effect: Hinders or kills susceptible bacteria.

Available forms

clindamycin hydrochloride
Capsules: 75 mg, 150 mg, 300 mg
clindamycin palmitate hydrochloride
Oral solution: 75 mg/5 ml
clindamycin phosphate
Foam, topical: 1%
Gel, lotion, topical suspension: 1%
Injection: 150 mg/ml

Vaginal cream: 2%
Vaginal suppository: 100 mg

Assessment

• Assess patient's infection before and regularly throughout therapy.
• Before giving first dose, obtain specimen for culture and sensitivity tests. Begin therapy pending results.
• Monitor renal, hepatic, and hematopoietic functions during prolonged therapy.
• Be alert for adverse reactions and drug interactions.
• If adverse GI reactions occur, monitor patient's hydration.
• Assess patient's and family's knowledge of drug therapy.

Nursing diagnoses

• Infection related to presence of bacteria susceptible to drug
• Risk for deficient fluid volume related to drug-induced adverse GI reactions
• Deficient knowledge related to drug therapy

Planning and implementation

• Don't refrigerate reconstituted oral solution because it will thicken. Drug is stable for 2 weeks at room temperature.
• Give capsule form with full glass of water to prevent dysphagia.
• For I.M. injection, inject deeply. Rotate sites. Warn patient that I.M. injection may be painful. Doses over 600 mg per injection aren't recommended.
• I.M. injection may raise CK in response to muscle irritation.
ALERT: Don't give opioid antidiarrheals to treat drug-induced diarrhea; they may prolong and worsen diarrhea.
ALERT: Because of a link to severe and even fatal colitis, give clindamycin only for serious infections.
Patient teaching
• Teach patient how to store oral solution.
• Tell patient to take entire amount prescribed even after he feels better.
• Warn patient that I.M. injection may be painful.
ALERT: Inform patient that vaginal cream contains mineral oil, which may weaken the rubber

latex of condoms or contraceptive diaphragms. Tell patient not to rely on such products while taking drug and for 5 days afterward. Contraceptive and sexually transmitted disease protection may be impaired.
• Instruct patient to report diarrhea and to avoid self-treatment because of the risk of life-threatening pseudomembranous colitis.
• Tell patient receiving drug I.V. to report discomfort at infusion site.

☑ Evaluation

• Patient is free from infection after drug therapy.
• Patient maintains adequate hydration during drug therapy.
• Patient and family state understanding of drug therapy.

clobetasol propionate
(kloh-BAY-tah-sol PRO-pee-uh-nayt)
Cormax, Dermovate*, Embeline E, Temovate, Temovate Emollient, Olux

Pharmacologic class: topical corticosteroid
Therapeutic class: anti-inflammatory
Pregnancy risk category: C

Indications and dosages

▶ **Inflammation and pruritus from moderate to severe corticosteroid-responsive dermatoses.** *Adults:* Apply a thin layer to affected skin areas b.i.d., once in the morning and once at night. Limit therapy to 14 days, with no more than 50 g cream or ointment or 50 ml lotion (25 mg total) weekly.
▶ **Inflammation and pruritus from moderate to severe corticosteroid-responsive dermatoses of the scalp; short-term topical therapy for mild to moderate plaque-type psoriasis of nonscalp regions, excluding the face and intertriginous areas.** *Adults:* Apply a small amount of Olux foam, up to a maximum of a golf ball-sized dollop, to affected skin b.i.d., once in the morning and once at night. Limit therapy to 14 days, with no more than 50 g of foam weekly.

Contraindications and cautions

• Contraindicated in patients hypersensitive to corticosteroids. Also contraindicated for acne,

rosacea, perioral dermatitis, or as monotherapy for widespread plaque psoriasis.
• Use caution when applying drug to face, groin, or axillae because these areas are at an increased risk for atrophic changes.
• Use cautiously in patients with glaucoma and diabetes.
☀ Lifespan: In pregnant women, avoid use because of possibility of teratogenic effects. In breast-feeding women, use cautiously and avoid applying to breasts because it's unknown whether drug appears in breast milk. In patients younger than age 12, drug isn't recommended. In elderly patients, begin at the low end of the dosage range and adjust carefully.

Adverse reactions

GU: glucosuria.
Metabolic: hyperglycemia.
Skin: burning and stinging sensation, pruritus, irritation, dryness and cracking, erythema, folliculitis, perioral dermatitis, allergic contact dermatitis, hypopigmentation, hypertrichosis, acneiform eruptions, skin atrophy, telangiectasia (dilatation of capillaries), striae.
Other: *hypothalamic-pituitary-adrenal axis suppression,* Cushing's syndrome, numbness of fingers.

Interactions

None reported.

Effects on lab test results

• May increase glucose level.
• May cause false-positive results with adrenocorticotropic hormone (ACTH) stimulation, a.m. cortisol, and urine-free cortisol tests.

Pharmacokinetics

Absorption: Variable, mainly by skin. Increases in areas of skin damage, inflammation, or occlusion. Small amount is systemic.
Distribution: Throughout the local skin. Any drug absorbed systemically is rapidly removed from the blood and goes to muscle, liver, skin, intestines, and kidneys.
Metabolism: Mainly in skin. Small amount in liver to inactive compounds.
Excretion: Drug and active metabolites, in the liver and bile. Inactive metabolites, by the kidneys, mainly as glucuronides and sulfates but also as unconjugated products. Small amounts

of the metabolites are also in urine and feces.
Half-life: Unknown.

Route	Onset	Peak	Duration
Topical	Unknown	Unknown	Unknown

Action

Chemical effect: Unknown. Drug is a high-potency group I fluorinated corticosteroid usually reserved for severe dermatoses that haven't responded to a less potent formulation.
Therapeutic effect: Decreases inflammation and itching.

Available forms

Cream: 0.05%
Foam: 0.05%
Gel: 0.05%
Ointment: 0.05%
Solution: 0.05%

NURSING PROCESS

⚕ Assessment

• Assess patient before and during therapy. Topical corticosteroid therapy may adversely affect and worsen symptoms in patients with diabetes or glaucoma.
• Monitor patient for adverse effects of corticosteroid therapy.
• If applied to face, groin, or axillae, observe often for skin atrophy.
• During long-term use, obtain ACTH stimulation, a.m. cortisol, and urine-free cortisol tests to monitor patient for hypothalamic-pituitary-adrenal (HPA) axis suppression.
• Assess patient's and family's knowledge of drug therapy.

⊕ Nursing diagnoses

• Risk of infection related to prolonged and very potent corticosteroid therapy.
• Impaired skin integrity related to underlying skin disease process
• Situational low self-esteem from underlying skin disease process
• Deficient knowledge related to topical corticosteroid therapy

▶ Planning and implementation

• When applying foam to the scalp, move hair away from the affected area so that the foam can be applied to each affected area.

• Don't use longer than 2 weeks.
• Drug is for external use only. Avoid rubbing eyes during and after application. If drug gets into the eyes, flush affected eye with copious amounts of water.
• Don't dispense directly onto hand because cream and foam will begin to melt immediately upon contact with warm skin. When using foam, invert can and dispense foam into can cap or directly onto the lesion.
• Apply sparingly in light film; then massage into skin gently until foam disappears.
• Don't use occlusive dressings or bandages. Don't cover or wrap treated area unless instructed by prescriber.
• If skin infection develops, give antifungal or antibacterial drugs. If infection doesn't respond promptly, stop drug until infection is under control.
• If irritation, skin infection, striae, or atrophy occurs, stop drug and notify prescriber.
• Drug can suppress HPA axis at doses as low as 2 g daily. If HPA axis suppression occurs, stop giving the drug, reduce the dosage, or substitute a less potent steroid.
• If no improvement occurs within 2 weeks, reassess diagnoses.
• Don't refrigerate. Store drug at room temperature.
Patient teaching
• Advise patient that drug is for external use only and to avoid contact with eyes.
• Instruct patient to use medication only as prescribed.
• Teach patient proper application of the topical steroid to affected area(s). Explain that occlusive dressings aren't recommended and may increase absorption and skin atrophy.
• Inform patient of potential adverse reactions and of signs and symptoms of infection and impaired healing. Urge patient to immediately notify prescriber if any occur.
• Warn patient not to use drug for longer than 14 days.
• Caution patient that foam formulation is flammable and to avoid flames or smoking during and immediately after application.
• Instruct patients using Olux foam that the contents are under pressure and container shouldn't be punctured or incinerated. Also, tell patient not to expose to heat or store at temperatures above 120° F (49° C).

Reactions may be *common*, uncommon, *life-threatening*, or COMMON AND LIFE-THREATENING.

☑ Evaluation
• Patient doesn't suffer from any infection caused by drug therapy.
• Patient is relieved of symptoms and remains free from any adverse effects of drug therapy.
• Patient's self-esteem increases as patient's skin improves.
• Patient and family state understanding of drug therapy.

clofarabine
kloh-FAR-uh-been
Clolar

Pharmacologic classification: purine nucleoside antimetabolite
Therapeutic classification: antineoplastic
Pregnancy risk category: D

Indications and dosages

▶ **Relapsed or refractory acute lymphoblastic leukemia after at least two previous regimens.** *Children ages 1 to 21:* 52 mg/m² by I.V. infusion over 2 hours daily for 5 consecutive days. Repeat about every 2 to 6 weeks based on recovery or return to baseline of organ function. May also give hydrocortisone 100 mg/m² I.V. on days 1 to 3 of cycle to help prevent capillary leak syndrome.

▽ I.V. administration

• Draw up the calculated dose through a 0.2-micron syringe filter and further dilute with D₅W or normal saline solution before infusion.
• Infuse drug within 24 hours of preparing it.
• Give over 2 hours with I.V. fluids.
• Store undiluted vials and resulting infusion solution at room temperature.
⊗ **Incompatibilities**
Don't give drug with other drugs through the same I.V. line.

Contraindications and cautions

• There are no known contraindications.
• Use very cautiously in patients with hepatic or renal dysfunction.
☀ **Lifespan:** In pregnant women, drug may cause fetal harm. Women of childbearing potential should avoid becoming pregnant while receiving this drug. It isn't known whether drug

appears in breast milk. Women shouldn't breast-feed while receiving drug.

Adverse reactions

CNS: *anxiety, depression, dizziness, fatigue, headache, irritability, lethargy, somnolence, tremor.*
CV: *edema, flushing, hypertension, hypotension, left ventricular systolic dysfunction, pericardial effusion, tachycardia.*
EENT: *epistaxis, mucosal inflammation, sore throat.*
GI: *abdominal pain, anorexia, constipation, decreased appetite, decreased weight, diarrhea, gingival bleeding, oral candidiasis, nausea, vomiting.*
GU: *hematuria.*
Hematologic: *bone marrow suppression,* FEBRILE NEUTROPENIA, NEUTROPENIA.
Hepatic: *hepatomegaly, jaundice.*
Musculoskeletal: *arthralgia, back pain, limb pain, myalgia.*
Respiratory: *pneumonia, cough, dyspnea, pleural effusion,* RESPIRATORY DISTRESS.
Skin: *contusion, dermatitis, dry skin, erythema, hand-foot syndrome, petechiae, pruritus.*
Other: BACTEREMIA, *capillary leak syndrome, cellulitis, herpes simplex, injection site pain, pain, pyrexia, rigors,* SEPSIS, *staphylococcal infections, systemic inflammatory response syndrome, transfusion reaction.*

Interactions

Drug-drug. *Blood pressure or cardiac drugs:* May increase the risk of adverse effects. Monitor patient closely.
Hepatotoxic drugs: May increase the risk of hepatic toxicity. Avoid use together.
Nephrotoxic drugs: May decrease excretion of clofarabine. Avoid use during the 5 days of clofarabine treatment.

Effects on lab test results

• May increase ALT, AST, bilirubin, creatinine, and hemoglobin levels and hematocrit.
• May decrease WBC counts and platelet counts.

Pharmacokinetics

Absorption: Given I.V.
Distribution: 47% bound to plasma proteins, mainly albumin.
Metabolism: Limited hepatic metabolism.

Excretion: 49% to 60% in urine unchanged.
Elimination half-life: about 5¼ hours.

Route	Onset	Peak	Duration
I.V.	Unknown	Unknown	Unknown

Action

Chemical effect: Inhibits DNA synthesis and repair and disrupts integrity of mitochondrial membranes, leading to programmed cell death.
Therapeutic effect: Kills selected cancer cells.

Available forms

Injection: 1 mg/ml in 20-ml vials

NURSING PROCESS

Assessment
• Assess patient's underlying condition before therapy and regularly throughout therapy.
• Assess patient for signs and symptoms of tumor lysis syndrome, cytokine release (tachypnea, tachycardia, hypotension, pulmonary edema) that could develop into systemic inflammatory response syndrome, capillary leak syndrome, and organ dysfunction.
• Monitor patient's respiratory status and blood pressure closely during treatment.
• Obtain CBC and platelet counts, and monitor hepatic and renal function regularly during treatment.
• Assess patient's and family's knowledge of drug therapy.

Nursing diagnoses
• Ineffective health maintenance related to underlying condition
• Risk for injury related to drug-induced adverse hematologic reactions
• Deficient knowledge related to drug therapy

Planning and implementation
• Monitor the patient for dehydration. Give I.V. fluids continuously during the 5-day treatment period.
• If you suspect hyperuricemia, give allopurinol.
• If the patient has signs and symptoms of systemic inflammatory response syndrome or capillary leak syndrome, stop drug immediately.
• If hypotension develops, stop the drug. If it resolves without treatment, restart clofarabine at a lower dose.

Patient teaching
• Tell patient and caregiver that adverse effects are common. The patient will need close monitoring during treatment.
• Tell patient and caregiver to report dizziness, light-headedness, fainting, decreased urine output, bruising, flulike symptoms, and infection immediately.
• Urge patient and caregiver to report yellowing of skin or eyes, darkened urine, or abdominal pain.
• Tell a patient of childbearing potential to avoid pregnancy and breast-feeding during therapy.

☑ Evaluation
• Patient demonstrates positive response to drug therapy.
• Patient doesn't experience injury as a result of drug therapy.
• Patient and family state understanding of drug therapy.

clomiphene citrate
(KLOH-meh-feen SIGH-trayt)
Clomid, Milophene, Serophene

Pharmacologic class: chlorotrianisene derivative
Therapeutic class: ovulation stimulant
Pregnancy risk category: X

Indications and dosages

▶ **To induce ovulation.** *Women:* 50 mg P.O. daily for 5 days starting on day 5 of menstrual cycle if bleeding occurs (first day of menstrual flow is day 1), or at any time if woman hasn't had recent uterine bleeding. If ovulation doesn't occur, may increase dosage to 100 mg P.O. daily for 5 days as soon as 30 days after previous course. Repeat until conception occurs or until three courses of therapy are completed.
▶ **Infertility‡.** *Men:* 50 to 400 mg P.O. daily for 2 to 12 months.

Contraindications and cautions

• Contraindicated in patients with undiagnosed abnormal genital bleeding, ovarian cyst not caused by polycystic ovarian syndrome, hepatic disease or dysfunction, uncontrolled thyroid or

adrenal dysfunction, or organic intracranial lesion (such as pituitary tumor).
Lifespan: In pregnant women, drug is contraindicated.

Adverse reactions

CNS: depression, dizziness, fatigue, headache, insomnia, light-headedness, restlessness, tension, *vasomotor flushes.*
CV: hypertension.
EENT: blurred vision, diplopia, photophobia, scotoma.
GI: bloating, distention, nausea, vomiting.
GU: *ovarian enlargement and cyst formation,* which regress spontaneously when drug is stopped; urinary frequency and polyuria.
Metabolic: *hyperglycemia,* increased appetite, weight gain.
Skin: dermatitis, rash, reversible alopecia, urticaria.
Other: breast discomfort.

Interactions

None significant.

Effects on lab test results

- May increase blood glucose level.

Pharmacokinetics

Absorption: Good.
Distribution: May undergo enterohepatic recirculation or may be stored in fat.
Metabolism: By liver.
Excretion: Mainly in feces via biliary elimination. *Half-life:* 5 days.

Route	Onset	Peak	Duration
P.O.	Unknown	Unknown	Unknown

Action

Chemical effect: May stimulate release of pituitary gonadotropins, follicle-stimulating hormone, and luteinizing hormone, resulting in maturation of ovarian follicle, ovulation, and development of corpus luteum.
Therapeutic effect: Induces ovulation.

Available forms

Tablets: 50 mg

NURSING PROCESS

Assessment

- Assess patient's underlying condition before therapy and regularly thereafter.
- Monitor drug's effectiveness by assessing ovulation through biphasic body temperature measurement, postovulatory pregnanediol level in urine, estrogen excretion, and changes in endometrial tissues.
- Be alert for adverse reactions.
- Assess patient's and family's knowledge of drug therapy.

Nursing diagnoses

- Excess fluid volume related to drug-induced fluid retention
- Sexual dysfunction related to underlying condition
- Deficient knowledge related to drug therapy

Planning and implementation

- Prepare administration instructions for patient: Begin daily dose on fifth day of menstrual flow and take for 5 consecutive days.
- Don't give more than three courses of therapy to attempt conception.

Patient teaching

- Tell patient about risk of multiple births and that risk increases with larger doses.
- Teach patient how to take and chart basal body temperature and to ascertain whether ovulation has occurred.
- Reassure woman that ovulation typically occurs after first course of therapy. If pregnancy doesn't occur, course of therapy may be repeated twice.

ALERT: Advise woman to stop taking drug and to contact prescriber immediately if pregnancy is suspected, because drug may have teratogenic effect on fetus.

- Advise woman to stop taking drug and to contact prescriber immediately if abdominal symptoms or pain occur; they may indicate ovarian enlargement or ovarian cyst.
- Tell patient to immediately report signs of impending visual toxicity, such as blurred vision, diplopia, scotoma, or photophobia.
- Warn patient to avoid hazardous activities until the drug's CNS effects are known; drug may cause dizziness or visual disturbances.

☑ Evaluation

- Patient is free from fluid retention at end of therapy.
- Woman ovulates with drug therapy.
- Patient and family state understanding of drug therapy.

clomipramine hydrochloride
(kloh-MIH-pruh-meen high-droh-KLOR-ighd)
Anafranil

Pharmacologic class: tricyclic antidepressant (TCA)
Therapeutic class: obsessive-compulsive disorder (OCD) drug
Pregnancy risk category: C

Indications and dosages

▶ **OCD.** *Adults:* Initially, 25 mg P.O. daily in divided doses with meals, gradually increase to 100 mg daily during first 2 weeks. Then increase to maximum dosage of 250 mg daily in divided doses with meals p.r.n. After adjusting dosage, give total daily dosage at h.s.
Children ages 10 to 18: Initially, 12.5 mg P.O. b.i.d. with meals, gradually increase to daily maximum of 3 mg/kg or 100 mg P.O., whichever is smaller. After adjusting dosage, give total daily dosage at h.s. Reassess and adjust periodically.
▶ **Panic disorder‡.** *Adults:* 12.5 to 150 mg (maximum, 200 mg) daily.

Contraindications and cautions

- Contraindicated in patients hypersensitive to drug or other TCAs, in patients in acute recovery period after MI, and within 14 days of MAO inhibitor therapy.
- Use cautiously in patients with history of seizure disorders or with brain damage; in those receiving other seizure-threshold–lowering drugs; in patients at risk for suicide; in patients with history of urine retention or angle-closure glaucoma, increased intraocular pressure, CV disease, impaired hepatic or renal function, or hyperthyroidism; in patients with tumors of the adrenal medulla; in patients receiving thyroid drug or electroconvulsive therapy; and in those undergoing elective surgery.
- ⚠ **Lifespan:** In pregnant and breast-feeding women, use cautiously.

Adverse reactions

CNS: aggressiveness, asthenia, dizziness, EEG changes, extrapyramidal reactions, fatigue, headache, insomnia, nervousness, myoclonus, *seizures,* somnolence, tremors.
CV: orthostatic hypotension, palpitations, tachycardia.
EENT: abnormal vision, laryngitis, otitis media in children, pharyngitis, rhinitis.
GI: abdominal pain, anorexia, constipation, diarrhea, dry mouth, dyspepsia, eructation, *nausea.*
GU: dysmenorrhea, impaired ejaculation, impotence, urinary hesitancy, UTI.
Hematologic: anemia, bone marrow suppression.
Metabolic: increased appetite, *weight gain.*
Musculoskeletal: *myalgia.*
Skin: *diaphoresis,* dry skin, photosensitivity, pruritus, rash.
Other: altered libido.

Interactions

Drug-drug. *Barbiturates:* May decrease TCA level. Monitor patient for decreased antidepressant effect.
Cimetidine, methylphenidate: May increase TCA level. Monitor patient for increased antidepressant effect.
Clonidine: May cause loss of blood pressure control and potentially life-threatening elevations in blood pressure. Avoid using together.
CNS depressants: May enhance CNS depression. Avoid using together.
Epinephrine, norepinephrine: May increase hypertensive effect. Use with caution, and monitor blood pressure.
MAO inhibitors: May cause hyperpyretic crisis, seizures, coma, or death. Don't use together or within 14 days of each other.
Drug-herb. *St. John's wort:* May raise serotonin level, causing serotonin syndrome. Discourage using together.
Drug-lifestyle. *Alcohol use:* May increase CNS depression. Discourage using together.
Smoking: May increase metabolism and decrease effectiveness. Discourage smoking.
Sun exposure: May cause photosensitivity. Urge patient to avoid sun exposure and to wear protective clothing and sunblock.

Reactions may be *common,* uncommon, *life-threatening*, or COMMON AND LIFE-THREATENING.

Effects on lab test results
• May decrease hemoglobin level and hematocrit.

Pharmacokinetics
Absorption: Good, but extensive first-pass metabolism limits bioavailability to about 50%.
Distribution: Into lipophilic tissues; about 98% bound to proteins.
Metabolism: Mainly hepatic with several metabolites.
Excretion: 66% in urine; remainder in feces.
Half-life: Parent compound, 32 hours; active metabolite, 69 hours.

Route	Onset	Peak	Duration
P.O.	≥ 2 wk	Unknown	Unknown

Action
Chemical effect: Selectively inhibits serotonin reuptake.
Therapeutic effect: Reduces OCD behaviors.

Available forms
Capsules: 25 mg, 50 mg, 75 mg

NURSING PROCESS

Assessment
• Assess patient's underlying condition before therapy and regularly thereafter.
• Assess patient's and family's knowledge of drug therapy.

Nursing diagnoses
• Ineffective coping related to patient's underlying condition
• Risk for injury related to drug-induced adverse reactions
• Deficient knowledge related to drug therapy

Planning and implementation
• During dosage adjustment, divide dose and give with meals to minimize GI effects. After dosage adjustment, give total daily dosage h.s.
• Don't abruptly stop giving the drug.
• Because hypertensive episodes may occur during surgery, taper off drug several days before surgery.
⑤ **ALERT:** Don't confuse clomipramine with chlorpromazine or clomiphene; don't confuse Anafranil with enalapril, nafarelin, or alfentanil.

Patient teaching
• Warn patient to avoid hazardous activities requiring alertness and good psychomotor coordination, especially during dosage adjustment. Daytime sedation and dizziness may occur.
• Tell patient to avoid alcohol while taking drug.
• Warn patient not to abruptly stop taking the drug.
• Advise patient to use sunblock, wear protective clothing, and avoid prolonged exposure to strong sunlight.

☑ Evaluation
• Patient's behavior and communication indicate improvement of obsessive-compulsive pattern.
• Patient doesn't experience injury from drug-induced adverse CNS reactions.
• Patient and family state understanding of drug therapy.

clonazepam
(kloh-NEH-zuh-pam)
Klonopin, Rivotril ♦ ◇

Pharmacologic class: benzodiazepine
Therapeutic class: anticonvulsant, antianxiety drug
Pregnancy risk category: D
Controlled substance schedule: IV

Indications and dosages
▶ **Lennox-Gastaut syndrome; atypical absence seizures; akinetic and myoclonic seizures.** *Adults:* Initially, not to exceed 1.5 mg P.O. t.i.d. May increase by 0.5 to 1 mg q 3 days until seizures are controlled. If given in unequal doses, give largest dose h.s. Maximum daily dosage is 20 mg.
Children age 10 and younger or weighing 30 kg (66 lb) or less: Initially, 0.01 to 0.03 mg/kg P.O. daily (maximum, 0.05 mg/kg daily) in two or three divided doses. Increase by 0.25 to 0.5 mg q third day to maximum maintenance dosage of 0.1 to 0.2 mg/kg daily p.r.n.
▶ **Panic disorder.** *Adults:* Initially, 0.25 mg P.O. b.i.d.; increase to target dose of 1 mg daily after 3 days. Some patients may benefit from doses up to maximum of 4 mg daily. To achieve 4 mg daily, increase dosage in increments of

0.125 to 0.25 mg b.i.d. q 3 days as tolerated until panic disorder is controlled. Stop drug gradually by decreases of 0.125 mg b.i.d. q 3 days until stopped.

▶ **Restless legs syndrome; adjunct in schizophrenia‡.** *Adults:* 0.5 to 2 mg P.O. q h.s.
▶ **Parkinsonian dysarthria‡.** *Adults:* 0.25 to 0.5 mg P.O. daily.
▶ **Acute manic episodes‡.** *Adults:* 0.75 to 16 mg P.O. daily.
▶ **Multifocal tic disorders‡.** *Adults:* 1.5 to 12 mg P.O. daily.
▶ **Neuralgia‡.** *Adults:* 2 to 4 mg P.O. daily.

Contraindications and cautions

• Contraindicated in patients hypersensitive to benzodiazepines and in those with acute angle-closure glaucoma or significant hepatic disease.
• Use cautiously in patients with mixed type of seizure because drug may precipitate generalized tonic-clonic seizures. Also, use cautiously in patients with chronic respiratory disease, or open-angle glaucoma not well controlled.
⚘ **Lifespan:** In pregnant women, use only when benefits to mother outweigh risks to fetus. Breast-feeding women should stop breast-feeding because drug appears in breast milk. In children, use cautiously. In elderly patients, use cautiously and start with low doses because of possible reduced hepatic and renal function.

Adverse reactions

CNS: agitation, *ataxia, behavioral disturbances* (especially in children), confusion, *drowsiness,* migraine, nightmares, psychosis, sleep disorders, slurred speech, **suicidal ideation,** tremor, vertigo.
EENT: abnormal eye movements, diplopia, earache, *increased salivation,* nystagmus, otitis, rhinitis, sinusitis, sore gums.
CV: chest pain, facial and ankle edema, palpitations, postural hypotension, thrombophlebitis.
GI: abnormal thirst, appetite changes, constipation, diarrhea, gastritis, nausea.
GU: dysuria, enuresis, nocturia, urine retention.
Hematologic: eosinophilia, *leukopenia, thrombocytopenia.*
Metabolic: change in appetite.
Musculoskeletal: muscle weakness, pain.
Respiratory: *respiratory depression,* upper respiratory tract infection.
Skin: acne flare, alopecia, contact dermatitis, flushing, rash.

Interactions

Drug-drug. *CNS depressants:* May increase CNS depression. Monitor patient closely.
Fluconazole, ketoconazole, itraconazole, miconazole: May increase and prolong levels, CNS depression, and psychomotor impairment. Don't use together.
Drug-herb. *Catnip, kava, lady's slipper, lemon balm, passion flower, sassafras, skullcap, valerian:* May enhance sedative effects of clonazepam. Discourage using together.
Drug-lifestyle. *Alcohol use:* May cause additive CNS effects. Strongly discourage alcohol use.

Effects on lab test results

• May increase liver function test values and eosinophil count. May decrease WBC and platelet counts.

Pharmacokinetics

Absorption: Good.
Distribution: Wide; 85% protein-bound.
Metabolism: By liver to several metabolites.
Excretion: In urine. *Half-life:* 18 to 50 hours.

Route	Onset	Peak	Duration
P.O.	Unknown	1–2 hr	Unknown

Action

Chemical effect: May act by facilitating effects of inhibitory neurotransmitter GABA.
Therapeutic effect: Prevents or stops seizure activity.

Available forms

Orally disintegrating tablets: 0.125 mg, 0.25 mg, 0.5 mg, 1 mg, 2 mg
Tablets: 0.5 mg, 1 mg, 2 mg

NURSING PROCESS

📋 **Assessment**

• Assess patient's seizure condition before therapy and regularly thereafter.
• Monitor level. Therapeutic level for anticonvulsant effects has been reported to be 20 to 80 nanograms/ml.
• Monitor CBC and liver function tests.
• Be alert for adverse reactions and drug interactions.
• Assess patient's and family's knowledge of drug therapy.

Reactions may be *common,* uncommon, *life-threatening,* or COMMON AND LIFE-THREATENING.

⊕ Nursing diagnoses
• Risk for injury related to potential for seizure activity
• Activity intolerance related to drug-induced sedation
• Deficient knowledge related to drug therapy

⊠ Planning and implementation
• Increase dose gradually.
⊛ **ALERT:** Never stop drug abruptly because seizures may worsen. Follow weaning protocol for safety.
• Withdrawal symptoms are similar to those of barbiturates (insomnia, dysphoria; then abdominal and muscle cramps, tremor, behavioral disorder; progressing to hallucinations, psychosis, convulsions).
• If adverse reactions develop, immediately call prescriber.
• Maintain seizure precautions.
⊛ **ALERT:** Don't confuse Klonopin or clonazepam with clonidine, clozapine, or clomiphene.
Patient teaching
• Advise patient to avoid driving or other potentially hazardous activities until drug's CNS effects are known.
• Instruct parents to monitor child's school performance because drug may interfere with attentiveness.
• Instruct patients using orally disintegrating tablets to use dry hands to peel back foil blister pouch and to place tablet in mouth immediately. The tablet disintegrates rapidly in saliva.
• Instruct patient or family to notify prescriber if oversedation or other adverse reaction develops or questions arise about therapy.
• Advise patients with panic disorder to continue psychotherapeutic interventions in addition to drug therapy.

✓ Evaluation
• Patient is free from seizure activity during drug therapy.
• Patient is able to meet daily activity needs.
• Patient and family state understanding of drug therapy.

---

clonidine hydrochloride
(KLON-uh-deen high-droh-KLOR-ighd)
**Catapres, Catapres-TTS, Dixarit♦ ◇,
Duraclon**

Pharmacologic class: centrally acting sympatholytic
Therapeutic class: antihypertensive
Pregnancy risk category: C

Indications and dosages
▶ **Essential, renal, and malignant hypertension.** *Adults:* Initially, 0.1 mg P.O. b.i.d. Then, increase by 0.1 to 0.2 mg daily q week. Usual dosage range is 0.1 to 0.3 mg b.i.d.; infrequently, dosages as high as 2.4 mg daily are used. Or transdermal patch applied to nonhairy area of intact skin on upper arm or torso q 7 days. Start with 0.1-mg system and adjust after 1 to 2 weeks with another 0.1-mg system or larger system if increases are needed to maintain normal blood pressure.
▶ **Severe pain.** *Adults:* Starting dosage for continuous epidural infusion is 30 mcg/hour. Adjust according to patient's response.
▶ **Prophylaxis for vascular headache‡.**
Adults: 0.025 mg P.O. b.i.d. to q.i.d., up to 0.15 mg P.O. daily in divided doses.
▶ **Adjunctive therapy for nicotine withdrawal‡.** *Adults:* Initially, 0.1 mg P.O. b.i.d., then gradually increase dose by 0.1 mg daily q week, up to 0.75 mg P.O. daily, as tolerated. Alternatively, apply transdermal patch (0.1 to 0.2 mg/24 hours) and replace weekly for the first 2 or 3 weeks after smoking cessation.
▶ **Adjunct in opioid withdrawal‡.** *Adults:* 5 to 17 mcg/kg P.O. daily in divided doses for up to 10 days. Adjust dosage to avoid hypotension and excessive sedation, and slowly withdraw drug.
▶ **Adjunct in menopausal symptoms‡.**
Adults: 0.025 to 0.2 mg P.O. b.i.d. Or apply transdermal patch (0.1 mg/24 hours) and replace weekly.
▶ **Dysmenorrhea‡.** *Adults:* 0.025 mg P.O. b.i.d. for 14 days before onset of menses and during menses.
▶ **Ulcerative colitis‡.** *Adults:* 0.3 mg P.O. t.i.d.
▶ **Diabetic diarrhea‡.** *Adults:* 0.15 to 1.2 mg P.O. daily. Or 1 to 2 patches q week (0.3 mg/24 hours).

▶ **Attention deficit hyperactivity disorder‡.**
Children: Initially, 0.05 mg P.O. q h.s. Increase
cautiously over 2 to 4 weeks to reach maintenance dosage of 0.05 to 0.4 mg daily depending
on the patient's weight and tolerance.

Contraindications and cautions

• Contraindicated in patients hypersensitive to
drug. Transdermal form is contraindicated in patients hypersensitive to any component of adhesive layer. Injectable form is contraindicated in
patients receiving anticoagulation therapy and
patients with a bleeding diathesis or injection-
site infection.
• Use cautiously in patient with severe coronary
insufficiency, recent MI, cerebrovascular disease, and chronic renal or hepatic impairment.
⚖ **Lifespan:** In pregnant women, safety and effectiveness haven't been established. In breast-
feeding women, use cautiously. In children,
safety and effectiveness haven't been established. In children with severe intractable pain
from malignancy that is unresponsive to epidural or spinal opioids or other conventional analgesic techniques, injectable form is restricted.

Adverse reactions

CNS: *anxiety, confusion, dizziness, drowsiness,*
fatigue, headache, nervousness, sedation, *som-
nolence,* vivid dreams.
CV: *bradycardia,* hypotension, orthostatic hy-
potension, *severe rebound hypertension.*
GI: *constipation, dry mouth, nausea, vomiting.*
GU: urine retention, impotence, UTI.
Metabolic: transient glucose intolerance.
Skin: *pruritus and dermatitis* with transdermal
patch.

Interactions

Drug-drug. *Amitriptyline, amoxapine, clomipramine, desipramine, doxepin, imipramine,
nortriptyline, protriptyline, trimipramine:* May
cause loss of blood pressure control with potentially life-threatening elevations in blood pressure. Don't use together.
Beta blockers, such as propranolol: May cause
severe rebound hypertension. Monitor patient
carefully.
CNS depressants: May enhance CNS depression. Use together cautiously.
MAO inhibitors: May decrease antihypertensive
effect. Use together cautiously.

Drug-herb. *Capsicum, yohimbe:* May reduce
antihypertensive effectiveness. Discourage using together.

Effects on lab test results

• May increase glucose and CK levels.

Pharmacokinetics

Absorption: Good.
Distribution: Wide.
Metabolism: Nearly 50% is transformed to in-
active metabolites.
Excretion: 65% in urine; 20% in feces. *Half-
life:* 6 to 20 hours.

Route	Onset	Peak	Duration
P.O.	15–30 min	1½–2½ hr	6–8 hr
Epidural	Immediate	19 min	Unknown
Transdermal	2–3 days	2–3 days	Several days

Action

Chemical effect: May inhibit central vasomotor
centers, decreasing sympathetic outflow to
heart, kidneys, and peripheral vasculature, resulting in decreased peripheral vascular resistance, decreased systolic and diastolic blood
pressure, and decreased heart rate. Produces
analgesia by mimicking the activation of de-
scending pain-suppressing pathways arising
from supraspinal control centers. Also inhibits
the release of substance P, an inflammatory neuropeptide.
Therapeutic effect: Lowers blood pressure and
decreases neurogenic pain.

Available forms

Injectable: 100 mcg/ml, 500 mcg/ml
Tablets: 0.025 mg, 0.1 mg, 0.2 mg, 0.3 mg
Transdermal: TTS-1 (releases 0.1 mg/24
hours), TTS-2 (releases 0.2 mg/24 hours),
TTS-3 (releases 0.3 mg/24 hours)

NURSING PROCESS

📝 **Assessment**
• Assess patient's blood pressure before therapy
and regularly thereafter.
• Antihypertensive effects of transdermal clonidine may take 2 to 3 days to become apparent.
Oral antihypertensive therapy may have to be
continued in interim.
• Be alert for adverse reactions and drug interactions.

Reactions may be *common,* uncommon, *life-threatening*, or COMMON AND LIFE-THREATENING.

- Observe patient for tolerance to drug's therapeutic effects; increase dosage if needed.
- Periodic eye examinations are recommended.
- Monitor site of transdermal patch for dermatitis. Ask patient about pruritus.
- Assess patient's and family's knowledge of drug therapy.

Nursing diagnoses
- Risk for injury related to presence of hypertension
- Ineffective protection related to severe rebound hypertension caused by abrupt cessation of drug
- Deficient knowledge related to drug therapy

Planning and implementation
- Drug may be given to lower blood pressure rapidly in some hypertensive emergency situations.
- Adjust dosage to patient's blood pressure and tolerance.
- Give last dose of day at bedtime.
- Epidural clonidine is more likely to be effective in patients with neuropathic pain than somatic or visceral pain.
- **ALERT:** Injection form is for epidural use only. The 500-mcg/ml dose must be diluted in normal saline for injection to provide a final concentration of 100 mcg/ml.
- When giving by epidural route, carefully monitor infusion pump and inspect catheter tubing for obstruction or dislodgement. Monitor access site for signs of infection or inflammation.
- Monitor patient closely, especially during the first few days of therapy. Respiratory depression or deep sedation may occur.
- To improve adherence of patch, apply adhesive overlay. Place patch at different site each week.
- Remove transdermal patch before defibrillation to prevent arcing.
- When stopping therapy in patients receiving both clonidine and beta blocker, gradually withdraw beta blocker first to minimize adverse reactions.
- Don't stop giving clonidine before surgery.
- **ALERT:** Don't confuse clonidine with quinidine, clozapine, Klonopin, clonazepam, or clomiphene; or Catapres with Cetapred or Combipres.

Patient teaching
- Advise patient not to stop drug abruptly because doing so may cause severe rebound hypertension. Explain that dose must be reduced gradually over 2 to 4 days.
- Tell patient to take the last daily dose immediately before bedtime.
- Reassure patient that transdermal patch usually adheres despite showering and other routine daily activities. Teach him how to use adhesive overlay to improve skin adherence. Also tell patient to place patch at different site each week.
- Caution patient that drug can cause drowsiness, but that he will develop tolerance to this adverse effect.
- Urge patient to rise slowly and avoid sudden position changes to reduce orthostatic hypotension.

Evaluation
- Patient's blood pressure is normal with drug therapy.
- Patient understands not to stop drug abruptly.
- Patient and family state understanding of drug therapy.

clopidogrel bisulfate
(kloh-PIH-doh-grel bigh-SUL-fayt)
Plavix

Pharmacologic class: inhibitor of adenosine diphosphate (ADP)–induced platelet aggregation
Therapeutic class: antiplatelet
Pregnancy risk category: B

Indications and dosages
▶ **Reduce atherosclerotic events in patients with atherosclerosis documented by recent stroke, MI, or peripheral arterial disease.** *Adults:* 75 mg P.O. daily.
▶ **Reduce atherosclerotic events in patients with acute coronary syndrome (unstable angina, non–Q-wave MI), including those managed medically and those who are to be managed with percutaneous coronary intervention (with or without stent) or coronary artery bypass graft.** *Adults:* Start therapy with a single 300-mg P.O. loading dose, then continue at 75 mg P.O. once daily. Also, give 75 to 325 mg aspirin once daily during therapy.

Contraindications and cautions

• Contraindicated in patients hypersensitive to drug or any of its components, and in those with pathologic bleeding, such as peptic ulcer or intracranial hemorrhage.
• Use cautiously in patients with hepatic impairment and in those at risk for increased bleeding from trauma, surgery, or other conditions.
☀ **Lifespan:** In breast-feeding women, drug is contraindicated. In children, safety and effectiveness haven't been established.

Adverse reactions

CNS: depression, dizziness, fatigue, headache, pain.
CV: chest pain, edema, hypertension.
EENT: epistaxis, rhinitis.
GI: abdominal pain, constipation, diarrhea, dyspepsia, gastritis, *hemorrhage,* ulcers.
GU: UTI.
Hematologic: purpura.
Musculoskeletal: arthralgia, back pain.
Respiratory: bronchitis, cough, dyspnea, upper respiratory tract infection.
Skin: rash, pruritus.
Other: flulike symptoms.

Interactions

Drug-drug. *Aspirin, NSAIDs:* May increase risk of GI bleeding. Monitor patient for signs of GI bleeding, such as abdominal pain or blood in vomitus or stool.
Heparin, warfarin: Safety hasn't been established. Use together cautiously, and monitor patient for bleeding.
Drug-herb. *Dong quai, feverfew, garlic, ginger, horse chestnut, red clover:* May increase risk of bleeding. Monitor patient closely.

Effects on lab test results

• May decrease platelet count.

Pharmacokinetics

Absorption: At least 50% and rapid.
Distribution: Highly bound to protein (94% to 98%).
Metabolism: Extensive.
Excretion: 50% in urine and 46% in feces.
Half-life: 8 hours.

Route	Onset	Peak	Duration
P.O.	2 hr	Unknown	5 days

Action

Chemical effect: Inhibits binding of ADP to its platelet receptor, which inhibits ADP-mediated activation and subsequent platelet aggregation. Because drug acts by irreversibly modifying the platelet ADP receptor, platelets exposed to drug are affected for their lifespan.
Therapeutic effect: Prevents clot formation.

Available forms

Tablets: 75 mg

NURSING PROCESS

🕮 Assessment
• Assess current use of OTC drugs, such as aspirin or NSAIDs, and herbal remedies.
• Assess patient for increased bleeding or bruising tendencies before and during drug therapy.
• Assess patient's and family's knowledge of drug therapy.

🔁 Nursing diagnoses
• Risk for injury related to potential for atherosclerotic events from underlying condition
• Ineffective protection related to increased risk of bleeding
• Deficient knowledge related to drug therapy

▶ Planning and implementation
• Five days after stopping drug, expect platelet aggregation to return to normal.
• Don't give drug to a patient with hepatic impairment or an increased risk of bleeding from trauma, surgery, or other pathologic conditions.
⊛ **ALERT:** Don't confuse Plavix with Paxil.
Patient teaching
• Tell patient it may take longer than usual to stop bleeding. Urge him to refrain from activities thatincrease the risk of trauma and bleeding.
• Instruct patient to notify prescriber about unusual bleeding or bruising.
• Tell patient to inform prescriber or dentist that he's taking drug before having surgery or starting new drug therapy.
• Inform patient that drug may be taken with or without food.

✅ Evaluation
• Patient has less risk of stroke, MI, and vascular death.
• Patient states appropriate bleeding precautions to take.

Reactions may be *common,* uncommon, *life-threatening*, or COMMON AND LIFE-THREATENING.

• Patient and family state understanding of drug therapy.

clorazepate dipotassium
(klor-AYZ-eh-payt digh-po-TAH-see-um)
Apo-Clorazepate ♦ , ClorazeCaps, GenENE, Novo-Clopate ♦ , Tranxene, Tranxene-SD, Tranxene T-Tab

Pharmacologic class: benzodiazepine
Therapeutic class: anxiolytic, anticonvulsant, sedative-hypnotic
Pregnancy risk category: D
Controlled substance schedule: IV

Indications and dosages

▶ **Acute alcohol withdrawal.** *Adults:* Day 1 dosage is 30 mg P.O. initially, followed by 30 to 60 mg P.O. in divided doses; day 2 dosage is 45 to 90 mg P.O. in divided doses; day 3 dosage is 22.5 to 45 mg P.O. in divided doses; day 4 dosage is 15 to 30 mg P.O. in divided doses; then gradually reduce dosage to 7.5 to 15 mg daily. Maximum daily dosage is 90 mg.
▶ **Anxiety.** *Adults:* 15 to 60 mg P.O. daily. *Elderly patients:* Initially, 7.5 to 15 mg daily in divided doses or as a single dose.
▶ **Adjunct in partial seizure disorder.** *Adults and children older than age 12:* Maximum recommended initial dosage is 7.5 mg P.O. in divided doses t.i.d. Maximum dosage increase is 7.5 mg weekly; maximum dosage is 90 mg daily.
Children ages 9 to 12: Maximum recommended initial dosage is 7.5 mg P.O. b.i.d. Maximum dosage increase is 7.5 mg weekly; maximum dosage is 60 mg daily.

Contraindications and cautions

• Contraindicated in patients hypersensitive to drug and in those with acute angle-closure glaucoma.
• Use cautiously in patients with suicidal tendencies, renal or hepatic impairment, or history of drug abuse.
• Reduce dosage in debilitated patients.
🜊 **Lifespan:** In pregnant women, especially those in their first trimester, avoid drug. For children younger than age 9, safety and effectiveness haven't been established. In elderly patients, reduce dosage.

Adverse reactions

CNS: *drowsiness,* fainting, *hangover, lethargy,* psychosis, restlessness.
CV: transient hypotension.
EENT: visual disturbances.
GI: abdominal discomfort, dry mouth, nausea, vomiting.
GU: incontinence, urine retention.

Interactions

Drug-drug. *Cimetidine:* May increase sedation. Monitor patient carefully.
CNS depressants: May increase CNS depression. Avoid using together.
Digoxin: May increase digoxin level and risk of toxicity. Monitor digoxin level.
Drug-herb. *Catnip, kava, lady's slipper, lemon balm, passion flower, sassafras,* skullcap, valerian: May enhance sedative effects. Avoid using together.
Drug-lifestyle. *Alcohol use:* May cause additive CNS effects. Strongly discourage alcohol use with these drugs.
Smoking: May increase benzodiazepine clearance. Monitor patient for lack of effect, and discourage smoking.

Effects on lab test results

• May increase liver function test values.

Pharmacokinetics

Absorption: Complete and rapid.
Distribution: Wide. 80% to 95% bound to protein.
Metabolism: In liver to oxazepam.
Excretion: Inactive glucuronide metabolites in urine. *Half-life:* 30 to 200 hours.

Route	Onset	Peak	Duration
P.O.	Unknown	½–2 hr	Unknown

Action

Chemical effect: May facilitate action of inhibitory neurotransmitter GABA. Depresses CNS at limbic and subcortical levels of brain and suppresses spread of seizure activity produced by epileptogenic foci in cortex, thalamus, and limbic structures.
Therapeutic effect: Relieves anxiety, prevents seizure activity, and promotes sleep and calmness.

C

Available forms

Tablets: 3.75 mg, 7.5 mg, 11.25 mg, 15 mg, 22.5 mg

NURSING PROCESS

📖 Assessment

• Assess patient's underlying condition before therapy and regularly thereafter.
• Monitor liver, renal, and hematopoietic function studies periodically in patients receiving repeated or prolonged therapy.
• Be alert for adverse reactions and drug interactions.
• Assess patient's and family's knowledge of drug therapy.

🔷 Nursing diagnoses

• Anxiety related to patient's underlying condition
• Risk of injury related to drug-induced adverse CNS reactions
• Deficient knowledge related to drug therapy

📎 Planning and implementation

• Possibility of abuse and addiction exists. Don't stop drug abruptly after prolonged use. Withdrawal symptoms may occur.
⊗ ALERT: Don't confuse clorazepate with clofibrate.

Patient teaching

• Warn patient to avoid activities that require alertness and good psychomotor coordination until the drug's CNS effects are known.
• Tell patient to avoid alcohol while taking drug.
• Suggest sugarless chewing gum or hard candy to relieve dry mouth.
• Warn patient to take drug only as directed and not to stop without prescriber's approval. Inform patient of drug's potential for dependence if taken longer than directed.

☑ Evaluation

• Patient says he's less anxious after taking drug.
• Patient doesn't experience injury as a result of drug-induced adverse CNS reactions.
• Patient and family state understanding of drug therapy.

clozapine
(KLOH-zuh-peen)
Clozaril, Fazaclo

Pharmacologic class: tricyclic dibenzodiazepine derivative
Therapeutic class: antipsychotic
Pregnancy risk category: B

Indications and dosages

▶ **Schizophrenia in severely ill patients unresponsive to other therapies; reduction in risk of recurrent suicidal behavior in schizophrenia or schizoaffective disorder.** *Adults:* Initially, 12.5 mg P.O. once daily or b.i.d.; increase by 25 to 50 mg daily (if tolerated) to 300 to 450 mg daily by end of 2 weeks. Base dosage on response, patient tolerance, and adverse reactions. Don't increase subsequent doses more than once or twice weekly, and don't exceed 100 mg. Many patients respond to 300 to 600 mg daily, but some may need as much as 900 mg daily. Don't exceed 900 mg daily.
⊘ Adjust-a-dose: In geriatric patients, use lowest recommended dose when starting therapy.

Contraindications and cautions

• Contraindicated in patients taking drugs that suppress bone marrow function and in those with uncontrolled epilepsy, history of drug-induced agranulocytosis, myelosuppressive disorders, severe CNS depression or coma, paralytic ileus, or WBC count below 3,500/mm^3.
• Use cautiously in patients with prostatic hyperplasia, urinary retention, or angle-closure glaucoma because clozapine has potent anticholinergic effects. Also use cautiously in patients receiving general anesthesia and in those with hepatic, renal, or cardiac disease.
🔆 Lifespan: In pregnant women, use cautiously. In breast-feeding women, drug is contraindicated. In children younger than age 12, safety and effectiveness haven't been established. In elderly patients, use cautiously and at lowest recommended dose.

Adverse reactions

CNS: agitation, akathisia, anxiety, ataxia, confusion, depression, disturbed sleep or nightmares, *dizziness, drowsiness,* fatigue, fever, headache, hyperkinesia, hypokinesia or akine-

sia, insomnia, myoclonus, rigidity, *sedation, seizures,* slurred speech, *syncope,* tremor, *vertigo,* weakness.
CV: *cardiomyopathy,* chest pain, ECG changes, hypertension, hypotension, orthostatic hypotension, tachycardia.
GI: constipation, dry mouth, *excessive salivation,* heartburn, nausea, vomiting.
GU: abnormal ejaculation, incontinence, urinary frequency, urinary urgency, urine retention.
Hematologic: *agranulocytosis, leukopenia.*
Metabolic: *severe hyperglycemia,* weight gain.
Musculoskeletal: muscle pain or spasm, muscle weakness.
Skin: rash.

Interactions

Drug-drug. *Anticholinergics:* May increase anticholinergic effects of clozapine. Avoid using together.
Antihypertensives: May increase hypotensive effects. Monitor blood pressure.
Bone marrow suppressants: May increase bone marrow toxicity. Don't use together.
Digoxin, warfarin, other highly protein-bound drugs: May increase levels of these drugs. Monitor patient closely for adverse reactions.
Psychoactive drugs: May produce additive effects. Use together cautiously.
Drug-herb. *St. John's wort:* May reduce drug level, causing a loss of symptom control in patients taking an antipsychotic. Discourage using together.
Drug-food. *Caffeine:* May increase clozapine level. Large fluctuations in caffeine consumption may affect therapeutic response to drug. Advise patient to limit caffeine.
Drug-lifestyle. *Alcohol use:* May increase CNS depression. Discourage using together.
Smoking: May increase metabolism of drug and decrease its effectiveness. Discourage smoking.

Effects on lab test results

• May increase ALT, AST, LDH, and alkaline phosphatase levels. May increase or decrease glucose level.
• May decrease WBC and granulocyte counts.

Pharmacokinetics

Absorption: Rapid.
Distribution: 95% bound to proteins.
Metabolism: Extensive.

Excretion: 50% of drug appears in urine and 30% in feces, mostly as metabolites. *Half-life:* Appears proportional to dose and may range from 8 to 12 hours.

Route	Onset	Peak	Duration
P.O.	Unknown	2½ hr	4–12 hr
P.O. orally disintegrating	Unknown	2½ hr	Unknown

Action

Chemical effect: Unknown. Binds to dopaminergic receptors (both D1 and D2) within limbic system of CNS and may interfere with adrenergic, cholinergic, histaminergic, and serotoninergic receptors.
Therapeutic effect: Relieves psychotic signs and symptoms.

Available forms

Orally disintegrating tablets: 25 mg, 100 mg
Tablets: 12.5 mg, 25 mg, 100 mg

NURSING PROCESS

Assessment
• Assess patient's psychotic condition before therapy and regularly thereafter.
• Monitor patient's baseline WBC and differential counts before therapy and weekly thereafter.
• Be alert for adverse reactions and drug interactions.
• Assess patient for risk factors of diabetes, and obtain baseline fasting blood glucose level. Routinely reassess patient for signs and symptoms of hyperglycemia, and obtain repeat laboratory work.
• After stopping drug, monitor WBC counts weekly for at least 4 weeks, and monitor patient closely for recurrence of psychotic symptoms.
• Assess patient's and family's knowledge of drug therapy.

Nursing diagnoses
• Disturbed thought processes related to patient's underlying condition
• Risk of infection related to potential for drug-induced agranulocytosis
• Deficient knowledge related to drug therapy

⟩ Planning and implementation

• Drug carries significant risk of agranulocytosis. If possible, give at least two trials of a standard antipsychotic before giving this drug.

⑤ **ALERT:** Watch for signs and symptoms of cardiomyopathy, including exertional dyspnea, fatigue, orthopnea, paroxysmal nocturnal dyspnea, and peripheral edema, and report them immediately.

• Use WBC count to help determine if therapy is safe. If WBC count drops below 3,500/mm³ after therapy starts or count drops substantially from baseline, monitor patient closely for signs of infection. If WBC count is 3,000 to 3,500/mm³ and granulocyte count is above 1,500/mm³, obtain WBC and differential counts twice weekly. If WBC count drops below 3,000/mm³ and granulocyte count drops below 1,500/mm³, interrupt therapy, notify prescriber, and monitor patient for signs of infection. If WBC count returns to above 3,000/mm³ and granulocyte count returns to above 1,500/mm³, restart therapy cautiously. Continue monitoring WBC and differential counts twice weekly until WBC count is above 3,500/mm³.

• If WBC count drops below 2,000/mm³ and granulocyte count drops below 1,000/mm³, patient may need protective isolation. If patient develops infection, prepare cultures according to institutional policy and give antibiotics. The prescriber may perform bone marrow aspiration to assess bone marrow function. Future therapy is contraindicated in such patients.

⑤ **ALERT:** Drug may increase risk of fatal myocarditis, especially during, but not limited to, the first month of therapy. In patients in whom myocarditis is suspected (unexplained fatigue, dyspnea, tachypnea, chest pain, tachycardia, fever, palpitations, and other signs or symptoms of heart failure or ECG abnormalities such as ST-T wave abnormalities or arrhythmias), stop therapy immediately and don't rechallenge.

⑤ **ALERT:** If drug must be stopped, withdraw gradually over a 1- to 2-week period. However, changes in patient's medical condition (including development of leukopenia) may require abruptly stopping the drug. Abruptly stopping long-term therapy may cause a sudden recurrence of psychotic symptoms.

• If therapy is restarted, follow usual guidelines for dosage increase. Reexposure to drug may increase severity and risk of adverse reactions. If therapy was stopped for WBC counts below 2,000/mm³ or granulocyte counts below 1,000/mm³, don't restart therapy.

⑤ **ALERT:** If dose has been set for a patient already taking St. John's wort, stopping the herb could increase drug level and cause dangerous toxic symptoms.

• Severe hypoglycemia may occur in a patient without a history of hypoglycemia. Drug may also cause hyperglycemia. Monitor diabetic patient regularly.

• Give patient no more than a 1-week supply of the drug.

• Orally disintegrating tablets contain phenylalanine.

Patient teaching

• Warn patient about risk of agranulocytosis. Tell him drug is available only through special monitoring program that requires weekly blood tests to monitor patient for agranulocytosis. Advise patient to report flulike symptoms, fever, sore throat, lethargy, malaise, or other signs of infection.

• Warn patient that while taking drug he should avoid activities that require alertness and good psychomotor coordination.

• Tell patient to rise slowly to avoid orthostatic hypotension.

• Advise patient to check with prescriber before taking OTC medicines, herbal remedies, or alcohol.

• Teach patient signs and symptoms of hyperglycemia (increased thirst and urination, increased appetite, weakness) and risks of diabetes, which may not resolve when drug is stopped.

• Recommend ice chips or sugarless candy or gum to help relieve dry mouth.

• Tell patient to store orally disintegrating tablets in blister packs and immediately place in his mouth after opening pack. He only needs to allow the tablet to disintegrate and then swallow it, with no need for water.

☑ Evaluation

• Patient demonstrates reduction in psychotic symptoms with drug therapy.

• Patient doesn't develop infection throughout drug therapy.

• Patient and family state understanding of drug therapy.

codeine phosphate
(KOH-deen FOS-fayt)
Paveral ♦

codeine sulfate

Pharmacologic class: opioid
Therapeutic class: analgesic, antitussive
Pregnancy risk category: C
Controlled substance schedule: II

Indications and dosages

▶ **Mild-to-moderate pain.** *Adults:* 15 to 60 mg
P.O. or 15 to 60 mg codeine phosphate by subcutaneous, I.M., or I.V. route q 4 to 6 hours,
p.r.n.
Children older than age 1: 0.5 mg/kg P.O., I.M.,
or subcutaneously q 4 hours, p.r.n.
▶ **Nonproductive cough.** *Adults:* 10 to 20 mg
P.O. q 4 to 6 hours. Maximum daily dosage is
120 mg.
Children ages 6 to 12: 5 to 10 mg P.O. q 4 to
6 hours. Maximum daily dosage is 60 mg.
Children ages 2 to 6: 2.5 to 5 mg P.O. q 4 to
6 hours. Maximum daily dosage is 30 mg.

▼ I.V. administration

• Keep opioid antagonist (naloxone) and resuscitative equipment available.
• Give drug very slowly by direct injection into
large vein.
• Don't give drug to children by I.V. route.
⊗ **Incompatibilities**
Aminophylline, ammonium chloride, amobarbital, bromides, chlorothiazide, heparin, iodides,
pentobarbital, phenobarbital, phenytoin, salts of
heavy metals, sodium bicarbonate, sodium
iodide, thiopental. Don't mix with other drugs.

Contraindications and cautions

• Contraindicated in patients hypersensitive to
drug.
• Use cautiously in debilitated patients and in
patients with head injury, increased intracranial
pressure, increased CSF pressure, hepatic or renal disease, hypothyroidism, Addison's disease,
acute alcoholism, seizures, severe CNS depression, bronchial asthma, COPD, respiratory depression, and shock.

⚹ **Lifespan:** In pregnant and breast-feeding
women, use cautiously. In children, use cautiously. In elderly patients, use cautiously.

Adverse reactions

CNS: *clouded sensorium, dizziness, euphoria,
sedation, seizures.*
CV: *bradycardia,* flushing, hypotension.
GI: *constipation, dry mouth,* ileus, *nausea,
vomiting.*
GU: urine retention.
Respiratory: *respiratory depression.*
Skin: pruritus.
Other: physical dependence.

Interactions

Drug-drug. *CNS depressants, general anesthetics, hypnotics, MAO inhibitors, other opioid
analgesics, sedatives, tranquilizers, tricyclic antidepressants:* May have additive effects. Use
together cautiously. Monitor patient response.
Drug-lifestyle. *Alcohol use:* May have additive
effects. Discourage using together.

Effects on lab test results

• May increase amylase and lipase levels.

Pharmacokinetics

Absorption: Good. Two-thirds as potent orally
as parenterally.
Distribution: Wide.
Metabolism: Mainly in liver.
Excretion: Mainly in urine. *Half-life:* 2½ to
4 hours.

Route	Onset	Peak	Duration
P.O.	10–30 min	1–2 hr	4–6 hr
I.V.	Immediate	Immediate	4–6 hr
I.M.	10–30 min	½–2 hr	4–6 hr
SubQ	10–30 min	Unknown	4–6 hr

Action

Chemical effect: Binds with opiate receptors in
CNS, altering perception of and emotional re-
sponse to pain through unknown mechanism.
Also suppresses cough reflex by direct action on
cough center in medulla.
Therapeutic effect: Relieves pain and cough.

Available forms

codeine phosphate
Injection: 15 mg/ml, 30 mg/ml, 60 mg/ml
Oral solution: 15 mg/5 ml, 10 mg/ml

Soluble tablets: 30 mg, 60 mg
codeine sulfate
Tablets: 15 mg, 30 mg, 60 mg

NURSING PROCESS

℞ Assessment
• Assess patient's pain or cough before and after drug therapy.
• Be alert for adverse reactions and drug interactions.
• Assess patient's and family's knowledge of drug therapy.

⊕ Nursing diagnoses
• Acute pain related to patient's underlying condition
• Fatigue related to presence of cough
• Deficient knowledge related to drug therapy

▶ Planning and implementation
• For full analgesic effect, give drug before patient has intense pain.
• **ALERT:** Codeine is metabolized to morphine by CYP 2D6; this gene may be absent in up to 7% of the population who experience reduced analgesic effect.
• Don't use drug when cough is valuable diagnostic sign or is beneficial (as after thoracic surgery).
• Give drug with food or milk to minimize adverse GI reactions.
• Don't inject discolored solution.
• Codeine is often prescribed with aspirin or acetaminophen to increase pain relief.
• Codeine's abuse potential is much lower than morphine's.
• If patient doesn't experience pain or cough relief, notify prescriber.
• **ALERT:** Don't confuse codeine with Cardene, Lodine, or Cordran.
Patient teaching
• Instruct patient to monitor bowel movements while increasing dietary fiber, fruit, and fluids if possible. Begin stool softener promptly if stool hardens. Patient should notify prescriber of first missed bowel movement and secure instructions for laxative use.
• Advise patient to take oral drug with milk or meals to minimize GI distress.
• Urge patient to ask for or take drug (if at home) before pain becomes severe.

• Warn ambulatory patient that he may feel dizzy when getting out of bed or walking. Tell outpatient to avoid driving and other hazardous activities until drug's CNS effects are known.
• Tell patient to report adverse drug reactions.

☑ Evaluation
• Patient is free of pain after drug administration.
• Patient's cough is suppressed after drug administration.
• Patient and family state understanding of drug therapy.

colchicine
(KOHL-chih-seen)
Colgout ◊

Pharmacologic class: *Colchicum autumnale* alkaloid
Therapeutic class: antigout drug
Pregnancy risk category: C (P.O.), D (I.V.)

Indications and dosages

▶ **To prevent acute gout attacks as prophylactic or maintenance therapy.** *Adults:* 0.6 mg P.O. daily. Give drug 3 to 4 days per week to patients who normally have one attack per year or fewer; give drug daily to patients who have more than one attack per year. In severe cases, 1.2 to 1.8 mg daily.
▶ **To prevent gout attacks in patients undergoing surgery.** *Adults:* 0.6 mg P.O. t.i.d. 3 days before and 3 days after surgery.
▶ **Acute gout, acute gouty arthritis.** *Adults:* Initially, 1.2 mg P.O.; then 0.6 mg q 1 to 2 hours until pain is relieved; nausea, vomiting, or diarrhea ensues; or a maximum dose of 8 mg is reached. Or 2 mg I.V. followed by 0.5 mg I.V. q 6 hours if needed. Or an initial dose of 1 mg I.V. followed by 0.5 mg once or twice daily if needed. Some prescribers prefer to give a single injection of 3 mg I.V. Don't give more than 4 mg for total I.V. dosage over 24 hours (one course). Don't give any further drug (I.V. or P.O.) for 7 days or more.
▶ **Familial Mediterranean fever‡.** *Adults:* 1 to 2 mg P.O. daily in divided doses.
▶ **Hepatic cirrhosis‡.** *Adults:* 1 mg P.O. 5 days weekly.

Reactions may be *common*, uncommon, **life-threatening**, or COMMON AND LIFE-THREATENING.

⧐ **Adjust-a-dose:** For patients with hepatic impairment or creatinine clearance of 10 to 50 ml/minute, decrease dosage by 50%.

▼ I.V. administration

- Don't dilute injection with D_5W injection or other fluids that might change pH of solution. If lower concentration is needed, dilute with normal saline solution or sterile water for injection.
- Preferably, inject into tubing of free-flowing I.V. solution. If diluted solution becomes turbid, don't inject.
- Give drug by slow I.V. push over 2 to 5 minutes. Monitor patient for signs of extravasation.
⊗ **Incompatibilities**
Dextrose 5% injection, bacteriostatic normal saline injection.

Contraindications and cautions

- Contraindicated in patients with serious cardiac disease, renal disease, or GI disorders.
- Use cautiously in debilitated patients, and in patients with early evidence of cardiac, renal, or GI disease.
⚖ **Lifespan:** In pregnant women, use cautiously if at all because fetal harm may occur. In breast-feeding women and in children, safety and effectiveness haven't been established. In elderly patients, use cautiously.

Adverse reactions

CNS: peripheral neuritis.
GI: *abdominal pain, diarrhea, nausea, vomiting.*
Hematologic: *agranulocytosis* (with prolonged use), *aplastic anemia,* nonthrombocytopenic purpura, *thrombocytopenia.*
Hepatic: *hepatic necrosis.*
Skin: alopecia, dermatitis, urticaria.
Other: *anaphylaxis, hypersensitivity reactions,* severe local irritation (if extravasation occurs).

Interactions

Drug-drug. *Loop diuretics:* May decrease effectiveness of colchicine prophylaxis. Avoid using together.
Phenylbutazone: May increase risk of leukopenia or thrombocytopenia. Don't use together.
Vitamin B_{12}: May impair absorption of vitamin B_{12}. Avoid using together.
Drug-lifestyle. *Alcohol use:* May impair effectiveness of drug prophylaxis. Discourage using together.

Effects on lab test results

- May increase alkaline phosphatase, AST, and ALT levels. May decrease carotene, cholesterol, and hemoglobin levels and hematocrit.
- May decrease platelet and granulocyte counts.
- May cause false-positive results in urine tests for hemoglobin and erythrocytes. May interfere with urinary determinations of 17-hydroxycorticosteroids using the Reddy, Jenkins, and Thorn procedure.

Pharmacokinetics

Absorption: Rapid. Unchanged drug may be reabsorbed from intestine by biliary processes.
Distribution: Rapid. Concentrated in leukocytes and distributed into kidneys, liver, spleen, and intestinal tract, but absent in heart, skeletal muscle, and brain.
Metabolism: Partially in liver and also slowly in other tissues.
Excretion: Mainly in feces, with lesser amounts in urine. *Half-life:* 1 to 10½ hours.

Route	Onset	Peak	Duration
P.O.	≤ 12 hr	½–2 hr	Unknown
I.V.	6–12 hr	½–2 hr	Unknown

Action

Chemical effect: May decrease WBC motility, phagocytosis, and lactic acid production, decreasing urate crystal deposits and reducing inflammation. As antiosteolytic drug, apparently inhibits mitosis of osteoprogenitor cells and decreases osteoclast activity.
Therapeutic effect: Relieves gout signs and symptoms.

Available forms

Injection: 0.5 mg/ml
Tablets: 0.5 mg (½₀ grain), 0.6 mg (¹⁄₁₀₀ grain) as sugar-coated granules

NURSING PROCESS

▨ **Assessment**
- Assess patient's underlying condition before therapy and regularly thereafter.
- Before therapy, obtain baseline laboratory studies, including CBC and uric acid level. Repeat regularly.
- Be alert for adverse reactions and drug interactions.

Rapid onset *Liquid form contains alcohol. ◆ Canada ◇ Australia †OTC ✐Photoguide ‡Off-label use

• Assess patient's and family's knowledge of drug therapy.

🔁 Nursing diagnoses
• Acute pain related to presence of gout
• Ineffective protection related to drug-induced hematologic adverse reactions
• Deficient knowledge related to drug therapy

⚡ Planning and implementation
• Give oral form of drug with meals to reduce GI effects. May be used with uricosurics.
• ⚡ ALERT: After a full course of 4 mg I.V., don't give drug by any other route for at least 7 days. Drug is toxic and death can result from overdose.
• Don't give I.M. or subcutaneously because severe local irritation occurs.
• Store drug in tightly closed, light-resistant container.
• Stop drug as soon as gout pain is relieved or at first sign of GI symptoms.
• Force fluids to maintain output at 2,000 ml daily.
Patient teaching
• Teach patient how to take drug.
• Advise patient to report rash, sore throat, fever, unusual bleeding, bruising, fatigue, weakness, numbness, or tingling.
• Tell patient when to stop drug.
• Urge patient not to drink alcohol during drug therapy because it may inhibit drug action.
• Advise patient to avoid all aspirin-containing drugs because they may precipitate gout.

📋 Evaluation
• Patient becomes pain free after drug therapy.
• Patient's CBC and platelet counts remain normal throughout drug therapy.
• Patient and family state understanding of drug therapy.

colesevelam hydrochloride
(koh-leh-SEV-eh-lam high-droh-KLOR-ighd)
Welchol

Pharmacologic class: polymeric bile acid sequestrant
Therapeutic class: antilipemic
Pregnancy risk category: B

Indications and dosages
▶ **Reduction of elevated LDL cholesterol level in patients with primary hypercholesterolemia (Frederickson Type IIa). May be given either alone or with an HMG-CoA reductase inhibitor.** *Adults:* If given alone, give 3 tablets (1,875 mg) P.O. twice daily with meals and liquid or 6 tablets (3,750 mg) once daily with a meal and liquid. Maximum dose is 7 tablets (4,375 mg). If used with an HMG-CoA reductase inhibitor (atorvastatin, fluvastatin, lovastatin, pravastatin, simvastatin), recommended dose is 4 to 6 tablets P.O. daily.

Contraindications and cautions
• Contraindicated in patients hypersensitive to drug or any of its components and in patients with bowel obstruction.
• Use cautiously in patients susceptible to vitamin K deficiency or deficiencies of fat-soluble vitamins. Also use cautiously in patients with dysphagia, swallowing disorders, severe GI motility disorders, and major GI tract surgery. Use cautiously in patients with triglyceride levels above 300 mg/dl because effects aren't known.
❄ **Lifespan:** In pregnant women, use only if clearly needed for risk of fat-soluble vitamin deficiency. In breast-feeding women, use cautiously; drug probably doesn't appear in breast milk because of lack of systemic absorption. In children, safety and effectiveness haven't been established.

Adverse reactions
CNS: asthenia, headache, pain.
EENT: pharyngitis, rhinitis, sinusitis.
GI: abdominal pain, *constipation,* diarrhea, *dyspepsia, flatulence,* nausea.
Musculoskeletal: back pain, myalgia.
Respiratory: increased cough.
Other: accidental injury, *flulike syndrome, infection.*

Interactions
None reported.

Effects on lab test results
• May increase HDL cholesterol and triglyceride levels. May decrease total cholesterol, LDL cholesterol, and apolipoprotein B levels.

Reactions may be *common,* uncommon, *life-threatening,* or COMMON AND LIFE-THREATENING.

Pharmacokinetics

Absorption: Not absorbed.
Distribution: None.
Metabolism: None.
Excretion: Mainly in feces as a complex bound to bile acids. Less than 0.05% of drug in urine.

Route	Onset	Peak	Duration
P.O.	Unknown	2 wk	Unknown

Action

Chemical effect: Binds to bile acids in the intestines and forms a nonabsorbable complex that's eliminated in feces. Partial removal of bile acids from the enterohepatic circulation results in an increased conversion of cholesterol to bile acids in the liver in an attempt to restore the depleted bile acids. The resulting increase in cholesterol causes systemic clearance of circulating LDL level.
Therapeutic effect: Lowers LDL and total cholesterol levels.

Available forms

Tablets: 625 mg

NURSING PROCESS

Assessment

• Rule out secondary causes of hypercholesterolemia before starting drug, such as poorly controlled diabetes, hypothyroidism, nephrotic syndrome, dysproteinemias, obstructive liver disease, other drug therapy, and alcoholism.
• Monitor total cholesterol, LDL, and triglyceride levels before and periodically during therapy.
• Monitor patient's bowel habits. If severe constipation develops, lower the dose and add a stool softener, or stop giving the drug.
• Assess patient's compliance with restricted diet and exercise program adjunctive to antilipemic therapy.
• Evaluate patient's and family's knowledge of drug therapy and importance of diet and exercise regimen.

Nursing diagnoses

• Imbalanced nutrition: more than body requirements of saturated fat and cholesterol related to dietary intake and lack of exercise program

• Risk for constipation related to drug-induced adverse gastrointestinal reactions
• Risk for injury related to presence of elevated LDL cholesterol level
• Deficient knowledge related to antilipemic drug therapy

Planning and implementation

• Give drug with a meal and a liquid.
• If given with an HMG-CoA reductase inhibitor, separate HMG-CoA reductase inhibitor and colesevelam.
• Store drug at room temperature but protect from moisture.

Patient teaching

• Instruct patient to take drug with a meal and a liquid.
• Teach patient to monitor bowel habits. Encourage a diet high in fiber and fluids. Instruct patient to notify prescriber promptly if severe constipation develops.
• Urge patient to follow prescribed diet that's restricted in saturated fat and cholesterol and high in vegetables and fiber. Also discuss and encourage an appropriate exercise program.
• Discuss with patient the importance of regularly monitoring lipid levels.
• Tell patient to notify prescriber if she's pregnant or breast-feeding.

Evaluation

• Patient begins a balanced diet and exercise regimen that's approved by prescriber.
• Patient doesn't suffer adverse GI effect from drug therapy.
• Patient's LDL cholesterol and total cholesterol levels are within normal limits.
• Patient and family state understanding of drug therapy.

corticotropin
(adrenocorticotropic hormone, ACTH)
(kor-teh-koh-TROH-pin)
ACTH, Acthar

repository corticotropin
H.P. Acthar Gel

Pharmacologic class: anterior pituitary hormone
Therapeutic class: diagnostic aid, replacement hormone
Pregnancy risk category: C

Indications and dosages

▶ **Diagnostic test of adrenocortical function.**
Adults and children: 40 units repository form I.M. or subcutaneously q 12 hours for 1 to 2 days. Or, 10 to 25 units aqueous form in 500 ml D_5W I.V. over 8 hours, between blood samplings. Individual dosages vary with adrenal glands' sensitivity to stimulation and with specific disease. Infants and younger children need larger doses per kilogram than older children and adults.

▶ **Inflammation, immunosuppression.**
Adults: 20 units aqueous form subcutaneously or I.M. in four divided doses. Or 40 to 80 units q 24 to 72 hours (repository form).

▼ I.V. administration

• Use aqueous form. Dilute in 500 ml D_5W.
• Infuse over 8 hours.
⊗ **Incompatibilities**
None reported.

Contraindications and cautions

• Contraindicated in patients hypersensitive to pork and pork products and in patients with peptic ulcer, scleroderma, osteoporosis, systemic fungal infections, ocular herpes simplex, peptic ulceration, heart failure, hypertension, adrenocortical hyperfunction or primary insufficiency, or Cushing's syndrome. Also contraindicated in those who have had recent surgery.
• Use cautiously in patients being immunized and in those with latent tuberculosis or tuberculin reactivity, hypothyroidism, cirrhosis, acute gouty arthritis, psychotic tendencies, renal insufficiency, diverticulitis, nonspecific ulcerative colitis, thromboembolic disorders, seizures, uncontrolled hypertension, or myasthenia gravis.
⚘ **Lifespan:** In pregnant women and women of childbearing age, use cautiously. In breast-feeding women, either stop drug or breast-feeding because of risks of ACTH to infant. In children, use cautiously because prolonged use of drug will inhibit skeletal growth. Intermittent administration is recommended.

Adverse reactions

CNS: depression, dizziness, euphoria, headache, *increased intracranial pressure,* insomnia, mood swings, *papilledema,* personality changes, psychosis, *seizures.*
CV: *heart failure,* hypertension, *shock.*
EENT: cataracts, glaucoma.
GI: abdominal distention, nausea, *pancreatitis,* peptic ulceration *(with perforation and hemorrhage),* ulcerative esophagitis, vomiting.
GU: menstrual irregularities.
Metabolic: *activation of latent diabetes mellitus,* calcium and potassium loss, hypokalemic alkalosis, negative nitrogen balance, *sodium and fluid retention,* suppression of growth in children.
Musculoskeletal: loss of muscle mass, muscle weakness, osteoporosis, steroid myopathy, vertebral compression fractures.
Skin: acne, allergic skin reactions, diaphoresis, ecchymoses, facial erythema, hirsutism, hyperpigmentation, impaired wound healing, petechiae, thin and fragile skin.
Other: cushingoid symptoms, *hypersensitivity reactions* (rash, *bronchospasm*), loss of corticotropin stimulatory effect, progressive increase in antibodies.

Interactions

Drug-drug. *Anticonvulsants, barbiturates, rifampin:* May increase metabolism of corticotropin and decrease effectiveness. Monitor patient for lack of effect.
Estrogens: May potentiate cortisol effects. Adjust dosage p.r.n.
NSAIDs, salicylates: May increase risk of GI bleeding. Avoid using together.
Oral anticoagulants: May alter PT. Monitor PT and INR. Adjust dosage p.r.n.
Potassium-wasting diuretics: May increase risk of hypokalemia. Monitor potassium level.

Reactions may be *common,* uncommon, *life-threatening,* or COMMON AND LIFE-THREATENING.

Effects on lab test results

• May increase glucose level. May decrease potassium and calcium levels.

Pharmacokinetics

Absorption: For repository injection, 8 to 16 hours.
Distribution: Unknown.
Metabolism: Unknown.
Excretion: By kidneys. *Half-life:* 15 minutes.

Route	Onset	Peak	Duration
I.V., I.M., SubQ			
aqueous	Rapid	1–2 hr	Unknown
repository	Unknown	3–12 hr	3 days

Action

Chemical effect: By replacing body's own tropic hormone, drug stimulates secretion of adrenal cortex hormones.
Therapeutic effect: Diagnoses or treats adrenocortical hormonal deficiency.

Available forms

Aqueous injection: 25 units/vial, 40 units/vial
Repository injection: 80 units/ml

NURSING PROCESS

Assessment

• Assess patient's underlying condition before and regularly during therapy.
• Before therapy, verify adrenal responsiveness and test for hypersensitivity and allergic reactions.
• Be alert for adverse reactions and drug interactions.
• Note and record weight changes, fluid exchange, and resting blood pressures until minimal effective dosage is achieved.
• Watch neonates of corticotropin-treated mothers for signs of hypoadrenalism.
• Monitor patient for stress.
• Assess patient's and family's knowledge of drug therapy.

Nursing diagnoses

• Ineffective protection related to underlying condition
• Risk for injury related to drug-induced adverse reactions
• Deficient knowledge related to drug test or therapy

Planning and implementation

• Use as adjunct, not sole, therapy. Use oral form in long-term therapy.
• If giving gel, warm it to room temperature, draw into large needle, and give slowly as deep I.M. injection with 21G or 22G needle. Warn patient that injection is painful.
ALERT: Check product label to be certain medication is for I.V. use; corticotropin repository injection is for I.M. or subcutaneous use only.
• Refrigerate reconstituted solution and use within 24 hours.
• Counteract edema with low-sodium, high-potassium intake; nitrogen loss with a high-protein diet; and psychotic changes with a reduction in corticotropin dosage or use of sedatives.
• Unusual stress may require additional use of rapidly acting corticosteroids. Gradually reduce corticotropin dosage to smallest effective dose to minimize induced adrenocortical insufficiency. If stressful situation (trauma, surgery, severe illness) occurs shortly after stopping drug, restart therapy.
ALERT: Don't confuse corticotropin with cosyntropin.

Patient teaching

• Instruct patient to tell physicians and health care professionals besides the prescriber about corticotropin use because stressful situations, such as trauma, surgery, or severe illness, may require adding rapidly acting corticosteroids.
• Tell patient to restrict sodium intake and consume high-protein, high-potassium diet.
• Advise patient to have close follow-up care.
• Warn patient that injections, especially I.M. injections, are painful.

Evaluation

• Patient's underlying condition improves with drug therapy.
• Patient doesn't experience injury as a result of drug-induced adverse reactions.
• Patient and family state understanding of drug therapy.

co-trimoxazole
(sulfamethoxazole-trimethoprim)
(koh-trigh-MOX-uh-zohl)
Apo-Sulfatrim♦, Apo-Sulfatrim DS♦,
Bactrim*, Bactrim DS, Bactrim I.V., Cotrim,
Cotrim DS, Novo-Trimel♦, Novo-Trimel
D.S.♦, Resprim◇, Roubac♦, Septra*,
Septra DS, Septra-I.V., Septrin◇, SMZ-TMP

Pharmacologic class: sulfonamide and folate
antagonist
Therapeutic class: antibiotic
Pregnancy risk category: C (X at term)

Indications and dosages

▶ **UTI, shigellosis.** *Adults:* 160 mg trimetho-
prim/800 mg sulfamethoxazole (double-strength
tablet) P.O. q 12 hours for 10 to 14 days in UTIs
and for 5 days in shigellosis. If indicated, I.V.
infusion is given at 8 to 10 mg/kg daily (based
on trimethoprim component) in two to four
divided doses q 6, 8, or 12 hours for up to
14 days. Maximum trimethoprim dosage is
960 mg daily.
Children age 2 months and older: 8 mg/kg
trimethoprim/40 mg/kg sulfamethoxazole P.O.
daily, in two divided doses q 12 hours (10 days
for UTI; 5 days for shigellosis). If indicated, I.V.
infusion is given at 8 to 10 mg/kg daily (based
on trimethoprim component) in two to four divided doses q 6, 8, or 12 hours. Don't exceed
adult dose.
⃠ **Adjust-a-dose:** In patients with impaired
renal function, if creatinine clearance is 15 to
30 ml/minute, reduce dosage by 50%. Don't use
if creatinine clearance is less than 15 ml/minute.
▶ **Otitis media in patients with penicillin
allergy or penicillin-resistant infection.**
Children and infants age 2 months and older:
8 mg/kg daily (based on trimethoprim component) P.O., in two divided doses q 12 hours for
10 days.
▶ *Pneumocystis jiroveci (carinii)* **pneumonia.**
*Adults, children, and infants age 2 months and
older:* 20 mg/kg trimethoprim/100 mg/kg sulfamethoxazole P.O. daily, in equally divided
doses q 6 hours for 14 days. If indicated, I.V. infusion may be given 15 to 20 mg/kg daily
(based on trimethoprim component) in three or
four divided doses q 6 to 8 hours for up to
14 days.

▶ **Chronic bronchitis.** *Adults:* 160 mg
trimethoprim/800 mg sulfamethoxazole P.O. q
12 hours for 10 to 14 days.
▶ **Traveler's diarrhea.** *Adults:* 160 mg
trimethoprim/800 mg sulfamethoxazole P.O.
b.i.d. for 3 to 5 days. Some patients may require
2 days of therapy or less.
▶ **UTI in men with prostatitis‡.** *Adults:*
160 mg trimethoprim/800 mg sulfamethoxazole
P.O. b.i.d. for 3 to 6 months.
▶ **Prophylaxis of chronic UTI‡.** *Adults:*
40 mg trimethoprim/200 mg sulfamethoxazole
or 80 mg trimethoprim/400 mg sulfamethoxazole P.O. daily or three times weekly for 3 to
6 months.
▶ **Septic agranulocytosis‡.** *Adults:* 2.5 mg/kg
I.V. q.i.d.; for prophylaxis, 80 to 160 mg b.i.d.
▶ **Nocardia infection‡.** *Adults:* 640 mg P.O.
(as trimethoprim component) daily for 7
months.
▶ **Pharyngeal gonococcal infection‡.** *Adults:*
720 mg P.O. (as trimethoprim component) daily
for 5 days.
▶ **Chancroid‡.** *Adults:* 160 mg P.O. b.i.d. (as
trimethoprim component) for 7 days.
▶ **Pertussis‡.** *Adults:* 320 mg P.O. daily (as
trimethoprim component) in two divided doses.
Children: 40 mg/kg P.O. daily in two divided
doses.
▶ **Cholera‡.** *Adults:* 160 mg P.O. b.i.d. (as
trimethoprim component) for 3 days.
⃠ **Adjust-a-dose:** For patients with renal impairment, if creatinine clearance is 15 to 30 ml/
minute, reduce daily dose by 50%. Don't use if
creatinine clearance is less than 15 ml/minute.

▼ I.V. administration

● Dilute contents of 5-ml ampule of drug in
125 ml D_5W before giving. If patient is on a fluid restriction, dilute 5 ml of drug in 75 ml D_5W.
● Infuse slowly over 60 to 90 minutes. Don't
give by rapid infusion or bolus injection.
● Don't refrigerate. Use within 6 hours if diluted in 125 ml and within 2 hours if diluted in
75 ml. If cloudiness or evidence of crystalliza-
tion is noted after mixing, discard solution.
⊗ **Incompatibilities**
All I.V. solutions except D_5W, other I.V. drugs.

Contraindications and cautions

● Contraindicated in patients with megaloblastic
anemia caused by folate deficiency, porphyria,
severe renal impairment (creatinine clearance

less than 15 ml/minute), or hypersensitivity to trimethoprim or sulfonamides.
• Use cautiously and reduce dose in patient with hepatic impairment, a creatinine clearance of 15 to 30 ml/minute, severe allergy or bronchial asthma, G6PD deficiency, or blood dyscrasia.
⚱ **Lifespan:** In pregnant women at term and in breast-feeding women, drug is contraindicated. In infants younger than age 2 months, safety and effectiveness haven't been established.

Adverse reactions

CNS: ataxia, fatigue, hallucinations, headache, insomnia, mental depression, nervousness, *seizures,* vertigo.
CV: thrombophlebitis.
GI: abdominal pain, anorexia, *diarrhea, nausea, stomatitis, vomiting.*
GU: crystalluria, hematuria, *toxic nephrosis with oliguria and anuria.*
Hematologic: *agranulocytosis,* aplastic anemia, hemolytic anemia, *leukopenia,* megaloblastic anemia, *thrombocytopenia.*
Hepatic: *hepatic necrosis,* jaundice.
Musculoskeletal: muscle weakness.
Skin: *epidermal necrolysis, erythema multiforme,* exfoliative dermatitis, generalized skin eruption, photosensitivity, pruritus, *Stevens-Johnson syndrome,* urticaria.
Other: *hypersensitivity reactions* (serum sickness, drug fever, *anaphylaxis*).

Interactions

Drug-drug. *Hormonal contraceptives:* May decrease contraceptive effectiveness and increase risk of breakthrough bleeding. Suggest nonhormonal contraception.
Oral anticoagulants: May increase anticoagulant effect. Monitor patient for bleeding.
Oral antidiabetics: May increase hypoglycemic effect. Monitor glucose level.
Phenytoin: May inhibit hepatic metabolism of phenytoin. Monitor phenytoin level.
Drug-herb. *Dong quai, St. John's wort:* May increase risk of photosensitivity. Advise patient to avoid unprotected exposure to sunlight.
Drug-lifestyle. *Sun exposure:* May cause photosensitivity reactions. Urge patient to avoid sun exposure and wear protective clothing and sunblock.

Effects on lab test results

• May increase BUN, creatinine, aminotransferase, and bilirubin levels. May decrease hemoglobin level and hematocrit.
• May decrease granulocyte, platelet, and WBC counts.

Pharmacokinetics

Absorption: Good.
Distribution: Wide (including middle ear fluid, prostatic fluid, bile, aqueous humor, and CSF). Protein binding is 44% for trimethoprim, 70% for sulfamethoxazole.
Metabolism: By liver.
Excretion: Mainly in urine. *Half-life:* Trimethoprim, 8 to 11 hours; sulfamethoxazole, 10 to 13 hours.

Route	Onset	Peak	Duration
P.O.	Unknown	1–4 hr	Unknown
I.V.	Immediate	Immediate	Unknown

Action

Chemical effect: Sulfamethoxazole inhibits formation of dihydrofolic acid from PABA; trimethoprim inhibits dihydrofolate reductase. Both decrease bacterial folic acid synthesis.
Therapeutic effect: Inhibits susceptible bacteria.

Available forms

Injection: trimethoprim 16 mg and sulfamethoxazole 80 mg/ml (5 ml/ampule)
Oral suspension: trimethoprim 40 mg and sulfamethoxazole 200 mg/5 ml
Tablets: trimethoprim 80 mg and sulfamethoxazole 400 mg; trimethoprim 160 mg and sulfamethoxazole 800 mg

NURSING PROCESS

☑ Assessment

• Assess patient's infection before therapy and regularly thereafter.
• Before giving first dose, obtain specimen for culture and sensitivity tests. Begin therapy pending results.
• Be alert for adverse reactions and drug interactions.
• If adverse GI reaction occurs, monitor patient's hydration.
• Monitor intake and output. Make sure urine output is at least 1,500 ml daily to ensure proper

hydration. Inadequate urine output can lead to crystalluria or tubular deposits of drug.
• Assess patient's and family's knowledge of drug therapy.

✪ Nursing diagnoses
• Infection related to presence of bacteria susceptible to drug
• Risk for deficient fluid volume related to drug-induced adverse GI reactions
• Deficient knowledge related to drug therapy

▷ Planning and implementation
• For maximum absorption, give drug with full glass of water at least 1 hour before or 2 hours after meals. Shake oral suspension thoroughly before giving.
• Never give I.M.
⊛ **ALERT:** Double-check dosage, which may be written as trimethoprim component.
• Note that DS in product name means double strength.
⊛ **ALERT:** Adverse reactions, especially hypersensitivity reactions, rash, and fever, occur more frequently in patients with AIDS.
Patient teaching
• Tell patient to take entire amount of drug exactly as prescribed, even if he feels better.
• Tell patient to take drug with full glass of water and to drink at least 3 to 4 L of water daily.
• Advise patient to avoid exposure to direct sunlight because of risk of photosensitivity reaction.
• Tell patient to report signs of rash, sore throat, fever, or mouth sores because drug may need to be stopped.

☑ Evaluation
• Patient is free from infection after drug therapy.
• Patient maintains adequate hydration after drug therapy.
• Patient and family state understanding of drug therapy.

cyanocobalamin (vitamin B_{12})
(sigh-an-oh-koh-BAH-luh-meen)
Anacobin ♦ , Bedoz ♦ , Big Shot B-$_{12}$, Crystamine, Crysti 1000, Cyanoject, Cyomin, Nascobal

hydroxocobalamin (vitamin B_{12})
Hydro-Cobex, LA-$_{12}$

Pharmacologic class: water-soluble vitamin
Therapeutic class: vitamin, nutrition supplement
Pregnancy risk category: A (C if used in doses above RDA)

Indications and dosages

▶ **RDA for cyanocobalamin.** *Adults and children ages 11 and older:* 2 mcg
Pregnant women: 2.2 mcg
Breast-feeding women: 2.6 mcg
Children ages 7 to 10: 1.4 mcg
Children ages 4 to 6: 1 mcg
Children ages 1 to 3: 0.7 mcg
Infants ages 6 months to 1 year: 0.5 mcg
Neonates and infants younger than age 6 months: 0.3 mcg
▶ **Vitamin B_{12} deficiency caused by inadequate diet, subtotal gastrectomy, or any other condition, disorder, or disease except malabsorption related to pernicious anemia or other GI disease.** *Adults:* 30 mcg hydroxocobalamin I.M. daily for 5 to 10 days, depending on severity of deficiency. Maintenance dosage is 100 to 200 mcg I.M. once monthly. Or 500 mcg intranasally once weekly. For subsequent prophylaxis, advise adequate nutrition and daily RDA vitamin B_{12} supplements.
Children: 1 to 5 mg hydroxocobalamin spread over 2 or more weeks in doses of 100 mcg I.M., depending on severity of deficiency. Maintenance dosage is 30 to 50 mcg I.M. monthly. For subsequent prophylaxis, advise adequate nutrition and daily RDA vitamin B_{12} supplements.
▶ **Pernicious anemia or vitamin B_{12} malabsorption.** *Adults:* Initially, 100 mcg cyanocobalamin I.M. or subcutaneously daily for 6 to 7 days; then 100 mcg I.M. or subcutaneously once monthly.
Children: 30 to 50 mcg I.M. or subcutaneously daily over 2 or more weeks; then 100 mcg I.M. or subcutaneously monthly for life.

▶ **Maintenance treatment for remission of pernicious anemia following I.M. vitamin B_{12} therapy in patients with no nervous system involvement; dietary deficiency, malabsorption disorders, inadequate secretion of intrinsic factor.** *Adults:* Initially, 1 spray in one nostril once weekly. Give at least 1 hour before or 1 hour after ingestion of hot foods or liquids.
▶ **Methylmalonic aciduria.** *Neonates:* 1,000 mcg cyanocobalamin I.M. daily.
▶ **Schilling test flushing dose.** *Adults and children:* 1,000 mcg hydroxocobalamin I.M. as a single dose.

Contraindications and cautions

• Contraindicated in patients with early Leber's disease or hypersensitivity to vitamin B_{12} or cobalt.
• Use cautiously in anemic patients with cardiac, pulmonary, or hypertensive disease and in those with severe vitamin B_{12}-dependent deficiencies.
⚠ **Lifespan:** In premature infants, use cautiously because some products contain benzyl alcohol, which may cause gasping syndrome.

Adverse reactions

CV: *heart failure,* peripheral vascular thrombosis, *pulmonary edema.*
GI: transient diarrhea.
Skin: itching, transitory exanthema, urticaria.
Other: *anaphylactoid reactions, anaphylaxis* (with parenteral use); burning, pain (at subcutaneous or I.M. injection sites).

Interactions

Drug-drug. *Aminoglycosides, chloramphenicol, colchicine, para-aminosalicylic acid and salts:* May cause malabsorption of vitamin B_{12}. Don't use together.
Drug-lifestyle. *Alcohol use:* May cause malabsorption of vitamin B_{12}. Discourage using together.

Effects on lab test results

• May decrease potassium level.
• May cause false-positive results for intrinsic factor antibody test.

Pharmacokinetics

Absorption: After oral use, irregular and dependent on sufficient intrinsic factor and calci-

um. After intranasal, I.M., and subcutaneous use, rapid. Vitamin B_{12} is protein-bound.
Distribution: Into liver, bone marrow, and other tissues.
Metabolism: In liver.
Excretion: Amount of vitamin B_{12} needed by body is reabsorbed; excess in urine. *Half-life:* 6 days.

Route	Onset	Peak	Duration
P.O.	Unknown	8–12 hr	Unknown
I.M.	Unknown	60 min	Unknown
SubQ	Unknown	Unknown	Unknown
Intranasal	Unknown	1–2 hr	Unknown

Action

Chemical effect: Acts as a coenzyme that stimulates metabolic functions. Needed for cell replication, hematopoiesis, and nucleoprotein and myelin synthesis.
Therapeutic effect: Increases vitamin B_{12} level.

Available forms

cyanocobalamin
Injection: 100 mcg/ml, 1,000 mcg/ml
Intranasal: 500 mcg/0.1 ml
Tablets: 25 mcg†, 50 mcg†, 100 mcg†, 250 mcg†, 500 mcg†, 1,000 mcg†
hydroxocobalamin
Injection: 1,000 mcg/ml

NURSING PROCESS

📝 Assessment
• Assess patient's vitamin B_{12} deficiency before therapy.
• Determine reticulocyte count, hematocrit, and B_{12}, iron, and folate levels before therapy starts.
• Monitor drug's effectiveness by assessing patient for improvement in signs and symptoms of vitamin B_{12} deficiency. Also, monitor reticulocyte count, hematocrit, and B_{12}, iron, and folate levels between fifth and seventh day of therapy and periodically thereafter.
• Infection, tumors, and renal, hepatic, or other debilitating diseases may reduce therapeutic response.
• Closely monitor potassium level for first 48 hours. Be alert for adverse reactions and drug interactions.
• Assess patient's and family's knowledge of drug therapy.

🕭 Nursing diagnoses

• Ineffective health maintenance related to underlying vitamin B$_{12}$ deficiency
• Risk for injury related to parenteral administration and drug-induced hypersensitivity reactions
• Deficient knowledge related to drug therapy

⧁ Planning and implementation

• Don't mix parenteral liquids in same syringe with other drugs.
• Drug is physically incompatible with dextrose solutions, alkaline or strongly acidic solutions, oxidizing or reducing drugs, heavy metals, chlorpromazine, phytonadione, prochlorperazine, and many other drugs.
• Hydroxocobalamin is approved for I.M. or deep subcutaneous use only. Its only advantage over cyanocobalamin is its longer duration.
• Don't give large oral doses of vitamin B$_{12}$ routinely because drug is lost through excretion.
• Protect vitamin from light. Don't refrigerate or freeze.
• Give potassium supplement, if needed.
• For intranasal form, prime the nasal device before first use. Repriming between doses isn't needed if the unit is upright.
• Give intranasal spray to one nostril weekly, at least 1 hour before or 1 hour after ingestion of hot foods or liquids.

Patient teaching
• Stress need for patient with pernicious anemia to return for monthly injections. Although total body stores may last 3 to 6 years, anemia will recur without monthly therapy.
• Emphasize importance of well-balanced diet.
• Tell patient to store oral tablets in tightly closed container at room temperature.

☑ Evaluation

• Patient's vitamin B$_{12}$ deficiency is resolved with drug therapy.
• Patient doesn't experience hypersensitivity reactions following parenteral administration of drug.
• Patient and family state understanding of drug therapy.

cyclobenzaprine hydrochloride
(sigh-kloh-BEN-zah-preen high-droh-KLOR-ighd)
Flexeril

Pharmacologic class: tricyclic antidepressant derivative
Therapeutic class: skeletal muscle relaxant
Pregnancy risk category: B

Indications and dosages

▶ **Adjunct to rest and physical therapy for relief of muscle spasm associated with acute, painful musculoskeletal conditions.** *Adults and children 15 and older:* 5 mg P.O. t.i.d. May increase to 10 mg P.O. t.i.d. Usual daily dose range is 20 to 40 mg, to a maximum of 60 mg. Use of cyclobenzaprine for periods longer than 3 weeks isn't recommended.
☒ **Adjust-a-dose:** In elderly patients and in patients with mild hepatic impairment, start with 5 mg and increase slowly. In patients with moderate to severe hepatic impairment, drug isn't recommended.
▶ **Fibrositis‡.** *Adults:* 10 to 40 mg P.O. daily.

Contraindications and cautions

• Contraindicated in patients hypersensitive to drug; in patients in the acute recovery phase of MI; in patients with hyperthyroidism, heart block, arrhythmias, conduction disturbances, or heart failure. Also contraindicated within 14 days of MAO inhibitor therapy.
• Use cautiously in debilitated patients and in patients with history of urine retention, acute angle-closure glaucoma, or increased intraocular pressure. Also use cautiously in patients taking anticholinergics.
⚘ **Lifespan:** In pregnant and breast-feeding women, and in children younger than age 15, safety and effectiveness haven't been established. In elderly patients, use cautiously.

Adverse reactions

CNS: depression, *dizziness, drowsiness,* euphoria, headache, insomnia, nightmares, paresthesia, *seizures,* visual disturbances, weakness.
CV: *arrhythmias,* tachycardia.
EENT: blurred vision.
GI: abdominal pain, abnormal taste, constipation, *dry mouth,* dyspepsia.
GU: urine retention.

Reactions may be *common,* uncommon, *life-threatening*, or COMMON AND LIFE-THREATENING.

Skin: pruritus, rash, urticaria.

Interactions

Drug-drug. *Anticholinergics:* May have additive anticholinergic effects. Avoid using together.
CNS depressants: May cause additive CNS depression. Avoid using together.
MAO inhibitors: May worsen CNS depression or anticholinergic effects. Don't give within 14 days after stopping an MAO inhibitor.
Drug-lifestyle. *Alcohol use:* May cause additive CNS depression. Discourage using together.

Effects on lab test results

None reported.

Pharmacokinetics

Absorption: Almost complete.
Distribution: 93% protein-bound.
Metabolism: During first pass, drug and metabolites undergo enterohepatic recycling.
Excretion: Mainly in urine as conjugated metabolites; also in feces via bile as unchanged drug. *Half-life:* 1 to 3 days.

Route	Onset	Peak	Duration
P.O.	≤1 hr	3–8 hr	12–24 hr

Action

Chemical effect: Unknown.
Therapeutic effect: Relieves muscle spasms.

Available forms

Tablets: 5 mg, 10 mg

NURSING PROCESS

⚖ Assessment
• Assess patient's underlying condition before therapy.
• Monitor the drug's effectiveness by assessing severity and frequency of the patient's muscle spasms.
• If drug is stopped abruptly after long-term use, watch for nausea, headache, and malaise.
• Assess patient's and family's knowledge of drug therapy.

⊞ Nursing diagnoses
• Acute pain related to presence of muscle spasms

• Risk for injury related to potential for drug-induced CNS adverse reactions
• Deficient knowledge related to drug therapy

▶ Planning and implementation
⊛ **ALERT:** Watch for symptoms of overdose, including cardiac toxicity. If you suspect toxicity, keep physostigmine available, and notify prescriber immediately.
• Don't give drug with other CNS depressants.
• With high doses, watch for adverse reactions similar to those of other TCAs.
⊛ **ALERT:** Don't confuse cyclobenzaprine with cyproheptadine.

Patient teaching
• Advise patient to report urinary hesitancy or urine retention. If constipation occurs, tell patient to increase fluid intake and suggest use of a stool softener.
• Caution patient not to split generic 10-mg tablets because the active ingredient may not split evenly.
• Warn patient to avoid activities that require alertness until drug's CNS effects are known.
• Warn patient to avoid using alcohol or other CNS depressants.
• Suggest sugarless chewing gum or hard candy to relieve dry mouth.

☑ Evaluation
• Patient is free from pain with drug therapy.
• Patient doesn't experience injury as a result of drug-induced adverse CNS reactions.
• Patient and family state understanding of drug therapy.

cyclophosphamide
(sigh-kloh-FOS-fuh-mighd)
Cycloblastin ◇ , Cytoxan, Cytoxan Lyophilized, Endoxan-Asta ◇ , Neosar, Procytox ◆

Pharmacologic class: alkylating drug
Therapeutic class: antineoplastic
Pregnancy risk category: D

Indications and dosages

▶ **Breast, head, neck, prostate, lung, and ovarian cancers; Hodgkin's disease; chronic lymphocytic leukemia; chronic myelocytic leukemia; acute lymphoblastic leukemia;**

acute myelocytic leukemia; neuroblastoma; retinoblastoma; malignant lymphoma; multiple myeloma; mycosis fungoides; sarcoma. *Adults and children:* Initially, 40 to 50 mg/kg I.V. in divided doses over 2 to 5 days. Or 10 to 15 mg/kg I.V. q 7 to 10 days, 3 to 5 mg/kg I.V. twice weekly, or 1 to 5 mg/kg P.O. daily, based on patient tolerance. Adjust dosage according to evidence of antitumor activity or leukopenia.

▶ **"Minimal change" nephrotic syndrome in children.** *Children:* 2.5 to 3 mg/kg P.O. daily for 60 to 90 days.

▶ **Polymyositis** ‡. *Adults:* 500 mg I.V. over 1 hour every 1 to 3 weeks, alone or with corticosteroids.

▶ **Rheumatoid arthritis**‡. *Adults:* 1.5 to 3 mg/kg P.O. daily.

▶ **Wegener's granulomatosis**‡. *Adults:* 1 to 2 mg/kg P.O. daily (usually given with prednisone).

▼ I.V. administration

● Preparing and giving I.V. form of drug cause carcinogenic, mutagenic, and teratogenic risks. Follow facility policy to reduce risks.
● Reconstitute powder using sterile water for injection or bacteriostatic water for injection that contains only parabens. For nonlyophilized product, add 5 ml to 100-mg vial, 10 ml to 200-mg vial, 25 ml to 500-mg vial, 50 ml to 1-g vial, or 100 ml to 2-g vial to produce solution containing 20 mg/ml. Shake to dissolve. Shaking may take up to 6 minutes because it may be difficult to completely dissolve drug. Lyophilized preparation is much easier to reconstitute. Check package insert for quantity of diluent needed to reconstitute drug.
● Check reconstituted solution for small particles. Filter solution if needed.
● Give by direct I.V. injection or infusion. For I.V. infusion, further dilute with D_5W, dextrose 5% in normal saline solution, dextrose 5% in Ringer's injection, lactated Ringer's injection, sodium lactate injection, or half-normal saline solution for injection.
● Reconstituted solution is stable for 6 days refrigerated or 24 hours at room temperature. However, use stored solutions cautiously because drug contains no preservatives.
⊗ **Incompatibilities**
None known.

Contraindications and cautions

● Contraindicated in patients with severe bone marrow depression.
● Use cautiously in patients who have recently undergone radiation therapy or chemotherapy and in patients with leukopenia, thrombocytopenia, malignant cell infiltration of bone marrow, or hepatic or renal disease.
☀ **Lifespan:** In pregnant women, use cautiously, if at all, because fetal harm may occur. In breast-feeding women, drug is contraindicated.

Adverse reactions

CV: *cardiotoxicity* (with very high doses and with doxorubicin).
GI: anorexia, mucositis, nausea and vomiting beginning within 6 hours, stomatitis.
GU: bladder fibrosis, gonadal suppression (may be irreversible), STERILE HEMORRHAGIC CYSTITIS.
Hematologic: *anemia; leukopenia,* nadir between days 8 and 15, recovery in 17 to 28 days; *thrombocytopenia.*
Metabolic: hyperuricemia.
Respiratory: *pulmonary fibrosis* (with high doses).
Skin: reversible alopecia in 50% of patients, especially with high doses.
Other: *anaphylaxis, secondary malignancies,* SIADH (with high doses), sterility.

Interactions

Drug-drug. *Barbiturates:* May increase drug effect and cyclophosphamide toxicity by inducing hepatic enzymes. Avoid using together.
Cardiotoxic drugs: May cause additive adverse cardiac effects. Avoid using together.
Chloramphenicol, corticosteroids: May reduce activity of cyclophosphamide. Use cautiously and monitor patient.
Digoxin: May decrease digoxin level. Monitor level closely and adjust dosage p.r.n.
Succinylcholine: May prolong neuromuscular blockade. Avoid using together.

Effects on lab test results

● May increase uric acid level. May decrease pseudocholinesterase and hemoglobin levels and hematocrit.
● May decrease WBC, RBC, and platelet counts.

Pharmacokinetics

Absorption: Almost complete with doses of 100 mg or less. Higher doses are 75% absorbed.
Distribution: Throughout body, with minimal amounts in saliva, sweat, and synovial fluid. Active metabolites are about 50% bound to proteins.
Metabolism: Metabolized to its active form by hepatic microsomal enzymes.
Excretion: Mainly in urine, with 5% to 30% as unchanged drug. *Half-life:* 3 to 12 hours.

Route	Onset	Peak	Duration
P.O., I.V.	Unknown	1 hr	Unknown

Action

Chemical effect: Cross-links strands of cellular DNA and interferes with RNA transcription, causing imbalance of growth that leads to cell death.
Therapeutic effect: Kills specific types of cancer cells; improves renal function in mild nephrotic syndrome in children.

Available forms

Injection: 100-mg, 200-mg, 500-mg, 1-g, 2-g vials
Tablets: 25 mg, 50 mg

NURSING PROCESS

Assessment

• Assess patient's underlying condition before and regularly during therapy.
• Monitor CBC, uric acid level, and renal and liver function tests.
• If corticosteroid therapy is stopped, monitor patient for cyclophosphamide toxicity.
• Be alert for adverse reactions and drug interactions.
• Assess patient's and family's knowledge of drug therapy.

Nursing diagnoses

• Ineffective health maintenance related to underlying condition
• Risk for injury related to drug-induced adverse reactions
• Deficient knowledge related to drug therapy

Planning and implementation

• Tablets are used for children with "minimal change" nephrotic syndrome, not to treat neoplastic disease.
• To prevent hyperuricemia with resulting uric acid nephropathy, allopurinol may be used with adequate hydration.

Patient teaching

• Warn patient that alopecia is likely to occur but is reversible.
• Warn patient to watch for evidence of infection (fever, sore throat, fatigue) and bleeding (easy bruising, nosebleeds, bleeding gums, melena) and to take temperature daily.
• Instruct patient to avoid OTC products that contain aspirin.
• Encourage patient to void every 1 to 2 hours while awake and to drink at least 3 L of fluid daily to minimize risk of hemorrhagic cystitis. Tell patient not to take drug at bedtime because infrequent urination during night may increase possibility of cystitis. If cystitis occurs, tell patient to stop drug and notify prescriber. Cystitis can occur months after therapy ends. Mesna may be given to lower risk and severity of bladder toxicity.
• Advise both men and women to practice contraception while taking drug and for 4 months after because drug is potentially teratogenic.
• Advise women of childbearing age to avoid becoming pregnant during therapy. Also recommend consulting with prescriber before becoming pregnant.

Evaluation

• Patient shows positive response to drug therapy.
• Patient doesn't experience injury as a result of drug-induced adverse reactions.
• Patient and family state understanding of drug therapy.

cycloserine
(sigh-kloh-SER-een)
Seromycin

Pharmacologic class: isoxazoline, D-alanine analogue
Therapeutic class: antituberculotic
Pregnancy risk category: C

Indications and dosages

▶ **Adjunct in pulmonary or extrapulmonary tuberculosis.** *Adults:* Initially, 250 mg P.O. q 12 hours for 2 weeks; then, if level is below 25 to 30 mcg/ml and no toxicity has developed, 250 mg q 8 hours for 2 weeks. If optimum blood level isn't achieved and no toxicity has developed, increase to 250 mg q 6 hours. Maximum dosage is 1 g daily. If CNS toxicity occurs, stop drug for 1 week and then resume at 250 mg daily for 2 weeks. If no serious toxic effects occur, increase by 250-mg increments q 10 days until level is 25 to 30 mcg/ml.

Contraindications and cautions

• Contraindicated in patients hypersensitive to drug, patients who consume excessive amounts of alcohol, and patients with seizure disorders, depression, severe anxiety, psychosis, or severe renal insufficiency.
• Use cautiously in patients with renal impairment, and reduce dosage.
⚘ **Lifespan:** In pregnant and breast-feeding women, use cautiously. In children, safety and effectiveness haven't been established.

Adverse reactions

CNS: *coma,* confusion, *depression,* drowsiness, dysarthria, *hallucinations,* headache, hyperirritability, hyperreflexia, memory loss, *nervousness,* paresis, paresthesia, *seizures, suicidal tendencies* and other psychotic symptoms, tremor, vertigo.
Other: hypersensitivity reactions (allergic dermatitis).

Interactions

Drug-drug. *Ethionamide, isoniazid:* May increase risk of CNS toxicity (seizures, dizziness, or drowsiness). Monitor patient closely.
Phenytoin: May increase phenytoin level. Adjust phenytoin dosage p.r.n.
Drug-lifestyle. *Alcohol use:* May increase risk of CNS toxicity. Advise patient to refrain from alcohol consumption during therapy.

Effects on lab test results

• May increase transaminase level.

Pharmacokinetics

Absorption: About 80%.
Distribution: Widely into body tissues and fluids, including CSF. Doesn't bind to proteins.

Metabolism: Possibly partial.
Excretion: Mainly in urine. *Half-life:* 10 hours.

Route	Onset	Peak	Duration
P.O.	Unknown	3–4 hr	Unknown

Action

Chemical effect: Inhibits cell-wall biosynthesis by interfering with bacterial use of amino acids (bacteriostatic).
Therapeutic effect: Aids in eradicating tuberculosis.

Available forms

Capsules: 250 mg

NURSING PROCESS

▨ **Assessment**
• Assess patient's underlying condition before therapy.
• Obtain specimen for culture and sensitivity tests before therapy begins and periodically thereafter to detect resistance.
• Monitor drug's effectiveness by evaluating culture and sensitivity results; watch for improvement in patient's underlying condition.
• Monitor cycloserine level periodically, especially in patients receiving high doses (more than 500 mg daily) because toxic reactions may occur with blood level above 30 mcg/ml.
• Monitor results of hematologic tests and renal and liver function studies.
• Be alert for adverse reactions and drug interactions.
• Assess patient's and family's knowledge of drug therapy.

▦ **Nursing diagnoses**
• Ineffective health maintenance related to presence of tuberculosis
• Risk for injury related to drug-induced CNS adverse reactions
• Deficient knowledge related to drug therapy

▷ **Planning and implementation**
• Always give with other antituberculotics to prevent development of resistant organisms. Drug is considered second-line treatment for tuberculosis
• Adjust dose according to level, toxicity, or effectiveness.

• Give pyridoxine, anticonvulsants, tranquilizers, or sedatives to relieve adverse reactions.
• Pyridoxine may prevent neurotoxicity.
⑤ ALERT: Don't confuse cycloserine with cyclophosphamide or cyclosporine.

Patient teaching
• Warn patient to avoid alcohol, which may cause serious neurologic reactions.
• Instruct patient to take drug exactly as prescribed, and warn against stopping drug without prescriber's approval.
• Stress importance of having laboratory studies done to monitor drug effectiveness and toxicity.

☑ Evaluation
• Patient maintains health after drug therapy.
• Patient has no injury as a result of drug-induced adverse reactions.
• Patient and family state understanding of drug therapy.

cyclosporine (cyclosporin)
(sigh-kloh-SPOOR-een)
Neoral, Sandimmun◇, Sandimmune

cyclosporine, modified
Gengraf

Pharmacologic class: polypeptide antibiotic
Therapeutic class: immunosuppressant
Pregnancy risk category: C

Indications and dosages

▶ **To prevent organ rejection in kidney, liver, or heart transplantation.** *Adults and children:* 15 mg/kg P.O. 4 to 12 hours before transplantation and continued daily postoperatively for 1 to 2 weeks. Reduce dosage by 5% each week to maintenance level of 5 to 10 mg/kg daily. Or 5 to 6 mg/kg I.V. concentrate 4 to 12 hours before transplantation. Postoperatively, repeat dosage daily until patient can tolerate P.O. forms. When converting from Sandimmune to Gengraf, use same daily dose as previously used for Sandimmune. Monitor level q 4 to 7 days after converting, and monitor blood pressure and creatinine level q 2 weeks during the first 2 months.
▶ **Severe, active rheumatoid arthritis that hasn't adequately responded to methotrexate.** *Adults:* 1.25 mg/kg Gengraf or Neoral P.O.

b.i.d. Increase dosage by 0.5 to 0.75 mg/kg daily after 8 weeks and again after 12 weeks to a maximum of 4 mg/kg daily. If no response is seen after 16 weeks, stop therapy.
▶ **Recalcitrant plaque psoriasis that isn't adequately responsive to at least one systemic therapy or in patients for whom other systemic therapy is contraindicated or isn't tolerated.** *Adults:* Initially, 2.5 mg/kg Gengraf or Neoral P.O. daily divided b.i.d. Maintain initial dose for 4 weeks. Increase by 0.5 mg/kg daily to a maximum of 4 mg/kg daily at 2-week intervals, p.r.n.
🔲 **Adjust-a-dose:** For patients with hypertension, a creatinine level 30% above pretherapy level, or abnormal CBC or liver function test results, decrease dosage by 25% to 50%. If creatinine level is 25% above pretherapy level, repeat creatinine measurement within 2 weeks. If creatinine level stays 25% to 50% above baseline, reduce dosage by 25% to 50%. If creatinine level 50% above baseline, reduce dosage by 25% to 50%. If creatinine level isn't reversed after two dosage modifications, stop therapy.

▼ I.V. administration
• Give drug I.V. to patients who can't tolerate oral drugs.
• Dilute each milliliter of concentrate in 20 to 100 ml of D_5W or normal saline solution for injection. Dilute immediately before infusion; infuse over 2 to 6 hours.
• Give I.V. concentrate at one-third oral dose and dilute before use.
• Protect I.V. solution from light.
⊗ **Incompatibilities**
None reported.

Contraindications and cautions
• Contraindicated in patients hypersensitive to drug or to polyoxyethylated castor oil (found in injectable form). Neoral and Gengraf are contraindicated in patients with psoriasis or rheumatoid arthritis who also have renal impairment, uncontrolled hypertension, or malignancies.
🔆 **Lifespan:** In pregnant women, use cautiously. In breast-feeding women, safety and effectiveness haven't been established.

Adverse reactions
CNS: headache, *seizures,* tremor.
CV: flushing, hypertension.

EENT: sinusitis.
GI: diarrhea, *gum hyperplasia,* nausea, oral thrush, vomiting.
GU: NEPHROTOXICITY.
Hematologic: anemia, LEUKOPENIA, THROMBOCYTOPENIA.
Hepatic: *hepatotoxicity.*
Skin: acne, *hirsutism.*
Other: *anaphylaxis,* infections.

Interactions

Drug-drug. *Aminoglycosides, amphotericin B, co-trimoxazole, NSAIDs:* May increase risk of nephrotoxicity. Monitor patient for toxicity.
Amphotericin B, cilastatin, cimetidine, diltiazem, erythromycin, imipenem, ketoconazole, metoclopramide, prednisolone: May increase level of cyclosporine. Monitor patient for increased toxicity.
Azathioprine, corticosteroids, cyclophosphamide, verapamil: May increase immunosuppression. Monitor patient closely for infection.
Carbamazepine, isoniazid, phenobarbital, phenytoin, rifampin: May decrease immunosuppressant effect. Increase cyclosporine dosage.
Vaccines: May decrease immune response. Postpone routine immunization.
Drug-food. *Grapefruit:* May increase drug level and cause toxicity. Discourage using together.
Drug-herb. *Pill-bearing spurge:* May inhibit CYP 3A enzymes affecting drug metabolism. Discourage using together.
St. John's wort: May significantly lower drug level and contribute to organ rejection. Discourage using together.

Effects on lab test results

• May increase BUN, creatinine, LDL, bilirubin, AST, ALT, and glucose levels. May decrease hemoglobin level and hematocrit.
• May decrease WBC and platelet counts.

Pharmacokinetics

Absorption: Varies widely. Only 30% of Sandimmune oral dose reaches systemic circulation, while 60% of Neoral reaches systemic circulation. Gengraf absorption is 10% to 89%, depending on patient population.
Distribution: Wide. 90% is protein-bound.
Metabolism: Extensive, in liver.

Excretion: Mainly in feces. *Half-life:* 10 to 27 hours.

Route	Onset	Peak	Duration
P.O.	Unknown	1½–3 hr	Unknown
I.V.	Unknown	Unknown	Unknown

Action

Chemical effect: Inhibits proliferation of T lymphocytes.
Therapeutic effect: Prevents organ rejection.

Available forms

Capsules: 25 mg, 50 mg, 100 mg
Capsules for microemulsion: 25 mg, 100 mg.
Injection: 50 mg/ml
Oral solution: 100 mg/ml

NURSING PROCESS

⚖ Assessment
• Assess patient's organ transplant before therapy.
• Monitor drug effectiveness by evaluating patient for signs and symptoms of organ rejection.
• Check drug level at regular intervals.
• Monitor BUN and creatinine levels because nephrotoxicity may develop 2 to 3 months after transplant surgery and require reducing the dose.
• Monitor liver function tests for hepatotoxicity, which usually occurs during first month after transplant.
• Monitor CBC and platelet counts regularly.
• Be alert for adverse reactions and drug interactions.
• Assess patient's and family's knowledge of drug therapy.

⊞ Nursing diagnoses
• Risk for injury related to potential for organ rejection
• Ineffective protection related to drug-induced immunosuppression
• Deficient knowledge related to drug therapy

▶ Planning and implementation
• Don't give psoralen plus ultraviolet A or ultraviolet B therapy, methotrexate, other immunosuppressants, coal tar, or radiation therapy to psoriasis patient taking Neoral or Gengraf.
• Always give drug with adrenal corticosteroids.

Reactions may be *common,* uncommon, *life-threatening,* or COMMON AND LIFE-THREATENING.

• Measure oral dose carefully in oral syringe. To increase palatability, mix with whole milk, chocolate milk, or fruit juice (except grapefruit juice). Oral solution for emulsion is less palatable when mixed with milk. Use glass container to minimize adherence to container walls.

• Give drug with meals to minimize GI distress.

🖲 **ALERT:** Sandimmune and Neoral aren't bioequivalent and can't be used interchangeably without prescriber supervision. When switching from Neoral to Sandimmune, increase monitoring to detect inadequate doses. Gengraf is bioequivalent to and interchangeable with Neoral capsules.

• Before giving drug to patient with rheumatoid arthritis, measure blood pressure at least twice and obtain two creatinine levels to estimate baseline. Evaluate patient's blood pressure and creatinine level every 2 weeks during first 3 months, then monthly if patient is stable. Monitor blood pressure and creatinine level after an increase in NSAID dosage or introduction of a new NSAID. If hypertension occurs, decrease dosage of Gengraf or Neoral by 25% to 50%. If hypertension persists, decrease dosage further or control blood pressure with antihypertensives.

• If patient also receives methotrexate, monitor CBC and liver function tests monthly.

• For patient with psoriasis, watch for occult infection and tumors before and throughout therapy.

• Before starting therapy in psoriasis patient, take blood pressure at least twice and obtain two creatinine levels. Also, obtain CBC and BUN, magnesium, uric acid, potassium, and lipid levels. Evaluate blood pressure, CBC, uric acid, creatinine, BUN, potassium, lipid, and magnesium levels every 2 weeks for the first 3 months, then monthly if patient is stable, or more frequently when adjusting dose. Reduce dose by 25% to 50% in case of significant abnormality.

• Monitor blood pressure and creatinine level after an increase in NSAID dosage or introduction of a new NSAID.

🖲 **ALERT:** Don't confuse cyclosporine with cyclophosphamide or cycloserine.

🖲 **ALERT:** Don't confuse Sandimmune with Sandoglobulin or Sandostatin.

Patient teaching

• Encourage patient to take drug at the same time each day.

• Advise patient to take Neoral on an empty stomach and not to mix with grapefruit juice.

• Advise patient to take with meals if drug causes nausea. Anorexia, nausea, and vomiting are usually transient and most common at the start of therapy.

• Tell patient not to stop taking drug without prescriber's approval.

• Instruct patient to swish and swallow nystatin four times daily to prevent oral thrush.

• Instruct patient on infection control and bleeding precautions, as indicated by CBC and platelet count results.

🗹 **Evaluation**

• Patient doesn't experience organ rejection while taking drug.

• Patient is free from infection and serious bleeding episodes throughout drug therapy.

• Patient and family state understanding of drug therapy.

cytarabine
(ara-C, cytosine arabinoside)
(sigh-TAR-uh-been)
Cytosar♦, Cytosar-U, Tarabine PFS

Pharmacologic class: antimetabolite
Therapeutic class: antineoplastic
Pregnancy risk category: D

Indications and dosages

▶ **Acute nonlymphocytic leukemia.** *Adults and children:* 100 mg/m²/day by continuous I.V. infusion (days 1 to 7) or 100 mg/m² I.V. q 12 hours (days 1 to 7). Give with other anticancer drugs.

▶ **Acute lymphocytic leukemia.** Consult literature for current recommendations.

▶ **Refractory acute leukemia.** *Adults and children:* 3 g/m² I.V. over 2 hours q 12 hours for 4 to 12 doses (repeated at 2- to 3-week intervals).

▶ **Meningeal leukemia.** *Adults and children:* Highly variable from 5 to 75 mg/m² intrathecally. Frequency also varies from once a day for 4 days to once q 4 days. Most common dosage is 30 mg/m², q 4 days until CSF is normal, followed by one more dose.

▼ I.V. administration

• Preparing and giving I.V. form are linked to carcinogenic, mutagenic, and teratogenic risks. Follow facility policy to reduce risks.
• To reduce nausea, give antiemetic before drug. Nausea and vomiting are more frequent when large doses are given rapidly by I.V. push. These reactions are less frequent when given by infusion. Dizziness may occur with rapid infusion.
• Reconstitute drug using provided diluent, which is bacteriostatic water for injection containing benzyl alcohol. Avoid this diluent when preparing drug for neonates or for intrathecal use. Reconstitute 100-mg vial with 5 ml of diluent or 500-mg vial with 10 ml of diluent. Reconstituted solution is stable for 48 hours. Discard cloudy reconstituted solution.
• For I.V. infusion, further dilute using normal saline solution for injection, D_5W, or sterile water for injection.

⊗ **Incompatibilities**
Allopurinol sodium, fluorouracil, ganciclovir sodium, heparin sodium, insulin (regular), methylprednisolone sodium succinate, nafcillin, oxacillin, penicillin.

Contraindications and cautions

• Contraindicated in patients hypersensitive to drug.
• Use cautiously in patients with hepatic disease.
⚖ **Lifespan:** In pregnant women, drug isn't recommended because fetal harm may occur. In breast-feeding women, drug is contraindicated.

Adverse reactions

CNS: neurotoxicity, including ataxia and cerebellar dysfunction (with high doses).
EENT: keratitis, nystagmus.
GI: *anal ulceration, anorexia, constipation,* diarrhea, *nausea, vomiting,* dysphagia, projectile vomiting from large I.V. dose given rapidly, reddened area at juncture of lips followed by sore mouth and oral ulcers in 5 to 10 days.
GU: urate nephropathy.
Hematologic: anemia; *leukopenia,* with initial WBC count nadir 7 to 9 days after drug is stopped and second (more severe) nadir 15 to 24 days after drug is stopped; reticulocytopenia; *thrombocytopenia,* with platelet count nadir occurring on day 10; *megaloblastosis.*
Hepatic: *hepatotoxicity* (usually mild and reversible).
Metabolic: hyperuricemia.

Skin: rash.
Other: *anaphylaxis,* flulike syndrome.

Interactions

Drug-drug. *Digoxin:* May decrease digoxin level. Monitor digoxin level.
Flucytosine: May decrease flucytosine activity. Monitor patient closely.
Gentamicin: May decrease activity against *Klebsiella pneumoniae.* Avoid using together.

Effects on lab test results

• May increase uric acid level. May decrease hemoglobin level and hematocrit.
• May increase megaloblasts. May decrease WBC, RBC, platelet, and reticulocyte counts.

Pharmacokinetics

Absorption: Good.
Distribution: Rapid and wide; 13% of drug is bound to proteins. Drug penetrates the blood–brain barrier only slightly after rapid I.V. dose; however, when drug is given by continuous I.V. infusion, CSF level reaches 40% to 60% of plasma level.
Metabolism: Mainly in liver but also in kidneys, GI mucosa, and granulocytes.
Excretion: In urine. Less than 10% of dose as unchanged drug in urine. *Half-life:* Initial, 8 minutes; terminal, 1 to 3 hours; in CSF, 2 hours.

Route	Onset	Peak	Duration
I.V., intrathecal	Unknown	Unknown	Unknown
SubQ	Unknown	20–60 min	Unknown

Action

Chemical effect: Inhibits DNA synthesis.
Therapeutic effect: Kills selected cancer cells.

Available forms

Injection: 100-mg, 500-mg, 1-g, 2-g vials

NURSING PROCESS

🗒 **Assessment**
• Assess patient's underlying condition before and regularly throughout therapy.
• Monitor uric acid level, hepatic and renal function studies, and CBC.
• Be alert for adverse reactions and drug interactions.

• If patient receives high doses, watch for neurotoxicity, which may first appear as nystagmus but can progress to ataxia and cerebellar dysfunction.
• Assess patient's and family's knowledge of drug therapy.

⊕ Nursing diagnoses
• Ineffective health maintenance related to underlying condition
• Risk for injury related to drug-induced adverse hematologic reactions
• Deficient knowledge related to drug therapy

▶ Planning and implementation
• When giving intrathecally, use preservative-free normal saline solution. Add 5 ml to 100-mg vial or 10 ml to 500-mg vial. Use immediately after reconstitution. Discard unused drug.
• Maintain high fluid intake and give allopurinol to avoid urate nephropathy in leukemia induction therapy.
• If granulocyte count is below 1,000/mm³ or if platelet count is below 50,000/mm³, modify or stop therapy.
• Corticosteroid eyedrops are prescribed to prevent drug-induced keratitis.
• Potential benefit must be judged against known adverse effects.
Patient teaching
• Warn patient to watch for signs of infection (fever, sore throat, fatigue) and bleeding (easy bruising, nosebleeds, bleeding gums, melena). Tell patient to take temperature daily.
• Instruct patient on infection control and bleeding precautions.
• Advise woman of childbearing age to avoid becoming pregnant during therapy. Also recommend consulting with prescriber before becoming pregnant.
• Encourage patient to drink at least 3 L of fluids daily.
• Instruct patient about need for frequent oral hygiene.

☑ Evaluation
• Patient demonstrates positive response to drug therapy.
• Patient doesn't experience injury as result of drug therapy.
• Patient and family state understanding of drug therapy.

cytomegalovirus immune globulin, intravenous (CMV-IGIV)
(sigh-toh-meh-GEH-loh-VIGH-rus ih-MYOON GLOH-byoo-lin)
CytoGam

Pharmacologic class: immune globulin
Therapeutic class: immune serum
Pregnancy risk category: C

Indications and dosages

▶ To attenuate primary CMV disease in seronegative kidney transplant recipients who receive kidney from a CMV seropositive donor. *Adults:* Give I.V. based on time after transplantation:
Within 72 hours: 150 mg/kg
2 weeks after: 100 mg/kg
4 weeks after: 100 mg/kg
6 weeks after: 100 mg/kg
8 weeks after: 100 mg/kg
12 weeks after: 50 mg/kg
16 weeks after: 50 mg/kg.
Give first dose at 15 mg/kg/hour. If no adverse reactions occur after 30 minutes, increase to 30 mg/kg/hour. If no adverse reactions occur after another 30 minutes, increase to 60 mg/kg/hour. Don't exceed 75 ml/hour. Subsequent doses may be given at 15 mg/kg/hour for 15 minutes, increasing at 15-minute intervals in stepwise fashion to 60 mg/kg/hour. Don't exceed 75 ml/hour. Monitor patient closely during and after rate change.
▶ Prophylaxis of CMV disease related to lung, liver, pancreas, and heart transplants. *Adults:* Use with ganciclovir in organ transplants from CMV seropositive donors into seronegative recipients. Maximum total dose per infusion is 150 mg/kg I.V. Give as follows based on time after transplantation:
Within 72 hours: 150 mg/kg
2 weeks after: 150 mg/kg
4 weeks after: 150 mg/kg
6 weeks after: 150 mg/kg
8 weeks after: 150 mg/kg
12 weeks after: 100 mg/kg
16 weeks after: 100 mg/kg.
Give first dose at 15 mg/kg/hour. If no adverse reactions occur after 30 minutes, increase rate to 30 mg/kg/hour. If no adverse reactions occur after another 30 minutes, increase infu-

sion to 60 mg/kg/hour. (Don't exceed 75 ml/hour.) Subsequent doses may be given at 15 mg/kg/hour for 15 minutes, increasing q 15 minutes in a stepwise fashion to a maximum of 60 mg/kg/hour. (Don't exceed 75 ml/hour.) Monitor patient closely during and after each rate change.

▼ I.V. administration

• Remove tab portion of vial cap and clean rubber stopper with 70% alcohol or equivalent. Don't shake vial; avoid foaming. Don't infuse if the solution has color or particulate matter or is turbid. Don't predilute.
• Give through separate I.V. line using constant infusion pump. Filters aren't needed. If unable to give through separate line, piggyback into existing line of saline solution injection or one of the following dextrose solutions with or without saline solution: dextrose 2.5% in water, D_5W, dextrose 10% in water, or dextrose 20% in water. Don't dilute more than 1:2 with any of these solutions.
• Begin infusion within 6 hours of entering vial; finish within 12 hours.
• Refrigerate drug at 36° to 46° F (2° to 8° C).
⊗ **Incompatibilities**
Other I.V. drugs.

Contraindications and cautions

• Contraindicated in patients with selective immunoglobulin (Ig)A deficiency or history of sensitivity to other human immunoglobulin preparations.
🌿 **Lifespan:** In pregnant women, use cautiously. In breast-feeding women and in children, safety and effectiveness haven't been established.

Adverse reactions

CNS: fever.
CV: flushing, hypotension.
GI: nausea, vomiting.
Musculoskeletal: back pain, muscle cramps.
Respiratory: wheezing.
Other: *anaphylaxis,* chills.

Interactions

Drug-drug. *Live-virus vaccines:* May interfere with immune response to live-virus vaccines. Defer vaccination for at least 3 months.

Effects on lab test results

None reported.

Pharmacokinetics

Absorption: Given I.V.
Distribution: Unknown.
Metabolism: Unknown.
Excretion: Unknown. *Half-life:* Immediately after transplantation, 8 days; 60 or more days after transplantation, 13 to 15 days.

Route	Onset	Peak	Duration
I.V.	Unknown	Unknown	Unknown

Action

Chemical effect: Supplies relatively high concentration of IgG antibodies against CMV. Increasing these antibody levels in CMV-exposed patients may reduce risk of serious CMV disease.
Therapeutic effect: Provides passive immunity to CMV.

Available forms

Solution for injection: 50 (± 10) mg (of protein) per ml

NURSING PROCESS

🔖 Assessment

• Assess patient's underlying condition before therapy starts.
• Take vital signs before starting therapy, mid-infusion, post-infusion, and before any increase in infusion rate.
• Monitor drug's effectiveness by evaluating kidney function.
• Be alert for adverse reactions and drug interactions.
• Assess patient's and family's knowledge of drug therapy.

🔷 Nursing diagnoses

• Risk for injury related to potential for organ rejection
• Decreased cardiac output related to drug-induced hypotension
• Deficient knowledge related to drug therapy

▶ Planning and implementation

• If patient develops anaphylaxis or if blood pressure drops, stop infusion, notify prescriber, and give CPR and drugs, such as diphenhydramine and epinephrine.
Patient teaching
• Teach patient about drug therapy.

Reactions may be *common,* uncommon, *life-threatening*, or COMMON AND LIFE-THREATENING.

• Instruct patient to notify prescriber immediately if adverse reactions develop.

☑ **Evaluation**
• Patient doesn't reject transplanted kidney during drug therapy.
• Patient maintains normal cardiac output throughout drug therapy.
• Patient and family state understanding of drug therapy.

dacarbazine
(deh-KAR-buh-zeen)
DTIC-Dome ♦

Pharmacologic class: alkylating drug
Therapeutic class: antineoplastic
Pregnancy risk category: C

Indications and dosages
▶ **Metastatic malignant melanoma.** *Adults:* 2 to 4.5 mg/kg I.V. daily for 10 days; then q 4 weeks, as tolerated. Or, 250 mg/m² I.V. daily for 5 days; repeat at 3-week intervals.
▶ **Hodgkin's disease.** *Adults:* 150 mg/m² I.V. daily (with other drugs) for 5 days; repeat q 4 weeks. Or, 375 mg/m² on first day of combined regimen; repeat q 15 days.

▼ I.V. administration
• Preparing and giving drug raises risk of carcinogenic, mutagenic, and teratogenic effects for staff. Follow facility policy to reduce risks.
• Reconstitute drug with sterile water for injection. Add 9.9 ml to 100-mg vial or 19.7 ml to 200-mg vial. Solution should be colorless to clear yellow. For infusion, further dilute, using up to 250 ml of normal saline solution or D₅W. Infuse over 30 minutes.
• During infusion, protect bag from direct sunlight to avoid drug breakdown. Dilute solution further or slow infusion to decrease pain at infusion site.
• If infiltration occurs, stop infusion immediately, apply ice to area for 24 to 48 hours, and notify prescriber.

• Reconstituted solutions are stable for 8 hours at room temperature under normal lighting conditions and up to 3 days if refrigerated. Diluted solutions are stable for 8 hours at room temperature under normal light and up to 24 hours if refrigerated. If solutions turn pink, this is a sign of decomposition. Discard drug.
⊗ **Incompatibilities**
Allopurinol sodium, cefepime, hydrocortisone sodium succinate, piperacillin with tazobactam.

Contraindications and cautions
• Contraindicated in patients hypersensitive to drug.
• Use cautiously in impaired bone marrow function.
⚹ **Lifespan:** In pregnant women, use cautiously and only when absolutely needed because fetal harm may occur. In breast-feeding women, drug is contraindicated. In children, safety and effectiveness haven't been established.

Adverse reactions
GI: *anorexia, severe nausea and vomiting.*
Hematologic: *leukopenia, thrombocytopenia* (nadir at 3 to 4 weeks).
Metabolic: hyperuricemia.
Skin: alopecia, phototoxicity.
Other: *anaphylaxis, flulike syndrome,* severe pain with concentrated solution or extravasation, tissue damage.

Interactions
Drug-drug. *Allopurinol:* May have additive hypouricemic effects. Monitor patient closely.
Anticoagulants, aspirin: May increase risk of bleeding. Avoid using together.
Bone marrow suppressants: May increase toxicity. Monitor hematologic studies closely.
Phenobarbital, phenytoin, and other drugs that induce hepatic metabolism: May increase dacarbazine metabolism. Adjust dosage.
Drug-lifestyle. *Sun exposure:* May cause photosensitivity reactions, especially during the first 2 days of therapy. Advise patient to avoid prolonged sun exposure and to wear protective clothing and sunblock.

Effects on lab test results
• May increase BUN and liver enzyme levels.
• May decrease WBC, RBC, and platelet counts.

Pharmacokinetics

Absorption: Given I.V.
Distribution: May localize in body tissues, especially the liver; minimally bound to proteins.
Metabolism: Rapid to several compounds, some of which may be active.
Excretion: About 30% to 45% in urine. *Half-life:* Initial, 19 minutes; terminal, 5 hours.

Route	Onset	Peak	Duration
I.V.	Unknown	Unknown	Unknown

Action

Chemical effect: May cross-link strands of cellular DNA and interfere with RNA transcription, causing imbalance of growth that leads to cell death.
Therapeutic effect: Kills selected cancer cells.

Available forms

Injection: 100-mg, 200-mg, 500-mg, 600-mg ♦ vials

NURSING PROCESS

Assessment
• Obtain history of patient's underlying disease before therapy, and reassess regularly throughout therapy.
• Monitor CBC, platelet count, and liver enzyme levels.
• Look for adverse reactions and drug interactions.
• Assess patient's and family's knowledge of drug therapy.

Nursing diagnoses
• Ineffective health maintenance related to presence of neoplastic disease
• Risk for injury related to risk of drug-induced adverse reactions
• Deficient knowledge related to drug therapy

Planning and implementation
• For Hodgkin's disease, drug usually is given with other antineoplastic drugs.
• To help decrease nausea, give antiemetics before use. Nausea and vomiting may subside after several doses.
• To prevent bleeding, avoid all I.M. injections when platelet count is below 50,000/mm³.

• Use blood transfusions to combat anemia. Patient may receive injections of RBC colony-stimulating factors to promote RBC production and decrease need for blood transfusions.
⚠ **ALERT:** Don't confuse dacarbazine with Dicarbosil, carbamazepine, or procarbazine.

Patient teaching
• Warn patient to watch for signs of infection (fever, sore throat, fatigue) and bleeding (easy bruising, nosebleeds, bleeding gums, melena). Tell patient to take temperature daily.
• Instruct patient to avoid OTC products containing aspirin.
• Advise patient to avoid sunlight and sunlamps for first 2 days after therapy.
• Reassure patient that flulike syndrome may be treated with mild antipyretics, such as acetaminophen.

✓ Evaluation
• Patient exhibits positive response to therapy, as evidenced on follow-up diagnostic studies and overall physical condition.
• Patient has no injury from drug-induced adverse reactions.
• Patient and family state understanding of drug therapy.

daclizumab
(da-KLIZ-yoo-mab)
Zenapax

Pharmacologic class: humanized immunoglobulin G1 monoclonal antibody
Therapeutic class: immunosuppressant
Pregnancy risk category: C

Indications and dosages

▶ **To prevent acute organ rejection in renal transplant patients receiving an immunosuppressive regimen that includes cyclosporine and corticosteroids.** *Adults:* 1 mg/kg I.V. Standard course of therapy is five doses. Give first dose no more than 24 hours before transplantation; give remaining four doses at 14-day intervals.

▽ I.V. administration

• Don't give drug in a direct I.V. injection. Dilute in 50 ml of sterile normal saline solution before administration. To avoid foaming, don't shake. Inspect for particulates and discoloration before use.

• Infuse over 15 minutes via a central or peripheral line. Don't add or infuse other drugs simultaneously through the same line.

• Drug may be refrigerated at 36° to 46° F (2° to 8° C) for 24 hours and is stable at room temperature for 4 hours. Discard solution if not used within 24 hours.

• Protect undiluted solution from direct light.

⊗ **Incompatibilities**
Other drugs infused through same I.V. line.

Contraindications and cautions

• Contraindicated in patients hypersensitive to drug or any of its components.

⚕ **Lifespan:** In pregnant or breast-feeding women, use cautiously. Tell women of child-bearing age to use contraception before, during, and for 4 months after drug therapy.

Adverse reactions

CNS: *anxiety,* depression, dizziness, fatigue, fever, generalized weakness, headache, insomnia, pain, prickly sensation, tremors.
CV: aggravated hypertension, chest pain, edema, fluid overload, hypertension, hypotension, tachycardia.
EENT: blurred vision, pharyngitis, rhinitis.
GI: abdominal distention, *abdominal pain, constipation, diarrhea, dyspepsia,* epigastric pain, flatulence, gastritis, hemorrhoids, *nausea, pyrosis,* vomiting.
GU: dysuria, hydronephrosis, *oliguria,* renal damage, renal insufficiency, *renal tubular necrosis,* urinary tract bleeding, urinary tract disorder, urine retention.
Hematologic: bleeding, lymphocele.
Metabolic: dehydration, diabetes mellitus.
Musculoskeletal: arthralgia, leg cramps, musculoskeletal or back pain, myalgia.
Respiratory: abnormal breath sounds, atelectasis, congestion, coughing, dyspnea, *hypoxia,* pleural effusion, *pulmonary edema,* rales.
Skin: acne, cellulitis, hirsutism, impaired wound healing without infection, *increased sweating,* night sweats, *pruritus, rash,* wound infections.
Other: limb edema, *severe infection,* shivering.

Interactions

Drug-drug. *Corticosteroids, cyclosporine, mycophenolate mofetil:* May increase mortality.

Monitor patient closely for lymphoproliferative disorders and opportunistic infections.

Effects on lab test results

• May increase BUN and creatinine levels.

Pharmacokinetics

Absorption: Given I.V.
Distribution: Unknown.
Metabolism: Unknown.
Excretion: Unknown. *Half-life:* 20 days.

Route	Onset	Peak	Duration
I.V.	Unknown	Unknown	Unknown

Action

Chemical effect: Inhibits interleukin-2 (IL-2) binding to prevent IL-2 from activating lymphocytes. Once in circulation, drug impairs response of immune system.
Therapeutic effect: Prevents organ rejection.

Available forms

Injection: 25 mg/5 ml

NURSING PROCESS

❧ Assessment
• Obtain history of patient's underlying condition before therapy, and reassess regularly.
• Check for opportunistic infections.
⑤ ALERT: Monitor patient for severe, acute hypersensitivity reactions when giving each dose (includes anaphylaxis, hypotension, bronchospasm, loss of consciousness, injection site reactions, edema, and arrhythmias). Stop drug if severe reaction occurs.
• Assess patient's and family's knowledge of drug therapy.

⊞ Nursing diagnoses
• Risk for injury related to potential for organ rejection
• Ineffective protection related to drug-induced immunosuppression
• Deficient knowledge related to drug therapy

⧉ Planning and implementation
• Use only with a prescriber experienced in immunosuppressant therapy and management of organ transplantation.

• Drug is used as part of an immunosuppressant regimen that includes corticosteroids and cyclosporine.

Patient teaching

• Tell patient to consult prescriber before taking other drugs during therapy.

• Advise patient to take precautions against infection.

• Inform patient that neither he nor any household member should receive vaccinations unless medically approved.

• Tell patient to immediately report wounds that fail to heal, unusual bruising or bleeding, or fever.

• Advise patient to drink plenty of fluids during therapy and to report painful urination, blood in the urine, or a decrease in urine output.

• Instruct women of childbearing age to use effective contraception before starting therapy, during therapy, and to continue until 4 months after completing therapy.

☑ Evaluation

• Patient doesn't experience organ rejection while taking drug.

• Patient is free from infection and serious bleeding episodes throughout drug therapy.

• Patient and family state understanding of drug therapy.

dalteparin sodium
(dal-TEH-peh-rin SOH-dee-um)
Fragmin

Pharmacologic class: low–molecular-weight heparin
Therapeutic class: anticoagulant
Pregnancy risk category: B

Indications and dosages

▶ **To prevent deep vein thrombosis (DVT) in patients undergoing abdominal or hip replacement surgery.** *Adults:* 2,500 international units subcutaneously daily. Start 1 to 2 hours before surgery and repeat once daily for 5 to 10 days until patient is mobile. Or, 5,000 international units subcutaneously the evening before surgery. Repeat q evening for 5 to 10 days until patient is mobile.

▶ **To decrease risk of thromboembolism in patients with severely restricted mobility during acute illness.** *Adults:* 5,000 international units subcutaneously daily for 12 to 14 days.

▶ **Unstable angina, non–Q wave MI.** *Adults:* 120 international units/kg up to 10,000 international units subcutaneously q 12 hours with oral aspirin (75 to 165 mg/day) therapy. Continue until patient is stable. Usual duration of treatment is 5 to 8 days.

Contraindications and cautions

• Contraindicated in patients hypersensitive to drug, heparin, or pork products, and in those with major bleeding or thrombocytopenia with positive in vitro tests for antiplatelet antibody in presence of drug.

• Use cautiously in patients with a history of heparin-induced thrombocytopenia; in patients with an increased risk of hemorrhage, such as those with severe uncontrolled hypertension, bacterial endocarditis, congenital or acquired bleeding disorders, active ulceration, angiodysplastic GI disease, or hemorrhagic stroke; and in those who recently underwent brain, spinal, or ophthalmologic surgery.

• Also use cautiously in patients with bleeding diathesis, thrombocytopenia, platelet defects, severe liver or kidney insufficiency, hypertensive or diabetic retinopathy, or recent GI bleeding.

⚘ Lifespan: In pregnant and breast-feeding women, use cautiously. In children, safety and effectiveness haven't been established.

Adverse reactions

CNS: fever.
Hematologic: bleeding complications, ***hemorrhage, thrombocytopenia.***
Skin: ecchymosis, pruritus, rash.
Other: *anaphylaxis, hematoma at injection site* (when given with heparin), pain at injection site.

Interactions

Drug-drug. *Antiplatelet drugs, oral anticoagulants:* May increase risk of bleeding. Use together cautiously; monitor patient for bleeding.

Effects on lab test results

• May increase ALT and AST levels.
• May decrease platelet count.

Pharmacokinetics

Absorption: Absolute bioavailability of anti-factor Xa is 87%.
Distribution: Volume is 40 to 60 ml/kg.
Metabolism: Unknown.
Excretion: In urine. *Half-life:* 3 to 5 hours.

Route	Onset	Peak	Duration
SubQ	Unknown	4 hr	Unknown

Action

Chemical effect: Enhances inhibition of factor Xa and thrombin by antithrombin.
Therapeutic effect: Prevents DVT.

Available forms

Multidose vial: 10,000 anti-factor Xa international units/ml
Syringe: 2,500 anti-factor Xa international units/0.2 ml; 5,000 anti-factor Xa international units/0.2 ml

NURSING PROCESS

⚖ Assessment
• Obtain history of patient's underlying condition before starting therapy.
• Those at risk for DVT include obese patients older than age 40 who are having surgery under general anesthesia that lasts longer than 30 minutes. Other risk factors include cancer and a history of DVT or pulmonary embolism.
• Monitor effectiveness by assessing patient for evidence of DVT.
• Perform routine CBCs (including platelet count) and fecal occult blood tests.
⚠ **ALERT:** Low–molecular-weight heparins used during neuraxial anesthesia or spinal puncture increase risk of epidural or spinal hematoma. Monitor patient closely for neurologic impairment.
• Look for adverse reactions and drug interactions.
• Assess patient's and family's knowledge of drug therapy.

⊞ Nursing diagnoses
• Risk for injury related to risk of DVT as result of underlying condition
• Ineffective protection related to drug-induced adverse hematologic reactions
• Deficient knowledge related to drug therapy

⊠ Planning and implementation
• Place patient in sitting or supine position when giving drug. Give by deep subcutaneous injection. Injection sites include U-shaped area below navel, upper outer side of thigh, and upper outer quadrangle of buttock. Rotate sites daily.
⚠ **ALERT:** Drug should never be given I.M. or I.V.
• Don't mix with other injections or infusions unless specific compatibility data are available that support such mixing.
⚠ **ALERT:** Drug isn't interchangeable (unit for unit) with unfractionated heparin or other low–molecular-weight heparin derivatives.
• Stop drug and notify prescriber if a thromboembolism occurs despite therapy.
Patient teaching
• Instruct patient and family to immediately notify the prescriber if signs of bleeding occur.
• Tell patient to avoid OTC medications containing aspirin or other salicylates.

☑ Evaluation
• Patient doesn't develop DVT.
• Patient maintains stable hematologic function.
• Patient and family state understanding of drug therapy.

dantrolene sodium
(DAN-troh-leen SOH-dee-um)
Dantrium, Dantrium Intravenous

Pharmacologic class: hydantoin derivative
Therapeutic class: skeletal muscle relaxant
Pregnancy risk category: C

Indications and dosages

▶ **Spasticity and sequelae from severe chronic disorders (such as multiple sclerosis, cerebral palsy, spinal cord injury, stroke).** *Adults:* 25 mg P.O. daily. Increase in 25-mg increments up to 100 mg b.i.d. to q.i.d. Maximum, 400 mg daily. Maintain each dosage level for 4 to 7 days to determine response.
Children: Initially, 0.5 mg/kg P.O. b.i.d., increase to t.i.d. and then to q.i.d. Increase dosage p.r.n. by 0.5 mg/kg daily to 3 mg/kg b.i.d. to q.i.d. Maximum, 100 mg q.i.d.

▶ **To manage malignant hyperthermic crisis.**
Adults and children: 1 mg/kg I.V. initially, then
repeat p.r.n. up to a total dosage of 10 mg/kg.
▶ **To prevent or lessen malignant hyperthermia in susceptible patients who need surgery.**
Adults: 4 to 8 mg/kg P.O. daily in three or four
divided doses for 1 or 2 days before procedure.
Final dose 3 to 4 hours before procedure. Or
2.5 mg/kg I.V. infused over 1 hour about 1 hour
before anesthesia. Additional doses, which must
be individualized, may be given intraoperatively.
▶ **To prevent recurrence of malignant hyperthermia.** *Adults:* 4 to 8 mg/kg P.O. daily in four
divided doses for up to 3 days after hyperthermic crisis.
▶ **To reduce succinylcholine-induced muscle
fasciculations and postoperative muscle
pain‡.** *Adults weighing less than 45 kg (99 lb):*
100 mg P.O. 2 hours before succinylcholine.
Adults weighing more than 45 kg: 150 mg P.O.
2 hours before succinylcholine.

▼ I.V. administration

• Give as soon as malignant hyperthermia reaction is recognized.
• Reconstitute each vial with 60 ml of sterile
water for injection, and shake vial until clear.
Don't use diluent that contains bacteriostatic
agent.
• Protect contents from light and use within
6 hours.
• Monitor patient for extravasation.
⊗ **Incompatibilities**
D_5W, normal saline solution, other I. V. drugs
mixed in a syringe.

Contraindications and cautions

• Contraindicated in patients whose spasticity is
used to maintain motor function and in patients
with upper motor neuron disorders, spasms
from rheumatic disorders, or active hepatic disease.
• Use cautiously in women, and in patients with
hepatic disease or severely impaired cardiac or
pulmonary function.
⚖ **Lifespan:** In pregnant women and patients
older than age 35, use cautiously. In breastfeeding women, drug is contraindicated.

Adverse reactions

CNS: confusion, *dizziness, drowsiness,* fever,
hallucinations, headache, insomnia, lightheadedness, *malaise,* nervousness, *seizures.*
CV: blood pressure changes, tachycardia.
EENT: auditory or visual disturbances, excessive tearing.
GI: anorexia, *bleeding,* constipation, cramping,
drooling, dysphagia, metallic taste, severe diarrhea.
GU: crystalluria, difficulty achieving erection,
dysuria, hematuria, incontinence, nocturia, urinary frequency.
Hepatic: hepatitis.
Musculoskeletal: *muscle weakness,* myalgia.
Respiratory: pleural effusion.
Skin: abnormal hair growth, diaphoresis,
eczematous eruption, photosensitivity, pruritus,
urticaria.
Other: chills.

Interactions

Drug-drug. *CNS depressants:* May increase
CNS depression. Avoid using together.
Estrogens: May increase risk of hepatotoxicity.
Use together cautiously.
I.V. verapamil: May cause CV collapse when
used together in anesthetized patients. Manufacturer recommends stopping verapamil before
giving I.V. dantrolene based on animal studies
Drug-lifestyle. *Alcohol use:* May increase CNS
depression. Avoid using together.
Sun exposure: Photosensitivity may occur. Urge
patient to avoid prolonged and unprotected sun
exposure.

Effects on lab test results

• May increase BUN, ALT, AST, and bilirubin
levels.

Pharmacokinetics

Absorption: 35% of P.O. dose.
Distribution: Substantially bound to protein,
mainly albumin.
Metabolism: In liver to its less active
5-hydroxy derivatives and to its amino derivative by reductive pathways.
Excretion: In urine as metabolites. *Half-life:*
P.O., 9 hours; I.V., 4 to 8 hours.

Route	Onset	Peak	Duration
P.O.	≤ 1 wk	5 hr	Unknown
I.V.	Unknown	Unknown	Unknown

Reactions may be *common,* uncommon, **life-threatening**, or COMMON AND LIFE-THREATENING.

Action

Chemical effect: Acts directly on skeletal muscle to interfere with intracellular calcium movement.
Therapeutic effect: Relieves muscle spasms.

Available forms

Capsules: 25 mg, 50 mg, 100 mg
Injection: 20 mg/vial

NURSING PROCESS

☲ Assessment

• Obtain history of patient's disorder before therapy.
• Obtain liver function tests at start of therapy.
• Monitor effectiveness by evaluating severity of spasticity.
• Be alert for adverse reactions and drug interactions.
• Assess patient's and family's knowledge of drug therapy.

⊕ Nursing diagnoses

• Acute pain related to presence of spasticity
• Risk for injury related to drug-induced adverse reactions
• Deficient knowledge related to drug therapy

⊇ Planning and implementation

• For optimum drug effect, divide daily dose into four doses.
• Give drug with meals or milk to prevent GI distress.
• Prepare oral suspension for each dose by dissolving capsule contents in juice or other suitable liquid. For multiple doses, use acid vehicle, such as citric acid in USP syrup. Refrigerate, and use within several days.
• Amount of relief determines whether dose can be reduced.
• If hepatitis, severe diarrhea, severe weakness, or sensitivity reaction occurs, don't give the drug, and immediately notify prescriber.
⊛ **ALERT:** Don't confuse Dantrium with Daraprim.
Patient teaching
• Tell patient to use caution when eating to avoid choking. Some patients may have trouble swallowing during therapy.
• Warn patient to avoid hazardous activities until the drug's full CNS effects are known.

• Advise patient to avoid combining dantrolene with alcohol or other CNS depressants.
• Tell patient to use sunblock and wear protective clothing, to report GI problems immediately, and to follow prescriber's orders regarding rest and physical therapy.

☑ Evaluation

• Patient states that pain from muscle spasticity has lessened.
• Patient has no injury from drug-induced adverse reactions.
• Patient and family state understanding of drug therapy.

daptomycin
(dap-toh-MY-sin)
Cubicin

Pharmacologic class: cyclic lipopeptide antibacterial
Therapeutic class: antibiotic
Pregnancy risk category: B

Indications and dosages

▶ **Complicated skin and skin structure infections caused by susceptible strains of** *Staphylococcus aureus* **(including methicillin-resistant strains),** *Streptococcus pyogenes,* *Streptococcus agalactiae, Streptococcus dysgalactiae,* **and** *Enterococcus faecalis* **(vancomycin-susceptible strains only).** *Adults:* 4 mg/kg by I.V. infusion over 30 minutes q 24 hours for 7 to 14 days.
⊠ **Adjust-a-dose:** For patients with renal impairment, including those receiving hemodialysis or continuous ambulatory peritoneal dialysis, if creatinine clearance is below 30 ml/minute, give 4 mg/kg I.V. q 48 hours. Whenever possible, give drug after hemodialysis.

▽ I.V. administration

• Reconstitute 250-mg vial with 5 ml of normal saline solution and 500-mg vial with 10 ml. Further dilute admixture with normal saline solution. Vials are for single use. Discard excess.
• Compatible with normal saline solution and lactated Ringer's injection. Flush line also used for other drugs with compatible fluids.
• For intermittent infusion, give drug over 30 minutes.

• Refrigerate vials at 36° to 46° F (2° to 8° C). Reconstituted and diluted solutions are stable 12 hours at room temperature or 48 hours at 36° to 46° F.

⊗ **Incompatibilities**
Dextrose-containing solutions. Any other I.V. drugs and solutions.

Contraindications and cautions

• Contraindicated in patients hypersensitive to drug or any of its components.
• Use cautiously in those with renal insufficiency.
⚮ **Lifespan:** In pregnant women, use cautiously. In breast-feeding women, use cautiously because it's unknown if drug appears in breast milk. In children, safety and effectiveness haven't been established. In patients older than age 65, use cautiously because drug may be less effective and cause more adverse reactions.

Adverse reactions

CNS: anxiety, confusion, dizziness, fever, headache, insomnia.
CV: chest pain, edema, *heart failure,* hypertension, hypotension.
EENT: sore throat.
GI: abdominal pain, constipation, decreased appetite, diarrhea, nausea, *pseudomembranous colitis,* vomiting.
GU: *renal failure,* UTI.
Hematologic: anemia.
Metabolic: hyperglycemia, *hypoglycemia,* hypokalemia.
Musculoskeletal: limb and back pain.
Respiratory: cough, dyspnea.
Skin: cellulitis, pruritus, rash.
Other: injection site reactions, fungal infections.

Interactions

Drug-drug. *HMG-CoA reductase inhibitors:* May increase risk of myopathy. Consider stopping these drugs while giving daptomycin.
Tobramycin: May affect levels of both drugs. Use together cautiously.
Warfarin: May alter anticoagulant activity. Monitor PT and INR for the first several days of daptomycin therapy.

Effects on lab test results

• May increase CK and alkaline phosphatase levels. May decrease potassium and hemoglobin

levels and hematocrit. May increase or decrease glucose level.
• May increase liver function test values.

Pharmacokinetics

Absorption: Given I.V.
Distribution: 92% protein bound, mainly to albumin.
Metabolism: Unknown.
Excretion: Mainly by kidneys. *Half-life:* About 8 hours.

Route	Onset	Peak	Duration
I.V.	Rapid	< 1 hr	Unknown

Action

Chemical effect: Binds to and depolarizes bacterial membranes to inhibit protein, DNA, and RNA synthesis.
Therapeutic effect: Kills bacteria in susceptible organisms.

Available forms

Powder for injection: 250-mg vial, 500-mg vial

NURSING PROCESS

📖 **Assessment**
• Monitor CBC and renal and liver function tests periodically.
• Monitor patient for superinfection because drug may cause overgrowth of nonsusceptible organisms.
• Watch for evidence of pseudomembranous colitis, and treat accordingly.
• Assess patient's and family's knowledge of drug therapy.

✦ **Nursing diagnoses**
• Risk for infection related to bacteria
• Impaired urine elimination related to daptomycin-induced renal impairment
• Deficient knowledge related to drug therapy

▷ **Planning and implementation**
• Obtain specimen for culture and sensitivity tests before giving the first dose. Begin therapy pending test results.
🔔 **ALERT:** Because drug may increase the risk of myopathy, monitor CK levels weekly. If they rise, monitor them more often. Stop giving the drug to a patient with evidence of myopathy

and CK levels over 1,000 units/L. Also stop giving the drug to a patient with CK levels more than 10 times the upper limit of normal. Consider stopping all other drugs linked with myopathy (such as HMG-CoA reductase inhibitors).

Patient teaching
• Advise patient to immediately report muscle weakness and infusion site irritation.
• Tell patient to report severe diarrhea, rash, and infection.
• Inform patient about adverse reactions.

☑ **Evaluation**
• Patient's infection is eradicated.
• Patient's renal function test values remain unchanged.
• Patient and family state understanding of drug therapy.

darbepoetin alfa
(dar-be-POE-e-tin AL-fa)
Aranesp

Pharmacologic class: hematopoietic
Therapeutic class: antianemic
Pregnancy risk category: C

Indications and dosages

▶ **Anemia related to chronic renal impairment.** *Adults:* Initially, 0.45 mcg/kg I.V. or subcutaneously once weekly. Adjust dose to achieve and maintain a target hemoglobin level not exceeding 12 g/dl. Don't increase dose more often than monthly. In patients being converted from epoetin alfa, starting dosage should be based on the previous epoetin alfa dosage, according to this table.

Previous weekly epoetin alfa dose (units/wk)	Weekly darbepoetin alfa dose (mcg/wk)
< 2,500	6.25
2,500–4,999	12.5
5,000–10,999	25
11,000–17,999	40
18,000–33,999	60
34,000–89,999	100
> 90,000	200

Give drug less often than epoetin alfa because its half-life is three times longer. If patient was receiving epoetin alfa two to three times a week, he should receive darbepoetin alfa once a week. If patient was receiving epoetin alfa once a week, he should receive darbepoetin alfa once q 2 weeks.

❊ **Adjust-a-dose:** If hemoglobin level is increasing and approaching 12 g/dl, reduce dose by 25%. If level continues to increase, withhold dose until level begins to decrease, and restart at a dose 25% below the previous dose. If level increases by more than 1 g/dl over 2 weeks, decrease dose by 25%. If increase is less than 1 g/dl over 4 weeks and iron stores are adequate, increase the dose by 25% of previous dose. Further increases can be made at 4-week intervals until target level is reached.

Patients who don't need dialysis may need lower maintenance doses because predialysis patients may be more responsive to the effects of darbepoetin alfa and thus may need close monitoring of blood pressure, hemoglobin level, renal function, and electrolyte balance.

Drug decreases plasma volume, thereby reducing dialysis efficiency. Thus, patients who are on dialysis may need adjustments in their dialysis prescription.

▶ **Anemia related to chemotherapy in patients with nonmyeloid malignancies.** *Adults:* 2.25 mcg/kg subcutaneously once weekly.

❊ **Adjust-a-dose:** If hemoglobin level increases less than 1 g/dl after 6 weeks of therapy, increase dose to 4.5 mcg/kg. If level increases by more than 1 g/dl in a 2-week period, or if it exceeds 12 g/dl, reduce dose by 25%. If level exceeds 13 g/dl, withhold drug until level drops to 12 g/dl and restart dose at 25% below the previous dose.

▼ **I.V. administration**

• Don't shake drug because doing so can denature it.
• Drug is provided in single-dose vials without a preservative. Don't pool or retain unused portions.
• If drug has particulate matter or is discolored, don't use.
• Give undiluted by I.V. injection.
• Store drug in refrigerator; don't freeze. Protect drug from light.

⊗ Incompatibilities
Other I.V. drugs and solutions.

Contraindications and cautions

- Contraindicated in patients hypersensitive to drug or any of its components and in patients with uncontrolled hypertension.
- Use cautiously in patients with underlying hematologic disease, such as hemolytic anemia, sickle cell anemia, thalassemia, or porphyria, because safety and effectiveness haven't been established.

Lifespan: In pregnant women and in children, safety and effectiveness haven't been established. With breast-feeding women, use cautiously because it's unknown whether drug appears in breast milk. Elderly patients may have greater sensitivity to the drug.

Adverse reactions

CNS: asthenia, dizziness, fatigue, fever, headache, seizures.
CV: *acute MI,* angina, CARDIAC ARREST, CARDIAC ARRHYTHMIA, chest pain, *edema,* fluid overload, ***heart failure,*** *hypertension, hypotension, thrombosis.*
GI: abdominal pain, constipation, diarrhea, nausea, vomiting.
Metabolic: dehydration.
Musculoskeletal: arthralgia, back pain, limb pain, myalgia.
Respiratory: bronchitis, cough, dyspnea, pneumonia, ***pulmonary embolism,*** upper respiratory tract infection.
Skin: hemorrhage at access site, pruritus, rash.
Other: flulike symptoms, *infection.*

Interactions

None reported.

Effects on lab test results

- May increase hemoglobin level and hematocrit. May decrease ferritin level.
- May increase RBC count.

Pharmacokinetics

Absorption: Slow and rate limiting. Bioavailability ranges from 30% to 50% (mean: 37%).
Distribution: Mostly to vascular space.
Metabolism: Unknown.
Excretion: Steady-state levels occur within 4 weeks. *Half-life:* 21 hours (I.V.); 49 hours (subcutaneous).

Route	Onset	Peak	Duration
I.V.	Unknown	Unknown	21 hr
SubQ	Unknown	34 hr	49 hr

Action

Chemical effect: Stimulates erythropoiesis the same way as endogenous erythropoietin produced by the kidneys. In a healthy patient, erythropoiesis increases the number of RBCs.
Therapeutic effect: Corrects anemia in patients with chronic renal impairment.

Available forms

Injection (albumin solution): 25 mcg/ml, 40 mcg/ml, 60 mcg/ml, 100 mcg/ml, 200 mcg/ml single-dose vials
Injection (polysorbate solution): 25 mcg/ml, 40 mcg/ml, 60 mcg/ml, 100 mcg/ml, 200 mcg/ml single-dose vials

NURSING PROCESS

Assessment

- Drug may increase blood pressure. Blood pressure should be controlled before starting therapy. Obtain baseline blood pressure before therapy, and carefully monitor and control patient's blood pressure during therapy.
- Monitor renal function and electrolytes in predialysis patients.

ALERT: Hemoglobin level may not increase until 2 to 6 weeks after therapy starts. Monitor level weekly until stabilized. Don't exceed the target level of 12 g/dl in patients with chronic renal impairment.

- Drug may increase risk of CV events, so carefully monitor and assess patient.
- Patient may have seizures. Follow patient closely, especially during the first several months of therapy.

Nursing diagnoses

- Risk for injury related to drug-induced adverse cardiac events
- Fatigue related to underlying anemia
- Deficient knowledge related to darbepoetin alfa therapy

▶ **Planning and implementation**

🕒 **ALERT:** If hemoglobin level increases 1 g/dl in any 2-week period, decrease dose. Any increase greater than 1 g/dl within a 2-week period will increase the risk of adverse CV reactions, such as seizures, stroke, exacerbation of hypertension, heart failure, acute MI, fluid overload, edema, or vascular thrombosis, infarction, or ischemia. If symptoms occur, decrease drug dose by 25%.

• Monitor iron before and during therapy. If ferritin level is less than 100 mcg/L and transferrin saturation is less than 20%, provide supplemental iron.

• Serious allergic reactions, including rash and urticaria, may occur. If an anaphylactic reaction occurs, stop giving drug and provide appropriate therapy.

• The maximum safe dose isn't known. Although doses greater than 3 mcg/kg/week for up to 28 weeks can be given, an excessive rise or rate of rise of hemoglobin level leads to adverse reactions. If patient has polycythemia, don't give drug.

• If patient doesn't respond to therapy, reevaluate patient for other etiologies that may inhibit erythropoiesis, such as folic acid or vitamin B_{12} deficiencies, infections, inflammatory or malignant processes, osteofibrosis cystica, occult blood loss, hemolysis, severe aluminum toxicity, and bone marrow fibrosis.

Patient teaching

• Teach patient how to give drug properly, including how to use and dispose of needles.

• Advise patient of adverse effects and allergic reactions.

• Inform patient of need to frequently monitor blood pressure, hemoglobin level, and hematocrit. Advise him to comply with antihypertensive therapy and dietary restrictions to keep blood pressure under control. Uncontrolled blood pressure is believed to cause seizures and hypertensive encephalopathy in patients with chronic renal impairment.

📋 **Evaluation**

• Patient's hemoglobin level increases to no more than 12 g/dl.

• Patient's blood pressure remains adequately controlled, and patient doesn't suffer any adverse reactions related to drug therapy.

• Patient and family state understanding of drug therapy.

darifenacin
dah-ree-PHEN-uh-sin
Enablex⌀

Pharmacologic classification: muscarinic receptor antagonist
Therapeutic classification: anticholinergic
Pregnancy risk category: C

Indications and dosages

▶ **Symptoms of urge incontinence, urgency, and frequency from an overactive urinary bladder.** *Adults:* Initially, 7.5 mg P.O. once daily. If needed, may increase to 15 mg P.O. once daily after 2 weeks.

⛒ **Adjust-a-dose:** If patient has moderate hepatic impairment (Child-Pugh class B) or takes a potent CYP 3A4 inhibitor (such as clarithromycin, itraconazole, ketoconazole, nefazodone, nelfinavir, ritonavir), don't exceed 7.5 mg P.O. once daily.

Contraindications and cautions

Contraindicated in patients hypersensitive to drug or its ingredients. Also contraindicated in patients with or at risk for urine retention, gastric retention, or uncontrolled narrow-angle glaucoma. Avoid use in patients with severe hepatic impairment (Child-Pugh C).

Use cautiously in patients with bladder outflow obstruction, decreased GI motility, GI obstruction, ulcerative colitis, myasthenia gravis, severe constipation, controlled narrow-angle glaucoma, or moderate hepatic impairment (Child-Pugh B).

☀ **Lifespan:** In pregnant women, use only if benefit to mother outweighs risk to fetus. In breast-feeding women, use cautiously; it isn't known if drug appears in breast milk. In children, safety and effectiveness haven't been established.

Adverse reactions

CNS: asthenia, dizziness.
CV: hypertension.
EENT: abnormal vision, dry eyes, pharyngitis, rhinitis, sinusitis.
GI: abdominal pain, *constipation,* diarrhea, *dry mouth,* dyspepsia, nausea, vomiting.
GU: urinary tract disorder, UTI, vaginitis.
Metabolic: weight gain.

Musculoskeletal: arthralgia, back pain.
Respiratory: bronchitis.
Skin: dry skin, pruritus, rash.
Other: accidental injury, flu syndrome, pain, peripheral edema.

Interactions

Drug-drug. *Anticholinergics:* May increase anticholinergic effects, such as dry mouth, blurred vision, and constipation. Monitor patient closely.
Digoxin: May increase digoxin level. Monitor digoxin level.
Drugs metabolized by CYP 2D6 (such as flecainide, thioridazine, tricyclic antidepressants): May increase levels of these drugs. Use together cautiously.
Drugs that are potent CYP 3A4 inhibitors (such as clarithromycin, itraconazole, ketoconazole, nefazodone, nelfinavir, ritonavir): May increase darifenacin levels. Maximum darifenacin dose is 7.5 mg P.O. daily.
Midazolam: May increase midazolam level. Monitor patient carefully.
Drug-lifestyle. *Hot weather:* May cause heat prostration from decreased sweating. Advise caution.

Effects on lab test results

None reported.

Pharmacokinetics

Absorption: Level peaks 7 hours after multiple doses.
Distribution: 98% plasma protein-bound, mainly to alpha$_1$-acid-glycoprotein.
Metabolism: Extensive, in liver (CYP 2D6, CYP 3A4).
Excretion: 60% in urine, 40% in feces; 3% unchanged. *Half-life:* 13 to 19 hours.

Route	Onset	Peak	Duration
P.O.	Unknown	7 hr	Unknown

Action

Chemical effect: Antagonizes muscarinic (M3) receptors, increasing bladder capacity and decreasing unstable detrusor contractions.
Therapeutic effect: Relieves symptoms of overactive bladder.

Available forms

Tablets (extended-release): 7.5 mg, 15 mg

NURSING PROCESS

Assessment
● Assess bladder function prior to initiating therapy.
● Monitor drug effects.
● If patient has bladder outlet obstruction, watch for urine retention.
● Assess patient for decreased gastric motility and constipation.
● Assess patient's and family's knowledge of drug therapy.

Nursing diagnoses
● Impaired urinary elimination related to underlying medical condition
● Risk for injury related to drug-induced adverse effects
● Deficient knowledge related to drug therapy

Planning and implementation
● If patient has a UTI, give antibiotics.
● Reduce GI distress by giving drug with food.
● If patient experiences urine retention, notify physician and prepare for urinary catheterization.
Patient teaching
● Tell patient to swallow tablet whole with plenty of liquid; caution against crushing or chewing the tablets.
● Inform patient that drug may be taken with or without food.
● Explain that drug may cause blurred vision. Tell patient to use caution, especially when performing hazardous tasks, until drug effects are known.
● Tell patient to report blurred vision, constipation, and urine retention.
● Discourage use of other drugs that may cause dry mouth, constipation, urine retention, or blurred vision.
● Tell patient that drug decreases sweating. Advise caution in hot environments and during strenuous activity.

Evaluation
● Patient experiences improved bladder function with drug therapy.
● Patient sustains no injuries from drug-induced effects.
● Patient and family state understanding of drug therapy.

daunorubicin citrate liposomal
(daw-noh-roo-BYE-sin SIH-trayt li-po-SOE-mul)
DaunoXome

Pharmacologic class: anthracycline
Therapeutic class: antineoplastic
Pregnancy risk category: D

Indications and dosages

▶ **First-line cytotoxic therapy for advanced HIV-related Kaposi's sarcoma.** *Adults:* 40 mg/m² I.V. over 60 minutes once q 2 weeks. Continue therapy unless patient shows signs of progressive disease or until drugs has to be stopped from other complications of HIV.
⊠ **Adjust-a-dose:** For patients with renal or hepatic impairment, if bilirubin is 1.2 to 3 mg/dl, give ¾ of normal dose; if bilirubin or creatinine level is greater than 3 mg/dl, give ½ of normal dose.

▼ I.V. administration

• Preparing and giving drug raises carcinogenic, mutagenic, and teratogenic risks. Follow institutional policy to reduce risks.
• Dilute drug with D₅W only. Withdraw the calculated volume of drug from the vial, and transfer it into an equivalent amount of D₅W for a concentration of 1 mg/ml.
• After dilution, immediately give I.V. over 60 minutes. If unable to use drug immediately, refrigerate at 36° to 46° F (2° to 8° C) for a maximum of 6 hours.
• Don't use in-line filters for I.V. infusion.
• Because local tissue necrosis may occur, monitor I.V. site closely to avoid extravasation. If extravasation occurs, stop I.V., apply ice, and notify prescriber.
• Monitor patient for adverse reactions. A triad of back pain, flushing, and chest tightness may occur within the first 5 minutes of the infusion. These symptoms subside after stopping the infusion and typically don't recur when the infusion resumes at a slower rate.
• Follow facility policy for handling and disposing of antineoplastics.
⊗ **Incompatibilities**
Bacteriostatic agents, other I.V. drugs, saline and other solutions.

Contraindications and cautions

• Contraindicated in patients hypersensitive to drug or any of its components.
• Use cautiously in patients with myelosuppression, cardiac disease, previous radiotherapy involving the heart, previous anthracycline use (doxorubicin > 300 mg/m² or equivalent), or hepatic or renal impairment.
⚘ **Lifespan:** In pregnant women, avoid use because the drug may harm the fetus. In children and the elderly, safety and effectiveness haven't been established.

Adverse reactions

CNS: abnormal gait, abnormal thinking, amnesia, anxiety, ataxia, confusion, depression, dizziness, emotional lability, *fatigue, fever,* hallucinations, *headache,* hyperkinesia, hypertonia, insomnia, malaise, meningitis, *neuropathy, seizures,* somnolence, syncope, tremor.
CV: angina pectoris, *arrhythmias, cardiac arrest,* cardiac tamponade, cardiomyopathy, chest pain, edema, flushing, hypertension, *MI,* palpitations, pericardial effusion, pulmonary hypertension, tachycardia.
EENT: abnormal vision, conjunctivitis, deafness, dry mouth, earache, eye pain, gingival bleeding, *rhinitis,* sinusitis, taste disturbance, tinnitus, tooth caries.
GI: *abdominal pain, anorexia,* constipation, *diarrhea,* dysphagia, gastritis, **hemorrhage,** hemorrhoids, increased appetite, melena, *nausea,* stomatitis, tenesmus, vomiting.
GU: dysuria, nocturia, polyuria.
Hematologic: lymphadenopathy, NEUTROPENIA, splenomegaly.
Hepatic: hepatomegaly.
Metabolic: dehydration.
Musculoskeletal: arthralgia, *back pain,* myalgia, *rigors.*
Respiratory: cough, *dyspnea,* hemoptysis, hiccups, increased sputum, pulmonary infiltration.
Skin: alopecia, dry skin, folliculitis, increased sweating, pruritus, seborrhea.
Other: *allergic reactions,* flulike symptoms, injection site inflammation, *opportunistic infections,* thirst.

Interactions

None reported.

Effects on lab test results

• May decrease neutrophil and platelet counts.

Pharmacokinetics

Absorption: Given I.V.
Distribution: Probably mainly in vascular fluid volume.
Metabolism: By the liver into active metabolites.
Excretion: Unknown. *Half-life:* 4½ hours.

Route	Onset	Peak	Duration
I.V.	Unknown	Unknown	Unknown

Action

Chemical effect: Exerts cytotoxic effects by intercalating between DNA base pairs and uncoiling the DNA helix. This inhibits DNA synthesis and DNA-dependent RNA synthesis. Also inhibits polymerase activity. The liposomal preparation maximizes the selectivity of daunorubicin for solid tumors in situ.
Therapeutic effect: Decreases tumor growth for advanced HIV-related Kaposi's sarcoma.

Available forms

Injection: 2 mg/ml (equivalent to 50 mg daunorubicin base)

NURSING PROCESS

⚡ Assessment
• Obtain history of patient's underlying condition before therapy, and reassess regularly thereafter.
• Obtain hepatic and renal studies before therapy.
• Monitor cardiac function regularly, especially immediately before giving a dose, because of the risk of cardiac toxicity and heart failure. Determine left ventricular ejection fraction at a total cumulative dose of 320 mg/m^2 and every 160 mg/m^2 thereafter.
• Monitor patient closely for signs of opportunistic infections.
• Be alert for adverse reactions and drug interactions.
• Assess patient's and family's knowledge of drug therapy.

🔄 Nursing diagnoses
• Risk for injury related to drug-induced adverse reactions
• Risk for infection related to myelosuppression
• Deficient knowledge related to drug therapy

▷ Planning and implementation
• Drug causes less nausea, vomiting, alopecia, neutropenia, thrombocytopenia, and potentially less cardiotoxicity than conventional daunorubicin.
• Give only under the supervision of a prescriber specializing in cancer chemotherapy.
• Monitor hematology closely because severe myelosuppression may occur. Obtain and check blood counts before each dose. If absolute granulocyte count is below 750 cells/mm^3, withhold drug.
⚕ ALERT: Drug has unique kinetic properties that are different from the conventional daunorubicin hydrochloride. Don't substitute or interchange the drugs on a milligram-to-milligram basis.
Patient teaching
• Inform patient that alopecia may occur, but that it's usually reversible.
• Tell patient to notify prescriber about sore throat, fever, or other signs of infection. Tell patient to avoid exposure to people with infections.
• Advise patient to report suspected or known pregnancy during therapy.
• Tell patient to report back pain, flushing, and chest tightness during the infusion.

✓ Evaluation
• Patient has no injury as a result of drug-induced adverse reactions.
• Patient remains free of infection.
• Patient and family state understanding of drug therapy.

daunorubicin hydrochloride
(daw-noh-ROO-buh-sin high-droh-KLOR-ighd)
Cerubidine

Pharmacologic class: anthracycline antineoplastic
Therapeutic class: antineoplastic
Pregnancy risk category: D

Indications and dosages

▶ **To induce remission in acute nonlymphocytic (myelogenous, monocytic, erythroid) leukemia.** *Adults younger than age 60:* When given with other drugs, 45 mg/m^2 I.V. daily on days 1, 2, and 3 of first course and on days 1 and 2 of subsequent courses with cytarabine infusions.

Adults age 60 or older: When given with other drugs, 30 mg/m² I.V. daily on days 1, 2, and 3 of first course and on days 1 and 2 of subsequent courses with cytarabine infusions.

▶ **To induce remission in acute lymphocytic leukemia.** *Adults:* 45 mg/m² I.V. daily on days 1, 2, and 3.

Children age 2 and older: 25 mg/m² I.V. on day 1 q week for up to 6 weeks, if needed.

Children younger than age 2 or with body surface area of less than 0.5 m²: Calculate dose based on body weight (1 mg/kg).

◻ **Adjust-a-dose:** For patients with impaired hepatic or renal function, reduce dosage as follows: If bilirubin level is 1.2 to 3 mg/dl, give 75% of normal dose; if bilirubin or creatinine level exceeds 3 mg/dl, give 50% of the normal dose.

▼ I.V. administration

• Preparing and giving drug raises carcinogenic, mutagenic, and teratogenic risks. Follow institutional policy to reduce risks.

• Reconstitute drug using 4 ml of sterile water for injection to produce a 5 mg/ml solution.

• Withdraw desired dose into syringe containing 10 to 15 ml of normal saline solution for injection. Over 2 to 3 minutes, inject into I.V. line containing free-flowing D₅W or normal saline solution.

• Monitor I.V. site for extravasation. If it occurs, stop I.V. injection immediately, notify prescriber, and apply ice to area for 24 to 48 hours.

• Don't inject with dexamethasone or heparin because a precipitate may form.

• Use within 8 hours of preparation. Reconstituted undiluted solution is stable 24 hours at room temperature, 48 hours if refrigerated.

⊗ **Incompatibilities**
Other I.V. drugs.

Contraindications and cautions

• Use cautiously in patients with myelosuppression and in those with impaired cardiac, renal, or hepatic function.

⚘ **Lifespan:** In pregnant women, avoid use due to potential fetal abnormality or death. Women of childbearing age should avoid becoming pregnant while on drug. Males being treated have increased risk of fertility impairment. Breast-feeding isn't recommended during ther-

apy due to possible increased risk of breast tumors. In children and the elderly, cardiotoxicity may be more frequent and occur at lower cumulative doses.

Adverse reactions

CNS: fever.
CV: *arrhythmias,* ECG changes, *irreversible cardiomyopathy,* myocarditis, *pericarditis.*
GI: anorexia, diarrhea, esophagitis, nausea, stomatitis, vomiting.
GU: red urine.
Hematologic: *bone marrow suppression.*
Hepatic: *hepatotoxicity.*
Metabolic: hyperuricemia.
Skin: *generalized alopecia,* pigmentation of fingernails and toenails, rash, *tissue sloughing with extravasation.*
Other: *anaphylaxis,* chills, severe cellulites.

Interactions

Drug-drug. *Bone marrow suppressants:* May increase risk of myelosuppression. Monitor patient closely.
Cyclophosphamide: May increase risk of cardiotoxicity. Monitor patient closely.
Doxorubicin: May increase risk of cardiotoxicity. Monitor patient closely.
Hepatotoxic drugs: May increase risk of hepatotoxicity. Monitor hepatic function closely.

Effects on lab test results

• May increase uric acid level.

Pharmacokinetics

Absorption: Given I.V. only.
Distribution: Wide; drug doesn't cross blood–brain barrier.
Metabolism: Extensive. One of metabolites has cytotoxic activity.
Excretion: Mainly in bile, with small portion in urine. *Half-life:* Initial, 45 minutes; terminal, 18½ hours.

Route	Onset	Peak	Duration
I.V.	Unknown	Unknown	Unknown

Action

Chemical effect: May interfere with DNA-dependent RNA synthesis by intercalation.
Therapeutic effect: Kills selected cancer cells.

Available forms

Injection: 20 mg/vial

Assessment
• Obtain history of patient's underlying disease before therapy, and reassess regularly throughout therapy.
• Check ECG before therapy.
• Monitor CBC and liver function tests; monitor ECG every month (or more frequently if needed) during therapy.
• Monitor pulse rate closely.
• Look for adverse reactions and drug interactions.
• Monitor patient for nausea and vomiting, which may be severe and may last 24 to 48 hours. Monitor patient's hydration during episodes of nausea and vomiting.
• Assess patient's and family's knowledge of drug therapy.

Nursing diagnoses
• Risk for injury related to presence of neoplastic disease
• Risk for deficient fluid volume related to drug-induced nausea and vomiting
• Deficient knowledge related to drug therapy

Planning and implementation
⑧ **ALERT:** Never give drug by I.M. or subcutaneous route.
• Cumulative dosage is limited to 500 to 600 mg/m^2 (450 mg/m^2 if patient also receives or has received cyclophosphamide or radiation therapy to cardiac area).
⑧ **ALERT:** Color is similar to that of doxorubicin. Don't confuse these two drugs.
• If signs of heart failure or cardiomyopathy develop, stop giving the drug and immediately notify the prescriber.
⑧ **ALERT:** The risk of myocardial toxicity increases after a total cumulative dose higher than 400 to 550 mg/m^2 in adults, 300 mg/m^2 in children older than age 2, and 10 mg/kg in children younger than age 2.
• Give antiemetics to help control nausea and vomiting.
Patient teaching
• Warn patient to watch for signs of infection and bleeding.

• Advise patient that red urine for 1 to 2 days is normal and doesn't indicate blood in urine.
• Inform patient that alopecia may occur, but that it's usually reversible.
• Advise women of childbearing age to avoid becoming pregnant during therapy.
• Instruct patient about need for protective measures, including conservation of energy, balanced diet, adequate rest, personal hygiene, clean environment, and avoidance of people with infections.

Evaluation
• Patient shows positive response to therapy as evidenced by reports of follow-up diagnostic tests and improved physical condition.
• Patient maintains adequate hydration throughout therapy.
• Patient and family state understanding of drug therapy.

delavirdine mesylate
(deh-luh-VEER-deen MES-ih-layt)
Rescriptor

Pharmacologic class: nonnucleoside reverse transcriptase inhibitor
Therapeutic class: antiretroviral
Pregnancy risk category: C

Indications and dosages
▶ **HIV-1 infection.** *Adults:* 400 mg P.O. t.i.d. with other appropriate antiretrovirals.

Contraindications and cautions
• Contraindicated in patients hypersensitive to drug or any of its components.
• Use cautiously in patients with impaired hepatic function.
⚖ **Lifespan:** In pregnant women, use only if potential benefits to the woman outweigh risks to the fetus. Breast-feeding women can transmit HIV to their infants. In children younger than age 16, safety and effectiveness haven't been established.

Adverse reactions
CNS: anxiety, *asthenia,* depression, *fatigue,* fever, *headache,* insomnia, localized pain.
EENT: pharyngitis, sinusitis.

Reactions may be *common,* uncommon, *life-threatening*, or COMMON AND LIFE-THREATENING.

GI: abdominal pain (generalized or localized), diarrhea, nausea, vomiting.
Respiratory: bronchitis, cough, upper respiratory tract infection.
Skin: *rash.*
Other: flulike syndrome.

Interactions

Drug-drug. *Amphetamines, antihistamines (nonsedating), benzodiazepines, calcium channel blockers, clarithromycin, dapsone, ergot alkaloids, indinavir, quinidine, rifabutin, sedative hypnotics, warfarin:* May increase or prolong therapeutic and adverse effects of these drugs. Avoid using together; however, reduced doses of indinavir and clarithromycin may be used.
Antacids: May reduce absorption of delavirdine. Separate doses by at least 1 hour.
Carbamazepine, phenobarbital, phenytoin: May decrease delavirdine level; use together cautiously.
Clarithromycin, fluoxetine, ketoconazole: May cause a 50% increase in delavirdine bioavailability. Monitor patient. Reduce dose of clarithromycin.
Didanosine: May decrease absorption of both drugs by 20%. Separate doses by at least 1 hour.
H$_2$-receptor antagonists: May increase gastric pH, reducing absorption of delavirdine. Long-term use together isn't recommended.
HMG-CoA reductase inhibitors, such as atorvastatin, lovastatin, and simvastatin: May increase levels of these drugs, raising risk for myopathy, including rhabdomyolysis. Avoid using together.
Rifabutin, rifampin: May decrease delavirdine levels. Rifabutin levels are increased by 100%. Avoid using together.
Saquinavir: May increase bioavailability of saquinavir fivefold. Monitor AST and ALT levels frequently when used together.
Sildenafil: May increase sildenafil level and risk of hypotension, visual changes, and priapism. Tell patient not to exceed 25 mg of sildenafil in a 48-hour period.

Effects on lab test results

• May increase ALT, GGT, amylase, bilirubin, and AST levels. May decrease hemoglobin level and hematocrit. May increase or decrease glucose level.

• May increase PT, PTT, and eosinophil count. May decrease granulocyte, neutrophil, WBC, RBC, and platelet counts.

Pharmacokinetics

Absorption: Rapid.
Distribution: 98% bound to protein.
Metabolism: Extensive, to inactive metabolites. Mainly in liver by cytochrome enzyme systems.
Excretion: 51% in the urine (less than 5% unchanged), 44% in the feces. *Half-life:* 5¼ hours.

Route	Onset	Peak	Duration
P.O.	Unknown	1 hr	Unknown

Action

Chemical effect: Drug binds directly to reverse transcriptase and blocks RNA- and DNA-dependent DNA polymerase activities.
Therapeutic effect: Inhibits HIV replication.

Available forms

Tablets: 100 mg, 200 mg

NURSING PROCESS

Assessment
• Assess patient's underlying condition before therapy and regularly thereafter.
• Be alert for adverse reactions and drug interactions.
• Monitor patient for drug-induced rash.
• Assess patient's and family's knowledge of drug therapy.

Nursing diagnoses
• Risk for impaired skin integrity related to potential adverse effects of medication
• Risk for infection related to patient's underlying condition
• Deficient knowledge related to drug therapy

Planning and implementation
• If rash develops, give diphenhydramine, hydroxyzine, or topical corticosteroids to relieve symptoms.
• Resistance develops rapidly when drug is used as monotherapy. Always give with appropriate antiretroviral therapy.
• If patient has trouble swallowing pills, add tablets to at least 3 oz (89 ml) of water, let stand for a few minutes, then stir well. Have patient

drink promptly, rinse the glass, and swallow the rinse to make sure entire dose is consumed.

Patient teaching

• Tell patient to stop taking the drug and to call prescriber if he develops a severe rash or rash accompanied by symptoms such as fever, blistering, oral lesions, conjunctivitis, swelling, or muscle or joint aches.

• Tell patient that drug doesn't cure HIV-1 infection and that he may continue to acquire illnesses related to HIV-1 infection.

• Urge patient to remain under medical supervision when taking drug because long-term effects aren't known.

• Advise patient to take drug as prescribed and not to alter doses without prescriber's approval. If a dose is missed, tell him to take the next dose as soon as possible but not to double the next dose.

• Inform patient that drug may be taken with or without food.

• Tell patient with achlorhydria to take drug with an acidic beverage, such as orange or cranberry juice.

• Advise patient taking sildenafil of increased risk for sildenafil-associated adverse events, including hypotension, vision changes, and priapism. Tell him to promptly report any symptoms to prescriber. Tell him not to exceed 25 mg of sildenafil in a 48-hour period.

• Advise patient to report use of other prescription drugs, OTC medicines, or herbal remedies.

☑ Evaluation

• Patient's skin integrity is maintained.

• Patient is free from opportunistic infections.

• Patient and family state understanding of drug therapy.

desipramine hydrochloride
(deh-SIP-rah-meen high-droh-KLOR-ighd)
Norpramin

Pharmacologic class: tricyclic antidepressant (TCA)
Therapeutic class: antidepressant
Pregnancy risk category: C

Indications and dosages

▶ **Depression.** *Adults:* Initially, 100 to 200 mg P.O. daily in divided doses; increase to maxi-

mum, 300 mg daily. Or, entire dose can be given h.s.

Elderly patients and adolescents: 25 to 100 mg P.O. daily in divided doses; increase gradually to maximum, 150 mg daily, if needed.

Contraindications and cautions

• Contraindicated in patients hypersensitive to drug or any of its components, in those in acute recovery phase of MI, and within 14 days of MAO inhibitor therapy.

• Use cautiously in patients taking thyroid medication and in those with CV disease, seizure disorder, glaucoma, thyroid disorder, or history of urine retention.

☀ Lifespan: In pregnant and breast-feeding women, use cautiously. In children younger than age 12, use is contraindicated.

Adverse reactions

CNS: confusion, *dizziness, drowsiness,* EEG changes, excitation, extrapyramidal reactions, headache, nervousness, *seizures,* tremors, weakness.

CV: ECG changes, hypertension, orthostatic hypotension, tachycardia.

EENT: *blurred vision,* mydriasis, tinnitus.

GI: anorexia, *constipation, dry mouth,* nausea, paralytic ileus, vomiting.

GU: urine retention.

Skin: *diaphoresis,* photosensitivity, rash, urticaria.

Other: hypersensitivity reaction, *sudden death.*

Interactions

Drug-drug. *Anticholinergics:* May enhance anticholinergic effects. Monitor patient closely.

Barbiturates, CNS depressants: May enhance CNS depression. Avoid using together.

Cimetidine, methylphenidate: May increase desipramine levels. Monitor patient for adverse reactions.

Clonidine: May cause loss of blood pressure control with potentially life threatening elevations in blood pressure. Don't use together.

Epinephrine, norepinephrine: May increase hypertensive effect. Use together cautiously.

MAO inhibitors: May cause severe excitation, hyperpyrexia, or seizures, usually with high dosage. Contraindicated within 14 days of MAO inhibitor therapy.

SSRIs: May inhibit the metabolism of TCAs, causing toxicity. Symptoms of TCA toxicity

---

may persist for several weeks after stopping SSRI. At least 5 weeks may be needed when switching from fluoxetine to a tricyclic antidepressant because of the long half-life of the active and parent metabolite.

Drug-lifestyle. *Alcohol use:* May enhance CNS depression. Discourage using together.

Smoking: May lower desipramine level. Monitor patient for lack of effect; encourage smoking cessation.

Sun exposure: May increase risk of photosensitivity. Advise against unprotected or prolonged sun exposure.

Effects on lab test results
• May increase or decrease glucose level.
• May increase liver function test values.

Pharmacokinetics
Absorption: Rapid.
Distribution: Wide, including CNS; 90% protein-bound.
Metabolism: By the liver; significant first-pass effect may explain different levels in patients taking same dosage.
Excretion: Mainly in urine. *Half-life:* Unknown.

Route	Onset	Peak	Duration
P.O.	2–4 wk	4–6 hr	Unknown

Action
Chemical effect: May increase amount of norepinephrine, serotonin, or both in the CNS by blocking their reuptake by neurons.
Therapeutic effect: Relieves depression.

Available forms
Tablets: 10 mg, 25 mg, 50 mg, 75 mg, 100 mg, 150 mg

NURSING PROCESS

Assessment
• Obtain history of patient's depression before therapy, and reassess regularly.
• Be alert for adverse reactions and drug interactions.
• Assess patient's and family's knowledge of drug therapy.

Nursing diagnoses
• Ineffective individual coping related to depression
• Risk for injury related to drug-induced adverse reactions
• Deficient knowledge related to drug therapy

Planning and implementation
• Don't abruptly stop giving the drug. Abruptly stopping long-term therapy may cause nausea, headache, and malaise.
• Because drug produces fewer anticholinergic effects than other TCAs, it's prescribed often for patients with cardiac problems.
• Because hypertensive episodes may occur during surgery, stop drug gradually several days before surgery.
ALERT: This drug may cause sudden death in children, although the cause isn't clearly defined.
• If signs of psychosis occur or increase, reduce dosage.

Patient teaching
• Warn patient to avoid hazardous activities until the drug's CNS effects are known. Drowsiness and dizziness usually subside after a few weeks.
• Tell patient to avoid alcohol during therapy because it may antagonize drug effects.
• Warn patient not to abruptly stop taking the drug.
• Advise patient to consult prescriber before taking other prescription drugs, OTC medications, or herbal remedies.
• Instruct patient to use sunblock, wear protective clothing, and avoid prolonged exposure to strong sunlight.

Evaluation
• Patient behavior and communication indicate improvement of depression.
• Patient has no injury as a result of drug-induced adverse reactions.
• Patient and family state understanding of drug therapy.

desloratadine

(des-lor-AT-a-deen)
Clarinex✓, Clarinex Reditabs

Pharmacologic class: selective H₁-receptor antagonist
Therapeutic class: antihistamine
Pregnancy risk category: C

Indications and dosages

▶ **To relieve symptoms of allergic rhinitis (seasonal and perennial); to relieve pruritus, and to reduce the number and size of hives in patients with chronic idiopathic urticaria.**
Adults and children age 12 and older: 5 mg P.O. daily via regular tablet, Reditabs, or 10 ml (2 tsp) syrup.
Children ages 6 to 11 years: 2.5 mg (5 ml) syrup P.O. daily.
Children ages 1 to 5 years: 1.25 mg (2.5 ml) syrup P.O. daily.
Children ages 6 to 11 months: 1 mg (2 ml) syrup P.O. daily.
Ⓢ Adjust-a-dose: In patients with hepatic or renal impairment, start dosage at 5 mg P.O. q other day.

Contraindications and cautions

• Contraindicated in patients hypersensitive to drug or any of its components, or loratadine. Drug can't be eliminated by hemodialysis.
⚘ Lifespan: Breast-feeding women should stop nursing or stop taking the drug because drug appears in breast milk. In children younger than age 6 months, safety and effectiveness haven't been established. In elderly patients, use cautiously because they may have decreased hepatic, renal, or cardiac function or other diseases and may be taking other drugs.

Adverse reactions

CNS: dizziness, *fatigue,* headache, somnolence.
CV: tachycardia.
EENT: pharyngitis.
GI: *dry mouth,* dyspepsia, nausea, *sore throat.*
GU: dysmenorrhea.
Musculoskeletal: myalgia.
Other: flulike symptoms, *hypersensitivity reaction* (including rash, edema, or ***anaphylaxis***).

Interactions

None reported.

Effects on lab test results

• May increase liver enzyme and bilirubin levels.

Pharmacokinetics

Absorption: Readily absorbed in plasma. Doesn't cross the blood–brain barrier. All forms equal in pharmacokinetics.
Distribution: 82% to 87% bound to proteins. Active metabolite is 85% to 89% protein bound.
Metabolism: Extensive, to inactive metabolite.
Excretion: Equal in urine and feces, mainly as metabolites. *Half-life:* 27 hours.

Route	Onset	Peak	Duration
P.O.	1 hr	3 hr	4 hr

Action

Chemical effect: Inhibits histamine release from human mast cells in vitro.
Therapeutic effect: Relieves allergy symptoms.

Available forms

Orally disintegrating tablets (Reditabs): 5 mg
Syrup: 0.5 mg/ml
Tablets: 5 mg

NURSING PROCESS

🕮 Assessment
• Assess patient's condition before therapy and regularly thereafter.
• Be alert for adverse reactions.
• Assess patient's and family's knowledge of drug therapy.

⊞ Nursing diagnoses
• Ineffective health maintenance related to underlying allergic condition
• Fatigue related to drug-induced reaction
• Deficient knowledge related to drug therapy

🕮 Planning and implementation
• Drug may be taken with or without food.
• Overdose may cause somnolence and increased heart rate. If these symptoms occur, consider removing unabsorbed drug through standard measures, treat symptoms and provide supportive therapy.

Patient teaching

• Advise patient not to exceed prescribed dosage. Doses of more than 5 mg don't increase effectiveness and may cause somnolence.
• Tell patient to report adverse effects.
• Store all forms at room temperature, not to exceed 86° F (30° C), and avoid exposure to light and moisture.
• Inform patient that orally disintegrating tablet may be taken with or without water.
• Instruct patient to remove a tablet from the blister pack and immediately place it on his tongue. The tablet will dissolve.
• Teach parents to use properly calibrated 5- to 10-ml dropper or syringe for syrup administration, not household measuring devices.

☑ Evaluation

• Patient's allergic symptoms are relieved.
• Patient doesn't suffer any drug-induced adverse effects.
• Patient and family state understanding of drug therapy.

desmopressin acetate
(dez-moh-PREH-sin AS-ih-tayt)
DDAVP, Stimate

Pharmacologic class: posterior pituitary hormone
Therapeutic class: antidiuretic, hemostatic
Pregnancy risk category: B

Indications and dosages

▶ **Nonnephrogenic diabetes insipidus, temporary polyuria, and polydipsia from pituitary trauma.** *Adults:* 10 to 40 mcg intranasally daily in one to three divided doses. Adjust morning and evening doses separately for adequate diurnal rhythm of water turnover. Or 0.05 mg P.O. b.i.d. Adjust each dose separately for an adequate diurnal rhythm of water turnover. Increase or decrease total oral daily dosage p.r.n. to achieve desired response. Dosage may range from 0.1 to 1.2 mg, divided into two or three daily doses. Start oral therapy 12 hours after last intranasal dose. Or, give 2 to 4 mcg I.V. or subcutaneously daily, usually in two equally divided doses.
Children ages 3 months to 12 years: 0.05 to 0.3 ml intranasally daily in one or two doses.

Children age 4 and older: Begin with 0.05 mg oral form P.O. b.i.d. Adjust each dose separately for an adequate diurnal rhythm of water turnover. Increase or decrease total oral daily dosage to achieve desired response. Dosages may range from 0.1 to 1.2 mg, divided into two or three daily doses. Start oral therapy 12 hours after the last intranasal dose.
Children younger than age 4: Adjust dosage of oral form individually to prevent an excessive decrease in blood osmolality.
▶ **Hemophilia A and von Willebrand's disease.** *Adults and children:* 0.3 mcg/kg diluted in normal saline solution and infused I.V. over 15 to 30 minutes. May repeat dose, if needed, based on laboratory response and patient's condition. Intranasal dose is 1 spray (of solution containing 1.5 mg/ml) into each nostril to provide total of 300 mcg.
Adults and children weighing less than 50 kg (110 lb): 1 spray into a single nostril (150 mcg).
▶ **Primary nocturnal enuresis.** *Children age 6 and older:* Initially, 20 mcg intranasally h.s. Adjust dosage according to response. Maximum, 40 mcg daily. Or 0.2 mg P.O. h.s. Adjust dose up to 0.6 mg P.O. to achieve desired response. Oral therapy may start 24 hours after last intranasal dose.

▽ I.V. administration

• For adults and children weighing more than 10 kg (22 lb), dilute with 50 ml sterile physiologic saline solution. For children weighing 10 kg or less, use 10 ml of diluent.
• Inspect for particulate matter and discoloration before infusing drug.
• Monitor blood pressure and pulse during infusion.
⊗ **Incompatibilities**
None reported.

Contraindications and cautions

• Contraindicated in patients hypersensitive to drug (or any of its components), and in those with type IIB von Willebrand's disease.
• Use cautiously in patients with coronary artery insufficiency or hypertensive CV disease and in those with conditions linked to fluid and electrolyte imbalance, such as cystic fibrosis, because these patients are prone to hyponatremia.
⚜ **Lifespan:** In pregnant and breast-feeding women, use cautiously. In infants younger than age 3 months, use of drug isn't recommended

because of their increased tendency to develop fluid imbalance. In children younger than age 12, safety of parenteral form of drug hasn't been established for management of diabetes insipidus.

Adverse reactions

CNS: headache.
CV: slight rise in blood pressure.
EENT: epistaxis, nasal congestion, rhinitis, sore throat.
GI: abdominal cramps, nausea.
GU: vulvar pain.
Respiratory: cough.
Other: flushing, local erythema, swelling or burning after injection.

Interactions

Drug-drug. *Demeclocycline, epinephrine, heparin, lithium:* May decrease response to desmopressin. Monitor patient closely.
Drug-lifestyle. *Alcohol use:* May increase risk of adverse effects. Discourage using together.

Effects on lab test results

None reported.

Pharmacokinetics

Absorption: After intranasal use, 10% to 20% by nasal mucosa. After subcutaneous use, unknown. After P.O. use, minimal.
Distribution: Unknown.
Metabolism: Unknown.
Excretion: Unknown. *Half-life:* Fast phase, about 8 minutes; slow phase, 114 hours.

Route	Onset	Peak	Duration
P.O.	1 hr	4–7 hr	8–12 hr
I.V.	15–30 min	½–2 hr	4–12 hr
SubQ	Unknown	Unknown	Unknown
Intranasal	≤ 1 hr	1–5 hr	8–12 hr

Action

Chemical effect: Increases flow of adenosine monophosphate and water through the kidneys, promoting reabsorption of water and producing concentrated urine (ADH effect). Releases factor VIII from plasma.
Therapeutic effect: Decreases diuresis and promotes clotting.

Available forms

Injection: 4 mcg/ml
Nasal solution: 0.1 mg/ml, 1.5 mg/ml
Tablets: 0.1 mg, 0.2 mg.

NURSING PROCESS

Assessment

- Obtain history of patient's underlying condition before therapy.
- Monitor effectiveness for diabetes insipidus or relief of symptoms of other disorders by checking patient's fluid intake and output, serum and urine osmolality, and urine specific gravity.
- Be alert for adverse reactions and drug interactions.
- Monitor patient carefully for hypertension during high-dose therapy.
- Assess patient's and family's knowledge of drug therapy.

Nursing diagnoses

- Deficient fluid volume related to underlying condition
- Acute pain related to drug-induced headache
- Deficient knowledge related to drug therapy

Planning and implementation

- When giving drug subcutaneously, rotate injection sites.
- Follow manufacturer's instructions exactly for intranasal administration.
- Ensure nasal passages are intact, clean, and free of obstruction before intranasal use.
- Intranasal use can cause changes in nasal mucosa, resulting in erratic, unreliable absorption. Report worsening condition to prescriber, who may prescribe injectable DDAVP.
- Don't use drug to treat severe cases of von Willebrand's disease or hemophilia A with factor VIII levels of 0% to 5%.
- Patients may be switched from intranasal to subcutaneous form, such as during episodes of rhinorrhea. Give ⅒ or ¼ of their usual nasal dose subcutaneously.
- When drug is used to treat diabetes insipidus, adjust dosage according to patient's fluid output. Adjust morning and evening doses separately for adequate diurnal rhythm of water turnover.

ALERT: Don't confuse desmopressin with vasopressin.

Patient teaching

- Instruct patient to clear nasal passages before using intranasal form of the drug.

• Teach patient and caregiver correct method of administration. Patient may have trouble measuring and inhaling drug into nostrils.
• Advise patient to report conditions such as nasal congestion, allergic rhinitis, or upper respiratory tract infection because dose adjustment may be required.
• Teach patient using subcutaneous desmopressin to rotate injection sites to avoid tissue damage.
• Warn patient to drink only enough water to satisfy thirst.
• Inform patient that when treating hemophilia A and von Willebrand's disease, giving desmopressin may avoid hazards of using blood products.
• Advise patient to wear or carry medical identification indicating use of drug.

☑ **Evaluation**
• Patient achieves normal fluid and electrolyte balance.
• Patient states that headache is relieved with mild analgesic.
• Patient and family state understanding of drug therapy.

dexamethasone
(deks-ah-METH-uh-sohn)
Decadron*, Dexamethasone Intensol*, Dexasone ♦, Dexone 0.5, Dexone 0.75, Dexone 1.5, Dexone 4, Hexadrol*, Maxidex, Mymethasone*, Oradexon ♦

dexamethasone acetate
Cortastat LA, Dalalone D.P., Decaject-L.A., Dexasone L.A., Dexone L.A., Solurex-LA

dexamethasone sodium phosphate
AK-Dex, Cortastat, Cortastat 10, Dalalone, Decadrol, Decadron, Decadron Phosphate, Decaject, Dexacen-4, Dexacorten, Dexone, Hexadrol Phosphate, Primethasone, Solurex

Pharmacologic class: glucocorticoid
Therapeutic class: anti-inflammatory, immunosuppressant
Pregnancy risk category: NR

Indications and dosages

▶ **Cerebral edema.** *Adults:* Initially, 10 mg dexamethasone sodium phosphate I.V. Then 4 mg I.M. q 6 hours until symptoms subside (usually 2 to 4 days). Then taper down over 5 to 7 days.
▶ **Inflammatory conditions, allergic reactions, neoplasias.** *Adults:* 4 mg dexamethasone sodium phosphate I.M. as a single dose. Continue maintenance therapy with dexamethasone tablets, 1.5 mg P.O. b.i.d. for 2 days; then 0.75 mg P.O. b.i.d. for 1 day; then 0.75 mg P.O. once daily for 2 days; then stop drug. Or 4 to 16 mg dexamethasone acetate I.M. into joint or soft tissue q 1 to 3 weeks. Or 0.8 to 1.6 mg into lesions q 1 to 3 weeks.
▶ **Shock.** *Adults:* 1 to 6 mg/kg dexamethasone sodium phosphate I.V. as single dose or 40 mg I.V. q 2 to 6 hours, p.r.n. Or 20 mg I.V. as a single dose, followed by continuous infusion of 3 mg/kg q 24 hours.
▶ **Suppression test for Cushing's syndrome.** *Adults:* After determining baseline 24-hour urine levels of 17-hydroxycorticosteroids, 0.5 mg P.O. q 6 hours for 48 hours; 24-hour urine collection made for determination of 17-hydroxycorticosteroid excretion again during second 24 hours of dexamethasone administration. Or 1 mg P.O. as a single dose at 11 PM. Draw blood for cortisol level at 8 AM the following day.
▶ **To prevent hyaline membrane disease in premature infants‡.** *Adults:* 5 mg dexamethasone sodium phosphate I.M. t.i.d. to mother for 2 days before delivery.
▶ **To prevent chemotherapy-induced nausea and vomiting‡.** *Adults:* 10 to 20 mg I.V. before giving chemotherapy. Additional doses (individualized for each patient and usually lower than initial dose) may be given I.V. or P.O. for 24 to 72 hours following cancer chemotherapy.

▼ I.V. administration

• When giving as direct injection, inject undiluted over at least 1 minute.
• When giving as intermittent or continuous infusion, dilute solution in normal saline solution or D_5W. For continuous infusion, change solution every 24 hours.
⊗ **Incompatibilities**
Ciprofloxacin, daunorubicin, diphenhydramine, doxapram, doxorubicin, glycopyrrolate, idarubicin, midazolam, vancomycin.

Contraindications and cautions

• Contraindicated in patients hypersensitive to drug or any of its components and in those with systemic fungal infections.

• Use cautiously in patients with seizures, emotional instability, psychotic tendencies, recent MI, thromboembolic disorders, heart failure, hypertension, GI ulcer, diverticulitis, nonspecific ulcerative colitis, recent intestinal anastomoses, renal disease, ocular herpes simplex, cirrhosis, diabetes mellitus, hypothyroidism, myasthenia gravis, osteoporosis, or tuberculosis. Because some forms contain sulfite preservatives, use cautiously in patients sensitive to sulfites.

⚞ **Lifespan:** In pregnant women, use cautiously. In breast-feeding women, drug isn't recommended. In children, long-term use of drug may delay growth and maturation.

Adverse reactions

CNS: *euphoria, insomnia,* pseudotumor cerebri, psychotic behavior, *seizures.*
CV: *arrhythmias,* edema, *heart failure,* hypertension, *thromboembolism.*
EENT: cataracts, glaucoma.
GI: GI irritation, increased appetite, *pancreatitis, peptic ulceration.*
GU: menstrual irregularities.
Metabolic: carbohydrate intolerance, hyperglycemia, hypokalemia.
Musculoskeletal: growth suppression in children, muscle weakness, osteoporosis.
Skin: acne, atrophy at I.M. injection sites, delayed wound healing, hirsutism, skin eruptions.
Other: acute adrenal insufficiency (may follow abrupt withdrawal after long-term therapy or such increased stress as infection, surgery, or trauma), cushingoid state (moonface, buffalo hump, central obesity), susceptibility to infections.

Interactions

Drug-drug. *Antidiabetics, including insulin:* May decrease corticosteroid response. May need dosage adjustment.
Aspirin, indomethacin, other NSAIDs: May increase risk of GI distress and bleeding. Give together cautiously.
Barbiturates, phenytoin, rifampin: May decrease corticosteroid effect. Increase corticosteroid dosage.

Digoxin: May increase risk of arrhythmia from hypokalemia. May need dosage adjustment.
Oral anticoagulants: May alter dosage requirements. Monitor PT and INR closely.
Potassium-depleting drugs: May enhance potassium-wasting effects of dexamethasone. Monitor potassium levels.
Salicylates: May decrease salicylate levels. Monitor patient for lack of therapeutic effects.
Skin-test antigens: May decrease response of skin-test antigens. Defer skin testing until therapy is completed.
Toxoids, vaccines: May decrease antibody response and increase risk of neurologic complications. Avoid using together.
Drug-lifestyle. *Alcohol use:* May increase risk of gastric irritation and GI ulceration. Discourage using together.

Effects on lab test results

• May increase glucose and cholesterol levels. May decrease potassium, calcium, T_3, and T_4 levels.

Pharmacokinetics

Absorption: For P.O. use, good. For injections, depends on location.
Distribution: To muscle, liver, skin, intestines, and kidneys. Bound weakly to transcortin and albumin. Only unbound portion is active.
Metabolism: In liver to inactive glucuronide and sulfate metabolites.
Excretion: Inactive metabolites and small amounts of unmetabolized drug by kidneys. Insignificant in feces. *Half-life:* About 1 to 2 days.

Route	Onset	Peak	Duration
P.O.	1–2 hr	1–2 hr	2½ days
I.V., I.M.	≤ 1 hr	1 hr	2 days–3 wk

Action

Chemical effect: May stabilize leukocyte lysosomal membranes; stimulate bone marrow; and influence protein, fat, and carbohydrate metabolism.
Therapeutic effect: Relieves cerebral edema, reduces inflammation and immune response, and reverses shock.

Available forms

dexamethasone
Elixir: 0.5 mg/5 ml

Reactions may be *common,* uncommon, *life-threatening,* or COMMON AND LIFE-THREATENING.

Oral solution: 0.5 mg/5 ml, 1 mg/ml
Tablets: 0.25 mg, 0.5 mg, 0.75 mg, 1 mg, 1.5 mg, 2 mg, 4 mg, 6 mg
dexamethasone acetate
Injection: 8 mg/ml, 16 mg/ml suspension
dexamethasone sodium phosphate
Injection: 4 mg/ml, 10 mg/ml, 20 mg/ml, 24 mg/ml

NURSING PROCESS

Assessment
- Obtain history of patient's underlying condition before therapy.
- Monitor patient's weight, blood pressure, glucose level, and electrolyte levels.
- Look for adverse reactions and drug interactions. Most adverse reactions to corticosteroids are dosage-dependent.
- Watch for depression or psychotic episodes, especially in high-dose therapy.
- Assess patient's and family's knowledge of drug therapy.

Nursing diagnoses
- Ineffective health maintenance related to underlying condition
- Risk for injury related to drug-induced adverse reactions
- Deficient knowledge related to drug therapy

Planning and implementation
- For better results and less toxicity, give once-daily dose in the morning.
- Give with food when possible.
- Give I.M. deeply into gluteal muscle. Rotate injection sites to prevent muscle atrophy.
- If possible, avoid giving drug subcutaneously because atrophy and sterile abscesses may occur.
- Always adjust to lowest effective dose.

ALERT: When stopping drug after long-term use, reduce dose gradually. Stopping drug abruptly may cause rebound inflammation, fatigue, weakness, arthralgia, fever, dizziness, lethargy, depression, fainting, orthostatic hypotension, dyspnea, anorexia, or hypoglycemia, or may be fatal.

ALERT: Give patient low-sodium diet high in potassium and protein. Also, give potassium supplements as directed.

- If patient's stress level (physical or psychological) increases, notify prescriber and increase dose.
- If patient has adverse reaction, notify prescriber, treat symptoms, and provide supportive therapy.

ALERT: Don't confuse dexamethasone with desoximetasone.

Patient teaching
- Tell patient not to abruptly stop taking the drug because this may be fatal.
- Teach patient the early signs of adrenal insufficiency (fatigue, muscle weakness, joint pain, fever, anorexia, nausea, dyspnea, dizziness, and fainting).
- Instruct patient to wear or carry medical identification that indicates need for supplemental systemic glucocorticoids during stress, especially as dose is decreased.
- Warn patient receiving long-term therapy about cushingoid symptoms and the need to notify prescriber about sudden weight gain or swelling.
- Warn patient about easy bruising.
- Advise patient receiving long-term therapy to consider exercise or physical therapy. Give vitamin D or calcium supplements.
- Advise patient receiving long-term therapy to have periodic ophthalmologic examinations.

Evaluation
- Patient's condition improves with drug therapy.
- Patient has no injury as a result of drug therapy.
- Patient and family state understanding of drug therapy.

dexmedetomidine hydrochloride
(DEX-meh-dih-TOE-mih-deen high-droh-KLOR-ighd)
Precedex

Pharmacologic class: selective $alpha_2$-adrenoreceptor agonist with sedative properties
Therapeutic class: sedative
Pregnancy risk category: C

Indications and dosages
▶ **Sedation of initially intubated and mechanically ventilated patients in the ICU.**
Adults: Loading infusion of 1 mcg/kg I.V. over

10 minutes; then a maintenance infusion of 0.2 to 0.7 mcg/kg/hour for up to 24 hours; adjust to achieve the desired level of sedation.
Adjust-a-dose: In elderly patients and those with renal or hepatic failure, reduce dosage.

I.V. administration

- Dilute in normal saline solution. To prepare the infusion, withdraw 2 ml of drug and add to 48 ml of normal saline injection to a total of 50 ml. Shake gently to mix well.
- Don't give through the same I.V. line with blood or plasma because physical compatibility hasn't been established.
- Infusion is compatible with lactated Ringer's solution, D_5W, normal saline solution, 20% mannitol, many anesthetic agents, atropine sulfate, morphine sulfate, and plasma substitute.
- Don't give infusion for longer than 24 hours.

⊗ **Incompatibilities**
Blood, plasma.

Contraindications and cautions

- Contraindicated in patients with hypersensitivity to dexmedetomidine.
- Use cautiously in patients with chronic hypertension, diabetes mellitus, advanced heart block, or renal or hepatic impairment.

Lifespan: In pregnant women, use only if potential benefits to the woman outweigh risks to the fetus because drug may be toxic to fetus. In breast-feeding women, use cautiously. In children, use isn't recommended. In elderly patients, use cautiously.

Adverse reactions

CNS: pain.
CV: ***arrhythmias, bradycardia,*** hypotension.
GI: *nausea,* thirst.
GU: oliguria.
Hematologic: anemia, leukocytosis.
Respiratory: ***hypoxia,*** pleural effusion, ***pulmonary edema.***
Other: infection.

Interactions

Drug-drug. *Anesthetics, hypnotics, opioids, sedatives:* May enhance effects. May need to reduce dexmedetomidine dose.

Effects on lab test results

- May decrease hemoglobin level and hematocrit.
- May increase WBC count.

Pharmacokinetics

Absorption: Given I.V.
Distribution: Rapid and wide. 94% protein-bound.
Metabolism: Almost complete.
Excretion: 95% in urine and 4% in feces. *Half-life:* About 2 hours.

Route	Onset	Peak	Duration
I.V.	Unknown	Unknown	Unknown

Action

Chemical effect: Selectively stimulates $alpha_2$-adrenoceptor in the CNS.
Therapeutic effect: Produces sedation of initially intubated and mechanically ventilated patients.

Available forms

Injection: 100 mcg/ml in 2-ml vials and 2-ml ampules

NURSING PROCESS

Assessment

- Assess renal and hepatic function before administration, particularly in elderly patients.
- Assess patient's response to drug. Some patients may stir and be alert when stimulated. This doesn't necessarily indicate lack of effectiveness.
- Look for adverse reactions and drug interactions.
- Assess patient's and family's knowledge of drug therapy.

Nursing diagnoses

- Risk for injury related to drug-induced adverse reactions
- Impaired spontaneous ventilation related to underlying disease process
- Deficient knowledge related to drug therapy

Planning and implementation

ALERT: Use a controlled infusion device at the rate calculated for patient's body weight.
- Continuously monitor cardiac condition.

• Drug can be continuously infused in mechanically ventilated patients before, during, and after extubation. Drug doesn't need to be stopped before extubation.

Patient teaching

• Tell patient that he'll be sedated while the drug is given, but that he may awake when stimulated.

• Tell patient that he'll be closely monitored and attended while sedated.

☑ **Evaluation**

• Patient has no injury as a result of drug-induced adverse reactions.

• Patient regains spontaneous ventilation.

• Patient and family state understanding of drug therapy.

---

dexmethylphenidate hydrochloride
(dex-meth-il-FEN-uh-date high-droh-KLOR-ighd)
Focalin, Focalin XR

Pharmacologic class: CNS stimulant
Therapeutic class: CNS stimulant
Pregnancy risk category: C
Controlled substance schedule: II

Indications and dosages

▶ **Attention deficit hyperactivity disorder (ADHD).**
Immediate-release tablets
Children age 6 and older: For patients who aren't taking racemic methylphenidate or who are taking another stimulant, start with 2.5 mg P.O. twice daily, at least 4 hours apart. For patients who are being switched from methylphenidate, start with one-half of the current methylphenidate dosage. Additionally, adjust dose weekly in increments of 2.5 to 5 mg daily to maximum of 20 mg daily in two divided doses.
Extended-release capsules
Adults: If patient takes neither dexmethylphenidate nor methylphenidate or takes a stimulant other than methylphenidate, 10 mg P.O. once daily in the morning. May adjust by 10 mg weekly. If patient takes methylphenidate, start with half the total daily methylphenidate dose. If patient takes immediate-release dexmethyl-

phenidate, may switch to same daily dose of extended-release form. Maximum, 20 mg daily.
Children age 6 and older: If patient takes neither dexmethylphenidate nor methylphenidate, or takes a stimulant other than methylphenidate, 5 mg P.O. once daily in the morning. May adjust by 5 mg weekly. If patient takes methylphenidate, start with half the total daily methylphenidate dose. If patient takes immediate-release dexmethylphenidate, may switch to same daily dose of extended-release form. Maximum, 20 mg daily.

Contraindications and cautions

• Contraindicated in patients hypersensitive to drug or any of its components. Also contraindicated in patients with severe anxiety, tension, agitation, or glaucoma and in those who have motor tics or a family history or diagnosis of Tourette syndrome. Also contraindicated within 14 days of MAO inhibitor therapy because hypertensive crisis may occur. Don't use to treat severe depression or to prevent or treat normal fatigue states.

• Use cautiously in patients with a history of drug abuse, alcoholism, psychosis, seizures, hypertension, hyperthyroidism, heart failure, or recent MI.

⚑ **Lifespan:** In pregnant women, use only if the potential benefits to the woman outweigh the risks to the fetus. In breast-feeding women, use cautiously because it's unknown if drug appears in breast milk. In children younger than age 6, don't use.

Adverse reactions

CNS: blurred vision, fever, growth suppression, insomnia, nervousness, psychosis.
CV: hypertension, tachycardia.
GI: *abdominal pain,* anorexia, nausea.
Hematologic: anemia, *leukopenia.*
Metabolic: weight loss.
Musculoskeletal: arthralgia, twitching (motor or vocal tics).

Interactions

Drug-drug. *Anticoagulants, anticonvulsants, SSRIs, tricyclic antidepressants:* May inhibit metabolism of these drugs. May need to decrease dosage of these drugs; monitor drug levels.

Antihypertensives: May decrease effectiveness of these drugs. Use together cautiously; monitor blood pressure.

Clonidine, other centrally acting alpha$_2$ agonists: May cause serious adverse effects. Use together cautiously.

MAO inhibitors: May increase risk of hypertensive crisis. Avoid use within 14 days of using MAO inhibitors.

Effects on lab test results

• May decrease hemoglobin level and hematocrit.

• May increase liver function test values. May decrease WBC count.

Pharmacokinetics

Absorption: Food delays rate of peak level but doesn't affect the amount absorbed.
Distribution: Rapid.
Metabolism: Extensive via de-esterification. Doesn't inhibit the CYP system. No active metabolites.
Excretion: 90% in urine. *Half-life:* About 2 hours.

Route	Onset	Peak	Duration
P.O.			
immediate-release	Unknown	1–1½ hr	Unknown
extended-release	Unknown	1–4 hr; 4½–7 hr	Unknown

Action

Chemical effect: May block presynaptic reuptake of norepinephrine and dopamine and increase the release of these neurotransmitters.
Therapeutic effect: Increases attention span and decreases hyperactivity and impulsiveness related to ADHD.

Available forms

Capsules (extended-release): 5 mg, 10 mg, 20 mg
Tablets: 2.5 mg, 5 mg, 10 mg

NURSING PROCESS

🕮 Assessment

• Diagnosis must be based on complete history and evaluation of the child in consultation with psychological, educational, and social specialists.

• Monitor blood pressure and pulse routinely during drug therapy.

• Look for adverse reactions.

• Check CBC with differential and platelet counts during long-term use.

✛ Nursing diagnoses

• Ineffective health maintenance related to underlying condition

• Ineffective coping by family due to patient's underlying hyperactivity condition

• Deficient knowledge of drug therapy

⟫ Planning and implementation

• Drug is meant to be an adjunct to comprehensive therapy program that includes psychological, educational, and social support.

• Drug contains only the active isomer required to effectively manage the symptoms of ADHD, at half the dose of Ritalin.

• Growth may be suppressed with long-term stimulant use. Monitor children for growth and weight gain. If growth is suppressed or if weight gain is lower than expected, stop giving the drug.

• If symptoms are aggravated or adverse reactions occur, reduce dosage or stop drug.

• If seizures occur, stop giving the drug.

• Symptoms of overdose include vomiting, agitation, tremors, hyperreflexia, muscle twitching, convulsions, euphoria, confusion, hallucinations, delirium, sweating, flushing, headache, hyperpyrexia, tachycardia, palpitations, cardiac arrhythmias, hypertension, mydriasis, and dry mucous membranes. Give supportive care and protection against self-injury and additional overstimulation.

• Stop drug if symptoms don't improve after 1 month.

Patient teaching

• Advise parents to monitor child's height and weight and to tell prescriber if they suspect any growth suppression.

• If patient can't swallow capsules, tell him to empty the contents onto a spoonful of applesauce and eat immediately.

⊛ ALERT: Tell patient not to cut, crush, or chew contents of extended-release capsules.

• Advise patient to take drug at the same time every day at the prescribed dose. Tell patient to

---

report any adverse reactions to prescriber immediately.

☑ Evaluation
• Patient responds positively to drug therapy.
• Patient and family are effectively coping with patient's underlying condition.
• Patient and family state understanding of drug therapy.

dextran, high-molecular-weight (dextran 70, dextran 75)
(DEKS-tran, high moh-LEH-kyoo-ler wayt)
Dextran 70, Dextran 75, Gentran 70, Gendex 75, Macrodex

Pharmacologic class: glucose polymer
Therapeutic class: plasma volume expander
Pregnancy risk category: C

Indications and dosages
▶ **Plasma expander.** *Adults:* 30 g (500 ml of 6% solution) I.V. In emergencies, may give 1.2 to 2.4 g (20 to 40 ml)/minute. In normovolemic or nearly normovolemic patients, don't infuse faster than 240 mg (4 ml)/minute. Don't give more than 1.2 g/kg during the first 24 hours of therapy. Actual dosage depends on amount of fluid loss and resulting hemoconcentration and must be determined for each patient.

▽ I.V. administration
• Use D₅W instead of normal saline solution because drug is hazardous for patients with heart failure, especially when given in normal saline solution.
• Give 20 ml of dextran 1 (containing 150 mg/ml) I.V. over 60 seconds 1 to 2 minutes before I.V. infusion of dextran, to protect against drug-induced anaphylaxis.
• Observe patient closely during early phase of infusion, when most anaphylactic reactions occur.
• Store drug at constant 77° F (25° C). Precipitate may form in storage. Heat to dissolve.
⊗ **Incompatibilities**
Any other I.V. drug added to a bottle of dextran, ascorbic acid, phytonadione, promethazine, protein hydrolysate.

Contraindications and cautions
• Contraindicated in patients hypersensitive to drug and in those with marked hemostatic defects, marked cardiac decompensation, renal disease with severe oliguria or anuria, hypervolemic conditions, or severe bleeding disorders.
• Use cautiously in patients with active hemorrhage, thrombocytopenia, impaired renal clearance, chronic liver disease, or abdominal conditions, and in patients undergoing bowel surgery.
☀ **Lifespan:** In pregnant women, use cautiously. Breast-feeding women should stop nursing or stop the drug. In children, safety and effectiveness haven't been established.

Adverse reactions
CNS: fever.
CV: fluid overload, thrombophlebitis.
EENT: nasal congestion.
GI: nausea, vomiting.
GU: anuria, increased specific gravity and viscosity of urine, oliguria, tubular stasis and blocking.
Musculoskeletal: arthralgia.
Skin: urticaria.
Other: *anaphylaxis,* hypersensitivity reactions.

Interactions
Drug-drug. *Abciximab, aspirin, heparin, thrombolytics, warfarin:* May increase bleeding. Use together cautiously; monitor patient for bleeding.

Effects on lab test results
• May increase ALT and AST levels. May decrease hemoglobin level and hematocrit.
• May increase bleeding time.

Pharmacokinetics
Absorption: Given I.V.
Distribution: Throughout vascular system.
Metabolism: Drug molecules with molecular weights above 50,000 are degraded to glucose at rate of about 70 to 90 mg/kg/day.
Excretion: Drug molecules with molecular weights below 50,000 in urine. *Half-life:* Unknown.

Route	Onset	Peak	Duration
I.V.	Immediate	Immediate	Unknown

Action

Chemical effect: Expands plasma volume by way of colloidal osmotic effect, drawing fluid from interstitial to intravascular space, providing fluid replacement.
Therapeutic effect: Expands plasma volume.

Available forms

Injection: Dextran 70 in normal saline solution or D_5W; 6% dextran 75 in normal saline solution or D_5W

⚡ Assessment

• Obtain history of patient's underlying condition and hydration before therapy, and reassess regularly. Frequently assess vital signs, fluid intake and output, and urine or serum osmolarity levels.
• Be alert for adverse reactions.
• Watch for circulatory overload and rise in central venous pressure. Plasma expansion is slightly greater than volume infused.
• Monitor hemoglobin level and hematocrit.
• Assess patient's and family's knowledge of drug therapy.

🔀 Nursing diagnoses

• Decreased cardiac output related to underlying condition
• Risk for injury related to potential for drug-induced hypersensitivity reaction
• Deficient knowledge related to drug therapy

🔢 Planning and implementation

• May significantly suppress platelet function with doses of 15 ml/kg.
• If oliguria or anuria occurs or isn't relieved by infusion, stop dextran and give loop diuretic.
• If hematocrit values fall below 30% by volume, notify prescriber.
• Drug may interfere with analyses of blood grouping, crossmatching, and bilirubin, glucose, and protein levels.
• **⊗ ALERT:** Low– and high–molecular-weight dextrans aren't interchangeable. Verify preparation before use.
Patient teaching
• Inform patient or family about drug therapy.
• Instruct patient to notify prescriber if adverse reactions, such as itching, occur.

☑ Evaluation

• Patient's vital signs and urine output return to normal.
• Patient doesn't develop hypersensitivity reaction to drug.
• Patient and family state understanding of drug therapy.

dextran, low–molecular-weight (dextran 40)

(DEKS-tran, LOH moh-LEH-kyoo-ler wayt)
Dextran 40, Gentran 40, 10% LMD, Rheomacrodex

Pharmacologic class: glucose polymer
Therapeutic class: plasma volume expander
Pregnancy risk category: C

Indications and dosages

▶ **Plasma volume expansion.** *Adults:* Dosage by I.V. infusion depends on amount of fluid loss. Initially, 10 ml/kg of dextran infused rapidly with central venous pressure monitoring; remainder of dose given slowly. Total dosage not to exceed 20 ml/kg in the first 24 hours. If therapy is continued longer than 24 hours, don't exceed 10 ml/kg daily. Continue for no longer than 5 days.
▶ **To prevent venous thrombosis.** *Adults:* 10 ml/kg (500 to 1,000 ml) I.V. on day of procedure; 500 ml on days 2 and 3.
▶ **Hemodiluent in extracorporeal circulation.** *Adults:* 10 to 20 ml/kg added to perfusion circuit. Total dosage not to exceed 20 ml/kg.

▼ I.V. administration

• Use D_5W solution instead of normal saline solution because drug is hazardous for patients with heart failure, especially when given in normal saline solution.
• Prescriber may order dextran 1, a dextran adjunct, to protect against drug-induced anaphylaxis. Give 20 ml of dextran 1 (containing 150 mg/ml) I.V. over 60 seconds, 1 to 2 minutes before I.V. infusion of dextran.
• Observe patient closely during early phase of infusion, when most anaphylactic reactions occur.

• Store at constant 77° F (25° C). Precipitate may form during storage. Heat to dissolve.
• Discard partially used containers.

⊗ **Incompatibilities**

Any other I.V. drug added to a bottle of dextran, ascorbic acid, phytonadione, promethazine, protein hydrolysate.

Contraindications and cautions

• Contraindicated in patients hypersensitive to drug and in those with marked hemostatic defects, marked cardiac decompensation, and renal disease with severe oliguria or anuria.
• Use cautiously in patients with active hemorrhage, thrombocytopenia, or diabetes mellitus.
❉ **Lifespan:** In pregnant women, use cautiously. Breast-feeding women should stop breast-feeding or not use the drug. In children, safety and effectiveness haven't been established.

Adverse reactions

CV: thrombophlebitis.
GI: nausea, vomiting.
GU: increased urine viscosity, tubular stasis and blocking.
Hematologic: anemia.
Skin: urticaria.
Other: *anaphylaxis,* hypersensitivity reactions.

Interactions

None significant.

Effects on lab test results

• May increase ALT and AST levels. May decrease hemoglobin level and hematocrit.
• May increase bleeding time.

Pharmacokinetics

Absorption: Given I.V.
Distribution: Throughout vascular system.
Metabolism: Drug molecules with molecular weights above 50,000 are degraded to glucose at about 70 to 90 mg/kg/day.
Excretion: By kidneys for drug molecules with molecular weights below 50,000. *Half-life:* Unknown.

Route	Onset	Peak	Duration
I.V.	Immediate	Immediate	≤ 3 hr

Action

Chemical effect: Expands plasma volume by colloidal osmotic effect, drawing fluid from interstitial to intravascular space, providing fluid replacement.
Therapeutic effect: Expands plasma volume.

Available forms

Injection: 10% dextran 40 in D_5W or normal saline solution

D

NURSING PROCESS

ᴿˣ Assessment
• Obtain history of patient's underlying condition and hydration before therapy, and reassess regularly. Frequently assess vital signs, fluid intake and output, and urine or serum osmolarity levels.
• Be alert for adverse reactions.
• Watch for circulatory overload and rise in central venous pressure. Plasma expansion is slightly greater than volume infused.
• Check hemoglobin level and hematocrit.
• Assess patient's and family's knowledge of drug therapy.

Nursing diagnoses
• Decreased cardiac output related to underlying condition
• Risk for injury related to potential for drug-induced hypersensitivity reaction
• Deficient knowledge related to drug therapy

Planning and implementation
• If oliguria or anuria occurs or isn't relieved by infusion, stop dextran and give loop diuretic.
• If hematocrit falls below 30% by volume, notify prescriber.
• Drug may interfere with analyses of blood grouping, crossmatching, and bilirubin, glucose, and protein levels.
🛈 **ALERT:** Low– and high–molecular-weight dextrans aren't interchangeable. Verify preparation before use.

Patient teaching
• Tell patient and family about therapy.
• Instruct patient to notify prescriber if adverse reactions, such as itching, occur.

☑ Evaluation

• Patient's vital signs and urine output return to normal.
• Patient has no hypersensitivity reaction to drug.
• Patient and family state understanding of drug therapy.

dextroamphetamine sulfate

(deks-troh-am-FET-uh-meen SUL-fayt)
Dexedrine*, Dexedrine Spansule, DextroStat, Ferndex, Oxydess II, Spancap #1

Pharmacologic class: amphetamine
Therapeutic class: CNS stimulant
Pregnancy risk category: C
Controlled substance schedule: II

Indications and dosages

► **Narcolepsy.** *Adults:* 5 to 60 mg P.O. daily in divided doses.
Children age 12 and older: 10 mg P.O. daily; increase by 10-mg increments weekly until desired response occurs or adult dose is reached.
Children ages 6 to 11: 5 mg P.O. daily; increase by 5-mg increments weekly until desired response occurs. Give first dose on awakening, additional doses (one or two) at intervals of 4 to 6 hours.
► **Attention deficit hyperactivity disorder.**
Children age 6 and older: 5 mg P.O. once daily or b.i.d.; increase by 5-mg increments weekly, p.r.n.
Children ages 3 to 5: 2.5 mg P.O. daily; increase by 2.5-mg increments weekly, p.r.n. In rare cases, more than 40 mg daily is needed.
► **Short-term adjunct in exogenous obesity‡.**
Adults: 5 to 30 mg P.O. daily 30 to 60 minutes before meals in divided doses of 5 to 10 mg. Or one 10- or 15-mg sustained-released capsule daily as a single dose in the morning.

Contraindications and cautions

• Contraindicated in patients hypersensitive to sympathomimetic amines and those with idiosyncratic reactions to them; within 14 days of MAO inhibitor use; and in those with hyperthyroidism, moderate-to-severe hypertension, symptomatic CV disease, glaucoma, advanced arteriosclerosis, or a history of drug abuse.
• Use cautiously in patients with motor and phonic tics, Tourette syndrome, and agitated states.
⚖ **Lifespan:** In pregnant women, use cautiously. In breast-feeding women, safety and effectiveness haven't been established.

Adverse reactions

CNS: dizziness, dysphoria, headache, *insomnia*, overstimulation, *restlessness,* tremors.
CV: arrhythmias, hypertension, palpitations, tachycardia.
GI: anorexia, constipation, diarrhea, dry mouth, other GI disturbances, unpleasant taste, weight loss.
GU: impotence.
Skin: urticaria.
Other: altered libido, chills.

Interactions

Drug-drug. *Acetazolamide, alkalizing drugs, antacids, sodium bicarbonate:* May increase renal reabsorption. Monitor patient for enhanced amphetamine effects.
Acidifying drugs, ammonium chloride, ascorbic acid: May decrease level and increase renal clearance of dextroamphetamine. Monitor patient for decreased amphetamine effects.
Adrenergic blockers: May be inhibited by amphetamines. Avoid using together.
Antihistamines: May counteract sedative effects of antihistamines. Monitor patient for loss of therapeutic effects.
Chlorpromazine: May inhibit central stimulant effects of amphetamines, and may be used to treat amphetamine poisoning. Monitor patient closely.
Haloperidol, phenothiazines, tricyclic antidepressants: May decrease amphetamine effect. Increase dose p.r.n.
Insulin, oral antidiabetics: May decrease antidiabetic requirement. Monitor glucose levels.
Lithium carbonate: May inhibit antiobesity and stimulating effects of amphetamines. Monitor patient closely.
MAO inhibitors: May cause severe hypertension; possibly hypertensive crisis. Don't use within 14 days of MAO inhibitor therapy.
Meperidine: Amphetamines may potentiate analgesic effect. Use together cautiously.

Reactions may be *common*, uncommon, *life-threatening*, or COMMON AND LIFE-THREATENING.

Methenamine: May increase urinary excretion and reduces effectiveness of amphetamines. Monitor effects.

Norepinephrine: May enhance adrenergic effect of norepinephrine. Monitor patient closely.

Phenobarbital, phenytoin: May delay absorption of dextroamphetamine. Monitor patient closely.

Propoxyphene: In cases of propoxyphene overdose, amphetamine CNS stimulation may be potentiated and fatal seizures can occur. Don't use together.

Drug-food. *Caffeine:* May increase amphetamine and related amine effects. Monitor patient closely.

Effects on lab test results
• May increase corticosteroid level.

Pharmacokinetics
Absorption: Rapid; for sustained-release capsules, more slowly.
Distribution: Wide.
Metabolism: Unknown.
Excretion: In urine. *Half-life:* 10 to 12 hours.

Route	Onset	Peak	Duration
P.O.	Unknown	Unknown	Unknown

Action
Chemical effect: Unknown; probably promotes nerve impulse transmission by releasing stored norepinephrine from nerve terminals in brain. Main sites of activity appear to be the cerebral cortex and reticular activating system.
Therapeutic effect: Helps prevent sleep and calms hyperactive children.

Available forms
Capsules (sustained-release): 5 mg, 10 mg, 15 mg
Tablets: 5 mg, 10 mg

NURSING PROCESS

▧ Assessment
• Obtain history of patient's underlying condition before therapy, and reassess regularly throughout therapy.
• Be alert for adverse reactions and drug interactions.
• Monitor sleeping pattern, and observe patient for signs of excessive stimulation.

• Assess patient's and family's knowledge of drug therapy.

⊕ Nursing diagnoses
• Ineffective health maintenance related to underlying condition
• Disturbed sleep pattern related to drug-induced insomnia
• Deficient knowledge related to drug therapy

▷ Planning and implementation
• Give at least 6 hours before bedtime to avoid sleep interference.
• Prolonged use may cause psychological dependence or habituation, especially in patients with history of drug addiction. After prolonged use, reduce dose gradually to prevent acute rebound depression.
Patient teaching
• Warn patient to avoid hazardous activities until the drug's CNS effects are known.
• Tell patient to avoid drinks containing caffeine, which increases the effects of amphetamines and related amines.
• Inform patient that fatigue may result as drug effects wear off.
• Instruct patient to report signs of excessive stimulation.
• Inform patient that when tolerance to anorexigenic effect develops, he should stop the drug, not increase the dose. Tell him to report decreased effectiveness of drug. Warn patient against stopping drug abruptly.

☑ Evaluation
• Patient shows improvement in underlying condition.
• Patient can sleep without difficulty.
• Patient and family state understanding of drug therapy.

dextromethorphan hydrobromide

(deks-troh-meth-OR-fan high-droh-BROH-mighd)
Balminil DMI, Benylin Adult†, Benylin Pediatric†, Broncho-Grippol-DM ♦, Hold DM†, DexAlone†, Koffex ♦, Robitussin Pediatric†, Trocal†, Vicks Formula 44 Cough Relief†

More commonly available in combination products such as Anti-Tuss DM Expectorant†, Cheracol D Cough†, Extra Action Cough†, Glycotuss DM†, Guiamid D.M. Liquid† Guiatuss-DM†, Halotussin-DM Expectorant†, Kolephrin GG/DM†, Mytussin DM†, Naldecon Senior DX†, Pertussin All-Night CS†, Rhinosyn-DMX Expectorant†, Robitussin-DM†, Silexin Cough†, Tolu-Sed DM†, Tuss-DM†, Unproco†, Vicks Children's Cough Syrup†, Vicks DayQuil LiquiCaps†

Pharmacologic class: levorphanol derivative (dextrorotatory methyl ether)
Therapeutic class: antitussive (nonopioid)
Pregnancy risk category: C

Indications and dosages

▶ **Nonproductive cough.** *Adults and children older than age 12:* 10 to 30 mg P.O. q 4 hours, or 30 mg gelcaps q 6 to 8 hours. Or 60-mg extended-release liquid b.i.d. Maximum, 120 mg daily.
Children ages 6 to 12: 5 to 10 mg P.O. q 4 hours, or 15 mg q 6 to 8 hours. Or 30-mg extended-release liquid b.i.d. Maximum, 60 mg daily.
Children ages 2 to 5: 2.5 to 5 mg P.O. q 4 hours, or 7.5 mg q 6 to 8 hours. Or 15-mg extended-release liquid b.i.d. Maximum, 30 mg daily. Dosages for children younger than age 2 must be individualized.

Contraindications and cautions

• Contraindicated within 14 days of MAO inhibitor therapy.
• Use cautiously in sedated or debilitated patients and in patients confined to supine position. Also, use cautiously in patients with aspirin sensitivity.
※ **Lifespan:** In pregnant women, use cautiously. In breast-feeding women, safety and effec-

tiveness haven't been established. In atopic children, use cautiously.

Adverse reactions

CNS: dizziness, drowsiness.
GI: stomach pain, nausea, vomiting.

Interactions

Drug-drug. *MAO inhibitors:* May increase risk of hypotension, coma, hyperpyrexia, and death. Don't use within 2 weeks of dextromethorphan hydrobromide therapy.
Selegiline: May increase risk of confusion, coma, hyperpyrexia. Avoid using together.
Drug-herb. *Parsley:* May cause serotonin syndrome. Discourage using together.

Effects on lab test results

None reported.

Pharmacokinetics

Absorption: Good.
Distribution: Unknown.
Metabolism: Extensive.
Excretion: Small amount unchanged. Metabolites mainly in urine; about 7% to 10% in feces.
Half-life: About 11 hours.

Route	Onset	Peak	Duration
P.O.	≤ 30 min	Unknown	3–12 hr

Action

Chemical effect: Suppresses cough reflex by direct action on cough center in medulla.
Therapeutic effect: Prevents cough.

Available forms

Gelcaps: 30 mg†
Liquid (extended-release): 30 mg/5 ml
Lozenges: 2.5 mg, 5 mg†, 7.5 mg†, 15 mg†
Solution: 3.5 mg/5 ml, 5 mg/5 ml*†, 7.5 mg/5 ml*†, 10 mg/5 ml*†, 15 mg/5 ml*†, 10 mg/15 ml*

NURSING PROCESS

☞ **Assessment**
• Obtain history of patient's cough before giving the drug, and reassess after giving the drug.
• Look for adverse reactions and drug interactions.
• Assess patient's and family's knowledge of drug therapy.

Reactions may be *common,* uncommon, *life-threatening,* or COMMON AND LIFE-THREATENING.

⊞ Nursing diagnoses
• Fatigue related to presence of nonproductive cough
• Risk for injury related to drug-induced adverse CNS reactions
• Deficient knowledge related to drug therapy

▷ Planning and implementation
• Don't use drug when cough is valuable diagnostic sign or is beneficial (such as after thoracic surgery).
• As an antitussive, 15 to 30 mg of dextromethorphan is equivalent to 8 to 15 mg of codeine.
• Use drug with chest percussion and vibration.
• If cough isn't relieved, notify prescriber.
Patient teaching
• Instruct patient to follow directions on medication bottle exactly; stress importance of not taking more drug than directed.
• Tell patient to call prescriber if cough persists more than 7 days.
• Suggest sugarless throat lozenges to decrease throat irritation and resulting cough.
• Advise patient to use humidifier to moisten air and ionizer or air filter to filter dust, smoke, and air pollutants.

✓ Evaluation
• Patient's cough is relieved.
• Patient has no injury as a result of therapy.
• Patient and family state understanding of drug therapy.

diazepam
(digh-AZ-uh-pam)
Apo-Diazepam ♦ , Diastat, Diazemuls ♦ ◇ , Diazepam Intensol, Novo-Dipam ♦ , PMSDiazepam ♦ , Valium✐, Vivol ♦

Pharmacologic class: benzodiazepine
Therapeutic class: anxiolytic, skeletal muscle relaxant, anticonvulsant, sedative-hypnotic
Pregnancy risk category: D
Controlled substance schedule: IV

Indications and dosages
▶ **Anxiety.** *Adults:* Depending on severity, 2 to 10 mg P.O. b.i.d. to q.i.d. Or 2 to 10 mg I.M. or I.V. q 3 to 4 hours, if needed.

Elderly patients: 2 to 2.5 mg P.O. once or twice daily; increase gradually, p.r.n.
Children age 6 months and older: 1 to 2.5 mg P.O. t.i.d. or q.i.d.; increase gradually, as needed and tolerated.
▶ **Acute alcohol withdrawal.** *Adults:* 10 mg P.O. t.i.d. or q.i.d. for the first 24 hours and reduce to 5 mg P.O. t.i.d. or q.i.d., p.r.n. Or, initially, 10 mg I.M. or I.V.; then 5 to 10 mg I.M. or I.V. in 3 to 4 hours, if needed.
▶ **Before endoscopic procedures.** *Adults:* Titrate I.V. dose to desired sedative response (up to 20 mg). Or 5 to 10 mg I.M. 30 minutes before procedure.
▶ **Muscle spasm.** *Adults:* 2 to 10 mg P.O. b.i.d. to q.i.d. daily. Or 5 to 10 mg I.M. or I.V. initially; then 5 to 10 mg I.M. or I.V. in 3 to 4 hours, p.r.n. For tetanus, larger doses may be required.
Elderly patients: 2 to 2.5 mg I.M. or I.V. once or twice daily; increase p.r.n.
Children age 5 and older: 5 to 10 mg I.M. or I.V. q 3 to 4 hours, p.r.n.
Infants older than age 30 days and younger than age 5: 1 to 2 mg I.M. or I.V. slowly repeated q 3 to 4 hours, p.r.n.
▶ **Preoperative sedation.** *Adults:* 10 mg I.M. (preferred) or I.V. before surgery.
▶ **Cardioversion.** *Adults:* 5 to 15 mg I.V. 5 to 10 minutes before procedure.
▶ **Adjunct in seizure disorders.** *Adults:* 2 to 10 mg P.O. b.i.d. to q.i.d.
Elderly patients: 2 to 2.5 mg P.O. once or twice daily; increase p.r.n.
Children and infants age 6 months and older: 1 to 2.5 mg P.O. t.i.d. or q.i.d. initially; increase as tolerated and needed.
▶ **Status epilepticus.** *Adults:* 5 to 10 mg I.V. (preferred) or I.M. initially. Repeat q 10 to 15 minutes, p.r.n., to maximum, 30 mg. Repeat in 2 to 4 hours, p.r.n.
Children age 5 and older: 1 mg I.V. q 2 to 5 minutes to maximum, 10 mg. Repeat in 2 to 4 hours, p.r.n.
Infants older than age 30 days and younger than age 5: 0.2 to 0.5 mg I.V. slowly q 2 to 5 minutes to maximum, 5 mg. Repeat in 2 to 4 hours, p.r.n.
▶ **To control acute repetitive seizure activity in patients already taking anticonvulsants.** *Adults and children age 12 and older:* 0.2 mg/kg P.R. using applicator. A second dose may be given 4 to 12 hours after the first dose, if needed.

Children ages 6 to 11: 0.3 mg/kg P.R. using applicator. A second dose may be given 4 to 12 hours after the first dose, if needed.
Children ages 2 to 5: 0.5 mg/kg P.R. using applicator. A second dose may be given 4 to 12 hours after the first dose, if needed.

▽ I.V. administration

• Give drug I.V. at no more than 5 mg/minute.
• Inject drug directly into vein. If this is impossible, inject slowly through infusion tubing as near to venous insertion site as possible. Watch closely for phlebitis at injection site.
• To avoid extravasation, don't inject into small veins.
• Monitor respirations every 5 to 15 minutes and before each I.V. dose. Have emergency resuscitation equipment and oxygen at bedside when giving drug I.V.

⊗ **Incompatibilities**
All other I.V. drugs, most I.V. solutions.

Contraindications and cautions

• Contraindicated in patients hypersensitive to drug or any of its components and in those with angle-closure glaucoma, shock, coma, or acute alcohol intoxication (parenteral form).
• Use cautiously in patients with hepatic or renal impairment, depression, or chronic open-angle glaucoma.

❧ **Lifespan:** In pregnant women (especially during the first trimester) and in breast-feeding women, avoid using the drug. In infants younger than age 6 months, oral form of drug is contraindicated. In elderly and debilitated patients, use cautiously and give a lower dose because these patients may be more susceptible to adverse CNS effects of drug.

Adverse reactions

CNS: anterograde amnesia, *ataxia,* depression, *drowsiness,* fainting, *hangover,* headache, insomnia, *lethargy, pain,* psychosis, restlessness, slurred speech, tremors.
CV: *bradycardia, CV collapse,* transient hypotension.
EENT: blurred vision, diplopia, nystagmus.
GI: abdominal discomfort, constipation, nausea, vomiting.
GU: incontinence, urine retention.
Respiratory: respiratory depression.
Skin: desquamation, rash, urticaria.

Other: *acute withdrawal syndrome* after stopping drug suddenly in physically dependent person, *phlebitis at injection site,* physical or psychological dependence.

Interactions

Drug-drug. *Cimetidine:* May increase sedation. Monitor patient carefully.
CNS depressants: May increase CNS depression. Avoid using together.
Digoxin: May increase digoxin level and toxicity. Monitor digoxin level.
Diltiazem: May increase CNS depression and prolong effects of diazepam. Use lower dose of diazepam.
Fluconazole, ketoconazole, itraconazole, miconazole: May increase and prolong diazepam level, CNS depression, and psychomotor impairment. Don't use together.
Phenobarbital: May increase effects of both drugs. Use together cautiously.
Phenytoin: May increase level of phenytoin. Monitor patient for toxicity.
Ranitidine: May decrease absorption. Monitor patient for decreased effect.
Drug-herb. *Kava, sassafras, valerian:* Sedative effects may be enhanced. Discourage using together.
Drug-lifestyle. *Alcohol use:* May cause additive CNS effects. Strongly discourage alcohol use with these drugs.
Smoking: May increase benzodiazepine clearance. Monitor patient for lack of drug effect.

Effects on lab test results

• May increase liver function test values. May decrease neutrophil count.

Pharmacokinetics

Absorption: For I.M. use, erratic.
Distribution: Wide; about 85% to 95% bound to plasma protein.
Metabolism: In liver to active metabolite, desmethyldiazepam.
Excretion: Most metabolites in urine, with small amount in feces. *Half-life:* About 1 to 12 days.

Route	Onset	Peak	Duration
P.O.	30 min	½–2 hr	3–8 hr
I.V.	1–5 min	≤ 15 min	15–60 min
I.M.	Unknown	2 hr	Unknown
P.R.	Unknown	1–5 hr	Unknown

Action

Chemical effect: May depress CNS at limbic and subcortical levels of brain; suppresses spread of seizure activity produced by epileptogenic foci in cortex, thalamus, and limbic system.

Therapeutic effect: Relieves anxiety, muscle spasms, and seizures (parenteral form); promotes calmness and sleep.

Available forms

Injection: 5 mg/ml
Oral solution: 5 mg/ml, 5 mg/5 ml
Rectal gel: 2.5 mg*, 5 mg*, 10 mg*, 15 mg*, 20 mg*
Sterile emulsion for injection: 5 mg/ml*
Tablets: 2 mg, 5 mg, 10 mg

NURSING PROCESS

🖉 Assessment

• Obtain history of patient's underlying condition before therapy, and reassess regularly thereafter.
• Periodically monitor liver, kidney, and hematopoietic function studies in patient receiving repeated or prolonged therapy.
• Look for adverse reactions and drug interactions.
• Assess patient's and family's knowledge of drug therapy.

🏵 Nursing diagnoses

• Ineffective health maintenance related to underlying condition
• Risk for injury related to drug-induced adverse CNS reactions
• Deficient knowledge related to drug therapy

▶ Planning and implementation

• When oral concentrate solution is used, dilute dose just before giving. Use water, juice, or carbonated beverages, or mix with semisolid food such as applesauce or pudding.
• Avoid P.R. use of Diastat for more than 5 episodes per month or one episode every 5 days.
• 🕲 **ALERT:** Drug should be given only by caregivers who can distinguish the distinct cluster of seizures or events from the patient's ordinary seizure activity, who can give the drug competently, who understand which seizure characteristics can be treated with drug, and who can

monitor the patient's response and recognize when immediate professional help is needed.
• Give drug I.M. only when giving I.V. or P.O. isn't possible because absorption is variable and injection is painful.
• Don't mix injectable form with other drugs because diazepam is incompatible with most drugs.
• Don't store parenteral solution in plastic syringes.
• Parenteral emulsion—a stabilized oil-in-water emulsion—should appear milky white and uniform. Avoid mixing with any other drugs or solutions, and avoid infusion sets or containers made from polyvinyl chloride. If diluting, mix drug with I.V. fat emulsion. Use admixture within 6 hours.
• Possibility of abuse and addiction exists. Don't withdraw drug abruptly after long-term use. Withdrawal symptoms may occur.
• 🕲 **ALERT:** Don't confuse diazepam with diazoxide.

Patient teaching
• Warn patient to avoid hazardous activities until the drug's CNS effects are known.
• Tell patient to avoid using alcohol during therapy.
• Warn patient to take drug only as directed and not to stop it without prescriber's approval.
• Warn patient about risk of physical and psychological dependence.

☑ Evaluation

• Patient shows improvement in underlying condition.
• Patient has no injury as result of drug-induced adverse CNS reactions.
• Patient and family state understanding of drug therapy.

diazoxide
(digh-uz-OKS-ighd)
Hyperstat IV, Proglycem

Pharmacologic class: peripheral vasodilator, insulin release inhibitor
Therapeutic class: antihypertensive, antihypoglycemic
Pregnancy risk category: C

Indications and dosages

▶ **Hypertensive crisis.** *Adults and children:*
1 to 3 mg/kg by I.V. bolus (maximum, 150 mg)
q 5 to 15 minutes until adequate response occurs. Repeat at 4- to 24-hour intervals, p.r.n.
▶ **Hypoglycemia from hyperinsulinism.**
Adults and children: 3 to 8 mg/kg P.O. daily in
2 or 3 divided doses q 8 to 12 hours.
Infants and neonates: 8 to 15 mg/kg P.O. daily
in two or three divided doses q 8 to 12 hours.

▼ I.V. administration

● Protect I.V. solutions from light. Don't use
darkened I.V. solutions because they aren't potent.
● Place patient in supine position during and for
1 hour after infusion.
● Keep dopamine or norepinephrine available in
case of severe hypotension.
● Give drug through peripheral vein only. Don't
give drug I.M., subcutaneously, or into body
cavities.
● Monitor blood pressure and ECG continuously. If severe hypotension develops, notify prescriber immediately and place patient in a
supine position.
● Watch for infiltration and irritation. Extravasation can cause tissue damage and necrosis.
⊗ **Incompatibilities**
Hydralazine, propranolol.

Contraindications and cautions

● Contraindicated in patients hypersensitive to
drug, other thiazides, or other sulfonamide-
derived drugs. Also contraindicated in compensatory hypertension (as in coarctation of the
aorta or arteriovenous shunt).
● Use cautiously in patients with impaired cerebral or cardiac function or uremia.
⚖ **Lifespan:** In pregnant women, use cautiously. In breast-feeding women, drug isn't recommended.

Adverse reactions

CNS: *cerebral ischemia,* dizziness, euphoria,
headache, light-headedness, *paralysis.*
CV: angina, arrhythmias, ECG changes, flushing, *MI,* myocardial ischemia, orthostatic hypotension, *shock,* warmth.
GI: abdominal discomfort, constipation, diarrhea, dry mouth, *nausea, vomiting.*
Hematologic: *thrombocytopenia.*

Metabolic: hyperglycemia, hyperuricemia,
sodium and water retention.
Skin: diaphoresis.
Other: inflammation, pain (with extravasation).

Interactions

Drug-drug. *Antihypertensives:* May cause severe hypotension. Use together cautiously, and
monitor blood pressure closely.
Hydantoins: May decrease hydantoin level and
anticonvulsant action. Monitor patient closely.
Insulin, oral antidiabetics: May alter insulin
and oral antidiabetic requirements in previously
stable patients. Monitor glucose level.
Sulfonylureas: May cause hyperglycemia. Monitor glucose level.
Thiazide diuretics: May increase diazoxide effects. Use together cautiously.

Effects on lab test results

● May increase glucose and uric acid levels.
● May decrease platelet count.

Pharmacokinetics

Absorption: After P.O. use, hyperglycemic effect begins in 1 hour. After I.V. use, blood pressure should decrease promptly, with maximum
effect in 1 hour.
Distribution: Throughout body; about 90%
protein-bound.
Metabolism: Partially in liver.
Excretion: Drug and metabolites slowly by kidneys. *Half-life:* 21 to 36 hours.

Route	Onset	Peak	Duration
P.O.	≤ 1 hr	Unknown	< 8 hr
I.V.	≤ 1 min	2–5 min	2–12 hr

Action

Chemical effect: Directly relaxes arteriolar
smooth muscle and decreases peripheral vascular resistance. Increases glucose levels by inhibiting pancreatic release of insulin, stimulating catecholamine release or increasing hepatic
release of glucose.
Therapeutic effect: Lowers blood pressure; increases blood sugar.

Available forms

Capsules: 50 mg
Injection: 15 mg/ml
Oral suspension: 50 mg/ml

✍ Assessment
• Obtain history of patient's blood pressure before therapy.
• Weigh patient daily.
• Monitor glucose levels daily; watch closely for signs of severe hyperglycemia or hyperosmolar nonketotic syndrome.
• Check patient's uric acid levels frequently.
• Look for adverse reactions and drug interactions.
• Assess patient's and family's knowledge of drug therapy.

🏥 Nursing diagnoses
• Risk for injury related to presence of hypertension
• Excess fluid volume related to drug-induced fluid retention
• Deficient knowledge related to drug therapy

▷ Planning and implementation
• Check patient's standing blood pressure before you stop giving the drug.
• If fluid or sodium retention develops, prescriber may order diuretics.
ⓢ **ALERT:** Don't confuse diazoxide with Dyazide or diazepam, Hyperstat with Nitrostat, Hyper-Tet, or HyperHep.
Patient teaching
• Inform patient that orthostatic hypotension can be minimized by rising slowly and avoiding sudden position changes.
• Instruct patient to remain in supine position for 30 minutes after injection.

☑ Evaluation
• Patient's blood pressure returns to normal.
• Patient maintains normal fluid and electrolyte balance during therapy.
• Patient and family state understanding of drug therapy.

diclofenac potassium
(digh-KLOH-fen-ek poh-TAH-see-um)
Cataflam

diclofenac sodium
Solaraze, Voltaren, Voltaren SR ♦ ,
Voltaren-XR

Pharmacologic class: NSAID
Therapeutic class: antiarthritic, antiinflammatory
Pregnancy risk category: B

Indications and dosages
▶ **Ankylosing spondylitis.** *Adults:* 25-mg delayed-release tablets P.O. q.i.d. (may give another 25 mg h.s., p.r.n.).
▶ **Osteoarthritis.** *Adults:* 50-mg immediate- or delayed-release tablets P.O. b.i.d. or t.i.d. Or 75 mg P.O. b.i.d. Or 100-mg extended-release tablets P.O. daily.
▶ **Rheumatoid arthritis.** *Adults:* 50-mg immediate- or delayed-release tablets P.O. t.i.d. or q.i.d. Or 75 mg P.O. b.i.d. Or 50 to 100 mg P.R. (where available) h.s. as substitute for last P.O. dose of day. Not to exceed 225 mg daily. Or 100-mg extended-release tablets P.O. daily or b.i.d.
▶ **Analgesia and primary dysmenorrhea.** *Adults:* 50 mg diclofenac potassium P.O. t.i.d. If needed, 100 mg may be given for first dose only.
▶ **Actinic keratosis.** *Adults:* Apply gel to lesion b.i.d.

Contraindications and cautions
• Contraindicated in patients hypersensitive to drug or any of its components and in those with hepatic porphyria or a history of asthma, urticaria, or other allergic reactions after taking aspirin or other NSAIDs.
• Use cautiously in patients with history of peptic ulcer disease, hepatic dysfunction, cardiac disease, hypertension, conditions that cause fluid retention, or impaired kidney function.
⚠ **Lifespan:** For women in late pregnancy or who are breast-feeding, drug isn't recommended. In children, safety and effectiveness haven't been established.

Adverse reactions

CNS: anxiety, depression, dizziness, drowsiness, headache, insomnia, irritability, migraine, myoclonus.
CV: edema, fluid retention, *heart failure,* hypertension.
EENT: blurred vision, epistaxis, eye pain, *laryngeal edema,* night blindness, reversible hearing loss, swelling of lips and tongue, tinnitus.
GI: abdominal distention, *abdominal pain or cramps,* appetite change, *bleeding,* bloody diarrhea, colitis, *constipation, diarrhea,* flatulence, *indigestion,* melena, *nausea,* peptic ulceration, taste disorder.
GU: *acute renal failure,* azotemia, *fluid retention,* interstitial nephritis, nephrotic syndrome, *oliguria,* papillary necrosis, proteinuria.
Hepatic: *hepatitis, hepatotoxicity,* jaundice.
Metabolic: hyperglycemia, *hypoglycemia.*
Musculoskeletal: back, leg, or joint pain.
Respiratory: *asthma.*
Skin: allergic purpura, alopecia, bullous eruption, dermatitis, eczema, photosensitivity, pruritus, rash, *Stevens-Johnson syndrome,* urticaria.
Other: *anaphylaxis, angioedema.*

Interactions

Drug-drug. *Anticoagulants, including warfarin:* May increase risk of bleeding. Monitor patient closely for bleeding.
Aspirin: May increase risk of bleeding. Don't use together.
Beta blockers: Antihypertensive effect of beta blocker may be blunted. Monitor blood pressure closely.
Cyclosporine, digoxin, lithium, methotrexate: May reduce renal clearance of these drugs and increase risk of toxicity. Monitor patient closely; monitor drug levels if appropriate.
Diuretics: May decrease diuretic effectiveness. Monitor patient for fluid retention.
Insulin, oral antidiabetics: May alter antidiabetic requirement. Monitor glucose level.
Potassium-sparing diuretics: May enhance potassium retention and increases potassium levels. Monitor patient for hyperkalemia.
Drug-herb. *Dong quai, feverfew, garlic, ginger, horse chestnut, red clover:* May increase risk of bleeding. Discourage using together.
St. John's wort: May increase risk of photosensitivity. Advise against unprotected and prolonged exposure to sunlight.

Drug-lifestyle. *Sun exposure:* May cause photosensitivity reactions. Urge patient to wear protective clothing and sunblock.

Effects on lab test results

• May increase ALT, AST, alkaline phosphatase, bilirubin, BUN, creatinine, and LDH levels. May increase or decrease glucose level.

Pharmacokinetics

Absorption: Rapid and almost complete. Delayed by food.
Distribution: Highly (nearly 100%) protein-bound.
Metabolism: Undergoes first-pass metabolism, with 60% of unchanged drug reaching systemic circulation.
Excretion: About 40% to 60% in urine; balance in bile. *Half-life:* 1 to 2 hours.

Route	Onset	Peak	Duration
P.O., P.R.	30 min	Unknown	8 hr
P.O. enteric-coated	30 min	2–3 hr	8 hr

Action

Chemical effect: Produces anti-inflammatory, analgesic, and antipyretic effects, possibly by inhibiting prostaglandin synthesis.
Therapeutic effect: Relieves inflammation, pain, and fever.

Available forms

diclofenac potassium
Tablets: 50 mg
diclofenac sodium
Suppositories: 50 mg ♦, 100 mg ♦
Tablets (delayed-release/enteric-coated): 25 mg, 50 mg, 75 mg
Tablets (extended-release): 100 mg ♦

NURSING PROCESS

🔲 Assessment
• Obtain history of patient's underlying condition before therapy.
• Monitor effectiveness by assessing patient for pain relief.
• Liver enzyme level may elevate. Monitor transaminase level, especially ALT level, periodically in a patient undergoing long-term ther-

---

Reactions may be *common,* uncommon, *life-threatening*, or COMMON AND LIFE-THREATENING.

apy. Take first level within the first 8 weeks of therapy.
- Look for adverse reactions and drug interactions.
- Assess patient's and family's knowledge of drug therapy.

🔲 Nursing diagnoses
- Acute pain related to underlying condition
- Risk for injury related to drug-induced adverse reactions
- Deficient knowledge related to drug therapy

▷ Planning and implementation
- If drug causes GI distress. Give with milk or food.
- Notify prescriber immediately if patient develops signs of GI bleeding, hepatotoxicity, or other adverse reactions.
- Rectal preparation isn't commercially available in the United States. Elsewhere, it may be substituted for the last oral dose of the day to decrease GI distress if can't take with food.

Patient teaching
- Tell patient to take drug with milk or food to minimize GI distress.
- Instruct patient not to crush, break, or chew enteric-coated tablets.
- Teach patient signs and symptoms of GI bleeding, and tell him to contact prescriber immediately if they occur.
- Teach patient signs and symptoms of hepatotoxicity, including nausea, fatigue, lethargy, pruritus, jaundice, right upper quadrant tenderness, and flulike symptoms. Tell him to contact prescriber immediately if these symptoms appear.

☑ Evaluation
- Patient is free from pain.
- Patient has no injury as result of drug-induced adverse reactions.
- Patient and family state understanding of drug therapy.

dicyclomine hydrochloride
(digh-SIGH-kloh-meen high-droh-KLOR-ighd)
Antispas, Bemote, Bentyl, Bentylol ♦,
Byclomine, Dibent, Dilomine, Di-Spaz,
Formulex ♦, Lomine ♦, Merbentyl ◇,
Or-Tyl, Spasmoban ♦

Pharmacologic class: anticholinergic
Therapeutic class: antimuscarinic, GI antispasmodic
Pregnancy risk category: B

Indications and dosages
▶ **Irritable bowel syndrome and other functional GI disorders.** *Adults:* Initially, 20 mg P.O. q.i.d.; increase to 40 mg q.i.d. Or 20 mg I.M. q 4 to 6 hours.
Children age 2 and older: 10 mg P.O. t.i.d. or q.i.d.
Infants ages 6 months to 2 years: 5 to 10 mg P.O. t.i.d. or q.i.d.
▶ **Colic‡.** *Infants age 6 months and older.* 5 to 10 mg P.O. t.i.d. or q.i.d. Adjust dosage according to patient's needs and response.

Contraindications and cautions
- Contraindicated in patients hypersensitive to anticholinergics and in those with obstructive uropathy, obstructive disease of GI tract, reflux esophagitis, severe ulcerative colitis, myasthenia gravis, unstable CV status in acute hemorrhage, or glaucoma.
- Use cautiously in patients with autonomic neuropathy, hyperthyroidism, coronary artery disease, arrhythmias, heart failure, hypertension, hiatal hernia, hepatic or renal disease, prostatic hypertrophy, or ulcerative colitis.
- ❊ **Lifespan:** In pregnant patients, use cautiously. In breast-feeding women and in infants younger than age 6 months, drug is contraindicated.

Adverse reactions
CNS: *dizziness;* drowsiness; fever; *headache;* insomnia; nervousness, confusion, and excitement in elderly patients.
CV: *palpitations,* tachycardia.
EENT: blurred vision, increased intraocular pressure, mydriasis.

GI: abdominal distention, *constipation, dry mouth,* heartburn, nausea, paralytic ileus, vomiting.
GU: impotence, urinary hesitancy, urine retention.
Skin: decreased sweating or possibly anhidrosis, other dermal changes, urticaria.
Other: allergic reactions.

Interactions

Drug-drug. *Amantadine, antihistamines, antiparkinsonians, disopyramide, glutethimide, meperidine, phenothiazines, procainamide, quinidine, tricyclic antidepressants:* May cause additive adverse effects. Avoid using together.
Antacids: May decrease absorption of oral anticholinergics. Separate doses by 2 to 3 hours.
Ketoconazole: May interfere with ketoconazole absorption. Give at least 2 hours after ketoconazole.

Effects on lab test results

None reported.

Pharmacokinetics

Absorption: 67% of P.O. dose.
Distribution: Unknown.
Metabolism: Unknown.
Excretion: 80% of P.O. dose in urine and 10% in feces. *Half-life:* Initial, about 2 hours; secondary, 9 to 10 hours.

Route	Onset	Peak	Duration
P.O.	Unknown	1–1½ hr	Unknown
I.M.	Unknown	Unknown	Unknown

Action

Chemical effect: Appears to exert nonspecific, indirect spasmolytic action on smooth muscle. Dicyclomine also possesses local anesthetic properties that may be partly responsible for spasmolysis.
Therapeutic effect: Relieves GI spasms.

Available forms

Capsules: 10 mg, 20 mg
Injection: 10 mg/ml
Syrup: 5 mg/5 ml ◊, 10 mg/5 ml
Tablets: 10 mg ◊, 20 mg

NURSING PROCESS

⚖ Assessment

• Obtain history of patient's underlying condition before therapy.
• Monitor the drug's effectiveness by regularly assessing patient for pain relief and improvement of underlying condition.
• Look for adverse reactions and drug interactions.
• Assess patient's and family's knowledge of drug therapy.

⊕ Nursing diagnoses

• Acute pain related to underlying condition
• Risk for injury related to drug-induced adverse CNS reactions
• Deficient knowledge related to drug therapy

▶ Planning and implementation

• Drug is synthetic tertiary derivative that may cause atropine-like adverse reactions. Overdose may cause curare-like effects, such as respiratory paralysis.
• High environmental temperatures may induce heatstroke during drug use. If symptoms occur, stop giving the drug.
• Give 30 to 60 minutes before meals and at bedtime. Bedtime dose can be larger; give at least 2 hours after last meal of the day.
⚠ **ALERT:** Don't give drug subcutaneously or I.V.
• Adjust dosage according to patient's needs and response. Up to 40 mg P.O. q.i.d. may be used in adults, but safety and effectiveness for more than 2 weeks haven't been established.
⚠ **ALERT:** The dicyclomine label may be misleading. The ampule label reads 10 mg/ml, but doesn't indicate that the ampule contains 2 ml of solution (20 mg of drug).
⚠ **ALERT:** Don't confuse dicyclomine with dyclonine or doxycycline; don't confuse Bentyl with Aventyl or Benadryl.
Patient teaching
• Instruct patient to refrain from driving and performing other hazardous activities if he's drowsy or dizzy or has blurred vision.
• Tell him to drink plenty of fluids to help prevent constipation.
• Urge patient to report rash or skin eruption.
• Tell patient to use sugarless gum or hard candy to relieve dry mouth.

☑ Evaluation

- Patient is free from pain.
- Patient doesn't experience injury as a result of drug-induced adverse CNS reactions.
- Patient and family state understanding of drug therapy.

didanosine (ddI)

(digh-DAN-uh-zeen)
Videx, Videx EC

Pharmacologic class: nucleoside reverse transcriptase inhibitor
Therapeutic class: antiretroviral
Pregnancy risk category: B

Indications and dosages

▶ **HIV infection when antiretroviral therapy is warranted.** *Adults weighing 60 kg (132 lb) and more:* 200-mg tablets P.O. q 12 hours or 400-mg tablets P.O. daily. Or 250-mg buffered powder q 12 hours. Or 400-mg delayed-release capsules P.O. daily.
Adults weighing less than 60 kg: 125 mg P.O. q 12 hours or 250 mg P.O. once daily. Or 167-mg buffered powder q 12 hours. Or 250-mg delayed-release capsules P.O. daily.
Children older than age 8 months: 120 mg/m^2 P.O. q 12 hours.
Children ages 2 weeks to 8 months: 100 mg/m^2 P.O. q 12 hours.
Adjust-a-dose: In adults who weigh 60 kg or more with creatinine clearance of 30 to 59 ml/minute, give 100-mg tablet b.i.d., 200-mg tablet or 200-mg delayed-release capsule once daily, or 100-mg buffered powder b.i.d. For clearance of 10 to 29 ml/minute, give 150-mg tablet, 125-mg delayed-release capsule, or 167-mg buffered powder once daily. For clearance less than 10 ml/minute, give 100-mg tablet, 125-mg delayed-release capsule, or 100-mg buffered powder once daily.

In adults who weigh less than 60 kg and have a clearance of 30 to 59 ml/minute, give 75-mg tablet b.i.d., 150-mg tablet or 125-mg delayed-release capsule once daily, or 100-mg buffered powder b.i.d. For clearance of 10 to 29 ml/minute, give 100-mg tablet, 125-mg delayed-release capsule, or 100-mg buffered powder once daily. For clearance less than 10 ml/minute or patients on dialysis, give 75-mg tablet or 100-mg buffered powder once daily. Capsules aren't indicated for these patients. No additional dose is needed after hemodialysis.

Contraindications and cautions

- Contraindicated in patients hypersensitive to drug or any of its components.
- Use cautiously in patients with a history of pancreatitis and in patients with peripheral neuropathy, renal or hepatic impairment, or hyperuricemia.

Lifespan: In pregnant women, use cautiously. In breast-feeding women, drug isn't recommended.

Adverse reactions

CNS: abnormal thinking, asthenia, anxiety, confusion, depression, *dizziness, fever, headache,* hypertonia, insomnia, nervousness, pain, *peripheral neuropathy,* ***seizures,*** twitching.
CV: edema, ***heart failure,*** hyperlipidemia, hypertension.
GI: abdominal pain, diarrhea, dry mouth, dyspepsia, flatulence, nausea, pancreatitis, vomiting.
Hematologic: anemia, granulocytosis, ***leukopenia, thrombocytopenia.***
Hepatic: ***hepatic failure,*** liver abnormalities, ***severe hepatomegaly.***
Metabolic: ***lactic acidosis.***
Musculoskeletal: arthritis, myalgia, myopathy.
Respiratory: cough, dyspnea, pneumonia.
Skin: alopecia, pruritus, rash.
Other: ***anaphylactoid reaction,*** chills, infection, sarcoma.

Interactions

Drug-drug. *Amprenavir, delavirdine, indinavir, nelfinavir, ritonavir, saquinavir:* May alter pharmacokinetics. Separate doses.
Antacids containing magnesium or aluminum hydroxides: Enhances adverse effects of antacid component (including diarrhea or constipation) when given with didanosine tablets or pediatric suspension. Avoid using together.
Dapsone, ketoconazole, drugs that require gastric acid for adequate absorption: May decrease absorption from buffering action. Give these drugs 2 hours before didanosine.
Fluoroquinolones, tetracyclines: May decrease absorption because of buffers in didanosine tablets or antacids in pediatric solution. Monitor patient for decreased effectiveness.

Itraconazole: May decrease levels of itraconazole. Avoid using together.

Tenofovir: May cause high rate of early virologic failure and emerging resistance. Don't use together. Switch patients currently on this regimen to eliminate tenofovir.

Drug-food. *Any food:* May increase rate of absorption. Give drug on an empty stomach.

Drug-herb. *St. John's wort:* May decrease drug levels, decreasing therapeutic effect. Discourage using together.

Effects on lab test results

• May increase uric acid, AST, ALT, alkaline phosphatase, and bilirubin levels. May decrease hemoglobin level and hematocrit.

• May decrease WBC, granulocyte, and platelet counts.

Pharmacokinetics

Absorption: Rapid. Commercially available forms contain buffers to raise stomach pH. Bioavailability averages 33%; tablets may be more bioavailable than buffered powder for oral solution. Food decreases absorption by 50%.

Distribution: Wide; drug penetration into CNS varies, but CSF levels average 46% of blood levels.

Metabolism: Probably similar to that of endogenous purines.

Excretion: In urine. *Half-life:* 48 minutes.

Route	Onset	Peak	Duration
P.O.	Unknown	30 min–1 hr	Unknown

Action

Chemical effect: Unknown; appears to inhibit replication of HIV by preventing DNA replication.

Therapeutic effect: Inhibits replication of HIV.

Available forms

Delayed-release capsules: 125 mg, 200 mg, 250 mg, 400 mg

Powder for oral solution (buffered): 100 mg/packet, 167 mg/packet, 250 mg/packet

Powder for oral solution (pediatric): 10 mg/ml in 2- and 4-g bottles

Tablets (chewable): 25 mg, 50 mg, 100 mg, 150 mg, 200 mg

NURSING PROCESS

☞ Assessment

• Obtain history of patient's underlying condition before therapy, and reassess regularly thereafter.

• Be alert for adverse reactions and drug interactions.

• Assess patient's and family's knowledge of drug therapy.

✛ Nursing diagnoses

• Infection related to presence of HIV infection

• Diarrhea related to drug-induced adverse effect on bowel

• Deficient knowledge related to drug therapy

❱ Planning and implementation

• Give drug on empty stomach at least 30 minutes before or 2 hours after meals, regardless of dosage form used, because giving drug with meals can decrease absorption by 50%.

• Give patient two tablets of the appropriate strength at each dose to provide adequate buffering.

• To give single-dose packets containing buffered powder for oral solution, pour contents into 4 oz of water. Don't use fruit juice or other beverages that may be acidic. Stir for 2 to 3 minutes until powder dissolves completely. Give immediately.

• Use care when preparing powder or crushing tablets to avoid putting excessive amounts of powder into air.

• Pharmacist must prepare pediatric powder for oral solution. It must be constituted with purified water, USP, and then diluted with antacid (either Mylanta Double Strength Liquid or Maalox TC Suspension) to final concentration of 10 mg/ml. The admixture is stable for 30 days if refrigerated (at 36° to 46° F [2° to 8° C]). Shake solution well before measuring dose.

• If pancreatitis is suspected, stop drug and don't continue until pancreatitis is ruled out.

• If patient has diarrhea while using powdered form, consider switching to tablet form.

Patient teaching

• Instruct patient to chew tablets thoroughly before swallowing and to drink at least 1 oz of water with each dose because tablets contain buffers that raise stomach pH to levels that prevent drug from breaking down. If tablets are

---

Reactions may be *common*, uncommon, *life-threatening*, or COMMON AND LIFE-THREATENING.

manually crushed, stir them thoroughly in 1 oz of water to disperse particles uniformly; then have patient drink mixture immediately.
• Inform patient on sodium-restricted diet that each two-tablet dose contains 529 mg of sodium; each single packet of buffered powder for oral solution contains 1.38 g of sodium.
• Warn patient about adverse CNS reactions, and tell patient to take safety precautions.
• Tell patient to notify prescriber if adverse GI reaction occurs.

☑ Evaluation

• Patient improves with therapy.
• Patient regains normal bowel pattern.
• Patient and family state understanding of drug therapy.

diflunisal
(digh-FLOO-neh-sol)
Dolobid

Pharmacologic class: NSAID
Therapeutic class: analgesic, antipyretic, anti-inflammatory
Pregnancy risk category: C

Indications and dosages

▶ **Mild to moderate pain.** *Adults:* Initially, 500 mg to 1 g P.O., followed by 250 to 500 mg q 8 to 12 hours.
▶ **Osteoarthritis, rheumatoid arthritis.** *Adults:* 500 mg to 1 g P.O. daily in two divided doses, usually q 12 hours. Maximum, 1,500 mg daily.
Adjust-a-dose: For patients older than age 65, give half the usual adult dose.

Contraindications and cautions

• Contraindicated in patients hypersensitive to drug or any of its components and in those who develop acute asthmatic attacks, urticaria, or rhinitis after taking aspirin or other NSAIDs.
• Use cautiously in patients with GI bleeding, history of peptic ulcer disease, renal impairment, compromised cardiac function, hypertension, or other conditions predisposing patient to fluid retention.
Lifespan: In breast-feeding women, drug isn't recommended. In children and teenagers with chickenpox or flulike illness, salicylates aren't recommended because of epidemiologic connection to Reye's syndrome.

Adverse reactions

CNS: *dizziness,* fatigue, *headache,* insomnia, somnolence.
EENT: *tinnitus,* visual disturbances.
GI: constipation, *diarrhea, dyspepsia,* flatulence, *GI pain, nausea,* vomiting.
GU: hematuria, interstitial nephritis, renal impairment.
Skin: ***erythema multiforme,*** pruritus, rash, ***Stevens-Johnson syndrome,*** stomatitis, sweating.
Other: dry mucous membranes.

Interactions

Drug-drug. *Acetaminophen, hydrochlorothiazide, indomethacin:* May substantially increase levels of these drugs, increasing risk of toxicity. Avoid using together.
Antacids: May decrease diflunisal level. Monitor patient for decreased therapeutic effect.
Aspirin: May increase adverse effects. Monitor patient closely.
Cyclosporine: May increase nephrotoxicity of cyclosporine. Avoid using together.
Methotrexate: May increase toxicity of methotrexate. Avoid using together.
Oral anticoagulants, thrombolytics: May enhance effects of these drugs. Use together cautiously.
Sulindac: May decrease level of sulindac's active metabolite. Monitor patient for decreased effect.
Drug-herb. *Dong quai, feverfew, garlic, ginger, horse chestnut, red clover:* May increase risk of bleeding. Discourage using together.

Effects on lab test results

None reported.

Pharmacokinetics

Absorption: Rapid and complete.
Distribution: Highly protein-bound.
Metabolism: In liver.
Excretion: In urine. *Half-life:* 8 to 12 hours.

Route	Onset	Peak	Duration
P.O.	1 hr	2–3 hr	8–12 hr

Action

Chemical effect: May inhibit prostaglandin synthesis.
Therapeutic effect: Relieves inflammation and pain; reduces body temperature.

Available forms

Tablets: 250 mg, 500 mg

NURSING PROCESS

⚗ Assessment

• Obtain history of patient's underlying condition before therapy, and reassess regularly thereafter.
• Look for adverse reactions and drug interactions.
• Assess patient's and family's knowledge of drug therapy.

🔅 Nursing diagnoses

• Acute pain related to underlying condition
• Risk for deficient fluid volume related to drug-induced adverse reactions
• Deficient knowledge related to drug therapy

▷ Planning and implementation

• Give drug with milk or food to minimize adverse GI reactions.
• **ALERT:** Don't confuse Dolobid with Slo-bid.
Patient teaching
• Advise patient to take with water, milk, or meals.
• Warn patient to avoid drug interactions by checking with prescriber or pharmacist before taking OTC drugs or herbal remedies, such as those containing aspirin or salicylates.

☑ Evaluation

• Patient is free from pain.
• Patient maintains adequate hydration throughout therapy.
• Patient and family state understanding of drug therapy.

digoxin
(dih-JOKS-in)
Digitek, Digoxin, Lanoxicaps, Lanoxin*◆

Pharmacologic class: cardiac glycoside
Therapeutic class: antiarrhythmic, inotropic
Pregnancy risk category: C

Indications and dosages

▶ **Heart failure, paroxysmal supraventricular tachycardia, atrial fibrillation and flutter.**
Tablets, elixir
Adults: For rapid digitalization, give 0.75 to 1.25 mg P.O. over 24 hours in two or more divided doses q 6 to 8 hours. For slow digitalization, give 0.125 to 0.5 mg daily for 5 to 7 days. Maintenance dose is 0.125 to 0.5 mg daily.
Children age 10 and older: 10 to 15 mcg/kg P.O. over 24 hours in two or more divided doses q 6 to 8 hours. Maintenance dose is 25% to 35% of total digitalizing dose.
Children ages 5 to 10: 20 to 35 mcg/kg P.O. over 24 hours in two or more divided doses q 6 to 8 hours. Maintenance dose is 25% to 35% of total digitalizing dose.
Children ages 2 to 5: 30 to 40 mcg/kg P.O. over 24 hours in two or more divided doses q 6 to 8 hours. Maintenance dose is 25% to 35% of total digitalizing dose.
Infants ages 1 month to 2 years: 35 to 60 mcg/kg P.O. over 24 hours in two or more divided doses q 6 to 8 hours. Maintenance dose is 25% to 35% of total digitalizing dose.
Neonates: 25 to 35 mcg/kg P.O. over 24 hours in two or more divided doses q 6 to 8 hours. Maintenance dose is 25% to 35% of total digitalizing dose.
Premature infants: 20 to 30 mcg/kg P.O. over 24 hours in two or more divided doses q 6 to 8 hours. Maintenance dose is 20% to 30% of total digitalizing dose.
Capsules
Adults: For rapid digitalization, give 0.4 to 0.6 mg P.O. initially, followed by 0.1 to 0.3 mg q 6 to 8 hours, as needed and tolerated, for 24 hours. For slow digitalization, give 0.05 to 0.35 mg daily in two divided doses for 7 to 22 days until therapeutic levels are reached. Maintenance dose is 0.05 to 0.35 mg daily in one or two divided doses.

D

◙ **Adjust-a-dose:** In children, digitalizing dose is based on child's age and is given in three or more divided doses over the first 24 hours. First dose is 50% of the total dose; subsequent doses are given q 4 to 8 hours as needed and tolerated. *Children age 10 and older:* For rapid digitalization, give 8 to 12 mcg/kg P.O. over 24 hours, divided as above. Maintenance dose is 25% to 35% of total digitalizing dose, given daily as a single dose.
Children ages 5 to 10: For rapid digitalization, give 15 to 30 mcg/kg P.O. over 24 hours, divided as above. Maintenance dose is 25% to 35% of total digitalizing dose, divided and given in two or three equal portions daily.
Children ages 2 to 5: For rapid digitalization, give 25 to 35 mcg/kg P.O. over 24 hours, divided as above. Maintenance dose is 25% to 35% of total digitalizing dose, divided and given in two or three equal portions daily.
Injection
Adults: For rapid digitalization, give 0.4 to 0.6 mg I.V. initially, followed by 0.1 to 0.3 mg I.V. q 4 to 8 hours, as needed and tolerated, for 24 hours. For slow digitalization, give appropriate daily maintenance dose for 7 to 22 days as needed until therapeutic levels are reached. Maintenance dose is 0.125 to 0.5 mg I.V. daily in one or two divided doses.
Children: Digitalizing dose is based on child's age and is given in three or more divided doses over the first 24 hours. First dose is 50% of total dose; subsequent doses are given q 4 to 8 hours as needed and tolerated.
Children age 10 and older: For rapid digitalization, give 8 to 12 mcg/kg I.V. over 24 hours, divided as above. Maintenance dose is 25% to 35% of total digitalizing dose, given daily as a single dose.
Children ages 5 to 10: For rapid digitalization, give 15 to 30 mcg/kg I.V. over 24 hours, divided as above. Maintenance dose is 25% to 35% of total digitalizing dose, divided and given in two or three equal portions daily.
Children ages 2 to 5: For rapid digitalization, give 25 to 35 mcg/kg I.V. over 24 hours, divided as above. Maintenance dose is 25% to 35% of total digitalizing dose, divided and given in two or three equal portions daily.
Infants ages 1 month to 2 years: For rapid digitalization, give 30 to 50 mcg/kg I.V. over 24 hours, divided as above. Maintenance dose is

25% to 35% of total digitalizing dose, divided and given in two or three equal portions daily.
Neonates: For rapid digitalization, give 20 to 30 mcg/kg I.V. over 24 hours, divided as above. Maintenance dose is 25% to 35% of the total digitalizing dose, divided and given in two or three equal portions daily.
Premature infants: For rapid digitalization, give 15 to 25 mcg/kg I.V. over 24 hours, divided as above. Maintenance dose is 20% to 30% of the total digitalizing dose, divided and given in two or three equal portions daily.
◙ **Adjust-a-dose:** In all dosage forms, give smaller loading and maintenance doses to patients with impaired renal function.
   For patients with renal impairment, decrease dosage. For patients with hyperthyroidism, may need to increase dosage.

▼ I.V. administration

• Dilute fourfold with D_5W, normal saline solution, or sterile water for injection to reduce the chance of precipitation.
• Infuse drug slowly over at least 5 minutes.
• Protect prepared drug from light.
⊗ **Incompatibilities**
Amiodarone, dobutamine, doxapram, drugs or solutions given through the same I.V. line, fluconazole, foscarnet, other I.V. drugs, propofol.

Contraindications and cautions

• Contraindicated in patients hypersensitive to the drug or any of its components and in those with digitalis-induced toxicity, ventricular fibrillation, or ventricular tachycardia unless caused by heart failure.
• Use cautiously in patients with acute MI, incomplete AV block, sinus bradycardia, PVCs, chronic constrictive pericarditis, hypertrophic cardiomyopathy, renal insufficiency, severe pulmonary disease, or hypothyroidism.
▲ **Lifespan:** In pregnant women, use cautiously. In breast-feeding women, use cautiously; it's unknown if the drug appears in breast milk. In elderly patients, use cautiously.

Adverse reactions

CNS: agitation, dizziness, fatigue, generalized muscle weakness, hallucinations, headache, malaise, paresthesia, stupor, vertigo.
CV: *arrhythmias, heart failure,* hypotension.

EENT: blurred vision, diplopia, light flashes, photophobia, yellow-green halos around visual images.
GI: anorexia, diarrhea, nausea, vomiting.

Interactions

Drug-drug. *Amiloride:* May inhibit digoxin effect and increase digoxin excretion. Monitor patient for altered digoxin effect.
Amiodarone, diltiazem, nifedipine, quinidine, verapamil: May increase digoxin level. Monitor patient for digoxin toxicity.
Amphotericin B, carbenicillin, corticosteroids, diuretics (including loop diuretics, chlorthalidone, metolazone, and thiazides), ticarcillin: May decrease potassium level, predisposing patient to digitalis toxicity. Monitor potassium levels.
Antacids, kaolin-pectin: May decrease digoxin absorption. Schedule doses as far as possible from P.O. digoxin administration.
Cholestyramine, colestipol, metoclopramide: May decrease absorption of P.O. digoxin. Monitor patient for decreased effect and low blood levels. Increase dosage.
Parenteral calcium, thiazides: May increase calcium level and decrease magnesium level, predisposing patient to digitalis toxicity. Monitor calcium and magnesium levels.
Drug-herb. *Betel palm, fumitory, goldenseal, lily of the valley, motherwort, rue, shepherd's purse:* May increase cardiac effect. Discourage using together.
Horsetail, licorice: May deplete potassium stores, leading to digitalis toxicity. Monitor potassium level closely.
Oleander, Siberian ginseng, squill: May enhance toxicity. Discourage using together.
St. John's wort: May reduce therapeutic effect of digoxin, requiring an increased dosage. Monitor patient for loss of therapeutic effect, and advise patient to avoid this herb.
Drug-lifestyle. *Alcohol use:* May increase CNS effects. Discourage using together.

Effects on lab test results

None reported.

Pharmacokinetics

Absorption: For tablet or elixir, 60% to 85%. For capsule, 90% to 100%.
Distribution: Wide; about 20% to 30% bound to plasma proteins.

Metabolism: Small amount in liver and gut by bacteria. This varies and may be substantial in some patients. Drug undergoes some enterohepatic recirculation (also variable). Metabolites have minimal cardiac activity.
Excretion: Mostly by kidneys as unchanged drug, although a substantial amount of metabolized or reduced drug may be excreted. In patients with renal impairment, biliary excretion is most important. *Half-life:* 30 to 40 hours.

Route	Onset	Peak	Duration
P.O.	30 min–2 hr	2–6 hr	3–4 days
I.V.	5–30 min	1–4 hr	3–4 days

Action

Chemical effect: Inhibits sodium-potassium-activated adenosine triphosphatase, thereby promoting movement of calcium from extracellular to intracellular cytoplasm and strengthening myocardial contraction. Also acts on CNS to enhance vagal tone, slowing conduction through SA and AV nodes and providing antiarrhythmic effect.
Therapeutic effect: Strengthens myocardial contractions and slows conduction through SA and AV nodes.

Available forms

Capsules: 0.05 mg, 0.1 mg, 0.2 mg
Elixir: 0.05 mg/ml
Injection: 0.05 mg/ml, 0.1 mg/ml (pediatric), 0.25 mg/ml
Tablets: 0.125 mg, 0.25 mg

NURSING PROCESS

🦋 Assessment

• Obtain history of patient's underlying condition before therapy.
• Monitor effectiveness by taking apical pulse for 1 full minute before giving a dose. Evaluate ECG, and regularly assess patient's cardiopulmonary condition for signs of improvement.
• Monitor drug level. Therapeutic level ranges from 0.5 to 2 nanograms/ml. Take level 8 hours after last P.O. dose.
• Monitor potassium level carefully.
• Look for adverse reactions and drug interactions.
• Assess patient's and family's knowledge of drug therapy.

Nursing diagnoses

- Decreased cardiac output related to underlying condition
- Ineffective protection related to digoxin toxicity caused by drug
- Deficient knowledge related to drug therapy

Planning and implementation

- Adjust dosages as needed. Hypothyroid patients are extremely sensitive to drug, and hyperthyroid patients may need a larger dosage. Reduce the dosage in patients with renal impairment.
- Before giving loading dose, obtain baseline data (heart rate and rhythm, blood pressure, and electrolyte levels) and question patient about use of drug within the previous 2 to 3 weeks.
- Loading dose is always divided over first 24 hours unless patient's condition indicates otherwise.
- Before giving drug, take apical pulse for 1 full minute. Record and report to prescriber significant changes (sudden increase or decrease in pulse rate, pulse deficit, irregular beats, and regularization of previously irregular rhythm). If these changes occur, check blood pressure and obtain 12-lead ECG.
- **ALERT:** If pulse rate slows to 60 beats/minute or less, withhold drug and notify prescriber.
- Reduce dosage by 20% to 25% when changing from tablets or elixir to liquid-filled capsules or injection because the new forms are better absorbed.
- For digoxin toxicity, give drugs that bind drug in intestine (for example, colestipol or cholestyramine). Treat arrhythmias with phenytoin I.V. or lidocaine I.V., and treat potentially life-threatening toxicity with specific antigen-binding fragments (such as digoxin immune Fab).
- Withhold drug for 1 to 2 days before elective cardioversion. Adjust dose after cardioversion.
- **ALERT:** Be careful when calculating doses. A tenfold miscalculation of a child's dose can easily occur.
- **ALERT:** Don't confuse digoxin with doxepin.

Patient teaching
- Instruct patient and caregiver about drug action, dosage regimen, pulse taking, reportable signs, and follow-up plans.
- Instruct patient not to substitute one brand of digoxin for another.
- Tell patient to eat potassium-rich foods.

Evaluation

- Patient has adequate cardiac output.
- Patient has no digoxin toxicity.
- Patient and family state understanding of drug therapy.

digoxin immune Fab (ovine)
(dih-JOKS-in ih-MYOON Fab)
Digibind, DigiFab

Pharmacologic class: antibody fragment
Therapeutic class: cardiac glycoside antidote
Pregnancy risk category: C

Indications and dosages

▶ **Life-threatening digoxin toxicity.** *Adults and children:* Dosage based on ingested amount or level of digoxin. When calculating amount of antidote, round up to the nearest whole number.

For digoxin tablets, find the number of antidote vials by multiplying the ingested amount by 0.8 and dividing answer by 0.5. For example, if patient takes 25 tablets of 0.25-mg digoxin, the ingested amount is 6.25 mg. Multiply 6.25 mg by 0.8 and divide answer by 0.5 to obtain 10 vials of antidote.

For digoxin capsules, find the number of antidote vials by dividing the ingested dose in mg by 0.5. For example, if patient takes 50 of 0.2-mg capsules, the ingested amount is 10 mg. Divide 10 mg by 0.5 to obtain 20 vials of antidote.

If the digoxin level is known, determine the number of antidote vials as follows: multiply the digoxin level in nanograms/ml by patient's weight in kg, divide by 100. For example, if digoxin is 4 nanograms/ml, and patient weighs 60 kg, multiply together to obtain 240. Divide by 100 to obtain 2.4 vials; then round up to 3 vials.

▶ **Acute toxicity or if estimated ingested amount or digoxin level is unknown.** *Adults and children:* Consider giving 10 vials of digoxin immune Fab and observing patient's response. Follow with another 10 vials. Dose is effective in most life-threatening ingestions in adults and children but may cause volume overload in young children.

▼ I.V. administration

• Reconstitute with 4 ml of sterile water for injection. For infusion, further dilute solution with normal saline. For children or other patients who need small doses, reconstitute Digibind in 38-mg vial with 34 ml of normal saline for 1 mg/ml concentration; reconstitute DigiFab in 40-mg vial with 36 ml of normal saline for 1 mg/ml concentration.

• Infuse over 30 minutes. If cardiac arrest is imminent, give as a bolus injection. Infuse via a 0.22-micron membrane filter to ensure no undissolved particulate matter is infused.

• Use reconstituted solution promptly. If not used immediately, refrigerate for up to 4 hours.

⊗ **Incompatibilities**
None reported.

Contraindications and cautions

• Use cautiously in patients allergic to ovine proteins. In these high-risk patients, perform skin test because drug is derived from digoxin-specific antibody fragments obtained from immunized sheep.

⚕ **Lifespan:** In pregnant women, use cautiously. In breast-feeding women, use cautiously; it's unknown if the drug appears in breast milk.

Adverse reactions

CV: *heart failure,* rapid ventricular rate.
Metabolic: hypokalemia.
Other: *anaphylaxis,* hypersensitivity reactions.

Interactions

None reported.

Effects on lab test results

• May decrease potassium level.

Pharmacokinetics

Absorption: Given I.V.
Distribution: Unknown.
Metabolism: Unknown.
Excretion: In urine. *Half-life:* 15 to 20 hours.

Route	Onset	Peak	Duration
I.V.	Varies	End of dose	2–6 hr

Action

Chemical effect: Binds molecules of digoxin, making them unavailable for binding at site of action on cells.
Therapeutic effect: Reverses digitalis toxicity.

Available forms

Injection: 38-mg vial (Digibind) and 40-mg vial (DigiFab)

▨ Assessment

• Obtain history of patient's digitalis intoxication before therapy.

• Monitor effectiveness by watching for decreased signs and symptoms of digitalis toxicity. In most patients, signs of digitalis toxicity disappear within a few hours.

• Because drug interferes with digitalis immunoassay measurements, standard digoxin levels are misleading until drug is cleared from body (about 2 days).

• Look for adverse reactions.

• Assess patient's and family's knowledge of drug therapy.

⊞ Nursing diagnoses

• Ineffective health maintenance related to digitalis intoxication

• Decreased cardiac output related to drug-induced heart failure

• Deficient knowledge related to drug therapy

▷ Planning and implementation

• Drug is used only for life-threatening overdose in patients with shock or cardiac arrest; ventricular arrhythmias, such as ventricular tachycardia or fibrillation; progressive bradycardia, such as severe sinus bradycardia; or second- or third-degree AV block not responsive to atropine.

• Give oxygen. Keep resuscitation equipment nearby.

Patient teaching

• Instruct patient to report respiratory difficulty, chest pain, or dizziness immediately.

☑ Evaluation

• Patient exhibits improved health with alleviation of digitalis toxicity.

• Patient demonstrates adequate cardiac output through normal vital signs and urine output and clear mental condition.

• Patient and family state understanding of drug therapy.

diltiazem hydrochloride
(dil-TIGH-uh-zem high-droh-KLOR-ighd)
Cardizem◊, Cardizem CD◊, Cardizem LA◊,
Cardizem SR, Cartia XT, Dilacor XR,
Diltia XT, Taztia XT, Tiazac

Pharmacologic class: calcium channel blocker
Therapeutic class: antianginal
Pregnancy risk category: C

Indications and dosages

▶ **Vasospastic angina (Prinzmetal's [variant]
angina), classic chronic stable angina pectoris.** *Adults:* 30 mg P.O. t.i.d. or q.i.d. before
meals and h.s. Increase dosage gradually to
maximum, 360 mg daily in divided doses. Or
120- to 180-mg extended-release capsules P.O.
once daily. Adjust dosage up to 480 mg once
daily.
▶ **Chronic stable angina.** *Adults:* Initially,
180 mg (Cardizem LA, Cardizem CD, or
extended-release capsules) once daily in the
morning or evening. May increase at intervals of
1 to 2 weeks if needed to maximum 360 mg.
▶ **Hypertension.** *Adults:* 60- to 120-mg
sustained-release capsules P.O. b.i.d. Adjust to
effect. Maximum, 360 mg daily. Or 180- to
240-mg extended-release capsules daily initially. Adjust dosage p.r.n. As monotherapy, 120 to
240 mg Cardizem LA P.O. once daily at the
same time each day, either in the morning or at
bedtime. Adjust dosage about q 14 days. Maximum, 540 mg daily.
▶ **Atrial fibrillation or flutter; paroxysmal
supraventricular tachycardia.** *Adults:*
0.25 mg/kg as I.V. bolus injection over 2 minutes. If response is inadequate, 0.35 mg/kg I.V.
after 15 minutes, followed with continuous infusion of 10 mg/hour. May increase in increments
of 5 mg/hour. Maximum, 15 mg/hour.

▼ I.V. administration

• For direct I.V. injection, no dilution of 5 mg/
ml injection is needed.
• For continuous I.V. infusion, add 5 mg/ml injection to 100, 200, or 500 ml of normal saline
solution, D_5W, or 5% dextrose and half-normal
saline solution to produce a final concentration
of 1, 0.83, or 0.45 mg/ml, respectively.
• Reconstitute drug in monovials and store up
to 24 hours in PVC bag as directed.

• For direct injection or continuous infusion,
give slowly while continuously monitoring ECG
and blood pressure.
• Don't give reconstituted solutions stored
longer than 24 hours or those with discoloration
or visible particulate matter.
⊗ **Incompatibilities**
Acetazolamide, acyclovir, aminophylline, ampicillin, cefoperazone, diazepam, furosemide,
heparin, hydrocortisone, insulin (regular),
methylprednisolone, nafcillin, phenytoin, rifampin, sodium bicarbonate, thiopental.

Contraindications and cautions

• Contraindicated in patients hypersensitive to
drug and in those with sick sinus syndrome,
second- or third-degree AV block without artificial pacemaker, hypotension (systolic blood
pressure below 90 mm Hg), acute MI, or pulmonary congestion (documented by X-ray).
• Use cautiously in patients with heart failure
and those with impaired liver or kidney function.
⚕ **Lifespan:** In pregnant women, use cautiously. Women who are breast-feeding should stop
breast-feeding or not use this drug. In children,
safety and effectiveness haven't been established. In elderly patients, use cautiously.

Adverse reactions

CNS: asthenia, dizziness, *headache,* insomnia,
somnolence.
CV: abnormal ECG, *arrhythmias, AV block,
bradycardia,* conduction abnormalities, *edema,*
flushing, *heart failure,* hypotension.
GI: abdominal discomfort, constipation, diarrhea, nausea, vomiting.
GU: nocturia, polyuria.
Skin: photosensitivity, pruritus, rash.

Interactions

Drug-drug. *Anesthetics:* May potentiate effects.
Monitor patient.
Cimetidine: May inhibit diltiazem metabolism.
Monitor patient for toxicity.
Cyclosporine: May increase cyclosporine levels
by decreasing its metabolism, leading to in-
creased risk of cyclosporine toxicity. Avoid us-
ing together.
Diazepam, midazolam, triazolam: May increase
CNS depression and prolong effects of these
drugs. Use lower dose of these benzodiazepines.

Digoxin: May increase levels of digoxin. Monitor patient and digoxin levels.

Propranolol, other beta blockers: May precipitate heart failure or prolong cardiac conduction time. Use together cautiously.

Drug-lifestyle. *Sun exposure:* May cause photosensitivity reactions. Advise patient to avoid unprotected or prolonged sun exposure.

Effects on lab test results

• May cause transient increase in liver enzyme levels.

Pharmacokinetics

Absorption: 80%. 40% of drug enters systemic circulation because of significant first-pass effect in liver.

Distribution: 70% to 85% of circulating drug is bound to plasma proteins.

Metabolism: In liver.

Excretion: 35% in urine and 65% in bile as unchanged drug and inactive and active metabolites. *Half-life:* 3 to 9 hours.

Route	Onset	Peak	Duration
P.O.	30 min–4 hr	2–18 hr	6–24 hr
I.V.			
bolus	3 min	Immediate	1–3 hr
infusion	3 min	Immediate	< 10 hr

Action

Chemical effect: Inhibits calcium ion influx across cardiac and smooth muscle cells, decreasing myocardial contractility and oxygen demand; also dilates coronary arteries and arterioles.

Therapeutic effect: Relieves anginal pain, lowers blood pressure, and restores normal sinus rhythm.

Available forms

Cardizem
Injection: 5 mg/ml (25 mg and 50 mg)
Tablets: 30 mg, 60 mg, 90 mg, 120 mg
Cardizem CD
Capsules (extended-release): 120 mg, 180 mg, 240 mg, 300 mg, 360 mg
Cardizem LA
Tablets (extended-release): 120 mg, 180 mg, 240 mg, 300 mg, 360 mg, 420 mg
Cardizem SR
Capsules (sustained-release): 60 mg, 90 mg, 120 mg

Cartia XT
Capsules (extended-release): 120 mg, 180 mg, 240 mg, 300 mg
Dilacor XR
Capsules (extended-release) containing multiple units of 60 mg: 120 mg, 180 mg, 240 mg
Diltia XT
Capsules (extended-release) containing multiple units of 60 mg: 120 mg, 180 mg, 240 mg
Tiazac
Capsules (sustained-release): 120 mg, 180 mg, 240 mg, 300 mg, 360 mg, 420 mg

NURSING PROCESS

℞ Assessment

• Obtain history of patient's underlying condition before therapy, and reassess regularly thereafter.

• Monitor blood pressure when therapy starts and when dosage changes.

• Monitor patient's ECG and heart rate and rhythm regularly.

• Be alert for adverse reactions and drug interactions.

• Assess patient's and family's knowledge of drug therapy.

🏵 Nursing diagnoses

• Ineffective health maintenance related to underlying condition

• Decreased cardiac output related to drug-induced adverse reactions

• Deficient knowledge related to drug therapy

⟩ Planning and implementation

• Give tablets before meals and at bedtime.

• Patients controlled on diltiazem alone or with other medications may be switched to Cardizem LA tablets once a day at the nearest equivalent total daily dose.

🟡 **ALERT:** If systolic blood pressure is below 90 mm Hg or heart rate is below 60 beats/minute, don't give the dose and notify prescriber.

• Assist patient with ambulation during start of therapy because dizziness may occur.

• To minimize edema, restrict the patient's fluid and sodium intake.

🟡 **ALERT:** Don't confuse Cardizem SR with Cardene SR.

Patient teaching

• If nitrate therapy is prescribed during adjustment of diltiazem dosage, urge patient compliance. Tell patient that S.L. nitroglycerin may be taken p.r.n. and as directed when angina is acute.
• Instruct patient to call prescriber if he experiences chest pain, shortness of breath, dizziness, palpitations, or swelling of the limbs.
• Tell patient to swallow extended- and sustained-release capsules whole and not to open, crush, or chew them.
• Instruct patient to take drug exactly as prescribed, even when feeling better.
• Advise patient to minimize exposure to direct sunlight and to take precautions when in sun because of drug-induced photosensitivity.
• Instruct patient to limit fluid and sodium intake to minimize edema.

☑ Evaluation

• Patient exhibits improvement in underlying condition.
• Patient maintains adequate cardiac output throughout therapy.
• Patient and family state understanding of drug therapy.

dimercaprol
(digh-mer-KAP-rohl)
BAL in Oil

Pharmacologic class: chelating drug
Therapeutic class: heavy metal antagonist
Pregnancy risk category: C

Indications and dosages

▶ **Severe arsenic or gold poisoning.** *Adults and children:* 3 mg/kg deep I.M. q 4 hours for 2 days; then q.i.d. on third day; then b.i.d. for 10 days.
▶ **Mild arsenic or gold poisoning.** *Adults and children:* 2.5 mg/kg deep I.M. q.i.d. for 2 days; then b.i.d. on third day; then once daily for 10 days.
▶ **Mercury poisoning.** *Adults and children:* Initially, 5 mg/kg deep I.M.; then 2.5 mg/kg daily or b.i.d. for 10 days.
▶ **Acute lead encephalopathy or lead level exceeding 100 mcg/dl.** *Adults and children:* 4 mg/kg deep I.M.; then q 4 hours with edetate

calcium disodium (250 mg/m^2 I.M.). Use separate sites. Maximum, 5 mg/kg per dose.

Contraindications and cautions

• Contraindicated in patients with hepatic dysfunction (except jaundice caused by arsenic).
• Use cautiously in patients with hypertension or oliguria.
⚠ **Lifespan:** In pregnant and breast-feeding women, safety and effectiveness haven't been established.

Adverse reactions

CNS: *fever,* headache, paresthesia.
CV: tachycardia, transient increase in blood pressure.
EENT: blepharospasm, conjunctivitis, excessive salivation, lacrimation, rhinorrhea.
GI: abdominal pain; burning sensation in lips, mouth, and throat; halitosis; nausea; vomiting.
GU: *dysuria,* renal damage.
Musculoskeletal: muscle pain or weakness.
Skin: diaphoresis, sterile abscess.
Other: decreased iodine uptake; *pain at injection site;* pain in teeth; pain or tightness in throat, chest, or hands.

Interactions

Drug-drug. *Iron:* May form a toxic metal complex; therefore, using together is contraindicated. Wait 24 hours after last dimercaprol dose.

Effects on lab test results

None reported.

Pharmacokinetics

Absorption: Unknown.
Distribution: To all tissues, mainly in intracellular space.
Metabolism: Rapid, to inactive products.
Excretion: Most metal complexes and inactive metabolites in urine and feces. *Half-life:* Unknown.

Route	Onset	Peak	Duration
I.M.	Unknown	30–60 min	4 hr

Action

Chemical effect: Forms complexes with heavy metals.
Therapeutic effect: Treats heavy metal intoxication.

Available forms

Injection: 100 mg/ml

NURSING PROCESS

◢ Assessment

• Obtain history of patient's toxicity before therapy.
• Assess the drug's effectiveness by monitoring the level of metallic substance ingested and by improvement in patient's condition.
• Look for adverse reactions and drug interactions.
• If adverse GI reactions occur, monitor patient's hydration.
• Observe injection site for local reaction.
• Assess patient's and family's knowledge of drug therapy.

◢ Nursing diagnoses

• Risk for poisoning related to exposure to toxic substance
• Risk for deficient fluid volume related to drug-induced nausea and vomiting
• Deficient knowledge related to drug therapy

◢ Planning and implementation

⊗ **ALERT:** Don't give I.V. Only give deep I.M., and then massage injection site.
• Be careful not to let drug come in contact with skin because it may cause skin reaction.
• Don't schedule patient for 131I uptake thyroid tests during therapy because drug decreases results.
• Solution with slight sediment is usable.
• Drug is ineffective in arsine gas poisoning.
⊗ **ALERT:** Don't use for iron, cadmium, or selenium toxicity. Complex form is highly toxic, even fatal.
• Use ephedrine or antihistamine to prevent or relieve mild adverse reactions.
• Keep urine alkaline to prevent renal damage; give oral sodium bicarbonate.
• Apply ice or cold compresses to injection site to alleviate local discomfort.
Patient teaching
• Warn patient that drug has unpleasant garlic-like odor.
• Advise patient that drug may cause pain at injection site.
• Instruct patient to report changes in urine output, fever, pain, nausea, or vomiting immediately.

◢ Evaluation

• Patient's toxicity is eliminated.
• Patient maintains adequate hydration throughout therapy.
• Patient and family state understanding of drug therapy.

diphenhydramine hydrochloride

(digh-fen-HIGH-drah-meen high-droh-KLOR-ighd)
Allerdryl ◆ †, AllerMax Caplets†, Banophen†, Banophen Caplets†, Beldin†, Benadryl†, Benadryl 25†, Benadryl Kapseals, Benylin Cough†, Bydramine Cough†, Compoz†, Diphenadryl†, Diphen Cough†, Diphenhist†, Diphenhist Captabs†, Genahist†, Hyrexin-50, Nytol Maximum Strength†, Nytol with DPH†, Sleep-Eze 3†, Sominex Formula 2†, Tusstat†, Twilite Caplets†, Uni-Bent Cough†

Pharmacologic class: nonselective ethanolamine derivative antihistamine
Therapeutic class: antihistamine (H_1-receptor antagonist), antitussive, sleep aid
Pregnancy risk category: B

Indications and dosages

▶ **Rhinitis, allergy symptoms, motion sickness, Parkinson's disease.** *Adults and children age 12 and older:* 25 to 50 mg P.O. t.i.d. or q.i.d. Or 10 to 50 mg deep I.M. or I.V. Maximum I.M. or I.V. dosage, 400 mg daily.
Children younger than age 12: 5 mg/kg daily P.O., deep I.M., or I.V. in divided doses q.i.d. Maximum, 300 mg daily.
▶ **Sedation.** *Adults:* 25 to 50 mg P.O. or deep I.M., p.r.n.
▶ **Nighttime sleep aid.** *Adults:* 50 mg P.O. h.s.
▶ **Nonproductive cough.** *Adults:* 25 mg P.O. q 4 to 6 hours (up to 150 mg daily).
Children ages 6 to 11: 12.5 mg P.O. q 4 to 6 hours (up to 75 mg daily).
Children ages 2 to 5: 6.25 mg P.O. q 4 to 6 hours (up to 25 mg daily).

▽ I.V. administration

• Make sure I.V. site is patent, and monitor it for irritation.
• Don't give I.V. drug faster than 25 mg/minute.

⊗ **Incompatibilities**
Allopurinol, amobarbital, amphotericin B, cefepime, dexamethasone, foscarnet, haloperidol lactate, pentobarbital, phenytoin, phenobarbital, thiopental.

Contraindications and cautions

• Contraindicated in patients hypersensitive to drug and in patients having acute asthmatic attacks.
• Use cautiously in patients with CV disease, hypertension, angle-closure glaucoma, increased intraocular pressure, stenosing peptic ulcer, pyloroduodenal and bladder-neck obstruction, prostatic hyperplasia, hyperthyroidism, asthma, or COPD.
⚘ Lifespan: In pregnant women, use cautiously. In neonates, premature neonates, and breast-feeding women, drug is contraindicated. In children younger than age 12, safety and effectiveness as a night-time sleep aid haven't been established. Children younger than age 6 should use only when directed by prescriber. Age restrictions for topical preparations vary depending on drug's formulation and manufacturer.

Adverse reactions

CNS: confusion, *dizziness, drowsiness,* fatigue, headache, incoordination, insomnia, nervousness, restlessness, *sedation, **seizures,** sleepiness,* tremor, vertigo.
CV: hypotension, palpitations, tachycardia.
EENT: blurred vision, diplopia, nasal congestion, tinnitus.
GI: anorexia, constipation, diarrhea, *dry mouth, epigastric distress, nausea,* vomiting.
GU: dysuria, urinary frequency, urine retention.
Hematologic: *agranulocytosis,* hemolytic anemia, ***thrombocytopenia.***
Respiratory: thickening of bronchial secretions.
Skin: photosensitivity, rash, urticaria.
Other: *anaphylactic shock.*

Interactions

Drug-drug. *CNS depressants:* May increase sedation. Use together cautiously; monitor patient for increased sedation.
MAO inhibitors: May increase anticholinergic effects. Don't use together.
Other products containing diphenhydramine, including topical forms: May increase risk of adverse reactions. Avoid using together.

Drug-lifestyle. *Alcohol use:* May increase adverse CNS effects. Discourage using together.
Sun exposure: May cause photosensitivity reactions. Urge patient to wear protective clothing and sunblock.

Effects on lab test results

• May decrease hemoglobin level and hematocrit.
• May decrease platelet and granulocyte counts.

Pharmacokinetics

Absorption: Good after P.O. use.
Distribution: Wide, including CNS; about 82% protein-bound.
Metabolism: In liver.
Excretion: Drug and metabolites mainly in urine. *Half-life:* About 3½ hours.

Route	Onset	Peak	Duration
P.O.	≤ 15 min	1–4 hr	6–8 hr
I.V.	Immediate	1–4 hr	6–8 hr
I.M.	Unknown	1–4 hr	6–8 hr

Action

Chemical effect: Competes with histamine for H_1-receptor sites on effector cells. Prevents but doesn't reverse histamine-mediated responses, particularly histamine's effects on smooth muscle of bronchial tubes, GI tract, uterus, and blood vessels. Provides local anesthesia by preventing initiation and transmission of nerve impulses, and suppresses cough reflex by direct effect in medulla of brain.
Therapeutic effect: Relieves allergy symptoms, motion sickness, and cough; improves voluntary movement; and promotes sleep and calmness.

Available forms

Capsules: 25 mg†, 50 mg†
Chewable tablets: 12.5 mg†
Elixir: 12.5 mg/5 ml*†
Injection: 10 mg/ml, 50 mg/ml
Syrup: 12.5 mg/5 ml†, 6.25 mg/5 ml†
Tablets: 25 mg†, 50 mg†

NURSING PROCESS

▨ Assessment
• Obtain history of patient's underlying condition before therapy, and reassess regularly thereafter.

- Be alert for adverse reactions and drug interactions.
- Assess patient's and family's knowledge of drug therapy.

Nursing diagnoses
- Ineffective health maintenance related to underlying condition
- Risk for injury related to drug-induced adverse CNS reactions
- Deficient knowledge related to drug therapy

Planning and implementation
- Reduce GI distress by giving drug with food or milk.
- Alternate injection sites to prevent irritation. Give I.M. injection deep into large muscle.
- If tolerance is observed, notify prescriber because another antihistamine may need to be substituted.
ALERT: Don't confuse diphenhydramine with dicyclomine, or Benadryl with Bentyl or Benylin.
Patient teaching
- Instruct patient to take drug 30 minutes before travel, to prevent motion sickness.
- Warn patient to avoid alcohol and to refrain from driving or performing other hazardous activities that require alertness.
- Tell patient that coffee or tea may reduce drowsiness.
- Inform patient that ice chips, sugarless gum, or hard candy may relieve dry mouth.
- Advise patient to stop taking the drug 4 days before allergy skin tests to preserve test accuracy.
- Tell patient to notify prescriber if tolerance develops because different antihistamine may need to be prescribed.
- Warn patient that he may be photosensitive. Advise use of sunblock or protective clothing.
- Warn patient to avoid using other products containing diphenhydramine, including topical forms, because of risk of adverse reactions.

Evaluation
- Patient shows improvement in underlying condition.
- Patient has no injury as result of therapy.
- Patient and family state understanding of drug therapy.

diphenoxylate hydrochloride and atropine sulfate
(digh-fen-OKS-ul-ayt high-droh-KLOR-ighd and AH-troh-peen SUL-fayt)
Logen, Lomanate, Lomotil*, Lonox

Pharmacologic class: opioid
Therapeutic class: antidiarrheal
Pregnancy risk category: C
Controlled substance schedule: V

Indications and dosages
▶ **Acute, nonspecific diarrhea.** *Adults:* Initially, 5 mg P.O. q.i.d.; then reduce dosage as soon as initial control is achieved. Maximum, 20 mg P.O. daily.
Children ages 2 to 12: 0.3 to 0.4 mg/kg liquid form P.O. daily in four divided doses. Maintenance dosage may be as low as 25% of initial dosage. Maximum, 20 mg P.O. daily.

Contraindications and cautions
- Contraindicated in patients hypersensitive to drug or any of its components and in those with acute diarrhea from poison (until toxic material is eliminated), acute diarrhea caused by organisms that penetrate the intestinal mucosa, or diarrhea from antibiotic-induced pseudomembranous enterocolitis. Also contraindicated in jaundiced patients.
- Use cautiously in patients with hepatic disease, opioid dependence, or acute ulcerative colitis. If abdominal distention or other signs of toxic megacolon develop, stop therapy immediately and notify prescriber.
⚖ **Lifespan:** In pregnant women, use cautiously. In breast-feeding women, drug isn't recommended. In children ages 2 to 12, use cautiously and in liquid form only. In children younger than age 2, drug is contraindicated.

Adverse reactions
CNS: confusion, depression, *dizziness,* drowsiness, euphoria, headache, lethargy, malaise, numbness in limbs, restlessness, *sedation.*
CV: tachycardia.
EENT: mydriasis.
GI: abdominal discomfort or distention, anorexia, *dry mouth,* fluid retention in bowel, nausea, *pancreatitis,* paralytic ileus, vomiting.
GU: urine retention.

Reactions may be *common,* uncommon, *life-threatening,* or COMMON AND LIFE-THREATENING.

Respiratory: respiratory depression.
Skin: pruritus, rash.
Other: *angioedema, anaphylaxis,* possible physical dependence with long-term use.

Interactions

Drug-drug. *Barbiturates, CNS depressants, opioids, tranquilizers:* May increase CNS depression. Monitor patient closely for increased sedation.
MAO inhibitors: May cause a hypertensive crisis. Don't use together.
Drug-lifestyle. *Alcohol use:* May increase CNS depression. Discourage using together.

Effects on lab test results

None reported.

Pharmacokinetics

Absorption: 90%.
Distribution: Unknown.
Metabolism: Extensive.
Excretion: Metabolites mainly in feces with lesser amounts in urine. *Half-life:* Diphenoxylate, 2½ hours; its major metabolite, diphenoxylic acid, 4½ hours; atropine, 2½ hours.

Route	Onset	Peak	Duration
P.O.	45–60 min	3 hr	3–4 hr

Action

Chemical effect: Unknown; probably increases smooth-muscle tone in GI tract, inhibits motility and propulsion, and diminishes secretions.
Therapeutic effect: Relieves diarrhea.

Available forms

Liquid: 2.5 mg/5 ml (with atropine sulfate 0.025 mg/5 ml)*
Tablets: 2.5 mg (with atropine sulfate 0.025 mg)

NURSING PROCESS

Assessment
- Assess patient's diarrhea before beginning therapy, and regularly during therapy.
- Be alert for adverse reactions and drug interactions.
- Assess patient's and family's knowledge of drug therapy.

Nursing diagnoses
- Diarrhea related to underlying condition
- Ineffective breathing pattern related to drug-induced respiratory depression
- Deficient knowledge related to drug therapy

Planning and implementation
- Fluid retention in the bowel may mask depletion of extracellular fluid and electrolytes, especially in young children with acute gastroenteritis. Correct fluid and electrolyte disturbances before starting therapy. Dehydration may increase risk of delayed toxicity.
- A 2.5-mg dose is as effective as 5 ml of camphorated opium tincture.
- Drug isn't indicated for treating antibiotic-induced diarrhea.
- Drug is unlikely to be effective if patient doesn't respond within 48 hours.
- Risk of physical dependence increases with high dosage and long-term use. Atropine sulfate helps discourage abuse.
- Use naloxone to treat respiratory depression caused by overdose.
- **ALERT:** Don't confuse Lomotil (diphenoxylate hydrochloride and atropine sulfate) with Lamictal (lamotrigine).

Patient teaching
- Tell patient not to exceed prescribed dosage.
- Warn patient not to use drug to treat acute diarrhea for longer than 2 days. Encourage him to seek medical attention if diarrhea persists.
- Advise patient to avoid hazardous activities, such as driving, until CNS effects of drug are known.

Evaluation
- Patient regains normal bowel pattern.
- Patient maintains normal breathing pattern throughout therapy.
- Patient and family state understanding of drug therapy.

D

dipyridamole

(digh-peer-IH-duh-mohl)
**Apo-Dipyridamole ♦ , Novo-Dipiradol ♦ ,
Persantin ◇ , Persantin 100 SR ◇ , Persantine**

Pharmacologic class: pyrimidine analogue
Therapeutic class: coronary vasodilator,
platelet aggregation inhibitor
Pregnancy risk category: B

Indications and dosages

▶ **To inhibit platelet adhesion in prosthetic
heart valves.** *Adults:* 75 to 100 mg P.O. q.i.d.
(with warfarin or aspirin).
▶ **Alternative to exercise in evaluation of
coronary artery disease during thallium-201
myocardial perfusion scintigraphy.** *Adults:*
0.57 mg/kg as I.V. infusion at constant rate over
4 minutes (0.142 mg/kg/minute).
▶ **Chronic angina pectoris‡.** *Adults:* 50 mg
P.O. t.i.d. at least 1 hour before meals; 2 to
3 months of therapy may be required to achieve
therapeutic response.
▶ **To prevent thromboembolic complications
in patients with various thromboembolic disorders other than prosthetic heart valves‡.**
Adults: 150 to 400 mg P.O. daily (with warfarin
or aspirin).

▽ I.V. administration

● If giving drug as a diagnostic agent, dilute in
half-normal or normal saline solution or D₅W in
at least a 1:2 ratio for total volume of 20 to
50 ml.
● Inject thallium-201 within 5 minutes of completing 4-minute infusion.
● Avoid freezing and protect from direct light.
⊗ **Incompatibilities**
Other I.V. drugs.

Contraindications and cautions

● Use cautiously in patients with hypotension.
✻ **Lifespan:** In pregnant women, use cautiously. In breast-feeding women and in children,
safety and effectiveness haven't been established.

Adverse reactions

CNS: dizziness, headache, weakness.

CV: blood pressure lability, chest pain, ECG abnormalities, fainting, flushing, hypertension
(with I.V. infusion), hypotension.
GI: abdominal distress, diarrhea, nausea, vomiting.
Skin: irritation (with undiluted injection), pruritus, rash.

Interactions

Drug-drug. *Heparin:* May increase bleeding.
Monitor patient closely for increased bleeding;
monitor PTT.
Theophylline: May prevent coronary vasodilation by I.V. dipyridamole. Avoid using together.
Drug-herb. *Dong quai, feverfew, garlic, ginger,
horse chestnut, red clover:* May increase risk of
bleeding. Discourage using together.

Effects on lab test results

None reported.

Pharmacokinetics

Absorption: Variable and slow; 27% to 59%.
Distribution: Wide. 91% to 97% protein
bound.
Metabolism: By liver.
Excretion: By way of biliary excretion of glucuronide conjugates. Some dipyridamole and
conjugates may undergo enterohepatic circulation and fecal excretion; small amount in urine.
Half-life: 1 to 12 hours.

Route	Onset	Peak	Duration
P.O.	Unknown	45–150 min	Unknown
I.V.	Unknown	2 min after therapy	Unknown
I.M.	Unknown	Unknown	Unknown

Action

Chemical effect: May involve its ability to increase adenosine, which is a coronary vasodilator and platelet aggregation inhibitor.
Therapeutic effect: Dilates coronary arteries
and helps prevent clotting.

Available forms

Injection: 10 mg/2 ml
Tablets: 25 mg, 50 mg, 75 mg

NURSING PROCESS

🔧 Assessment

• Obtain history of patient's underlying condition before therapy, and reassess regularly thereafter.
• Be alert for adverse reactions and drug interactions.
• Assess patient's and family's knowledge of drug therapy.

🔧 Nursing diagnoses

• Ineffective cardiopulmonary tissue perfusion related to underlying condition
• Acute pain related to drug-induced headache
• Deficient knowledge related to drug therapy

🔧 Planning and implementation

• Give drug 1 hour before meals. If patient develops adverse GI reactions, give drug with meals.
• The value of dipyridamole as part of an antithrombotic regimen is controversial; its use may not provide significantly better results than aspirin alone.
🔧 **ALERT:** Don't confuse dipyridamole with disopyramide; or Persantine with Periactin.

Patient teaching
• Instruct patient when to take drug.
• Tell patient to have his blood pressure checked frequently.
• Advise patient to take mild analgesic if headache occurs.
• Instruct patient to notify prescriber if chest pain occurs.

🔧 Evaluation

• Patient maintains adequate tissue perfusion and cellular oxygenation.
• Patient obtains relief from drug-induced headache with use of mild analgesic.
• Patient and family state understanding of drug therapy.

disopyramide
(digh-so-PEER-uh-mighd)
Rythmodan ◆ ◇

disopyramide phosphate
Norpace, Norpace CR, Rythmodan LA ◆

Pharmacologic class: pyridine derivative
Therapeutic class: antiarrhythmic
Pregnancy risk category: C

Indications and dosages

▶ **Symptomatic PVCs (unifocal, multifocal, or coupled); ventricular tachycardia not severe enough to require cardioversion.** *Adults:* For parenteral use, initially give 2 mg/kg I.V. slowly (over not less than 15 minutes). Give drug until arrhythmia is gone or patient has received 150 mg. If conversion is successful but arrhythmia returns, repeat dosage. Total I.V. dosage shouldn't exceed 300 mg in first hour. Follow with I.V. infusion of 0.4 mg/kg/hour (usually 20 to 30 mg/hour) to maximum, 800 mg daily.
Adults weighing more than 50 kg (110 lb): Initial loading dose is 300 mg P.O. for rapid control of ventricular arrhythmia. Follow with 150 mg q 6 hours or 300 mg q 12 hours with controlled-release capsules.
Adults weighing 50 kg or less: Initial loading dose is 200 mg P.O., then 100 mg P.O. q 6 hours as conventional capsules or 200 mg P.O. q 12 hours with controlled-release capsules.
Children ages 12 to 18: 6 to 15 mg/kg P.O. daily, divided into equal amounts and given q 6 hours.
Children ages 4 to 12: 10 to 15 mg/kg P.O. daily, divided into equal amounts and given q 6 hours.
Children ages 1 to 4: 10 to 20 mg/kg P.O. daily, divided into equal amounts and given q 6 hours.
Children younger than age 1: 10 to 30 mg/kg P.O. daily, divided into equal amounts and given q 6 hours.
🔧 **Adjust-a-dose:** For patients with renal impairment, if creatinine clearance is 30 to 40 ml/minute, give 100 mg q 8 hours; if creatinine clearance is 15 to 30 ml/minute, give 100 mg q 12 hours; if creatinine clearance is less than 15 ml/minute, give 100 mg q 24 hours.

▼ I.V. administration

• Add 200 mg to 500 ml of compatible solution, such as normal saline solution or D_5W.
• Use an infusion pump. Don't mix with other drugs.
• Give slowly over at least 15 minutes.
• Switch to P.O. therapy as soon as possible.
⊗ **Incompatibilities**
Other I.V. drugs.

Contraindications and cautions

• Contraindicated in patients hypersensitive to the drug or any of its components and in those with cardiogenic shock or second- or third-degree heart block without an artificial pacemaker.
• Use cautiously or avoid using, if possible, in patients with heart failure.
• Use cautiously in patients with underlying conduction abnormalities, urinary tract diseases (especially prostatic hypertrophy), hepatic or renal impairment, myasthenia gravis, or acute angle-closure glaucoma.
※ **Lifespan:** In pregnant women, use cautiously. In breast-feeding women, drug isn't recommended.

Adverse reactions

CNS: *acute psychosis,* agitation, depression, dizziness, fatigue, headache, syncope.
CV: *arrhythmias,* chest pain, edema, *heart block, heart failure,* hypotension.
EENT: blurred vision, dry eyes, dry nose.
GI: abdominal pain, anorexia, bloating, constipation, diarrhea, dry mouth, nausea, vomiting.
GU: urinary hesitancy, urine retention.
Hepatic: cholestatic jaundice.
Metabolic: weight gain.
Musculoskeletal: aches, muscle weakness, pain.
Respiratory: shortness of breath.
Skin: dermatosis, pruritus, rash.

Interactions

Drug-drug. *Antiarrhythmics:* May cause additive or antagonized antiarrhythmic effects. Monitor patient ECG closely.
Erythromycin: May increase disopyramide level, causing arrhythmias and prolonged QTc interval. Monitor ECG closely.
Phenytoin: May increase metabolism of disopyramide. Monitor patient for decreased antiarrhythmic effect.

Rifampin: May decrease disopyramide level. Monitor patient for decreased effectiveness.
Drug-herb. *Jimson weed:* May adversely affect CV function. Discourage using together.

Effects on lab test results

None reported.

Pharmacokinetics

Absorption: Rapid and good.
Distribution: Throughout extracellular fluid but not extensively bound to tissues. Protein-binding is typically 50% to 65%.
Metabolism: In liver.
Excretion: In urine. *Half-life:* 7 hours.

Route	Onset	Peak	Duration
P.O.	½–3½ hr	2–2½ hr	1½–8½ hr
I.V.	Unknown	Unknown	Unknown

Action

Chemical effect: May depress phase 0 and prolong action potential. All class I drugs have membrane-stabilizing effects.
Therapeutic effect: Restores normal sinus rhythm.

Available forms

disopyramide
Capsules: 100 mg ♦, 150 mg ♦
disopyramide phosphate
Capsules: 100 mg, 150 mg
Capsules (controlled-release): 100 mg, 150 mg
Injection: 10 mg/ml ♦ ◊
Tablets (sustained-release): 150 mg ♦

NURSING PROCESS

≋ Assessment

• Obtain history of patient's arrhythmia before therapy.
• Monitor the drug's effectiveness by assessing patient's ECG pattern and apical pulse rate.
• Be alert for adverse reactions and drug interactions.
• Assess patient's and family's knowledge of drug therapy.

⊞ Nursing diagnoses

• Decreased cardiac output related to underlying arrhythmia

- Ineffective protection related to drug-induced proarrhythmias
- Deficient knowledge related to drug therapy

⊠ **Planning and implementation**

- Correct any underlying electrolyte abnormalities before therapy begins.
- Check apical pulse before therapy. Notify prescriber if pulse rate is slower than 60 beats/minute or faster than 120 beats/minute.
- Don't use sustained- and controlled-release preparations for rapid control of ventricular arrhythmias, when therapeutic levels must be rapidly attained; in patients with cardiomyopathy or suspected cardiac decompensation; or in those with severe renal impairment.
- For administration to young children, pharmacist may prepare disopyramide suspension from 100-mg capsules using cherry syrup. Suspension should be dispensed in amber glass bottles and protected from light.
- If heart block develops, QRS complex widens by more than 25%, or QT interval is prolonged by more than 25% above baseline; stop the drug and notify the prescriber.

Patient teaching
- When switching patient from immediate- to sustained-release capsules, advise him to take sustained-release capsule 6 hours after last immediate-release capsule was taken.
- Teach patient importance of taking drug on time and exactly as prescribed. This may require use of alarm clock for night doses.
- Advise patient to use sugarless gum or hard candy to relieve dry mouth.
- Tell patient not to crush or chew extended-release tablets.

☑ **Evaluation**
- Patient's ECG reveals that arrhythmia has been corrected.
- Patient develops no new arrhythmias as result of therapy.
- Patient and family state understanding of drug therapy.

disulfiram
(digh-SUL-fih-ram)
Antabuse

Pharmacologic class: aldehyde dehydrogenase inhibitor
Therapeutic class: alcohol deterrent
Pregnancy risk category: C

Indications and dosages

▶ **Adjunct to manage alcohol dependence.**
Adults: 250 to 500 mg P.O. as single dose in morning for 1 to 2 weeks. If drowsiness occurs, give in the evening. Maintenance dosage is 125 to 500 mg P.O. daily (average dosage, 250 mg) until permanent self-control is established. Therapy may continue for months or years.

Contraindications and cautions

- Contraindicated during alcohol intoxication and within 12 hours of alcohol ingestion. Also contraindicated in patients hypersensitive to disulfiram or thiram derivatives used in pesticides and rubber vulcanization; patients with psychoses, myocardial disease, or coronary occlusion; and patients receiving metronidazole, paraldehyde, alcohol, or alcohol-containing preparations.
- Use cautiously in patients receiving phenytoin therapy and in patients with diabetes mellitus, hypothyroidism, seizure disorder, cerebral damage, nephritis, or hepatic cirrhosis or insufficiency.
※ **Lifespan:** In pregnant women, don't use. In breast-feeding women, use cautiously. In children, safety and effectiveness haven't been established.

Adverse reactions

CNS: delirium, depression, drowsiness, fatigue, headache, neuritis, peripheral neuritis, polyneuritis, psychotic reactions, restlessness.
EENT: optic neuritis.
GI: metallic or garlic aftertaste.
GU: impotence.
Skin: acneiform or allergic dermatitis.
Other: *disulfiram reaction.*

Interactions

Drug-drug. *Alfentanil:* May prolong duration of effect. Monitor patient closely.
Anticoagulants: May increase anticoagulant effect. Adjust dosage of anticoagulant accordingly; monitor patient for bleeding.
CNS depressants: May increase CNS depression. Use together cautiously.
Isoniazid: May cause ataxia or marked change in behavior. Avoid using together.
Metronidazole: May cause psychotic reaction. Avoid using together; wait for 2 weeks following disulfiram.
Midazolam: May increase plasma levels of midazolam. Use together cautiously.
Paraldehyde: May cause toxic level of acetaldehyde. Don't use together.
Phenytoin: May increase toxic effects of phenytoin. Monitor phenytoin levels closely and adjust dose.
Tricyclic antidepressants, especially amitriptyline: May cause transient delirium. Monitor patient closely.
Drug-herb. *Passion flower, pill-bearing spurge, pokeweed, squaw vine, squill, sundew, sweet flag, tormentil, valerian, yarrow:* May cause disulfiram reaction if herb contains alcohol. Discourage using together.
Drug-lifestyle. *Alcohol use:* May cause disulfiram reaction, including flushing, tachycardia, bronchospasm, sweating, nausea, and vomiting. Death may also occur. Warn patients against using products containing alcohol or drinking alcohol.
Cocaine use: May increase adverse cardiovascular effects of cocaine. Discourage use together.

Effects on lab test results

• May increase cholesterol level.

Pharmacokinetics

Absorption: Complete.
Distribution: Highly lipid soluble and initially localized in fat.
Metabolism: Mostly oxidized in liver.
Excretion: Mainly in urine; 5% to 20% in feces. *Half-life:* Unknown.

Route	Onset	Peak	Duration
P.O.	1–2 hr	Unknown	< 14 days

Action

Chemical effect: Blocks oxidation of ethanol at acetaldehyde stage. Excess acetaldehyde produces highly unpleasant reaction in presence of even small amounts of ethanol.
Therapeutic effect: Deters alcohol consumption.

Available forms

Tablets: 250 mg, 500 mg

NURSING PROCESS

☰ Assessment
• Obtain history of patient's alcoholism before therapy.
• Do a complete physical examination and laboratory studies, including CBC, chemistry panel, and transaminase determination before therapy. Repeat physical examination and laboratory studies regularly.
• Monitor the drug's effectiveness by assessing patient's abstinence from alcohol.
• Measure blood alcohol level weekly.
• Be alert for adverse reactions and drug interactions. Disulfiram reaction is precipitated by alcohol use and may include flushing, throbbing headache, dyspnea, nausea, copious vomiting, diaphoresis, thirst, chest pain, palpitations, hyperventilation, hypotension, syncope, anxiety, weakness, blurred vision, and confusion. In severe reactions, patient may experience respiratory depression, CV collapse, arrhythmias, MI, acute heart failure, seizures, unconsciousness, and death.
• Mild reactions may occur in sensitive patients with blood alcohol levels of 5 to 10 mg/dl; symptoms are fully developed at 50 mg/dl; unconsciousness typically occurs at 125- to 150-mg/dl level. Reaction may last from 30 minutes to several hours or as long as alcohol remains in blood.
• Assess patient's and family's knowledge of drug therapy.

▣ Nursing diagnoses
• Ineffective health maintenance related to alcoholism
• Acute pain related to drug-induced headache
• Deficient knowledge related to drug therapy

▶ Planning and implementation

• Use only under close medical and nursing supervision. Only give drug to patient who hasn't used alcohol for at least 12 hours. Make sure that patient clearly understands consequences of therapy and gives permission for its use. Use drug only if patient is cooperative, well-motivated, and receiving supportive psychiatric therapy.

• Drug is usually given during the day, although it may be given at night if drowsiness occurs. Establish lowered maintenance dose until permanent self-control is practiced. Therapy may continue for months or years.

Patient teaching

• Caution patient's family that drug should never be given to the patient without his knowledge because severe reaction or death could result if the patient ingests alcohol.

• Warn patient to avoid all sources of alcohol (for example, sauces and cough syrups). Even external application of liniments, shaving lotion, and back-rub preparations may precipitate disulfiram reaction. Tell patient that alcohol reaction may occur as long as 2 weeks after single dose of disulfiram, and that the longer he remains on drug, the more sensitive he becomes to alcohol.

• Tell patient to wear or carry medical identification identifying him as a disulfiram user.

• Reassure patient that drug-induced adverse reactions (unrelated to alcohol use), such as drowsiness, fatigue, impotence, headache, peripheral neuritis, and metallic or garlic taste, subside after about 2 weeks of therapy.

☑ Evaluation

• Patient abstains from alcohol consumption.

• Patient's headache is relieved with mild analgesic therapy.

• Patient and family state understanding of drug therapy.

dobutamine hydrochloride
(doh-BYOO-tuh-meen high-droh-KLOR-ighd)
Dobutrex

Pharmacologic class: adrenergic, beta$_1$ agonist
Therapeutic class: inotropic drug
Pregnancy risk category: B

Indications and dosages

▶ **To increase cardiac output in short-term treatment of cardiac decompensation caused by depressed contractility, such as during refractory heart failure, and as adjunct in cardiac surgery.** *Adults:* 2 to 20 mcg/kg/minute I.V. infusion. Usual dosage range is 2.5 to 10 mcg/kg/minute. Rarely, rates up to 40 mcg/kg/minute may be needed; however, such doses may worsen ischemia.

▼ I.V. administration

• Dilute concentrate for injection to no more than 5 mg/ml. Compatible solutions include D$_5$W, half-normal saline solution injection, normal saline solution injection, and lactated Ringer's injection. The contents of one vial (250 mg) diluted with 1,000 ml of solution yield 250 mcg/ml; diluted with 500 ml, 500 mcg/ml; diluted with 250 ml, 1,000 mcg/ml.

• Oxidation of drug may slightly discolor admixtures containing dobutamine. This doesn't indicate significant loss of potency, provided drug is used within 24 hours of reconstitution.

• Don't mix with sodium bicarbonate injection because drug is incompatible with alkaline solutions.

• Don't give in same I.V. line with other drugs. Drug is incompatible with heparin, hydrocortisone sodium succinate, cefazolin, neutral cephalothin, penicillin, and ethacrynate sodium.

• Give drug using central venous catheter or large peripheral vein. Titrate infusion according to patient's condition per prescriber's guidelines. Use infusion pump.

• Watch for irritation and infiltration. Extravasation can cause inflammation, tissue damage, and necrosis. Change I.V. sites regularly to avoid phlebitis.

• Solutions remain stable for 24 hours.

⊗ **Incompatibilities**
Acyclovir, alkaline solutions, alteplase, aminophylline, bretylium, bumetanide, calcium chloride, calcium gluconate, cefepime, diazepam, digoxin, doxapram, furosemide, heparin, indomethacin, insulin (regular), magnesium sulfate, midazolam, piperacillin with tazobactam, phenytoin, phytonadione, potassium chloride, sodium bicarbonate, thiopental, verapamil, warfarin.

Contraindications and cautions

• Contraindicated in patients hypersensitive to drug or any of its components and in those with idiopathic hypertrophic subaortic stenosis.
• Use cautiously in patients with history of hypertension. Drug may cause exaggerated pressor response.
⚠ Lifespan: In pregnant and breast-feeding women and in children, safety and effectiveness haven't been established.

Adverse reactions

CNS: headache.
CV: angina, *hypertension, hypotension, increased heart rate,* nonspecific chest pain, phlebitis, *PVCs.*
GI: nausea, vomiting.
Musculoskeletal: mild leg cramps or tingling sensation.
Respiratory: *asthma attacks,* shortness of breath.
Other: *anaphylaxis.*

Interactions

Drug-drug. *Beta blockers:* May antagonize dobutamine effects. Don't use together.
Bretylium: May potentiate action of vasopressors on adrenergic receptors; arrhythmias may result. Monitor ECG closely.
General anesthetics: May increase risk of ventricular arrhythmias. Monitor patient closely.
Tricyclic antidepressants: May potentiate the pressor response and cause arrhythmias. Use with caution.
Drug-herb. *Rue:* May increase inotropic potential. Monitor vital signs closely.

Effects on lab test results

• May decrease potassium level.

Pharmacokinetics

Absorption: Given I.V.
Distribution: Wide.
Metabolism: By liver.
Excretion: Mainly in urine with minor amounts in feces. *Half-life:* 2 minutes.

Route	Onset	Peak	Duration
I.V.	1–2 min	≤ 10 min	Unknown

Action

Chemical effect: Directly stimulates beta$_1$ receptors to increase myocardial contractility and stroke volume. Decreases peripheral vascular resistance (afterload), reduces ventricular filling pressure (preload), and may facilitate AV node conduction.
Therapeutic effect: Increases cardiac output.

Available forms

Injection: 12.5 mg/ml in 20-ml vials.
Premixed: 0.5 mg/ml (125 mg or 250 mg) in D$_5$W, 1 mg/ml (250 mg or 500 mg) in D$_5$,W 2 mg/ml (500 mg) in D5W, 4 mg/ml (1000 mg) in D$_5$W

NURSING PROCESS

✒ Assessment

• Assess patient's condition before therapy and regularly thereafter.
• Continuously monitor ECG, blood pressure, pulmonary capillary wedge pressure, cardiac condition, and urine output.
• Monitor electrolyte level.
• Be alert for adverse reactions and drug interactions.
• Assess patient's and family's knowledge of drug therapy.

⊕ Nursing diagnoses

• Decreased cardiac output related to underlying condition
• Acute pain related to headache
• Deficient knowledge related to drug therapy

▶ Planning and implementation

• Before starting therapy, correct hypovolemia with plasma volume expanders.
• Give digoxin before giving this drug. Because drug increases AV node conduction, patients with atrial fibrillation may develop rapid ventricular rate.
⚠ ALERT: Don't confuse dobutamine with dopamine.

Patient teaching
• Tell patient to report chest pain, shortness of breath, and headache.

✔ Evaluation

• Patient regains adequate cardiac output exhibited by stable vital signs, normal urine output, and clear mental condition.
• Patient's headache is relieved with analgesic administration.

Reactions may be *common,* uncommon, *life-threatening*, or COMMON AND LIFE-THREATENING.

• Patient and family state understanding of drug therapy.

docetaxel
(doks-uh-TAKX-ul)
Taxotere

Pharmacologic class: taxoid antineoplastic
Therapeutic class: antineoplastic
Pregnancy risk category: D

Indications and dosages

▶ **Locally advanced or metastatic breast cancer for which prior chemotherapy has failed.** *Adults:* 60 to 100 mg/m² I.V. over 1 hour q 3 weeks.

⊠ **Adjust-a-dose:** If patient initially receives 100 mg/m² and develops febrile neutropenia, neutrophils less than 500 cells/mm³ for more than 1 week, or severe or cumulative cutaneous reactions, decrease dose to 75 mg/m². If reactions continue, decrease dose to 55 mg/m² or stop therapy.

If patient receives 60 mg/m² initially and doesn't develop febrile neutropenia, neutrophils less than 500 cells/mm³, severe or cumulative cutaneous reactions, or severe peripheral neuropathy, increase dosage. Stop therapy if patient develops grade 3 peripheral neuropathy.

▶ **Locally advanced or metastatic non–small-cell lung cancer after failure of platinum-based chemotherapy.** *Adults:* 75 mg/m² I.V. over 1 hour q 3 weeks.

⊠ **Adjust-a-dose:** For patients with febrile neutropenia, neutrophils less than 500 cells/mm³ for more than 1 week, severe or cumulative cutaneous reactions, or other grade 3 or 4 nonhematologic toxicity, stop drug until toxicity is resolved; then restart at 55 mg/m². For patients who develop grade 3 or higher peripheral neuropathy, stop drug entirely.

▶ **Unresectable, locally advanced, or metastatic non–small-cell lung cancer in patient who has not previously received chemotherapy for this condition with cisplatin.** *Adults:* 75 mg/m² I.V. over 1 hour immediately followed by cisplatin 75 mg/m² I.V. over 30 to 60 minutes q 3 weeks.

⊠ **Adjust-a-dose:** For patients whose lowest platelet count during the previous course of therapy was less than 25,000 cells/mm³, those

with febrile neutropenia, and those with serious nonhematologic toxicities, decrease dosage to 65 mg/m². In patients who require a further dose reduction, give 50 mg/m². For cisplatin dosage adjustments, see manufacturers' prescribing information.

▶ **Androgen-independent metastatic prostate cancer in combination with prednisone.** *Men:* 75 mg/m² I.V. as a 1-hour infusion q 3 weeks given with prednisone, 5 mg P.O. b.i.d. continuously. Premedicate with dexamethasone 8 mg P.O. at 12 hours, 3 hours, and 1 hour before the infusion.

⊠ **Adjust-a-dose:** In patients who develop febrile neutropenia, neutrophils < 500 cells/mm³ for more than 1 week, severe or cumulative cutaneous reactions, or moderate neurosensory signs or symptoms, reduce subsequent dose to 60 mg/m². In patients who continue to have reactions with the decreased dose, stop treatment.

▶ **Adjuvant post-surgery treatment of operable node-positive breast cancer.** *Adults:* 75 mg/m² I.V. as a 1-hour infusion given 1 hour after doxorubicin 50 mg/m² and cyclophosphamide 500 mg/m² q 3 weeks for 6 cycles. Patient's neutrophil count should be 1,500 cells/mm³ or higher.

⊠ **Adjust-a-dose:** Patients who develop febrile neutropenia should receive granulocyte-colony stimulating factor in all subsequent cycles. If febrile neutropenia doesn't resolve, it will continue and docetaxel dose will be reduced to 60 mg/m². For patients who develop severe or cumulative cutaneous reactions or moderate neurosensory signs and symptoms, reduce dose to 60 mg/m². If these reactions persist at the reduced dosage, stop treatment.

▼ I.V. administration

• Premedicate with oral corticosteroids for 3 days, starting 1 day before treatment to reduce fluid retention and hypersensitivity reactions.
• Wear gloves while preparing and giving drug. If solution contacts skin, wash immediately and thoroughly with soap and water. If drug contacts mucous membranes, flush thoroughly with water. Mark all waste materials with chemotherapy hazard labels.
• Prepare and store infusion solutions in bottles (glass or polypropylene) or plastic bags, and give through polyethylene-lined administration sets.

• Dilute drug with diluent supplied. Allow drug and diluent to stand at room temperature for 5 minutes before mixing. After adding diluent contents to vial, rotate vial gently for 15 seconds. Let solution stand for a few minutes for foam to dissipate.
• To prepare solution for infusion, withdraw required amount of premixed solution from vial and add it to 250 ml normal saline solution or D_5W to yield 0.3 to 0.9 mg/ml. Doses exceeding 240 mg need a larger volume of infusion solution to stay below 0.9 mg/ml of drug. Mix infusion thoroughly by manual rotation.
• Give drug as a 1-hour infusion; store unopened vials in the refrigerator.
• If solution isn't clear or if it contains precipitates, discard it. Use infusion solution within 8 hours.

⊗ **Incompatibilities**
None reported.

Contraindications and cautions

• Contraindicated in patients hypersensitive to drug or other drugs containing polysorbate 80 and in those with neutrophil counts below 1,500 cells/mm^3.
• Don't give drug to patients with severe hepatic impairment, bilirubin level higher than the upper limits of normal (ULN) or with AST or ALT level higher than 1.5 times ULN concomitant with alkaline phosphatase level higher than 2.5 times ULN.
Lifespan: In pregnant and breast-feeding women, drug is contraindicated. In children younger than age 16, safety and effectiveness haven't been established.

Adverse reactions

CNS: *asthenia,* dysesthesia, pain, paresthesia, weakness.
CV: *fluid retention,* hypotension.
GI: diarrhea, nausea, stomatitis, vomiting.
Hematologic: *anemia, **febrile neutropenia, leukopenia, myelosuppression, neutropenia, thrombocytopenia.***
Musculoskeletal: arthralgia, back pain, *myalgia.*
Respiratory: dyspnea.
Skin: *alopecia,* desquamation, flushing, nail pain, nail pigment changes, rash, skin eruptions.
Other: chest tightness, chills, drug fever, HYPERSENSITIVITY REACTIONS, infection, ***septic and nonseptic death.***

Interactions

Drug-drug. *Drugs that are induced, inhibited, or metabolized by CYP 3A4 (cyclosporin, ketoconazole, erythromycin, troleandomycin):* May modify docetaxel metabolism. Use together cautiously.

Effects on lab test results

• May increase ALT, AST, bilirubin, and alkaline phosphatase levels. May decrease hemoglobin level and hematocrit.
• May decrease WBC and platelet counts.

Pharmacokinetics

Absorption: Given I.V.
Distribution: 94% is protein-bound.
Metabolism: Partly by liver.
Excretion: Mainly in feces. *Half-life:* About 12 hours.

Route	Onset	Peak	Duration
I.V.	Immediate	Unknown	Unknown

Action

Chemical effect: Disrupts the microtubular network essential for mitotic and interphase cellular functions.
Therapeutic effect: Inhibits mitosis, producing antineoplastic effect.

Available forms

Injection: 20 mg, 80 mg

NURSING PROCESS

Assessment

• Monitor blood count frequently during therapy.
• Assess patient's and family's knowledge of drug therapy.

Nursing diagnoses

• Ineffective health maintenance related to neoplastic disease
• Deficient knowledge related to drug therapy

Planning and implementation

• Don't give drug to patients with baseline neutrophil count less than 1,500/mm^3.
ALERT: Don't confuse Taxotere with Taxol.

Patient teaching

• Warn patient that alopecia occurs in almost 80% of patients.

• Tell patient to promptly report sore throat, fever, unusual bruising or bleeding, or signs of fluid retention.

☑ **Evaluation**
• Patient shows positive response to drug.
• Patient and family state understanding of drug therapy.

---

docusate calcium
(dioctyl calcium sulfosuccinate)
(DOK-yoo-sayt KAL-see-um)
DC Softgels, Pro-Cal-Sof, Surfak

docusate potassium
(dioctyl potassium sulfosuccinate)
Diocto-K†, Kasof†

docusate sodium
(dioctyl sodium sulfosuccinate)
Colace†, Coloxyl ◇, Coloxyl Enema
Concentrate1!, Dialose†, Diocto†, Dioeze†,
Disonate†, DOK†, DOS Softgels†,
Doxinate†, D-S-S†, Modane Soft†, Pro-Sof†,
Regulax SS†, Regulex ♦ †, Regutol†,
Therevac-SB†

Pharmacologic class: surfactant
Therapeutic class: emollient laxative
Pregnancy risk category: C

Indications and dosages

▶ **Stool softener.** *Adults and children age 12 and older:* 50 to 360 mg P.O. daily until bowel movements are normal. Or give enema (where available). Dilute 1:24 with sterile water before administration, and give 100 to 150 ml (retention enema), 300 to 500 ml (evacuation enema), or 0.5 to 1.5 liters (flushing enema).
Children ages 6 to 12: 40 to 120 mg docusate sodium P.O. daily.
Children ages 3 to 6: 20 to 60 mg docusate sodium P.O. daily.
Children younger than age 3: 10 to 40 mg docusate sodium P.O. daily. Higher dosages used for initial therapy. Adjust dosage to individual response.
Adults and children: Usual dosage 240 mg docusate calcium P.O. daily until bowel movements are normal.

Contraindications and cautions

• Contraindicated in patients hypersensitive to drug or any of its components and in those with intestinal obstruction, undiagnosed abdominal pain, signs of appendicitis, fecal impaction, or acute surgical abdomen.
⚯ **Lifespan:** In pregnant women, use cautiously.

Adverse reactions

EENT: throat irritation.
GI: bitter taste, diarrhea, laxative dependence with long-term or excessive use, mild abdominal cramping.

Interactions

Drug-drug. *Mineral oil:* May increase mineral oil absorption and cause toxicity and lipoid pneumonia. Separate doses.

Effects on lab test results

None reported.

Pharmacokinetics

Absorption: Minimal.
Distribution: Mainly local.
Metabolism: None.
Excretion: In feces. *Half-life:* Unknown.

Route	Onset	Peak	Duration
P.O.	Varies	Varies	24–72 hr
P.R.	Unknown	Unknown	Unknown

Action

Chemical effect: Reduces surface tension of interfacing liquid contents of bowel. This detergent activity promotes incorporation of additional liquid into stool, thus forming softer mass.
Therapeutic effect: Softens stool.

Available forms

docusate calcium
Capsules: 50 mg†, 240 mg†
docusate potassium
Capsules: 100 mg†, 240 mg†
docusate sodium
Capsules: 50 mg† 60 mg†, 100 mg†, 240 mg†, 250 mg†
Enema concentrate: 18 g/100 ml (must be diluted) ◇
Oral liquid: 150 mg/15 ml†
Oral solution: 50 mg/ml†

Syrup: 20 mg/5 ml*†, 50 mg/15 ml†, 60 mg/
15 ml†, 100 mg/30 ml†
Tablets: 100 mg†

NURSING PROCESS

⚖ Assessment
• Obtain history of patient's bowel patterns before therapy, and reassess regularly thereafter.
• Before giving drug for constipation, determine if patient has adequate fluid intake, exercise, and diet.
• Be alert for adverse reactions and drug interactions.
• Assess patient's and family's knowledge of drug therapy.

⊕ Nursing diagnoses
• Constipation related to underlying condition
• Diarrhea related to prolonged or excessive use of drug
• Deficient knowledge related to drug therapy

⟩ Planning and implementation
• Give liquid in milk, fruit juice, or infant formula to mask bitter taste.
• Drug is the laxative of choice for patients who shouldn't strain during defecation, including patients recovering from MI or rectal surgery, patients with a rectal or anal disease that makes passage of firm stool difficult, or patients with postpartum constipation.
• Store drug at 59° to 86° F (15° to 30° C), and protect liquid from light.
• If abdominal cramping occurs, stop drug and notify prescriber.
• Drug doesn't stimulate intestinal peristaltic movements.
⊛ **ALERT:** Don't confuse Colace and Calan.
Patient teaching
• Teach patient about dietary sources of bulk, which include bran and other cereals, fresh fruit, and vegetables.
• Instruct patient to use only occasionally and not to use for more than 1 week without prescriber's knowledge.
• Tell patient to stop taking the drug and to notify the prescriber if severe cramping occurs.

☑ Evaluation
• Patient's constipation is relieved.
• Patient remains free from diarrhea during therapy.

• Patient and family state understanding of drug therapy.

dofetilide
(doh-FET-eh-lighd)
Tikosyn

Pharmacologic class: antiarrhythmic
Therapeutic class: class III antiarrhythmic
Pregnancy risk category: C

Indications and dosages
▶ **To maintain normal sinus rhythm in patients with symptomatic atrial fibrillation or atrial flutter for longer than 1 week who have been converted to normal sinus rhythm; to convert atrial fibrillation and atrial flutter to normal sinus rhythm.** *Adults:* Dosage is individualized and is based on creatinine clearance and QT interval, which must be obtained before first dose. (If pulse is less than 60 beats/minute, use QT interval.) Usual dosage is 500 mcg P.O. b.i.d. for patients with creatinine clearance above 60 ml/minute.
☒ **Adjust-a-dose:** For patients with renal impairment, if creatinine clearance is 40 to 60 ml/minute, give 250 mcg P.O. b.i.d. If creatinine clearance is 20 to 39 ml/minute, give 125 mcg P.O. b.i.d. If creatinine clearance is less than 20 ml/minute, drug is contraindicated.
For patients who develop prolonged QT interval, adjust dosage or stop drug.

Contraindications and cautions
• Contraindicated in patients with congenital or acquired prolonged QT-interval syndromes. Also contraindicated in patients with baseline QTc interval greater than 440 msec (500 msec in patients with ventricular conduction abnormalities). Also contraindicated in patients with creatinine clearance below 20 ml/min and in patients hypersensitive to drug and in those receiving verapamil, cimetidine, trimethoprim (alone or with sulfamethoxazole), or ketoconazole.
• Use cautiously in patients with severe hepatic impairment.
❀ **Lifespan:** In pregnant women, use cautiously. In breast-feeding women, drug isn't recommended. In children, safety and effectiveness haven't been established.

Adverse reactions

CNS: anxiety, asthenia, *cerebral ischemia,* dizziness, *headache,* insomnia, migraine, paresthesia, *stroke,* syncope.
CV: angina, atrial fibrillation, AV block, *brady-cardia,* bundle branch block, *cardiac arrest,* chest pain, edema, heart block, hypertension, *MI,* palpitations, peripheral edema, *torsades de pointes, ventricular fibrillation, ventricular tachycardia.*
EENT: facial paralysis.
GI: abdominal pain, diarrhea, nausea.
GU: UTI.
Hepatic: liver damage.
Musculoskeletal: arthralgia, back pain.
Respiratory: dyspnea, increased cough, respiratory tract infection.
Skin: rash, sweating.
Other: *angioedema,* flulike syndrome.

Interactions

Drug-drug. *Amiloride, metformin, triamterene:* May increase dofetilide level. Use together cautiously.
Cimetidine, ketoconazole, sulfamethoxazole, trimethoprim, verapamil: May increase dofetilide level. Don't use together.
Inhibitors of CYP 3A4 (amiodarone, azole antifungals, cannabinoids, diltiazem, macrolide antibiotics, nefazodone, norfloxacin, protease inhibitors, quinine, serotonin reuptake inhibitors, zafirlukast): May decrease metabolism and increase dofetilide level. Use together cautiously; monitor patient for toxicity.
Inhibitors of renal cationic secretion (megestrol, prochlorperazine): May increase dofetilide level. Avoid using together.
Drug-food. *Grapefruit juice:* May decrease dofetilide's hepatic metabolism and increase its level. Avoid using together.

Effects on lab test results

None reported.

Pharmacokinetics

Absorption: More than 90%; levels peak at 2 to 3 hours. Steady-state levels are achieved in 2 to 3 days. Unaffected by food or antacid.
Distribution: Wide with a volume of distribution of 3 L/kg. Protein-binding is 60% to 70%.
Metabolism: Small, by the CYP 3A4 isoenzyme in the liver.

Excretion: 80% in urine, of which 80% is unchanged drug while the rest is inactive or minimally active metabolites. *Half-life:* 10 hours.

Route	Onset	Peak	Duration
P.O.	Unknown	2–3 hr	Unknown

Action

Chemical effect: Prolongs repolarization without affecting conduction velocity by blocking the cardiac ion channel carrying potassium current.
Therapeutic effect: Converts atrial fibrillation and atrial flutter to normal sinus rhythm, and maintains normal rhythm.

Available forms

Distributed only to hospitals and other institutions with dosage and treatment initiation programs. Inpatient and subsequent outpatient discharge and refills of prescriptions are allowed only with confirmation that prescriber has access to these programs.
Capsules: 125 mcg (0.125 mg), 250 mcg (0.25 mg), 500 mcg (0.5 mg)

NURSING PROCESS

⏏ Assessment

• Obtain accurate medication list (prescription, OTC, and herbal) from patient before starting drug; stop antiarrhythmic under careful monitoring for at least 2 days before giving second antiarrhythmic. Don't give drug within 3 months of amiodarone unless level is below 0.3 mcg/ml.
• Assess patient's QTc interval, cardiac rhythm, creatinine clearance, and vital signs before starting medication. Prolongation of the QTc interval requires subsequent dosage adjustments or discontinuation. Continuous ECG monitoring is required for a minimum of 3 days for maintenance therapy, or 12 hours after conversion to normal sinus rhythm.
• Obtain potassium level before starting therapy and regularly thereafter. Hypokalemia and hypomagnesemia may occur when giving potassium-depleting diuretics, increasing the risk of torsades de pointes. Achieve and maintain normal potassium level.
• Monitor patient for prolonged diarrhea, sweating, and vomiting, and report any such symp-

toms to the prescriber because electrolyte imbalance may increase the risk of arrhythmias.
• Monitor renal function and QTc interval every 3 months.
• Assess patient's and family's knowledge of drug therapy.

⊕ Nursing diagnoses
• Decreased cardiac output related to underlying arrhythmia
• Risk for injury related to drug-induced adverse reactions
• Deficient knowledge related to drug therapy

▷ Planning and implementation
• If patient doesn't convert to normal sinus rhythm within 24 hours after starting drug, use electrical cardioversion.
• Drug must be given by specially certified prescriber in an acute care facility due to potentially high risk of torsades de pointes.
• If drug must be stopped to allow administration of other interacting drugs, allow washout period of at least 2 days before starting other drug.
Patient teaching
• Instruct patient to notify prescriber about any change in prescription drugs, OTC medications, or herbal remedies.
• Urge patient to immediately report excessive or prolonged diarrhea, sweating, vomiting, or loss of appetite or thirst to prescriber.
• Inform patient that dofetilide can be taken without regard to meals or antacids.
• Tell patient not to take drug with grapefruit juice.
• Warn patient not to use OTC Tagamet-HB for ulcers or heartburn. Explain that antacids and OTC acid reducers such as Zantac 75 mg, Pepcid, Axid, and Prevacid are acceptable.
• Instruct woman to notify prescriber about planned, suspected, or known pregnancy.
• Advise patient not to breast-feed while taking dofetilide.
• If patient misses a dose, tell him to skip it and wait for the next scheduled dose. Caution against doubling the dose.

☑ Evaluation
• Patient maintains normal sinus rhythm.
• Patient has no injury as a result of drug-induced adverse reactions.

• Patient and family state understanding of drug therapy.

dolasetron mesylate
(doh-LEH-seh-trohn MES-ih layt)
Anzemet

Pharmacologic class: selective serotonin (5-HT3) receptor antagonist
Therapeutic class: antiemetic
Pregnancy risk category: B

Indications and dosages
▶ **To prevent nausea and vomiting after cancer chemotherapy.** *Adults:* 100 mg P.O. given as a single dose 1 hour before chemotherapy. Or 1.8 mg/kg (or a fixed dose of 100 mg) as a single I.V. dose given 30 minutes before chemotherapy.
Children ages 2 to 16: 1.8 mg/kg P.O. 1 hour before chemotherapy. Or 1.8 mg/kg as single I.V. dose 30 minutes before chemotherapy. Injectable form can be mixed with apple juice and given P.O. Maximum dose, 100 mg.
▶ **To prevent postoperative nausea and vomiting.** *Adults:* 100 mg P.O. within 2 hours before surgery. Or 12.5 mg as single I.V. dose about 15 minutes before cessation of anesthesia.
Children ages 2 to 16: 1.2 mg/kg P.O. given within 2 hours before surgery, to maximum, 100 mg. Or 0.35 mg/kg (up to 12.5 mg) as single I.V. dose about 15 minutes before cessation of anesthesia. Injectable form can be mixed with apple juice and given P.O.
▶ **Postoperative nausea and vomiting.** *Adults:* 12.5 mg as a single I.V. dose as soon as nausea or vomiting begins.
Children ages 2 to 16: 0.35 mg/kg to maximum, 12.5 mg, as a single I.V. dose as soon as nausea or vomiting begins.

▼ I.V. administration
• Drug can be injected as rapidly as 100 mg in 30 seconds, or diluted in 50 ml of compatible solution and infused over 15 minutes.
• If an arrhythmia develops, stop the drug and notify prescriber immediately.
• After dilution, solution is stable for 24 hours at room temperature or 48 hours if refrigerated.
⊗ **Incompatibilities**
Injection shouldn't be mixed with other drugs.

Contraindications and cautions

• Contraindicated in patients hypersensitive to drug or any of its components.

• Give cautiously to patients who have or may develop prolonged cardiac conduction intervals, such as those with electrolyte abnormalities, history of arrhythmias, and cumulative high-dose anthracycline therapy.

⚞ **Lifespan:** In breast-feeding women, use cautiously because it's unknown if drug appears in breast milk. In infants, drug isn't recommended.

Adverse reactions

CNS: dizziness, drowsiness, fatigue, fever, *headache.*
CV: *arrhythmias, bradycardia,* ECG changes, hypertension, hypotension, tachycardia.
GI: abdominal pain, anorexia, constipation, *diarrhea,* dyspepsia.
GU: oliguria, urine retention.
Skin: pruritus, rash.
Other: chills, pain at injection site.

Interactions

Drug-drug. *Drugs that induce CYP enzymes (such as rifampin):* May decrease hydrodolasetron level. Monitor patient for decreased effectiveness of drug.
Drugs that inhibit CYP enzymes (such as cimetidine): May increase hydrodolasetron level. Monitor patient for adverse effects.
Drugs that prolong ECG intervals (such as antiarrhythmics): May increase risk of arrhythmia. Monitor patient closely.

Effects on lab test results

• May increase ALT and AST levels.

Pharmacokinetics

Absorption: Rapid for hydrodolasetron, an active metabolite that has an absolute bioavailability of 75%.
Distribution: Wide, with 69% to 77% bound to plasma protein.
Metabolism: Rapid and complete.
Excretion: Two-thirds of hydrodolasetron is in urine; rest in feces. *Half-life:* 8 hours.

Route	Onset	Peak	Duration
P.O.	Rapid	1 hr	8 hr
I.V.	Rapid	36 min	7 hr

Action

Chemical effect: Blocks the action of serotonin, thereby preventing serotonin from stimulating the vomiting reflex.
Therapeutic effect: Prevents nausea and vomiting.

Available forms

Injection: 20 mg/ml as 12.5 mg/0.625 ml-ampule or 100 mg/5 ml-vial
Tablets: 50 mg, 100 mg

D

NURSING PROCESS

⧗ Assessment

• Assess patient for history of nausea and vomiting related to chemotherapy or postoperative recovery.
• Be alert for adverse reactions and drug interactions.
• Monitor ECG carefully in patients who have or may develop prolonged cardiac conduction intervals.
• Assess patient's and family's knowledge of drug therapy.

⧗ Nursing diagnoses

• Imbalanced nutrition: less than body requirements, related to nausea and vomiting
• Risk for injury related to drug-induced adverse CNS reaction
• Deficient knowledge related to drug therapy

⧉ Planning and implementation

• Injection for P.O. use is stable in apple juice for 2 hours at room temperature.
⚠ **ALERT:** Don't confuse Anzemet with Avandamet.
Patient teaching
• Tell patient about potential adverse effects.
• Instruct patient not to mix injection in juice for P.O. use until just before taking the dose.
• Tell patient to report nausea or vomiting.

⧗ Evaluation

• Patient has no nausea and vomiting.
• Patient is free from injury.
• Patient and family state understanding of drug therapy.

Rapid onset   *Liquid form contains alcohol.   ◆Canada   ◇Australia   †OTC   ⦿Photoguide   ‡Off-label use*

donepezil hydrochloride
(doh-NEH-peh-zil high-droh-KLOR-ighd)
Aricept, Aricept ODT

Pharmacologic class: reversible inhibitor of acetylcholinesterase
Therapeutic class: psychotherapeutic drug for Alzheimer's disease
Pregnancy risk category: C

Indications and dosages
▶ **Mild to moderate dementia of the Alzheimer's type.** *Adults:* Initially, 5 mg P.O. daily h.s. After 4 to 6 weeks, may increase dosage to 10 mg daily.

Contraindications and cautions
• Contraindicated in patients hypersensitive to drug or to piperidine derivatives.
• Use cautiously in patients with history of ulcer disease, CV disease, asthma or COPD, or urinary outflow impairment. Also use cautiously in patients currently taking NSAIDs.
≋ **Lifespan:** In pregnant women, use only if benefits to the woman outweigh risks to the fetus. Breast-feeding women shouldn't nurse during therapy. In children, safety and effectiveness haven't been established.

Adverse reactions
CNS: abnormal crying, abnormal dreams, aggression, aphasia, ataxia, depression, dizziness, fatigue, *headache,* insomnia, irritability, nervousness, pain, paresthesia, restlessness, *seizures,* somnolence, syncope, tremor, vertigo.
CV: atrial fibrillation, chest pain, hypertension, hypotension, vasodilation.
EENT: blurred vision, cataracts, eye irritation, sore throat.
GI: anorexia, bloating, *diarrhea,* epigastric pain, fecal incontinence, *GI bleeding, nausea,* vomiting.
GU: frequent urination.
Metabolic: dehydration, weight decrease.
Musculoskeletal: arthritis, bone fracture, muscle cramps, toothache.
Respiratory: bronchitis, dyspnea.
Skin: diaphoresis, ecchymosis, pruritus, urticaria.

Other: accident, hot flushes, increased libido, influenza.

Interactions
Drug-drug. *Anticholinergics:* May interfere with anticholinergic activity. Monitor patient for effects.
Bethanechol, succinylcholine: May have additive effects. Monitor patient closely.
Carbamazepine, dexamethasone, phenytoin, phenobarbital, rifampin: May increase rate of donepezil elimination. Monitor patient for effects.
Cholinomimetics, cholinesterase inhibitors: May have synergistic effect. Monitor patient closely.
Drug-herb. *Jaborandi tree, pill-bearing spurge:* May cause additive effect and increased risk of toxicity. Discourage using together.

Effects on lab test results
None reported.

Pharmacokinetics
Absorption: Good.
Distribution: 96% plasma protein-bound, mainly to albumin.
Metabolism: Extensive.
Excretion: In urine and feces. *Half-life:* 70 hours.

Route	Onset	Peak	Duration
P.O.	Unknown	3–4 hr	Unknown

Action
Chemical effect: Reversibly inhibits acetylcholinesterase in the CNS, thereby increasing the acetylcholine level.
Therapeutic effect: Temporarily improves cognitive function in patients with Alzheimer's disease.

Available forms
Tablets: 5 mg, 10 mg

NURSING PROCESS
▨ **Assessment**
• Monitor patient for symptoms of active or occult GI bleeding.
• Assess patient's and family's knowledge of drug therapy.

Reactions may be *common,* uncommon, *life-threatening*, or COMMON AND LIFE-THREATENING.

🔁 Nursing diagnoses
• Risk for injury related to adverse effects of drug
• Deficient knowledge related to drug therapy

▶ Planning and implementation
• Give drug h.s., with or without food.
• If cholinergic crisis (severe nausea, vomiting, salivation, sweating, bradycardia, hypotension, respiratory depression, convulsions, and collapse) occurs, treat with an anticholinergic such as atropine.

Patient teaching
• Explain that drug doesn't alter underlying degenerative disease but can alleviate symptoms.
• Tell caregiver to give drug in the evening, just before bedtime.
• Advise patient and caregiver to immediately report significant adverse effects or changes in overall health condition.
• Tell caregiver to inform health care team that patient is taking drug before patient receives anesthesia.

☑ Evaluation
• Patient remains free from injury.
• Patient and family state understanding of drug therapy.

dopamine hydrochloride
(DOH-puh-meen high-droh-KLOR-ighd)
Intropin, Revimine ♦

Pharmacologic class: adrenergic
Therapeutic class: inotropic, vasopressor
Pregnancy risk category: C

Indications and dosages

▶ **To treat shock and correct hemodynamic imbalances; to improve perfusion to vital organs; to increase cardiac output; to correct hypotension.** *Adults:* Initially, 1 to 5 mcg/kg/minute by I.V. infusion. Adjust dosage to desired hemodynamic or renal response, increase by 1 to 4 mcg/kg/minute at 10- to 30-minute intervals.

▼ I.V. administration
• Dilute with D₅W, normal saline solution, or combination of D₅W and normal saline solution. Mix just before use.

• Use continuous infusion pump to regulate flow rate.
• Use central line or large vein, such as in antecubital fossa, to minimize risk of extravasation. If extravasation occurs, stop infusion immediately and call prescriber. Extravasation may require treatment by infiltration of area with 5 to 10 mg of phentolamine and 10 to 15 ml of normal saline solution.
• If solution is discolored, discard within 24 hours.

⊗ Incompatibilities
Acyclovir sodium, additives with a dopamine and dextrose solution, alteplase, amphotericin B, cefepime, furosemide, gentamicin, indomethacin sodium trihydrate, iron salts, insulin, oxidizing agents, penicillin G potassium, sodium bicarbonate or other alkaline solutions, thiopental.

Contraindications and cautions
• Contraindicated in patients with uncorrected tachyarrhythmias, pheochromocytoma, or ventricular fibrillation.
• Use cautiously in patients with occlusive vascular disease, cold injuries, diabetic endarteritis, and arterial embolism, and in those taking MAO inhibitors.
🜲 **Lifespan:** In pregnant women, use cautiously. In breast-feeding women and in children, safety and effectiveness haven't been established.

Adverse reactions
CNS: headache.
CV: anginal pain, *arrhythmias, bradycardia,* conduction disturbances, ectopic beats, hypertension, *hypotension,* palpitations, tachycardia, vasoconstriction, *widening of QRS complex.*
GI: nausea, vomiting.
GU: azotemia.
Respiratory: *asthma attacks,* dyspnea.
Skin: necrosis, piloerection, tissue sloughing with extravasation.
Other: *anaphylaxis.*

Interactions
Drug-drug. *Alpha and beta blockers:* May antagonize dopamine effects. Monitor patient for effect.
Ergot alkaloids: May increase blood pressure. Don't use together.

Inhaled anesthetics: May increase risk of arrhythmias or hypertension. Monitor vital signs and ECG closely.

Oxytocic drugs: May potentiate pressor effect, resulting in severe hypertension. Avoid using together, if possible.

Phenelzine, tranylcypromine: May cause severe headache, hypertension, fever, and hypertensive crisis. Avoid using together.

Phenytoin: May lower blood pressure in dopamine-stabilized patients. Monitor blood pressure carefully.

Tricyclic antidepressants: May decrease pressor response. Monitor patient closely.

Effects on lab test results

● May increase glucose and urea levels.

Pharmacokinetics

Absorption: Given I.V.
Distribution: Wide; doesn't cross blood–brain barrier.
Metabolism: To inactive compounds in liver, kidneys, and plasma.
Excretion: In urine, mainly as its metabolites.
Half-life: 9 minutes.

Route	Onset	Peak	Duration
I.V.	≤ 5 min	Unknown	≤ 10 min

Action

Chemical effect: Stimulates dopaminergic, beta-adrenergic, and alpha-adrenergic receptors of sympathetic nervous system.
Therapeutic effect: Increases cardiac output, blood pressure, and renal perfusion (in low doses).

Available forms

Injection: 40 mg/ml, 80 mg/ml, 160 mg/ml as concentrate for injection for I.V. infusion; 0.8 mg/ml (200 or 400 mg) in D_5W; 1.6 mg/ml (400 or 800 mg) in D_5W; 3.2 mg/ml (800 mg) in D_5W as parenteral injection for I.V. infusion

NURSING PROCESS

⚗ Assessment

● Obtain history of patient's underlying condition before therapy.
● During infusion, frequently monitor ECG, blood pressure, cardiac output, central venous pressure, pulmonary capillary wedge pressure,

pulse rate, urine output, and color and temperature of limbs.
● Be alert for adverse reactions and drug interactions.
● Be aware that acidosis decreases effectiveness of dopamine.
● After drug is stopped, watch closely for sudden drop in blood pressure.
● Assess patient's and family's knowledge of drug therapy.

⚕ Nursing diagnoses

● Ineffective tissue perfusion (cerebral, cardiopulmonary, and renal) related to underlying condition
● Risk for injury related to drug-induced adverse reactions
● Deficient knowledge related to drug therapy

▶ Planning and implementation

● Be aware that dosages of 0.5 to 2 mcg/kg/minute mainly stimulate dopamine receptors and dilate renal vasculature increasing urine output. Dosages of 2 to 10 mcg/kg/minute stimulate beta receptors for increased cardiac output. Higher dosages also stimulate alpha-adrenergic receptors, causing vasoconstriction and increased blood pressure. Most patients are satisfactorily maintained on dosages below 20 mcg/kg/minute.
● Drug isn't used to treat blood or fluid volume deficit. If deficit exists, replace fluid before giving vasopressors.
● Taper dosage slowly to evaluate stability of blood pressure.
● If patient receiving dopamine has disproportionate rise in diastolic pressure (a marked decrease in pulse pressure), decrease infusion rate, and watch carefully for further evidence of predominant vasoconstrictor activity, unless such effect is desired.
● If an adverse reaction develops, notify prescriber, who will reduce the dosage or stop the drug.
● If urine flow decreases without hypotension, notify prescriber and reduce dosage.
● **ALERT:** Don't confuse dopamine with dobutamine.

Patient teaching

● Emphasize importance of reporting discomfort at I.V. site immediately.
● Explain to patient the need for drug therapy.

☑ Evaluation

• Patient regains adequate cerebral, cardiopulmonary, and renal tissue perfusion.
• Patient doesn't experience injury as result of drug-induced adverse reactions.
• Patient and family state understanding of drug therapy.

dorzolamide hydrochloride
(dor-ZOLE-uh-mighd high-droh-KLOR-ighd)
Trusopt

Pharmacologic class: carbonic anhydrase inhibitor, sulfonamide
Therapeutic class: antiglaucoma drug
Pregnancy risk category: C

Indications and dosages

▶ **Increased intraocular pressure (IOP) in patients with ocular hypertension or open-angle glaucoma.** *Adults and children:* Instill 1 drop in the conjunctival sac of affected eye t.i.d.

Contraindications and cautions

• Contraindicated in patients hypersensitive to drug or any of its components Also contraindicated in those with renal impairment.
• Use cautiously in patients with impaired hepatic function.
♨ **Lifespan:** In pregnant women, use only if potential benefits to the woman outweigh the risks to the fetus. In breast-feeding women, drug isn't recommended because it's unknown if it appears in breast milk. In elderly patients, use cautiously because they may have greater sensitivity to drug.

Adverse reactions

CNS: asthenia, dizziness, fatigue, headache, paresthesia.
EENT: blurred vision; dryness; eyelid crusting; iridocyclitis; lacrimation; ocular allergic reactions, including conjunctivitis, itching, and lid reactions; ocular burning, stinging, and discomfort; ocular pain; photophobia; redness; superficial punctate keratitis; throat irritation; transient myopia.
GI: bitter taste, nausea.
GU: urolithiasis.

Respiratory: *bronchospasm,* dyspnea.
Skin: contact dermatitis, pruritus, rash, urticaria.
Other: *angioedema.*

Interactions

Drug-drug. *Oral carbonic anhydrase inhibitors:* May cause additive effects. Don't use together.
Topical beta blockers: May cause additive effects. Give drugs 10 minutes apart.

Effects on lab tests results

• May decrease potassium and pH levels.

Pharmacokinetics

Absorption: Systemic.
Distribution: 33% bound to plasma proteins. Accumulates in RBCs during regular therapy.
Metabolism: In the liver by CYP isoenzymes.
Excretion: Primarily unchanged in urine. *Half-life:* 4 months.

Route	Onset	Peak	Duration
Ophthalmic	1–2 hr	2–3 hr	8 hr

Action

Chemical effect: Inhibits carbonic anhydrase in the ciliary processes of the eye. This action reduces aqueous humor secretion, presumably by slowing the formation of bicarbonate ions with subsequent reduction in sodium and fluid transport.
Therapeutic effect: Reduces IOP.

Available forms

Ophthalmic solution: 2%

NURSING PROCESS

☞ Assessment

• Assess patient before starting therapy.
• Because drug is a sulfonamide that is absorbed systemically, the adverse reactions caused by sulfonamides, such as Stevens-Johnson syndrome, agranulocytosis, and aplastic anemia, may occur. Although these symptoms haven't been shown with this drug, monitor for them during therapy.
• Overdose may result in electrolyte imbalance, acidosis, and CNS effects. Monitor electrolyte

levels (especially potassium) and pH levels. Provide supportive therapy for any overdose.
• Assess patient's and family's understanding of drug therapy.

🔬 Nursing diagnoses
• Risk for infection to the eyes related to inadvertent contamination of the multidose container
• Disturbed visual perception related to underlying ocular condition
• Deficient knowledge related to drug therapy

⟩⟩ Planning and implementation
• If patient is wearing contact lenses, remove lenses before giving the drug. Contact lenses may be reinserted 15 minutes after the drug is given.
• Instruct patient not to blink after administration, just close eyes. Apply light finger pressure on lacrimal sac for 1 minute after instillation to minimize systemic absorption of drug.
• If more than one topical ophthalmic drug is being used, give drugs at least 10 minutes apart.
Patient teaching
• Teach patient how to instill drops properly. Advise him to wash hands before and after instilling solution, and warn him not to touch dropper or tip to eye or surrounding tissue, to prevent contamination to the dropper.
• If patient wears contact lenses, instruct him to remove them before instilling the drops and to reinsert them 15 minutes after instillation.
• Advise patient to report ocular reactions, particularly conjunctivitis and lid reactions, immediately to prescriber and to stop drug.

✓ Evaluation
• Patient doesn't suffer from any infection related to drug administration.
• Patient's underlying condition is resolved with drug therapy.
• Patient and family state understanding of drug therapy.

doxapram hydrochloride
(DOKS-uh-prahm high-droh-KLOR-ighd)
Dopram

Pharmacologic class: analeptic
Therapeutic class: CNS and respiratory stimulant
Pregnancy risk category: B

Indications and dosages
▶ **Postanesthesia respiratory stimulation, drug-induced CNS depression, chronic pulmonary disease with acute hypercapnia.**
Adults: 0.5 to 1 mg/kg of body weight (up to 2 mg/kg in CNS depression) by I.V. injection or infusion. Repeat q 5 minutes, if needed. Maximum, 4 mg/kg, up to 3 g daily
▶ **COPD.** *Adults:* 1 to 2 mg/minute by I.V. infusion. Maximum, 3 mg/minute for maximum duration of 2 hours.

▽ I.V. administration
• For I.V. infusion, add 250 mg of drug to 250 ml of 5% or 10% dextrose or normal saline solution injection; concentration equals 1 mg/ml.
• For acute hypercapnia related to COPD, add 400 mg of drug to 180 ml of dextrose or normal saline solution to equal 2 mg/ml. Infuse at 1 to 3 mg/minute.
• Give drug slowly because rapid infusion may cause hemolysis.
• Watch for irritation and infiltration.
⊗ **Incompatibilities**
Aminophylline, ascorbic acid, cefoperazone, cefotaxime, cefotetan, cefuroxime sodium, dexamethasone sodium phosphate, diazepam, digoxin, dobutamine, folic acid, furosemide, hydrocortisone sodium phosphate, hydrocortisone sodium succinate, ketamine, methylprednisolone sodium succinate, minocycline, thiopental, ticarcillin disodium.

Contraindications and cautions
• Contraindicated in patients with seizure disorders; head injury; CV disorders; frank, uncompensated heart failure; severe hypertension; stroke; respiratory failure or incompetence secondary to neuromuscular disorders, muscle paresis, flail chest, obstructed airway, pulmonary embolism, pneumothorax, restrictive respi-

ratory disease, acute bronchial asthma, or dyspnea; or hypoxia not related to hypercapnia.
• Don't use in patients with severe hypotension. If sudden hypotension occurs, stop drug.
• Use cautiously in patients with bronchial asthma, severe tachycardia or arrhythmias, cerebral edema or increased CSF pressure, hyperthyroidism, pheochromocytoma, or metabolic disorders.
≋ Lifespan: In pregnant women, use cautiously. In breast-feeding women and in children, safety and effectiveness haven't been established.

Adverse reactions

CNS: apprehension, bilateral Babinski's signs, disorientation, dizziness, fever, *headache,* paresthesia, pupil dilation, *seizures.*
CV: *arrhythmias,* chest pain and tightness, depressed T waves, flushing, increased blood pressure, variations in heart rate.
EENT: *laryngospasm,* sneezing.
GI: diarrhea, nausea, vomiting.
GU: bladder stimulation with incontinence, urine retention.
Musculoskeletal: muscle spasms.
Respiratory: *bronchospasm,* cough, dyspnea, hiccups, rebound hypoventilation.
Skin: diaphoresis, pruritus.

Interactions

Drug-drug. *MAO inhibitors, sympathomimetics:* May potentiate adverse CV effects. Use together cautiously.

Effects on lab test results

• May increase BUN and hemoglobin levels and hematocrit.
• May decrease erythrocyte, WBC, and RBC counts.

Pharmacokinetics

Absorption: Given I.V.
Distribution: Wide.
Metabolism: 99% by liver.
Excretion: In urine. *Half-life:* 2½ to 4 hours.

Route	Onset	Peak	Duration
I.V.	20–40 sec	1–2 min	5–12 min

Action

Chemical effect: Not clearly defined; acts either directly on central respiratory centers in medulla or indirectly on chemoreceptors.
Therapeutic effect: Stimulates respirations.

Available forms

Injection: 20 mg/ml (benzyl alcohol 0.9%)

D

NURSING PROCESS

⬚ Assessment
• Obtain history of patient's underlying condition before beginning therapy.
• Assess blood pressure, heart rate, deep tendon reflexes, and arterial blood gases before giving drug, and monitor closely throughout therapy.
• Monitor the drug's effectiveness by observing patient for improvement in CNS and respiratory function.
• Be alert for adverse reactions and drug interactions.
• Assess patient's and family's knowledge of drug therapy.

⬚ Nursing diagnoses
• Ineffective breathing pattern related to underlying condition
• Risk for trauma related to potential for drug-induced seizure activity
• Deficient knowledge related to drug therapy

⬚ Planning and implementation
• Don't use in patients with severe hypotension. If sudden hypotension occurs or dyspnea develops, stop giving the drug.
• Establish adequate airway before giving the drug. Prevent patient from aspirating vomitus by placing him on his side. Have suction equipment nearby.
• Drug is used only in surgical- or emergency-department situations.
• If patient shows increase in arterial carbon dioxide or oxygen tension or if mechanical ventilation is started, stop drug and notify prescriber.
⚠ **ALERT:** Don't confuse doxapram with doxorubicin, doxepin, doxacurium, or doxazosin.
Patient teaching
• If patient is alert, instruct him to report chest pain or tightness immediately.

☑ Evaluation
• Patient regains normal respiratory pattern.
• Patient has no seizures as result of therapy.
• Patient and family state understanding of drug therapy.

doxazosin mesylate
(doks-AY-zoh-sin MES-ih-layt)
Cardura

Pharmacologic class: alpha blocker
Therapeutic class: antihypertensive
Pregnancy risk category: C

Indications and dosages
▶ **Essential hypertension.** *Adults:* Initially, 1 mg P.O. daily. Increase to 2 mg daily, then 4 mg daily, then 8 mg. Maximum, 16 mg daily, but dosage above 4 mg daily increases risk of adverse reactions. To minimize adverse reactions, adjust dosage slowly (typically increase only q 2 weeks).
▶ **BPH.** *Adults:* Initially, 1 mg P.O. once daily, morning or evening; may increase to 2 mg and, thereafter, to 4 mg and to 8 mg once daily p.r.n. Adjust dosage in 1- to 2-week intervals.

Contraindications and cautions
• Contraindicated in patients hypersensitive to drug and to quinazoline derivatives (including prazosin and terazosin).
• Use cautiously in patients with impaired liver function.
⚕ **Lifespan:** In pregnant women, use cautiously. In breast-feeding women, drug isn't recommended because it appears in breast milk at levels about 20 times greater than those in maternal plasma. In children, safety and effectiveness haven't been established.

Adverse reactions
CNS: *asthenia, dizziness,* drowsiness, *headache,* pain, somnolence, vertigo.
CV: *arrhythmias,* edema, hypotension, palpitations, *orthostatic hypotension,* tachycardia.
EENT: abnormal vision, pharyngitis, rhinitis.
GI: constipation, diarrhea, nausea, vomiting.
Musculoskeletal: arthralgia, myalgia.
Respiratory: dyspnea.
Skin: pruritus, rash.

Interactions
Drug-drug. *Clonidine:* May decrease clonidine effects. Adjust dosage.
Drug-herb. *Butcher's broom:* May reduce drug effects. Discourage using together.

Effects on lab test results
• May decrease WBC and neutrophil counts.

Pharmacokinetics
Absorption: Good.
Distribution: 98% protein-bound.
Metabolism: Extensive.
Excretion: 63% in bile and feces; 9% in urine.
Half-life: 19 to 22 hours.

Route	Onset	Peak	Duration
P.O.	1–2 hr	5–6 hr	24 hr

Action
Chemical effect: Acts on peripheral vasculature to produce vasodilation.
Therapeutic effect: Lowers blood pressure.

Available forms
Tablets: 1 mg, 2 mg, 4 mg, 8 mg

NURSING PROCESS

☲ Assessment
• Obtain history of patient's blood pressure before beginning therapy, and reassess regularly thereafter.
• Determine effect on standing and supine blood pressure at 2 to 6 hours and 24 hours after giving the drug.
• Be alert for adverse reactions.
• Monitor patient's ECG for arrhythmias.
• Assess patient's and family's knowledge of drug therapy.

⊕ Nursing diagnoses
• Risk for injury related to presence of hypertension
• Decreased cardiac output related to drug-induced adverse CV reactions
• Deficient knowledge related to drug therapy

▷ Planning and implementation
• Increase dosage gradually, with adjustments every 2 weeks for hypertension and every 1 to 2 weeks for BPH.

Reactions may be *common*, uncommon, *life-threatening*, or COMMON AND LIFE-THREATENING.

• If syncope occurs, place patient in recumbent position and provide supportive therapy. A transient hypotensive response isn't considered a contraindication to continued therapy.
ALERT: Don't confuse doxazosin with doxapram, doxorubicin, or doxepin. Don't confuse Cardura with Coumadin, K-Dur, Cardene, or Cordarone.

Patient teaching

• Advise patient that he's susceptible to a first-dose effect similar to that produced by other alpha blockers: marked orthostatic hypotension, accompanied by dizziness or syncope. Orthostatic hypotension is most common after first dose, but it can also occur when stopping therapy or adjusting dosage.
• Warn patient that dizziness or fainting may occur. Advise patient to refrain from driving and performing other hazardous activities until drug's adverse CNS effects are known.
• Stress importance of regular follow-up visits.

Evaluation

• Patient's blood pressure becomes normal.
• Patient maintains adequate cardiac output throughout therapy.
• Patient and family state understanding of drug therapy.

doxepin hydrochloride

(DOKS-eh-pin high-droh-KLOR-ighd)
Novo-Doxepin ♦, Sinequan, Triadapin ♦

Pharmacologic class: tricyclic antidepressant
Therapeutic class: antidepressant
Pregnancy risk category: C

Indications and dosages

▶ **Depression, anxiety.** *Adults and children age 12 and older:* Initially, 25 to 75 mg P.O. daily in divided doses to maximum, 300 mg daily. Or, give entire maintenance dosage once daily. Maximum, 150 mg.
Adjust-a-dose: Reduce dosage in elderly or debilitated patients, adolescents, and those receiving other drugs (especially anticholinergics).

Contraindications and cautions

• Contraindicated in patients hypersensitive to the drug or any of its components and in those with glaucoma or a tendency for urine retention.
Lifespan: In pregnant women and in children younger than age 12, safety and effectiveness haven't been established. In breast-feeding women, drug isn't recommended.

Adverse reactions

CNS: ataxia, confusion, *dizziness, drowsiness,* EEG changes, excitation, extrapyramidal reactions, hallucinations, headache, nervousness, paresthesia, ***seizures,*** tremors, weakness.
CV: ECG changes, hypertension, orthostatic hypotension, tachycardia.
EENT: *blurred vision,* mydriasis, tinnitus.
GI: anorexia, constipation, dry mouth, glossitis, nausea, vomiting.
GU: urine retention.
Hematologic: ***bone marrow depression, including agranulocytosis, aplastic anemia, leukopenia, and thrombocytopenia;*** eosinophilia.
Skin: *diaphoresis,* photosensitivity, rash, urticaria.
Other: hypersensitivity reaction.

Interactions

Drug-drug. *Barbiturates, CNS depressants:* May increase CNS depression. Avoid using together.
Cimetidine, fluoxetine, methylphenidate, sertraline: May increase doxepin level. Monitor patient for increased adverse reactions.
Clonidine: May cause loss of blood pressure control with potentially life-threatening elevations in blood pressure. Don't use together.
Epinephrine, norepinephrine: May increase hypertensive effect. Use cautiously; monitor blood pressure closely.
MAO inhibitors: May cause severe excitation, hyperpyrexia, or seizures, usually with high dosage. Avoid using together.
Drug-herb. *St. John's wort, SAMe, yohimbe:* May elevate serotonin level. Discourage using together.
Drug-food. *Carbonated beverages, grape juice:* May be incompatible. Avoid using together.
Drug-lifestyle. *Alcohol use:* May increase CNS depression. Discourage using together.
Sun exposure: May increase risk of photosensitivity reactions. Discourage unprotected or prolonged exposure to the sun.

Effects on lab test results

• May increase liver enzyme levels. May decrease hemoglobin level and hematocrit. May increase or decrease glucose level.
• May increase eosinophil count. May decrease RBC, WBC, granulocyte, and platelet counts.

Pharmacokinetics

Absorption: Rapid.
Distribution: Wide, including CNS; 90% protein-bound.
Metabolism: By liver. A significant first-pass effect may explain varying levels in patients with same dosage.
Excretion: Mainly in urine. *Half-life:* 6 to 8 hours.

Route	Onset	Peak	Duration
P.O.	Unknown	≤ 2 hr	Unknown

Action

Chemical effect: Unknown; increases amount of norepinephrine, serotonin, or both in CNS by blocking their reuptake by presynaptic neurons.
Therapeutic effect: Relieves depression and anxiety.

Available forms

Capsules: 10 mg, 25 mg, 50 mg, 75 mg, 100 mg, 150 mg
Oral concentrate: 10 mg/ml

NURSING PROCESS

✏ Assessment

• Assess patient's depression or anxiety before and during therapy.
• Be alert for adverse reactions and drug interactions.
• Assess patient's and family's knowledge of drug therapy.

🔄 Nursing diagnoses

• Ineffective individual coping related to underlying condition
• Risk for injury related to drug-induced adverse CNS reactions
• Deficient knowledge related to drug therapy

⟩ Planning and implementation

• Dilute oral concentrate with 120 ml of water, milk, or juice (except grape juice). Don't mix

with carbonated beverages because they are incompatible.
• Don't abruptly stop giving the drug. Abruptly stopping long-term therapy may cause nausea, headache, and malaise, which don't indicate addiction.
• Stop drug gradually several days before surgery because hypertensive episodes may occur.
• If signs of psychosis occur or increase, notify prescriber and reduce dosage.
⚠ **ALERT:** Don't confuse doxepin with doxazosin, digoxin, doxapram, or Doxidan; don't confuse Sinequan with saquinavir.

Patient teaching

• Tell patient to dilute oral concentrate with 120 ml of water, milk, or juice (orange, grapefruit, tomato, prune, or pineapple). Drug is incompatible with carbonated beverages and grape juice.
• Advise patient to take full dose at bedtime, but warn him that he may have morning orthostatic hypotension.
• Warn patient to avoid hazardous activities that require alertness and good psychomotor coordination until the drug's CNS effects are known. Drowsiness and dizziness usually subside after a few weeks.
• Tell patient to avoid using alcohol while taking the drug.
• Warn patient not to stop drug therapy suddenly.
• Advise patient to consult prescriber before taking prescription drugs, OTC medications, or herbal remedies.
• Advise patient to use sunblock, wear protective clothing, and avoid prolonged exposure to strong sunlight.

✓ Evaluation

• Patient behavior and communication indicate improvement of depression or anxiety.
• Patient has no injury as result of drug-induced adverse CNS reactions.
• Patient and family state understanding of drug therapy.

doxercalciferol
(dox-er-kal-SIF-eh-rol)
Hectorol

Pharmacologic class: synthetic vitamin D analogue
Therapeutic class: parathyroid hormone antagonist
Pregnancy risk category: B

Indications and dosages

▶ **To reduce intact parathyroid hormone (iPTH) levels to manage secondary hyperparathyroidism in patients undergoing long-term renal dialysis.** *Adults:* Initially, 10 mcg P.O. three times weekly at dialysis. Adjust dosage p.r.n. to lower intact PTH levels to 150 to 300 picograms per milliliter (pg/ml). Increase dosage by 2.5 mcg at 8-week intervals if the intact PTH level doesn't go down by 50% and fails to reach target range. Maximum, 20 mcg P.O. three times weekly. If intact PTH levels fall below 100 pg/ml, stop drug for 1 week and then resume at a dose that's at least 2.5 mcg lower than the last dose.

▶ **Secondary hyperparathyroidism in pre-dialysis patients with Stage 3 or 4 chronic kidney disease.** *Adults:* 1 mcg P.O. daily. Adjust dosage p.r.n. to lower blood iPTH levels to target range. Target range for stage 3 is 35 to 70 pg/ml. Target range for stage 4 is 70 to 110 pg/ml. Increase dosage at 2-week intervals by 0.5 mcg if levels are above 70 pg/ml (stage 3) or above 110 pg/ml (stage 4). If level falls below 35 pg/ml for stage 3 or 70 pg/ml for stage 4, stop drug for 1 week, then resume at a dose at least 0.5 mcg lower than prior dose. Maximum, 3.5 mcg daily.

Contraindications and cautions

• Contraindicated in patients with a recent history of hypercalcemia, hyperphosphatemia, or vitamin D toxicity.
• Use cautiously in patients with hepatic insufficiency, and frequently monitor calcium, phosphorus, and intact PTH levels in these patients.
⚠ **Lifespan:** In breast-feeding women, and in children younger than age 12, drug isn't recommended. In elderly patients, use cautiously because adverse CNS reactions, orthostatic hy-

potension, and GI and GU distresses are more likely to develop.

Adverse reactions

CNS: dizziness, headache, malaise, sleep disorder.
CV: *bradycardia,* edema.
GI: anorexia, constipation, dyspepsia, *nausea, vomiting.*
Metabolic: weight gain or loss.
Musculoskeletal: arthralgia.
Respiratory: *dyspnea.*
Skin: pruritus.
Other: abscess.

Interactions

Drug-drug. *Calcium-containing or non–aluminum-containing phosphate binders:* May cause hypercalcemia or hyperphosphatemia and decrease effectiveness of doxercalciferol. Use together cautiously, and adjust dosage of phosphate binders as directed.
Cholestyramine, mineral oil: May decrease intestinal absorption of doxercalciferol. Avoid using together.
Glutethimide, phenobarbital, and other enzyme inducers; phenytoin and other enzyme inhibitors: May affect doxercalciferol metabolism. Adjust dosage as directed.
Magnesium-containing antacids: May cause hypermagnesemia. Monitor patient for toxicity.
Orlistat: May interfere with intestinal absorption of vitamin D analogues. Give drug at least 2 hours before or 2 hours after Orlistat administration.
Vitamin D supplements: May cause additive effects and hypercalcemia. Monitor patient for toxicity.

Effects on lab test results

None reported.

Pharmacokinetics

Absorption: Good.
Distribution: Unknown.
Metabolism: To its active forms in the liver.
Excretion: Major metabolite attains peak levels at 11 to 12 hours after repeated doses. *Half-life:* 32 to 37 hours, with a range of up to 96 hours.

Route	Onset	Peak	Duration
P.O.	Unknown	11–12 hr	Unknown

Action

Chemical effect: Regulates calcium levels. Acts directly on the parathyroid glands to suppress PTH synthesis and secretion.
Therapeutic effect: Reduces elevated intact PTH levels.

Available forms

Capsules: 0.5 mcg, 2.5 mcg

NURSING PROCESS

�☰ Assessment

• Assess hepatic function before starting therapy.
• Monitor calcium, phosphorus, and intact PTH levels. Monitor them more frequently in patients with hepatic insufficiency.
• Be alert for adverse reactions and drug interactions.
• Assess patient's and family's knowledge of drug therapy.

⊕ Nursing diagnoses

• Imbalanced nutrition: less than body requirements related to adverse GI effects
• Risk for injury related to adverse CNS effects
• Deficient knowledge related to drug therapy

▷ Planning and implementation

• Give drug with dialysis (about q other day). Individualize doses based on intact PTH levels, with monitoring of calcium and phosphorus levels before therapy and weekly thereafter.
• If patient has hypercalcemia or hyperphosphatemia, or if the calcium level multiplied by the phosphorus level (Ca × P) is greater than 70, immediately stop doxercalciferol until these values decrease.
• Progressive hypercalcemia from vitamin D overdose may require emergency attention. Acute hypercalcemia may worsen arrhythmias and seizures and affect the action of digoxin. Chronic hypercalcemia can lead to vascular and soft-tissue calcification.
• Calcium-based or non–aluminum-containing phosphate binders and a low-phosphate diet are used to control phosphorus levels in patients undergoing dialysis. Adjust dosage of this drug and other therapies to maintain PTH suppression and calcium and phosphorus levels.

Patient teaching

• Inform patient that dosage will be adjusted over several months to achieve satisfactory PTH suppression.
• Tell patient to adhere to a low-phosphorus diet and to follow instructions regarding calcium supplements.
• Tell patient to obtain prescriber's approval before using OTC drugs, including antacids and vitamin preparations containing calcium or vitamin D.
• Inform patient that early signs and symptoms of hypercalcemia include weakness, headache, somnolence, nausea, vomiting, dry mouth, constipation, muscle pain, bone pain, and metallic taste. Late signs and symptoms include polyuria, polydipsia, anorexia, weight loss, nocturia, conjunctivitis, pancreatitis, photophobia, rhinorrhea, pruritus, hyperthermia, decreased libido, hypertension, and arrhythmias.

☑ Evaluation

• Patient has no nausea and vomiting.
• Patient remains free from injury.
• Patient and family state understanding of drug therapy.

doxorubicin hydrochloride
(doks-oh-ROO-bih-sin high-droh-KLOR-ighd)
Adriamycin◇, Adriamycin PFS, Adriamycin RDF, Rubex

Pharmacologic class: anthracycline antibiotic
Therapeutic class: antineoplastic
Pregnancy risk category: D

Indications and dosages

▶ **Bladder, breast, lung, ovarian, stomach, testicular, and thyroid cancers; Hodgkin's disease; acute lymphoblastic and myeloblastic leukemia; Wilms' tumor; neuroblastoma; lymphoma; sarcoma.** *Adults:* 60 to 75 mg/m² I.V. as single dose q 3 weeks; or 30 mg/m² I.V. in single daily dose on days 1 through 3 of 4-week cycle. Alternatively, 20 mg/m² I.V. once weekly. Maximum cumulative dosage, 550 mg/m².
⊠ Adjust-a-dose: In elderly patients and those with myelosuppression or impaired cardiac or hepatic function, dosage may need adjustment.

If bilirubin level increases, decrease dosage: 50% of dosage when bilirubin level is 1.2 to 3 mg/dl; 25% of dosage when bilirubin level is greater than 3 mg/dl.

▽ I.V. administration

• Preparing and giving drug carry carcinogenic, mutagenic, and teratogenic risks. Follow facility policy to reduce risks.
• Reconstitute using preservative-free normal saline solution injection. Add 5 ml to 10-mg vial, 10 ml to 20-mg vial, or 25 ml to 50-mg vial. Shake vial, and allow drug to dissolve; final concentration is 2 mg/ml.
• Give by direct injection into I.V. line of free-flowing compatible I.V. solution containing D_5W or normal saline solution injection in no less than 3 minutes.
• Drug is a severe vesicant, and extravasation may cause tissue necrosis. To avoid extravasation, don't place I.V. line over joints or in limbs with poor venous or lymphatic drainage.
• If extravasation occurs, stop I.V. injection immediately, notify prescriber, and apply ice to area for 24 to 48 hours. Monitor area closely because extravasation reaction may be progressive. Early consultation with plastic surgeon may be advisable.
• If vein streaking occurs, slow administration rate. If welts occur, stop administration and notify prescriber.
• Refrigerated, reconstituted solution is stable for 48 hours; at room temperature, it's stable for 24 hours.
⊗ **Incompatibilities**
Allopurinol, aluminum, aminophylline, bacteriostatic diluents, cefepime, cephalothin, dexamethasone sodium phosphate, diazepam, fluorouracil, furosemide, ganciclovir, heparin sodium, hydrocortisone sodium succinate, piperacillin with tazobactam

Contraindications and cautions

• Contraindicated in patients with marked myelosuppression induced by previous therapy with other antitumor drugs or radiotherapy and in those who have received lifetime cumulative dosage of 550 mg/m².
⚘ **Lifespan:** In pregnant and breast-feeding women, drug isn't recommended. In children, safety and effectiveness haven't been established.

Adverse reactions

CV: *arrhythmias;* cardiac depression, seen in ECG changes, such as sinus tachycardia, T-wave flattening, ST-segment depression, voltage reduction; *irreversible cardiomyopathy.*
EENT: conjunctivitis.
GI: anorexia, diarrhea, esophagitis, *nausea, stomatitis, vomiting.*
GU: transient red urine.
Hematologic: *leukopenia* during days 10 through 15, with recovery by day 21; MYELO-SUPPRESSION; *thrombocytopenia.*
Skin: *complete alopecia;* facial flushing; *hyperpigmentation of nails, dermal creases,* or skin (especially in previously irradiated areas); urticaria.
Other: *anaphylaxis,* hyperuricemia, severe cellulitis or tissue sloughing if drug extravasates.

Interactions

Drug-drug. *Calcium channel blockers:* May potentiate cardiotoxic effects. Monitor patient closely.
Digoxin: May decrease digoxin level. Monitor patient closely.
Paclitaxel: May decrease doxorubicin clearance. Monitor patient for toxicity.
Phenobarbital: May increase doxorubicin clearance. Monitor patient closely.
Phenytoin: May decrease phenytoin level. Check level.
Streptozocin: May increase and prolong blood level of doxorubicin HCl. Dosage may need adjustment.
Drug-herb. *Green tea:* May enhance antitumor effects of drug. Urge patient to discuss with prescriber before using together.

Effects on lab test results

• May increase bilirubin, uric acid, and glucose levels. May decrease calcium and hemoglobin levels and hematocrit.
• May decrease WBC, neutrophil, and platelet counts.

Pharmacokinetics

Absorption: Given I.V.
Distribution: Wide; doesn't cross blood–brain barrier.
Metabolism: Extensive, by hepatic microsomal enzymes to several metabolites, one of which has cytotoxic activity.

Excretion: Mainly in bile, minimally in urine.
Half-life: Initial, 30 minutes; terminal,
16½ hours.

Route	Onset	Peak	Duration
I.V.	Unknown	Unknown	Unknown

Action

Chemical effect: May interfere with DNA-
dependent RNA synthesis by intercalation.
Therapeutic effect: Hinders or kills certain
cancer cells.

Available forms

Injection (preservative-free): 2 mg/ml
Powder for injection: 10-mg, 20-mg, 50-mg,
100-mg, 150-mg vials

NURSING PROCESS

🔖 Assessment

• Obtain history of patient's neoplastic dis-
order before therapy, and reassess regularly
thereafter.
• Assess ECG before therapy.
• Monitor CBC and liver function tests; monitor
ECG monthly during therapy.
• Be alert for adverse reactions and drug inter-
actions.
• Assess patient's and family's knowledge of
drug therapy.

🔲 Nursing diagnoses

• Ineffective health maintenance related to presence of neoplastic disease
• Decreased cardiac output related to drug-
induced cardiotoxicity
• Deficient knowledge related to drug therapy

⬗ Planning and implementation

• To reduce nausea, premedicate with antiemetic.
• If skin or mucosal contact occurs, immediately wash area with soap and water.
• In case of leak or spill, inactivate drug with
5% sodium hypochlorite solution (household
bleach).
• Never give drug I.M. or subcutaneously.
• If tachycardia develops, stop giving the drug
or slow infusion rate, and notify the prescriber.
• If signs of heart failure develop, stop drug immediately and notify prescriber. Limit cumulative dose to 550 mg/m² (400 mg/m² when pa-

tient also receives or has received cyclophosphamide or radiation therapy to cardiac area) to
prevent heart failure.
• Alternate dosage schedule (once weekly) to
lower the risk of cardiomyopathy.
• Provide adequate hydration. Alkalinizing
urine or giving allopurinol may prevent or minimize uric acid nephropathy.
• Report adverse reactions to prescriber and
provide supportive care.
⚠ **ALERT:** Avoid confusing doxorubicin and
daunorubicin. Red color is similar.
⚠ **ALERT:** Liposomal doxorubicin and conventional doxorubicin aren't interchangeable.
Clearance of liposomal form is significantly less
than with the conventional form. Decrease liposomal doxorubicin dose.
Patient teaching
• Warn patient to watch for signs of infection
(fever, sore throat, fatigue) and bleeding (easy
bruising, nosebleed, bleeding gums, melena).
Have patient take temperature daily.
• Advise patient that orange to red urine for 1 to
2 days is normal and doesn't indicate presence
of blood in urine.
• Tell patient that total alopecia may occur
within 3 to 4 weeks. Hair may regrow 2 to
5 months after drug is stopped.
• Instruct patient to report symptoms of heart
failure and other cardiac signs and symptoms
promptly to prescriber.
• Tell patient to use safety precautions to prevent injury.

☑ Evaluation

• Patient exhibits positive response to therapy,
as noted on improved follow-up studies.
• Patient maintains adequate cardiac output
throughout therapy.
• Patient and family state understanding of drug
therapy.

doxorubicin hydrochloride liposomal
(doks-oh-ROO-bih-sin high-droh-KLOR-ighd ly-puh-SOE-mull)
Doxil

Pharmacologic class: anthracycline antibiotic
Therapeutic class: antineoplastic
Pregnancy risk category: D

Indications and dosages

▶ **Metastatic ovarian cancer in women with disease refractory to paclitaxel- and platinum-based chemotherapy regimens.** *Women:* 50 mg/m² (doxorubicin hydrochloride equivalent) I.V. at an initial infusion rate of 1 mg/minute once q 4 weeks for at least 4 courses. Continue as long as patient doesn't progress, shows no evidence of cardiotoxicity, and continues to tolerate treatment. If no infusion-related adverse events occur, increase infusion rate to complete administration over 1 hour.

▶ **AIDS-related Kaposi's sarcoma in patients with disease that has progressed with previous combination chemotherapy or in patients who are intolerant to such therapy.** *Adults:* 20 mg/m² (doxorubicin hydrochloride equivalent) I.V. over 30 minutes, once q 3 weeks, for as long as patient responds satisfactorily and tolerates therapy.

⎕ **Adjust-a-dose:** For patients with impaired hepatic function, if bilirubin level is 1.2 to 3 mg/dl, give one-fourth of the normal dose; if bilirubin level is more than 3 mg/dl, give one-half of the normal dose. Consult package insert for dose modifications for hand-foot syndrome, hematologic toxicity, and stomatitis.

▽ I.V. administration

• Follow facility procedures for proper handling and disposal of antineoplastics.
• Dilute dose (maximum, 90 mg) in 250 ml of D₅W using aseptic technique.
• Carefully check label on the I.V. bag before giving drug. Accidentally substituting Doxil for conventional doxorubicin hydrochloride can cause severe adverse effects.
• Infuse I.V. over 30 to 60 minutes, depending on the dose. Don't use with in-line filters.

• Monitor patient carefully during infusion. Flushing, shortness of breath, facial swelling, headache, chills, back pain, tightness in the chest or throat, or hypotension may occur. These reactions resolve over several hours to a day once the infusion is stopped; they may also resolve by slowing the infusion rate.
• If extravasation occurs, stop infusion immediately and restart in another vein. Applying ice over the extravasation site for about 30 minutes may help to alleviate the local reaction.
• Refrigerate diluted solution at 36° to 46° F (2° to 8° C), and give within 24 hours.
⊗ **Incompatibilities**
Other I.V. drugs

Contraindications and cautions

• Contraindicated in patients hypersensitive to the conventional form of doxorubicin hydrochloride or any component in the liposomal form. Also contraindicated in patients with marked myelosuppression or those who have received a lifetime cumulative dosage of 550 mg/m² (400 mg/m² if patient received radiotherapy to the mediastinal area or simultaneous therapy with other cardiotoxic drugs, such as cyclophosphamide).
• Use in patients with a history of CV disease only when the potential benefits of the drug outweigh the risks.
• Use cautiously in patients who have received another anthracycline.
⚖ **Lifespan:** In women of child-bearing age, avoid pregnancy during therapy; don't start drug if patient is pregnant. In breast-feeding women, use cautiously because it's unknown if it appears in breast milk. In children, safety and effectiveness haven't been established. In elderly patients, use cautiously because they may have greater sensitivity to the drug.

Adverse reactions

CNS: anxiety, *asthenia,* depression, dizziness, emotional lability, fatigue, fever, headache, insomnia, malaise, paresthesia, somnolence.
CV: *arrhythmias, cardiomyopathy,* chest pain, *heart failure,* hypotension, *pericardial effusion,* peripheral edema, tachycardia.
EENT: conjunctivitis, mouth ulceration, mucous membrane disorder, optic neuritis, pharyngitis, retinitis, rhinitis.
GI: abdominal pain, anorexia, constipation, diarrhea, dyspepsia, dysphagia, enlarged ab-

domen, esophagitis, glossitis, *nausea,* oral candidiasis, *stomatitis,* taste disturbance, vomiting.
GU: albuminuria.
Hematologic: *anemia, leukopenia,* NEUTROPENIA, THROMBOCYTOPENIA.
Hepatic: hyperbilirubinemia.
Metabolic: dehydration, hyperglycemia, hypocalcemia, weight loss.
Musculoskeletal: back pain, myalgia.
Respiratory: dyspnea, increased cough, pneumonia.
Skin: *alopecia,* dry skin, exfoliative dermatitis, hand-foot syndrome, herpes zoster, pruritus, *rash,* skin discoloration, skin disorder, sweating.
Other: *allergic reaction,* chills, *infection,* infusion-related reactions, *sepsis.*

Interactions

No drug interactions have been reported; however, doxorubicin hydrochloride liposomal may interact with drugs known to interact with the conventional form of doxorubicin hydrochloride.

Effects on lab test results

• May increase bilirubin and glucose levels. May decrease calcium and hemoglobin levels and hematocrit.
• May increase PT. May decrease WBC, neutrophil, and platelet counts.

Pharmacokinetics

Absorption: Given I.V.
Distribution: Mostly to vascular fluid.
Metabolism: Doxorubicinol, the major metabolite, is detected at very low levels.
Excretion: Slow, in two phases. *Half-life:* 5 hours in the first phase, 55 hours in the second phase with doses of 10 to 20 mg/m^2.

Route	Onset	Peak	Duration
I.V.	Unknown	Unknown	Unknown

Action

Chemical effect: Doxil is doxorubicin hydrochloride encapsulated in liposomes that, because of their small size and persistence in circulation, can penetrate the altered vasculature of tumors. The mechanism of action of doxorubicin hydrochloride is probably related to its ability to bind DNA and inhibit nucleic acid synthesis.

Therapeutic effect: Hinders or kills certain cancer cells in patients with ovarian cancer or AIDS-related Kaposi's sarcoma.

Available forms

Injection: 2 mg/ml

NURSING PROCESS

🕮 Assessment
• Obtain an accurate medication list from patient, including previous or current chemotherapeutic drugs.
• Evaluate patient's hepatic function before beginning therapy, and adjust dose accordingly.
• Monitor cardiac function closely by endomyocardial biopsy, echocardiography, or gated radionuclide scans. If results indicate that the patient may have cardiac injury, the benefit of continued therapy must be weighed against the risk of myocardial injury.
• Be alert for adverse reactions.
• Assess patient's and family's knowledge of drug therapy.

🔲 Nursing diagnoses
• Risk for infection related to myelosuppression
• Risk for injury related to drug-induced adverse reactions
• Deficient knowledge related to drug therapy

❯ Planning and implementation
• Don't give drug I.M. or subcutaneously.
⚠ **ALERT:** Don't substitute on a milligram-per-milligram basis with conventional doxorubicin hydrochloride.
• Drug may increase the toxicity of other antineoplastic therapies.
• Take into account any earlier or simultaneous therapy with related compounds, such as daunorubicin, when giving total dose. Heart failure and cardiomyopathy may occur after therapy stops.
• Monitor CBC, including platelets, before each dose and frequently throughout therapy. Leukopenia is usually transient. Hematologic toxicity may require dosage reduction or suspension or delay of therapy. Persistent severe myelosuppression may result in superinfection or hemorrhage. Patient may need granulocyte colony-stimulating factor (or granulocyte-macrophage colony-stimulating factor) to support blood counts.

Reactions may be *common,* uncommon, *life-threatening*, or COMMON AND LIFE-THREATENING.

Patient teaching

• Tell patient to notify prescriber about symptoms of hand-foot syndrome, such as tingling or burning, redness, flaking, bothersome swelling, small blisters, or small sores on the palms of hands or soles of feet.

• Advise patient to report symptoms of stomatitis, such as painful redness, swelling, or sores in the mouth.

• Advise patient to avoid exposure to people with infections. Tell patient to report fever of 100.5° F (38° C) or higher.

• Urge patient to report nausea, vomiting, tiredness, weakness, rash, or mild hair loss.

• Advise woman of childbearing age to avoid pregnancy during therapy.

☑ **Evaluation**

• Patient has no infection.

• Patient has no injury as a result of drug-induced adverse reactions.

• Patient and family state understanding of drug therapy.

doxycycline
(docks-ih-SYE-kleen)

doxycycline hyclate
Apo-Doxy♦, Doryx, Doxy-100, Doxy-200, Doxycin♦, Doxytec♦, Novo-♦oxylinl, Nu-Doxycycline♦, Periostat, Vibramycin, Vibra-Tabs

doxycycline hydrochloride◇
Doryx◇, Doxylin◇, Doxy Tablets◇, Vibramycin◇, Vibra-Tabs◇

doxycycline monohydrate
Adoxa, Monodox, Vibramycin

Pharmacologic class: tetracycline
Therapeutic class: antibiotic
Pregnancy risk category: D

Indications and dosages

▶ **Infections caused by sensitive gram-negative and gram-positive organisms, *Chlamydia*, *Mycoplasma*, *Rickettsia*, and organisms that cause trachoma.** *Adults and children weighing more than 45 kg (99 lb):* 100 mg P.O. q 12 hours on first day; then 100 mg P.O. daily. Or, 200 mg I.V. on first day in one or two infusions; then 100 to 200 mg I.V. daily. For severe infections, 100 mg P.O. q 12 hours may be used.

Children older than age 8 and weighing less than 45 kg: 4.4 mg/kg P.O. or I.V. daily in divided doses q 12 hours on first day, then 2.2 to 4.4 mg/kg daily.

▶ **Gonorrhea in patients allergic to penicillin.** *Adults:* 100 mg P.O. b.i.d. for 7 days. Or 300 mg P.O. initially; repeat dose in 1 hour.

▶ **Primary or secondary syphilis in patients allergic to penicillin.** *Adults and children older than age 8:* 100 mg P.O. b.i.d. for 2 weeks (early detection) or for 4 weeks (if more than 1 year's duration).

▶ **Uncomplicated urethral, endocervical, or rectal infection caused by *Chlamydia trachomatis* or *Ureaplasma urealyticum*.** *Adults:* 100 mg P.O. b.i.d. for at least 7 days.

▶ **To prevent malaria.** *Adults:* 100 mg P.O. daily.

Children older than age 8: 2 mg/kg P.O. once daily. Don't exceed adult dose. Begin 1 to 2 days before travel to malarious area and continue throughout travel and for 4 weeks thereafter.

▶ **Adjunct to scaling and root planing to promote attachment level gain and to reduce pocket depth in patients with adult periodontitis.** *Adults:* 20 mg Periostat P.O. b.i.d. more than 1 hour before or 2 hours after the morning and evening meals and after scaling and root planing. Effective for 9 months.

▶ **Adjunct to other antibiotics for inhalation, GI, and oropharyngeal anthrax.** *Adults:* 100 mg I.V. q 12 hours initially until susceptibility test results are known. Switch to 100 mg P.O. b.i.d. when appropriate. Treat for 60 days total.

Children older than age 8 and weighing more than 45 kg: 100 mg I.V. q 12 hours, then switch to 100 mg P.O. b.i.d. when appropriate. Treat for 60 days total.

Children older than age 8 and weighing 45 kg or less: 2.2 mg/kg I.V. q 12 hours, then switch to 2.2 mg/kg P.O. b.i.d. when appropriate. Treat for 60 days total.

Children age 8 and younger: 2.2 mg/kg I.V. q 12 hours, then switch to 2.2 mg/kg P.O. b.i.d. when appropriate. Treat for 60 days total.

D

▶ **Cutaneous anthrax.** *Adults:* 100 mg P.O. b.i.d. for 60 days.
Children older than age 8 and weighing more than 45 kg: 100 mg P.O. q 12 hours for 60 days.
Children older than age 8 and weighing 45 kg or less: 2.2 mg/kg P.O. q 12 hours for 60 days.
Children age 8 and younger: 2.2 mg/kg P.O. q 12 hours for 60 days.

▶ **Adjunct to severe acne.** *Adults:* 200 mg Adoxa P.O. on day 1 (give as 100 mg q 12 hours or 50 mg q 6 hours); follow with a maintenance dose of 100 mg P.O. daily, or 50 mg P.O. b.i.d.

▶ **To prevent traveler's diarrhea commonly caused by enterotoxigenic** *Escherichia coli*‡.
Adults: 100 mg P.O. daily for up to 3 days.

▶ **To prevent sexually transmitted diseases in rape victims**‡. *Adults and adolescents:* 100 mg Adoxa P.O. b.i.d. for 7 days after a single 2-g oral dose of metronidazole is given with a single 125-mg I.M. dose of ceftriaxone.

▶ **Lyme disease**‡. *Adults and children older than age 9:* 100 mg Adoxa P.O. b.i.d. or t.i.d. for 10 to 30 days.

▶ **Pleural effusions related to cancer**‡.
Adults: 500 mg of doxycycline diluted in 250 ml of normal saline solution and instilled into pleural space via chest tube.

▼ I.V. administration

● Reconstitute powder for injection with sterile water for injection. Use 10 ml in 100-mg vial and 20 ml in 200-mg vial. Dilute solution to 100 to 1,000 ml for I.V. infusion.
● Don't expose drug to light or heat. Protect it from sunlight during infusion.
● Don't infuse solutions that are more concentrated than 1 mg/ml.
● Depending on the dose, infusion lasts typically 1 to 4 hours. Complete infusion within 12 hours.
● Monitor I.V. infusion site for signs of thrombophlebitis.
● Monitor for infiltration or irritation.
● Reconstituted injectable solution is stable for 72 hours if refrigerated.
⊗ **Incompatibilities**
Allopurinol; drugs unstable in acidic solutions, such as barbiturates; erythromycin lactobionate; heparin; meropenem; nafcillin; penicillin G potassium; piperacillin with tazobactam; riboflavin; and sulfonamides.

Contraindications and cautions

● Contraindicated in patients hypersensitive to drug or other tetracyclines.
● Use cautiously in patients with impaired kidney or liver function.
⚖ **Lifespan:** In breast-feeding women, avoid using due to risk of adverse reactions in infant. Pregnant women, children younger than age 8, and immunocompromised patients may receive the usual dose and regimen for anthrax. In children younger than age 8 and in the fetus during last half of pregnancy, these drugs may cause permanent discoloration of teeth, enamel defects, and bone growth retardation. These effects are dose limited; therefore, drug may be used for a short time (7 to 14 days) if short courses are not repeated. In pregnant women, drug isn't recommended unless other options aren't available due to potential risk of bone growth retardation and neural tube defects.

Adverse reactions

CNS: intracranial hypertension (pseudotumor cerebri).
CV: pericarditis, thrombophlebitis.
EENT: dysphagia, glossitis.
GI: anogenital inflammation, anorexia, *diarrhea,* enterocolitis, *epigastric distress,* nausea, oral candidiasis, vomiting.
Hematologic: eosinophilia, hemolytic anemia, **neutropenia, thrombocytopenia.**
Musculoskeletal: bone growth retardation if used in children younger than age 8.
Skin: increased pigmentation, maculopapular and erythematous rash, photosensitivity, urticaria.
Other: *anaphylaxis,* enamel defects, hypersensitivity reactions, permanent discoloration of teeth, superinfection.

Interactions

Drug-drug. *Antacids (including sodium bicarbonate) and laxatives containing aluminum, magnesium, or calcium; antidiarrheals:* May decrease antibiotic absorption. Give antibiotic 1 hour before or 2 hours after these drugs.
Carbamazepine, phenobarbital: May decrease antibiotic effect. Avoid using together, if possible.
Ferrous sulfate and other iron products, zinc: May decrease antibiotic absorption. Give drug 3 hours after or 2 hours before iron.

Reactions may be *common,* uncommon, **life-threatening**, or COMMON AND LIFE-THREATENING.

Hormonal contraceptives: May decrease contraceptive effectiveness and increase risk of breakthrough bleeding. Recommend nonhormonal form of birth control.

Methoxyflurane: May cause nephrotoxicity with tetracyclines. Avoid using together.

Oral anticoagulants: May increase anticoagulant effect. Monitor PT and INR, and adjust dosage.

Penicillins: May interfere with bactericidal action of penicillins. Avoid using together.

Drug-lifestyle. *Alcohol use:* May decrease antibiotic effect. Avoid using together.

Sun exposure: May cause photosensitivity reactions. Urge patient to avoid unprotected and prolonged sun exposure.

Effects on lab test results

• May increase BUN and liver enzyme levels. May decrease hemoglobin level and hematocrit.

• May increase eosinophil count. May decrease platelet, neutrophil, and WBC counts.

• May cause false-negative reading of glucose oxidase reagent (Diastix or Chemstrip uG). May cause false-positive reading of copper sulfate tests (Clinitest) with parenteral form.

Pharmacokinetics

Absorption: 90% to 100%.

Distribution: Wide, but poor in CSF; 25% to 93% protein-bound.

Metabolism: Insignificant; some hepatic degradation occurs.

Excretion: Mainly unchanged in urine; some in feces. *Half-life:* About 1 day after multiple doses.

Route	Onset	Peak	Duration
P.O.	Unknown	1½–4 hr	Unknown
I.V.	Immediate	Unknown	Unknown

Action

Chemical effect: May exert bacteriostatic effect by binding to 30S ribosomal subunit of microorganisms, thus inhibiting protein synthesis.

Therapeutic effect: Hinders bacterial growth.

Available forms

doxycycline calcium
Syrup: 50 mg/5 ml
doxycycline hyclate
Capsules: 20 mg, 50 mg, 100 mg
Capsules (coated pellets): 75 mg, 100 mg

Injection: 100 mg, 200 mg
Tablets: 20 mg, 100 mg
doxycycline hydrochloride ◇
Capsules: 50 mg ◇, 100 mg ◇
Tablets: 50 mg ◇, 100 mg ◇
doxycycline monohydrate
Capsules: 50 mg, 100 mg
Oral suspension: 25 mg/5 ml
Tablets: 50 mg, 75 mg, 100 mg

NURSING PROCESS

Assessment

• Obtain history of patient's infection before therapy, and reassess regularly thereafter.

• Obtain specimen for culture and sensitivity tests before giving the first dose. Begin therapy pending test results.

• Be alert for adverse reactions and drug interactions.

• If patient has adverse GI reactions, monitor his hydration.

• Assess patient's and family's knowledge of drug therapy.

Nursing diagnoses

• Infection related to presence of susceptible bacteria

• Risk for deficient fluid volume related to drug-induced adverse GI reactions

• Deficient knowledge related to drug therapy

Planning and implementation

• Check expiration date. Outdated or deteriorated tetracyclines may cause reversible nephrotoxicity (Fanconi's syndrome).

• If drug causes adverse GI reaction, may give with milk or food.

• Follow current Centers for Disease Control and Prevention recommendations for anthrax.

• Ciprofloxacin and doxycycline are first-line therapy for anthrax; 500 mg amoxicillin P.O. t.i.d. for adults and 80 mg/kg/day divided q 8 hours for children is an option for completing therapy after improvement.

• Cutaneous anthrax with signs of systemic involvement, extensive edema, or lesions on the head or neck requires I.V. therapy and a multidrug approach.

• Additional antimicrobials for anthrax multidrug regimens can include rifampin, vancomycin, penicillin, ampicillin, chloramphenicol, imipenem, clindamycin, and clarithromycin.

• Steroids may be considered as adjunctive therapy for anthrax patients with severe edema and for meningitis, based on experience with bacterial meningitis of other etiologies.

• If meningitis is suspected, doxycycline would be less optimal because of poor CNS penetration.

• Notify prescriber of adverse reactions. Some adverse reactions, such as superinfection, may necessitate substitution of another antibiotic.

⚠ **ALERT:** Don't confuse doxycycline with doxylamine or dicyclomine.

Patient teaching

• Tell patient to take entire amount of medication exactly as prescribed, even after he feels better.

• Instruct patient to take oral drug with milk or food but not with antacids if adverse GI reaction develops. Tell patient to take drug no less than 1 hour before bedtime to prevent irritation from esophageal reflux.

• Advise parent giving drug to a child that tablets may be crushed and mixed with low-fat milk, low-fat chocolate milk, regular (whole) chocolate milk, chocolate pudding, or apple juice mixed with sugar in equal proportions. Store mixtures in refrigerator, except apple juice mixture (which can be stored at room temperature), and discard after 24 hours.

• Tell patient to use sunscreen and avoid strong sunlight during therapy to prevent photosensitivity reactions.

• Stress good oral hygiene.

• Tell patient to check expiration dates and to discard outdated doxycycline because it may become toxic.

• Advise patient taking hormonal contraceptive to use alternative means of contraception within 1 week of therapy.

☑ **Evaluation**

• Patient is free from infection.

• Patient maintains adequate hydration throughout therapy.

• Patient and family state understanding of drug therapy.

dronabinol
(delta-9-tetrahydrocannabinol)
(droh-NAB-eh-nohl)
Marinol

Pharmacologic class: cannabinoid
Therapeutic class: antiemetic, appetite stimulant
Pregnancy risk category: C
Controlled substance schedule: III

Indications and dosages

▶ **Nausea and vomiting from chemotherapy.**
Adults: 5 mg/m^2 P.O. 1 to 3 hours before administration of chemotherapy. Then same dose q 2 to 4 hours after chemotherapy for total of four to six doses daily. If needed, increase dosage in increments of 2.5 mg/m^2 to maximum dose, 15 mg/m^2.

▶ **Anorexia and weight loss in patients with AIDS.** *Adults:* 2.5 mg P.O. b.i.d. before lunch and dinner, increase p.r.n. to maximum, 20 mg daily.

Contraindications and cautions

• Contraindicated in patients hypersensitive to sesame oil or cannabinoids.

• Use cautiously in patients with heart disease, psychiatric illness, or history of drug abuse.

⚘ **Lifespan:** In breast-feeding women, drug isn't recommended. In children, safety and effectiveness haven't been established. In elderly patients, use cautiously.

Adverse reactions

CNS: amnesia, asthenia, ataxia, confusion, depersonalization, disorientation, *dizziness, drowsiness, euphoria,* hallucinations, headache, muddled thinking, *paranoia, somnolence.*
CV: orthostatic hypotension, palpitations, tachycardia, vasodilation.
EENT: visual disturbances.
GI: abdominal pain, diarrhea, dry mouth, nausea, vomiting.

Interactions

Drug-drug. *CNS depressants, psychotomimetic substances, sedatives:* May have additive effects. Avoid using together.
Drug-lifestyle. *Alcohol use:* May have additive effects. Discourage using together.

Reactions may be *common,* uncommon, *life-threatening*, or COMMON AND LIFE-THREATENING.

Effects on lab test results
None reported.

Pharmacokinetics
Absorption: 95%.
Distribution: Rapid; 97% to 99% protein-bound.
Metabolism: Extensive.
Excretion: Mainly in feces. *Half-life:* 1 to 1½ days.

Route	Onset	Peak	Duration
P.O.	Unknown	2–4 hr	4–6 hr

Action
Chemical effect: Unknown.
Therapeutic effect: Relieves nausea and vomiting caused by chemotherapy and stimulates appetite.

Available forms
Capsules: 2.5 mg, 5 mg, 10 mg

NURSING PROCESS

🔁 Assessment
• Obtain history of patient's underlying condition before therapy.
• Monitor the drug's effectiveness by assessing for nausea, vomiting, or weight gain. Drug effects may persist for days after therapy ends.
• Be alert for adverse reactions and drug interactions.
• Monitor patient for dependence. Dronabinol is the principal active substance in *Cannabis sativa* (marijuana). It can produce physical and psychological dependence and has high potential for abuse.
• Monitor patient's hydration, weight, and nutrition regularly.
• Assess patient's and family's knowledge of drug therapy.

🔲 Nursing diagnoses
• Risk for deficient fluid volume related to nausea and vomiting from chemotherapy
• Disturbed thought processes related to drug-induced adverse CNS reactions
• Deficient knowledge related to drug therapy

▷ Planning and implementation
• Give drug only to patients who haven't responded satisfactorily to other antiemetics.

• Give drug 1 to 3 hours before chemotherapy starts and again 2 to 4 hours after chemotherapy.
Patient teaching
• Inform patient that drug may cause unusual changes in mood or other adverse behavioral effects.
• Caution patient to avoid hazardous activities until the drug's CNS effects are known.
• Warn family members to make sure patient is supervised by a responsible person during and immediately after therapy.

🔳 Evaluation
• Patient maintains adequate hydration.
• Patient regains normal thought processes after effects of drug therapy have dissipated.
• Patient and family state understanding of drug therapy.

drotrecogin alfa (activated)
(droh-truh-KO-jin AL-fah)
Xigris

Pharmacologic class: recombinant protease of human activated protein C
Therapeutic class: antithrombotic
Pregnancy risk category: C

Indications and dosages
▶ **Reduction of mortality in patients with severe sepsis (sepsis from acute organ dysfunction).** *Adults:* 24 mcg/kg/hour I.V. infusion for a total of 96 hours.

▼ I.V. administration
• Reconstitute 5-mg vials with 2.5 ml sterile water for injection, USP, and 20-mg vials with 10 ml of sterile water for injection, USP. The resulting concentration is 2 mg/ml. Gently swirl each vial until powder is completely dissolved; avoid inverting or shaking the vial.
• If the reconstituted vial isn't used immediately, it may be held at controlled room temperature of 59° to 86° F (15° to 30° C) for up to 3 hours, or stored in a refrigerator at 36° to 46° F (2° to 8° C).
• Further dilute the reconstituted solution with sterile normal saline injection. Withdraw appropriate amount of reconstituted drug into a prepared infusion bag of sterile normal saline solution. When adding the drug, direct the stream to

the side of the bag to minimize agitation of the solution.
• Gently invert the infusion bag to obtain a homogenous solution. Don't transport the infusion bag between locations using mechanical delivery systems.
• Inspect for particulate matter and discoloration before giving.
• Give drug within 12 hours of preparing solution for infusion. Don't freeze. Avoid heat and direct sunlight.
• For an I.V. pump, the solution of reconstituted drug is typically diluted into an infusion bag containing sterile normal saline solution to a final concentration between 100 mcg/ml and 200 mcg/ml.
• For a syringe pump, the reconstituted solution is typically diluted with sterile normal saline solution to a final concentration between 100 mcg/ml and 1,000 mcg/ml. When giving less than 200 mcg/ml at less than 5 ml/hour, the infusion set must be primed for about 15 minutes at a flow rate of about 5 ml/hour.
• Give via a dedicated I.V. line or lumen of a multilumen central venous catheter. The only other solutions that can be given through the same line are normal saline solution, lactated Ringer's injection, dextrose, or dextrose and saline mixtures.
⊗ **Incompatibilities**
Other I.V. drugs.

Contraindications and cautions

• Contraindicated in patients with active internal bleeding, hemorrhagic stroke within 3 months, intracranial or intraspinal surgery within 2 months, severe head trauma, trauma with an increased risk of life-threatening bleeding, an epidural catheter, intracranial neoplasm or mass lesion, or evidence of cerebral herniation. Drug is also contraindicated in patients hypersensitive to drotrecogin alfa (activated) or any of its components.
• Use cautiously in patients with a high risk of bleeding, such as those who are taking heparin (15 units/kg/hour or more); those with a platelet count of less than $30,000 \times 10^6$/L (even if the platelet count increases after transfusions), those with an INR greater than 3; those who have experienced GI bleeding within 6 weeks; those who have had thrombolytic therapy within 3 days; those who have been given oral anticoagulants, glycoprotein IIb/IIIa inhibitors, aspirin

(more than 650 mg/day) or other platelet inhibitors within 7 days; those who have had ischemic stroke within 3 months; those who have had intracranial arteriovenous malformation or aneurysm, bleeding diathesis, chronic severe hepatic disease, or any other condition in which bleeding constitutes a significant hazard or would be particularly difficult to manage because of its location.
• Use only after careful consideration of the risk versus benefit in patients with single organ dysfunction and recent surgery as they may not be at a high risk of death.
⚠ **Lifespan:** In pregnant women, drug should be used only if benefit to patient exceeds risk to the fetus. Breast-feeding women should stop nursing or stop taking the drug because it's unknown whether drug appears in breast milk. In children, safety and effectiveness haven't been established.

Adverse reactions

Hematologic: HEMORRHAGE.

Interactions

Drug-drug. *Drugs that affect hemostasis:* May increase risk of bleeding. Use together cautiously; monitor patient for bleeding.

Effects on lab test results

• May increase APTT and PT.
• May interfere with one-stage coagulation assays based on APTT (such as factors VIII, IX, and XI assays), causing inconclusive results.

Pharmacokinetics

Absorption: Given I.V.
Distribution: Steady-state levels within 2 hours.
Metabolism: Unknown.
Excretion: Unknown. *Half-life:* Unknown.

Route	Onset	Peak	Duration
I.V.	Rapid	Unknown	Unknown

Action

Chemical effect: Inhibits monocytes from producing human tumor necrosis factor, by blocking leukocyte from adhering to selectins, and by limiting the thrombin-induced inflammatory response.
Therapeutic effect: Prevents clots and blocks cell death.

Available forms

Injection: 5 mg; 20 mg

⚖ Assessment

• Assess patient before starting and during drug therapy for risk of bleeding or contraindications.
• Monitor patient closely for bleeding. If significant bleeding occurs, immediately stop the infusion.
• Because drug may prolong APTT, it can't be used to reliably assess the condition of the coagulopathy during infusion. Because drug has minimal effect on PT, PT can be used instead.

⊞ Nursing diagnoses

• Risk for injury caused by increased bleeding potential related to drug therapy.
• Deficient knowledge related to drug therapy.

≫ Planning and implementation

• If the infusion is interrupted, restart at the baseline 24-mcg/kg/hour infusion rate. Dose escalation, bolus doses, and dose adjustment based on observation or laboratory parameters aren't recommended.
• Stop drug 2 hours before an invasive surgical procedure with a risk of bleeding. After hemostasis is reached, drug may be restarted 12 hours after major invasive procedures or surgery or immediately after uncomplicated, less-invasive procedures.

Patient teaching

• Inform patient of potential adverse reactions.
• Instruct patient to report signs of bleeding promptly.
• Advise patient that bleeding may occur for up to 28 days after therapy.

☑ Evaluation

• Patient doesn't experience any hemorrhaging during and 28 days after drug therapy.
• Patient and family state understanding of drug therapy.

duloxetine hydrochloride

(dull-OX-uh-teen high-droh-KLOR-idgh)
Cymbalta✒

D

Pharmacologic class: selective serotonin and norepinephrine reuptake inhibitor
Therapeutic class: antidepressant, central pain inhibitor
Pregnancy risk category: C

Indications and dosages

▶ **Major depressive disorder.** *Adults:* Initially, 20 mg P.O. bid to 60 mg P.O. once daily or in two divided doses. Maximum, 60 mg daily.
▶ **Neuropathic pain from diabetic peripheral neuropathy.** *Adults:* 60 mg P.O. once daily.
⧄ **Adjust-a-dose:** Patients with renal impairment may need a lower initial dose and gradual dose increases.

Contraindications and cautions

• Contraindicated in patients hypersensitive to drug or its ingredients, those taking MAO inhibitors, and those with uncontrolled narrow angle-closure glaucoma or a creatinine clearance less than 30 ml/minute. Drug isn't recommended for patients with hepatic dysfunction, or end-stage renal disease or those who drink substantial amounts of alcohol.
• Use cautiously in patients with a history of mania or seizures and those with hypertension, controlled narrow angle-closure glaucoma, or conditions that slow gastric emptying.
☝ **Lifespan:** In pregnant women, use during third trimester may cause complications for the neonate, including respiratory distress, cyanosis, apnea, seizures, vomiting, hypoglycemia, and hyperreflexia, that may require prolonged hospitalization, respiratory support, and tube feeding. Weigh potential benefit for the mother versus risks to the fetus. Breast-feeding women shouldn't use. Safety and effectiveness in children haven't been established.

Adverse reactions

CNS: anxiety, asthenia, *dizziness, fatigue,* fever, *headache,* hypoesthesia, initial insomnia, *insomnia,* irritability, lethargy, nervousness, nightmares, restlessness, sleep disorder, *somnolence, suicidal ideation,* tremor.

CV: hot flushes, hypertension, increased heart rate.
EENT: blurred vision, nasopharyngitis, pharyngolaryngeal pain.
GI: *constipation, diarrhea, dry mouth,* dyspepsia, gastritis, nausea, vomiting.
GU: abnormal orgasm, abnormally increased frequency of urination, delayed or dysfunctional ejaculation, dysuria, erectile dysfunction, urinary hesitancy.
Metabolic: *decreased appetite, hypoglycemia,* increased appetite, weight gain or loss.
Musculoskeletal: muscle cramps, myalgia.
Respiratory: cough.
Skin: increased sweating, night sweats, pruritus, rash.
Other: decreased libido, rigors.

Interactions

Drug-drug. *CNS drugs:* May increase adverse effects. Use cautiously together.
CYP 1A2 inhibitors (cimetidine, fluvoxamine, certain quinolones): May increase duloxetine level. Avoid use together.
CYP 2D6 inhibitors (fluoxetine, paroxetine, quinidine): May increase duloxetine level. Use together cautiously.
Drugs that reduce gastric acidity: May cause premature breakdown of duloxetine's protective coating and early release of the drug. Monitor patient for effects.
MAO inhibitors: May cause hyperthermia, rigidity, myoclonus, autonomic instability, rapid fluctuations of vital signs, agitation, and eventually, delirium and coma. Wait at least 14 days after stopping an MAO inhibitor before starting duloxetine; wait at least 5 days after stopping duloxetine before starting an MAO inhibitor.
Thioridazine: May prolong the QT interval and increase the risk of serious ventricular arrhythmias and sudden death. Avoid use together.
Tricyclic antidepressants (amitriptyline, nortriptyline, imipramine): May increase levels of these drugs. Tricyclic antidepressant dose may need to be reduced and levels monitored closely.
Type 1C antiarrhythmics (flecainide, propafenone), phenothiazines (except thioridazine): May increase levels of these drugs. Use cautiously together.
Drug-lifestyle. *Alcohol use:* May increase the risk of liver damage. Discourage alcohol use.

Effects on lab test results

● May increase alkaline phosphatase, ALT, AST, bilirubin, and CK levels.

Pharmacokinetics

Absorption: Compared with the morning dose, the evening dose has a 3-hour delay in absorption and a one-third increase in clearance.
Distribution: More than 90% protein-bound to albumin and alpha$_1$-acid glycoprotein.
Metabolism: Numerous metabolites by the liver via CYP 2D6 and 1A2.
Excretion: 70% in urine and 20% in feces as metabolites. *Half-life:* 12 hours.

Route	Onset	Peak	Duration
P.O.	Unknown	6 hr	Unknown

Action

Chemical effect: May inhibit serotonin and norepinephrine reuptake in the CNS.
Therapeutic effect: Relieves depression. Relieves neuropathic pain in patients with diabetic peripheral neuropathy.

Available forms

Capsules (delayed-release): 20 mg, 30 mg, 60 mg

NURSING PROCESS

⚖ Assessment
● Monitor patient for worsening depression or suicidal behavior, especially during dosage initiation or changes.
● Monitor blood pressure periodically during therapy.
● Reassess patient periodically to determine whether therapy needs to continue.
● Assess patient's and family's knowledge of drug therapy.

🔁 Nursing diagnoses
● Disturbed thought processes related to presence of depression
● Chronic pain related to underlying disease process and neuropathic pain
● Deficient knowledge related to drug therapy

➤ Planning and implementation
● Monitor older patient for increased effect, and adjust dosage. Old and young adults respond

---

similarly, but older patients may be more sensitive to drug effects.
• Decrease dosage gradually, and watch for symptoms such as dizziness, nausea, headache, *previous dose and decrease even more gradually.

Patient teaching
⚠ **ALERT:** Warn families or caregivers to report signs of worsening depression (such as agitation, irritability, insomnia, hostility, impulsivity) and signs of suicidal behavior to prescriber immediately.
• Tell patient to consult his prescriber or pharmacist if he plans to take other prescription or OTC drugs or an herbal or other dietary supplement.
• Instruct patient to swallow capsules whole and not to chew, crush, or open them because they have an enteric coating.
• Urge patient to avoid activities that are hazardous or require mental alertness until he knows the drug's effects.
• Warn against drinking substantial amounts of alcohol due to risk of severe liver toxicity.
• If patient takes drug for depression, explain that it may take 1 to 4 weeks to take effect.

☑ Evaluation
• Patient's behavior and communication indicate improved thought processes.
• Patient reports decreased pain.
• Patient and family state understanding of drug therapy.

---

dutasteride
(doo-TAS-teer-ighd)
Avodart

Pharmacologic class: 5-alpha-reductase enzyme inhibitor
Therapeutic class: BPH drug
Pregnancy risk category: X

Indications and dosages
▶ **BPH.** *Men:* 0.5 mg P.O. once daily.

Contraindications and cautions
• Contraindicated in patients hypersensitive to drug, its components, or other 5-alpha-reductase inhibitors.

• Use cautiously in patients with hepatic disease and in those taking long-term potent CYP 3A4 inhibitors.
⚠ **Lifespan:** In pregnant and breast-feeding women and in children, drug is contraindicated. It's unknown if drug appears in breast milk.

Adverse reactions
GU: decreased libido, ejaculation disorder, impotence.
Other: gynecomastia.

Interactions
Drug-drug. *CYP 3A4 inhibitors (cimetidine, diltiazem, itraconazole, ketoconazole, macrolide antibiotics, protease inhibitors, ritonavir, verapamil):* May increase dutasteride level. Use together cautiously.

Effects on lab test results
• May decrease prostate-specific antigen (PSA) level.

Pharmacokinetics
Absorption: Bioavailability of about 60%.
Distribution: 99% bound to albumin and 96.6% bound to alpha$_1$-acid glycoprotein.
Metabolism: Extensive, by CYP 3A4.
Excretion: Mainly in feces, 5% unchanged and 40% as metabolites, trace amounts in urine.
Half-life: 5 weeks.

Route	Onset	Peak	Duration
P.O.	Unknown	2–3 hr	Unknown

Action
Chemical effect: Inhibits conversion of testosterone to dihydrotestosterone, the androgen mainly responsible for initial development and later enlargement of the prostate gland.
Therapeutic effect: Resolves BPH.

Available forms
Capsules: 0.5 mg

NURSING PROCESS

☲ Assessment
• Before therapy, assess patient to rule out other urologic diseases.

• Carefully monitor patients with a large residual urine volume, severely diminished urine flow, or both, for obstructive uropathy.
• Perform digital rectal examinations and other evaluations for prostate cancer on patients with BPH before starting therapy, and reassess periodically thereafter.
• Be alert for adverse effects.
• Assess patient's and family's knowledge of drug therapy.

✪ Nursing diagnoses
• Impaired urinary elimination related to underlying condition
• Sexual dysfunction related to adverse effects of medication
• Deficient knowledge related to drug therapy

❯ Planning and implementation
• Because drug may be absorbed through the skin, don't allow women who are or may become pregnant to handle the drug.
• If capsule leaks onto skin, wash the area immediately with soap and water.
• Patient shouldn't donate blood within 6 months of last dose.
• Establish new baseline PSA level in men treated for 3 to 6 months, and use it to assess potentially cancer-related changes in PSA level.
• To interpret PSA level in men treated for 6 months or more, double the PSA level for comparison with normal levels in untreated men.
Patient teaching
• Tell patient to swallow the capsule whole and to take with or without food.
• Inform patient that ejaculate volume may decrease, but sexual function will remain normal.
• Tell patient that pregnant women shouldn't handle drug. A boy born to a woman who was exposed to the drug during pregnancy may have abnormal sex organs.
• Tell patient not to donate blood within 6 months of his final dose.

☑ Evaluation
• Patient has normal urinary flow without urinary residual volume.
• Patient doesn't experience adverse effects.
• Patient and family state understanding of drug therapy.

edetate calcium disodium
(calcium EDTA)
(ED-eh-tayt KAL-see-um digh-SOH-dee-um)
Calcium Disodium Versenate

Pharmacologic class: chelating drug
Therapeutic class: heavy metal antagonist
Pregnancy risk category: B

Indications and dosages

▶ **Acute lead encephalopathy or lead levels above 70 mcg/dl.** *Adults and children:* 1.5 g/m^2 I.V. or I.M. daily in divided doses at 12-hour intervals for 3 to 5 days, usually with dimercaprol. Give a second course in 5 to 7 days.
▶ **Lead poisoning without encephalopathy, or asymptomatic patient with lead levels between 20 mcg/dl and 70 mcg/dl.** *Children:* 1 g/m^2 I.V. or I.M. daily in divided doses for 5 days. Give second course after 2 to 4 days, as needed.
◪ **Adjust-a-dose:** In patients with lead nephropathy, decrease dosage and frequency as follows: for serum creatinine level of 2 to 3 mg/dl, give 500 mg/m^2/day for 5 days; for serum creatinine level of 3 to 4 mg/dl, give 500 mg/m^2/day q 48 hours for three doses; for serum creatinine level greater than 4 mg/dl, give 500 mg/m^2 once weekly.

▽ I.V. administration

• I.V. use may increase intracranial pressure. To treat lead encephalopathy, give by I.M. route instead.
• Dilute drug with 250 to 500 ml of D_5W or normal saline injection.
• Infuse half of daily dose over 1 hour in asymptomatic patients or over 2 hours in symptomatic patients. Give rest of infusion at least 6 hours later. Or give by slow infusion over 4 to 24 hours.
⊗ **Incompatibilities**
Amphotericin B, dextrose 10% in water, hydralazine hydrochloride, invert sugar 10% in normal saline solution, invert sugar 10% in

water, lactated Ringer's solution, Ringer's injection, 1/6 M sodium lactate.

Contraindications and cautions

• Contraindicated in patients with anuria, acute renal disease, or hepatitis.
• Use cautiously in patients with mild renal disease. Reduce dosages.
⚖ **Lifespan:** In pregnant and breast-feeding women, use cautiously.

Adverse reactions

CNS: sudden fever, headache, paresthesia, numbness, fatigue.
CV: *arrhythmias,* hypotension.
EENT: sneezing and nasal congestion.
GI: anorexia, nausea, vomiting.
GU: proteinuria, hematuria, *nephrotoxicity.*
Metabolic: hypercalcemia, zinc deficiency.
Musculoskeletal: arthralgia, myalgia.
Other: chills, excessive thirst.

Interactions

Drug-drug. *Zinc insulin:* May interfere with action of insulin by binding with zinc. Monitor patient closely.
Zinc supplements: May decrease effectiveness of edetate calcium disodium and zinc supplements because of chelation. Withhold zinc supplements until therapy is complete.

Effects on lab test results

• May increase AST, ALT, and calcium levels. May decrease zinc and hemoglobin levels and hematocrit.

Pharmacokinetics

Absorption: Well absorbed after I.M. administration.
Distribution: Primarily in extracellular fluid.
Metabolism: None.
Excretion: In urine. *Half-life:* 20 minutes to 1¼ hours.

Route	Onset	Peak	Duration
I.V., I.M.	1 hr	1–2 days	Unknown

Action

Chemical effect: Forms stable, soluble complexes with metals, particularly lead.
Therapeutic effect: Abolishes effects of lead poisoning.

Available forms

Injection: 200 mg/ml

NURSING PROCESS

☡ Assessment

• Obtain history of patient's underlying condition before therapy.
• Monitor the drug's effectiveness by checking lead level and observing for decreasing signs and symptoms of lead poisoning.
• Monitor fluid intake and output; conduct urinalysis, BUN, and ECG daily.
• Be alert for adverse reactions.
• Assess patient's and family's knowledge of drug therapy.

✤ Nursing diagnoses

• Risk for injury related to lead poisoning
• Ineffective renal tissue perfusion related to drug-induced fatal nephrosis
• Deficient knowledge related to drug therapy

▷ Planning and implementation

• When giving I.M., add procaine hydrochloride to I.M. solution to minimize pain. Watch for local reactions.
• Use I.M. route for children and patients with lead encephalopathy.
• Force fluids to facilitate lead excretion, except in patients with lead encephalopathy.
• To avoid toxicity, use with dimercaprol.
• Apply ice or cold compresses to injection site to ease local reaction.
Ⓢ **ALERT:** Don't confuse edetate calcium disodium with edetate disodium, which is used to treat hypercalcemia.
Patient teaching
• Warn patient that some adverse reactions, such as fever, chills, thirst, and nasal congestion, may occur 4 to 8 hours after use.
• Encourage patient and family to identify and remove source of lead in home.

☑ Evaluation

• Patient sustains no injury as a result of lead poisoning.
• Patient has no signs of altered renal tissue perfusion.
• Patient and family state understanding of drug therapy.

edetate disodium
(ED-eh-tayt digh-SOH-dee-um)
Disodium EDTA, Endrate, Sodium Edetate

Pharmacologic class: chelating drug
Therapeutic class: heavy metal antagonist
Pregnancy risk category: C

Indications and dosages
▶ **Hypercalcemic crisis.** *Adults:* 50 mg/kg/day by slow I.V. infusion for 5 days; no drug for 2 days; then repeat course, as needed. Maximum, 3 g I.V. daily and 15 doses total. *Children:* 40 to 70 mg/kg/day by slow I.V. infusion. Maximum, 70 mg/kg I.V. daily.
▶ **Digoxin-induced arrhythmias.** *Adults and children:* 15 mg/kg/hour I.V. daily. Maximum, 60 mg/kg I.V. daily.

▼ I.V. administration
• Drug isn't recommended for direct or intermittent injection.
• Keep I.V. calcium available to treat hypocalcemia.
• Dilute before use. For adults, add dose to 500 ml of D_5W or normal saline solution and give over 3 or more hours. For children, dilute to maximum of 30 mg/ml in D_5W or normal saline solution and give over 3 or more hours.
• Don't exceed recommended dose or rate of administration.
• Avoid rapid I.V. infusion, which may result in profound hypocalcemia and lead to tetany, seizures, arrhythmias, and respiratory arrest.
• Extravasation can cause tissue damage and necrosis; watch for irritation and infiltration.
• Record I.V. site used and avoid repeated use of same site to decrease likelihood of thrombophlebitis.
• Keep patient in bed for 15 minutes after infusion to avoid orthostatic hypotension.
⊗ **Incompatibilities**
None reported.

Contraindications and cautions
• Contraindicated in patients hypersensitive to the drug or any of its components and in those with anuria, known or suspected hypocalcemia, significant renal disease, active or healed tubercular lesions, or a history of seizures or intracranial lesions.

• Use cautiously in patients with limited cardiac reserve, heart failure, or hypokalemia.
❉ **Lifespan:** In pregnant and breast-feeding women, use cautiously.

Adverse reactions
CNS: circumoral paresthesia, numbness, headache.
CV: hypertension, thrombophlebitis, orthostatic hypotension.
GI: nausea, vomiting, diarrhea, anorexia, abdominal cramps.
GU: *nephrotoxicity,* urinary urgency, nocturia, dysuria, polyuria, proteinuria, renal insufficiency, *renal failure, tubular necrosis.*
Metabolic: hypocalcemia, *hypomagnesia.*
Skin: dermatitis, erythema.
Other: infusion site pain.

Interactions
Drug-drug. *Digoxin:* Drop in calcium caused by edetate disodium may reverse effects of digoxin overdose. Monitor patient closely for renewed digoxin toxicity if hypercalcemia recurs.
Zinc insulins: May decrease glucose and chelate zinc in some insulin. Dosage adjustments of insulin may be required.

Effects on lab test results
• May increase uric acid level. May decrease calcium, magnesium, potassium, zinc, and hemoglobin levels and hematocrit.

Pharmacokinetics
Absorption: Administered I.V.
Distribution: Distributed widely throughout body but doesn't enter CSF in significant amounts.
Metabolism: None.
Excretion: In urine. *Half-life:* Unknown.

Route	Onset	Peak	Duration
I.V.	Unknown	Unknown	Unknown

Action
Chemical effect: Chelates with metals, such as calcium, to form stable, soluble complex.
Therapeutic effect: Lowers calcium level and stabilizes heart rhythm in emergency conditions.

Available forms
Injection: 150 mg/ml

NURSING PROCESS

🕮 Assessment

• Obtain history of patient's calcium level before therapy.
• Monitor drug's effectiveness by obtaining calcium level after each dose. If drug is used to treat digoxin-induced arrhythmias, evaluate patient's ECG frequently.
• Monitor kidney function tests frequently.
• Be alert for adverse reactions.
• Assess patient's and family's knowledge of drug therapy.

🔳 Nursing diagnoses

• Risk for injury related to hypercalcemia
• Ineffective protection related to drug-induced hypocalcemia
• Deficient knowledge related to drug therapy

🔲 Planning and implementation

• If generalized systemic reactions (fever, chills, back pain, emesis, muscle cramps, urinary urgency) occur 4 to 8 hours after infusion, report them to prescriber. Treatment is usually symptomatic. Effects usually subside within 12 hours.
• Other drugs for hypercalcemia are safer and more effective than edetate disodium.
⊙ **ALERT:** Don't confuse edetate disodium with edetate calcium disodium, which is used to treat lead toxicity.
Patient teaching
• Instruct patient to immediately report respiratory difficulty, dizziness, and muscle cramping.
• Advise patient to move from sitting or lying position slowly to avoid dizziness.
• Reassure patient that generalized systemic reaction usually subsides within 12 hours.
• If treating digoxin toxicity, instruct patient on correct usage of drug and required laboratory follow-up.

☑ Evaluation

• Patient sustains no injury as result of hypercalcemia.
• Patient's calcium level doesn't fall below normal after edetate disodium therapy.
• Patient and family state understanding of drug therapy.

efalizumab
(eh-fah-LEE-zoo-mab)
Raptiva

Pharmacologic class: immunosuppressant
Therapeutic class: antipsoriatic
Pregnancy risk category: C

Indications and dosages

▶ **Chronic moderate-to-severe plaque psoriasis when systemic therapy or phototherapy is appropriate.** *Adults:* Single dose of 0.7 mg/kg subcutaneously; follow with weekly doses of 1 mg/kg subcutaneously. Maximum single dose, 200 mg.

Contraindications and cautions

• Contraindicated in patients hypersensitive to drug or any of its components and in patients with significant infection.
• Use cautiously in patients with chronic infection or a history of recurrent infection. Also use cautiously in patients with a history of or high risk for malignancy.
☀ **Lifespan:** In pregnant women, use cautiously; it isn't known whether drug harms fetus. Tell breast-feeding women to stop breast-feeding or to stop using the drug because risk to the infant is unknown. In children, safety and effectiveness haven't been established. In elderly patients, use cautiously because of their increased risk of infection.

Adverse reactions

CNS: fever, *headache, pain, stroke.*
GI: *nausea.*
Hematologic: *thrombocytopenia.*
Musculoskeletal: back pain, myalgia.
Skin: acne.
Other: chills, flulike syndrome, hypersensitivity reaction, *infection,* malignancy.

Interactions

Drug-drug. *Other immunosuppressants:* May increase risk of infection and malignancy. Avoid use together.
Vaccines: May decrease or eliminate immune response to vaccine. Avoid use together.

Effects on lab test results

• May increase alkaline phosphatase level.

• May increase lymphocyte and leukocyte counts. May decrease platelet count.

Pharmacokinetics

Absorption: 50% bioavailable.
Distribution: Unknown.
Metabolism: Unknown.
Excretion: Unknown. *Half-life:* Unknown.

Route	Onset	Peak	Duration
SubQ	1–2 days	Unknown	25 days

Action

Chemical effect: Binds to a leukocyte function antigen and decreases its expression, thus inhibiting the action of T lymphocytes at sites of inflammation, including psoriatic skin.
Therapeutic effect: Decreases inflammation of psoriatic skin.

Available forms

Injection: 125-mg single-use vial

NURSING PROCESS

⚗ Assessment
• Watch for thrombocytopenia. Check patient's platelet count monthly before start of treatment, monthly until laboratory effects are stable, and then every 3 months.
• Monitor patient for worsening of psoriasis during or after therapy.
• Assess patient's and family's knowledge of drug therapy.

⊕ Nursing diagnoses
• Impaired skin integrity related to underlying condition
• Ineffective protection related to drug-induced thrombocytopenia
• Deficient knowledge related to drug therapy

⟫ Planning and implementation
• To reconstitute, inject 1.3 ml of sterile water for injection into the vial. Swirl gently to dissolve the powder, which takes less than 5 minutes. Don't shake the vial.
• Reconstitute the drug immediately before use.
• Don't use any other diluent besides sterile water, and use a vial only once.
• The reconstituted solution should be colorless to pale yellow and free of particulates. Don't

use the solution if it contains particulates or is discolored.
• Use reconstituted solution immediately, or store reconstituted solution at room temperature and use within 8 hours.
• Rotate injection sites.
• Don't add other drugs to solution.
• Keep powder refrigerated, and protect vials from light.
• Stop drug if patient develops severe infection or malignancy.
• Don't give vaccines to patients taking this drug because the immune response may be inadequate.
• If patient becomes pregnant while taking the drug or within 6 weeks after stopping it, enroll her in the Raptiva Pregnancy Registry by calling 1-877-727-8482).

Patient teaching
• Tell patient to take drug exactly as prescribed.
• Explain that platelet counts will be monitored during therapy.
• Urge patient to immediately report evidence of severe thrombocytopenia, such as bleeding gums, bruising, or petechiae.
• Tell patient to report weight changes because the dosage may need to be changed.
• Advise patient to report any newly diagnosed infection or malignancy.
• Tell patient to report worsening psoriasis.
• Caution patient to immediately report pregnancy or suspected pregnancy while taking drug or within 6 weeks of stopping drug.

☑ Evaluation
• Patient's underlying condition improves with drug therapy.
• Patient develops no serious complications from drug-induced thrombocytopenia.
• Patient and family state understanding of drug therapy.

efavirenz
(eh-FAH-veer-enz)
Sustiva

Pharmacologic class: nonnucleoside reverse transcriptase inhibitor (NNRTI)
Therapeutic class: antiretroviral
Pregnancy risk category: D

Indications and dosages

▶ **HIV-1 infection.** *Adults:* 600 mg P.O. daily with a protease inhibitor or nucleoside analog reverse transcriptase inhibitors.
Children age 3 and older weighing 10 to less than 15 kg (22 to less than 33 lb): 200 mg P.O. daily.
Children weighing 15 to less than 20 kg (33 to less than 44 lb): 250 mg P.O. daily.
Children weighing 20 to less than 25 kg (44 to less than 55 lb): 300 mg P.O. daily.
Children weighing 25 to less than 32.5 kg (55 to less than 72 lb): 350 mg P.O. daily.
Children weighing 32.5 to less than 40 kg (72 to less than 88 lb): 400 mg P.O. daily.
Children weighing 40 kg (88 lb) or more: 600 mg P.O. once daily.

Contraindications and cautions

• Contraindicated in patients hypersensitive to drug or any of its components.
• Use cautiously in patients with hepatic impairment or in those receiving hepatotoxic drugs.
⚠ **Lifespan:** In pregnant and breast-feeding women, drug is contraindicated. In children and elderly patients, use cautiously.

Adverse reactions

CNS: abnormal dreams or thinking, agitation, amnesia, confusion, depersonalization, depression, *dizziness,* euphoria, fatigue, hallucinations, headache, hypoesthesia, impaired concentration, insomnia, somnolence, nervousness, fever.
GI: abdominal pain, anorexia, diarrhea, dyspepsia, flatulence, nausea, vomiting.
GU: hematuria, renal calculi.
Skin: increased sweating, *erythema multiforme, Stevens-Johnson syndrome, toxic epidermal necrolysis,* rash, pruritus.

Interactions

Drug-drug. *Amprenavir, indinavir, lopinavir:* May decrease levels of these drugs. Consider alternative therapy or dosage adjustment.
Clarithromycin: May decrease level of clarithromycin and increase level of main metabolite. Also increases risk of rash. Consider using azithromycin instead.
Drugs that induce the CYP enzyme system (such as phenobarbital, rifampin): May increase clearance of efavirenz, resulting in lower level. Avoid use together.

Ergot derivatives, midazolam, triazolam: May inhibit metabolism of these drugs through competition for the CYP enzyme system, possibly causing serious or life-threatening adverse events (such as arrhythmias, prolonged sedation, or respiratory depression). Avoid use together.
Ethinyl estradiol: May increase level of ethinyl estradiol. Advise use of a reliable method of barrier contraception in addition to hormonal contraceptive.
Psychoactive drugs: May cause additive CNS effects. Avoid use together.
Rifabutin: May decrease rifabutin level. Increase dosage of rifabutin to 450 to 600 mg once daily or 600 mg two to three times a week.
Ritonavir: May increase levels of efavirenz and ritonavir. Monitor patient closely.
Saquinavir: May significantly decrease saquinavir level. Don't use with saquinavir as sole protease inhibitor.
Voriconazole: May significantly decrease voriconazole level while significantly increasing efavirenz level. Avoid use together.
Warfarin: May increase or decrease level and effects of warfarin. Monitor INR.
Drug-herb. *St. John's wort:* May decrease efavirenz level. Discourage use together.
Drug-food. *High-fat meals:* May increase absorption of drug, increasing risk of adverse effects. Instruct patient to maintain a low-fat diet.
Drug-lifestyle. *Alcohol use:* Enhances CNS effects. Discourage alcohol use.

Effects on lab test results

• May increase ALT, AST, and cholesterol levels.

Pharmacokinetics

Absorption: Steady-state levels reached in 6 to 10 days. Food increases amount of drug in body.
Distribution: Highly bound to proteins, predominantly albumin.
Metabolism: Primarily by CYP system to metabolites that are inactive against HIV-1.
Excretion: Primarily in feces. *Half-life:* 40 to 76 hours.

Route	Onset	Peak	Duration
P.O.	Unknown	3–5 hr	Unknown

Action

Chemical effect: An NNRTI that inhibits the transcription of HIV-1 RNA to DNA, a critical step in the viral replication process.
Therapeutic effect: Lowers viral load of HIV in the blood and increases CD4+ lymphocytes.

Available forms

Capsules: 50 mg, 100 mg, 200 mg
Tablets: 600 mg

NURSING PROCESS

🔬 Assessment

• Monitor liver function test results in a patient with a history of hepatitis B or C and in those taking ritonavir.
• Monitor cholesterol level.
• Children may be more susceptible to adverse reactions, especially diarrhea, nausea, vomiting, and rash.
• Observe skin before starting drug and regularly thereafter for signs of rash.
• Assess patient's and family's knowledge of drug therapy.

🔧 Nursing diagnoses

• Risk for infection related to patient's underlying condition
• Risk for impaired skin integrity related to potential adverse effects of drug
• Deficient knowledge related to drug therapy

▷ Planning and implementation

• Use drug with other antiretrovirals and not as monotherapy because resistant viruses emerge rapidly when it's used alone. Don't add on as a single drug to a failing regimen.
• Using drug with ritonavir may cause a higher occurrence of adverse effects, such as dizziness, nausea, paresthesia, and elevated liver enzyme levels.
• Rule out pregnancy before starting therapy in women of childbearing age.
• Give drug h.s. on an empty stomach to decrease adverse effects.
Patient teaching
• Instruct patient to take drug on an empty stomach, preferably at bedtime, and to take it with water, juice, milk, or soda.
• Inform patient about need for scheduled blood tests to monitor liver function and cholesterol levels.

• Tell patient to use reliable method of barrier contraception in addition to hormonal contraceptives, and to notify prescriber immediately if pregnancy is suspected. Drug is a known risk to the fetus.
• Inform patient that drug doesn't cure HIV infection and that it won't affect the complications of HIV. Explain that it doesn't reduce the risk of HIV transmission through sexual contact or blood contamination.
• Instruct patient to take drug at the same time each day and always with other antiretrovirals.
• Tell patient to take drug exactly as prescribed and not to stop without medical approval.
• Inform patient that rash is the most common adverse effect. Tell patient to immediately report any rash or any other adverse effects. Rash may be serious in rare cases.
• Instruct patient to report use of other drugs.
• Advise patient that dizziness, difficulty sleeping or concentrating, drowsiness, or unusual dreams may occur during the first few days of therapy. Reassure patient that these symptoms typically resolve after 2 to 4 weeks and that it may help to take drug h.s.
• Tell patient not to use alcohol and not to drive or operate machinery until drug's effects are known.

✓ Evaluation

• Patient is free of opportunistic infections.
• Patient's skin integrity is maintained.
• Patient and family state understanding of drug therapy.

eletriptan hydrobromide
(el-eh-TRIP-tan high-dro-BRO-mighd)
Relpax

Pharmacologic class: serotonin receptor agonist
Therapeutic class: antimigraine
Pregnancy risk category: C

Indications and dosages

▶ **Acute migraine with or without aura.**
Adults: 20 to 40 mg P.O. at the first migraine symptom. If headache recurs after initial relief, repeat dose at least 2 hours later. Maximum, 80 mg daily.

Contraindications and cautions

• Contraindicated in patients hypersensitive to drug or any of its components and in those with severe hepatic impairment; ischemic heart disease, such as angina pectoris, a history of MI, or silent ischemia; coronary artery vasospasm, including Prinzmetal's variant angina; and other CV conditions. Also contraindicated in patients with cerebrovascular disorders, such as stroke or transient ischemic attack; peripheral vascular disease, including ischemic bowel disease; uncontrolled hypertension; or hemiplegic or basilar migraine.

• Avoid use within 24 hours of another serotonin agonist or an ergotamine-containing or ergot-type drug.

⚓ **Lifespan:** In pregnant women, use drug only when benefits outweigh risks to the fetus. In breast-feeding women, use cautiously because drug appears in breast milk. In children, safety and effectiveness haven't been established. In elderly patients, use cautiously because they may have 15% lower drug clearance, the half-life of the drug is prolonged to about 6 hours, and these patients may develop higher blood pressure than younger patients.

Adverse reactions

CNS: *asthenia,* dizziness, headache, hypertonia, hypesthesia, pain, paresthesia, somnolence, vertigo.
CV: chest tightness, pain, and pressure; flushing; palpitations.
EENT: transient corneal opacity, conjunctivitis, photophobia, dry eyes, abnormal accommodation, eye hemorrhage, melanin toxicity, *lacrimation disorder,* abnormal vision.
GI: abdominal pain, discomfort, or cramps; dry mouth; dyspepsia; dysphagia; nausea.
Musculoskeletal: back pain.
Respiratory: pharyngitis.
Skin: increased sweating.
Other: chills.

Interactions

Drug-drug. *CYP 3A4 inhibitors, such as clarithromycin, itraconazole, ketoconazole, nefazodone, nelfinavir, ritonavir, and troleandomycin:* May decrease eletriptan metabolism. Avoid use within 72 hours of these drugs.
Ergotamine-containing or ergot-type drugs, such as dihydroergotamine or methysergide, and other serotonin agonists: May prolong vasospastic reactions. Avoid use within 24 hours of these drugs.
Propranolol: May increase bioavailability of eletriptan. No dosage adjustment is needed.

Effects on lab test results

None reported.

Pharmacokinetics

Absorption: Oral bioavailability is 50%. Drug level peaks in 1.5 to 2 hours.
Distribution: About 85% protein bound.
Metabolism: Primarily by the CYP 3A4 enzyme. The metabolite of eletriptan is active but without therapeutic effect.
Excretion: Clearance is 10% renal and 90% nonrenal. *Half-life:* About 4 hours.

Route	Onset	Peak	Duration
P.O.	½ hr	1½–2 hr	Unknown

Action

Chemical effect: Binds to serotonin receptors and may constrict intracranial blood vessels and inhibit proinflammatory neuropeptide release.
Therapeutic effect: Relieves migraine symptoms.

Available forms

Tablets: 20 mg, 40 mg

NURSING PROCESS

▨ **Assessment**
• Obtain history of patient's underlying condition before therapy.
• Assess patient for medical history or risk factors for liver disease, heart disease, cerebrovascular disease, peripheral vascular disease, ischemic bowel, or uncontrolled hypertension.
• Be alert for adverse reactions.
• Assess patient's and family's knowledge of drug therapy.

▨ **Nursing diagnoses**
• Recurrent acute pain related to migraine headaches
• Risk for injury related to adverse reactions
• Deficient knowledge related to drug therapy

▷ **Planning and implementation**
• Use only in patients with a clear diagnosis of migraine, not for prevention.

• If first use produces no response, reconsider diagnosis; a second dose will probably not be effective if the first dose causes no response.
• The safety of treating more than three migraines in 30 days hasn't been established.
⊛ **ALERT:** Serious cardiac events, including acute MI, arrhythmias, and death, occur rarely—usually within a few hours after use.
• Don't use in patient with risk factors for coronary artery disease, in a postmenopausal woman, or in a man older than age 40, unless patient is reasonably free of underlying CV disease. If drug must be used because of intractable migraine pain unresponsive to other drugs, give the first dose under medical supervision.
• Ophthalmologic effects, such as melanin-binding and toxicity, and corneal opacities, may occur with long-term use.

Patient teaching
• Instruct patient to take dose at the first sign of a migraine headache. If the headache returns after the first dose, he may take a second dose after 2 hours. Caution patient not to take more than 80 mg in 24 hours.
• Warn patient to avoid driving and operating machinery if he feels dizzy or fatigued after taking drug.
• Tell patient to immediately report pain, tightness, heaviness, or pressure in the chest, throat, neck, or jaw.

☑ Evaluation
• Patient experiences relief from migraine headache.
• Patient has no signs of adverse reaction to the drug.
• Patient and family state understanding of drug therapy and conditions that are contraindications for use of this drug.

emtricitabine
(em-trih-SIGH-tah-been)
Emtriva

Pharmacologic class: nucleoside reverse transcriptase inhibitor (NRTI)
Therapeutic class: antiretroviral
Pregnancy risk category: B

Indications and dosages

▶ **HIV-1 infection with other antiretrovirals.**
Adults: 200 mg capsule P.O. daily or 240 mg (24 ml) oral solution
Children age 3 months to 18 years: For children who weigh more than 33 kg (73 lb) and can swallow intact capsule, give one 200-mg capsule P.O. once daily. Otherwise, give 6 mg/kg oral solution, up to a maximum dose of 240 mg once daily.
⧠ **Adjust-a-dose:** For adults who have baseline creatinine clearance of 30 to 49 ml/minute, give 200-mg capsule q 48 hours or 120 mg oral solution q 24 hours; if creatinine clearance is 15 to 29 ml/minute, give 200-mg capsule q 72 hours or 80-mg oral solution q 24 hours; if clearance is less than 15 ml/minute (including patients requiring dialysis), give 200-mg capsule q 96 hours or 60-mg oral solution q 24 hours. If dose is scheduled on the day of hemodialysis, give it after dialysis. For children with renal insufficiency, there's no established dosage reduction. Consider reducing the dose and increasing the interval.

Contraindications and cautions

• Contraindicated in patients hypersensitive to drug or any of its components.
• Lower the dose and use cautiously in patients with renal impairment.
• Drug isn't indicated for chronic hepatitis B virus infection, and the safety and effectiveness of the drug hasn't been established in patients infected with hepatitis B virus and HIV.
⚘ **Lifespan:** In pregnant women, use cautiously because there are no adequate and well-controlled studies in this group. Women should avoid breast-feeding to prevent transmitting HIV to infants. In children younger than age 3 months, safety and effectiveness haven't been established.

Adverse reactions

CNS: *headache, asthenia,* nightmares, depression, insomnia, peripheral neuropathy, neuritis, paresthesia.
EENT: rhinitis.
GI: *diarrhea, nausea,* abdominal pain, dyspepsia, vomiting.
Hepatic: *severe hepatomegaly, steatosis.*
Metabolic: *lactic acidosis.*
Musculoskeletal: arthralgia, myalgia.
Respiratory: *cough.*

Reactions may be *common,* uncommon, *life-threatening*, or COMMON AND LIFE-THREATENING.

Interactions

None reported.

Effects on lab test results

● May increase ALT, AST, bilirubin, triglyceride, amylase, lipase, CK, and glucose levels.

Pharmacokinetics

Absorption: Rapid.
Distribution: At peak level, the mean plasma-to-blood ratio is about 1, and the mean semen-to-plasma ratio is about 4.
Metabolism: Not metabolized by CYP enzymes. Less than 15% undergoes oxidation and glucuronidation by the liver.
Excretion: Primarily in urine. *Half-life:* About 10 hours.

Route	Onset	Peak	Duration
P.O.	Unknown	1–2 hr	Unknown

Action

Chemical effect: Inhibits activity of HIV-1 reverse transcriptase by competing with natural substrate and being incorporated into new viral DNA chains, which results in their destruction.
Therapeutic effect: Helps block HIV replication.

Available forms

Capsules: 200 mg
Oral solution: 10 mg/ml

NURSING PROCESS

☲ Assessment

● Monitor liver and renal function tests.
● Assess all HIV-positive patients for chronic HBV infection before starting therapy.
● In a patient infected with both HBV and HIV, hepatitis B may worsen after therapy. Closely monitor patient for at least several months.
● Assess patient's and family's knowledge of drug therapy.

⊞ Nursing diagnoses

● Risk for infection related to patient's underlying condition
● Risk for disturbed body image related to redistribution of body fat due to antiretroviral therapy
● Deficient knowledge related to drug therapy

⊡ Planning and implementation

● If patient develops symptoms of lactic acidosis or pronounced hepatotoxicity, stop drug.
● Redistribution or accumulation of body fat, including central obesity, dorsocervical fat enlargement (buffalo hump), peripheral wasting, facial wasting, breast enlargement, and cushingoid appearance, may occur.
● Effects of higher doses aren't known; overdose can be treated with hemodialysis.
Patient teaching
● Tell patient that drug doesn't cure HIV infection and doesn't reduce the risk of transmitting HIV to others through sexual contact or blood contamination.
● Tell patient that drug must be taken for life.
● Stress importance of compliance and of planning compliance strategies in advance.
● Inform patient of potential adverse reactions, including lactic acidosis, hepatotoxicity, and redistribution or accumulation of body fat.
● Tell patient to contact prescriber immediately if she suspects she is pregnant.
● Instruct patient or family to refrigerate the oral solution. If stored at room temperature, they should use it within 3 months.

☑ Evaluation

● Patient remains free of opportunistic infection.
● Patient experiences no adverse drug effects.
● Patient and family state understanding of drug therapy.

enalaprilat
(eh-NAH-leh-prel-at)

enalapril maleate
Amprace ◇, Renitec ◇, Vasotec✐

Pharmacologic class: ACE inhibitor
Therapeutic class: antihypertensive
Pregnancy risk category: C (D in second and third trimesters)

Indications and dosages

▶ **Hypertension.** *Adults:* Initially 5 mg P.O. once daily; adjust according to response. Usual dosage range is 10 to 40 mg daily as single dose or two divided doses. Or 1.25 mg I.V. over 5 minutes q 6 hours.

▢ **Adjust-a-dose:** For patient taking a diuretic, initially 2.5 mg P.O. once daily. Or 0.625 mg I.V. over 5 minutes, repeated in 1 hour, if needed, and followed by 1.25 mg I.V. q 6 hours. In patients with creatinine clearance of 30 ml/minute or less, initial dose is 2.5 mg P.O. daily, increased gradually to maximum of 40 mg daily. Or give 0.625 mg I.V. and repeat in 1 hour if needed. Then give 1.25 mg I.V. q 6 hours. In hemodialysis patients, give 2.5 mg P.O. on dialysis days and adjust dose on nondialysis days based on blood pressure. Or give 0.625 mg I.V. q 6 hours.

▶ **Heart failure.** *Adults:* Initially 2.5 mg P.O. daily. Increase dosage after a few days or weeks according to response. Recommended range is 2.5 to 20 mg twice daily.

▢ **Adjust-a-dose:** In patients with hyponatremia (serum sodium level less than 130 mEq/L) or severe renal impairment (creatinine clearance 30 ml/minute or less), initial dose is 2.5 mg P.O. daily given under close supervision. Increase at intervals of 4 or more days to 2.5 mg twice daily, then 5 mg twice daily, to a maximum of 40 mg daily.

▶ **Asymptomatic left ventricular dysfunction.** *Adults:* 2.5 mg P.O. b.i.d.; adjust as tolerated to target of 20 mg P.O. daily in divided doses.

▽ I.V. administration

• Giving doses greater than 1.25 mg isn't more effective.
• Compatible solutions include D₅W, normal saline solution, dextrose 5% in lactated Ringer's solution, and D₅W in normal saline solution.
• Inject drug slowly over at least 5 minutes, or dilute in 50 ml of compatible solution and infuse over 15 minutes.
⊗ **Incompatibilities**
Amphotericin B, phenytoin sodium.

Contraindications and cautions

• Contraindicated in patients hypersensitive to drug or any of its components and in those with a history of angioedema from ACE inhibitor.
• Use cautiously in patients with renal impairment, especially those with bilateral renal artery stenosis or unilateral renal artery stenosis in a single functioning kidney.
⚘ **Lifespan:** In pregnant women, use only when benefits outweigh risks to the fetus. In

breast-feeding women and in children, safety hasn't been established.

Adverse reactions

CNS: *headache, dizziness, fatigue,* vertigo, asthenia, syncope.
CV: *hypotension,* chest pain.
GI: diarrhea, nausea, abdominal pain, vomiting.
GU: decreased renal function.
Hematologic: *neutropenia, thrombocytopenia, agranulocytosis.*
Metabolic: *hyperkalemia.*
Respiratory: dry, persistent, tickling, nonproductive cough; dyspnea.
Skin: rash.
Other: *angioedema.*

Interactions

Drug-drug. *Diuretics:* May cause excessive reduction of blood pressure. Monitor patient.
Insulin, oral antidiabetics: May increase risk of hypoglycemia, especially at start of enalapril therapy. Monitor patient and glucose levels closely.
Lithium: May increase risk of lithium toxicity. Monitor lithium levels.
NSAIDs: May reduce antihypertensive effect. Monitor blood pressure.
Potassium supplements, potassium-sparing diuretics: May increase risk of hyperkalemia. Avoid these drugs unless hypokalemic blood levels are confirmed.
Drug-herb. *Licorice:* May cause sodium retention and increase blood pressure, interfering with therapeutic effects of ACE inhibitors. Discourage licorice intake during drug therapy.
Drug-lifestyle. *Alcohol use:* May produce additive hypotensive effect. Discourage use together.
Sun exposure: Photosensitivity reaction may occur. Urge patient to avoid unprotected or prolonged sun exposure.

Effects on lab test results

• May increase ALT, AST, bilirubin, BUN, creatinine, and potassium levels. May decrease sodium and hemoglobin levels and hematocrit.
• May decrease neutrophil, granulocyte, and platelet counts.

Pharmacokinetics

Absorption: About 60% of P.O. dose absorbed from GI tract.
Distribution: Unknown.

E

Metabolism: Metabolized extensively to active metabolite.
Excretion: About 94% in urine and feces as enalaprilat and enalapril. *Half-life:* 12 hours.

Route	Onset	Peak	Duration
P.O.	1 hr	4–6 hr	24 hr
I.V.	15 min	1–4 hr	6 hr

Action

Chemical effect: May inhibit ACE, preventing conversion of angiotensin I to angiotensin II, a potent vasoconstrictor. Reduced formation of angiotensin II decreases peripheral arterial resistance, thus decreasing aldosterone secretion.
Therapeutic effect: Lowers blood pressure.

Available forms

Injection: 1.25 mg/ml
Tablets: 2.5 mg, 5 mg, 10 mg, 20 mg

NURSING PROCESS

☞ Assessment
• Obtain history of patient's blood pressure before starting therapy, and reassess regularly.
• Monitor CBC with differential counts before therapy, every 2 weeks for first 3 months of therapy, and periodically thereafter.
• Monitor potassium intake and serum potassium level.
• Be alert for adverse reactions and drug interactions.
• Assess patient's and family's knowledge of drug therapy.

🔡 Nursing diagnoses
• Risk for injury related to presence of hypertension
• Risk for infection related to drug-induced adverse hematologic reactions
• Deficient knowledge related to drug therapy

▷ Planning and implementation
• If patient has hypotension after first dose, adjust dose as long as patient is under medical supervision.
• If CBC becomes abnormal or if evidence of infection arises, notify prescriber immediately.
• If angioedema (including laryngeal edema) occurs, notify prescriber and stop drug immediately. Institute appropriate therapy (epinephrine

solution 1:1,000 [0.3 to 0.5 ml] subcutaneously), and take measures to ensure patent airway.
Patient teaching
• Advise patient to report evidence of angioedema, such as breathing difficulty and swelling of face, eyes, lips, or tongue.
• Instruct patient to report signs of infection, such as fever and sore throat.
• Advise patient that light-headedness can occur, especially during first few days of therapy. Tell patient to rise slowly to minimize this effect and to report symptoms to prescriber. If patient experiences syncope, tell him to stop taking drug and to call prescriber immediately.
• Tell patient to use caution in hot weather and during exercise. Inadequate fluid intake, vomiting, diarrhea, and excessive perspiration can lead to light-headedness and syncope.
• Advise patient to avoid sodium substitutes; these products may contain potassium, which can cause hyperkalemia.
• Tell patient to notify prescriber if pregnancy occurs. Drug will probably need to be changed.

☑ Evaluation
• Patient's blood pressure becomes normal.
• Patient's CBC remains normal throughout therapy.
• Patient and family state understanding of drug therapy.

enfuvirtide
(ehn-FOO-ver-tighd)
Fuzeon

Pharmacologic class: fusion inhibitor
Therapeutic class: antiretroviral
Pregnancy risk category: B

Indications and dosages

▶ **HIV-1 infection, with other antiretrovirals, in patients with continued HIV-1 replication despite antiretroviral therapy.** *Adults:* 90 mg subcutaneously b.i.d., injected into the upper arm, anterior thigh, or abdomen.
Children ages 6 to 16: 2 mg/kg subcutaneously b.i.d.; maximum dose, 90 mg.

Contraindications and cautions

• Contraindicated in patients hypersensitive to drug or any of its components.

≋ **Lifespan:** In pregnant women, use only when benefits outweigh risks to the fetus. Breast-feeding women should stop breast-feeding to prevent transmitting HIV to infants. In children younger than age 6, safety and effectiveness haven't been established.

Adverse reactions

CNS: anxiety, asthenia, depression, *insomnia,* peripheral neuropathy.
EENT: conjunctivitis, sinusitis, taste disturbance.
GI: abdominal pain, constipation, *diarrhea, nausea,* **pancreatitis.**
Hematologic: lymphadenopathy.
Metabolic: anorexia, weight decrease.
Musculoskeletal: myalgia.
Respiratory: *bacterial pneumonia,* cough.
Skin: pruritus, skin papilloma, *ecchymosis.*
Other: herpes simplex, influenza, flulike illness, *injection-site reactions.*

Interactions

None reported.

Effects on lab test results

• May increase triglyceride, amylase, lipase, ALT, AST, CK, and GGT levels. May decrease hemoglobin level and hematocrit.
• May decrease eosinophil count.

Pharmacokinetics

Absorption: Absorbed well after subcutaneous administration into arm, thigh, or abdomen.
Distribution: 92% protein bound.
Metabolism: May undergo catabolism to its constituent amino acids; hydrolyzed to a metabolite detectable in plasma.
Excretion: Unknown. *Half-life:* 4 hours.

Route	Onset	Peak	Duration
SubQ	Unknown	4–8 hr	Unknown

Action

Chemical effect: Interferes with entry of HIV-1 into cells by inhibiting fusion of HIV-1 to cell membranes.
Therapeutic effect: Controls symptoms of HIV infection.

Available forms

Injection: 108-mg single-use vials (90 mg/ml after reconstitution)

NURSING PROCESS

🗒 Assessment
• Use drug only in patients who are HIV-positive.
• Assess patient for evidence of bacterial pneumonia.
• Observe injection site for local reaction.
• Assess patient's and family's knowledge of drug therapy.

⊕ Nursing diagnoses
• Risk for infection related to underlying condition
• Deficient knowledge related to drug therapy

▶ Planning and implementation
• Reconstitute vial with 1.1 ml sterile water for injection. Tap vial for 10 seconds, and then gently roll it between hands to prevent foaming. Let drug stand for up to 45 minutes to ensure reconstitution. Or gently roll vial between hands until product is completely dissolved. Then draw up correct dose and inject drug.
• If drug isn't used immediately after reconstitution, refrigerate in original vial and use within 24 hours. Don't inject drug until it's at room temperature.
• Store vials that haven't been reconstituted at room temperature.
• Vial is for single use; discard unused portion.
• Rotate injection sites. Don't inject into same site for two consecutive doses, and don't inject into moles, scar tissue, bruises, or the navel.
• Injection site reactions (pain, discomfort, induration, erythema, pruritus, nodules, cysts, ecchymosis) are common and may require analgesics or rest.
• ⓢ **ALERT:** Monitor patient closely for bacterial pneumonia. Patients at high risk include those with a low initial CD4+ count or high initial viral load, those who use I.V. drugs or smoke, and those with a history of lung disease.
• Hypersensitivity may occur with the first dose or later doses. If symptoms occur, stop drug.
• Register pregnant women in the Antiretroviral Pregnancy Registry by phoning 1-800-258-4263.
Patient teaching
• Teach patient how to prepare and give drug and how to safely dispose of used needles and syringes.

Reactions may be *common,* uncommon, **life-threatening**, or **COMMON AND LIFE-THREATENING**.

• Tell patient to rotate injection sites and to watch for cellulitis or local infection.

• Urge patient to immediately report evidence of pneumonia, such as cough with fever, rapid breathing, or shortness of breath.

• Tell patient to stop taking drug and seek medical attention if evidence of hypersensitivity develops, such as rash, fever, nausea, vomiting, chills, rigors, and hypotension.

• Inform patient that drug doesn't cure HIV infection and that it must be taken with other antiretrovirals.

• Tell patient to inform prescriber if she's pregnant, plans to become pregnant, or is breast-feeding while taking this drug.

• Tell patient that drug may impair the ability to drive or operate machinery.

☑ **Evaluation**

• Patient is free from opportunistic infections.

• Patient and family state understanding of drug therapy.

enoxaparin sodium

(eh-NOKS-uh-pah-rin SOH-dee-um)
Lovenox

Pharmacologic class: low–molecular-weight heparin derivative
Therapeutic class: anticoagulant
Pregnancy risk category: B

Indications and dosages

▶ **To prevent deep vein thrombosis (DVT) following hip or knee replacement surgery.** *Adults:* 30 mg subcutaneously q 12 hours for 7 to 10 days. Initial dose given 12 to 24 hours after surgery, provided hemostasis has been established. Or, for hip replacement surgery, 40 mg subcutaneously once daily given initially 9 to 15 hours before surgery. May continue with 40 mg subcutaneously once daily or 30 mg subcutaneously q 12 hours for 3 weeks.

▶ **To prevent DVT following abdominal surgery.** *Adults:* 40 mg subcutaneously once daily for 7 to 10 days with initial dose given 2 hours before surgery.

▶ **To prevent ischemic complications of unstable angina and non–Q-wave MI.** *Adults:* 1 mg/kg subcutaneously q 12 hours for 2 to

8 days with oral aspirin therapy (100 to 325 mg daily).

▶ **Inpatient with acute DVT with or without pulmonary embolism.** *Adults:* 1 mg/kg subcutaneously q 12 hours. Or 1.5 mg/kg subcutaneously once daily (at same time every day) for 5 to 7 days until therapeutic oral anticoagulant effect (INR of 2 to 3) is achieved. Warfarin therapy usually starts within 72 hours of enoxaparin injection.

▶ **Outpatient with acute DVT and without pulmonary embolism.** *Adults:* 1 mg/kg subcutaneously q 12 hours for 5 to 7 days until INR of 2 to 3 is achieved. Warfarin therapy is usually started within 72 hours of the enoxaparin injection.

▶ **Immobile patients during an acute illness.** *Adults:* 40 mg subcutaneously given once daily for 6 to 11 days. Up to 14 days may be tolerated.

⚠ **Adjust-a-dose:** In patients with a creatinine clearance less than 30 ml/minute receiving drug as prophylaxis following abdominal surgery or hip or knee replacement surgery, and in medical patients for prophylaxis during acute illness, decrease dosage to 30 mg subcutaneously daily. In patients with creatinine clearance less than 30 ml/minute receiving drug for acute DVT or prophylaxis of ischemic complications of unstable angina and non–Q-wave MI, give 1 mg/kg subcutaneously daily.

Contraindications and cautions

• Contraindicated in patients hypersensitive to drug or any of its components, to heparin, or to pork products; in those with active major bleeding or thrombocytopenia; and in those who have antiplatelet antibodies in presence of drug.

• Not recommended for thromboprophylaxis in patients with prosthetic heart valves.

• Use cautiously in patients with postoperative indwelling epidural catheters and patients who have had epidural or spinal anesthesia. Epidural and spinal hematomas may result in long-term or permanent paralysis. Also use cautiously in patients with a history of heparin-induced thrombocytopenia; in patients with conditions that increase their risk of hemorrhage (such as bacterial endocarditis); and in patients with congenital or acquired bleeding disorders, ulcer disease, angiodysplastic GI disease, hemorrhagic stroke, or recent spinal, eye, or brain surgery.

E

※ **Lifespan:** In pregnant women, use cautiously, and only when benefits outweigh risks to the fetus. In breast-feeding women, use cautiously because it's unknown if the drug appears in breast milk. In children, safety and effectiveness haven't been established.

Adverse reactions

CNS: fever, pain, confusion.
CV: edema, peripheral edema.
GI: nausea.
Hematologic: *anemia, thrombocytopenia, hemorrhage, bleeding complications.*
Skin: irritation, pain, hematoma, or erythema at injection site; rash; urticaria, ecchymosis.
Other: *angioedema, anaphylaxis.*

Interactions

Drug-drug. *Anticoagulants, antiplatelet drugs, NSAIDs:* May increase risk of bleeding. Don't use together.
Plicamycin, valproic acid: May cause hypoprothrombinemia and inhibit platelet aggregation. Monitor patient closely.

Effects on lab test results

• May increase ALT and AST levels. May decrease hemoglobin level and hematocrit.
• May decrease platelet count.

Pharmacokinetics

Absorption: Unknown.
Distribution: Unknown.
Metabolism: Unknown.
Excretion: Unknown. *Half-life:* 4½ hours.

Route	Onset	Peak	Duration
SubQ	Unknown	3–5 hr	< 24 hr

Action

Chemical effect: Accelerates formation of antithrombin IIIB–thrombin complex and deactivates thrombin, preventing conversion of fibrinogen to fibrin.
Therapeutic effect: Prevents pulmonary embolism and DVT.

Available forms

Ampules: 30 mg/0.3 ml
Syringes (prefilled, graduated): 60 mg/0.6 ml, 80 mg/0.8 ml, 100 mg/ml, 120 mg/0.8 ml, 150 mg/ml

Syringes (prefilled): 30 mg/0.3 ml, 40 mg/0.4 ml
Vial (multidose): 300 mg/3 ml (contains 15 mg/ml of benzyl alcohol)

NURSING PROCESS

Assessment
• Obtain history of patient's coagulation parameters before starting therapy.
• Monitor the drug's effectiveness by evaluating patient for signs and symptoms of pulmonary embolism or DVT.
• Monitor platelet counts regularly. Patient with normal coagulation doesn't require regular monitoring of PT, INR, or PTT.
• Frequently monitor neurologic condition of patients who have had spinal or epidural anesthesia. If abnormalities are discovered, alert prescriber immediately.
• Be alert for adverse reactions and drug interactions.
• Assess patient's and family's knowledge of drug therapy.

Nursing diagnoses
• Risk for injury related to risk for pulmonary embolism or DVT after knee or hip replacement surgery
• Ineffective protection related to drug-induced bleeding complications
• Deficient knowledge related to drug therapy

Planning and implementation
⑤ **ALERT:** To avoid drug loss, don't expel air bubble from 30- or 40-mg prefilled syringes.
⑤ **ALERT:** Never give drug I.M.
• Don't massage after subcutaneous injection. Rotate sites among the left and right anterolateral and the left and right posterolateral abdominal walls.
⑤ **ALERT:** Drug can't be used interchangeably (unit for unit) with unfractionated heparin or other low–molecular-weight heparins.
• Avoid excessive I.M. injections of other drugs to prevent or minimize hematomas. Don't give I.M. injections when patient is anticoagulated.
• To treat severe overdose, give protamine sulfate (a heparin antagonist) by slow I.V. infusion at concentration of 1% to equal dosage of enoxaparin injected.

Reactions may be *common*, uncommon, *life-threatening*, or COMMON AND LIFE-THREATENING.

Patient teaching

• Instruct patient and family to watch for signs of bleeding and to notify prescriber immediately.
• Tell patient to avoid OTC drugs that contain aspirin or other salicylates.
• Tell pregnant women and women of childbearing potential about the potential hazard to fetus and mother if drug is used during pregnancy.

☑ Evaluation

• Patient doesn't develop pulmonary embolism or DVT.
• Patient has no bleeding complications during therapy.
• Patient and family state understanding of drug therapy.

entacapone

(en-TAK-uh-pohn)
Comtan

Pharmacologic class: COMT inhibitor
Therapeutic class: antiparkinsonian
Pregnancy risk category: C

Indications and dosages

▶ **Adjunct to levodopa and carbidopa in idiopathic Parkinson's disease in patients who experience end-of-dose wearing-off.**
Adults: 200 mg P.O. with each dose of levodopa and carbidopa up to eight times daily. Maximum, 1,600 mg daily. Reducing daily levodopa dose or extending interval between doses may optimize patient's response.

Contraindications and cautions

• Contraindicated in patients hypersensitive to the drug or any of its components.
• Use cautiously in patients with hepatic impairment, biliary obstruction, or orthostatic hypotension.
⚞ **Lifespan:** In pregnant women, use drug only when benefits outweigh risks to the fetus. In breast-feeding women, use cautiously because it's unknown if the drug appears in breast milk.

Adverse reactions

CNS: *dyskinesia, hyperkinesia,* hypokinesia, dizziness, anxiety, somnolence, agitation, fatigue, asthenia, hallucinations.
GI: *nausea, diarrhea,* abdominal pain, constipation, vomiting, dry mouth, dyspepsia, flatulence, gastritis, taste perversion.
GU: urine discoloration.
Hematologic: purpura.
Musculoskeletal: back pain, *rhabdomyolysis.*
Respiratory: dyspnea.
Skin: sweating.
Other: bacterial infection.

Interactions

Drug-drug. *Ampicillin, chloramphenicol, cholestyramine, erythromycin, probenecid, rifampin:* May block biliary excretion, resulting in higher levels of entacapone. Use cautiously.
CNS depressants: May have additive effects. Use cautiously.
Drugs metabolized by COMT, such as bitolterol, dobutamine, dopamine, epinephrine, isoetharine, isoproterenol, and norepinephrine: May cause higher levels of these drugs, which may increase heart rate, change blood pressure, or cause arrhythmias. Use cautiously.
Nonselective MAO inhibitors, such as phenelzine and tranylcypromine: May inhibit normal catecholamine metabolism. Don't use together.
Drug-lifestyle. *Alcohol use:* May cause additive CNS effects. Discourage use together.

Effects on lab test results

None reported.

Pharmacokinetics

Absorption: Rapid, with level peaking in about 1 hour. Food doesn't affect absorption.
Distribution: About 98% protein-bound, mainly to albumin, and doesn't distribute widely into tissues.
Metabolism: Almost completely metabolized by glucuronidation before elimination.
Excretion: About 10% in urine; the remainder in bile and feces. *Half-life:* 0.4 to 0.7 hours for first phase and 2.4 hours for second phase.

Route	Onset	Peak	Duration
P.O.	1 hr	1 hr	6 hr

Action

Chemical effect: Drug is a reversible inhibitor of peripheral COMT, which is responsible for elimination of various catecholamines, including dopamine. Blocking this pathway when giving levodopa and carbidopa may result in higher levels of levodopa, thereby allowing greater dopaminergic stimulation in the CNS and leading to a greater effect on parkinsonian symptoms.

Therapeutic effect: Controls idiopathic Parkinson's disease signs and symptoms.

Available forms

Tablets: 200 mg

NURSING PROCESS

🕮 Assessment
• Assess hepatic and biliary function before starting therapy.
• Monitor blood pressure closely. Watch for orthostatic hypotension.
• Monitor patient for hallucinations.
• Assess patient's and family's knowledge of drug therapy.

🕮 Nursing diagnoses
• Impaired physical mobility related to presence of parkinsonism
• Disturbed thought processes related to drug-induced adverse reactions
• Deficient knowledge related to drug therapy

🕮 Planning and implementation
• Use with levodopa and carbidopa. Drug isn't effective when given as monotherapy.
• Drug may be given with immediate- or sustained-release levodopa and carbidopa and may be taken with or without food.
• Lower levodopa and carbidopa dosage or increase dosing interval to avoid adverse effects.
• Drug may cause or worsen dyskinesia despite reduction of levodopa dosage.
• Watch for diarrhea, which usually begins 4 to 12 weeks after therapy starts but may begin as early as the first week or as late as many months after therapy starts.
• Abruptly stopping the drug or lowering the dosage could lead to sudden worsening of Parkinson's disease; it may also lead to hyperpyrexia and confusion, a symptom complex resembling neuroleptic malignant syndrome. Ta-

per off dose and monitor patient closely. Adjust other antiparkinson drugs as required.
• Observe for urine discoloration.
• Rarely, rhabdomyolysis has occurred with drug use.

Patient teaching
• Instruct patient not to crush or break tablet and to take it at same time as levodopa and carbidopa.
• Warn patient to avoid hazardous activities until drug's CNS effects are known.
• Advise patient not to use alcohol.
• Instruct patient to use caution when standing after a prolonged period of sitting or lying down because dizziness may occur. This effect is more common early in therapy.
• Warn patient that hallucinations, dyskinesia, nausea, diarrhea, and urine discoloration may occur.
• Inform patient that abruptly stopping drug therapy can cause sudden severe symptoms.
• Advise female patient to notify prescriber if she's pregnant or breast-feeding or if she plans to become pregnant.

✓ Evaluation
• Patient exhibits improved physical mobility.
• Patient maintains normal thought process.
• Patient and family state understanding of drug therapy.

entecavir
(ehn-TECK-ah-veer)
Baraclude

Pharmacologic class: guanosine nucleoside analog
Therapeutic class: antiviral
Pregnancy risk category: C

Indications and dosages

▶ **Chronic hepatitis B infection in patients with active viral replication and either persistently increased serum aminotransferase levels or histologically active disease.** *Adults and adolescents age 16 and older who have had no previous nucleoside treatment:* 0.5 mg P.O. once daily on an empty stomach.
Adults and adolescents age 16 and older who have a history of viremia and are taking lamivu-

dine or have resistance mutations: 1 mg P.O. once daily on an empty stomach.

Adjust-a-dose: *Patients with no previous nucleoside treatment:* If creatinine clearance is 30 to 49 ml/minute, give 0.25 mg P.O. once daily. If clearance is 10 to 29 ml/minute, give 0.15 mg P.O. once daily. If clearance is less than 10 ml/minute or patient is undergoing hemodialysis or continuous ambulatory peritoneal dialysis, give 0.05 mg P.O. once daily.

Patients with lamivudine resistance: If creatinine clearance is 30 to 49 ml/minute, give 0.5 mg P.O. once daily. If clearance is 10 to 29 ml/minute, give 0.3 mg P.O. once daily. If clearance is less than 10 ml/minute or patient is undergoing hemodialysis or continuous ambulatory peritoneal dialysis, give 0.1 mg P.O. once daily.

Contraindications and cautions

- Contraindicated in patients hypersensitive to drug or its components.
- Use cautiously in patients with renal impairment and after liver transplantation.
- **Lifespan:** In pregnant women, use only when benefits outweigh risks to the fetus. In breast-feeding women, avoid use; it's unknown if the drug appears in breast milk. In patients younger than age 16, safety and effectiveness haven't been established. In elderly patients, adjust dosage for age-related decreases in renal function.

Adverse reactions

CNS: dizziness, fatigue, headache.
GI: diarrhea, dyspepsia, nausea.
GU: hematuria, glycosuria.
Hepatic: *hepatomegaly with steatosis.*
Other: *lactic acidosis.*

Interactions

Drug-drug. *Cyclosporine, tacrolimus:* May further decrease renal function. Monitor renal function carefully.
Drugs that reduce renal function or compete for active tubular secretion: May increase serum levels of either drug. Monitor renal function, and watch for adverse effects.
Drug-food. *Food:* May delay absorption and decrease serum drug level. Give drug on an empty stomach, at least 2 hours before or after a meal.

Effects on lab test results

- May increase ALT, amylase, AST, blood glucose, creatinine, lipase, and total bilirubin levels.
- May decrease platelet count.

Pharmacokinetics

Absorption: Absorbed through the GI tract. Food delays and decreases absorption.
Distribution: Extensive in tissues. Drug is 13% bound to plasma proteins.
Metabolism: Drug isn't a substrate, inhibitor, or inducer of the CYP enzyme system.
Excretion: By kidneys, 62% to 73% unchanged. *Half-life:* 128 to 149 hours.

Route	Onset	Peak	Duration
P.O.	Unknown	½–1½ hr	Unknown

Action

Chemical effect: Inhibits hepatitis B virus polymerase and reduces viral DNA levels.
Therapeutic effect: Reduces symptoms of hepatitis B infection.

Available forms

Oral solution: 0.05 mg/ml
Tablets: 0.5 mg, 1 mg

NURSING PROCESS

Assessment
- Assess patient's condition before therapy and regularly thereafter.
- Monitor renal and liver function tests during therapy.
- **ALERT:** Hepatitis B may worsen severely after entecavir therapy stops.
- Monitor hepatic function for several months in patients who stop therapy. If appropriate, restart therapy for hepatitis B.
- Assess patient's and family's knowledge of drug therapy.

Nursing diagnoses
- Risk for injury related to development of lactic acidosis and severe hepatomegaly with steatosis secondary to drug therapy
- Ineffective therapeutic regimen management secondary to long-term drug therapy
- Deficient knowledge related to drug therapy

▷ Planning and implementation

⚠ **ALERT:** The drug may cause life-threatening lactic acidosis and severe hepatomegaly with steatosis.

• To monitor fetal outcome, call the Pregnancy Registry at 1-800-258-4263.
• The optimal duration of treatment hasn't been established.

Patient teaching

• Tell patient that drug should be taken on an empty stomach at least 2 hours before or after a meal.
• Caution against mixing or diluting oral solution with any other substances. Teach proper use of spoon used to measure dose.
• Advise patient to report new adverse effects or new therapy with another drug.
• Explain that drug doesn't reduce the risk of hepatitis B virus transmission to others.
• Teach patient the signs and symptoms of lactic acidosis, such as muscle pain, weakness, dyspnea, GI distress, cold extremities, dizziness, and fast or irregular heartbeat.
• Teach patient the signs and symptoms of hepatotoxicity, such as jaundice, dark urine, light-colored stool, loss of appetite, nausea, and lower stomach pain.
• Warn patient not to stop drug abruptly.

☑ Evaluation

• Patient remains free from lactic acidosis and severe hepatomegaly with steatosis during therapy.
• Patient maintains therapeutic regimen as shown by improvement of hepatitis B viral infection.
• Patient and family state understanding of drug therapy.

ephedrine sulfate
(eh-FED-rihn SUL-fayt)
Kondon's Nasal†, Pretz-D†

Pharmacologic class: adrenergic
Therapeutic class: bronchodilator, vasopressor (parenteral form), nasal decongestant
Pregnancy risk category: C

Indications and dosages

▶ **Hypotension.** *Adults:* 25 to 50 mg I.M. or subcutaneously, or 10 to 25 mg I.V. infusion, or 5 to 25 mg by slow I.V. bolus injection, p.r.n., up to maximum of 150 mg/24 hours.
Children: 3 mg/kg or 100 mg/m² subcutaneously or I.V. daily in four to six divided doses.
▶ **Bronchodilation, nasal decongestion.**
Adults and children older than age 12: 25 to 50 mg P.O. q 3 to 4 hours p.r.n. For use as a bronchodilator, 12.5 to 25 mg P.O. q 4 hours. Maximum, 150 mg in 24 hours. As a nasal decongestant, 0.5% solution applied topically to nasal mucosa as drops or nasal pack. Instill no more often than q 4 hours.
Children ages 2 to 12: 2 to 3 mg/kg or 100 mg/m² P.O. daily in four to six divided doses.

▽ I.V. administration

• Compatible with most common I.V. solutions.
• For vasopressor action, use I.V. route initially. Give slowly until systolic blood pressure is 30 to 40 mm Hg below patient's normal systolic pressure or 80 to 100 mm Hg.

⊗ **Incompatibilities**
Fructose 10% in normal saline solution; hydrocortisone sodium succinate; Ionosol B, D-CM, and D solutions; pentobarbital sodium; phenobarbital sodium; thiopental.

Contraindications and cautions

• Contraindicated in patients hypersensitive to drug, to any of its components, or to other sympathomimetic drugs; in those with porphyria, severe coronary artery disease, arrhythmias, angle-closure glaucoma, psychoneurosis, angina pectoris, substantial organic heart disease, or CV disease; and in those taking MAO inhibitors.
• Use cautiously in patients with hypertension, hyperthyroidism, nervous or excitable states, diabetes, or prostatic hyperplasia.
✷ **Lifespan:** In pregnant women, in children, and in older men, use cautiously. In breastfeeding women, drug is contraindicated.

Adverse reactions

CNS: *insomnia, nervousness,* dizziness, headache, euphoria, confusion, delirium.
CV: *palpitations,* tachycardia, hypertension, precordial pain.
EENT: dryness of nose and throat.
GI: nausea, vomiting, anorexia.
GU: urine retention, painful urination from visceral sphincter spasm.

Musculoskeletal: muscle weakness.
Skin: diaphoresis.

Interactions

Drug-drug. *Acetazolamide:* May increase ephedrine level. Monitor patient for toxicity.
Alpha blockers: Doesn't counteract beta blocker effects, resulting in hypotension. Monitor blood pressure.
Antihypertensives: May decrease effects. Monitor blood pressure.
Beta blockers: Doesn't counteract alpha-adrenergic effects, resulting in hypertension. Monitor blood pressure.
Digoxin, general anesthetics (halogenated hydrocarbons): May increase risk of ventricular arrhythmias. Monitor patient closely.
Ergot alkaloids: May enhance vasoconstrictor activity. Monitor patient closely.
Guanadrel, guanethidine: May enhance pressor effects of ephedrine. Monitor patient closely.
Isocarboxazid: When given with sympathomimetics, may cause hypertensive crisis. Don't use together.
Methyldopa, reserpine: May inhibit effects of ephedrine. Use together cautiously.
Phenelzine, tranylcypromine: May cause severe headache, hypertension, fever, and hypertensive crisis. Avoid use together.
Tricyclic antidepressants: May decrease pressor response. Monitor patient's blood pressure closely.

Effects on lab test results

None reported.

Pharmacokinetics

Absorption: Rapid and complete after P.O., I.M., or subcutaneous administration; unknown after nasal and I.V. administration.
Distribution: Widely distributed throughout body.
Metabolism: Slow, in liver.
Excretion: Unchanged in urine. Rate of excretion depends on urine pH. *Half-life:* 3 to 6 hours.

Route	Onset	Peak	Duration
P.O.	15–60 min	Unknown	3–5 hr
I.V.	≤ 5 min	Unknown	1 hr
I.M.	10–20 min	Unknown	1 hr
SubQ	Unknown	Unknown	1 hr
Intranasal	Unknown	Unknown	Unknown

Action

Chemical effect: Stimulates alpha and beta receptors; direct- and indirect-acting sympathomimetic.
Therapeutic effect: Raises blood pressure, causes bronchodilation, and relieves nasal congestion.

Available forms

Capsules: 25 mg, 50 mg
Injection: 25 mg/ml, 50 mg/ml
Nasal solution: 0.25%†, 0.5%†, 1%†
Tablets: 30 mg†

NURSING PROCESS

⚡ Assessment

• Obtain history of patient's underlying condition before starting therapy, and reassess regularly.
• Be alert for adverse reactions and drug interactions.
• Assess patient's and family's knowledge of drug therapy.

⊕ Nursing diagnoses

• Ineffective health maintenance related to underlying condition
• Risk for deficient fluid volume related to drug-induced adverse GI reactions
• Deficient knowledge related to drug therapy

⟩ Planning and implementation

• Hypoxia, hypercapnia, and acidosis, which may reduce drug effectiveness or increase adverse reactions, must be identified and corrected before or during ephedrine administration for shock.
• Volume deficit must be corrected before giving vasopressors. This drug isn't a substitute for blood or fluid volume replenishment.
• To prevent insomnia, avoid giving within 2 hours of bedtime.
• When effectiveness decreases, notify prescriber. Effectiveness decreases after 2 to 3 weeks, as tolerance develops. Drug isn't addictive.

Patient teaching
• Warn patient not to take OTC drugs that contain ephedrine without consulting prescriber.
• Teach patient how to instill nose drops, and warn him not to exceed recommended dose.

Rapid onset   *Liquid form contains alcohol.   ♦ Canada   ◇ Australia   †OTC   ⟋Photoguide   ‡Off-label use

• Advise patient to notify prescriber if effectiveness decreases and to adjust dosage as instructed.
• Instruct patient to notify prescriber if adverse reactions occur.
• Caution patient not to perform hazardous activities if adverse CNS reactions occur.

☑ **Evaluation**
• Patient exhibits improvement in underlying condition.
• Patient maintains adequate hydration throughout therapy.
• Patient and family state understanding of drug therapy.

epinastine hydrochloride
(eh-pin-AH-stein high-droh-KLOR-ighd)
Elestat

Pharmacologic class: histamine antagonist and mast cell stabilizer
Therapeutic class: ophthalmic antihistamine
Pregnancy risk category: C

Indications and dosages
▶ **To prevent itching in allergic conjunctivitis.** *Adults and children age 3 and older:* Instill 1 drop into each eye twice daily. Continue drug as long as allergen is present, even if patient has no symptoms.

Contraindications and cautions
• Contraindicated in patients hypersensitive to the drug or any of its components.
⚠ **Lifespan:** In pregnant women, use cautiously. In breast-feeding women, use cautiously because it's unknown if the drug appears in breast milk. In children younger than age 3, safety and effectiveness haven't been established.

Adverse reactions
CNS: headache.
EENT: burning eyes, hyperemia, enlarged lymph nodes near eyes, pharyngitis, pruritus, rhinitis, sinusitis.
Respiratory: increased cough, upper respiratory tract infection.
Other: cold symptoms, infection.

Interactions
None reported.

Effects on lab test results
None reported.

Pharmacokinetics
Absorption: Immediate.
Distribution: 64% bound to proteins.
Metabolism: Less than 10% of drug.
Excretion: Mainly unchanged in urine. *Half-life:* About 12 hours.

Route	Onset	Peak	Duration
Ophthalmic	Immediate	Unknown	8 hr

Action
Chemical effect: Inhibits release of mediators from cells involved in hypersensitivity reactions.
Therapeutic effect: Temporarily prevents eye itching.

Available forms
Ophthalmic solution: 0.05% in 5-and 10-ml bottles

NURSING PROCESS

☑ **Assessment**
• Drug is for ophthalmic use only. Don't inject or give orally.
• Monitor patient for infection.
• Assess patient's and family's knowledge of drug therapy.

☑ **Nursing diagnoses**
• Ineffective health maintenance related to underlying condition
• Risk for infection related to adverse effects of drug
• Deficient knowledge related to drug therapy

▷ **Planning and implementation**
• Don't use for contact lens–related eye irritation.
• Preservative in drug may be absorbed by soft contact lenses. If patient wears soft lenses, wait at least 10 minutes after instillation to have him insert his lenses.
Patient teaching
• Teach patient proper instillation technique. To avoid contaminating the drops, warn patient not

to touch the dropper tip to eyelids, skin around the eyes, or anything else.
• Caution patient not to use drops to treat contact lens–related eye irritation and not to wear contact lenses if eyes are red.
• Advise patient to report adverse reactions.
• Tell patient to keep bottle tightly closed when not in use.

☑ **Evaluation**
• Patient responds well to therapy.
• Patient remains free from infection during drug therapy.
• Patient and family state understanding of drug therapy.

epinephrine (adrenaline)
(eh-pih-NEF-rin)
**Adrenalin, Bronkaid Mistometer♦,
MicroNefrin†, Nephron†, Primatene Mist†**

epinephrine bitartrate
**AsthmaHaler Mist†, Bronitin Mist†,
Bronkaid Suspension Mist†**

epinephrine hydrochloride
**Adrenalin Chloride†, Ana-Guard, EpiPen
Auto-Injector, EpiPen Jr. Auto-Injector**

Pharmacologic class: adrenergic
Therapeutic class: bronchodilator, vasopressor, cardiac stimulant, topical antihemorrhagic
Pregnancy risk category: C

Indications and dosages
▶**Bronchospasm, hypersensitivity reactions, anaphylaxis.** *Adults:* 0.1 to 0.5 ml of 1:1,000 subcutaneously or I.M.; repeat q 10 to 15 minutes, p.r.n. Or 1 to 2.5 ml of 1:10,000 injection I.V. slowly over 5 to 10 minutes.
Children: 0.01 ml (10 mcg) of 1:1,000/kg subcutaneously; repeat q 20 minutes to 4 hours, p.r.n.
▶**Hemostasis.** *Adults:* 1:50,000 to 1:1,000 applied topically.
▶**Acute asthma attacks.** *Adults and children age 4 and older:* 160 to 250 mcg (metered aerosol), which is equivalent to one inhalation, repeat once if needed after at least 1 minute; don't give subsequent doses for at least 3 hours. Or give 1% (1:100) solution of epinephrine or

2.25% solution of racepinephrine by hand-bulb nebulizer as one to three deep inhalations; repeat q 3 hours, p.r.n.
▶**Prolonging local anesthetic effect.** *Adults and children:* Mix 1:500,000 to 1:50,000 with local anesthetic.
▶**Restoring cardiac rhythm in cardiac arrest.** *Adults:* 1 to 10 ml of 1:10,000 solution by slow I.V., q 3 to 5 minutes, as needed. Or 2 to 25 ml with 10 ml normal saline solution or D₅W for injection via endotracheal tube. If no I.V. route or intratracheal route is available, give drug intracardiac. Intracardiac dose is 0.3 to 0.5 mg (1:10,000 solution). Up to 5 mg may be given, especially in patients who don't respond to usual I.V. dose. After initial I.V. bolus administration, drug may be infused I.V. at 1 to 4 mcg/minute.
Children: 10 mcg/kg I.V., or 5 to 10 mcg (0.05 to 0.1 ml of 1:10,000)/kg intracardiac.

▼I.V. administration
• Use D₅W, normal saline injection, lactated Ringer's injection, or combinations of dextrose in sodium chloride. Mix just before use.
• Give 1:10,000 dilution prepared by diluting 1 ml of commercially available 1:1,000 injection with 10 ml of water for injection or normal saline injection.
• In emergency situations, epinephrine hydrochloride may be injected slowly as a dilute solution or infused slowly I.V. Injection can be repeated in 5 to 10 minutes, as needed. Dosages in emergencies are controversial; some researchers may use higher than usual dosages for cardiac resuscitation.
• Follow peripheral administration with a 20-ml flush, and elevate the site for 10 to 20 seconds to ensure delivery to the central circulation.
• Discard solution after 24 hours or if solution is discolored or contains precipitate. Keep solution in light-resistant container, and don't remove before use.
⊗ **Incompatibilities**
Aminophylline; ampicillin sodium; cephapirin; furosemide; Ionosol D-CM, PSL, and T solutions with D₅W; mephentermine. Rapidly destroyed by alkaline solutions or oxidizing drugs, including halogens, nitrates, nitrites, permanganates, sodium bicarbonate, and salts of easily reducible metals, such as iron, copper, and zinc.

E

Contraindications and cautions

• Contraindicated in patients with angle-closure glaucoma, shock (other than anaphylactic shock), organic brain damage, cardiac dilation, arrhythmias, coronary insufficiency, or cerebral arteriosclerosis. Also contraindicated in patients receiving general anesthesia with halogenated hydrocarbons or cyclopropane and in patients in labor (may delay second stage).

• Some commercial products contain sulfites and are contraindicated in patients with sulfite allergies except when drug is used for serious allergic reactions or in other emergency situations.

• In conjunction with local anesthetics, epinephrine is contraindicated for use in fingers, toes, ears, nose, or genitalia.

• Use cautiously in patients with long-standing bronchial asthma or emphysema who have developed degenerative heart disease and in those with hyperthyroidism, CV disease, hypertension, psychoneurosis, or diabetes.

⚠ **Lifespan:** In pregnant women in labor, drug is contraindicated. In pregnant women not in labor, in children, and in elderly patients, use cautiously. In breast-feeding women, stop breast-feeding or don't use the drug.

Adverse reactions

CNS: *nervousness, tremors,* euphoria, anxiety, cold limbs, vertigo, *headache, drowsiness,* diaphoresis, disorientation, agitation, fear, weakness, ***cerebral hemorrhage,*** increased rigidity and tremors in patients with Parkinson's disease, ***stroke.***
CV: *palpitations,* widened pulse pressure, *hypertension, tachycardia,* ***ventricular fibrillation, shock,*** anginal pain, ECG changes.
GI: nausea, vomiting.
Metabolic: hyperglycemia, glycosuria.
Respiratory: dyspnea.
Skin: urticaria, pain.
Other: pallor, hemorrhage at injection site.

Interactions

Drug-drug. *Alpha blockers:* May cause hypotension from unopposed beta blocker effects. Monitor blood pressure.
Antihistamines, thyroid hormones: When given with sympathomimetics, may cause severe adverse cardiac effects. Avoid giving together.
Carteolol, nadolol, penbutolol, pindolol, propranolol, timolol: May cause an initial hyper-

tensive episode followed by bradycardia. Stop the beta blocker 3 days before anticipated epinephrine use. Monitor patient closely.
Digoxin, general anesthetics (halogenated hydrocarbons): May increase risk of ventricular arrhythmias. Monitor patient closely.
Doxapram, methylphenidate: May increase CNS stimulation or pressor effects. Monitor patient closely.
Ergot alkaloids: May increase vasoconstrictor activity. Monitor patient closely.
Guanadrel, guanethidine: May increase pressor effects of epinephrine. Monitor the patient closely.
Levodopa: May increase risk of cardiac arrhythmias. Monitor patient closely.
MAO inhibitors: May increase risk of hypertensive crisis. Don't use together.
Tricyclic antidepressants: May increase the pressor response and cause arrhythmias. Use cautiously.

Effects on lab test results

• May increase BUN, glucose, and lactic acid levels.

Pharmacokinetics

Absorption: Well absorbed after subcutaneous or I.M. injection. Rapidly absorbed after inhalation administration.
Distribution: Distributed widely throughout body.
Metabolism: Metabolized at sympathetic nerve endings, liver, and other tissues to inactive metabolites.
Excretion: Excreted in urine. *Half-life:* Unknown.

Route	Onset	Peak	Duration
I.V.	Immediate	≤ 5 min	1–4 hr
I.M.	Varies	Unknown	1–4 hr
SubQ	6–15 min	≤ 30 min	1–4 hr
Inhalation	3–5 min	Unknown	1–3 hr

Action

Chemical effect: Stimulates alpha and beta receptors in sympathetic nervous system.
Therapeutic effect: Relaxes bronchial smooth muscle, causes cardiac stimulation, relieves allergic signs and symptoms, helps stop local bleeding, and decreases pain sensation.

Reactions may be *common,* uncommon, ***life-threatening***, or COMMON AND LIFE-THREATENING.

Available forms

Aerosol inhaler: 220 mcg/metered spray†
Injection: 0.01 mg/ml (1:100,000), 0.1 mg/ml (1:10,000), 0.5 mg/ml (1:2,000), 1 mg/ml (1:1,000)
Nebulizer inhaler: 1% (1:100) ♦ †, 2.25% (rac-epinephrine) ◊ †
Parenteral: 5 mg/ml (1:200) parenteral suspension

NURSING PROCESS

⚗ Assessment
• Obtain history of patient's underlying condition before starting therapy; reassess regularly.
• When administering I.V., monitor blood pressure, heart rate, and ECG when therapy starts and frequently thereafter.
• Be alert for adverse reactions and drug interactions.
• Assess patient's and family's knowledge of drug therapy.

Nursing diagnoses
• Ineffective health maintenance related to underlying condition
• Decreased cardiac output related to drug-induced adverse CV effects
• Deficient knowledge related to drug therapy

Planning and implementation
ⓈALERT: 1 mg of epinephrine is equal to 1 ml of 1:1,000 or 10 ml of 1:10,000.
• Epinephrine is drug of choice in emergency treatment of anaphylactic reaction.
• Avoid I.M. administration of parenteral suspension into buttocks. Gas gangrene may occur because epinephrine reduces oxygen tension of tissues, encouraging growth of contaminating organisms.
• Massage site after I.M. injection to counteract vasoconstriction. Repeated local injection can cause necrosis, resulting from vasoconstriction at injection site.
• Wait 2 minutes between bronchodilator inhalations. Always give bronchodilator first and wait 5 minutes before giving a different inhalant. Don't give patient more than 12 bronchodilator inhalations in 24 hours.
• Giving drug on time is important.
• If adverse reactions develop, notify prescriber, and adjust dosage or stop the drug. If patient's

pulse increases by 20% or more when drug is given, notify prescriber.
• If blood pressure rises sharply, rapid-acting vasodilators, such as nitrites or alpha blockers, can be given to counteract marked pressor effect of large doses of epinephrine.

Patient teaching
• Tell patient to take drug exactly as prescribed and to take it around the clock.
• Teach patient to perform oral inhalation correctly. Give the following instructions for using metered-dose inhaler:
1. Clear nasal passages and throat.
2. Breathe out, expelling as much air from lungs as possible.
3. Place mouthpiece 1 inch in front of mouth, and inhale deeply as dose from inhaler is released.
4. Hold breath for several seconds, remove mouthpiece, and exhale slowly.
• Tell patient to wait at least 2 minutes between inhalations.
• Tell patient who also is using corticosteroid inhaler to use bronchodilator first, then wait about 5 minutes before using corticosteroid. This allows bronchodilator to open air passages for maximum effectiveness.
• Instruct patient who has acute hypersensitivity reactions, such as to bee stings, to self-inject epinephrine at home.
• Tell patient to reduce intake of foods containing caffeine, such as coffee, colas, and chocolates, when taking bronchodilator.
• Instruct patient to contact prescriber immediately if he experiences fluttering of heart, rapid beating of heart, shortness of breath, or chest pain.
• Tell patient to obtain approval from prescriber before taking OTC medicines or herbal remedies.
• Show patient how to check pulse. Instruct him to check pulse before and after using bronchodilator and to call prescriber if pulse rate increases by more than 20 beats/minute.

☑ Evaluation
• Patient shows improvement in underlying condition.
• Patient maintains adequate cardiac output throughout therapy.
• Patient and family state understanding of drug therapy.

epirubicin hydrochloride
(ep-uh-ROO-bih-sin high-droh-KLOR-ighd)
Ellence

Pharmacologic class: anthracycline
Therapeutic class: antineoplastic
Pregnancy risk category: D

Indications and dosages

▶ **Adjuvant therapy for breast cancer with lymph node metastasis after resection.**
Adults: 100 to 120 mg/m² I.V. infusion over 3 to 5 minutes via a free-flowing I.V. solution on day 1 of each cycle q 3 to 4 weeks; or divided equally in two doses on days 1 and 8 of each cycle. Maximum cumulative (lifetime) dosage is 900 mg/m².

⊠ **Adjust-a-dose:** Dosage change after the first cycle is based on toxicity. For patient with platelet count below 50,000/mm³, absolute neutrophil count (ANC) below 250/mm³, neutropenic fever, or grade 3 or 4 nonhematologic toxicity, reduce day 1 dose in subsequent cycles to 75% of the day 1 dose in the current cycle. Delay day 1 therapy in subsequent cycles until platelet count is 100,000/mm³ or above, ANC is 1,500/mm³ or above, and nonhematologic toxicities recover to grade 1.

For patients receiving divided doses (days 1 and 8), give 75% of the day 1 dose on day 8 if platelet count is 75,000 to 100,000/mm³ and ANC is 1,000 to 1,499/mm³. If day 8 platelet count is below 75,000/mm³, ANC is below 1,000/mm³, or grade 3 or 4 nonhematologic toxicity occurs, skip the day 8 dose.

In patients with bone marrow impairment, start dose at 75 to 90 mg/m². Give lower dosages to patients with hepatic or severe renal impairment.

▼ I.V. administration

● Drug is a vesicant. Never give I.M. or subcutaneously. Always give through free-flowing I.V. solution of normal saline solution or D₅W over 3 to 5 minutes.
● Give prophylactic antibiotic therapy with trimethoprim and sulfamethoxazole or a fluoroquinolone to patients receiving 120 mg/m² dose.
● Give antiemetics before giving drug to reduce nausea and vomiting.

● Avoid veins over joints or in limbs with compromised venous or lymphatic drainage.
● If burning or stinging occurs, immediately stop infusion and restart in another vein.
● Facial flushing and local erythematous streaking along the vein may indicate too-rapid administration.
● Discard unused solution in vial 24 hours after vial is penetrated.
⊗ **Incompatibilities**
Fluorouracil, heparin, other I.V. drugs.

Contraindications and cautions

● Contraindicated in patients hypersensitive to the drug or any of its components, other anthracyclines, or anthracenediones. Also contraindicated in patients with baseline neutrophil counts below 1,500/mm³, in those with severe myocardial insufficiency or recent MI, in those previously treated with anthracyclines to total cumulative dosages, and in those with severe hepatic dysfunction.
● Use cautiously in patients with active or dormant cardiac disease, previous or simultaneous radiotherapy to the mediastinal and pericardial area, or previous therapy with other anthracyclines or anthracenediones. Also use cautiously with other cardiotoxic drugs.
🜹 **Lifespan:** In pregnant and breast-feeding women, drug is contraindicated. In children, safety and effectiveness haven't been established. In elderly patients, especially women older than age 70, use cautiously because of greater chance of toxicity.

Adverse reactions

CNS: *lethargy,* fever.
CV: ***cardiomyopathy, heart failure.***
EENT: *conjunctivitis, keratitis.*
GI: *nausea, vomiting, diarrhea,* anorexia, *mucositis.*
GU: *amenorrhea.*
Hematologic: LEUKOPENIA, NEUTROPENIA, *anemia,* THROMBOCYTOPENIA.
Skin: *alopecia,* rash, itch, skin changes.
Other: *infection, local toxicity, hot flushes.*

Interactions

Drug-drug. *Calcium channel blockers, other cardioactive compounds:* May increase risk of heart failure. Monitor cardiac function closely.

Reactions may be *common,* uncommon, *life-threatening,* or COMMON AND LIFE-THREATENING.

Cimetidine: May increase epirubicin level (by 50%) and decrease clearance. Avoid use together.
Cytotoxic drugs: May result in additive toxicities (especially hematologic and GI). Monitor patient closely.
Radiation therapy: May enhance effects. Monitor patient carefully.

Effects on lab test results

- May decrease hemoglobin level and hematocrit.
- May decrease WBC, neutrophil, and platelet counts.

Pharmacokinetics

Absorption: Administered I.V.
Distribution: Rapid and widely distributed into tissues. Protein-binding is about 77%, mainly to albumin, and appears to concentrate in RBCs.
Metabolism: Extensive and rapid.
Excretion: Mostly biliary. *Half-life:* 31 to 35 hours.

Route	Onset	Peak	Duration
I.V.	Unknown	Unknown	Unknown

Action

Chemical effect: The precise mechanism of drug's cytotoxic effects isn't completely known. It's thought to form a complex with DNA by intercalation between nucleotide base pairs, thereby inhibiting DNA, RNA, and protein synthesis, resulting in cytocidal activity. Drug may also interfere with replication and transcription of DNA.
Therapeutic effect: Kills certain cancer cells.

Available forms

Injection: 2 mg/ml

NURSING PROCESS

Assessment

- Obtain baseline total bilirubin, AST, creatinine, and CBC (including ANC). Evaluate cardiac function by obtaining an ECG and measuring left ventricular ejection fraction (LVEF) before therapy.
- Monitor LVEF regularly during therapy, and stop drug at first sign of cardiac impairment. Monitor patient for early signs of cardiac toxicity, including sinus tachycardia, ECG abnormalities, tachyarrhythmias, bradycardia, AV block, and bundle branch block.
- Obtain total and differential WBC, RBC, and platelet counts before and during each therapy cycle.
- Assess patient's and family's knowledge of drug therapy.

Nursing diagnoses

- Risk for injury related to drug-induced adverse reactions
- Risk for infection related to myelosuppression
- Deficient knowledge related to drug therapy

Planning and implementation

- Give drug under supervision of a prescriber experienced in the use of cancer chemotherapy.
- Wear protective clothing (goggles, gown, disposable gloves) when handling this drug. Pregnant health care providers shouldn't handle this drug because of risks to fetus.
- Cardiac toxicity may occur 2 to 3 months after stopping drug, causing reduced LVEF, evidence of heart failure (tachycardia, dyspnea, pulmonary edema, dependent edema, hepatomegaly, ascites, pleural effusion, and gallop rhythm). Delayed cardiac toxicity depends on the cumulative dosage of epirubicin. Don't exceed a cumulative dose of 900 mg/m^2.
- Monitor uric acid, potassium, calcium phosphate, and creatinine levels immediately after initial chemotherapy in patients susceptible to tumor lysis syndrome. Hydration, urine alkalinization, and prophylaxis with allopurinol may prevent hyperuricemia and minimize complications of tumor lysis syndrome.
- Lowest WBC count usually occurs 10 to 14 days after drug administration and returns to normal by day 21.
- Anthracycline-induced leukemia may occur.
- Administration of drug after previous radiation therapy may induce an inflammatory cell reaction at the site of irradiation.

ALERT: Don't confuse epirubicin with other anthracyclines, such as daunorubicin, doxorubicin, or idarubicin.

Patient teaching

- Advise patient to report nausea, vomiting, stomatitis, dehydration, fever, evidence of infection, symptoms of heart failure (tachycardia, dyspnea, edema), or injection-site pain.
- Inform patient of the risk of cardiac damage and drug-related leukemia.

• Tell women of childbearing age not to become pregnant. Tell men to use effective contraception.
• Advise women that irreversible amenorrhea or premature menopause may occur.
• Advise patient about probable hair loss. Tell patient that hair usually regrows 2 to 3 months after therapy is stopped.
• Advise patient that urine may appear red 1 to 2 days after administration of the drug.

✓ Evaluation
• Patient sustains no injury from drug-induced adverse reactions.
• Patient remains free of infection.
• Patient and family state understanding of drug therapy.

eplerenone
(eh-PLAIR-eh-nown)
Inspra

Pharmacologic class: aldosterone receptor antagonist
Therapeutic class: antihypertensive
Pregnancy risk category: B

Indications and dosages

▶ **Heart failure post-MI.** *Adults:* Initially 25 mg P.O. daily or every other day. Increase to 50 mg P.O. daily if needed within 4 weeks, according to potassium level.
⑤ **Adjust-a-dose:** In patients with potassium level less than 5 mEq/L, increase dosage from 25 mg every other day to 25 mg daily, or increase dosage from 25 mg daily to 50 mg daily. For potassium level of 5 to 5.4 mEq/L, no dosage adjustment needed. For potassium level of 5.5 to 5.9 mEq/L, decrease dosage from 50 mg daily to 25 mg daily, or decrease dosage from 25 mg daily to 25 mg every other day; or if dosage was 25 mg every other day, withhold drug. For potassium level greater than 6 mEq/L, withhold drug. May restart drug at 25 mg every other day when potassium level is less than 5.5 mEq/L.
▶ **Hypertension.** *Adults:* 50 mg P.O. once daily. If response is inadequate after 4 weeks, increase dosage to 50 mg P.O. b.i.d. Maximum, 100 mg daily.

⑤ **Adjust-a-dose:** For either indication, patients who are also receiving a weak CYP 3A4 inhibitor (such as erythromycin, verapamil, fluconazole) need a reduced starting dose of 25 mg P.O. daily.

Contraindications and cautions

• Contraindicated in patients with potassium level greater than 5.5 mEq/L at start of treatment, type 2 diabetes with microalbuminuria, serum creatinine level greater than 2 mg/dl in men or greater than 1.8 mg/dl in women, or creatinine clearance less than 30 ml/minute (less than 50 ml/minute if patient is being treated for high blood pressure). Also contraindicated in patients treated simultaneously with potassium supplements, potassium-sparing diuretics (amiloride, spironolactone, or triamterene), or strong CYP 3A4 inhibitors, such as ketoconazole, itraconazole, clarithromycin, nefazodone, nelfinavir, and ritonavir.
• Use cautiously in patients with mild to moderate hepatic impairment.
☀ **Lifespan:** In pregnant women, use only if the benefits outweigh risks to the fetus. In breast-feeding women, use cautiously because it's unknown whether drug appears in breast milk. In children, safety and effectiveness haven't been established.

Adverse reactions

CNS: dizziness, fatigue.
GI: diarrhea, abdominal pain.
GU: albuminuria, abnormal vaginal bleeding.
Metabolic: *hyperkalemia.*
Respiratory: cough.
Other: flulike syndrome, gynecomastia.

Interactions

Drug-drug. *ACE inhibitors, angiotensin II receptor antagonists:* May increase risk of hyperkalemia. Use together cautiously.
Lithium: May increase risk of lithium toxicity. Monitor lithium level.
NSAIDs: May reduce the antihypertensive effect and cause severe hyperkalemia in patients with renal impairment. Monitor blood pressure and potassium level.
Potassium supplements, potassium-sparing diuretics (amiloride, spironolactone, triamterene): May increase risk of hyperkalemia and sometimes fatal arrhythmias. Avoid use together.

Strong CYP 3A4 inhibitors (clarithromycin, itraconazole, ketoconazole, nefazodone, nelfinavir, ritonavir, troleandomycin): May increase eplerenone level. Avoid use together.

Weak CYP 3A4 inhibitors (erythromycin, fluconazole, saquinavir, verapamil): May increase eplerenone level. Reduce eplerenone starting dose to 25 mg P.O. once daily.

Drug-herb. *St. John's wort:* May decrease eplerenone level over time. Discourage use together.

Effects on lab test results

• May increase potassium, creatinine, BUN, triglyceride, cholesterol, ALT, and GGT levels. May decrease sodium level.

Pharmacokinetics

Absorption: Bioavailability of drug is unknown.
Distribution: Protein binding is about 50%.
Metabolism: Predominantly by CYP 3A4 pathway.
Excretion: Primarily in urine. *Half-life:* 4 to 6 hours.

Route	Onset	Peak	Duration
P.O.	Unknown	1½ hr	Unknown

Action

Chemical effect: Binds to mineralocorticoid receptors and blocks aldosterone. Aldosterone may increase blood pressure through induction of sodium reabsorption and other mechanisms.
Therapeutic effect: Lowers blood pressure.

Available forms

Tablets: 25 mg, 50 mg, 100 mg

NURSING PROCESS

Assessment
• Obtain history of patient's underlying condition before starting therapy.
• Obtain patient's baseline blood pressure and potassium levels and reassess regularly.
• Assess patient's and family's knowledge of drug therapy.

Nursing diagnoses
• Risk for ineffective health maintenance related to hypertension

• Risk for injury related to the presence of hypertension
• Deficient knowledge related to drug therapy

Planning and implementation
• Drug may be used alone or with other antihypertensives.
• The drug's full therapeutic effect occurs within 4 weeks.
• Monitor patient for signs and symptoms of hyperkalemia.
• Overdose may cause hypotension and hyperkalemia. Treat symptoms and provide support. Drug binds extensively to charcoal but can't be removed by hemodialysis.
ALERT: Don't confuse Inspra (eplerenone) with Spiriva (tiotropium bromide).

Patient teaching
• Tell patient drug can be taken with or without food.
• Advise patient to avoid potassium supplements and salt substitutes.
• Tell patient to report adverse reactions.

Evaluation
• Patient's blood pressure remains within normal limits.
• Patient's potassium remains within normal limits.
• Patient and family state understanding of drug therapy.

epoetin alfa (erythropoietin)
(ee-POH-eh-tin AL-fah)
Epogen, Eprex◇, Procrit

Pharmacologic class: glycoprotein
Therapeutic class: hematopoietic
Pregnancy risk category: C

Indications and dosages

▶ **Anemia caused by chronic renal disease.**
Adults: Starting dosage is 50 to 100 units/kg I.V. or subcutaneously three times weekly. Maintenance dosage is highly individualized.
Infants and children ages 1 month to 16 years who are on dialysis: 50 units/kg I.V. or subcutaneously three times weekly. Maintenance dosage is highly individualized to keep hemoglobin level in target range.

◩ **Adjust-a-dose:** When target hemoglobin level approaches 12 g/dl or if it rises more than 1 g/dl in any 2-week period, reduce dosage. If hemoglobin level doesn't increase by 2 g/dl after 8 weeks of therapy and is below the target range, increase dosage.

▶ **Anemia from zidovudine therapy in HIV-infected patients.** *Adults:* 100 units/kg I.V. or subcutaneously three times weekly for 8 weeks or until target hemoglobin level is reached. If response isn't satisfactory after 8 weeks, increase dosage by 50 to 100 units/kg I.V. or subcutaneously three times weekly. After 4 to 8 weeks, further increase dosage in increments of 50 to 100 units/kg three times weekly, up to a maximum of 300 units/kg three times weekly. *Infants and children ages 8 months to 17 years‡:* 50 to 400 units/kg subcutaneously or I.V. two to three times weekly.

▶ **Anemia from cancer chemotherapy.** *Adults:* 150 units/kg subcutaneously three times weekly for 8 weeks or until target hemoglobin level is reached. If response isn't satisfactory after 8 weeks, increase dosage up to 300 units/kg subcutaneously three times weekly. Or 40,000 units subcutaneously once weekly. If hemoglobin level hasn't increased by at least 1 g/dl in the absence of RBC transfusion, increase dose to 60,000 units weekly. *Infants and children ages 6 months to 18 years‡:* 25 to 300 units/kg subcutaneously or I.V. three to seven times weekly.

◩ **Adjust-a-dose:** Withhold drug if hemoglobin level exceeds 13 g/dl. Reduce dose by 25% and resume therapy when hemoglobin level is less than 12 g/dl. If hemoglobin level increases by more than 1 g/dl in any 2-week period, reduce dose by 25%.

▶ **To reduce need for allogenic blood transfusion in anemic patients undergoing elective, noncardiac, nonvascular surgery.** *Adults:* 300 units/kg subcutaneously once daily for 10 days before surgery, on the day of surgery, and for 4 days after surgery. Or 600 units/kg subcutaneously in once-weekly doses (21, 14, and 7 days before surgery), plus a fourth dose on day of surgery.

▶ **Anemia related to rheumatoid arthritis and rheumatic disease‡.** *Adults:* 50 to 200 units/kg subcutaneously three times weekly.

▶ **Anemia related to prematurity‡.** *Neonates:* 25 to 100 units/kg subcutaneously three times weekly.

▼ I.V. administration

● Don't shake.
● Give drug by direct injection without dilution.
● If patient is having dialysis, drug may be given into venous return line after dialysis session. To keep drug from adhering to tubing, inject drug with blood still in the line; then flush with normal saline solution.

⊗ **Incompatibilities**
Other I.V. drugs.

Contraindications and cautions

● Contraindicated in patients with uncontrolled hypertension and in patients with hypersensitivity to mammal-cell–derived products or albumin.

⚯ **Lifespan:** In pregnant women, use cautiously. In breast-feeding women, use cautiously because it's unknown if the drug appears in breast milk. In children younger than age 1 month, safety and effectiveness haven't been established.

Adverse reactions

CNS: headache, *seizures,* paresthesia, fatigue, fever, dizziness, asthenia.
CV: increased clotting of arteriovenous grafts, *hypertension, edema.*
GI: nausea, vomiting, diarrhea, abdominal pain and constipation in children.
Hematologic: iron deficiency, thrombocytosis.
Metabolic: hyperuricemia, *hyperkalemia,* hyperphosphatemia.
Musculoskeletal: *arthralgia.*
Respiratory: cough, shortness of breath.
Skin: *rash,* urticaria.
Other: injection-site reaction.

Interactions

None significant.

Effects on lab test results

● May increase BUN, creatinine, uric acid, potassium, phosphate, and hemoglobin levels and hematocrit.
● May increase platelet count.

Pharmacokinetics

Absorption: After subcutaneous administration, systemic absorption is delayed, incomplete, and variable compared with I.V. administration.
Distribution: Unknown.

Reactions may be *common,* uncommon, *life-threatening,* or COMMON AND LIFE-THREATENING.

Metabolism: Unknown.
Excretion: Unknown. *Half-life:* 4 to 13 hours.

Route	Onset	Peak	Duration
I.V.	1 wk	Immediate	Unknown
SubQ	1–6 wk	5–24 hr	Unknown

Action

Chemical effect: Mimics effects of erythropoietin, a naturally occurring hormone produced by the kidneys. It functions as both growth and differentiating factors, enhancing the rate of RBC production.
Therapeutic effect: Corrects anemia.

Available forms

Injection: 2,000 units/ml, 3,000 units/ml, 4,000 units/ml, 10,000 units/ml, 20,000 units/ ml, 40,000 units/ml

NURSING PROCESS

Assessment
• Assess patient's CBC and blood pressure before starting therapy.
• Assess effectiveness by monitoring CBC results. Suggested target hemoglobin range is 10 to 12 g/dl. Hematocrit may rise and cause excessive clotting. Watch for evidence of blood clot formation, such as shortness of breath and cold, swollen, or pulseless limb.
• Patient's response depends on amount of endogenous erythropoietin. Patients with 500 units/L or more usually have transfusion-dependent anemia and probably won't respond to drug. Those with levels below 500 units/L usually respond well.
• Before and during therapy, monitor patient's serum iron level. Most patients will require supplemental iron to support erythropoiesis.
• Monitor blood pressure closely. Up to 80% of patients with chronic renal impairment have hypertension. Blood pressure may rise, especially when hematocrit is increasing in early part of therapy.
• After injection (usually within 2 hours), some patients complain of pain or discomfort in their limbs (long bones) and pelvis and of coldness and sweating. Symptoms may persist for up to 12 hours and then disappear.
• If adverse GI reaction occurs, monitor patient's hydration.

• Assess patient's and family's knowledge of drug therapy.

Nursing diagnoses
• Ineffective protection related to reduced production of endogenous erythropoietin
• Risk for deficient fluid volume related to drug-induced adverse GI reactions
• Deficient knowledge related to drug therapy

Planning and implementation
• When used in an HIV-infected patient, individualize the dose based on the response. Dosage recommendations are for patients with endogenous erythropoietin levels of 500 units/L or less and cumulative zidovudine doses of 4.2 g per week or less.
• Patient may need additional heparin to prevent clotting during dialysis.
• Start diet restrictions or drug therapy to control blood pressure.
Patient teaching
• Advise patient that blood specimens will be drawn weekly for blood counts and that dose adjustments may be made based on results.
• Warn patient to avoid hazardous activities, such as driving or operating heavy machinery, early in therapy; excessively rapid rise in hematocrit may increase the risk of seizures.
• Tell patient to notify prescriber if adverse reactions occur.

Evaluation
• Patient's blood count is normal.
• Patient maintains adequate hydration throughout therapy.
• Patient and family state understanding of drug therapy.

eprosartan mesylate
(eh-proh-SAR-ten MEH-sih-layt)
Teveten

Pharmacologic class: angiotensin II receptor antagonist
Therapeutic class: antihypertensive
Pregnancy risk category: C (D in second and third trimesters)

Indications and dosages

▶ **Hypertension.** *Adults:* Initially 600 mg P.O. daily. Daily dosage ranges from 400 to 800 mg given as single daily dose or two divided doses. Drug can be given alone or with other antihypertensives.

Contraindications and cautions

• Contraindicated in patients hypersensitive to drug or any of its components.
• Use cautiously in patients with an activated renin-angiotensin system, such as volume- or salt-depleted patients, and in patients whose renal function may depend on the activity of the renin-angiotensin-aldosterone system, such as patients with severe heart failure. Use cautiously in patients with renal artery stenosis.
⚜ **Lifespan:** In pregnant and breast-feeding women, drug is contraindicated. In children, safety and effectiveness haven't been established. In elderly patients, use cautiously because of decreased response to drug.

Adverse reactions

CNS: depression, fatigue, headache, dizziness.
CV: chest pain, dependent edema, hypertriglyceridemia.
EENT: pharyngitis, rhinitis, sinusitis.
GI: abdominal pain, dyspepsia, diarrhea.
GU: UTI.
Hematologic: *neutropenia.*
Musculoskeletal: arthralgia, myalgia.
Respiratory: cough, upper respiratory tract infection, bronchitis.
Other: injury, viral infection.

Interactions

None significant.

Effects on lab test results

• May increase BUN and triglyceride levels. May decrease hemoglobin level and hematocrit.
• May decrease neutrophil count.

Pharmacokinetics

Absorption: Absolute bioavailability of single oral dose is about 13%.
Distribution: Protein-binding is about 98%.
Metabolism: No active metabolites.
Excretion: Eliminated by biliary and renal excretion. *Half-life:* 5 to 9 hours.

Route	Onset	Peak	Duration
P.O.	1–2 hr	1–3 hr	24 hr

Action

Chemical effect: Blocks vasoconstrictor and aldosterone-secreting effects of angiotensin II by selectively blocking binding of angiotensin II to its receptor sites in many tissues, such as vascular smooth muscle and the adrenal gland.
Therapeutic effect: Lowers blood pressure.

Available forms

Tablets: 400 mg, 600 mg

NURSING PROCESS

⚗ Assessment
• Monitor blood pressure closely at start of therapy. If hypotension occurs, place patient in supine position and give normal saline solution I.V.
• Determine patient's fluid balance and sodium level before starting drug therapy.
• In elderly patients, watch for a slightly decreased response to drug.
• Be alert for adverse reactions.
• Assess patient's and family's knowledge of drug therapy.

⊕ Nursing diagnoses
• Risk for injury related to presence of hypertension
• Risk for infection related to neutropenia
• Deficient knowledge related to drug therapy

▷ Planning and implementation
• Correct hypovolemia and hyponatremia before starting therapy to reduce risk of symptomatic hypotension.
• A transient episode of hypotension isn't cause for stopping therapy altogether. Restart once patient's blood pressure is stabilized.
• Drug may be used alone or with other antihypertensives, such as diuretics and calcium channel blockers. Maximum blood pressure response may take 2 to 3 weeks.
• Monitor patient for facial or lip swelling because angioedema has occurred with other angiotensin II antagonists.
Patient teaching
• Advise woman of childbearing age to use reliable form of contraception and to notify pre-

scriber immediately if pregnancy is suspected. Stop drug under medical supervision.

• Advise patient to report facial or lip swelling and signs and symptoms of infection, such as fever or sore throat.

• Tell patient to notify prescriber before taking OTC product to treat a dry cough.

• Inform patient that drug may be taken without regard to meals.

• Tell patient to store drug at a controlled room temperature (68° to 77° F [20° to 25° C]).

☑ **Evaluation**
• Patient's blood pressure is well controlled, and patient remains free of injury.
• WBC count is normal.
• Patient and family state understanding of drug therapy.

eptifibatide
(ep-tih-FY-beh-tide)
Integrilin

Pharmacologic class: glycoprotein IIb/IIIa inhibitor
Therapeutic class: antiplatelet
Pregnancy risk category: B

Indications and dosages

▶ **Acute coronary syndrome (unstable angina or non–ST segment elevation MI) in patients with serum creatinine level below 2 mg/dl, being managed medically and in those undergoing percutaneous coronary intervention (PCI).** *Adults:* 180 mcg/kg I.V. bolus as soon as possible after diagnosis, followed by a continuous I.V. infusion of 2 mcg/kg per minute until hospital discharge or start of coronary artery bypass graft surgery, up to 72 hours. If undergoing PCI, continue infusion until hospital discharge, or for up to 18 to 24 hours after the procedure, whichever comes first, up to 96 hours. Give patients weighing more than 121 kg (267 lb) a maximum bolus of 22.6 mg followed by a maximum infusion rate of 15 mg/hour.
◎ **Adjust-a-dose:** For adults with creatinine clearance less than 50 ml/minute or a creatinine level between 2 and 4 mg/dl, give 180 mcg/kg I.V. bolus as soon as possible after diagnosis, followed by an infusion rate of 1 mcg/kg per minute. For patients weighing more than 121 kg

(267 lb), the maximum bolus dose is 22.6 mg and the maximum infusion rate is 7.5 mg/hour.
▶ **Patients with serum creatinine level below 2 mg/dl, undergoing PCI.** *Adults:* 180 mcg/kg I.V. bolus given immediately before the procedure, immediately followed by an infusion of 2 mcg/kg/minute and a second I.V. bolus of 180 mcg/kg given 10 minutes after the first bolus. Continue infusion until hospital discharge or for up to 18 to 24 hours, whichever comes first; a minimum of 12 hours of eptifibatide infusion is recommended. Give patients weighing more than 121 kg a maximum bolus of 22.6 mg followed by a maximum of 15 mg/hour.
◎ **Adjust-a-dose:** For adults with creatinine clearance less than 50 ml/minute or a creatinine level between 2 and 4 mg/dl, give 180 mcg/kg immediately before the procedure, immediately followed by an infusion of 1 mcg/kg per minute and a second bolus of 180 mcg/kg given 10 minutes after the first bolus. Give patients weighing more than 121 kg a maximum of 22.6 mg/bolus followed by a maximum rate of 7.5 mg/hour.

▼ I.V. administration

• Drug is intended for use with heparin and aspirin.
• Inspect solution for particulate matter before use. If particles are visible, the sterility is suspect. Discard the solution.
• Drug may be given in same I.V. line with normal saline solution or normal saline and 5% dextrose; main infusion may also contain up to 60 mEq/L of potassium chloride.
• Drug may be given in same I.V. line as alteplase, atropine, dobutamine, heparin, lidocaine, meperidine, metoprolol, midazolam, morphine, nitroglycerin, or verapamil.
• When obtaining I.V. access, avoid use of noncompressible sites (such as subclavian or jugular veins).
• Withdraw bolus dose from 10-ml vial into a syringe and give by I.V. push over 1 to 2 minutes. Give I.V. infusion undiluted directly from 100-ml vial using an infusion pump.
• If patient requires thrombolytic therapy, stop infusion.
• Refrigerate vials at 36° to 46° F (2° to 8° C). Protect from light until administration.
⊗ **Incompatibilities**
Furosemide.

Contraindications and cautions

• Contraindicated in patients hypersensitive to drug or any of its components and in those with a history of bleeding diathesis, evidence of active abnormal bleeding within previous 30 days, severe hypertension (systolic blood pressure over 200 mm Hg or diastolic blood pressure over 110 mm Hg) not adequately controlled with antihypertensives, major surgery within previous 6 weeks, history of stroke within 30 days, history of hemorrhagic stroke, current or planned use of another parenteral GP IIb/IIIa inhibitor, or platelet count below 100,000/mm^3. Also contraindicated in patients whose creatinine level is 2 mg/dl or higher (for the 180-mcg/kg bolus and 2-mcg/kg/minute infusion) or 4 mg/dl or higher (for the 135-mcg/kg bolus and 0.5-mcg/kg/minute infusion) and in patients dependent on dialysis.

☆ Lifespan: In pregnant women, use cautiously. In breast-feeding women, use cautiously because it's unknown if the drug appears in breast milk. In children, safety and effectiveness haven't been established.

Adverse reactions

CV: hypotension.
GU: hematuria.
Hematologic: BLEEDING, *thrombocytopenia*.
Other: bleeding at femoral artery access site.

Interactions

Drug-drug. *Clopidogrel, dipyridamole, NSAIDs, warfarin, thrombolytics, ticlopidine:* May increase risk of bleeding. Monitor patient closely.
Other inhibitors of platelet receptor IIb/IIIa: May have potential for serious bleeding. Don't give together.

Effects on lab test results

• May decrease platelet count.

Pharmacokinetics

Absorption: Administered I.V.
Distribution: 25% bound to proteins.
Metabolism: None reported. No major metabolites are detected.
Excretion: 50% of drug is excreted in urine.
Half-life: 2½ hours.

Route	Onset	Peak	Duration
I.V.	Immediate	Immediate	4–6 hr after therapy

Action

Chemical effect: Reversibly binds to the glycoprotein IIb/IIIa receptor on human platelets and inhibits platelet aggregation.
Therapeutic effect: Prevents clot formation.

Available forms

Injection: 10-ml (2 mg/ml), 100-ml (0.75 mg/ml, 2 mg/ml) vials

NURSING PROCESS

⏱ Assessment

• Obtain history of patient's underlying medical conditions, especially conditions that put patient at risk for bleeding.
• Obtain accurate patient weight. Use drug cautiously in patients weighing more than 143 kg (315 lb).
• Determine creatinine and hemoglobin levels, hematocrit, platelet count, PT, INR, and PTT before start of therapy and regularly thereafter.
• Monitor patient for bleeding.
• Assess patient's and family's knowledge of drug therapy.

⊕ Nursing diagnoses

• Ineffective cardiopulmonary tissue perfusion related to presence of acute coronary syndrome
• Risk for injury related to increased bleeding tendencies
• Deficient knowledge related to drug therapy

▷ Planning and implementation

• Stop this drug and heparin, and achieve sheath hemostasis by standard compressive techniques at least 4 hours before hospital discharge.
• In patients undergoing coronary artery bypass graft surgery, stop infusion before surgery.
• Minimize use of arterial and venous punctures, I.M. injections, urinary catheters, and nasotracheal and nasogastric tubes.
• If platelet count is less than 100,000/mm^3, notify prescriber and stop both this drug and heparin.
Patient teaching
• Explain that drug is a blood thinner used to prevent heart attack.

E

- Explain that the benefits of the drug far outweigh the risk of serious bleeding.
- Instruct patient to report chest discomfort or other adverse events immediately.

☑ **Evaluation**
- Patient maintains adequate cardiopulmonary tissue perfusion.
- Patient has no life-threatening bleeding episode.
- Patient and family state understanding of drug therapy.

erlotinib
(ur-LOE-tie-nib)
Tarceva

Pharmacologic class: human epidermal growth factor receptor 1 (HER1)/epidermal growth factor receptor (EGFR)–tyrosine kinase inhibitor
Therapeutic class: antineoplastic
Pregnancy risk category: D

Indications and dosages

▶ **Locally advanced or metastatic non–small-cell lung cancer after failure of at least one other chemotherapeutic.** *Adults:* 150 mg P.O. once daily taken at least 1 hour before or 2 hours after meals. Continue until disease progresses or intolerable toxicity occurs.
⎯**Adjust-a-dose:** In patients with severe skin reactions or severe diarrhea refractory to loperamide, reduce dose in 50-mg decrements or stop therapy.

Contraindications and cautions

- Use cautiously in patients with pulmonary disease or liver impairment and those who have received or are receiving chemotherapy because it may worsen adverse pulmonary effects.
⚘ **Lifespan:** In pregnant women, use only if benefits outweigh risks to the fetus. If patient becomes pregnant during therapy, drug may harm fetus and increase risk of miscarriage. Women shouldn't breast-feed while taking this drug. In children, safety and effectiveness haven't been established.

Adverse reactions

CNS: *fatigue.*
EENT: *conjunctivitis, keratoconjuctivitis sicca.*

GI: abdominal pain, *anorexia, diarrhea, nausea,* stomatitis, *vomiting.*
Respiratory: cough, dyspnea, ***pulmonary toxicity.***
Skin: *dry skin,* pruritus, *rash, acne.*
Other: *infection.*

Interactions

Drug-drug. *Anticoagulants, such as warfarin:* May increase risk of bleeding. Monitor PT and INR.
Atazanavir, clarithromycin, indinavir, itraconazole, ketoconazole, nefazodone, nelfinavir, ritonavir, saquinavir, telithromycin, troleandomycin, voriconazole: May decrease erlotinib metabolism. Use together cautiously, and consider reducing erlotinib dosage.
Carbamazepine, phenobarbital, phenytoin, rifampicin, rifabutin: May increase erlotinib metabolism. Erlotinib dosage may need to be increased.
Drug-herb. *St. John's wort:* May increase erlotinib metabolism. Erlotinib dosage may need to be increased. Discourage use together.

Effects on lab test results

- May increase ALT, AST, and bilirubin levels.
- May increase PT and INR.

Pharmacokinetics

Absorption: About 60%.
Distribution: About 93% protein bound to albumin and alpha$_1$-acid glycoprotein.
Metabolism: Mainly by CYP 3A4 and partly by CYP 1A2 and CYP 1A1.
Excretion: 83% in feces. *Half-life:* 36 hours.

Route	Onset	Peak	Duration
P.O.	Unknown	4 hr	Unknown

Action

Chemical effect: Probably inhibits tyrosine kinase activity in EGFR, which is expressed on the surface of normal and cancer cells, and is particularly selective for HER1.
Therapeutic effect: Increases survival of patients with locally advanced or metastatic non–small-cell lung cancer.

Available forms

Tablets: 25 mg, 100 mg, 150 mg

NURSING PROCESS

⚕ Assessment
• Assess patient's underlying condition before drug therapy.
• Monitor liver function tests periodically during therapy. If values change dramatically, consider reducing dosage or stopping drug.
• Monitor patient for severe diarrhea, and give loperamide if needed.
• Assess patient's and family's knowledge of drug therapy.

✚ Nursing diagnoses
• Ineffective health maintenance related to presence of neoplastic disease
• Risk for deficient fluid volume related to drug-induced adverse GI reactions
• Deficient knowledge related to drug therapy

❯ Planning and implementation
• Rarely, serious interstitial lung disease may occur. If patient develops dyspnea, cough, or fever, withhold therapy. Stop drug if interstitial lung disease develops.
• Overdose may cause diarrhea, rash, and liver transaminase elevations. If overdose occurs, withhold drug and treat symptoms.

Patient teaching
• Tell woman of childbearing age to use contraception while taking this drug and for 2 weeks afterward.
• Tell patient to immediately report new or worsened cough, shortness of breath, eye irritation, or severe or persistent diarrhea, nausea, anorexia, or vomiting.
• Instruct patient to take drug 1 hour before or 2 hours after food.
• Explain the likelihood of serious interactions with other drugs and herbal supplements and the need to tell prescriber about any change in drugs and supplements taken.

✔ Evaluation
• Patient responds to drug therapy.
• Patient maintains adequate hydration.
• Patient and family state understanding of drug therapy.

ertapenem sodium
(ur-tah-PEN-uhm SOH-dee-um)
Invanz

Pharmacologic class: carbapenem
Therapeutic class: antibiotic
Pregnancy risk category: B

Indications and dosages

▶ **Complicated intraabdominal infections caused by *Escherichia coli, Clostridium clostridiiforme, Eubacterium lentum, Peptostreptococcus, Bacteroides fragilis, B. distasonis, B. ovatus, B. thetaiotaomicron, B. uniformis*.** *Adults and children age 13 and older:* 1 g I.V. or I.M. once daily for 5 to 14 days.
Infants and children age 3 months to 13 years: 15 mg/kg I.V. q 12 hours for 5 to 14 days. Don't exceed 1 g daily.
▶ **Complicated skin and skin-structure infections caused by *Staphylococcus aureus* (methicillin-susceptible strains), *Streptococcus pyogenes, E. coli, Peptostreptococcus* species.** *Adults and children age 13 and older:* 1 g I.V. or I.M. once daily for 7 to 14 days.
Infants and children age 3 months to 13 years: 15 mg/kg I.V. q 12 hours for 7 to 14 days. Don't exceed 1 g daily.
▶ **Community-acquired pneumonia caused by *Streptococcus pneumoniae* (penicillin-susceptible strains), *Haemophilus influenzae* (beta-lactamase–negative strains), *Moraxella catarrhalis*.** *Adults and children age 13 and older:* 1 g I.V. or I.M. once daily for 10 to 14 days. If improvement occurs after at least 3 days of therapy, appropriate oral therapy may be used to complete the full course of therapy.
Infants and children age 3 months to 13 years: 15 mg/kg I.V. q 12 hours for 10 to 14 days. Don't exceed 1 g daily. If patient improves after at least 3 days of treatment, use appropriate oral therapy to complete the full course of treatment.
▶ **Complicated UTI, including pyelonephritis, caused by *E. coli, Klebsiella pneumoniae*.** *Adults and children age 13 and older:* 1 g I.V. or I.M. once daily for 10 to 14 days. If improvement occurs after at least 3 days, appropriate oral therapy may be used to complete the full course of therapy.

Infants and children age 3 months to 13 years: 15 mg/kg I.V. q 12 hours for 10 to 14 days. Don't exceed 1 g daily. If patient improves after at least 3 days of treatment, use appropriate oral therapy to complete the full course of treatment.

► **Acute pelvic infections, including postpartum endomyometritis, septic abortion, and postsurgical gynecologic infections caused by *Streptococcus agalactiae, E. coli, B. fragilis, Porphyromonas asaccharolytica, Peptostreptococcus species, Prevotella bivia.*** *Adults and children age 13 and older:* 1 g I.V. or I.M. once daily for 3 to 10 days.

Infants and children age 3 months to 13 years: 15 mg/kg I.V. q 12 hours for 3 to 10 days. Don't exceed 1 g daily.

⧉ **Adjust-a-dose:** In adult patients, if creatinine clearance is 30 ml/minute or less, give 500 mg daily. A supplementary dose of 150 mg is recommended after a hemodialysis session only in patients who are given the recommended daily ertapenem dose of 500 mg within 6 hours before hemodialysis. If ertapenem is given 6 hours or more before hemodialysis, no supplementary dose is needed.

▼ I.V. administration

• Reconstitute the contents of a 1-g drug vial with 10 ml of water for injection, normal saline injection, or bacteriostatic water for injection. Don't use diluents containing dextrose. Shake well to dissolve, and immediately transfer contents of the reconstituted vial to 50 ml of normal saline injection.
• Infuse over 30 minutes. Complete the infusion within 6 hours of reconstitution.
• Don't store lyophilized powder above 77° F (25° C). The reconstituted solution, immediately diluted in normal saline injection, may be stored at room temperature and used within 6 hours or stored for 24 hours under refrigeration (41° F [5° C]) and used within 4 hours after removal from refrigeration. Don't freeze solutions of ertapenem.

⊗ **Incompatibilities**
Diluents containing dextrose (alpha-D-glucose), other I.V. drugs.

Contraindications and cautions

• Contraindicated in patients hypersensitive to the drug or any of its components or to other drugs in the same class; also contraindicated in patients who have had anaphylactic reactions to

beta-lactams. I.M. use is contraindicated in patients hypersensitive to local anesthetics of the amide type. (Lidocaine hydrochloride is used as the diluent.)
• Use cautiously in patients with CNS disorders or compromised renal function because seizures may occur. Ertapenem sodium may be removed by hemodialysis, if needed.

❦ **Lifespan:** In pregnant women, use only if benefits outweigh risks to the fetus. In breastfeeding women, drug appears in breast milk. In elderly patients with renal impairment, select dose carefully and monitor renal function.

Adverse reactions

CNS: asthenia, fatigue, anxiety, altered mental status, dizziness, headache, insomnia, *seizures,* fever, pain.
CV: edema, swelling, chest pain, hypertension, hypotension, tachycardia.
EENT: pharyngitis.
GI: abdominal pain, acid regurgitation, oral candidiasis, constipation, *diarrhea,* dyspepsia, nausea, *vomiting,* abdominal distention, *pseudomembranous colitis.*
GU: vaginitis, renal dysfunction, hematuria, urine retention.
Hematologic: coagulation abnormalities, eosinophilia, anemia, *neutropenia, leukopenia, thrombocytopenia,* thrombocytosis.
Hepatic: jaundice.
Metabolic: hyperglycemia, *hyperkalemia,* hypernatremia.
Musculoskeletal: leg pain.
Respiratory: cough, dyspnea, rales, rhonchi, *respiratory distress.*
Skin: erythema, pruritus, rash, extravasation, infused vein complication, phlebitis, thrombophlebitis, infusion site pain and redness.
Other: *septicemia,* chills, hypersensitivity reactions.

Interactions

Drug-drug. *Probenecid:* May reduce renal clearance and increase half-life. Avoid use together.

Effects on lab test results

• May increase ALT, AST, alkaline phosphatase, BUN, creatinine, glucose, potassium, sodium, and bilirubin levels. May decrease albumin, sodium bicarbonate, and hemoglobin levels and hematocrit.

E

• May increase PT, PTT, eosinophil count, and urinary RBC and WBC counts. May decrease segmented neutrophil and WBC counts. May increase or decrease platelet count.

Pharmacokinetics

Absorption: Almost completely absorbed after I.M. administration. Mean bioavailability of 90%.
Distribution: Highly bound to proteins, primarily albumin.
Metabolism: Doesn't inhibit metabolism mediated by any of the CYP isoforms. Stable against hydrolysis by a variety of beta-lactamases, including penicillinase, cephalosporinase, and extended-spectrum beta-lactamase. Hydrolyzed by metallo-beta-lactamases.
Excretion: Primarily by the kidneys. *Half-life:* 4 hours.

Route	Onset	Peak	Duration
I.V.	Immediate	30 min	24 hr
I.M.	Unknown	2 hr	24 hr

Action

Chemical effect: Inhibition of cell wall synthesis is mediated through ertapenem binding to penicillin-binding proteins.
Therapeutic effect: Kills susceptible bacteria.

Available forms

Injection: 1 g

NURSING PROCESS

🔬 Assessment
• Check for previous penicillin, cephalosporin, or other beta-lactam hypersensitivity.
• If giving I.M., check for hypersensitivity to local, amide-type anesthetics.
• Obtain specimens for culture and sensitivity testing before giving first dose. Therapy may start before results are available.
• Monitor renal, hepatic, and hematopoietic function during prolonged therapy.
• Be alert for adverse reactions, particularly diarrhea, seizures, and superinfection.
• Assess patient's and family's knowledge of drug therapy.

🔵 Nursing diagnoses
• Diarrhea related to drug-induced adverse reaction

• Ineffective health maintenance related to underlying infectious disease process
• Deficient knowledge related to anti-infective therapy

❯ Planning and implementation
🔕 **ALERT:** Don't mix or infuse with other drugs.
• When giving I.M., reconstitute the contents of a 1-g vial of drug with 3.2 ml of 1% lidocaine hydrochloride injection (without epinephrine). Refer to prescribing information for lidocaine hydrochloride. Shake vial thoroughly to form solution. Immediately withdraw the contents of the vial and give by deep I.M. injection into a large muscle, such as the gluteal muscles or lateral part of the thigh. Use reconstituted I.M. solution within 1 hour of preparing. Don't give reconstituted solution I.V.
• Avoid inadvertent injection into a blood vessel during I.M. administration.
• If diarrhea persists during therapy, stop drug and collect stool specimen for culture to rule out pseudomembranous colitis.
• Vomiting is more common in children than in adults.
• If allergic reaction occurs, stop drug immediately and give immediate treatment with airway management, epinephrine, oxygen, and I.V. steroids.
• Continue anticonvulsants in patients with known seizure disorders. If focal tremors, myoclonus, or seizures occur, evaluate patient neurologically and give anticonvulsants if not given before. Decrease or stop drug after reexamining dosage.
• Signs and symptoms of overdose may include nausea, diarrhea, and dizziness. If an overdose occurs, stop drug and treat supportively until drug has been eliminated from the body.
🔕 **ALERT:** Don't confuse Avinza with Invanz.
Patient teaching
• Inform patient of potential adverse reactions and urge him to notify prescriber immediately if they occur.
• Tell patient to alert prescriber if he develops diarrhea.

✅ Evaluation
• Patient tolerates and responds well to drug therapy.
• Patient doesn't develop colitis or any other adverse reactions from drug therapy.

Reactions may be *common,* uncommon, *life-threatening,* or COMMON AND LIFE-THREATENING.

• Patient and family state understanding of drug therapy.

erythromycin base
(eh-rith-roh-MIGH-sin bays)
Apo-Erythro♦, E-Base, E-Mycin, Erybid♦, Eryc∅, Ery-Tab, Erythromycin Delayed-Release, Erythromycin Filmtabs, PCE Dispertab

erythromycin estolate
Ilosone, Ilosone Pulvules

erythromycin ethylsuccinate
Apo-Erythro-ES♦, E.E.S., E.E.S. Granules, EryPed, EryPed 200, EryPed 400

erythromycin lactobionate
Erythrocin Lactobionate

erythromycin stearate
Apo-Erythro-S♦, Erythrocin Stearate

Pharmacologic class: macrolide
Therapeutic class: antibiotic
Pregnancy risk category: B

Indications and dosages

▶ **Acute pelvic inflammatory disease caused by** *Neisseria gonorrhoeae. Adults:* 500 mg erythromycin lactobionate I.V. q 6 hours for 3 days; then 250 mg erythromycin base, estolate, or stearate P.O. q 6 hours or 333 mg q 8 hours for 7 days. Or 400 mg ethylsuccinate P.O. q 6 hours for 7 days.
▶ **Endocarditis prophylaxis for dental procedures in patients allergic to penicillin.** *Adults:* Initially 800 mg ethylsuccinate or 1 g stearate P.O. 1 hour before procedure; then 400 mg ethylsuccinate or 500 mg stearate P.O. 6 hours later.
Children: Initially 20 mg/kg ethylsuccinate or stearate P.O. 1 hour before procedure; then 10 mg/kg 6 hours later.
▶ **Intestinal amebiasis.** *Adults:* 250 mg erythromycin base, estolate, or stearate, or 400 mg ethylsuccinate, P.O. q 6 hours, or 333 mg erythromycin base q 8 hours, or 500 mg q 12 hours for 10 to 14 days.

Children: 30 to 50 mg/kg erythromycin base, estolate, ethylsuccinate, or stearate P.O. daily in divided doses q 6 hours for 10 to 14 days.
▶ **Mild to moderately severe respiratory tract, skin, and soft-tissue infections caused by sensitive** *Streptococcus pyogenes, Bordetella pertussis, Corynebacterium diphtheriae, Diplococcus pneumoniae, Listeria monocytogenes, Mycoplasma pneumoniae. Adults:* 250 to 500 mg erythromycin base, estolate, or stearate P.O. q 6 hours; or 400 to 800 mg erythromycin ethylsuccinate P.O. q 6 hours; or 15 to 20 mg/kg I.V. daily as continuous infusion or in divided doses q 6 hours for 10 to 21 days, depending on severity and source of infection, until oral dosage can be taken.
Children: 20 to 50 mg/kg oral erythromycin salts P.O. daily in divided doses q 6 hours; or 15 to 20 mg/kg I.V. daily in divided doses q 4 to 6 hours.
▶ **Syphilis.** *Adults:* 500 mg erythromycin base, estolate, or stearate P.O. q.i.d. for 15 days.
▶ **Legionnaires' disease.** *Adults:* 1 to 4 g P.O. or I.V. daily in divided doses for 10 to 14 days.
▶ **Uncomplicated urethral, endocervical, or rectal infections when tetracyclines are contraindicated.** *Adults:* 500 mg erythromycin base, estolate, or stearate or 800 mg ethylsuccinate P.O. q.i.d. or 666 mg erythromycin base P.O. q 8 hours for at least 7 days.
▶ **Urogenital** *Chlamydia trachomatis* **infections during pregnancy.** *Adults:* 500 mg erythromycin base, estolate, or stearate P.O. q.i.d. or 666 mg q 8 hours for at least 7 days; or 250 mg erythromycin base, estolate, or stearate, or 333 mg q 8 hours, or 500 mg q 12 hours, or 400 mg ethylsuccinate P.O. q.i.d. for at least 14 days.
▶ **Conjunctivitis caused by** *C. trachomatis* **in neonates.** *Neonates:* 50 mg/kg P.O. daily in four divided doses for 14 days or more.
▶ **Pneumonia of infancy caused by** *C. trachomatis. Infants:* 50 mg/kg P.O. daily in four divided doses for at least 2 but usually 3 weeks; a second course may be needed.
▶ **Early form of Lyme disease in persons allergic to penicillins and cephalosporins and in whom tetracyclines are contraindicated‡.** *Adults and children age 8 and older:* 250 to 500 mg erythromycin base P.O. t.i.d. or q.i.d. Or 30 to 40 mg/kg P.O. daily in divided doses for 10 to 30 days.

Children younger than age 8: 30 to 40 mg/kg erythromycin base P.O. daily in divided doses (not to exceed adult dose) for 10 to 30 days.
▶ **Early Lyme disease manifested as erythema migrans‡.** *Adults:* 500 mg erythromycin base P.O. q.i.d. for 14 to 21 days.
Children: 12.5 mg/kg erythromycin base P.O. q.i.d. (maximum, 500 mg/dose) for 14 to 21 days.
▶ **Diarrhea caused by** *Campylobacter jejuni‡.* *Adults:* 500 mg erythromycin base P.O. q.i.d. for 7 days.
▶ **Genital, inguinal, or anorectal lymphogranuloma venereum‡.** *Adults:* 500 mg erythromycin base P.O. q.i.d. for 21 days.
▶ **Chancroid caused by** *Haemophilus ducreyi‡.* *Adults:* 500 mg P.O. q.i.d. for 7 days, until ulcers or lymph nodes are healed.
▶ **Tetanus caused by** *Clostridium tetani‡.* *Adults:* 500 mg P.O. q 6 hours for 10 days.
▶ **Granuloma inguinale‡.** *Adults:* 500 mg P.O. q.i.d. for at least 21 days.

▼ I.V. administration

• Prepare the initial solution by adding 10 ml sterile water for injection to the 500-mg vial or 20 ml diluent to the 1-g vial. All other diluents may cause precipitation. Use only preservative-free sterile water for injection. Dilute each 250 mg in at least 100 ml of normal saline solution, lactated Ringer's injection, or Normosol-R.
• Don't administer by I.V. bolus.
• Infuse over 1 hour or by continuous infusion.
⊗ **Incompatibilities**
Ascorbic acid injection, colistimethate, dextrose 2.5% in half-strength Ringer's lactate, dextrose 5% in lactated Ringer's solution, dextrose 5% in normal saline solution, D_5W, dextrose 10% in water, floxacillin, furosemide, heparin sodium, linezolid, metoclopramide, dextrose 5% in Normosol-M, Ringer's injection, vitamin B complex with C. Manufacturer recommends not administering with other I.V. drugs.

Contraindications and cautions

• Contraindicated in patients hypersensitive to drug, any of its components, or other macrolides. Also contraindicated in patients taking pimozide. Erythromycin estolate is contraindicated in patients with hepatic disease.
• Use other erythromycin salts cautiously in patients with impaired liver function.

🕮 **Lifespan:** In pregnant women, use cautiously. In breast-feeding women, use cautiously because the drug appears in breast milk. The American Academy of Pediatrics considers erythromycin compatible with breast-feeding. In neonates, avoid I.V.drug because it may contain benzyl alcohol.

Adverse reactions

CNS: fever, dizziness, headache.
CV: *ventricular arrhythmias,* venous irritation or thrombophlebitis after I.V. injection.
EENT: hearing loss.
GI: abdominal pain and cramping, nausea, vomiting, diarrhea, *pseudomembranous colitis.*
Hepatic: cholestatic hepatitis.
Skin: urticaria, rash, eczema.
Other: overgrowth of nonsusceptible bacteria or fungi, *anaphylaxis.*

Interactions

Drug-drug. *Carbamazepine:* May increase carbamazepine level and risk of toxicity. Avoid use together.
Clindamycin, lincomycin: May be antagonistic. Don't use together.
Cyclosporine: May increase cyclosporine level. Monitor patient closely for toxicity.
Digoxin: May increase digoxin level. Monitor patient for digoxin toxicity.
Disopyramide: May increase disopyramide level; may result, in some cases, in arrhythmias and prolonged QT intervals. Monitor ECG.
Ergot alkaloids: May cause acute ergot toxicity. Monitor carefully.
HMG-CoA reductase inhibitors: May increase risk of myopathy and rhabdomyolysis. Avoid use together.
Midazolam, triazolam: May increase effects of these drugs. Monitor patient closely.
Oral anticoagulants: May increase anticoagulant effects. Monitor PT and INR closely; monitor patient for bleeding.
Strong CYP 3A inhibitors (such as diltiazem or verapamil): May increase risk of life-threatening cardiac condition. Don't use together.
Tacrolimus: May increase tacrolimus level and risk of adverse reactions, such as nephrotoxicity. Use together cautiously.
Theophylline: May decrease erythromycin level and increase risk of theophylline toxicity. Use together cautiously.

Reactions may be *common,* uncommon, *life-threatening,* or COMMON AND LIFE-THREATENING.

Vinblastine: May increase risk of vinblastine toxicity. Use together cautiously.

Drug-herb. *Pill-bearing spurge:* May inhibit CYP 3A enzymes and alter drug metabolism. Discourage use together.

Effects on lab test results

• May increase CK, ASP, ALT, alkaline phosphatase, and biliribin levels. May decrease bicarbonate level.

• May increase eosinophil, neutrophil, and platelet counts.

• May falsely elevate urinary catecholamines, 17-hydroxycorticosterone, and 17-ketosteroids. May interfere with colorimetric assays, resulting in falsely elevated AST and ALT levels.

Pharmacokinetics

Absorption: Most erythromycin salts are absorbed in duodenum. Because erythromycin base is acid-sensitive, it must be buffered or have enteric coating to prevent destruction by gastric acid. Acid salts and esters (estolate, ethylsuccinate, and stearate) aren't affected by gastric acidity; they're unaffected or may even be enhanced by food. Give erythromycin base and stearate preparations on empty stomach.

Distribution: Widely distributed in most body tissues and fluids except CSF, where it appears at low levels. About 80% of erythromycin base and 96% of erythromycin estolate are protein-bound.

Metabolism: Partially metabolized in liver.

Excretion: Mainly unchanged in bile. *Half-life:* 1.6 hours.

Route	Onset	Peak	Duration
P.O.	Unknown	1–4 hr	Unknown
I.V.	Immediate	Immediate	Unknown

Action

Chemical effect: Inhibits bacterial protein synthesis by binding to 50S subunit of ribosome.

Therapeutic effect: Inhibits bacterial growth.

Available forms

erythromycin base
Capsules (delayed-release): 250 mg
Tablets (enteric-coated): 250 mg, 333 mg, 500 mg
Tablets (filmtabs): 250 mg, 500 mg
erythromycin estolate
Capsules: 250 mg

Oral suspension: 125 mg/5 ml, 250 mg/5 ml
Tablets: 500 mg
erythromycin ethylsuccinate
Oral suspension: 100 mg/2.5 ml, 200 mg/5 ml, 400 mg/5 ml
Powder for oral suspension: 200 mg/5 ml, 400 mg/5ml
Tablets: 400 mg
erythromycin lactobionate
Injection: 500-mg, 1-g vials
erythromycin stearate
Tablets (film-coated): 250 mg, 500 mg

NURSING PROCESS

☆ Assessment

• Obtain history of patient's infection before starting therapy, and reassess regularly.

• Obtain appropriate specimen for culture and sensitivity tests before starting therapy. Begin therapy pending test results.

• Be alert for adverse reactions and drug interactions.

• If adverse GI reaction occurs, monitor patient's hydration.

• Monitor liver function. Drug may increase levels of alkaline phosphatase, ALT, AST, and bilirubin. Erythromycin estolate (most frequently used of all forms of erythromycin) may cause serious hepatotoxicity in adults (reversible cholestatic jaundice). A patient who develops hepatotoxicity may react similarly to other erythromycin forms.

• Monitor hearing for losses if high doses given I.V.

• Assess patient's and family's knowledge of drug therapy.

💠 Nursing diagnoses

• Infection related to presence of susceptible bacteria

• Risk for deficient fluid volume related to potential for drug-induced adverse GI reactions

• Deficient knowledge related to drug therapy

▷ Planning and implementation

⚠ ALERT: The American Heart Association no longer recommends using erythromycin to prevent bacterial endocarditis. However, practitioners who have successfully used the drug as prophylaxis in individual patients may continue to do so.

• When giving suspension, note concentration.

• For best absorption, give oral form with full glass of water 1 hour before or 2 hours after meals. Coated tablets may be taken with meals. Tell patient not to drink fruit juice with drug.
• Coated tablets or encapsulated pellets cause less GI upset; they may be more tolerable in patients who can't tolerate drug.

Patient teaching

• Tell patient how to take oral drug.
• Tell patient to take entire amount of drug exactly as prescribed, even after he feels better.
• Instruct patient to notify prescriber if adverse reaction occurs, especially nausea, abdominal pain, and fever.

⚫ Evaluation

• Patient is free from infection.
• Patient maintains adequate hydration with therapy.
• Patient and family state understanding of drug therapy.

escitalopram oxalate
(ES-sigh-TAL-uh-pram ocks-UH-layt)
Lexapro⌀

Pharmacologic class: SSRI
Therapeutic class: anxiolytic, antidepressant
Pregnancy risk category: C

Indications and dosages

▶ **Major depressive disorder; generalized anxiety disorder.** *Adults:* Initially 10 mg P.O. daily, increasing to 20 mg, if needed, after at least 1 week.
▶ **Panic disorder‡.** *Adults:* 10 mg P.O. daily.
⧗ **Adjust-a-dose:** For elderly patients and those with hepatic impairment, 10 mg P.O. daily initially and as maintenance dosage.

Contraindications and cautions

• Contraindicated in patients hypersensitive to drug or its components or to citalopram. Also contraindicated within 14 days of MAO inhibitor therapy.
• Use cautiously in patients with suicidal ideation, a history of mania, seizure disorders, or renal or hepatic impairment. Also use cautiously in patients with diseases that produce altered metabolism or hemodynamic responses.

❄ **Lifespan:** In pregnant women, use drug only if the benefits to the woman outweigh the risks to the fetus. Breast-feeding women should stop breast-feeding or stop drug. Drug appears in breast milk. In children, safety and effectiveness haven't been established. In elderly patients, use cautiously because they may have greater sensitivity to drug.

Adverse reactions

CNS: fever, *headache, insomnia,* dizziness, *somnolence,* paresthesia, light-headedness, migraine, tremor, vertigo, abnormal dreams, irritability, impaired concentration, fatigue, lethargy.
CV: palpitations, hypertension, flushing, chest pain.
EENT: rhinitis, sinusitis, blurred vision, tinnitus, earache.
GI: *nausea,* diarrhea, constipation, indigestion, abdominal pain, vomiting, increased or decreased appetite, dry mouth, flatulence, heartburn, cramps, gastroesophageal reflux.
GU: *ejaculation disorder,* impotence, anorgasmia, menstrual cramps, UTI, urinary frequency.
Metabolic: weight gain or loss.
Musculoskeletal: arthralgia, myalgia, muscle cramps, extremity pain.
Respiratory: bronchitis, cough.
Skin: rash, increased sweating.
Other: decreased libido, yawning, flulike symptoms, toothache.

Interactions

Drug-drug. *Carbamazepine:* May increase escitalopram clearance caused by CYP induction. Monitor patient for expected antidepressant effect and adjust dose p.r.n.
Cimetidine: May increase escitalopram level. Monitor patient for adverse reactions to escitalopram.
Citalopram: May cause additive effects. Avoid use together.
CNS drugs: May cause additive effects. Use together cautiously.
Desipramine, other drugs metabolized by CYP 2D6: May increase levels of these drugs. Use together cautiously.
Lithium: May enhance serotonergic effect of escitalopram. Use together cautiously, and monitor lithium level.

MAO inhibitors: May cause serious, sometimes fatal, reactions. Avoid using drug within 14 days of MAO inhibitor.

Sumatriptan: May increase serotonergic effects, leading to weakness, enhanced reflex response, and incoordination. Use these drugs together cautiously.

Tricyclic antidepressants: May increase antidepressant level. Use together cautiously. Monitor antidepressant level. Reduce antidepressant dose if needed.

Drug-lifestyle. *Alcohol use:* May increase CNS effects. Discourage using together.

Effects on lab test results

None reported.

Pharmacokinetics

Absorption: Absolute bioavailability is 80%.
Distribution: Protein binding is about 56%.
Metabolism: Extensive, primarily by CYP 3A4 and CYP 2C19 to inactive metabolites.
Excretion: About 8% unchanged in urine. *Half-life:* 27 to 32 hours.

Route	Onset	Peak	Duration
P.O.	Unknown	5 hr	Unknown

Action

Chemical effect: May increase serotonergic activity in the CNS by inhibiting neuronal reuptake of serotonin.
Therapeutic effect: Relieves depressive symptoms and anxiety.

Available forms

Oral solution: 5 mg/5 ml
Tablets: 5 mg, 10 mg, 20 mg

NURSING PROCESS

Assessment

• Obtain history of patient's medical condition before starting therapy.
• Closely monitor patients at high risk of suicide.
• Assess patient for history of drug abuse, and observe for signs of misuse or abuse.
• Assess patient's and family's knowledge of drug therapy.

Nursing diagnoses

• Ineffective individual coping related to underlying condition
• Risk for interrupted family processes related to underlying condition
• Deficient knowledge related to drug therapy

Planning and implementation

• In case of overdose, establish and maintain an airway, induce vomiting, and give activated charcoal. Closely observe and monitor vital signs and cardiac health, and maintain supportive care. Dialysis isn't effective, and no known antidote exists.

ALERT: Don't confuse Lexapro with Celexa or Loxitane.

Patient teaching

• Inform patient that symptoms will improve gradually over several weeks rather than immediately.
• Tell patient to continue taking drug as prescribed even though improvement may not occur for 1 to 4 weeks.
• Tell patient to use caution while driving or operating hazardous machinery because of drug's potential to impair judgment, thinking, and motor skills.
• Advise patient to consult prescriber before taking other prescription or OTC drugs.
• Tell patient that drug may be taken in the morning or evening with or without food.
• Encourage patient to avoid alcohol while taking drug.
• Tell patient to notify prescriber if she's pregnant or breast-feeding.

Evaluation

• Patient is able to carry out activities vital to usual role performance.
• Patient doesn't experience interrupted family processes.
• Patient and family state understanding of drug therapy.

E

esmolol hydrochloride
(EZ-moh-lohl high-droh-KLOR-ighd)
Brevibloc

Pharmacologic class: beta blocker
Therapeutic class: antiarrhythmic
Pregnancy risk category: C

Indications and dosages

▶ **Supraventricular tachycardia; control of ventricular rate in patients with atrial fibrillation or flutter in perioperative, postoperative, or other emergent circumstances; noncompensatory sinus tachycardia when heart rate requires specific interventions.** *Adults:* Loading dose is 500 mcg/kg/minute by I.V. infusion over 1 minute, followed by 4-minute maintenance infusion of 50 mcg/kg/minute. If adequate response doesn't occur within 5 minutes, repeat loading dose and infuse 100 mcg/kg/minute for 4 minutes. Repeat loading dose and increase maintenance infusion stepwise, p.r.n. Maximum maintenance infusion for tachycardia is 200 mcg/kg/minute.
▶ **Management of perioperative and postoperative tachycardia or hypertension.** *Adults:* For perioperative therapy, 80 mg (about 1 mg/kg) I.V. bolus over 30 seconds, followed by 150 mcg/kg/minute I.V., if needed. Adjust infusion rate, p.r.n., to maximum of 300 mcg/kg/minute. Postoperative therapy is the same as for supraventricular tachycardia, although dosages adequate for control may be as high as 300 mcg/kg/minute.

▼ I.V. administration

• Don't give by I.V. push; use infusion-control device. The 10-mg/ml single-dose vial may be used without diluting, but injection concentrate (250 mg/ml) must be diluted to no more than 10 mg/ml before infusion. Remove 20 ml from 500 ml of D_5W, lactated Ringer's solution, or half-normal or normal saline solution, and add two ampules of drug.
• Doses greater than 200 mcg/kg/minute aren't recommended.
• When patient's heart rate becomes stable, replace drug with a longer-acting antiarrhythmic, such as propranolol, digoxin, or verapamil; 30 minutes after giving the first dose of a replacement, reduce infusion rate by 50%. Moni-

tor patient response, and if pulse is controlled for 1 hour after giving second dose of replacement, stop infusion.
• If local reaction develops at infusion site, change to another site. Avoid using butterfly needles.
• Don't abruptly stop giving the drug because withdrawal effects may occur. If immediate withdrawal is needed, use caution.
• Drug is intended for short-term use, no longer than 48 hours.
• Watch for irritation and infiltration because extravasation may cause tissue damage or necrosis.
⊗ **Incompatibilities**
Diazepam, furosemide, procainamide, thiopental sodium, warfarin sodium, 5% sodium bicarbonate injection.

Contraindications and cautions

• Contraindicated in patients with sinus bradycardia, heart block greater than first-degree, cardiogenic shock, or overt heart failure.
• Use cautiously in patients with impaired kidney function, diabetes, or bronchospasm.
⚖ **Lifespan:** In pregnant women, use cautiously. In breast-feeding women, use cautiously because it's unknown if the drug appears in breast milk. In children, safety and effectiveness haven't been established.

Adverse reactions

CNS: dizziness, somnolence, headache, agitation, fatigue, confusion.
CV: HYPOTENSION, peripheral ischemia.
EENT: nasal congestion.
GI: *nausea,* vomiting.
Respiratory: *bronchospasm,* wheezing, dyspnea.
Other: inflammation, induration at infusion site.

Interactions

Drug-drug. *Digoxin:* Esmolol may increase digoxin level by 10% to 20%. Monitor digoxin level.
Morphine: May increase esmolol level. Adjust esmolol carefully.
Prazosin: May increase the risk of orthostatic hypotension in the early phases of use together. Assist patient to stand slowly until effects are known.

Reserpine, other catecholamine-depleting drugs: May cause additive bradycardia and hypotension. Adjust esmolol carefully.
Succinylcholine: Esmolol may prolong neuromuscular blockade. Monitor patient.
Verapamil: May increase the effects of both drugs. Monitor cardiac function closely, and decrease dosages p.r.n.

Effects on lab test results
• May increase LDH level. May decrease hemoglobin level.

Pharmacokinetics
Absorption: Administered I.V.
Distribution: Rapid; 55% protein-bound.
Metabolism: Rapid.
Excretion: By kidneys as metabolites. *Half-life:* About 9 minutes.

Route	Onset	Peak	Duration
I.V.	Immediate	30 min	< 30 min

Action
Chemical effect: Decreases heart rate, myocardial contractility, and blood pressure.
Therapeutic effect: Restores normal sinus rhythm.

Available forms
Injection: 10 mg/ml, 250 mg/ml

NURSING PROCESS

☰ Assessment
• Obtain history of patient's arrhythmias before starting therapy.
• Monitor ECG and blood pressure continuously during infusion. Up to 50% of patients develop hypotension. Monitor patient closely, especially if blood pressure was low before therapy.
• Be alert for adverse reactions and drug interactions.
• Assess patient's and family's knowledge of drug therapy.

☷ Nursing diagnoses
• Decreased cardiac output related to presence of arrhythmias
• Ineffective cerebral tissue perfusion related to drug-induced hypotension
• Deficient knowledge related to drug therapy

⯮ Planning and implementation
• If patient develops severe dose-related hypotension, decrease dose or stop infusion and immediately notify prescriber. Hypotension will reverse within 30 minutes.
• If patient develops symptoms of heart failure (shortness of breath, night cough, swelling of the limbs), notify prescriber.
Patient teaching
• Inform patient of need for continuous ECG, blood pressure, and heart rate monitoring to assess effectiveness of drug and detect adverse reactions.

☑ Evaluation
• Patient regains normal cardiac output with correction of arrhythmias.
• Patient's blood pressure remains normal throughout therapy.
• Patient and family state understanding of drug therapy.

esomeprazole magnesium
(ee-soh-MEP-rah-zohl mag-NEEZ-ee-uhm)
Nexium

esomeprazole sodium
Nexium I.V.

Pharmacologic class: proton pump inhibitor
Therapeutic class: antisecretory
Pregnancy risk category: B

Indications and dosages

▶ **Gastroesophageal reflux disease (GERD), healing of erosive esophagitis.** *Adults:* 20 or 40 mg P.O. daily for 4 to 8 weeks. If symptoms persist, use for an additional 4 to 8 weeks.
▶ **Long-term maintenance of healing in erosive esophagitis.** *Adults:* 20 mg P.O. daily for no more than 6 months.
▶ **Eradication of *Helicobacter pylori* to reduce duodenal ulcer recurrence.** *Adults:* Combination triple therapy with esomeprazole magnesium 40 mg P.O. daily plus amoxicillin 1,000 mg P.O. b.i.d. and clarithromycin 500 mg P.O. b.i.d., all for 10 days.
▶ **Short-term treatment of GERD in patients with a history of erosive esophagitis who are unable to take drug orally.** *Adults:* 20 or 40 mg I.V. once daily by direct injection over

3 minutes or by I.V. infusion over 10 to 30 minutes for up to 10 days. Switch patient to oral therapy as soon as possible.

▶ **Reduced risk of gastric ulcers in patients on continuous NSAID therapy.** *Adults:* 20 to 40 mg P.O. once daily for up to 6 months.

⧄ **Adjust-a-dose:** For patients with severe hepatic impairment, the maximum dose is 20 mg P.O. daily.

I.V. administration

• Reconstitute 20- or 40-mg vial with 5 ml of D_5W, normal saline solution, or lactated Ringer's injection and give by I.V. bolus over 3 minutes. Or further dilute to a total volume of 50 ml and give I.V. over 10 to 30 minutes.
• Flush I.V. line with D_5W, normal saline solution, or lactated Ringer's injection before and after administration.
• Store reconstituted solution and admixture at room temperature. Reconstituted solution should be used within 12 hours. For admixture diluted with D_5W, give within 6 hours. If diluted with normal saline solution or lactated Ringer's injection, use within 12 hours.
⊗ **Incompatibilities**
Don't infuse with other I.V. drugs.

Contraindications and cautions

• Contraindicated in patients hypersensitive to any component of esomeprazole or omeprazole. Combination triple therapy for the eradication of *H. pylori* is contraindicated in patients hypersensitive to clarithromycin, macrolide antibiotics, amoxicillin, or penicillin.
• Use cautiously in patients with severe hepatic insufficiency.
⚘ **Lifespan:** In pregnant women, use only if benefits outweigh risks to the fetus. In breast-feeding women, use cautiously because it's unknown whether drug appears in breast milk. In children, safety and effectiveness haven't been established.

Adverse reactions

CNS: headache.
GI: diarrhea, abdominal pain, nausea, flatulence, dry mouth, vomiting, constipation.

Interactions

Drug-drug. *Amoxicillin, clarithromycin:* May increase esomeprazole levels. Monitor patient for toxicity.

Diazepam: May decrease diazepam clearance and increase level of diazepam. Monitor patient for diazepam toxicity.
Digoxin, iron salts, ketoconazole: May interfere with drug absorption. Monitor patient closely.
Other drugs metabolized by CYP 2C19: May alter esomeprazole clearance. Monitor patient closely, especially elderly patient or patient with hepatic insufficiency.
Warfarin: May prolong PT and INR causing abnormal bleeding. Monitor the patient and PT and INR carefully.
Drug-food. *Any food:* May reduce bioavailability. Advise patient to take drug 1 hour before eating.

Effects on lab test results

• May increase creatinine, uric acid, bilirubin, alkaline phosphatase, ALT, AST, potassium, sodium, thyroxine, thyroid-stimulating hormone, and hemoglobin levels and hematocrit.
• May increase WBC and platelet counts.

Pharmacokinetics

Absorption: The level following a 40-mg dose is three times higher than after a 20-mg dose. Repeated daily dosing of 40 mg yields systemic bioavailability of 90% compared with a single 40-mg dose, which yields 64%. Giving drug with food reduces mean level by 33% to 53%.
Distribution: About 97% protein-bound.
Metabolism: Extensive in the liver by CYP 2C19 to form hydroxy and desmethyl metabolites. CYP 2C19 exhibits polymorphism. About 3% of whites and 15% to 20% of Asians who lack CYP 2C19 may have decreased levels. CYP 3A4 metabolizes the remaining amount.
Excretion: About 80% excreted as inactive metabolites in urine. Systemic clearance of esomeprazole decreases with multiple-dose administration. *Half-life:* 1 to 1½ hours.

Route	Onset	Peak	Duration
P.O.	Unknown	1½ hr	13–17 hr
I.V.	Unknown	Unknown	Unknown

Action

Chemical effect: Suppresses gastric secretion through proton pump inhibition. Inhibits the $H^+-K^+-ATPase$ pump in gastric parietal cells, thereby reducing gastric acidity by blocking the final step in acid production.
Therapeutic effect: Decreases gastric acid.

Available forms

Capsules (delayed-release containing enteric-coated pellets): 20 mg, 40 mg
Powder for injection: 20 mg, 40 mg in single-use vials

NURSING PROCESS

⚕ Assessment

• Assess patient's condition before and during drug therapy. Patients with a history of gastric ulcers or those who are age 60 and older on continuous NSAID therapy have increased risk of gastric ulcers.
• Monitor liver function test results because drug is extensively metabolized by CYP 2C19. In patients with hepatic insufficiency, drug increases liver function test values.
• Long-term therapy with omeprazole has caused atrophic gastritis. Be alert for adverse reactions.
• Assess patient's and family's knowledge of drug therapy.

⊞ Nursing diagnoses

• Impaired tissue integrity related to underlying gastroesophageal condition
• Imbalanced nutrition: less than body requirements related to decreased oral intake due to underlying gastroesophageal disorder
• Deficient knowledge related to drug therapy

⊳ Planning and implementation

• Give esomeprazole at least 1 hour before meals because food decreases the extent of absorption.
• Overdose may result in confusion, drowsiness, blurred vision, tachycardia, nausea, diaphoresis, dry mouth, and headache. Provide supportive care. Dialysis is not effective.
• Urge patient to avoid alcohol and foods that increase gastric secretions.
Patient teaching
• Tell patient to take drug exactly as prescribed and at least 1 hour before meals.
• If patient has trouble swallowing capsule, suggest that he open it, sprinkle contents into applesauce, and swallow applesauce immediately. Warn against crushing or chewing the drug pellets.
• Tell patient to report continued or worsened symptoms or any adverse reaction.

☑ Evaluation

• Patient responds positively to drug therapy.
• Patient is able to tolerate liquids and foods orally without any nausea or vomiting.
• Patient and family state understanding of drug therapy.

estazolam

(eh-STAZ-uh-lam)
ProSom

Pharmacologic class: benzodiazepine
Therapeutic class: hypnotic
Pregnancy risk category: X
Controlled substance schedule: IV

Indications and dosages

▶ **Insomnia.** *Adults:* 1 mg P.O. h.s. Some patients may need 2 mg.
⟡ **Adjust-a-dose:** For elderly patients, give 1 mg P.O. h.s.; use higher doses cautiously. Frail, elderly, or debilitated patients may take 0.5 mg, but this low dose may be only marginally effective.

Contraindications and cautions

• Contraindicated in patients hypersensitive to drug or any of its components.
• Use cautiously in patients with hepatic, renal, or pulmonary disease; depression; or suicidal tendencies.
⚘ **Lifespan:** In pregnant or breast-feeding women, drug is contraindicated. In children, safety and effectiveness haven't been established.

Adverse reactions

CNS: fatigue, dizziness, daytime drowsiness, somnolence, asthenia, hypokinesia, headache, abnormal thinking.
GI: dyspepsia, abdominal pain.
Musculoskeletal: back pain, stiffness.
Respiratory: cold symptoms, pharyngitis.

Interactions

Drug-drug. *Cimetidine, disulfiram, isoniazid, hormonal contraceptives:* May impair metabolism and clearance of benzodiazepines and prolong their half-life. Monitor patient for CNS depression.

Rapid onset   *Liquid form contains alcohol.   ◆ Canada   ◇ Australia   †OTC   ✐Photoguide   ‡Off-label use

CNS depressants, including antihistamines, opioid analgesics, benzodiazepines: May increase CNS depression. Avoid use together.

Digoxin, phenytoin: May increase levels of these drugs, resulting in toxicity. Monitor levels closely.

Fluconazole, ketoconazole, itraconazole, miconazole: May increase and prolong drug level, CNS depression, and psychomotor impairment. Don't use together.

Rifampin: May increase metabolism and clearance and decrease half-life. Watch for decreased effectiveness.

Theophylline: May act as a drug antagonist. Watch for decreased effectiveness.

Drug-herb. *Catnip, kava, lady's slipper, lemon balm, passionflower, sassafras, skullcap, valerian:* May enhance sedative effects. Discourage use together.

Drug-lifestyle. *Alcohol use:* May increase CNS and respiratory depression. Strongly discourage use together.

Smoking: May increase drug metabolism and clearance and decrease half-life. Monitor patient for decreased effectiveness.

Effects on lab test results

● May increase ALT and AST levels.

Pharmacokinetics

Absorption: Rapid and complete.
Distribution: 93% protein-bound.
Metabolism: Extensive.
Excretion: Metabolites excreted primarily in urine. *Half-life:* 10 to 24 hours.

Route	Onset	Peak	Duration
P.O.	Unknown	1–3 hr	Unknown

Action

Chemical effect: May act on limbic system and thalamus of CNS by binding to specific benzodiazepine receptors.
Therapeutic effect: Promotes sleep.

Available forms

Tablets: 1 mg, 2 mg

NURSING PROCESS

Assessment

● Obtain history of patient's sleep pattern before starting therapy, and reassess regularly.

● Monitor liver and kidney function and CBC periodically during long-term therapy.

● Be alert for adverse reactions and drug interactions.

● Watch for withdrawal symptoms. If drug is stopped suddenly, patients who have received 6 weeks of continuous therapy may experience withdrawal.

● Assess patient's and family's knowledge of drug therapy.

Nursing diagnoses

● Disturbed sleep pattern related to underlying condition
● Risk for trauma related to drug-induced adverse CNS reactions
● Deficient knowledge related to drug therapy

Planning and implementation

● Before leaving bedside, make sure patient has swallowed drug.
● Take precautions to prevent hoarding by depressed, suicidal, or drug-dependent patient, or patient who has history of drug abuse.

Patient teaching

● Tell patient not to increase drug dose on his own, but to inform prescriber if he thinks that drug is no longer effective.
● Warn patient to avoid hazardous activities that require mental alertness or physical coordination. For inpatient (particularly elderly patient), supervise walking and raise side rails.
● Warn patient that additive depressant effects can occur if alcohol is consumed while taking drug or within 24 hours afterward.
● If patient uses a hormonal contraceptive, recommend an alternative birth-control method during therapy because drug may enhance contraceptive hormone metabolism and decrease its effect.

Evaluation

● Patient is able to sleep.
● Patient's safety is maintained.
● Patient and family state understanding of drug therapy.

---

estradiol (oestradiol)

(eh-stray-DYE-ol)
**Alora, Climara, Esclim, Estrace⌀,
Estrace Vaginal Cream, Estraderm,
Estraderm MX◇, Estring, FemPatch,
Femtran◇, Gynodiol, Menorest◇,
Menostar, Oesclim◆, Vivelle, Vivelle-Dot**

estradiol acetate
Femring Vaginal Ring

estradiol cypionate
Depo-Estradiol

estradiol gel
EstroGel

estradiol hemihydrate
Estrasorb, Vagifem

estradiol valerate (oestradiol valerate)
Delestrogen

Pharmacologic class: hormone
Therapeutic class: estrogen replacement, anti-neoplastic
Pregnancy risk category: X

Indications and dosages

▶ **Vasomotor symptoms, vulvar and vaginal atrophy, hypoestrogenism from hypogonadism, castration, or primary ovarian failure.** *Adults:* 1 to 2 mg estradiol P.O. daily in cycles of 21 days on and 7 days off or cycles of 5 days on and 2 days off. Or 0.025-mg daily Esclim transdermal system applied to a clean, dry area of the trunk twice weekly. Adjust dose, if needed, after the first 2 or 3 weeks of therapy, then at 3 to 6 months, p.r.n. Or 1 Estraderm transdermal system delivering 0.05 mg/24 hours applied twice weekly. Or, the Vivelle transdermal system delivering either 0.05 mg/24 hours or 0.0375 mg/24 hours applied twice weekly. Or, the Climara system delivering 0.05 mg/24 hours or 0.1 mg/24 hours applied transdermally once weekly in cycles of 3 weeks on and 1 week off. Or, 1 to 5 mg estradiol cypionate I.M. q 3 to 4 weeks. Or 10 to 20 mg estradiol valerate I.M. q 4 weeks, p.r.n. Or Estrasorb topical emulsion delivering 0.05 mg estradiol/day:

Apply contents of two 1.74-g foil pouches daily, using one pouch for each thigh and calf.
▶ **Atrophic vaginitis, kraurosis vulvae.**
Women: 2 to 4 g estradiol intravaginal applications of cream daily for 1 to 2 weeks. When vaginal mucosa is restored, maintenance dosage of 1 g one to three times weekly in a cycle. Or 0.05 mg/24 hours Climara applied weekly in a cycle. Or 0.05 mg/24 hours Estraderm applied twice weekly in a cycle. Or 10 to 20 mg estradiol valerate I.M. q 4 weeks, p.r.n.
▶ **Palliative therapy for advanced, inoperable breast cancer.** *Men and postmenopausal women:* 10 mg estradiol P.O. t.i.d. for 3 months.
▶ **Palliative therapy for advanced inoperable prostate cancer.** *Men:* 1 to 2 mg estradiol P.O. t.i.d. Or 30 mg estradiol valerate I.M. q 1 to 2 weeks.
▶ **To prevent postmenopausal osteoporosis in high-risk patients for whom non-estrogen therapy is inappropriate.** *Women:* 0.025 mg daily Vivelle-Dot, or Alora, or 0.5 mg daily Estraderm applied to a clean, dry area of the trunk twice weekly. Or 0.025 mg daily Climara patch applied once weekly, continuously. Or 0.014 mg daily Menostar patch applied to clean, dry area of the lower abdomen once weekly.
▶ **Vasomotor symptoms.** *Women:* 0.05 mg daily Climara patch applied once weekly, continuously. Or 1.25 EstroGel applied to skin in thin layer, wrist to shoulder, once daily.
▶ **Moderate to severe vulvar and vaginal atrophy unresponsive to vaginal products.** *Women:* 1.25 EstroGel applied to skin in thin layer, wrist to shoulder, once daily.

Contraindications and cautions

• Contraindicated in patients with thrombophlebitis, thromboembolic disorders, estrogen-dependent neoplasia, breast or reproductive organ cancer (except as palliative therapy), or undiagnosed abnormal genital bleeding. Also contraindicated in patients with history of thrombophlebitis or thromboembolic disorders linked to estrogen use (except as palliative therapy of breast and prostate cancer) and in patients with liver dysfunction or disease.
• Use cautiously in patients with cerebrovascular or coronary artery disease, asthma, bone diseases, migraine, seizures, or cardiac or renal dysfunction and in women with strong family history of breast cancer or who have breast nod-

ules, fibrocystic disease, or abnormal mammogram findings. Use the lowest effective dose.
• This drug has not been approved for the prevention of cognitive disorders or memory loss.
⚫ **Lifespan:** In pregnant and breast-feeding women, drug is contraindicated. In children, use is contraindicated except in some adolescents with pubertal delay because of risk of early epiphyseal closure, breast enlargement, vaginal cornification or bleeding, and male pubertal abnormalities.

Adverse reactions

CNS: headache, *dizziness,* chorea, depression, seizures.
CV: thrombophlebitis, *thromboembolism,* hypertension, edema.
EENT: worsening of myopia or astigmatism, intolerance of contact lenses.
GI: *nausea,* vomiting, abdominal cramps, bloating, diarrhea, constipation, *pancreatitis.*
GU: breakthrough bleeding, altered menstrual flow, dysmenorrhea, amenorrhea, *endometrial cancer,* cervical erosion, altered cervical secretions, enlargement of uterine fibromas, vaginal candidiasis, testicular atrophy, impotence.
Hepatic: cholestatic jaundice, gallbladder disease, *hepatic adenoma.*
Metabolic: increased appetite, weight changes, hyperglycemia, hypercalcemia, hyperthyroidism.
Respiratory: upper respiratory infection.
Skin: melasma, urticaria, erythema nodosum, dermatitis, hair loss, pruritus.
Other: *breast cancer,* breast changes (tenderness, enlargement, secretion), gynecomastia, flulike syndrome, abnormal Pap smear.

Interactions

Drug-drug. *Bromocriptine:* May cause amenorrhea, interfering with bromocriptine effects. Avoid use together.
Carbamazepine, phenobarbital, rifampin: May decrease effectiveness of estrogen therapy. Monitor patient closely.
Corticosteroids: May enhance effects. Monitor patient closely.
Cyclosporine: May increase risk of toxicity. Frequently monitor cyclosporine levels.
Dantrolene, other hepatotoxic drugs: May increase risk of hepatotoxicity. Monitor patient closely.

Hydantoins: Use together may cause loss of seizure control and increase risk of breakthrough bleeding, spotting, and pregnancy. Monitor patient closely.
Itraconazole, ketoconazole, macrolides, ritonavir: May increase concentration of estrogens. Watch for increased adverse effects.
Oral anticoagulants: May decrease anticoagulant effects. Dosage adjustments may be needed. Monitor PT and INR.
Tamoxifen: Estrogens may interfere with effectiveness of tamoxifen. Avoid use together.
Thyroid hormones: May alter serum thyroxine and thyrotropin concentrations. Increase thyroid hormone dose as needed.
Topiramate: May increase the metabolism of estrogens and decrease effectiveness. Monitor patient closely.
Drug-herb. *St. John's wort:* May decrease concentrations of estrogens. Monitor patient for decreased effectiveness and changes in bleeding patterns.
Drug-food. *Caffeine:* May increase caffeine levels. Monitor effects.
Drug-lifestyle. *Smoking:* May increase risk of CV effects. If smoking continues, may need alternative therapy. Urge patient to stop smoking.

Effects on lab test results

• May increase total T_4, thyroid-binding globulin, triglyceride, and clotting factor VII, VIII, IX, and X levels.
• May increase PT and norepinephrine-induced platelet aggregation.

Pharmacokinetics

Absorption: Well absorbed but substantially inactivated by liver after P.O. use. Absorbed rapidly and lasts days after I.M. use. Readily absorbed into systemic circulation after transdermal use.
Distribution: Highest levels in fat. About 50% to 80% protein-bound.
Metabolism: Primarily in liver.
Excretion: Primarily through kidneys. *Half-life:* Unknown.

Route	Onset	Peak	Duration
P.O., I.M., vaginal	Unknown	Unknown	Unknown
Transdermal			
Esclim	Unknown	27–30 hr	Unknown
Estrasorb	Immediate	Unknown	Unknown
EstroGel	Immediate	1 hr	24–36 hr

Action

Chemical effect: Increases synthesis of DNA, RNA, and protein and reduces release of follicle-stimulating hormone and luteinizing hormone from pituitary gland.
Therapeutic effect: Replaces estrogen in women and treats some male prostate and breast cancers.

Available forms

estradiol
Tablets (micronized): 0.5 mg, 1 mg, 1.5 mg, 2 mg
Transdermal patch: 0.014 mg/day, 0.025 mg/ 24 hours, 0.0375 mg/24 hours, 0.05 mg/ 24 hours, 0.06 mg/day, 0.075 mg/24 hours, 0.1 mg/24 hours
Transdermal gel: 0.06%
Vaginal cream (in nonliquefying base): 0.01%
Vaginal ring: 0.0075 mg/24 hours
estradiol acetate
Vaginal ring: 0.05 mg/24 hours, 0.1 mg/ 24 hours
estradiol cypionate
Injection (in oil): 5 mg/ml
estradiol hemihydrate
Topical emulsion: 4.35 mg hemihydrate/1.74 g; 3.48 g of emulsion delivers 0.05 mg estradiol/day
Vaginal tablets: 25 mcg
estradiol valerate
Injection (in oil): 10 mg/ml, 20 mg/ml, 40 mg/ml

NURSING PROCESS

⚕ Assessment
● Obtain history of patient's underlying condition before starting therapy, and reassess regularly.
● Make sure patient has thorough physical examination before starting estrogen therapy.
● Ask patient about allergies, especially to foods or plants. Estradiol is available as aqueous solution or as solution in peanut oil; estradiol cypionate, as solution in cottonseed oil or vegetable oil; estradiol valerate, as solution in castor oil, sesame oil, or vegetable oil.
● Patient receiving long-term therapy should have yearly gynecologic and physical examinations. Periodically monitor lipid level, blood pressure, body weight, and liver function.
● Assess patient's and family's knowledge of drug therapy.

⚕ Nursing diagnoses
● Ineffective health maintenance related to underlying condition
● Ineffective tissue perfusion (cerebral, peripheral, pulmonary, or myocardial) related to drug-induced thromboembolism
● Deficient knowledge related to drug therapy

≥ Planning and implementation
● Give oral drug at mealtimes or h.s. (for once-daily dose) to minimize nausea.
● To give as I.M. injection, make sure drug is well-dispersed in solution by rolling vial between palms. Inject deep into large muscle. Rotate injection sites to prevent muscle atrophy. Never give drug I.V.
● Apply transdermal patch to clean, dry, hairless, intact skin on abdomen or buttocks. Don't apply to breasts, waistline, or other areas where clothing can loosen patch. When applying, ensure good contact with skin, especially around edges, and hold in place with palm for about 10 seconds. Rotate application sites.
● Begin transdermal patch 1 week after withdrawal of oral therapy, or sooner if menopausal symptoms appear before end of week.
⚠ **ALERT:** EstroGel dries in 2 to 5 minutes. Avoid fire, flame, or smoking until gel is dry because gel contains alcohol.
● Because of risk of thromboembolism, stop therapy at least 1 month before procedures that increase risk of prolonged immobilization or thromboembolism, such as knee or hip surgery. If you suspect thromboembolism, withhold drug and notify prescriber.
⚠ **ALERT:** Estrogen preparations aren't interchangeable.
Patient teaching
● Inform patient about adverse effects of estrogen.
● Emphasize importance of regular physical examinations. In postmenopausal women, estro-

gen replacement therapy for longer than 5 years may increase risk of endometrial cancer. Tell patient that risk is reduced by using cyclic rather than continuous therapy and lowest dosages of estrogen. Drug probably doesn't increase risk of breast cancer.

• Teach patient how to use vaginal cream. Tell her to wash vaginal area with soap and water before applying. Tell her to apply drug h.s. or to lie flat for 30 minutes after application to minimize drug loss.

• Warn patient to immediately report abdominal pain; pain, numbness, or stiffness in legs or buttocks; pressure or pain in chest; shortness of breath; severe headaches; visual disturbances, such as blind spots, flashing lights, or blurriness; vaginal bleeding or discharge; breast lumps; swelling of hands or feet; yellow skin or sclera; dark urine; and light-colored stools.

• Explain to patient receiving cyclic therapy for postmenopausal symptoms that, although withdrawal bleeding may occur during week off drug, fertility hasn't been restored. Pregnancy can't occur because she hasn't ovulated.

• Teach patient using Estrasorb topical emulsion to rub into thigh and calf until thoroughly absorbed, rub excess on hands into buttocks, and let dry before covering with clothing. Tell patient to wash hands thoroughly.

• Teach patient using transdermal gel (Estro-Gel) to apply in a thin layer on one arm and let dry before smoking, nearing flames, dressing, or letting someone touch that arm. Recommend bathing before application to maintain full dosage.

• Tell diabetic patient to report elevated glucose test results so antidiabetic dosage can be adjusted.

• Teach woman how to perform routine breast self-examination.

☑ Evaluation

• Patient shows improvement in underlying condition.

• Patient has no thromboembolic event during therapy.

• Patient and family state understanding of drug therapy.

estradiol and norgestimate
(eh-stray-DYE-ol and nor-JESS-tih-mayt)
Prefest

estrogens, conjugated, and medroxyprogesterone
(ESS-troh-jenz, KAHN-jih-gayt-ed, and med-roks-ee-proh-JESS-ter-ohn)
Premphase, Prempro

Pharmacologic class: hormones
Therapeutic class: combined estrogen and progestin
Pregnancy risk category: X

Indications and dosages

▶ **Moderate to severe vasomotor symptoms and vulvar and vaginal atrophy caused by menopause; prevention of osteoporosis in women with an intact uterus.** *Women:* 1 mg estradiol (pink tablet) P.O. daily for 3 days; then 1 mg estradiol/0.09 mg norgestimate (white tablet) P.O. daily for 3 days. Repeat cycle until blister card is empty. Or 0.625 mg/2.5 mg (Prempro) P.O. once daily; can increase to 0.625 mg/5 mg tablet if needed. Or 0.625 mg conjugated estrogens (maroon tablet) P.O. once daily on days 1 through 14 and 0.625 mg conjugated estrogen/5 mg medroxyprogesterone (light blue tablet) P.O. once daily on days 15 through 28.

Contraindications and cautions

• Contraindicated in patients hypersensitive to any component of drugs and in patients with cancer of the breast, estrogen-dependent neoplasia, undiagnosed abnormal vaginal bleeding, or active or previous thrombophlebitis or thromboembolic disorders. Hormone replacement therapy is contraindicated for cardiac disease prevention.

• Use cautiously in women who have had a hysterectomy, are overweight, or have abnormal lipid profiles, gallbladder disease, or impaired liver function.

⑤ **ALERT:** Don't use estrogens and progestins to prevent CV disease. The Women's Health Initiative study reported increased risks of MI, stroke, invasive breast cancer, pulmonary emboli, and deep vein thrombosis in postmenopausal women during 5 years of combination therapy.

Because of these risks, give estrogens and progestins at the lowest effective dose and for the shortest duration.

⚠ **Lifespan:** In women who are or may be pregnant, drug is contraindicated.

Adverse reactions

CNS: depression, dizziness, fatigue, pain, *headache, seizures, stroke.*
CV: edema, *thromboembolism, pulmonary embolism, MI.*
EENT: pharyngitis, sinusitis, worsening of myopia or astigmatism, intolerance of contact lenses.
GI: flatulence, *nausea,* abdominal pain, weight changes.
GU: dysmenorrhea, vaginal bleeding, vaginitis, decreased libido, *endometrial cancer.*
Hepatic: gallbladder disease, *hepatic adenoma.*
Musculoskeletal: arthralgia, myalgia, *back pain.*
Respiratory: cough, upper respiratory tract infection.
Other: flulike symptoms, viral infection, breast pain, *breast cancer,* tooth disorder.

Interactions

Drug-drug. *Bromocriptine:* May cause amenorrhea, interfering with bromocriptine effects. Avoid use together.
Carbamazepine, phenobarbital, rifampin: May decrease effectiveness of estrogen therapy. Monitor patient closely.
Corticosteroids: May enhance effects. Monitor patient closely.
Cyclosporine: May increase risk of toxicity. Frequently monitor cyclosporine level.
Dantrolene, other hepatotoxic drugs: May increase risk of hepatotoxicity. Monitor patient closely.
Hydantoins: Use together may cause loss of seizure control and increased risk of breakthrough bleeding, spotting, and pregnancy. Monitor patient closely.
Itraconazole, ketoconazole, macrolides, ritonavir: May increase concentration of estrogens. Monitor patient for increased adverse effects.
Oral anticoagulants: May decrease anticoagulant effects. Dosage adjustments may be needed. Monitor PT and INR.
Tamoxifen: Estrogens may interfere with effectiveness of tamoxifen. Avoid use together.

Thyroid hormones: May alter serum thyroxine and thyrotropin levels. Increase thyroid hormone dose as needed.
Topiramate: May increase the metabolism of estrogens and decrease effectiveness. Monitor patient closely.
Drug-herb. *St. John's wort:* May decrease concentrations of estrogens. Watch for decreased effectiveness and changes in bleeding patterns.
Drug-food. *Caffeine:* May increase caffeine level. Monitor effects.
Drug-lifestyle. *Smoking:* May increase risk of CV effects. If smoking continues, patient may need alternative therapy. Urge patient to stop smoking.

Effects on lab test results

● May increase glucose, calcium, thyroxine-binding globulin, LDL, triglyceride, total circulating corticosteroid and sex steroid, total plasma cortisol, fibrinogen, plasminogen antigen, and blood clotting factor VII, VIII, IX, and X levels. May decrease folate, metyrapone, HDL, and antithrombin III levels.
● May increase PT, PTT, platelet aggregation time, and platelet count. May decrease T_3 resin uptake, glucose tolerance, and cortisol secretion rate.

Pharmacokinetics

Absorption: Unknown.
Distribution: Wide, highly protein bound.
Metabolism: Mainly metabolized in the liver.
Excretion: Mainly in the urine. *Half-life:* About 16 hours for estrogens and 8 to 9 hours for progestins in postmenopausal women.

Route	Onset	Peak	Duration
P.O.			
estrogens	Unknown	Varies	Unknown
progestins	Rapid	1–2 hr	Several days

Action

Chemical effect: Circulating estrogens modulate pituitary secretion of gonadotropins, luteinizing hormone, and follicle-stimulating hormone. Estrogen-replacement therapy reduces elevated levels of these hormones in postmenopausal women. Estrogens also contribute to the reduction of the rate of bone turnover. Progestins counter estrogenic effects by decreasing the number of nuclear estradiol receptors and suppressing epithelial DNA synthesis in endometrial tissue.

Therapeutic effect: Relieves menopausal vasomotor symptoms and vaginal dryness; reduces the severity of osteoporosis.

Available forms

Prefest
Blister card of 15 pink and 15 white tablets. Pink tablets are 1 mg estradiol; white tablets are 1 mg estradiol and 0.09 mg norgestimate.

Premphase
Dial pack of 14 maroon and 14 light blue tablets. Maroon tablets are 0.625 mg estrogen; light blue tablets are 0.625 mg estrogen and 5 mg medroxyprogesterone.

Prempro
Dial pack of 28 tablets, available in these doses: 0.3 mg estrogen and 1.5 mg medroxyprogesterone, 0.45 mg and 1.5 mg, 0.625 mg and 2.5 mg, 0.625 mg and 5 mg.

NURSING PROCESS

⚗ Assessment
• Obtain history of patient's underlying condition before therapy, and reassess regularly thereafter.
• Make sure patient has a thorough physical examination before starting drug therapy.
• Assess patient's risks for venous thromboembolism.
• Assess patient's risk for cancer because hormone replacement therapy may increase the risk of breast cancer in postmenopausal women.
• Be alert for adverse reactions.
• Assess patient's and family's knowledge of drug therapy.

✥ Nursing diagnoses
• Ineffective peripheral tissue perfusion related to drug-induced thromboembolism
• Ineffective health maintenance related to underlying condition
• Deficient knowledge related to drug therapy

▷ Planning and implementation
⑤ ALERT: Combined product may increase risk of MI, stroke, invasive breast cancer, pulmonary embolism, and deep vein thrombosis in postmenopausal women ages 50 to 79. There's also an increased risk of probable dementia in postmenopausal women age 65 and older.

• Reassess patient at 6-month intervals to make sure treatment is still needed.
• Monitor patient for hypercalcemia if she has breast cancer and bone metastases. If severe hypercalcemia occurs, notify the prescriber and stop the drug; take the appropriate measures to reduce calcium level.

Patient teaching
• Explain the risks of estrogen therapy, including breast cancer, uterine cancer, abnormal blood clotting, gallbladder disease, heart disease, and stroke.
• Tell patient to immediately report any undiagnosed, persistent, or recurring abnormal vaginal bleeding.
• Instruct women to perform monthly breast examinations and have a yearly breast examination by a health care provider. Also recommend annual mammogram if patient is older than age 50.
• Tell patient to immediately report pain in the calves or chest, sudden shortness of breath, coughing blood, severe headache, vomiting, dizziness, faintness, changes in vision or speech, and weakness or numbness in arms or legs. These are warning signals of blood clots.
• Urge patient to report evidence of liver problems, such as yellowing of skin or eyes and upper right quadrant pain.
• Instruct patient to report pain, swelling, or tenderness in abdomen, which may indicate gallbladder problems.
• Tell patient to store drug at room temperature away from excessive heat and moisture. It remains stable for 18 months.

☑ Evaluation
• Patient has no thromboembolic event during therapy.
• Patient's underlying condition improves.
• Patient and family state understanding of drug therapy.

estrogens, conjugated (estrogenic substances, conjugated; oestrogens, conjugated)

(ESS-troh-jenz, KAHN-jih-gayt-ed)
C.E.S.♦, Cenestin, Premarin, Premarin Intravenous

Pharmacologic class: hormone
Therapeutic class: estrogen, antineoplastic, antiosteoporotic
Pregnancy risk category: X

Indications and dosages

▶ **Abnormal uterine bleeding caused by hormonal imbalance.** *Women:* 25 mg I.V. or I.M. Repeat dose in 6 to 12 hours, if needed.
▶ **Vulvar or vaginal atrophy.** *Women:* 0.5 to 2 g cream intravaginally once daily in cycles of 3 weeks on, 1 week off. Or 0.3 mg P.O. daily.
▶ **Castration, primary ovarian failure.** *Adults:* Initially 1.25 mg P.O. daily in cycles of 3 weeks on, 1 week off. Adjust dose p.r.n.
▶ **Hypogonadism.** *Women:* 0.3 to 0.625 mg P.O. daily, given cyclically 3 weeks on, 1 week off.
▶ **Moderate to severe vasomotor symptoms with or without moderate to severe symptoms of vulvar and vaginal atrophy related to menopause.** *Women:* 0.3 mg P.O. daily, or cyclically 25 days on, 5 days off for atrophy; 0.45 mg P.O. daily for vasomotor symptoms.
▶ **Palliative therapy for inoperable prostatic cancer.** *Men:* 1.25 to 2.5 mg P.O. t.i.d.
▶ **Palliative therapy for breast cancer.** *Adults:* 10 mg P.O. t.i.d. for 3 months or more.
▶ **To prevent osteoporosis in women with an increased risk but for whom non-estrogen therapy is inappropriate.** *Adults:* 0.3 to 0.625 mg P.O. daily, or cyclically, 25 days on, 5 days off.

▼ I.V. administration

• Refrigerate before reconstituting.
• Withdraw 5 ml of air from vial before adding diluent.
• Reconstitute powder for injection with diluent provided (sterile water for injection with benzyl alcohol). Gently agitate to mix drug. Avoid shaking container.

• When giving by direct I.V. injection, give slowly to avoid flushing.
⊗ **Incompatibilities**
Acidic solutions, ascorbic acid.

Contraindications and cautions

• Contraindicated in patients with thrombophlebitis, thromboembolic disorders, estrogen-dependent neoplasia, breast or reproductive organ cancer (except for palliative therapy), or undiagnosed abnormal genital bleeding.
• Use cautiously in patients with cerebrovascular or coronary artery disease, asthma, bone disease, migraine, seizures, or cardiac, hepatic, or renal dysfunction and in women with a close family history of breast or genital tract cancer or who have breast nodules, fibrocystic disease, or abnormal mammogram findings.
☀ **Lifespan:** In children and in pregnant or breast-feeding women, drug is contraindicated.

Adverse reactions

CNS: headache, dizziness, chorea, depression, lethargy, *seizures, stroke.*
CV: thrombophlebitis, *thromboembolism,* hypertension, edema, *pulmonary embolism, MI.*
EENT: worsening of myopia or astigmatism, intolerance of contact lenses.
GI: *nausea,* vomiting, abdominal cramps, bloating, diarrhea, constipation, anorexia, *pancreatitis.*
GU: breakthrough bleeding, altered menstrual flow, dysmenorrhea, amenorrhea, *endometrial cancer,* cervical erosion, altered cervical secretions, enlargement of uterine fibromas, vaginal candidiasis, testicular atrophy, impotence.
Hepatic: gallbladder disease, cholestatic jaundice, *hepatic adenoma.*
Metabolic: increased appetite, weight changes, hyperglycemia, hypercalcemia.
Skin: melasma, urticaria, erythema nodosum, dermatitis, flushing (with rapid I.V. administration), hirsutism, hair loss.
Other: breast changes (tenderness, enlargement, secretion), *breast cancer,* gynecomastia.

Interactions

Drug-drug. *Bromocriptine:* May cause amenorrhea, interfering with bromocriptine effects. Avoid use together.
Carbamazepine, phenobarbital, rifampin: May decrease estrogen effectiveness. Monitor patient closely.

Corticosteroids: May enhance effects. Monitor patient closely.
Cyclosporine: May increase risk of toxicity. Frequently monitor cyclosporine levels.
Dantrolene, other hepatotoxic drugs: May increase risk of hepatotoxicity. Monitor patient closely.
Hydantoins: Use together may cause loss of seizure control and increased risk of breakthrough bleeding, spotting, and pregnancy. Monitor patient closely.
Itraconazole, ketoconazole, macrolides, ritonavir: May increase concentration of estrogens. Monitor patient for increased adverse effects.
Oral anticoagulants: May decrease anticoagulant effects. Dosage adjustments may be needed. Monitor PT and INR.
Tamoxifen: Estrogens may interfere with effectiveness of tamoxifen. Avoid use together.
Thyroid hormones: May alter serum thyroxine and thyrotropin concentrations. Increase thyroid hormone dose as needed.
Topiramate: May increase the metabolism of estrogens and decrease effectiveness. Monitor patient closely.
Drug-herb. *St. John's wort:* May decrease concentrations of estrogens. Watch for decreased effectiveness and changes in bleeding patterns.
Drug-food. *Caffeine:* May increase caffeine level. Monitor effects.
Drug-lifestyle. *Smoking:* May increase risk of CV effects. If smoking continues, patient may need alternative therapy. Urge patient to stop smoking.

Effects on lab test results

• May increase glucose, calcium, total T_4, thyroid-binding globulin, phospholipid, triglyceride, and clotting factor VII, VIII, IX, and X levels.
• May increase PT and norepinephrine-induced platelet aggregation.

Pharmacokinetics

Absorption: Rapid, continuing for days after I.M. use.
Distribution: Highest levels in fat; about 50% to 80% protein-bound.
Metabolism: Primarily in liver.
Excretion: Majority through kidneys. *Half-life:* Unknown.

Route	Onset	Peak	Duration
P.O., I.V., I.M., vaginal	Unknown	Unknown	Unknown

Action

Chemical effect: Increases synthesis of DNA, RNA, and protein in responsive tissues; also reduces release of follicle-stimulating hormone and luteinizing hormone from pituitary gland.
Therapeutic effect: Provides estrogen replacement, relieves vasomotor menopausal symptoms and vaginal dryness, helps prevent severity of osteoporosis, and provides palliation for prostate and breast cancer.

Available forms

Injection: 25 mg/5 ml
Tablets: 0.3 mg, 0.45 mg, 0.625 mg, 0.9 mg, 1.25 mg
Vaginal cream: 0.625 mg/g

NURSING PROCESS

⚕ Assessment
• Obtain history of patient's underlying condition before starting therapy, and reassess regularly.
• Make sure patient has thorough physical examination before starting estrogen therapy.
• Patient receiving long-term therapy should have yearly examinations. Periodically monitor lipid levels, blood pressure, body weight, and liver function.
• Be alert for adverse reactions and drug interactions.
• Assess patient's and family's knowledge of drug therapy.

⚕ Nursing diagnoses
• Ineffective health maintenance related to underlying condition
• Ineffective tissue perfusion (cerebral, peripheral, pulmonary, or myocardial) related to drug-induced thromboembolism
• Deficient knowledge related to drug therapy

▷ Planning and implementation
• Give oral forms at mealtimes or h.s. (for once-daily dose) to minimize nausea.
• When giving I.M., inject deep into large muscle. Rotate injection sites to prevent muscle atrophy.

• Use I.M. or I.V. to rapidly treat dysfunctional uterine bleeding or to reduce surgical bleeding.
• Because of risk of thromboembolism, stop therapy at least 1 month before procedures that may prolong immobilization, such as knee or hip surgery. If thromboembolism is suspected, withhold drug, notify prescriber, and provide supportive care.
ALERT: Estrogens aren't interchangeable.

Patient teaching

• Inform patient about adverse effects.
• Emphasize importance of regular physical examinations. In postmenopausal women, using the drug for longer than 5 years may increase risk of endometrial carcinoma. This risk is reduced by using cyclic rather than continuous therapy and lowest dosages. Drug probably doesn't increase risk of breast cancer.
• Teach patient how to use vaginal cream. Tell her to wash vaginal area with soap and water before applying. Tell her to apply drug h.s. or to lie flat for 30 minutes after application to minimize drug loss.
• Explain to patient on cyclic therapy for postmenopausal symptoms that, although withdrawal bleeding may occur during week off drug, fertility hasn't been restored. Pregnancy can't occur because she hasn't ovulated.
• Warn patient to immediately report abdominal pain; pain, numbness, or stiffness in legs or buttocks; pressure or pain in chest; shortness of breath; severe headaches; visual disturbances, such as blind spots, flashing lights, or blurriness; vaginal bleeding or discharge; breast lumps; swelling of hands or feet; yellow skin or sclera; dark urine; and light-colored stools.
• Tell diabetic patient to report elevated glucose test results so antidiabetic dosage can be adjusted.
• Teach woman how to perform routine breast self-examination.

Evaluation

• Patient shows improvement in underlying condition.
• Patient has no thromboembolic event during therapy.
• Patient and family state understanding of drug therapy.

estrogens, esterified

(ESS-troh-jenz, ESS-tehr-eh-fighd)
Estratab, Menest, Neo-Estrone

Pharmacologic class: hormone
Therapeutic class: antineoplastic, estrogen
Pregnancy risk category: X

Indications and dosages

▶ **Inoperable prostate cancer.** *Men:* 1.25 to 2.5 mg P.O. t.i.d.
▶ **Breast cancer with metastasis.** *Men and postmenopausal women:* 10 mg P.O. t.i.d. for 3 or more months.
▶ **Hypogonadism.** *Women:* 2.5 to 7.5 mg P.O. daily in divided doses in cycles of 20 days on, 10 days off.
▶ **Castration, primary ovarian failure.** *Women:* 2.5 mg P.O. daily to t.i.d. in cycles of 3 weeks on, 1 week off.
▶ **Vasomotor menopausal symptoms.** *Women:* Average dosage is 1.25 mg P.O. daily in cycles of 3 weeks on, 1 week off.
▶ **Atrophic vaginitis or urethritis.** *Women:* 0.3 to 1.25 mg P.O. daily in cycles of 3 weeks on, 1 week off.
▶ **Prevention of osteoporosis in women at significant risk for whom non-estrogen therapy is inappropriate.** *Women:* Initially 0.3 mg P.O. daily; may increase to maximum, 1.25 mg daily.

Contraindications and cautions

• Contraindicated in patients with breast cancer (except when metastatic disease is present), estrogen-dependent neoplasia, active thrombophlebitis or thromboembolic disorders, undiagnosed abnormal genital bleeding, hypersensitivity to drug, or history of thromboembolic disease.
• Use cautiously in patients with history of hypertension, depression, cardiac or renal dysfunction, liver impairment, bone diseases, migraine, seizures, or diabetes mellitus.
Lifespan: In children and in pregnant or breast-feeding women, drug is contraindicated.

Adverse reactions

CNS: headache, dizziness, chorea, depression, lethargy, ***seizures, stroke.***
CV: thrombophlebitis, ***thromboembolism,*** hypertension, edema, ***pulmonary embolism, MI.***

EENT: worsening of myopia or astigmatism, intolerance of contact lenses.
GI: nausea, vomiting, abdominal cramps, bloating, diarrhea, constipation, anorexia, *pancreatitis.*
GU: breakthrough bleeding, altered menstrual flow, dysmenorrhea, amenorrhea, *breast and endometrial cancers,* cervical erosion, altered cervical secretions, enlargement of uterine fibromas, vaginal candidiasis, testicular atrophy, impotence.
Hepatic: cholestatic jaundice, *hepatic adenoma,* gallbladder disease.
Metabolic: increased appetite, weight changes, hypercalcemia.
Skin: melasma, rash, erythema nodosum, dermatitis, hirsutism, hair loss.
Other: gynecomastia, breast changes (tenderness, enlargement, secretion).

Interactions

Drug-drug. *Bromocriptine:* May cause amenorrhea, interfering with bromocriptine effects. Avoid use together.
Carbamazepine, phenobarbital, rifampin: May decrease estrogen effectiveness. Monitor patient closely.
Corticosteroids: May enhance effects. Monitor patient closely.
Cyclosporine: May increase risk of toxicity. Frequently monitor cyclosporine level.
Dantrolene, other hepatotoxic drugs: May increase risk of hepatotoxicity. Monitor patient closely.
Hydantoins: Use together may cause loss of seizure control and increased risk of breakthrough bleeding, spotting, and pregnancy. Monitor patient closely.
Itraconazole, ketoconazole, macrolides, ritonavir: May increase concentration of estrogens. Watch for increased adverse effects.
Oral anticoagulants: May decrease anticoagulant effects. Dosage adjustments may be needed. Monitor PT and INR.
Tamoxifen: Estrogens may interfere with effectiveness of tamoxifen. Avoid use together.
Thyroid hormones: May alter serum thyroxine and thyrotropin concentrations. Increase thyroid hormone dose as needed.
Topiramate: May increase the metabolism of estrogens and decrease effectiveness. Monitor patient closely.

Drug-herb. *St. John's wort:* May decrease concentrations of estrogens. Watch for decreased effectiveness and changes in bleeding patterns.
Drug-food. *Caffeine:* May increase caffeine level. Monitor effects.
Drug-lifestyle. *Smoking:* May increase risk of CV effects. Urge patient to stop smoking. If smoking continues, patient may need alternative therapy.

Effects on lab test results

• May increase glucose, calcium, total T_4, thyroid-binding globulin, phospholipid, triglyceride, and clotting factor VII, VIII, IX, and X levels.
• May increase PT and norepinephrine-induced platelet aggregation.

Pharmacokinetics

Absorption: Well absorbed but substantially inactivated by liver.
Distribution: Highest levels in fat; about 50% to 80% protein-bound.
Metabolism: Primarily in liver.
Excretion: Primarily by kidneys. *Half-life:* Unknown.

Route	Onset	Peak	Duration
P.O.	Unknown	Unknown	Unknown

Action

Chemical effect: Increases synthesis of DNA, RNA, and protein and reduces release of follicle-stimulating hormone and luteinizing hormone from pituitary gland.
Therapeutic effect: Provides estrogen replacement, hinders prostate and breast cancer cell growth, and relieves menopausal vasomotor symptoms and vaginal dryness.

Available forms

Tablets: 0.3 mg, 0.625 mg, 1.25 mg, 2.5 mg
Tablets (film-coated): 0.3 mg, 0.625 mg, 1.25 mg, 2.5 mg

NURSING PROCESS

⚗ Assessment

• Obtain history of patient's underlying condition before starting therapy, and reassess regularly thereafter.
• Make sure patient has thorough physical examination before starting drug therapy.

• Patient receiving long-term therapy should have yearly examinations. Periodically monitor lipid levels, blood pressure, body weight, and liver function.
• Be alert for adverse reactions and drug interactions.
• Assess patient's and family's knowledge of drug therapy.

🔹 **Nursing diagnoses**
• Ineffective health maintenance related to underlying condition
• Ineffective tissue perfusion (cerebral, peripheral, pulmonary, or myocardial) related to drug-induced thromboembolism
• Deficient knowledge related to drug therapy

▶ **Planning and implementation**
• Give oral forms at mealtimes or bedtime (for once-daily dose) to minimize nausea.
• Because of risk of thromboembolism, stop therapy at least 1 month before procedures that may cause prolonged immobilization or thromboembolism, such as knee or hip surgery. If thromboembolism is suspected, withhold drug, notify prescriber, and provide supportive care.
⑤ **ALERT:** Estrogens aren't interchangeable.
Patient teaching
• Inform patient about adverse effects.
• Emphasize importance of regular physical examinations. Tell postmenopausal women who use the drug for more than 5 years that it may increase their risk for endometrial carcinoma, but that this risk is reduced by using cyclic rather than continuous therapy and the lowest dosages of estrogen. Also inform her that the drug probably doesn't increase risk of breast cancer.
• Explain to patient on cyclic therapy for postmenopausal symptoms that although withdrawal bleeding may occur during the week off, fertility hasn't been restored. Pregnancy can't occur because she hasn't ovulated.
• Warn patient to immediately report abdominal pain; pain, numbness, or stiffness in legs or buttocks; pressure or pain in chest; shortness of breath; severe headaches; visual disturbances, such as blind spots, flashing lights, or blurriness; vaginal bleeding or discharge; breast lumps; swelling of hands or feet; yellow skin or sclera; dark urine; and light-colored stools.

• Tell diabetic patient to report elevated glucose test results so antidiabetic dosage can be adjusted.
• Teach woman how to perform routine breast self-examination.

☑ **Evaluation**
• Patient shows improvement in underlying condition.
• Patient has no thromboembolic event during therapy.
• Patient and family state understanding of drug therapy.

estropipate (piperazine estrone sulfate)
(ess-troh-PIH-payt)
Ogen, Ortho-Est

Pharmacologic class: hormone
Therapeutic class: estrogen
Pregnancy risk category: X

Indications and dosages

▶ **Management of moderate-to-severe vasomotor symptoms, vulvar and vaginal atrophy.** *Women:* 0.75 to 6 mg P.O. daily 3 weeks on, 1 week off, or 2 to 4 g of vaginal cream daily. Typically dosage given on cyclic, short-term basis.
▶ **Primary ovarian failure, castration, hypogonadism.** *Women:* Given on cyclic basis with 1.5 to 9 mg P.O. daily for first 3 weeks and then rest period of 8 to 10 days. If bleeding doesn't occur by end of rest period, repeat cycle.
▶ **To prevent osteoporosis.** *Women:* 0.625 mg P.O. daily for 25 days of 31-day cycle. Repeat cycle p.r.n.

Contraindications and cautions

• Contraindicated in patients with active thrombophlebitis, thromboembolic disorders, estrogen-dependent neoplasia, undiagnosed genital bleeding, or breast, reproductive organ, or genital cancer.
• Use cautiously in patients with cerebrovascular or coronary artery disease, asthma, depression, bone disease, migraine, seizures, or cardiac, hepatic, or renal dysfunction and in women with family history (mother, grandmoth-

er, sister) of breast or genital tract cancer or who have breast nodules, fibrocystic disease, or abnormal mammogram findings. Use the lowest effective dose for the shortest duration.

• This drug has not been approved for the prevention of cognitive disorders or memory loss.

⚞ **Lifespan:** In children and in pregnant or breast-feeding women, drug is contraindicated.

Adverse reactions

CNS: depression, headache, dizziness, migraine, *seizure, stroke.*
CV: edema, thrombophlebitis, *pulmonary embolism, thromboembolism, MI.*
GI: *nausea,* vomiting, abdominal cramps, bloating.
GU: increased size of uterine fibromas, *endometrial and breast cancers,* vaginal candidiasis, cystitis-like syndrome, dysmenorrhea, amenorrhea, breakthrough bleeding.
Hepatic: cholestatic jaundice.
Metabolic: hypercalcemia, weight changes.
Skin: hemorrhagic eruption, erythema nodosum, *erythema multiforme,* hirsutism, melasma, hair loss.
Other: breast engorgement or enlargement, libido changes, aggravation of porphyria.

Interactions

Drug-drug. *Bromocriptine:* May cause amenorrhea, interfering with bromocriptine effects. Avoid use together.
Carbamazepine, phenobarbital, rifampin: May decrease estrogen effectiveness. Monitor patient closely.
Corticosteroids: May enhance effects. Monitor patient closely.
Cyclosporine: May increase risk of toxicity. Frequently monitor cyclosporine level.
Dantrolene, other hepatotoxic drugs: May increase risk of hepatotoxicity. Monitor patient closely.
Hydantoins: Use together may cause loss of seizure control and increased risk of breakthrough bleeding, spotting, and pregnancy. Monitor patient closely.
Itraconazole, ketoconazole, macrolides, ritonavir: May increase concentration of estrogens. Watch for increased adverse effects.
Oral anticoagulants: May decrease anticoagulant effects. Dosage adjustments may be needed. Monitor PT and INR.

Tamoxifen: Estrogens may interfere with effectiveness of tamoxifen. Avoid use together.
Thyroid hormones: May alter serum thyroxine and thyrotropin concentrations. Increase thyroid hormone dose as needed.
Topiramate: May increase the metabolism of estrogens and decrease effectiveness. Monitor patient closely.
Drug-herb. *St. John's wort:* May decrease concentrations of estrogens. Watch for decreased effectiveness and changes in bleeding patterns.
Drug-food. *Caffeine:* May increase caffeine level. Monitor effects.
Drug-lifestyle. *Smoking:* May increase risk of CV effects. Urge patient to stop smoking. If smoking continues, patient may need alternate therapy.

Effects on lab test results

• May increase calcium, total T_4, thyroid-binding globulin, phospholipid, triglyceride, and clotting factor VII, VIII, IX, and X levels.
• May increase PT and norepinephrine-induced platelet aggregation.

Pharmacokinetics

Absorption: Not well characterized after P.O. or intravaginal administration.
Distribution: Highest levels in fat; about 50% to 80% protein-bound.
Metabolism: Primarily in liver.
Excretion: Primarily by kidneys. *Half-life:* Unknown.

Route	Onset	Peak	Duration
P.O., vaginal	Unknown	Unknown	Unknown

Action

Chemical effect: Increases synthesis of DNA, RNA, and protein and reduces release of follicle-stimulating hormone and luteinizing hormone from pituitary gland.
Therapeutic effect: Provides estrogen replacement, relieves menopausal vasomotor symptoms, and helps reduce severity of osteoporosis.

Available forms

Tablets: 0.75 mg, 1.5 mg, 3 mg, 6 mg
Vaginal cream: 1.5 mg/g (0.15%)

NURSING PROCESS

☷ Assessment
• Obtain history of patient's underlying condition before starting therapy, and reassess regularly.
• Make sure patient has thorough physical examination before starting drug therapy.
• Patient receiving long-term therapy should have yearly examinations. Periodically monitor lipid level, blood pressure, body weight, and liver function.
• Be alert for adverse reactions and drug interactions.
• Assess patient's and family's knowledge of drug therapy.

⊕ Nursing diagnoses
• Ineffective health maintenance related to underlying condition
• Ineffective tissue perfusion (cerebral, peripheral, pulmonary, or myocardial) related to drug-induced thromboembolism
• Deficient knowledge related to drug therapy

❯ Planning and implementation
• Give oral forms with meals or h.s. (for once-daily dose) to minimize nausea.
• Because of risk of thromboembolism, stop therapy at least 1 month before procedures that may cause prolonged immobilization or thromboembolism, such as knee or hip surgery. If thromboembolism is suspected, withhold drug, notify prescriber, and provide supportive care.
⚠ ALERT: Estrogens aren't interchangeable.
Patient teaching
• Inform patient about adverse effects.
• Emphasize importance of regular physical examinations. Tell postmenopausal women who use the drug for more than 5 years that it may increase their risk of endometrial carcinoma, but that the risk is reduced by using cyclic rather than continuous therapy and the lowest dosages of estrogen. Also inform her that the drug probably doesn't increase risk of breast cancer.
• Teach patient how to use vaginal cream. Tell her to wash vaginal area with soap and water before applying. Tell her to use drug h.s. or to lie flat for 30 minutes after application to minimize drug loss.
• Explain to patient on cyclic therapy for postmenopausal symptoms that although withdrawal bleeding may occur during the week off, fertili-

ty hasn't been restored. Pregnancy can't occur because she hasn't ovulated.
• Explain to patient being treated for hypogonadism that therapy length depends on her endometrial response to drug. If satisfactory withdrawal bleeding doesn't occur, oral progestin may be added. Explain to patient that despite return of withdrawal bleeding, pregnancy can't occur because she isn't ovulating.
• Warn patient to immediately report abdominal pain; pain, numbness, or stiffness in legs or buttocks; pressure or pain in chest; shortness of breath; severe headaches; visual disturbances, such as blind spots, flashing lights, or blurriness; vaginal bleeding or discharge; breast lumps; swelling of hands or feet; yellow skin or sclera; dark urine; and light-colored stools.
• Tell diabetic patient to report elevated glucose test results so antidiabetic dosage can be adjusted.
• Teach woman how to perform routine breast self-examination.

☑ Evaluation
• Patient shows improvement in underlying condition.
• Patient has no thromboembolic event during therapy.
• Patient and family state understanding of drug therapy.

eszopiclone
(ess-zoe-PICK-lone)
Lunesta◆

Pharmacologic class: pyrrolopyrazine derivative
Therapeutic class: hypnotic
Pregnancy risk category: C
Controlled substance schedule: IV

Indications and dosages
▶ **Insomnia.** *Adults:* 2 mg P.O. immediately h.s. Increase to 3 mg p.r.n.
Elderly patients having trouble falling asleep: 1 mg P.O. immediately h.s. Increase to 2 mg p.r.n.
Elderly patients having trouble staying asleep: 2 mg P.O. immediately h.s.
☒ **Adjust-a-dose:** In patients with severe hepatic impairment, start with 1 mg P.O. In patients

who also take a potent CYP 3A4 inhibitor, start with 1 mg and increase to 2 mg if needed.

Contraindications and cautions

• Use cautiously in patients with diseases or conditions that could affect metabolism or hemodynamic responses. Also use cautiously in patients with compromised respiratory function, severe hepatic impairment, or signs and symptoms of depression.

⚜ **Lifespan:** In pregnant women, use only if benefits outweigh risk to the fetus. In breastfeeding women, use cautiously because it isn't known if drug appears in breast milk. In children, safety and effectiveness haven't been established. Elderly patients may be more sensitive to drug effects.

Adverse reactions

CNS: abnormal dreams, anxiety, confusion, depression, dizziness, hallucinations, *headache,* nervousness, pain, *somnolence,* neuralgia.
EENT: unpleasant taste.
GI: diarrhea, dry mouth, dyspepsia, nausea, vomiting.
GU: UTI.
Respiratory: respiratory infection.
Skin: pruritus, rash.
Other: accidental injury, decreased libido, viral infection.

Interactions

Drug-drug. *CNS depressants:* May have additive CNS effects. Adjust dosage of either drug as needed.
CYP 3A4 inhibitors (clarithromycin, itraconazole, ketoconazole, nefazodone, nelfinavir, ritonavir, troleandomycin): May decrease eszopiclone elimination, increasing the risk of toxicity. Use together cautiously.
Olanzapine: May impair cognitive function or memory. Use together cautiously.
Rifampicin: May decrease eszopiclone activity. Don't use together.
Drug-food. *High-fat meals:* May decrease eszopiclone absorption and decrease drug effects. Discourage high-fat meals with or just before taking drug.
Drug-lifestyle. *Alcohol:* May decrease psychomotor ability. Discourage use together.

Effects on lab test results

None reported.

Pharmacokinetics

Absorption: Rapid.
Distribution: In plasma; about 50% to 60% protein-bound.
Metabolism: By CYP 3A4 in the liver, with two mainly inactive metabolites.
Excretion: In urine, mainly as metabolites.
Half-life: 6 hours.

Route	Onset	Peak	Duration
P.O.	Rapid	1 hr	Unknown

Action

Chemical effect: Drug probably interacts with gamma amino-butyric acid receptors at binding sites close to or connected to benzodiazepine receptors.
Therapeutic effect: Promotes sleep.

Available forms

Tablets: 1 mg, 2 mg, 3 mg

NURSING PROCESS

⚗ Assessment
• Evaluate patient for physical and psychiatric disorders before treatment.
• Be alert for drug interactions and adverse reactions.
• If patient is still having trouble sleeping after using drug for short-term therapy, check for other psychological disorders.
• Monitor patient for changes in behavior, including those that suggest depression or suicidal thinking.
• Assess patient's and family's knowledge of drug therapy.

▣ Nursing diagnoses
• Disturbed sleep pattern related to presence of insomnia
• Risk for injury related to drug-induced adverse CNS reactions
• Deficient knowledge related to drug therapy

▷ Planning and implementation
⊕ ALERT: Give drug immediately before patient goes to bed or after patient has gone to bed and has trouble falling asleep.
• Use the lowest effective dose.
• Use only for short periods (for example, 7 to 10 days).

Reactions may be *common,* uncommon, *life-threatening,* or COMMON AND LIFE-THREATENING.

E

• Overdose may cause impaired consciousness, hypotension, and CNS depression.

• Treat overdose symptomatically and supportively; flumazenil may be helpful. It isn't known if eszopiclone is removed by dialysis.

Patient teaching

• Urge patient to take drug immediately before going to bed because drug may cause dizziness or light-headedness.

• Caution patient not to take eszopiclone unless he can get a full night's sleep.

• Advise patient to avoid taking drug after a high-fat meal.

• Tell patient to avoid activities that require mental alertness until the drug's effects are known.

• Advise patient to avoid alcohol while taking drug.

• Urge patient to immediately report changes in behavior and thinking.

• Warn patient not to stop drug abruptly or change dose without consulting the prescriber.

• Inform patient that tolerance or dependence may develop if drug is taken for a prolonged period.

☑ Evaluation

• Patient no longer experiences insomnia with drug therapy.

• Patient does not experience injury from adverse CNS reactions.

• Patient and family state understanding of drug therapy.

etanercept
(ee-TAN-er-sept)
Enbrel

Pharmacologic class: tumor necrosis factor (TNF) blocker
Therapeutic class: antirheumatic
Pregnancy risk category: B

Indications and dosages

▶ **Psoriatic arthritis, ankylosing spondylitis, moderately to severely active rheumatoid arthritis.** *Adults:* 25 mg subcutaneously twice weekly, on same day or 72 to 96 hours apart, or 50 mg subcutaneously from prefilled syringe once weekly. Continue methotrexate, glucocor-

ticoids, salicylates, NSAIDs, or analgesics during therapy.

▶ **Moderately to severely active polyarticular-course juvenile rheumatoid arthritis in patients who have had an inadequate response to one or more disease-modifying antirheumatic drugs.** *Children ages 4 to 17:* 0.4 mg/kg (maximum, 25 mg/dose) subcutaneously twice weekly, on same day or 72 to 96 hours apart.

▶ **Chronic moderate to severe plaque psoriasis in patients who are candidates for systemic therapy or phototherapy.** *Adults:* 50 mg subcutaneously twice weekly, 3 to 4 days apart for 3 months. Then, reduce dosage to 50 mg subcutaneously once weekly.

Contraindications and cautions

• Contraindicated in patients hypersensitive to drug or any of its components and in those with sepsis. Stop giving the drug to a patient who develops a serious infection or sepsis. Use of live vaccines during drug therapy is contraindicated.

• Use cautiously in patients with a history of recurring infections and in those with underlying diseases that predispose them to infection, such as diabetes or heart failure. Also use cautiously in patients with CNS demyelinating disorders and in those with a history of significant hematologic abnormalities.

🌢 **Lifespan:** In pregnant women, use cautiously. Breast-feeding women should stop drug or stop breast-feeding. In children younger than age 4, safety and effectiveness haven't been established.

Adverse reactions

CNS: asthenia, *headache,* dizziness.
EENT: rhinitis, pharyngitis, sinusitis.
GI: abdominal pain, dyspepsia.
Respiratory: *upper respiratory tract infections,* cough, respiratory disorder.
Skin: rash.
Other: infections, *malignancies,* injection site reaction.

Interactions

Drug-drug. *Live-virus vaccinations:* Transmission of infection remains unknown. Avoid use together.

Effects on lab test results

• May cause positive antinuclear antibody or positive anti–double-stranded DNA antibodies measured by radioimmunoassay and *Crithidia luciliae* assay.

Pharmacokinetics

Absorption: Level peaks in 72 hours.
Distribution: Unknown.
Metabolism: Unknown.
Excretion: Unknown. *Half-life:* 115 hours.

Route	Onset	Peak	Duration
SubQ	Unknown	3 days	Unknown

Action

Chemical effect: Binds specifically to TNF and blocks its action, reducing inflammatory and immune responses found in rheumatoid arthritis.
Therapeutic effect: Reduces signs and symptoms of rheumatoid arthritis.

Available forms

Injection: 25-mg single-use vial, 50-mg/ml prefilled syringe

NURSING PROCESS

🔢 Assessment

• Obtain history of patient's underlying condition before starting therapy, and reassess regularly.
• Obtain accurate immunization history from parents or guardians of juvenile rheumatoid arthritis patients. Patient should be brought up-to-date with all immunizations before starting drug.
• Monitor patient for infection.
• Assess patient's and family's knowledge of drug therapy.

🔵 Nursing diagnoses

• Acute pain related to underlying condition
• Risk for infection related to drug-induced adverse reactions
• Deficient knowledge related to drug therapy

▶ Planning and implementation

• Drug is for subcutaneous injection only.
• Reconstitute aseptically with 1 ml of supplied sterile bacteriostatic water for injection, USP (0.9% benzyl alcohol). Don't filter reconstituted solution during preparation or administration. Inject diluent slowly into vial. Minimize foaming by gently swirling during dissolution rather than shaking. Dissolution takes less than 5 minutes.

• Inspect solution for particulates and discoloration before use. Reconstituted solution should be clear and colorless. Don't use solution if it's discolored or cloudy, or if particulates exist.
• Don't add other drugs or diluents to reconstituted solution.
• Use reconstituted solution as soon as possible. Solution may be refrigerated in vial for up to 6 hours at 36° to 46° F (2° to 8° C).
• Inject at least 1 inch from another injection site; don't use areas where skin is tender, bruised, red, or hard. Recommended sites include the thigh, abdomen, and upper arm. Rotate sites regularly.
• Don't give live vaccines during therapy.
• Drug may affect defenses against infection. If serious infection occurs, notify prescriber and stop therapy.
• Needle cover of diluent syringe contains dry natural rubber (latex). Don't allow those sensitive to latex to handle cover.
• **ALERT:** Don't confuse Enbrel with Levbid.

Patient teaching

• If patient will be administering drug, teach mixing and injection techniques, including rotation of injection sites.
• Instruct patient to use puncture-resistant container to dispose of needles and syringes.
• Tell patient that injection site reactions typically occur within first month of therapy and decrease thereafter.
• Urge patient to avoid live vaccines during therapy. Stress importance of alerting other health care providers of etanercept use.
• Instruct patient to promptly report evidence of infection to prescriber.

✔ Evaluation

• Patient's pain decreases.
• Patient is free from infection.
• Patient and family state understanding of drug therapy.

ethacrynate sodium

(eth-uh-KRIH-nayt SOH-dee-um)
Sodium Edecrin

ethacrynic acid

Edecril◊, Edecrin

Pharmacologic class: loop diuretic
Therapeutic class: diuretic
Pregnancy risk category: B

Indications and dosages

▶ **Acute pulmonary edema.** *Adults:* 50 mg or
0.5 to 1 mg/kg I.V. to maximum dose of
100 mg. Usually, only one dose is needed; occasionally, second dose may be required.
▶ **Edema.** *Adults:* 50 to 200 mg P.O. daily. Refractory cases may require up to 200 mg b.i.d.
Children age 1 and older: Initial dose is 25 mg
P.O.; increase cautiously in 25-mg increments
daily until desired effect is achieved.
▶ **Hypertension‡.** *Adults:* Initially 25 mg P.O.
daily. Adjust dosage p.r.n. Maximum maintenance dosage is 200 mg P.O. daily in two divided doses.

▼ I.V. administration

• Reconstitute vacuum vial with 50 ml of D_5W
or normal saline solution.
• Give slowly through I.V. line of running infusion or by direct injection over several minutes.
• If more than one I.V. dose is needed, use new
injection site to avoid thrombophlebitis.
• Discard unused solution after 24 hours. Don't
use cloudy or opalescent solutions.
⊗ Incompatibilities
Hydralazine, Normosol-M, procainamide, ranitidine, reserpine, solutions or drugs with pH below 5, tolazoline, triflupromazine, whole blood
and its derivatives.

Contraindications and cautions

• Contraindicated in patients hypersensitive to
the drug or any of its components and in those
with anuria.
• Use cautiously in patients with electrolyte abnormalities, advanced cirrhosis of the liver, hepatic encephalopathy, or renal impairment.
⚕ Lifespan: In pregnant women, use cautiously. In breast-feeding women, it's unknown if
drug is present in breast milk. In infants, drug is
contraindicated.

Adverse reactions

CNS: fever, malaise, confusion, fatigue, vertigo,
headache, nervousness.
CV: volume depletion and dehydration, orthostatic hypotension.
EENT: transient deafness (with too-rapid I.V.
injection), blurred vision, tinnitus, hearing loss.
GI: cramping, diarrhea, anorexia, nausea, vomiting, GI bleeding, *pancreatitis.*
GU: nocturia, polyuria, frequent urination, oliguria, hematuria.
Hematologic: *agranulocytosis, neutropenia,
thrombocytopenia, azotemia.*
Metabolic: hyperuricemia, hypochloremic alkalosis, dilutional hyponatremia, hypokalemia,
hypocalcemia, *hypomagnesemia,* hyperglycemia, and impairment of glucose tolerance.
Skin: dermatitis, rash.
Other: chills.

Interactions

Drug-drug. *Aminoglycoside antibiotics:* May
potentiate ototoxic adverse reactions of both
drugs. Use together cautiously.
Antihypertensives: May increase risk of hypotension. Use together cautiously.
Chlorothiazide, chlorthalidone, hydrochlorothiazide, indapamide, metolazone: May cause
excessive diuretic response, resulting in serious
electrolyte abnormalities or dehydration. Adjust
doses carefully while monitoring patient closely
for excessive diuretic responses.
Cisplatin: May increase risk of ototoxicity.
Avoid use together.
Digoxin: May increase risk of digoxin toxicity
from ethacrynate-induced hypokalemia. Monitor potassium and digoxin levels.
Lithium: May decrease lithium clearance, increasing risk of lithium toxicity. Monitor lithium level.
Metolazone: May cause profound diuresis and
enhance electrolyte loss. Use together cautiously.
NSAIDs: May decrease diuretic effectiveness.
Use together cautiously.
Warfarin: May potentiate anticoagulant effect.
Use together cautiously.
Drug-herb. *Licorice root:* May contribute to
potassium depletion caused by diuretics. Discourage licorice root intake.

Drug-lifestyle. *Sun exposure:* Photosensitivity may occur. Discourage prolonged or unprotected exposure to sunlight.

Effects on lab test results

• May increase glucose, BUN, and uric acid levels. May decrease potassium, sodium, calcium, and magnesium levels.
• May decrease granulocyte, neutrophil, and platelet counts.

Pharmacokinetics

Absorption: Ethacrynic acid is absorbed rapidly from GI tract. Ethacrynate sodium is administered I.V.
Distribution: Unknown.
Metabolism: Unknown.
Excretion: Unknown. *Half-life:* 1 hour.

Route	Onset	Peak	Duration
P.O.	30 min	2 hr	6–8 hr
I.V.	5 min	15–30 min	2 hr

Action

Chemical effect: Inhibits sodium and chloride reabsorption at renal tubules and ascending loop of Henle.
Therapeutic effect: Promotes sodium and water excretion.

Available forms

Injection: 50 mg (with 62.5 mg of mannitol and 0.1 mg of thimerosal)
Tablets: 25 mg, 50 mg

NURSING PROCESS

℞ Assessment

• Obtain history of patient's underlying condition before starting therapy.
• Monitor effectiveness by regularly checking urine output, weight, peripheral edema, and breath sounds.
• Monitor fluid intake, blood pressure, and electrolyte levels.
• Monitor uric acid levels, especially in patients with history of gout.
• Be alert for adverse reactions and drug interactions.
• Assess patient's and family's knowledge of drug therapy.

Nursing diagnoses

• Excess fluid volume related to underlying condition
• Impaired urinary elimination related to diuretic therapy
• Deficient knowledge related to drug therapy

Planning and implementation

• Give drug with food or milk because P.O. use may cause GI upset.
• To prevent nocturia, give P.O. doses in morning.
• Don't mix with whole blood or its derivatives.
• Don't give subcutaneously or I.M. because of local pain and irritation.
• Potassium chloride and sodium supplements may be needed.
• If diarrhea occurs, notify prescriber because severe diarrhea may warrant stopping drug.
Patient teaching
• Advise patient to avoid sudden posture changes and to rise slowly to avoid orthostatic hypotension.
• Advise diabetic patient to closely monitor glucose level.
• Teach patient and family to identify and report signs of hypersensitivity or fluid and electrolyte disturbances.
• Teach patient to monitor fluid volume by daily weight and intake and output.
• Tell patient to take oral drug early in day to avoid interruption of sleep by nocturia.

Evaluation

• Patient is free from edema.
• Patient demonstrates adjustment of lifestyle to deal with altered patterns of urinary elimination.
• Patient and family state understanding of drug therapy.

ethambutol hydrochloride
(ee-THAM-byoo-tall high-droh-KLOR-ighd)
Etibi ♦ , Myambutol

Pharmacologic class: semisynthetic antituberculotic
Therapeutic class: antituberculotic
Pregnancy risk category: B

Indications and dosages

▶ **Adjunct therapy for pulmonary tuberculosis.** *Adults and children age 13 and older:* For patients who haven't received previous antitubercular therapy, 15 mg/kg P.O. daily. For patients who have received previous antitubercular therapy, 25 mg/kg P.O. daily for 60 days until cultures are negative; then decrease to 15 mg/kg P.O. daily.

▶ **Adjunct therapy for pulmonary *Mycobacterium avium* complex infections in patients without HIV‡.** *Adults:* 25 mg/kg P.O. daily for 2 months followed by 15 mg/kg P.O. daily until cultures are negative for 1 year.

▶ **Adjunct therapy for disseminated *Mycobacterium avium* complex infections‡.** *Adults:* 15 mg/kg P.O. daily for patient's lifetime.

Contraindications and cautions

• Contraindicated in patients hypersensitive to drug and in patients with optic neuritis.
• Use cautiously in patients with impaired kidney function, cataracts, recurrent eye inflammations, gout, or diabetic retinopathy.
⚠ **Lifespan:** In pregnant women, use cautiously. In breast-feeding women, use cautiously because it's unknown if the drug appears in breast milk. In children younger than age 13, drug is contraindicated.

Adverse reactions

CNS: fever, malaise, headache, dizziness, confusion, hallucinations, peripheral neuritis.
EENT: dose-related optic neuritis, vision loss, loss of color discrimination, especially red and green.
GI: anorexia, nausea, vomiting, abdominal pain.
Hematologic: *thrombocytopenia.*
Respiratory: bloody sputum.
Skin: dermatitis, pruritus, *toxic epidermal necrolysis.*
Other: *anaphylactoid reactions,* precipitation of gout.

Interactions

Drug-drug. *Aluminum salts:* May delay and reduce absorption of ethambutol. Separate doses by several hours.

Effects on lab test results

• May increase ALT, AST, bilirubin, and uric acid levels. May decrease glucose level.
• May decrease platelet count.

Pharmacokinetics

Absorption: Rapid.
Distribution: Wide; 8% to 22% protein-bound.
Metabolism: Undergoes partial hepatic metabolism.
Excretion: After 24 hours, about 50% of unchanged drug and 8% to 15% of its metabolites in urine; 20% to 25% in feces. *Half-life:* About 3½ hours.

Route	Onset	Peak	Duration
P.O.	Unknown	2–4 hr	Unknown

Action

Chemical effect: May interfere with synthesis of one or more metabolites of susceptible bacteria, altering cellular metabolism during cell division.
Therapeutic effect: Hinders bacterial growth.

Available forms

Tablets: 100 mg, 400 mg

NURSING PROCESS

⬛ Assessment
• Obtain history of patient's infection before starting therapy.
• Perform visual acuity and color discrimination tests before and during therapy (monthly when dose is 25 mg/kg or more).
• Monitor the drug's effectiveness by regularly assessing for improvement in patient's condition and evaluating culture and sensitivity test results.
• Obtain AST and ALT levels before starting therapy. Then monitor AST and ALT levels every 2 to 4 weeks.
• Monitor uric acid level; observe patient for symptoms of gout.
• Be alert for adverse reactions and drug interactions.
• Assess patient's and family's knowledge of drug therapy.

⬛ Nursing diagnoses
• Infection related to presence of susceptible bacteria

• Disturbed sensory perception (visual) related to drug-induced adverse reactions
• Deficient knowledge related to drug therapy

⊠ **Planning and implementation**
• Anticipate the need for a lower dose in a patient with impaired kidney function.
• Always give ethambutol with other antituberculotics to prevent development of resistant organisms.
⊛ **ALERT:** Don't confuse ethambutol with Ethmozine.
Patient teaching
• Reassure patient that visual disturbances will disappear several weeks to months after the therapy ends.
• Warn patient not to perform hazardous activities if visual disturbances or adverse CNS reactions occur.
• Emphasize need for regular follow-up care.

⊠ **Evaluation**
• Patient is free from infection.
• Patient regains pretreatment vision.
• Patient and family state understanding of drug therapy.

ethinyl estradiol and desogestrel
(ETH-ih-nill es-truh-DIGH-ol and DAY-so-jest-rul)
monophasic: Apri, Desogen, Ortho-Cept
biphasic: Kariva, Mircette
triphasic: Cyclessa, Velivet

ethinyl estradiol and ethynodiol diacetate
monophasic: Demulen 1/35, Demulen 1/50, Zovia 1/35E, Zovia 1/50E

ethinyl estradiol and levonorgestrel
emergency: Preven
monophasic: Alesse, Aviane, Lessina, Levlen, Levlite, Levora, Nordette, Portia
triphasic: Climara Pro, Enpresse, Tri-Levlen, Triphasil, Trivora

ethinyl estradiol and norethindrone
monophasic: Balziva, Brevicon, Genora 0.5/35, Genora 1/35, ModiCon, Norethin 1/35E, Norinyl 1+35, Ortho-Novum 1/35, Ovcon-35, Ovcon-50
biphasic: Necon 10/11, Nortrel, Ortho-Novum 10/11
triphasic: Necon 7/7/7, Nortrel 7/7/7, Ortho-Novum 7/7/7, Tri-Norinyl

ethinyl estradiol and norethindrone acetate
monophasic: Junel 1/20, Junel 1.5/30, Loestrin 21 1/20, Loestrin 21 1.5/30, Necon 1/35, Nortrel 1/35
triphasic: Estrostep

ethinyl estradiol and norgestimate
monophasic: MonoNessa, Ortho-Cyclen, Sprintec
triphasic: Ortho Tri-Cyclen, Ortho Tri-Cyclen Lo, Tri-Sprintec

ethinyl estradiol and norgestrel
monophasic: Cryselle, Low-Ogestrel, Lo/Ovral, Lo/Ovral 28, Ogestrel 0.5/50, Ovral

ethinyl estradiol, norethindrone acetate, and ferrous fumarate
monophasic: Junel Fe 1/20, Junel Fe 1/5/30, Loestrin Fe 1/20, Loestrin Fe 1.5/30, Microgestin Fe 1/20, Microgestin Fe 1.5/30

mestranol and norethindrone
monophasic: Necon 1/50, Norinyl 1+50, Ortho-Novum 1/50
triphasic: Estrostep Fe, Estrostep 21

Pharmacologic class: hormonal contraceptive
Therapeutic class: estrogen with progestin
Pregnancy risk category: X

Indications and dosages
▶ **Contraception.** *Women:* 1 monophasic tablet P.O. daily, beginning on day 5 of menstrual cycle (first day of menstrual flow is day 1). With 20- and 21-tablet packages, new cycle begins 7 days after last tablet taken. With 28-tablet

packages, dosage is 1 tablet daily without interruption; extra tablets are placebos or contain
iron. Or first-color biphasic tablet P.O. daily for
10 days; then next color tablet for 11 days. Or 1
triphasic tablet P.O. daily in sequence specified
by brand. Or 1 transdermal patch, changed
weekly.
► **Moderate acne vulgaris in women and
girls age 15 and older who have no known
contraindications to hormonal contraceptive
therapy, desire hormonal contraception, have
achieved menarche, and are unresponsive to
topical antiacne drugs.** *Women and girls age
15 and older:* 1 tablet Estrostep, Ortho Tri-
Cyclen, or Tri-Sprintec P.O. daily. (Twenty-one
tablets contain active ingredients, and seven are
inert.)

Contraindications and cautions

• Contraindicated in patients with thromboembolic disorders, cerebrovascular or coronary artery disease, diplopia or ocular lesion arising
from ophthalmic vascular disease, classic migraine, MI, known or suspected breast cancer,
known or suspected estrogen-dependent neoplasia, benign or malignant liver tumors, active liver disease or history of cholestatic jaundice with
pregnancy or prior use of hormonal contraceptives, or undiagnosed abnormal vaginal bleeding.
• Use cautiously in patients with cardiac, renal,
or hepatic insufficiency; hyperlipidemia; hypertension; migraine; seizure disorders; or asthma.
⚠ **Lifespan:** In adolescents, hormonal contraception isn't advised until after at least 2 years
of well-established menstrual cycles and completion of physiologic maturation to avoid later
fertility and menstrual problems. In women who
are pregnant or suspect they may be pregnant
and in breast-feeding women, drug is contraindicated.

Adverse reactions

CNS: *headache, dizziness,* depression, lethargy,
migraine, ***stroke.***
CV: thromboembolism, hypertension, edema,
pulmonary embolism.
EENT: worsening of myopia or astigmatism,
intolerance of contact lenses, exophthalmos,
diplopia.
GI: granulomatous colitis, nausea, vomiting,
abdominal cramps, bloating, diarrhea, constipation, anorexia, ***pancreatitis.***

GU: *breakthrough bleeding,* dysmenorrhea,
amenorrhea, cervical erosion or abnormal secretions, enlargement of uterine fibromas, vaginal
candidiasis.
Hepatic: gallbladder disease, cholestatic jaundice, ***liver tumors.***
Metabolic: changes in appetite, weight gain,
hyperglycemia, hypercalcemia.
Skin: rash, acne, ***erythema multiforme.***
Other: breast changes (tenderness, enlargement, secretion).

Interactions

Drug-drug. *Alprazolam, chlordiazepoxide, diazepam, temazepam:* May prolong the half-life
of these drugs. Watch for adverse effects.
Atorvastatin: May increase level of estrogens.
Monitor patient closely.
*Beta blockers, corticosteroids, theophyllines,
tricyclic antidepressants:* May enhance effects
of these drugs. Monitor patient closely.
Bromocriptine: May cause amenorrhea, interfering with bromocriptine effects. Avoid use together.
*Carbamazepine, phenobarbital, phenytoin, ri-
fampin:* May decrease effectiveness of estrogen
therapy. Monitor patient closely.
Cyclosporine: May inhibit cyclosporine metabolism, increasing the risk of toxicity. Avoid use
together, if possible. If given together, monitor
cyclosporine level and renal and hepatic function. Adjust cyclosporine dose as needed.
Dantrolene, other hepatotoxic drugs: May increase risk of hepatotoxicity. Monitor patient
closely.
*Griseofulvin, penicillins, sulfonamides, tetracy-
clines:* May decrease effectiveness of hormonal
contraceptives. Avoid use together, or suggest
barrier contraception for the duration of therapy.
*Lamotrigine, lorazepam, oxazepam, temaze-
pam:* May increase clearance of these drugs.
Monitor patient for lack of effect.
Oral anticoagulants: May decrease anticoagulant effects. Dosage adjustments may be needed.
Monitor PT and INR.
Selegiline: May increase selegiline levels. Monitor patient closely.
Tamoxifen: May interfere with effectiveness of
tamoxifen. Avoid use together.
Drug-herb. *St. John's wort:* May decrease level
of estrogens. Watch for decreased effectiveness
and changes in bleeding patterns.

E

Drug-food. *Caffeine:* May increase caffeine level. Monitor effects.

Drug-lifestyle. *Smoking:* May increase risk of CV effects and thrombosis. Discourage patient from smoking. If smoking continues, patient may need a different form of contraception.

Effects on lab test results

• May increase glucose, calcium, fibrinogen, triglyceride, phospholipid, total T_4, thyroid-binding globulin, plasminogen, liver enzyme, and clotting factor II, VII, VIII, IX, X, and XII levels.

• May increase PT and norepinephrine-induced platelet aggregation.

Pharmacokinetics

Absorption: Mostly well absorbed.
Distribution: Wide; extensively bound to proteins.
Metabolism: Mainly in liver.
Excretion: In urine and feces. *Half-life:* 6 to 20 hours.

Route	Onset	Peak	Duration
P.O., transdermal	Unknown	Varies	Unknown

Action

Chemical effect: Inhibits ovulation through negative feedback mechanism directed at hypothalamus. Estrogen suppresses secretion of follicle-stimulating hormone, blocking follicle development and ovulation. Progestin suppresses secretion of luteinizing hormone so ovulation can't occur. Progestin thickens cervical mucus, which interferes with sperm migration and prevents implantation.

Therapeutic effect: Prevents pregnancy and relieves signs and symptoms of endometriosis.

Available forms

monophasic
ethinyl estradiol and desogestrel
Tablets: ethinyl estradiol 30 mcg and desogestrel 0.15 mg (Apri, Desogen, Ortho-Cept); ethinyl estradiol 25 mcg and desogestrel 0.1 mg
ethinyl estradiol and ethynodiol diacetate
Tablets: ethinyl estradiol 35 mcg and ethynodiol diacetate 1 mg (Demulen 1/35, Zovia 1/35E); ethinyl estradiol 50 mcg and ethynodiol diacetate 1 mg (Demulen 1/50, Zovia 1/50E)

ethinyl estradiol and levonorgestrel
Tablets: ethinyl estradiol 30 mcg and levonorgestrel 0.15 mg (Levlen, Levora, Nordette, Portia); ethinyl estradiol 20 mcg, levonorgestrel 0.1 mg (Alesse, Aviane, Lessina, Levlite)
ethinyl estradiol and norethindrone
Tablets: ethinyl estradiol 35 mcg and norethindrone 0.4 mg (Balziva, Ovcon-35); ethinyl estradiol 35 mcg and norethindrone 0.5 mg (Brevicon, Necon, Nortrel, ModiCon); ethinyl estradiol 35 mcg and norethindrone 1 mg (Necon 1/35, Nortrel 1/35, Norinyl 1+35, Ortho-Novum 1/35); ethinyl estradiol 50 mcg and norethindrone 1 mg (Ovcon-50)
ethinyl estradiol and norethindrone acetate
Tablets: ethinyl estradiol 20 mcg and norethindrone acetate 1 mg (Loestrin 21 1/20); ethinyl estradiol 30 mcg and norethindrone acetate 1.5 mg (Loestrin 21 1.5/30)
ethinyl estradiol and norgestimate
Tablets: ethinyl estradiol 35 mcg and norgestimate 0.25 mg (Ortho-Cyclen)
ethinyl estradiol and norgestrel
Tablets: ethinyl estradiol 30 mcg and norgestrel 0.3 mg (Cryselle, Lo/Ovral, Lo/Ovral 28, Low-Ogestrel); ethinyl estradiol 50 mcg and norgestrel 0.5 mg (Ovral, Ovral 28, Ogestrel 0.5/50)
ethinyl estradiol, norethindrone acetate, and ferrous fumarate
Tablets: ethinyl estradiol 20 mcg, norethindrone acetate 1 mg, and ferrous fumarate 75 mg (Loestrin Fe 1/20, Microgestin Fe 1/20); ethinyl estradiol 30 mcg, norethindrone acetate 1.5 mg, and ferrous fumarate 75 mg (Loestrin Fe 1.5/30, Microgestin Fe 1.5/30)
mestranol and norethindrone
Tablets: mestranol 50 mcg and norethindrone 1 mg (Necon 1/50, Norinyl 1+50, Ortho-Novum 1/50)

biphasic
ethinyl estradiol and desogestrel
Tablets: ethinyl estradiol 20 mcg and desogestrel 0.15 mg (Kariva, Mircette)
ethinyl estradiol and norethindrone
Tablets: ethinyl estradiol 35 mcg and norethindrone 0.5 mg during phase 1 (10 days); ethinyl estradiol 35 mcg and norethindrone 1 mg during phase 2 (11 days) (Necon 10/11, Ortho-Novum 10/11)

Reactions may be *common*, uncommon, *life-threatening*, or COMMON AND LIFE-THREATENING.

triphasic

ethinyl estradiol and desogestrel
Tablets: desogestrel 0.1 mg and ethinyl estradiol 25 mcg (7 tablets); desogestrel 0.125 mg and ethinyl estradiol 25 mcg (7 tablets); desogestrel 0.15 mg and ethinyl estradiol 25 mcg (7 tablets) (Cyclessa); 0.1 mg desogestrel and 0.025 mg ethinyl estradiol (7 tablets); 0.125 mg desogestrel and 0.025 mg ethinyl estradiol (7 tablets); and 0.15 mg desogestrel and 0.025 mg ethinyl estradiol (7 tablets) (Velivet)

ethinyl estradiol and levonorgestrel
Tablets: ethinyl estradiol 30 mcg and levonorgestrel 0.05 mg during phase 1 (6 days); ethinyl estradiol 40 mcg and levonorgestrel 0.075 mg during phase 2 (5 days); ethinyl estradiol 30 mcg and levonorgestrel 0.125 mg during phase 3 (10 days) (Tri-Levlen, Triphasil, Trivora-28, Enpresse)
Transdermal patch: ethinyl estradiol 0.045 mg and levonorgestrel 0.015 mg

ethinyl estradiol and norethindrone
Tablets: ethinyl estradiol 35 mcg and norethindrone 0.5 mg during phase 1 (7 days); ethinyl estradiol 35 mcg and norethindrone 1 mg during phase 2 (9 days); ethinyl estradiol 35 mcg and norethindrone 0.5 mg during phase 3 (5 days) (Tri-Norinyl); ethinyl estradiol 35 mcg and norethindrone 0.5 mg during phase 1 (7 days); ethinyl estradiol 35 mcg and norethindrone 0.75 mg during phase 2 (7 days); ethinyl estradiol 35 mcg and norethindrone 1 mg during phase 3 (7 days) (Necon 7/7/7, Nortrel 7/7/7, Ortho-Novum 7/7/7)

ethinyl estradiol and norethindrone acetate
Tablets: ethinyl estradiol 0.02 mg and norethindrone acetate 1 mg (5 tablets), ethinyl estradiol 0.03 mg and norethindrone acetate 1 mg (7 tablets), ethinyl estradiol 0.035 mg and norethindrone acetate 1 mg (9 tablets) (Estrostep Fe, Estrostep 21)

ethinyl estradiol and norgestimate
Tablets: ethinyl estradiol 35 mcg and norgestimate 0.18 mg during phase 1 (7 days); ethinyl estradiol 35 mcg and norgestimate 0.215 mg during phase 2 (7 days); ethinyl estradiol 35 mcg and norgestimate 0.25 mg during phase 3 (7 days) (Ortho Tri-Cyclen)

NURSING PROCESS

⚗ Assessment
• Obtain history of patient's fertility or underlying endometriosis before starting therapy.
• Monitor the drug's effectiveness by determining if pregnancy test is negative or if patient with endometriosis has diminished signs and symptoms.
• Periodically monitor lipid levels, blood pressure, body weight, and liver function.
• Be alert for adverse reactions and drug interactions.
• Assess patient's and family's knowledge of drug therapy.

⊕ Nursing diagnoses
• Health-seeking behavior (prevention of pregnancy) related to family planning
• Acute pain related to drug-induced headache
• Deficient knowledge related to drug therapy

▷ Planning and implementation
• Make sure patient has been properly instructed about prescribed hormonal contraceptive before she takes first dose.
🅢 **ALERT:** Make sure patient has negative pregnancy test before therapy starts.
• If patient develops granulomatous colitis, stop therapy and notify prescriber.
• Stop drug at least 1 week before surgery to decrease risk of thromboembolism. Tell patient to use other, nonhormonal method of birth control.
🅢 **ALERT:** Don't confuse Nortrel 7/7/7 with Nortrel 0.5/35 or Nortrel 1/35.
🅢 **ALERT:** Don't confuse Necon 7/7/7 with Nortrel 7/7/7.
Patient teaching
• Tell patient to take tablets at same time each day; nighttime dosing may reduce nausea and headaches.
• Advise patient to use barrier method of birth control for first week of first cycle.
• Tell patient that missed doses in midcycle greatly increase likelihood of pregnancy.
• If 1 pill is missed, take pill as soon as possible; if remembered on the next day, take 2 pills, then continue regular dosage schedule. Use additional method of contraception for remainder of cycle.
• If 2 consecutive pills are missed, take 2 pills a day for next 2 days; then resume regular dosage

schedule. Use additional method of contraception for the next 7 days or preferably for the remainder of cycle.

• If 2 consecutive pills are missed in the third week or if patient misses 3 consecutive pills, tell patient to contact prescriber for dosage instructions.

• Warn patient that headache, nausea, dizziness, breast tenderness, spotting, and breakthrough bleeding are common at first. Effects will diminish after 3 to 6 months.

• Instruct patient to weigh herself at least twice weekly and to report sudden weight gain or edema to prescriber.

• Warn patient to avoid exposure to ultraviolet light or prolonged exposure to sunlight.

⊛ **ALERT:** Warn patient to immediately report abdominal pain; numbness, stiffness, or pain in legs or buttocks; pressure or pain in chest; shortness of breath; severe headache; visual disturbances, such as blind spots, blurriness, or flashing lights; undiagnosed vaginal bleeding or discharge; two consecutive missed menstrual periods; lumps in breast; swelling of hands or feet; or severe pain in abdomen.

• Advise patient that smoking while using hormonal contraceptives increases risks of thromboembolic events.

• Teach patient how to perform breast self-examination.

• If one menstrual period is missed and tablets have been taken on schedule, tell patient to continue taking them. If two consecutive menstrual periods are missed, tell patient to stop drug and have pregnancy test. Progestins may cause birth defects if taken early in pregnancy.

• Advise patient not to take same drug for longer than 12 months without consulting prescriber. Stress importance of Papanicolaou test and annual gynecologic examination.

• Advise patient to check with prescriber about how soon pregnancy may be attempted after hormonal therapy is stopped.

• Warn patient that she may not be able to become pregnant immediately after drug is stopped.

• Advise women on prolonged contraceptive therapy to stop drug and use other nonhormonal birth control methods. Periodically reassess patient while off hormone therapy.

☑ **Evaluation**
• Patient doesn't become pregnant.

• Patient obtains relief from drug-induced headache with administration of mild analgesic.
• Patient and family state understanding of drug therapy.

ethinyl estradiol and drospirenone
(ETH-ih-nill es-truh-DIGH-ol and droh-SPEER-ih-nohn)
Yasmin

Pharmacologic class: hormonal contraceptive
Therapeutic class: estrogen and progestin
Pregnancy risk category: X

Indications and dosages

▶ **Contraception.** *Women and postpubertal girls:* 1 yellow tablet P.O. daily beginning on day 1 of menstrual cycle (first day of menstruation). Continue 1 yellow tablet P.O. daily for 21 consecutive days; then 1 white inert tablet should be taken P.O. daily on days 22 through 28. Begin the next and all subsequent 28-day regimens on the same day of the week that the first regimen began, following the same schedule. Restart yellow tablets on the next day after the last white tablet. Or 1 yellow tablet P.O. daily, beginning on the first Sunday after the onset of menstruation. Continue 1 yellow tablet P.O. daily for 21 consecutive days; then take 1 white inert tablet P.O. daily on days 22 through 28. Begin the next and all subsequent 28-day regimens on the same day of the week that the first regimen began, following the same schedule. Restart yellow tablets on the next day after taking the last white tablet.

Contraindications and cautions

• Contraindicated in women with hepatic dysfunction, tumor, or disease; renal or adrenal insufficiency; thrombophlebitis, thromboembolic disorders, or history of deep vein thrombosis or thromboembolic disorders; cerebrovascular or coronary artery disease; known or suspected breast cancer, endometrial cancer, or other estrogen-dependent neoplasia; unexplained vaginal bleeding; or cholestatic jaundice of pregnancy or jaundice with other contraceptive pill use. Also contraindicated in women older than age 35 who smoke 15 or more cigarettes daily.

• Use cautiously in patients with risk factors for CV disease, such as hypertension, hyperlipidemias, obesity, and diabetes.

⚖ **Lifespan:** In women who are pregnant or suspect they may be pregnant, drug is contraindicated. In breast-feeding women, drug is contraindicated. In girls who haven't reached menarche, drug is contraindicated.

Adverse reactions

CNS: asthenia, *stroke,* depression, dizziness, emotional lability, headache, migraine, nervousness.
CV: *thromboembolism,* hypertension, edema, *mesenteric thrombosis, MI,* thrombophlebitis.
EENT: cataracts, steepening of corneal curvature, intolerance to contact lenses, pharyngitis, retinal thrombosis, sinusitis.
GI: abdominal pain, abdominal cramping, bloating, changes in appetite, colitis, diarrhea, gastroenteritis, nausea, vomiting.
GU: amenorrhea, breakthrough bleeding, change in cervical erosion and secretion, change in menstrual flow, cystitis, cystitis-like syndrome, dysmenorrhea, *hemolytic uremic syndrome,* renal impairment, leukorrhea, menstrual disorder, premenstrual syndrome, spotting, temporary infertility, UTI, vaginal candidiasis, vaginitis.
Hepatic: *Budd-Chiari syndrome,* cholestatic jaundice, gallbladder disease, *hepatic adenomas,* benign liver tumors.
Metabolic: reduced tolerance to carbohydrates, porphyria, weight gain.
Musculoskeletal: back pain.
Respiratory: bronchitis, *pulmonary embolism,* upper respiratory tract infection.
Skin: acne, *erythema multiforme,* erythema nodosum, hemorrhagic eruption, hirsutism, loss of scalp hair, melasma, pruritus, rash.
Other: changes in libido, breast changes, decreased lactation.

Interactions

Drug-drug. *ACE inhibitors, aldosterone antagonists, angiotensin II receptor antagonists, NSAIDs, potassium-sparing diuretics, heparin:* May increase risk of hyperkalemia. Monitor potassium level.
Acetaminophen: May decrease acetaminophen level. Adjust acetaminophen dose p.r.n.
Ampicillin, griseofulvin, tetracycline: May decrease contraceptive effect. Encourage use of additional method of birth control while taking the antibiotic.
Ascorbic acid, atorvastatin: May increase contraceptive level. Monitor patient for adverse effects.
Carbamazepine, phenobarbital, phenytoin: May increase metabolism of ethinyl estradiol and decrease contraceptive effectiveness. Encourage use of alternative method of birth control.
Clofibrate, morphine, salicylic acid, temazepam: May decrease levels and increase clearance of these drugs. Monitor effectiveness.
Cyclosporine, prednisolone, theophylline: May increase levels of these drugs. Monitor patient for adverse effects and toxicity.
Phenylbutazone, rifampin: May decrease contraceptive effectiveness and increase breakthrough bleeding. Encourage use of alternative method of birth control.
Drug-herb. *St. John's wort:* May decrease contraceptive effect and increase breakthrough bleeding. Encourage use of additional method of birth control, or discourage use together.
Drug-lifestyle. *Smoking:* May increase risk of CV adverse effects and thromboembolism. Warn patient to avoid smoking and tobacco products while taking hormonal contraceptives.

Effects on lab test results

• May increase circulating total thyroid hormone, triglyceride, other binding protein, sex hormone–binding globulin, total circulating endogenous sex steroid, corticoid, potassium, folate, liver enzyme, and clotting factors VII, VIII, IX, and X levels.
• May increase PT. May decrease glucose tolerance.

Pharmacokinetics

Absorption: Steady-state level occurs after 10 days for drospirenone and during second half of treatment cycle for ethinyl estradiol.
Distribution: Wide. Drospirenone is about 97% bound to nonspecific proteins. Ethinyl estradiol is about 98% bound to albumin and other nonspecific proteins.
Metabolism: Drospirenone is metabolized mainly by metabolites in plasma and to a minor extent in the liver by CYP 3A4 to inactive metabolites. Ethinyl estradiol is mainly metabolized by hydroxylation and subject to presystemic conjugation in the small bowel and the liver.

Excretion: Small amounts of drospirenone unchanged in urine and feces. Ethinyl estradiol as metabolites in urine and feces. *Half-life:* drospirenone, 30 hours; ethinyl estradiol, 24 hours.

Route	Onset	Peak	Duration
P.O.	Unknown	1–3 hr	Unknown

Action

Chemical effect: Suppresses gonadotropins, follicle-stimulating hormone, and luteinizing hormone, thereby preventing ovulation, changing the cervical mucus to increase the difficulty of penetration by sperm and changing the endometrium to increase the difficulty of implantation.
Therapeutic effect: Reduces the opportunity for conception.

Available forms

Tablets: 21 yellow tablets containing 3 mg drospirenone and 0.03 mg ethinyl estradiol, and 7 inert white tablets

NURSING PROCESS

✒ Assessment

• Determine if patient is pregnant before giving the drug.
• Find out if the patient smokes, and investigate her medical history, CV health, and potassium level before starting drug.
• Assess and be alert for adverse reactions. The use of contraceptives increases the risk of MI, thromboembolism, stroke, hepatic neoplasia, gallbladder disease, and hypertension, especially in patients with hypertension, diabetes, hyperlipidemia, and obesity.
• Monitor patient's laboratory results during drug therapy.
• Assess patient's and family's knowledge of contraception and drug therapy.

⊕ Nursing diagnoses

• Risk for injury related to drug-induced adverse reactions
• Health seeking behavior for the prevention of pregnancy related to family planning
• Deficient knowledge of contraceptive drug therapy

▶ Planning and implementation

• Because of the postpartum risk of thromboembolism, don't start drug earlier than 4 to 6 weeks after delivery.
• If patient misses two consecutive periods, tell her to obtain a negative pregnancy test result before continuing contraceptive. If pregnancy test is positive, tell her to immediately stop taking the drug.
• In patients scheduled to have elective surgery that may increase the risk of thromboembolism, stop contraceptive use from at least 4 weeks before until 2 weeks after surgery. Also avoid use during and after prolonged immobilization. Advise patient to use alternative methods of birth control.
• Overdose may cause nausea and withdrawal bleeding. Monitor potassium and sodium levels, and watch for signs of metabolic acidosis.
• If loss of vision, proptosis, diplopia, papilledema, or retinal vascular lesions occur, stop use and evaluate patient. Recommend that contact lens wearers be evaluated by an ophthalmologist if they have changes in vision or lens intolerance.
• Evaluate patient who experiences unusual breakthrough bleeding for malignancy or pregnancy.
• If patient suffers from sharp or crushing chest pains, hemoptysis, sudden shortness of breath, calf pain, breast lumps, severe stomach pains, difficulty sleeping, weakness, fatigue, or jaundice, stop drug. Notify prescriber immediately and offer supportive treatment p.r.n.
Patient teaching
• Inform patient that pills are used to prevent pregnancy and don't protect against HIV and other sexually transmitted diseases.
• Advise patient of the dangers of smoking while taking hormonal contraceptives. Suggest that she choose a different form of birth control if she continues smoking.
• Tell patient to schedule gynecologic examinations yearly and perform breast self-examination monthly.
• Inform patient that spotting, light bleeding, or stomach upset may occur during the first one to three packs of pills. Tell her to continue taking the pills and to notify prescriber if these symptoms persist.
• Tell patient to take the pill at the same time each day, preferably during the evening or h.s.

Reactions may be *common*, uncommon, *life-threatening*, or COMMON AND LIFE-THREATENING.

• Tell patient to immediately report sharp chest pain, coughing of blood, or sudden shortness of breath, pain in the calf, crushing chest pain or chest heaviness, sudden severe headache or vomiting, dizziness or fainting, visual or speech disturbances, weakness or numbness in an arm or leg, loss of vision, breast lumps, severe stomach pain or tenderness, difficulty sleeping, lack of energy, fatigue, change in mood, jaundice with fever, loss of appetite, dark urine, or light-colored bowel movements.

• Tell patient to notify prescriber if she wears contact lenses and notices a change in vision or has difficulty wearing the lenses.

• Advise patient to use additional method of birth control during the first 7 days of the first cycle of hormonal contraceptive.

• Tell patient that the risk of pregnancy increases with each active yellow tablet she forgets to take.

• If patient misses 1 tablet, tell her to take it as soon as she remembers and to take the next pill at the regular time.

• If patient misses 2 tablets during week 1 or 2 of the pack, tell her to use an additional method of birth control for 7 days. Instruct her to take 2 pills on the day she remembers and 2 pills the next day, and then to resume the normal schedule.

• If patient misses 2 tablets during week 3, tell her to use an additional method of birth control for 7 days. If she uses day 1 start, tell her to throw away the rest of the pack and start a new pack the same day. If she uses Sunday start, tell her to keep taking 1 pill each day until Sunday, then to throw away the pack, and start a new pack that day. Tell patient that she may miss her period this month, but to notify prescriber if she misses it 2 months in a row because it may mean she's pregnant.

• If patient misses 3 or more tablets during the first 3 weeks, tell her to use an additional method of birth control for 7 days. If she uses day 1 start, tell her to throw away the rest of the pack and start a new pack the same day. If she uses Sunday start, tell her to keep taking 1 pill each day until Sunday, then to throw away the pack, and start a new pack that day. Tell patient that she may miss her period this month, but to notify prescriber if she misses it 2 months in a row because it may mean she's pregnant.

• If patient misses any of the white tablets, tell her to throw away the missed pills and keep taking 1 pill each day until the pack is empty. She doesn't need to use an additional method of birth control.

• Tell patient to use an additional method of birth control and notify prescriber if she isn't sure what to do about missed pills.

✓ Evaluation

• Patient doesn't suffer from any drug-induced adverse reactions.

• Patient doesn't become pregnant.

• Patient and family state understanding of drug therapy.

ethinyl estradiol and etonogestrel vaginal ring
(ETH-ih-nill es-truh-DIGH-ol and et-oh-noe-JESS-trel)
NuvaRing

Pharmacologic class: intravaginal hormonal contraceptive
Therapeutic class: progestin and estrogen
Pregnancy risk category: X

Indications and dosages

▶ **Contraception.** *Women:* Insert one ring vaginally, and leave in place for 3 weeks. Insert new ring exactly 1 week after the previous ring was removed, even if still menstruating.

Contraindications and cautions

• Contraindicated in patients hypersensitive to the drug or any of its components and in patients older than age 35 who smoke 15 or more cigarettes daily. Also contraindicated in patients with thrombophlebitis, thromboembolic disorder, history of deep vein thrombophlebitis, cerebral vascular or coronary artery disease (current or previous), valvular heart disease with complications, severe hypertension, diabetes with vascular complications, headache with focal neurologic symptoms, major surgery with prolonged immobilization, known or suspected cancer of the endometrium or breast, estrogen-dependent neoplasia, abnormal undiagnosed vaginal bleeding, jaundice related to pregnancy or previous use of hormonal contraceptive, active liver disease, or benign or malignant hepatic tumors.

• Use cautiously in patients with hypertension, hyperlipidemias, obesity, diabetes, a condition that could be aggravated by fluid retention, a history of depression, or impaired liver function.

🔆 **Lifespan:** In women who are or may be pregnant, drug is contraindicated. In breast-feeding women, drug isn't recommended; tell patient to use alternative forms of contraception until baby is weaned. In women who choose not to breast-feed, don't start drug earlier than 4 weeks after delivery. In girls who haven't reached menarche, drug is contraindicated. In postmenopausal women, don't use.

Adverse reactions

CNS: *headache,* emotional lability.
EENT: sinusitis.
GI: nausea.
GU: *vaginitis, leukorrhea,* device-related events (such as foreign body sensation, coital difficulties, device expulsion), vaginal discomfort.
Metabolic: weight gain.
Respiratory: upper respiratory tract infection.

Interactions

Drug-drug. *Acetaminophen, ascorbic acid, atorvastatin, itraconazole:* May increase ethinyl estradiol level. Monitor patient for adverse effects.

Ampicillin, barbiturates, carbamazepine, felbamate, griseofulvin, oxcarbazepine, phenylbutazone, phenytoin, rifampin, tetracyclines, topiramate: May decrease contraceptive effectiveness and increase risk of pregnancy, breakthrough bleeding, or both. Tell patient to use an additional form of contraception while taking these drugs.

Anti-HIV protease inhibitors: May increase or decrease the bioavailability of estrogen or progestin. Suggest other methods of birth control.

Clofibric acid, morphine, salicylic acid, temazepam: May increase clearance of these drugs. Monitor patient for effectiveness.

Cyclosporine, prednisolone, theophylline: May increase levels of these drugs. Monitor cyclosporine and theophylline levels, and adjust dosages p.r.n.

Drug-herb. *St. John's wort:* May reduce contraceptive effectiveness, increase risk of pregnancy, and increase risk of breakthrough bleeding. Discourage use together.

Drug-lifestyle. *Smoking:* May increase risk of serious CV side effects and thromboembolism,

especially in women age 35 and older who smoke 15 or more cigarettes daily. Urge patient to quit smoking.

Effects on lab test results

• May increase prothrombin, thyroid-binding globulin (leading to increased circulating total thyroid hormone levels), other binding protein, sex hormone–binding globulin, triglyceride, lipoprotein, other lipid, and clotting factor VII, VIII, IX, and X levels. May decrease antithrombin III and folate levels.

• May increase norepinephrine-induced platelet aggregation. May decrease T_3 resin uptake and glucose tolerance.

Pharmacokinetics

Absorption: Both hormonal components are rapidly absorbed. Bioavailability of etonogestrel and ethinyl estradiol is 100% and 55.6%, respectively.

Distribution: Etonogestrel is 66% protein-bound and 32% bound to sex hormone–binding globulin. Ethinyl estradiol is about 98% nonspecific protein-bound and increases levels of sex hormone–binding globulin.

Metabolism: Both components of drug are metabolized in the liver by CYP 3A4.

Excretion: Both components are mainly in urine, bile, and feces. *Half-life:* ethinyl estradiol, 45 hours; etonogestrel, 29 hours.

Route	Onset	Peak	Duration
Vaginal	Immediate	Unknown	Unknown

Action

Chemical effect: Suppresses gonadotropins, which inhibits ovulation, increases the viscosity of cervical mucus (decreasing the ability of sperm to enter the uterus), and alters the endometrial lining (reducing potential for implantation).

Therapeutic effect: Decreases risk of pregnancy.

Available forms

Vaginal ring: Delivers 0.120 mg etonogestrel and 0.015 mg ethinyl estradiol daily

NURSING PROCESS

🔬 Assessment
• Assess patient for pregnancy before giving the drug.
• Find out if the patient smokes, and investigate her medical history, CV health, and risk factors before starting drug.
• Be alert for adverse reactions.
• Use of contraceptives increases the risk of MI, thromboembolism, stroke, hepatic neoplasia, gallbladder disease, and hypertension, especially in patients with hypertension, diabetes, hyperlipidemia, and obesity. Monitor patient for related signs and symptoms.
• Monitor patient's laboratory results during drug therapy.
• Assess patient's and family's knowledge of contraception and drug therapy.

🔲 Nursing diagnoses
• Risk for injury related to drug-induced adverse reactions
• Health seeking behavior for the prevention of pregnancy related to family planning
• Deficient knowledge of contraceptive drug therapy

❱ Planning and implementation
• Stop drug at least 4 weeks before and for 2 weeks after procedures that may increase the risk of thromboembolism and during and after prolonged immobilization.
• If patient develops unexplained partial or complete loss of vision, proptosis, diplopia, papilledema, or retinal vascular lesions, stop drug.
• If patient has hypertension or renal disease, monitor blood pressure closely. If blood pressure rises, stop drug.
• If migraine begins or worsens or if patient has recurrent, persistent, or severe headaches, stop drug.
• If jaundice occurs, stop drug. The hormones may be poorly metabolized in patients with liver disease.
• If patient has persistent or severe abnormal menstrual bleeding, look for cause. If amenorrhea occurs, rule out pregnancy.
• If depression occurs, stop drug to determine whether depression is drug-related.
• If patient hasn't adhered to the prescribed regimen and a menstrual period is missed, if prescribed regimen is adhered to and two periods

are missed, or if the patient has retained the ring for longer than 4 weeks, rule out pregnancy.
• Overdose may cause nausea, vomiting, vaginal bleeding, or other menstrual irregularities. Offer supportive treatment.

Patient teaching
• If no hormonal contraceptive is used in the preceding month, tell patient to insert ring on day 5 of the menstrual cycle (counting the first day of menstruation as day 1). For the first cycle of use, tell her to use an additional form of birth control within 7 days of inserting ring.
• When switching from other combination (estrogen plus progestin) hormonal contraceptives, tell patient to insert the ring within 7 days of the last dose of combined hormonal contraceptive, no later than the day that a new cycle of tablets would have begun. No backup form of contraception is needed.
• When switching from a progestin-only form of contraception, tell patient to use a backup form of contraception for the first 7 days of using the ring. Provide these instructions: If switching from progestin-only tablets, insert ring on any day of the month; don't skip any days between the last oral dose and insertion of the ring. If switching from progestin-only implants (such as Norplant), insert the vaginal ring on the same day that the implants are removed. If switching from progestin-only intrauterine device (IUD), insert the vaginal ring on the same day that the IUD is removed. If switching from contraceptive injections (such as Depo-Provera), insert the vaginal ring on the same day that the next injection would be due. Begin use within the first 5 days after complete first-trimester abortion, 4 weeks postpartum if not breast-feeding, or 4 weeks after a second-trimester abortion.
• Teach patient or provide patient with instructions for proper placement of vaginal ring. Also encourage proper handwashing before and after ring insertion to prevent vaginal infections.
• If the ring is removed or expelled (for example, while removing a tampon or moving the bowels), tell patient to wash with cool to luke-warm water and reinsert immediately. If the ring stays out for more than 3 hours, contraceptive may not be effective, and a backup method of contraception should be recommended until the reinserted ring is used continuously for 7 days.

E

• Emphasize the importance of having annual physical examinations to check for adverse effects or developing contraindications.
• Tell patient that drug doesn't protect against HIV and other sexually transmitted diseases.
• Advise patient not to smoke while using contraceptive.
• Tell patient not to use a diaphragm if a backup method of birth control is needed.
• Tell patient who wears contact lenses to contact an ophthalmologist if vision or lens tolerance changes.

☑ **Evaluation**
• Patient doesn't suffer from any drug-induced adverse reactions or vaginal infections.
• Patient doesn't become pregnant.
• Patient and family state understanding of drug therapy.

ethinyl estradiol and norelgestromin transdermal system
(ETH-ih-nill es-truh-DIGH-ol and nor-el-GESS-troh-min)
Ortho Evra

Pharmacologic class: transdermal hormonal contraceptive
Therapeutic class: estrogen and progestin
Pregnancy risk category: X

Indications and dosages

▶ **Contraception.** *Women:* Apply one patch weekly for 3 weeks. Week 4 is patch-free. On the day after week 4 ends, apply a new patch to start a new 4-week cycle. Apply each new patch on the same day of the week.

Contraindications and cautions

• Contraindicated in patients hypersensitive to the drug or any of its components and in those with a history of deep vein thrombosis or related disorder, history of cerebrovascular or coronary artery disease, past or current known or suspected breast cancer, endometrial cancer or other known or suspected estrogen-dependent neoplasia, hepatic adenoma or carcinoma, or known or suspected pregnancy. Also contraindicated in patients with thrombophlebitis, thromboembolic disorders, valvular heart disease with complica-

tions, severe hypertension, diabetes with vascular involvement, headaches with focal neurologic symptoms, major surgery with prolonged immobilization, undiagnosed abnormal genital bleeding, cholestatic jaundice of pregnancy or jaundice with previous hormonal contraceptive use, or acute or chronic hepatocellular disease with abnormal liver function.
• Use cautiously in patients with CV disease risk factors, with conditions that might be aggravated by fluid retention, or with a history of depression.
⚖ **Lifespan:** In breast-feeding women, safety and effectiveness haven't been established; advise an alternative method of birth control. In girls who haven't reached menarche, safety and effectiveness haven't been evaluated; don't use.

Adverse reactions

CNS: *headache,* emotional lability, ***cerebral hemorrhage.***
CV: ***thromboembolic events, MI,*** hypertension, edema.
EENT: contact lens intolerance.
GI: nausea, abdominal pain, vomiting.
GU: menstrual cramps, changes in menstrual flow, vaginal candidiasis.
Hepatic: *hepatic adenomas,* benign liver tumors, gallbladder disease.
Metabolic: weight changes.
Respiratory: upper respiratory tract infection.
Skin: application site reaction.
Other: breast tenderness, enlargement, or secretion.

Interactions

Drug-drug. *Acetaminophen, clofibric acid, morphine, salicylic acid, temazepam:* May decrease levels or increase clearance of these drugs. Monitor patient closely for lack of drug effect.
Ampicillin, barbiturates, carbamazepine, felbamate, griseofulvin, oxcarbazepine, phenylbutazone, phenytoin, rifampin, topiramate: Contraceptive effectiveness may be reduced, resulting in unintended pregnancy or breakthrough bleeding. If used together, encourage backup method of contraception.
Anti-HIV protease inhibitors: Effectiveness and safety of contraceptives may be affected. Use together cautiously.

Ascorbic acid, atorvastatin, itraconazole, keto-conazole: May increase hormone levels. Use together cautiously.
Cyclosporine, prednisolone, theophylline: May increase levels of these drugs. Monitor patient for adverse effects.
Drug-herb. *St. John's wort:* May reduce effectiveness of contraceptive and cause breakthrough bleeding. Discourage use together.
Drug-lifestyle. *Smoking:* May increase risk of serious CV side effects, especially in those older than age 35 who smoke 15 or more cigarettes daily. Urge patient to quit smoking.

Effects on lab test results

● May increase clotting factor VII, VIII, IX, and X; prothrombin; circulating total thyroid hormone; triglyceride; other binding protein; sex hormone-binding globulin; total circulating endogenous sex steroid; and corticoid levels. May decrease antithrombin III and folate levels.
● May decrease free T_3 resin uptake and glucose tolerance.

Pharmacokinetics

Absorption: Rapid. Maintained at a steady state while the patch is worn.
Distribution: Norelgestromin and norgestrel (a metabolite) are more than 97% protein bound. Ethinyl estradiol is extensively bound to albumin.
Metabolism: In the liver.
Excretion: Norelgestromin and ethinyl estradiol are eliminated in 28 hours and 17 hours, respectively. The metabolites are eliminated in the urine and feces. *Ethinyl estradiol half-life:* 6 to 45 hours. *Norelgestromin half-life:* 28 hours.

Route	Onset	Peak	Duration
Transdermal	Rapid	2 days	Unknown

Action

Chemical effect: Suppresses gonadotropins and inhibits ovulation. Changes cervical mucus, complicating entry of sperm into the uterus, and changes endometrium, decreasing the likelihood of implantation.
Therapeutic effect: Reduces risk of pregnancy.

Available forms

Transdermal patch: norelgestromin 6 mg and ethinyl estradiol 0.75 mg (releases 150 mcg of norelgestromin and 20 mcg of ethinyl estradiol every 24 hours)

NURSING PROCESS

✍ Assessment
● Rule out pregnancy before giving drug to the patient.
● Find out if the patient smokes, and investigate her medical history and CV health before starting drug.
● Be alert for any drug-induced adverse reactions.
● Monitor patient for signs and symptoms related to use of contraceptives: increased risk of MI, thromboembolism, stroke, hepatic neoplasia, gallbladder disease, and hypertension, especially in patients with hypertension, diabetes, hyperlipidemia, and obesity.
● Monitor patient's laboratory results during drug therapy.
● Assess patient's knowledge of contraception and drug therapy.

Nursing diagnoses
● Risk for injury related to drug-induced adverse reactions
● Health seeking behavior for the prevention of pregnancy related to family planning
● Deficient knowledge of contraceptive drug therapy

Planning and implementation
● Encourage women with a history of hypertension or renal disease to use a different method of contraception. If Ortho Evra is used, monitor blood pressure closely; if hypertension occurs, stop use.
● Drug may be less effective in women weighing 90 kg (198 lb) or more.
● Cigarette smoking increases the risk of serious CV adverse effects. This risk increases especially in women age 35 and older who smoke 15 or more cigarettes per day.
● A woman starting the patch for the first time should wait until the day she begins her menstrual period. She will then choose a first-day start or a Sunday start.
● If woman chooses a first-day start, the patch should be applied during the first 24 hours of her menstrual period. If therapy starts after day 1 of the menstrual cycle, a nonhormonal backup

method of birth control should be used for the first week of the first treatment cycle.

• If the woman chooses a Sunday start, the patch should be applied on the first Sunday after her menstrual period starts. She must use backup contraception for the first week of her cycle. If the woman's menstrual period begins on a Sunday, she should apply the first patch on that day, and no backup contraception is needed.

• When switching from an oral contraceptive, apply patch on the first day of withdrawal bleeding. If applied after this time, backup contraception should be used for the first week.

• Therapy should be started no sooner than 4 weeks after childbirth. If the woman hasn't had a menstrual period, rule out pregnancy, and have her use backup contraception for the first week.

• After abortion or miscarriage in the first trimester, the patch may be started immediately. If it isn't started within 5 days of a first-trimester abortion, follow directions for a woman starting therapy for the first time.

• Patch shouldn't be started earlier than 4 weeks after a second-trimester abortion or miscarriage.

• If used postpartum or postabortion, risk of thromboembolic disease increases.

• If breakthrough bleeding occurs for more than a few cycles, remove patch and assess cause.

• If no withdrawal bleeding occurs on patch-free week, resume on the next scheduled patch-change day. If withdrawal bleeding fails to occur for two consecutive cycles, rule out pregnancy.

• If skin becomes irritated, the patch may be removed and a new patch applied at a different site until the next patch-change day.

• Stop use at least 4 weeks before and for 2 weeks after elective surgery that increases risk of thromboembolism and during and after prolonged immobilization.

• If patient has vision loss, proptosis, diplopia, papilledema, retinal vascular lesions, or recurrent, persistent, or severe headaches, stop use.

• If jaundice occurs, stop use.

• If patient becomes severely depressed, stop use and evaluate whether the depression is drug related.

Patient teaching

• Emphasize the importance of having annual physical examinations to check for adverse effects or developing contraindications.

• Tell patient that the contraceptive patch doesn't protect against HIV and other sexually transmitted diseases.

• Advise patient to immediately apply a new patch once the used patch is removed, on the same day of the week, every 7 days for 3 weeks. Week 4 is patch-free. Tell patient to expect bleeding to occur during this time.

• Advise patient to start a new cycle, applying a new patch on the usual patch-change day, regardless of when the menstrual period starts or ends.

• Teach patient how to properly apply the patch.

• Tell patient to apply each patch to a new clean, dry area of the skin on the buttocks, abdomen, upper outer arm, or upper torso to avoid irritation. Tell patient not to apply to the breasts or to skin that's red, irritated, or cut. Instruct patient to avoid creams, oils, powder, or makeup on or near the skin where the patch will be placed because it may cause the patch to become loose.

• Tell patient what to do if a patch is partially or completely detached:

– *If patch is detached for less than 24 hours:* Try to reapply it to the same place or replace it with a new patch immediately. No backup contraception is needed.

– *If the patch is detached for 24 hours or more, or if the woman isn't sure how long the patch has been detached:* Stop the current cycle and start a new cycle immediately by applying a new patch. A backup form of contraception must be used for the first week of the new cycle because the patient may not be protected from pregnancy.

– *If the patch is no longer sticky, if it has become stuck to itself or another surface, if it has other material stuck to it, or if it has previously become loose or fallen off:* Tell patient not to attempt to reapply patch that is no longer sticky. If she can't reapply patch, she must apply a new one immediately. She shouldn't use adhesives or wraps to hold the patch in place.

• Tell patient what to do if she forgets to change her patch:

– *At the start of the cycle:* Apply the first patch of the new cycle as soon as she remembers and to use backup contraception for the first week of the new cycle.

– *In the middle of the patch cycle for 1 or 2 days:* Apply a new patch immediately. Apply

the next patch on the usual patch-change day. No backup contraception is needed.
– *In the middle of the patch cycle for more than 2 days:* Stop the current contraceptive cycle, and start a new 4-week cycle immediately by applying a new patch. Use backup contraception for 1 week.
– *At the end of a patch cycle:* If the patient forgets to take off her patch, tell her to remove it as soon as she remembers and to start the next cycle on the usual patch-change day, the day after day 28. No backup contraception is needed.
• If patient wants to change her patch-change day, tell her to complete her current cycle and apply a new patch on the desired day during the patch-free week. There shouldn't be more than 7 consecutive patch-free days.
• Tell patient what to do if she misses a menstrual period:
– If patient hasn't adhered to the prescribed schedule, pregnancy should be ruled out at the time of the first missed period.
– If patient adhered to the prescribed regimen and missed one period, she should continue using the patches. If she adhered to the prescribed regimen and missed two consecutive periods, pregnancy should be ruled out.
• Tell patient to immediately stop drug if pregnancy is confirmed.
• Tell patient who wears contact lenses to contact an ophthalmologist if visual changes or changes in lens tolerance develop.
• Stress that if patient isn't sure what to do about mistakes with patch use, she should use a backup method of birth control, such as a condom, spermicide, or diaphragm. She should contact her prescriber for further instructions.

☑ **Evaluation**
• Patient doesn't have any drug-induced adverse reactions.
• Patient doesn't become pregnant.
• Patient and family state understanding of drug therapy.

etodolac (ultradol)
(eh-toh-DOH-lak)
Lodine, Lodine XL

Pharmacologic class: NSAID
Therapeutic class: analgesic, antiarthritic
Pregnancy risk category: C (D in third trimester)

Indications and dosages
▶ **Acute pain.** *Adults:* 200 to 400 mg P.O. of film-coated tablets or capsules q 6 to 8 hours. Maximum dose is 1,200 mg daily.
▶ **Acute or long-term management of osteoarthritis or rheumatoid arthritis.** *Adults:* 600 to 1,000 mg P.O. daily of film-coated tablets or capsules in two divided doses. For extended-release tablets, usual dosage is 400 to 1,000 mg P.O. once daily. Maximum dose is 1,200 mg daily.

Contraindications and cautions
• Contraindicated in patients hypersensitive to the drug or any of its components and in those with history of aspirin- or NSAID-induced asthma, rhinitis, urticaria, or other allergic reactions.
• Use cautiously in patients with history of GI bleeding, ulceration, and perforation; in patients with renal or hepatic impairment, heart failure, hypertension, or cardiac function impairments; and in those predisposed to fluid retention.
⚖ Lifespan: In pregnant women during first and second trimesters, use cautiously. During third trimester, drug is contraindicated. In breast-feeding women, use cautiously because it's unknown if the drug appears in breast milk. In children younger than age 18, safety and effectiveness haven't been established.

Adverse reactions
CNS: *asthenia, malaise, dizziness,* depression, drowsiness, nervousness, insomnia, headache, fever, syncope.
CV: hypertension, *heart failure,* flushing, palpitations, edema, fluid retention.
EENT: blurred vision, tinnitus, photophobia, dry mouth.
GI: *dyspepsia,* flatulence, abdominal pain, diarrhea, nausea, constipation, gastritis, melena, vomiting, anorexia, peptic ulceration, *GI bleeding, perforation,* ulcerative stomatitis, thirst.

GU: dysuria, urinary frequency, *renal impairment.*
Hematologic: hemolytic anemia, *leukopenia, thrombocytopenia,* agranulocytosis.
Hepatic: hepatitis.
Metabolic: weight gain.
Respiratory: *asthma.*
Skin: pruritus, rash, photosensitivity, *Stevens-Johnson syndrome.*
Other: chills.

Interactions

Drug-drug. *ACE inhibitors, beta blockers, diuretics:* May blunt the effects of these drugs. Monitor patient closely.
Antacids: May decrease peak levels of drug. Monitor patient for decreased etodolac effect.
Aspirin: May reduce protein-binding of etodolac without altering its clearance. Significance isn't known. Avoid use together.
Cyclosporine: May impair elimination and increase risk of nephrotoxicity. Avoid use together.
Digoxin, lithium, methotrexate: May impair elimination of these drugs, increasing levels and risk of toxicity. Monitor blood levels.
Phenytoin: May increase levels of phenytoin. Monitor patient and levels for toxicity.
Warfarin: May decrease protein-binding of warfarin but doesn't change its clearance. Although no dosage adjustment is needed, monitor PT and INR closely, and watch for bleeding.
Drug-herb. *Dong quai, feverfew, garlic, ginger, horse chestnut, red clover:* May increase risk of bleeding. Discourage use together.
St. John's wort: May increase risk of photosensitivity. Discourage use together.
Drug-lifestyle. *Alcohol use:* May increase chance of adverse effects. Discourage use together.
Sun exposure: May cause photosensitivity reactions. Urge patient to avoid unprotected or prolonged exposure to sunlight.

Effects on lab test results

• May increase BUN and creatinine levels. May decrease uric acid and hemoglobin levels and hematocrit.
• May increase liver function test values. May decrease platelet, granulocyte, and WBC counts.
• May cause false-positive test for urinary bilirubin.

Pharmacokinetics

Absorption: Well absorbed from GI tract.
Distribution: To liver, lungs, heart, and kidneys.
Metabolism: Extensive.
Excretion: In urine primarily as metabolites; 16% is excreted in feces. *Half-life:* 7¼ hours.

Route	Onset	Peak	Duration
P.O.	≤ 30 min	1–2 hr	4–12 hr

Action

Chemical effect: May inhibit prostaglandin synthesis.
Therapeutic effect: Relieves inflammation and pain.

Available forms

Capsules: 200 mg, 300 mg
Tablets (extended-release): 400 mg, 500 mg, 600 mg
Tablets (film-coated): 400 mg, 500 mg

NURSING PROCESS

▨ Assessment
• Obtain history of patient's underlying condition before starting therapy.
• Be alert for adverse reactions and drug interactions.
• Assess patient's and family's knowledge of drug therapy.

▣ Nursing diagnoses
• Acute pain related to underlying condition
• Risk for injury related to drug-induced adverse reactions
• Deficient knowledge related to drug therapy

▷ Planning and implementation
• Give drug with milk or meals to minimize GI discomfort.
⊛ ALERT: Don't confuse Lodine with iodine.
Patient teaching
• Advise patient that serious GI toxicity, including peptic ulceration and bleeding, can occur as a result of taking NSAIDs, despite absence of GI symptoms. Teach patient the signs and symptoms of GI bleeding, such as dark tarry stools, generalized weakness, and coffee-ground emesis, and tell him to contact prescriber immediately if they occur.
• Tell patient to take drug with milk or food.

Reactions may be *common*, uncommon, *life-threatening*, or COMMON AND LIFE-THREATENING.

• Instruct patient to notify prescriber if other adverse reactions occur or if drug doesn't relieve pain.

• Advise patient to use sunblock, wear protective clothing, and avoid prolonged exposure to sunlight to prevent photosensitivity reactions.

• Tell patient not to use drug during last trimester of pregnancy.

☑ Evaluation

• Patient is free from pain.

• Patient has no injury as result of drug-induced adverse reactions.

• Patient and family state understanding of drug therapy.

etoposide (VP-16)
(eh-toh-POH-sighd)
Etopophos, Toposar, VePesid

Pharmacologic class: podophyllotoxin
Therapeutic class: antineoplastic
Pregnancy risk category: D

Indications and dosages

▶ **Testicular cancer.** *Adults:* 50 to 100 mg/m² I.V. on 5 consecutive days q 3 to 4 weeks; or 100 mg/m² on days 1, 3, and 5 q 3 to 4 weeks for three to four courses of therapy.

▶ **Small-cell carcinoma of lung.** *Adults:* 35 mg/m²/day I.V. for 4 days; or 50 mg/m²/day I.V. for 5 days. P.O. dose is two times I.V. dose rounded to nearest 50 mg.

▶ **AIDS-related Kaposi's sarcoma‡.** *Adults:* 150 mg/m² I.V. for 3 consecutive days q 4 weeks. Repeat cycles, p.r.n.

▼ I.V. administration

• Keep diphenhydramine, hydrocortisone, epinephrine, and needed emergency equipment available to establish airway in case of anaphylaxis.

• Don't give through membrane-type in-line filter because diluent may dissolve filter.

• Dilute drug for infusion in either D₅W or normal saline solution to 0.2 or 0.4 mg/ml. Higher concentrations may crystallize.

• Give drug by slow I.V. infusion (over at least 30 minutes) to prevent severe hypotension.

• If systolic blood pressure falls below 90 mm Hg, stop infusion and notify prescriber.

• Solutions diluted to 0.2 mg/ml are stable 96 hours at room temperature in plastic or glass unprotected from light; solutions diluted to 0.4 mg/ml are stable 48 hours under same conditions.

⊗ **Incompatibilities**
Cefepime hydrochloride, filgrastim, gallium nitrate, idarubicin.

Contraindications and cautions

• Contraindicated in patients hypersensitive to the drug or any of its components.

• Use cautiously in patients who have had cytotoxic or radiation therapy.

🎐 **Lifespan:** In pregnant women, use cautiously and only when benefits outweigh risks to the fetus. In breast-feeding women, drug is contraindicated. In children, safety and effectiveness haven't been established.

Adverse reactions

CNS: peripheral neuropathy.
CV: hypotension.
GI: nausea, vomiting, anorexia, diarrhea, abdominal pain, stomatitis.
Hematologic: anemia, *myelosuppression* (dose-limiting), LEUKOPENIA, THROMBOCYTOPENIA.
Skin: reversible alopecia.
Other: *anaphylaxis,* rash.

Interactions

Drug-drug. *Warfarin:* May further prolong PT. Monitor patient for bleeding, and monitor PT and INR.

Effects on lab test results

• May decrease hemoglobin level and hematocrit.

• May decrease WBC, RBC, platelet, and neutrophil counts.

Pharmacokinetics

Absorption: Only moderately absorbed across GI tract after P.O. administration. Bioavailability ranges from 25% to 75%, with average of 50% of dose being absorbed.
Distribution: Distributed widely in body tissues; crosses blood-brain barrier to limited and variable extent. Etoposide is about 94% protein-bound.
Metabolism: Only small portion of dose is metabolized in liver.

Excretion: Excreted primarily in urine as unchanged drug; smaller portion excreted in feces. *Half-life:* Initial, 30 minutes to 2 hours; terminal, 5¼ to 11 hours.

Route	Onset	Peak	Duration
P.O., I.V.	Unknown	Unknown	Unknown

Action

Chemical effect: Unknown.
Therapeutic effect: Inhibits selected cancer cell growth.

Available forms

Capsules: 50 mg
Injection: 20 mg/ml
Powder for injection: 100 mg

NURSING PROCESS

⚕ Assessment
• Obtain history of patient's underlying condition before starting therapy.
• Obtain baseline blood pressure before therapy, and monitor blood pressure at 30-minute intervals during infusion.
• Monitor effectiveness by noting results of follow-up diagnostic tests and overall physical health and by regularly checking tumor size and rate of growth through appropriate studies. Etoposide has produced complete remission in small-cell lung cancer and testicular cancer.
• Monitor CBC. Observe patient for signs of bone marrow suppression.
• Be alert for adverse reactions and drug interactions.
• Assess patient's and family's knowledge of drug therapy.

⚕ Nursing diagnoses
• Ineffective health maintenance related to presence of neoplastic disease
• Ineffective protection related to drug induced adverse hematologic reactions
• Deficient knowledge related to drug therapy

⚕ Planning and implementation
• Follow facility policy to reduce risks. Preparation and administration of parenteral form creates carcinogenic, mutagenic, and teratogenic risks for staff.
• Store capsules in refrigerator.

Patient teaching
• Warn patient to watch for signs of infection and bleeding. Teach patient how to take infection-control and bleeding precautions.
• Tell patient that reversible hair loss may occur.
• Instruct patient to report discomfort, pain, or burning at I.V. insertion site.

⚕ Evaluation
• Patient exhibits positive response to therapy.
• Patient's immune function returns to normal when therapy stops.
• Patient and family state understanding of drug therapy.

exemestane
(ecks-eh-MES-tayn)
Aromasin

Pharmacologic class: aromatase inhibitor
Therapeutic class: antineoplastic
Pregnancy risk category: D

Indications and dosages

▶ **Advanced breast cancer in postmenopausal women whose disease has progressed after tamoxifen therapy.** *Women:* 25 mg P.O. once daily after a meal.
▶ **Adjuvant treatment of postmenopausal women with estrogen-receptor–positive early breast cancer after 2 to 3 years of tamoxifen therapy, to complete 5 consecutive years of adjuvant hormonal therapy.** *Women:* 25 mg P.O. once daily after a meal.

Contraindications and cautions

• Contraindicated in patients hypersensitive to drug or any of its components.
⚕ **Lifespan:** In premenopausal women, drug is contraindicated.

Adverse reactions

CNS: *fever, depression, insomnia, anxiety, fatigue, pain,* dizziness, headache, paresthesia, generalized weakness, asthenia, confusion, hypoesthesia.
CV: *hot flushes,* hypertension, edema, chest pain.
EENT: sinusitis, rhinitis, pharyngitis.

GI: nausea, vomiting, abdominal pain, anorexia, constipation, diarrhea, dyspepsia.
GU: UTI.
Metabolic: increased appetite.
Musculoskeletal: pathologic fractures, arthralgia, back pain, skeletal pain.
Respiratory: *dyspnea,* bronchitis, coughing, upper respiratory tract infection.
Skin: rash, increased sweating, alopecia, itching.
Other: infection, flulike syndrome, lymphedema.

Interactions

Drug-drug. *Drugs that contain estrogen:* May interact. Don't give together.
Drugs that induce CYP 3A4, such as rifampicin, phenytoin: May decrease exemestane level; increase dose to 50 mg once daily.

Effects on lab test results

None reported.

Pharmacokinetics

Absorption: Rapidly absorbed, with about 42% of dose absorbed from the GI tract following P.O. administration. Level increases by 40% after a high-fat meal.
Distribution: Extensively distributed in tissues and 90% bound to proteins.
Metabolism: Extensively metabolized by the liver. Main liver isoenzyme is CYP 3A4.
Excretion: Excreted equally in urine and feces. *Half-life:* 24 hours.

Route	Onset	Peak	Duration
P.O.	Unknown	1–2 hr	Unknown

Action

Chemical effect: Acts as a false substrate for the aromatase enzyme, the principal enzyme that converts androgens to estrogens in premenopausal and postmenopausal women. Results in lower levels of circulating estrogens.
Therapeutic effect: Hinders growth of estrogen-dependent breast cancer cells.

Available forms

Tablets: 25 mg

NURSING PROCESS

◈ Assessment
• Assess patient's breast cancer before starting therapy and regularly thereafter.
• Monitor patient for adverse reactions.
• If adverse GI reactions occur, monitor patient's hydration.
• Assess patient's and family's knowledge of drug therapy.

◈ Nursing diagnoses
• Ineffective health maintenance related to presence of breast cancer
• Risk for impaired physical mobility related to potential adverse musculoskeletal effects
• Deficient knowledge related to drug therapy

◈ Planning and implementation
• Give drug only to postmenopausal women.
• Don't give with drugs that contain estrogen because doing so could interfere with intended action.
• Continue until tumor regression is evident.
⚠ ALERT: Don't confuse exemestane with estramustine.
Patient teaching
• Tell patient to take drug after a meal.
• Inform patient that she may need to take drug for a long period.
• Advise patient to report adverse effects to prescriber.

◈ Evaluation
• Patient responds well to drug.
• Patient has no musculoskeletal adverse reactions.
• Patient and family state understanding of drug therapy.

exenatide
(ecks-EHN-uh-tighd)
Byetta

Pharmacologic class: incretin mimetic
Therapeutic class: antidiabetic
Pregnancy risk category: C

Indications and dosages

▶ Adjunctive therapy to improve glycemic control in patients with type 2 diabetes who

take metformin, a sulfonylurea, or both.
Adults: 5 mcg subcutaneously b.i.d. within
60 minutes before morning and evening meals.
Increase to 10 mcg b.i.d. after 1 month p.r.n.

Contraindications and cautions

• Contraindicated in patients hypersensitive to
drug or its components. Don't give to patients
with type 1 diabetes or diabetic ketoacidosis.
Avoid in patients with end-stage renal disease,
creatinine clearance less than 30 ml/minute, or
severe GI disease.
⚕ **Lifespan:** In pregnant women, use only if
benefits justify risks to the fetus. In breast-feeding women, use cautiously because it isn't
known if drug appears in breast milk. In children, safety and effectiveness haven't been established.

Adverse reactions

CNS: dizziness, headache, jittery feeling.
GI: diarrhea, dyspepsia, nausea, vomiting.
Metabolic: *hypoglycemia.*
Skin: excessive sweating.
Other: injection site reaction.

Interactions

Drug-drug. *Drugs that are rapidly absorbed:*
May slow gastric emptying and reduce absorption of some oral drugs. Use cautiously together.
*Oral drugs that need to maintain a threshold
level to maintain effectiveness (antibiotics, hormonal contraceptives):* May reduce rate and extent of absorption of these drugs. Give these
drugs at least 1 hour before giving exenatide.
Sulfonylureas: May increase the risk of hypoglycemia. Reduce sulfonylurea dose as needed,
and monitor patient closely.

Effects on lab test results

None reported.

Pharmacokinetics

Absorption: Peaks in plasma in about 2 hours.
Distribution: Volume of about 28.3 L after a
single dose.
Metabolism: Not metabolized.
Excretion: Mainly by glomerular filtration.
Half-life: 2.4 hours.

Route	Onset	Peak	Duration
SubQ	Unknown	2 hr	10 hr

Action

Chemical effect: Reduces fasting and postprandial glucose levels in type 2 diabetes by stimulating insulin production in response to elevated
glucose levels, inhibiting glucagon release after
meals and slowing gastric emptying.
Therapeutic effect: Lowers glucose level.

Available forms

Injection: 5 mcg/dose in 1.2-ml prefilled pen,
10 mcg/dose in 2.4-ml prefilled pen (60 doses).

NURSING PROCESS

✍ Assessment
• Assess GI function before treatment starts.
• Monitor blood glucose level regularly and
glycosylated hemoglobin level periodically.
• Monitor patient for adverse reactions and drug
interactions.
• Assess patient's and family's knowledge of
drug therapy.

✪ Nursing diagnoses
• Risk for injury related to drug-induced hypo-
glycemia
• Ineffective health maintenance related to hy-
perglycemia
• Deficient knowledge related to drug therapy

▶ Planning and implementation
• Drug comes in two strengths; check cartridge
carefully before use.
• Overdose may cause rapid decline in blood
glucose levels, leading to severe nausea and
vomiting, tachycardia, restlessness, and dizziness.
• Provide symptomatic care for hypoglycemia.
If patient is responsive, give fast-acting oral carbohydrate. If unresponsive, give I.V. glucose.
• Store drug in refrigerator at 36° to 46° F (2° to
8° C).
⑤ **ALERT:** Don't confuse exenatide (Byetta) with
ezetimibe (Zetia).
Patient teaching
• Explain the risks of exenatide.
• Review proper use and storage of dosage pen,
particularly the one-time setup for each new
pen.
• Inform patient that prefilled pen doesn't include a needle; explain which needle length and
gauge is appropriate.

Reactions may be *common,* uncommon, *life-threatening*, or COMMON AND LIFE-THREATENING.

- Instruct patient to inject drug in the thigh, abdomen, or upper arm within 60 minutes before morning and evening meals. Caution against injecting drug after a meal.
- Advise patient that drug may decrease appetite, food intake, and body weight and that these changes don't warrant a change in dosage.
- Review steps for managing hypoglycemia, especially if patient takes a sulfonylurea.
- Stress importance of proper storage (refrigerated), infection prevention, and timing of exenatide dose in relation to other oral drugs.

☑ **Evaluation**
- Patient sustains no injury.
- Patient's glucose level is normal with drug therapy.
- Patient and family state understanding of drug therapy.

ezetimibe
(eh-ZET-eh-mighb)
Zetia◊

Pharmacologic class: selective cholesterol absorption inhibitor
Therapeutic class: antilipemic
Pregnancy risk category: C

Indications and dosages
▶ **Primary hypercholesterolemia, alone or with HMG-CoA reductase inhibitors; adjunct to atorvastatin or simvastatin in patients with homozygous familial hypercholesterolemia; homozygous sitosterolemia to reduce sitosterol and campesterol levels.**
Adults: 10 mg P.O. daily.

Contraindications and cautions
- Contraindicated in patients allergic to any component of the drug. Use with a HMG-CoA reductase inhibitor is contraindicated in patients with active hepatic disease or unexplained increase in transaminase levels.
- ⚛ Lifespan: In pregnant women, use only if benefits outweigh risks to the fetus. If used in pregnant women, don't give with an HMG-CoA reductase inhibitor. In breast-feeding women, use cautiously because it's unknown if drug appears in breast milk. In children, safety and effectiveness haven't been established. In elderly

patients, use cautiously because they may have a greater sensitivity to drug.

Adverse reactions
CNS: dizziness, headache, fatigue.
CV: chest pain.
EENT: pharyngitis, sinusitis.
GI: abdominal pain, diarrhea.
Musculoskeletal: back pain, arthralgia, myalgia.
Respiratory: cough, upper respiratory tract infection.
Other: viral infection.

Interactions
Drug-drug. *Bile acid sequestrant (cholestyramine):* May decrease ezetimibe level. Give ezetimibe at least 2 hours before or 4 hours after cholestyramine.
Cyclosporine, fenofibrate, gemfibrozil: May increase ezetimibe level. Monitor patient closely for adverse effects.
Fibrates: May increase excretion of cholesterol into the gallbladder bile. Avoid use together.

Effects on lab test results
- May increase liver function test values.

Pharmacokinetics
Absorption: Absorbed and conjugated to an active metabolite.
Distribution: More than 90% bound to proteins.
Metabolism: Primarily and rapidly metabolized in the small intestine and liver via glucuronide conjugation.
Excretion: Biliary and renal. *Half-life:* 22 hours.

Route	Onset	Peak	Duration
P.O.	Unknown	4–12 hr	Unknown

Action
Chemical effect: Inhibits absorption of cholesterol by the small intestine. Decreases hepatic cholesterol stores and increases cholesterol clearance.
Therapeutic effect: Lowers cholesterol levels.

Available forms
Tablets: 10 mg

NURSING PROCESS

⊅ Assessment
● Obtain history of patient's underlying condition before starting therapy.
● Monitor total cholesterol, LDL, HDL, and triglyceride levels before and during therapy.
● Assess patient's and family's knowledge of drug therapy.

⊞ Nursing diagnoses
● Risk for injury related to elevated cholesterol levels
● Deficient knowledge related to drug therapy

⊠ Planning and implementation
● Use drug only after diet and other nondrug therapy prove ineffective. Have patient follow a standard low-cholesterol diet before and during therapy.
● Before starting drug, evaluate patient for secondary causes of dyslipidemia.
● When drug is used with an HMG-CoA reductase inhibitor, check liver function test results at start of therapy and thereafter according to the recommendations relevant to the HMG-CoA reductase inhibitor being used.
● Use with an HMG-CoA reductase inhibitor significantly reduces total cholesterol, LDL, apolipoprotein B, and triglyceride levels and (except with pravastatin) increases HDL level more than use of an HMG-CoA reductase inhibitor alone.
● **ALERT:** Don't confuse Zetia with Zebeta, Zestril, or Zyrtec.
Patient teaching
● Emphasize importance of following a cholesterol-lowering diet.
● Tell patient he may take drug without regard to meals.
● Advise patient to notify prescriber of unexplained muscle pain, weakness, or tenderness.
● Urge patient to tell prescriber if he's taking herbal or dietary supplements.
● Advise patient to visit his prescriber for routine follow-up and blood tests.
● Tell patient to notify prescriber if she becomes pregnant.

⊠ Evaluation
● Patient's cholesterol level is within normal limits.

● Patient and family state understanding of drug therapy.

famciclovir
(fam-SIGH-kloh-veer)
Famvir

Pharmacologic class: synthetic acyclic guanine derivative
Therapeutic class: antiviral
Pregnancy risk category: B

Indications and dosages

▶ **Acute herpes zoster.** *Adults:* 500 mg P.O. q 8 hours for 7 days.
⧄ Adjust-a-dose: For patients with renal impairment, if creatinine clearance is 40 to 59 ml/minute, give 500 mg q 12 hours; if creatinine clearance is 20 to 39 ml/minute, give 500 mg q 24 hours; if creatinine clearance is less than 20 ml/minute, give 250 mg q 48 hours.
▶ **Recurrent episodes of genital herpes.**
Adults: 125 mg P.O. b.i.d. for 5 days. Therapy begins as soon as symptoms occur.
⧄ Adjust-a-dose: For patients with renal impairment, if creatinine clearance is 20 to 39 ml/minute, give 125 mg q 24 hours; if creatinine clearance is less than 20 ml/minute, give 125 mg q 48 hours.
▶ **Long-term suppressive therapy of recurrent episodes of genital herpes.** *Adults:* 250 mg P.O. q 12 hours for up to 1 year.
⧄ Adjust-a-dose: For patients with renal impairment, if creatinine clearance is 20 to 39 ml/minute, give 125 mg q 12 hours; if creatinine clearance is less than 20 ml/minute, give 125 mg q 24 hours.
▶ **Recurrent herpes simplex virus infections in HIV-infected patients.** *Adults:* 500 mg P.O. b.i.d. for 7 days.
⧄ Adjust-a-dose: For patients with renal impairment, if creatinine clearance is 20 to 39 ml/minute, give 500 mg q 24 hours; if creatinine clearance is less than 20 ml/minute, give 250 mg q 24 hours.

Contraindications and cautions

• Contraindicated in patients hypersensitive to drug or any of its components.
• Use cautiously in patients with renal or hepatic impairment. Dosage adjustment may be needed.
⚠ **Lifespan:** In pregnant women, use only if benefits outweigh risks to the fetus. In breast-feeding women, use cautiously because it's unknown if drug appears in breast milk. In men, use cautiously because of risk of decreased fertility. In children, safety and effectiveness haven't been established.

Adverse reactions

CNS: *headache,* fatigue, dizziness, paresthesia, somnolence.
EENT: pharyngitis, sinusitis.
GI: diarrhea, *nausea,* vomiting, constipation, anorexia, abdominal pain.
Musculoskeletal: back pain, arthralgia.
Skin: pruritus; zoster-related signs, symptoms, and complications.

Interactions

Drug-drug. *Probenecid:* May increase level of famciclovir. Monitor patient for increased adverse effects.

Effects on lab test results

• May increase AST, ALT, total bilirubin, creatinine, amylase, and lipase levels. May decrease hemoglobin level and hematocrit.
• May decrease WBC and neutrophil counts.

Pharmacokinetics

Absorption: Absolute bioavailability is 77%.
Distribution: Less than 20% is bound to proteins.
Metabolism: Extensive, in liver to active drug, penciclovir, and inactive metabolites.
Excretion: Primarily in urine. *Half-life:* 2 to 3 hours.

Route	Onset	Peak	Duration
P.O.	Unknown	≤ 1 hr	Unknown

Action

Chemical effect: Converted to penciclovir, which enters viral cells and inhibits DNA polymerase and viral DNA synthesis.
Therapeutic effect: Inhibits viral replication. Spectrum of activity includes herpes simplex types 1 and 2 and varicella zoster viruses.

Available forms

Tablets: 125 mg, 250 mg, 500 mg

NURSING PROCESS

▨ Assessment
• Assess patient's viral infection before starting therapy, and reassess regularly throughout therapy.
• Be alert for adverse reactions and drug interactions.
• If adverse GI reactions occur, monitor patient's hydration.
• Assess patient's and family's knowledge of drug therapy.

▨ Nursing diagnoses
• Infection related to presence of virus susceptible to famciclovir
• Risk for deficient fluid volume related to drug's adverse GI reactions
• Deficient knowledge related to drug therapy

▷ Planning and implementation
• Give a lower dose in patients with renal insufficiency.
• Drug may be taken with or without food.
Patient teaching
• Teach patient how to prevent spread of infection to others.
• Urge patient to recognize and report early symptoms of herpes infection, such as tingling, itching, or pain.

☑ Evaluation
• Patient is free from infection.
• Patient maintains adequate hydration.
• Patient and family state understanding of drug therapy.

famotidine
(fam-OH-tih-deen)
Pepcid†✐, Pepcid AC†, Pepcid RPD, Pepcidine ◇

Pharmacologic class: H$_2$-receptor antagonist
Therapeutic class: antisecretory
Pregnancy risk category: B

Indications and dosages

▶ **Duodenal ulcer (short-term therapy).**
Adults: For acute therapy, 40 mg P.O. once daily
h.s. or 20 mg P.O. b.i.d. Maintenance, 20 mg
P.O. once daily h.ś.
▶ **Benign gastric ulcer (short-term therapy).**
Adults: 40 mg P.O. daily h.s. for 8 weeks.
▶ **Pathologic hypersecretory conditions
(such as Zollinger-Ellison syndrome).** *Adults:*
20 mg P.O. q 6 hours up to 160 mg q 6 hours.
▶ **Gastroesophageal reflux disease (GERD).**
Adults: 20 mg P.O. b.i.d. for up to 6 weeks. For
esophagitis caused by GERD, 20 to 40 mg b.i.d.
for up to 12 weeks.
Children ages 1 to 16: 1 mg/kg/day P.O. in divided doses b.i.d. up to 80 mg daily.
▶ **Peptic ulcer in children.** *Children ages 1 to
16:* 0.5 mg/kg/day P.O. h.s. or divided twice
daily up to 40 mg daily.
▶ **Heartburn, prevention of heartburn.**
Adults: 10 mg Pepcid AC P.O. 1 hour before
meals (prevention) or 10 mg Pepcid AC P.O.
with water when symptoms occur. Maximum,
20 mg daily. Drug shouldn't be taken daily for
more than 2 weeks without prescriber authoriza-
tion.
▶ **Hospitalized patients with intractable
ulcerations or hypersecretory conditions or
patients who can't take oral drugs.** *Adults:*
20 mg I.V. q 12 hours.
Children ages 1 to 16: 0.25 mg/kg I.V. q
12 hours, up to 40 mg daily.
◩ **Adjust-a-dose:** Patients with moderate (creatinine clearance less than 50 ml/minute) or
severe (creatinine clearance less than 10 ml/
minute) renal insufficiency may have dosages
reduced to half-strength, or the interval prolonged to 36 to 48 hours, p.r.n., to avoid excess
drug accumulation.

▽ I.V. administration

● For I.V. injection, dilute 2 ml (20 mg) with
compatible I.V. solution to total volume of either 5 or 10 ml. Compatible solutions include
sterile water for injection, normal saline injection, D_5W or dextrose 10% in water injection,
5% sodium bicarbonate injection, and lactated
Ringer's injection. Inject over at least 2 minutes.
● For intermittent I.V. infusion, dilute 20 mg
(2 ml) drug in 100 ml of compatible solution.
Solution is stable for 48 hours at room temperature after dilution. Infuse over 15 to 30 minutes.

● If infiltration or phlebitis occurs, apply warm
compresses and use different site for next dose.
● Store premixed injection at room temperature.
Store unmixed injection in refrigerator at 36° to
46° F (2° to 8° C).
⊗ **Incompatibilities**
Amphotericin B cholesterol complex, azithro-
mycin, cefepime, piperacillin with tazobactam.

Contraindications and cautions

● Contraindicated in patients hypersensitive to
drug or any of its components. Injection may
contain benzyl alcohol as a preservative; some
preparations contain phenylalanine.
🔥 **Lifespan:** In pregnant women, use cautiously. In breast-feeding women, use cautiously because it's unknown if the drug appears in breast
milk. In children younger than 1 year old, drug
is contraindicated.

Adverse reactions

CNS: *headache,* dizziness, vertigo, malaise,
paresthesia, fever.
CV: palpitations, flushing.
EENT: tinnitus, orbital edema.
GI: diarrhea, constipation, anorexia, taste disor-
der, dry mouth.
Musculoskeletal: musculoskeletal pain.
Skin: acne, dry skin.
Other: transient irritation at I.V. site.

Interactions

None significant.

Effects on lab test results

● May increase BUN, creatinine, and liver enzyme levels.

Pharmacokinetics

Absorption: 40% to 45%.
Distribution: Wide.
Metabolism: 30% to 35% by liver.
Excretion: Mostly unchanged in urine. *Half-
life:* 2½ to 3½ hours.

Route	Onset	Peak	Duration
P.O.	≤ 1 hr	1–3 hr	10–12 hr
I.V.	≤ 1 hr	20 min	10–12 hr

Action

Chemical effect: Competitively inhibits action of H_2 at receptor sites of parietal cells, decreasing gastric acid secretion.
Therapeutic effect: Decreases gastric acid levels and prevents heartburn.

Available forms

Gelcaps: 10 mg
Injection: 10 mg/ml, 20 mg/50 ml (premixed)
Powder for oral suspension: 40 mg/5 ml after reconstitution
Tablets: 10 mg†, 20 mg, 40 mg
Tablets (chewable): 10 mg†
Tablets (orally disintegrating): 20 mg, 40 mg

NURSING PROCESS

Assessment

• Assess creatinine clearance before treatment.
• Assess patient's GI disorder before starting therapy and reassess regularly.
• Be alert for adverse reactions.
• Determine if patient has phenylalanine sensitivity.
• Assess patient's and family's knowledge of drug therapy.

Nursing diagnoses

• Impaired tissue integrity related to underlying GI disorder
• Deficient knowledge related to drug therapy

Planning and implementation

• Give daily doses or last dose of the day at bedtime.
• Store reconstituted oral suspension below 86° F (30° C). Discard after 30 days.
Patient teaching
• Tell patient to take drug with food. Remind him that drug is most effective if taken h.s. Tell patient taking 20 mg b.i.d. to take one dose h.s.
• With prescriber's knowledge, allow patient to take antacids, especially at beginning of therapy when pain is severe.
• Urge patient not to smoke because it may increase gastric acid secretion and worsen disease.
• Advise patient not to take drug for more than 8 weeks unless specifically ordered by prescriber. Tell patient not to self-medicate for heartburn longer than 2 weeks without prescriber's knowledge.

✓ Evaluation

• Patient reports decrease in or relief of GI pain with drug.
• Patient and family state understanding of drug therapy.

felodipine
(feh-LOH-dih-peen)
Agon ◇, Agon SR ◇, Plendil, Plendil ER ◇, Renedil ◆

F

Pharmacologic class: calcium channel blocker
Therapeutic class: antihypertensive
Pregnancy risk category: C

Indications and dosages

▶ **Hypertension.** *Adults:* Initially, 5 mg P.O. daily. Adjust dosage based on response, usually at no less than 2-week intervals. Usual dosage is 2.5 to 10 mg daily.
Elderly patients: 2.5 mg P.O. daily; adjust as for adults. Maximum, 10 mg daily.

Contraindications and cautions

• Contraindicated in patients hypersensitive to drug or any of its components.
• Use cautiously in patients with heart failure, particularly those receiving beta blockers, and in patients with impaired hepatic function.
≋ **Lifespan:** In pregnant and breast-feeding women, use cautiously. In children, safety and effectiveness haven't been established.

Adverse reactions

CNS: *headache,* dizziness, paresthesia, asthenia.
CV: *flushing, peripheral edema,* chest pain, palpitations.
EENT: rhinorrhea, pharyngitis, gingival hyperplasia.
GI: abdominal pain, nausea, constipation, diarrhea.
Musculoskeletal: muscle cramps, back pain.
Respiratory: upper respiratory infection, cough.
Skin: rash.

Interactions

Drug-drug. *Anticonvulsants:* May decrease felodipine level. Avoid use together.

Cimetidine, erythromycin, itraconazole, ketoconazole: May decrease felodipine clearance. Give lower doses of felodipine.
Metoprolol: May alter pharmacokinetics of metoprolol. No dosage adjustment needed. Monitor patient for adverse effects.
Tacrolimus: May increase tacrolimus level. Monitor tacrolimus level and adjust dose as needed.
Theophylline: May slightly decrease theophylline level. Monitor patient's response carefully.
Drug-herb. *St. John's wort:* May increase metabolism of felodipine. Discourage use together.
Drug-food. *Grapefruit, lime:* May increase level and adverse effects of drug. Discourage use together.

Effects on lab test results

None reported.

Pharmacokinetics

Absorption: Almost complete, but extensive first-pass metabolism reduces absolute bioavailability to about 20%.
Distribution: More than 99% bound to proteins.
Metabolism: Possibly hepatic.
Excretion: More than 70% in urine and 10% in feces as metabolites. *Half-life:* 11 to 16 hours.

Route	Onset	Peak	Duration
P.O.	2–5 hr	2½–5 hr	24 hr

Action

Chemical effect: Prevents entry of calcium ions into vascular smooth muscle and cardiac cells.
Therapeutic effect: Lowers blood pressure.

Available forms

Tablets: 5 mg ◇
Tablets (extended-release): 2.5 mg, 5 mg, 10 mg

NURSING PROCESS

Assessment

- Assess patient's blood pressure before starting therapy, and reassess regularly.
- Be alert for adverse reactions and drug interactions.
- Assess patient's and family's knowledge of drug therapy.

Nursing diagnoses

- Risk for injury related to presence of hypertension
- Excessive fluid volume related to drug-induced peripheral edema
- Deficient knowledge related to drug therapy

Planning and implementation

- Drug may be given with or without food.

ALERT: Don't confuse Plendil with Isordil.

Patient teaching

- Instruct patient to swallow tablets whole and not to crush or chew them.
- Tell patient to take drug even when he feels better, to watch his diet, and to check with prescriber or pharmacist before taking other drugs, including OTC and herbal remedies.
- Advise patient to practice good oral hygiene and to see dentist regularly.

Evaluation

- Patient's blood pressure is normal.
- Patient doesn't develop complications from peripheral edema.
- Patient and family state understanding of drug therapy.

fenofibrate

(feh-noh-FIGH-brayt)

Antara, Lofibra, Tricor, Triglide

Pharmacologic class: fibric acid derivative
Therapeutic class: antilipemic
Pregnancy risk category: C

Indications and dosages

▶ **Adjunct to diet for patients with very high triglyceride levels (type IV and V hyperlipidemia) who are at high risk of pancreatitis and who don't respond adequately to diet alone.** *Adults:* For Antara, initial dose is 43 to 130 mg P.O. daily. Maximum, 130 mg daily. For Lofibra, 67 to 200 mg P.O. daily. Maximum, 200 mg daily. For Tricor, 48 to 145 mg P.O. daily. Maximum, 145 mg daily. For Triglide, 50 to 160 mg P.O. daily. Maximum, 160 mg daily. Based on results of repeat triglyceride level tests at 4- to 8-week intervals, increase dosage p.r.n. to maximum.

▶ **Adjunct to diet for the reduction of LDL, total cholesterol, triglyceride, and apolipo-**

protein B levels and to increase HDL level in patients with primary hypercholesterolemia or mixed dyslipidemia (Frederickson types IIa and IIb). *Adults:* For Antara, initial dose is 130 mg P.O. daily. For Lofibra, initial dose is 200 mg P.O. daily. For Tricor, initial dose is 145 mg P.O. daily. For Triglide, initial dose is 160 mg P.O. daily. May reduce dose if lipid levels fall significantly below the target range.

Adjust-a-dose: For patients with creatinine clearance less than 50 ml/minute and elderly patients, initially give 43 mg daily for Antara, 67 mg daily for Lofibra, 48 mg daily for Tricor, or 50 mg daily for Triglide. Increase dose only after evaluating effects on renal function and triglyceride level.

Contraindications and cautions

• Contraindicated in patients hypersensitive to drug or any of its components and in those with gallbladder disease, hepatic dysfunction, primary biliary cirrhosis, severe renal dysfunction, or unexplained persistent liver function abnormalities.

• Use cautiously in patients with history of pancreatitis.

Lifespan: In pregnant women, use only if benefits outweigh risks to the fetus. Breast-feeding women should stop the drug or stop breast-feeding. In children, safety and effectiveness haven't been established. In elderly patients, start with lower dosage.

Adverse reactions

CNS: *dizziness,* pain, asthenia, fatigue, paresthesia, insomnia, *headache.*
CV: *arrhythmias.*
EENT: eye irritation, eye floaters, earache, conjunctivitis, blurred vision, rhinitis, sinusitis.
GI: dyspepsia, eructation, flatulence, nausea, vomiting, abdominal pain, constipation, diarrhea, *pancreatitis,* increased appetite.
GU: polyuria, vaginitis.
Hepatic: cholelithiasis.
Musculoskeletal: arthralgia, myalgia, *rhabdomyolysis,* myositis.
Respiratory: cough.
Skin: pruritus, rash.
Other: hypersensitivity reaction, *infection,* flu-like syndrome, decreased libido.

Interactions

Drug-drug. *Bile acid sequestrants:* May bind drug and inhibit absorption. Give drug 1 hour before or 4 to 6 hours after bile acid sequestrants.
Coumarin-type anticoagulants: May increase anticoagulant effect. Monitor PT and INR closely. Reduce anticoagulant dosage p.r.n.
Cyclosporine, immunosuppressants, nephrotoxic drugs: May cause renal dysfunction, which may compromise the elimination of drug. Use together cautiously.
HMG-CoA reductase inhibitors: Because of risk of myopathy, rhabdomyolysis, and acute renal impairment from use of HMG-CoA reductase inhibitors with gemfibrozil (another fibrate derivative), don't use together.
Drug-food. *Any food:* May increase absorption. Give drug with meals.
Drug-lifestyle. *Alcohol use:* May elevate triglyceride levels. Discourage use together.

Effects on lab test results

• May increase BUN, creatinine, ALT, and AST levels. May decrease uric acid and hemoglobin levels and hematocrit.
• May decrease WBC count.

Pharmacokinetics

Absorption: Good.
Distribution: 99% bound to proteins.
Metabolism: Rapidly hydrolyzed by esterases to active metabolite, fenofibric acid.
Excretion: 60% in urine, mainly as metabolites, and 25% in feces. *Half-life:* 20 hours.

Route	Onset	Peak	Duration
P.O.	Unknown	6–8 hr	Unknown

Action

Chemical effect: May inhibit triglyceride synthesis, decreasing amount of very–low-density lipoproteins released into circulation. May stimulate breakdown of triglyceride-rich protein.
Therapeutic effect: Decreases triglyceride levels.

Available forms

Micronized capsules: 43 mg, 67 mg, 87 mg, 130 mg, 134 mg, 200 mg
Tablets: 48 mg, 50 mg, 54 mg, 145 mg, 160 mg

☙ Assessment
• Assess baseline lipid levels and liver function test results before starting therapy and periodically thereafter.
• Be alert for adverse reactions and drug interactions.
• Assess patient's and family's knowledge of drug therapy.

⊕ Nursing diagnoses
• Impaired tissue integrity: muscular related to adverse drug reaction
• Risk for infection related to adverse drug reactions
• Deficient knowledge related to drug therapy

▷ Planning and implementation
• Stop giving the drug to a patient who doesn't have an adequate response after 2 months of therapy with maximum dose.
• Give tablets with meals to increase bioavailability.
• Evaluate renal function and triglyceride levels in patient with severe renal impairment before increasing dose.
• Counsel patient on importance of adhering to triglyceride-lowering diet.
⊛ **ALERT:** Don't confuse Tricor with Tracleer.
Patient teaching
• Advise patient to promptly report symptoms of unexplained muscle weakness, pain, or tenderness, especially if accompanied by malaise or fever.
• Urge patient to take drug with meals to optimize drug absorption.
• Advise patient to continue weight-control measures, including diet and exercise, and to reduce alcohol intake before starting therapy.
• Instruct patient who also takes bile acid resin to take fenofibrate 1 hour before or 4 to 6 hours after bile acid resin.

☑ Evaluation
• Patient remains free of myositis and rhabdomyolysis.
• Patient remains free from infection.
• Patient and family state understanding of drug therapy.

fentanyl citrate
(FEN-tuh-nihl SIGH-trayt)
Sublimaze

fentanyl transdermal system
Duragesic-12, Duragesic-25, Duragesic-50, Duragesic-75, Duragesic-100

fentanyl transmucosal
Actiq

Pharmacologic class: opioid
Therapeutic class: analgesic, anesthetic
Pregnancy risk category: C
Controlled substance schedule: II

Indications and dosages

▶ **Adjunct to general anesthetic.** *Adults and children older than age 12:* For low-dose therapy, 2 mcg/kg I.V. For moderate-dose therapy, 2 to 20 mcg/kg I.V.; then 25 to 100 mcg I.V. or I.M., p.r.n. For high-dose therapy, 20 to 50 mcg/kg I.V.; then 25 mcg to one-half initial loading dose I.V., p.r.n.
Children ages 2 to 12: 2 to 3 mcg/kg I.V. or I.M. during induction and maintenance phases of general anesthesia.
▶ **Adjunct to regional anesthesia.** *Adults:* 50 to 100 mcg I.M. or slow I.V. over 1 to 2 minutes.
▶ **Postoperative pain.** *Adults:* 50 to 100 mcg I.M. q 1 to 2 hours, p.r.n.
▶ **To manage persistent, moderate to severe chronic pain in opioid-tolerant patients who require continuous, around-the-clock opioid analgesics for an extended period of time.**
Adults and children age 2 or older: When converting to Duragesic, the initial dose is based on the daily dose, potency and characteristics of the current opioid therapy, the reliability of the relative potency estimates used to calculate the needed dose of fentanyl, the degree of opioid tolerance, and the condition of the patient. Each system may be worn for 72 hours, although some adult patients may need systems to be applied q 48 hours during the initial period. May increase dose 3 days after the first dose and then q 6 days thereafter.
▶ **Breakthrough cancer pain in opioid-tolerant patients.** *Adults and adolescents age 16 and older:* 200 mcg Actiq P.O. transmucosal-

ly initially; adjust dose based on response. Have patient suck on each unit for 15 minutes. An additional unit may be given 30 minutes after start of the previous dose. Don't use more than 2 units per episode of breakthrough pain.

▼ I.V. administration

• Only staff trained in giving I.V. anesthetics and managing their adverse effects should give drug I.V.
• Keep naloxone and resuscitation equipment available when giving drug I.V.
• Drug is commonly used I.V. with droperidol to produce neuroleptanalgesia.

⊗ **Incompatibilities**

Azithromycin, fluorouracil, lidocaine, methohexital, pentobarbital sodium, phenytoin, thiopental.

Contraindications and cautions

• Contraindicated in patients intolerant of drug. Transdermal fentanyl is contraindicated in patients hypersensitive to adhesives; patients who need postoperative pain management; patients who have acute, mild, or intermittent pain that can be managed with nonopioid drugs; and patients who aren't opioid tolerant. Don't use in patients with increased intracranial pressure, impaired consciousness, or coma.
• Use cautiously in debilitated patients and in patients with brain tumors, increased CSF pressure, COPD, decreased respiratory reserve, potentially compromised respirations, hepatic or renal disease, or bradyarrhythmias.
� **Lifespan:** In pregnant women, use cautiously. In breast-feeding women, use cautiously because it's unknown if the drug appears in breast milk. Actiq is contraindicated for use during labor and delivery. In children younger than age 2, safety and effectiveness of I.V. drug haven't been established. In children younger than age 16, safety and effectiveness of Actiq haven't been established. In children younger than age 12 and children younger than age 18 weighing less than 50 kg (110 lb), transdermal system is contraindicated. In elderly patients, use all forms cautiously because dosages may have prolonged CNS and respiratory effects.

Adverse reactions

CNS: *sedation, somnolence, clouded sensorium, euphoria,* dizziness, headache, *confusion, asthenia,* nervousness, hallucinations, anxiety, depression.

CV: hypotension, hypertension, *arrhythmias,* chest pain, *bradycardia.*
EENT: dry mouth.
GI: nausea, vomiting, constipation, ileus, abdominal pain.
GU: urine retention.
Respiratory: *respiratory depression,* hypoventilation, dyspnea, *apnea.*
Skin: pruritus, diaphoresis.
Other: physical dependence, reaction at application site (erythema, papules, edema).

Interactions

Drug-drug. *CNS depressants, general anesthetics, hypnotics, MAO inhibitors, other opioid analgesics, sedatives, tricyclic antidepressants:* May have additive effects. Use together cautiously. Reduce fentanyl dose by one-fourth or one-third. Reduce dosages of other drugs.
Diazepam: May cause CV depression when given with high doses of fentanyl. Monitor patient closely.
Potent CYP 3A4 inhibitors (clarithromycin, erythromycin, itraconazole, ketoconazole, nelfinavir, nefazodone, ritonavir, troleandomycin): May increase analgesia, CNS depression, and hypotensive effects. Monitor patient's respiratory status and vital signs.
Protease inhibitors: May increase CNS and respiratory depression. Monitor patient closely.
Droperidol: May cause hypotension and decreased pulmonary arterial pressure. Monitor patient closely.
Drug-lifestyle. *Alcohol use:* May have additive effects. Discourage use together.

Effects on lab test results

None reported.

Pharmacokinetics

Absorption: Varies with drug route.
Distribution: Accumulates in adipose tissue and skeletal muscle.
Metabolism: In liver.
Excretion: In urine. *Half-life:* 3½ hours after parenteral use, 5 to 15 hours after transmucosal use, 18 hours after transdermal use.

Route	Onset	Peak	Duration
I.V.	1–2 min	3–5 min	30–60 min
I.M.	7–15 min	20–30 min	1–2 hr
Transmucosal	15 min	20–30 min	Unknown
Transdermal	12–24 hr	1–3 days	Varies

Action

Chemical effect: May bind with opioid receptors in CNS, altering both perception of and emotional response to pain.
Therapeutic effect: Relieves pain.

Available forms

Injection: 50 mcg/ml
Transdermal system: patches designed to release 25, 50, 75, or 100 mcg of fentanyl per hour
Transmucosal: 200 mcg, 400 mcg, 600 mcg, 800 mcg, 1,200 mcg, 1,600 mcg

NURSING PROCESS

Assessment

• Assess patient's underlying condition before starting therapy.
• Evaluate degree of pain relief provided by each dose.
• Periodically monitor postoperative vital signs and bladder function. Because drug decreases both rate and depth of respirations, monitoring of arterial oxygen saturation (Sao_2) may help assess respiratory depression.
ALERT: Transdermal fentanyl levels peak between 24 and 72 hours after initial application and dose increases. Monitor patients for life-threatening hypoventilation, especially during these times.
• Be alert for adverse reactions and drug interactions.
• Assess patient's and family's knowledge of drug therapy.

Nursing diagnoses

• Acute pain related to underlying condition
• Ineffective breathing pattern related to respiratory depression
• Deficient knowledge related to drug therapy

Planning and implementation

• For better analgesic effect, give drug before patient has intense pain.
• To give Actiq transmucosal lozenge:
– Open childproof foil package with scissors immediately before use.
– Place lozenge in patient's mouth between the cheek and the lower gums, occasionally switching sides using the handle.
– Make sure patient sucks the lozenge, rather than chewing and swallowing, which may cause lower peak concentrations.
– Make sure patient consumes the lozenge in 15 minutes. Faster or slower consumption may reduce its effects.
– If signs of excess opioid effects appear before the entire lozenge dissolves, remove the lozenge from the patient's mouth and decrease future doses.
– Dispose of Actiq, particularly any unused portions, in the storage container provided in Actiq's welcome kit.
ALERT: Ask patient and caregivers about the presence of children in the home because Actiq lozenges may be fatal to a child. Make sure they know how to dispose of lozenges properly.
• Transdermal drug isn't recommended for postoperative pain.
• Use dosage equivalency charts to calculate transdermal dose based on daily morphine intake—for example, for every 90 mg of oral morphine or 15 mg of I.M. morphine daily, give 25 mcg/hour of transdermal drug.
• Adjust dose gradually in patient using transdermal system. Delay dose adjustment until after at least two applications. Reaching steady-state levels of new dosage may take up to 6 days.
• High doses can produce muscle rigidity, which can be reversed with neuromuscular blockers; however, patient must be artificially ventilated.
• Immediately report respiratory rate below 12 breaths/minute or decreased respiratory volume or Sao_2.
• When drug is used postoperatively, encourage patient to turn, cough, and breathe deeply to prevent atelectasis.
• Most patients have good control of pain for 3 days while wearing transdermal system, but a few may need a new application after 48 hours. Because drug level rises for first 24 hours after application, analgesic effect can't be evaluated on the first day. Make sure patient has adequate supplemental analgesic to prevent breakthrough pain.
• When reducing opioid therapy or switching to a different analgesic, withdraw transdermal system gradually. Because drug level drops gradually after removal, give half of equianalgesic dose of new analgesic 12 to 18 hours after removal.

(£) **ALERT:** Don't confuse fentanyl with sufentanil.

Patient teaching

• Teach patient proper application of transdermal patch. Instruct patient to clip hair at application site, but to avoid razors, which may irritate skin. Tell him to wash area with clear water if needed, but not with soaps, oils, lotions, alcohol, or other substances that may irritate skin or prevent adhesion. Urge him to dry area completely before application.

• Tell patient to remove transdermal system from package just before applying, to hold in place for 10 to 20 seconds, and to be sure edges of patch adhere to the skin.

• Teach patient to dispose of transdermal patch by folding so that adhesive side adheres to itself, and then flushing it down toilet.

• If patient needs another patch after 72 hours, tell him to apply it to new site.

• Inform patient that heat from fever or environment may increase transdermal delivery and cause toxicity, which requires dosage adjustment. Instruct patient to notify prescriber if fever occurs or if he will be spending time in hot climate.

(£) **ALERT:** Strongly warn patient to keep drug safely secured, away from children.

• Advise parent or caregiver to place transdermal patch on the upper back for a child or a patient who's cognitively impaired, to reduce the chance the patch will be removed and placed in the mouth.

• Teach patient how to properly take transmucosal Actiq, and to apply transdermal systems.

(£) **ALERT:** Teach patient proper disposal of transmucosal Actiq units.

☑ Evaluation

• Patient is free from pain.

• Patient maintains adequate ventilation throughout drug therapy.

• Patient and family state understanding of drug therapy.

ferrous fumarate
(FEH-rus FYOO-muh-rayt)

Femiron†, Feostat†, Feostat Drops†, Ferretts†, Fumasorb†, Fumerin†, Hemocyte†, Ircon†, Neo-Fer♦†, Nephro-Fer†, Novofumar♦†, Palafer♦† Span-FF†

ferrous gluconate

Fergon†, Fertinic♦, Novoferrogluc♦

ferrous sulfate

Apo-Ferrous Sulfate, ED-IN-SOL, Feosol*†, Feratab, Fer-Gen-Sol Drops†, Fer-In-Sol*†, Fer-Iron Drops†, Fero-Grad♦, Fero-Gradumet†, Irospan†, Mol-Iron

ferrous sulfate, dried

Feosol, Fer-In-Sol, Fe50, Slow-Fe†

Pharmacologic class: oral iron supplement
Therapeutic class: hematinic
Pregnancy risk category: A

Indications and dosages

▶ **Iron deficiency.** *Adults:* 150 to 300 mg elemental iron P.O. daily given in three divided doses.
Children: 3 to 6 mg/kg P.O. daily given in one to three divided doses.
Premature infants: 2 to 4 mg/kg P.O. daily given in one to two divided doses. Maximum dose is 15 mg/day.

Contraindications and cautions

• Contraindicated in patients hypersensitive to drug or its ingredients; patients with primary hemochromatosis, hemosiderosis, hemolytic anemia (unless iron deficiency anemia is also present), peptic ulcer disease, regional enteritis, or ulcerative colitis; and patients receiving repeated blood transfusions.

• Use cautiously on long-term basis.

☀ **Lifespan:** In breast-feeding women, iron supplements usually are recommended. In children, use cautiously. Extended-release forms aren't recommended for children. In elderly patients, may cause constipation.

Adverse reactions

GI: nausea, epigastric pain, vomiting, constipation, diarrhea, black stools, anorexia.

Other: temporary staining of teeth (suspension, drops).

Interactions

Drug-drug. *Antacids, cholestyramine resin, levodopa, tetracycline, vitamin E:* May decrease iron absorption. Separate doses by 2 to 4 hours.
Chloramphenicol: May increase iron response. Watch patient carefully.
Fluoroquinolones, penicillamine, tetracyclines: May decrease GI absorption of these drugs, possibly decreasing levels and effectiveness. Separate doses by 2 to 4 hours.
L-thyroxine: May decrease L-thyroxine absorption. Separate doses by at least 2 hours. Monitor thyroid function.
Levodopa, methyldopa: May decrease absorption and effectiveness of levodopa and methyldopa. Monitor patient for decreased effects of these drugs.
Vitamin C: May increase iron absorption. Suggest patient take vitamin C with drug.
Drug-food. *Cereals, cheese, coffee, eggs, milk, tea, whole-grain breads, yogurt:* May impair oral iron absorption. Advise against using together.

Effects on lab test results

None reported.

Pharmacokinetics

Absorption: Primarily at duodenum and proximal jejunum. For enteric coating and some extended-release formulas, may be decreased. With food, may decrease by 33% to 50%.
Distribution: Binds immediately to carrier protein, transferrin, then to bone marrow for incorporation into hemoglobin.
Metabolism: Liberated by destruction of hemoglobin but is conserved and reused by body.
Excretion: Healthy people lose only small amounts of mineral each day. Men and postmenopausal women lose about 1 mg daily, and premenopausal women about 1.5 mg daily. The loss usually occurs in nails, hair, feces, and urine. *Half-life:* Unknown.

Route	Onset	Peak	Duration
P.O.	≤ 4 days	7–10 days	2–4 mo

Action

Chemical effect: Provides elemental iron, an essential component in formation of hemoglobin.
Therapeutic effect: Relieves iron deficiency.

Available forms

ferrous fumarate
(Each 100 mg provides 33 mg of elemental iron.)
Drops: 45 mg/0.6 ml†
Oral suspension: 100 mg/5 ml†
Tablets: 200 mg, 324 mg, 325 mg, 350 mg
Tablets (chewable): 100 mg†
ferrous gluconate
(Each 100 mg provides 11.6 mg of elemental iron.)
Capsules: 86 mg†
Tablets: 240 mg, 300 mg†, 320 mg† (contains 37 mg elemental iron), 325 mg†
ferrous sulfate
(About 20% elemental iron; dried and powdered, it's about 32% elemental iron.)
Capsules: 150 mg†, 159 mg (dried), 190 mg (dried), 250 mg†, 390 mg†
Capsules (extended-release): 150 mg (dried), 160 mg (dried)
Drops: 75 mg/0.6 ml, 125 mg/ml
Elixir: 220 mg/5 ml*†
Solution: 75 mg/0.6 ml, 300 mg/5 ml
Syrup: 90 mg/5 ml*†
Tablets: 195 mg†, 300 mg†, 325 mg†, 187 mg (dried), 200 mg (dried)
Tablets (extended-release): 160 mg (dried)†, 525 mg

NURSING PROCESS

⚕ Assessment
• Obtain baseline assessment of patient's iron deficiency before starting therapy.
• Evaluate hemoglobin level, hematocrit, and reticulocyte count during therapy.
• Be alert for adverse reactions and drug interactions.
• Assess patient's and family's knowledge of drug therapy.

⊞ Nursing diagnoses
• Fatigue related to iron deficiency
• Constipation related to adverse effect of drug therapy on GI tract
• Deficient knowledge related to drug therapy

▷ Planning and implementation
• Give tablets with juice or water, but not with milk or antacids.
• Dilute liquid forms in juice or water, but not in milk or antacids.

- To avoid staining teeth, give suspension or elixir with straw and place drops at back of throat.
- Don't crush or allow patient to chew extended-release forms.
- GI upset may be related to dose. Preferably give drug between meals, but if GI upset continues, may give with food, except eggs, milk products, coffee, and tea, which may impair absorption. Enteric-coated or sustained-release forms reduce GI upset but also reduce amount absorbed.
- Oral iron may turn stools black. Although this unabsorbed iron is harmless, it could mask presence of melena. Have stools tested for presence of blood.

Patient teaching
- **ALERT:** Inform parents that as few as three tablets can cause poisoning in children.
- If patient misses a dose, tell him to take it as soon as he remembers but not to double the dose.
- Advise patient to avoid taking drug with certain foods that may impair oral iron absorption, including yogurt, cheese, eggs, milk, wholegrain breads and cereals, tea, and coffee.
- Teach dietary measures for preventing constipation.

Evaluation
- Patient reports fatigue is no longer a problem in daily life.
- Patient states appropriate measures to prevent or relieve constipation.
- Patient and family state understanding of drug therapy.

fexofenadine hydrochloride
(feks-oh-FEN-uh-deen high-droh-KLOR-ighd)
Allegra, Telfast ◆

Pharmacologic class: H₁-receptor antagonist
Therapeutic class: antihistamine
Pregnancy risk category: C

Indications and dosages
▶ **Seasonal allergic rhinitis.** *Adults and children age 12 and older:* 60 mg P.O. b.i.d. or 180 mg P.O. once daily.
Children ages 6 to 11: 30 mg P.O. b.i.d.
▶ **Chronic idiopathic urticaria.** *Children age 12 and older:* 60 mg P.O. b.i.d.

Children ages 6 to 11: 30 mg P.O. b.i.d.
Adjust-a-dose: For patients with renal impairment, if creatinine clearance is less than 80 ml/minute, increase dosage interval to q 24 hours.

Contraindications and cautions
- Contraindicated in patients hypersensitive to the drug or any of its components.
- Use cautiously in patients with renal impairment.
Lifespan: In pregnant women, use only if benefits outweigh risks to the fetus, and avoid use in the third trimester. In breast-feeding women, use cautiously because it's unknown if drug appears in breast milk. In children younger than age 6, safety and effectiveness haven't been established.

Adverse reactions
CNS: fatigue, drowsiness, *headache.*
GI: nausea, dyspepsia.
GU: dysmenorrhea.
Musculoskeletal: back pain.
Respiratory: cough, sinusitis.
Other: viral infection.

Interactions
Drug-drug. *Aluminum- or magnesium-containing antacids:* May interfere with absorption of fexofenadine. Separate administration times.
Erythromycin, ketoconazole: May increase fexofenadine levels. Prolonged QT interval has occurred with other antihistamines. Monitor patient closely.
Drug-lifestyle. *Alcohol:* May increase sedative effects. Discourage use together.
Drug-food. *Apple, grapefruit, and orange juice:* May decrease GI absorption of drug, reducing effects. Discourage use together.

Effects on lab test results
None reported.

Pharmacokinetics
Absorption: Rapid.
Distribution: Protein-binding is 60% to 70%.
Metabolism: Unknown.
Excretion: Mainly in feces. *Half-life:* 14½ hours.

Route	Onset	Peak	Duration
P.O.	Unknown	3 hr	14 hr

Action

Chemical effect: Selectively inhibits peripheral H_1-receptors.
Therapeutic effect: Relieves symptoms of seasonal allergies.

Available forms

Capsules: 60 mg
Tablets: 30 mg, 60 mg, 120 mg, 180 mg

NURSING PROCESS

🖉 Assessment
• Assess patient's seasonal allergy symptoms before starting therapy and regularly thereafter.
• Monitor patient for adverse reactions.
• Assess patient's and family's knowledge of drug therapy.

🖏 Nursing diagnoses
• Risk for injury related to fatigue and drowsiness caused by drug
• Ineffective health maintenance related to underlying condition
• Deficient knowledge related to drug therapy

⧁ Planning and implementation
• Reduce daily dosage in patient with renal impairment or currently on dialysis.
• Avoid giving with apple, orange, or grapefruit juice.
⧁ ALERT: Don't confuse Allegra with Viagra.
Patient teaching
• Instruct patient not to exceed prescribed dose and to take drug only when affected by seasonal allergy symptoms.
• Warn patient not to drink alcohol and to avoid hazardous activities that require alertness until the drug's CNS effects are known.
• Tell patient that coffee or tea may reduce drowsiness. Suggest sugarless gum, hard candy, or ice chips to relieve dry mouth.
• Tell patient to avoid taking drug with apple, orange, or grapefruit juice.

☑ Evaluation
• Patient experiences limited fatigue and drowsiness caused by the drug.
• Patient responds well to the drug.
• Patient and family state understanding of drug therapy.

filgrastim (granulocyte colony-stimulating factor; G-CSF)
(fil-GRAH-stem)
Neupogen

Pharmacologic class: biologic response modifier
Therapeutic class: colony-stimulating factor, hematopoietic
Pregnancy risk category: C

Indications and dosages

▶ **To decrease risk of infection in patients with nonmyeloid cancers receiving myelosuppressive antineoplastics followed by bone marrow transplant.** *Adults and children:* 10 mcg/kg I.V. or subcutaneously daily at least 24 hours after cytotoxic chemotherapy and bone marrow infusion. Adjust subsequent doses according to neutrophil response.
▶ **Congenital neutropenia.** *Adults:* 6 mcg/kg subcutaneously b.i.d. Adjust dosage based on response.
▶ **Idiopathic or cyclic neutropenia.** *Adults:* 5 mcg/kg subcutaneously daily. Adjust dosage based on response.
▶ **Peripheral blood progenitor cell collection.** *Adults:* 10 mcg/kg subcutaneously daily for at least 4 days before first leukapheresis and continuing until the last leukapheresis is completed.
▶ **To decrease risk of infection in patients with nonmyeloid cancers receiving myelosuppressive antineoplastics, agranulocytosis‡, pancytopenia with colchicine overdose‡, acute leukemia‡, hematologic toxicity with zidovudine therapy‡.** *Adults and children:* 5 mcg/kg I.V. or subcutaneously daily as single dose. May increase in increments of 5 mcg/kg for each chemotherapy cycle, depending on duration and severity of nadir of absolute neutrophil count (ANC).
▶ **Myelodysplasia‡.** *Adults:* 0.3 to 10 mcg/kg subcutaneously daily.
▶ **Neutropenia from HIV infection‡.** *Adults and adolescents:* 5 to 10 mcg/kg subcutaneously or I.V. daily for 2 to 4 weeks.

▽ I.V. administration

• Dilute in 50 to 100 ml of D_5W. If final concentration will be 2 to 15 mcg/ml, add albumin

---

at 2 mg/ml (0.2%) to minimize binding of drug to plastic containers or tubing.
• Give by intermittent infusion over 15 to 60 minutes or continuous infusion over 24 hours.
• Refrigerate drug at 36° to 46° F (2° to 8° C). Don't freeze; avoid shaking. Store at room temperature for maximum of 6 hours; discard after 6 hours.

⊗ **Incompatibilities**
Amphotericin B, cefepime, cefonicid, cefotaxime, cefoxitin, ceftizoxime, ceftriaxone, cefuroxime, clindamycin, dactinomycin, etoposide, fluorouracil, furosemide, heparin sodium, mannitol, methylprednisolone sodium succinate, metronidazole, mitomycin, piperacillin, prochlorperazine edisylate, sodium solutions, thiotepa.

Contraindications and cautions

• Contraindicated in patients hypersensitive to proteins derived from *Escherichia coli* or to the drug or any of its components.
⚕ **Lifespan:** In pregnant women, use cautiously. In breast-feeding women, use cautiously because it's unknown if the drug appears in breast milk.

Adverse reactions

CNS: *fever, fatigue,* headache, weakness.
CV: *MI, arrhythmias,* chest pain.
GI: *nausea, vomiting, diarrhea, mucositis,* stomatitis, constipation.
GU: hematuria, proteinuria.
Hematologic: *thrombocytopenia,* leukocytosis.
Musculoskeletal: *skeletal pain.*
Respiratory: dyspnea, cough.
Skin: *alopecia,* rash, cutaneous vasculitis.
Other: hypersensitivity reactions.

Interactions

Drug-drug. *Chemotherapeutics:* May cause sensitivity in rapidly dividing myeloid cells. Don't use filgrastim within 24 hours of chemotherapy.

Effects on lab test results

• May increase creatinine, uric acid, alkaline phosphatase, and LDH levels.
• May increase WBC count. May decrease platelet count.

Pharmacokinetics

Absorption: Rapid.
Distribution: Unknown.
Metabolism: Unknown.
Excretion: Unknown. *Half-life:* About 3½ hours.

Route	Onset	Peak	Duration
I.V.	5–60 min	24 hr	1–7 days
SubQ	5–60 min	2–8 hr	1–7 days

Action

Chemical effect: Stimulates proliferation and differentiation of hematopoietic cells. Drug is specific for neutrophils.
Therapeutic effect: Raises WBC count.

Available forms

Injection: 300 mcg/ml in 1-ml and 1.6-ml single-use vials; 300 mcg/0.5 ml, 480 mcg/0.8 ml in prefilled syringes

NURSING PROCESS

🔍 **Assessment**
• Assess patient's underlying condition before starting therapy.
• Obtain baseline CBC and platelet count before and during therapy.
• Be alert for adverse reactions and drug interactions.
• Ask patient about skeletal pain.
• Assess patient's and family's knowledge of drug therapy.

📋 **Nursing diagnoses**
• Ineffective protection related to underlying condition or treatment
• Acute pain related to adverse drug effects on skeletal muscle
• Deficient knowledge related to drug therapy

▶ **Planning and implementation**
• Don't give drug within 24 hours of cytotoxic chemotherapy.
• Once dose is withdrawn from vial, discard the unused portion. Vials are for single-dose use and contain no preservatives.
• Give daily for up to 2 weeks, or until ANC has returned to 10,000/mm³ after expected chemotherapy-induced neutrophil nadir.
🔔 **ALERT:** Rare cases of splenic rupture have occurred.

⑤ ALERT: Don't confuse Neupogen with Neumega.

Patient teaching
• Teach patient how to give drug and how to dispose of used needles, syringes, drug containers, and unused drug.
• Tell patient to report bruising or spontaneous bleeding, such as frequent nosebleeds.
• Teach patient how to manage skeletal pain.
• Tell patient to immediately report upper left abdominal or shoulder pain, because these may be signs of splenic rupture.

☑ Evaluation
• Patient's WBC count is normal.
• Patient reports skeletal pain is bearable or relieved with analgesic administration and comfort measures.
• Patient and family state understanding of drug therapy.

finasteride
(fin-ES-teh-righd)
Propecia, Proscar

Pharmacologic class: steroid derivative
Therapeutic class: androgen synthesis inhibitor
Pregnancy risk category: X

Indications and dosages

▶ **To reduce the progression of BPH symptoms.** *Men:* 5 mg Proscar P.O. daily with doxazosin.
▶ **To reduce risk of acute urine retention and need for surgery, including prostatectomy and transurethral resection of prostate; symptomatic BPH; adjunct therapy after radical prostatectomy‡, first-stage prostate cancer‡, acne‡, or hirsutism‡.** *Adults:* 5 mg Proscar P.O. daily.
▶ **Male pattern baldness.** *Men:* 1 mg Propecia P.O. daily.

Contraindications and cautions

• Contraindicated in patients hypersensitive to drug or any of its components or to other 5-alpha-reductase inhibitors, such as dutasteride. Use cautiously in patients with liver dysfunction.
⚠ **Lifespan:** In women and children, drug is contraindicated.

Adverse reactions

GU: impotence, decreased volume of ejaculate.
Other: decreased libido.

Interactions

None significant.

Effects on lab test results

• May decrease prostate-specific antigen (PSA) level.

Pharmacokinetics

Absorption: Not clearly defined, but average bioavailability may be as high as 63%.
Distribution: 90% bound to proteins; crosses blood-brain barrier.
Metabolism: Extensive.
Excretion: 39% in urine as metabolites; 57% in feces. *Half-life:* Unknown.

Route	Onset	Peak	Duration
P.O.	Unknown	1–2 hr	2 wk

Action

Chemical effect: Competitively inhibits steroid 5-reductase, an enzyme that forms potent androgen 5-dihydrotestosterone (DHT) from testosterone. Because DHT influences development of the prostate gland, lower levels will relieve symptoms of BPH. For male pattern baldness, a balding scalp contains higher amounts of DHT; drug lowers scalp and serum DHT levels.
Therapeutic effect: Relieves symptoms of BPH, reduces hair loss, and promotes hair growth.

Available forms

Tablets: 1 mg, 5 mg

NURSING PROCESS

⚕ Assessment
• Before starting therapy, assess patient's BPH and evaluate him for conditions that could mimic BPH, including hypotonic bladder; prostate cancer, infection, or stricture; and neurologic conditions. Carefully monitor patients with large residual urine volume or severely diminished urine flow. These patients may not be candidates for therapy.
• Assess patient for improvement in BPH symptoms.
• Perform periodic digital rectal examinations.

• Be alert for adverse reactions and drug inter-actions.
• Carefully evaluate sustained increases in PSA levels, which could indicate noncompliance or disease progression.
• Assess patient's and family's knowledge of drug therapy.

⊕ Nursing diagnoses
• Impaired urinary elimination related to BPH
• Ineffective sexuality patterns related to drug-induced impotence
• Deficient knowledge related to drug therapy

⊵ Planning and implementation
• Because it's impossible to identify which patients will respond to therapy, keep in mind that a minimum of 6 months of therapy may be needed.
Patient teaching
• Warn woman who is or may become pregnant not to handle crushed or broken tablets because of risk of adverse effects on fetus.
• Reassure patient that, although drug may decrease volume of ejaculate, it doesn't appear to impair normal sexual function. Impotence and decreased libido have occurred in less than 4% of patients.
• Tell patient taking drug for male pattern baldness that he may not notice any effects for 3 months or more.
• Warn patient not to donate blood until at least 1 month after final dose.
• Tell patient that drug may be taken without regard to meals.

☑ Evaluation
• Patient's BPH symptoms diminish.
• Patient states appropriate ways to manage sexual dysfunction.
• Patient and family state understanding of drug therapy.

flecainide acetate
(FLEH-kay-nighd AS-ih-tayt)
Tambocor

Pharmacologic class: benzamide derivative
Therapeutic class: antiarrhythmic
Pregnancy risk category: C

Indications and dosages
▶ **Paroxysmal supraventricular tachycardia; paroxysmal atrial fibrillation or flutter in patients without structural heart disease.**
Adults: 50 mg P.O. q 12 hours. Increase in increments of 50 mg b.i.d. q 4 days until effectiveness is achieved. Maximum, 300 mg daily.
▶ **Life-threatening ventricular arrhythmias, such as sustained ventricular tachycardia.**
Adults: 100 mg P.O. q 12 hours. Increase in increments of 50 mg b.i.d. q 4 days until effectiveness is achieved. Maximum, 400 mg daily for most patients. Or, where available (Australia), give 2 mg/kg I.V. push over at least 10 minutes; or dilute dose and give as infusion.
⊠ **Adjust-a-dose:** For patients with renal impairment, if creatinine clearance is 35 ml/minute or less, initial dose is 100 mg once daily or 50 mg b.i.d.; if more than 35 ml/minute, initial dose is 100 mg q 12 hours. Adjust doses cautiously for all renally impaired patients. When flecainide is used with amiodarone, decrease flecainide dose by 50%.

▼ I.V. administration ◇
• For I.V. infusion, mix only with D_5W.
• When giving by I.V. push, give over at least 10 minutes.
⊗ **Incompatibilities**
Saline solutions.

Contraindications and cautions
• Contraindicated in patients hypersensitive to the drug or any of its components and in those with cardiogenic shock, second- or third-degree AV block, recent MI, or right bundle branch block related to left hemiblock (in absence of artificial pacemaker).
• Use cautiously in patients with heart failure, cardiomyopathy, severe renal or hepatic disease, prolonged QT interval, sick sinus syndrome, or blood dyscrasia.
⚹ **Lifespan:** In pregnant women, use cautiously. Breast-feeding women should stop breast-feeding or not use the drug. In children, safety and effectiveness haven't been established.

Adverse reactions
CNS: *dizziness, headache,* fatigue, tremor, anxiety, insomnia, depression, malaise, paresthesia, ataxia, vertigo, *light-headedness, syncope,* asthenia, fever.

CV: edema, *arrhythmias,* chest pain, *heart failure, cardiac arrest,* palpitations, flushing.
EENT: blurred vision and other visual disturbances.
GI: nausea, constipation, abdominal pain, dyspepsia, vomiting, diarrhea, anorexia.
Respiratory: *dyspnea.*
Skin: rash.

Interactions

Drug-drug. *Amiodarone, cimetidine:* May alter pharmacokinetics. Watch for toxicity. Decrease flecainide dose by 50%.
Digoxin: May increase digoxin level by 15% to 25%. Monitor digoxin level; watch for toxicity.
Disopyramide, verapamil: Negative inotropic properties may be additive with flecainide. Avoid giving together.
Propranolol, other beta blockers: May increase both flecainide and propranolol levels by 20% to 30%. Monitor patient for propranolol and flecainide toxicity.
Urine acidifying and alkalinizing drugs: May substantially alter excretion of flecainide. Monitor patient for flecainide toxicity or decreased effectiveness.
Drug-lifestyle. *Smoking:* May lower drug level. Discourage smoking.

Effects on lab test results

None reported.

Pharmacokinetics

Absorption: Rapid and almost complete; bioavailability is 85% to 90%.
Distribution: Possibly wide; 40% binds to proteins.
Metabolism: In liver to inactive metabolites; 30% escapes metabolism.
Excretion: In urine. *Half-life:* 12 to 27 hours.

Route	Onset	Peak	Duration
P.O.	Unknown	2–3 hr	Unknown
I.V.	Immediate	Immediate	Unknown

Action

Chemical effect: Decreases excitability, conduction velocity, and automaticity as result of slowed atrial, AV node, His-Purkinje system, and intraventricular conduction and causes slight but significant prolongation of refractory periods in these tissues.

Therapeutic effect: Restores normal sinus rhythm.

Available forms

Injection: 10 mg/ml ◊
Tablets: 50 mg, 100 mg, 150 mg

NURSING PROCESS

Assessment
• Assess patient's arrhythmia before starting therapy.
• Monitor effectiveness by continuous ECG monitoring initially; long-term oral administration requires regular ECG readings.
• Monitor level, especially in patient with renal impairment or heart failure. Therapeutic level ranges from 0.2 to 1 mcg/ml. Risk of adverse effects increases when trough level exceeds 1 mcg/ml.
• Monitor potassium level regularly.
• Be alert for adverse reactions and drug interactions.
• Assess patient's and family's knowledge of drug therapy.

Nursing diagnoses
• Decreased cardiac output related to underlying arrhythmia
• Ineffective protection related to drug-induced new arrhythmias
• Deficient knowledge related to drug therapy

Planning and implementation
• If used to prevent ventricular arrhythmias, give drug only to patient with documented life-threatening arrhythmias.
• If patient has pacemaker, check that pacing threshold was determined 1 week before and after starting therapy because drug can alter endocardial pacing thresholds.
• Correct hypokalemia or hyperkalemia before giving drug because these electrolyte disturbances may alter effect.
• Twice-daily administration enhances patient compliance.
• Because of drug's long half-life, its full effect may take 3 to 5 days. Give I.V. lidocaine with drug for first several days.
• Keep emergency equipment nearby when giving drug.

• If ECG disturbances occur, withhold drug, obtain rhythm strip, and notify prescriber immediately.
Patient teaching
• Stress importance of taking oral drug exactly as prescribed.
• Warn patient to avoid hazardous activities that require alertness or good vision if adverse CNS or visual reaction occurs.
• Tell patient to limit fluid and sodium intake to minimize heart failure or fluid retention and to weigh himself daily on the same scale at around the same time. Urge him to report promptly sudden weight gain.

☑ **Evaluation**
• Patient regains normal cardiac output with abolishment of underlying arrhythmia after drug therapy.
• Patient doesn't develop new arrhythmias.
• Patient and family state understanding of drug therapy.

fluconazole
(floo-KON-uh-zohl)
Diflucan◊

Pharmacologic class: bis-triazole derivative
Therapeutic class: antifungal
Pregnancy risk category: C

Indications and dosages

▶ **Oropharyngeal and esophageal candidiasis.** *Adults:* 200 mg P.O. or I.V. on first day, followed by 100 mg daily. Higher doses (up to 400 mg daily) may be used for esophageal disease. Continue for 2 weeks after symptoms resolve.
Children: 6 mg/kg P.O. or I.V. on first day, followed by 3 mg/kg daily for at least 2 weeks.
▶ **Systemic candidiasis.** *Adults:* 400 mg P.O. or I.V. on first day, followed by 200 mg daily. Continue at least 4 weeks or for 2 weeks after symptoms resolve.
Children: 6 to 12 mg/kg P.O. or I.V. daily.
▶ **Cryptococcal meningitis.** *Adults:* 400 mg P.O. or I.V. on first day, followed by 200 mg once daily. Higher doses (up to 400 mg daily) may be used. Continue for 10 to 12 weeks after CSF culture is negative.

Children: 12 mg/kg P.O. or I.V. on first day; follow with 6 mg/kg P.O. or I.V. daily for 10 to 12 weeks after CSF culture becomes negative.
▶ **To prevent candidiasis in bone marrow transplant.** *Adults:* 400 mg. P.O. or I.V. once daily. Start prophylaxis several days before anticipated granulocytopenia. Continue therapy for 7 days after neutrophil count rises above 1,000/mm³.
▶ **To suppress relapse of cryptococcal meningitis in patients with AIDS.** *Adults:* 200 mg P.O. or I.V. daily.
Children: 3 to 6 mg/kg P.O. daily.
▶ **Vulvovaginal candidiasis.** *Adults:* 150 mg P.O. as a single dose.
▶ **Candidal infection, long-term suppression in patients with HIV infection‡.** *Adults:* 100 to 200 mg P.O. or I.V. daily.
▶ **To prevent mucocutaneous candidiasis, cryptococcosis, coccidioidomycosis, or histoplasmosis in patients with HIV infection‡.**
Adults: 200 to 400 mg P.O. or I.V. daily.
Children and infants: 2 to 8 mg/kg P.O. daily.
◫ **Adjust-a-dose:** For patients with renal impairment, give an initial loading dose of 50 to 400 mg. If creatinine clearance is 50 ml/minute or less, reduce dose by 50% in patients not receiving dialysis. For patients on hemodialysis, give 100% of usual dose after each dialysis session.

▽ **I.V. administration**
• Don't remove protective overwrap from I.V. bags until just before use to ensure product sterility. Plastic container may show some opacity from moisture absorbed during sterilization. This is normal; it won't affect the drug and will dissipate over time.
• Give by continuous infusion at no more than 200 mg/hour. Use infusion pump. To prevent air embolism, don't connect in series with other infusions.
⊗ **Incompatibilities**
Amphotericin B, amphotericin B cholesteryl sulfate complex, ampicillin sodium, calcium gluconate, cefotaxime sodium, ceftazidime, ceftriaxone, cefuroxime sodium, chloramphenicol sodium succinate, clindamycin phosphate, co-trimoxazole, diazepam, digoxin, erythromycin lactobionate, furosemide, haloperidol lactate, hydroxyzine hydrochloride, imipenem and cilastatin sodium, pentamidine, piperacillin

sodium, ticarcillin disodium, trimethoprim-sulfamethoxazole. Don't add other drugs.

Contraindications and cautions

• Contraindicated in patients hypersensitive to drug or any of its components.
• Although no information exists regarding cross-sensitivity, use cautiously in patients hypersensitive to other antifungal azole compounds.
≊ **Lifespan:** In pregnant women, use cautiously. In breast-feeding women, drug isn't recommended.

Adverse reactions

CNS: headache.
GI: *nausea,* vomiting, abdominal pain, diarrhea.
Hepatic: *hepatotoxicity.*
Skin: rash, *Stevens-Johnson syndrome.*
Other: *anaphylaxis.*

Interactions

Drug-drug. *Alprazolam, chlordiazepoxide, clonazepam, clorazepate, diazepam, estazolam, flurazepam, midazolam, quazepam, triazolam:* May increase and prolong level, CNS depression, and psychomotor impairment. Don't use together.
Amitriptyline: May increase amitriptyline levels. Avoid combining, if possible.
Atorvastatin, fluvastatin, lovastatin, pravastatin, simvastatin: May increase levels and adverse effects of these HMG-CoA reductase inhibitors. Avoid use together. If they must be given together, reduce dose of HMG-CoA reductase inhibitor.
Carbamazepine: May increase carbamazepine level. Monitor levels closely.
Cyclosporine, phenytoin, tacrolimus: May increase levels of these drugs. Monitor cyclosporine or phenytoin level, and watch for drug toxicity.
Isoniazid, phenytoin, oral sulfonylureas, rifampin, valproic acid: May increase risk of elevated hepatic transaminases. Monitor patient and level closely.
Oral antidiabetics (tolbutamide, glyburide, glipizide): May increase levels of these drugs. Monitor patient for enhanced hypoglycemic effect.
Rifampin: May enhance fluconazole metabolism. Monitor patient for lack of response.
Theophylline: May decrease theophylline clearance. Monitor level.

Warfarin: May increase risk of bleeding. Monitor PT and INR.
Zidovudine: May increase zidovudine activity. Monitor patient closely.
Drug-lifestyle. *Alcohol use:* May increase risk of hepatotoxicity. Discourage use together.

Effects on lab test results

• May increase alkaline phosphatase, ALT, AST, bilirubin, and GGT levels.
• May decrease WBC and platelet counts.

Pharmacokinetics

Absorption: Rapid and complete.
Distribution: Wide; 12% protein-bound.
Metabolism: Partial.
Excretion: Primarily by kidneys; more than 80% unchanged in urine. *Half-life:* 20 to 50 hours.

Route	Onset	Peak	Duration
P.O.	Unknown	1–2 hr	Unknown
I.V.	Immediate	Immediate	Unknown

Action

Chemical effect: Inhibits fungal CYP, an enzyme responsible for fungal sterol synthesis, and weakens fungal cell walls.
Therapeutic effect: Hinders fungal growth.

Available forms

Injection: 200 mg/100 ml, 400 mg/200 ml
Powder for oral suspension: 10 mg/ml, 40 mg/ml
Tablets: 50 mg, 100 mg, 150 mg, 200 mg

NURSING PROCESS

⚝ Assessment
• Assess patient's fungal infection before starting therapy, and reassess regularly.
• Periodically monitor liver function during prolonged therapy. Although adverse hepatic effects are rare, they can be serious.
• Be alert for adverse reactions and drug interactions.
• If adverse GI reactions occur, monitor patient's hydration.
• Assess patient's and family's knowledge of drug therapy.

⬡ Nursing diagnoses
• Infection related to presence of susceptible fungi
• Risk for deficient fluid volume related to adverse GI reactions
• Deficient knowledge related to drug therapy

⟫ Planning and implementation
• If patient develops mild rash, monitor him closely. If lesions progress, stop drug and notify prescriber.
Patient teaching
• Urge patient to adhere to regimen and to return for follow-up.
• Tell patient to report adverse reactions to prescriber.

☑ Evaluation
• Patient is free from infection.
• Patient maintains adequate hydration.
• Patient and family state understanding of drug therapy.

---

flucytosine (5-fluorocytosine, 5FC)
(floo-SIGH-toh-seen)
Ancobon, Ancotil ◇

Pharmacologic class: fluorinated pyrimidine
Therapeutic class: antifungal
Pregnancy risk category: C

Indications and dosages
▶ **Severe fungal infections caused by susceptible strains of *Candida* (including septicemia, endocarditis, urinary tract and pulmonary infections) and *Cryptococcus* (meningitis, pulmonary infection, and possible UTIs).** *Adults:* 50 to 150 mg/kg P.O. daily in divided doses given q 6 hours.
▶ **Chromomycosis‡.** *Adults:* 150 mg/kg P.O. daily.

Contraindications and cautions
• Contraindicated in patients hypersensitive to the drug or any of its components.
• Use cautiously in those with hepatic or renal impairment or bone marrow suppression.
☀ **Lifespan:** In pregnant women, use cautiously. Breast-feeding women should stop breast-feeding or not use the drug. In children, safety and effectiveness haven't been established.

Adverse reactions
CNS: dizziness, confusion, headache, vertigo, sedation, fatigue, weakness, hallucinations, psychosis, ataxia, paresthesia, parkinsonism, peripheral neuropathy.
CV: chest pain, *cardiac arrest.*
EENT: hearing loss.
GI: nausea, vomiting, diarrhea, abdominal pain, dry mouth, duodenal ulcer, *hemorrhage,* ulcerative colitis.
GU: azotemia, crystalluria, *renal impairment.*
Hematologic: anemia, eosinophilia, *leukopenia, bone marrow suppression, thrombocytopenia,* agranulocytosis, *aplastic anemia.*
Hepatic: jaundice.
Metabolic: *hypoglycemia,* hypokalemia.
Respiratory: *respiratory arrest,* dyspnea.
Skin: occasional rash, pruritus, urticaria, photosensitivity.

Interactions
Drug-drug. *Amphotericin B:* May have synergistic effects and enhance toxicity when used together. Monitor patient.
Cytosine: May inactivate the antifungal activity of flucytosine. Monitor patient.

Effects on lab test results
• May increase urine urea, alkaline phosphatase, ALT, AST, bilirubin, creatinine, and BUN levels. May decrease glucose, potassium, and hemoglobin levels and hematocrit.
• May increase eosinophil count. May decrease WBC, platelet, and granulocyte counts.

Pharmacokinetics
Absorption: 75% to 90%; food decreases absorption rate.
Distribution: Wide. CSF levels vary from 60% to 100% of blood levels; 2% to 4% bound to proteins.
Metabolism: Only small amounts.
Excretion: 75% to 95% unchanged in urine.
Half-life: 2½ to 6 hours.

Route	Onset	Peak	Duration
P.O.	Unknown	1–2 hr	Unknown

F

Action

Chemical effect: May penetrate fungal cells where it's converted to fluorouracil—a known metabolic antagonist—and causes defective protein synthesis.
Therapeutic effect: Hinders fungal growth, including some strains of *Cryptococcus* and *Candida.*

Available forms

Capsules: 250 mg, 500 mg

NURSING PROCESS

☑ Assessment

• Assess patient's fungal infection before starting therapy, and reassess regularly.
• Before starting therapy, obtain hematologic tests and renal and liver function studies. Make sure susceptibility tests showing that organism is flucytosine-sensitive are on chart.
• Monitor blood, liver, and renal function studies frequently; obtain susceptibility tests weekly to monitor drug resistance.
• If possible, regularly perform blood level assays of drug to maintain flucytosine at therapeutic level (25 to 120 mcg/ml). Higher levels may be toxic.
• Be alert for adverse reactions and drug interactions.
• If adverse GI reaction occurs, monitor patient's hydration.
• Assess patient's and family's knowledge of drug therapy.

⊕ Nursing diagnoses

• Infection related to presence of susceptible fungi
• Risk for deficient fluid volume related to adverse GI reactions
• Deficient knowledge related to drug therapy

❱ Planning and implementation

• Give capsules over 15 minutes to reduce adverse GI reactions.
Patient teaching
• Inform patient that therapeutic response may take weeks or months.
• Tell patient how to take capsules.
• Warn patient to avoid activities requiring mental alertness if adverse CNS reactions occur.

☑ Evaluation

• Patient is free from infection.
• Patient maintains adequate hydration throughout drug therapy.
• Patient and family state understanding of drug therapy.

fludarabine phosphate
(floo-DAR-uh-been FOS-fayt)
Fludara

Pharmacologic class: antimetabolite, purine antagonist
Therapeutic class: antineoplastic
Pregnancy risk category: D

Indications and dosages

▶ **B-cell chronic lymphocytic leukemia in patients who either haven't responded or have responded inadequately to at least one standard alkylating drug regimen, mycosis fungoides‡, hairy cell leukemia‡, and Hodgkin's and malignant lymphoma‡.** *Adults:* 25 mg/m^2 I.V. over 30 minutes for 5 consecutive days. Repeat cycle q 28 days.
◩ **Adjust-a-dose:** For patients with renal impairment, if creatinine clearance is 30 to 70 ml/minute, decrease dose by 20%. Don't give if creatinine clearance is less than 30 ml/minute.
▶ **Chronic lymphocytic leukemia‡.** *Adults:* Usually, 18 to 30 mg/m^2 I.V. over 30 minutes for 5 consecutive days q 28 days. Therapy is based on patient's response and tolerance.

▽ I.V. administration

• Preparing and giving the drug create mutagenic, teratogenic, and carcinogenic risks. Follow facility policy to reduce risks.
• To prepare solution from lyophilized powder, add 2 ml of sterile water for injection to solid cake of drug. Drug will dissolve within 15 seconds; each ml will contain 25 mg of drug. Dilute this solution or injection further in 100 or 125 ml of D$_5$W or normal saline injection.
• Check injection for particulate matter or discoloration; reconstituted solution should be clear.
• Use within 8 hours of reconstitution.
• Store drug in refrigerator at 36° to 46° F (2° to 8° C).

⊗ **Incompatibilities**

Acyclovir sodium, amphotericin B, chlorpromazine, daunorubicin, ganciclovir, hydroxyzine hydrochloride, prochlorperazine edisylate.

Contraindications and cautions

• Contraindicated in patients hypersensitive to the drug or any of its components.
• Use cautiously in patients with renal insufficiency.
⚠ **Lifespan:** In pregnant women, use only if benefits outweigh risks to the fetus. In breastfeeding women and in children, safety and effectiveness haven't been established.

Adverse reactions

CNS: *fever, fatigue, malaise, weakness, paresthesia,* headache, peripheral neuropathy, sleep disorder, depression, pain, cerebellar syndrome, **stroke,** transient ischemic attack, agitation, *confusion, coma.*
CV: edema, angina, phlebitis, *arrhythmias, heart failure, MI, supraventricular tachycardia,* deep venous thrombosis, aneurysm, *hemorrhage.*
EENT: *visual disturbances,* hearing loss, delayed blindness (with high doses), sinusitis, pharyngitis, epistaxis.
GI: *nausea, vomiting, diarrhea,* constipation, *anorexia,* stomatitis, GI BLEEDING, esophagitis, mucositis.
GU: dysuria, *UTIs,* urinary hesitancy, proteinuria, hematuria, *renal impairment.*
Hematologic: anemia, myelosuppression, *neutropenia, thrombocytopenia.*
Hepatic: *liver failure,* cholelithiasis.
Metabolic: hyperglycemia, dehydration, hyperuricemia, hyperphosphatemia.
Musculoskeletal: myalgia.
Respiratory: *cough, pneumonia, dyspnea, upper respiratory infection,* allergic pneumonitis, hemoptysis, *hypoxia,* bronchitis, *pulmonary toxicity.*
Skin: alopecia, diaphoresis, *rash,* pruritus, seborrhea.
Other: chills, INFECTION, tumor lysis syndrome, *anaphylaxis.*

Interactions

Drug-drug. *Anticoagulants:* May interfere with anticoagulant response. Monitor PT; adjust dose as needed.

Estrogens: May decrease metabolism of fludarabine. Monitor patient.
Other myelosuppressants: May increase toxicity. Avoid use together.
Pentostatin: May increase risk of pulmonary toxicity. Avoid use together.
Salicylates: May decrease effect of salicylates and increase ulcerogenic effects. Avoid use together.

Effects on lab test results

• May increase glucose, phosphate, potassium, and uric acid levels. May decrease hemoglobin level and hematocrit.
• May decrease platelet and neutrophil counts.

Pharmacokinetics

Absorption: Administered I.V.
Distribution: Unknown.
Metabolism: Rapidly dephosphorylated and then phosphorylated intracellularly to its active metabolite.
Excretion: 23% in urine as unchanged active metabolite. *Half-life:* About 10 hours.

Route	Onset	Peak	Duration
I.V.	7–21 hr	Unknown	Unknown

Action

Chemical effect: Unknown; actions may be multifaceted. After conversion to its active metabolite, fludarabine interferes with DNA synthesis by inhibiting DNA polymerase alpha, ribonucleotide reductase, and DNA primase.
Therapeutic effect: Kills susceptible cancer cells.

Available forms

Injection: 50 mg/2 ml
Powder for injection: 50 mg

NURSING PROCESS

⚕ Assessment

• Assess patient's underlying condition before starting therapy, and reassess regularly.
• Careful hematologic monitoring is needed, especially of neutrophil and platelet counts, because bone marrow suppression can be severe.
• Be alert for adverse reactions and drug interactions.
• Assess patient's and family's knowledge of drug therapy.

🔷 Nursing diagnoses

- Ineffective health maintenance related to presence of leukemia
- Ineffective protection related to drug-induced immunosuppression
- Deficient knowledge related to drug therapy

🔷 Planning and implementation

- Optimum duration of therapy isn't known. Recommendations suggest three additional cycles after achieving maximum response.

Patient teaching

- Warn patient to watch for evidence of infection and bleeding.
- Tell patient to notify prescriber if adverse reactions occur.

🔷 Evaluation

- Patient shows positive response to fludarabine therapy.
- Patient develops no serious infections or bleeding complications.
- Patient and family state understanding of drug therapy.

---

fludrocortisone acetate
(floo-droh-KOR-tuh-sohn AS-ih-tayt)
Florinef

Pharmacologic class: mineralocorticoid, glucocorticoid
Therapeutic class: adrenocortical steroid
Pregnancy risk category: C

Indications and dosages

▶ **Adrenal insufficiency (partial replacement), adrenogenital syndrome.** *Adults:* 0.1 to 0.2 mg P.O. daily.
▶ **Orthostatic hypotension‡.** *Adults:* 0.1 to 0.4 mg P.O. daily.

Contraindications and cautions

- Contraindicated in patients hypersensitive to drug or any of its components and in those with systemic fungal infections.
- Use cautiously in patients with hypothyroidism, cirrhosis, ocular herpes simplex, emotional instability with psychotic tendencies, nonspecific ulcerative colitis, diverticulitis, fresh intestinal anastomoses, active or latent peptic ulcer, re-

nal insufficiency, hypertension, osteoporosis, and myasthenia gravis.
⚖ **Lifespan:** In pregnant women, use only if benefits outweigh risks to the fetus. In breast-feeding women, use cautiously because it's unclear if the drug appears in breast milk. In children, long-term use may delay growth and maturation.

Adverse reactions

CNS: headache, dizziness, *seizures.*
CV: *sodium and water retention,* hypertension, cardiac hypertrophy, *edema,* **heart failure.**
EENT: glaucoma, cataracts.
GI: peptic ulcer.
Metabolic: hypokalemia, hyperglycemia.
Musculoskeletal: weakness.
Skin: bruising, diaphoresis, urticaria, allergic rash, **anaphylaxis.**

Interactions

Drug-drug. *Amphotericin B, drugs that deplete potassium (such as thiazide diuretics):* May enhance potassium-wasting effects of fludrocortisone. Monitor potassium levels.
Barbiturates, phenytoin, rifampin: May increase clearance of fludrocortisone acetate. Monitor patient for effect.
Drug-food. *Food containing sodium:* May increase blood pressure. Advise patient to limit sodium intake.

Effects on lab test results

- May increase glucose level. May decrease potassium level.

Pharmacokinetics

Absorption: Good.
Distribution: To muscle, liver, skin, intestines, and kidneys. Extensively bound to proteins. Only unbound portion is active.
Metabolism: In liver to inactive metabolites.
Excretion: In urine; insignificant amount in feces. *Half-life:* 18 to 36 hours.

Route	Onset	Peak	Duration
P.O.	Varies	Varies	1–2 days

Action

Chemical effect: Increases sodium reabsorption and potassium and hydrogen secretion at distal convoluted tubule of nephron.

Therapeutic effect: Increases sodium level and decreases potassium and hydrogen levels.

Available forms

Tablets: 0.1 mg

NURSING PROCESS

⏱ Assessment
- Assess patient's underlying condition before starting therapy, and reassess regularly.
- Monitor patient's blood pressure, weight, and electrolyte levels.
- Be alert for adverse reactions and drug interactions.
- Assess patient's and family's knowledge of drug therapy.

⊕ Nursing diagnoses
- Ineffective health maintenance related to underlying adrenal condition
- Excessive fluid volume related to drug-induced adverse reactions
- Deficient knowledge related to drug therapy

⧁ Planning and implementation
- Drug is used with cortisone or hydrocortisone in patients with adrenal insufficiency.
- If hypertension occurs, notify prescriber, who may lower dose by 50%.
- Potassium supplements may be needed for excessive potassium loss.
- Signs of overdose include excessive weight gain, edema, hypertension, hypokalemia, and enlarged heart. Stop therapy for a few days until symptoms subside, and then resume drug at a lower dose.

Patient teaching
- Tell patient to notify prescriber about worsened symptoms, such as hypotension, weakness, cramping, and palpitations.
- Warn patient that mild peripheral edema is common.

✓ Evaluation
- Patient's health is improved.
- Patient develops no sodium and water retention.
- Patient and family state understanding of drug therapy.

flumazenil
(floo-MAZ-ih-nil)
Romazicon

Pharmacologic class: benzodiazepine antagonist
Therapeutic class: antidote
Pregnancy risk category: C

Indications and dosages

▶ **Complete or partial reversal of sedative effects of benzodiazepines after anesthesia or short diagnostic procedures (conscious sedation).** *Adults:* Initially, 0.2 mg I.V. over 15 seconds. If patient doesn't reach desired level of consciousness (LOC) after 45 seconds, repeat dose. Repeat at 1-minute intervals until cumulative dose of 1 mg has been given (initial dose plus four more doses), if needed. Most patients respond after 0.6 to 1 mg of drug. In case of resedation, repeat dose after 20 minutes, but don't give more than 1 mg at any one time and no more than 3 mg/hour.
▶ **Suspected benzodiazepine overdose.** *Adults:* Initially, 0.2 mg I.V. over 15 seconds. If patient doesn't reach desired LOC after 30 seconds, give 0.3 mg over 30 seconds. If patient still doesn't respond adequately, give 0.5 mg over 30 seconds; repeat 0.5-mg doses p.r.n. at 1-minute intervals up to a cumulative dose of 3 mg. Most patients with benzodiazepine overdose respond to cumulative doses between 1 and 3 mg; rarely, patients who respond partially after 3 mg may need additional doses. Don't give more than 5 mg over 5 minutes initially. Sedation that persists after this dosage is unlikely to be caused by benzodiazepines. In case of resedation, repeat dose after 20 minutes, but don't give more than 1 mg at any one time and no more than 3 mg/hour.

▽ I.V. administration
- Compatible solutions include D_5W, lactated Ringer's injection, and normal saline solution.
- Give drug into I.V. line in large vein with free-flowing I.V. solution to minimize pain at injection site.
- Discard within 24 hours any unused drug that has been drawn into syringe or diluted.
⊗ **Incompatibilities**
None reported.

Contraindications and cautions

• Contraindicated in patients hypersensitive to drug, any of its components, or benzodiazepines; patients who show evidence of serious cyclic antidepressant overdose; and those who received a benzodiazepine to treat a potentially life-threatening condition (such as status epilepticus).

• Use cautiously in patients at high risk for developing seizures; patients who recently have received multiple doses of parenteral benzodiazepine; patients displaying signs of seizure activity; patients who may be at risk for unrecognized benzodiazepine dependence, such as ICU patients; and patients with head injury, psychiatric, or alcohol-dependency problems.

⚘ **Lifespan:** In pregnant women, use cautiously. In breast-feeding women, use cautiously because it's unknown if the drug appears in breast milk. In children, safety and effectiveness haven't been established.

Adverse reactions

CNS: *dizziness, headache, seizures,* agitation, emotional lability, tremor, insomnia.
CV: *arrhythmias,* cutaneous vasodilation, palpitations.
EENT: abnormal or blurred vision.
GI: nausea, vomiting.
Respiratory: dyspnea, hyperventilation.
Skin: diaphoresis.
Other: pain at injection site.

Interactions

Drug-drug. *Antidepressants, drugs that can cause seizures or arrhythmias:* May cause seizures or arrhythmias after effect of benzodiazepine overdose is removed. Use with caution, if at all, in cases of mixed overdose.

Effects on lab test results

None reported.

Pharmacokinetics

Absorption: Administered I.V.
Distribution: Rapid; 50% bound to proteins.
Metabolism: By liver.
Excretion: 90% to 95% appears in urine as metabolites. *Half-life:* 54 minutes.

Route	Onset	Peak	Duration
I.V.	Unknown	Unknown	Unknown

Action

Chemical effect: Competitively inhibits actions of benzodiazepines on GABA-benzodiazepine receptor complex.
Therapeutic effect: Awakens patient from sedative effects of benzodiazepines.

Available forms

Injection: 0.1 mg/ml in 5- and 10-ml multiple-dose vials.

NURSING PROCESS

🍴 **Assessment**
• Assess patient's sedation before starting therapy.
• Assess patient's LOC frequently.
• Be alert for adverse reactions and drug interactions.
⚠ **ALERT:** Monitor patient closely for resedation that may occur after reversal of benzodiazepine effects because drug's duration of action is shorter than that of benzodiazepines. Monitor patient closely after long-acting benzodiazepines, such as diazepam, or high doses of short-acting benzodiazepines, such as 10 mg of midazolam. In most cases, severe resedation is unlikely in patient who shows no signs of resedation 2 hours after 1-mg dose of flumazenil.
• Monitor patient's ECG for evidence of arrhythmias.
• Assess patient's and family's knowledge of drug therapy.

💬 **Nursing diagnoses**
• Ineffective protection related to sedated state
• Decreased cardiac output related to drug-induced seizures
• Deficient knowledge related to drug therapy

▸ **Planning and implementation**
• If arrhythmias or other adverse reactions occur, notify prescriber and treat accordingly.
Patient teaching
• Warn patient to avoid hazardous activities within 24 hours.
• Tell patient not to use alcohol, CNS depressants, or OTC drugs for 24 hours.
• Give family members important instructions or provide patient with written instructions.

✔ **Evaluation**
• Patient is awake and alert.

Reactions may be *common,* uncommon, *life-threatening*, or COMMON AND LIFE-THREATENING.

• Patient maintains adequate cardiac output.
• Patient and family state understanding of drug therapy.

fluorouracil (5-fluorouracil, 5-FU)
(floo-roh-YOOR-uh-sil)
Adrucil, Carac, Efudex, Fluoroplex

Pharmacologic class: antimetabolite
Therapeutic class: antineoplastic
Pregnancy risk category: D (injection); X (topical)

Indications and dosages

▶ **Colon, rectal, breast, stomach, and pancreatic cancers.** *Adults:* 12 mg/kg I.V. daily for 4 days; if no toxicity, give 6 mg/kg on days 6, 8, 10, and 12; then begin single weekly maintenance dose of 10 to 15 mg/kg I.V. after toxicity (if any) from initial course subsides. Dosages based on lean body weight. Maximum single dose, 800 mg.

▶ **Palliative therapy of advanced colorectal cancer.** *Adults:* 425 mg/m² I.V. daily for 5 consecutive days. Give with 20 mg/m² of leucovorin I.V. Repeat at 4-week intervals for two additional courses; then repeat at intervals of 4 to 5 weeks, as tolerated.

▶ **Multiple actinic (solar) keratoses; superficial basal cell carcinoma.** *Adults:* Apply cream or topical solution b.i.d.

▶ **Multiple actinic (solar) keratosis of the face and anterior scalp.** *Adults:* Apply a thin layer of cream or topical solution to the washed and dried affected area daily for up to 4 weeks.

▼ I.V. administration

• Give antiemetic to reduce nausea before giving drug.
• Preparing and giving drug create carcinogenic, mutagenic, and teratogenic risks for staff. Follow facility policy to reduce risks.
• Drug may be given by direct injection without dilution.
• For I.V. infusion, drug may be diluted with D₅W, sterile water for injection, or normal saline injection.
• Infuse slowly over 2 to 8 hours. Don't use cloudy solution. If crystals form, dissolve by warming.

• Use plastic I.V. containers for giving continuous infusions. Solution is more stable in plastic I.V. bags than in glass bottles.

⊗ **Incompatibilities**
Aldesleukin, amphotericin B cholesterol complex, carboplatin, cisplatin, cytarabine, diazepam, doxorubicin, droperidol, epirubicin, fentanyl citrate, filgrastim, gallium nitrate, leucovorin calcium, metoclopramide, morphine sulfate, ondansetron, topotecan, vinorelbine tartrate.

Contraindications and cautions

• Contraindicated in patients hypersensitive to the drug or any of its components; in those with poor nutrition, bone marrow suppression (WBC counts of 5,000/mm³ or less or platelet counts of 100,000/mm³ or less), or potentially serious infections; and in those who have had major surgery within the previous month.
• Use cautiously after high-dose pelvic radiation therapy and in patients who have received alkylating drugs. Also use cautiously in patients who have impaired hepatic or renal function or widespread neoplastic infiltration of bone marrow.
▲ **Lifespan:** In pregnant and breast-feeding women, drug is contraindicated. In children, safety and effectiveness haven't been established.

Adverse reactions

CNS: acute cerebellar syndrome, ataxia, confusion, disorientation, euphoria, headache, nystagmus, *weakness, malaise.*
CV: thrombophlebitis, *myocardial ischemia,* angina.
EENT: epistaxis, photophobia, lacrimation, lacrimal duct stenosis, visual changes.
GI: stomatitis, GI ulcer, nausea and vomiting, diarrhea, anorexia, *GI bleeding.*
Hematologic: *leukopenia, thrombocytopenia, agranulocytosis,* anemia.
Skin: *reversible alopecia; dermatitis; erythema; scaling; pruritus;* contact dermatitis; nail changes; pigmented palmar creases; erythematous, desquamative rash of hands and feet; photosensitivity; *pain, burning,* soreness, suppuration, and swelling with topical use.
Other: *anaphylaxis.*

Interactions

Drug-drug. *Leucovorin calcium, previous therapy with alkylating drugs:* May increase fluorouracil toxicity. Use cautiously.
Drug-lifestyle. *Sun exposure:* Photosensitivity reactions may occur. Urge patient to avoid unprotected or prolonged sun exposure.

Effects on lab test results

• May increase alkaline phosphatase, AST, ALT, bilirubin, LDH, and urine 5-hydroxyindole-acetic acid levels. May decrease hemoglobin level and hematocrit.
• May decrease WBC, RBC, platelet, and granulocyte counts.

Pharmacokinetics

Absorption: Unknown for topical forms.
Distribution: Wide; crosses blood-brain barrier.
Metabolism: Majority of drug degraded in liver; small amount converted in tissues to active metabolite.
Excretion: Metabolites primarily through lungs as carbon dioxide. *Half-life:* 20 minutes.

Route	Onset	Peak	Duration
I.V., topical	Unknown	Unknown	Unknown

Action

Chemical effect: Inhibits DNA synthesis.
Therapeutic effect: Inhibits cell growth of selected cancers.

Available forms

Cream: 1%, 5%
Injection: 50 mg/ml
Topical solution: 1%, 2%, 5%

NURSING PROCESS

▨ Assessment

• Assess patient's condition before starting therapy and reassess regularly.
• Monitor fluid intake and output, CBC, platelet count, and renal and hepatic function tests.
• Be alert for adverse reactions and interactions.
• Fluorouracil toxicity may be delayed for 1 to 3 weeks. Lowest WBC count is 9 to 14 days after each dose; lowest platelet count is 7 to 14 days after each dose .
• Monitor patient receiving topical form for serious adverse reaction. Ingestion and systemic absorption may cause leukopenia, thrombocy-topenia, stomatitis, diarrhea, or GI ulceration, bleeding, and hemorrhage. Application to large ulcerated areas may cause systemic toxicity.
• Watch for stomatitis or diarrhea (signs of toxicity).
• Assess patient's and family's knowledge of drug therapy.

⊕ Nursing diagnoses

• Ineffective health maintenance related to underlying neoplastic condition
• Ineffective protection related to adverse hematologic reactions
• Deficient knowledge related to drug therapy

⧉ Planning and implementation

⟳ **ALERT:** Drug sometimes is ordered as 5-fluorouracil or 5-FU. The numeral 5 is part of drug name and shouldn't be confused with dosage units.
• When giving topically, apply cautiously near eyes, nose, and mouth.
• Avoid occlusive dressings because they increase risk of inflammatory reactions in adjacent normal skin.
• Wash hands immediately after handling topical form.
• Wash and dry affected area; wait 10 minutes. Apply thin layer of cream to affected area.
• Use 1% topical form on face. Higher concentrations are used for thicker-skinned areas or resistant lesions.
• Use 5% topical form for superficial basal cell carcinoma confirmed by biopsy.
• May apply sunscreen and moisturizer 2 hours after application.
• Risk of local irritation isn't increased by extending therapy from 2 to 4 weeks; irritation typically resolves within 2 weeks of stopping drug.
• Don't refrigerate fluorouracil.
• Use sodium hypochlorite 5% (household bleach) to inactivate drug if it spills.
• If diarrhea occurs, stop giving the drug and notify prescriber.
• If WBC count is less than 2,000/mm³, consider protective isolation.

Patient teaching
• Warn patient that alopecia may occur, but it's reversible.
• Advise patient to avoid prolonged exposure to sunlight or ultraviolet light when topical form is used.

Reactions may be *common,* uncommon, *life-threatening,* or COMMON AND LIFE-THREATENING.

• Tell patient to use sunblock to avoid inflammatory erythematous dermatitis. Long-term use of drug may cause erythematous, desquamative rash of hands and feet, which may be treated with pyridoxine (50 to 150 mg P.O. daily) for 5 to 7 days.

• Warn patient that topically treated area may be unsightly during therapy and for several weeks after. Full healing may take 1 to 2 months. Local irritation typically resolves 2 weeks after drug is stopped.

• Inform patient that sunscreen and a moisturizer may be applied 2 hours after drug application.

☑ Evaluation

• Patient shows positive response to fluorouracil therapy.

• Patient develops no serious adverse hematologic reactions.

• Patient and family state understanding of drug therapy.

fluoxetine hydrochloride
(floo-OKS-eh-teen high-droh-KLOR-ighd)
Prozac*❢*, Prozac-20 ◇ , Prozac Weekly, Sarafem Pulvules

Pharmacologic class: SSRI
Therapeutic class: antidepressant
Pregnancy risk category: C

Indications and dosages

▶ **Depression, obsessive-compulsive disorder (OCD).** *Adults:* Initially, 20 mg P.O. in morning; increase by patient's response. May be given b.i.d. in morning and at noon. Maximum, 80 mg daily.
Children ages 7 to 17: For OCD, 10 mg P.O. daily. After 2 weeks, increase dose to 20 mg daily to maximum of 60 mg daily. In lower-weight children, increase dose to 20 to 30 mg daily after several weeks. Maximum, 60 mg daily.
Children ages 8 to 18: For depression, 10 to 20 mg P.O. daily. After 1 week, increase to 20 mg daily. Start lower-weight children at 10 mg daily and increase dose to 20 mg daily after several weeks.
▶ **Maintenance therapy for depression in stabilized patients.** *Adults:* 90 mg Prozac Weekly P.O. once weekly. Start 7 days after the last daily dose of Prozac 20 mg.
▶ **Moderate to severe bulimia nervosa.** *Adults:* 60 mg daily P.O. in the morning.
▶ **Premenstrual dysphoric disorder (PMDD).** *Adults:* 20 mg Sarafem P.O. daily every day of the menstrual cycle or starting 14 days before the anticipated onset of menstruation through the first full day of menses and repeating with each new cycle. Maximum, 80 mg daily.
▶ **Panic disorder with or without agoraphobia.** *Adults:* 10 mg P.O. daily. May increase in 10-mg increments at intervals of no less than 1 week to maximum dosage of 60 mg.
▶ **Anorexia nervosa‡.** *Adults:* 40 mg P.O. daily in weight-restored patients.
▶ **Depression linked to bipolar disorder‡.** *Adults:* 20 to 60 mg P.O. daily.
▶ **Cataplexy‡.** *Adults:* 20 mg P.O. daily or b.i.d. in conjunction with CNS stimulant therapy.
▶ **Alcohol dependence‡.** *Adults:* 60 mg P.O. daily.
▶ **To prevent migraine headaches‡.** *Adults:* 10 to 40 mg P.O. daily.
▶ **Posttraumatic stress disorder‡, Raynaud phenomenon‡.** *Adults:* 20 to 60 mg P.O. daily.
▶ **Generalized anxiety disorder‡, hot flashes‡.** *Adults:* 20 mg P.O. daily.

Contraindications and cautions

• Contraindicated in patients hypersensitive to the drug or any of its components and in those taking MAO inhibitors within 14 days of starting therapy. Don't give MAO inhibitors or thioridazine within 5 weeks of discontinuing fluoxetine.

• Use cautiously in patients at high risk for suicide and in those with history of mania, seizures, diabetes mellitus, or hepatic, renal, or CV disease.

⚠ **Lifespan:** In pregnant women, use cautiously. In breast-feeding women, it's unknown if drug appears in breast milk. In children younger than age 7, safety and effectiveness in OCD haven't been established. In children younger than age 8, safety and effectiveness in major depressive disorder haven't been established. In children, safety and effectiveness for panic disorder, PMDD, and bulimia nervosa haven't been established. In adults age 65 and older treated for depression, start with lower dosage.

Adverse reactions

CNS: fever, nervousness, anxiety, insomnia, somnolence, headache, drowsiness, fatigue, tremor, dizziness, asthenia.
CV: palpitations.
EENT: nasal congestion, pharyngitis, sinusitis.
GI: *nausea, diarrhea, dry mouth, anorexia,* dyspepsia, constipation, abdominal pain, vomiting, flatulence, increased appetite.
Metabolic: weight loss.
Musculoskeletal: muscle pain.
Respiratory: cough, upper respiratory infection, *respiratory distress.*
Skin: rash, pruritus, urticaria.
Other: flulike syndrome, hot flushes, sexual dysfunction.

Interactions

Drug-drug. *Amphetamines, dextromethorphan, dihydroergotamine, meperidine, SSRIs, sumatriptan, tramadol, trazodone:* May increase risk of serotonin syndrome. Avoid use together.
Benzodiazepines, tricyclic antidepressants: May increase CNS effects. Monitor patient and level closely; adjust doses, p.r.n.
Carbamazepine, clozapine, cyclosporine, flecainide, haloperidol, propafenone, ritonavir, vinblastine: May increase levels of these drugs. Monitor levels and patient for adverse effects.
Cyproheptadine: May reverse or decrease pharmacologic effect. Monitor patient closely.
Insulin, oral antidiabetics: May alter glucose levels and need for antidiabetic. Adjust dosage.
Lithium: May alter lithium level. Monitor lithium level closely.
Phenelzine, selegiline, tranylcypromine: May cause serotonin syndrome (CNS irritability, shivering, and altered consciousness). Don't give drug within 2 weeks of an SSRI.
Phenytoin: May increase phenytoin level and risk of toxicity. Monitor phenytoin level and adjust dosage.
Sumatriptan: May cause weakness, hyperreflexia, and incoordination. Monitor the patient closely.
Thioridazine: May raise level of thioridazine, leading to a higher risk of serious ventricular arrhythmias and sudden death. Don't give within 5 weeks of each other.
Tryptophan: May increase toxic reaction with agitation, GI distress, and restlessness. Don't use together.

Warfarin, other highly protein-bound drugs: May increase level of fluoxetine or other highly protein-bound drugs. Monitor level of these drugs closely.
Drug-herb. *St. John's wort:* May increase the risk of serotonin syndrome. Discourage use together.
Drug-lifestyle. *Alcohol use:* May increase CNS depression. Discourage use together.

Effects on lab test results

None reported.

Pharmacokinetics

Absorption: Good.
Distribution: 95% protein-bound.
Metabolism: Primarily in liver to active metabolites.
Excretion: By kidneys. *Half-life:* 2 to 3 days.

Route	Onset	Peak	Duration
P.O.	1–4 wk	6–8 hr	Unknown

Action

Chemical effect: May inhibit CNS neuronal uptake of serotonin.
Therapeutic effect: Relieves depression and obsessive-compulsive behaviors.

Available forms

Capsules: 90 mg (Prozac Weekly)
Oral solution: 20 mg/5 ml
Pulvules: 10 mg, 20 mg, 40 mg
Tablets: 10 mg

NURSING PROCESS

⚕ Assessment
• Assess patient's condition before starting therapy, and reassess regularly.
• Be alert for adverse reactions and drug interactions.
• Observe closely for evidence of suicidal thoughts or behaviors until depression is relieved.
• Assess patient's and family's knowledge of drug therapy.

⚕ Nursing diagnoses
• Ineffective individual coping related to patient's underlying condition
• Disturbed sleep pattern related to drug-induced insomnia

Reactions may be *common*, uncommon, **life-threatening**, or COMMON AND LIFE-THREATENING.

• Deficient knowledge related to drug therapy

▷ Planning and implementation
• An elderly or debilitated patient, or a patient with renal or hepatic dysfunction, may need a lower dose or less frequent administration.
• Give drug in morning to prevent insomnia.
• Give antihistamines or topical corticosteroids to treat rashes or pruritus.
• Low-weight children may need several weeks between dosage increases.
🛇 **ALERT:** Don't confuse Prozac with Prilosec.
🛇 **ALERT:** Don't confuse Sarafem with Serophene.

Patient teaching
• Tell patient not to take drug in afternoon or evening because fluoxetine commonly causes nervousness and insomnia.
• Instruct patient to take drug with or without food.
• Warn patient to avoid hazardous activities that require alertness and psychomotor coordination until the drug's CNS effects are known.
• Advise patient to consult prescriber before taking any other prescription or OTC drugs.

☑ Evaluation
• Patient behavior and communication indicate an improvement of depression with drug therapy.
• Patient has no insomnia with drug use.
• Patient and family state understanding of drug therapy.

---

fluphenazine decanoate
(floo-FEN-uh-zeen deh-kuh-NOH-ayt)
Modecate ♦ ◇ , Modecate Concentrate, Prolixin Decanoate

fluphenazine hydrochloride
Anatensol ◇ *, Apo-Fluphenazine ♦ ,
Modecate Concentrate ♦ , Moditen HCl ♦ ,
Prolixin*

Pharmacologic class: phenothiazine (piperazine derivative)
Therapeutic class: antipsychotic
Pregnancy risk category: C

Indications and dosages
▶ **Psychotic disorders.** *Adults:* Initially, 2.5 to 10 mg hydrochloride P.O. daily in divided doses q 6 to 8 hours; may increase cautiously to 20 mg. Maintenance, 1 to 5 mg P.O. daily. Or 1.25 mg hydrochloride I.M. initially; then 2.5 to 10 mg I.M. daily in divided doses q 6 to 8 hours. Or 12.5 to 25 mg decanoate I.M. or subcutaneously q 4 to 6 weeks. Maximum dose, 100 mg. *Elderly patients:* Initially 1 to 2.5 mg P.O. daily. Adjust according to response.

Contraindications and cautions
• Contraindicated in patients hypersensitive to drug or any of its components and in those with CNS depression, bone marrow suppression, other blood dyscrasia, subcortical damage, liver damage, or coma.
• Use cautiously in debilitated patients and those with pheochromocytoma, severe CV disease, peptic ulcer, fever, exposure to extreme heat or cold or phosphorous insecticides, respiratory disorder, hypocalcemia, seizure disorder, severe reactions to insulin or electroconvulsive therapy, mitral insufficiency, glaucoma, or prostatic hyperplasia. Use parenteral form cautiously in patients with asthma and patients allergic to sulfites.
⚘ **Lifespan:** In pregnant women, use cautiously. In breast-feeding women, use cautiously because it's unknown if the drug appears in breast milk. In children, safety and effectiveness haven't been established. In elderly patients, use cautiously.

Adverse reactions
CNS: extrapyramidal reactions, tardive dyskinesia, sedation, pseudoparkinsonism, EEG changes, drowsiness, *seizures,* dizziness, *neuroleptic malignant syndrome.*
CV: orthostatic hypotension, tachycardia, ECG changes.
EENT: *dry mouth,* ocular changes, *blurred vision,* nasal congestion.
GI: constipation.
GU: *urine retention,* dark urine, menstrual irregularities, inhibited ejaculation.
Hematologic: *leukopenia, agranulocytosis, aplastic anemia,* eosinophilia, hemolytic anemia.
Hepatic: cholestatic jaundice.
Metabolic: weight gain, increased appetite.
Skin: mild photosensitivity.
Other: gynecomastia, allergic reactions.

Interactions

Drug-drug. *Antacids:* May inhibit absorption of oral phenothiazines. Separate doses by at least 2 hours.
Anticholinergics: May increase anticholinergic effects. Avoid use together.
Barbiturates, lithium: May decrease phenothiazine effect. Observe patient.
Centrally acting antihypertensives: May decrease antihypertensive effect. Monitor blood pressure.
CNS depressants: May increase CNS depression. Avoid use together.
Drug-lifestyle. *Alcohol use:* May increase CNS depression, particularly psychomotor skills. Strongly discourage use together.
Sun exposure: May increase risk of photosensitivity. Discourage prolonged or unprotected exposure to sun.

Effects on lab test results

• May decrease hemoglobin level and hematocrit.
• May increase eosinophil count. May decrease WBC, granulocyte, and platelet counts. May alter liver function test values.

Pharmacokinetics

Absorption: For tablet, erratic and variable.
Distribution: Wide. CNS levels are usually higher than those in blood; 91% to 99% protein-bound.
Metabolism: Extensive.
Excretion: Mostly in urine. *Half-life:* Hydrochloride, 15 hours; decanoate, 7 to 10 days.

Route	Onset	Peak	Duration
P.O.	≤ 1 hr	30 min	6–8 hr
I.M., SubQ	1–3 days	Unknown	1–6 wk

Action

Chemical effect: Unknown; may block dopamine receptors in brain.
Therapeutic effect: Relieves psychotic signs and symptoms.

Available forms

fluphenazine decanoate
Depot injection: 25 mg/ml, 100 mg/ml ◆
fluphenazine hydrochloride
Elixir: 2.5 mg/5 ml*
I.M. injection: 2.5 mg/ml

Oral concentrate: 5 mg/ml*
Tablets: 1 mg, 2.5 mg, 5 mg, 10 mg

NURSING PROCESS

⚗ Assessment

• Assess patient's condition before starting therapy and regularly thereafter.
• Monitor therapy with weekly bilirubin tests during first month, periodic blood tests (CBC and liver function), and periodic renal function and ophthalmic tests (long-term use).
• Be alert for adverse reactions and drug interactions.
• Monitor patient for tardive dyskinesia, which may occur after prolonged use. Reaction may not appear until months or years later and may disappear spontaneously or persist for life despite no longer taking the drug.
• Assess patient's and family's knowledge of drug therapy.

⊕ Nursing diagnoses

• Impaired thought processes related to psychosis
• Impaired physical mobility related to extrapyramidal reactions
• Deficient knowledge related to drug therapy

▶ Planning and implementation

⑨ ALERT: The oral concentrate forms are up to 10 times more concentrated than elixir form. Check dosage order carefully.
• Dilute liquid concentrate with water, fruit juice (except apple), milk, or semisolid food just before administration.
• When giving I.M. or subcutaneously, for long-acting oil preparation form (decanoate), use dry needle of at least 21G. Allow 24 to 96 hours for onset of action. Note and report adverse reactions in patient taking these drug forms.
• Oral liquid and parenteral forms can cause contact dermatitis. Wear gloves when preparing solutions, and avoid contact with skin and clothing.
• Protect drug from light. Slight yellowing of liquid or concentrate is common and doesn't affect potency. Discard markedly discolored solutions.
• If patient, especially a pregnant woman or a child, develops symptoms of blood dyscrasia (fever, sore throat, infection, cellulitis, weakness) or extrapyramidal reactions for longer

than a few hours, don't give the next dose. Notify prescriber.

• Acute dystonic reactions may be treated with diphenhydramine.

• Don't abruptly stop the drug unless a severe adverse reaction occurs. After abruptly stopping long-term therapy, patient may experience gastritis, nausea, vomiting, dizziness, tremor, feeling of warmth or cold, diaphoresis, tachycardia, headache, and insomnia.

Patient teaching

• Warn patient to avoid activities that require alertness and psychomotor coordination until the drug's CNS effects are known.

• Tell patient not to mix concentrate with beverages containing caffeine, tannics (such as tea), or pectinates (such as apple juice).

• Tell patient not to drink alcohol during therapy.

• Advise patient to relieve dry mouth with sugarless gum or hard candy.

• Have patient report urine retention or constipation.

• Tell patient to use sunblock and to wear protective clothing.

• Inform patient that drug may discolor urine.

• Stress importance of not stopping drug suddenly.

Ⅴ Evaluation

• Patient demonstrates decrease in psychotic behavior.

• Patient maintains pretreatment physical mobility.

• Patient and family state understanding of drug therapy.

flurazepam hydrochloride
(floo-RAH-zuh-pam high-droh-KLOR-ighd)
Apo-Flurazepam ♦, Dalmane, Novo-
Flupam ♦, Somnol ♦

Pharmacologic class: benzodiazepine
Therapeutic class: sedative-hypnotic
Pregnancy risk category: X
Controlled substance schedule: IV

Indications and dosages

▶ **Insomnia.** *Adults:* 15 to 30 mg P.O. h.s.
Dose repeated once, p.r.n.

Contraindications and cautions

• Contraindicated in patients hypersensitive to drug or any of its components and in pregnancy.

• Use cautiously in patients with impaired hepatic or renal function, chronic pulmonary insufficiency, mental depression, suicidal tendencies, or history of drug abuse.

⚥ Lifespan: In pregnant women, drug is contraindicated. In breast-feeding women, drug is contraindicated because it isn't known if drug appears in breast milk. In children younger than age 15, safety and effectiveness haven't been established. In elderly patients, use cautiously and at a lower dose because they're more susceptible to CNS effects of drug.

Adverse reactions

CNS: *daytime sedation, dizziness, drowsiness, disturbed coordination,* lethargy, confusion, *headache,* light-headedness, nervousness, hallucinations, staggering, ataxia, disorientation, *coma.*
GI: nausea, vomiting, heartburn, diarrhea, abdominal pain.
Other: physical or psychological dependence.

Interactions

Drug-drug. *Cimetidine:* May increase sedation from decreased hepatic metabolism of benzodiazepines. Monitor patient carefully.
CNS depressants, including opioid analgesics: May cause excessive CNS depression. Use together cautiously.
Digoxin: May increase digoxin level and risk of digoxin toxicity. Monitor patient and digoxin level closely.
Disulfiram, hormonal contraceptives, isoniazid: May decrease metabolism of benzodiazepines, leading to toxicity. Monitor patient closely.
Fluconazole, itraconazole, ketoconazole, miconazole: May increase and prolong level, CNS depression, and psychomotor impairment. Don't use together.
Phenytoin: May increase phenytoin level. Monitor patient for toxicity.
Rifampin: May enhance metabolism of benzodiazepines. Monitor patient for decreased effectiveness.
Theophylline: May antagonize flurazepam. Monitor patient for decreased effectiveness.
Drug-herb. *Catnip, kava, lady's slipper, lemon balm, passionflower, sassafras, skullcap, valer-*

ian: May enhance sedative effects. Discourage use together.
Drug-lifestyle. *Alcohol use:* May cause additive CNS and respiratory depression. Strongly discourage use together.
Smoking: May enhance metabolism of benzodiazepines. Discourage use together.

Effects on lab test results

• May increase AST, ALT, total and direct bilirubin, and alkaline phosphatase levels.

Pharmacokinetics

Absorption: Rapid.
Distribution: Wide; about 97% bound to protein.
Metabolism: In liver to active metabolite.
Excretion: In urine. *Half-life:* 2 to 4 days.

Route	Onset	Peak	Duration
P.O.	Unknown	30 min–1 hr	Unknown

Action

Chemical effect: Unknown; may act on limbic system, thalamus, and hypothalamus of CNS to produce hypnotic effects.
Therapeutic effect: Promotes sleep and calmness.

Available forms

Capsules: 15 mg, 30 mg
Tablets: 15 mg ♦, 30 mg ♦

NURSING PROCESS

Assessment

• Assess patient's sleep patterns and CNS before starting therapy.
• Evaluate patient's ability to sleep. Drug is more effective on second, third, and fourth nights of use.
• Be alert for adverse reactions and drug interactions.
• Assess patient's and family's knowledge of drug therapy.

Nursing diagnoses

• Disturbed sleep pattern related to underlying patient problem
• Risk for trauma related to drug-induced adverse CNS reactions
• Deficient knowledge related to drug therapy

Planning and implementation

• Before leaving bedside, make sure patient has swallowed capsule.
Patient teaching
• Encourage patient to continue drug, even if it doesn't relieve insomnia on the first night.
• Warn patient to avoid activities that require alertness or physical coordination. For inpatient, particularly for elderly patient, supervise walking and raise bed rails.
• Advise patient that physical and psychological dependence is possible with long-term use.

Evaluation

• Patient notes drug-induced sleep.
• Patient's safety is maintained.
• Patient and family state understanding of drug therapy.

flutamide
(FLOO-tuh-mighd)
Euflex ♦ , Eulexin

Pharmacologic class: nonsteroidal antiandrogen
Therapeutic class: antineoplastic
Pregnancy risk category: D

Indications and dosages

▶ **Locally advanced (stage B2) or metastatic (stage D2) prostatic carcinoma.** *Adults:*
250 mg P.O. q 8 hours. Used with luteinizing hormone–releasing hormone analogs such as leuprolide acetate.
▶ **Hirsutism in women‡.** *Adults:* 250 mg P.O. daily.

Contraindications and cautions

• Contraindicated in patients hypersensitive to the drug or any of its components and in those with severe hepatic impairment.
Lifespan: In women and girls, drug is contraindicated. In boys, safety and effectiveness haven't been established. In elderly patients, use drug cautiously because its half-life is prolonged.

Adverse reactions

CNS: drowsiness, confusion, depression, anxiety, nervousness, paresthesia.
CV: peripheral edema, hypertension.

Reactions may be *common,* uncommon, *life-threatening,* or COMMON AND LIFE-THREATENING.

GI: diarrhea, nausea, vomiting, anorexia.
GU: impotence, urine discoloration.
Hematologic: *thrombocytopenia, leukopenia,* anemia, hemolytic anemia.
Hepatic: hepatitis, *hepatic encephalopathy.*
Skin: rash, photosensitivity.
Other: hot flashes, loss of libido, gynecomastia.

Interactions

Drug-drug. *Warfarin:* May increase PT. Monitor patient's PT and INR.
Drug-lifestyle. *Sun exposure:* May cause sensitivity reactions. Warn patient to avoid unprotected or prolonged sun exposure.

Effects on lab test results

• May increase BUN, creatinine, and liver enzyme levels. May decrease hemoglobin level and hematocrit.
• May decrease WBC and platelet counts.

Pharmacokinetics

Absorption: Rapid and complete.
Distribution: Concentrates in prostate; 95% protein-bound.
Metabolism: More than 97% occurs rapidly, with at least six metabolites.
Excretion: More than 95% in urine. *Half-life:* 6 hours.

Route	Onset	Peak	Duration
P.O.	Unknown	2 hr	Unknown

Action

Chemical effect: Inhibits androgen uptake or prevents androgen binding in cell nuclei in target tissues.
Therapeutic effect: Hinders prostatic cancer cell activity.

Available forms

Capsules: 125 mg
Tablets: 250 mg ◆

NURSING PROCESS

Assessment
• Assess patient's prostatic cancer before starting therapy.
• Monitor liver function test results periodically.
• Be alert for adverse reactions.
• If adverse GI reaction occurs, monitor hydration.

• Assess patient's and family's knowledge of drug therapy.

Nursing diagnoses
• Ineffective health maintenance related to presence of prostatic cancer
• Risk for deficient fluid volume related to adverse GI reactions
• Deficient knowledge related to drug therapy

Planning and implementation
• Drug may be given with or without meals.
• Give with luteinizing hormone–releasing antagonist (such as leuprolide acetate).
Patient teaching
• Make sure patient knows that flutamide must be taken continuously with drug used for medical castration (such as leuprolide acetate) to allow full benefit of therapy. Leuprolide suppresses testosterone production, and flutamide inhibits testosterone action at cellular level. Together they can impair growth of androgen-responsive tumors. Advise patient not to stop either drug.
• Tell patient to notify prescriber if adverse reactions occur.
• Instruct patient to avoid prolonged exposure to sun and other UV light. Use sunscreens and protective clothing until tolerance is determined.

Evaluation
• Patient responds well to drug.
• Patient maintains adequate hydration throughout drug therapy.
• Patient and family state understanding of drug therapy.

fluticasone propionate
(FLOO-tih-ka-sohn proh-PIGH-oh-nayt)
Flonase, Flovent Diskus ◆ , Flovent HFA, Flovent Inhalation Aerosol

Pharmacologic class: corticosteroid
Therapeutic class: intranasal and inhalation anti-inflammatory
Pregnancy risk category: C

Indications and dosages

▶ **Asthma prevention and chronic asthma in patients who need oral corticosteroids.** *Adults and children age 12 and older previously taking* *bronchodilators alone:* Initially 88 mcg Flovent HFA or Inhalation Aerosol b.i.d. to maximum of 440 mcg b.i.d. Or 100 mcg Flovent Diskus b.i.d. to maximum of 500 mcg b.i.d.

Adults and children age 12 and older previously taking inhaled corticosteroids: Initially 88 to 220 mcg Flovent HFA or Inhalation Aerosol b.i.d. to maximum of 440 mcg b.i.d. In patients with poor asthma control, initial doses of Flovent HFA or Inhalation Aerosol may be above 88 mcg b.i.d. Or 100 to 250 mcg Flovent Diskus b.i.d. to maximum of 500 mcg b.i.d. In patients with poor asthma control, initial doses of Flovent Diskus may be above 100 mcg b.i.d.

Adults and children age 12 and older previously taking oral corticosteroids: 440 mcg to a maximum of 880 mcg Flovent HFA or Inhalation Aerosol b.i.d. Or 500 to 1,000 mcg Flovent Diskus b.i.d. to maximum of 1,000 mcg b.i.d.

Adults and children age 12 and older starting HFA or inhalation aerosol therapy who are receiving oral corticosteroid therapy: Reduce prednisone dose to no more than 2.5 mg daily on a weekly basis, beginning after at least 1 week of therapy with fluticasone.

Children ages 4 to 11 previously taking bronchodilators alone: Initially 50 mcg Flovent Diskus b.i.d. to maximum of 100 mcg b.i.d.

Children ages 4 to 11 previously taking inhaled corticosteroids: Initially 50 mcg Flovent Diskus b.i.d. to maximum of 100 mcg b.i.d. In patients with poor asthma control, initial doses may be above 50 mcg b.i.d.

▶ **Management of nasal symptoms of seasonal and perennial allergic and nonallergic rhinitis.** *Adults:* 2 sprays (100 mcg) Flonase in each nostril once daily or 1 spray (50 mcg) b.i.d. Reduce dosage to 1 spray in each nostril daily for maintenance therapy. Or, for seasonal allergic rhinitis, 2 sprays (100 mcg) in each nostril once daily p.r.n. for symptom control, although greater symptom control may be achieved with regular use.

Children age 4 and older: Initially 1 spray (50 mcg) Flonase in each nostril once daily. If patient doesn't respond, increase to 2 sprays (100 mcg) in each nostril daily. Once adequate control is achieved, decrease dose to 1 spray in each nostril daily. Maximum dosage is 2 sprays in each nostril daily.

Contraindications and cautions

● Contraindicated in patients hypersensitive to any of the components of these preparations. Also contraindicated as primary therapy for patients with status asthmaticus or other acute episodes of asthma in whom intensive measures are needed.

● Use cautiously in patients with ocular herpes simplex or untreated systemic, bacterial, viral, fungal, or parasitic infection, and in those with active or quiescent pulmonary tuberculosis.

⚖ **Lifespan:** In pregnant women, use only if benefits outweigh risks to the fetus. In breast-feeding women, use cautiously because it's unknown if the drug appears in breast milk. In children younger than age 12, safety and effectiveness of the HFA and inhalation aerosols haven't been studied. In children younger than age 4, safety and effectiveness of the nasal formulation hasn't been studied.

Adverse reactions

CNS: fever, *headache,* dizziness, migraine, nervousness.

EENT: conjunctivitis, eye irritation, mouth irritation, *oral candidiasis, pharyngitis,* acute nasopharyngitis, nasal congestion, sinusitis, dysphonia, rhinitis, otitis media, tonsillitis, nasal discharge, earache, laryngitis, epistaxis, sneezing, hoarseness.

GI: diarrhea, abdominal pain, viral gastroenteritis, colitis, abdominal discomfort, nausea, vomiting.

GU: dysmenorrhea, candidiasis of vagina, pelvic inflammatory disease, vaginitis, vulvovaginitis, irregular menstrual cycle.

Metabolic: cushingoid features, weight gain.

Musculoskeletal: growth retardation in children, pain in joints, aches and pains, disorder or symptoms of neck sprain or strain, sore muscles.

Respiratory: *upper respiratory tract infection,* bronchitis, chest congestion, dyspnea, irritation from inhalant.

Skin: dermatitis, urticaria.

Other: dental problems, influenza.

Interactions

Drug-drug. *Ketoconazole:* May increase mean fluticasone level. Use care when giving fluticasone with long-term ketoconazole and other known CYP 3A4 inhibitors.

Reactions may be *common,* uncommon, *life-threatening,* or COMMON AND LIFE-THREATENING.

Effects on lab test results

• May increase glucose level.
• May cause an abnormal response to the 6-hour cosyntropin stimulation test with high doses.

Pharmacokinetics

Absorption: Mostly systemic, with 30% of the delivered dose reaching the lungs. Less than 2% from the nasal mucosa.
Distribution: 91% protein-bound.
Metabolism: Via CYP 3A4 pathway.
Excretion: In feces primarily as unchanged drug and metabolites. *Half-life:* 3 hours.

Route	Onset	Peak	Duration
Inhalation	24 hr	1–2 wk	Several days
Nasal	12 hr–3 days	4–7 days	Several days

Action

Chemical effect: Inhibits many cell types and mediator production or secretion involved in asthma.
Therapeutic effect: Improves breathing ability by reducing inflammation.

Available forms

Nasal suspension: 50-mcg metered inhaler
Oral HFA and inhalation aerosol: 44 mcg, 110 mcg, 220 mcg
Oral inhalation powder: 50 mcg/actuation, 100 mcg/actuation, 250 mcg/actuation

NURSING PROCESS

Assessment
• Obtain history of patient's underlying condition before starting therapy, and reassess regularly.
• Because of risk of systemic absorption of inhaled corticosteroids, observe patient carefully for evidence of systemic corticosteroid effects.
• Monitor patient, especially postoperatively or during periods of stress, for evidence of inadequate adrenal response.
• Monitor growth in children closely because growth suppression may occur.
• Assess patient's and family's knowledge of drug therapy.

Nursing diagnoses
• Ineffective breathing pattern related to respiratory condition

• Impaired oral mucous membrane related to potential adverse effect of oral candidiasis
• Deficient knowledge related to drug therapy

Planning and implementation
• During withdrawal from oral corticosteroids, patient may have symptoms of systemically active corticosteroid withdrawal, such as joint or muscle pain, lethargy, and depression, despite maintenance or even improvement of respiratory function.
• Bronchospasm may occur with an immediate increase in wheezing after a dose. If bronchospasm occurs following inhalation, treat immediately with a fast-acting inhaled bronchodilator.
• If patient is using a bronchodilator regularly, administer it at least 5 minutes before corticosteroid.
ALERT: Use lowest effective dose in children to minimize growth suppression.
Patient teaching
• Tell patient that drug isn't intended to relieve acute bronchospasm.
• For proper use of drug and to attain maximum improvement, tell patient to use drug at regular intervals as directed.
• Instruct patient not to increase dosage but to contact prescriber if symptoms don't improve or if condition worsens.
• Instruct patient to contact prescriber immediately if episodes of asthma aren't responsive to bronchodilators. During such episodes, patients may need therapy with oral corticosteroids.
• Warn patient to avoid exposure to chickenpox or measles, and if exposed to immediately consult prescriber.
• Tell patient to carry or wear medical identification indicating that he may need supplementary corticosteroids during stress or a severe asthma attack.
• During periods of stress or a severe asthma attack, instruct patient who has been withdrawn from systemic corticosteroids to immediately resume oral corticosteroids (in large doses) and to contact prescriber for further instruction. Instruct him to rinse his mouth after inhalation.
• Instruct patient to shake canister well before using inhalation aerosol or HFA and to avoid spraying either into the eyes.
• Inform patient that inhalation aerosol is being replaced with the HFA version for environmen-

F

tal reasons; doses and effectiveness remain the same.

☑ Evaluation
• Patient has normal breathing pattern.
• Patient doesn't develop oral candidiasis.
• Patient and family state understanding of drug therapy.

fluticasone propionate and salmeterol inhalation powder
(FLOO-tih-ka-sohn proh-PIGH-oh-nayt and sal-MEH-teh-rohl)
Advair Diskus 100/50, Advair Diskus 250/50, Advair Diskus 500/50

Pharmacologic class: corticosteroid, long-acting beta$_2$ agonist
Therapeutic class: anti-inflammatory, bronchodilator
Pregnancy risk category: C

Indications and dosages

▶ **Chronic asthma.** *Adults and children age 12 and older:* 1 oral inhalation twice daily, morning and evening, at least 12 hours apart. Maximum oral inhalation of Advair Diskus 500/50 is twice daily.
Adults and children older than age 12 not taking an inhaled corticosteroid: 1 oral inhalation of Advair Diskus 100/50 twice daily.
Adults and children older than age 12 taking beclomethasone dipropionate: If daily dosage of beclomethasone dipropionate is 420 mcg or less, start with 1 oral inhalation of Advair Diskus 100/50 twice daily. If beclomethasone dipropionate daily dosage is 462 to 840 mcg, start with one oral inhalation of Advair Diskus 250/50 twice daily.
Adults and children older than age 12 taking budesonide: If daily dosage of budesonide is 400 mcg or less, start with 1 oral inhalation of Advair Diskus 100/50 twice daily. If budesonide daily dose is 800 to 1,200 mcg, start with 1 oral inhalation of Advair Diskus 250/50 twice daily. If budesonide daily dose is 1,600 mcg, start with 1 oral inhalation of Advair Diskus 500/50 twice daily.
Adults and children older than age 12 taking flunisolide: If daily dose of flunisolide is 1,000

mcg or less, start with 1 oral inhalation of Advair Diskus 100/50 twice daily. If flunisolide daily dose is 1,250 to 2,000 mcg, start with 1 oral inhalation of Advair Diskus 250/50 twice daily.
Adults and children older than age 12 taking fluticasone propionate inhalation aerosol: If daily dose of fluticasone propionate inhalation aerosol is 176 mcg or less, start with 1 oral inhalation of Advair Diskus 100/50 twice daily. If fluticasone propionate inhalation aerosol daily dose is 440 mcg, start with 1 oral inhalation of Advair Diskus 250/50 twice daily. If fluticasone propionate inhalation aerosol daily dose is 660 to 880 mcg, start with 1 oral inhalation of Advair Diskus 500/50 twice daily.
Adults and children older than age 12 taking fluticasone propionate inhalation powder: If fluticasone propionate inhalation powder daily dose is 200 mcg or less, start with 1 oral inhalation of Advair Diskus 100/50 twice daily. If fluticasone propionate inhalation powder daily dose is 500 mcg, start with 1 oral inhalation of Advair Diskus 250/50 twice daily. If fluticasone propionate inhalation powder daily dose is 1,000 mcg, start with 1 oral inhalation of Advair Diskus 500/50 twice daily.
Adults and children older than age 12 taking triamcinolone acetonide: If triamcinolone acetonide daily dose is 1,000 mcg or less, start with 1 oral inhalation of Advair Diskus 100/50 twice daily. If triamcinolone acetonide daily dose is 1,100 to 1,600 mcg, start with 1 oral inhalation of Advair Diskus 250/50 twice daily.
Children ages 4 to 11: 1 oral inhalation of Advair Diskus 100/50 twice daily, morning and evening, at least 12 hours apart.
☒ **Adjust-a dose:** In all patients, after asthma has been controlled, adjust to lowest effective dosage.
▶ **Maintenance therapy for airflow obstruction in patients with COPD from chronic bronchitis.** *Adults:* 1 inhalation 250/50 twice daily, about 12 hours apart.

Contraindications and cautions

• Contraindicated in patients hypersensitive to the drug or any of its components. Also contraindicated as primary therapy for status asthmaticus or other potentially life-threatening acute asthmatic episodes.
• Drug isn't indicated for exercise-induced bronchospasms.

• Use cautiously in patients with active or quiescent respiratory tuberculosis infection; untreated systemic fungal, bacterial, viral, or parasitic infection; or ocular herpes simplex. Also use cautiously in patients with CV disorders, especially coronary insufficiency, cardiac arrhythmias, and hypertension; in patients with seizure disorders or thyrotoxicosis; in patients unusually responsive to sympathomimetic amines; and in patients with hepatic impairment (because salmeterol is metabolized mainly in the liver).

★ **Lifespan:** In pregnant women, use only if benefits outweigh risks to the fetus. In breastfeeding women, use cautiously; it isn't known if drug is found in breast milk. In children younger than age 4, safety and effectiveness haven't been established. Closely monitor growth in children because growth suppression may occur. Maintain child on lowest effective dose to minimize potential for growth suppression.

Adverse reactions

CNS: pain, sleep disorder, tremor, hypnagogic effects, fever, compressed nerve syndromes, *headache,* agitation, nervousness.
CV: palpitations, chest pains, fluid retention, rapid heart rate, *arrhythmias.*
EENT: *pharyngitis,* sinusitis, hoarseness, dysphonia, oral candidiasis, rhinorrhea, rhinitis, sneezing, nasal irritation, blood in nasal mucosa, keratitis, conjunctivitis, eye redness, viral eye infections, congestion.
GI: nausea, vomiting, abdominal pain and discomfort, diarrhea, gastroenteritis, oral discomfort and pain, constipation, oral ulcerations, oral erythema and rashes, appendicitis, unusual taste.
Musculoskeletal: muscle pain, arthralgia, articular rheumatism, muscle stiffness, tightness, rigidity, bone and cartilage disorders, back pain.
Respiratory: upper respiratory tract infection, lower viral respiratory infections, bronchitis, cough, pneumonia, *paradoxical bronchospasms, severe asthma or asthma-related deaths.*
Skin: viral skin infections, urticaria, skin flakiness, disorders of sweat and sebum, sweating.
Other: dental discomfort and pain, bacterial infections, allergies, allergic reactions, influenza.

Interactions

Drug-drug. *Beta blockers:* May block pulmonary effect of salmeterol, producing severe bronchospasm in patients with asthma. Avoid use together. If needed, use a cardioselective beta blocker cautiously.
Ketoconazole, other inhibitors of CYP: May increase fluticasone level and adverse effects. Use together cautiously.
Loop diuretics, thiazide diuretics: May cause or worsen ECG changes or hypokalemia. Use together cautiously.
MAO inhibitors, tricyclic antidepressants: May potentiate the action of salmeterol on the vascular system. Avoid use within 2 weeks of these drugs.

Effects on lab test results

• May increase or decrease liver function test values.

Pharmacokinetics

Absorption: *Fluticasone propionate:* systemic. *Salmeterol:* local. With long-term therapy, salmeterol is found in blood within 45 minutes.
Distribution: *Fluticasone:* 91% bound to proteins and weakly and reversibly bound to erythrocytes. *Salmeterol:* 96% bound to proteins.
Metabolism: Mainly by CYP 3A4.
Excretion: *Fluticasone:* less than 5% of a dose in urine as metabolites, with remainder in feces as an unchanged drug and metabolite. *Salmeterol xinafoate:* 25% and 60% in urine and feces, respectively, over a period of 7 days. *Fluticasone half-life:* 8 hours; *salmeterol half-life:* 5½ hours.

Route	Onset	Peak	Duration
Inhalation			
salmeterol	Unknown	5 min	Unknown
fluticasone	Unknown	1–2 hr	Unknown

Action

Chemical effect: Fluticasone's action is unknown. Salmeterol xinafoate stimulates intracellular adenyl cyclase, the enzyme that catalyzes conversion of adenosine triphosphate (ATP) to cAMP. Increased cAMP levels relax bronchial smooth muscle and inhibit release of mediators of immediate hypersensitivity from cells, especially mast cells.

F

Therapeutic effect: Reduces inflammation in the lungs and opens airways to improve pulmonary function.

Available forms

Inhalation powder: 100 mcg fluticasone and 50 mcg salmeterol, 250 mcg fluticasone and 50 mcg salmeterol, 500 mcg fluticasone and 50 mcg salmeterol

NURSING PROCESS

⚕ Assessment

• Obtain patient's medical history, and assess patient before starting therapy.
⚠ **ALERT:** Chronic overdose of fluticasone may cause signs and symptoms of hypercorticism. Salmeterol overdose may cause seizures, angina, hypertension, hypotension, tachycardia, arrhythmias, nervousness, headache, tremor, muscle cramps, dry mouth, palpitations, nausea, prolonged QT interval, ventricular arrhythmia, hypokalemia, hyperglycemia, cardiac arrest, and death. Stop drug and give a cardioselective beta blocker. Monitor cardiac condition.
• Monitor patient for urticaria, angioedema, rash, bronchospasm, or other signs of hypersensitivity, which may occur immediately after a dose of Advair Diskus.
• Monitor patient for increased use of inhaled short-acting beta$_2$-agonist. The dose of Advair Diskus may need to be increased.
• Monitor patient for hypercorticism and adrenal suppression. If these occur, reduce dosage slowly.
• Monitor patient for eosinophilia, vasculitic rash, worsening pulmonary symptoms, cardiac complications, or neuropathy, which may be signs of a serious eosinophilic condition.
• Monitor patient for signs or symptoms of thrush.
• Assess patient's and family's knowledge of drug therapy.

⚕ Nursing diagnoses

• Ineffective airway clearance related to underlying asthmatic condition
• Activity intolerance related to underlying asthmatic condition
• Deficient knowledge related to proper inhalation with the device and drug therapy

▶ Planning and implementation

⚠ **ALERT:** Don't switch patient directly from systemic corticosteroids to Advair Diskus. Hypothalamic-pituitary-adrenal axis suppression from corticosteroid therapy requires gradual weaning of steroid before replacement with inhaled steroid to avoid risk of death from adrenal insufficiency.
• After asthma has been controlled, adjust to the lowest effective dose.
⚠ **ALERT:** Don't start Advair Diskus therapy during rapidly deteriorating or potentially life-threatening episodes of asthma. Serious acute respiratory events, including death, can occur, especially in blacks.
⚠ **ALERT:** When a patient uses Advair Diskus, make sure the patient has an inhaled, short-acting beta$_2$-agonist (such as albuterol) for acute symptoms that occur between doses of Advair Diskus.
⚠ **ALERT:** Advair Diskus can produce paradoxical bronchospasm. If it does, treat immediately with a short-acting, inhaled bronchodilator (such as albuterol) and stop Advair Diskus therapy.
• If patient is exposed to chickenpox, give varicella zoster immune globulin as prophylaxis. If chickenpox develops, give an antiviral.
• If patient is exposed to measles, give pooled I.M. immunoglobulin as prophylaxis.
• Store at controlled room temperature (68° F to 77° F [20° to 25° C]) in a dry place away from direct heat or sunlight. Discard the device 1 month after removal from the moisture-protective overwrap pouch or after every foil-wrapped blister has been used, whichever comes first. Don't attempt to take the device apart.
Patient teaching
• Instruct patient on most effective use of the Advair Diskus.
• Instruct patient to keep the Advair Diskus in a dry place, to avoid washing the mouthpiece or other parts of the device, and to avoid taking the Diskus apart.
• Tell patient to stop taking an oral or inhaled long-acting beta$_2$-agonist simultaneously when beginning Advair Diskus.
⚠ **ALERT:** Explain to patient that Advair Diskus is used only for long-term maintenance and not for acute symptoms of asthma or for prevention of exercise-induced bronchospasm. Urge patient to use a short-acting beta$_2$-agonist (such as albuterol) for relief of acute symptoms.

Reactions may be *common,* uncommon, *life-threatening,* or COMMON AND LIFE-THREATENING.

• Instruct patient to rinse mouth after each inhalation to prevent oral candidiasis.

• Inform patient that improvement may be seen within 30 minutes after an Advair dose; however, the full benefit may not occur for 1 week or more.

⊛ **ALERT:** Instruct patient not to exceed prescribed dose under any circumstances.

• Instruct patient to report decreasing effects or increasing use of the short-acting beta$_2$-agonist inhaler immediately to his prescriber.

• Instruct patient not to use Advair Diskus with a spacer device.

• Tell patient to report palpitations, chest pain, rapid heart rate, tremor, or nervousness immediately to prescriber. Also instruct patient to avoid stimulants, such as caffeine, while on Advair Diskus therapy because they may increase these adverse reactions.

• Instruct patient to contact prescriber immediately if exposed to chickenpox or measles.

☑ **Evaluation**
• Patient's activity tolerance increases.
• Patient has a normal breathing pattern and optimal air exchange.
• Patient and family state understanding of drug therapy.

fluvastatin sodium
(floo-vuh-STAH-tin SOH-dee-um)
Lescol, Lescol XL

Pharmacologic class: HMG-CoA reductase inhibitor
Therapeutic class: cholesterol inhibitor
Pregnancy risk category: X

Indications and dosages

▶ **To reduce LDL and total cholesterol levels in patients with primary hypercholesterolemia (types IIa and IIb) or to slow progression of coronary atherosclerosis in patients with coronary artery disease; elevated triglyceride and apolipoprotein B levels in patients with primary hypercholesterolemia and mixed dyslipidemia whose response to dietary restriction and other nonpharmacologic measures has been inadequate.** *Adults:* Initially, 20 to 40 mg P.O. h.s. Increase dosage

p.r.n. to maximum of 80 mg daily (in divided doses).

▶ **To reduce the risk of undergoing coronary revascularization procedures.** *Adults:* For patients requiring LDL cholesterol reduction of 25% or more, initially 40 mg (regular-release) P.O. or 80 mg (extended-release) P.O. as a single dose in the evening. Or 40 mg (regular-release) P.O. b.i.d. For patients requiring LDL cholesterol reduction of less than 25%, initially 20 mg P.O. daily. The recommended range is 20 to 80 mg daily.

◨ **Adjust-a-dose:** If levels of ALT or AST persist at least three times the upper limit of normal, stop giving the drug. Drug is primarily cleared hepatically, so dosage adjustments for mild to moderate renal impairment aren't needed. Exercise caution with severe renal impairment.

Contraindications and cautions

• Contraindicated in patients hypersensitive to drug or any of its components and in those with active liver disease or conditions that cause unexplained, persistent elevations of transaminase levels. Also contraindicated during pregnancy.

• Use cautiously in patients with severe renal impairment or with history of liver disease or heavy alcohol use.

❀ **Lifespan:** In pregnant and breast-feeding women and women of childbearing age, drug is contraindicated. In children, safety and effectiveness haven't been established.

Adverse reactions

CNS: headache, fatigue, dizziness, insomnia.
EENT: sinusitis, rhinitis, pharyngitis.
GI: dyspepsia, diarrhea, nausea, vomiting, abdominal pain, constipation, flatulence.
Hematologic: *leukopenia, thrombocytopenia,* hemolytic anemia.
Musculoskeletal: arthropathy, myalgia, arthralgia.
Respiratory: *upper respiratory infection,* cough, bronchitis.
Skin: rash.
Other: tooth disorder, hypersensitivity reactions.

Interactions

Drug-drug. *Cholestyramine, colestipol:* May bind with fluvastatin in GI tract and decrease absorption. Separate administration times by at least 4 hours.

Cimetidine, omeprazole, ranitidine: May decrease fluvastatin metabolism. Monitor patient for enhanced effects.

Cyclosporine and other immunosuppressants, erythromycin, gemfibrozil, niacin: May increase risk of polymyositis and rhabdomyolysis. Avoid use together.

Digoxin: May increase digoxin level. Monitor digoxin levels carefully.

Fluconazole, itraconazole, ketoconazole: May increase level and adverse effects of fluvastatin. Avoid use together. If they must be given together, reduce dose of fluvastatin.

Rifampin: May enhance rifampin metabolism and decrease level. Monitor patient for lack of effect.

Drug-herb. *Red yeast rice:* May increase the risk of adverse events or toxicity. Discourage use together.

Drug-lifestyle. *Alcohol use:* May increase risk of hepatotoxicity. Discourage use together.

Effects on lab test results

• May increase ALT, AST, bilirubin, and CK levels. May decrease hemoglobin level and hematocrit.
• May decrease platelet and WBC counts.

Pharmacokinetics

Absorption: Rapid and almost complete on empty stomach.
Distribution: More than 98% protein-bound.
Metabolism: Complete.
Excretion: About 5% in urine, 90% in feces as metabolites. *Half-life:* Less than 1 hour.

Route	Onset	Peak	Duration
P.O.	Unknown	30–45 min	Unknown

Action

Chemical effect: Inhibits HMG-CoA reductase, an early (and rate-limiting) step in synthetic pathway of cholesterol.
Therapeutic effect: Lowers blood LDL and cholesterol levels.

Available forms

Capsules: 20 mg, 40 mg
Tablets (extended release): 80 mg

NURSING PROCESS

⚗ Assessment

• Assess patient's LDL and total cholesterol levels before starting therapy, and evaluate regularly.
• Perform liver function tests periodically.
• Be alert for adverse reactions and drug interactions.
• Assess patient's and family's knowledge of drug therapy.

⊕ Nursing diagnoses

• Risk for injury related to elevated LDL and cholesterol blood levels
• Diarrhea related to adverse effect of drug on GI tract
• Deficient knowledge related to drug therapy

▶ Planning and implementation

• Start drug only after diet and other nondrug therapies have proven ineffective.
• Give drug h.s. to enhance effectiveness.
• Maintain standard low-cholesterol diet during therapy.

Patient teaching
• Tell patient that drug may be taken with or without food; effectiveness is enhanced if taken in evening.
• Teach patient about proper dietary management, weight control, and exercise. Explain their importance in controlling lipid levels.
• Warn patient to restrict alcohol consumption.
• Tell patient to inform prescriber of any adverse reactions, particularly muscle aches and pains.
• Tell patient to stop drug and notify prescriber about planned, suspected, or known pregnancy.

☑ Evaluation

• Patient's LDL and total cholesterol levels are within normal limits.
• Patient maintains normal bowel pattern.
• Patient and family state understanding of drug therapy.

---

fluvoxamine maleate
(floo-VOKS-uh-meen MAL-ee-ayt)
Luvox

Pharmacologic class: SSRI
Therapeutic class: antidepressant
Pregnancy risk category: C

Indications and dosages

▶ **Obsessive-compulsive disorder (OCD),**
depression‡. *Adults:* Initially, 50 mg P.O. daily
h.s. Increase in 50-mg increments q 4 to 7 days
until maximum benefit occurs. Maximum,
300 mg daily. If total daily amount exceeds
100 mg, divide and give in two doses.
Children ages 8 to 17: 25 mg P.O. q h.s. Maximum daily dose for children ages 8 to 11 is
200 mg. Maximum daily dose for children ages
12 to 17 is 300 mg. Increase initial dosage q
4 to 7 days, p.r.n. Divide doses greater than
50 mg b.i.d.
❊ **Adjust-a-dose:** For elderly patients and patients with hepatic impairment, initially 25 mg
P.O. daily then increase gradually to a maximum daily dose of 200 mg.

Contraindications and cautions

• Contraindicated in patients hypersensitive to
SSRIs or any of their ingredients and within
2 weeks of an MAO inhibitor. Use with thioridazine or pimozide is contraindicated because
ventricular arrhythmias and death may occur.
• Use cautiously in patients with hepatic dysfunction, suicidal ideation, conditions that may
affect hemodynamic responses or metabolism,
or history of mania or seizures.
⚥ **Lifespan:** In pregnant women and in breast-
feeding women, use cautiously. In children
younger than age 8, drug is contraindicated for
OCD. In children, drug is contraindicated for
major depressive disorder. In elderly patients,
use cautiously and start at a lower dose.

Adverse reactions

CNS: headache, asthenia, *somnolence, insomnia, nervousness, dizziness,* tremor, anxiety, hypertonia, agitation, depression, CNS stimulation.
CV: palpitations, vasodilation.
EENT: amblyopia.

GI: *nausea, diarrhea,* constipation, dyspepsia,
anorexia, vomiting, flatulence, dysphagia, taste
perversion, *dry mouth.*
GU: abnormal ejaculation, urinary frequency,
impotence, anorgasmia, urine retention.
Respiratory: upper respiratory tract infection,
dyspnea, yawning.
Skin: sweating.
Other: decreased libido, flulike syndrome,
chills, tooth disorder.

Interactions

Drug-drug. *Benzodiazepines, theophylline,
warfarin:* May reduce clearance of these drugs.
Use together cautiously (except for diazepam,
which shouldn't be given with fluvoxamine).
Adjust dosage p.r.n.
*Carbamazepine, clozapine, haloperidol,
methadone, metoprolol, propranolol, tricyclic
antidepressants:* May elevate levels of these
drugs. Use together cautiously. Monitor patient
closely for adverse reactions. Adjust dosage if
needed.
Diltiazem: May cause bradycardia. Monitor
heart rate.
Lithium, tryptophan: May enhance fluvoxamine
effects. Use together cautiously.
Phenelzine, selegiline, tranylcypromine: May
cause serotonin syndrome, which may include
CNS irritability, shivering, and altered consciousness. Use together may also cause severe
excitation, hyperpyrexia, myoclonus, delirium,
and coma. Don't give an MAO inhibitor within
2 weeks of an SSRI.
Pimozide, thioridazine: May prolong QT interval. Avoid use together.
Sumatriptan: May cause weakness, hyperreflexia, and incoordination. Monitor patient closely.
Drug-herb. *St. John's wort:* May cause serotonin syndrome. Discourage use together.
Drug-food. *Caffeine:* May decrease caffeine
elimination and increase caffeine effects. Discourage use together.
Drug-lifestyle. *Alcohol use:* May increase CNS
effects. Discourage use together.
Smoking: May decrease effectiveness of drug.
Discourage patient from smoking.
Sun exposure: May cause photosensitivity. Discourage prolonged or unprotected exposure to
sunlight.

Effects on lab test results

None reported.

F

Pharmacokinetics

Absorption: Good.
Distribution: 77% protein-bound.
Metabolism: In liver.
Excretion: In urine. *Half-life:* 17 hours.

Route	Onset	Peak	Duration
P.O.	3–10 wk	3–8 hr	Unknown

Action

Chemical effect: May selectively inhibit neuronal uptake of serotonin, which is thought to reduce obsessive-compulsive disorders.
Therapeutic effect: Decreases obsessive-compulsive behavior.

Available forms

Tablets: 25 mg, 50 mg, 100 mg

NURSING PROCESS

Assessment
• Assess patient's condition before starting therapy, and reassess regularly. Patient may need several weeks of therapy before having a positive response.
• Be alert for adverse reactions and drug interactions.
• Assess child with OCD for signs of depression, including suicidal thoughts and behaviors.
• Assess patient's and family's knowledge of drug therapy.

Nursing diagnoses
• Ineffective individual coping related to underlying condition
• Diarrhea related to adverse effect of drug on GI tract
• Deficient knowledge related to drug therapy

Planning and implementation
• Don't give drug within 14 days of MAO inhibitor therapy.
• Give drug h.s., with or without food.
⚠ **ALERT:** Don't confuse Luvox with Lasix.
⚠ **ALERT:** Don't confuse fluvoxamine with fluvoxate or fluoxetine.
Patient teaching
• Instruct patient not to stop drug abruptly but to first consult prescriber.
• Warn patient to avoid hazardous activities until the drug's CNS effects are known.

• Advise patient not to drink alcoholic beverages during therapy.
• Inform patient that smoking may decrease effectiveness of drug.
• Tell patient that drug may be taken with or without food.
• Instruct woman to notify prescriber about planned, suspected, or known pregnancy.
• Tell patient who develops rash, hives, or related allergic reaction to notify prescriber.
• Inform patient that several weeks of therapy may be needed to obtain full antidepressant effect. Once improved, advise patient not to stop drug unless directed by prescriber.
• Advise patient to check with prescriber before taking OTC drugs or herbal remedies because interactions can occur.

Evaluation
• Patient's obsessive-compulsive behaviors are diminished.
• Patient maintains normal bowel patterns.
• Patient and family state understanding of drug therapy.

folic acid (vitamin B₉)

(FOH-lek AS-id)
Apo-Folic ♦, Folvite, Novo-Folacid ♦

Pharmacologic class: folic acid derivative
Therapeutic class: vitamin
Pregnancy risk category: A

Indications and dosages

▶ **To maintain health.** *Infants:* Up to 0.1 mg P.O. daily.
Children younger than age 4: Up to 0.3 mg P.O. daily.
Adults and children age 4 and older: 0.4 mg P.O. daily.
Pregnant or lactating women: 0.8 mg P.O. daily.
▶ **Megaloblastic or macrocytic anemia caused by folic acid or other nutritional deficiency, hepatic disease, alcoholism, intestinal obstruction, excessive hemolysis.** *Adults and children age 4 and older:* 0.4 mg to 1 mg P.O., subcutaneously, or I.M. daily. After anemia caused by folic acid deficiency is corrected, proper diet and supplements are needed to prevent recurrence.

Children younger than age 4: Up to 0.3 mg P.O., subcutaneously, or I.M. daily.
Pregnant and breast-feeding women: 0.8 mg P.O., subcutaneously, or I.M. daily.
▶ **Prevention of megaloblastic anemia in pregnancy.** *Adults:* Up to 1 mg P.O., subcutaneously, or I.M. daily throughout pregnancy.
▶ **Nutritional supplement.** *Adults:* 0.1 mg P.O., subcutaneously, or I.M. daily.
Children: 0.05 mg P.O. daily.
▶ **To test folic acid deficiency in patients with megaloblastic anemia without masking pernicious anemia.** *Adults and children:* 0.1 to 0.2 mg P.O. or I.M. for 10 days with diet low in folate and vitamin B_{12}.
▶ **Tropical sprue.** *Adults:* 3 to 15 mg P.O. daily.

Contraindications and cautions

● Contraindicated in patients with vitamin B_{12} deficiency or undiagnosed anemia.
❅ **Lifespan:** In pregnant women, folic acid therapy is recommended to prevent fetal neural tube defects.

Adverse reactions

CNS: general malaise.
GI: bitter taste, anorexia, nausea, flatulence.
Respiratory: *bronchospasm.*
Other: allergic reactions (rash, pruritus, erythema).

Interactions

Drug-drug. *Aminosalicylic acid, chloramphenicol, methotrexate, sulfasalazine, trimethoprim:* May antagonize folic acid. Monitor patient for decreased folic acid effect. Use together cautiously.
Anticonvulsants (such as phenobarbital, phenytoin): May increase anticonvulsant metabolism and decrease anticonvulsant blood levels. Monitor patient closely.

Effects on lab test results

● May decrease RBC count.

Pharmacokinetics

Absorption: Rapid after P.O. use.
Distribution: Complete; liver contains about half of total body stores. Concentrated actively in CSF.
Metabolism: In liver.

Excretion: Excess is unchanged in urine; small amounts in feces. *Half-life:* Unknown.

Route	Onset	Peak	Duration
P.O., I.M., SubQ	Unknown	30–60 min	Unknown

Action

Chemical effect: Stimulates normal erythropoiesis and nucleoprotein synthesis.
Therapeutic effect: Nutritional supplement.

Available forms

Injection: 5 mg/ml with 1.5% benzyl alcohol
Tablets: 0.1 mg†, 0.4 mg†, 0.8 mg†, 1 mg

NURSING PROCESS

☲ Assessment
● Assess patient's folic acid deficiency before starting therapy.
● Evaluate CBC and assess patient's physical status throughout therapy.
● Be alert for adverse reactions and drug interactions.
● Assess patient's and family's knowledge of drug therapy.

⬢ Nursing diagnoses
● Imbalanced nutrition: less than body requirements related to presence of folic acid deficiency
● Deficient knowledge related to drug therapy

▷ Planning and implementation
● Patient with small-bowel resection and intestinal malabsorption may need parenteral administration.
● Don't mix with other drugs in same syringe for I.M. injections.
● Protect from light and heat; store at room temperature.
● Give vitamin B_{12} with this therapy if needed.
● Make sure patient is getting properly balanced diet.
Ⓢ **ALERT:** Some preparations contain benzyl alcohol. Don't use in infants and children.
Ⓢ **ALERT:** Don't confuse folic acid with folinic acid.
Patient teaching
● Teach patient proper nutrition to prevent recurrence of anemia.

Rapid onset   *Liquid form contains alcohol.   ◆ Canada   ◇ Australia   †OTC   ✐ Photoguide   ‡ Off-label use

- Tell patient to report hypersensitivity reactions or breathing difficulty.
- Urge patient to avoid alcohol because it increases folic acid requirements.

☑ **Evaluation**
- Patient's CBC is normal.
- Patient and family state understanding of drug therapy.

fondaparinux sodium
(fon-duh-PAIR-in-ux SOH-dee-uhm)
Arixtra

Pharmacologic class: inhibitor of activated factor X (Xa)
Therapeutic class: anticoagulant
Pregnancy risk category: B

Indications and dosages

▶ **To prevent deep vein thrombosis in patients undergoing abdominal surgery or surgery for hip fracture, hip replacement, or knee replacement.** *Adults weighing 50 kg (110 lb) or more:* 2.5 mg subcutaneously once daily for 5 to 9 days. Give initial dose after hemostasis is established, 6 to 8 hours after surgery. Giving the dose earlier than 6 hours after surgery increases the risk for major bleeding. In patients undergoing hip fracture surgery, an extended prophylaxis course of up to 24 additional days is recommended, and a total of 32 days (perioperative and extended prophylaxis) has been tolerated.
▶ **Acute deep vein thrombosis with warfarin; acute pulmonary embolism with warfarin when therapy is initiated in the hospital.**
Adults weighing more than 100 kg (220 lb): 10 mg subcutaneously daily for 5 to 9 days.
Adults weighing 50 to 100 kg: 7.5 mg subcutaneously daily for 5 to 9 days.
Adults weighing less than 50 kg: 5 mg subcutaneously daily for 5 to 9 days.

For all patients, begin oral anticoagulant therapy as soon as possible, usually within 72 hours.

Contraindications and cautions

- Contraindicated in patients with creatinine clearance less than 30 ml/minute; in those who are hypersensitive to the drug or as prophylaxis

for abdominal, hip, or knee surgery in patients who weigh less than 50 kg; and in those with active major bleeding, bacterial endocarditis, or thrombocytopenia with a positive test result for antiplatelet antibody during therapy.
- Use cautiously in patients also being treated with platelet inhibitors and in those at increased risk for bleeding, such as patients who have congenital or acquired bleeding disorders, a bleeding diathesis, active ulcerative and angiodysplastic GI disease, or hemorrhagic stroke; and patients who recently had brain, spinal, or ophthalmologic surgery. Also use cautiously in patients who have had epidural or spinal anesthesia or spinal puncture because they have an increased risk of epidural or spinal hematoma (which may cause permanent paralysis). Use cautiously in patients undergoing elective hip surgery with mild or moderate renal impairment. Also use caution in patients with a creatinine clearance of 30 to 50 ml/minute, a history of heparin-induced thrombocytopenia, uncontrolled arterial hypertension, or a history of recent GI ulceration, diabetic retinopathy, or hemorrhage.
⚹ **Lifespan:** In pregnant women, use only if benefits outweigh risks to the fetus. In breastfeeding women, use cautiously because it's unknown if drug appears in breast milk. In children, safety and effectiveness haven't been established. In elderly patients, use cautiously because the risk of major bleeding increases with age.

Adverse reactions

CNS: insomnia, dizziness, confusion, pain, headache, *fever, spinal and epidural hematomas.*
CV: hypotension, edema.
GI: *nausea,* constipation, vomiting, diarrhea, dyspepsia.
GU: UTI, urine retention.
Hematologic: *hemorrhage,* anemia, hematoma, *postoperative hemorrhage, thrombocytopenia.*
Metabolic: hypokalemia.
Skin: mild local irritation (injection site bleeding, rash, pruritus), bullous eruption, purpura, increased wound drainage, rash.

Interactions

Drug-drug. *Drugs that increase risk of bleeding (NSAIDs, platelet inhibitors, salicylates, anticoagulants):* May increase risk of hemorrhage.

Reactions may be *common*, uncommon, *life-threatening*, or COMMON AND LIFE-THREATENING.

If drugs must be used together, monitor patient closely.

Effects on lab results

• May increase creatinine, AST, ALT, and bilirubin levels. May decrease potassium and hemoglobin levels and hematocrit.
• May decrease platelet count.

Pharmacokinetics

Absorption: Rapid and complete; 100% bioavailability.
Distribution: Mainly in blood. At least 94% bound to antithrombin III (AT-III).
Metabolism: Not studied.
Excretion: Up to 77% in urine unchanged in 72 hours. *Half-life:* 17 to 21 hours.

Route	Onset	Peak	Duration
SubQ	Unknown	2–3 hr	Unknown

Action

Chemical effect: Binds to AT-III and potentiates the natural neutralization of factor Xa by AT-III. Neutralization of factor Xa interrupts the coagulation cascade, thereby inhibiting formation of thrombin and thrombus development.
Therapeutic effect: Prevents the formation of blood clots.

Available forms

Injection: 2.5 -mg/0.5 ml prefilled syringe

NURSING PROCESS

⬛ Assessment

• Assess patient's underlying condition before starting therapy.
• Be alert for adverse reactions and drug interactions.
• Patient who has received epidural or spinal anesthesia is at increased risk for epidural or spinal hematoma, which may result in long-term or permanent paralysis. Monitor patient closely for neurological impairment.
• Monitor renal function periodically, and stop drug in patient who develops unstable renal function or severe renal impairment.
• Routinely assess patient for signs and symptoms of bleeding, and regularly monitor CBC, platelet count, creatinine level, and stool occult blood test results. If platelet count is less than 100,000/mm³, stop drug.

• Effect may last for 2 to 4 days after stopping drug in patient with normal renal function.
• Don't use PT and APTT tests to measure effectiveness.
• Assess patient's and family's knowledge of drug therapy.

⬛ Nursing diagnoses

• Risk for injury related to potential for thrombosis or pulmonary emboli development from underlying condition
• Increased risk for trauma related to increased risk of bleeding and hemorrhaging due to drug therapy
• Deficient knowledge related to anticoagulant therapy

⬛ Planning and implementation

• Give by subcutaneous injection only, in fatty tissue only, rotating injection sites.
• Visually inspect the single-dose prefilled syringe for particulate matter and discoloration before administration.
• Don't mix with other injections.
⬥ **ALERT:** Don't use interchangeably with heparin, low–molecular-weight heparins, or heparinoids.
• To avoid loss of drug, don't expel air bubble from the syringe.
• If patient begins to overtly bleed while being given the drug, apply strong pressure to the injection area and immediately notify the prescriber.
• Overdose may lead to hemorrhagic complications. Stop giving the drug and treat bleeding appropriately.
⬥ **ALERT:** Don't confuse Arixtra with the lab test anti-factor Xa, sometimes written anti-Xa.
⬥ **ALERT:** Don't confuse Arixtra with Bextra.
Patient teaching
• Teach patient signs and symptoms of bleeding. If any occur, patient should immediately contact the prescriber.
• Instruct patient to avoid OTC products that contain aspirin, other salicylates, or NSAIDs and other prescribed anticoagulants.
• Teach patient the correct way to give drug to himself subcutaneously.
• Show patient the different sites for injection, and explain that he must alternate injection sites to prevent hardening of fatty tissues.
• Teach patient the proper disposal of the syringe.

✓ Evaluation

• Patient has no pulmonary embolus or thrombus during drug therapy.
• Patient is free from any injury or bleeding.
• Patient and family state understanding of drug therapy.

formoterol fumarate inhalation powder

(for-MOE-tur-all FOO-muh-rayt)
Foradil Aerolizer

Pharmacologic class: selective beta$_2$ agonist
Therapeutic class: bronchodilator
Pregnancy risk category: C

Indications and dosages

▶ **Preventive and maintenance therapy for bronchospasm in patients with reversible obstructive airway disease or nocturnal asthma who usually need short-acting inhaled beta$_2$ agonists.** *Adults and children age 5 and older:* One 12-mcg capsule by inhalation via Aerolizer inhaler q 12 hours. Don't give more than one capsule twice daily (24 mcg daily). If symptoms are present between doses, use a short-acting beta$_2$ agonist for immediate relief.
▶ **To prevent exercise-induced bronchospasm.** *Adults and children age 12 and older:* One 12-mcg capsule by inhalation via Aerolizer inhaler at least 15 minutes before exercise, given occasionally, p.r.n. Avoid giving additional doses within 12 hours of first dose.
▶ **Maintenance therapy for COPD.** *Adults:* One 12-mcg capsule by inhalation via Aerolizer inhaler q 12 hours. Total daily dosage of greater than 24 mcg isn't recommended.

Contraindications and cautions

• Contraindicated in patients hypersensitive to drug or any of its components.
• Use cautiously in patients with CV disease, particularly coronary insufficiency, cardiac arrhythmias, and hypertension; in those who are unusually responsive to sympathomimetic amines; and in those with diabetes mellitus because hyperglycemia and ketoacidosis have occurred rarely with use of beta agonists. Also use cautiously in patients with lactose or milk allergy, seizure disorders, or thyrotoxicosis.

• Do not use to treat acute asthma attack or bronchospasm.
※ **Lifespan:** In pregnant women, use cautiously because drug may interfere with uterine contractility. In breast-feeding women, use cautiously because it isn't known if drug appears in breast milk. In children younger than age 5, safety and effectiveness haven't been established for asthma. In children younger than age 12, safety and effectiveness haven't been established for exercise-induced bronchospasm.

Adverse reactions

CNS: tremor, dizziness, insomnia, nervousness, headache, fatigue, malaise.
CV: chest pain, angina, hypertension, hypotension, tachycardia, *arrhythmias,* palpitations.
EENT: dry mouth, tonsillitis, dysphonia.
GI: nausea.
Metabolic: hypokalemia, hyperglycemia, *metabolic acidosis.*
Musculoskeletal: muscle cramps.
Respiratory: bronchitis, chest infection, dyspnea.
Skin: rash.
Other: viral infection.

Interactions

Drug-drug. *Adrenergics:* May potentiate sympathetic effects of formoterol. Use together cautiously.
Beta blockers: May antagonize effects of beta agonists, causing bronchospasm in asthmatic patients. Avoid use except when benefits outweigh risks. Use cardioselective beta blockers cautiously to minimize risk of bronchospasm.
Corticosteroids, diuretics, xanthine derivatives: May potentiate hypokalemic effect of formoterol. Use together cautiously.
Loop or thiazide diuretics: May worsen ECG changes or hypokalemia with beta agonists. Use together cautiously, and monitor patient closely.
MAO inhibitors, tricyclic antidepressants, and other drugs that prolong the QT interval: May increase risk of ventricular arrhythmias. Use together cautiously.

Effects on lab test results

• May decrease potassium level. May increase glucose level.

Pharmacokinetics

Absorption: Rapid. Drug levels peak within 5 minutes after a 120-mcg dose.
Distribution: 61% to 64% bound to proteins.
Metabolism: Primarily involving CYP 2D6, 2C19, 2C9, and 2A6. Doesn't appear to inhibit CYP enzymes at therapeutic levels.
Excretion: 59% to 62% in urine and 32% to 34% in feces over 5 days. *Half-life:* Unknown.

Route	Onset	Peak	Duration
Inhalation	1–3 min	½-1½ hr	12 hr

Action

Chemical effect: Relaxes bronchial and cardiac smooth muscle by acting on beta$_2$-adrenergic receptors; stimulates intracellular adenyl cyclase, the enzyme responsible for catalyzing the conversion of adenosine triphosphate (ATP) to cAMP. Increase in cAMP leads to relaxation of bronchial smooth muscle and inhibition of mediator release from mast cells.
Therapeutic effect: Prevents and controls bronchospasm.

Available forms

Capsules for inhalation: 12 mcg

NURSING PROCESS

⚗ Assessment
● Assess patient's underlying condition before starting therapy, and reassess regularly.
● Evaluate patient's use of short-acting beta$_2$ agonists for immediate relief of bronchospasm. Drug may be used with short-acting beta$_2$ agonists, inhaled corticosteroids, and theophylline therapy to manage asthma.
● Assess patient's and family's knowledge of drug therapy.

📋 Nursing diagnoses
● Impaired gas exchange related to underlying pulmonary condition
● Risk for activity intolerance related to underlying pulmonary condition
● Knowledge deficit related to formoterol fumarate therapy

❯ Planning and implementation
● Before use, store drug in refrigerator. After use, drug may be stored at room temperature.

Don't remove capsule from unopened blister until immediately before use.
● Give capsules only by oral inhalation and only with the Aerolizer inhaler.
● Don't use Foradil Aerolizer with a spacer device.
● For patient using drug twice daily, don't give additional doses to prevent exercise-induced bronchospasm.
● Don't use as a substitute for short-acting beta$_2$ agonists for immediate relief of bronchospasm, or as a substitute for inhaled or oral corticosteroids.
● Don't begin use in patients with rapidly deteriorating or significantly worsening asthma.
● If usual dose doesn't control symptoms of bronchoconstriction and the patient's short-acting beta$_2$ agonist becomes less effective, reevaluate patient and therapy.
● For patient who formerly used regularly scheduled short-acting beta$_2$ agonists, decrease use of these drugs to an as-needed basis when long-acting therapy starts.
● Don't let the patient exhale into the device.
● Pierce capsules only once. To minimize risk of shattering capsule, strictly follow storage and use instructions. The Aerolizer contains a screen that will catch any broken pieces of the capsule before they enter the patient's mouth or lungs.
● Drug may cause life-threatening paradoxical bronchospasm. If this occurs, immediately stop giving the drug and use a different drug.
● Monitor patient for tachycardia, hypertension, and other adverse CV effects. If they occur, stop drug.
● Watch for immediate hypersensitivity reactions, such as anaphylaxis, urticaria, angioedema, rash, and bronchospasm.
● Signs and symptoms of overdose include excessive beta blocker stimulation (tachycardia, tremor, hypotension) and exaggerated adverse effects, leading to cardiac arrest and death. To treat overdose, stop drug, monitor cardiac condition, give appropriate symptomatic relief or supportive therapy, and use cardioselective beta blockers cautiously. It's unknown whether dialysis is beneficial.
⚕ ALERT: Capsules shouldn't be swallowed.
⚕ ALERT: Don't confuse Foradil with Toradol.
Patient teaching
● Tell patient not to increase the dosage or frequency of use without medical advice.

• Warn patient not to stop or reduce other drugs taken for asthma.

• Advise patient that drug isn't for acute asthmatic episodes; instead, he should use short-acting beta$_2$ agonist.

• Advise patient to report worsening symptoms, decreasing effectiveness, or increasing use of short-acting beta$_2$ agonist.

• Tell patient to report nausea, vomiting, shakiness, headache, fast or irregular heartbeat, chest pain, or sleeplessness.

• Tell patient being treated for exercise-induced bronchospasm to take drug at least 15 minutes before exercise. Additional doses can't be taken for 12 hours.

• Tell patient not to use the Foradil Aerolizer with a spacer device or to exhale or blow into the inhaler.

• Advise patient to avoid washing the Aerolizer and to always keep it dry. Advise patient to use the new device that comes with each refill.

• Tell patient to avoid exposing capsules to moisture and to handle them only with dry hands.

☑ **Evaluation**

• Patient's pulmonary symptoms improve.
• Patient's activity intolerance improves.
• Patient and family state understanding of drug therapy.

fosamprenavir calcium
(foss-am-PREH-nuh-veer CAL-see-um)
Lexiva

Pharmacologic class: protease inhibitor
Therapeutic class: antiretroviral
Pregnancy risk category: C

Indications and dosages

▶ **HIV infection with other antiretrovirals.**
Adults: In patients previously untreated, 1,400 mg P.O. twice daily (without ritonavir). Or 1,400 mg P.O. once daily and ritonavir 200 mg P.O. once daily. Or 700 mg P.O. b.i.d. and ritonavir 100 mg P.O. b.i.d. In patients previously treated with a protease inhibitor, 700 mg P.O. b.i.d. plus ritonavir 100 mg P.O. b.i.d.
◩ **Adjust-a-dose:** If the patient takes efavirenz, fosamprenavir, and ritonavir once daily, give an additional 100 mg daily of ritonavir (300 mg to-

tal). If the patient has mild or moderate hepatic impairment and takes fosamprenavir without ritonavir, reduce the dosage to 700 mg P.O. b.i.d. Avoid use in patients with severe hepatic impairment because dose can't be reduced below 700 mg.

Contraindications and cautions

• Contraindicated in patients hypersensitive to amprenavir or any of its components. Also contraindicated with dihydroergotamine, ergonovine, ergotamine, flecainide, methylergonovine, midazolam, pimozide, propafenone, and triazolam.

• Use cautiously in patients allergic to sulfonamides and those with mild to moderate hepatic impairment. Avoid use in patients with severe hepatic impairment.

⚞ **Lifespan:** In pregnant women, breastfeeding women, and children, safety and effectiveness haven't been established.

Adverse reactions

CNS: depression, fatigue, headache, oral paresthesia.
GI: abdominal pain, diarrhea, nausea, vomiting.
Skin: pruritus, *rash.*

Interactions

Drug-drug. *Amitriptyline, cyclosporine, imipramine, tacrolimus:* May increase levels of these drugs. Monitor drug levels.
Antiarrhythmics (amiodarone, lidocaine, quinidine): May increase antiarrhythmic level. Use together cautiously and monitor antiarrhythmic levels.
Atorvastatin: May increase atorvastatin level. Give 20 mg daily or less of atorvastatin and monitor patient carefully. Or consider other HMG-CoA reductase inhibitors, such as fluvastatin, pravastatin, or rosuvastatin.
Benzodiazepines (alprazolam, clorazepate, diazepam, flurazepam): May increase benzodiazepine level. Decrease benzodiazepine dosage p.r.n.
Calcium channel blockers (amlodipine, diltiazem, felodipine, isradipine, nicardipine, nifedipine, nimodipine, nisoldipine, verapamil): May increase calcium channel blocker level. Use together cautiously.
Carbamazepine, dexamethasone, H$_2$-receptor antagonists, phenobarbital, phenytoin, proton-pump inhibitors: May decrease amprenavir level. Use together cautiously.

Delavirdine: May cause loss of virologic response and resistance to delavirdine. Avoid use together.

Dihydroergotamine, ergonovine, ergotamine, flecainide, methylergonovine, midazolam, pimozide, propafenone, triazolam: May cause serious adverse reactions. Avoid use together.

Efavirenz, nevirapine, saquinavir: May decrease amprenavir level. Appropriate combination doses haven't been established.

Efavirenz with ritonavir: May decrease amprenavir level. Increase ritonavir by 100 mg daily (300 mg total) when giving efavirenz, fosamprenavir, and ritonavir once daily. No change needed in ritonavir when giving efavirenz, fosamprenavir, and ritonavir twice daily.

Ethinyl estradiol and norethindrone: May increase ethinyl estradiol and norethindrone levels. Recommend nonhormonal contraception.

Indinavir, nelfinavir: May increase amprenavir level. Appropriate combination doses haven't been established.

Ketoconazole, itraconazole: May increase ketoconazole and itraconazole levels. Reduce ketoconazole or itraconazole dosage as needed if patient takes more than 400 mg daily of fosamprenavir. Don't give more than 200 mg daily.

Lopinavir with ritonavir: May decrease amprenavir and lopinavir levels. Appropriate combination doses haven't been established.

Lovastatin, simvastatin: May increase risk of myopathy, including rhabdomyolysis. Avoid use together.

Methadone: May decrease methadone level. Increase methadone dosage p.r.n.

Rifabutin: May increase rifabutin level. Obtain CBC weekly to watch for neutropenia and decrease rifabutin dosage by at least half. If patient takes ritonavir, decrease dosage by at least 75% from the usual 300 mg daily. Maximum, 150 mg q other day or three times weekly.

Rifampin: May decrease amprenavir level and drug effect. Avoid use together.

Sildenafil, vardenafil: May increase sildenafil and vardenafil levels. Recommend cautious use of sildenafil at 25 mg q 48 hours or vardenafil at no more than 2.5 mg q 24 hours. If patient takes ritonavir, recommend cautious use of vardenafil at no more than 2.5 mg q 72 hours. Tell patient to report adverse events.

Warfarin: May alter warfarin level. Monitor INR.

Drug-herb. *St. John's wort:* May cause loss of virologic response and resistance to fosamprenavir or its class of protease inhibitors. Discourage use together.

Effects on lab test results
• May increase lipase, triglyceride, AST, and ALT levels.
• May decrease neutrophil count.

Pharmacokinetics
Absorption: Food has no effect.
Distribution: 90% protein-bound.
Metabolism: Rapid and almost complete via CYP 3A4 pathway.
Excretion: Unknown. *Half-life:* 7¼ hours.

Route	Onset	Peak	Duration
P.O.	Unknown	1½–4 hr	Unknown

Action
Chemical effect: Converts rapidly to amprenavir, which binds to the active site of HIV-1 protease and causes formation of immature noninfectious viral particles.
Therapeutic effect: Hinders HIV activity.

Available forms
Tablets: 700 mg

NURSING PROCESS

🔲 Assessment
• Monitor patient with hemophilia for spontaneous bleeding.
• During initial therapy, monitor patient for such opportunistic infections as *Mycobacterium avium* complex, CMV, *Pneumocystis jiroveci (carinii)* pneumonia, and tuberculosis.
• Assess patient for redistribution or accumulation of body fat, as in central obesity, dorsocervical fat enlargement (buffalo hump), peripheral wasting, facial wasting, breast enlargement, and a cushingoid appearance.
• Assess patient's and family's knowledge of drug therapy.

🔲 Nursing diagnoses
• Infection related to presence of HIV
• Risk for deficient fluid volume related to adverse GI reactions
• Deficient knowledge related to drug therapy

▷ Planning and implementation

• Patient with hepatitis B or C, or noticeable increase in transaminase level before therapy, may have an increased risk of transaminase elevation. Monitor patient.

Patient teaching

• Tell patient that drug doesn't reduce the risk of transmitting HIV to others.

• Inform patient that the drug may reduce the risk of progression to AIDS and death.

• Explain that drug must be used with other antiretrovirals.

• Tell patient not to alter the dosage or stop taking drug without consulting the prescriber.

• Urge patient to inform the prescriber about sulfa allergy.

• Because this drug may interact with many drugs, urge patient to tell the prescriber about any prescription or OTC drugs and herbal products that he takes (especially St. John's wort).

• Explain that body fat may redistribute or accumulate.

▓ Evaluation

• Patient responds well to therapy.

• Patient maintains adequate hydration.

• Patient and family state understanding of drug therapy.

foscarnet sodium (phosphonoformic acid)
(fos-KAR-net SOH-dee-um)
Foscavir

Pharmacologic class: pyrophosphate analog
Therapeutic class: antiviral
Pregnancy risk category: C

Indications and dosages

▶ **CMV retinitis in patients with AIDS.**
Adults: Initially, 60 mg/kg I.V. over 1 hour q 8 hours for 2 to 3 weeks, depending on response. Or 90 mg/kg I.V. q 12 hours over 1.5 to 2 hours for 2 to 3 weeks, depending on response. Follow with maintenance infusion of 90 mg/kg I.V. daily over 2 hours; if disease progresses, increase dosage as needed and tolerated to 120 mg/kg daily.
◊ **Adjust-a-dose:** In patients with renal impairment, adjust dosage for creatinine clearance less

than 1.5 ml/kg/minute. If creatinine clearance is less than 0.4 ml/kg/minute, stop drug.

▶ **Mucocutaneous acyclovir-resistant herpes simplex virus infections.** *Adults:* 40 mg/kg I.V. infused over at least 1 hour, either q 8 or 12 hours for 2 to 3 weeks or until healed.
◊ **Adjust-a-dose:** In patients with renal impairment, if creatinine clearance is less than 1.5 ml/kg/minute, adjust dosage. If creatinine clearance is less than 0.4 ml/kg/minute, stop drug.

▶ **Varicella zoster infection‡.** *Adults:* 40 mg/kg I.V. q 8 hours for 14 to 21 days.

▼ I.V. administration

• If infusing via central venous access, the standard 24-mg/ml solution may or may not be diluted. When a peripheral venous catheter is used, dilute solution to 12 mg/ml with D_5W or normal saline solution.

• To reduce the risk of nephrotoxicity, give 750 to 1,000 ml of normal saline solution or D_5W before first dose and then concurrently with each subsequent dose.

• Don't exceed recommended dosage, infusion rate, or frequency of administration. All doses must be individualized based on patient's renal function.

• Use infusion pump to give drug over at least 1 hour.

• Use solution within 24 hours of first entry into sealed bottle.

⊗ **Incompatibilities**
Acyclovir, amphotericin B, co-trimoxazole, dextrose 30%, diazepam, digoxin, diphenhydramine, dobutamine, droperidol, ganciclovir, haloperidol, lactated Ringer's solution, leucovorin, lorazepam, midazolam, pentamidine, phenytoin, prochlorperazine, promethazine, solutions containing calcium (such as total parenteral nutrition), trimetrexate, vancomycin.

Contraindications and cautions

• Contraindicated in patients hypersensitive to drug or any of its components.

• Use cautiously and at a lower dose in a patient with abnormal renal function because drug will accumulate and toxicity will increase. Because drug is nephrotoxic, it may worsen renal impairment. Some nephrotoxicity occurs in most patients treated with drug.

♨ **Lifespan:** In pregnant women, use cautiously. In breast-feeding women, use cautiously because it's unknown if the drug appears in breast milk. In children, safety and effectiveness haven't been established. In elderly patients, use cautiously because they are more likely to have decreased renal function.

Adverse reactions

CNS: *fever,* pain, *headache, seizures, fatigue, malaise, asthenia, paresthesia, dizziness, hypoesthesia, neuropathy,* tremor, ataxia, cerebrovascular disorder, generalized spasms, dementia, stupor, sensory disturbances, meningitis, aphasia, abnormal coordination, EEG abnormalities, depression, confusion, anxiety, insomnia, somnolence, nervousness, amnesia, agitation, aggressive reaction.
CV: hypertension, palpitations, ECG abnormalities, sinus tachycardia, first-degree AV block, hypotension, flushing, edema, facial edema.
EENT: visual disturbances, eye pain, conjunctivitis, sinusitis, pharyngitis, rhinitis.
GI: taste perversion, dry mouth, *nausea, diarrhea, vomiting, abdominal pain, anorexia,* constipation, dysphagia, *rectal hemorrhage,* melena, flatulence, ulcerative stomatitis, *pancreatitis.*
GU: abnormal renal function, albuminuria, dysuria, polyuria, urethral disorder, urine retention, UTI, *acute renal impairment, nephrotoxicity,* candidiasis.
Hematologic: anemia, *granulocytopenia, leukopenia, bone marrow suppression, thrombocytopenia, thrombosis,* lymphadenopathy.
Hepatic: abnormal hepatic function.
Metabolic: hypokalemia, *hypomagnesemia,* hypophosphatemia or hyperphosphatemia, hypocalcemia, hyponatremia.
Musculoskeletal: leg cramps, arthralgia, myalgia.
Respiratory: *cough, dyspnea,* pneumonic respiratory insufficiency, pulmonary infiltration, *stridor, pneumothorax, bronchospasm,* hemoptysis.
Skin: *rash, increased sweating,* pruritus, skin ulceration, erythematous rash, seborrhea, skin discoloration.
Other: *sepsis,* rigors, inflammation, pain at infusion site, lymphoma-like disorder, sarcoma, back or chest pain, bacterial or fungal infections, abscess, flulike symptoms.

Interactions

Drug-drug. *Nephrotoxic drugs (such as aminoglycosides, amphotericin B):* May increase risk of nephrotoxicity. Avoid use together.

Pentamidine: May increase risk of nephrotoxicity and severe hypocalcemia. Don't use together.
Zidovudine: May increase risk or severity of anemia. Monitor blood counts.

Effects on lab test results

● May increase BUN, creatinine, phosphate, ALT, AST, alkaline phosphatase, and bilirubin levels. May decrease calcium, magnesium, phosphate, potassium, sodium, and hemoglobin levels and hematocrit.
● May decrease granulocyte and WBC counts. May increase or decrease platelet count.

Pharmacokinetics

Absorption: Administered I.V.
Distribution: 14% to 17% protein-bound.
Metabolism: None.
Excretion: 80% to 90% unchanged in urine.
Half-life: 3 hours.

Route	Onset	Peak	Duration
I.V.	Immediate	Immediate	Unknown

Action

Chemical effect: Blocks pyrophosphate binding sites on DNA polymerases and reverse transcriptases.
Therapeutic effect: Kills virus.

Available forms

Injection: 24 mg/ml in 250- and 500-ml bottles

NURSING PROCESS

Assessment

● Assess patient's infection before therapy and regularly thereafter.
● Obtain electrolyte levels and creatinine clearance before therapy, two or three times weekly during induction and at least once every 1 or 2 weeks during maintenance.
● Drug may cause dose-related transient decrease in ionized calcium, which may not show up in laboratory values. Watch for tetany and seizures with abnormal electrolyte levels.
● Monitor patient's hemoglobin level and hematocrit. Patient may develop anemia severe enough that he needs transfusions.
● Be alert for adverse reactions and drug interactions.
● Assess patient's and family's knowledge of drug therapy.

⊕ Nursing diagnoses

• Infection related to presence of herpes virus susceptible to drug
• Disturbed sensory perception (tactile) related to drug's adverse effect
• Deficient knowledge related to drug therapy

⊠ Planning and implementation

• Because drug is highly toxic and toxicity is probably dose-related, use lowest effective maintenance dosage.

Patient teaching
• Advise patient to report circumoral tingling, numbness in limbs, and paresthesia.

☑ Evaluation

• Patient is free from infection.
• Patient has no adverse neurologic reactions.
• Patient and family state understanding of drug therapy.

fosinopril sodium

(foh-SIN-oh-pril SOH-dee-um)
Monopril✿

Pharmacologic class: ACE inhibitor
Therapeutic class: antihypertensive
Pregnancy risk category: C (D in second and third trimesters)

Indications and dosages

▶ **Hypertension.** *Adults:* Initially, 10 mg P.O. daily. Adjust dosage based on blood pressure at peak and trough levels. Usual dosage, 20 to 40 mg daily. Maximum, 80 mg daily. May divide dosage.
Children ages 6 to 16, weighing 50 kg (110 lb) or more: Give 5 to 10 mg P.O. daily.
▶ **Adjunct therapy for heart failure.** *Adults:* Initially, 10 mg P.O. once daily. Increase dosage over several weeks to maximum tolerable, but no more than 40 mg P.O. daily. If possible, stop diuretic therapy.
◣ **Adjust-a-dose:** For patients who have heart failure with moderate to severe renal impairment or who are being vigorously diuresed, give initial dose of 5 mg P.O. daily.

Contraindications and cautions

• Contraindicated in patients hypersensitive to drug or any of its components or to other ACE

inhibitors, including patients with a history of ACE inhibitor–induced angioedema and patients with hereditary or idiopathic angioedema. Avoid use in patients with renal artery stenosis.
• Use cautiously in patients with impaired renal or hepatic function.
❋ **Lifespan:** In pregnant women, use only if benefits outweigh risks to the fetus. In breast-feeding women, drug is contraindicated. In children younger than age 6 or those weighing less than 50 kg, safety and effectiveness haven't been established.

Adverse reactions

CNS: headache, dizziness, fatigue, syncope, paresthesia, sleep disturbance, *stroke.*
CV: chest pain, angina, *MI*, rhythm disturbances, palpitations, hypotension, orthostatic hypotension.
EENT: tinnitus, sinusitis.
GI: dry mouth, nausea, vomiting, diarrhea, *pancreatitis,* abdominal distention, abdominal pain, constipation.
GU: renal insufficiency.
Hepatic: *hepatitis.*
Metabolic: *hyperkalemia.*
Musculoskeletal: arthralgia, musculoskeletal pain, myalgia.
Respiratory: dry, persistent, tickling, nonproductive cough; *bronchospasm.*
Skin: urticaria, rash, photosensitivity, pruritus.
Other: decreased libido, sexual dysfunction, gout, *angioedema.*

Interactions

Drug-drug. *Antacids:* May impair absorption. Separate administration times by at least 2 hours.
Diuretics, other antihypertensives: May increase risk of excessive hypotension. Stop diuretic or lower fosinopril dosage.
Lithium: May increase lithium levels and lithium toxicity. Avoid use together.
Potassium-sparing diuretics, potassium supplements, sodium substitutes containing potassium: May increase risk of hyperkalemia. Monitor potassium levels.
Drug-herb. *Licorice:* May cause sodium retention and increase blood pressure, interfering with therapeutic effect of ACE inhibitor. Discourage ingestion of licorice during drug therapy.

Drug-food. *Salt substitutes containing potassium:* May increase risk of hyperkalemia. Monitor potassium closely.
Drug-lifestyle. *Alcohol use:* May have additive hypotensive effects. Discourage use together.

Effects on lab test results

• May increase BUN, creatinine, and potassium levels. May decrease hemoglobin level and hematocrit.
• May increase liver function test values.

Pharmacokinetics

Absorption: Slow, primarily in proximal small intestine.
Distribution: More than 95% protein-bound.
Metabolism: Mainly in liver and gut.
Excretion: 50% in urine; remainder in feces.
Half-life: 11½ hours.

Route	Onset	Peak	Duration
P.O.	≤ 1 hr	2–6 hr	24 hr

Action

Chemical effect: Inhibits ACE, preventing conversion of angiotensin I to angiotensin II, a potent vasoconstrictor, which decreases peripheral arterial resistance, and aldosterone secretion.
Therapeutic effect: Lowers blood pressure.

Available forms

Tablets: 10 mg, 20 mg, 40 mg

NURSING PROCESS

Assessment
• Assess blood pressure before starting therapy and regularly thereafter.
• Assess renal and hepatic function before starting therapy and regularly thereafter.
• Monitor potassium intake and potassium level. Diabetic patients, those with renal impairment, and those receiving drugs that can increase potassium levels may develop hyperkalemia.
• Other ACE inhibitors have been linked to agranulocytosis and neutropenia. Monitor CBC with differential counts before therapy, every 2 weeks for first 3 months of therapy, and periodically thereafter.
• If adverse GI reaction occurs, monitor patient's hydration.

• Assess patient's and family's knowledge of drug therapy.

Nursing diagnoses
• Risk for injury related to presence of hypertension
• Risk for deficient fluid volume related to adverse GI reactions
• Deficient knowledge related to drug therapy

Planning and implementation
• Drug may be taken with food, but it slows absorption.
Patient teaching
• Tell patient to avoid salt substitutes because they may contain potassium, which increases the risk of hyperkalemia.
• Urge patient to report signs of infection (such as fever and sore throat); easy bruising or bleeding; swelling of tongue, lips, face, eyes, mucous membranes, or limbs; difficulty swallowing or breathing; and hoarseness.
• Tell patient to use caution in hot weather and during exercise. Inadequate fluid intake, vomiting, diarrhea, and excessive perspiration can lead to light-headedness and syncope.
• Tell woman to notify prescriber about planned, suspected, or known pregnancy. Drug will probably need to be stopped.

Evaluation
• Patient's blood pressure is normal.
• Patient maintains adequate hydration throughout drug therapy.
• Patient and family state understanding of drug therapy.

fosphenytoin sodium
(fahs-FEN-eh-toyn SOH-dee-um)
Cerebyx

Pharmacologic class: hydantoin
Therapeutic class: anticonvulsant
Pregnancy risk category: D

Indications and dosages

▶ **Status epilepticus.** *Adults:* 15 to 20 mg phenytoin sodium equivalent (PE)/kg I.V. at 100 to 150 mg PE/minute as loading dose; then 4 to 6 mg PE/kg I.V. daily as maintenance dose.

(Phenytoin may be used instead of fosphenytoin as maintenance, using the appropriate dose.)
▶ **To prevent and treat seizures during neurosurgery (nonemergent loading or maintenance doses).** *Adults:* Loading dose of 10 to 20 mg PE/kg I.M. or I.V. at infusion rate not exceeding 150 mg PE/minute. Maintenance dosage is 4 to 6 mg PE/kg I.V. or I.M. daily.
▶ **Short-term substitution for oral phenytoin therapy.** *Adults:* Same total daily dosage equivalent as oral phenytoin sodium therapy given as a single daily dose I.M. or I.V. at infusion rate not exceeding 150 mg PE/minute. Some patients may need more frequent doses.

▽ I.V. administration

• Dilute drug in D_5W or normal saline solution for injection to a level ranging from 1.5 to 25 mg PE/ml.
• Don't exceed 150 mg PE/minute.
• Monitor patient's ECG, blood pressure, and respirations throughout period of highest phenytoin levels—about 10 to 20 minutes after end of fosphenytoin infusion.
• Refrigerate at 36° to 46° F (2° C to 8° C). Don't keep at room temperature for longer than 48 hours.
⊗ **Incompatibilities**
Other I.V. drugs.

Contraindications and cautions

• Contraindicated in patients hypersensitive to drug or any of its components, phenytoin, or other hydantoins. Also contraindicated in patients with sinus bradycardia, SA block, second- or third-degree AV block, Adams-Stokes syndrome, or acute hepatotoxicity. Drug isn't indicated for absence seizures.
• Use cautiously in patients with renal and hepatic disease or in those with hypoalbuminemia.
⚞ **Lifespan:** In pregnant women, use drug only if nature, frequency, and severity of seizures pose a serious threat to the patient. In breast-feeding women, use cautiously. In children, safety and effectiveness haven't been established. In elderly patients, use a lower dose because of their decreased metabolism and decreased phenytoin clearance.

Adverse reactions

CNS: abnormal thinking, agitation, asthenia, *ataxia,* **brain edema,** decreased reflexes, *dizziness,* dysarthria, headache, extrapyramidal syndrome, fever, hypoesthesia, increased reflexes, incoordination, *intracranial hypertension,* nervousness, paresthesia, speech disorder, *somnolence,* stupor, vertigo.
CV: hypotension, hypertension, tachycardia, tremor, facial edema, vasodilation, *severe CV reactions, ventricular fibrillation.*
EENT: amblyopia, deafness, diplopia, *nystagmus,* tinnitus.
GI: constipation, dry mouth, nausea, taste perversion, tongue disorder, vomiting.
Hepatic: *hepatotoxicity.*
Metabolic: hypokalemia.
Musculoskeletal: back pain, myasthenia, pelvic pain.
Respiratory: pneumonia.
Skin: ecchymosis, *pruritus,* rash.
Other: accidental injury, chills, infection, injection-site reaction and pain.

Interactions

Drug-drug. *Amiodarone, chloramphenicol, chlordiazepoxide, cimetidine, diazepam, dicumarol, disulfiram, estrogens, ethosuximide, fluoxetine, H_2-receptor antagonists, halothane, isoniazid, methylphenidate, phenothiazines, phenylbutazone, salicylates, succinimides, sulfonamides, tolbutamide, trazodone:* May increase phenytoin level and thus its therapeutic effects. Use together cautiously.
Carbamazepine, reserpine: May decrease phenytoin level. Monitor patient.
Coumarin, digitoxin, doxycycline, estrogens, furosemide, hormonal contraceptives, rifampin, quinidine, theophylline, vitamin D: May decrease effectiveness of these drugs because of increased hepatic metabolism. Monitor patient closely.
Phenobarbital, sodium valproate, valproic acid: May increase or decrease phenytoin level. Monitor patient.
Tricyclic antidepressants: May lower seizure threshold and require adjustments in phenytoin dosage. Use cautiously.
Drug-lifestyle. *Acute alcohol use:* May increase phenytoin level and toxic effects. Discourage alcohol use.
Chronic alcohol use: May decrease phenytoin level. Monitor patient; discourage alcohol use.

Reactions may be *common,* uncommon, *life-threatening*, or COMMON AND LIFE-THREATENING.

Effects on lab test results

• May increase alkaline phosphatase, GGT, and glucose levels. May decrease potassium and T_4 levels.

• May decrease platelet, WBC, granulocyte, leukocyte, and RBC counts.

Pharmacokinetics

Absorption: Complete.
Distribution: Wide; 95% to 99% protein-bound.
Metabolism: In the liver; undergoes rapid hydrolysis to phenytoin.
Excretion: In the urine as phenytoin metabolites. *Half-life:* 15 minutes.

Route	Onset	Peak	Duration
I.V.	Unknown	Immediate	Unknown
I.M.	Unknown	30 min	Unknown

Action

Chemical effect: Because fosphenytoin is a prodrug of phenytoin, their action is the same: stabilizing neuronal membranes.
Therapeutic effect: Prevents and controls seizures.

Available forms

Injection: 2 ml (150 mg fosphenytoin sodium equivalent to 100 mg phenytoin sodium), 10 ml (750 mg fosphenytoin sodium equivalent to 500 mg phenytoin sodium)

NURSING PROCESS

🔡 Assessment

• Don't give drug I.M. for status epilepticus because therapeutic phenytoin levels may not occur as rapidly as with I.V. administration.

• Don't monitor phenytoin level until about 2 hours after the end of I.V. infusion or 4 hours after I.M. injection.

• Assess patient's and family's knowledge of drug therapy.

🔢 Nursing diagnoses

• Risk for trauma related to seizures
• Deficient knowledge related to drug therapy

🔳 Planning and implementation

• Drug should always be prescribed and dispensed in PE units. Don't make any adjustments in recommended dose when substituting fosphenytoin for phenytoin, or vice versa.

• I.M. use generates systemic phenytoin levels similar to oral phenytoin sodium, allowing essentially interchangeable use.

🛇 **ALERT:** Abruptly stopping the drug may cause status epilepticus. Substitute another drug, or reduce the dosage of this drug gradually.

🛇 **ALERT:** Don't confuse Cerebyx with Celexa or Celebrex.

Patient teaching

• Warn patient that sensory disturbances may occur with I.V. use.

• Instruct patient to immediately report adverse reactions, especially rash.

🗹 Evaluation

• Patient is free from seizures.
• Patient and family state understanding of drug therapy.

---

frovatriptan succinate
(froh-vah-TRIP-tan SUK-seh-nayt)
Frova⌀

Pharmacologic class: serotonin 5-HT$_1$ receptor agonist
Therapeutic class: antimigraine drug
Pregnancy risk category: C

Indications and dosages

▶ **Migraine attacks with or without aura.**
Adults: 2.5 mg P.O. taken at the first sign of migraine attack. If the headache recurs after initial relief, a second tablet may be given after waiting for at least 2 hours. Don't give more than 3 tablets daily.

Contraindications and cautions

• Contraindicated in patients hypersensitive to drug or any of the inactive ingredients. Also contraindicated in patients with history of or current ischemic heart disease, coronary artery vasospasm (including Prinzmetal's variant angina), or other significant underlying CV conditions. Don't use in patients with cerebrovascular syndromes, such as stroke of any type or transient ischemic attacks, or in patients with peripheral vascular disease, including, but not limited to, ischemic bowel disease. Contraindicated

---

in patients with uncontrolled hypertension and in patients with hemiplegic or basilar migraine.
☂ Lifespan: In pregnant women, use drug only if benefits outweigh risks to the fetus. In breast-feeding women, use cautiously because it's unknown if drug appears in breast milk. In children, safety and effectiveness haven't been established. In elderly patients, no special dosage has been suggested, but experience is limited.

Adverse reactions

CNS: dizziness, headache, fatigue, pain, paresthesia, insomnia, anxiety, somnolence, dysesthesia, hypoesthesia, *stroke.*
CV: flushing, palpitations, chest pain, *MI, cardiac arrhythmias,* hypertension.
EENT: abnormal vision, tinnitus, sinusitis, rhinitis.
GI: dry mouth, dyspepsia, vomiting, abdominal pain, diarrhea, nausea.
Musculoskeletal: skeletal pain.
Skin: increased sweating.
Other: hot or cold sensation.

Interactions

Drug-drug. *Ergotamine or ergot-type drugs (such as dihydroergotamine or methysergide):* May cause prolonged vasospastic reactions. Don't use within 24 hours of each other.
5-HT$_{1B/1D}$ agonists: May have additive effects. Use of other 5-HT$_1$ agonists within 24 hours of frovatriptan isn't recommended.
Hormonal contraceptives, propranolol: May increase bioavailability of frovatriptan. Monitor patient for adverse effects.
SSRIs (such as citalopram, fluoxetine, fluvoxamine, paroxetine, sertraline): May cause weakness, hyperreflexia, and incoordination. Monitor patient closely.

Effects on lab test results

None reported.

Pharmacokinetics

Absorption: Oral bioavailability of 20% in men and 30% in women. Food delays the time to peak, but not the bioavailability of the drug.
Distribution: 15% protein-bound.
Metabolism: In the liver, by CYP 1A2. Drug doesn't appear to be an inducer or inhibitor of CYP.

Excretion: In the urine and feces. *Half-life:* 26 hours.

Route	Onset	Peak	Duration
P.O.	Unknown	2–4 hr	Unknown

Action

Chemical effect: May inhibit excessive dilation of extracerebral intracranial arteries in migraine headaches.
Therapeutic effect: Relieves pain caused by migraines.

Available forms

Tablets: 2.5 mg

NURSING PROCESS

✑ Assessment
• Assess underlying condition before starting therapy, and reassess regularly throughout therapy.
• Obtain complete medical history, paying particular attention to history of CV and cerebrovascular disease.
• Assess patient's and family's knowledge of drug therapy.

✑ Nursing diagnoses
• Acute pain related to migraine headache
• Activity intolerance related to migraine headache
• Knowledge deficit related to frovatriptan succinate therapy

▷ Planning and implementation
⚠ ALERT: Don't give within 24 hours of another 5-HT$_1$ agonist or an ergotamine or ergotlike drug.
⚠ ALERT: Serious cardiac events, including acute MI and life-threatening cardiac rhythm disturbances may occur within a few hours of giving 5-HT$_1$ agonists.
• Drug may bind to the melanin of the eye and cause ophthalmic effects. No specific ophthalmic monitoring is recommended.
• The safety of treating an average of more than four migraine attacks in a 30-day period hasn't been established.
• If used in a patient with risk factors for unrecognized coronary artery disease (such as hypertension, hypercholesterolemia, smoking, obesity, strong family history of coronary artery

---

Reactions may be *common,* uncommon, *life-threatening*, or COMMON AND LIFE-THREATENING.

disease, woman with surgical or physiologic menopause, man older than age 40), give the first dose in a medically staffed and equipped facility. Obtain an ECG after the first dose. Periodically assess cardiac condition in intermittent, long-term users of 5-HT$_1$ agonists or those who have or acquire risk factors during therapy.

Patient teaching

• Instruct patient to take the dose at the first sign of a migraine headache. If the headache comes back after the first dose, a second dose may be taken after 2 hours. Tell patient not to take more than 3 tablets in a 24-hour period.

• Inform patient that, in rare cases, patients have experienced serious heart problems, stroke, or high blood pressure after taking the drug.

• Advise patient to take extra care or avoid driving and operating machinery if dizziness or fatigue develops.

• Emphasize importance of immediately reporting rash, itching, or pain, tightness, heaviness, or pressure in the chest, throat, neck, or jaw after taking the drug.

• Instruct patient not to take drug within 24 hours of taking another serotonin receptor agonist or ergotamine-type drugs.

☑ Evaluation

• Patient is relieved of pain.

• Patient's activity tolerance returns to baseline.

• Patient and family state understanding of drug therapy.

fulvestrant

(full-VESS-trant)
Faslodex

Pharmacologic class: estrogen receptor antagonist
Therapeutic class: antineoplastic
Pregnancy risk category: D

Indications and dosages

▶ **Hormone-receptor–positive metastatic breast cancer in postmenopausal women with disease progression following antiestrogen therapy.** *Adults:* 250 mg by slow I.M. injection into buttock once monthly.

Contraindications and cautions

• Contraindicated in patients hypersensitive to drug or any of its components.

• Use cautiously in patients with moderate or severe hepatic impairment.

⚠ Lifespan: In pregnant women, drug is contraindicated. Women of childbearing age should avoid getting pregnant while taking the drug. Breast-feeding women should stop breast-feeding or not take the drug. In children, safety and effectiveness haven't been established.

Adverse reactions

CNS: *pain,* dizziness, *asthenia, headache,* insomnia, fever, paresthesia, depression, anxiety.
CV: *vasodilation,* chest pain, peripheral edema.
EENT: *pharyngitis.*
GI: *nausea, vomiting, constipation, abdominal pain, diarrhea,* anorexia.
GU: UTI.
Hematologic: anemia.
Musculoskeletal: *bone pain, back pain,* pelvic pain, arthritis.
Respiratory: *dyspnea, cough.*
Skin: rash, sweating.
Other: accidental injury, flulike syndrome, *injection-site pain.*

Interactions

None reported.

Effects on lab test results

• May decrease hemoglobin level and hematocrit.

Pharmacokinetics

Absorption: Unknown.
Distribution: Extensive and rapid. 99% bound to proteins.
Metabolism: Extensive, via several pathways.
Excretion: Hepatically cleared, 90% in feces.
Half-life: 29 to 51 days.

Route	Onset	Peak	Duration
I.M.	Unknown	7 days	1 mo

Action

Chemical effect: Competitively binds estrogen receptors and down-regulates estrogen-receptor protein in breast cancer cells.
Therapeutic effect: Fights cancer cells.

Available forms

Injection: 50 mg/ml in 2.5-ml and 5-ml pre-filled syringes

NURSING PROCESS

⚕ Assessment
• Monitor hemoglobin level and hematocrit before starting therapy and during therapy.
• Confirm that patient isn't pregnant before starting therapy.
• Observe injection site for local reaction.
• Assess patient's and family's knowledge of drug therapy.

✣ Nursing diagnoses
• Risk for imbalanced nutrition: less than body requirements, related to side effects of therapy
• Risk for acute pain related to side effects of therapy
• Deficient knowledge related to drug therapy

▷ Planning and implementation
• Because drug is given I.M., don't use in patients with bleeding diatheses or thrombocytopenia or in those taking anticoagulants.
• **ALERT:** The drug is packaged in one 5-ml prefilled syringe or two 2.5-ml prefilled syringes. If using the 2.5-ml syringes, both syringes must be given to achieve the full 250-mg recommended monthly dose.
• Expel the gas bubble from syringe before administration.

Patient teaching
• Tell patient the most common adverse reactions are GI symptoms, headache, back pain, hot flushes, and sore throat.
• Advise women of childbearing age to avoid pregnancy and to report suspected pregnancy immediately. Drug crosses the placenta after a single I.M. dose and harms the fetus.

✓ Evaluation
• Patient maintains adequate nutrition during therapy.
• Patient doesn't experience pain as an adverse effect.
• Patient and family state understanding of therapy.

furosemide (frusemide)
(fyoo-ROH-seh-mighd)
**Apo-Furosemide ♦ , Furoside ♦ , Lasix⌀ ,
Lasix Special ♦ , Novosemide ♦ ,
Uritol ♦**

Pharmacologic class: loop diuretic
Therapeutic class: diuretic, antihypertensive
Pregnancy risk category: C

Indications and dosages
▶ **Acute pulmonary edema.** *Adults:* 40 mg I.V. injected slowly over 1 to 2 minutes; then 80 mg I.V. in 1 to 1½ hours, if needed.
Infants and children: 1 mg/kg I.M. or I.V. If desired results don't occur after 2 hours, may increase initial dose by 1 mg/kg. Separate doses by at least 2 hours.
▶ **Edema.** *Adults:* 20 to 80 mg P.O. daily in morning; second dose in 6 to 8 hours. Carefully adjust up to 600 mg daily if needed. Or 20 to 40 mg I.M. or I.V.; increase by 20 mg q 2 hours until desired response occurs. Give I.V. dose slowly over 1 to 2 minutes.
Infants and children: 2 mg/kg P.O. daily; increase by 1 to 2 mg/kg in 6 to 8 hours, if needed. Carefully adjust up to 6 mg/kg daily, if needed. Or 1 mg/kg slow IV; increase by 1 mg/kg q 2 hours until desired response.
▶ **Heart failure and chronic renal impairment.** *Adults:* 2 to 2.5 g daily P.O. or I.V. Maximum I.V. injection, 1 g daily over 30 minutes.
▶ **Hypertension.** *Adults:* 40 mg P.O. b.i.d. Adjust dosage according to response.
▶ **Hypercalcemia‡.** *Adults:* 80 to 100 mg I.V. q 1 to 2 hours. Or 120 mg P.O. daily.

▽ I.V. administration
• Dilute with D₅W, normal saline solution, or lactated Ringer's solution,
• Infuse no more than 4 mg/minute to avoid ototoxicity.
• Give drug by direct injection over 1 to 2 minutes.
• Avoid exposing injection to light; it may discolor and become useable.
• Use prepared infusion solution within 24 hours.
⊗ **Incompatibilities**
Acidic solutions, aminoglycosides, amiodarone, ascorbic acid, bleomycin, buprenorphine, chlor-

promazine, diazepam, dobutamine, doxapram, doxorubicin, droperidol, epinephrine, erythromycin, esmolol, fluconazole, fructose 10% in water, gentamicin, hydralazine, idarubicin, invert sugar 10% in electrolyte #2, isoproterenol, meperidine, metoclopramide, milrinone, morphine, netilmicin, norepinephrine, ondansetron, prochlorperazine, promethazine, quinidine, vinblastine, vincristine.

Contraindications and cautions

• Contraindicated in patients hypersensitive to drug or any of its components and in those with anuria.
• Use cautiously in patients with hepatic cirrhosis.
• Patients with allergy to sulfonamides may also be allergic to furosemide.
✿ Lifespan: In pregnant women, use only if benefits outweigh risks to the fetus. In breastfeeding women, don't use drug.

Adverse reactions

CNS: fever, vertigo, headache, dizziness, paresthesia, restlessness, weakness.
CV: orthostatic hypotension, thrombophlebitis (with I.V. use), volume depletion, dehydration.
EENT: transient deafness, blurred or yellow vision.
GI: *pancreatitis,* anorexia, abdominal discomfort, diarrhea, nausea, vomiting, constipation.
GU: azotemia, nocturia, polyuria, frequent urination, oliguria.
Hematologic: *agranulocytosis, leukopenia, thrombocytopenia,* anemia, *aplastic anemia.*
Hepatic: hepatic dysfunction.
Metabolic: asymptomatic hyperuricemia, hyperglycemia and glucose intolerance, hypochloremic alkalosis, hypokalemia, fluid and electrolyte imbalances, including dilutional hyponatremia, hypocalcemia, and hypomagnesemia.
Musculoskeletal: muscle spasm.
Skin: dermatitis, purpura, photosensitivity.
Other: gout, transient pain at I.M. injection site.

Interactions

Drug-drug. *Aminoglycoside antibiotics, cisplatin:* May potentiate ototoxicity. Use together cautiously.
Amphotericin B, corticosteroids, corticotropin: May increase risk of hypokalemia. Monitor potassium level closely.

Antidiabetics: May decrease hypoglycemic effects. Monitor glucose level.
Antihypertensives: May increase risk of hypotension. Use together cautiously.
Chlorothiazide, chlorthalidone, hydrochlorothiazide, indapamide, metolazone: May cause excessive diuretic response, resulting in serious electrolyte abnormalities or dehydration. Adjust doses carefully while monitoring patient closely.
Digoxin, neuromuscular blockers: May increase toxicity from furosemide-induced hypokalemia. Monitor potassium level closely.
Ethacrynic acid: May increase risk of ototoxicity. Don't use together.
Lithium: May decrease lithium excretion, resulting in lithium toxicity. Monitor lithium level.
NSAIDs: May inhibit diuretic response. Use together cautiously.
Salicylates: May cause salicylate toxicity. Use together cautiously.
Drug-herb. *Aloe.* May increase drug effects. Monitor patient for dehydration.
Licorice: May cause rapid potassium loss. Monitor patient for hypokalemia; discourage licorice intake.
Drug-lifestyle. *Alcohol use:* May cause additive hypotensive and diuretic effect. Discourage use together.
Sun exposure: May cause photosensitivity reactions. Urge patient to avoid unprotected or prolonged sun exposure.

Effects on lab test results

• May increase glucose, cholesterol, and uric acid levels. May decrease potassium, sodium, calcium, magnesium, and hemoglobin levels and hematocrit.
• May decrease granulocyte, WBC, and platelet counts.

Pharmacokinetics

Absorption: 60% after P.O. use; unknown after I.M. use.
Distribution: 95% protein-bound.
Metabolism: Minimal.
Excretion: 50% to 80% in urine. *Half-life:* 30 minutes.

Route	Onset	Peak	Duration
P.O.	20–60 min	1–2 hr	6–8 hr
I.V.	5 min	30 min	2 hr
I.M.	Unknown	Unknown	Unknown

Action

Chemical effect: Inhibits sodium and chloride reabsorption at proximal and distal tubules and ascending loop of Henle.
Therapeutic effect: Promotes water and sodium excretion.

Available forms

Injection: 10 mg/ml
Oral solution: 40 mg/5 ml, 10 mg/ml
Tablets: 20 mg, 40 mg, 80 mg, 500 mg ♦

NURSING PROCESS

☑ Assessment
• Assess patient's underlying condition before starting therapy.
• Monitor weight, peripheral edema, breath sounds, blood pressure, fluid intake and output, and electrolyte, glucose, BUN, and carbon dioxide levels.
• Monitor uric acid level, especially if patient has a history of gout.
• Be alert for adverse reactions and drug interactions.
• Assess patient's and family's knowledge of drug therapy.

⊕ Nursing diagnoses
• Excessive fluid volume related to presence of edema
• Impaired urinary elimination related to diuretic therapy
• Deficient knowledge related to drug therapy

▶ Planning and implementation
• Give a P.O. or I.M. dose in the morning to prevent nocturia. Give a second dose in early afternoon.
• Store tablets in light-resistant container to prevent discoloration. Don't use yellowed injectable preparation.
• Refrigerate oral furosemide solution to ensure drug stability.
• If oliguria or azotemia develops or increases, notify prescriber.
Patient teaching
• Advise patient to stand slowly to prevent dizziness, not to drink alcohol, and to minimize strenuous exercise in hot weather.
• Instruct patient to report ringing in ears, severe abdominal pain, or sore throat and fever because they may indicate toxicity.

⊛ **ALERT:** Discourage patient from storing different drugs in same container because this increases risk of errors. The most popular strengths of furosemide and digoxin are white tablets of similar size.
• Tell patient to check with prescriber before taking OTC drugs or herbal remedies.

☑ Evaluation
• Patient is free from edema.
• Patient demonstrates adjustment of lifestyle to cope with altered patterns of urinary elimination.
• Patient and family state understanding of drug therapy.

gabapentin
(geh-buh-PEN-tin)
Neurontin✍

Pharmacologic class: anticonvulsant
Therapeutic class: anticonvulsant
Pregnancy risk category: C

Indications and dosages

▶ **Adjunct therapy of partial seizures with and without secondary generalization in patients with epilepsy.** *Adults and children older than age 12:* Initially, 300 mg P.O. t.i.d. Increase dosage gradually based on response. Dosages of 900 to 1,800 mg daily in three divided doses are effective for most patients. Dosages up to 3,600 mg daily are well tolerated.
Children ages 3 to 12: Starting dosage, 10 to 15 mg/kg P.O. daily in three divided doses; adjust over 3 days to reach effective dosage.
Children ages 5 to 12: Effective dosage, 25 to 35 mg/kg P.O. daily in three divided doses.
Children ages 3 to 4: Effective dosage, 40 mg/kg P.O. daily in three divided doses.
⊠ **Adjust-a-dose:** For adults and children age 12 and older with renal impairment or undergoing hemodialysis, if creatinine clearance is 30 to 59 ml/minute, give 400 to 1,400 mg P.O. daily, divided b.i.d. If creatinine clearance is 15 to 29 ml/minute, give 200 to 700 mg P.O. daily. If

creatinine clearance is less than 15 ml/minute, give 100 to 300 mg P.O. daily; reduce dose in proportion to creatinine clearance (for example, for patients with a creatinine clearance of 7.5 ml/minute, give one-half the dose that a patient with 15 ml/minute would receive).

For dialysis patients, maintenance dosages are based on estimated creatinine clearance. Give supplemental postdialysis dose of 125 to 350 mg after each 4 hours of dialysis.
▶ **Postherpetic neuralgia.** *Adults:* 300 mg P.O. once daily on day 1, then 300 mg b.i.d. on day 2, and 300 mg t.i.d. on day 3. Adjust p.r.n. for pain relief to maximum daily dosage, 1,800 mg, divided t.i.d.

Contraindications and cautions

● Contraindicated in patients hypersensitive to the drug or any of its components.
⚡ **Lifespan:** In pregnant women, use cautiously. In breast-feeding women and in children younger than age 3, safety and effectiveness haven't been established. In children ages 3 to 12, use cautiously; drug may cause mild to moderate emotional lability, hostility, aggressive behavior, and hyperkinesias.

Adverse reactions

CNS: *somnolence, dizziness, ataxia, fatigue, nystagmus, tremor,* nervousness, dysarthria, amnesia, depression, abnormal thinking, twitching, abnormal coordination.
CV: peripheral edema, vasodilation.
EENT: *diplopia, rhinitis,* pharyngitis, dry throat, *amblyopia.*
GI: nausea, vomiting, dyspepsia, dry mouth, constipation.
GU: impotence.
Hematologic: *leukopenia.*
Metabolic: increased appetite, weight gain.
Musculoskeletal: back pain, myalgia, fractures.
Respiratory: cough.
Skin: pruritus, abrasion.
Other: dental abnormalities.

Interactions

Drug-drug. *Antacids:* May decrease gabapentin absorption. Separate administration times by at least 2 hours.
Morphine: May increase gabapentin level and risk of CNS depression. Decrease dose of either drug.

Drug-lifestyle. *Alcohol use:* May increase CNS depression. Discourage use together.

Effects on lab test results

● May decrease WBC count.
● May cause false-positive tests for urine protein when Ames-N-Multistix SG dipstick test is used.

Pharmacokinetics

Absorption: Bioavailability isn't dose-proportional but averages 60%.
Distribution: Circulates largely unbound to protein.
Metabolism: Insignificant.
Excretion: By kidneys as unchanged drug.
Half-life: 5 to 7 hours.

Route	Onset	Peak	Duration
P.O.	Unknown	2–4 hr	Unknown

Action

Chemical effect: Unknown; although structurally related to GABA, drug doesn't interact with GABA receptors and isn't converted metabolically into GABA or a GABA agonist.
Therapeutic effect: Prevents and treats partial seizures and treats postherpetic neuralgia.

Available forms

Capsules: 100 mg, 300 mg, 400 mg, 800 mg
Solution: 250 mg/5 ml
Tablets (film-coated): 100 mg, 300 mg, 400 mg, 600 mg, 800 mg

NURSING PROCESS

Assessment
● Assess patient's disorder before starting therapy and regularly thereafter.
● Routine monitoring of level isn't needed. Drug doesn't appear to alter levels of other anticonvulsants.
● Be alert for adverse reactions and drug interactions.
● Assess patient's and family's knowledge of drug therapy.

Nursing diagnoses
● Risk for trauma related to seizures
● Risk for injury related to drug-induced adverse CNS reactions
● Deficient knowledge related to drug therapy

▶ Planning and implementation

- Give first dose h.s. to minimize drowsiness, dizziness, fatigue, and ataxia.

ALERT: If stopping drug or substituting another drug, do so gradually over at least 1 week to minimize risk of seizures. Don't abruptly stop other anticonvulsants when starting therapy.

- Take seizure precautions.

ALERT: Don't confuse Neurontin with Noroxin.

Patient teaching

- Tell patient drug can be taken with or without food.
- Warn patient to avoid hazardous activities until the drug's CNS effects are known.

✓ Evaluation

- Patient is free from seizures.
- Patient has no injury from adverse CNS reactions.
- Patient and family state understanding of drug therapy.

galantamine hydrobromide

(gah-LAN-tah-meen high-droh-BROH-mide)
Razadyne, Razadyne ER

Pharmacologic class: reversible, competitive acetylcholinesterase inhibitor
Therapeutic class: cholinomimetic
Pregnancy risk category: B

Indications and dosages

▶ **Mild to moderate dementia of Alzheimer's type.** *Adults:* Initially, 4 mg P.O. b.i.d., preferably with morning and evening meals. If dose is well tolerated after minimum of 4 weeks of therapy, increase to 8 mg b.i.d. A further increase to 12 mg b.i.d. may be attempted only after at least 4 weeks of the previous dose. Recommended dosage range is 16 to 24 mg daily in two divided doses. Or if using the extended-release form, 8 mg P.O. once daily in the morning with food. Increase to 16 mg P.O. once daily after a minimum of 4 weeks. May further increase to 24 mg once daily after a minimum of 4 weeks, based on patient response and tolerability.

Adjust-a-dose: For patients with hepatic impairment with a Child-Pugh score of 7 to 9, don't exceed 16 mg daily. For patients with a Child-Pugh score of 10 to 15, don't give drug. For patients with moderate renal impairment, don't exceed 16 mg daily. For patients with creatinine clearance less than 9 ml/minute, don't give drug.

Contraindications and cautions

- Contraindicated in patients hypersensitive to the drug or any of its components.
- Use cautiously in patients with supraventricular cardiac conduction disorders and in those taking other drugs that significantly slow the heart rate. Use cautiously before or during procedures involving anesthesia with succinylcholine-type or other similar neuromuscular blockers. Use cautiously in patients with a history of peptic ulcer disease and in those taking NSAIDs. Because of the potential for cholinomimetic effects, use cautiously in patients with bladder outflow obstruction, seizures, asthma, or COPD.

Lifespan: In pregnant women, use only if benefits outweigh risks to the fetus. In breast-feeding women, use cautiously because it's unknown if drug appears in breast milk. In children, safety and effectiveness haven't been established.

Adverse reactions

CNS: dizziness, headache, tremor, depression, insomnia, somnolence, fatigue, syncope.
CV: ***bradycardia,*** heart block.
EENT: rhinitis.
GI: *nausea, vomiting,* anorexia, *diarrhea,* abdominal pain, dyspepsia.
GU: UTI, hematuria.
Hematologic: anemia.
Metabolic: weight loss.

Interactions

Drug-drug. *Amitriptyline, fluoxetine, fluvoxamine, quinidine:* May decrease galantamine clearance. Monitor patient closely.
Anticholinergics: May antagonize activity of anticholinergics. Monitor patient.
Cholinergics (such as bethanechol, succinylcholine): May have a synergistic effect. Monitor patient closely. May need to avoid use before procedures using general anesthesia with succinylcholine-type neuromuscular blockers.
Cimetidine, erythromycin, ketoconazole, paroxetine: May increase bioavailability of galantamine. Monitor patient closely.

Effects on lab test results

• May decrease hemoglobin level and hematocrit.

Pharmacokinetics

Absorption: Rapid and good, with an oral bioavailability of about 90%. Levels peak in 1 hour. In elderly patients, levels are 30% to 40% higher than in young, healthy people.
Distribution: Primarily to blood. Protein binding isn't significant.
Metabolism: In liver by CYP 2D6 and CYP 3A4 and glucuronidated. Using with inhibitors of these enzyme systems may result in modest increases in drug bioavailability.
Excretion: In urine, unchanged as glucuronide and metabolites. *Half-life:* About 7 hours.

Route	Onset	Peak	Duration
P.O.	Unknown	1 hr	Unknown

Action

Chemical effect: Unknown; may enhance cholinergic function by increasing the level of acetylcholine in the brain.
Therapeutic effect: Improves cognition in patients with Alzheimer's disease.

Available forms

Oral solution: 4 mg/ml
Tablets: 4 mg, 8 mg, 12 mg
Capsules (extended-release): 8 mg, 16 mg, 24 mg
Oral solution and tablets are bioequivalent.

NURSING PROCESS

Assessment

• Assess underlying condition before starting therapy, and reassess regularly.
• Bradycardia and heart block have been reported in patients with and without underlying cardiac conduction abnormalities. Consider all patients at risk for adverse effects on cardiac conduction.
• Patients are at increased risk for gastric ulcers because of the potential for increased gastric acid secretion. Monitor patient closely for symptoms of active or occult GI bleeding.
• Assess patient's and family's knowledge of drug therapy.

Nursing diagnoses

• Risk for injury due to wandering related to Alzheimer's disease
• Risk for imbalanced fluid volume related to drug-induced adverse GI reactions
• Deficient knowledge related to drug therapy

Planning and implementation

• Give drug with food and ensure adequate fluid intake to decrease the risk of nausea and vomiting.
• If drug is stopped for several days, restart at the lowest dose and increase, at a minimum of 4-week intervals, to the previous dose.
• Use proper technique when dispensing the oral solution with the pipette. Dispense measured amount in a liquid and give right away.
• Don't give more than 16 mg daily in patients with moderate hepatic or renal impairment.
• In case of overdose, contact a poison control center. Treat symptoms and provide support. Atropine I.V. may be used as an antidote; give an initial dose of 0.5 to 1 mg and base subsequent doses on response. It's unknown if drug is removed by dialysis.

Patient teaching
• Advise patient or his caregiver that the conventional tablets should be taken with morning and evening meals and the extended-release capsules should be taken with the morning meal.
• Inform patient or caregiver that dosage increases should occur at no more than 4-week intervals.
• Explain that nausea and vomiting occur in less than 25% of patients.
• Advise patient or caregiver that following the recommended dosing and administration schedule can minimize common adverse effects.
• Tell patient or caregiver, if therapy is interrupted for several days or longer, to restart the drug at the lowest dose and increase based on the prescriber's dosing schedule.
• Advise patient or caregiver to report signs and symptoms of bradycardia immediately to the prescriber.
• Advise patient or caregiver that drug may enhance cognitive function, but may not alter the underlying disease process.

Evaluation

• Patient's cognition improves and tendency to wander decreases.

• Patient and family state that drug-induced adverse GI reactions haven't occurred.
• Patient and family state understanding of drug therapy.

ganciclovir (DHPG)
(jan-SIGH-kloh-veer)
Cytovene, Cytovene-IV

Pharmacologic class: synthetic nucleoside
Therapeutic class: antiviral
Pregnancy risk category: C

Indications and dosages

▶ **CMV retinitis in immunocompromised patients, including those with AIDS.** *Adults:* 5 mg/kg I.V. over 1 hour q 12 hours for 14 to 21 days, followed by 5 mg/kg I.V. daily for 7 days weekly, or 6 mg/kg I.V. daily for 5 of 7 days weekly. Or, following I.V. induction therapy, give 1,000 mg P.O. t.i.d. with food or 500 mg P.O. six times a day q 3 hours with food while awake.
▶ **To prevent CMV disease in transplant recipients at risk for CMV disease.** *Adults:* 5 mg/kg I.V. over 1 hour q 12 hours for 7 to 14 days, followed by 5 mg/kg I.V. once daily, or 6 mg/kg I.V. once daily for 5 of 7 days weekly. Alternatively, 1,000 mg P.O. t.i.d. with food. Length of therapy in transplant recipients depends on duration and degree of immunosuppression.
▶ **To prevent CMV disease in patients with advanced HIV infection at risk for development of CMV disease.** *Adults:* 1,000 mg P.O. t.i.d. with food.
▶ **Other CMV infections‡.** *Adults:* 5 mg/kg I.V. over 1 hour q 12 hours for 14 to 21 days. Or 2.5 mg/kg I.V. over 1 hour q 8 hours for 14 to 21 days.
§ **Adjust-a-dose:** For patients with renal impairment, adjust dosage according to the table at the top of page 625. For patients receiving hemodialysis, see dosages for creatinine clearance greater than 10 ml/minute.

▼ I.V. administration

• Reconstitute with 10 ml sterile water for injection. Shake vial to dissolve drug.

• Further dilute appropriate dose in normal saline solution, D_5W, Ringer's lactate, or Ringer's solution (typically 100 ml).
• Use caution when preparing alkaline solution.
• Infuse over 1 hour. Faster infusions will cause increased toxicity. Never exceed recommended infusion rate. Use infusion pump. Don't give as I.V. bolus or by rapid infusion.
• Infusion concentrations greater than 10 mg/ml aren't recommended.

⊗ **Incompatibilities**
Aldesleukin, amifostine, aztreonam, cefepime, cytarabine, doxorubicin hydrochloride, fludarabine, foscarnet, ondansetron, paraben (bacteriostatic agent), piperacillin sodium with tazobactam, sargramostim, vinorelbine. Manufacturer recommends not giving with other I.V. drugs.

Contraindications and cautions

• Contraindicated in patients hypersensitive to ganciclovir or acyclovir. Patients with allergies to acyclovir may also react to ganciclovir. Also contraindicated in those with absolute neutrophil count below $500/mm^3$ or platelet count below $25,000/mm^3$.
• Use cautiously and at a lower dosage in patients with renal impairment.
⚠ **Lifespan:** In pregnant women, use only if benefits outweigh risks to the fetus. In breastfeeding women, use cautiously because it isn't known if drug appears in breast milk. In children, safety and effectiveness haven't been established.

Adverse reactions

CNS: *seizures, coma,* altered dreams, confusion, ataxia, dizziness, headache, pain, behavioral changes.
CV: *arrhythmias,* hypotension, hypertension.
EENT: retinal detachment in CMV retinitis.
GI: nausea, vomiting, diarrhea, anorexia.
GU: hematuria.
Hematologic: *thrombocytopenia, agranulocytosis, leukopenia, granulocytopenia,* anemia.
Other: inflammation, phlebitis at injection site.

Interactions

Drug-drug. *Cytotoxic drugs:* May increase toxic effects, especially hematologic effects and stomatitis. Monitor patient closely.
Imipenem and cilastatin: May heighten seizure activity. Monitor patient closely.

Creatinine clearance (ml/min)	Initial I.V. dosage		Maintenance I.V. dosage		P.O. dosage	
	Dose (mg/kg)	Interval	Dose (mg/kg)	Interval	Dose (mg)	Interval
50–69	2.5	12 hr	2.5	24 hr	1,500	24 hr
					500	8 hr
25–49	2.5	24 hr	1.25	24 hr	1,000	24 hr
					500	12 hr
10–24	1.25	24 hr	0.625	24 hr	500	24 hr
< 10	1.25	3 times/wk	0.625	3 times/wk	500	3 times/wk

Immunosuppressants (such as azathioprine, corticosteroids, cyclosporine): May enhance immune and bone marrow suppression. Use together cautiously.
Probenecid: May increase ganciclovir level. Monitor patient closely.
Zidovudine: May increase risk of granulocytopenia. Monitor patient closely.

Effects on lab test results

• May increase creatinine, ALT, AST, GGT, and alkaline phosphatase levels. May decrease hemoglobin level and hematocrit.
• May decrease granulocyte, platelet, neutrophil, and WBC counts.

Pharmacokinetics

Absorption: Poor. Bioavailability is about 5% under fasting conditions.
Distribution: Preferentially concentrates in CMV-infected cells.
Metabolism: Less than 10%.
Excretion: Mostly unchanged. *Half-life:* About 3 hours.

Route	Onset	Peak	Duration
P.O.	Unknown	3 hr	Unknown
I.V.	Immediate	Immediate	Unknown

Action

Chemical effect: Unknown, may inhibit viral DNA synthesis of CMV.
Therapeutic effect: Inhibits CMV.

Available forms

Capsules: 250 mg, 500 mg
Injection: 500 mg/vial

NURSING PROCESS

G

✍ Assessment
• Assess patient's condition before starting therapy and regularly thereafter.
• Obtain CBC, neutrophil, and platelet counts every 2 days during twice-daily ganciclovir use and at least weekly thereafter.
• Monitor hydration if adverse GI reaction occurs with oral drug.
• Be alert for adverse reactions and drug interactions.
• Assess patient's and family's knowledge of drug therapy.

⊕ Nursing diagnoses
• Infection related to CMV retinitis
• Ineffective protection related to adverse hematologic reactions
• Deficient knowledge related to drug therapy

▷ Planning and implementation
• Give oral form of drug with food.
• **ALERT:** Don't give drug subcutaneously or I.M. because severe tissue irritation could result.
• **ALERT:** Encourage fluid intake; ensure adequate hydration during drug infusion.
• Alert prescriber to signs of renal impairment because the dosage will need adjustment.
• Capsules are linked to a risk of rapid progression of CMV retinitis. Don't use capsules for induction therapy; use only as maintenance therapy in patients who benefit from not taking drug I.V.

Patient teaching
• Tell patient to take oral form of drug with food.
• Stress importance of drinking adequate fluids throughout therapy.
• Advise patient to report pain or discomfort at I.V. site.

• Instruct patient about infection-control and bleeding precautions.

☑ Evaluation
• Patient is free from infection.
• Patient has no serious adverse hematologic reactions.
• Patient and family state understanding of drug therapy.

ganirelix acetate
(gan-eh-REL-iks AS-ih-tayt)
Antagon

Pharmacologic class: gonadotropin-releasing hormone (Gn-RH) antagonist
Therapeutic class: fertility drug
Pregnancy risk category: X

Indications and dosages

▶ **To inhibit premature luteinizing hormone (LH) surges in women undergoing medically supervised, controlled ovarian hyperstimulation.** *Women:* 250 mcg subcutaneously once daily during early to midfollicular phase of menstrual cycle. Continue daily until enough follicles of sufficient size are confirmed by ultrasound; human chorionic gonadotropin will then be given to induce final maturation of follicles.

Contraindications and cautions

• Contraindicated in patients hypersensitive to the drug or any of its components or to Gn-RH or Gn-RH analog.
• Use cautiously in patients with potential hypersensitivity to Gn-RH and in those with latex allergies because the product packaging contains natural rubber latex.
⚠ **Lifespan:** In pregnant women, drug is contraindicated. In breast-feeding women, avoid using drug. In children, drug is contraindicated.

Adverse reactions

CNS: headache.
GI: abdominal pain, nausea.
GU: vaginal bleeding, gynecologic abdominal pain, ovarian hyperstimulation syndrome, miscarriage.
Other: injection-site reaction.

Interactions
None reported.

Effects on lab test results
• May decrease bilirubin and hemoglobin levels and hematocrit.
• May increase WBC count.

Pharmacokinetics
Absorption: Rapid, with an average of 91% absorbed.
Distribution: 82% bound to proteins.
Metabolism: Drug is found essentially unchanged in urine up to 24 hours after dose. Two metabolites have been detected in feces.
Excretion: Primarily in feces. *Half-life:* 13 to 16 hours.

Route	Onset	Peak	Duration
SubQ	Unknown	1 hr	Unknown

Action
Chemical effect: Blocks pituitary Gn-RH receptors and suppresses LH and follicle-stimulating hormone (FSH) secretion. This suppression in the early- to mid-menstrual cycle stops premature gonadotropin surges that could interfere with medically supervised ovarian hyperstimulation.
Therapeutic effect: Increases fertility.

Available forms
Injection: 250 mcg/0.5 ml in prefilled syringes

NURSING PROCESS

☞ Assessment
• Before starting therapy, make sure patient isn't pregnant.
• Carefully monitor a patient who reports previous potential hypersensitivity to Gn-RH; monitor patient closely after first injection.
• Assess patient's and family's knowledge of drug therapy.

⊞ Nursing diagnoses
• Disturbed self-esteem related to infertility
• Acute pain secondary to drug-induced adverse reactions
• Deficient knowledge related to drug therapy

Reactions may be *common*, uncommon, *life-threatening*, or COMMON AND LIFE-THREATENING.

⊠ Planning and implementation
• Only prescribers experienced in infertility therapy should prescribe this drug.
• Natural rubber latex packaging of this product may cause allergic reactions in a hypersensitive patient.

Patient teaching
• Tell patient that the correct use of drug injection is extremely important to the success of the fertility therapy. Patient must be able to follow a strict administration schedule.
• Teach patient proper technique for subcutaneous injection of drug.
• Advise patient to use the abdomen or upper thigh for injection and to alternate injection sites with each dose.
• Advise patient to store drug at room temperature, away from heat and light, and out of children's reach.

☑ Evaluation
• Patient becomes pregnant.
• Patient has no adverse reactions.
• Patient and family state understanding of drug therapy.

gatifloxacin
(gah-tih-FLOCKS-ah-sin)
Tequin

Pharmacologic class: fluoroquinolone
Therapeutic class: antibiotic
Pregnancy risk category: C

Indications and dosages
▶ **Acute bacterial exacerbation of chronic bronchitis caused by** *Streptococcus pneumoniae, Haemophilus influenzae, Haemophilus parainfluenzae, Moraxella catarrhalis,* **or** *Staphylococcus aureus. Adults:* 400 mg I.V. or P.O. daily for 5 days.
▶ **Complicated UTI caused by** *Escherichia coli, Klebsiella pneumoniae,* **or** *Proteus mirabilis;* **acute pyelonephritis caused by** *E. coli. Adults:* 400 mg I.V. or P.O. daily for 7 to 10 days.
▶ **Acute sinusitis caused by** *S. pneumoniae* **or** *H. influenzae. Adults:* 400 mg I.V. or P.O. daily for 10 days.
▶ **Community-acquired pneumonia caused by** *S. pneumoniae, H. influenzae, H. parain-*

fluenzae, M. catarrhalis, S. aureus, Mycoplasma pneumoniae, Chlamydia pneumoniae, **or** *Legionella pneumophila. Adults:* 400 mg I.V. or P.O. daily for 7 to 14 days.
▶ **Uncomplicated urethral gonorrhea in men and cervical gonorrhea or acute uncomplicated rectal infections in women caused by** *Neisseria gonorrhoeae. Adults:* 400 mg P.O. as single dose.
▶ **Uncomplicated UTI caused by** *E. coli, K. pneumoniae,* **or** *P. mirabilis. Adults:* 400 mg I.V. or P.O. as single dose, or 200 mg I.V. or P.O. daily for 3 days.
▶ **Uncomplicated skin and skin-structure infections caused by** *S. aureus* **(methicillin-susceptible strains only) or** *Streptococcus pyogenes. Adults:* 400 mg I.V. or P.O. daily for 7 to 10 days.
▶ **Postexposure to inhalation anthrax, inhalation anthrax‡, prevention or treatment when parenteral therapy isn't available.** *Adults:* 400 mg P.O. once daily for 60 days.
⑤ **Adjust-a-dose:** For patients with renal impairment, if creatinine clearance is less than 40 ml/minute or if the patient is on hemodialysis or continuous peritoneal dialysis, give initial dose of 400 mg P.O., followed by 200 mg P.O. daily.

▼ I.V. administration
• Dilute drug in single-use vials with D_5W or normal saline solution to 2 mg/ml.
• Infuse over 60 minutes.
• Discard any unused portion of single-dose vials.
• Diluted solutions are stable for 14 days at room temperature or refrigerated. Frozen solutions are stable for up to 6 months, except for 5% sodium bicarbonate solutions. Thaw at room temperature. After thawing, solutions are stable for 14 days when stored at room temperature or refrigerated.
⊗ **Incompatibilities**
Other I.V. drugs.

Contraindications and cautions
• Contraindicated in patients hypersensitive to fluoroquinolones or in patients with prolonged QTc interval or uncorrected hypokalemia.
• Use cautiously in patients with significant bradycardia, acute myocardial ischemia, known or suspected CNS disorders, or renal insufficiency.

✳ **Lifespan:** In pregnant women, use only if benefits outweigh risks to the fetus. Breast-feeding women should either stop nursing or not take the drug, taking into account the importance of the drug to the mother. In children, safety and effectiveness haven't been established.

Adverse reactions

CNS: headache, dizziness, abnormal dreams, insomnia, paresthesia, tremor, fever, vertigo.
CV: palpitations, hypertension, chest pain, peripheral edema.
EENT: tinnitus, abnormal vision, pharyngitis.
GI: nausea, diarrhea, abdominal pain, constipation, dyspepsia, oral candidiasis, *pseudomembranous colitis,* glossitis, stomatitis, mouth ulcer, vomiting, disturbed taste.
GU: dysuria, hematuria, vaginitis.
Metabolic: hyperglycemia.
Musculoskeletal: arthralgia, myalgia, back pain, tendon rupture.
Respiratory: dyspnea.
Skin: rash, sweating.
Other: *anaphylaxis,* chills, redness at injection site, hypersensitivity.

Interactions

Drug-drug. *Aluminum hydroxide, aluminum-magnesium hydroxide, calcium carbonate, magnesium hydroxide:* May decrease effects of gatifloxacin. Give antacid at least 4 hours before or 2 hours after gatifloxacin.
Antidiabetics (glyburide, insulin): May cause symptoms of hypoglycemia or hyperglycemia. Monitor glucose level.
Antipsychotics, cisapride, erythromycin, tricyclic antidepressants: May prolong QT interval. Use cautiously.
Class IA antiarrhythmics (procainamide, quinidine), class III antiarrhythmics (amiodarone, sotalol): May prolong QT interval. Avoid use together.
NSAIDs: May increase risk of CNS stimulation and seizures. Use together cautiously.
Probenecid: May increase gatifloxacin level and prolong its half-life. Monitor patient closely.
Warfarin: May enhance effects of warfarin. Monitor PT and INR.
Drug-lifestyle. *Sun exposure:* Photosensitivity reactions may occur. Urge patient to avoid unprotected or prolonged sun exposure.

Effects on lab test results

● May increase ALT, AST, and LDH levels.

Pharmacokinetics

Absorption: Good.
Distribution: Wide. 20% protein-bound.
Metabolism: Limited biotransformation.
Excretion: More than 70% excreted unchanged by the kidneys. *Half-life:* 7 to 14 hours.

Route	Onset	Peak	Duration
P.O.	Unknown	1–2 hr	Unknown
I.V.	Unknown	Unknown	Unknown

Action

Chemical effect: Inhibits DNA gyrase and topoisomerase, preventing cell replication and division. It's active against gram-positive and gram-negative organisms.
Therapeutic effect: Kills susceptible bacteria.

Available forms

Injection: 200 mg/20-ml vial, 400 mg/40-ml vial; 200 mg in 100 ml D_5W, 400 mg in 200 ml D_5W
Tablets: 200 mg, 400 mg

NURSING PROCESS

⚚ **Assessment**
● In patient being treated for gonorrhea, test for syphilis and chlamydia at time of diagnosis.
● In patient with renal insufficiency, monitor kidney function.
● In patient with diabetes, monitor glucose level.
● Monitor patient on digoxin for digoxin toxicity.
● Be alert for adverse reactions and drug interactions.
● Assess patient's and family's knowledge of drug therapy.

⊕ **Nursing diagnoses**
● Infection related to presence of bacteria susceptible to drug
● Risk for injury related to drug-induced adverse reactions
● Deficient knowledge related to drug therapy

▷ **Planning and implementation**
● Give oral form of drug 4 hours before antacids containing aluminum or magnesium, didanosine

buffered solution tablets or buffered powder, or products containing zinc, magnesium, or iron.
• If patient has seizures, increased intracranial pressure, psychosis, or CNS stimulation leading to tremors, restlessness, light-headedness, confusion, hallucinations, paranoia, depression, nightmares, or insomnia, stop giving drug and notify prescriber.
• If patient has a rash or other signs of hypersensitivity, stop giving drug and notify prescriber.
• If patient has pain, inflammation, or rupture of a tendon, stop giving drug and notify prescriber.
• Monitor patient for diarrhea because pseudomembranous colitis may occur in patients taking antibiotics.
⑤ **ALERT:** Don't confuse Tequin with Ticlid or Tegretol.

Patient teaching
• Tell patient to take drug as prescribed and to finish all the medication even if symptoms disappear.
• Advise patient to take drug 4 hours before products containing aluminum, magnesium, zinc, or iron.
• Advise patient to use sunblock and protective clothing when exposed to excessive sunlight.
• Warn patient to avoid hazardous tasks until adverse CNS effects of drugs are known.
• Advise diabetic patient to monitor glucose level and to notify prescriber if hypoglycemia occurs.
• Advise patient to immediately report palpitations; fainting spells; rash; hives; difficulty swallowing or breathing; swelling of the lips, tongue, or face; tightness in throat; hoarseness; or other symptoms of allergic reaction.
• Advise patient to stop drug, refrain from exercise, and notify prescriber about pain, inflammation, or rupture of a tendon.

☑ Evaluation
• Patient is free from infection after drug therapy.
• Patient has no injury as a result of drug-induced adverse reactions.
• Patient and family state understanding of drug therapy.

gatifloxacin ophthalmic solution
(gah-ti-FLOCKS-ah-sin off-THAL-mick suh-LOO-shun)
Zymar

Pharmacologic class: fluoroquinolone
Therapeutic class: antibiotic
Pregnancy risk category: C

Indications and dosages
▶ **Bacterial conjunctivitis.** *Adults and children age 1 and older:* While patient is awake, instill 1 drop into affected eyes q 2 hours up to eight times daily for 2 days. Then, instill 1 drop up to four times daily for 5 more days.

Contraindications and cautions
• Contraindicated in patients hypersensitive to the drug or any of its components or to quinolones or any of their components.
⚕ **Lifespan:** In pregnant women, use cautiously. In breast-feeding women, use cautiously because it's unknown if the drug appears in breast milk. In children younger than age 1 year, drug is contraindicated.

Adverse reactions
CNS: headache.
EENT: chemosis, conjunctival hemorrhage, *conjunctival irritation,* discharge, dry eyes, eye irritation, eyelid edema, *increased lacrimation, keratitis,* pain, *papillary conjunctivitis,* red eyes, reduced visual acuity.
GI: taste disturbance.

Interactions
None reported.

Effects on lab test results
None reported.

Pharmacokinetics
Absorption: Unknown.
Distribution: Unknown.
Metabolism: Unknown.
Excretion: Unknown. *Half-life:* Unknown.

Route	Onset	Peak	Duration
Ophthalmic	Unknown	Unknown	Unknown

Action

Chemical effect: Inhibits DNA gyrase and topoisomerase, preventing cell replication and division.
Therapeutic effect: Kills susceptible bacteria.

Available forms

Solution: 0.3% in 2.5- and 5-ml bottles

NURSING PROCESS

⚎ Assessment
• Monitor therapy for effectiveness.
• Monitor patient for adverse reactions.
• Assess patient's and family's knowledge of drug therapy.

⊕ Nursing diagnoses
• Disturbed visual perception related to eye infection
• Deficient knowledge related to drug therapy

▷ Planning and implementation
• Don't inject solution subconjunctivally or into the anterior chamber of the eye.
• Systemic drug causes serious hypersensitivity reactions. If allergic reaction occurs, stop giving the drug and treat symptoms.
• Monitor patient for superinfection.
Patient teaching
• Tell patient to immediately stop taking the drug and seek medical treatment if evidence of a serious allergic reaction develops, such as itching, rash, swelling of the face or throat, or difficulty breathing.
• Tell patient not to wear contact lenses.
• Warn patient to avoid touching the applicator tip to anything, including eyes and fingers.
• Teach patient that prolonged use may encourage infections with nonsusceptible bacteria.

▨ Evaluation
• Patient recovers from infection.
• Patient and family state understanding of drug therapy.

gemfibrozil
(jem-FIGH-broh-zil)
Apo-Gemfibrozil ◆ , Gen-Fibro ◆ , Lopid, Novo-Gemfibrozil ◆ , Nu-Gemfibrozil ◆

Pharmacologic class: fibric acid derivative
Therapeutic class: antilipemic
Pregnancy risk category: C

Indications and dosages

▶ **Type IV and V hyperlipidemia unresponsive to diet and other drugs; reduction of risk of coronary heart disease in patients with type IIb hyperlipidemia who can't tolerate or who are refractory to therapy with bile acid sequestrants or niacin.** *Adults:* 1,200 mg P.O. daily in two divided doses, 30 minutes before morning and evening meals. If no benefit occurs after 3 months, stop drug.

Contraindications and cautions

• Contraindicated in patients hypersensitive to the drug or any of its components and in those with hepatic or severe renal dysfunction (including primary biliary cirrhosis) or gallbladder disease.
⚖ **Lifespan:** In pregnant women, use cautiously. In breast-feeding women and in children, safety and effectiveness haven't been established.

Adverse reactions

CNS: blurred vision, headache, dizziness, fatigue.
GI: *abdominal and epigastric pain,* diarrhea, nausea, vomiting, flatulence, *dyspepsia,* taste perversion.
Hematologic: *severe anemia, leukopenia, thrombocytopenia, bone marrow hypoplasia.*
Hepatic: bile duct obstruction, gallstones.
Musculoskeletal: painful limbs, *rhabdomyolysis.*
Skin: rash, dermatitis, pruritus.

Interactions

Drug-drug. *Cyclosporine:* May decrease cyclosporine effects. Monitor cyclosporine level.
HMG-CoA reductase inhibitors: Myopathy with rhabdomyolysis may occur. Don't use together.
Oral anticoagulants: May enhance effects of oral anticoagulants. Monitor patient.

Reactions may be *common,* uncommon, *life-threatening*, or COMMON AND LIFE-THREATENING.

Repaglinide: May increase repaglinide level. Avoid use together.

Effects on lab test results

• May increase ALT, AST, and CK levels. May decrease potassium and hemoglobin levels and hematocrit.

• May decrease eosinophil, WBC, and platelet counts.

Pharmacokinetics

Absorption: Good.
Distribution: 95% protein-bound.
Metabolism: By liver.
Excretion: Primarily in urine. *Half-life:* 1¼ hours.

Route	Onset	Peak	Duration
P.O.	2–5 days	> 4 wk	Unknown

Action

Chemical effect: Inhibits peripheral lipolysis and also reduces triglyceride synthesis in liver.
Therapeutic effect: Lowers triglyceride levels and raises HDL levels.

Available forms

Tablets: 600 mg

NURSING PROCESS

Assessment

• Obtain patient's triglyceride and HDL levels before starting therapy and regularly thereafter.

• Obtain CBC and liver function tests periodically during first 12 months of therapy.

• Be alert for adverse reactions and drug interactions.

• Assess patient's and family's knowledge of drug therapy.

Nursing diagnoses

• Risk for injury related to elevated blood lipids and cholesterol levels

• Diarrhea related to drug's adverse effect on GI tract

• Deficient knowledge related to drug therapy

Planning and implementation

• Give drug 30 minutes before breakfast and dinner.

• Make sure patient is following standard low-cholesterol diet.

Patient teaching

• Instruct patient to take drug 30 minutes before breakfast and dinner.

• Teach patient dietary management of lipids (restricting total fat and cholesterol intake) and measures to control other cardiac disease risk factors. If appropriate, suggest weight control, exercise, and smoking cessation programs.

• Advise patient to avoid driving or other potentially hazardous activities until drug's CNS effects are known.

• Tell patient to observe bowel movements and to report signs of steatorrhea or bile duct obstruction (nausea, vomiting, abdominal or epigastric pain, and diarrhea).

Evaluation

• Patient's triglyceride and cholesterol levels are normal.

• Patient regains normal bowel patterns.

• Patient and family state understanding of drug therapy.

gemifloxacin mesylate
(geh-mih-FLOCKS-a-sin MESS-ih-late)
Factive

Pharmacologic class: fluoroquinolone
Therapeutic class: antibacterial
Pregnancy risk category: C

Indications and dosages

▶ **Acute bacterial exacerbation of chronic bronchitis caused by** *Streptococcus pneumoniae, Haemophilus influenzae, Haemophilus parainfluenzae, Moraxella catarrhalis. Adults:* 320 mg P.O. once daily for 5 days.

▶ **Mild to moderate community-acquired pneumonia caused by** *S. pneumoniae* (including penicillin-resistant strains), *H. influenzae, M. catarrhalis, Mycoplasma pneumoniae, Chlamydia pneumoniae, Klebsiella pneumoniae. Adults:* 320 mg P.O. once daily for 7 days.

Adjust-a-dose: For patients with renal impairment, if creatinine clearance is 40 ml/minute or less or if patient receives routine hemodialysis or continuous ambulatory peritoneal dialysis, reduce dosage to 160 mg P.O. once daily.

G

Contraindications and cautions

• Contraindicated in patients hypersensitive to fluoroquinolones or any of their components, those with a history of prolonged QT interval, those with uncorrected electrolyte disorders, and those taking a class IA or III antiarrhythmic.
• Use cautiously in patients with epilepsy, predisposition to seizures, or renal impairment.
⚠ Lifespan: In pregnant women, use only if benefits outweigh risks to the fetus. In breastfeeding women, use cautiously because it isn't known if drug appears in breast milk. In children, safety and effectiveness of drug haven't been established.

Adverse reactions

CNS: headache, dizziness, fatigue.
GI: abdominal pain, diarrhea, nausea, *pseudomembranous colitis,* vomiting.
Musculoskeletal: ruptured tendons.
Skin: rash.
Other: *hypersensitivity reactions.*

Interactions

Drug-drug. *Antacids (magnesium or aluminum), didanosine (chewable tablets, buffered tablets, or pediatric powder for oral solution), iron, multivitamins containing metal cations (such as zinc), sucralfate:* May decrease gemifloxacin level. Give gemifloxacin at least 3 hours before or 2 hours after these drugs.
Antiarrhythmics (amiodarone, procainamide, quinidine, sotalol): May increase risk of prolonged QT interval. Avoid use together.
Drugs that affect QT interval (such as antidepressants, antipsychotics, and erythromycin): May increase risk of prolonged QT interval. Use together cautiously.
Probenecid: May increase gemifloxacin level. Use together cautiously.
Warfarin: May increase anticoagulation effects. Monitor patient's PT and INR.
Drug-lifestyle. *Sun exposure:* May increase risk of photosensitivity. Discourage excessive or unprotected exposure to ultraviolet light or sunlight.

Effects on lab test results

• May increase ALT and AST levels.

Pharmacokinetics

Absorption: Rapid and unaffected by food.

Distribution: Wide, especially to lung tissue and fluids; 60% to 70% protein-bound.
Metabolism: Limited, mainly hepatic; some minor metabolites formed.
Excretion: In feces and urine as unchanged drug and metabolites. *Half-life:* 4 to 12 hours.

Route	Onset	Peak	Duration
P.O.	Unknown	½–2 hr	Unknown

Action

Chemical effect: Prevents cell growth by inhibiting DNA gyrase and topoisomerase IV, which interferes with DNA synthesis.
Therapeutic effect: Kills susceptible bacteria.

Available forms

Tablets: 320 mg

NURSING PROCESS

⚚ Assessment
• Serious and occasionally fatal hypersensitivity reaction may occur. Monitor patient carefully.
• Drug may cause CNS effects, such as tremors and anxiety. Monitor patient carefully.
• Carefully monitor patient's liver enzyme levels. Liver enzyme levels may rise during therapy but will resolve afterward.
• Assess patient's and family's knowledge of drug therapy.

⊕ Nursing diagnoses
• Infection related to presence of bacteria susceptible to drug.
• Risk for injury related to adverse effects of drug therapy
• Deficient knowledge related to drug therapy

▷ Planning and implementation
• Rash is more likely to appear in a patient younger than age 40, especially women and those taking hormone therapy. Stop giving drug if rash appears.
• Drug may cause tendon rupture, arthropathy, or osteochondrosis. Stop drug if patient reports pain, inflammation, or signs of muscle rupture.
• If patient has a photosensitivity reaction, stop giving drug.
• Serious diarrhea may indicate pseudomembranous colitis. Stop drug if needed.
• Keep patient adequately hydrated to avoid concentration of urine.

Reactions may be *common*, uncommon, **life-threatening**, or COMMON AND LIFE-THREATENING.

• In acute overdose, empty patient's stomach by inducing vomiting or performing gastric lavage. Hydrate patient if needed, and continue treating symptoms. Hemodialysis removes 20% to 30% of a dose.

Patient teaching
• Instruct patient to finish full course of therapy, even if symptoms improve.
• Tell patient to stop drug and seek medical care if evidence of hypersensitivity reaction develops.
• Tell patient to report serious diarrhea.
• Instruct patient to drink fluids liberally.
• Warn patient against taking OTC drugs or dietary supplements with this drug without consulting prescriber.
• Tell patient to avoid excessive exposure to sunlight or ultraviolet light.
• Urge patient to report pain, inflammation, or rupture of tendons.
• Warn patient to avoid driving or other hazardous activities until effects of drug are known.

☑ Evaluation
• Patient is free from infection after drug treatment.
• Patient remains free from injury from adverse reactions.
• Patient and family state understanding of drug therapy.

gemtuzumab ozogamicin
(gem-TOO-zuh-mab oh-zoh-GAM-ih-sin)
Mylotarg

Pharmacologic class: monoclonal antibody
Therapeutic class: chemotherapeutic drug
Pregnancy risk category: D

Indications and dosages

▶ **Patients with CD33-positive acute myeloid leukemia in first relapse who are not considered candidates for cytotoxic chemotherapy.**
Adults age 60 and older: 9 mg/m^2 I.V. infusion over 2 hours q 14 days for a total of two doses. One hour before the infusion, give 50 mg of diphenhydramine P.O. and 650 to 1,000 mg of acetaminophen P.O. Additional doses of acetaminophen 650 to 1,000 mg P.O. can be given q 4 hours, p.r.n.

▼ I.V. administration

• During preparation and administration, protect from direct and indirect sunlight and unshielded fluorescent light.
• Administer in 100 ml of normal saline injection. Place the 100-ml I.V. bag into an ultraviolet light protectant bag. Use drug solution in I.V. bag immediately.
• Use a separate I.V. line equipped with a low–protein-binding 1.2-micron terminal filter for administration of drug. May be infused by central or peripheral line.
• Don't give I.V. push or bolus.
• Monitor vital signs during infusion and for 4 hours after infusion.
⊗ Incompatibilities
None reported.

Contraindications and cautions

• Contraindicated in patients hypersensitive to drug or any of its components.
• Use cautiously in patients with hepatic impairment.
✳ Lifespan: Drug is indicated only for adults age 60 and older. In pregnant women, avoid using drug. Advise women of childbearing age not to become pregnant. Breast-feeding women should stop nursing or stop taking drug. It's unknown whether drug appears in breast milk. In children, safety and effectiveness haven't been established.

Adverse reactions

CNS: *asthenia, depression, dizziness, headache, insomnia, pain, fever.*
CV: *hypertension, hypotension, tachycardia.*
EENT: *epistaxis, pharyngitis, rhinitis.*
GI: *enlarged abdomen, abdominal pain, anorexia, constipation, diarrhea, dyspepsia, nausea, stomatitis, vomiting.*
GU: *hematuria,* VAGINAL HEMORRHAGE.
Hematologic: *anemia,* BLEEDING, LEUKOPENIA, NEUTROPENIA, NEUTROPENIC FEVER, THROMBOCYTOPENIA, SEVERE MYELOSUPPRESSION.
Hepatic: *hepatotoxicity, hyperbilirubinemia, veno-occlusive disease.*
Metabolic: hyperglycemia, hypokalemia, *hypomagnesemia.*
Musculoskeletal: arthralgia, back pain.

G

Respiratory: *increased cough,* dyspnea, *hypoxia, acute respiratory distress syndrome,* pneumonia, *pulmonary edema.*
Skin: *rash.*
Other: herpes simplex, chills, SEPSIS, *severe hypersensitivity reactions.*

Interactions

None reported.

Effects on lab test results

• May increase liver enzyme, LDH, and glucose levels. May decrease potassium, magnesium, and hemoglobin levels and hematocrit.
• May decrease leukocyte, neutrophil, and platelet counts.

Pharmacokinetics

Absorption: Administered I.V.
Distribution: Unknown.
Metabolism: Unknown. Liver microsomal enzymes may be involved.
Excretion: Unknown. *Half-life:* Total and unconjugated calicheamicin, 45 and 100 hours, respectively, after the first dose. After the second dose, total calicheamicin, 60 hours.

Route	Onset	Peak	Duration
I.V.	Unknown	Unknown	Unknown

Action

Chemical effect: May bind to the CD33 antigen expressed on the surface of leukemic blasts in patients with acute myeloid leukemia, resulting in the formation of a complex that is internalized by the cell. The calicheamicin derivative is then released inside the cell, causing DNA double strand breaks and cell death.
Therapeutic effect: Kills cancer cells.

Available forms

Powder for injection: 5 mg

NURSING PROCESS

Assessment
• Monitor CBC and platelets before starting and during therapy.
• Monitor liver enzymes before and during therapy.
• Monitor patient for postinfusion reactions and tumor lysis syndrome.
• Monitor I.V. site for local reactions.

• Assess patient's and family's knowledge of drug therapy.

Nursing diagnoses
• Risk for injury related to adverse effects of drug
• Risk for infection related to drug-induced adverse hematologic reactions
• Deficient knowledge related to drug therapy

Planning and implementation
• Use only under the supervision of a prescriber experienced in the use of cancer drugs.
• Drug may produce a postinfusion symptom complex in the 24 hours immediately after the infusion; symptoms include chills, fever, hypotension, hypertension, hyperglycemia, hypoxia, or dyspnea.
• Tumor lysis syndrome may occur. Provide adequate hydration, and treat with allopurinol to prevent hyperuricemia.
• Drug isn't dialyzable.
• Severe myelosuppression will occur in all patients given the recommended dose. Careful hematologic monitoring is required.
• Monitor electrolytes, hepatic function, CBC, and platelets during therapy.
Patient teaching
• Inform patient about postinfusion symptoms, and instruct him to continue to take acetaminophen 650 to 1,000 mg q 4 hours p.r.n.
• Tell patient to watch for signs of infection (fever, sore throat, and fatigue) and bleeding (easy bruising, nosebleeds, bleeding gums, and melena). Tell patient to take temperature daily, before acetaminophen dose.

Evaluation
• Patient remains free from infection.
• Patient's laboratory values remain above critical levels throughout course of therapy.
• Patient and family state understanding of drug therapy.

gentamicin sulfate
(jen-tuh-MIGH-sin SUL-fayt)
Cidomycin ♦ , Garamycin, Gentamicin
Sulfate ADD-Vantage, Jenamicin

Pharmacologic class: aminoglycoside
Therapeutic class: antibiotic
Pregnancy risk category: D

Indications and dosages

▶ **Serious infections caused by sensitive
strains of** *Pseudomonas aeruginosa, Escherichia coli, Proteus, Klebsiella, Serratia, Enterobacter, Citrobacter, Staphylococcus. Adults:*
3 mg/kg daily in divided doses I.M. or I.V. q
8 hours. For life-threatening infections, patient
may receive up to 5 mg/kg daily in three to four
divided doses. Reduce dosage to 3 mg/kg daily
as soon as indicated.
Children: 2 to 2.5 mg/kg I.M. or I.V. q 8 hours.
Neonates older than age 1 week and infants:
2.5 mg/kg daily I.M. or I.V. q 8 hours.
*Preterm infants and neonates age 1 week and
younger:* 2.5 mg/kg I.V. q 12 hours.
▶ **Meningitis.** *Adults:* 3 mg/kg daily in
divided doses I.M. or I.V. q 8 hours. For life-
threatening infections, patient may receive up to
5 mg/kg daily in three to four divided doses. Reduce dosage to 3 mg/kg daily as soon as indicated. Or 4 to 8 mg intrathecally daily may be
used.
Children and infants older than age 3 months:
2 to 2.5 mg/kg I.M. or I.V. q 8 hours. Or 1 to
2 mg intrathecally daily may be used.
▶ **Endocarditis prophylaxis for GI or GU
procedure or surgery.** *Adults:* 1.5 mg/kg to
maximum dose, 80 mg, I.M. or I.V. 30 to
60 minutes before procedure or surgery. Give
separately with ampicillin I.M. or I.V. followed
in 6 hours by ampicillin or amoxicillin alone.
Children: 2 mg/kg I.M. or I.V. 30 to 60 minutes
before procedure or surgery. Give separately
with ampicillin I.M. or I.V. followed in 6 hours
by ampicillin or amoxicillin alone.
▶ **Posthemodialysis to maintain therapeutic
level.** *Adults:* 1 to 1.7 mg/kg I.M. or I.V. after
each dialysis session.
Children: 2 to 2.5 mg/kg I.M. or by I.V. infusion after each dialysis session.

▼ I.V. administration

● When giving drug by intermittent I.V. infusion, dilute with 50 to 200 ml of D_5W or normal
saline injection.
● Infuse over 30 minutes to 2 hours.
● After infusion, flush line with normal saline
solution or D_5W.
⊗ **Incompatibilities**
Allopurinol, amphotericin B, ampicillin,
azithromycin, cefazolin, cefepime, cefotaxime,
ceftazidime, ceftriaxone sodium, cefuroxime,
cephapirin, certain parenteral nutrition formulations, cytarabine, dopamine, fat emulsions,
furosemide, heparin, hetastarch, idarubicin, indomethacin sodium trihydrate, nafcillin, propofol, ticarcillin, warfarin.

Contraindications and cautions

● Contraindicated in patients hypersensitive to
the drug or other aminoglycosides.
● Use cautiously in patients with renal impairment or neuromuscular disorders.
⚕ **Lifespan:** In pregnant women, don't use because drug is teratogenic. Beast-feeding women
should stop the drug or stop breast-feeding. In
neonates, infants, and the elderly, use drug cautiously.

Adverse reactions

CNS: headache, lethargy, numbness, paresthe-
sias, twitching, peripheral neuropathy, *seizures,
neurotoxicity.*
EENT: *ototoxicity.*
GU: NEPHROTOXICITY.
Hematologic: *thrombocytopenia, leukopenia,
agranulocytosis.*
Other: hypersensitivity reactions.

Interactions

Drug-drug. *Acyclovir, amphotericin B, cisplatin, methoxyflurane, other aminoglycosides,
vancomycin:* May increase ototoxicity and
nephrotoxicity. Use together cautiously.
*Atracurium, doxacurium, mivacurium, pancuro-
nium, rocuronium, tubocurarine, vecuronium:*
May increase neuromuscular blockade. Monitor
patient closely.
Cephalothin: May increase nephrotoxicity. Use
together cautiously; monitor renal function.
Dimenhydrinate: May mask symptoms of ototoxicity. Use with caution.
Diuretics: May increase ototoxicity. Avoid use
together.

G

General anesthetics: May increase effects of nondepolarizing muscle relaxant, including prolonged respiratory depression. Use together only when necessary.
Indomethacin: May decrease renal clearance of gentamicin, leading to increased risk of toxicity.
I.V. loop diuretics (such as furosemide): May increase ototoxicity. Use cautiously.
Neurotoxic drugs: May increase neurotoxicity. Avoid use together.
Parenteral penicillins (such as ampicillin, ticarcillin): May inactivate gentamicin in vitro. Don't mix together.

Effects on lab test results

- May increase BUN, creatinine, nonprotein nitrogen, ALT, AST, bilirubin, and LDH levels. May decrease hemoglobin level and hematocrit.
- May increase eosinophil count. May decrease WBC, platelet, and granulocyte counts.

Pharmacokinetics

Absorption: Rapid and complete after I.M. use.
Distribution: Wide. CSF penetration is low even in adults with inflamed meninges. Higher CSF levels are achieved in neonates than in adults. Protein binding is minimal.
Metabolism: None.
Excretion: Primarily in urine. *Half-life:* 2 to 3 hours.

Route	Onset	Peak	Duration
I.V.	Immediate	15–30 min	Unknown
I.M.	Unknown	30–90 min	Unknown
Intrathecal	Unknown	Unknown	Unknown

Action

Chemical effect: Inhibits protein synthesis by binding to ribosomes.
Therapeutic effect: Kills susceptible bacteria (many aerobic gram-negative organisms and some aerobic gram-positive organisms). Drug may act against some aminoglycoside-resistant bacteria.

Available forms

Injection: 40 mg/ml (adult), 10 mg/ml (pediatric), 2 mg/ml (intrathecal)
I.V. infusion (premixed): 40 mg, 60 mg, 70 mg, 80 mg, 90 mg, 100 mg, 120 mg, 160 mg, 180 mg available in normal saline solution

NURSING PROCESS

Assessment

- Assess patient's infection and hearing before starting therapy and regularly thereafter.
- Obtain specimen for culture and sensitivity tests before giving the first dose. Begin therapy pending test results.
- Weigh patient and review baseline renal function studies before therapy and regularly during therapy. Notify prescriber of any changes; adjust dosage.
- Obtain blood for peak drug level 1 hour after I.M. injection and 30 minutes to 1 hour after I.V. infusion; for trough levels, draw blood just before next dose. Don't collect blood in heparinized tube because heparin is incompatible with aminoglycosides.
- Peak level above 12 mcg/ml and trough level above 2 mcg/ml may increase risk of toxicity.
- Be alert for adverse reactions and drug interactions.
- Assess patient's and family's knowledge of drug therapy.

Nursing diagnoses

- Infection related to presence of susceptible bacteria
- Impaired urinary elimination related to nephrotoxicity
- Deficient knowledge related to drug therapy

Planning and implementation

- Give I.M. injection deep into large muscle mass (gluteal or midlateral thigh); rotate injection sites. Don't inject more than 2 g of drug per site.

ALERT: Use preservative-free forms of gentamicin for intrathecal route.

- Hemodialysis (8 hours) removes up to 50% of drug.
- Notify prescriber about signs of decreasing renal function or changes in hearing.
- Therapy usually continues for 7 to 10 days. If no response occurs in 3 to 5 days, therapy may be stopped and new specimens obtained for culture and sensitivity testing.
- Therapeutic peak and trough levels are 4 to 12 mcg/ml and less than 2 mcg/ml, respectively.
- Make sure patient is well hydrated to minimize chemical irritation of renal tubules.

Patient teaching
• Instruct patient to notify prescriber about adverse reactions, such as changes in hearing.
• Emphasize importance of drinking at least 2 L of fluids daily, if not contraindicated.

☑ Evaluation
• Patient is free from infection.
• Patient maintains normal renal function throughout drug therapy.
• Patient and family state understanding of drug therapy.

glimepiride
(gligh-MEH-peh-righd)
Amaryl

Pharmacologic class: sulfonylurea
Therapeutic class: antidiabetic
Pregnancy risk category: C

Indications and dosages
▶ **Type 2 (non–insulin-dependent) diabetes mellitus when hyperglycemia can't be managed by diet and exercise alone.** *Adults:* Initially, 1 to 2 mg P.O. once daily with first main meal of day. Usual maintenance dosage is 1 to 4 mg P.O. once daily. After reaching 2 mg, increase dosage in increments not exceeding 2 mg q 1 to 2 weeks, based on patient's response. Maximum, 8 mg daily.
▶ **Adjunct to insulin therapy in patients with type 2 (non–insulin-dependent) diabetes mellitus whose hyperglycemia can't be managed by diet and exercise with oral hypoglycemics.** *Adults:* 8 mg P.O. once daily with first main meal of day with low-dose insulin. Adjust insulin upward weekly p.r.n., based on patient's response.
▶ **Adjunct to metformin therapy in patients with type 2 (non–insulin-dependent) diabetes mellitus whose hyperglycemia can't be managed by diet, exercise, and glimepiride or metformin alone.** *Adults:* 8 mg P.O. once daily with first main meal of the day with metformin. Adjust dosages based on patient's blood glucose response to determine minimum effective dosage of each drug.
▧ **Adjust-a-dose:** For patients with renal or hepatic impairment, initial dose is 1 mg P.O. daily

with breakfast; then adjust based on the patient's fasting glucose levels.

Contraindications and cautions
• Contraindicated in patients hypersensitive to the drug or any of its components, in those with diabetic ketoacidosis, and in those with allergies to sulfonamides or thiazide diuretics.
• Use cautiously in debilitated or malnourished patients and in those with adrenal, pituitary, hepatic, or renal insufficiency.
⚖ **Lifespan:** In pregnant and breast-feeding women, drug is contraindicated. In children, safety and effectiveness haven't been established. In elderly patients, use cautiously because they might be more sensitive to the drug.

Adverse reactions
CNS: dizziness, asthenia, headache.
EENT: changes in accommodation.
GI: nausea.
Hematologic: *leukopenia,* hemolytic anemia, *agranulocytosis, thrombocytopenia, aplastic anemia, pancytopenia.*
Hepatic: cholestatic jaundice.
Metabolic: *hypoglycemia.*
Skin: allergic skin reactions.

Interactions
Drug-drug. *Beta blockers:* May mask symptoms of hypoglycemia. Monitor glucose level carefully.
Drugs that produce hyperglycemia, thiazides and other diuretics: May lead to loss of glucose control. May require dosage adjustment.
Insulin: May increase potential for hypoglycemia. Monitor glucose level closely.
NSAIDs, other highly protein-bound drugs: May increase hypoglycemic action of sulfonylureas, such as glimepiride. Monitor patient carefully.
Drug-herb. *Aloe, bitter melon, bilberry leaf, burdock, dandelion, fenugreek, garlic, ginseng:* May improve glucose control, which may allow reduction of oral hypoglycemic. Tell patient to discuss herbs with prescriber before use.
Drug-lifestyle. *Alcohol use:* May alter glycemic control, most commonly toward hypoglycemia. May cause disulfiram-like reaction. Discourage use together.

G

Sun exposure: May cause photosensitivity. Discourage prolonged or unprotected exposure to the sun.

Effects on lab test results

• May increase BUN, creatinine, alkaline phosphatase, ALT, and AST levels. May decrease glucose, sodium, and hemoglobin levels and hematocrit.
• May decrease WBC, RBC, platelet, and granulocyte counts.

Pharmacokinetics

Absorption: Complete.
Distribution: Almost completely protein-bound.
Metabolism: Complete.
Excretion: In urine and feces. *Half-life:* 9 hours.

Route	Onset	Peak	Duration
P.O.	≤ 1 hr	2–3 hr	24 hr

Action

Chemical effect: Stimulates release of insulin from pancreatic beta cells; increases sensitivity of peripheral tissues to insulin.
Therapeutic effect: Lowers glucose levels.

Available forms

Tablets: 1 mg, 2 mg, 4 mg

NURSING PROCESS

☰ Assessment
• Monitor fasting glucose periodically to determine therapeutic response. Also monitor glycosylated hemoglobin level, usually every 3 to 6 months, to more precisely assess long-term glycemic control.
• Assess patient's and family's knowledge of drug therapy.

☰ Nursing diagnoses
• Ineffective health maintenance related to hyperglycemia
• Risk for injury related to drug-induced hypoglycemia
• Deficient knowledge related to drug therapy

☰ Planning and implementation
• Oral hypoglycemic drugs have been linked to an increased risk of CV mortality compared with diet alone or with diet and insulin therapy.

• Give drug with the first meal of the day.
Patient teaching
• Tell patient to take drug with first meal of day.
• Stress importance of adhering to diet, weight-reduction, exercise, and personal hygiene programs.
• Explain to patient and family how to monitor glucose levels, identify signs and symptoms, and treat hyperglycemia and hypoglycemia.
• Advise patient to wear or carry medical identification that describes his condition.
• Instruct patient to avoid alcohol consumption during therapy.

☑ Evaluation
• Patient's glucose level is normal.
• Patient recognizes hypoglycemia early and treats it before injury occurs.
• Patient and family state understanding of drug therapy.

glipizide
(GLIH-pih-zighd)
Glucotrol◆, Glucotrol XL◆, Minidiab ◇

Pharmacologic class: sulfonylurea
Therapeutic class: antidiabetic
Pregnancy risk category: C

Indications and dosages

▶ **Adjunct to diet to lower glucose level in patients with type 2 (non–insulin-dependent) diabetes mellitus.** *Adults:* Initially 5 mg immediate-release P.O. daily 30 minutes before breakfast. Maximum recommended total daily dose, 40 mg. Or 5-mg extended-release tablets P.O. daily. Adjust in 5-mg increments q 3 months depending on level of glycemic control. Maximum daily dose for extended-release tablets, 20 mg.
☰ Adjust-a-dose: In elderly patients with liver disease, 2.5 mg immediate-release or 5 mg extended-release. Maximum once-daily dose is 15 mg.
▶ **To replace insulin therapy.** *Adults:* If insulin dosage is more than 20 units daily, patient is started at usual dosage in addition to 50% of insulin. If insulin dosage is less than 20 units, stop insulin.

Contraindications and cautions

• Contraindicated in patients hypersensitive to the drug or any of its components, in those with diabetic ketoacidosis, and in those with allergies to sulfonamides or thiazide diuretics.
• Use cautiously in patients with renal and hepatic disease and in debilitated or malnourished patients.
⚠ Lifespan: In pregnant and breast-feeding women, drug is contraindicated. In children, safety and effectiveness haven't been established because of the rarity of type 2 diabetes mellitus in this population. In elderly patients, use cautiously.

Adverse reactions

CNS: dizziness, drowsiness, headache.
CV: facial flushing.
GI: nausea, vomiting, constipation.
Hematologic: *agranulocytosis, thrombocytopenia, aplastic anemia.*
Hepatic: cholestatic jaundice.
Metabolic: *hypoglycemia.*
Skin: rash, pruritus.

Interactions

Drug-drug. *Anabolic steroids, chloramphenicol, clofibrate, guanethidine, MAO inhibitors, phenylbutazone, probenecid, salicylates, sulfonamides:* May increase hypoglycemic activity. Monitor glucose level.
Beta blockers: May prolong hypoglycemic effect and mask symptoms of hypoglycemia. Use together cautiously.
Corticosteroids, glucagon, rifampin, thiazide diuretics: May decrease hypoglycemic response. Monitor glucose level.
Hydantoins: May increase levels of hydantoins. Monitor levels.
Oral anticoagulants: May increase hypoglycemic activity or enhance anticoagulant effect. Monitor glucose level, PT, and INR.
Drug-herb. *Aloe, bilberry leaf, bitter melon, burdock, dandelion, fenugreek, garlic, ginseng:* May improve glucose control, which may allow reduction of oral hypoglycemic. Tell patient to discuss herbs with prescriber before use.
Drug-lifestyle. *Alcohol use:* May alter glycemic control, most commonly toward hypoglycemia. May also cause disulfiram-like reaction. Discourage use together.
Sun exposure: May cause photosensitivity. Discourage prolonged or unprotected sun exposure.

Effects on lab test results

• May increase BUN, creatinine, alkaline phosphatase, AST, and LDH levels. May decrease glucose and hemoglobin levels and hematocrit.
• May decrease granulocyte and platelet counts.

Pharmacokinetics

Absorption: Rapid and complete.
Distribution: In extracellular fluid; 98% to 99% protein-bound.
Metabolism: By liver to inactive metabolites.
Excretion: Primarily in urine. *Half-life:* 2 to 4 hours.

Route	Onset	Peak	Duration
P.O.	15–30 min	1–3 hr	10–24 hr

Action

Chemical effect: May stimulate insulin release from pancreas, reduce glucose output by liver, and increase peripheral sensitivity to insulin.
Therapeutic effect: Lowers glucose level.

Available forms

Tablets: 5 mg, 10 mg
Tablets (extended-release): 2.5 mg, 5 mg, 10 mg

NURSING PROCESS

▨ Assessment
• Assess glucose level before starting therapy and regularly thereafter.
• Patient transferring from insulin therapy to oral antidiabetic needs glucose monitoring at least three times daily before meals.
• During periods of increased stress, such as from infection, fever, surgery, or trauma, patient may need insulin therapy. Monitor patient closely for hyperglycemia in these situations.
• Be alert for adverse reactions and drug interactions.
• Assess patient's and family's knowledge of drug therapy.

▨ Nursing diagnoses
• Ineffective health maintenance related to hyperglycemia
• Risk for injury related to drug-induced hypoglycemia
• Deficient knowledge related to drug therapy

▶ Planning and implementation

• Give drug about 30 minutes before meals.
• Some patients may attain effective control with once-daily dose; others show better response with divided doses.
• For a hypoglycemic reaction, give oral form of fast-acting carbohydrates or glucagon or I.V. glucose (if patient can't swallow or is comatose). Then give patient a complex carbohydrate snack when he awakens, and determine cause of the reaction.
• Make sure adjunct therapies, such as diet and exercise, are being used appropriately.
⑨ **ALERT:** Don't confuse glipizide with glyburide.

Patient teaching
• Teach patient about diabetes and the importance of following a therapeutic regimen: adhering to specific diet, weight reduction, exercise and personal hygiene programs, and avoiding infection.
• Explain how to monitor glucose level and how to recognize and treat hypoglycemia and hyperglycemia.
• Tell patient not to change dosage without prescriber's consent and to report any adverse reactions.
• Advise patient not to take other drugs, including OTC drugs or herbal remedies, without first checking with prescriber.
• Instruct patient not to drink alcohol during drug therapy.
• Advise patient to carry medical identification at all times.

✓ Evaluation

• Patient's glucose level is normal with drug therapy.
• Patient doesn't experience hypoglycemia or hyperglycemia.
• Patient and family state understanding of drug therapy.

glipizide and metformin hydrochloride
(GLIH-pih-zighd and met-FOR-min high-droh-KLOR-ighd)
Metaglip

Pharmacologic class: sulfonylurea and biguanide
Therapeutic class: antidiabetic
Pregnancy risk category: C

Indications and dosages

▶ **First-line therapy, as adjunct to diet and exercise, to improve glycemic control in patients with type 2 (non–insulin-dependent) diabetes.** *Adults:* Initially, 2.5 mg/250 mg P.O. once daily with a meal. In patients whose fasting glucose level is 280 to 320 mg/dl, start with 2.5 mg/500 mg P.O. b.i.d. Increase dosage in increments of 1 tablet per day q 2 weeks to maximum, 10 mg/1,000 mg or 10 mg/2,000 mg daily in divided doses.
▶ **Second-line therapy in type 2 diabetes when diet, exercise, and initial therapy with a sulfonylurea or metformin can't provide adequate glycemic control.** *Adults:* Initially, 2.5 mg/500 mg or 5 mg/500 mg P.O. b.i.d. with the morning and evening meals. Increase in increments of no more than 5 mg/500 mg daily, to minimum effective dose needed to adequately control glucose, or to maximum daily dose, 20 mg/2,000 mg.

Contraindications and cautions

• Contraindicated in patients hypersensitive to the drug or any of its components and in those with renal disease, creatinine level at least 1.5 mg/dl in men and at least 1.4 mg/dl in women, abnormal creatinine clearance, heart failure, shock, acute MI, septicemia, or acute or chronic metabolic acidosis, including diabetic ketoacidosis. Also contraindicated after surgery.
• Use cautiously in patients with hepatic dysfunction, malnourished or debilitated patients, and those with adrenal or pituitary insufficiency. Also use cautiously in patients with abnormal vitamin B_{12} levels or hypoglycemia, and in those who consume alcohol.
⚞ **Lifespan:** In pregnant women, use is not recommended. If the drug is used, stop therapy at least 1 month before delivery. In breast-feeding women, use cautiously. In children, safety and

effectiveness haven't been established. In elderly patients, use cautiously because aging causes reduced renal function. Don't start drug in patients age 80 or older unless renal function is normal, and don't give older patients the maximum dosage.

Adverse reactions

CNS: *headache,* dizziness.
CV: hypertension.
GI: nausea, *diarrhea,* vomiting, abdominal pain.
GU: UTI.
Metabolic: *hypoglycemia, lactic acidosis.*
Musculoskeletal: muscle pain.
Respiratory: *upper respiratory tract infection.*

Interactions

Drug-drug. *Azoles, beta blockers, chloramphenicol, coumarin, MAO inhibitors, NSAIDs, probenecid, salicylates, sulfonamides:* May increase the effect of sulfonylureas. Monitor patient closely for hypoglycemia. May increase loss of glucose control when these drugs are withdrawn.
Calcium channel blockers, corticosteroids, estrogens, highly protein-bound drugs, isoniazid, hormonal contraceptives, nicotinic acid, phenytoin, phenothiazines, sympathomimetics, thyroid products, thiazides and other diuretics: May increase risk of hyperglycemia and loss of glucose control. May increase risk of hypoglycemia when these drugs are withdrawn. Monitor glucose level.
Cationic drugs (amiloride, digoxin, morphine, procainamide, quinidine, quinine, ranitidine, triamterene, trimethoprim, vancomycin): May increase metformin level. Monitor patient carefully.
Furosemide: May increase metformin level and decrease furosemide level. Monitor patient closely.
Iodinated contrast material used in radiologic studies: May increase risk of acute renal impairment. Stop drug for 48 hours before and after such tests.
Nifedipine: May increase metformin level. Decrease metformin dose if needed.
Drug-herb. *Juniper berries, ginseng, garlic, fenugreek, coriander, dandelion root, celery:* May increase risk of hypoglycemia. Discourage use together.

Drug-lifestyle. *Alcohol use:* May increase risk of hypoglycemia and lactic acidosis. Discourage use together.

Effects on lab test results

• May decrease glucose and vitamin B_{12} levels.

Pharmacokinetics

Absorption: For glipizide, rapid and complete. For metformin, delayed by food.
Distribution: For glipizide, extensively protein bound. For metformin, negligibly bound.
Metabolism: For glipizide, extensive with inactive primary metabolites. For metformin, none.
Excretion: For glipizide, inactive metabolites and unchanged in the urine. For metformin, unchanged in the urine. *Glipizide half-life:* 2 to 4 hours. *Metformin half-life:* 6 hours.

Route	Onset	Peak	Duration
P.O.			
glipizide	15–30 min	1–3 hr	Unknown
metformin	Unknown	Unknown	Unknown

Action

Chemical effect: Glipizide appears to lower glucose levels by stimulating the pancreas to release insulin. Metformin decreases hepatic glucose production and intestinal absorption of glucose and improves insulin sensitivity.
Therapeutic effect: Lowers glucose levels.

Available forms

Tablets: 2.5 mg glipizide and 250 mg metformin hydrochloride; 2.5 mg and 500 mg; 5 mg and 500 mg

NURSING PROCESS

⚕ Assessment
• Monitor CBC and renal function annually.
• Periodically monitor fasting glucose level and glycosylated hemoglobin level.
• If laboratory abnormalities or vague, poorly defined illness occurs, evaluate patient for ketoacidosis or lactic acidosis. If acidosis occurs, stop giving drug immediately.
• Assess patient's and family's knowledge of drug therapy.

✠ Nursing diagnoses
• Risk for ineffective health maintenance related to underlying disease

• Risk for deficient fluid volume related to high glucose levels
• Deficient knowledge related to drug therapy

≫ Planning and implementation
• Temporarily stop drug in patients undergoing radiologic studies involving iodinated contrast materials or any surgical procedure.
• Lactic acidosis is a rare but serious complication that can result from metformin accumulation. The risk of lactic acidosis increases with the degree of renal impairment and patient's age. Early symptoms of lactic acidosis may include malaise, myalgias, respiratory distress, increasing somnolence, and nonspecific abdominal distress. GI symptoms that occur after a patient is stabilized with Metaglip are unlikely to be drug-related and could be from lactic acidosis or other serious disease. Suspect lactic acidosis in any diabetic patient with metabolic acidosis lacking evidence of ketoacidosis.
• To reduce the risk of lactic acidosis, use the minimum effective dose and monitor renal function regularly.
• If CV collapse, acute heart failure, acute MI, or other conditions characterized by hypoxemia occur, stop drug because these conditions may be related to lactic acidosis and may cause prerenal azotemia.
• Stop giving the drug to a patient with any condition linked to hypoxemia, dehydration, or sepsis.
• Overdose of glipizide may produce hypoglycemia. Patient taking more than 100 g of metformin may develop hypoglycemia and lactic acidosis, but no proof exists that taking the drug causes this.
• For mild hypoglycemia, give oral glucose and adjust drug dosage or meal patterns. Severe hypoglycemia with coma, seizures, or other neurologic impairment requires immediate hospitalization. If hypoglycemic coma is diagnosed or suspected, give a rapid I.V. injection of 50% glucose solution, followed by a continuous infusion of a 10% solution at a rate that will maintain a glucose level above 100 mg/dl. Monitor patient closely for 24 to 48 hours because hypoglycemia may recur.
• Hemodialysis may remove metformin but not glipizide.

Patient teaching
• Tell patient to take once daily with breakfast or twice daily with breakfast and dinner.
• Tell patient to immediately report signs of lactic acidosis, including unexplained hyperventilation, myalgia, malaise, unusual drowsiness, suddenly developing a slow or irregular heartbeat, or feeling cold, dizzy, or light-headed.
• Tell patient that GI symptoms are common during initial therapy but should resolve. Tell patient to report persistent or new onset of GI symptoms.
• Advise patient to avoid drinking alcohol.

✓ Evaluation
• Patient's glucose level remains normal during drug therapy.
• Patient doesn't suffer from fluid volume deficit.
• Patient and family state understanding of drug therapy.

glucagon
(GLOO-kuh-gon)

Pharmacologic class: pancreatic hormone
Therapeutic class: antihypoglycemic
Pregnancy risk category: B

Indications and dosages
▶ **Hypoglycemia.** *Adults and children weighing more than 20 kg (44 lb):* 1 mg I.V., I.M., or subcutaneously.
Children weighing 20 kg or less: 0.5 mg I.V., I.M., or subcutaneously.
▶ **Diagnostic aid for radiologic examination.** *Adults:* 0.25 to 2 mg I.V. or I.M. before start of radiologic procedure.

▽ I.V. administration
• Reconstitute drug in 1-unit vial with 1 ml of diluent; reconstitute drug in 10-unit vial with 10 ml of diluent. Use only diluent supplied by manufacturer when preparing doses of 2 mg or less. For larger doses, dilute with sterile water for injection.
• Don't exceed concentration of 1 mg/ml (1 unit/ml).
• For I.V. drip infusion, use dextrose solution, which is compatible with glucagon. Drug forms precipitate in chloride solutions.

• Inject directly into vein or into I.V. tubing of free-flowing compatible solution over 2 to 5 minutes. Interrupt primary infusion during glucagon injection (if using same I.V. line). Repeat in 15 minutes if needed.
• If patient fails to respond, give I.V. glucose. When patient responds, give supplemental carbohydrate promptly.
⊗ Incompatibilities
Sodium chloride solution, solutions with pH of 3 to 9.5.

Contraindications and cautions

• Contraindicated in patients hypersensitive to the drug or any or its components and in those with pheochromocytoma.
• Use cautiously in patients with history of insulinoma or pheochromocytoma.
⚘ Lifespan: In pregnant women, use only if benefits outweigh risks to the fetus. In breast-feeding women, use cautiously because it's unknown if the drug appears in breast milk. In children, safety and effectiveness as a diagnostic aid haven't been established.

Adverse reactions

CV: hypotension.
GI: nausea, vomiting.
Respiratory: *respiratory distress.*
Skin: urticaria.
Other: *allergic reactions.*

Interactions

Drug-drug. *Oral anticoagulants:* May increase anticoagulant effect. Monitor PT and INR closely; monitor patient for bleeding.

Effects on lab test results

• May decrease potassium level.

Pharmacokinetics

Absorption: Unknown.
Distribution: Unknown.
Metabolism: Extensive by liver, in kidneys and plasma, and at its tissue receptor sites in plasma membranes.
Excretion: By kidneys. *Half-life:* 8 to 18 minutes.

Route	Onset	Peak	Duration
I.V., I.M., SubQ	Immediate	≤ 30 min	1–2 hr

Action

Chemical effect: Promotes catalytic depolymerization of hepatic glycogen to glucose.
Therapeutic effect: Raises glucose level.

Available forms

Powder for injection: 1 mg (1 unit)/vial

NURSING PROCESS

🔎 Assessment
• Assess patient's glucose level before starting therapy and after giving the drug.
• Be alert for adverse reactions and drug interactions.
• If patient vomits, monitor his hydration.
• Assess patient's and family's knowledge of drug therapy.

G

Nursing diagnoses
• Risk for injury related to hypoglycemia
• Risk for deficient fluid volume related to drug-induced vomiting
• Deficient knowledge related to drug therapy

Planning and implementation
• For I.M use, reconstitute drug in 1-unit vial with 1 ml of diluent; reconstitute drug in 10-unit vial with 10 ml of diluent. Use only diluent supplied by manufacturer when preparing doses of 2 mg or less. For larger doses, dilute with sterile water for injection.
• Arouse lethargic patient as quickly as possible and give additional carbohydrates orally to prevent secondary hypoglycemic reactions. Notify prescriber that patient's hypoglycemic episode required glucagon use. If patient doesn't respond to drug, provide emergency intervention. Unstable hypoglycemic diabetic patient may not respond to drug. Give glucose I.V. instead.
• If patient can't retain some form of sugar for 1 hour because of nausea or vomiting, notify prescriber.
Patient teaching
• Instruct patient and family in proper drug administration.
• Teach them to recognize signs and symptoms of hypoglycemia, and tell them to notify prescriber immediately in emergencies.

☑ Evaluation
• Patient's glucose level returns to normal.
• Patient remains well hydrated.
• Patient and family state understanding of drug therapy.

glyburide (glibenclamide)
(GLIGH-byoo-righd)
Albert Glyburide ♦, Apo-Glyburide ♦, DiaBeta◈, Euglucon ♦, Gen-Glybe ♦, Glynase PresTab, Micronase◈, Novo-Glyburide ♦, Nu-Glyburide ♦

Pharmacologic class: sulfonylurea
Therapeutic class: antidiabetic
Pregnancy risk category: B (for Micronase, Glynase); C (for DiaBeta)

Indications and dosages
▶ **Adjunct to diet to lower glucose level in patients with type 2 (non–insulin-dependent) diabetes mellitus.** *Adults:* Initially, 1.25- to 5-mg regular tablets P.O. once daily with breakfast. For maintenance, 1.25 to 20 mg daily as single dose or in divided doses. Or, initially, 0.75- to 3-mg micronized formulation P.O. daily. For maintenance, 0.75 to 12 mg P.O. daily in single or divided doses.
▶ **To replace insulin therapy.** *Adults:* Initially, if insulin dosage is more than 40 units daily, 5-mg regular tablets or 3-mg micronized form P.O. once daily in addition to 50% of insulin dosage. If insulin dosage is 20 to 40 units daily, 5-mg regular tablets or 3-mg micronized form P.O. once daily while abruptly stopping insulin. If insulin dosage is less than 20 units daily, 2.5- to 5-mg regular tablets or 1.5- to 3-mg micronized form P.O. once daily while abruptly stopping insulin.

Contraindications and cautions
• Contraindicated in patients hypersensitive to the drug or any of its components, in those with diabetic ketoacidosis, and in those with allergies to sulfonamides or thiazide diuretics.
• Use cautiously in patients with hepatic or renal impairment and in debilitated or malnourished patients.
❀ **Lifespan:** In pregnant women, breastfeeding women, and children, drug is contraindicated. In elderly patients, use cautiously.

Adverse reactions
CV: facial flushing.
GI: nausea, epigastric fullness, heartburn.
Hematologic: *agranulocytosis, thrombocytopenia, aplastic anemia.*
Hepatic: cholestatic jaundice.
Metabolic: *hypoglycemia.*
Skin: rash, pruritus.

Interactions
Drug-drug. *Anabolic steroids, chloramphenicol, clofibrate, guanethidine, MAO inhibitors, phenylbutazone, salicylates, sulfonamides:* May increase hypoglycemic activity. Monitor glucose level.
Beta blockers: May prolong hypoglycemic effect and mask symptoms of hypoglycemia. Use together cautiously.
Corticosteroids, glucagon, rifampin, thiazide diuretics: May decrease hypoglycemic response. Monitor glucose level.
Hydantoins: May increase level of hydantoins. Monitor level.
Oral anticoagulants: May increase hypoglycemic activity or enhance anticoagulant effect. Monitor glucose level, PT, and INR.
Drug-herb. *Aloe, bitter melon, bilberry leaf, burdock, dandelion, fenugreek, garlic, ginseng:* Improvement in glucose control may allow reduction of oral hypoglycemic. Tell patient to discuss herbs with prescriber before use.
Drug-lifestyle. *Alcohol use:* May alter glycemic control, most commonly hypoglycemia. May also cause disulfiram-like reaction. Discourage use together.
Sun exposure: May cause photosensitivity. Discourage prolonged or unprotected exposure to sunlight.

Effects on lab test results
• May increase BUN, alkaline phosphatase, bilirubin, AST, ALT, and LDH levels. May decrease glucose and hemoglobin levels and hematocrit.
• May decrease WBC, platelet, and granulocyte counts.

Pharmacokinetics
Absorption: Almost complete.
Distribution: 99% protein-bound.
Metabolism: Complete.
Excretion: As metabolites in urine and feces in equal proportions. *Half-life:* 10 hours.

Route	Onset	Peak	Duration
P.O.	45–60 min	2–4 hr	24 hr

Action

Chemical effect: May stimulate insulin release from pancreas, reduce glucose output by liver, increase peripheral sensitivity to insulin, and cause mild diuresis.
Therapeutic effect: Lowers glucose levels.

Available forms

Tablets: 1.25 mg, 2.5 mg, 5 mg
Tablets (micronized): 1.5 mg, 3 mg, 4.5 mg, 6 mg

NURSING PROCESS

Assessment

- Assess glucose level before starting therapy and regularly thereafter.
- Patient transferring from insulin therapy to oral antidiabetic needs glucose monitoring at least three times daily before meals.
- During periods of increased stress, such as from infection, fever, surgery, or trauma, patient may need insulin therapy. Monitor patient closely for hyperglycemia in these situations.
- Be alert for adverse reactions and drug interactions.
- Assess patient's and family's knowledge of drug therapy.

Nursing diagnoses

- Ineffective health maintenance related to hyperglycemia
- Risk for injury related to drug-induced hypoglycemia
- Deficient knowledge related to drug therapy

Planning and implementation

- Micronized glyburide (Glynase PresTab) contains drug in smaller particle size and isn't bioequivalent to regular tablets. Adjust dose in a patient who has been taking Micronase or DiaBeta.
- Although most patients take drug once daily, patient taking more than 10 mg daily may achieve better results with twice-daily dosage.
- For hypoglycemic reaction, give oral form of fast-acting carbohydrates or, if patient can't swallow or is comatose, glucagon or I.V. glucose. Then give patient a complex carbohydrate snack when patient is conscious, and determine cause of reaction.
- Make sure that adjunct therapy, such as diet and exercise, is appropriate.

ALERT: Don't confuse glyburide with glipizide.

Patient teaching

- Teach patient about diabetes and the importance of following therapeutic regimen by adhering to specific diet, weight reduction, exercise, and personal hygiene programs and by avoiding infection.
- Explain how to monitor glucose level and recognize and treat hypoglycemia and hyperglycemia.
- Tell patient not to change dosage without prescriber's consent and to report any adverse reactions.
- Advise patient not to take OTC drugs or herbal remedies without first checking with prescriber.
- Instruct patient not to drink alcohol during drug therapy.
- Advise patient to wear or carry medical identification at all times.

Evaluation

- Patient's glucose level is normal with drug therapy.
- Patient doesn't experience hypoglycemia.
- Patient and family state understanding of drug therapy.

glyburide and metformin hydrochloride

(GLIGH-byoo-righd and met-FOR-min high-droh-KLOR-ighd)
Glucovance

Pharmacologic class: sulfonylurea and biguanide
Therapeutic class: antidiabetic
Pregnancy risk category: B

Indications and dosages

▶ **Type 2 (non–insulin-dependent) diabetes when hyperglycemia can't be controlled with diet and exercise alone.** *Adults:* Initially 1.25 mg/250 mg P.O. once daily or b.i.d. with meals.

▧ **Adjust-a-dose:** In patients with glycosylated hemoglobin level above 9% or a fasting glucose level above 200 mg/dl, start with 1.25 mg/ 250 mg twice daily with morning and evening meals. Increase daily dosage in increments of 1.25 mg/250 mg per day q 2 weeks up to the minimum dosage needed to adequately control glucose level. Maximum, 20 mg glyburide and 2,000 mg metformin daily.
▶ **Second-line therapy in patients with type 2 diabetes when diet, exercise, and initial therapy with a sulfonylurea or metformin don't provide adequate glycemic control.** *Adults:* Initially 2.5 mg/500 mg or 5 mg/500 mg twice daily with meals. Increase in increments of no more than 5 mg/500 mg up to the minimum effective dosage needed to adequately control glucose level. Maximum, 20 mg glyburide and 2,000 mg metformin daily.

Contraindications and cautions

• Contraindicated in patients hypersensitive to drugs and in patients with renal disease, renal dysfunction, or metabolic acidosis (including diabetic ketoacidosis). Also contraindicated in patients receiving drugs for heart failure.
• Use cautiously in hepatically impaired, debilitated, or malnourished patients and in those with adrenal or pituitary insufficiency because of increased risk of hypoglycemia.
☙ **Lifespan:** In pregnant women, use is not recommended. Insulin is the recommended method for glycemic control during pregnancy. In breast-feeding women, drug is contraindicated. In children, safety and effectiveness haven't been established. In elderly patients, use cautiously. Monitor their renal function and don't give the maximum dosage of Glucovance. In patients age 80 and older, don't start drug unless creatinine clearance shows that renal function isn't reduced.

Adverse reactions

CNS: headache, dizziness.
GI: *diarrhea,* nausea, vomiting, abdominal pain.
Metabolic: HYPOGLYCEMIA, *lactic acidosis.*
Respiratory: *upper respiratory infection.*

Interactions

Drug-drug. *Beta blockers, chloramphenicol, ciprofloxacin, coumarins, highly protein-bound drugs, MAO inhibitors, miconazole, NSAIDs,*

probenecid, salicylates, sulfonamides: May increase hypoglycemic activity of glyburide. Monitor glucose level.
Calcium channel blockers, corticosteroids, estrogens, hormonal contraceptives, isoniazid, nicotinic acid, phenothiazines, phenytoin, sympathomimetics, thiazides and other diuretics, thyroid drugs: May increase risk of hyperglycemia. Monitor patient's glucose level.
Cationic drugs (such as amiloride, cimetidine, digoxin, morphine, procainamide, quinidine, quinine, ranitidine, triamterene, trimethoprim, vancomycin): May increase metformin level. Monitor patient.
Furosemide: May increase metformin level and decrease furosemide level. Monitor patient closely.
Nifedipine: May increase metformin level. Decrease metformin dosage if needed.
Drug-lifestyle. *Alcohol use:* May alter glycemic control, most commonly toward hypoglycemia. May also cause disulfiram-like reaction with glyburide component. Also may increase metformin effects on lactate metabolism. Avoid use together.

Effects on lab test results

• May increase lactate level. May decrease glucose level.

Pharmacokinetics

Absorption: For glyburide, almost complete. For metformin, food decreases extent and slightly delays rate.
Distribution: For glyburide, extensively protein-bound. For metformin, negligibly bound to proteins.
Metabolism: For glyburide, complete, to weakly active metabolites. For metformin, none.
Excretion: For glyburide, as metabolites in urine and bile in equal proportions. For metformin, unchanged in urine. *Glyburide half-life:* 10 hours. *Metformin half-life:* About 6 hours.

Route	Onset	Peak	Duration
P.O.			
glyburide	1 hr	4 hr	24 hr
metformin	Unknown	Unknown	Unknown

Action

Chemical effect: Glyburide stimulates the release of insulin from the pancreas. Metformin decreases hepatic glucose production and intes-

tinal absorption of glucose and improves insulin sensitivity.
Therapeutic effect: Lowers glucose level.

Available forms

Tablets: 1.25 mg glyburide and 250 mg metformin, 2.5 mg glyburide and 500 mg metformin, 5 mg glyburide and 500 mg metformin

NURSING PROCESS

⏱ Assessment
• Assess underlying condition before starting therapy, and reassess regularly.
• Obtain a list of the patient's current and past drugs. For patients previously treated with glyburide or metformin, don't give a starting dose of Glucovance that exceeds the daily dose of the glyburide (or equivalent dose of another sulfonylurea) and metformin already being taken.
• Assess glucose level before starting therapy and regularly thereafter. Monitor glycosylated hemoglobin level to assess long-term therapy.
• Obtain baseline renal function studies, and don't start drug if creatinine levels are 1.5 mg/dl or more for men or 1.4 mg/dl or more for women. Monitor renal function at least once yearly while the patient takes drug and more often in those with increased risk of renal dysfunction. If renal impairment is detected, stop drug.
• Monitor patient closely during times of increased stress, such as infection, fever, surgery, or trauma. Insulin therapy may be needed.
• Monitor patient's lab test results for megaloblastic anemia. Patient with inadequate vitamin B_{12} or calcium intake or absorption is predisposed to developing subnormal vitamin B_{12} levels when taking metformin.
• Assess patient's and family's knowledge of drug therapy.

⊕ Nursing diagnoses
• Ineffective tissue perfusion, peripheral, related to presence of hyperglycemia
• Risk for injury related to drug-induced hypoglycemia
• Deficient knowledge related to glyburide and metformin hydrochloride therapy

▶ Planning and implementation
• Make sure that adjunct therapy, such as diet and exercise, is appropriate.

• Temporarily stop giving the drug to a patient undergoing radiologic studies with intravascular iodinated contrast materials, because use of such products may result in acute alteration of renal function.
• Temporarily stop giving the drug to a patient having surgery that requires restricted intake of food and fluids, and don't restart until restriction is lifted.
• For mild hypoglycemia, give oral glucose immediately and adjust dosage and meal patterns. Severe hypoglycemic reactions with coma, seizure, or other neurologic impairment are rare but demand immediate hospitalization. If hypoglycemic coma is diagnosed or suspected, give patient a rapid I.V. injection of 50% glucose solution followed by continuous infusion of 10% glucose solution at a rate that will maintain glucose at a level above 100 mg/dl. Monitor patient with hypoglycemia closely until out of danger and, if the reaction is severe, for a minimum of 24 to 48 hours, because hypoglycemia may recur.
• For a patient requiring additional glycemic control, add a thiazolidinedione.
• Lactic acidosis is a rare but serious complication that can result from metformin accumulation. The risk of lactic acidosis increases with the degree of renal impairment and patient's age. Early symptoms of lactic acidosis may include malaise, myalgias, respiratory distress, increasing somnolence, and nonspecific abdominal distress. GI symptoms that occur after a patient is stabilized with Glucovance are unlikely to be drug-related and could be from lactic acidosis or other serious disease. Suspect lactic acidosis in any diabetic patient with metabolic acidosis lacking evidence of ketoacidosis.
• If CV collapse, acute heart failure, acute MI, or other conditions characterized by hypoxemia occur, stop drug because these conditions may be related to lactic acidosis and may cause prerenal azotemia.
• Assess patient for evidence of ketoacidosis or lactic acidosis, including electrolyte, ketone, glucose, pH, lactate, pyruvate, and metformin levels. If evidence of acidosis occurs, stop drug.
Patient teaching
• Tell patient to take once-daily dose with breakfast or twice-daily doses with breakfast and dinner.
• Teach patient about diabetes and the importance of following therapeutic regimen by ad-

G

hering to diet, weight reduction, regular exercise, and hygiene programs and by avoiding infection.

• Explain how and when to monitor glucose level and how to differentiate between hypoglycemia and hyperglycemia.

• Tell patient that his vitamin B_{12} level will be tested every 2 to 3 years.

• Instruct patient to stop drug and report unexplained hyperventilation, myalgia, malaise, unusual somnolence, or other symptoms of early lactic acidosis.

• Tell patient that GI symptoms are common early in drug therapy. GI symptoms that occur after prolonged therapy may be related to lactic acidosis or other serious disease and should be reported promptly.

• Advise patient against excessive alcohol intake, either acute or chronic.

• Advise patient not to take any other drugs, including OTC drugs, without checking with prescriber.

• Instruct patient to wear or carry medical identification.

☑ Evaluation
• Patient's glucose level is normal with drug therapy.
• Patient doesn't experience hypoglycemia.
• Patient and family state understanding of drug therapy.

goserelin acetate
(GOH-seh-reh-lin AS-ih-tayt)
Zoladex, Zoladex 3-Month

Pharmacologic class: luteinizing hormone–releasing hormone (LH-RH) analog
Therapeutic class: antineoplastic
Pregnancy risk category: X (for endometriosis); D (for advanced breast cancer)

Indications and dosages

▶ **Endometriosis, advanced breast cancer.**
Adults: One 3.6-mg implant subcutaneously q 28 days into upper abdominal wall for 6 months in endometriosis, longer in breast cancer. For endometriosis, maximum duration of therapy is 6 months.

▶ **Palliative therapy of advanced carcinoma of the prostate.** *Men:* One 10.8-mg implant

subcutaneously q 12 weeks into upper abdominal wall, given with radiotherapy and Flutamide.

▶ **Endometrial thinning before endometrial ablation for dysfunctional uterine bleeding.**
Adults: One or two 3.6-mg implants subcutaneously into upper abdominal wall. Give each implant 4 weeks apart.

Contraindications and cautions

• Contraindicated in patients hypersensitive to LH-RH, LH-RH agonist analogs, goserelin acetate, or any of its components.
• The 10.8-mg implant is contraindicated for use in women.
• Use cautiously in patients with risk factors for osteoporosis, such as family history of osteoporosis, chronic alcohol or tobacco abuse, or use of drugs that affect bone density.
⚖ **Lifespan:** In pregnant women, breastfeeding women, and children, drug is contraindicated.

Adverse reactions

CNS: *stroke,* lethargy, pain, dizziness, insomnia, anxiety, depression, headache, emotional lability, fever.
CV: edema, *heart failure, arrhythmias,* hypertension, *MI,* peripheral vascular disorder, chest pain.
GI: nausea, vomiting, diarrhea, constipation, ulcer.
GU: *impotence, lower urinary tract symptoms,* renal insufficiency, urinary obstruction, UTI, amenorrhea, vaginal dryness.
Hematologic: anemia.
Metabolic: hyperglycemia, weight increase.
Musculoskeletal: loss of bone mineral density.
Respiratory: COPD, upper respiratory tract infection.
Skin: rash, diaphoresis.
Other: chills, *hot flushes,* breast swelling and tenderness, changes in breast size, *sexual dysfunction,* gout.

Interactions

None reported.

Effects on lab test results

• May increase ALT, AST, LDL, HDL, cholesterol, triglyceride, calcium, and glucose levels. May decrease hemoglobin level and hematocrit.

Reactions may be *common*, uncommon, *life-threatening*, or COMMON AND LIFE-THREATENING.

Pharmacokinetics
Absorption: Slow.
Distribution: Low protein-binding.
Metabolism: Hydrolysis of C-terminal amino acids.
Excretion: Mostly via the kidneys with 20% unchanged. *Half-life:* About 4 hours.

Route	Onset	Peak	Duration
SubQ	2–4 wk	12–15 days	Throughout therapy

Action
Chemical effect: Acts on pituitary to decrease release of follicle-stimulating hormone and LH, resulting in dramatically lowered levels of sex hormones.
Therapeutic effect: Decreases effects of sex hormones on tumor growth in prostate gland and tissue growth in uterus.

Available forms
Implants: 3.6 mg, 10.8 mg

NURSING PROCESS

Assessment
● Assess patient's condition before starting therapy and regularly thereafter.
● When used for prostate cancer, drug may initially worsen symptoms because it initially increases testosterone levels. Patient may have increased bone pain. Rarely, disease (spinal cord compression or ureteral obstruction) may worsen.
● Be alert for adverse reactions.
● Assess patient's and family's knowledge of drug therapy.

Nursing diagnoses
● Ineffective health maintenance related to underlying condition
● Acute pain related to drug's adverse effect
● Deficient knowledge related to drug therapy

Planning and implementation
● Give under supervision of prescriber.
● Give drug into upper abdominal wall. After cleaning area with alcohol swab (and injecting local anesthetic), stretch patient's skin with one hand while grasping barrel of syringe with the other. Insert needle into subcutaneous fat; then change direction of needle so that it parallels

abdominal wall. Push in needle until hub touches patient's skin, and then withdraw about 1 cm (this creates a gap for drug to be injected) before depressing plunger completely.
● To avoid need for new syringe and injection site, don't aspirate after inserting needle.
● Implant comes in preloaded syringe. If package is damaged, don't use syringe. Make sure drug is visible in translucent chamber.
● After implantation, area requires bandage after needle is withdrawn.
● If implants require removal, schedule patient for ultrasound to locate them.
● Notify prescriber of adverse reactions, and provide supportive care.
Patient teaching
● Advise patient to report every 28 days for new implant. A delay of a couple of days is permissible.
● Tell patient to call prescriber if menstruation persists or breakthrough bleeding occurs. Menstruation should stop during therapy.
● After therapy ends, inform patient that she may experience delayed return of menses. Persistent amenorrhea is rare.
● Warn patient that pain may occur.

Evaluation
● Patient responds well to drug.
● Patient has no pain.
● Patient and family state understanding of drug therapy.

granisetron hydrochloride
(grah-NEEZ-eh-trohn high-droh-KLOR-ighd)
Kytril

Pharmacologic class: selective 5-hydroxytryptamine (5-HT$_3$) receptor antagonist
Therapeutic class: antiemetic, antinauseant
Pregnancy risk category: B

Indications and dosages
▶ **Prevention of nausea and vomiting caused by emetogenic chemotherapy.** *Adults and children age 2 and older:* 10 mcg/kg undiluted and given by direct injection over 30 seconds, or diluted and infused over 5 minutes. Begin infusion within 30 minutes before chemotherapy starts. Or, for adults, 1 mg P.O. up to 1 hour before chemotherapy and repeated 12 hours later.

Or, for adults, 2 mg P.O. daily within 1 hour before chemotherapy.

▶ **Prevention of nausea and vomiting from radiation, including total body irradiation and fractionated abdominal radiation.** *Adults:* 2 mg P.O. once daily within 1 hour of radiation.

▶ **Postoperative nausea and vomiting.** *Adults:* 1 mg I.V. undiluted and given over 30 seconds. For prevention, give before anesthesia induction or immediately before reversal.

▼ I.V. administration

• Dilute drug with normal saline injection or D_5W to make 20 to 50 ml.

• Infuse over 5 minutes, beginning within 30 minutes before chemotherapy starts and only on days chemotherapy is given.

• Diluted solutions are stable for 24 hours at room temperature.

⊗ **Incompatibilities**
Other I.V. drugs.

Contraindications and cautions

• Contraindicated in patients hypersensitive to the drug or any of its components.

� **Lifespan:** In pregnant women, use cautiously. In breast-feeding women, use cautiously because it's unknown if the drug appears in breast milk. In children, safety and effectiveness haven't been established for postoperative nausea and vomiting. In children younger than age 2, safety and effectiveness haven't been established for nausea and vomiting from chemotherapy. Safety and effectiveness of oral drug haven't been established in children of any age.

Adverse reactions

CNS: *headache, asthenia,* somnolence, agitation, anxiety, CNS stimulation, insomnia, *fever, pain, dizziness.*
CV: hypertension, *hypotension, bradycardia.*
GI: *nausea, vomiting,* diarrhea, *constipation,* taste disorder, abdominal pain, flatulence, dyspepsia, decreased appetite.
GU: UTI, *oliguria.*
Hematologic: anemia, *leukocytosis, leukopenia, thrombocytopenia.*
Respiratory: cough, increased sputum, *dyspnea.*
Skin: rash, dermatitis, alopecia, *urticaria.*
Other: *hypersensitivity reactions, anaphylaxis,* infection.

Interactions

Drug-herb. *Horehound:* May enhance serotonergic effects. Discourage use together.

Effects on lab test results

• May increase ALT and AST levels. May decrease hemoglobin level and hematocrit.
• May decrease WBC and platelet counts.

Pharmacokinetics

Absorption: Unknown.
Distribution: Distributed freely between plasma and RBCs; protein binding about 65%.
Metabolism: By liver.
Excretion: In urine and feces. *Half-life:* 5 to 9 hours.

Route	Onset	Peak	Duration
P.O., I.V.	Unknown	Unknown	Unknown

Action

Chemical effect: Located in the CNS at the area postrema (chemoreceptor trigger zone) and in the peripheral nervous system on nerve terminals of the vagus nerve. Drug's blocking action may occur at both sites.
Therapeutic effect: Prevents nausea and vomiting from chemotherapy.

Available forms

Injection: 1 mg/ml (contains benzyl alcohol)
Oral solution: 1 mg/5 ml
Tablets: 1 mg

NURSING PROCESS

🔖 **Assessment**
• Assess patient's chemotherapy and GI reactions before starting therapy.
• Monitor patient for nausea and vomiting.
• Be alert for adverse reactions.
• If drug is ineffective or diarrhea occurs, monitor hydration.
• Assess patient's and family's knowledge of drug therapy.

⊕ **Nursing diagnoses**
• Risk for deficient fluid volume related to nausea and vomiting
• Acute pain related to drug-induced headache
• Deficient knowledge related to drug therapy

Reactions may be *common*, uncommon, *life-threatening*, or COMMON AND LIFE-THREATENING.

⊠ Planning and implementation
• Give oral form of drug 1 hour before chemotherapy; repeat in 12 hours.
⊕ **ALERT:** Don't mix with other drugs. Compatibility data are limited.
• If patient has nausea or vomits, alert prescriber.
Patient teaching
• Tell patient to notify prescriber if adverse drug reactions occur.

☑ Evaluation
• Patient has no nausea or vomiting with chemotherapy.
• Patient's headache is relieved with mild analgesic.
• Patient and family state understanding of drug therapy.

---

guaifenesin (glyceryl guaiacolate)
(gwah-FEH-nih-sin)
Diabetic Tussin EX, Guiatuss*†, Hytuss†, Hytuss-2X†, Mucinex†, Mucinex ER, Naldecon Senior EX†, Organidin NR, Robitussin*†

Pharmacologic class: propanediol derivative
Therapeutic class: expectorant
Pregnancy risk category: C

Indications and dosages
▶ **Expectorant.** *Adults and children age 12 and older:* 200 to 400 mg P.O. q 4 hours, or 600 to 1,200 mg extended-release capsules q 12 hours. Maximum, 2,400 mg daily.
Children ages 6 to 11: 100 to 200 mg P.O. q 4 hours. Maximum, 1,200 mg daily.
Children ages 2 to 5: 50 to 100 mg P.O. q 4 hours. Maximum, 600 mg daily.

Contraindications and cautions
• Contraindicated in patients hypersensitive to the drug or any of its components.
🔅 **Lifespan:** In pregnant women, use cautiously. In breast-feeding women, safety and effectiveness haven't been established. In children younger than age 2 years, safety and effectiveness haven't been established. For children younger than age 12, don't give extended-release form.

Adverse reactions
CNS: drowsiness.
GI: stomach pain, diarrhea, vomiting, nausea (with large doses).
Skin: rash.

Interactions
None significant.

Effects on lab test results
• May cause false 5-hydroxyindoleacetic acid and vanillylmandelic acid results.

Pharmacokinetics
Absorption: Good.
Distribution: Unknown.
Metabolism: Unknown.
Excretion: Renal, as inactive metabolites. *Half-life:* Unknown.

Route	Onset	Peak	Duration
P.O.	Unknown	Unknown	Unknown

Action
Chemical effect: Increases production of respiratory tract fluids to help liquefy and reduce viscosity of tenacious secretions.
Therapeutic effect: Thins respiratory secretions for easier removal.

Available forms
Capsules: 200 mg†
Liquid: 100 mg/5 ml, 200 mg/5 ml
Syrup: 100 mg/5 ml†
Tablets: 100 mg†, 200 mg†, 200 mg, 400 mg
Tablets (extended-release): 600 mg†, 1,200 mg†

NURSING PROCESS

☒ Assessment
• Assess patient's sputum production before and after giving drug.
• Be alert for adverse reactions.
• If adverse GI reactions occur, monitor patient's hydration.
• Assess patient's and family's knowledge of drug therapy.

🔲 Nursing diagnoses
• Ineffective airway clearance related to underlying condition

---

• Risk for deficient fluid volume related to adverse GI reactions
• Deficient knowledge related to drug therapy

▷ **Planning and implementation**
• Give drug with a full glass of water.
Patient teaching
• Inform patient that persistent cough may indicate a serious condition. Tell him to contact prescriber if cough lasts longer than 1 week, recurs frequently, or accompanies a high fever, rash, or severe headache.
• Advise patient to take each dose with a full glass of water before and after dose. Increasing fluid intake may prove beneficial.
③ **ALERT:** Advise patient not to break, crush, or chew extended-release tablets.
• Encourage patient to perform deep-breathing exercises.

✔ **Evaluation**
• Patient's lungs are clear and respiratory secretions are normal.
• Patient maintains adequate hydration.
• Patient and family state understanding of drug therapy.

haloperidol
(hal-oh-PER-uh-dol)
Apo-Haloperidol ◆ , Haldol, Novo-Peridol ◆ ,
Peridol ◆ , PMS-Haloperidol ◆ , Serenace ◇

haloperidol decanoate
Haldol Decanoate, Haldol LA ◆

haloperidol lactate
Haldol

Pharmacologic class: butyrophenone derivative
Therapeutic class: antipsychotic
Pregnancy risk category: C

Indications and dosages

▶ **Psychotic disorders.** *Adults and children age 12 and older:* Initial range is 0.5 to 5 mg P.O. b.i.d. or t.i.d. Or 2 to 5 mg I.M. q 4 to 8

hours, although hourly administration may be needed until control is obtained. Maximum, 100 mg P.O. daily.
Children ages 3 to 11: 0.05 to 0.15 mg/kg P.O. given b.i.d. or t.i.d. Severely disturbed children may need higher doses.
▶ **Chronically psychotic patients who need prolonged therapy.** *Adults:* Initially, 10 to 20 times previous daily dosage of oral haloperidol equivalent up to a maximum of 100 mg decanoate given I.M. q 4 weeks. Usual maintenance dosage, 10 to 15 times previous daily dosage in oral haloperidol equivalents.
▶ **Nonpsychotic behavior disorders.** *Children ages 3 to 12:* 0.05 to 0.075 mg/kg P.O. b.i.d. or t.i.d. Maximum, 6 mg P.O. daily.
▶ **Tourette syndrome.** *Adults:* 0.5 to 1.5 mg P.O. t.i.d. Some patients may require up to 10 mg/day in two or three divided doses. *Children ages 3 to 12:* 0.05 to 0.075 mg/kg P.O. b.i.d. or t.i.d.
▶ **Delirium‡.** *Adults:* 1 to 2 mg I.V. q 2 to 4 hours.

▼ **I.V. administration**
• I.V. form not recommended; best I.V. dosage hasn't been established.
⊗ **Incompatibilities**
Allopurinol, amphotericin B, benztropine, cefepime, diphenhydramine, fluconazole, foscarnet, heparin, hydromorphone, hydroxyzine, ketorolac, morphine, nitroprusside, piperacillin and tazobactam.

Contraindications and cautions

• Contraindicated in patients hypersensitive to the drug or any of its components and in those with parkinsonism, coma, or CNS depression.
• Use cautiously in debilitated patients; in patients who take anticonvulsants, anticoagulants, antiparkinsonians, or lithium; and in patients with a history of seizures or EEG abnormalities, severe CV disorders, allergies, glaucoma, or urine retention.
⚘ **Lifespan:** In pregnant women, use only if benefits outweigh risks to the fetus. In breast-feeding women, drug is contraindicated. In elderly patients, use cautiously. Elderly patients need a lower initial dose and a more gradual dosage adjustment. In children younger than age 3 or those who weigh less than 15 kg (33 lb), use is contraindicated.

Adverse reactions

CNS: ***severe extrapyramidal reactions,*** tardive dyskinesia, sedation, ***seizures, neuroleptic malignant syndrome.***
CV: tachycardia, ECG changes, ***torsades de pointes,*** hypotension, hypertension, ***bradycardia.***
EENT: blurred vision.
GU: urine retention, menstrual irregularities.
Hematologic: ***leukopenia,*** leukocytosis.
Hepatic: jaundice.
Skin: rash.
Other: gynecomastia.

Interactions

Drug-drug. *Carbamazepine:* May decrease haloperidol level. Monitor patient.
CNS depressants: May increase CNS depression. Avoid use together.
Fluoxetine: May cause severe extrapyramidal reaction. Don't use together.
Lithium: May cause lethargy and confusion with high doses. Monitor patient.
Methyldopa: May cause symptoms of dementia or psychosis to appear. Monitor patient.
Phenytoin: May decrease haloperidol level. Monitor patient.
Drug-herb. *Nutmeg:* May cause loss of symptom control or interference with therapy for psychiatric illness. Discourage use together.
Drug-lifestyle. *Alcohol use:* May increase CNS depression. Discourage use together.

Effects on lab test results

• May increase liver function test values. May increase or decrease WBC count.

Pharmacokinetics

Absorption: 60% after P.O. use; 70% of I.M. dose within 30 minutes. I.M. route provides 4 to 10 times more active drug than oral route.
Distribution: Wide, with high levels in adipose tissue; 91% to 99% protein-bound.
Metabolism: Extensive.
Excretion: 40% in urine within 5 days; 15% in feces by way of biliary tract. *Half-life:* P.O., 24 hours; I.M., 21 hours.

Route	Onset	Peak	Duration
P.O.	Unknown	3–6 hr	Unknown
I.M.			
lactate	Unknown	10–20 min	Unknown
decanoate	Unknown	3–9 days	Unknown

Action

Chemical effect: May block postsynaptic dopamine receptors in brain.
Therapeutic effect: Decreases psychotic behaviors.

Available forms

haloperidol
Tablets: 0.5 mg, 1 mg, 2 mg, 5 mg, 10 mg, 20 mg
haloperidol decanoate
Injection: 50 mg/ml, 100 mg/ml
haloperidol lactate
Injection: 5 mg/ml
Oral concentrate: 2 mg/ml

H

NURSING PROCESS

Assessment

• Assess patient's disorder before starting therapy and regularly thereafter.
• Be alert for adverse reactions and drug interactions.
• Monitor patient for tardive dyskinesia, which may not appear until months or years later and may disappear spontaneously or persist for life despite stopping use of the drug.
• Assess patient's and family's knowledge of drug therapy.

Nursing diagnoses

• Disturbed thought processes related to underlying condition
• Impaired physical mobility related to extrapyramidal effects
• Deficient knowledge related to drug therapy

Planning and implementation

ALERT: Give drug by deep I.M. injection in gluteal region, using a 21G needle. Don't exceed 3 ml for each injection.
ALERT: I.V. form not recommended; optimum I.V. dosage has not been established.
• When changing from oral to injection form, give patient 10 to 15 times oral dose once monthly (maximum, 100 mg).
• Protect drug from light. Slight yellowing of liquid or concentrate is common and doesn't affect potency. Discard markedly discolored solutions.
• Don't abruptly stop giving the drug unless severe adverse reaction occurs.

• Acute dystonic reactions may be treated with diphenhydramine.

Patient teaching
• Warn patient to avoid activities that require alertness and psychomotor coordination until the drug's CNS effects are known.
• Tell patient not to drink alcohol while taking drug.
• Tell patient to relieve dry mouth with sugarless gum or hard candy.
• Instruct patient to take drug exactly as prescribed and not to double doses to compensate for missed ones.

☑ Evaluation
• Patient demonstrates decreased psychotic behavior and agitation.
• Patient maintains physical mobility.
• Patient and family state understanding of drug therapy.

heparin sodium
(HEH-prin SOH-dee-um)
Hepalean ♦ , Heparin Leo ♦ , Heparin Lock Flush Solution (with Tubex), Hep-Lock, Uniparin ◇

Pharmacologic class: anticoagulant
Therapeutic class: heparin
Pregnancy risk category: C

Indications and dosages

Heparin dosage is highly individualized depending on patient's disease state, age, and renal and hepatic health.
▶ **Deep vein thrombosis, pulmonary embolism.** *Adults:* Initially, 10,000 units as I.V. bolus; then adjust according to PTT and give I.V. q 4 to 6 hours (5,000 to 10,000 units). Or 5,000 units as I.V. bolus; then 20,000 to 40,000 units in 24 hours by I.V. infusion pump. Adjust hourly rate 4 to 6 hours after bolus dose according to PTT.
Children: Initially, 50 units/kg I.V. drip. Maintenance dosage is 100 units/kg I.V. drip over 4 hours. Constant infusion: 20,000 units/m² daily. Adjust dosages according to PTT.
▶ **Embolism prevention.** *Adults:* 5,000 units subcutaneously q 8 to 12 hours. In surgical patients, give first dose 2 hours before procedure; follow with 5,000 units subcutaneously q 8 to

12 hours for 5 to 7 days or until patient is fully ambulatory.
▶ **Open-heart surgery.** *Adults:* (total body perfusion) 150 to 400 units/kg continuous I.V. infusion.
▶ **DIC.** *Adults:* 50 to 100 units/kg I.V. q 4 hours as a single injection or constant infusion. If no improvement in 4 to 8 hours, stop drug.
Children: 25 to 50 units/kg I.V. q 4 hours as a single injection or constant infusion. If no improvement in 4 to 8 hours, stop drug.
▶ **Maintaining patency of I.V. indwelling catheters.** *Adults:* 10 to 100 units I.V. flush. Use sufficient volume to fill device. Not intended for therapeutic use.
▶ **Unstable angina‡.** *Adults:* 70 to 80 units/kg I.V. loading dose; follow by infusion maintaining PTT at 1.5 to 2 times control level during first week of anginal pain.
▶ **Post MI, cerebral thrombosis in evolving stroke, left ventricular thrombi, heart failure, history of embolism, and atrial fibrillation‡.** *Adults:* 5,000 units subcutaneously q 12 hours empirically. Or 75 units/kg continuous infusion to maintain PTT at 1.5 to 2 times control value; follow by warfarin sodium.

▼ I.V. administration

• Check order and vial carefully. Heparin comes in various concentrations.
• Give drug I.V. using infusion pump to provide maximum safety because of long-term effects and irregular absorption when given subcutaneously.
• Check constant I.V. infusions regularly, even when pumps are in good working order, to prevent giving too much or too little.
• Never piggyback other drugs into infusion line while heparin infusion is running. Many antibiotics and other drugs deactivate heparin. Never mix any drug with heparin in syringe when bolus therapy is used.
• If I.V. bag is empty, restart it as soon as possible and reschedule bolus dose immediately. Don't skip dose or increase rate to catch up.
⊗ **Incompatibilities**
Alteplase, amikacin, amiodarone, ampicillin sodium, atracurium, chlorpromazine, ciprofloxacin, codeine phosphate, cytarabine, dacarbazine, daunorubicin, dextrose 4.3% in sodium chloride solution 0.18%, diazepam, diltiazem, dobutamine, doxorubicin, doxycycline hyclate,

droperidol, ergotamine, erythromycin gluceptate or lactobionate, filgrastim, gentamicin, haloperidol lactate, hydrocortisone sodium succinate, hydroxyzine hydrochloride, idarubicin, kanamycin, labetalol, levorphanol, meperidine, methadone, methotrimeprazine, methylprednisone sodium succinate, morphine sulfate, netilmicin, nicardipine, penicillin G potassium, penicillin G sodium, pentazocine lactate, phenytoin sodium, polymyxin B sulfate, prochlorperazine edisylate, promethazine hydrochloride, quinidine gluconate, 1/6 M sodium lactate, streptomycin, tobramycin sulfate, trifluoperazine, triflupromazine, vancomycin, vinblastine, warfarin; solutions containing a phosphate buffer, sodium carbonate, or sodium oxalate.

Contraindications and cautions

• Contraindicated in patients hypersensitive to the drug or any of its components.
• Use very cautiously in patients with active bleeding; blood dyscrasia; bleeding tendencies, such as hemophilia, thrombocytopenia, or hepatic disease with hypoprothrombinemia; suspected intracranial hemorrhage; suppurative thrombophlebitis; inaccessible ulcerative lesions (especially of GI tract) and open ulcerative wounds; extensive denudation of skin; ascorbic acid deficiency and other conditions causing increased capillary permeability; subacute bacterial endocarditis; shock; advanced renal disease; threatened abortion; and severe hypertension. Also use very cautiously during or after brain, eye, or spinal cord surgery; during spinal tap or spinal anesthesia; and during continuous tube drainage of stomach or small intestine. Although heparin is clearly hazardous in these conditions, risk versus benefits must be evaluated. Use cautiously in patients with mild hepatic or renal disease, alcoholism, an occupation with a risk of physical injury, or a history of allergies, asthma, or GI ulcerations.
⚠ **Lifespan:** In pregnant women who need anticoagulation, most clinicians use heparin. Use it cautiously, especially during the last trimester and immediately postpartum, because of the increased risk of maternal hemorrhage. Heparin doesn't appear in breast milk. In neonates, safety and effectiveness haven't been established. In elderly patients, use cautiously and at a lower dose.

Adverse reactions

CNS: fever.
EENT: rhinitis, conjunctivitis, lacrimation.
Hematologic: *hemorrhage, overly prolonged clotting time, thrombocytopenia.*
Skin: irritation, mild pain, hematoma, ulceration, pruritus, urticaria, cutaneous or subcutaneous necrosis.
Other: *white clot syndrome, hypersensitivity reactions,* chills, burning of feet, *anaphylaxis.*

Interactions

Drug-drug. *Aspirin, other salicylates and antiplatelet drugs:* May increase the risk of bleeding. Monitor coagulation tests and patient closely for bleeding.
Oral anticoagulants: May cause additive anticoagulation. Monitor PT, INR, and PTT; monitor patient for bleeding.
Thrombolytics: May increase risk of hemorrhage. Monitor patient closely for bleeding.
Drug-herb. *Dong quai, feverfew, garlic, ginger, horse chestnut, motherwort, red clover:* May increase risk of bleeding. Monitor patient closely for bleeding.

Effects on lab test results

• May increase ALT and AST levels.
• May increase INR, PT, and PTT. May decrease platelet count.

Pharmacokinetics

Absorption: Peak level varies.
Distribution: Extensively bound to lipoprotein, globulins, and fibrinogen.
Metabolism: Thought to be removed by reticuloendothelial system, with some metabolism occurring in liver.
Excretion: Small amount in urine as unchanged drug. *Half-life:* 1 to 2 hours. Half-life is dose-dependent and nonlinear and may be disproportionately prolonged at higher doses.

Route	Onset	Peak	Duration
I.V.	Immediate	Unknown	Unknown
SubQ	20–60 min	2–4 hr	Unknown

Action

Chemical effect: Accelerates formation of antithrombin III–thrombin complex and deactivates thrombin, preventing conversion of fibrinogen to fibrin.

Therapeutic effect: Decreases ability of blood to clot.

Available forms

Products are derived from beef lung or porcine intestinal mucosa.

heparin sodium
Carpuject: 5,000 units/ml
Disposable syringes: 1,000 units/ml;
2,500 units/ml; 5,000 units/ml; 7,500 units/ml;
10,000 units/ml; 15,000 units/ml; 20,000 units/ml; 40,000 units/ml
Premixed I.V. solutions: 1,000 units in 500 ml of normal saline solution; 2,000 units in 1,000 ml of normal saline solution; 12,500 units in 250 ml of half-normal saline solution; 25,000 units in 250 ml of half-normal saline solution; 25,000 units in 500 ml of half-normal saline solution; 10,000 units in 100 ml of D_5W; 12,500 units in 250 ml of D_5W; 25,000 units in 250 ml of D_5W; 25,000 units in 500 ml of D_5W; 20,000 units in 500 ml of D_5W
Unit-dose ampules: 1,000 units/ml;
5,000 units/ml; 10,000 units/ml
Vials: 1,000 units/ml; 2,500 units/ml;
5,000 units/ml; 7,500 units/ml; 10,000 units/ml;
15,000 units/ml; 20,000 units/ml; 40,000 units/ml
heparin sodium flush
Disposable syringes: 10 units/ml, 100 units/ml
Vials: 10 units/ml, 100 units/ml

NURSING PROCESS

Assessment
• Assess patient's underlying condition before starting therapy.
• Draw blood to establish baseline coagulation values before starting therapy.
• Monitor the drug's effectiveness by measuring PTT carefully and regularly. Anticoagulation is present when PTT values are 1½ to 2 times control values.
• To avoid falsely elevated PTT, always draw blood 30 minutes before next dose. Draw blood for PTT 8 hours after start of continuous I.V. heparin therapy. Don't draw blood for PTT from I.V. tubing of heparin infusion; draw blood from opposite arm.
• Be alert for adverse reactions and drug interactions.
• Monitor platelet counts regularly. Thrombocytopenia caused by heparin may be linked to a type of arterial thrombosis known as white clot syndrome.
• Solutions more concentrated than 100 units/ml can irritate blood vessels.
• Assess patient's and family's knowledge of drug therapy.

Nursing diagnoses
• Risk for injury related to potential for thrombosis or emboli development from underlying condition
• Ineffective protection related to increased bleeding risks
• Deficient knowledge related to drug therapy

Planning and implementation
• Give low-dose injections sequentially between iliac crests in lower abdomen deep into subcutaneous fat. Inject drug slowly. Leave needle in place for 10 seconds after injection, then withdraw. Don't massage after subcutaneous injection. Watch for bleeding at injection site. Alternate sites every 12 hours.
• Drug requirements are higher in early phases of thrombogenic diseases and febrile states, lower when patient's condition stabilizes.
• Place notice above patient's bed to inform I.V. team or laboratory staff to apply pressure dressings after taking blood.
• Take precautions to reduce bleeding.
• To minimize the risk of hematoma, avoid excessive I.M. injection of other drugs. If possible, don't give I.M. injections at all.
⑤ ALERT: To treat severe overdose, use protamine sulfate, a heparin antagonist. Base dosage on heparin dose, the route used, and time elapsed since it was given. As a general rule, 1 to 1.5 units of protamine/100 units of heparin are given if only a few minutes have elapsed; 0.5 to 0.75 mg protamine/100 units heparin if 30 to 60 minutes have elapsed; and 0.25 to 0.375 mg protamine/100 units heparin if 2 or more hours have elapsed.
• Abruptly stopping the drug may increase coagulability, and heparin therapy is usually followed by oral anticoagulants for prophylaxis.
⑤ ALERT: Don't give heparin with low–molecular-weight heparins.
⑤ ALERT: Spell out units instead of abbreviating as "U" to reduce the risk of error by misreading it as a zero (0).
⑤ ALERT: Don't confuse heparin with Hespan.

Reactions may be *common*, uncommon, *life-threatening*, or COMMON AND LIFE-THREATENING.

Patient teaching
• Instruct patient and family to watch for signs of bleeding and to immediately notify the prescriber.
• Tell patient to avoid OTC drugs containing aspirin, other salicylates, some herbal remedies, and other drugs that may interact with heparin.

☑ Evaluation
• Patient's PTT reflects goal of heparin therapy.
• Patient has no injury from bleeding.
• Patient and family state understanding of drug therapy.

hepatitis B immune globulin, human
(hep-uh-TIGH-tus bee ih-MYOON GLOH-byoo-lin, HYOO-mun)
BayHep B, HBIG, Nabi-HB

Pharmacologic class: immunoglobulin
Therapeutic class: hepatitis B prophylaxis
Pregnancy risk category: C

Indications and dosages

▶ **Hepatitis B exposure in high-risk patients.**
Adults and children: 0.06 ml/kg I.M. within 7 days after exposure (preferably within first 24 hours). If patient refuses hepatitis B vaccine, repeat dosage 28 days after exposure.
Neonates born to patients who test positive for hepatitis B surface antigen (HBsAg): 0.5 ml I.M. within 12 hours of birth.

Contraindications and cautions

• Contraindicated in patients with a history of anaphylactic reactions to immune serum.
• Use cautiously in patients with severe thrombocytopenia or any coagulation disorder that would contraindicate I.M. injections.
☙ **Lifespan:** In pregnant women, use cautiously. In breast-feeding women, use cautiously because it's unknown if drug appears in breast milk.

Adverse reactions

CNS: *headache.*
Musculoskeletal: *myalgia.*
Skin: urticaria.

Other: *anaphylaxis, angioedema, injection-site reactions.*

Interactions

Drug-drug. *Live-virus vaccines:* May interfere with response to live-virus vaccines. Defer routine immunization for 3 months.

Effects on lab test results

None reported.

Pharmacokinetics

Absorption: Slow.
Distribution: Unknown.
Metabolism: Unknown.
Excretion: Unknown. *Half-life:* Antibodies to HBsAg, 21 days.

Route	Onset	Peak	Duration
I.M.	1–6 days	3–11 days	≥ 2 mo

Action

Chemical effect: Provides passive immunity to hepatitis B.
Therapeutic effect: Prevents hepatitis B.

Available forms

Injection: 1-ml, 4-ml, 5-ml vials

NURSING PROCESS

☡ Assessment
• Assess patient's allergies and reaction to immunizations before starting therapy.
• Monitor effectiveness by checking patient's antibody titers.
• Be alert for anaphylaxis.
• Assess patient's and family's knowledge of drug therapy.

⊞ Nursing diagnoses
• Ineffective protection related to lack of immunity to hepatitis B
• Deficient knowledge related to drug therapy

▷ Planning and implementation
• Inject drug into anterolateral aspect of thigh or deltoid muscle in older children and adults; inject into anterolateral aspect of thigh for neonates and children younger than age 3.
• Make sure epinephrine 1:1,000 is available in case anaphylaxis occurs.

• For postexposure prophylaxis (for example, needle stick, direct contact), drug is usually given with hepatitis B vaccine.

Patient teaching
• Instruct patient to immediately report respiratory difficulty.

☑ **Evaluation**
• Patient exhibits passive immunity to hepatitis B.
• Patient and family state understanding of drug therapy.

high–molecular-weight hyaluronan
(HI–mow-LECK-yuh-lerr-wait high-al-your-RON-ann)
Hyalgan, Orthovisc, Supartz, Synvisc

Pharmacologic class: hyaluronic acid derivative
Therapeutic class: viscosupplement; analgesic
Pregnancy risk category: NR

Indications and dosages

▶ **To reduce pain caused by osteoarthritis of the knee in patients who haven't responded to nondrug therapy or simple analgesics.**
Adults: Intra-articular injection (one syringe) into affected knee once weekly for a total of three to four injections.

Contraindications and cautions

• Contraindicated in patients allergic to hyaluronate preparations, birds, eggs, feathers, and poultry.
• Contraindicated in patients with infection or skin disease in area of injection site or joint.
⚠ **Lifespan:** In pregnant women, use only if benefits outweigh risks to the fetus. In breast-feeding women and in children, safety and effectiveness haven't been established.

Adverse reactions

CNS: *headache,* pain, dizziness.
CV: *hypotensive crisis*
Musculoskeletal: *arthralgia,* back pain, bursitis.
Other: injection-site pain, anaphylactoid reaction.

Interactions

Drug-drug. *Skin preparation disinfectants that contain quaternary ammonium salts:* May cause hyaluronan to precipitate. Don't use together.

Effects on lab test results

None reported.

Pharmacokinetics

Absorption: None.
Distribution: None.
Metabolism: None.
Excretion: None. *Half-life:* Unknown.

Route	Onset	Peak	Duration
Intra-articular	Unknown	Unknown	Unknown

Action

Chemical effect: Supplements body's natural supply of hyaluronan, which acts as a shock absorber and lubricant in the joints.
Therapeutic effect: Relief of pain in knee joints in osteoarthritis patients.

Available forms

Injection: 30 mg/2 ml

NURSING PROCESS

▨ **Assessment**
• Assess patient for joint effusion before giving the drug. Remove joint effusion before injecting drug.
• Evaluate patient's degree of pain relief. Pain may not be relieved until after the third injection.
• Assess patient for injection-site reactions. Inflammation may increase briefly in affected knee in a patient with inflammatory osteoarthritis.
• Assess patient's and family's knowledge of drug therapy.

▨ **Nursing diagnoses**
• Acute pain related to underlying medical condition
• Impaired physical mobility related to underlying medical condition
• Deficient knowledge related to drug therapy

▷ **Planning and implementation**
• Drug should be given by staff trained in intra-articular administration.

Reactions may be *common*, uncommon, *life-threatening*, or COMMON AND LIFE-THREATENING.

• Use an 18G to 21G needle. Inject contents of one syringe into one knee. If needed, use a second syringe for the second knee.

• Don't give less than three injections in a treatment cycle.

• Safety and effectiveness of drug use for more than one treatment cycle or in joints other than the knee aren't known.

• Give drug immediately after opening. Store in original package at room temperature (lower than 77° F [25° C]); don't freeze. Discard unused drug.

Patient teaching

• Tell patient that pain and inflammation may increase briefly after the injection.

• Urge patient to avoid strenuous or weight-bearing activity, such as running or tennis, for more than an hour within 48 hours of an injection.

• Tell patient to report injection-site reactions, such as pain, swelling, itching, heat, rash, bruising, or redness.

• Inform patient that a treatment cycle includes at least three injections and that pain may not be relieved until after the third injection.

• Caution patient to report planned or suspected pregnancy.

☑ Evaluation

• Patient is free from pain.

• Patient has full physical mobility.

• Patient and family state understanding of drug therapy.

hydralazine hydrochloride
(high-DRAL-uh-zeen high-droh-KLOR-ighd)
Alphapress ◊, **Apresoline, Novo-Hylazin** ◆

Pharmacologic class: peripheral vasodilator
Therapeutic class: antihypertensive
Pregnancy risk category: C

Indications and dosages

▶ **Essential hypertension (orally, alone or with other antihypertensives); severe essential hypertension (parenterally, to lower blood pressure quickly).** *Adults:* Initially, 10 mg P.O. q.i.d.; gradually increase to 50 mg q.i.d., p.r.n. Maximum recommended dosage is 200 mg daily, but some patients may need 300 to 400 mg daily. Or give 10 to 20 mg I.V.

slowly and repeat p.r.n. Switch to P.O. antihypertensives as soon as possible. Or 10 to 50 mg I.M.; repeat p.r.n. Switch to P.O. form as soon as possible.

▶ **To manage hypertensive emergencies related to pregnancy (preeclampsia, eclampsia).** *Adults:* 5 to 10 mg I.V.; repeat q 20 to 30 minutes p.r.n., to achieve adequate blood pressure control. Or, infuse at 0.5 to 10 mg/hour.

▶ **To manage severe heart failure‡.** *Adults:* Initially 50 to 75 mg P.O.; then adjust according to patient's response. Most patients respond to 200 to 600 mg daily, divided q 6 to 12 hours, but daily dosages as high as 3 g have been given.

▽ I.V. administration

• Drug is compatible with normal saline solution, Ringer's and lactated Ringer's solutions, and several other common I.V. solutions. Manufacturer doesn't recommend mixing drug in infusion solutions.

• Drug changes color in most infusion solutions, but the change doesn't indicate loss of potency.

• Give drug slowly and repeat p.r.n., usually every 4 to 6 hours.

• Monitor blood pressure closely.

⊗ Incompatibilities
Aminophylline, ampicillin sodium, chlorothiazide, dextrose 10% in lactated Ringer's solution, dextrose 10% in normal saline solution, D_5W, diazoxide, doxapram, edetate calcium disodium, ethacrynate, fructose 10% in normal saline solution, fructose 10% in water, furosemide, hydrocortisone sodium succinate, mephentermine, metaraminol bitartrate, methohexital, nitroglycerin, phenobarbital sodium, verapamil.

Contraindications and cautions

• Contraindicated in patients hypersensitive to the drug or any of its components and in those with coronary artery disease or mitral valvular rheumatic heart disease.

• Use cautiously in patients with suspected cardiac disease, stroke, or severe renal impairment, and in those taking other antihypertensives.

⚕ Lifespan: In pregnant women, use cautiously. In breast-feeding women and in children, safety and effectiveness haven't been established.

Adverse reactions

CNS: peripheral neuritis, *headache,* dizziness.
CV: orthostatic hypotension, tachycardia, *arrhythmias,* angina, palpitations.
GI: nausea, vomiting, diarrhea, anorexia.
Hematologic: *neutropenia, leukopenia, agranulocytopenia.*
Metabolic: *weight gain,* sodium retention.
Skin: rash.
Other: *lupus-like syndrome.*

Interactions

Drug-drug. *Diazoxide, MAO inhibitors:* May cause severe hypotension. Use together cautiously.
Indomethacin: May decrease hydralazine effects. Monitor patient.
Metoprolol, propranolol: May increase levels and effects of these drugs. Monitor patient closely; adjust dose of either drug p.r.n.

Effects on lab test results

• May decrease hemoglobin level and hematocrit.
• May decrease neutrophil, WBC, RBC, granulocyte, and platelet counts.

Pharmacokinetics

Absorption: Rapid after P.O. use; food enhances absorption. Unknown after I.M. administration.
Distribution: Wide; 88% to 90% protein-bound.
Metabolism: Extensive, in GI mucosa and liver.
Excretion: Primarily in urine. *Half-life:* 3 to 7 hours.

Route	Onset	Peak	Duration
P.O.	20–30 min	1–2 hr	2–4 hr
I.V.	≤ 5 min	15–30 min	2–6 hr
I.M.	10–30 min	1 hr	2–6 hr

Action

Chemical effect: Unknown. As a direct-acting vasodilator, it relaxes arteriolar smooth muscle.
Therapeutic effect: Lowers blood pressure.

Available forms

Injection: 20 mg/ml
Tablets: 10 mg, 25 mg, 50 mg, 100 mg

NURSING PROCESS

◈ Assessment

• Assess blood pressure before starting therapy and regularly thereafter.
• Monitor CBC, lupus erythematosus cell preparation, and antinuclear antibody titer determination during long-term therapy.
• Be alert for adverse reactions and drug interactions, especially lupus-like reactions at high drug dosages.
• Assess patient's and family's knowledge of drug therapy.

◈ Nursing diagnoses

• Risk for injury related to presence of hypertension
• Excessive fluid volume related to sodium retention
• Deficient knowledge related to drug therapy

◈ Planning and implementation

• Give oral form of drug with meals to increase absorption.
• Some clinicians combine hydralazine therapy with diuretics and beta blockers to decrease sodium retention and tachycardia and to prevent angina.
• Compliance may be improved by giving drug twice daily. Check with prescriber.
◈ **ALERT:** Don't confuse hydralazine with hydroxyzine.
Patient teaching
• Instruct patient to take oral form with meals.
• Inform patient that orthostatic hypotension can be minimized by rising slowly and not changing position suddenly.
• Tell patient not to abruptly stop taking the drug, but to call prescriber if adverse reactions occur.
• Tell patient to limit sodium intake.

◈ Evaluation

• Patient's blood pressure is normal.
• Fluid retention doesn't develop.
• Patient and family state understanding of drug therapy.

Reactions may be *common,* uncommon, *life-threatening,* or COMMON AND LIFE-THREATENING.

hydrochlorothiazide
(high-droh-klor-oh-THIGH-uh-zighd)
Apo-Hydro ◆, Aquazide-H, Dichlotride ◇,
Dithiazide ◇, Diuchlor HI, Esidrix, Ezide,
HydroDIURIL, Hydro-Par, Microzide, Neo-
Codema ◆, Novo-Hydrazide ◆, Nu-Hydro ◆,
Oretic, Urozide ◆

Pharmacologic class: thiazide diuretic
Therapeutic class: diuretic, antihypertensive
Pregnancy risk category: B

Indications and dosages

▶ **Edema.** *Adults:* 25 to 100 mg P.O. daily or
intermittently.
▶ **Hypertension.** *Adults:* 12.5 to 50 mg P.O.
once daily. May increase or decrease daily
dosage based on blood pressure.
Children ages 2 to 12: 2.2 mg/kg or 60 mg/m^2
P.O. daily in two divided doses. Usual dosage
range is 37.5 to 100 mg P.O. daily.
*Infants and children ages 6 months to younger
than 2 years:* 2.2 mg/kg or 60 mg/m^2 P.O. daily
in two divided doses. Usual dosage range is
12.5 to 37.5 mg P.O. daily.
Infants younger than age 6 months: Up to
3.3 mg/kg daily in two divided doses.

Contraindications and cautions

• Contraindicated in patients with anuria and in
patients hypersensitive to other thiazides or sulfonamide derivatives.
• Use cautiously in patients with severe renal
disease, impaired hepatic function, and progressive hepatic disease.
☀ **Lifespan:** In pregnant women, drug isn't recommended. In breast-feeding women, safety
and effectiveness haven't been established. In
elderly patients, use lower initial dose.

Adverse reactions

CV: volume depletion and dehydration, ortho-
static hypotension.
GI: anorexia, nausea, *pancreatitis.*
GU: nocturia, polyuria, frequent urination, *re-
nal impairment.*
Hematologic: *aplastic anemia, agranulocyto-
sis, leukopenia, thrombocytopenia.*
Hepatic: *hepatic encephalopathy.*
Metabolic: hypokalemia, asymptomatic hyper-
uricemia, hyperglycemia and impairment of glu-

cose tolerance, fluid and electrolyte imbalances,
dilutional hyponatremia, hypochloremia, *metabolic alkalosis,* and hypercalcemia.
Skin: dermatitis, photosensitivity, rash.
Other: gout, *anaphylactic reactions,* hypersensitivity reactions, such as pneumonitis and vasculitis.

Interactions

Drug-drug. *Antidiabetics:* May decrease effectiveness of hypoglycemics. Adjust dosage p.r.n.;
monitor glucose level.
Antihypertensives: May have additive antihypertensive effect. Use together cautiously; monitor
blood pressure closely.
Barbiturates, opioids: May increase orthostatic
hypotensive effect. Monitor patient closely.
*Bumetanide, ethacrynic acid, furosemide,
torsemide:* May cause excessive diuretic response resulting in serious electrolyte abnormalities or dehydration. Adjust doses while monitoring patient for excessive diuretic responses.
Cholestyramine, colestipol: May decrease intestinal absorption of thiazides. Give drugs separately.
Diazoxide: May increase antihypertensive, hyperglycemic, and hyperuricemic effects. Use together cautiously.
Digoxin: May increase risk of digoxin toxicity
from hydrochlorothiazide-induced hypokalemia.
Monitor potassium and digoxin levels.
Lithium: May decrease lithium excretion, increasing risk of lithium toxicity. Monitor level.
NSAIDs: May increase risk of NSAID-induced
renal impairment. Monitor patient closely.
Drug-herb. *Dandelion:* May interfere with diuretic activity. Discourage use together.
Licorice root: May contribute to the potassium
depletion caused by thiazides. Discourage use
together.
Drug-lifestyle. *Alcohol use:* May increase orthostatic hypotensive effect. Discourage use together.
Sun exposure: May increase photosensitivity.
Urge patient to avoid unprotected or prolonged
sun exposure.

Effects on lab test results

• May increase glucose, cholesterol, triglyceride, calcium, and uric acid levels. May decrease potassium, sodium, chloride, and hemoglobin levels and hematocrit.

H

• May decrease granulocyte, WBC, and platelet counts.

Pharmacokinetics

Absorption: Varies with different forms of drug.
Distribution: Protein binding is 40% to 68%.
Metabolism: None.
Excretion: Unchanged in urine. *Half-life:* 5½ to 15 hours.

Route	Onset	Peak	Duration
P.O.	2 hr	4–6 hr	6–12 hr

Action

Chemical effect: Increases sodium and water excretion by inhibiting sodium and chloride reabsorption in the distal segment of the nephron.
Therapeutic effect: Promotes sodium and water excretion, thereby lowering blood pressure.

Available forms

Capsules: 12.5 mg
Oral solution: 50 mg/5 ml
Tablets: 25 mg, 50 mg, 100 mg

NURSING PROCESS

Assessment
• Assess patient's edema or blood pressure before starting therapy.
• Monitor the drug's effectiveness by regularly checking blood pressure, urine output, and weight. In a patient with hypertension, therapeutic response may be delayed several days.
• Monitor electrolyte levels.
• Monitor creatinine and BUN levels regularly. If these levels are more than twice normal, monitor patient for decreased effectiveness.
• Monitor uric acid level, especially in patient with history of gout.
• Be alert for adverse reactions and drug interactions.
• Assess patient's and family's knowledge of drug therapy.

Nursing diagnoses
• Ineffective health maintenance related to presence of edema or hypertension
• Impaired urinary elimination related to diuretic effect of drug

• Deficient knowledge related to drug therapy

Planning and implementation
• Give drug in morning to prevent nocturia.
• If nausea occurs, give drug with food.
• Drug may be used with potassium-sparing diuretic to prevent potassium loss.
Patient teaching
• Advise patient to take drug with food to minimize GI upset.
• Warn patient not to change position suddenly and to rise slowly to avoid orthostatic hypotension.
• Instruct patient not to drink alcohol during drug therapy.
• Advise patient to use sunblock to prevent photosensitivity reactions.
• Tell patient to check with prescriber before taking OTC drugs or herbal remedies.

Evaluation
• Patient's blood pressure is normal, and no edema is present.
• Patient demonstrates adjustment of lifestyle to accommodate altered patterns of urinary elimination.
• Patient and family state understanding of drug therapy.

hydrocortisone
(high-droh-KOR-tuh-sohn)
Cortef, Cortenema, Hydrocortone

hydrocortisone acetate
Cortifoam, Hydrocortone Acetate

hydrocortisone cypionate
Cortef

hydrocortisone sodium phosphate
Hydrocortone Phosphate

hydrocortisone sodium succinate
A-hydroCort, Solu-Cortef

Pharmacologic class: adrenocortical steroid
Therapeutic class: glucocorticoid
Pregnancy risk category: NR

Indications and dosages

▶ **Severe inflammation, adrenal insufficiency.** *Adults:* 20 to 240 mg hydrocortisone or cypionate P.O. daily. Or 5 to 75 mg acetate injected into joints or soft tissue. Give once q 2 to 3 weeks, although some conditions may require weekly injections. Dosage varies with degree of inflammation and size and location of the joint or soft tissues. Or 15 to 240 mg phosphate I.V., I.M., or subcutaneously daily, divided into 12-hour intervals. Or, initially, 100 to 500 mg succinate I.V. or I.M.; may repeat q 2 to 6 hours p.r.n.

▶ **Adjunct for ulcerative colitis and proctitis.** *Adults:* 1 enema (100 mg) hydrocortisone or acetate P.R. nightly for 21 days.

▶ **Shock.** *Adults:* Initially, 50 mg/kg succinate I.V. repeated in 4 hours or q 24 hours, p.r.n. Or 0.5 mg to 2 g I.V. q 2 to 6 hours, p.r.n. *Children:* 0.16 to 1 mg/kg or 6 to 30 mg/m² phosphate I.M. or succinate I.M. or I.V. daily or b.i.d.

▼ I.V. administration

• Don't use acetate or suspension form I.V.
• Hydrocortisone sodium phosphate may be added directly to D₅W or normal saline solution for I.V. administration.
• Reconstitute hydrocortisone sodium succinate with bacteriostatic water or bacteriostatic sodium chloride solution before adding to I.V. solutions. When giving by direct I.V. injection, inject over at least 30 seconds. For infusion, dilute with D₅W, normal saline solution, or D₅W in normal saline solution to 1 mg/ml or less.
• When giving as direct injection, inject directly into vein or I.V. line containing free-flowing compatible solution over 30 seconds to several minutes.
• When giving as intermittent or continuous infusion, dilute solution according to manufacturer's instructions and give over prescribed duration. If used for continuous infusion, change solution every 24 hours.

⊗ **Incompatibilities**
Hydrocortisone sodium phosphate: doxapram, mitoxantrone, sargramostim.
Hydrocortisone sodium succinate: amobarbital, ampicillin sodium, bleomycin, ciprofloxacin, colistimethate, cytarabine, dacarbazine, diazepam, dimenhydrinate, ephedrine, ergotamine, furosemide, heparin sodium, hydralazine, idarubicin, Ionosol B with invert sugar 10%,

kanamycin, methylprednisolone sodium succinate, midazolam, nafcillin, pentobarbital sodium, phenobarbital sodium, phenytoin, prochlorperazine edisylate, promethazine hydrochloride, sargramostim, vancomycin, vitamin B complex with C.

Contraindications and cautions

• Contraindicated in patients hypersensitive to drug or any of its components, and in those with systemic fungal infections. Hydrocortisone sodium succinate is contraindicated in premature infants.
• Use cautiously in patients with recent MI and in those with GI ulcer, renal disease, hypertension, osteoporosis, diabetes mellitus, hypothyroidism, cirrhosis, diverticulitis, nonspecific ulcerative colitis, recent intestinal anastomoses, thromboembolic disorders, seizures, myasthenia gravis, heart failure, tuberculosis, ocular herpes simplex, emotional instability, and psychotic tendencies.
❦ **Lifespan:** In pregnant women, use cautiously. In breast-feeding women, use cautiously. Drug isn't recommended in high doses. In children, use cautiously because long-term use may delay growth and maturation.

Adverse reactions

Most adverse reactions are dose- or duration-dependent.
CNS: *euphoria, insomnia,* psychotic behavior, pseudotumor cerebri, *seizures.*
CV: *heart failure,* hypertension, edema, *arrhythmias, thromboembolism.*
EENT: cataracts, glaucoma.
GI: peptic ulceration, GI irritation, increased appetite, *pancreatitis.*
Metabolic: hypokalemia, hyperglycemia, carbohydrate intolerance.
Musculoskeletal: muscle weakness, growth suppression in children, osteoporosis.
Skin: hirsutism, delayed wound healing, acne, various skin eruptions, easy bruising.
Other: susceptibility to infections, *acute adrenal insufficiency with increased stress (infection, surgery, or trauma) or abrupt withdrawal after long-term therapy.*

Interactions

Drug-drug. *Aspirin, indomethacin, other NSAIDs:* May increase risk of GI distress and bleeding. Give together cautiously.

H

Barbiturates, phenytoin, rifampin: May decrease corticosteroid effect; may require increased dosage.
Live-attenuated virus vaccines, other toxoids and vaccines: May decrease antibody response and increase risk of neurologic complications. Avoid use together.
Oral anticoagulants: May alter dosage requirements. Monitor PT and INR closely.
Potassium-depleting drugs (such as thiazide diuretics): May enhance potassium-wasting effects of hydrocortisone. Monitor potassium level.
Skin-test antigens: May decrease skin response. Defer skin testing until therapy is completed.
Drug-lifestyle. *Alcohol use:* May increase risk of GI effects. Discourage use together.

Effects on lab test results

• May increase glucose and cholesterol levels. May decrease potassium and calcium levels.

Pharmacokinetics

Absorption: Rapid after P.O. use. Variable after I.M. or intra-articular injection. Unknown after rectal use.
Distribution: Distributed to muscle, liver, skin, intestines, and kidneys. Extensively protein-bound. Only unbound portion is active.
Metabolism: Metabolized in liver.
Excretion: Inactive metabolites and small amounts of unmetabolized drug excreted in urine; insignificant quantities excreted in feces. *Half-life:* 8 to 12 hours.

Route	Onset	Peak	Duration
P.O., I.V., I.M., P.R.	Varies	Varies	Varies

Action

Chemical effect: Not clearly defined; may stabilize leukocyte lysosomal membranes, suppress immune response, stimulate bone marrow, and influence nutrient metabolism.
Therapeutic effect: Reduces inflammation, suppresses immune function, and raises adrenocorticoid hormonal levels.

Available forms

hydrocortisone
Enema: 100 mg/60 ml
Tablets: 5 mg, 10 mg, 20 mg

hydrocortisone acetate
Enema: 10% aerosol foam (provides 90 mg/application)
Injection: 25-mg/ml*, 50-mg/ml* suspension
Suppositories: 25 mg
hydrocortisone cypionate
Oral suspension: 10 mg/5 ml
hydrocortisone sodium phosphate
Injection: 50-mg/ml solution
hydrocortisone sodium succinate
Injection: 100 mg/vial*, 250 mg/vial*, 500 mg/vial*, 1,000 mg/vial*

NURSING PROCESS

⚗ Assessment
• Assess patient's condition before starting therapy and regularly thereafter.
• Monitor patient's weight, blood pressure, and electrolyte levels.
• Monitor patient for stress. Fever, trauma, surgery, and emotional problems may increase adrenal insufficiency.
• Periodically measure growth and development during high-dose or prolonged therapy in infants and children.
• Be alert for adverse reactions and drug interactions.
• Assess patient's and family's knowledge of drug therapy.

🔁 Nursing diagnoses
• Ineffective health maintenance related to underlying condition
• Ineffective protection related to immunosuppression
• Deficient knowledge related to drug therapy

⟩ Planning and implementation
• For better results and less toxicity, give once-daily dose in morning.
• Give oral dose with food.
• Give I.M. injection deep into gluteal muscle. Rotate injection sites to prevent muscle atrophy.
• Rectal suppositories may produce the same systemic effects as other forms of hydrocortisone. If therapy must exceed 21 days, stop gradually by giving every other night for 2 or 3 weeks.
• **ALERT:** Avoid subcutaneous injection because atrophy and sterile abscesses may occur.
• Injectable forms aren't used for alternate-day therapy.

• High-dose therapy usually doesn't continue beyond 48 hours.
• Always adjust to lowest effective dose, and gradually reduce dosage after long-term therapy.
• Give potassium supplements.
• If evidence of adrenal insufficiency appears, notify prescriber and increase dosage.
• Notify prescriber about adverse reactions. Provide supportive care.
⟁ **ALERT:** Avoid abbreviating drug as HCT, which can be misread as HCTZ (hydrochlorothiazide).
⟁ **ALERT:** Don't confuse Solu-Cortef with Solu-Medrol.

Patient teaching
• Teach patient signs of early adrenal insufficiency (fatigue, muscle weakness, joint pain, fever, anorexia, nausea, dyspnea, dizziness, and fainting).
• Instruct patient to carry or wear medical identification that identifies need for supplemental systemic glucocorticoids during stress.
⟁ **ALERT:** Tell patient not to abruptly stop taking the drug without prescriber's consent. Abruptly stopping therapy may lead to rebound inflammation, fatigue, weakness, arthralgia, fever, dizziness, lethargy, depression, fainting, orthostatic hypotension, dyspnea, anorexia, and hypoglycemia. After prolonged use, sudden withdrawal may be fatal.
• Warn patient receiving long-term therapy about cushingoid symptoms, and tell him to report sudden weight gain or swelling to prescriber.
• Advise him to consider exercise or physical therapy, to ask his prescriber about vitamin D or calcium supplements, and to have periodic ophthalmic examinations.
• Warn patient about easy bruising.

☑ Evaluation
• Patient's condition improves.
• Serious complications related to drug-induced immunosuppression don't develop.
• Patient and family state understanding of drug therapy.

hydromorphone hydrochloride (dihydromorphinone hydrochloride)
(high-droh-MOR-fohn high-droh-KLOR-ighd)
Dilaudid, Dilaudid-HP

Pharmacologic class: opioid
Therapeutic class: analgesic, antitussive
Pregnancy risk category: C
Controlled substance schedule: II

Indications and dosages
▶ **Moderate to severe pain.** *Adults:* 2 to 4 mg P.O. q 4 to 6 hours p.r.n. Or 1 to 2 mg I.M., subcutaneously, or I.V. (slowly over at least 2 to 3 minutes) q 4 to 6 hours p.r.n. Or 3-mg rectal suppository q 6 to 8 hours p.r.n.
▶ **Cough.** *Adults:* 1 mg P.O. q 3 to 4 hours p.r.n.
Children ages 6 to 12: 0.5 mg P.O. q 3 to 4 hours p.r.n.

▼ I.V. administration
• For infusion, drug may be mixed in D₅W, normal saline solution, D₅W in normal saline solution, D₅W in half-normal saline solution, or Ringer's or lactated Ringer's solutions.
• For direct injection, give over at least 2 minutes.
• Respiratory depression and hypotension may occur. Monitor respiration and circulation frequently.
⊗ **Incompatibilities**
Alkalines, amphotericin B cholesterol complex, ampicillin sodium, bromides, cefazolin, dexamethasone, diazepam, gallium nitrate, haloperidol, heparin sodium, iodides, minocycline, phenobarbital sodium, phenytoin sodium, prochlorperazine edisylate, sargramostim, sodium bicarbonate, sodium phosphate, thiopental.

Contraindications and cautions
• Contraindicated in patients hypersensitive to drug or any of its components, patients with intracranial lesions from increased intracranial pressure, patients with status asthmaticus, and whenever ventilatory function is depressed in the absence of resuscitative equipment. Also contraindicated as obstetric analgesia.
• Use with extreme caution in patients with COPD, cor pulmonale, a substantially decreased

respiratory reserve, hypoxia, hypercapnia, or respiratory depression. Use cautiously in debilitated patients and in patients with hepatic or renal disease, hypothyroidism, Addison's disease, prostatic hypertrophy, urethral stricture, CNS depression or coma, toxic psychosis, gallbladder disease, acute alcoholism, alcohol withdrawal, kyphoscoliosis, or sulfite sensitivity (because drug contains sodium metabisulfite and may cause allergic-type reactions, including anaphylactic symptoms or asthmatic episodes, especially in people with asthma). Also use cautiously after GI surgery.

☀ **Lifespan:** In pregnant women, use only if potential benefits to mother outweigh risks to the fetus. During labor and delivery, don't use drug. Women shouldn't breast-feed while receiving drug. In children, safety and effectiveness haven't been established except as listed for cough. In elderly patients, use cautiously.

Adverse reactions

CNS: *sedation, somnolence, clouded sensorium, dizziness, euphoria,* **seizures.**
CV: hypotension, **bradycardia.**
EENT: blurred vision, diplopia, nystagmus.
GI: nausea, vomiting, constipation, ileus.
GU: urine retention.
Respiratory: *respiratory depression, bronchospasm.*
Other: induration with repeated subcutaneous injections, physical dependence.

Interactions

Drug-drug. *CNS depressants, general anesthetics, hypnotics, MAO inhibitors, other opioid analgesics, sedatives, tranquilizers, tricyclic antidepressants:* May have additive effects. Use together cautiously. Reduce hydromorphone dose, and monitor patient response.
Drug-lifestyle. *Alcohol use:* May have additive effects. Discourage use together.

Effects on lab test results

• May increase amylase and lipase levels.

Pharmacokinetics

Absorption: Good.
Distribution: Unknown.
Metabolism: Primarily in liver.
Excretion: Primarily in urine. *Half-life:* 2½ to 4 hours.

Route	Onset	Peak	Duration
P.O.	30 min	30 min–2 hr	4–5 hr
I.V.	10–15 min	15–30 min	2–3 hr
I.M.	15 min	30–60 min	4–5 hr
SubQ	15 min	30–90 min	4 hr
P.R.	Unknown	Unknown	4 hr

Action

Chemical effect: Binds with opioid receptors in CNS, altering perception of and emotional response to pain. Suppresses cough reflex by direct action on cough center in medulla.
Therapeutic effect: Relieves pain and cough.

Available forms

Injection: 1 mg/ml, 2 mg/ml, 4 mg/ml, 10 mg/ml
Injection (lyophilized powder): 250 mg/vial
Liquid: 5 mg/5 ml
Suppositories: 3 mg
Tablets: 2 mg, 4 mg, 8 mg

NURSING PROCESS

⚗ Assessment

• Assess patient's pain or cough before and after giving drug.
• Drug may worsen or mask gallbladder pain.
• Drug is a commonly abused opioid. Be alert for addictive behavior or drug abuse.
• Be alert for adverse reactions and drug interactions.
• Assess patient's and family's knowledge of drug therapy.

⊕ Nursing diagnoses

• Acute pain related to underlying condition
• Ineffective breathing pattern related to respiratory depression
• Deficient knowledge related to drug therapy

⊳ Planning and implementation

• For better analgesic effect, give drug before patient's pain becomes intense.
• Dilaudid-HP, a highly concentrated form (10 mg/ml), may be given in smaller volumes to prevent discomfort caused by large-volume I.M. or subcutaneous injections. Check dosage carefully.
• To avoid induration with subcutaneous injection, rotate injection sites.

Reactions may be *common,* uncommon, *life-threatening,* or COMMON AND LIFE-THREATENING.

• Keep resuscitation equipment and opioid antagonist (naloxone) available.

• Postoperatively, encourage patient to turn, cough, and deep-breathe to avoid atelectasis.

• Recommend increased intake of fiber and fluids and a stool softener to prevent constipation during maintenance therapy.

• Signs and symptoms of overdose include respiratory depression, CNS depression progressing to stupor or coma, flaccid muscles, cold and clammy skin, bradycardia, hypotension, and constricted pupils. Severe overdose may include apnea, circulatory collapse, cardia arrest, and death.

• To treat overdose, ensure a patent airway and provide ventilation as needed. If patient is conscious and received the oral form of drug, gastric lavage or induced emesis may be useful in removing unabsorbed drug. If patient is unconscious and has a secure airway, activated charcoal may be given by NG tube; a saline cathartic or sorbitol may be added to the first dose. If patient has significant respiratory or circulatory depression, give naloxone; use caution if patient may be physically dependent on hydromorphone. Provide symptomatic and supportive treatment, including I.V. fluids, vasopressors, and other measures as needed.

Patient teaching

• Advise ambulatory patient to be careful when getting out of bed or walking. Warn patient to avoid activities that require mental alertness until the drug's CNS effects are known.

• Encourage patient to ask for drug before pain becomes severe.

• If patient's respiratory rate decreases, tell patient or caregiver to notify prescriber.

• Instruct patient to avoid alcohol consumption during drug therapy.

☑ Evaluation

• Patient is free from pain.

• Patient maintains adequate breathing patterns.

• Patient and family state understanding of drug therapy.

hydroxychloroquine sulfate
(high-droks-ee-KLOR-oh-kwin SUL-fayt)
Plaquenil

Pharmacologic class: 4-aminoquinoline
Therapeutic class: antimalarial, antiinflammatory
Pregnancy risk category: C

Indications and dosages

▶ **Suppressive prophylaxis of malaria attacks caused by** *Plasmodium vivax, P. malariae, P. ovale,* **and susceptible strains of** *P. falciparum. Adults:* 310 mg base P.O. weekly on same day of week. Begin 1 to 2 weeks before exposure and continue for 4 weeks after leaving endemic areas.
Children: 5 mg base/kg P.O. weekly, not to exceed 310 mg.
Patients untreated before exposure: Initial loading dose is doubled (620 mg for adults, 10 mg/kg for children) P.O. in two divided doses 6 hours apart.

▶ **Acute malarial attacks.** *Adults:* Initially, 620 mg base P.O.; then 310 mg base after 6 hours; then 310 mg base daily for 2 days.
Children: Initial dose, 10 mg base/kg (up to 620 mg base); second dose, 5 mg base/kg (up to 310 mg base) 6 hours after first dose; third dose, 5 mg base/kg 18 hours after second dose; fourth dose, 5 mg base/kg 24 hours after third dose.

▶ **Lupus erythematosus (chronic discoid and systemic).** *Adults:* 400 mg (sulfate) P.O. daily or b.i.d., continued for several weeks or months, depending on response. Prolonged maintenance dosage: 200 to 400 mg (sulfate) daily.

▶ **Rheumatoid arthritis.** *Adults:* Initially, 400 to 600 mg (sulfate) P.O. daily. When good response occurs (usually in 4 to 12 weeks), reduce dosage by 50% and continue at 200 to 400 mg daily.

Contraindications and cautions

• Contraindicated in patients hypersensitive to the drug or any of its components and in patients with retinal or visual field changes or porphyria.

• Use cautiously in patients with severe GI, neurologic, or blood disorders, and in patients with hepatic disease or alcoholism because drug concentrates in liver. Also use cautiously in

those with G6PD deficiency or psoriasis because drug may worsen these conditions.
❀ **Lifespan:** In pregnant women, use cautiously. In breast-feeding women, safety and effectiveness haven't been established. In children who need long-term therapy, drug is contraindicated.

Adverse reactions

CNS: irritability, nightmares, ataxia, *seizures,* psychic stimulation, toxic psychosis, vertigo, nystagmus, lassitude, fatigue, dizziness, hypoactive deep tendon reflexes.
EENT: serious visual disturbances, ototoxicity.
GI: anorexia, abdominal cramps, diarrhea, nausea, vomiting.
Hematologic: *agranulocytosis, leukopenia, thrombocytopenia, aplastic anemia, hemolysis in patients with G6PD deficiency.*
Metabolic: weight loss.
Musculoskeletal: skeletal muscle weakness.
Skin: pruritus, lichen planus eruptions, skin and mucosal pigmentary changes, pleomorphic skin eruptions, alopecia, bleaching of hair.

Interactions

Drug-drug. *Aluminum and magnesium salts, kaolin:* May decrease GI absorption. Separate administration times.
Cimetidine: May decrease hepatic metabolism of hydroxychloroquine. Monitor patient for toxicity.

Effects on lab test results

• May decrease hemoglobin level and hematocrit.
• May decrease granulocyte, WBC, and platelet counts.

Pharmacokinetics

Absorption: Good and almost complete.
Distribution: Concentrates in liver, spleen, kidneys, heart, and brain and is strongly bound in melanin-containing cells. Drug is bound to proteins.
Metabolism: By liver.
Excretion: Mostly unchanged in urine. *Half-life:* 32 to 50 days.

Route	Onset	Peak	Duration
P.O.	Unknown	2–4½ hr	Unknown

Action

Chemical effect: May bind to and alter properties of DNA in susceptible organisms.
Therapeutic effect: Prevents or hinders growth of *P. malariae, P. ovale, P. vivax,* and *P. falciparum.* Relieves inflammation.

Available forms

Tablets: 200 mg (equivalent to 155-mg base)

NURSING PROCESS

☞ Assessment
• Assess patient's condition before starting therapy and regularly thereafter.
• Make sure baseline and periodic ophthalmic examinations are performed because blindness can occur. Check periodically for ocular muscle weakness after long-term use.
• Obtain audiometric examinations before, during, and after therapy, and especially during long-term therapy.
• Monitor CBC and liver function studies periodically during long-term therapy.
• Assess patient for overdose, which can quickly lead to headache, drowsiness, visual disturbances, CV collapse, and seizures, followed by cardiopulmonary arrest. Children are extremely susceptible to toxicity, so don't give them long-term therapy.
• Be alert for adverse reactions and drug interactions.
• Assess patient's and family's knowledge of drug therapy.

⊕ Nursing diagnoses
• Infection related to susceptible organisms
• Disturbed sensory perception (visual and auditory) related to adverse reactions to drug
• Deficient knowledge related to drug therapy

❯ Planning and implementation
• Give drug right before or after meals on same day of each week.
• Notify prescriber immediately about severe blood disorder that can't be attributed to disease. Blood reaction may require stopping drug.
Patient teaching
• Advise patient to take drug immediately before or after meals on same day each week to enhance compliance for prophylaxis.

Reactions may be *common,* uncommon, *life-threatening,* or COMMON AND LIFE-THREATENING.

● If adverse CNS or visual disturbances occur, warn patient to avoid hazardous activities.
● Tell patient to promptly report visual or auditory changes.

☑ Evaluation
● Patient is free from infection.
● Patient maintains normal visual and auditory function.
● Patient and family state understanding of drug therapy.

hydroxyurea
(high-droks-ee-yoo-REE-uh)
Droxia, Hydrea, Mylocel

Pharmacologic class: antimetabolite
Therapeutic class: antineoplastic; antisickling drug
Pregnancy risk category: D

Indications and dosages

Dosage and indications for hydroxyurea may vary. Check current literature for recommended protocol.
▶ **Solid tumors.** *Adults:* 80 mg/kg Hydrea or Mylocel P.O. as a single dose q 3 days; or 20 to 30 mg/kg Hydrea or Mylocel P.O. as a single daily dose.
▶ **Head and neck cancers, excluding the lip.** *Adults:* 80 mg/kg Hydrea or Mylocel P.O. as a single dose q 3 days.
▶ **Resistant chronic myelocytic leukemia.** *Adults:* 20 to 30 mg/kg Hydrea or Mylocel P.O. as a single daily dose.
▶ **To reduce the frequency of painful crises and to reduce the need for blood transfusions in patients with sickle cell anemia with recurrent moderate-to-severe painful crises (typically at least 3 during the preceding 12 months).** *Adults:* Base dosage on the patient's actual or ideal weight, whichever is less. The initial dose is 15 mg/kg Droxia P.O. as a single daily dose. The patient's blood count must be monitored every 2 weeks; see package insert for dosage adjustment.

Contraindications and cautions

● Contraindicated in patients hypersensitive to the drug or any of its components and in those with marked bone marrow depression and severe anemia.
● Use cautiously in patients with renal dysfunction.
● **Lifespan:** In pregnant women, use only if benefits outweigh risks to the fetus. In breast-feeding women, drug is contraindicated. In children, safety and effectiveness haven't been established. Elderly patients may be more sensitive to the drug and require a lower dosage.

Adverse reactions

CNS: fever, malaise, drowsiness, hallucinations, headache, dizziness, disorientation, *seizures.*
GI: anorexia, nausea, vomiting, diarrhea, stomatitis.
GU: *renal toxicity.*
Hematologic: *leukopenia, thrombocytopenia,* anemia, *megaloblastosis, bone marrow suppression.*
Metabolic: hyperuricemia.
Skin: rash, pruritus, mucositis.
Other: chills.

Interactions

Drug-drug. *Cytotoxic drugs, radiation therapy:* May enhance toxicity of hydroxyurea. Use together cautiously.

Effects on lab test results

● May increase liver enzyme, BUN, creatinine, and uric acid levels. May decrease hemoglobin level and hematocrit.
● May decrease WBC, RBC, and platelet counts.

Pharmacokinetics

Absorption: Good. Level is higher with a large, single dose than with divided doses.
Distribution: Crosses blood-brain barrier.
Metabolism: 50% of dose degraded in liver.
Excretion: 50% of drug in urine as unchanged drug; metabolites excreted through lungs as carbon dioxide and in urine as urea. *Half-life:* 3 to 4 hours.

Route	Onset	Peak	Duration
P.O.	Unknown	2 hr	Unknown

Action

Chemical effect: Unknown; thought to inhibit DNA synthesis.

Therapeutic effect: Hinders growth of certain cancer cells.

Available forms

Capsules: 200 mg, 300 mg, 400 mg, 500 mg
Tablets: 1,000 mg

✍ Assessment
• Assess patient's condition before therapy and regularly thereafter.
• Measure CBC, BUN, uric acid, and creatinine levels.
• Auditory and visual hallucinations and hematologic toxicity increase with decreased renal function.
• Radiation therapy may increase risk or severity of GI distress or stomatitis.
• Be alert for adverse reactions and drug interactions.
• Assess patient's and family's knowledge of drug therapy.

🔁 Nursing diagnoses
• Ineffective health maintenance related to presence of neoplastic disease
• Ineffective protection related to adverse hematologic reactions
• Deficient knowledge related to drug therapy

▷ Planning and implementation
• Keep patient hydrated.
• Dosage modification may be needed after chemotherapy or radiation therapy.
• Bone marrow suppression is dose-limited and dose-related, with rapid recovery.
Patient teaching
• If patient can't swallow capsules, tell him to empty contents of capsules into water and drink immediately.
• Warn patient to watch for signs of infection (fever, sore throat, fatigue) and bleeding (easy bruising, nosebleed, bleeding gums, melena). Instruct patient to take infection-control and bleeding precautions. Tell patient to take temperature daily.
• Advise woman of childbearing age not to become pregnant during therapy and to consult with prescriber before becoming pregnant.

✔ Evaluation
• Patient responds well to drug therapy.

• Serious infections or bleeding complications don't develop.
• Patient and family state understanding of drug therapy.

hydroxyzine embonate ◇
(high-DROKS-ih-zeen EM-boh-nayt)
Atarax

hydroxyzine hydrochloride
Apo-Hydroxyzine ♦ , Atarax, Hydroxacen, Hyzine-50, Multipax ♦ , Neucalm, Novo-Hydroxyzin ♦ , QYS, Vistacon-50, Vistaject-50, Vistaril

hydroxyzine pamoate
Vistaril

Pharmacologic class: piperazine derivative
Therapeutic class: anxiolytic, sedative, antihistamine, antipruritic, antiemetic, antispasmodic
Pregnancy risk category: C

Indications and dosages

▶ **Anxiety.** *Adults:* 50 to 100 mg P.O. q.i.d.
Children age 6 and older: 50 to 100 mg P.O. daily in divided doses.
Children younger than age 6: 50 mg P.O. daily in divided doses.
▶ **Preoperative and postoperative adjunct therapy.** *Adults:* 25 to 100 mg I.M. q 4 to 6 hours.
Children: 1.1 mg/kg I.M. q 4 to 6 hours.
▶ **Pruritus from allergies.** *Adults:* 25 mg P.O. t.i.d. or q.i.d.
Children age 6 and older: 50 to 100 mg P.O. daily in divided doses.
Children younger than age 6: 50 mg P.O. daily in divided doses.
▶ **Psychiatric and emotional emergencies, including acute alcoholism.** *Adults:* 50 to 100 mg I.M. q 4 to 6 hours p.r.n.
▶ **Nausea and vomiting (excluding nausea and vomiting of pregnancy).** *Adults:* 25 to 100 mg I.M.
Children: 1.1 mg/kg I.M.
▶ **Prepartum and postpartum adjunct therapy.** *Adults:* 25 to 100 mg I.M.

Reactions may be *common*, uncommon, **life-threatening**, or COMMON AND LIFE-THREATENING.

Contraindications and cautions

● Contraindicated in patients hypersensitive to hydroxyzine or cetirizine

⚖ **Lifespan:** In early pregnancy, drug is contraindicated. In breast-feeding women, safety and effectiveness haven't been established. In elderly patients, use cautiously and at lower doses.

Adverse reactions

CNS: *drowsiness,* involuntary motor activity.
GI: *dry mouth.*
Other: marked discomfort at I.M. injection site, hypersensitivity reactions.

Interactions

Drug-drug. *CNS depressants:* May increase CNS depression. Avoid use together.
MAO inhibitors: May enhance anticholinergic effects. Use together cautiously.
Drug-lifestyle. *Alcohol use:* May increase CNS depression. Discourage use together.
Sun exposure: Photosensitivity may occur. Urge patient to avoid unprotected or prolonged sun exposure.

Effects on lab test results

● May cause false elevations of urine 17-hydroxycorticosteroids, depending on test method used.

Pharmacokinetics

Absorption: Rapid and complete after P.O. administration. Unknown for I.M. administration.
Distribution: Unknown.
Metabolism: Almost complete.
Excretion: Primarily in urine. *Half-life:* 3 hours.

Route	Onset	Peak	Duration
P.O.	15–30 min	2 hr	4–6 hr
I.M.	Unknown	Unknown	4–6 hr

Action

Chemical effect: Unknown; may suppress activity in key regions of subcortical area of CNS.
Therapeutic effect: Relieves anxiety and itching, promotes calmness, and alleviates nausea and vomiting.

Available forms

hydroxyzine embonate
Capsules: 25 mg, 50 mg

hydroxyzine hydrochloride
Capsules: 10 mg ◊ , 25 mg, 50 mg, 100 mg
Injection: 25 mg/ml*, 50 mg/ml*
Syrup: 10 mg/5 ml*
Tablets: 10 mg, 25 mg, 50 mg, 100 mg
Tablets (film-coated): 10 mg, 25 mg, 50 mg
hydroxyzine pamoate
Capsules: 25 mg, 50 mg, 100 mg
Oral suspension: 25 mg/5 ml

NURSING PROCESS

⚕ Assessment
● Assess patient's condition before therapy and regularly thereafter.
● Be alert for adverse reactions and drug interactions.
● Assess patient's and family's knowledge of drug therapy.

⊞ Nursing diagnoses
● Ineffective health maintenance related to underlying condition
● Risk for injury related to adverse CNS reactions
● Deficient knowledge related to drug therapy

▷ Planning and implementation
● Give a lower dose to an elderly or debilitated patient.
● Parenteral form (hydroxyzine hydrochloride) for I.M. use only; Z-track injection method is preferred. Aspirate I.M. injection carefully to prevent inadvertent intravascular injection. Inject deep into large muscle mass.
Ⓢ **ALERT:** Never give I.V.
Ⓢ **ALERT:** Don't confuse hydroxyzine with hydralazine.
Patient teaching
● Warn patient to avoid hazardous activities until CNS effects of drug are known.
● Tell patient to avoid alcohol during drug therapy.
● Suggest sugarless hard candy or gum to relieve dry mouth.

☑ Evaluation
● Patient exhibits improved health.
● Patient doesn't experience injury.
● Patient and family state understanding of drug therapy.

---

ibandronate sodium
(ih-BAN-druh-nayt SOH-dee-um)
Boniva

Pharmacologic classification: bisphosphonate
Therapeutic classification: bone resorption inhibitor
Pregnancy risk category: C

Indications and dosages

▶ **Treatment or prevention of postmenopausal osteoporosis.** *Adults:* 2.5 mg P.O. daily or 150 mg P.O. once monthly, taken first thing in the morning with a large glass of plain water 1 hour before any food or other drugs. Must maintain a standing or upright seated position for 60 minutes after ingestion.

Contraindications and cautions

• Contraindicated in patients hypersensitive to ibandronate and patients with uncorrected hypocalcemia or an inability to stand or sit upright for 60 minutes. Not recommended for patients with severe renal impairment (creatinine clearance less than 30 ml/minute).
• Use cautiously in patients with a history of GI disorders.
≋ **Lifespan:** In pregnant women, use only if benefits outweigh risks to the fetus. In breastfeeding women, use cautiously because it isn't known if drug appears in breast milk. In children, safety and effectiveness haven't been established.

Adverse reactions

CNS: asthenia, dizziness, headache, insomnia, nerve root lesion, vertigo.
CV: hypertension.
EENT: nasopharyngitis, pharyngitis.
GI: abdominal pain, constipation, diarrhea, *dyspepsia,* gastritis, nausea, vomiting.
GU: UTI.
Musculoskeletal: arthralgia, arthritis, *back pain,* joint disorder, limb pain, localized osteoarthritis, muscle cramps, myalgia, osteonecrosis.

Respiratory: bronchitis, pneumonia, upper respiratory tract infection.
Skin: rash.
Other: allergic reaction, infection, influenza, tooth disorder.

Interactions

Drug-drug. *Aspirin, NSAIDs:* May increase GI irritation. Use together cautiously.
Aluminum-, calcium-, magnesium-, or iron-containing products: May decrease ibandronate absorption. Give ibandronate 60 minutes before vitamins, minerals, or antacids.
Drug-food. *Food, milk, and beverages other than water:* May decrease ibandronate absorption. Give drug on an empty stomach with plain water.
Drug-lifestyle. *Alcohol use:* May decrease ibandronate absorption and increase risk of esophageal irritation. Discourage use together.

Effects on lab test results

• May increase cholesterol level. May decrease total alkaline phosphatase level.
• May interfere with bone-imaging agents.

Pharmacokinetics

Absorption: Drug is absorbed in the upper GI tract; bioavailability is low and is significantly impaired by food or non-water beverages.
Distribution: Rapidly binds to bone or is eliminated.
Metabolism: Not metabolized.
Excretion: Eliminated unchanged in urine and feces; 50% to 60% excreted by kidneys. *Half-life:* 37 to 157 hours in patients taking the 150-mg dose.

Route	Onset	Peak	Duration
P.O.	Unknown	½–2 hr	Unknown

Action

Chemical effect: Inhibits the osteoclast activity of bone breakdown and removal to reduce bone loss.
Therapeutic effect: Increases bone mass.

Available forms

Tablets: 2.5 mg, 150 mg

NURSING PROCESS

⚕ Assessment

• Assess patient for adequate intake of calcium and vitamin D.

• Monitor patient for signs or symptoms of esophageal irritation, including dysphagia, painful swallowing, retrosternal pain, and heartburn.

• Monitor patient for bone, joint, and muscle pain, which may be severe or incapacitating.

• Watch for signs and symptoms of uveitis and scleritis.

• Assess patient's and family's knowledge of drug therapy.

⊕ Nursing diagnoses

• Risk for injury related to decreased bone mass

• Risk for deficient fluid volume related to drug-induced GI upset

• Deficient knowledge related to drug therapy

⧉ Planning and implementation

• Correct hypocalcemia or other disturbances of bone and mineral metabolism before therapy.

• Administer drug in the morning 60 minutes before the first meal or fluid and before any other medicines.

• Bisphosphonates may lead to osteonecrosis, mainly in the jaw. Dental surgery may worsen the condition. Assess the risk of stopping ibandronate if the patient needs dental procedures.

• Signs of possible overdose include hypocalcemia, hypophosphatemia, upset stomach, dyspepsia, esophagitis, gastritis, or ulcer.

• Treatment of overdose includes giving milk or antacids to enhance binding of ibandronate. Avoid emesis to minimize gastric irritation. Keep patient upright during management of overdose. Dialysis isn't helpful.

Patient teaching

• Tell patient taking the monthly dose to take it on the same date each month and to wait at least 7 days between doses if she misses a scheduled dose.

• Instruct patient to take drug 60 minutes before eating or drinking in the morning and before any other drugs, including OTC products, such as calcium, antacids, and vitamins.

• Advise patient to swallow drug whole with a full glass of plain water while standing or sitting and to remain upright for at least 60 minutes after taking drug.

• Caution patient to take only with plain water and no other beverage.

• Instruct patient not to chew or suck on the tablet.

• Advise patient to take calcium and vitamin D supplements as directed by prescriber.

• Tell patient to report any bone, joint, or muscle pain.

• Advise patient to stop drug and immediately report signs and symptoms of esophageal irritation, such as dysphagia, painful swallowing, retrosternal pain, or heartburn.

✓ Evaluation

• Patient does not suffer any injury related to decreased bone mass.

• Patient maintains adequate hydration.

• Patient and family state understanding of drug therapy.

ibuprofen
(igh-byoo-PROH-fen)
ACT-3 ◇, Advil†, Advil Children's, Advil Infants' Drops†, Advil Junior Strength†, Advil Liqui-Gels†, Advil Migraine†, Apo-Ibuprofen ♦, Brufen ◇, Genpril Caplets†, Genpril Tablets†, Haltran†, IBU†, Ibu-Tab†, Junior Strength Motrin†, Menadol, Midol Cramp†, Midol IB, Motrin, Motrin Children's†, Motrin Drops†, Motrin IB Caplets†, Motrin IB Gelcaps†, Motrin IB Tablets† Motrin Infants' Drops†, Motrin Migraine Pain Caplets†, Novo-Profen, Nurofen, Rafen ◇, Saleto-200

Pharmacologic class: NSAID
Therapeutic class: analgesic, antipyretic, anti-inflammatory
Pregnancy risk category: B

Indications and dosages

▶ **Rheumatoid arthritis, osteoarthritis.**
Adults: 300 to 800 mg P.O. t.i.d. or q.i.d., not to exceed 3.2 g P.O. daily.
Children: 20 to 40 mg/kg P.O. daily, divided into three to four doses.
▶ **Mild to moderate pain, dysmenorrhea.**
Adults: 400 mg P.O. q 4 to 6 hours p.r.n.
Children ages 6 months to 12 years: 10 mg/kg per dose P.O. q 6 to 8 hours. Maximum, 40 mg/kg daily.

▶ **Fever, minor aches and pains.** *Adults and children older than age 12:* 200 to 400 mg P.O. q 4 to 6 hours p.r.n. Don't exceed 1.2 g P.O. daily or give for longer than 3 days for fever or 10 days for pain unless directed by prescriber. *Children ages 6 months to 12 years:* If temperature is below 102.5° F (39° C), recommended dosage is 5 mg/kg P.O. q 6 to 8 hours p.r.n. Treat higher temperatures with 10 mg/kg P.O. q 6 to 8 hours p.r.n. to maximum dosage of 40 mg/kg daily.

Contraindications and cautions

• Contraindicated in patients hypersensitive to the drug or any of its components and in those with nasal polyps, angioedema, and bronchospastic reaction to aspirin or other NSAIDs.
• Use cautiously in patients with GI disorders, history of peptic ulcer disease, hepatic or renal disease, cardiac decompensation, hypertension, or intrinsic coagulation defects.
🌼 **Lifespan:** In pregnant and breast-feeding women, use cautiously. In infants younger than age 6 months, safety and effectiveness haven't been established. In elderly patients, use with caution and at a lower dose because they are at greater risk for adverse GI effects.

Adverse reactions

CNS: *headache, drowsiness, dizziness,* cognitive dysfunction, aseptic meningitis.
CV: *peripheral edema,* edema, hypertension, *heart failure.*
EENT: visual disturbances, *tinnitus.*
GI: epigastric distress, nausea, *occult blood loss,* peptic ulceration.
GU: reversible renal failure.
Hematologic: prolonged bleeding time, anemia, *neutropenia, pancytopenia, thrombocytopenia, aplastic anemia, leukopenia,* agranulocytosis.
Respiratory: *bronchospasm.*
Skin: pruritus, rash, urticaria, photosensitivity reactions, *Stevens-Johnson syndrome.*

Interactions

Drug-drug. *Antihypertensives, furosemide, thiazide diuretics:* May decrease effectiveness of diuretics or antihypertensives. Monitor patient.
Aspirin: May decrease drug level and increase risk of adverse GI reactions. Avoid use together.
Corticosteroids: May increase risk of adverse GI reactions. Avoid use together.

Cyclosporine: May increase nephrotoxicity of both drugs. Avoid use together.
Digoxin: May increase digoxin level. Monitor level closely for digoxin toxicity.
Lithium, oral anticoagulants: May increase levels or effects of these drugs. Monitor patient for toxicity.
Methotrexate: May increase risk of methotrexate toxicity. Monitor patient closely.
Probenecid: Probenecid may increase level and toxicity of NSAIDs. Monitor patient for signs of toxicity.
Drug-herb. *Dong quai, feverfew, garlic, ginger, horse chestnut, red clover:* May increase risk of bleeding. Monitor patient closely for bleeding.
St. John's wort: May increase risk of photosensitivity reactions. Advise patient to avoid unprotected or prolonged exposure to sunlight.
Drug-lifestyle. *Alcohol use:* May increase risk of adverse GI reactions. Discourage use together.
Smoking: May increase risk for gastric ulceration. Discourage use together.
Sun exposure: May cause photosensitivity reactions. Advise patient to avoid unprotected or prolonged exposure to sunlight.

Effects on lab test results

• May increase BUN, creatinine, ALT, AST, potassium levels. May decrease glucose and hemoglobin levels and hematocrit.
• May decrease neutrophil, WBC, RBC, platelet, and granulocyte counts.

Pharmacokinetics

Absorption: Rapid and complete from GI tract.
Distribution: Highly protein-bound.
Metabolism: Undergoes biotransformation in liver.
Excretion: Mainly in urine, with some biliary excretion. *Half-life:* 2 to 4 hours.

Route	Onset	Peak	Duration
P.O.	≤ 30 min	2–4 hr	≥ 4 hr

Action

Chemical effect: May inhibit prostaglandin synthesis.
Therapeutic effect: Relieves pain, fever, and inflammation.

Available forms

Caplets: 200 mg†

Capsules (liquid-filled): 200 mg†
Oral drops: 40 mg/ml†
Oral suspension: 100 mg/5 ml†
Tablets: 100 mg†, 200 mg†, 400 mg†, 600 mg, 800 mg
Tablets (chewable): 50 mg†, 100 mg†
Tablets (film-coated): 100 mg†, 200 mg†, 400 mg†, 600 mg, 800 mg

NURSING PROCESS

⚚ Assessment
• Assess patient's underlying condition before starting therapy.
• Evaluate patient for relief from pain, fever, or inflammation. Full effects on arthritis may take 2 to 4 weeks.
• Check renal and hepatic function periodically in long-term therapy.
• Be alert for adverse reactions and drug interactions.
• Assess patient's and family's knowledge of drug therapy.

⊞ Nursing diagnoses
• Chronic pain related to underlying condition
• Risk for injury related to drug-induced adverse reactions
• Deficient knowledge related to drug therapy

⧁ Planning and implementation
• Give with meals or milk to reduce adverse GI reactions.
• If drug is ineffective, notify prescriber.
• If renal or hepatic abnormalities occur, stop drug and notify prescriber.
Patient teaching
• Tell patient to take drug with meals or milk to reduce adverse GI reactions.
• ⓢ ALERT: Tell adult patient using OTC drug not to exceed 1.2 g daily, not to give drug to children younger than age 12, and not to take drug for extended periods without consulting prescriber.
• Warn patient that using drug with aspirin, alcohol, or corticosteroids may increase the risk of adverse GI reactions.
• Serious GI toxicity, including peptic ulceration and bleeding, can occur in patients taking NSAIDs, despite absence of GI symptoms.
• Teach patient to recognize and report signs and symptoms of GI bleeding.

• Instruct patient not to drink alcohol during therapy.
• Instruct patient to use sunblock, wear protective clothing, and avoid prolonged exposure to sunlight.
• Inform patient that some ankle swelling may occur, but tell him to call prescriber promptly if weight increases by 3 to 5 lbs/week, or he develops shortness of breath, cough, or palpitations.

☑ Evaluation
• Patient is free from pain.
• Patient doesn't experience injury from adverse reactions.
• Patient and family state understanding of drug therapy.

ibutilide fumarate
(igh-BYOO-tih-lighd FYOO-muh-rayt)
Corvert

Pharmacologic class: ibutilide derivative
Therapeutic class: class III antiarrhythmic
Pregnancy risk category: C

Indications and dosages

▶ **Rapid conversion of recent atrial fibrillation or atrial flutter to sinus rhythm.** *Adults weighing 60 kg (132 lb) or more:* 1 mg I.V. over 10 minutes.
Adults weighing less than 60 kg (132 lb): 0.01 mg/kg I.V. over 10 minutes.

▽ I.V. administration

• Give undiluted or diluted in 50 ml of diluent. Add to normal saline solution for injection or D_5W injection before infusion. Add contents of one 10-ml vial (0.1 mg/ml) to a 50-ml infusion bag to form admixture of about 0.017 mg/ml ibutilide fumarate. Drug is compatible with polyvinyl chloride plastic bags and polyolefin bags.
• Admixtures with approved diluents are chemically and physically stable for 24 hours at room temperature or 48 hours if refrigerated.
• Inspect parenteral drugs for particles and discoloration before giving.
• Stop infusion if arrhythmia stops or if patient develops sustained or nonsustained ventricular tachycardia or significantly prolonged QT interval. If arrhythmia doesn't stop within 10 min-

utes after infusion ends, give a second 10-minute infusion of equal strength.

⊗ **Incompatibilities**
None reported.

Contraindications and cautions

• Contraindicated in patients hypersensitive to the drug or any of its components.
• Contraindicated for use in patients with history of polymorphic ventricular tachycardia, such as torsades de pointes.
• Use cautiously in patients with hepatic or renal dysfunction; usually, no dosage adjustments are needed.
🜲 **Lifespan:** In pregnant women, use cautiously. In breast-feeding women and in children, safety and effectiveness haven't been established.

Adverse reactions

CNS: headache, syncope.
CV: ventricular extrasystoles, *nonsustained ventricular tachycardia,* hypotension, bundle branch block, *sustained polymorphic ventricular tachycardia, AV block,* hypertension, *QT interval prolongation, bradycardia,* palpitations, tachycardia, *heart failure.*
GI: nausea.
GU: *renal failure.*

Interactions

Drug-drug. *Class IA antiarrhythmics (such as disopyramide, procainamide, quinidine), other class III drugs (such as amiodarone, sotalol):* May increase risk of prolonged refractory state. Avoid use together.
Digoxin: Supraventricular arrhythmias may mask cardiotoxicity from excessive digoxin levels. Use cautiously.
H₁-receptor antagonist antihistamines, phenothiazines, tetracyclic antidepressants, tricyclic antidepressants, other drugs that prolong QT interval: May increase risk of proarrhythmias. Monitor patient closely.

Effects on lab test results

None reported.

Pharmacokinetics

Absorption: Administered I.V.
Distribution: Highly distributed; about 40% protein-bound.
Metabolism: Not clearly defined.

Excretion: Excreted in urine and feces. *Half-life:* Averages about 6 hours.

Route	Onset	Peak	Duration
I.V.	Unknown	Unknown	Unknown

Action

Chemical effect: Prolongs action potential in isolated cardiac myocyte and increases atrial and ventricular refractoriness; has predominantly class III properties.
Therapeutic effect: Restores normal sinus rhythm.

Available forms

Injection: 0.1 mg/ml in 10-ml vials

NURSING PROCESS

Assessment
• Assess patient's arrhythmia before starting therapy.
⚠ **ALERT:** Monitor ECG continuously during therapy and for at least 4 hours afterward (or until QT interval returns to baseline) because drug can induce or worsen ventricular arrhythmias. If ECG shows arrhythmias, monitor it longer.
• Be alert for adverse reactions and drug interactions.
• Assess patient's and family's knowledge of drug therapy.

Nursing diagnoses
• Decreased cardiac output related to arrhythmias
• Risk for injury related to life-threatening arrhythmias
• Deficient knowledge related to drug therapy

Planning and implementation
• Drug should be given only by skilled personnel. During and after administration, have available proper equipment and facilities for a cardiac emergency, such as cardiac monitor, intracardiac pacer, cardioverter or defibrillator, and drugs for sustained ventricular tachycardia.
• Correct hypokalemia and hypomagnesemia before therapy to reduce risk of proarrhythmia.
Patient teaching
• Tell patient to promptly report adverse reactions, especially headaches, dizziness, weakness, palpitations, or chest pains.

• Instruct patient to report any discomfort at injection site.

☑ **Evaluation**
• Patient regains normal sinus rhythm.
• Life-threatening arrhythmia doesn't develop.
• Patient and family state understanding of drug therapy.

idarubicin hydrochloride
(igh-duh-ROO-bih-sin high-droh-KLOR-ighd)
Idamycin, Idamycin PFS

Pharmacologic class: anthracycline antibiotic
Therapeutic class: antineoplastic
Pregnancy risk category: D

Indications and dosages

▶ **Acute myeloid leukemia, including French-American-British classifications M1 through M7, with other approved antileukemic drugs.** *Adults:* 12 mg/m² by slow I.V. injection (over 10 to 15 minutes) daily for 3 days with 100 mg/m² of cytarabine by continuous I.V. infusion daily for 7 days or cytarabine as 25-mg/m² bolus followed by 200 mg/m² by continuous infusion daily for 5 days. Give second course, if needed. If patient develops severe mucositis, don't give until recovery is complete, and reduce dosage by 25%.

🔢 **Adjust-a-dose:** For patients with hepatic or renal impairment, reduce dosage. If bilirubin level is above 5 mg/dl, withhold drug.

▼ I.V. administration

• Preparation and administration of drug have carcinogenic, mutagenic, and teratogenic risks for personnel. Follow facility policy to reduce risks.
• Reconstitute to final concentration of 1 mg/ml using normal saline solution for injection. Add 5 ml to 5-mg vial or 10 ml to 10-mg vial. Don't use bacteriostatic saline solution. Vial is under negative pressure.
• Give over 10 to 15 minutes into free-flowing I.V. infusion of normal saline solution or D₅W running into large vein. If extravasation occurs, stop infusion immediately, elevate limb, and notify prescriber. Apply intermittent ice packs for 30 minutes immediately and then 30 minutes q.i.d. for 4 days. Consult plastic surgery

promptly if pain, erythema, edema, vesication, or ulceration occurs.
• Reconstituted solutions are stable for 72 hours at 59° to 86° F (15° to 30° C), 7 days if refrigerated. Label unused solutions with chemotherapy hazard label.

⊗ **Incompatibilities**
Acyclovir sodium, alkaline solutions, allopurinol, ampicillin sodium with sulbactam, cefazolin, cefepime, ceftazidime, clindamycin phosphate, dexamethasone sodium phosphate, etoposide, furosemide, gentamicin, heparin, hydrocortisone sodium succinate, lorazepam, meperidine, methotrexate sodium, piperacillin sodium with tazobactam, sodium bicarbonate, teniposide, vancomycin, vincristine.

Contraindications and cautions

• Use cautiously in patients with bone marrow suppression induced by previous drug therapy or radiotherapy and in patients with impaired hepatic or renal function, heart disease, or previous therapy with anthracyclines at high cumulative doses or other potentially cardiotoxic drugs.
Lifespan: In pregnant and breast-feeding women, use cautiously. In children, safety and effectiveness haven't been established.

Adverse reactions

CNS: *fever, headache, changed mental status,* peripheral neuropathy, *seizures.*
CV: *heart failure,* atrial fibrillation, chest pain, *MI,* myocardial insufficiency, *arrhythmias, myocardial toxicity, cardiomyopathy.*
GI: *nausea, vomiting, cramps, diarrhea, mucositis, severe enterocolitis with perforation.*
Hematologic: MYELOSUPPRESSION, HEMORRHAGE.
Skin: *alopecia,* rash, urticaria, bullous erythrodermatous rash on palms and soles, urticaria at injection site, erythema at previously irradiated sites, tissue necrosis at injection site if extravasation occurs.
Other: INFECTION.

Interactions

None reported.

Effects on lab test results

• May increase BUN, creatinine, and uric acid and levels. May decrease hemoglobin level and hematocrit.

• May increase liver function test values. May decrease RBC, WBC, and platelet counts.

Pharmacokinetics

Absorption: Administered I.V.
Distribution: 97% lipophilic and tissue-bound, with highest levels in nucleated blood and bone marrow cells.
Metabolism: Extensively outside of liver. Metabolite is cytotoxic.
Excretion: Primarily biliary. *Half-life:* 20 to 22 hours.

Route	Onset	Peak	Duration
I.V.	Unknown	≤ 3 min	Unknown

Action

Chemical effect: May inhibit nucleic acid synthesis by intercalation; interacts with enzyme topoisomerase II.
Therapeutic effect: Hinders growth of susceptible leukemic cells.

Available forms

Powder for injection: 1 mg/ml available in 5-, 10-, and 20-mg vials

NURSING PROCESS

🏷 Assessment

• Assess patient's condition before starting therapy and regularly thereafter.
• Assess patient for systemic infection, and control infection before therapy begins.
• Monitor CBC and hepatic and renal function test results frequently.
• Be alert for adverse reactions and drug interactions, especially signs of heart failure, infection, and hemorrhage.
• Assess patient's and family's knowledge of drug therapy.

🔀 Nursing diagnoses

• Ineffective health maintenance related to presence of underlying condition
• Ineffective protection related to adverse hematologic reactions
• Deficient knowledge related to drug therapy

❯ Planning and implementation

• Take appropriate preventive measures (including adequate hydration) before starting treatment.

🏵 **ALERT:** Never give drug I.M. or subcutaneously.
• Hyperuricemia may result from rapid destruction of leukemic cells. Give allopurinol.
🏵 **ALERT:** Don't confuse idarubicin with daunorubicin.
Patient teaching
• Teach patient to recognize and report signs of extravasation, infection, bleeding, and heart failure, such as shortness of breath and leg swelling.
• Advise patient that red urine for several days is normal and doesn't indicate blood in urine.
• Advise women of childbearing age to use a reliable contraceptive during therapy and to consult with prescriber before becoming pregnant.

☑ Evaluation

• Patient responds well to drug.
• Serious adverse hematologic reactions don't develop.
• Patient and family state understanding of drug therapy.

ifosfamide
(igh-FOHS-fuh-mighd)
IFEX

Pharmacologic class: alkylating drug
Therapeutic class: antineoplastic
Pregnancy risk category: D

Indications and dosages

▶ **Testicular cancer.** *Adults:* 1.2 g/m² I.V. daily for 5 consecutive days. Repeat q 3 weeks or after patient recovers from hematologic toxicity.
▶ **Lung cancer, Hodgkin's and malignant lymphoma, breast cancer, acute lymphocytic leukemia, ovarian cancer, gastric cancer, pancreatic cancer, sarcomas, cervical cancer, and uterine cancer‡.** *Adults:* 1.2 to 2.5 g/m² I.V. daily for 3 to 5 days, with cycles of therapy repeated p.r.n.

▼ I.V. administration

• Follow facility policy to reduce risks. Preparation and administration are linked to carcinogenic, mutagenic, and teratogenic risks for personnel.
• Reconstitute each gram of drug with 20 ml of diluent to yield 50 mg/ml. Use sterile water for

injection or bacteriostatic water for injection. Solutions may be further diluted with sterile water, dextrose 2.5% or 5% in water, half-normal or normal saline solution for injection, D_5W and normal saline solution for injection, or lactated Ringer's injection.

• Infuse each dose over at least 30 minutes.

• Ifosfamide and mesna are physically compatible and may be mixed in same I.V. solution.

• Reconstituted solution is stable for 1 week at room temperature or 6 weeks if refrigerated. If drug was reconstituted with sterile water, however, use solution within 6 hours.

⊗ Incompatibilities
Cefepime, methotrexate sodium.

Contraindications and cautions

• Contraindicated in patients hypersensitive to the drug or any of its components and in those with severely depressed bone marrow function.

• Use cautiously in patients with renal impairment or compromised bone marrow from leukopenia, granulocytopenia, extensive bone marrow metastases, previous radiation therapy, or previous therapy with cytotoxic drugs.

⚞ Lifespan: In pregnant and breast-feeding women, drug is contraindicated. In children, safety and effectiveness haven't been established.

Adverse reactions

CNS: lethargy, *somnolence, confusion, depressive psychosis,* **coma, seizures,** ataxia.
GI: *nausea, vomiting.*
GU: *hemorrhagic cystitis, hematuria,* **nephrotoxicity.**
Hematologic: **leukopenia, thrombocytopenia, myelosuppression.**
Metabolic: *metabolic acidosis.*
Skin: *alopecia.*
Other: infection.

Interactions

Drug-drug. *Anticoagulants, aspirin:* May increase risk of bleeding. Avoid use together.
Barbiturates, chloral hydrate, phenytoin: May increase ifosfamide toxicity by inducing hepatic enzymes that hasten formation of toxic metabolites. Monitor patient closely.
Mesna: May decrease ifosfamide-induced bladder toxicity. May be given together.
Myelosuppressants: May enhance hematologic toxicity. Dosage adjustment may be needed.

Effects on lab test results

• May increase BUN, creatinine, bilirubin, and liver enzyme levels. May decrease hemoglobin level and hematocrit.

• May decrease WBC, RBC, and platelet counts.

Pharmacokinetics

Absorption: Administered I.V.
Distribution: Crosses blood-brain barrier, but its metabolites don't, so alkylation doesn't occur in CSF.
Metabolism: About 50% of dose is metabolized in liver.
Excretion: Primarily in urine. *Half-life:* About 14 hours.

Route	Onset	Peak	Duration
I.V.	Unknown	Unknown	Unknown

Action

Chemical effect: Cross-links strands of cellular DNA and interferes with RNA transcription, which causes growth imbalance that leads to cell death.
Therapeutic effect: Kills cancer cells.

Available forms

Injection: 1 g (supplied with 200-mg ampule of mesna), 3 g (supplied with 400-mg ampule of mesna)

NURSING PROCESS

🔍 Assessment

• Assess patient's condition before starting therapy and regularly thereafter.

• Obtain urinalysis before each dose. If microscopic hematuria is present, evaluate patient for hemorrhagic cystitis. Adjust dosage of mesna, a protecting agent given with drug, if needed.

• Monitor CBC and renal and liver function test results.

• Be alert for adverse reactions and drug interactions.

• Assess patient for mental status changes. Dosage may need to be decreased or therapy stopped.

• Assess patient's and family's knowledge of drug therapy.

⊕ **Nursing diagnoses**
• Ineffective health maintenance related to presence of cancer
• Ineffective protection related to adverse CNS and hematologic reactions
• Deficient knowledge related to drug therapy

❯ **Planning and implementation**
• Give antiemetic before giving drug to decrease nausea.
• Give drug with mesna to prevent hemorrhagic cystitis. Give mesna with or before drug to prevent cystitis. Give at least 2 L of fluids daily, either P.O. or I.V.
• Don't give drug h.s.; infrequent voiding at night may increase risk of cystitis. If cystitis develops, stop giving drug and notify prescriber.
• Bladder irrigation with normal saline solution may decrease possibility of cystitis.
• Institute infection control and bleeding precautions.
⊛ **ALERT:** Don't confuse ifosfamide with cyclophosphamide.
Patient teaching
• Tell patient to void frequently to minimize contact of drug and its metabolites with bladder mucosa.
• Warn patient to watch for evidence of infection (fever, sore throat, fatigue), CNS effects (somnolence and dizziness), and bleeding (easy bruising, nosebleed , bleeding gums, melena). Teach patient about infection-control and bleeding precautions, and tell him to report adverse effects. Tell him to take his temperature daily.
• Instruct patient to avoid OTC drugs that contain aspirin.
• Stress importance of adequate fluid intake. Explain that it may help prevent hemorrhagic cystitis.
• Warn patient that hyperpigmentation may occur.

☑ **Evaluation**
• Patient responds well to drug.
• Serious infections and CNS and bleeding complications don't develop.
• Patient and family state understanding of drug therapy.

iloprost
(IGH-loe-prost)
Ventavis

Pharmacologic class: prostacyclin analog
Therapeutic class: vasodilator
Pregnancy risk category: C

Indications and dosages

▶ **Pulmonary arterial hypertension in patients with New York Heart Association Class III or IV symptoms.** *Adults:* Initially, 2.5 mcg inhaled using the Prodose AAD System. As tolerated, increase to 5 mcg inhaled six to nine times daily while awake, p.r.n., but no more than q 2 hours. Maximum, 5 mcg nine times daily.

Contraindications and cautions

• No known contraindications. Don't use in patients whose systolic blood pressure is less than 85 mm Hg.
• Use drug cautiously in patients who have hepatic or renal impairment and in patients with COPD, severe asthma, or acute pulmonary infection.
⚖ **Lifespan:** In pregnant women, use only if benefits outweigh risk to fetus. In breast-feeding women, breast-feeding should be stopped because it isn't known if drug appears in breast milk. In children, safety and effectiveness haven't been established. In elderly patients, use cautiously and start with a low dosage.

Adverse reactions

CNS: *headache,* insomnia, *syncope.*
CV: chest pain, *heart failure, hypotension,* palpitations, peripheral edema, *supraventricular tachycardia, vasodilation.*
EENT: tongue pain.
GI: *nausea,* vomiting.
GU: *renal failure.*
Musculoskeletal: back pain, muscle cramps, *trismus.*
Respiratory: *cough,* dyspnea, hemoptysis, pneumonia, *pulmonary edema.*
Other: *flulike syndrome.*

Interactions

Drug-drug. *Antihypertensive drugs, vasodilators:* May increase effects of these drugs. Monitor patient's blood pressure.
Anticoagulants: May increase the risk of bleeding. Monitor patient closely.

Effects on lab test results

• May increase alkaline phosphatase and GGT levels.

Pharmacokinetics

Absorption: No GI absorption.
Distribution: Protein-binding is 60%, mainly to albumin.
Metabolism: To inactive metabolites.
Excretion: Mainly in urine; some in feces.
Half-life: 20 to 30 minutes.

Route	Onset	Peak	Duration
Inhalation	Unknown	Unknown	30–60 min

Action

Chemical effect: Lowers pulmonary arterial pressure by dilating systemic and pulmonary arterial beds. Drug also affects platelet aggregation, although effect in pulmonary hypertension treatment isn't known.
Therapeutic effect: Improved exercise tolerance, fewer symptoms, and lack of deterioration.

Available forms

Inhalation solution: 20 mcg/2-ml single-use ampule

NURSING PROCESS

🔲 Assessment

• Assess patient's underlying condition, and assess regularly thereafter.
• Monitor patient's vital signs carefully at start of treatment.
• Monitor patient for syncope.
• Monitor patient for evidence of pulmonary edema; stop treatment immediately.
• Assess patient's and family's knowledge of drug therapy.

🔲 Nursing diagnoses

• Ineffective tissue perfusion (cardiopulmonary) related to underlying condition

• Risk for injury related to drug-induced syncope
• Deficient knowledge related to drug therapy

🔲 Planning and implementation

• Keep drug away from skin and eyes.
• Administer drug only through Prodose AAD device.
• Take care not to inhale drug while providing treatment.
• Overdose may cause hypotension, headache, flushing, nausea, vomiting, and diarrhea.
• To treat overdose, stop the inhalation session as needed. Monitor patient closely, and provide symptomatic treatment.

Patient teaching
• Advise patient to take drug exactly as prescribed using Prodose AAD.
• Urge patient to follow manufacturer's instructions for preparing and inhaling drug.
• Advise patient to keep a backup Prodose AAD in case the original malfunctions.
• Tell patient to keep drug away from skin and eyes and to rinse the area immediately if contact occurs.
• Caution patient not to ingest the drug solution.
• Inform patient that drug may cause dizziness and fainting. Urge him to stand up slowly from a sitting or lying position and to report worsening of symptoms.
• Tell patient to take drug before physical exertion but no more than every 2 hours.
• Discourage exposing other people—especially pregnant women and babies—to drug.
• Teach patient how to clean equipment and safely dispose of used ampules after each treatment. Caution patient not to save or use leftover solution.

🔲 Evaluation

• Patient's pulmonary artery pressure decreases and patient reaches pulmonary hemodynamic stability.
• Patient maintains a stable blood pressure and does not experience syncope.
• Patient and family state understanding of drug therapy.

imatinib mesylate
(i-MAH-tin-nib MEH-suh-layt)
Gleevec

Pharmacologic class: protein-tyrosine kinase inhibitor
Therapeutic class: antineoplastic
Pregnancy risk category: D

Indications and dosages

▶ **Chronic myeloid leukemia (CML) in blast crisis, in accelerated phase, or in chronic phase after failure of interferon-alpha therapy; newly diagnosed Philadelphia chromosome–positive chronic-phase CML.**
Adults: For chronic-phase CML, 400 mg P.O. daily as single dose with a meal and large glass of water. For accelerated-phase CML or blast crisis, 600 mg P.O. daily as single dose with a meal and large glass of water. Continue treatment as long as patient continues to benefit. May increase daily dose to 600 mg P.O. in chronic phase or to 800 mg P.O. (400 mg P.O. b.i.d.) in accelerated phase or blast crisis. Increase dosage only if no severe adverse reactions and no severe non–leukemia-related neutropenia or thrombocytopenia occur in the following circumstances: disease progression (at any time), failure to achieve a satisfactory hematologic response after at least 3 months of treatment, or loss of a previously achieved hematologic response.
▶ **Patients with kit (CD117)-positive unresectable or metastatic malignant GI stromal tumors (GIST).** *Adults:* 400 or 600 mg P.O. daily.
▶ **Philadelphia chromosome–positive chronic-phase CML in patients whose disease has recurred after stem cell transplant or who are resistant to interferon-alpha therapy.**
Children age 3 and older: 260 mg/m² P.O. as single daily dose or divided into two doses, taken with a meal and large glass of water. May increase dosage to 340 mg/m² daily.
⛔ Adjust-a-dose: For severe nonhematologic adverse reactions (severe hepatotoxicity or severe fluid retention), withhold drug until resolved; resume treatment based on initial severity of reaction.

For patient with bilirubin level higher than three times the institutional upper limit of normal (IULN) or liver transaminase levels higher than five times IULN, withhold drug until bilirubin level returns to less than 1½ IULN and transaminase levels to less than 2½ IULN. Then resume drug at reduced daily dose. (Adult dosages can be decreased from 400 mg to 300 mg or from 600 mg to 400 mg. Children's dosages can be decreased from 260 mg/m² daily to 200 mg/m² daily or from 340 mg/m² daily to 260 mg/m² daily.)

For severe hematologic reactions in patients with chronic-phase CML (starting dose 400 mg or 260 mg/m² in children) or GIST (starting dose 400 mg) and an absolute neutrophil count (ANC) less than 1 × 10⁹/L or platelet count less than 50 × 10⁹/L, take these steps:
1. Stop drug until ANC is 1.5 × 10⁹/L or greater and platelets are 75 × 10⁹/L or greater.
2. Resume treatment at original starting dose of 400 mg or 600 mg, or 260 mg/m² in children.
3. If patient has recurrence of ANC less than 1 × 10⁹/L or platelets less than 50 × 10⁹/L, repeat step 1 and resume drug at reduced dose (300 mg if starting dose was 400 mg; 400 mg if starting dose was 600 mg; or in children, 200 mg/m² if starting dose was 260 mg/m²).

For severe hematologic reactions in patients with accelerated-phase CML and blast crisis or GIST (starting dose 600 mg) and ANC less than 0.5 × 10⁹/L or platelets less than 10 × 10⁹/L occurring after at least 1 month of treatment, take these steps:
1. Check if cytopenia is related to leukemia via marrow aspirate or biopsy.
2. If cytopenia is unrelated to leukemia, reduce dose of drug to 400 mg.
3. If cytopenia persists 2 weeks, reduce further to 300 mg.
4. If cytopenia persists 4 weeks and is still unrelated to leukemia, stop Gleevec until ANC is 1 × 10⁹/L or greater and platelets are 20 × 10⁹/L or greater, and then resume at 300 mg.

Contraindications and cautions

• Contraindicated in patients hypersensitive to the drug or any of its components.
• Use cautiously in hepatically impaired patients.
⚘ Lifespan: In pregnant and breast-feeding women, drug is contraindicated. In children younger than age 3, safety and effectiveness haven't been established. In elderly patients, use

cautiously because they may have an increased risk of edema when taking drug.

Adverse reactions

CNS: *headache, insomnia,* CEREBRAL HEMORRHAGE, *fatigue,* weakness, *fever, dizziness.*
CV: *edema, **heart failure.***
EENT: nasopharyngitis, *epistaxis.*
GI: *anorexia, nausea, diarrhea, abdominal pain,* constipation, *vomiting, dyspepsia,* GI HEMORRHAGE.
GU: *renal failure.*
Hematologic: HEMORRHAGE, *neutropenia, thrombocytopenia, anemia.*
Hepatic: *liver toxicity.*
Metabolic: *hypokalemia, weight increase.*
Musculoskeletal: *myalgia, muscle cramps, musculoskeletal pain,* arthralgia.
Respiratory: *cough,* dyspnea, pneumonia, ***pulmonary edema,** pleural effusion, nasopharyngitis,* upper respiratory tract infection.
Skin: *rash,* pruritus, petechiae.
Other: night sweats.

Interactions

Drug-drug. *Acetaminophen:* May increase risk of liver toxicity. Monitor patient.
Cyclosporine, dihydropyridine calcium channel blockers, certain HMG-CoA reductase inhibitors, pimozide, triazolobenzodiazepines: May increase levels of these drugs. Monitor patient for toxicity and obtain levels.
CYP 3A4 inducers (carbamazepine, dexamethasone, phenobarbital, phenytoin, rifampin): May increase metabolism and decrease imatinib level. Use cautiously.
CYP 3A4 inhibitors (clarithromycin, erythromycin, itraconazole, ketoconazole): May decrease metabolism and increase imatinib level. Monitor patient for toxicity.
Warfarin: May alter metabolism of warfarin. Avoid use together; instead, use standard heparin or a low–molecular-weight heparin.
Drug-herb. *St. John's wort:* May decrease drug effects. Warn patient not to use together.

Effects on lab test results

• May increase creatinine, bilirubin, alkaline phosphatase, AST, and ALT levels. May decrease potassium and hemoglobin levels and hematocrit.
• May decrease neutrophil and platelet counts.

Pharmacokinetics

Absorption: Well absorbed.
Distribution: 98% protein-bound.
Metabolism: Primarily by CYP 3A4.
Excretion: Primarily in feces as metabolites.
Half-life: 18 to 40 hours.

Route	Onset	Peak	Duration
P.O.	Unknown	2–4 hr	Unknown

Action

Chemical effect: Inhibits Bcr-Abl tyrosine kinase, the abnormal tyrosine kinase created in CML. Inhibits tumor growth of Bcr-Abl–transfected murine myeloid cells and Bcr-Abl–positive leukemia lines derived from CML patients in blast crisis.
Therapeutic effect: Stops tumor growth.

Available forms

Tablets: 100 mg, 400 mg

NURSING PROCESS

⚚ Assessment

• Assess neoplastic disease before starting therapy, and reassess regularly.
• Obtain baseline weight before starting therapy, and then weigh patient daily. Evaluate and treat unexpected and rapid weight gain.
• Assess patient's and family's knowledge of drug therapy.
• Monitor patient closely for fluid retention, which can be severe.
• Monitor CBC weekly for first month, biweekly for second month, and periodically thereafter.
• Monitor liver function test results carefully because severe hepatotoxicity may occur. Decrease dosage as needed.
• Because the long-term safety of this drug isn't known, carefully monitor renal toxicity, liver toxicity, and immunosuppression.

⊞ Nursing diagnoses

• Ineffective health maintenance related to neoplastic disease
• Risk for falls related to drug-induced adverse reactions
• Deficient knowledge related to drug therapy

⊳ Planning and implementation

• For CML, increase dosage only if no severe adverse reactions and no severe non–leukemia-related neutropenia or thrombocytopenia has occurred under the following circumstances: disease progression (at any time), failure to achieve a satisfactory hematologic response after at least 3 months of treatment, or loss of a previously achieved hematologic response.

• Because GI irritation is common, give drug with food.

• For patients unable to swallow tablets, dissolve tablets in water or apple juice (50 ml for 100-mg tablet or 200 ml for 400-mg tablet). Stir and have patient drink immediately.

Patient teaching

• Instruct patient to take drug with food and a large glass of water.

• Urge patient to report to the prescriber any adverse effects, such as fluid retention, signs of bleeding, or infection.

• Advise patient to have periodic liver and kidney function tests and tests to determine blood counts.

• Tell patient to avoid OTC products with acetaminophen.

☑ Evaluation

• Patient shows positive response to drug therapy on follow-up studies.

• Patient doesn't experience falls.

• Patient and family state understanding of drug therapy.

imipenem and cilastatin sodium
(im-ih-PEN-em and sigh-luh-STAT-in SO-dee-um)
Primaxin IM, Primaxin IV

Pharmacologic class: carbapenem (thienamycin class); beta-lactam antibiotic
Therapeutic class: antibiotic
Pregnancy risk category: C

Indications and dosages

▶ **Mild to moderate lower respiratory tract, skin, skin structure, intra-abdominal, and gynecologic infections; serious lower respiratory and urinary tract, intra-abdominal, and gynecologic infections; bacterial septicemia; bone and joint infections; serious soft-tissue infections; endocarditis; polymicrobic infections.** *Adults weighing at least 70 kg (154 lb):* 500 to 750 mg I.M. q 12 hours. Or 250 mg to

1 g I.V. q 6 to 8 hours. Maximum I.V. dosage is 50 mg/kg or 4 g daily, whichever is less.
Children age 3 months and older: 15 to 25 mg/kg I.V. q 6 hours. Maximum dosage for fully susceptible organisms is 2 g daily and for moderately susceptible organisms, 4 g daily (based on adult studies).
Infants ages 4 weeks to 3 months and weighing at least 1.5 kg (3.3 lb): 25 mg/kg I.V. q 6 hours.
Neonates ages 1 to 4 weeks and weighing at least 1.5 kg: 25 mg/kg I.V. q 8 hours.
Neonates younger than 1 week and weighing at least 1.5 kg: 25 mg/kg I.V. q 12 hours.
◪ **Adjust-a-dose:** For patients who weigh less than 70 kg (154 lb), give lower dose or use longer intervals between doses if needed.

For patients with renal impairment, if creatinine clearance is 6 to 20 ml/minute, give 125 to 250 mg I.V. q 12 hours. If creatinine clearance is less then 5 ml/minute, withhold drug unless hemodialysis is instituted within 48 hours.

▼ I.V. administration

• When reconstituting powder, shake until solution is clear. Solutions may range from colorless to yellow; variations of color within this range don't affect drug's potency. After reconstitution, solution is stable for 10 hours at room temperature and for 48 hours when refrigerated.

• Don't give drug by direct I.V. bolus injection. Give 250- or 500-mg dose by I.V. infusion over 20 to 30 minutes. Infuse each 1-g dose over 40 to 60 minutes. If nausea occurs, slow infusion.

⊗ **Incompatibilities**

Antibiotics, dextrose 5% in lactated Ringer's injection, other I.V. drugs including allopurinol, amiodarone, amphotericin B cholesterol complex, azithromycin, etoposide, fluconazole, gemcitabine, lorazepam, meperidine, midazolam, milrinone, sargramostim, sodium bicarbonate.

Contraindications and cautions

• Contraindicated in patients hypersensitive to drug or any of its components.

• Use cautiously in patients allergic to penicillins or cephalosporins and in those with history of seizure disorders, especially if they also have compromised renal function.

☙ **Lifespan:** In pregnant women, use cautiously. In breast-feeding women, use cautiously because it's unknown if drug appears in breast milk. In children younger than age 12, I.M. safety and effectiveness haven't been established. In children with CNS infections, I.V. use isn't recommended because of risk of seizures. In children weighing less than 30 kg (66 lb) with renal impairment, use is contraindicated. In elderly patients, use cautiously because they may have decreased renal function.

Adverse reactions

CNS: ***seizures,*** dizziness, somnolence, fever.
CV: hypotension, thrombophlebitis.
GI: nausea, vomiting, diarrhea, ***pseudomembranous colitis.***
Skin: rash, urticaria, pruritus.
Other: hypersensitivity reactions ***(anaphylaxis),*** pain at injection site.

Interactions

Drug-drug. *Beta-lactam antibiotics:* May cause in vitro antagonism. Avoid use together.
Cyclosporine: May increase adverse CNS effects of both drugs, possibly because of additive or synergistic toxicity. Avoid use together.
Ganciclovir: May cause seizures. Avoid use together.
Probenecid: May increase cilastatin levels. Avoid use together.

Effects on lab test results

- May increase BUN, creatinine, ALT, AST, alkaline phosphatase, bilirubin, and LDH levels. May decrease hemoglobin level and hematocrit.
- May increase eosinophil count. May decrease WBC and platelet counts.

Pharmacokinetics

Absorption: Imipenem is about 75% bioavailable; cilastatin is about 95% bioavailable.
Distribution: Rapid and wide. About 20% of imipenem is protein-bound; 40% of cilastatin is protein-bound.
Metabolism: Imipenem is metabolized by kidney dehydropeptidase I, resulting in low urine levels. Cilastatin inhibits this enzyme, reducing imipenem metabolism.
Excretion: About 70% excreted unchanged by kidneys. *Half-life:* 1 hour after I.V. dose; 2 to 3 hours after I.M. dose.

Route	Onset	Peak	Duration
I.V.	Unknown	Immediate	Unknown
I.M.	Unknown	1–2 hr	Unknown

Action

Chemical effect: Imipenem is bactericidal and inhibits bacterial cell wall synthesis. Cilastatin inhibits enzymatic breakdown of imipenem in kidneys, making it effective in urinary tract.
Therapeutic effect: Kills susceptible organisms, including many gram-positive, gram-negative, and anaerobic bacteria.

Available forms

Powder for I.M. injection: 500- and 750-mg vials
Powder for I.V. injection: 250- and 500-mg vials

NURSING PROCESS

Assessment

- Assess patient's infection before starting therapy and regularly thereafter.
- Obtain urine specimen for culture and sensitivity tests before starting therapy. Start therapy pending test results.
- Be alert for adverse reactions and drug interactions.
- If adverse GI reaction occurs, monitor patient's hydration status.
- Assess patient's and family's knowledge of drug therapy.

Nursing diagnoses

- Infection related to presence of susceptible organisms
- Risk for deficient fluid volume related to adverse GI reactions
- Deficient knowledge related to drug therapy

Planning and implementation

- Reconstitute drug for I.M. injection with 1% lidocaine hydrochloride (without epinephrine) as directed.

ALERT: If seizures develop and persist despite anticonvulsants, notify prescriber, stop giving the drug, and institute seizure precautions and protocols.

Patient teaching

- Instruct patient to report adverse reactions because supportive therapy may be needed.
- Warn patient about pain at injection site.

Evaluation

- Patient is free from infection.

• Patient maintains adequate hydration throughout therapy.
• Patient and family state understanding of drug therapy.

imipramine hydrochloride
(ih-MIP-ruh-meen high-droh-KLOR-ighd)
Apo-Imipramine ♦ , Impril ♦ ,
Melipramine ◇ , Norfranil, Novopramine ♦ ,
Tipramine, Tofranil

imipramine pamoate
Tofranil-PM

Pharmacologic class: dibenzazepine-derivative tricyclic antidepressant
Therapeutic class: antidepressant
Pregnancy risk category: D

Indications and dosages

▶ **Depression.** *Adults:* 75 to 100 mg P.O. daily in divided doses; increase in 25- to 50-mg increments to maximum dosage. Or 25 mg P.O. daily; increase in 25-mg increments every other day. Or entire dosage may be given h.s. Maximum dosage is 200 mg P.O. daily for outpatients, 300 mg P.O. daily for inpatients, and 100 mg P.O. daily for elderly patients.
▶ **Enuresis.** *Children age 6 and older:* 25 mg P.O. 1 hour before bedtime. If no response within 1 week, increase dosage 50 mg nightly for children younger than age 12 or 75 mg nightly for children age 12 and older. Maximum, 2.5 mg/kg P.O. daily.
▶ **Attention-deficit/hyperactivity disorder‡.** *Children age 6 and older:* 2 to 5 mg/kg P.O. given in two to three divided daily doses.

Contraindications and cautions

• Contraindicated in patients hypersensitive to the drug or any of its components, patients receiving MAO inhibitors, and patients in acute recovery phase of MI.
• Use cautiously in patients at risk for suicide, those receiving thyroid drugs, and those with history of urine retention or angle-closure glaucoma, increased intraocular pressure, CV disease, impaired hepatic function, hyperthyroidism, seizure disorder, or renal impairment.
※ **Lifespan:** In pregnant and breast-feeding women, don't use. In children, safety and effec-

tiveness haven't been established for treating depression. In elderly patients, use lower dose and more gradual dose increases to avoid toxicity.

Adverse reactions

CNS: *drowsiness, dizziness,* excitation, tremor, weakness, confusion, headache, nervousness, EEG changes, *seizures, stroke,* extrapyramidal reactions.
CV: *orthostatic hypotension,* tachycardia, ECG changes, hypertension, *MI, arrhythmias, heart block.*
EENT: *blurred vision,* tinnitus, mydriasis.
GI: *dry mouth, constipation,* nausea, vomiting, anorexia, paralytic ileus.
GU: *urine retention,* impotence, testicular swelling.
Metabolic: *hypoglycemia,* hyperglycemia.
Skin: rash, urticaria, *diaphoresis,* photosensitivity reactions.
Other: hypersensitivity reactions, gynecomastia, galactorrhea and breast enlargement, altered libido, SIADH.

Interactions

Drug-drug. *Barbiturates, CNS depressants:* May enhance CNS depression. Avoid use together.
Cimetidine, methylphenidate: May increase imipramine level. Monitor patient for adverse reactions.
Clonidine: May cause loss of blood pressure control with potentially life-threatening elevations in blood pressure. Don't use together.
Epinephrine, norepinephrine: May cause life-threatening hypertensive effect. Use cautiously; monitor patient's blood pressure.
MAO inhibitors: May cause hyperpyretic crisis, severe seizures, and death. Don't use together.
SSRIs: May increase effects of tricyclic antidepressants; symptoms may persist several weeks after fluoxetine therapy stops. Monitor symptoms closely.
Drug-herb. *SAM-e, St. John's wort:* May elevate serotonin level. Discourage use together.
Yohimbe: May increase blood pressure effects. Avoid use together.
Drug-lifestyle. *Alcohol use:* May enhance CNS depression. Discourage use together.
Smoking: May decrease imipramine level. Monitor patient for lack of effect; discourage patient from smoking.

Reactions may be *common,* uncommon, *life-threatening,* or COMMON AND LIFE-THREATENING.

Sun exposure: May increase risk of photosensitivity reactions. Advise patient to avoid unprotected or prolonged exposure to sunlight.

Effects on lab test results

• May increase or decrease glucose level.
• May increase liver function test values.

Pharmacokinetics

Absorption: Rapid and complete.
Distribution: Wide. 90% protein-bound.
Metabolism: By liver. A significant first-pass effect may explain variable level in different patients taking same dose.
Excretion: Mostly in urine. *Half-life:* 11 to 25 hours.

Route	Onset	Peak	Duration
P.O.	Unknown	1–2 hr	Unknown

Action

Chemical effect: Increases amount of norepinephrine, serotonin, or both in CNS by blocking their reuptake by presynaptic neurons.
Therapeutic effect: Relieves depression and childhood enuresis (hydrochloride form).

Available forms

imipramine hydrochloride
Tablets: 10 mg, 25 mg, 50 mg
imipramine pamoate
Capsules: 75 mg, 100 mg, 125 mg, 150 mg

NURSING PROCESS

▓ Assessment

• Assess patient's condition before starting therapy and regularly thereafter.
• Observe patient closely for evidence of suicidal thoughts or behaviors until depression is relieved.
• Be alert for adverse reactions and drug interactions.
• Assess patient's and family's knowledge of drug therapy.

▓ Nursing diagnoses

• Ineffective individual coping related to depression
• Deficient knowledge related to drug therapy

▷ Planning and implementation

• Give a lower dose to an elderly or a debilitated patient, an adolescent, or a patient with aggravated psychotic symptoms.
• Although doses can be given up to four times daily, patients also may receive entire daily dose at one time because of drug's long action.
• Don't abruptly stop giving the drug. After abruptly stopping long-term therapy, the patient may experience nausea, headache, and malaise. These symptoms don't indicate addiction. Provide supportive treatment.
• Drug causes high risk of orthostatic hypotension. Check sitting and standing blood pressures after initial dose.
• Because of hypertensive episodes during surgery in patients receiving tricyclic antidepressants, gradually stop giving the drug over several days before surgery.
• If signs of psychosis occur or increase, notify prescriber, lower the dose, and institute safety precautions.
⟐ **ALERT:** Don't confuse imipramine with desipramine.
Patient teaching
• Advise patient to take full dose h.s., but warn about possible morning orthostatic hypotension.
• Suggest taking drug with food or milk if it causes stomach upset.
• Suggest relieving dry mouth with sugarless chewing gum or hard candy. Encourage good dental prophylaxis because persistent dry mouth may increase the risk of dental caries.
• Tell patient not to drink alcohol or smoke during therapy.
• Warn patient to avoid hazardous activities until the drug's CNS effects are known.
• Warn the patient not to abruptly stop taking the drug.
• Advise patient to consult prescriber before taking other prescription drugs, OTC drugs, or herbal remedies.
• Advise patient to use sunblock, wear protective clothing, and avoid prolonged exposure to sunlight to prevent photosensitivity reactions.

▓ Evaluation

• Patient behavior and communication show diminished depression.
• Patient and family state understanding of drug therapy.

immune globulin intramuscular (gamma globulin, IG, IGIM)
(ih-MYOON GLOB-yoo-lin in-truh-MUS-kyoo-ler)
BayGam

immune globulin intravenous (IGIV)
Carimune, Gamimune N, Gammagard S/D, Gammar-P IV, Iveegam EN, Octagam, Panglobulin, Polygam S/D, Venoglobulin-S

Pharmacologic class: immunologic drug
Therapeutic class: immune serum
Pregnancy risk category: C

Indications and dosages

▶ **Primary humoral immunodeficiency (IGIV); primary defective antibody synthesis, such as agammaglobulinemia or hypogammaglobulinemia, in patients who are at increased risk of infection.** *Adults and children:* 100 to 200 mg/kg I.V. Gamimune N or Octagam monthly, at 0.01 to 0.02 ml/kg/minute for 30 minutes. If no discomfort, rate can slowly be increased to a maximum of 0.08 ml/kg/minute. Or 200 to 400 mg/kg I.V. Gammagard S/D; then monthly doses of 100 mg/kg. Start infusion at 0.5 ml/kg/hour and increase to maximum of 4 ml/kg/hour. Dosage is related to patient response. Or 200 mg/kg I.V. Iveegam EN monthly. May increase dose to maximum of 800 mg/kg or give more frequently to produce desired effect. Infusion rate is 1 to 2 ml/minute for 5% solution. Or 200 mg/kg I.V. Panglobulin or Carimune monthly. Start with 0.5 to 1 ml/minute of 3% solution; gradually increase dose to 2.5 ml/minute after 15 to 30 minutes. Or 200 to 400 mg/kg I.V. Polygam S/D at 0.5 ml/kg/hour, increasing to a maximum of 4 ml/kg/hour. Subsequent dose is 100 mg/kg I.V. monthly. Or 200 mg/kg I.V. Venoglobulin-S monthly. Increase dose to 300 to 400 mg/kg and give more often than once monthly if immune globulin G levels aren't adequate. Infuse at 0.01 to 0.02 ml/kg/minute for 30 minutes; if tolerated, increase 5% solutions to 0.08 ml/kg/minute and 10% solutions to 0.05 ml/kg/minute. Or initially, 1.3 ml/kg I.M. BayGam. Maintenance dosage of 0.66 ml/kg (at least 100 mg/kg) q 3 to 4 weeks. Maximum single dose of IGIM is 30 to 50 ml in adults and 20 to 30 ml in infants and small children.
Adults: 200 to 400 mg/kg I.V. Gammar-P IV q 3 to 4 weeks. Infuse at 0.01 ml/kg/minute and increase to 0.02 ml/kg/minute after 15 to 30 minutes if no problems occur. Maximum infusion rate is 0.06 ml/kg/minute.
Adolescents and children: 200 to 400 mg/kg I.V. Gammar-P IV q 3 to 4 weeks.

▶ **Idiopathic thrombocytopenic purpura (IGIV).** *Adults and children:* 400 mg/kg 5% solution I.V. Gamimune N or Octagam for 5 days, or 1,000 mg/kg 10% solution I.V. for 1 to 2 days with maintenance dosage of 10% solution at 400 to 1,000 mg/kg I.V. single infusion to maintain 30,000/mm³ platelet count. Or 1,000 mg/kg I.V. Gammagard S/D or Polygam S/D as a single dose. Give up to three doses on alternate days, if needed. Or, 400 mg/kg I.V. Panglobulin or Carimune for 2 to 5 consecutive days, depending on platelet count and immune response. Or maximum of 2,000 mg/kg I.V. Venoglobulin-S over 5 days or less. Maintenance dosage, 1,000 mg/kg p.r.n.

▶ **Bone marrow transplant (IGIV).** *Adults older than age 20:* 500 mg/kg 5% or 10% solution I.V. Gamimune N or Octagam on days 7 and 2 before transplantation, and then weekly until 90 days after transplantation.

▶ **B-cell chronic lymphocytic leukemia (IGIV).** *Adults:* 400 mg/kg I.V. Gammagard S/D or Polygam S/D q 3 to 4 weeks.

▶ **Pediatric HIV infection (IGIV).** *Children:* 400 mg/kg I.V. Gamimune N q 28 days, at 0.01 to 0.02 ml/kg/minute for 30 minutes; increase to maximum of 0.08 ml/kg/minute.

▶ **Kawasaki syndrome (IGIV).** *Adults:* 400 mg/kg I.V. Iveegam EN daily over 2 hours for 4 consecutive days, or a single dose of 2,000 mg/kg I.V. over 10 to 12 hours. Start within 10 days of disease onset. Treat concurrently with aspirin (80 to 100 mg/kg P.O. daily through day 14; then 3 to 10 mg/kg P.O. daily for 5 weeks). Or either a single dose of 1g/kg or 400 mg/kg I.V. Gammagard S/D or Polygam S/D daily for 4 days beginning within 7 days of onset of fever. Treat concurrently with aspirin (80 to 100 mg/kg in 4 divided daily doses).

▶ **Hepatitis A exposure (IGIM).** *Adults and children:* 0.02 ml/kg I.M. as soon as possible after exposure. Up to 0.06 ml/kg may be given for prolonged or intense exposure.

Reactions may be *common*, uncommon, *life-threatening*, or COMMON AND LIFE-THREATENING.

► **Measles exposure (IGIM).** *Adults and children:* 0.02 ml/kg I.M. within 6 days after exposure.
► **Measles postexposure prophylaxis (IGIM).** *Immunocompromised children:* 0.5 ml/kg I.M. (maximum, 15 ml) within 6 days after exposure.
► **Chickenpox exposure (IGIM).** *Adults and children:* 0.6 to 1.2 ml/kg I.M. as soon as possible after exposure.
► **Rubella exposure in first trimester of pregnancy (IGIM).** *Women:* 0.55 ml/kg I.M. as soon as possible after exposure (within 72 hours).

▽ I.V. administration

• I.V. products aren't interchangeable. Gammagard requires a filter, which is supplied by the manufacturer.
• Most adverse effects are related to rapid infusion rate. Infuse slowly.
• In patients with a risk of a thrombotic event, don't give an infusion concentration higher than 5%, start infusion rate no faster than 0.5 ml/kg per hour, and speed up slowly only if well tolerated to a maximum rate of 4 ml/kg per hour.
⊗ **Incompatibilities**
Don't mix with other I.V. drugs.

Contraindications and cautions

• Contraindicated in patients hypersensitive to the drug or any of its components, in patients with a history of an allergic response to thimerosal, and in patients with selective immune globulin A deficiencies.
• I.M. administration contraindicated in patients with severe thrombocytopenia or other coagulation-bleeding disorders.
• Use Gammagard S/D cautiously in patients with renal impairment.
• Use caution when giving drug to patients with a history of CV disease or thrombotic episodes because I.V. drug may cause thrombotic events. The exact cause of this is unknown.
⚠ **Lifespan:** In pregnant women, use cautiously. In breast-feeding women, use cautiously because it's unknown if the drug appears in breast milk.

Adverse reactions

CNS: severe headache requiring hospitalization, faintness, malaise, fever.
CV: chest pain, *MI, heart failure* (Gammagard S/D).

GI: nausea, vomiting.
GU: *nephrotic syndrome, acute tubular necrosis,* osmotic nephrosis, *acute renal impairment.*
Musculoskeletal: muscle stiffness at injection site.
Respiratory: transfusion-related acute lung injury, *pulmonary embolism.*
Skin: urticaria, erythema.
Other: *anaphylaxis.*

Interactions

Drug-drug. *Live-virus vaccines:* Antibodies in the vaccine may interfere with drug therapy. Don't give within 6 months after giving immune globulin.

Effects on lab test results

• May increase BUN and creatinine levels.

Pharmacokinetics

Absorption: Slow.
Distribution: Evenly between intravascular and extravascular spaces.
Metabolism: Unknown.
Excretion: Unknown. *Half-life:* 21 to 24 days in immunocompromised patients.

Route	Onset	Peak	Duration
I.V.	Immediate	Immediate	Unknown
I.M.	Unknown	2–5 days	Unknown

Action

Chemical effect: Provides passive immunity by increasing antibody titer. The primary component is immune globulin G.
Therapeutic effect: Helps prevent infections.

Available forms

IGIM
Injection: 2-ml and 10-ml vials
IGIV
Injection: 5% and 10% in 10-ml, 50-ml, 100-ml, 200-ml, and 250-ml vials (Gamimune N); 5% in 1-g, 2.5-g, 5-g, and 10-g bottles (Octagam); 5% and 10% in 50-ml, 100-ml, and 200-ml vials (Venoglobulin-S); 5% in 1-g, 2.5-g, 5-g, and 10-g single-use bottles
Powder for injection: 50 mg protein/ml in 2.5-g, 5-g, and 10-g vials (Gammagard S/D); 1-g, 2.5-g, and 5-g vials (Gammar-P IV); 500-mg and 1-g, 2.5-g, and 5-g vials (Iveegam); 2.5-g, 5-g, and 10-g vials (Polygam S/D); 3-g, 6-g, and 12-g vials (Panglobulin, Carimune)

✍ Assessment
• Obtain history of allergies and reactions to immunizations.
• Observe patient for signs of anaphylaxis or other adverse reactions immediately after injection.
• Inspect injection site for local reactions.
• Monitor effectiveness by checking antibody titers after administration.
• Assess patient's and family's knowledge of drug therapy.

🔟 Nursing diagnoses
• Ineffective protection related to lack of or decreased immunity
• Ineffective breathing pattern related to anaphylaxis
• Deficient knowledge related to drug therapy

⊠ Planning and implementation
• Give I.M. injection in gluteal region. Divide any dose larger than 10 ml, and inject into several muscle sites to reduce local discomfort.
• If 6 weeks or more have passed since exposure or since symptoms have begun, don't give immune globulin to help prevent hepatitis A.
• Make sure epinephrine 1:1,000 is available in case of anaphylaxis.
• **⑧ ALERT:** I.V. and I.M. products aren't interchangeable.
Patient teaching
• Instruct patient to immediately report respiratory difficulty.
• Tell patient that local reactions may occur at injection site.
• Instruct patient to promptly notify prescriber if adverse reaction persists or becomes severe.

✅ Evaluation
• Patient exhibits increased passive immunity.
• Patient shows no signs of anaphylaxis.
• Patient and family state understanding of drug therapy.

indapamide
(in-DAP-uh-mighd)
Lozide ◆ Lozol, Natrilix ◇

Pharmacologic class: thiazide-like diuretic
Therapeutic class: diuretic, antihypertensive
Pregnancy risk category: B

Indications and dosages
▶ **Edema.** *Adults:* Initially, 2.5 mg P.O. daily in morning. Increase to 5 mg daily after 1 week, if needed.
▶ **Hypertension.** *Adults:* Initially, 1.25 mg P.O. daily in morning. Increase to 2.5 mg daily after 4 weeks. Increase to 5 mg daily after 4 more weeks.

Contraindications and cautions
• Contraindicated in patients hypersensitive to the drug, any of its components, or other sulfonamide-derived drugs. Also contraindicated in patients with anuria.
• Use cautiously in patients with severe renal disease, impaired hepatic function, and progressive hepatic disease.
• **⚡ Lifespan:** In pregnant women, use cautiously. In breast-feeding women and children, safety and effectiveness haven't been established.

Adverse reactions
CNS: *headache,* irritability, nervousness, *dizziness, light-headedness,* weakness.
CV: volume depletion and dehydration, orthostatic hypotension.
GI: nausea, *pancreatitis.*
GU: nocturia, polyuria, frequent urination.
Metabolic: anorexia, hypokalemia, hyperuricemia, metabolic alkalosis, hyponatremia, hypochloremia.
Musculoskeletal: muscle cramps and spasms.
Skin: dermatitis, photosensitivity reactions, rash.
Other: gout.

Interactions
Drug-drug. *Antihypertensives:* May cause severe hypotension. Use together cautiously. *Bumetanide, ethacrynic acid, furosemide, torsemide:* May cause excessive diuretic response, resulting in serious electrolyte abnormalities or dehydration. Adjust doses carefully

while monitoring the patient for excessive diuretic responses.

Diazoxide: May increase antihypertensive, hyperglycemic, and hyperuricemic effects. Use together cautiously.

Digoxin: May increase risk of digoxin toxicity from indapamide-induced hypokalemia. Monitor potassium and digoxin levels.

Lithium: May decrease lithium clearance and increase risk of lithium toxicity. Use together cautiously.

NSAIDs: May reduce the diuretic, natriuretic, and antihypertensive effects. Monitor patient.

Drug-lifestyle. *Sun exposure:* May cause photosensitivity reactions. Avoid prolonged and unprotected exposure to sunlight.

Effects on lab test results

• May increase glucose, cholesterol, triglyceride, and uric acid levels. May decrease potassium, sodium, and chloride levels.

Pharmacokinetics

Absorption: Complete.
Distribution: Wide because of its lipophilicity; 71% to 79% protein-bound.
Metabolism: Undergoes significant hepatic metabolism.
Excretion: Primarily in urine; smaller amounts in feces. *Half-life:* About 14 hours.

Route	Onset	Peak	Duration
P.O.	1–2 hr	≤ 2 hr	≤ 36 hr

Action

Chemical effect: Unknown; probably inhibits sodium reabsorption in distal segment of nephron. Also has direct vasodilating effect, possibly from calcium channel-blocking action.
Therapeutic effect: Promotes water and sodium excretion and lowers blood pressure.

Available forms

Tablets: 1.25 mg, 2.5 mg

NURSING PROCESS

Assessment

• Assess patient's underlying condition before starting therapy.
• Monitor effectiveness by assessing fluid intake and output, weight, and blood pressure. In hypertensive patient, therapeutic response may be delayed several days.
• Monitor electrolytes and glucose levels.
• Monitor creatinine and BUN levels regularly. If these levels are more than twice normal, drug is less effective.
• Monitor uric acid level, especially if patient has history of gout.
• Be alert for adverse reactions and drug interactions.
• Assess patient's and family's knowledge of drug therapy.

Nursing diagnoses

• Risk for injury related to presence of hypertension
• Excessive fluid volume related to presence of edema
• Deficient knowledge related to drug therapy

Planning and implementation

• To prevent nocturia, give drug in the morning.
• Drug may be used with potassium-sparing diuretic to prevent potassium loss.
Patient teaching
• Advise patient not to suddenly change position, and to rise slowly to avoid orthostatic hypotension.
• Advise patient to use sunblock and avoid prolonged exposure to sunlight to prevent photosensitivity reactions.
• Teach patient to monitor fluid volume by recording daily weight and intake and output.
• Tell patient to avoid high-sodium foods and to choose high-potassium foods.
• Advise patient to take drug early in day to avoid nocturia.

Evaluation

• Patient's blood pressure is normal.
• Patient is free from edema.
• Patient and family state understanding of drug therapy.

indinavir sulfate
(in-DIH-nuh-veer SUL-fayt)
Crixivan

Pharmacologic class: protease inhibitor
Therapeutic class: antiretroviral
Pregnancy risk category: C

Indications and dosages

▶ **HIV infection.** *Adults:* 800 mg P.O. q 8 hours.
⊠ **Adjust-a-dose:** For patients with mild to moderate hepatic insufficiency resulting in cirrhosis, reduce dosage to 600 mg P.O. q 8 hours.

Contraindications and cautions

• Contraindicated in patients hypersensitive to the drug or any of its components.
• Use cautiously and at a reduced dosage in patients with hepatic insufficiency.
⚘ **Lifespan:** In pregnant women, use only if benefits outweigh risks to the fetus. In breastfeeding women, use cautiously because it isn't known if drug appears in breast milk. In children, safety and effectiveness haven't been established.

Adverse reactions

CNS: headache, insomnia, dizziness, malaise, somnolence, asthenia, fatigue.
GI: *abdominal pain, nausea,* diarrhea, vomiting, acid regurgitation, anorexia, dry mouth, taste perversion.
GU: *nephrolithiasis, acute renal failure.*
Hematologic: *hemolytic anemia, neutropenia.*
Hepatic: hyperbilirubinemia, *hepatic failure.*
Metabolic: *hyperglycemia,* new onset diabetes mellitus.
Musculoskeletal: flank pain, back pain.
Other: redistribution and accumulation of body fat.

Interactions

Drug-drug. *Amprenavir, saquinavir:* May increase levels of these drugs. Dosage adjustments probably aren't needed.
Carbamazepine: May decrease indinavir level. Avoid use together.
Clarithromycin: May alter level of clarithromycin. Monitor patient.

Didanosine: May need normal gastric pH for optimal absorption of indinavir. Give these drugs and indinavir at least 1 hour apart on an empty stomach.
Efavirenz, nevirapine: May decrease indinavir level. Increase indinavir to 1,000 mg q 8 hours.
Ergot derivatives, pimozide: May result in life-threatening events. Avoid use together.
HMG-CoA reductase inhibitors: May increase levels of these drugs and increase risk of myopathy and rhabdomyolysis. Avoid use together.
Ketoconazole, itraconazole, delavirdine: May increase level of indinavir. Consider reducing indinavir dosage to 600 mg q 8 hours.
Midazolam, triazolam: Competition for CYP 3A4 by indinavir may inhibit metabolism of these drugs and increase risk of serious or life-threatening events, such as arrhythmias or prolonged sedation. Don't give together.
Nelfinavir: May increase levels of indinavir by 50% and nelfinavir by 80%. Monitor patient closely.
Rifabutin: May increase level of rifabutin and decrease level of indinavir. Give indinavir 1,000 mg q 8 hours and decrease the rifabutin dose to either 150 mg daily or 300 mg two to three times a week.
Rifampin: May significantly diminish level of indinavir because rifampin is a potent inducer of CYP 3A4. Avoid use together.
Ritonavir: May increase indinavir level by two to five times. Adjust dosage to indinavir 400 mg b.i.d. and ritonavir 400 mg b.i.d., or indinavir 800 mg b.i.d. and ritonavir 100 to 200 mg b.i.d.
Sildenafil, tadalafil, vardenafil: May increase levels of these drugs and the risk of adverse effects (hypotension, visual changes, priapism). Tell patient not to exceed 25 mg of sildenafil in a 48-hour period, 10 mg of tadalafil in a 72-hour period, or 2.5 mg vardenafil in a 24-hour period.
Drug-herb. *St. John's wort:* May reduce level of indinavir by more than 50%. Discourage use together.
Drug-food. *Any food:* May substantially decrease absorption of oral indinavir. Give drug on an empty stomach.
Grapefruit juice: May decrease level and therapeutic effect of indinavir. Advise patient to take drug with liquid other than grapefruit juice.

Effects on lab test results

• May increase ALT, AST, bilirubin, amylase, triglyceride, cholesterol, and glucose levels. May decrease hemoglobin level and hematocrit.
• May decrease neutrophil and platelet counts.

Pharmacokinetics

Absorption: Rapid.
Distribution: 60% bound to proteins.
Metabolism: By liver and kidneys.
Excretion: In urine. *Half-life:* 2 hours.

Route	Onset	Peak	Duration
P.O.	Unknown	< 1 hr	1–8 hr

Action

Chemical effect: Binds to and inhibits protease active sites. Prevents cleavage of viral polyproteins, resulting in formation of immature, noninfectious viral particles.
Therapeutic effect: Reduces symptoms of HIV.

Available forms

Capsules: 100 mg, 200 mg, 333 mg, 400 mg

NURSING PROCESS

Assessment

• Monitor adverse reactions and drug interactions.
• Assess patient's and family's knowledge of drug therapy.

Nursing diagnoses

• Infection related to presence of virus
• Risk for deficient fluid volume related to effect on kidneys
• Deficient knowledge related to drug therapy

Planning and implementation

• Give at least 48 oz (1.5 L) of fluids every 24 hours to maintain adequate hydration.
• Give drug on an empty stomach, 1 hour before or 2 hours after a meal.
Patient teaching
• Instruct patient to use barrier contraception.
• If patient misses a dose, advise him to take the next dose at regularly scheduled time and not to double the dose.
• Instruct patient to take drug on an empty stomach with water 1 hour before or 2 hours after a meal.

• Instruct patient to store capsules in the original container and to keep the desiccant in the bottle.
• Instruct patient to drink at least 48 oz (1.5 L) of fluid daily.
• Advise HIV-positive women to prevent transmitting virus to infant by not breast-feeding.
• Instruct patient to promptly report evidence of nephrolithiasis (flank pain, hematuria) or diabetes (increased thirst, polyuria)
• Advise patient taking sildenafil, tadalafil, or vardenafil that he may be at increased risk for adverse reactions, such as hypotension, visual changes, and priapism, and that he should promptly report any symptoms to prescriber. Patient shouldn't take more than 25 mg of sildenafil in a 48-hour period, 10 mg of tadalafil in a 72-hour period, or 2.5 mg of vardenafil in a 24-hour period.

Evaluation

• Patient's health improves, and signs and symptoms of underlying condition diminish with use of drug.
• Patient maintains adequate hydration.
• Patient and family state understanding of drug therapy.

indomethacin
(in-doh-METH-uh-sin)
Apo-Indomethacin♦, Arthrexin◇, Indocid♦◇, Indocid SR♦, Indocin*, Indocin SR, Indomethagan, Novo-Methacin♦

indomethacin sodium trihydrate
Apo-Indomethacin♦, Indocid PDA♦, Indocin I.V., Novo-Methacin♦

Pharmacologic class: NSAID
Therapeutic class: analgesic, antipyretic, anti-inflammatory
Pregnancy risk category: B (D in third trimester)

Indications and dosages

▶ **Moderate to severe rheumatoid arthritis or osteoarthritis, ankylosing spondylitis.**
Adults: 25 mg P.O. b.i.d. or t.i.d. with food or antacids. Increase by 25 mg or 50 mg daily q 7 days up to 200 mg daily. Or 50 mg P.R. q.i.d.

Or 75-mg sustained-release capsule P.O. to start, in morning or h.s., followed, if needed, by another 75 mg b.i.d.

▶ **Acute gouty arthritis.** *Adults:* 50 mg P.O. t.i.d. Reduce dose as soon as possible; then stop. Don't use sustained-release capsules.

▶ **Acute painful shoulders (bursitis or tendinitis).** *Adults:* 75 to 150 mg P.O. daily t.i.d. or q.i.d. with food or antacids for 7 to 14 days.

▶ **To close hemodynamically significant patent ductus arteriosus in premature infants.** *Neonates less than 48 hours old:* 0.2 mg/kg I.V. followed by two doses of 0.1 mg/kg at 12- to 24-hour intervals.

Neonates ages 2 to 7 days: 0.2 mg/kg I.V. followed by two doses of 0.2 mg/kg at 12- to 24-hour intervals.

Neonates more than 7 days old: 0.2 mg/kg I.V. followed by two doses of 0.25 mg/kg at 12- to 24-hour intervals.

▶ **Pericarditis‡.** *Adults:* 75 to 200 mg P.O. daily in three to four divided doses.

▶ **Dysmenorrhea‡.** *Adults:* 25 mg P.O. t.i.d. with food or antacids.

▶ **Bartter's syndrome‡.** *Adults:* 150 mg P.O. daily with food or antacids.

Children: 0.5 to 2 mg/kg P.O. in divided doses.

▼ I.V. administration

● Reconstitute powder for injection with sterile water for injection or normal saline solution. For each 1-mg vial, add 1 ml of diluent to yield 1 mg/ml; add 2 ml of diluent to yield 0.5 mg/ml.

● Use only preservative-free diluents to prepare I.V. injection. Never use diluents containing benzyl alcohol because it has been linked to fatal gasping syndrome in neonates. Because injection contains no preservatives, reconstitute immediately before administration and discard unused solution.

● Give by direct injection over 20 to 30 minutes per published literature although the optimum rate has not been established by the manufacturer.

● If patient has anuria or marked oliguria, don't give second or third scheduled I.V. dose; instead, notify prescriber.

⊗ **Incompatibilities**
Amino acid injection, calcium gluconate, cimetidine, dextrose injection, dobutamine, dopamine, gentamicin, levofloxacin, solutions with pH less than 6, tobramycin sulfate, tolazoline.

Contraindications and cautions

● Contraindicated in patients hypersensitive to the drug or any of its components and in those with a history of aspirin- or NSAID-induced asthma, rhinitis, or urticaria. Suppositories contraindicated in patients with a history of proctitis or recent rectal bleeding.

● Because of its high risk of adverse effects during prolonged use, don't use drug routinely as analgesic or antipyretic.

● Use cautiously in patients with epilepsy, parkinsonism, hepatic or renal disease, CV disease, infection, mental illness or depression, or history of GI disease.

⚖ **Lifespan:** In pregnant and breast-feeding women, drug is contraindicated. In children younger than age 14, safety and effectiveness haven't been established by manufacturer. In infants with untreated infection, active bleeding, coagulation defects, thrombocytopenia, congenital heart disease (in whom patency of ductus arteriosus is needed for satisfactory pulmonary or systemic blood flow), necrotizing enterocolitis, or renal impairment, drug is contraindicated. In elderly patients, use cautiously.

Adverse reactions

P.O. and P.R.
CNS: *headache, dizziness,* depression, drowsiness, confusion, peripheral neuropathy, *seizures,* psychic disturbances, syncope, vertigo.
CV: hypertension, edema, *heart failure.*
EENT: blurred vision, corneal and retinal damage, hearing loss, tinnitus.
GI: nausea, vomiting, anorexia, diarrhea, peptic ulceration, *GI bleeding.*
GU: hematuria, *acute renal failure.*
Hematologic: hemolytic anemia, *aplastic anemia, agranulocytosis, leukopenia, thrombocytopenic purpura,* iron-deficiency anemia.
Metabolic: *hyperkalemia.*
Respiratory: respiratory distress
Skin: rash, pruritus, urticaria, *Stevens-Johnson syndrome.*
Other: hypersensitivity reactions, *anaphylaxis, angioedema.*
I.V.
GI: *GI bleeding,* vomiting.
GU: renal dysfunction, azotemia.
Metabolic: hyponatremia, *hyperkalemia, hypoglycemia.*
Respiratory: *respiratory distress.*

Reactions may be *common,* uncommon, **life-threatening**, or COMMON AND LIFE-THREATENING.

Other: hypersensitivity reactions, rash, *anaphylaxis, angioedema.*

Interactions

Drug-drug. *Aminoglycosides, cyclosporine, methotrexate:* May enhance toxicity of these drugs. Avoid use together.
Antihypertensives: May reduce antihypertensive effect. Monitor blood pressure closely.
Aspirin: May decrease indomethacin level and increase the risk of GI toxicity. Avoid use together.
Corticosteroids: May increase risk of GI toxicity. Don't use together.
Diflunisal, probenecid: May decrease indomethacin excretion. Monitor patient for increased adverse reactions to indomethacin.
Digoxin: May prolong half-life of digoxin. Use together cautiously; monitor digoxin level.
Dipyridamole: May enhance fluid retention. Avoid use together.
Furosemide, thiazide diuretics: May impair response to both drugs. Avoid using together, if possible.
Lithium: May increase lithium levels. Monitor patient for lithium toxicity.
Triamterene: May cause nephrotoxicity. Monitor patient closely.
Drug-herb. *Dong quai, feverfew, garlic, ginger, horse chestnut, red clover:* May increase risk of bleeding. Monitor patient closely for bleeding.
Senna: May block laxative effects. Discourage use together.
St. John's wort: May increase risk of photosensitivity. Advise patient to avoid unprotected or prolonged exposure to sunlight.
Drug-lifestyle. *Alcohol use:* May increase risk of GI toxicity. Discourage use together.

Effects on lab test results

• May increase AST, ALT, BUN, creatinine, and potassium levels. May decrease glucose, sodium, and hemoglobin levels and hematocrit.
• May decrease WBC, granulocyte, and platelet counts.

Pharmacokinetics

Absorption: Rapid and complete.
Distribution: Highly protein-bound.
Metabolism: In liver.

Excretion: Mainly in urine, with some biliary excretion. *Half-life:* 4¼ hours.

Route	Onset	Peak	Duration
P.O.	30 min	1–4 hr	4–6 hr
I.V.	Immediate	Immediate	Unknown
P.R.	2–4 hr	Unknown	4–6 hr

Action

Chemical effect: Unknown; produces anti-inflammatory, analgesic, and antipyretic effects, possibly by inhibiting prostaglandin synthesis.
Therapeutic effect: Relieves pain, fever, and inflammation.

Available forms

indomethacin
Capsules: 25 mg, 50 mg
Capsules (sustained-release): 75 mg
Oral suspension: 25 mg/5 ml
Suppositories: 50 mg
indomethacin sodium trihydrate
Injection: 1-mg vials

NURSING PROCESS

☒ Assessment
• Assess patient's condition before starting therapy and regularly thereafter.
• Monitor patient carefully for bleeding and for reduced urine output during I.V. use.
• Be alert for adverse reactions and drug interactions.
• Assess patient's and family's knowledge of drug therapy.

☷ Nursing diagnoses
• Chronic pain related to underlying condition
• Risk for injury related to adverse reactions
• Deficient knowledge related to drug therapy

☵ Planning and implementation
• If GI upset occurs, give oral form of drug with food, milk, or antacid.
• If ductus arteriosus reopens, give second course of one to three doses. If ineffective, surgery may be needed.
• If patient has bleeding or reduced urine output, stop giving the drug and notify prescriber.
• Drug may enhance hypothalamic-pituitary-adrenal axis response to dexamethasone suppression test.
• Notify prescriber if drug is ineffective.

Rapid onset   *Liquid form contains alcohol.   ♦ Canada   ◇ Australia   †OTC   ✐ Photoguide   ‡Off-label use

Patient teaching
• Tell patient to take oral form of drug with food, milk, or antacid if GI upset occurs.
• Inform patient that use of oral form with aspirin, alcohol, or corticosteroids may increase risk of adverse GI reactions.
• Teach patient signs and symptoms of GI bleeding, and tell him to report them to prescriber. Serious GI toxicity, including peptic ulceration and bleeding despite absence of GI symptoms, can occur in patients taking oral NSAIDs.
• Instruct patient not to drink alcohol during therapy.
• Tell patient to notify prescriber immediately about visual or hearing changes. Patient receiving long-term oral therapy should have regular eye and hearing examinations, CBC, and renal function tests to detect toxicity.
• Advise patient to avoid hazardous activities if adverse CNS reactions occur.

☑ **Evaluation**
• Patient is free from pain.
• Patient doesn't experience injury from adverse reactions.
• Patient and family state understanding of drug therapy.

infliximab
(in-FLICKS-ih-mab)
Remicade

Pharmacologic class: monoclonal antibody
Therapeutic class: anti-inflammatory
Pregnancy risk category: B

Indications and dosages

▶ **Moderate to severe active Crohn's disease; to reduce the number of draining fistulas and maintain fistula closure in patients with Crohn's disease.** *Adults:* 5 mg/kg I.V. infusion (over at least 2 hours), given as an induction regimen at 0, 2, and 6 weeks, followed by a maintenance regimen of 5 mg/kg q 8 weeks thereafter. For patients who respond and then lose their response, consideration may be given to treatment with 10 mg/kg. Patients who don't respond by week 14 are unlikely to respond to continued therapy; consider stopping drug in these patients.

▶ **With methotrexate, for moderate to severe active rheumatoid arthritis.** *Adults:* 3 mg/kg I.V. infusion over at least 2 hours. Give additional doses of 3 mg/kg at 2 and 6 weeks after initial infusion and q 8 weeks thereafter. If response is inadequate, increase up to 10 mg/kg or give q 4 weeks.
▶ **Ankylosing spondylitis.** *Adults:* 5 mg/kg I.V. infusion over at least 2 hours. Give additional doses of 5 mg/kg at 2 and 6 weeks after first infusion and then q 6 weeks thereafter.
▶ **Psoriatic arthritis, with or without methotrexate.** *Adults:* 5 mg/kg I.V. infusion over at least 2 hours. Give additional doses of 5 mg/kg at 2 and 6 weeks after first infusion and then q 8 weeks thereafter.
▶ **Moderate to severe ulcerative colitis.** *Adults:* Induction dose, 5 mg/kg I.V. over 2 hours given at 0, 2, and 6 weeks, followed by a maintenance dose of 5 mg/kg q 8 weeks thereafter.

▽ **I.V. administration**

• Drug is incompatible with plasticized polyvinyl chloride equipment or devices; so prepare only in glass infusion bottles or polypropylene or polyolefin infusion bags.
• Give through polyethylene-lined administration sets with an in-line, sterile, nonpyrogenic, low–protein-binding filter (pore size of 1.2 mm or less).
• Reconstitute with 10 ml sterile solution for injection using syringe with 21G or smaller needle. Don't shake; gently swirl to dissolve powder. Solution should be colorless to light yellow and opalescent; it may contain a few translucent particles. If you see other particles or discoloration, don't use.
• Vials don't contain antibacterial preservatives; use reconstituted drug immediately.
• Dilute total volume of reconstituted drug to 250 ml with normal saline solution for injection. Infusion concentration range is 0.4 to 4 mg/ml.
• Infuse within 3 hours of preparation and for at least 2 hours after starting.
• If an infusion reaction occurs, stop giving the drug, notify prescriber, and give acetaminophen, antihistamines, corticosteroids, and epinephrine.
⊗ **Incompatibilities**
Other I.V. drugs.

Contraindications and cautions

• Contraindicated in patients hypersensitive to murine proteins or any other of the drug's components.

• In patients with mild heart failure (New York Heart Association [NYHA] Class I or II), use cautiously. Don't give this drug to patients with moderate to severe heart failure (NYHA Class III or IV).

• Use cautiously in patients with a history of hematologic abnormalities or those with CNS demyelinating or seizure disorders.

⚠ **Lifespan:** In pregnant women, give only if benefits outweigh risks to the fetus. In breast-feeding women, stop breast-feeding or don't use the drug. In children, safety and effectiveness haven't been established. In elderly patients, use cautiously.

Adverse reactions

CNS: pain, *headache, fatigue, fever,* depression, dizziness, malaise, insomnia, systemic and cutaneous vasculitis.

CV: *hypertension,* peripheral edema, ***pericardial effusion,*** hypotension, tachycardia, chest pain, flushing.

EENT: *pharyngitis,* rhinitis, *sinusitis,* conjunctivitis.

GI: *nausea, abdominal pain,* vomiting, constipation, *dyspepsia, diarrhea,* flatulence, intestinal obstruction, mouth pain, ulcerative stomatitis.

GU: dysuria, increased urinary frequency, *UTI.*

Hematologic: anemia, hematoma, ***leukopenia, neutropenia, pancytopenia.***

Musculoskeletal: myalgia, *arthralgia,* arthritis, *back pain.*

Respiratory: *upper respiratory tract infection, bronchitis, coughing,* dyspnea.

Skin: *rash,* pruritus, candidiasis, acne, alopecia, eczema, erythema, erythematous rash, maculopapular rash, papular rash, dry skin, increased sweating, urticaria, ecchymosis.

Other: chills, flulike syndrome, hot flushes, abscess, toothache, hypersensitivity reaction, ***severe opportunistic infections, tuberculosis.***

Interactions

Drug-drug. *Anakinra:* May increase the risk of serious infections and neutropenia. Avoid use together.

Live vaccines: No data are available on response to vaccines or on the secondary transmission of infection by live-virus vaccines. Don't use together.

Effects on lab test results

• May increase liver enzyme levels. May decrease hemoglobin level and hematocrit.

Pharmacokinetics

Absorption: Administered I.V.
Distribution: Primarily within the vascular compartment.
Metabolism: Unknown.
Excretion: Unknown. *Half-life:* 9½ days.

Route	Onset	Peak	Duration
I.V.	Unknown	Unknown	Unknown

Action

Chemical effect: Binds to tumor necrosis factor (TNF)-alpha to neutralize it and inhibit its binding with receptors, reducing the infiltration of inflammatory cells and production of TNF-alpha in inflamed areas of the intestine.
Therapeutic effect: Relieves inflammation.

Available forms

Injection: 100-mg vials

NURSING PROCESS

⚗ Assessment

• Obtain history of patient's underlying condition before starting therapy, and reassess regularly.

• Use in Crohn's disease and ulcerative colitis only after patient has had an inadequate response to conventional therapy.

• Observe patient for infusion-related reactions, including fever, chills, pruritus, urticaria, dyspnea, hypotension, hypertension, and chest pain, within 2 hours of infusion.

• Monitor liver function test results.

• Observe patient for development of lymphomas and infection. Patients with chronic Crohn's disease and long-term exposure to immunosuppressants are more likely to develop lymphomas and infections.

• Consider stopping treatment in patient who develops significant hematologic abnormalities or CNS adverse reactions.

• Drug may affect normal immune responses. Monitor patient for development of autoimmune antibodies and lupus-like syndrome; stop giving

the drug if symptoms develop. Symptoms should resolve.
• Tuberculosis, invasive fungal infections, and other fatal opportunistic infections may occur.
• In patient with heart failure, monitor patient's cardiac status.
• Assess patient's and family's knowledge of drug therapy.

🔃 Nursing diagnoses
• Chronic pain related to inflammation of the GI tract
• Imbalanced nutrition: less than body requirements related to underlying medical condition
• Deficient knowledge related to drug therapy

▷ Planning and implementation
• If patient develops new or worsening symptoms of heart failure, stop giving the drug.
• Patient may develop tuberculosis, invasive fungal infections, or other opportunistic infection. Test patient for latent tuberculosis infection with a tuberculin skin test. Start treatment of latent tuberculosis infection before therapy.
• Patient may develop histoplasmosis, listeriosis, and pneumocystosis. For patients who have lived in regions where histoplasmosis is endemic, carefully consider the benefits and risks before starting therapy.

Patient teaching
• Tell patient about infusion reaction symptoms and the need to report them to prescriber.
• Inform patient of postinfusion adverse effects, and tell him to promptly report them.
• Advise patient to seek immediate medical attention for signs and symptoms of infection or strange or unusual bleeding or bruising.

✓ Evaluation
• Patient is free from pain.
• Patient maintains adequate nutrition.
• Patient and family state understanding of drug therapy.

---

influenza virus vaccine live, intranasal
(inn-floo-EHN-zah VY-russ vack-SEEN LYV, inn-truh-NAZ-ul)
FluMist

Pharmacologic class: neuraminidase inhibitor
Therapeutic class: antiviral
Pregnancy risk category: C

Indications and dosages

▶ **Active immunization for influenza A and B viruses.** *Adults and children ages 9 to 49:* 0.5 ml per season.
Children ages 5 to 8 (not previously vaccinated with FluMist): Two doses of 0.5 ml each, 60 days apart (± 14 days for initial season).
Children ages 5 to 8 (previously vaccinated with FluMist): 0.5 ml per season.

Contraindications and cautions

• Contraindicated in patients hypersensitive to the drug or any of its components, including eggs or egg products. Also contraindicated in patients who may be immunosuppressed or have altered or compromised immune status as a consequence of treatment with systemic corticosteroids, alkylating drugs, antimetabolites, radiation, or other immunosuppressive therapies. Contraindicated in patients with known or suspected immune deficiency diseases, such as combined immunodeficiency, agammaglobulinemia, or thymic abnormalities; conditions such as HIV infection, malignancy, leukemia, or lymphoma; or a history of Guillain-Barré syndrome or asthma or reactive airway disease.
🜲 **Lifespan:** In pregnant women, drug is contraindicated. In breast-feeding women, use cautiously because it's unknown if drug appears in breast milk. In children ages 5 to 17 receiving aspirin or drugs that contain aspirin, drug is contraindicated because of the link with Reye's syndrome. In children younger than age 5 and adults age 50 and older, safety and effectiveness haven't been established.

Adverse reactions

CNS: irritability, headache, fever.
EENT: runny nose, nasal congestion, sore throat.
GI: vomiting.

Musculoskeletal: muscle aches.
Respiratory: cough.
Other: chills, decreased activity.

Interactions

Drug-drug. *Antivirals active against influenza A or B viruses:* May cause synergistic or decreased effect. Wait 48 hours after stopping antiviral therapy before giving vaccine. Don't give antivirals within 2 weeks of vaccine.
Aspirin: May cause Reye's syndrome. Avoid use together.

Effects on lab test results

None reported.

Pharmacokinetics

Absorption: Unknown.
Distribution: Unknown.
Metabolism: Unknown.
Excretion: Unknown. *Half-life:* Unknown.

Route	Onset	Peak	Duration
Intranasal	Unknown	Unknown	Unknown

Action

Chemical effect: May play a role in prevention and recovery from infection. Induces influenza strain-specific serum antibodies.
Therapeutic effect: Protects against influenza.

Available forms

Intranasal spray: 0.5 ml

NURSING PROCESS

Assessment
• Assess patient's health and immune status.
• To prevent allergic or other adverse reaction, review patient's history for possible sensitivity to influenza vaccine components, including eggs and egg products.
• Be alert for adverse reactions.
• Assess patient's and family's knowledge of therapy.

Nursing diagnoses
• Risk for infection related to influenza A and B virus
• Deficient knowledge related to vaccine therapy

Planning and implementation
⚠ ALERT: Keep epinephrine injection (1:1,000) or compatible treatment readily available in case of an acute anaphylactic reaction.
• Don't give drug until at least 72 hours after a patient's fever has started.
• Advise vaccine recipient and the parents of immunized child to avoid close contact within the same household with immunocompromised people for at least 21 days.
• Report adverse reactions. The U.S. Department of Health and Human Services has established a Vaccine Adverse Event Reporting System to manage reports of suspected adverse reactions for any vaccine (1-800-822-7967). Reporting forms may also be obtained at the FDA Web site (http://vaers.hhs.gov).
• Give drug before exposure to influenza. The peak of influenza varies from year to year, but typically occurs between late December and early March. Because the duration of protection from drug isn't known and yearly variation in the influenza strains is possible, revaccinate annually to increase the likelihood of protection.
• Don't give with other vaccines.
• Drug may not protect 100% of patients.
• Thaw drug before giving. To thaw, hold the sprayer in the palm of the hand and support the plunger rod with the thumb. Give the vaccine immediately. Or thaw drug in a refrigerator, and store at 36° to 46° F (2° to 8° C) for no more than 24 hours before use. When thawed, drug is a colorless to pale yellow liquid that's clear to slightly cloudy. Some particulates may be present, but they don't affect use.
• Give about 0.25 ml into each nostril while the recipient is in an upright position. Insert the tip of the sprayer just inside the nose, and depress the plunger to spray. The dose-divider clip is removed from the sprayer to give the second half of the dose into the other nostril.
Patient teaching
• Inform parents of children ages 5 to 8 that two doses of the drug are required the first time it's used.
• Tell patient to avoid close contact within the same household with immunocompromised people for at least 21 days.
• Instruct patient to report any suspected adverse reaction to the prescriber or clinic where the vaccine was given.
• Inform patient that annual revaccination may increase the likelihood of protection and that not

every person who receives the vaccine will be protected.

☑ Evaluation
• Patient remains free of adverse effects of the therapy.
• Patient does not contract influenza A or B virus.
• Patient and family state understanding of vaccine therapy.

insulin aspart (rDNA origin) injection
(IN-suh-lin AS-part)
NovoLog

insulin aspart (rDNA origin) protamine suspension and insulin aspart (rDNA origin) injection
NovoLog 70/30

Pharmacologic class: human insulin analog
Therapeutic class: antidiabetic
Pregnancy risk category: C

Indications and dosages

▶ **Control of hyperglycemia in diabetes mellitus.** *Adults and children age 2 and older:* 0.5 to 1 unit/kg NovoLog subcutaneously daily within 5 to 10 minutes of start of meal. About 50% to 70% of the daily insulin requirement may be provided by this drug and the remainder by intermediate-acting or long-acting insulin. Initially, dosage for NovoLog external insulin infusion pumps is based on the total daily insulin dosage of the previously used regimen. Give 50% of the total dosage as a bolus at mealtime and the remainder as basal infusion. Adjust dose as needed. Or give NovoLog 70/30 twice daily within 15 minutes of meals.

Contraindications and cautions

• Contraindicated during episodes of hypoglycemia and in patients hypersensitive to NovoLog or its excipients.
• Use cautiously in patients prone to hypoglycemia and hypokalemia, such as patients who are fasting, have autonomic neuropathy, or are using potassium-lowering drugs or drugs sensitive to potassium levels.

❀ **Lifespan:** In breast-feeding women, use cautiously because it's unknown if drug appears in breast milk. In children younger than age 2, safety and effectiveness haven't been established.

Adverse reactions
Metabolic: *hypoglycemia, hyperkalemia.*
Skin: lipodystrophy, pruritus, rash.
Other: allergic reactions, injection site reactions.

Interactions
Drug-drug. *ACE inhibitors, disopyramide, fibrates, fluoxetine, MAO inhibitors, oral antidiabetics, propoxyphene, salicylates, somatostatin analog (octreotide), and sulfonamide antibiotics:* May enhance the glucose-lowering effects of insulin and may increase likelihood of hypoglycemia. Monitor glucose level and signs of hypoglycemia. May require insulin dose adjustment.
Carteolol, nadolol, pindolol, propranolol, timolol: May mask symptoms of hypoglycemia as a result of beta blockade (such as tachycardia). Use cautiously in patients with diabetes.
Corticosteroids, danazol, diuretics, estrogens, isoniazid, niacin, phenothiazine derivatives, progestogens (hormonal contraceptives), somatropin, sympathomimetics (such as epinephrine, salbutamol, and terbutaline), thyroid hormones: May reduce the glucose-lowering effect of insulin and may cause hyperglycemia. Monitor glucose level. May require insulin dosage adjustment.
Guanethidine, reserpine: May mask signs and symptoms of hypoglycemia (may be reduced or absent). Monitor glucose level.
Lithium salts, pentamidine: May enhance or weaken glucose-lowering effect of insulin, causing hypoglycemia or hyperglycemia. Pentamidine may cause hypoglycemia, which may sometimes be followed by hyperglycemia. Monitor glucose level.
Drug-lifestyle. *Alcohol use:* May increase the glucose-lowering effects of insulin. Discourage use together.

Effects on lab test results
• May decrease glucose and potassium levels.

Pharmacokinetics

Absorption: Bioavailable as regular human insulin. Faster absorption and onset and shorter duration of action compared to regular human insulin.
Distribution: 0% to 9% protein-binding, similar to regular insulin.
Metabolism: Unknown.
Excretion: Unknown. *Half-life:* 81 minutes.

Route	Onset	Peak	Duration
SubQ			
NovoLog	15–30 min	1–3 hr	3–5 hr
NovoLog 70/30	Rapid	1–4 hr	24 hr

Action

Chemical effect: Binds to insulin receptors on muscle and fat cells, lowers glucose level, facilitates the cellular uptake of glucose, and inhibits the output of glucose from the liver.
Therapeutic effect: Lowers glucose level.

Available forms

10-ml vial for injection: 100 units of insulin aspart per ml (U-100)
3-ml PenFill cartridges: 100 units/ml

NURSING PROCESS

☒ Assessment
• Assess underlying condition before starting therapy, and reassess regularly.
• Monitor glucose level before starting therapy and regularly throughout therapy.
• Monitor patient's glycosylated hemoglobin level regularly.
• Monitor urine ketones when glucose level is elevated.
• Monitor patient for injection-site reactions.
• Monitor patient with an external insulin pump for erythematous, pruritic, or thickened skin at injection site.
• Assess patient's and family's knowledge of drug therapy.

⊕ Nursing diagnoses
• Risk for impaired skin integrity related to adverse drug effects
• Risk for injury related to drug-induced hypoglycemia
• Deficient knowledge related to insulin aspart therapy

▧ Planning and implementation
• Give NovoLog 5 to 10 minutes before the start of a meal. Give NovoLog 70/30 up to 15 minutes before the start of a meal. Because of drug's rapid onset and short duration of action, patients may require the addition of longer-acting insulins to prevent before-meal hyperglycemia.
• Give subcutaneously into the abdominal wall, thigh, or upper arm. Rotate sites to minimize lipodystrophies.
• Monitor patient for hypoglycemia, which may occur as a result of an excess of insulin relative to food intake, energy expenditure, or both. The warning signs and symptoms of hypoglycemia include shaking, sweating, dizziness, fatigue, hunger, irritability, confusion, blurred vision, headaches, or nausea and vomiting. Treat mild episodes of hypoglycemia with oral glucose. Adjust drug dosage, meal patterns, or exercise, if needed. Treat more severe episodes involving coma, seizure, or neurologic impairment with I.M. or subcutaneous glucagon or concentrated I.V. glucose. Sustain carbohydrate intake and observe because hypoglycemia may recur.
• Look at insulin vial before use. NovoLog should appear as a clear, colorless solution. It should never contain particulate matter, appear cloudy or viscous, or be discolored. NovoLog 70/30 should appear uniformly white and cloudy and should never contain particulate matter or be discolored.
• Don't use drug after its expiration date. Discard after expiration date.
• Store drug between 36° and 46° F (2° and 8° C). Don't freeze. Don't expose vials to excessive heat or sunlight. Open vials are stable at room temperature for 28 days.
⑤ ALERT: Pump or infusion-set malfunctions or insulin degradation can lead to hyperglycemia and ketosis in a short time because of a subcutaneous depot of fast-acting insulin.
• Don't dilute or mix insulin aspart with any other insulin when using an external insulin pump.
• Insulin aspart is recommended for use with Disetronic H-TRON plus V100 with Disetronic 3.15 plastic cartridges and Classic or Tender infusion sets, and MiniMed Models 505, 506, and 507 with MiniMed 3-ml syringes and Polyfin or Sof-set infusion sets. The use of insulin aspart

in quick-release infusion sets and cartridge
adapters has not been assessed.
• Replace infusion sets and insulin aspart in the
reservoir and choose a new infusion site every
48 hours or less to avoid insulin degradation and
infusion set malfunction.
• Discard drug exposed to temperatures higher
than 98.6° F (37° C). The temperature may exceed room temperature when the pump housing,
cover, tubing, or sport case is exposed to sunlight or radiant heat.
③ **ALERT:** Spell out "units" to reduce the risk of
error of misreading "U" as "0" (zero).
③ **ALERT:** Don't confuse Novolog 70/30 with
Novolin 70/30.
③ **ALERT:** Don't confuse Novolog with Novolin
or Humalog.
Patient teaching
• Inform patient of the drug's risks and benefits.
• Teach patient to recognize symptoms of hypoglycemia and hyperglycemia and how to treat
them.
• Instruct patient on injection techniques, timing of dose to meals, adherence to meal planning, importance of regular glucose monitoring
and periodic glycosylated hemoglobin testing,
and proper storage of insulin.
• Tell woman to notify prescriber if she plans to
become or becomes pregnant. Information on
drug in pregnancy or lactation isn't available.
• Instruct patient to report changes at injection
site, including redness, itchiness, or thickened
skin.
• Tell patient not to dilute or mix insulin aspart
with any other insulin when using an external
insulin pump.
• Teach patient how to properly use the external
insulin pump.

☑ **Evaluation**
• Patient doesn't experience adverse reactions
from drug.
• Patient's glucose level is within the normal
range.
• Patient and family state understanding of drug
therapy.

insulin detemir
(IN-suh-lin DEH-teh-meer)
Levemir

Pharmacologic class: insulin analog
Therapeutic class: antidiabetic
Pregnancy risk category: C

Indications and dosages

▶ **Hyperglycemia in patients with diabetes
mellitus who need basal (long-acting) insulin.**
Adults: Base dosage on patient response and
glucose level. In insulin-naive patients with type
2 diabetes, start with 0.1 to 0.2 units/kg subcutaneously once daily in the evening or 10 units
once or twice daily based on glucose level. Patients with type 1 or 2 diabetes receiving basal-
bolus treatment or basal insulin only may switch
to insulin detemir on a unit-to-unit basis adjusted to glycemic target.

Contraindications and cautions

• Contraindicated in patients hypersensitive to
insulin detemir or its excipients. Don't give drug
with an insulin infusion pump.
• Use cautiously in patients with hepatic or renal impairment; they may need dosage adjustment.
⚖ **Lifespan:** In pregnant women, use only if
benefits outweigh risks to the fetus. In breast-
feeding women, use cautiously; it isn't known
whether drug appears in breast milk. In children, safety and efficacy haven't been established. In elderly patients, starting dosage, increments of change, and maintenance dosage
should be conservative; hypoglycemia may be
harder to recognize in these patients.

Adverse reactions

CV: edema.
Metabolic: HYPOGLYCEMIA, sodium retention,
weight gain.
Skin: injection site reactions, lipodystrophy,
pruritus, rash.
Other: allergic reactions.

Interactions

Drug-drug. *Beta blockers, clonidine, guanethidine, reserpine:* May decrease or conceal signs
of hypoglycemia. Avoid use together if possible.

Reactions may be *common,* uncommon, *life-threatening*, or COMMON AND LIFE-THREATENING.

Beta blockers, clonidine, lithium salts: May increase or decrease blood glucose–lowering effect of insulin. Monitor blood glucose level carefully.

Corticosteroids, danazol, diuretics, estrogens, isoniazid, phenothiazines, progestogens (hormonal contraceptives), somatropin, sympathomimetics, thyroid hormones: May decrease blood glucose–lowering effect of insulin. Monitor blood glucose level carefully.

ACE inhibitors, antidiabetic drugs, disopyramide, fibrates, fluoxetine, MAO inhibitors, octreotide, propoxyphene, salicylates, sulfonamides: May increase blood glucose–lowering effect of insulin and risk of hypoglycemia. Monitor blood glucose carefully.

Insulin other than insulin detemir: May alter the action of one or both insulins if mixed together. Don't mix or dilute insulin detemir with other insulins.

Pentamidine: May cause initial hypoglycemia followed by hyperglycemia. Use together cautiously.

Drug-lifestyle. *Alcohol use:* May increase or decrease blood glucose–lowering effect of insulin. Discourage use together.

Effects on lab test results

• May decrease glucose level.

Pharmacokinetics

Absorption: Slow and prolonged.
Distribution: 98% bound to albumin.
Metabolism: Unknown.
Excretion: Unknown. *Half life:* 5 to 7 hours.

Route	Onset	Peak	Duration
SubQ	Unknown	6–8 hr	6–23 hr

Action

Chemical effect: Regulates glucose metabolism by binding to insulin receptors, facilitating cellular uptake of glucose into muscle and fat, and inhibiting release of glucose from liver.
Therapeutic effect: Lowers glucose level.

Available forms

Injection: 100 units/ml in 10-ml vials, 3-ml cartridges (PenFill), 3-ml prefilled syringes (InnoLet, FlexPen)

NURSING PROCESS

🕮 Assessment
• Monitor blood glucose level routinely in all patients receiving insulin.
• Measure patient's glycosylated hemoglobin level periodically.
• Watch for hyperglycemia, especially if patient's diet or exercise patterns change.
• Assess patient for signs and symptoms of hypoglycemia. Insulin doses may need adjustment.
• Assess patient's and family's knowledge of drug therapy.

🔟 Nursing diagnoses
Risk for injury related to drug-induced hypoglycemia
Ineffective health maintenance related to hyperglycemia
Deficient knowledge related to drug therapy

▶ Planning and implementation
🕲 **ALERT:** Don't give this drug by I.V. or I.M. route.
🕲 **ALERT:** Don't mix or dilute insulin detemir with other insulins.
• Early warning symptoms of hypoglycemia may be less pronounced in patients who take beta blockers and patients with long-standing diabetes, diabetic nerve disease, or intensified diabetes control. Monitor glucose level closely in these patients because severe hypoglycemia could develop before symptoms do.
• Insulin doses may need adjustment if patient experiences illness, emotional disturbance, or other stresses or if patient changes his usual meal plan or exercise level.
Patient teaching
• Teach diabetes management, including glucose monitoring, injection techniques, and continuous rotation of injection sites.
🕲 **ALERT:** Teach patient not to mix insulin detemir with any other insulin or solution.
• Instruct patient to use only solution that's clear and colorless, with no visible particles.
• Tell patient to recognize and report signs and symptoms of hyperglycemia, such as nausea, vomiting, drowsiness, flushed dry skin, dry mouth, increased urination, thirst, and loss of appetite.
• Urge patient to check blood glucose level often to achieve control and to avoid hyperglycemia and hypoglycemia.

I

• Teach patient to recognize and report signs and symptoms of hypoglycemia, such as sweating, dizziness, light-headedness, headache, drowsiness, and irritability.

• Advise patient to carry a quick source of simple sugar, such as hard candy or glucose tablets, in case of hypoglycemia.

• Caution patient not to stop insulin abruptly or change the amount or type of insulin used without consulting prescriber.

• Advise patient to avoid alcohol because it lowers the glucose level.

• Caution woman to consult prescriber before trying to become pregnant.

• Tell patient to store unused vials, cartridges, and prefilled syringes in the refrigerator at 36° to 46° F (2° to 8° C).

• After initial use, vials may be refrigerated or stored at room temperature, below 86° F (30° C), away from direct heat and light, for up to 42 days. Cartridges or prefilled syringes may be stored at room temperature, below 86° F (30° C). Tell patient not to store or refrigerate insulin with a needle in place.

• Caution against freezing insulin detemir and against using insulin detemir that has been frozen.

☑ **Evaluation**

• Patient does not experience drug-induced hypoglycemia.

• Patient's glucose level remains within normal limits with drug therapy.

• Deficient knowledge related to drug therapy.

insulin glargine (rDNA)
(IN-suh-lin glar-gene)
Lantus

Pharmacologic class: insulin analog
Therapeutic class: antidiabetic
Pregnancy risk category: C

Indications and dosages

▶ **Management of type 1 or type 2 diabetes mellitus in patients who need basal (long-acting) insulin for the control of hyperglycemia.** *Adults and children age 6 and older:* Individualize dosage. Start drug subcutaneously at the same dose as the current insulin dose at the same time each day.

▶ **Management of type 2 diabetes mellitus in patients previously treated with oral antidiabetics.** *Adults:* 10 units subcutaneously once daily h.s. Adjust as needed to total daily dosage of 2 units to 100 units subcutaneously at the same time each day.

Contraindications and cautions

• Contraindicated in patients hypersensitive to insulin glargine or its excipients. Don't use drug during episodes of hypoglycemia.

• Use cautiously in patients with renal or hepatic impairment, and adjust dosage as directed.

⚖ **Lifespan:** In breast-feeding women, use cautiously because it's unknown if the drug appears in breast milk. In children younger than age 6, safety and effectiveness of drug haven't been established. In elderly patients, use cautiously to avoid hypoglycemia.

Adverse reactions

EENT: retinopathy.
Metabolic: *hypoglycemia.*
Skin: lipodystrophy, pruritus, rash.
Other: allergic reactions, pain at injection site.

Interactions

Drug-drug. *ACE inhibitors, disopyramide, fibrates, fluoxetine, MAO inhibitors, octreotide, oral antidiabetics, propoxyphene, salicylates, sulfonamide antibiotics:* May cause hypoglycemia and increased insulin effect. Monitor glucose level. Insulin glargine dosage may need adjustment.

Carteolol, nadolol, pindolol, propranolol, timolol: May mask symptoms of hypoglycemia (such as tachycardia) as a result of beta blockade. Use cautiously in patients with diabetes.

Clonidine: May mask signs of hypoglycemia and may either strengthen or weaken glucose-lowering effect of insulin. Monitor glucose level carefully. Insulin glargine dosage may need adjustment.

Corticosteroids, danazol, diuretics, estrogens, isoniazid, phenothiazines (prochlorperazine, promethazine), progestins (hormonal contraceptives), sympathomimetics (albuterol, epinephrine, terbutaline), thyroid hormones: May reduce the glucose-lowering effect of insulin. Monitor glucose level. Insulin glargine dosage may need adjustment.

Guanethidine, reserpine: May mask signs of hypoglycemia. Avoid using together, if possible. Monitor glucose level carefully.

Lithium: May either enhance or weaken the glucose-lowering effect of insulin. Monitor glucose level. Insulin glargine dosage may need adjustment.

Pentamidine: May cause hypoglycemia, which may be followed by hyperglycemia. Avoid using together, if possible.

Drug-herb. *Aloe, bilberry leaf, bitter melon, burdock, dandelion, fenugreek, garlic, ginseng:* May improve glucose control and allow a reduced antidiabetic dosage. Tell patient to discuss the use of herbal remedies with prescriber before use.

Licorice root: May increase dosage requirements of insulin. Discourage use together.

Drug-lifestyle. *Alcohol use:* May increase the glucose-lowering effects of insulin. Discourage use together.

Emotional stress, exercise: May enhance or weaken the glucose-lowering effect of insulin. Monitor glucose level. Insulin glargine dosage may need adjustment.

Effects on lab test results

● May decrease glucose level.

Pharmacokinetics

Absorption: Slower, more prolonged absorption than NPH and a relatively constant level over 24 hours with no pronounced peak when compared with NPH insulin. After injection into subcutaneous tissue, the acidic solution is neutralized, leading to formation of microprecipitates. From these microprecipitates, small amounts of insulin glargine are slowly released.

Distribution: Unknown.

Metabolism: Partly metabolized to form two active metabolites similar to insulin.

Excretion: Unknown. *Half-life:* Unknown.

Route	Onset	Peak	Duration
SubQ	Slow	None	10¾–24 hr

Action

Chemical effect: Increases glucose transport across muscle and fat cell membranes to reduce glucose level. Promotes conversion of glucose to its storage form, glycogen.

Therapeutic effect: Lowers glucose level.

Available forms

Injection: 10-ml vial of 100 units/ml

NURSING PROCESS

📖 Assessment

● Obtain history of patient's underlying condition before starting therapy, and reassess regularly. As with any insulin, the desired glucose level and the doses and timing of antidiabetic drug must be determined individually.

● Monitor glucose level closely.

● Monitor patient for hypoglycemia. Early symptoms may be different or less pronounced in patients with long-standing diabetes, diabetic nerve disease, or intensified diabetes control.

● Assess patient's and family's knowledge of drug therapy.

💠 Nursing diagnoses

● Ineffective health maintenance related to hyperglycemia

● Risk for injury related to drug-induced hypoglycemia

● Deficient knowledge related to drug therapy

▶ Planning and implementation

● Drug isn't intended for I.V. use. Its prolonged action depends on injection into the subcutaneous space.

● Because of its prolonged duration, insulin glargine isn't the insulin of choice for diabetic ketoacidosis.

● The rate of absorption and onset and the duration of action may be affected by exercise and other circumstances, such as illness and emotional stress.

● Don't dilute drug or mix it with any other insulin or solution.

● As with any insulin therapy, lipodystrophy may occur at injection site and delay insulin absorption. Rotate injection sites to reduce lipodystrophy.

● 🔔 **ALERT:** Spell out units to reduce the risk of error by misreading "U" as "0" (zero).

● Store unopened vials at 36° F to 46° F (2° to 8° C). Don't freeze. Discard opened vials, whether refrigerated or not, after 28 days. May store opened vials at room temperature away from direct heat and light.

🔔 **ALERT:** Don't confuse Lantus with Lente.

Patient teaching

• Teach patient proper glucose-monitoring techniques and proper diabetes management.
• Teach diabetic patient signs and symptoms of hypoglycemia, such as fatigue, weakness, confusion, headache, and pale skin.
• Advise patient to treat mild episodes of hypoglycemia with oral glucose tablets. Encourage patient to always carry glucose tablets in case of a hypoglycemic episode.
• Teach patient the importance of maintaining a diabetic diet. Explain that adjustments in drug dosage, meal patterns, and exercise may be needed to regulate blood glucose.
• Tell patient that any change of insulin should be made cautiously and only under medical supervision. Changes in insulin strength, manufacturer, type (regular, NPH, insulin analogs), species (animal, human), or method of manufacture (ribosomal DNA versus animal source) may warrant a dosage change. Oral antidiabetic treatment may need to be adjusted.
• Tell patient to consult prescriber before using OTC drugs.
• Advise patient not to dilute or mix any other insulin or solution with insulin glargine. Tell patient to discard the vial if the solution is cloudy.
• Instruct patient to store insulin glargine vials in the refrigerator, if possible.

☑ Evaluation

• Patient's blood glucose level is normal.
• Patient doesn't experience hypoglycemic reactions.
• Patient and family state understanding of drug therapy.

insulin glulisine (rDNA origin)
(IN-suh-lin GLUE-lih-seen)
Apidra

Pharmacologic class: human insulin analog
Therapeutic class: antidiabetic
Pregnancy risk category: C

Indications and dosages

▶ **Diabetes mellitus.** *Adults:* Individualize dosage. Give subcutaneous injection within 15 minutes before a meal or within 20 minutes after meal starts if regimen also includes a longer-acting insulin or basal insulin analog. Or

give subcutaneous infusion using an external infusion pump.

Contraindications and cautions

• Contraindicated during periods of hypoglycemia and in patients hypersensitive to insulin glulisine or one of its excipients.
• Use cautiously in patients with moderate to severe renal or hepatic dysfunction.
🜚 **Lifespan:** In pregnant women, safety and effectiveness haven't been established. In breastfeeding women, use cautiously because it's unknown if the drug appears in breast milk. In children, safety and effectiveness haven't been established.

Adverse reactions

Metabolic: *hypoglycemia.*
Skin: *injection-site reactions,* lipodystrophy, pruritus, rash.
Other: allergic reactions, *anaphylaxis,* insulin antibody production.

Interactions

Drug-drug. *ACE inhibitors, disopyramide, fibrates, fluoxetine, MAO inhibitors, oral antidiabetics, pentoxifylline, propoxyphene, salicylates, sulfonamide antibiotics:* May increase glucose-lowering effects. Monitor glucose level, and watch for evidence of hypoglycemia.
Beta blockers, clonidine, lithium, pentamidine: May cause unpredictable response to insulin. Use together cautiously; monitor patient closely.
Clozapine, corticosteroids, danazol, diazoxide, diuretics, estrogens, glucagons, isoniazid, olanzapine, phenothiazines, progestogens, protease inhibitors, somatropin, sympathomimetics (such as epinephrine, albuterol, and terbutaline), thyroid hormones: May decrease glucose-lowering effects. Monitor glucose level carefully.
Drug-lifestyle. *Alcohol:* May increase or decrease drug effects, resulting in either hypoglycemia or hyperglycemia. Discourage alcohol use.

Effects on lab test results

• May decrease glucose level.

Pharmacokinetics

Absorption: Absorbed rapidly, faster than regular insulin.
Distribution: Wide.

Metabolism: Bound and inactivated in peripheral tissues plus primary metabolism in the liver.
Excretion: Renal filtration. *Half-life:* 42 minutes.

Route	Onset	Peak	Duration
SubQ	15 min	34–91 min	105–210 min

Action

Chemical effect: Increases peripheral glucose uptake by skeletal muscle and fat and decreases hepatic glucose production.
Therapeutic effect: Lowers glucose level.

Available forms

Injection: 10-ml vial of 100 units/ml

NURSING PROCESS

Assessment

• Monitor patient for signs and symptoms of hyperglycemia, including drowsiness, fruity breath, frequent urination, and thirst.
• Monitor patient for signs and symptoms of hypoglycemia, including cool, diaphoretic skin; shaking; trembling; confusion; headache; irritability; hunger; tachycardia; and nausea.
• Look for early warning signs of hypoglycemia. They may be different or less pronounced in patients who take beta blockers, who have had an oral antidiabetic added to the regimen, or who have long-term diabetes or diabetic nerve disease.
• Assess injection site for redness, swelling, or itching.
• Monitor patient for lipodystrophy at injection site. Lipodystrophy may delay insulin absorption.
• Assess patient's and family's knowledge of drug therapy.

Nursing diagnoses

• Ineffective health maintenance related to presence of underlying disease
• Risk for injury related to drug-induced hypoglycemia
• Deficient knowledge related to drug therapy

Planning and implementation

• Use with a longer-acting or basal insulin analog.
ALERT: Drug has a more rapid onset and shorter duration of action than regular human insulin.

Give within 15 minutes before or immediately after a meal.
• Don't mix drug in a syringe with other insulins except NPH.
• When drug is used in an external subcutaneous infusion pump, don't mix with other insulins or with a diluent.
• Adjust dosage for changes in insulin strength, manufacturer, or type.
• Adjust dosage for changes in physical activity or usual meal plan.
• Adjust dosage during illness, emotional disturbances, or stress.
Patient teaching
• Tell patient to take drug within 20 minutes of eating.
• Teach patient how to give subcutaneous insulin injections.
• Tell patient not to mix drug in a syringe with any insulin other than NPH.
• If patient is mixing drug with NPH, tell patient to use U-100 syringes, to draw insulin glulisine into the syringe before NPH insulin, and to inject the mixture immediately.
• Instruct patient to rotate injection sites to avoid injection-site reactions.
• If patient is using an external infusion pump, teach proper use of the device. Tell patient not to mix drug with other insulin or diluents. Instruct patient to change the infusion set, reservoir with insulin, and infusion site every 48 hours.
• Teach patient the signs and symptoms of hypoglycemia (sweating, rapid pulse, trembling, confusion, headache, irritability, and nausea). Advise the patient to treat these symptoms by eating or drinking something containing sugar.
• Tell the patient to contact his prescriber for dose adjustments if hypoglycemia occurs frequently.
• Show patient how to monitor and log his glucose levels to assess diabetes control.
• Explain the possible long-term complications of diabetes and the importance of regular preventive therapy. Urge patient to follow prescribed diet and exercise regimen. To further reduce the increased risk of heart disease, encourage patient to stop smoking and lose weight.
• Instruct patient to wear or carry identification showing that he has diabetes.
• Tell patient to store unopened vials in the refrigerator. Opened vials must be stored

below 77° F (25° C) and should be used within 28 days. Drug should be protected from direct heat and light.

☑ **Evaluation**
• Patient's glucose level is normal.
• Patient doesn't experience hypoglycemia.
• Patient and family state understanding of drug therapy.

insulins
(IN-suh-linz)

insulin (regular)
Actrapid ◇ , Actrapid Penfill ◇ , Humulin R, Humulin R Regular U-500 (concentrated), Hypurin Neutral ◇ , Novolin R, Novolin R PenFill, Novolin R Prefilled, Velosulin BR

insulin (lispro)
Humalog, NovoLog

insulin lispro protamine and insulin lispro
Humalog Mix25 ◇ , Humalog Mix 75/25, NovoLog 70/30

isophane insulin suspension (NPH)
Humulin N, Humulin NPH ◇ , Hypurin Isophane ◇ , Novolin N, Novolin N PenFill, Novolin N Prefilled, Protaphane ◇ , Protaphane Prefill

isophane insulin suspension and insulin injection (70% isophane insulin and 30% insulin injection)
Humulin 70/30, Novolin 70/30, Novolin 70/30 PenFill, Novolin 70/30 Prefilled, Mixtard 30/70 ◇ , Mixtard 30/70 Penfill ◇

isophane insulin suspension and insulin injection (50% isophane insulin and 50% insulin injection)
Humulin 50/50, Mixtard 50/50 ◇ , Mixtard Penfill 50/50 ◇

isophane insulin suspension and insulin injection (80% isophane insulin and 20% insulin injection)
Mixtard 80/20 ◇ , Mixtard Penfill 80/20 ◇

Pharmacologic class: pancreatic hormone
Therapeutic class: antidiabetic
Pregnancy risk category: B

Indications and dosages

▶ **Moderate to severe diabetic ketoacidosis or hyperosmolar hyperglycemia (regular insulin).** *Adults older than age 20:* Give loading dose of 0.15 units/kg I.V. by direct injection, followed by 0.1 unit/kg/hour as a continuous infusion. Decrease rate of insulin infusion to 0.05 to 0.1 unit/kg/hour when glucose level reaches 250 to 300 mg/dl. Start infusion of D_5W in half-normal saline solution separately from the insulin infusion when glucose level is 150 to 200 mg/dl in patients with diabetic ketoacidosis or 250 to 300 mg/dl in those with hyperosmolar hyperglycemia. Give dose of insulin subcutaneously 1 to 2 hours before stopping insulin infusion (intermediate-acting insulin is recommended).
Adults and children age 20 or younger: Loading dose isn't recommended. Start with 0.1 unit/kg/hour by I.V. infusion. Once condition improves, decrease rate of insulin infusion to 0.05 unit/kg/hour. Start infusion of D_5W in half-normal saline solution separately from the insulin infusion when glucose level is 250 mg/dl.
▶ **Mild diabetic ketoacidosis (regular insulin).** *Adults older than age 20:* Give loading dose of 0.4 to 0.6 unit/kg divided in two equal parts, with half the dose given by direct I.V. injection and half given I.M. or subcutaneously. Subsequent doses can be based on 0.1 unit/kg/hour I.M. or subcutaneously.
▶ **Newly diagnosed diabetes mellitus (regular insulin).** *Adults older than age 20:* Individualize therapy. Initially, 0.5 to 1 unit/kg/day subcutaneously as part of a regimen with short-acting and long-acting insulin therapy.
Adults and children age 20 or younger: Individualize therapy. Initially 0.1 to 0.25 unit/kg subcutaneously q 6 to 8 hours for 24 hours; then adjust accordingly.
▶ **Control of hyperglycemia with Humalog and longer-acting insulin in patients with type 1 diabetes mellitus.** *Adults:* Dosage varies

---

among patients and must be determined by prescriber familiar with patient's metabolic needs, eating habits, and other lifestyle variables. Inject subcutaneously within 15 minutes before or after a meal.

▶ **Control of hyperglycemia with Humalog and sulfonylureas in patients with type 2 diabetes mellitus.** *Adults and children older than age 3:* Dosage varies among patients and must be determined by prescriber familiar with patient's metabolic needs, eating habits, and other lifestyle variables. Inject subcutaneously within 15 minutes before or after a meal.

▶ **Hyperkalemia‡.** *Adults:* 50 ml of dextrose 50% given over 5 minutes, followed by 5 to 10 units of regular insulin by I.V. push.

▼ I.V. administration

• Give only regular insulin I.V. Inject directly into vein or into a port close to I.V. access site. Intermittent infusion isn't recommended. If given by continuous infusion, infuse drug diluted in normal saline solution at prescribed rate.
• Regular insulin is used in patients with circulatory collapse, diabetic ketoacidosis, or hyperkalemia.
• Don't use Humulin R (concentrated) U-500 I.V.
• Don't use intermediate- or long-acting insulins for coma or other emergency requiring rapid drug action.
• Ketosis-prone type 1, severely ill, and newly diagnosed diabetic patients with very high glucose levels may need hospitalization and I.V. treatment with regular fast-acting insulin.
⊗ **Incompatibilities**
Aminophylline, amobarbital, chlorothiazide, cytarabine, digoxin, diltiazem, dobutamine, dopamine, levofloxacin, methylprednisolone sodium succinate, nafcillin, norepinephrine, pentobarbital sodium, phenobarbital sodium, phenytoin sodium, ranitidine, sodium bicarbonate, thiopental.

Contraindications and cautions

• Contraindicated in hypoglycemia and in patients hypersensitive to insulin or any of its ingredients.
❧ **Lifespan:** In pregnant and breast-feeding women, insulin is drug of choice to treat diabetes.

Adverse reactions

Metabolic: *hypoglycemia,* hyperglycemia (rebound or Somogyi effect).
Skin: urticaria, itching, swelling, redness, stinging, warmth at injection site, rash.
Other: lipoatrophy, lipohypertrophy, hypersensitivity reactions, *anaphylaxis,* rash.

Interactions

Drug-drug. *AIDS antiretrovirals, corticosteroids, dextrothyroxine, epinephrine, thiazide diuretics:* May diminish insulin response. Monitor patient for hyperglycemia.
Anabolic steroids, clofibrate, guanethidine, MAO inhibitors, salicylates, tetracyclines: May prolong hypoglycemic effect. Monitor glucose level carefully.
Carteolol, nadolol, pindolol, propranolol, timolol: May mask symptoms of hypoglycemia (such as tachycardia) as a result of beta blockade. Use cautiously in patients with diabetes.
Hormonal contraceptives: May decrease glucose tolerance in diabetic patients. Monitor glucose level, and adjust insulin dosage carefully.
Drug-herb. *Basil, bay, bee pollen, burdock, ginseng, glucomannan, horehound, marshmallow, myrrh, sage:* May affect glycemic control. Monitor glucose level carefully.
Drug-lifestyle. *Alcohol use:* May increase the glucose-lowering effects of insulin. Discourage use together.
Marijuana use: May increase glucose level. Tell patient about this interaction.
Smoking: May increase glucose level and decrease response to insulin. Discourage patient from smoking; have patient monitor glucose level closely.

Effects on lab test results

• May decrease glucose, magnesium, and potassium levels.

Pharmacokinetics

Absorption: Highly variable after subcutaneous administration depending on insulin type and injection site.
Distribution: Wide.
Metabolism: Some is bound and inactivated by peripheral tissues, but most appears to be degraded in liver and kidneys.

Excretion: Filtered by renal glomeruli; undergoes some tubular reabsorption. *Half-life:* About 9 minutes after I.V. administration.

Route	Onset	Peak	Duration
I.V.	≤ 30 min	15–30 min	30 min–1 hr
SubQ	15 min–8 hr	2–30 hr	5–36 hr

Action

Chemical effect: Increases glucose transport across muscle and fat cell membranes to reduce glucose level. Promotes conversion of glucose to its storage form, glycogen.
Therapeutic effect: Lowers glucose level.

Available forms

Available without a prescription
insulin (regular)
Injection (human): 100 units/ml (Humulin R, Novolin R, Novolin R PenFill, Novolin R Prefilled, Velosulin BR)
isophane insulin suspension (NPH)
Injection (human): 100 units/ml (Humulin N, Novolin N, Novolin N PenFill, Novolin N Prefilled)
insulin zinc suspension (lente)
Injection (human): 100 units/ml (Novolin L)
isophane insulin suspension and insulin injection combinations
Injection (human): 100 units/ml (Humulin 70/30, Novolin 70/30, Novolin 70/30 PenFill, Novolin 70/30 Prefilled, Humulin 50/50)
Available by prescription only
insulin (regular)
Injection (human): 100 units/ml (Actrapid, Actrapid Penfill ◊), 500 units/ml (Humulin R Regular U-500 [concentrated])
Injection (bovine): 100 units/ml (Hypurin Neutral ◊)
insulin (lispro)
Injection (human): 100 units/ml (Humalog)
insulin lispro protamine and insulin lispro
Injection (human): 100 units/ml (Humalog Mix 25 ◊, Humalog Mix 50/50, Humalog Mix 75/25)
isophane insulin suspension (NPH)
Injection (human): 100 units/ml (Humulin NPH ◊, Protaphane ◊, Protaphane Prefill ◊)
Injection (bovine): 100 units/ml (Hypurin Isophane ◊)

isophane insulin suspension and insulin injection combinations
Injection (human): 100 units/ml (Mixtard 30/70 ◊, Mixtard 30/70 Penfill ◊, Mixtard 50/50 ◊, Mixtard Penfill 50/50 ◊, Mixtard 80/20 ◊, Mixtard Penfill 80/20 ◊)

NURSING PROCESS

⚚ Assessment

• Assess patient's glucose level before starting therapy and regularly thereafter. If patient is under stress, unstable, pregnant, recently diagnosed, or taking drugs that can interact with insulin, monitor level more frequently.
• Monitor patient's glycosylated hemoglobin level regularly.
• Monitor urine ketone level when glucose level is elevated.
• Be alert for adverse reactions and drug interactions.
• Monitor injection sites for local reactions.
• Assess patient's and family's knowledge of drug therapy.

⊕ Nursing diagnoses

• Ineffective health maintenance related to hyperglycemia
• Risk for injury related to drug-induced hypoglycemia
• Deficient knowledge related to drug therapy

⧉ Planning and implementation

ⓢ **ALERT:** Dose is always expressed in USP units. Use only syringes calibrated for particular concentration of insulin given (such as U-100 for 100 units/ml insulin).
• Insulin resistance may develop; large insulin doses are needed to control symptoms of diabetes in these patients. U-500 insulin is available as Regular (Concentrated) for such patients. Although not normally stocked in every pharmacy, it's readily available. Give hospital pharmacy sufficient notice before the need to refill in-house prescription. Never store U-500 insulin in same area with other insulin preparations because of danger of severe overdose if given accidentally to other patients.
• To mix insulin suspension, swirl vial gently or rotate between palms or between palm and thigh. Don't shake vigorously because doing so causes bubbling and air in syringe.

Reactions may be *common,* uncommon, *life-threatening*, or COMMON AND LIFE-THREATENING.

• Humalog insulin has a rapid onset of action. Give 15 minutes before meals.

• Regular insulin may be mixed with NPH insulins in any proportion.

• Switching from separate injections to prepared mixture may alter patient response. Whenever NPH is mixed with regular insulin in same syringe, give immediately to avoid loss of potency.

• Don't use insulin that has changed color or become clumped or granular.

• Check expiration date on vial before using.

• Usual route is subcutaneous. Pinch fold of skin with fingers starting at least 3 inches apart, and insert needle at 45- to 90-degree angle.

• Press but don't rub site after injection. Rotate and chart injection sites to avoid overuse of one area. Rotate injection sites within same anatomic region to help diabetic patients achieve better control.

• Ketosis-prone type 1, severely ill, and newly diagnosed diabetic patients with very high glucose levels may require hospitalization and I.V. treatment with regular fast-acting insulin.

• Store drug in cool area. Refrigeration is desirable but not essential except for concentrated regular insulin.

• Notify prescriber of sudden changes in glucose levels, dangerously high or low levels, or ketosis.

• If patient develops diabetic ketoacidosis or hyperglycemic hyperosmolar nonketotic coma, provide supportive treatment.

• Treat hypoglycemic reaction with oral form of rapid-acting glucose if patient can swallow, or with glucagon or I.V. glucose if patient can't be roused. Follow with complex carbohydrate snack when patient is awake, and determine cause of reaction.

• Make sure patient is following appropriate diet and exercise programs. Adjust insulin dosage when other aspects of regimen are changed.

• Discuss with prescriber how to deal with noncompliance.

• Treat lipoatrophy or lipohypertrophy according to prescribed protocol.

Ⓢ **ALERT:** Spell out units to reduce the risk of error by misreading the "U" as "0" (zero).

Patient teaching

• Tell patient that insulin relieves symptoms but doesn't cure disease.

• Inform patient about nature of disease; importance of following therapeutic regimen; adherence to specific diet, weight reduction, exercise, and personal hygiene programs; and ways of avoiding infection. Review timing of injections and eating, and explain that meals must not be skipped.

• Stress that accuracy of measurement is very important, especially with concentrated regular insulin. Aids, such as a magnifying sleeve or dose magnifier, may improve accuracy. Instruct patient and family how to measure and give insulin.

• Advise patient not to alter order of mixing insulins or change model or brand of syringe or needle.

• Tell patient that glucose monitoring and urine ketone tests are essential guides to dosage and success of therapy. Stress the importance of recognizing hypoglycemic symptoms because insulin-induced hypoglycemia is hazardous and may cause brain damage if prolonged. Most adverse effects are self-limiting and temporary.

• Teach patient about proper use of equipment for monitoring glucose level.

• Instruct patient not to drink alcohol during therapy.

• Advise patient not to smoke within 30 minutes after insulin injection. Smoking decreases absorption.

• Tell patient that marijuana use may increase insulin requirements.

• Advise patient to wear or carry medical identification at all times, to carry ample insulin supply and syringes on trips, to have carbohydrates (lump of sugar or candy) on hand for emergencies, and to note time-zone changes for dose scheduling when traveling.

☑ **Evaluation**

• Patient's glucose level is normal.

• Patient sustains no injury from drug-induced hypoglycemia.

• Patient and family state understanding of drug therapy.

interferon alfa-2a, recombinant (rIFN-A)
(in-ter-FEER-on AL-fuh too-ay ree-COM-bih-nent)
Roferon-A

interferon alfa-2b, recombinant (IFN-alpha 2)
Intron-A

Pharmacologic class: biological response modifier
Therapeutic class: antineoplastic, immunomodulator
Pregnancy risk category: C

Indications and dosages

▶ **Hairy cell leukemia.** *Adults:* For induction, 3 million international units alfa-2a subcutaneously or I.M. daily for 16 to 24 weeks. For maintenance, 3 million international units alfa-2a subcutaneously or I.M. three times weekly. Or 2 million international units /m² alfa-2b I.M. or subcutaneously three times weekly for induction and maintenance.
▶ **Condylomata acuminata.** *Adults:* 1 million international units alfa-2b per lesion, intralesionally, three times weekly for 3 weeks. May repeat after 12 to 16 weeks if results are not satisfactory
▶ **Kaposi's sarcoma.** *Adults:* For induction, 36 million international units alfa-2a subcutaneously or I.M. daily for 10 to 12 weeks; for maintenance, 36 million international units alfa-2a three times weekly. Doses may begin at 3 million international units and escalate every 3 days until patient is given 36 million international units daily, in order to decrease toxicity. Or 30 million international units/m² alfa-2b subcutaneously or I.M. three times weekly. Maintain dose unless disease progresses rapidly or intolerance occurs.
▶ **Chronic hepatitis C.** *Adults:* 3 million international units alfa-2a three times weekly subcutaneously or I.M. for 12 months (48 to 52 weeks). Alternatively, induction dose of 6 million international units alfa-2a three times weekly for the first 3 months (12 weeks) followed by 3 million international units alfa-2a three times weekly for 9 months (36 weeks). If no response after 3 months, stop therapy. Retreatment with either 3 or 6 million interna-

tional units alfa-2a three times weekly for 6 to 12 months may be considered. Or 3 million international units alfa-2b subcutaneously or I.M. three times weekly. In patients tolerating therapy with normalization of ALT at 16 weeks of treatment, extend therapy to 18 to 24 months. If no normalization of ALT at 16 weeks of treatment, consider stopping therapy.
▶ **Chronic hepatitis B.** *Adults:* 30 to 35 million international units alfa-2b subcutaneously or I.M. weekly either as 5 million international units daily or 10 million international units three times weekly for 16 weeks.
Children ages 1 to 17: 3 million international units/m² alfa-2b subcutaneously three times weekly for 1 week; then escalate dosage to 6 million international units/m² subcutaneously three times weekly (up to 10 million international units/m² subcutaneously three times weekly) for 16 to 24 weeks.
▶ **Chronic myelogenous leukemia.** *Adults:* 9 million international units alfa-2a daily I.M. or subcutaneously. An escalating dosage regimen, in which daily doses of 3 million and 6 million international units are given over 3 days followed by 9 million international units daily for remainder of therapy, may produce increased short-term tolerance.
Children: 2.5 to 5 million international units/m² alfa-2a I.M. daily.
▶ **Malignant melanoma.** *Adults:* 20 million international units/m² alfa-2b daily given as I.V. infusion 5 days in a row for 4 weeks. For maintenance therapy, 10 million international units/m² subcutaneously three times weekly for 48 weeks. If adverse effects occur, stop therapy until they subside, and then resume therapy at 50% of the previous dose. If intolerance persists, stop therapy.
▶ **Initial treatment of aggressive follicular malignant lymphoma in conjunction with combination chemotherapy containing anthracycline.** *Adults:* 5 million international units alfa-2b subcutaneously three times weekly for up to 18 months.
▶ **Metastatic renal cell carcinoma‡.** *Adults:* 5 to 20 million international units alfa-2b subcutaneously daily or three times weekly.

Contraindications and cautions

• Contraindicated in patients hypersensitive to the drug, any of its components, or mouse protein.

• Use cautiously in patients with severe hepatic or renal function impairment, seizure disorders, compromised CNS function, cardiac disease, or myelosuppression.

• Alpha interferons cause or aggravate fatal or life-threatening neuropsychiatric, autoimmune, ischemic, and infectious disorders. Monitor patient closely. Stop drug in patients with persistently severe or worsening signs or symptoms of these conditions.

⚞ Lifespan: In pregnant women, use cautiously. In breast-feeding women, stop drug or stop breast-feeding. In children, safety and effectiveness haven't been established.

Adverse reactions

CNS: *dizziness,* confusion, paresthesia, numbness, lethargy, *depression,* nervousness, difficulty in thinking or concentrating, *insomnia,* sedation, apathy, anxiety, *irritability,* syncope, fatigue, vertigo, gait disturbances, poor coordination, *headache.*
CV: hypotension, chest pain, *arrhythmias,* palpitations, *heart failure, cyanosis, hypertension,* edema, flushing, *MI.*
EENT: excessive salivation, visual disturbances, dry or inflamed oropharynx, rhinorrhea, sinusitis, conjunctivitis, earache, eye irritation, rhinitis.
GI: *anorexia, nausea, diarrhea,* vomiting, abdominal fullness, *abdominal pain,* flatulence, constipation, hypermotility, gastric distress, dysgeusia.
GU: transient impotence.
Hematologic: anemia, *leukopenia, neutropenia, mild thrombocytopenia.*
Hepatic: *hepatitis.*
Respiratory: *coughing, dyspnea,* tachypnea.
Skin: *rash,* dryness, *pruritus,* partial alopecia, *diaphoresis,* urticaria.
Other: *flulike syndrome,* hot flushes, *injection site reaction.*

Interactions

Drug-drug. *Aminophylline, theophylline:* May reduce theophylline clearance. Monitor level.
Cardiotoxic, hematotoxic, or neurotoxic drugs: Effects of previously or concurrently administered drugs may be increased by interferons. Monitor patient closely.
CNS depressants: May enhance CNS effects. Avoid use together.
Interleukin-2: May increase risk of renal impairment from interleukin-2. Monitor patient closely.

Live-virus vaccines: May increase risk of adverse reactions and decreased antibody response. Don't use together.
Zidovudine: May have synergistic adverse effects between alfa-2b and zidovudine. Carefully monitor WBC count.
Drug-lifestyle. *Alcohol use:* May increase risk of GI bleeding. Discourage use together.
Sun exposure: May cause photosensitivity reactions. Discourage prolonged or unprotected sun exposure.

Effects on lab test results

• May increase calcium, potassium, AST, ALT, alkaline phosphatase, LDH, triglyceride, and fasting glucose levels. May decrease hemoglobin level and hematocrit.

• May increase PT, INR, and PTT. May decrease WBC, neutrophil, and platelet counts.

Pharmacokinetics

Absorption: More than 80% absorbed after I.M. or subcutaneous injection.
Distribution: Wide and rapid.
Metabolism: Drug appears to be metabolized in liver and kidneys.
Excretion: Reabsorbed from glomerular filtrate with minor biliary elimination. *Half-life:* 3½ to 8½ hours.

Route	Onset	Peak	Duration
I.M.	Unknown	3¾ hr	Unknown
SubQ	Unknown	7¼ hr	Unknown
Intralesional	Unknown	Unknown	Unknown

Action

Chemical effect: May involve direct antiproliferative action against tumor cells or viral cells to inhibit replication and change immune response by enhancing phagocytic macrophages and by augmenting specific cytotoxicity of lymphocytes for target cells.
Therapeutic effect: Inhibits growth of certain tumor cells and viral cells.

Available forms

alfa-2a (Roferon-A)
Prefilled syringes for subcutaneous use only: 3 million international units/0.5 ml; 6 million international units/0.5 ml; 9 million international units/0.5 ml

Solution for injection: 18 million international units/multidose vial; 36 million international units/single-dose vial
alfa-2b (Intron A)
Powder for injection with diluent: 5 million international units/vial; 10 million international units/vial; 18 million international units/multidose vial; 25 million international units/vial; 50 million international units/vial
Solution for injection: 3 million international units/vial or syringe; 5 million international units/vial or syringe; 10 million international units/vial; 18 million international units/multidose vial; 25 million international units/vial
Multidose pens: 18 million international units (3 million international units per dose); 30 million international units (5 million international units per dose); 60 million international units (10 million international units per dose)

NURSING PROCESS

☞ Assessment
● Assess patient's condition before starting therapy and regularly thereafter.
● Obtain allergy history. Drug contains phenol as preservative and albumin as stabilizer.
● Assess patient for flulike symptoms before starting therapy; these tend to diminish with continued therapy.
● Alpha interferons may cause or aggravate fatal or life-threatening neuropsychiatric, autoimmune, ischemic, and infectious disorders. Monitor patients closely. Stop drug in patients with persistently severe or worsening signs or symptoms of these conditions. In many, but not all, cases, these disorders resolve after stopping therapy.
● Monitor blood studies. Tests include CBC with differential, platelet count, blood chemistry and electrolyte studies, liver function, and, if patient has cardiac disorder or advanced stages of cancer, ECGs. Any effects are dose-related and reversible. Recovery occurs within several days or weeks after withdrawal.
● Be alert for adverse reactions and drug interactions.
● Assess patient's and family's knowledge of drug therapy.

⊕ Nursing diagnoses
● Ineffective health maintenance related to underlying condition

● Risk for injury related to drug-induced adverse CNS reactions
● Deficient knowledge related to drug therapy

▷ Planning and implementation
● Premedicate patient with acetaminophen to minimize flulike symptoms.
● Give drug h.s. to minimize daytime drowsiness.
● Make sure patient is well hydrated, especially during initial stages of treatment.
● **ALERT:** Different brands of interferon may not be equivalent and may require different dosages.
● Use subcutaneous administration route in patients whose platelet count is below 50,000/mm³.
● When giving interferon alfa-2b for condylomata acuminata, use only 10 million–international units vial because dilution of other strengths for intralesional use results in hypertonic solution. Don't reconstitute 10 million–international units vial with more than 1 ml of diluent. Use tuberculin or similar syringe and 25G to 30G needle. Don't inject too deeply beneath lesion or too superficially. As many as five lesions can be treated at one time. To ease discomfort, give drug in evening with acetaminophen.
● Refrigerate drug.
● Notify prescriber of severe adverse reactions, which may require a lower dose or stopping the drug.
● Using drug with blood dyscrasia–causing drugs, bone marrow suppressants, or radiation therapy may increase bone marrow suppression. A lower dose may be needed.
Patient teaching
● Advise patient that laboratory tests will be performed before starting therapy and periodically thereafter.
● Instruct patient in proper oral hygiene because bone marrow–suppressant effects may lead to microbial infection, delayed healing, and gingival bleeding. Drug may decrease salivary flow.
● Emphasize need to follow prescriber's instructions about taking and recording temperature. Explain how and when to take acetaminophen.
● Advise patient to check with prescriber for instructions after missing dose.
● Tell patient that drug may cause temporary hair loss; explain that it will grow back when therapy ends.
● Teach patient how to prepare and give drug and how to dispose of used needles, syringes, containers, and unused drug. Give him a copy of

information for patients included with product, and make sure he understands it. Also provide information on drug stability.

• Warn patient not to receive any immunization without prescriber's approval and to avoid contact with people who have taken polio vaccine. Use with live-virus vaccine may increase adverse reactions and decrease patient's antibody response. Patient is at increased risk for infection.

• Instruct patient to avoid alcohol during drug therapy.

• Advise patient to report signs of depression.

☑ **Evaluation**
• Patient shows improved health.
• Patient sustains no injury from adverse CNS reactions.
• Patient and family state understanding of drug therapy.

interferon beta-1b, recombinant
(in-ter-FEER-on BAY-tuh WUN BEE ree-CAHM-bih-nehnt)
Betaseron

Pharmacologic class: biological response modifier
Therapeutic class: antiviral, immunoregulator
Pregnancy risk category: C

Indications and dosages

▶ **To reduce frequency of exacerbations in patients with relapsing forms of multiple sclerosis.** *Adults:* 0.0625 mg subcutaneously q other day for weeks 1 and 2; then 0.125 mg subcutaneously q other day for weeks 3 and 4; then 0.1875 mg subcutaneously q other day for weeks 5 and 6; then 0.25 mg subcutaneously q other day thereafter.

Contraindications and cautions

• Contraindicated in patients hypersensitive to interferon beta or human albumin.
🔥 **Lifespan:** In pregnant and breast-feeding women, use only if benefits outweigh risks to the fetus or infant. In children, safety and effectiveness haven't been established.

Adverse reactions

CNS: depression, anxiety, emotional lability, depersonalization, *malaise, suicidal tendencies,* confusion, somnolence, *seizures,* headache, dizziness.
CV: *hemorrhage.*
EENT: laryngitis.
GI: nausea, diarrhea, constipation.
GU: menstrual disorders.
Hematologic: *leukopenia, neutropenia.*
Hepatic: *liver failure.*
Respiratory: dyspnea.
Other: flulike symptoms, breast pain, pelvic pain, lymphadenopathy, hypersensitivity reaction, inflammation, pain, and necrosis at injection site.

Interactions

Drug-lifestyle. *Sun exposure:* May cause photosensitivity reactions. Discourage prolonged or unprotected sun exposure.

Effects on lab test results

• May increase ALT and bilirubin levels.
• May decrease WBC and neutrophil counts.

Pharmacokinetics

Absorption: Bioavailability is 50% after subcutaneous injection.
Distribution: Unknown.
Metabolism: Unknown.
Excretion: Unknown. *Half-life:* 8 minutes to 4¼ hours.

Route	Onset	Peak	Duration
SubQ	Unknown	1–8 hr	Unknown

Action

Chemical effect: Attaches to membrane receptors and causes cellular changes, including increased protein synthesis.
Therapeutic effect: Decreases exacerbations in multiple sclerosis.

Available forms

Powder for injection: 0.3 mg with separate 1.2-ml prefilled syringe of sodium chloride, 0.54% diluent.

NURSING PROCESS

🔬 **Assessment**
• Assess patient's underlying condition before starting therapy.
• Monitor frequency of exacerbations after drug therapy begins.

• Monitor WBC counts, platelet counts, and blood chemistries, including liver function test results.

⑤ **ALERT:** Serious liver damage can occur with therapy, including hepatic failure and need for liver transplant. Monitor liver function 1, 3, and 6 months after treatment starts, then periodically thereafter.

• Be alert for adverse reactions.
• Monitor patient for depression and suicidal ideation.
• Assess patient's and family's knowledge of drug therapy.

🔱 Nursing diagnoses
• Ineffective health maintenance related to exacerbations of multiple sclerosis
• Risk for injury related to drug-induced adverse CNS reactions
• Deficient knowledge related to drug therapy

⧆ Planning and implementation
• Premedicate patient with acetaminophen to minimize flulike symptoms.
• To reconstitute, inject 1.2 ml of supplied diluent (0.54% saline solution for injection) into vial and gently swirl to dissolve drug. Don't shake. Reconstituted solution will contain 8 million units (0.25 mg)/ml. Discard vials that contain particles or discolored solution.
• Inject preparation immediately.
• Store at room temperature. Once reconstituted, may refrigerate for up to 3 hours before use.
• Rotate injection sites to minimize local reactions.
Patient teaching
• Warn woman of childbearing age about dangers to fetus. Tell her to notify prescriber promptly if she becomes pregnant.
• Teach patient how to give subcutaneous injections, including solution preparation, use of aseptic technique, rotation of injection sites, and equipment disposal. Periodically reevaluate patient's technique.
• Advise patient to take drug h.s. to minimize mild flulike symptoms.
• Advise patient of need for blood testing to check liver status and need to report anorexia, fatigue, malaise, dark urine, light feces, or jaundice to prescriber promptly.
• Advise patient to report thoughts of depression or suicidal ideation.

☑ Evaluation
• Patient exhibits decreased frequency of exacerbations.
• Patient sustains no injury from adverse CNS reactions.
• Patient and family state understanding of drug therapy.

interferon gamma-1b
(in-ter-FEER-on GAH-muh wun bee)
Actimmune

Pharmacologic class: biological response modifier
Therapeutic class: immunomodulator; antineoplastic
Pregnancy risk category: C

Indications and dosages

▶ **To delay disease progression in patients with severe, malignant osteopetrosis; chronic granulomatous disease.** *Patients with body surface area greater than 0.5 m²:* 50 mcg/m² (1 million international units/m²) subcutaneously three times weekly in the deltoid or anterior thigh.
Patients with body surface area 0.5 m² or less: 1.5 mcg/kg/dose subcutaneously three times weekly in the deltoid or anterior thigh.

Contraindications and cautions

• Contraindicated in patients hypersensitive to the drug or any of its components or to genetically engineered products derived from *Escherichia coli.*
• Use cautiously in patients with cardiac disease, compromised CNS function, or seizure disorders.
• Drug metabolized by CYP metabolism. Use cautiously with other drugs using same system of metabolism.
⧱ Lifespan: In pregnant women, use cautiously. In breast-feeding women, use cautiously because it's unknown if drug appears in breast milk. In children younger than age 1, safety and effectiveness haven't been established.

Adverse reactions

CNS: fatigue, decreased mental status, gait disturbance.
GI: nausea, vomiting, diarrhea.

Hematologic: *neutropenia, thrombocytopenia.*
Skin: rash.
Other: flulike syndrome, erythema and tenderness at injection site.

Interactions

Drug-drug. *Myelosuppressive drugs:* May have additive myelosuppression. Monitor patient closely.
Zidovudine: May have additive bone marrow suppression. Consider reducing dosage.

Effects on lab test results

• May increase liver enzyme levels.
• May decrease neutrophil and platelet counts.

Pharmacokinetics

Absorption: About 90% absorbed after subcutaneous or I.M. administration.
Distribution: Unknown.
Metabolism: Unknown.
Excretion: Unknown. *Half-life:* 6 hours.

Route	Onset	Peak	Duration
SubQ	Unknown	≤ 7 hr	Unknown

Action

Chemical effect: Acts as interleukin-type lymphokine. Drug has potent phagocyte-activating properties and enhances oxidative metabolism of tissue macrophages.
Therapeutic effect: Promotes phagocytes.

Available forms

Injection: 100 mcg (2 million international units)/0.5-ml vial

NURSING PROCESS

Assessment

• Assess patient's condition before starting therapy and regularly thereafter.
• Be alert for adverse reactions and drug interactions. Flulike symptoms include headache, fever, chills, myalgia, and arthralgia.
• If adverse GI reactions occur, monitor patient's hydration status.
• Assess patient's and family's knowledge of drug therapy.

Nursing diagnoses

• Ineffective health maintenance related to underlying condition

• Risk for fluid volume deficit related to adverse GI reactions
• Deficient knowledge related to drug therapy

Planning and implementation

• Premedicate with acetaminophen to minimize symptoms at beginning of therapy. Flulike symptoms tend to diminish with continued therapy.
• Discard unused portion. Each vial is for single-dose use and doesn't contain preservative.
• Give drug h.s. to reduce discomfort from flulike symptoms.
• Refrigerate drug immediately. Vials must be stored at 36° to 46° F (2° to 8° C). Don't freeze. Don't shake vial; avoid excessive agitation. Discard vials that have been left at room temperature for more than 12 hours.
Patient teaching
• Teach patient and family how to give drug and how to dispose of used needles, syringes, containers, and unused drug. Give him a copy of patient information included with product, and make sure he understands it.
• Instruct patient to notify prescriber if adverse reaction occurs.

Evaluation

• Patient responds well to drug.
• Patient maintains adequate hydration.
• Patient and family state understanding of drug therapy.

ipratropium bromide
(ip-ruh-TROH-pee-um BROH-mighd)
Atrovent

Pharmacologic class: anticholinergic
Therapeutic class: bronchodilator
Pregnancy risk category: B

Indications and dosages

▶ Bronchospasm caused by COPD. *Adults and children age 12 and older:* 2 inhalations q.i.d. Additional inhalations may be needed. However, don't exceed 12 total inhalations in 24 hours. Or use inhalation solution, giving up to 500 mcg q 6 to 8 hours via oral nebulizer.
▶ Rhinorrhea linked to allergic and nonallergic perennial rhinitis. *Adults and children*

age 6 and older: 2 sprays of 0.03% nasal spray in each nostril b.i.d. or t.i.d.

▶ **Rhinorrhea caused by the common cold.** *Adults and children age 12 and older:* 2 sprays of 0.06% nasal spray per nostril t.i.d. or q.i.d. *Children ages 5 to 11:* 2 sprays of 0.06% nasal spray per nostril t.i.d.

▶ **Rhinorrhea linked to seasonal allergic rhinitis.** *Adults and children age 5 and older:* 2 sprays of 0.06% nasal spray per nostril q.i.d.

Contraindications and cautions

• Contraindicated in patients hypersensitive to the drug, any of its components, or atropine or its derivatives and in those hypersensitive to soya lecithin or related food products, such as soybeans and peanuts.
• Use cautiously in patients with angle-closure glaucoma, prostatic hyperplasia, or bladder-neck obstruction.
• Safety and effectiveness of use beyond 4 days for rhinorrhea from the common cold or 3 weeks for seasonal allergic rhinitis haven't been established.
⚠ **Lifespan:** In pregnant women, use cautiously. In breast-feeding women, use cautiously because it's unknown if the drug appears in breast milk. In children younger than age 12, safety of oral inhaler or nebulizer hasn't been established.

Adverse reactions

CNS: nervousness, dizziness, headache.
CV: palpitations.
EENT: blurred vision, epistaxis.
GI: nausea, GI distress, dry mouth.
Respiratory: cough, upper respiratory tract infection, bronchitis, ***bronchospasm.***
Skin: rash.

Interactions

Drug-drug. *Anticholinergics:* May increase anticholinergic effects. Avoid use together.
Cromolyn sodium: Will form precipitate if mixed in same nebulizer. Don't use together.
Drug-herb. *Jaborandi tree, pill-bearing spurge:* May decrease drug effects. Use cautiously.

Effects on lab test results

None reported.

Pharmacokinetics

Absorption: Not readily absorbed into systemic circulation.

Distribution: Not distributed.
Metabolism: Small amount that is absorbed is metabolized in liver.
Excretion: Absorbed drug excreted in urine and bile; remainder excreted unchanged in feces.
Half-life: About 2 hours.

Route	Onset	Peak	Duration
Inhalation	5–15 min	1–2 hr	3–6 hr

Action

Chemical effect: Inhibits vagally mediated reflexes by antagonizing acetylcholine.
Therapeutic effect: Relieves bronchospasms and symptoms of seasonal allergic rhinitis.

Available forms

Inhaler: Each metered dose supplies 18 mcg
Nasal spray: 0.03% (21 mcg/spray), 0.06% (42 mcg/spray)
Solution for inhalation: 0.02% (500-mcg vial)
Solution for nebulizer: 0.02% (200 mcg/ml), 0.025% (250 mcg/ml) ◊

NURSING PROCESS

⏱ Assessment
• Assess patient's condition before and after drug therapy; monitor peak expiratory flow.
• Be alert for adverse reactions and drug interactions.
• Assess patient's and family's knowledge of drug therapy.

🔟 Nursing diagnoses
• Ineffective breathing pattern related to patient's underlying condition
• Acute pain related to drug-induced headache
• Deficient knowledge related to drug therapy

▶ Planning and implementation
⚠ **ALERT:** Drug isn't effective for treating acute episodes of bronchospasm when rapid response is needed.
• Don't exceed 12 total inhalations in 24 hours; total nasal sprays shouldn't exceed 8 in each nostril in 24 hours.
• If giving more than one inhalation, let 2 minutes elapse between inhalations. If giving more than one type of inhalant, always give bronchodilator first and wait 5 minutes before giving the other.
• Give drug on time to ensure maximal effect.

Reactions may be *common,* uncommon, *life-threatening*, or COMMON AND LIFE-THREATENING.

● If drug fails to relieve bronchospasms, notify prescriber.

⊛ **ALERT:** Don't confuse Atrovent with Alupent.

Patient teaching

● Warn patient that drug isn't effective for treating acute episodes of bronchospasm where rapid response is needed.

● Give patient these instructions for using metered-dose inhaler: clear nasal passages and throat. Breathe out, expelling as much air from lungs as possible. Place mouthpiece well into mouth, and inhale deeply as you release dose from inhaler. Hold breath for several seconds, remove mouthpiece, and exhale slowly.

● Tell patient to avoid accidentally spraying into eyes. Temporary blurring of vision may result.

● Tell patient to wait at least 2 minutes before repeating when using more than one inhalation.

● If patient also uses a corticosteroid inhaler, tell him to use ipratropium first and then wait about 5 minutes before using the corticosteroid. This process allows bronchodilator to open air passages for maximum effectiveness of the corticosteroid.

● Tell patient to take a missed dose as soon as remembered, unless it's almost time for next dose. In that case, tell him to skip the missed dose and not to double the dose.

☑ Evaluation

● Patient's bronchospasms are relieved.

● Patient doesn't suffer from any drug-induced headaches.

● Patient and family state understanding of drug therapy.

irbesartan
(ir-buh-SAR-tun)
Avapro

Pharmacologic class: angiotensin II receptor antagonist
Therapeutic class: antihypertensive
Pregnancy risk category: C (D in second and third trimesters)

Indications and dosages

▶ **Hypertension.** *Adults and children age 13 and older:* Initially 150 mg P.O. daily; increase to a maximum of 300 mg daily, if needed.

Children ages 6 to 12 years: Initially, 75 mg P.O. daily; increase to a maximum of 150 mg daily, if needed.

▶ **Nephropathy in type 2 diabetic patients.**
Adults: 300 mg P.O. daily.

⊠ **Adjust-a-dose:** In patients who are volume- or salt-depleted, give lower initial dose of 75 mg P.O. daily.

Contraindications and cautions

● Contraindicated in patients hypersensitive to the drug or any of its components.

● Use cautiously in volume- or salt-depleted patients and in patients with renal impairment or renal artery stenosis.

❇ **Lifespan:** In pregnant women, drug should be stopped as soon as possible; use in the second and third trimesters can cause fetal death. Breast-feeding women should stop the drug or stop breast-feeding. In children younger than age 6, safety and effectiveness haven't been established.

Adverse reactions

CNS: fatigue, anxiety, dizziness, headache.
CV: chest pain, edema, tachycardia.
EENT: pharyngitis, rhinitis, sinus abnormality.
GI: diarrhea, dyspepsia, abdominal pain, nausea, vomiting.
GU: UTI.
Metabolic: *hyperkalemia.*
Musculoskeletal: musculoskeletal trauma or pain.
Respiratory: *upper respiratory tract infection.*
Skin: rash.

Interactions

Drug-drug. *Other potassium-sparing drugs and potassium supplements:* Use cautiously because of risk of hyperkalemia.

Effects on lab test results

● May increase potassium level.

Pharmacokinetics

Absorption: Rapid and complete, with an average absolute bioavailability of 60% to 80%.
Distribution: Wide; 90% bound to proteins.
Metabolism: Primarily by conjugation and oxidation.

Excretion: Biliary and renal. About 20% is recovered in urine and the rest in feces. *Half-life:* 11 to 15 hours.

Route	Onset	Peak	Duration
P.O.	Unknown	1½–2 hr	24 hr

Action

Chemical effect: Inhibits the vasoconstricting and aldosterone-secreting effects of angiotensin II by selectively blocking binding of angiotensin II to receptor sites in many tissues.
Therapeutic effect: Lowers blood pressure.

Available forms

Tablets: 75 mg, 150 mg, 300 mg

NURSING PROCESS

⚡ Assessment
• Monitor patient's blood pressure regularly. Dizziness and orthostatic hypotension may occur more frequently in patients with type 2 diabetes mellitus and renal disease.
• Monitor patient's electrolytes, particularly potassium, and assess patient for volume or salt depletion before starting drug therapy.
• Make sure a woman of childbearing age uses effective birth control before starting this drug because of danger to fetus in second and third trimesters.
• Assess patient's and family's knowledge of drug therapy.

⊕ Nursing diagnoses
• Risk for hypotension in volume- or salt-depleted patients
• Risk of injury related to the presence of hypertension
• Deficient knowledge related to drug therapy

⊠ Planning and implementation
• If drug is needed to control blood pressure, give with a diuretic or other antihypertensive.
• If patient becomes hypotensive, place in a supine position and give an I.V. infusion of normal saline solution.
Patient teaching
• Warn woman of childbearing age about consequences of exposing fetus to drug. Tell her to call prescriber immediately if she suspects she is pregnant.

• Tell patient that drug may be taken once daily with or without food.
• Instruct patient to avoid driving and hazardous activities until CNS effects of drug are known.

☑ Evaluation
• Patient doesn't experience hypotension as a result of volume or salt depletion.
• Patient's blood pressure remains within normal limits, and drug therapy doesn't cause injury.
• Patient and family state understanding of drug therapy.

iron dextran
(IGH-ern DEKS-tran)
DexFerrum, DexIron ♦ , InFeD

Pharmacologic class: parenteral iron supplement
Therapeutic class: hematinic
Pregnancy risk category: C

Indications and dosages

▶ **Iron deficiency anemia.** Total dose (in ml) is based on patient's weight and hemoglobin (Hgb) level using the following formula:

$$\text{Dose (ml)} = 0.0442 \text{ (desired Hgb – observed Hgb)} \times \text{weight}^{**} + (0.26 \times \text{weight})$$

**Ideal body weight (IBW) or actual body weight if less than IBW, in kilograms

For children 5 to 15 kg, use actual weight in kg.

One ml iron dextran provides 50 mg elemental iron.
Adults and children: For I.M. use, 0.5-ml test dose injected by Z-track method. If no reactions occur, maximum daily doses are 0.5 ml (25 mg) for infants weighing less than 5 kg (11 lb), 1 ml (50 mg) for children weighing less than 10 kg (22 lb), and 2 ml (100 mg) for heavier children and adults. For I.V. use, 0.5-ml test dose injected over 30 seconds for InFeD, but for DexFerrum, inject over at least 5 minutes. If no reactions occur in 1 hour, remainder of therapeutic dose is given I.V. Therapeutic dose repeated I.V. daily. Maximum single dose is 100 mg. Give slowly (1 ml/minute).

Reactions may be *common*, uncommon, *life-threatening*, or COMMON AND LIFE-THREATENING.

▼ I.V. administration

- Check facility policy before giving I.V.
- Use I.V. when patient has insufficient muscle mass for deep I.M. injection, impaired absorption from muscle as a result of stasis or edema, possibility of uncontrolled I.M. bleeding from trauma (as may occur in hemophilia), or massive and prolonged parenteral therapy (as may be needed in chronic substantial blood loss).
- When I.V. dose is complete, flush vein with 10 ml of normal saline solution. Have patient rest for 15 to 30 minutes after I.V. administration.

⊗ **Incompatibilities**
Other I.V. drugs, parenteral nutrition solutions for I.V. infusion.

Contraindications and cautions

- Contraindicated in patients hypersensitive to drug or any of its components and in those with acute infectious renal disease or anemia disorders (except iron deficiency anemia).
- Use cautiously in patients who have serious hepatic impairment, rheumatoid arthritis, or other inflammatory diseases, and in patients with history of significant allergies or asthma.

⚡ **Lifespan:** In pregnant women, use only when benefits outweigh the potential risks to the fetus. In breast-feeding women, use cautiously because it's unknown if the drug appears in breast milk. In children younger than age 4 months, safety and effectiveness haven't been studied.

Adverse reactions

CNS: headache, transitory paresthesia, arthralgia, myalgia, dizziness, malaise, syncope.
CV: chest pain, chest tightness, *shock,* hypertension, *arrhythmias,* hypotensive reaction, peripheral vascular flushing with overly rapid I.V. administration, tachycardia.
GI: nausea, vomiting, metallic taste, transient loss of taste, abdominal pain, diarrhea.
Respiratory: *bronchospasm.*
Skin: rash, urticaria, *brown discoloration* at I.M. injection site.
Other: *soreness, inflammation, and local phlebitis* at I.V. injection site; sterile abscess; necrosis; atrophy; fibrosis; *anaphylaxis;* delayed sensitivity reactions.

Interactions

Drug-drug. *Chloramphenicol:* May increase iron level because of decreased iron clearance and erythropoiesis. Consult prescriber about using together.

Effects on lab test results

- May increase bilirubin and hemoglobin levels and hematocrit. May decrease calcium level.
- May falsely increase bilirubin level. May falsely decrease calcium level. May interfere with bone scans involving 99m Tc-diphosphonate.

Pharmacokinetics

Absorption: In two stages: 60% after 3 days and up to 90% by 3 weeks. Remainder is absorbed over several months or longer.
Distribution: During first 3 days, local inflammation facilitates passage of drug into lymphatic system; drug is then ingested by macrophages, which enter lymph and blood.
Metabolism: Cleared from plasma by reticuloendothelial cells of liver, spleen, and bone marrow.
Excretion: Trace amounts in urine, bile, and feces. *Half-life:* 6 hours.

Route	Onset	Peak	Duration
I.V., I.M.	72 hr	Unknown	3–4 wk

Action

Chemical effect: Provides elemental iron, a component of hemoglobin.
Therapeutic effect: Increases level of iron, an essential component of hemoglobin.

Available forms

Injection: 50 mg elemental iron/ml

NURSING PROCESS

⊞ Assessment
- Assess patient's iron deficiency before starting therapy.
- Monitor the drug's effectiveness by evaluating hemoglobin level, hematocrit, and reticulocyte count, and monitor patient's health status.
- Be alert for adverse reactions and drug interactions.
- Observe patient for delayed reactions (1 to 2 days), which may include arthralgia, backache, chills, dizziness, headache, malaise, fever, myalgia, nausea, and vomiting.
- Assess patient's and family's knowledge of drug therapy.

⚕ Nursing diagnoses
• Ineffective health maintenance related to iron deficiency
• Risk for injury related to potential drug-induced anaphylaxis
• Deficient knowledge related to drug therapy

▶ Planning and implementation
• Don't give iron dextran with oral iron preparations.
• I.M. or I.V. injections of iron are recommended only for patients for whom oral administration is impossible or ineffective.
• **ALERT:** I.M. or I.V. test dose is required.
• When giving I.M., use a 19G or 20G needle that is 2 to 3 inches long. Inject drug deep into upper outer quadrant of buttock—never into arm or other exposed area. Use Z-track method to avoid leakage into subcutaneous tissue and staining of skin.
• Minimize skin staining by using separate needle to withdraw drug from its container.
• Keep epinephrine and resuscitation equipment readily available to treat anaphylaxis.
Patient teaching
• Warn patient to avoid OTC vitamins that contain iron.
• Teach patient to recognize and report symptoms of reaction or toxicity.

✔ Evaluation
• Patient's hemoglobin level, hematocrit, and reticulocyte count are normal.
• Patient doesn't experience anaphylaxis.
• Patient and family state understanding of drug therapy.

iron sucrose
(IGH-ern SOO-krohs)
Venofer

Pharmacologic classification: polynuclear iron (III)-hydroxide in sucrose
Therapeutic classification: hematinic
Pregnancy risk category: B

Indications and dosages
▶ **Iron deficiency anemia in patients undergoing long-term hemodialysis who are receiving supplemental erythropoietin therapy.**
Adults: 100 mg (5 ml) of elemental iron I.V.

directly in the dialysis line either by slow injection (1 ml per minute) or by infusion over 15 minutes during the dialysis session, one to three times weekly for a total of 1,000 mg in 10 doses. Repeat, if needed.
▶ **Iron deficiency anemia in chronic kidney disease patients not on dialysis.** *Adults:* 200 mg by slow I.V. injection undiluted over 2 to 5 minutes on five separate occasions during a 14-day period to a total cumulative dose of 1,000 mg.

▼ I.V. administration
• Inspect for particulate matter and discoloration before administration.
• For slow injection, administer at 1 ml (20 mg elemental iron) undiluted solution per minute, not exceeding one vial (100 mg elemental iron) per injection.
• For infusion, dilute to a maximum of 100 ml in normal saline solution immediately before infusion, and infuse 100 mg elemental iron over at least 15 minutes. Administering by infusion may reduce the risk of hypotension.
• Transferrin saturation values increase rapidly after I.V. administration of iron sucrose. Obtain iron level values 48 hours after I.V. dosing.
⊗ **Incompatibilities**
Other I.V. drugs, parenteral nutrition infusions.

Contraindications and cautions
• Contraindicated in patients with evidence of iron overload, patients hypersensitive to the drug or any of its inactive components, and in patients with anemia not caused by iron deficiency.
🕸 **Lifespan:** In pregnant women, use cautiously. In breast-feeding women, use cautiously because it's not known whether drug appears in breast milk. In children, safety and effectiveness of drug haven't been established. In elderly patients, make dose selection conservatively; these patients may have decreased hepatic, renal, and cardiac function and other diseases and drug therapies.

Adverse reactions
CNS: fever, headache, asthenia, malaise, dizziness, pain.
CV: *hypotension,* chest pain, **heart failure,** hypertension, fluid retention.
GI: nausea, vomiting, diarrhea, abdominal pain, taste perversion.
Musculoskeletal: *leg cramps,* bone and muscle pain.

Reactions may be *common,* uncommon, *life-threatening*, or COMMON AND LIFE-THREATENING.

Respiratory: dyspnea, pneumonia, cough.
Skin: pruritus.
Other: accidental injury, hypersensitivity reaction, *anaphylaxis, sepsis,* injection-site reaction.

Interactions

Drug-drug. *Oral iron preparations:* May reduce absorption of these compounds. Avoid use together.

Effects on lab test results

● May increase liver enzyme levels.

Pharmacokinetics

Absorption: Administered I.V.
Distribution: Mainly in blood and somewhat in extravascular fluid. A significant amount of iron is also distributed in the liver, spleen, and bone marrow.
Metabolism: Dissociated by the reticuloendothelial system into iron and sucrose.
Excretion: About 75% of sucrose and 5% of the iron component are eliminated by urinary excretion in 24 hours. *Half-life:* 6 hours.

Route	Onset	Peak	Duration
I.V.	Unknown	Unknown	Variable

Action

Chemical effect: Dissociated by the reticuloendothelial system into iron and sucrose. The released iron component eventually replenishes depleted body iron stores, resulting in significant increases in iron and ferritin levels and significant decreases in total iron binding capacity.
Therapeutic effect: Increases iron level.

Available forms

Injection: 20 mg/ml of elemental iron in 5-ml vial

NURSING PROCESS

Assessment
● Assess underlying condition before starting therapy, and reassess regularly.
● Monitor ferritin and hemoglobin levels, hematocrit, and transferrin saturation.
● Monitor patient for adverse reactions or hypersensitivity reactions to the drug.
● Assess patient's and family's knowledge of drug therapy.

Nursing diagnoses
● Acute pain related to adverse drug effects
● Ineffective health maintenance related to iron deficiency
● Deficient knowledge related to iron sucrose therapy

Planning and implementation
● Monitor patient for symptoms of overdose or too-rapid infusion, which include hypotension, headache, nausea, dizziness, joint aches, paresthesia, abdominal and muscle pain, edema, and CV collapse.
● Observe patient for rare but fatal hypersensitivity reactions characterized by anaphylaxis, loss of consciousness, collapse, hypotension, dyspnea, or seizures.
● Withhold dose in patient with evidence of iron overload.
Patient teaching
● Instruct patient to notify prescriber if symptoms of overdose occur, such as headache, nausea, dizziness, joint aches, paresthesia, or abdominal and muscle pain.
● Warn patient not to take OTC vitamins containing iron.

Evaluation
● Patient does not experience pain.
● Patient's hemoglobin level and hematocrit are normal.
● Patient and family state understanding of iron sucrose therapy.

isoniazid (isonicotinic acid hydride INH)
(igh-soh-NIGH-uh-sid)
Isotamine ◆, Laniazid, Nydrazid, PMS Isoniazid ◆

Pharmacologic class: isonicotinic acid hydrazine
Therapeutic class: antituberculotic
Pregnancy risk category: C

Indications and dosages

▶ **Actively growing tubercle bacilli with other antituberculotics.** *Adults and children age 15 and older:* 5 mg/kg P.O. or I.M. daily in single dose, maximum 300 mg P.O. or I.M.

daily, continued for 6 months to 2 years. Or 15 mg/kg (maximum dose 900 mg/daily) two to three times weekly.
Infants and children: 10 to 15 mg/kg P.O. or I.M. daily in single dose, maximum 300 mg P.O. or I.M. daily, continued for 18 months to 2 years. Or 20 to 40 mg/kg (maximum dose 900 mg/daily) two to three times weekly.
▶ **Prevention of tubercle bacilli in those closely exposed to tuberculosis or those with positive skin tests whose chest X-rays and bacteriologic studies are consistent with non-progressive tuberculosis.** *Adults:* 300 mg P.O. daily in single dose, for 6 months to 1 year.
Infants and children: 10 mg/kg P.O. daily in single dose. Maximum, 300 mg P.O. daily for 1 year.

Contraindications and cautions

• Contraindicated in patients with acute hepatic disease or isoniazid-related liver damage.
• Use cautiously in patients with chronic non–isoniazid-related liver disease, seizure disorders (especially in those taking phenytoin), severe renal impairment, or chronic alcoholism.
⚘ **Lifespan:** In pregnant women, use cautiously. In breast-feeding women, small amounts of drug appear in breast milk but aren't sufficient to cause harm or therapeutic benefit to the infant. In elderly patients, use cautiously.

Adverse reactions

CNS: *peripheral neuropathy,* paresthesias, psychosis, *seizures.*
GI: nausea, vomiting, epigastric distress, constipation, dry mouth.
Hematologic: *agranulocytosis,* hemolytic anemia, *aplastic anemia,* eosinophilia, *leukopenia, neutropenia, thrombocytopenia, methemoglobinemia,* pyridoxine-responsive hypochromic anemia.
Hepatic: *hepatitis.*
Metabolic: hyperglycemia, *metabolic acidosis.*
Other: rheumatic syndrome and lupuslike syndrome, hypersensitivity reactions, irritation at I.M. injection site.

Interactions

Drug-drug. *Acetaminophen:* May increase hepatotoxic effects of acetaminophen. Don't give together.

Antacids and laxatives containing aluminum: May decrease rate and amount of isoniazid absorbed. Give isoniazid at least 1 hour before antacid or laxative.
Carbamazepine: May increase risk of isoniazid hepatotoxicity. Use together cautiously.
Carbamazepine, phenytoin: May increase levels of these anticonvulsants. Monitor patient closely.
Corticosteroids: May decrease therapeutic effect of isoniazid. Monitor patient's need for larger isoniazid dose.
Cyclosporine: May increase adverse CNS effects of cyclosporine. Monitor patient closely.
Disulfiram: May cause neurologic symptoms, including changes in behavior and coordination. Avoid use together.
Ketoconazole: May decrease ketoconazole levels. Monitor patient closely.
Oral anticoagulants: May increase anticoagulation. Monitor patient for signs of bleeding.
Rifampin: May increase risk of hepatotoxicity. Monitor patient closely.
Theophylline: May increase theophylline level. Monitor level closely, and adjust theophylline dosage.
Drug-food. *Foods containing tyramine:* May cause hypertensive crisis. Tell patients to avoid such foods altogether.
Drug-lifestyle. *Alcohol use:* May increase risk of isoniazid-related hepatitis. Discourage use together.

Effects on lab test results

• May increase transaminase, glucose, and bilirubin levels. May decrease calcium, phosphate, and hemoglobin levels and hematocrit.
• May increase eosinophil count. May decrease WBC, granulocyte, neutrophil, and platelet counts.

Pharmacokinetics

Absorption: Complete and rapid after P.O. administration. Also absorbed readily after I.M. injection.
Distribution: Wide.
Metabolism: Primarily in liver. Rate of metabolism varies individually; fast acetylators metabolize drug five times as rapidly as others. About 50% of blacks and whites are slow acetylators, whereas more than 80% of Chinese, Japanese, and Eskimos are fast acetylators.

Excretion: Primarily in urine; some in saliva, sputum, feces, and breast milk. *Half-life:* 1 to 4 hours.

Route	Onset	Peak	Duration
P.O., I.M.	Unknown	1–2 hr	Unknown

Action

Chemical effect: May inhibit cell wall biosynthesis by interfering with lipid and DNA synthesis.
Therapeutic effect: Kills susceptible bacteria, such as *Mycobacterium tuberculosis, M. bovis,* and some strains of *M. kansasii.*

Available forms

Injection: 100 mg/ml
Oral solution: 50 mg/5 ml
Tablets: 100 mg, 300 mg

NURSING PROCESS

✎ Assessment
• Assess patient's infection before starting therapy by physical examination and culture and sensitivity testing.
• Monitor patient for improvement, and evaluate culture and sensitivity tests.
• Be alert for adverse reactions and drug interactions.
• Monitor hepatic function closely for changes.
• Monitor patient for paresthesia of hands and feet, which usually precedes peripheral neuropathy, especially in patients who are malnourished, alcoholic, diabetic, or slow acetylators.
• Assess patient's and family's knowledge of drug therapy.

✦ Nursing diagnoses
• Infection related to presence of susceptible bacteria
• Disturbed sensory perception (tactile) related to drug-induced peripheral neuropathy
• Deficient knowledge related to drug therapy

▷ Planning and implementation
• Give oral form of drug 1 hour before or 2 hours after meals to avoid decreased absorption.
• Switch from I.M. to P.O. form as soon as possible.

⊛ ALERT: Always give isoniazid with other antituberculotics to prevent development of resistant organisms.
• Give pyridoxine to prevent peripheral neuropathy, especially in malnourished patients.
Patient teaching
• Tell patient to take drug as prescribed; warn against stopping drug without prescriber's consent.
• Advise patient to take with food if GI irritation occurs.
• Instruct patient not to drink alcohol during therapy.
• Instruct patient to avoid certain foods (fish, such as skip jack and tuna, and foods containing tyramine, such as aged cheese, beer, and chocolate) because drug acts like an MAO inhibitor.
• Tell patient to notify prescriber immediately if symptoms of liver impairment occur (loss of appetite, fatigue, malaise, jaundice, dark urine).
• Urge patient to comply with treatment, which may last for months or years.

✓ Evaluation
• Patient is free from infection.
• Patient maintains normal peripheral nervous system function.
• Patient and family state understanding of drug therapy.

isoproterenol (isoprenaline)
(igh-soh-proh-TEER-uh-nol)
Isuprel

isoproterenol hydrochloride

isoproterenol sulfate
Medihaler-Iso

Pharmacologic class: adrenergic
Therapeutic class: bronchodilator, cardiac stimulant
Pregnancy risk category: C

Indications and dosages

▶ **Bronchospasm.** *Adults and children:* For acute dyspneic episodes, one inhalation of sulfate form initially. Repeat, if needed, after 2 to 5 minutes. Maintenance dosage is one to two inhalations four to six times daily. Repeat once more 10 minutes after second dose. Give no more than three doses for each attack.

▶**Bronchospasm in COPD.** Give by intermittent positive pressure breathing or for nebulization by compressed air or oxygen.

Adults: 2 ml of 0.125% or 2.5 ml of 0.1% solution (prepared by diluting 0.5 ml of 0.5% solution to 2 or 2.5 ml or by diluting 0.25 ml of 1% solution to 2 or 2.5 ml with water or half-normal or normal saline solution) up to five times daily.

Children: 2 ml of 0.125% solution or 2.5 ml of 0.1% solution up to five times daily.

▶**Heart block and ventricular arrhythmias.** *Adults:* Initially, 0.02 to 0.06 mg hydrochloride I.V. Subsequent doses 0.01 to 0.2 mg I.V. or 5 mcg/minute I.V. Or 0.2 mg I.M. initially; then 0.02 to 1 mg, p.r.n.

Children: Give half of initial adult dose of hydrochloride.

▶**Shock.** *Adults and children:* 0.5 to 5 mcg/minute hydrochloride by continuous I.V. infusion. Usual concentration is 1 mg (5 ml) in 500 ml D₅W. Infusion rate adjusted according to heart rate, central venous pressure, blood pressure, and urine flow.

▶**Postoperative cardiac patients with bradycardia‡.** *Children:* I.V. infusion of 0.029 mcg/kg/minute.

▶**As an aid in diagnosing the cause of mitral regurgitation‡.** *Adults:* 4 mcg/minute I.V. infusion.

▶**As an aid in diagnosing coronary artery disease or lesions‡.** *Adults:* 1 to 3 mcg/minute I.V. infusion.

▼ I.V. administration

• If injection solution is discolored or contains precipitate, don't use.

• Give drug by direct injection or I.V. infusion. For infusion, drug may be diluted with most common I.V. solutions.

• If heart rate exceeds 110 beats/minute with I.V. infusion, notify prescriber. Doses sufficient to increase heart rate to more than 130 beats/minute may induce ventricular arrhythmias.

• When giving I.V. isoproterenol to treat shock, closely monitor blood pressure, central venous pressure, ECG, arterial blood gas measurements, and urine output. Carefully adjust infusion rate according to these measurements. Use continuous infusion pump to regulate flow rate.

⊗ Incompatibilities

Alkalies, aminophylline, furosemide, metals, sodium bicarbonate.

Contraindications and cautions

• Contraindicated in patients with tachycardia caused by digitalis intoxication, in those with arrhythmias (other than those that may respond to treatment with isoproterenol), and in those with angina pectoris.

• Use cautiously in patients with renal or CV disease, coronary insufficiency, diabetes, hyperthyroidism, or history of sensitivity to sympathomimetic amines.

🐾 **Lifespan:** In pregnant and breast-feeding women, use cautiously. In children and elderly patients, use cautiously.

Adverse reactions

CNS: *headache,* mild tremor, weakness, dizziness, nervousness, insomnia, ***Adams-Stokes syndrome.***

CV: palpitations, tachycardia, angina, flushing of face, ***cardiac arrest,*** labile blood pressure, ***arrhythmias.***

GI: nausea, vomiting.

Metabolic: hyperglycemia.

Respiratory: ***bronchospasm.***

Skin: diaphoresis.

Interactions

Drug-drug. *Epinephrine, other sympathomimetics:* Increases risk of arrhythmias. Avoid use together.

Propranolol, other beta blockers: Blocks bronchodilating effect of isoproterenol. If used together, monitor patient carefully.

Effects on lab test results

• May increase glucose level.

Pharmacokinetics

Absorption: Rapid after P.O. inhalation.
Distribution: Wide.
Metabolism: By conjugation in GI tract and by enzymatic reduction in liver, lungs, and other tissues.
Excretion: Primarily in urine. *Half-life:* Unknown.

Route	Onset	Peak	Duration
I.V.	Immediate	Unknown	< 1 hr
Inhalation	2–5 min	Unknown	½–2 hr

Reactions may be *common,* uncommon, *life-threatening,* or COMMON AND LIFE-THREATENING.

Action

Chemical effect: Relaxes bronchial smooth muscle by acting on beta$_2$-adrenergic receptors. As cardiac stimulant, acts on beta$_1$-adrenergic receptors in heart.
Therapeutic effect: Relieves bronchospasms and heart block and restores normal sinus rhythm after ventricular arrhythmia.

Available forms

isoproterenol
Nebulizer inhaler: 0.25%, 0.5%, 1%
isoproterenol hydrochloride
Aerosol inhaler: 131 mcg/metered spray
Injection: 20 mcg/ml, 200 mcg/ml
Solution for inhalation: 0.5%, 1%
isoproterenol sulfate
Aerosol inhaler: 80 mcg/metered spray

NURSING PROCESS

Assessment
• Assess patient's underlying condition before starting therapy.
• Monitor cardiopulmonary status frequently.
• Be alert for adverse reactions and drug interactions.
• This drug may aggravate ventilation and perfusion abnormalities. Even when ease of breathing is improved, arterial oxygen tension may fall paradoxically.
• Assess patient's and family's knowledge of drug therapy.

Nursing diagnoses
• Ineffective health maintenance related to underlying condition
• Risk for injury related to drug-induced adverse reactions
• Deficient knowledge related to drug therapy

Planning and implementation
• Drug doesn't treat blood or fluid volume deficit. Correct volume deficit before giving vasopressors.
• If drug is given by inhalation with oxygen, make sure oxygen concentration won't suppress respiratory drive.
• Follow same instructions for metered powder nebulizer, although deep inhalation isn't needed.
• If adverse reactions occur, notify prescriber; adjust dosage or stop drug if needed.

• If precordial distress or angina occurs, stop drug immediately.
ALERT: Don't confuse Isuprel with Ismelin or Isordil.

Patient teaching
• Give patient the following instructions for using metered-dose inhaler: Clear nasal passages and throat. Breathe out, expelling as much air from lungs as possible. Place mouthpiece well into mouth, and inhale deeply as you release dose from inhaler. Hold breath for several seconds, remove mouthpiece, and exhale slowly.
• Tell patient to wait at least 2 minutes before repeating when using more than one inhalation.
• If patient also uses a corticosteroid inhaler, tell him to use bronchodilator first, and then wait about 5 minutes before using corticosteroid. This process allows bronchodilator to open air passages for maximum effectiveness of the corticosteroid.
• Warn patient using oral inhalant that this drug may turn sputum and saliva pink.
• Tell patient to stop drug and notify prescriber about chest tightness or dyspnea.
• Warn patient against overuse of drug. Tell him that tolerance can develop.
• Tell patient to reduce caffeine intake during therapy.

Evaluation
• Patient exhibits improved health.
• Patient doesn't experience injury from adverse reactions.
• Patient and family state understanding of drug therapy.

isosorbide dinitrate
(igh-soh-SOR-bighd digh-NIGH-trayt)
Apo-ISDN ♦, Cedocard SR ♦, Coronex ♦, Dilatrate-SR, Isochron, Isordil, Isordil Titradose, Isotrate, Sorbitrate

isosorbide mononitrate
IMDUR, ISMO, Isotrate ER, Monoket

Pharmacologic class: nitrate
Therapeutic class: antianginal, vasodilator
Pregnancy risk category: C

Indications and dosages

▶ **Acute angina, prophylaxis in situations likely to cause angina.** *Adults:* 2.5 to 10 mg isosorbide dinitrate S.L. for prompt relief of angina pain, repeated q 2 to 3 hours during acute phase, or q 4 to 6 hours for prophylaxis. Or 2.5 to 10 mg chewable tablets, p.r.n., for acute attack or q 2 to 3 hours for prophylaxis but only after initial test dose of 5 mg to determine risk of severe hypotension. Or, initially, 5 to 20 mg P.O.; then maintain on 10 to 40 mg P.O. q 6 hours. Or, initially, 40 mg extended-release tablets P.O.; then maintain on 40 to 80 mg P.O. q 8 to 12 hours. Use isosorbide mononitrate for prophylaxis only: 20 mg P.O. b.i.d. with doses 7 hours apart and first dose on awakening. For sustained-release form, 30 to 60 mg P.O. once daily on arising. After several days, dosage may be increased to 120 mg once daily; rarely, 240 mg may be needed.

▶ **Adjunctive treatment of heart failure‡.** *Adults:* 80 mg isosorbide dinitrate P.O. daily with hydralazine. Maximum dose is 160 mg isosorbide dinitrate and 300 mg hydralazine.

▶ **Diffuse esophageal spasm without gastroesophageal reflux‡.** *Adults:* 10 to 30 mg isosorbide dinitrate P.O. q.i.d.

Contraindications and cautions

• Contraindicated in patients hypersensitive to nitrates, in those with idiosyncratic reactions to nitrates, and in those with severe hypotension, shock, or acute MI with low left ventricular filling pressure.

• Use cautiously in patients with blood volume depletion (such as that resulting from diuretic therapy) or mild hypotension.

⚱ **Lifespan:** In pregnant women, use cautiously. In breast-feeding women, use cautiously because it's unknown if drug appears in breast milk. In children, safety and effectiveness haven't been established.

Adverse reactions

CNS: *headache,* dizziness, weakness.
CV: orthostatic hypotension, tachycardia, palpitations, ankle edema, fainting, *flushing.*
GI: nausea, vomiting.
Skin: cutaneous vasodilation.
Other: hypersensitivity reactions, S.L. burning.

Interactions

Drug-drug. *Antihypertensives:* Possibly increased hypotensive effects. Monitor patient closely during initial therapy.
Sildenafil, tadalafil, vardenafil: May increase hypotensive effects. Avoid use together.
Drug-lifestyle. *Alcohol use:* May increase hypotension. Discourage use together.

Effects on lab test results

None reported.

Pharmacokinetics

Absorption: Dinitrate is well absorbed from GI tract but undergoes first-pass metabolism, resulting in bioavailability of about 50% (depending on dosage form used). Mononitrate is also absorbed well, with almost 100% bioavailability.
Distribution: Distributed widely throughout body.
Metabolism: Metabolized in liver to active metabolites.
Excretion: Excreted in urine. *Half-life:* Dinitrate P.O., 5 to 6 hours; S.L., 2 hours; mononitrate, about 5 hours.

Route	Onset	Peak	Duration
P.O.	2–60 min	2–60 min	1–12 hr
S.L.	2–5 min	2–5 min	1–2 hr

Action

Chemical effect: May reduce cardiac oxygen demand by decreasing left ventricular end diastolic pressure (preload) and, to a lesser extent, systemic vascular resistance (afterload). May increase blood flow through collateral coronary vessels.
Therapeutic effect: Relieves angina.

Available forms

isosorbide dinitrate
Capsules (extended-release): 40 mg
Tablets: 5 mg, 10 mg, 20 mg, 30 mg, 40 mg
Tablets (chewable): 5 mg, 10 mg
Tablets (S.L.): 2.5 mg, 5 mg, 10 mg
Tablets (sustained-release): 40 mg
isosorbide mononitrate
Tablets: 10 mg, 20 mg
Tablets (extended-release): 30 mg, 60 mg, 120 mg

⚖ Assessment
- Assess patient's angina before starting therapy and regularly thereafter.
- Monitor blood pressure, heart rate and rhythm, and intensity and duration of drug response.
- Be alert for adverse reactions and drug interactions.
- Assess patient's and family's knowledge of drug therapy.

⊕ Nursing diagnoses
- Acute pain related to angina
- Risk for injury related to drug-induced adverse reactions
- Deficient knowledge related to drug therapy

❯ Planning and implementation
- To prevent development of tolerance, don't give drug during an 8- to 12-hour period daily. The dosage regimen for isosorbide mononitrate (one tablet on awakening with second dose in 7 hours, or one extended-release tablet daily) is intended to offer a nitrate-free period during the day to minimize nitrate tolerance.
- Give drug on empty stomach, either 30 minutes before or 1 to 2 hours after meals, and have patient swallow tablets whole. Have patient chew chewable tablets thoroughly before swallowing.
- Give S.L. form of drug at first sign of angina. Have patient wet tablet with saliva, place it under his tongue until completely absorbed, and sit down and rest. Dose may be repeated every 10 to 15 minutes for maximum of three doses.
- Ⓢ **ALERT:** Don't stop therapy abruptly because coronary vasospasm may occur.
- If patient's pain doesn't subside, notify prescriber immediately.
- Ⓢ **ALERT:** Don't confuse Isordil with Isuprel or Inderal.
- Ⓢ **ALERT:** Don't confuse Coronex (isosorbide dinitrate) with Coronex (the herbal supplement for male virility and vitality).

Patient teaching
- Advise patient to take drug regularly, as prescribed, and to keep it accessible at all times.
- Ⓢ **ALERT:** Advise patient that abrupt discontinuation causes coronary vasospasm.
- Tell patient to take S.L. tablet at first sign of attack. Explain that tablet should be wet with saliva and placed under tongue until completely absorbed, and that patient should sit down and rest

until pain subsides. Tell patient that dose may be repeated every 10 to 15 minutes for maximum of three doses. If drug doesn't provide relief, tell him to get medical help promptly.
- Tell patient who complains of tingling sensation with drug placed S.L. to try holding tablet in buccal pouch.
- Ⓢ **ALERT:** Warn patient not to confuse S.L. form with P.O. form.
- Instruct patient taking oral form to take tablet on empty stomach, either 30 minutes before or 1 to 2 hours after meals, and to swallow tablet whole or chew chewable tablet thoroughly before swallowing.
- Tell patient to minimize orthostatic hypotension by changing to upright position slowly. Tell him to go up and down stairs carefully and to lie down at first sign of dizziness.
- Instruct patient to avoid alcohol consumption during therapy.
- Tell patient to store drug in cool place, in tightly closed container, away from light.

☑ Evaluation
- Patient is free from pain.
- Patient doesn't experience injury from adverse reactions.
- Patient and family state understanding of drug therapy.

isotretinoin
(igh-soh-TREH-tih-noyn)
Accutane, Accutane Roche ♦ , Claravis, Roaccutane ◇ , Sotret

Pharmacologic class: retinoic acid derivative
Therapeutic class: antiacne drug
Pregnancy risk category: X

Indications and dosages

▶ **Severe recalcitrant nodular acne unresponsive to conventional therapy.** *Adults and children ages 12 to 17:* 0.5 to 1 mg/kg P.O. daily in two divided doses for 15 to 20 weeks. Maximum daily dosage, 2 mg/kg.
▶ **Keratinization disorders resistant to conventional therapy, prevention of skin cancer‡.** *Adults:* Dosage varies with specific disease and severity of the disorder. Dosages up to 2 to 4 mg/kg P.O. daily have been used. Consult literature for specific recommendations.

▶ **Squamous cell cancer of the head and neck‡.** *Adults:* 50 to 100 mg/m² P.O.

Contraindications and cautions

• Contraindicated in patients hypersensitive to parabens, which are used as preservatives.
• Use cautiously in patients with genetic predisposition or history of osteoporosis, osteomalacia, or other disorders of bone metabolism. Also use cautiously in patients with a history of mental illness or family history of psychiatric disorders, asthma, liver disease, diabetes, heart disease, osteoporosis, weak bones, or anorexia nervosa.
⚖ **Lifespan:** In women of childbearing age, drug is contraindicated unless patient has had negative serum pregnancy test within 2 weeks of beginning therapy, will begin drug therapy on second or third day of next menstrual period, and will comply with stringent contraceptive measures for 1 month before therapy, during therapy, and at least 1 month after therapy. In pregnant women, drug is contraindicated. In breast-feeding women, use cautiously. In children younger than age 12, safety and effectiveness haven't been established. In children ages 12 to 17, use cautiously.

Adverse reactions

CNS: *headache, fatigue,* psychosis, *suicide,* depression, psychosis, *aggressive and violent behavior,* emotional instability, pseudotumor cerebri (benign intracranial hypertension), *seizure, stroke.*
CV: hypertriglyceridemia.
EENT: *conjunctivitis,* corneal deposits, dry eyes, visual disturbances, hearing impairment, decreased night vision, intolerance to contact lenses.
GI: nonspecific GI symptoms, gum bleeding and inflammation, nausea, vomiting, *acute pancreatitis,* inflammatory bowel disease.
Hepatic: *hepatitis,* increased liver enzymes.
Hematologic: anemia.
Metabolic: hyperglycemia.
Musculoskeletal: skeletal hyperostosis, calcification of tendons and ligaments, premature epiphyseal closure, decreases in bone mineral density, musculoskeletal symptoms, back pain, *arthralgia,* arthritis, tendinitis, other types of bone abnormalities, *rhabdomyolysis.*
Skin: *cheilosis, rash, dry skin,* peeling of palms and toes, skin infection, thinning of hair, photosensitivity.

Interactions

Drug-drug. *Corticosteroids:* May increase risk of osteoporosis. Use together cautiously.
Medicated soaps and cleansers, medicated cover-ups, topical resorcinol peeling agents (benzoyl peroxide), and preparations containing alcohol: Cumulative drying effect. Use cautiously.
Microdosed progesterone birth control pills that don't contain estrogen: May decrease effectiveness of birth control. Advise patient to use alternative contraceptive methods.
Phenytoin: May increase risk of osteomalacia. Use together cautiously.
Tetracyclines: May increase the potential for the development of pseudotumor cerebri. Avoid use together.
Vitamin A products: May have additive toxic effect. Avoid use together.
Drug-food. *Any food:* May enhance absorption of drug. Have patient take drug with food.
Drug-lifestyle. *Alcohol use:* May increase risk of hypertriglyceridemia. Discourage use together.
Sun exposure: May increase photosensitivity reactions. Advise patient to use sunscreen and wear protective clothing.

Effects on lab test results

• May increase CK, ALT, AST, alkaline phosphatase, glucose, and triglyceride levels. May decrease hemoglobin level and hematocrit.
• May increase platelet count.

Pharmacokinetics

Absorption: Rapid.
Distribution: Wide; 99.9% protein-bound, primarily to albumin.
Metabolism: Metabolized in liver and possibly in gut wall.
Excretion: Unknown. *Half-life:* 30 minutes to 39 hours.

Route	Onset	Peak	Duration
P.O.	Unknown	3 hr	Unknown

Action

Chemical effect: May normalize keratinization, reversibly decrease size of sebaceous glands, and alter composition of sebum to less viscous form that is less likely to plug follicles.
Therapeutic effect: Improves skin integrity.

Reactions may be *common,* uncommon, *life-threatening,* or COMMON AND LIFE-THREATENING.

Available forms

Capsules: 10 mg, 20 mg, 30 mg, 40 mg

NURSING PROCESS

Assessment

- Assess patient's skin before starting therapy and regularly thereafter.
- Obtain baseline lipid studies, liver function test results, and pregnancy test before therapy. Monitor these values at regular intervals until response to drug is established (usually about 4 weeks).
- Monitor glucose and CK levels in patients who engage in vigorous physical activity.
- Be alert for adverse reactions and drug interactions.
- Osteoporosis, osteopenia, bone fractures, and delayed healing of bone fractures have been seen in patients taking isotretinoin. While a causal relationship hasn't been established, an effect can't be ruled out. Long-term effects haven't been studied. It's important not to exceed the recommended dose or duration.
- Most adverse reactions appear to be dose-related, occurring at dosages greater than 1 mg/kg daily. They're usually reversible when therapy is stopped or dosage reduced.
- To minimize the risk of fetal exposure, drug is only available through restricted distribution program approved by the FDA called iPLEDGE.
- Actively monitor mood and behavioral changes because of risk of significant psychological changes including suicidal thoughts and behavior.
- Assess patient's and family's knowledge of drug therapy.

Nursing diagnoses

- Impaired skin integrity related to underlying skin condition
- Impaired tissue integrity related to adverse reactions
- Deficient knowledge related to drug therapy

Planning and implementation

- Start second course of therapy at least 8 weeks after completion of first course because improvement may continue after stopping drug.
- Any suspected fetal exposure to drug must be immediately reported to the FDA's MedWatch program at 1-800-FDA-1088 and the iPLEDGE pregnancy registry at 1-866-495-0654 or www.ipledgeprogram.com.
- Give drug with meals or shortly thereafter to enhance absorption.

ALERT: Screen patient with headache, nausea and vomiting, or visual disturbances for papilledema. Signs and symptoms of pseudotumor cerebri require an immediate stop to therapy and prompt neurologic intervention.

Patient teaching

- Advise patient to take drug with milk, meals, or shortly after meals to ensure adequate absorption.
- Tell patient to immediately report visual disturbances and bone, muscle, or joint pain.
- Warn patient that contact lenses may feel uncomfortable during therapy.
- Warn patient against using abrasives, medicated soaps and cleansers, acne preparations containing peeling agents, and topical alcohol preparations (including cosmetics, after-shave, cologne) because these agents cause cumulative irritation or excessive drying of skin.
- Instruct patient not to drink alcohol during therapy.
- Inform patient to report mood changes, such as increased hostility or depression, and suicidal thinking immediately; these may be drug related.
- Tell patient to avoid prolonged exposure to sunlight, to use sunblock, and to wear protective clothing.

ALERT: Advise patient not to donate blood during or for 30 days after therapy; severe fetal abnormalities may occur if a pregnant woman receives blood containing isotretinoin.

- Advise women of childbearing age to use two reliable forms of contraception simultaneously within 1 month of treatment, during treatment and for 1 month after treatment as prescribed under the iPLEDGE program, and to report suspected pregnancy immediately.

Evaluation

- Patient has improved skin condition.
- Patient is free from conjunctivitis, corneal deposits, and dry eyes.
- Patient and family state understanding of drug therapy.

itraconazole
(ih-truh-KAHN-uh-zohl)
Sporanox

Pharmacologic class: synthetic triazole
Therapeutic class: antifungal
Pregnancy risk category: C

Indications and dosages

▶ **Pulmonary and extrapulmonary blasto-
mycosis, histoplasmosis.** *Adults:* 200 mg P.O.
(capsules) daily. Dosage may be increased as
needed and tolerated in 100-mg increments to
maximum of 400 mg daily. Divide doses
larger than 200 mg daily into two doses. Continue treatment for at least 3 months. In life-
threatening illness, loading dose of 200 mg t.i.d.
is given for 3 days. Or give 200 mg by I.V. infusion over 1 hour twice daily for four doses; then
200 mg I.V. once daily.
▶ **Aspergillosis.** *Adults:* 200 to 400 mg P.O.
(capsules) daily. Or give 200 mg by I.V. infusion over 1 hour twice daily for four doses; then
decrease to 200 mg I.V. once daily for up to
14 days.
▶ **Onychomycosis for toenails with or without fingernail involvement.** *Adults:* 200 mg
P.O. (capsules) once daily for 12 weeks.
▶ **Onychomycosis for fingernails.** *Adults:*
Two treatment phases, each consisting of
200 mg P.O. (capsules) b.i.d. for 1 week. Phases
are separated by a 3-week period without drug.
▶ **Esophageal candidiasis.** *Adults:* 100 to
200 mg P.O. (oral solution) swished in mouth
vigorously and swallowed daily for a minimum
of 3 weeks.
▶ **Oropharyngeal candidiasis.** *Adults:* 200 mg
P.O. (oral solution) swished in mouth vigorously and swallowed daily for 1 to 2 weeks. For patients unresponsive to fluconazole tablets, give
100 mg swished in mouth vigorously and swallowed twice daily for 2 to 4 weeks.

▼ I.V. administration

● Injection form should not be used in patients
with creatinine clearance below 30 ml/minute.
● Distributed in a kit that includes a 50-ml bag
of normal saline solution for injection and filtered infusion set.
● Do not administer by I.V. bolus injection.

● Infuse over 60 minutes, using an infusion set
with a filter.
● Flush I.V. line with 15 to 20 ml of normal
saline solution after each infusion.
⊗ **Incompatibilities**
● Dextrose solution, lactated Ringer's solution.

Contraindications and cautions

● Contraindicated in patients hypersensitive to
the drug or any of its components. Also contraindicated in patients with ventricular dysfunction, heart failure, or a history of heart failure.
Also contraindicated in patients receiving cisapride, oral midazolam, triazolam, pimozide,
dofetilide, or quinidine; HMG-CoA reductase
inhibitors metabolized by CYP 3A4 (lovastatin,
simvastatin); ergot alkaloids (dihydroergotamine, ergonovine, methylergonovine).
● Use cautiously in patients with hypochlorhydria (they may not absorb drug as readily as
patients with normal gastric acidity), in HIV-
infected patients (hypochlorhydria can accompany HIV infection), and in those with liver disease.
✦ **Lifespan:** In pregnant women, use cautiously. In breast-feeding women, drug is contraindicated because it appears in breast milk. In children, safety and effectiveness haven't been
established.

Adverse reactions

CNS: malaise, fatigue, *headache,* dizziness,
somnolence, fever, asthenia, pain, tremor, abnormal dreaming, anxiety, depression.
CV: edema, hypertension, orthostatic hypoten-
sion, *heart failure,* hypertriglyceridemia.
EENT: rhinitis, sinusitis, pharyngitis.
GI: *nausea,* vomiting, diarrhea, abdominal pain,
anorexia, dyspepsia, flatulence, increased ap-
petite, constipation, gastritis, gastroenteritis, ul-
cerative stomatitis, gingivitis.
GU: albuminuria, impotence, cystitis, UTI.
Hematologic: *neutropenia.*
Hepatic: *impaired hepatic function, hepato-
toxicity, liver failure.*
Metabolic: hypokalemia.
Musculoskeletal: myalgia.
Respiratory: upper respiratory tract infection,
pulmonary edema.
Skin: rash, pruritus.
Other: decreased libido, injury, herpes zoster,
hypersensitivity reactions, urticaria, *angio-
edema, Stevens-Johnson syndrome.*

Reactions may be *common,* uncommon, *life-threatening,* or COMMON AND LIFE-THREATENING.

Interactions

Drug-drug. *Alprazolam, chlordiazepoxide, clonazepam, clorazepate, diazepam, estazolam, flurazepam, midazolam, quazepam, triazolam:* May increase and prolong levels of these drugs, CNS depression, and psychomotor impairment. Don't use together.

Antacids, H$_2$-receptor antagonists, phenytoin, rifampin: May decrease itraconazole level. Avoid use together.

Antineoplastics (busulfan, docetaxel, vinca alkaloids): May inhibit metabolism of these drugs, resulting in toxicity. Avoid use together.

Aripiprazole: May increase levels of this drug. Decrease aripiprazole dose by 50%.

Atorvastatin, fluvastatin, lovastatin, pravastatin, simvastatin: May increase levels and adverse effects of these HMG-CoA reductase inhibitors. Don't use together.

Buspirone, carbamazepine, corticosteroids, cyclosporine, digoxin: May increase levels of these drugs. Monitor level closely.

Calcium channel blockers: May increase negative inotropic effect, causing edema. Use together with caution, and adjust dosages as necessary.

Cisapride, dofetilide, pimozide, quinidine: May increase levels of these drugs by CYP 3A4 metabolism, causing serious CV events, including torsades de pointes, prolonged QT interval, ventricular tachycardia, cardiac arrest, or sudden death. Use together is contraindicated.

Didanosine: May decrease therapeutic effect of itraconazole. Give itraconazole at least 2 hours before didanosine.

Isoniazid: May decrease itraconazole level. Monitor patient closely.

Macrolide antibiotics (clarithromycin, erythromycin): May increase concentrations of itraconazole. Adjust dosage accordingly.

Oral anticoagulants: May enhance anticoagulant effects. Monitor PT and INR closely.

Oral antidiabetics: May cause hypoglycemia. Monitor glucose level.

Protease inhibitors: May increase concentrations of protease inhibitors, resulting in toxicity. Use together with caution.

Rifamycin, rifabutin, rifampin: May reduce the effectiveness of itraconazole. Avoid use together.

Drug-food. *Cola:* May increase drug level and adverse effects. Advise patient to take drug with water.

Grapefruit: May delay absorption of drug. Advise patient to avoid grapefruit products.

Orange juice: May decrease level and therapeutic effects of drug. Advise patient to avoid taking drug with orange juice.

Effects on lab test results

• May increase alkaline phosphatase, ALT, AST, bilirubin, and GGT levels. May decrease potassium level.

Pharmacokinetics

Absorption: Bioavailability is maximal when oral solution is taken without food but maximal for capsules when taken with a full meal.
Distribution: Protein binding is 99.8%. Extensively distributed in tissues susceptible to infection.
Metabolism: Extensively metabolized by liver.
Excretion: In feces and urine. *Half-life:* 1 to 8¼ hours.

Route	Onset	Peak	Duration
P.O.			
fasting	Unknown	2 hr	Unknown
nonfasting	Unknown	5 hr	Unknown
I.V.	Unknown	Unknown	Unknown

Action

Chemical effect: Interferes with fungal cell wall synthesis by inhibiting formation of ergosterol and increasing cell wall permeability.
Therapeutic effect: Hinders fungi, including *Aspergillus* sp. and *Blastomyces dermatitidis.*

Available forms

Capsules: 100 mg
Injection: 10 mg/ml in a kit with 25-ml ampule, 50-ml bag of normal saline solution for injection, and a filtered infusion set
Oral solution: 10 mg/ml

NURSING PROCESS

Assessment
• Assess patient's infection before starting therapy and regularly thereafter.
• Before starting treatment, obtain nail specimens for potassium hydroxide preparation, fungal culture, or nail biopsy to confirm diagnosis of onychomycosis.
• Monitor liver and renal function test results.

• Be alert for adverse reactions and drug interactions.
• Assess patient's and family's knowledge of drug therapy.

⊕ **Nursing diagnoses**
• Infection related to presence of susceptible fungi
• Risk for deficient fluid volume related to adverse reactions
• Deficient knowledge related to drug therapy

▷ **Planning and implementation**
• Don't use in patient with baseline liver impairment, unless in a life-threatening situation where benefit exceeds risk. If signs of liver dysfunction occur, monitor liver function closely and stop therapy; don't restart unless the benefit exceeds the risk.
• Give capsules with food. Don't give oral solution with food.
⊛ **ALERT:** Oral solution and capsules aren't interchangeable.
• If signs and symptoms of heart failure occur, stop drug.
• Report signs and symptoms of liver disease and abnormal liver test results.
Patient teaching
• Teach patient to recognize and report signs and symptoms of liver disease (anorexia, dark urine, pale feces, unusual fatigue, or jaundice) and heart failure (weight gain more than 3-5 lbs in one week, ankle or leg swelling, new shortness of breath).
• Tell patient to take capsules with food to ensure maximum absorption.
• Instruct patient to swish oral solution vigorously in the mouth (10 ml at a time) for several seconds and then swallow. Oral solution should be taken without food, if possible.

☑ **Evaluation**
• Patient is free from infection.
• Patient maintains adequate fluid balance.
• Patient and family state understanding of drug therapy.

kaolin and pectin mixtures
(KAY-oh-lin and PEK-tin MIX-cherz)
K-Pek, Kaodene Non-Narcotic†, Kaolin w/Pectin†, Kao-Spen, Kapectolin†

Pharmacologic class: absorbent
Therapeutic class: antidiarrheal
Pregnancy risk category: NR

Indications and dosages

▶ **Mild, nonspecific diarrhea.** *Adults:* With regular-strength suspension, 60 to 120 ml P.O. after each bowel movement. With liquid, 45 ml P.O. one to three times daily or after each loose bowel movement.
Children ages 6 to 12: With regular-strength suspension, 30 to 60 ml P.O. after each bowel movement. With liquid, 22.5 ml P.O. one to three times daily or after each loose bowel movement.
Children ages 3 to 6: With regular-strength suspension, 15 to 30 ml P.O. after each bowel movement. With liquid, 15 ml P.O. one to three times daily or after each loose bowel movement.

Contraindications and cautions

• Don't use in patients with diarrhea linked to pseudomembranous colitis or caused by toxigenic bacteria.
• Use cautiously in patients with bleeding disorders or salicylate sensitivity.
❋ **Lifespan:** In pregnant women and in children, use cautiously.

Adverse reactions

GI: constipation; fecal impaction or ulceration (in infants and elderly or debilitated patients after long-term use).

Interactions

Drug-drug. *Oral drugs:* May decrease drug absorption. Separate administration times by at least 2 or 3 hours.

Effects on lab test results

None reported.

Reactions may be *common,* uncommon, *life-threatening,* or COMMON AND LIFE-THREATENING.

Pharmacokinetics

Absorption: None.
Distribution: None.
Metabolism: None.
Excretion: In stool. *Half-life:* Unknown.

Route	Onset	Peak	Duration
P.O.	Unknown	Unknown	Unknown

Action

Chemical effect: Decreases fluid content of feces, although total water loss seems to remain the same.
Therapeutic effect: Alleviates diarrhea.

Available forms

Liquid: 3.9 g kaolin and 194.4 mg pectin per 30 ml with bismuth subsalicylate (Kaodene)
Oral suspension: 5.2 g kaolin and 260 mg pectin per 30 ml† (Kao-Spen), 90 g kaolin and 2 g pectin per 30 ml† (Kapectolin†, Kaolin w/Pectin†)

NURSING PROCESS

☜ Assessment
• Assess patient's bowel patterns before and after therapy.
• Be alert for adverse GI reactions and drug interactions.
• Assess patient's and family's knowledge of drug therapy.

☷ Nursing diagnoses
• Diarrhea related to underlying condition
• Constipation related to long-term use of drug
• Deficient knowledge related to drug therapy

❱ Planning and implementation
• Read label carefully. Check dosage and strength.
• Give dose after each loose bowel movement.
• Don't use in place of specific therapy for underlying cause of diarrhea.
Patient teaching
• Warn patient not to use drug to replace therapy for underlying cause of the disease.
• Advise patient not to use drug for more than 2 days.

✓ Evaluation
• Patient reports decrease in or absence of loose stools.

• Patient doesn't have constipation.
• Patient and family state understanding of drug therapy.

ketoconazole
(kee-toh-KAHN-uh-zohl)
Nizoral, Nizoral A-D

Pharmacologic class: imidazole derivative
Therapeutic class: antifungal
Pregnancy risk category: C

Indications and dosages

▶ **Systemic candidiasis, chronic mucocandidiasis, oral thrush, candiduria, coccidioidomycosis, histoplasmosis, chromomycosis, paracoccidioidomycosis, severe cutaneous dermatophyte infection resistant to therapy with topical or oral griseofulvin.** *Adults and children who weigh more than 40 kg (88 lb):* Initially, 200 mg P.O. daily in single dose. Increase to 400 mg once daily in patients who don't respond to lower dosage.
Children age 2 and older: 3.3 to 6.6 mg/kg P.O. daily as single dose.
Note: Minimum treatment for candidiasis is 7 to 14 days; for other systemic fungal infections, 6 months; for resistant dermatophyte infections, at least 4 weeks.
▶ **Cutaneous candidiasis, tinea corporis, tinea pedis, tinea cruris, and tinea versicolor.** *Adults:* Apply cream once daily to cover the affected area and area immediately surrounding it. Treat candidal infection, tinea cruris, tinea corporis, and tinea versicolor for 2 weeks. Patients with tinea pedis require 6 weeks of treatment.
▶ **Seborrheic dermatitis.** *Adults:* Apply cream to affected area twice daily for 4 weeks or until resolved.
▶ **Dandruff.** *Adults:* Moisten hair and scalp with water. Gently massage shampoo over the entire scalp area for about 1 minute. Rinse thoroughly with warm water. Repeat, leaving shampoo on scalp for an additional 3 minutes. After second thorough rinse, dry hair with towel or warm air flow. Use shampoo twice weekly for 4 weeks with at least 3 days between each shampooing. Then use as needed.

K

Contraindications and cautions

• Contraindicated in patients hypersensitive to the drug or any of its components, and in those taking oral midazolam or triazolam.
• Use cautiously in patients with hepatic disease and in those taking other hepatotoxic drugs.
⚜ **Lifespan:** In pregnant women, use cautiously. Breast-feeding women should stop breast feeding or use another drug. Safety in children younger than age 2 hasn't been established.

Adverse reactions

CNS: headache, nervousness, dizziness, *suicidal tendencies.*
GI: *nausea, vomiting,* abdominal pain, diarrhea, constipation.
Hematologic: *thrombocytopenia.*
Hepatic: *hepatotoxicity.*
Skin: itching, stinging (cream).
Other: gynecomastia with tenderness.

Interactions

Drug-drug. *Alprazolam, chlordiazepoxide, clonazepam, clorazepate, diazepam, estazolam, flurazepam, midazolam, quazepam, triazolam:* May increase and prolong levels, CNS depression, and psychomotor impairment. Don't use together.
Antacids, anticholinergics, H₂-receptor antagonists, proton pump inhibitors, sucralfate: May decrease ketoconazole absorption. Wait at least 2 hours after ketoconazole dose before giving these drugs.
Atorvastatin, fluvastatin, lovastatin, pravastatin, simvastatin: May increase level and adverse effects of these HMG-CoA reductase inhibitors. Avoid this combination. If they must be given together, reduce dose of HMG-CoA reductase inhibitor.
Corticosteroids: May increase corticosteroid bioavailability and may decrease clearance, possibly resulting in toxicity. Monitor patient closely.
Cyclosporine, methylprednisolone, tacrolimus: May increase levels of these drugs. Adjust their dosages, and monitor their levels closely.
Didanosine: Therapeutic effects of ketoconazole may be decreased by the buffers in the chewable tablets
Isoniazid, rifampin: May increase ketoconazole metabolism. Monitor patient for decreased antifungal effect.

Oral anticoagulants: May enhance anticoagulant response may be enhanced. Monitor PT and INR.
Oral midazolam, triazolam: May elevate levels of these drugs, which may increase or prolong sedative or hypnotic effects. Avoid using together.

Effects on lab test results

• May increase lipid, alkaline phosphatase, ALT, and AST levels. May decrease hemoglobin level and hematocrit.
• May decrease platelet and WBC counts.

Pharmacokinetics

Absorption: Decreased by raised gastric pH and may be increased in extent and consistency by food.
Distribution: Into bile, saliva, cerumen, synovial fluid, and sebum. Penetration into CSF is erratic and probably minimal. 84% to 99% bound to proteins.
Metabolism: In liver.
Excretion: Primarily in feces, with smaller amount in urine. *Half-life:* 8 hours.

Route	Onset	Peak	Duration
P.O.	Unknown	1–2 hr	Unknown

Action

Chemical effect: Inhibits purine transport and DNA, RNA, and protein synthesis; increases cell wall permeability, making fungus more susceptible to osmotic pressure.
Therapeutic effect: Kills or hinders growth of susceptible fungi, including most pathogenic fungi.

Available forms

Cream: 2%
Shampoo: 1%†, 2%
Tablets: 200 mg

NURSING PROCESS

⚗ Assessment
• Assess patient's infection before starting therapy and regularly thereafter.
• Evaluate laboratory studies for eradication of fungi.
• Be alert for adverse reactions and drug interactions.

• If adverse GI reactions occur, monitor patient's hydration.
• Assess patient's and family's knowledge of drug therapy.

🔲 Nursing diagnoses
• Infection related to presence of susceptible fungi
• Risk for deficient fluid volume related to adverse GI reactions
• Deficient knowledge related to drug therapy

▷ Planning and implementation
• Because of risk of serious hepatotoxicity, don't use for less serious conditions, such as fungus infections of skin or nails.
• To minimize nausea, divide daily amount into two doses. Also, giving drug with meals helps to decrease nausea.
• Have patient dissolve each tablet in 4 ml aqueous solution of 0.2N hydrochloric acid and sip mixture through straw to avoid contact with teeth. Have patient drink full glass (8 oz) of water afterward.
⊛ ALERT: Cream contains sulfites, which can cause allergic reactions in susceptible individuals.
Patient teaching
• Instruct patient with achlorhydria to dissolve each tablet in 4 ml aqueous solution of 0.2N hydrochloric acid, sip mixture through a straw (to avoid contact with teeth), and drink a glass of water after the dose because drug requires gastric acidity to dissolve and absorb completely.
• Make sure patient understands that therapy will continue until all tests indicate that active fungal infection has subsided. If drug is stopped too soon, infection will recur.
• Reassure patient that nausea will subside.
• Tell patient that shampoo and cream are for external use only and to avoid contact with eyes.
• Instruct patient to separate doses of H₂-receptor antagonists, antacids, anticholinergics, proton pump inhibitors, and sucralfate at least 2 hours from drug, as drug requires stomach acidity to work properly.

✓ Evaluation
• Patient is free from infection.
• Patient maintains adequate hydration.
• Patient and family state understanding of drug therapy.

ketoprofen
(kee-toh-PROH-fen)
Actron†, Apo-Keto ♦, Apo-Keto-E ♦, Novo-Keto-EC ♦, Orudis, Orudis-E ♦, Orudis KT†, Orudis SR ♦ ◇, Oruvail, Rhodis ♦, Rhodis-EC ♦

Pharmacologic class: NSAID
Therapeutic class: analgesic, antipyretic, anti-inflammatory
Pregnancy risk category: B (D in third trimester)

Indications and dosages
▶ **Rheumatoid arthritis and osteoarthritis.**
Adults: 75 mg t.i.d., 50 mg q.i.d., or 200 mg as sustained-release tablet once daily. Maximum, 300 mg daily. Or, where suppository is available, 100 mg P.R. b.i.d. or one suppository h.s. (with ketoprofen P.O. during day).
▶ **Mild to moderate pain; dysmenorrhea.**
Adults: 25 to 50 mg P.O. q 6 to 8 hours, p.r.n. Maximum, 300 mg daily.
▶ **Minor aches and pain or fever†.** *Adults:* 12.5 mg with full glass of water q 4 to 6 hours. Don't exceed 25 mg in 4 hours or 75 mg in 24 hours.
🔲 Adjust-a-dose: In patients with mildly impaired renal function, the maximum total daily dose is 150 mg. In more severe renal impairment (GFR less than 25 ml/minute or end-stage renal impairment), the maximum total daily dose is 100 mg. In patients with impaired liver function and serum albumin level less than 3.5 g/dl, the maximum initial total daily dosage is 100 mg. Reduce initial dosage in patients age 75 and older.

Contraindications and cautions
• Contraindicated in patients hypersensitive to the drug or any of its components, and in those with a history of aspirin- or NSAID-induced asthma, urticaria, or other allergic reactions.
• Use cautiously in patients with a history of peptic ulcer disease, renal or liver dysfunction, hypertension, heart failure, or fluid retention.
⚹ Lifespan: In pregnant women, don't use drug during the third trimester. In breast-feeding women, don't use because drug appears in breast milk. In children, safety and effectiveness haven't been established. In children younger

K

than age 16, safety and effectiveness of OTC use haven't been established.

Adverse reactions

CNS: *headache, dizziness, excitation, depression, malaise, nervousness.*
EENT: tinnitus, visual disturbances, *laryngeal edema.*
GI: *nausea, abdominal pain, diarrhea, constipation, flatulence,* peptic ulceration, anorexia, vomiting, stomatitis.
GU: *nephrotoxicity.*
Hematologic: prolonged bleeding time, *thrombocytopenia, agranulocytosis.*
Metabolic: *edema.*
Respiratory: dyspnea, *bronchospasm.*
Skin: rash, photosensitivity, exfoliative dermatitis.

Interactions

Drug-drug. *Anticoagulants:* May increase anticoagulant effect. Monitor patient for signs and symptoms of bleeding.
Aspirin: May increase risk of adverse GI reactions and increase ketoprofen levels. Avoid using together.
Corticosteroids: May increase risk of adverse GI reactions. Avoid using together.
Hydrochlorothiazide, other diuretics: May decrease diuretic effectiveness. Monitor patient for lack of effect.
Lithium, methotrexate: May increase levels of these drugs, leading to toxicity. Monitor levels closely.
Other NSAIDS: May increase risk of bleeding. Monitor patient.
Probenecid: May increase ketoprofen level. Avoid using together.
Drug-herb. *Dong quai, feverfew, garlic, ginger, horse chestnut, red clover:* May increase risk of bleeding. Monitor patient closely.
St. John's wort: May increase risk of photosensitivity reactions. Advise patient to avoid unprotected or prolonged exposure to sunlight.
Drug-lifestyle. *Alcohol use:* May increase risk of GI toxicity. Discourage using together.
Sun exposure: May cause photosensitivity reactions. Advise patient to avoid unprotected or prolonged exposure to sunlight.

Effects on lab test results

- May increase BUN level.
- May increase liver function test values.

- May increase bleeding time. May decrease WBC and platelet counts.
- May interfere with glucose and iron levels, depending on test used.

Pharmacokinetics

Absorption: Rapid and complete.
Distribution: Highly protein-bound.
Metabolism: Extensive, in liver.
Excretion: In urine. *Half-life:* 2 to 5½ hours for extended-release forms.

Route	Onset	Peak	Duration
P.O., P.R.	1–2 hr	½–2 hr	3–4 hr
P.O.			
extended-release	2–3 hr	6–9 hr	24–48 hr

Action

Chemical effect: May inhibit prostaglandin synthesis.
Therapeutic effect: Relieves pain, fever, and inflammation.

Available forms

Capsules: 25 mg, 50 mg, 75 mg
Capsules (extended-release): 100 mg, 150 mg, 200 mg
Suppositories: 100 mg ♦
Tablets: 12.5 mg†
Tablets (enteric-coated): 50 mg ♦, 100 mg ♦
Tablets (sustained-release): 200 mg ♦

NURSING PROCESS

🔲 Assessment

- Assess patient's pain before and after giving the drug. Full effect may not occur for 2 to 4 weeks.
- Check renal and hepatic function every 6 months during long-term therapy.
- Be alert for adverse reactions and drug interactions.
- If adverse GI reactions occur, monitor patient's hydration.
- Assess patient's and family's knowledge of drug therapy.

🔲 Nursing diagnoses

- Chronic pain related to underlying condition
- Risk for deficient fluid volume related to adverse GI reactions
- Deficient knowledge related to drug therapy

Reactions may be *common,* uncommon, *life-threatening,* or COMMON AND LIFE-THREATENING.

❱ Planning and implementation

● Sustained-release form isn't recommended for patients in acute pain.

● May give drug with antacids, food, or milk to minimize adverse GI effects.

● Inform lab technician that patient is taking drug; it may interfere with tests for glucose and iron levels, depending on testing method used.

Patient teaching

● Patient may take drug with milk or meals if he experiences adverse GI effects.

● Tell patient that full therapeutic effect may be delayed for 2 to 4 weeks.

● Instruct patient to report adverse visual or auditory reactions immediately.

● Teach patient to recognize and immediately report evidence of GI bleeding. Explain that serious GI toxicity, including peptic ulceration and bleeding, can occur in patients taking NSAIDs even without GI symptoms.

● Inform patient that use with aspirin, alcohol, or corticosteroids may increase risk of adverse GI reactions.

● Advise patient to use sunblock, wear protective clothing, and avoid prolonged exposure to sunlight. Explain that drug may cause photosensitivity reactions.

☑ Evaluation

● Patient is free from pain.

● Patient maintains normal hydration.

● Patient and family state understanding of drug therapy.

---

ketorolac tromethamine
(KEE-toh-roh-lak troh-METH-uh-meen)
Acular, Acular LS, Toradol

Pharmacologic class: NSAID
Therapeutic class: analgesic, antiinflammatory
Pregnancy risk category: C (D in third trimester)

Indications and dosages

❱ **Short-term management of pain.** *Adults younger than age 65:* Base dosage on patient response. Initially, 60 mg I.M. or 30 mg I.V. as single dose or doses of 30 mg I.M. or I.V. q 6 hours. Maximum, 120 mg daily. To switch to P.O. route, initially give 20 mg P.O., and then

10 mg P.O. q 4 to 6 hours, p.r.n., up to 40 mg daily. Maximum combined use of drug not to exceed 5 days.

Adults age 65 and older, renally impaired patients, and those weighing less than 50 kg (110 lb): Initially, 30 mg I.M. or 15 mg I.V. as single dose or doses of 15 mg I.M. or I.V. q 6 hours. Maximum, 60 mg daily. To switch to P.O. route, 10 mg P.O. q 4 to 6 hours, p.r.n., up to 40 mg daily. Maximum combined use of drug not to exceed 5 days.

❱ **Ocular itching caused by seasonal allergic rhinitis.** *Adults:* 1 drop (0.25 mg) four times daily.

❱ **Postoperative inflammation following cataract surgery.** *Adults:* 1 drop to affected eye four times daily starting 24 hours after surgery and continuing for the first 2 postoperative weeks.

❱ **Pain and burning or stinging following corneal refractive surgery.** *Adults:* 1 drop in the operated eye four times daily as needed for up to 4 days.

▼ I.V. administration

● Injection solution contains alcohol.

● Give I.V. bolus over at least 15 seconds.

⊗ **Incompatibilities**
Haloperidol lactate; nalbuphine; solutions that result in a relatively low pH, such as hydroxyzine, meperidine, morphine sulfate, and prochlorperazine; thiethylperazine.

Contraindications and cautions

● Contraindicated in patients hypersensitive to the drug or any of its components; in those with a history of nasal polyps, angioedema, bronchospastic reactivity, or allergic reactions to aspirin or other NSAIDs; in patients receiving aspirin or other NSAIDs; in those with advanced renal impairment; and in those at risk for renal impairment as a result of volume depletion. Also contraindicated in patients with a high risk of bleeding and in those with suspected or confirmed cerebrovascular bleeding, hemorrhagic diathesis, and incomplete hemostasis.

● Not recommended for intrathecal or epidural administration because of its alcohol content.

● Use cautiously in patients in the perioperative period, and in patients with hepatic or renal impairment, history of serious GI events or peptic ulcer disease, cardiac decompensation, hypertension, or coagulation disorders.

K

Lifespan: In pregnant women, safety during first two trimesters hasn't been established; drug is contraindicated in third trimester. In breastfeeding women, use cautiously because trace amounts have been detected in breast milk. In children, safety of oral form hasn't been established; I.M. and I.V. use are safe in children age 2 and older; ophthalmic solutions are safe for children age 3 and older.

Adverse reactions

CNS: drowsiness, insomnia, syncope, dizziness, *headache.*
CV: edema, hypertension, palpitations.
EENT: *transient stinging and burning,* corneal edema, ocular irritation, keratitis (ocular form).
GI: *nausea, dyspepsia, GI pain,* diarrhea.
GU: hematuria, polyuria, *renal failure.*
Hematologic: purpura, eosinophilia, anemia.
Skin: sweating.
Other: pain at injection site.

Interactions

Drug-drug. *Antihypertensives, diuretics:* May decrease effectiveness of these drugs. Monitor reactions closely.
Cyclosporine: May increase risk of nephrotoxicity. Use together cautiously.
Lithium: May increase lithium level. Monitor level closely.
Low–molecular-weight heparin, salicylates, warfarin: May increase levels of free (unbound) salicylates or warfarin in blood. Significance is unknown.
Methotrexate: May decrease methotrexate clearance and increase toxicity. Don't use together.
Drug-herb. *Dong quai, feverfew, garlic, ginger, horse chestnut, red clover:* May increase risk of bleeding. Monitor patient closely.
St. John's wort: May increase risk of photosensitivity reactions. Advise patient to avoid unprotected or prolonged exposure to sunlight.

Effects on lab test results

• May decrease hemoglobin level and hematocrit.
• May increase eosinophil count and liver function test values.

Pharmacokinetics

Absorption: Complete after I.M. use. After P.O. use, food delays absorption but doesn't decrease amount absorbed.

Distribution: More than 99.9% protein-bound.
Metabolism: Mainly in liver.
Excretion: More than 90% in urine, with the remainder in feces. *Half-life:* 4 to 6 hours.

Route	Onset	Peak	Duration
P.O.	30–60 min	30–60 min	6–8 hr
I.V.	Immediate	Immediate	8 hr
I.M.	≤ 30 min	1–2 hr	6–8 hr

Action

Chemical effect: May inhibit prostaglandin synthesis.
Therapeutic effect: Relieves pain and inflammation.

Available forms

Injection: 15 mg/ml, 30 mg/ml
Ophthalmic solution: 0.4%, 0.5%
Tablets: 10 mg

NURSING PROCESS

Assessment
• Assess patient's pain before and after drug therapy.
• Be alert for adverse reactions and drug interactions.
• Assess patient's and family's knowledge of drug therapy.

Nursing diagnoses
• Acute pain related to underlying condition
• Risk for injury related to drug-induced adverse CNS reactions
• Deficient knowledge related to drug therapy

Planning and implementation
• When switching from I.M. to P.O., don't exceed 120 mg (including maximum of 40 mg P.O.) on day of transition.
• I.M. use may cause pain at injection site. Apply pressure to site for 15 to 30 seconds after injection to minimize local effects.
• If pain persists or worsens, notify prescriber.
③ ALERT: Don't confuse Toradol with Foradil.
Patient teaching
• Teach patient to recognize and immediately report signs and symptoms of GI bleeding. Explain that serious GI toxicity, even without any symptoms, can occur.
• Advise patient to report persistent or worsening pain.

Reactions may be *common,* uncommon, *life-threatening*, or COMMON AND LIFE-THREATENING.

- Explain that drug is intended only for short-term use.

☑ Evaluation
- Patient is free from pain.
- Patient sustains no injury from adverse reactions.
- Patient and family state understanding of drug therapy.

ketotifen fumarate
(kee-toe-TYE-fen FOO-muh-rayt)
Zaditor

Pharmacologic class: histamine antagonist and mast cell stabilizer
Therapeutic class: ophthalmic antihistamine
Pregnancy risk category: C

Indications and dosages
▶ **To temporarily prevent itching of eye caused by allergic conjunctivitis.** *Adults and children age 3 and older:* Instill 1 drop in affected eye q 8 to 12 hours.

Contraindications and cautions
- Contraindicated in patients hypersensitive to the drug or any of its components.
- ☀ **Lifespan:** In pregnant women, use cautiously. In breast-feeding women, use cautiously; it's unknown if topical ocular drug appears in breast milk. In children younger than age 3, safety and effectiveness haven't been established.

Adverse reactions
CNS: *headaches.*
EENT: *conjunctival infection, rhinitis,* ocular allergic reactions, burning or stinging of eyes, conjunctivitis, eye discharge, dry eyes, eye pain, eyelid disorder, itching of eyes, keratitis, lacrimation disorder, mydriasis, photophobia, ocular rash, pharyngitis.
Other: flulike syndrome.

Interactions
None reported.

Effects on lab test results
None reported.

Pharmacokinetics
Absorption: Unknown.
Distribution: Unknown.
Metabolism: Unknown.
Excretion: Unknown. *Half-life:* Unknown.

Route	Onset	Peak	Duration
Ophthalmic	Within min	Unknown	Unknown

Action
Chemical effect: Inhibits release of mediators from cells involved in hypersensitivity reactions.
Therapeutic effect: Temporary prevention of eye itching.

Available forms
Ophthalmic solution: 0.025% solution in 5-ml and 7.5-ml bottles

NURSING PROCESS

℞ Assessment
- Assess underlying condition before starting therapy, and reassess regularly during therapy.
- Monitor patient for sensitivity reactions.
- Monitor patient for signs of infection.
- Assess patient's and family's knowledge of drug therapy.

Nursing diagnoses
- Impaired tissue integrity related to drug-induced adverse EENT reactions
- Deficient knowledge related to ketotifen fumarate therapy

Planning and implementation
- Drug is for ophthalmic use only; not for injection or oral use.
- Drug isn't indicated for use with irritation related to contact lenses.
- Preservative in drug may be absorbed by soft contact lenses. Have patient remove contact lenses before giving drops, and tell him not to reinsert them for at least 10 minutes.
Patient teaching
- Teach patient proper instillation technique. Tell him to avoid contaminating dropper tip and solution and not to touch eyelids or surrounding areas with dropper tip of bottle.
- Tell patient not to wear contact lenses if eyes are red. Warn patient not to use drug to treat irritation related to contact lenses.

• Instruct patient who wears soft contact lenses and whose eyes aren't red to wait at least 10 minutes after instilling drug before inserting contact lenses.
• Advise patient to report adverse reactions to prescriber.
• Instruct patient to keep bottle tightly closed when not in use.

☑ **Evaluation**
• Patient demonstrates appropriate management of any adverse EENT reactions.
• Patient and family state understanding of therapy.

labetalol hydrochloride
(lah-BAY-tuh-lol high-droh-KLOR-ighd)
Normodyne, Presolol ◇, Trandate

Pharmacologic class: alpha and beta blocker
Therapeutic class: antihypertensive
Pregnancy risk category: C

Indications and dosages

▶ **Hypertension.** *Adults:* 100 mg P.O. b.i.d. with or without diuretic. Adjust dosage in increments of 100 mg b.i.d. q 2 or 3 days. Maintenance dosage, 200 to 400 mg b.i.d. Some patients may need 1.2 to 2.4 g/day.
▶ **Severe hypertension, hypertensive emergency.** *Adults:* 200 mg I.V. diluted for infusion at 2 mg/minute until obtaining satisfactory response; then stop infusion. Or give by repeated I.V. injection; initially, 20 mg I.V. slowly over 2 minutes. Then repeat injections of 40 to 80 mg q 10 minutes, p.r.n. to maximum dose, 300 mg.

▼ I.V. administration

• Dilute 200 mg in 160 ml for 1 mg/ml solution for infusion. May use 200 mg/250 ml solution.
• Dilute with D_5W, normal saline solutions, Ringer's solution, or lactated Ringer's solution.
• Give diluted infusion with infusion-control device.
• Give direct I.V. injection over 2 minutes at 10-minute intervals.

• Monitor blood pressure every 5 minutes for 30 minutes, then q 30 minutes for 2 hours, then every hour for 6 hours.
• When given I.V. for hypertensive emergency, drug produces rapid, predictable fall in blood pressure within 5 to 10 minutes.
• Have patient lie down for 3 hours after infusion.
• Store drug at 36° to 86° F (2° to 30° C) and protect from light.

⊗ **Incompatibilities**
Alkali solutions, cefoperazone, ceftriaxone, furosemide, heparin, nafcillin, sodium bicarbonate, thiopental, warfarin.

Contraindications and cautions

• Contraindicated in patients hypersensitive to the drug or any of its components and in those with bronchial asthma, overt cardiac failure, greater than first-degree heart block, cardiogenic shock, severe bradycardia, and other conditions linked to severe and prolonged hypotension.
• Use cautiously in patients with heart failure, hepatic impairment, chronic bronchitis, emphysema, peripheral vascular disease, or pheochromocytoma.
⚖ **Lifespan:** In pregnant and breast-feeding women, use cautiously. In children, safety and effectiveness haven't been established. Elderly patients typically need a lower maintenance dosage.

Adverse reactions

CNS: vivid dreams, *dizziness,* fatigue, headache, transient scalp tingling.
CV: *orthostatic hypotension,* peripheral vascular disease, ***bradycardia, ventricular arrhythmias.***
EENT: nasal stuffiness.
GI: nausea, vomiting, diarrhea.
GU: sexual dysfunction, urine retention.
Respiratory: increased airway resistance.
Skin: rash.

Interactions

Drug-drug. *Beta agonists:* May blunt the bronchodilator effect of these drugs in patients with bronchospasm. Increase dosage of these bronchodilators.
Cimetidine: May enhance labetalol's effect. Give together cautiously; monitor patient for adverse reactions.

Diuretics and other antihypertensives: May increase hypotension. Monitor patient and adjust dosage.
Glutethimide: May decrease effects of labetalol. Adjust labetalol dose carefully to reach optimal blood pressure control.
Halothane: May increase hypotension. Monitor blood pressure.
Insulin, oral antidiabetics: May change required dosage in previously stabilized diabetic patients. Observe patient carefully.
Tricyclic antidepressants: May increase risk of tremor. Monitor patient.

Effects on lab test results

● May increase glucose, transaminase, and blood urea levels.
● May cause false-positive result for amphetamines in urine drug screen.

Pharmacokinetics

Absorption: 90% to 100%, but drug undergoes extensive first-pass metabolism in liver and only about 25% reaches circulation unchanged.
Distribution: Wide; about 50% protein-bound.
Metabolism: Extensive, in liver and possibly GI mucosa.
Excretion: About 5% unchanged in urine; remainder as metabolites in urine and feces.
Half-life: About 5½ hours after I.V. use; 6 to 8 hours after P.O. use.

Route	Onset	Peak	Duration
P.O.	≤ 20 min	2–4 hr	8–12 hr
I.V.	2–5 min	5 min	2–4 hr

Action

Chemical effect: May be related to reduced peripheral vascular resistance as result of alpha-adrenergic blockade.
Therapeutic effect: Lowers blood pressure.

Available forms

Injection: 5 mg/ml
Tablets: 100 mg, 200 mg, 300 mg

NURSING PROCESS

Assessment

● Obtain history of patient's hypertension before starting therapy.
● Monitor blood pressure frequently. Drug masks common signs of shock.

● Be alert for adverse reactions and drug interactions.
● With oral form, full antihypertensive effect is usually seen within the first 1 to 3 hours of initial dose or dose change.
● Assess patient's and family's knowledge of drug therapy.

Nursing diagnoses

● Ineffective health maintenance related to presence of hypertension
● Risk for trauma related to drug-induced hypotension
● Deficient knowledge related to drug therapy

Planning and implementation

● If dizziness occurs, give h.s. or give smaller doses t.i.d. to help minimize this reaction.
ⓢ ALERT: Don't confuse Trandate with Tridrate or Trental.
Patient teaching
● Tell patient that abruptly stopping therapy can worsen angina and cause MI.
● Inform patient that rising slowly and avoiding sudden position changes can minimize dizziness.

Evaluation

● Patient's blood pressure is normal.
● Patient doesn't experience trauma caused by drug-induced hypotension.
● Patient and family state understanding of drug therapy.

lactulose
(LAK-tyoo-lohs)
Cephulac, Cholac, Chronulac, Constilac, Constulose, Duphalac, Enulose, Generlac, Kristalose, Lac-Dol ◇

Pharmacologic class: disaccharide
Therapeutic class: laxative
Pregnancy risk category: B

Indications and dosages

▶ **Constipation.** *Adults:* 10 to 20 g (15 to 30 ml) P.O. daily, increase to 60 ml/day, if needed.
▶ **To prevent and treat hepatic encephalopathy, including hepatic precoma and coma in patients with severe hepatic disease.** *Adults:*

Initially, 20 to 30 g (30 to 45 ml) P.O. t.i.d. or q.i.d. until two to three soft stools are produced daily. Usual dosage, 60 to 100 g total daily. Or 200 g (300 ml) diluted with 700 ml of water or normal saline solution and given as retention enema q 4 to 6 hours, p.r.n.

Adolescents and older children: 27 to 60 g (40 to 90 ml) daily in divided doses.

Infants: 1.67 to 6.67 g (2.5 to 10 ml) daily in divided doses.

For all patients, the desired effect is two to three stools per day. If diarrhea occurs with first dose, reduce dose immediately. If diarrhea persists, stop drug.

▶ **To induce bowel evacuation in geriatric patients with colonic retention of barium and severe constipation after a barium meal examination‡.** *Adults:* 3.3 to 6.7 g P.O. b.i.d. for 1 to 4 weeks.

▶ **To restore bowel movements after hemorrhoidectomy‡.** *Adults:* 10 g P.O. twice during day before surgery and for 5 days postoperatively.

Contraindications and cautions

• Contraindicated in patients on low-galactose diet.

• Use cautiously in patients with diabetes mellitus because drug contains lactose, galactose, and other sugars.

⚘ **Lifespan:** In pregnant women, use only when clearly needed. In breast-feeding women, use cautiously; it's unknown if the drug appears in breast milk. In children, use for chronic constipation is contraindicated. In elderly patients, use cautiously because they may be more susceptible to hyponatremia.

Adverse reactions

GI: *abdominal cramps, belching, diarrhea, distention, flatulence,* nausea, vomiting.

Interactions

Drug-drug. *Antacids, antibiotics, oral neomycin:* May decrease effectiveness of lactulose. Avoid using together.

Effects on lab test results

• May increase glucose level. May decrease ammonia, chloride, potassium, and sodium levels.

Pharmacokinetics

Absorption: Minimal.

Distribution: Local, primarily in colon.
Metabolism: By colonic bacteria.
Excretion: Mostly in feces; absorbed portion in urine.

Route	Onset	Peak	Duration
P.O.	24–48 hr	Varies	Varies
P.R.	Unknown	Unknown	Unknown

Action

Chemical effect: Produces osmotic effect in colon. Resulting distention promotes peristalsis. Decreases blood ammonia build-up that causes hepatic encephalopathy, probably as result of bacterial degradation, which lowers pH of colon contents.

Therapeutic effect: Relieves constipation, decreases blood ammonia concentration.

Available forms

Crystals for reconstitution: 10 g/packet, 20 g/packet
Solution: 10 g/15 ml, 3.33 g/5 ml

NURSING PROCESS

⚕ Assessment

• Assess patient's condition before starting therapy, and regularly thereafter to monitor the drug's effectiveness. If patient has hepatic encephalopathy, assess mental condition.

• Monitor patient's electrolyte levels during long-term use.

• Monitor ammonia levels in patient with hepatic disease.

• Be alert for adverse reactions and drug interactions.

• Assess patient's and family's knowledge of drug therapy.

⊕ Nursing diagnoses

• Constipation related to underlying condition

• Deficient knowledge related to drug therapy

▶ Planning and implementation

Ⓢ **ALERT:** Don't confuse lactulose with lactose.

• Replace fluid loss.

• Diarrhea may indicate overdose.

• To minimize sweet taste, dilute with water or fruit juice or give with food.

• If enema isn't retained for at least 30 minutes, repeat dose.

ALERT: For a patient undergoing electro-cautery procedures during proctoscopy or colonoscopy, the accumulation of hydrogen gas, combined with an electrical spark may cause an explosion. For a patient undergoing electro-cautery procedures, give an enema with a non-fermentable solution.
• Store drug at room temperature, preferably below 86° F (30° C); don't freeze.
Patient teaching
• Advise patient to dilute drug with juice or water, or to take with food to improve taste.
• Inform patient of adverse reactions and tell him to notify prescriber if reactions become bothersome or if having more than two or three soft stools daily.

☑ **Evaluation**
• Patient's constipation is relieved.
• Patient and family state understanding of drug therapy.

lamivudine (3TC)
(la-MI-vyoo-deen)
Epivir, Epivir-HBV

Pharmacologic class: nucleoside reverse transcriptase inhibitor
Therapeutic class: antiretroviral
Pregnancy risk category: C

Indications and dosages
▶ **HIV infection (with other antiretrovirals).**
Adults and children age 16 and older: 300 mg Epivir P.O. once daily or 150 mg P.O. b.i.d.
Children ages 3 months to 16 years: 4 mg/kg Epivir P.O. b.i.d. Maximum, 150 mg b.i.d.
Neonates age 30 days and younger‡: 2 mg/kg Epivir P.O. b.i.d.
⬛ **Adjust-a-dose:** For adults and adolescents with renal impairment, if creatinine clearance is 30 to 49 ml/minute, give 150 mg Epivir P.O. daily; if clearance is 15 to 29 ml/minute, give 150 mg P.O. on day 1, then 100 mg daily; if clearance is 5 to 14 ml/minute, give 150 mg on day 1, then 50 mg daily; if clearance is less than 5 ml/minute, give 50 mg on day 1, then 25 mg daily.
▶ **Chronic hepatitis B with evidence of hepatitis B virus (HBV) replication and active**

liver inflammation. *Adults:* 100 mg Epivir-HBV P.O. once daily.
Children ages 2 to 17: 3 mg/kg Epivir-HBV once daily. Maximum daily, 100 mg.
⬛ **Adjust-a-dose:** For adult patients with renal impairment, if creatinine clearance is 30 to 49 ml/minute, give 100 mg Epivir-HBV as first dose, then 50 mg P.O. daily; if clearance is 15 to 29 ml/minute, give 100 mg first dose, then 25 mg P.O. daily; if clearance is 5 to 14 ml/minute, give 35 mg first dose, then 15 mg P.O. daily; if clearance is less than 5 ml/minute, give 35 mg first dose, then 10 mg P.O. daily.

Contraindications and cautions
• Contraindicated in patients hypersensitive to the drug or any of its components, as well as in combination antiretroviral therapy with abacavir, lamivudine, and tenofovir, and with didanosine, lamivudine, and tenofovir because of early drug resistance in HIV-infected patients.
• Epivir-HBV is contraindicated for patients co-infected with HBV and HIV.
• Safety and effectiveness of Epivir-HBV in all patients for longer than 1 year haven't been established; ideal duration of therapy isn't known.
• Use cautiously in patients with decompensated liver disease or organ transplant. Use cautiously and at a reduced dosage in patients with renal impairment.
⚘ **Lifespan:** In pregnant women, use only if benefits outweigh risks to the fetus. Breast-feeding women should stop breast-feeding or take another drug. In children younger than age 2, safety and effectiveness in chronic hepatitis B haven't been established. In children with history of pancreatitis or other significant risk factors for pancreatitis, use cautiously, if at all.

Adverse reactions
For HIV-infected patients
CNS: *fever, headache, fatigue, neuropathy, malaise, dizziness, insomnia, sleep disorders,* depressive disorders.
EENT: *nasal symptoms.*
GI: *nausea, diarrhea, vomiting, anorexia,* abdominal pain, abdominal cramps, dyspepsia, **pancreatitis,** *hepatomegaly* (children).
Hematologic: **neutropenia,** anemia, **thrombocytopenia,** lymphadenopathy (in children).
Musculoskeletal: *musculoskeletal pain,* myalgia, arthralgia.
Respiratory: *cough.*

Skin: rash (*rashes* in children).
Other: *chills, lactic acidosis.*
For hepatitis B patients
CNS: *malaise, fatigue, headache, fever.*
EENT: ear, nose, and throat infections, sore throat.
GI: abdominal pain and discomfort, *nausea, vomiting, diarrhea.*
Musculoskeletal: *myalgia,* arthralgia.
Skin: rash.
Other: *lactic acidosis.*

Interactions

Drug-drug. *Co-trimoxazole:* May increase bioavailability of lamivudine. Dosage modification isn't needed. Avoid giving lamivudine with high doses of co-trimoxazole for *Pneumocystis jiroveci (carinii)* pneumonia and toxoplasmosis. *Zalcitabine:* May inhibit activation of one another. Avoid using together.

Effects on lab test results

• May increase ALT and bilirubin levels. May decrease hemoglobin level and hematocrit.
• May decrease neutrophil and platelet counts.

Pharmacokinetics

Absorption: Rapid, for HIV-infected patients.
Distribution: Possibly into extravascular spaces. Volume is independent of dose and doesn't correlate with body weight. Less than 36% is bound to proteins.
Metabolism: To trans-sulfoxide.
Excretion: Primarily unchanged in urine. *Half-life:* 5 to 7 hours.

Route	Onset	Peak	Duration
P.O.	Unknown	1–3 hr	Unknown

Action

Chemical effect: Inhibits HIV reverse transcription by viral DNA chain termination and RNA- and DNA-dependent DNA polymerase activities.
Therapeutic effect: Reduces the symptoms of HIV infection, reduces liver inflammation of chronic hepatitis B and may seroconvert some patients.

Available forms

Epivir
Oral solution: 10 mg/ml
Tablets: 150 mg, 300 mg

Epivir-HBV
Oral solution: 5 mg/ml
Tablets: 100 mg

NURSING PROCESS

Assessment

• Obtain history of patient's underlying condition before starting therapy, and reassess regularly thereafter to monitor the drug's effectiveness.
• Test patient with HBV for HIV before and throughout therapy, because drug isn't appropriate for those dually infected.
ALERT: Some patients with chronic HBV infection may have recurrent hepatitis on stopping the drug. Patients with liver disease may have more severe consequences; therefore, monitor liver function tests, markers of HBV replication, and clinical signs regularly after stopping the drug.
• Monitor renal function before and throughout therapy.
• Monitor patient's CBC, platelet count, and liver function. Report any abnormalities to prescriber.
• Assess patient's and family's knowledge of drug therapy.

Nursing diagnoses

• Risk for infection related to the presence of HIV
• Risk for injury related to drug-induced CNS adverse reactions
• Deficient knowledge related to drug therapy

Planning and implementation

• Safety and effectiveness of drug haven't been established for chronic hepatitis B in a patient infected with both HIV and HBV. Drug-resistant HBV variations may occur in such a patient; HIV drug resistance often occurs also.
ALERT: Lactic acidosis and severe hepatomegaly, including fatal cases, have been reported.
• If signs, symptoms, or laboratory abnormalities suggest pancreatitis, stop therapy immediately and notify prescriber.
• An Antiretroviral Pregnancy Registry has been established to monitor maternal-fetal outcomes of pregnant women exposed to drug.

To register a pregnant woman, call 1-800-258-4263, or register online at www.apregistry.com.
⊛ **ALERT:** Don't confuse lamivudine with lamotrigine.

Patient teaching
• Inform patient that long-term effects of drug are unknown.
• Stress importance of taking drug exactly as prescribed.
• Teach patient the signs and symptoms of pancreatitis. Advise him to report signs and symptoms immediately.

☑ **Evaluation**
• Patient responds well to drug therapy.
• Patient sustains no injury as a result of drug-induced CNS adverse reactions.
• Patient and family state understanding of drug therapy.

lamivudine and zidovudine
(la-MI-vyoo-deen and zye-DOE-vyoo-deen)
Combivir

Pharmacologic class: nucleoside reverse transcriptase inhibitor
Therapeutic class: antiretroviral
Pregnancy risk category: C

Indications and dosages

▶ **HIV infection.** *Adults and children age 12 and older who weigh more than 50 kg (110 lb):* One tablet P.O. b.i.d.

Contraindications and cautions

• Contraindicated in patients hypersensitive to the drug or any of its components, in those who need dosage adjustments (such as those who weigh less than 50 kg), in those with creatinine clearance less than 50 ml/minute, and in those with impaired hepatic function. Also contraindicated in patients with dose-limiting adverse effects.
• Safety and effectiveness of lamivudine haven't been established for patients infected with HIV and hepatitis B virus (HBV). Drug-resistant HBV variations may occur in these patients after receiving combination drug.
※ **Lifespan:** In pregnant women, use only if benefits outweigh risks to the fetus. Breast-feeding women should stop breast-feeding or use

another drug. In children younger than age 12, drug is contraindicated.

Adverse reactions

CNS: *fever, headache, malaise, fatigue, insomnia, dizziness, neuropathy,* depression.
EENT: *nasal signs and symptoms.*
GI: *nausea, diarrhea, vomiting, anorexia,* abdominal pain, abdominal cramps, dyspepsia.
Hematologic: *neutropenia,* severe anemia.
Hepatic: *severe hepatomegaly with steatosis.*
Musculoskeletal: *musculoskeletal pain,* myalgia, arthralgia.
Respiratory: *cough.*
Skin: rash.
Other: *chills,* **lactic acidosis.**

Interactions

Drug-drug. *Atovaquone, fluconazole, methadone, probenecid, valproic acid given with zidovudine:* May increase bioavailability of zidovudine. Dosage modification isn't needed.
Co-trimoxazole, nelfinavir: May increase bioavailability of lamivudine. Dosage modification isn't needed. Avoid giving lamivudine with high doses of co-trimoxazole for *Pneumocystis jiroveci (carinii)* pneumonia and toxoplasmosis.
Ganciclovir, interferon-alfa, and other bone marrow suppressive or cytotoxic drugs: May increase hematologic toxicity of zidovudine. Use cautiously as with other reverse transcriptase inhibitors.
Nelfinavir, ritonavir: May decrease bioavailability of zidovudine. Dosage modification isn't needed.
Zalcitabine: May inhibit intracellular phosphorylation of one another. Avoid using these drugs together.

Effects on lab test results

• May increase ALT, AST, and amylase levels. May decrease hemoglobin level and hematocrit.
• May decrease neutrophil count.

Pharmacokinetics

Absorption: Rapid for both drugs, with bioavailability of 86% and 64%, respectively.
Distribution: Extensive for both drugs with low protein binding.
Metabolism: About 5% for lamivudine; 74% for zidovudine.

L

Excretion: Primarily in the urine. *Half-lives of lamivudine and zidovudine:* 5 to 7 hours and ½ to 3 hours, respectively.

Route	Onset	Peak	Duration
P.O.	Unknown	Unknown	Unknown

Action

Chemical effect: Inhibits reverse transcriptase by DNA chain termination. Both drugs are also weak inhibitors of DNA polymerase. Together, they act synergistically by suppressing or delaying the emergence of resistant strains that can occur with retroviral monotherapy, because dual resistance requires multiple mutations.
Therapeutic effect: Reduces the symptoms of HIV infection.

Available forms

Tablets: 150 mg lamivudine and 300 mg zidovudine

NURSING PROCESS

Assessment
• Obtain history of patient's underlying condition before starting therapy, and reassess regularly thereafter to monitor the drug's effectiveness.
• Watch for hematologic toxicity by taking frequent blood counts, especially in patients with advanced HIV infection.
• Assess patient's fine motor skills and peripheral sensation for evidence of peripheral neuropathies.
⚠ ALERT: In a patient with chronic HBV infection, hepatitis may recur when drug is stopped. Patients with pre-existing liver disease may have more severe consequences. Periodically monitor liver function test results and markers of HBV replication in patient with liver disease and HBV.
• Assess patient's and family's knowledge of drug therapy.

Nursing diagnoses
• Risk for infection related to the presence of HIV
• Disturbed sensory perception (tactile) related to drug-induced peripheral neuropathy
• Deficient knowledge related to drug therapy

Planning and implementation
⚠ ALERT: Fatal lactic acidosis and severe hepatomegaly with steatosis may occur. If patient develops signs or symptoms of lactic acidosis or severe hepatotoxicity, stop drug.
• Use drug cautiously in patients with bone marrow suppression (granulocyte count below 1,000/mm^3 or hemoglobin level below 9.5 g/dl).
• An Antiretroviral Pregnancy Registry has been established to monitor maternal-fetal outcomes of pregnant women exposed to drug. To register a pregnant patient call 1-800-258-4263 or register online at www.apregistry.com.
Patient teaching
• Advise patient that therapy won't cure HIV infection and that he may continue to experience illness.
• Warn patient that HIV transmission can still occur with drug therapy. Educate patient about using barrier contraception when engaging in sexual activities to prevent disease transmission.
• Teach patient signs and symptoms of neutropenia and anemia (fever, chills, infection, fatigue), and instruct him to immediately report any occurrences to the prescriber.
• Tell patient to have blood counts followed closely while on drug, especially if he has advanced disease.
• Advise patient to consult prescriber or pharmacist before taking other drugs.
• Warn patient to report abdominal pain immediately.
• Instruct patient to report signs and symptoms of myopathy or myositis, such as muscle inflammation, pain, weakness, and a decrease in muscle size.
• Stress importance of taking combination drug therapy exactly as prescribed to reduce the development of drug resistance.
• Tell patient he may take combination with or without food.
• Inform woman that breast-feeding is contraindicated with an HIV infection, whether or not she is taking drug.

Evaluation
• Patient responds well to drug.
• Patient doesn't develop peripheral neuropathy.
• Patient and family state understanding of drug therapy.

lamotrigine

(lah-MOH-trigh-jeen)
Lamictal

Pharmacologic class: phenyltriazine
Therapeutic class: anticonvulsant, mood stabilizer
Pregnancy risk category: C

Indications and dosages

▶ **Adjunct therapy for partial seizures caused by epilepsy or generalized seizures of Lennox-Gastaut syndrome.** *Adults and children older than age 12:* For patients taking valproic acid with other enzyme-inducing anticonvulsants, 25 mg P.O. q other day for 2 weeks; then 25 mg P.O. daily for 2 weeks. Continue to increase, p.r.n., by 25 to 50 mg/day q 1 to 2 weeks until effective maintenance dosage of 100 to 400 mg daily, given in one or two divided doses, is reached. When added to valproic acid alone, maintenance dosage is 100 to 200 mg P.O. daily. For patients receiving enzyme-inducing anticonvulsants and not valproic acid, 50 mg P.O. daily for 2 weeks; then 100 mg P.O. daily in two divided doses for 2 weeks. Increase, p.r.n., by 100 mg daily q 1 to 2 weeks. Maintenance dosage, 300 to 500 mg P.O. daily in two divided doses.
Children ages 2 to 12 who weigh 6.7 to 40 kg (15 to 88 lb): For patients taking valproic acid with other enzyme-inducing anticonvulsants, 0.15 mg/kg P.O. daily in one or two divided doses (round down to nearest whole tablet) for 2 weeks, followed by 0.3 mg/kg daily in one or two divided doses for another 2 weeks. Then maintenance dosage, 1 to 5 mg/kg daily (maximum, 200 mg daily in one to two divided doses). For patients receiving enzyme-inducing anticonvulsants and not valproic acid, 0.6 mg/kg P.O. daily in two divided doses (round down to nearest whole tablet) for 2 weeks, followed by 1.2 mg/kg daily in two divided doses for another 2 weeks. Maintenance dosage, 5 to 15 mg/kg daily (maximum, 400 mg daily in two divided doses).
▶ **To convert patients from monotherapy with a hepatic enzyme-inducing anticonvulsant to lamotrigine.** *Adults and children age 16 and older:* Add 50 mg P.O. once daily to current therapy for 2 weeks, followed by 100 mg

P.O. daily in two divided doses for 2 weeks. Then increase daily dosage by 100 mg q 1 to 2 weeks until maintenance dosage of 500 mg daily in two divided doses is reached. Gradually withdraw hepatic enzyme-inducing anticonvulsant in 20% decrements weekly for 4 weeks.
🖿 Adjust-a-dose: For patients with severe renal impairment or moderate to severe hepatic impairment, use lower maintenance dosage.
▶ **Bipolar disorder.** *Adults not taking carbamazepine (or other enzyme-inducing drugs) or valproic acid:* Target dose, 200 mg/day. Initially, 25 mg daily for weeks 1 and 2; then 50 mg daily for weeks 3 and 4; then 100 mg daily for week 5; then 200 mg daily for weeks 6 and 7.
Adults taking carbamazepine (or other enzyme-inducing drugs) and not taking valproic acid: Target dose, 400 mg/day. Initially, 50 mg daily for weeks 1 and 2; then 100 mg daily in divided doses for weeks 3 and 4; then 200 mg daily in divided doses for week 5; then 300 mg daily in divided doses for week 6; and up to 400 mg daily in divided doses for week 7.
Adults taking valproic acid: Target dose, 100 mg/day. Initially, 25 mg q other day for weeks 1 and 2; then 25 mg daily for weeks 3 and 4; then 50 mg daily for week 5; then 100 mg daily for weeks 6 and 7.
🖿 Adjust-a-dose: If other psychotropic drugs are withdrawn following stabilization, adjust dosage.

Contraindications and cautions

• Contraindicated in patients hypersensitive to the drug or any of its components.
• Use cautiously in patients with renal, hepatic, or cardiac impairment.
⚐ Lifespan: In pregnant women, use only when benefits outweigh risks to the fetus. In breast-feeding women, use cautiously, it isn't known if drug appears in breast milk. In children, drug is only indicated as adjunctive therapy for the generalized seizures of Lennox-Gastaut syndrome. For other uses, safety and effectiveness haven't been established in children younger than age 16.

Adverse reactions

CNS: fever, *dizziness, headache, ataxia, somnolence,* incoordination, insomnia, tremor, depression, anxiety, *seizures,* irritability, speech disorder, decreased memory, aggravated reaction, concentration disturbance, sleep disorder, emo-

L

tional lability, vertigo, malaise, mind racing, ***suicide attempts.***
CV: palpitations.
EENT: *diplopia, blurred vision,* vision abnormality, nystagmus, rhinitis, pharyngitis.
GI: *nausea, vomiting,* diarrhea, dyspepsia, abdominal pain, constipation, anorexia, dry mouth.
GU: dysmenorrhea, vaginitis, amenorrhea.
Musculoskeletal: dysarthria, muscle spasm, neck pain.
Respiratory: cough, dyspnea.
Skin: ***Stevens-Johnson syndrome, toxic epidermal necrolysis,*** rash, pruritus, alopecia, acne.
Other: hot flushes, flulike syndrome, infection, chills, tooth disorder.

Interactions

Drug-drug. *Acetaminophen:* May reduce lamotrigine level, decreasing therapeutic effects. Monitor patient.
Carbamazepine, oxcarbazepine, phenobarbital, phenytoin, primidone, rifamycins: May decrease steady-state level of lamotrigine. Monitor patient closely for decreased effect.
Folate inhibitors (such as co-trimoxazole, methotrexate): May have additive effect because lamotrigine inhibits dihydrofolate reductase, an enzyme involved in folic acid synthesis. Monitor patient closely for adverse effects and toxicities.
Hormonal contraceptives, progestins: May reduce lamotrigine level. Adjust the dose of lamotrigine p.r.n.
Valproic acid: May decrease lamotrigine clearance, which increases steady-state levels. Monitor patient closely for toxicity.
Drug-herb. *Evening primrose oil:* May lower the seizure threshold. Discourage using together.
Drug-lifestyle. *Sun exposure:* May cause photosensitivity reactions. Urge patient to avoid unprotected or prolonged exposure to sunlight.

Effects on lab test results

None reported.

Pharmacokinetics

Absorption: Rapid and complete with negligible first-pass metabolism.
Distribution: 55% protein-bound.
Metabolism: Predominantly by glucuronic acid conjugation.
Excretion: Primarily in urine. *Half-life:* 14½ to 70¼ hours, depending on dosage schedule and use of other anticonvulsants.

Route	Onset	Peak	Duration
P.O.	Unknown	1½–4¾ hr	Unknown

Action

Chemical effect: May inhibit release of glutamate and aspartate, excitatory neurotransmitters in the brain, through action at sodium channels.
Therapeutic effect: Prevents partial seizures, stabilizes mood.

Available forms

Tablets: 25 mg, 100 mg, 150 mg, 200 mg
Tablets (chewable dispersible): 2 mg, 5 mg, 25 mg

NURSING PROCESS

Assessment

- Obtain history of patient's disorder before starting therapy.
- Evaluate patient for reduction in frequency and duration of seizures after therapy begins. Check adjunct anticonvulsant level periodically.
- Monitor signs and symptoms of bipolar disorder and suicidal thoughts.
- Assess patient's and family's knowledge of drug therapy.

Nursing diagnoses

- Risk for trauma related to seizures
- Risk for impaired skin integrity related to dermatologic reactions
- Deficient knowledge related to drug therapy

Planning and implementation

- If drug is added to therapy that includes valproic acid, lower dosage.

ALERT: Don't abruptly stop giving the drug because doing so increases the risk of seizures and unstable mood. Taper drug over at least 2 weeks.
ALERT: Rash may be life-threatening. If one develops, stop giving the drug and immediately notify prescriber. Don't restart.
ALERT: Don't confuse Lamictal with Lamisil.

Patient teaching

- Inform patient that drug may cause rash. Combination therapy with valproic acid and lamotrigine is more likely to cause a serious rash. Tell patient to immediately report rash or signs or symptoms of hypersensitivity because they could be life-threatening.

• Instruct patient to avoid prolonged exposure to sunlight, use sunblock, and wear protective clothing to avoid photosensitivity.
• Warn patient not to engage in hazardous activity until the drug's CNS effects are known.

☑ **Evaluation**
• Patient is seizure-free.
• Patient doesn't develop drug-induced skin reactions.
• Patient and family state understanding of drug therapy.

lansoprazole
(lan-soh-PRAY-zohl)
Prevacid⧸, Prevacid I.V., Prevacid SoluTab

Pharmacologic class: proton-pump inhibitor
Therapeutic class: gastric antisecretory
Pregnancy risk category: B

Indications and dosages

▶ **Short-term therapy for active duodenal ulcer.** *Adults:* 15 mg P.O. daily for 4 weeks.
▶ **Maintenance of healed duodenal ulcers; maintenance of healing erosive esophagitis.** *Adults:* 15 mg P.O. daily.
▶ **Short-term therapy for erosive esophagitis.** *Adults:* 30 mg P.O. daily for up to 8 weeks. If healing doesn't occur, give additional 8 weeks of therapy. Maintenance dosage for healing is 15 mg P.O. daily.
Children ages 12 to 17: 30 mg P.O. once daily for up to 8 weeks.
Children ages 1 to 11 who weigh 30 kg (66 lb) or less: 15 mg P.O. daily for up to 12 weeks.
Children ages 1 to 11 who weigh more than 30 kg: 30 mg P.O. daily for up to 12 weeks.
▶ **Short-term therapy for erosive esophagitis when the patient isn't able to take oral drug.** *Adults:* 30 mg I.V. daily, over 30 minutes, for up to 7 days. As soon as the patient can take oral drug, switch to P.O. and continue for 6 to 8 weeks.
▶ **Short-term therapy for active benign gastric ulcer.** *Adults:* 30 mg P.O. daily for up to 8 weeks.
Helicobacter pylori **eradication to reduce risk of duodenal ulcer recurrence.** *Adults:* For triple therapy, 30 mg P.O. lansoprazole with 500 mg P.O. clarithromycin and 1 g P.O. amoxi-

cillin, each given q 12 hours for 14 days. For dual therapy, 30 mg P.O. lansoprazole with 1 g P.O. amoxicillin, each given q 8 hours for 14 days.
▶ **Long-term therapy for pathologic hypersecretory conditions, including Zollinger-Ellison syndrome.** *Adults:* Initially, 60 mg P.O. daily. Increase dosage p.r.n. If more than 120 mg daily, give in divided doses.
▶ **Short-term therapy for symptomatic gastroesophageal reflux disease.** *Adults:* 15 mg P.O. daily for up to 8 weeks.
Children ages 12 to 17: 15 mg P.O. daily for up to 8 weeks.
Children ages 1 to 11 who weigh 30 kg (66 lb) or less: 15 mg P.O. daily for up to 12 weeks.
Children ages 1 to 11 who weigh more than 30 kg: 30 mg P.O. daily for up to 12 weeks.
▶ **NSAID-related ulcer in patients who are continuing NSAIDs.** *Adults:* 30 mg P.O. daily for 8 weeks.
▶ **To reduce risk of NSAID-related ulcer in a patient who has a history of gastric ulcer and needs NSAIDs.** *Adults:* 15 mg P.O. daily for up to 12 weeks.

▽ I.V. administration

• Reconstitute with 5 ml sterile water for injection only.
• Mix gently until the powder is dissolved.
• Infuse over 30 minutes using the provided 1.2 micron in-line filter, which will remove any precipitate that forms when reconstituted solution comes in contact with I.V. solutions.
⊗ **Incompatibilities**
Other I.V. drugs.

Contraindications and cautions

• Contraindicated in patients hypersensitive to the drug or any of its components.
• Drug isn't recommended as maintenance therapy for patients with active duodenal ulcers or erosive esophagitis.
⚕ **Lifespan:** In pregnant women, use only when benefits outweigh risks to the fetus. In breast-feeding women, don't use; it isn't known if drug appears in breast milk. In children younger than age 1, safety and effectiveness haven't been established.

Adverse reactions

GI: diarrhea, nausea, abdominal pain.

L

Interactions

Drug-drug. *Ampicillin esters, digoxin, iron salts, ketoconazole:* May interfere with absorption of these drugs. Monitor patient closely.
Sucralfate: May delay lansoprazole absorption. Give lansoprazole at least 30 minutes before sucralfate.
Theophylline: May slightly increase theophylline clearance. Use together cautiously. Adjust dosage, if needed when lansoprazole is started or stopped.
Drug-herb. *Male fern:* May inactivate drug in alkaline environments. Discourage using together.
St. John's wort: May increase risk of photosensitivity reactions. Advise patient to avoid unprotected or prolonged exposure to sunlight.
Drug-food. *Food:* May decrease absorption of drug when taken with meals. Take drug on an empty stomach, before meals.

Effects on lab test results

None reported.

Pharmacokinetics

Absorption: Rapid.
Distribution: 97% bound to proteins.
Metabolism: Extensive, in liver.
Excretion: Mainly in feces, minimally in urine.
Half-life: Less than 2 hours.

Route	Onset	Peak	Duration
P.O.	Unknown	2 hr	> 24 hr

Action

Chemical effect: Inhibits proton pump and binds to hydrogen or potassium adenosine triphosphatase, located at secretory surface of gastric parietal cells.
Therapeutic effect: Decreases gastric acid formation.

Available forms

Capsules (delayed-release): 15 mg, 30 mg
Injection: 30-mg single-use vial
Oral suspension (delayed-release): 15 mg/packet, 30 mg/packet
Tablets (orally disintegrating, delayed-release): 15 mg, 30 mg. Orally disintegrating tablets contain 2.5 mg phenylalanine/15 mg tablet and 5.1 mg phenylalanine/30 mg tablet

NURSING PROCESS

⚕ Assessment

- Assess patient's condition before starting therapy and regularly thereafter to monitor drug's effectiveness.
- Be alert for adverse reactions and drug interactions.
- Assess patient's and family's knowledge of drug therapy.

⊕ Nursing diagnoses

- Impaired tissue integrity related to underlying condition
- Ineffective health maintenance related to drug-induced adverse reactions
- Deficient knowledge related to drug therapy

❯ Planning and implementation

③ ALERT: Orally disintegrating tablets contain phenylalanine. Assess patient for sensitivity before starting therapy.
- Give drug on an empty stomach.
- If giving by NG tube, mix contents of capsule with 40 ml of apple juice in a syringe and give within 3 to 5 minutes. Flush with additional apple juice to ensure entire dose is given and to maintain patency of the tube.
- If giving capsule to a patient who has difficulty swallowing, empty contents of capsule into about 2 oz (60 ml) of apple, cranberry, grape, orange, pineapple, prune, tomato, or vegetable juice, mix briefly, and use within 30 minutes. To ensure complete dose, rinse glass with two or more servings of juice and have patient drink immediately. Or mix contents of capsule with 1 tbs of applesauce, pudding, cottage cheese, yogurt, or strained pears and have patient swallow immediately. Tell him not to chew or crush granules.
- For the oral suspension, empty packet contents into 30 ml of water. Stir well and have patient drink immediately. Tell patient not to chew or crush the contents of the capsules or the suspension. Don't use with other liquids or food. If any material remains after drinking, add more water, stir, and have patient drink immediately.
- Place orally disintegrating tablets on the patient's tongue and allow to dissolve completely. Water isn't needed. If using NG tube or oral syringe, dissolve 15-mg tablet in 4 ml water or 30mg tablet in 10 ml water.

⑨ ALERT: Don't crush drug or allow patient to chew it.

• If adverse reaction occurs, notify prescriber and provide supportive care.

• Adjust dosage in patients with severe liver disease.

Patient teaching

• Tell patient not to crush or chew drug and to take it before a meal.

• Explain how to mix drug with other liquids if patient has difficulty swallowing.

• Tell patient to allow orally disintegrating tablets to dissolve on tongue until the particles can be swallowed.

• Instruct patient to notify prescriber if any adverse reactions occur.

☑ Evaluation

• Patient regains normal GI tissue integrity.

• Patient doesn't experience serious adverse reactions.

• Patient and family state understanding of drug therapy.

leflunomide
(leh-FLOO-noh-mighd)
Arava

Pharmacologic class: pyrimidine synthesis inhibitor
Therapeutic class: immunomodulator
Pregnancy risk category: X

Indications and dosages

▶ **Active rheumatoid arthritis, to reduce signs and symptoms, to retard structural damage based on X-ray evidence of erosions and joint space narrowing, to improve physical function.** *Adults:* 100 mg P.O. q 24 hours for 3 days followed by 20 mg (daily maximum) P.O. q 24 hours. If this dosage isn't tolerated, decrease to 10 mg daily.

Contraindications and cautions

• Contraindicated in patients hypersensitive to the drug or any of its components.

• Use cautiously in patients with hepatic insufficiency, hepatitis B or C, severe immunodeficiency, bone marrow dysplasia, or severe uncontrolled infections.

• Use cautiously in patients with renal insufficiency.

🔥 **Lifespan:** In pregnant and breast-feeding women, drug is contraindicated. In children, safety and effectiveness haven't been established. In men attempting to father children, drug isn't recommended.

Adverse reactions

CNS: asthenia, dizziness, fever, headache, paresthesia, malaise, migraine, sleep disorder, vertigo, neuritis, anxiety, depression, insomnia, neuralgia.
CV: angina pectoris, *hypertension,* chest pain, peripheral edema, palpitations, tachycardia, vasculitis, vasodilation, varicose veins.
EENT: pharyngitis, rhinitis, sinusitis, epistaxis, enlarged salivary gland, blurred vision, cataracts, conjunctivitis, eye disorders.
GI: mouth ulcer, oral candidiasis, stomatitis, dry mouth, anorexia, *diarrhea,* dyspepsia, gastroenteritis, nausea, abdominal pain, vomiting, cholelithiasis, colitis, constipation, esophagitis, flatulence, gastritis, melena, gingivitis, taste perversion.
GU: UTI, albuminuria, cystitis, dysuria, hematuria, menstrual disorder, pelvic pain, vaginal candidiasis, prostate disorder, urinary frequency.
Hematologic: anemia, hyperlipidemia.
Metabolic: weight loss, *diabetes mellitus,* hyperglycemia, hyperthyroidism, hypokalemia.
Musculoskeletal: arthrosis, back pain, bursitis, muscle cramps, myalgia, bone necrosis, bone pain, arthralgia, leg cramps, joint disorder, neck pain, synovitis, tendon rupture, tenosynovitis.
Respiratory: bronchitis, increased cough, pneumonia, *respiratory infection,* **asthma,** dyspnea, lung disorders.
Skin: *alopecia,* eczema, pruritus, *rash,* dry skin, acne, contact dermatitis, fungal dermatitis, hair discoloration, hematoma, nail disorder, skin nodule, subcutaneous nodule, maculopapular rash, skin disorder, skin discoloration, skin ulcer, increased sweating, ecchymosis.
Other: allergic reaction, flulike syndrome, injury or accident, pain, abscess, cyst, hernia, tooth disorder, herpes simplex, herpes zoster.

Interactions

Drug-drug. *Cholestyramine, charcoal:* May decrease leflunomide level. Sometimes used for this effect in overdose.

Live vaccines: May alter immune response. Avoid live vaccines during therapy, and remember leflunomide's long half-life when considering a live vaccine after therapy stops.

Methotrexate, other hepatotoxic drugs: May increase risk of hepatotoxicity. Monitor liver enzyme levels.

NSAIDs (diclofenac, ibuprofen): May increase NSAID levels. Significance is unknown; monitor patient.

Rifampin: May increase active leflunomide metabolite level. Use together cautiously.

Tolbutamide: May increase tolbutamide levels. Significance is unknown; monitor patient.

Effects on lab test results

• May increase AST, ALT, glucose, lipid, T_4, and CK levels. May decrease potassium, TSH, and hemoglobin levels and hematocrit.

Pharmacokinetics

Absorption: 80%.

Distribution: Low; extensively bound to albumin.

Metabolism: Primary route hasn't been identified.

Excretion: Renal and biliary; 43% in urine, 48% in feces. *Half-life:* 15 to 18 days.

Route	Onset	Peak	Duration
P.O.	Unknown	6–12 hr	Unknown

Action

Chemical effect: Inhibits dihydroorotate dehydrogenase, an enzyme involved in pyrimidine synthesis, and is antiproliferative and anti-inflammatory.

Therapeutic effect: Reduces pain and inflammation related to rheumatoid arthritis.

Available forms

Tablets: 10 mg, 20 mg, 100 mg

NURSING PROCESS

⚕ Assessment

• Assess patient's condition before starting therapy, and regularly thereafter to monitor the drug's effectiveness.

• Be alert for adverse reactions and drug interactions.

• Monitor platelet and WBC counts, ALT and hemoglobin levels, and hematocrit, at baseline

and at monthly intervals during the first 6 months; if stable, continue monitoring q 6 to 8 weeks. If used with methotrexate or other immunosuppressant, monitor patient's AST, ALT, and albumin levels monthly.

⚕ ALERT: Severe liver damage, sometimes fatal, may rarely occur. Most cases of severe liver damage occur within 6 months of therapy in a patient with multiple risk factors for hepatotoxicity (liver disease, other hepatotoxins).

• Monitor for overlapping hematologic toxicity when switching to another antirheumatic.

• Because of drug's long half-life, carefully observe patient after reducing dosage because level may take several weeks to decline.

• Assess patient's and family's knowledge of drug therapy.

⊕ Nursing diagnoses

• Ineffective health maintenance related to underlying disease

• Deficient knowledge related to drug therapy

▷ Planning and implementation

• If ALT level increases to between two and three times the upper limit of normal (ULN), lower the dose to 10 mg/day. This may allow you to continue use under close monitoring. If ALT stays between two and three times ULN despite the lower dose, or if ALT level increases to more than three times ULN, stop giving the drug, give cholestyramine or charcoal, and monitor the patient closely. Give additional doses of cholestyramine or charcoal p.r.n.

⚕ ALERT: Drug can cause fetal harm when given during pregnancy. Stop giving the drug to a woman planning to become pregnant, and notify prescriber.

• Stop drug in a man who plans to father a child. Tell him to take 8 g cholestyramine P.O. t.i.d. for 11 days to remove drug. Check levels.

• If bone marrow suppression occurs, stop the drug and start cholestyramine or charcoal therapy.

• Some immunosuppressants, possibly including leflunomide, increase the risk of cancer, particularly lymphoproliferative disorders. Use drug only when benefits exceed risks.

Patient teaching

• Explain the need for frequent blood test monitoring.

Reactions may be *common,* uncommon, *life-threatening,* or COMMON AND LIFE-THREATENING.

• Instruct patient to use contraceptive measures during drug therapy and until drug is no longer active.
• If a patient suspects she is pregnant, advise her to immediately notify the prescriber.
• Advise breast-feeding woman not to breast-feed during therapy.
• Tell patient that he may continue taking aspirin, other NSAIDs, and low-dose corticosteroids, but that combined use of drug with antimalarials, I.M. or P.O. gold, penicillamine, azathioprine, or methotrexate hasn't been adequately studied. Instruct patient to review all drugs with prescriber before use.

☑ **Evaluation**
• Patient's symptoms of rheumatoid arthritis improve.
• Patient and family state understanding of drug therapy.

leucovorin calcium (citrovorum factor, folinic acid)
(loo-koh-VOR-in KAL-see-um)

Pharmacologic class: formyl derivative (active reduced form of folic acid)
Therapeutic class: vitamin, antidote
Pregnancy risk category: C

Indications and dosages
▶ **Overdose of folic acid antagonist.** *Adults and children:* P.O., I.M., or I.V. dose equivalent to weight of antagonist given.
▶ **Rescue after high methotrexate dose given as cancer therapy.** *Adults and children:* 10 mg/m² P.O., I.M., or I.V. q 6 hours until methotrexate level falls below 5×10^{-8} M.
▶ **Megaloblastic anemia caused by congenital enzyme deficiency.** *Adults and children:* 3 to 6 mg I.M. daily; then 1 mg P.O. or I.M. daily for life.
▶ **Folate-deficient megaloblastic anemia.** *Adults and children:* Up to 1 mg P.O. or I.M. daily. Duration of therapy depends on hematologic response.
▶ **Hematologic toxicity caused by pyrimethamine or trimethoprim therapy.** *Adults and children:* 5 to 15 mg P.O. or I.M. daily.

▶ **Palliative treatment of advanced colorectal carcinoma.** *Adults:* 20 mg/m² I.V., followed by fluorouracil, for 5 consecutive days. Repeat q 4 weeks for two additional courses; then q 4 to 5 weeks, if tolerated.

▼ I.V. administration
• Give leucovorin I.V. to patients with GI toxicity (diarrhea, stomatitis, vomiting) when doses exceed 25 mg.
• When using powder for injection, reconstitute drug in 50-mg vial with 5 ml, 100 mg vial with 10 ml, or 350-mg vial with 17 ml of sterile water or bacteriostatic water for injection. When doses are greater than 10 mg/m² don't use diluents containing benzyl alcohol, especially in neonates.
• Don't give faster than 160 mg/minute because of the calcium concentration.
• Protect drug from light and heat, especially reconstituted parenteral forms.
⊗ **Incompatibilities**
Droperidol, fluorouracil, foscarnet, sodium bicarbonate.

Contraindications and cautions
• Contraindicated in patients with pernicious anemia and other megaloblastic anemias caused by lack of vitamin B_{12}.
☕ **Lifespan:** In breast-feeding women, use cautiously; it's unknown if drug appears in breast milk. In children, use cautiously because drug may increase risk of seizures. In neonates, injection form is contraindicated because it contains benzyl alcohol.

Adverse reactions
Respiratory: *bronchospasm.*
Skin: hypersensitivity reactions (rash, pruritus, erythema).

Interactions
Drug-drug. *Anticonvulsants:* May decrease anticonvulsant effectiveness. Monitor patient closely.
Fluorouracil: May enhance fluorouracil toxicity. Adjust dosage of fluorouracil p.r.n.
Methotrexate: May decrease effectiveness of intrathecal methotrexate. Avoid using together.

Effects on lab test results
None reported.

Pharmacokinetics

Absorption: Rapid, after P.O. use.
Distribution: Throughout body; liver contains about one-half of total body folate stores.
Metabolism: In liver.
Excretion: By kidneys. *Half-life:* 6¼ hours.

Route	Onset	Peak	Duration
P.O.	20–30 min	2–3 hr	3–6 hr
I.V.	5 min	10 min	3–6 hr
I.M.	10–20 min	< 1 hr	3–6 hr

Action

Chemical effect: Readily converts to other folic acid derivatives.
Therapeutic effect: Raises folic acid level.

Available forms

Injection: 3 mg/ml in 1-ml ampule; 10 mg/ml in 5-ml vial
Powder for injection: 50-mg, 100-mg, and 350-mg vials for reconstitution
Tablets: 5 mg, 15 mg, 25 mg

NURSING PROCESS

⏲ Assessment

● Assess patient's condition before starting therapy and regularly thereafter to monitor the drug's effectiveness.
● Monitor creatinine level daily to detect renal dysfunction.
● Be alert for adverse reactions and drug interactions.
● Monitor patient for rash, wheezing, pruritus, and urticaria, which can be signs of drug allergy.
● Assess patient's and family's knowledge of drug therapy.

⊕ Nursing diagnoses

● Ineffective health maintenance related to underlying condition
● Deficient knowledge related to drug therapy

❯ Planning and implementation

● Drug may mask diagnosis of pernicious anemia.
● Follow leucovorin rescue schedule and protocol closely to maximize therapeutic response.
● Don't give simultaneously with systemic methotrexate.

⚠ **ALERT:** Don't confuse leucovorin (folinic acid) with folic acid. To avoid confusion, don't refer to leucovorin as folinic acid.
Patient teaching
● Explain to patient reasons for drug therapy.

☑ Evaluation

● Patient's condition improves.
● Patient and family state understanding of drug therapy.

leuprolide acetate
(loo-PROH-lighd AS-ih-tayt)
Eligard, Lucrin◇, Lupron, Lupron Depot, Lupron Depot-Ped, Lupron Depot-3 Month, Lupron Depot-4 Month, Lupron for Pediatric Use, Viadur

Pharmacologic class: synthetic analog of gonadotropin-releasing hormone
Therapeutic class: antineoplastic, luteinizing hormone-releasing hormone agonist
Pregnancy risk category: X

Indications and dosages

❯ **Advanced prostate cancer.** *Men:* 1 mg subcutaneously daily. Or 7.5 mg I.M. depot injection monthly. Or 7.5 mg Eligard subcutaneously once monthly. Or 22.5 mg I.M. q 3 months (84 days). Or 22.5 mg Eligard subcutaneously q 3 months. Or 30 mg I.M. depot injection q 4 months (16 weeks). Or 30 mg Eligard subcutaneously q 4 months. Or 45 mg Eligard subcutaneously q 6 months. Or 72 mg Viadur implant subcutaneously q 12 months
❯ **Endometriosis.** *Women:* 3.75 mg I.M. as single injection once monthly. Or 11.25 mg I.M. q 3 months (depot injection only). Recommended duration of treatment is 6 months.
❯ **Central precocious puberty.** *Children:* Initially, 0.3 mg/kg (minimum, 7.5 mg) I.M. depot injection as a single injection q 4 weeks. Increase dosage in increments of 3.75 mg q 4 weeks, if needed. This will be considered the maintenance dosage. Or 50 mcg/kg subcutaneously (injection form) daily. If total downregulation isn't achieved, increase dosage by 10 mcg/kg daily. This becomes the maintenance dosage. Stop drug before girls reach age 11 and before boys reach age 12.

▶ **Uterine leiomyomata (depot only).** *Women:* 3.75 mg I.M. monthly or one dose of 11.25 mg I.M. with iron therapy. Recommended duration of therapy is 3 months or less.

Contraindications and cautions

• Contraindicated in patients hypersensitive to the drug or any of its components, or other gonadotropin-releasing hormone analogs, and in women with undiagnosed vaginal bleeding. Viadur implant is contraindicated in women and children.
• Use cautiously in patients hypersensitive to benzyl alcohol.
⚖ **Lifespan:** In women, the 30-mg depot formulation is contraindicated. In pregnant and breast-feeding women, drug is contraindicated. In neonates, drug is contraindicated because it contains benzyl alcohol.

Adverse reactions

CNS: dizziness, *depression, headache, pain.*
CV: *arrhythmias,* angina, *MI, peripheral edema.*
GI: *nausea, vomiting.*
GU: impotence.
Musculoskeletal: transient bone pain (during first week of therapy), *decreased bone density.*
Respiratory: *pulmonary embolism.*
Skin: skin reactions at injection site.
Other: *hot flushes,* decreased libido, gynecomastia.

Interactions

None significant.

Effects on lab test results

• May increase BUN, creatinine, bilirubin, alkaline phosphatase, LDH, glucose, uric acid, albumin, calcium, phosphorus, total cholesterol, LDL, and triglyceride levels. May decrease potassium, HDL, and hemoglobin levels and hematocrit.
• May increase WBC count. May decrease PT, PTT, and RBC and platelet counts.
• May give inaccurate reading of pituitary gonadotropic and gonadal functions during therapy and for up to 12 weeks afterwards.

Pharmacokinetics

Absorption: Rapid and complete after subcutaneous use; unknown for I.M. use.

Distribution: Unknown; about 7% to 15% bound to proteins at therapeutic level.
Metabolism: Unknown.
Excretion: Unknown. *Half-life:* 3 hours.

Route	Onset	Peak	Duration
I.M., SubQ	Unknown	4 hr	1–3 mo
Implant	Unknown	4 hr	12 mo

Action

Chemical effect: Initially stimulates but then inhibits release of gonadotropin-releasing hormone, resulting in testosterone and estrogen suppression.
Therapeutic effect: Hinders prostatic cancer cell growth, eases signs and symptoms of endometriosis, and inhibits progression of puberty in children. Also decreases uterine and fibroid volume.

Available forms

Microspheres for injection, lyophilized: 3.75 mg, 7.5 mg, 11.25 mg, 15 mg, 22.5 mg, 30 mg
Implant: 72 mg
Injection: 5 mg/ml in 2.8-ml multiple-dose vial
Suspension for depot injection: 7.5 mg, 22.5 mg, 30 mg, 45 mg (single-use kit)

NURSING PROCESS

📋 **Assessment**
• Assess patient's condition before starting therapy and regularly thereafter to monitor the drug's effectiveness.
• Be alert for adverse reactions.
• Assess patient's and family's knowledge of drug therapy.

💠 **Nursing diagnoses**
• Ineffective health maintenance related to underlying condition
• Disturbed thought processes related to drug-induced depression
• Deficient knowledge related to drug therapy

▷ **Planning and implementation**
Ⓢ **ALERT:** Never give drug by I.V. injection.
Ⓢ **ALERT:** Different products have specific mixing and administration instructions. When using the two-syringe mixing system, after connecting the syringes, inject the liquid contents from syringe A into the powder in syringe B. Mix prod-

uct by pushing contents back and forth between syringes for about 45 seconds. (Shaking syringes won't provide adequate mixing.) The suspension will be colorless to pale yellow. The 7.5-mg suspension should be a light tan to tan color. Use immediately after mixing. Attach the needle provided in the kit and inject subcutaneously.

• Give once-monthly depot injection under medical supervision. Use supplied diluent to reconstitute. (Discard extra diluent that is provided.) Draw 1 ml into syringe with 22G needle. (When preparing Lupron Depot-3 Month 22.5 mg, use a 23G or larger needle.) Withdraw 1.5 ml from ampule for the 3-month formulation. Inject into vial and shake well. Suspension will appear milky. Although suspension is stable for 24 hours after reconstitution, it doesn't contain a bacteriostatic agent. Use immediately.

• When using prefilled dual-chamber syringes, screw white plunger into end stopper until stopper begins to turn. Remove and discard tab around base of needle. Hold syringe upright and release diluent by slowly pushing plunger until first stopper is at blue line in middle of barrel. Gently shake syringe to form a uniform milky suspension. If particles adhere to stopper, tap syringe. Remove needle guard and advance plunger to expel air from syringe. Inject entire contents I.M. as for a normal injection.

• Drug is a nonsurgical alternative to orchiectomy or estrogen therapy for advanced prostate cancer.

• The 12-month subcutaneous implant is surgically placed in the upper inner arm.

⑤ **ALERT:** A fractional dose of drug formulated to be given q 3 months isn't equivalent to same dose of once-monthly formulation.

Patient teaching

• Before starting therapy in child for central precocious puberty, make sure parents understand importance of continuous therapy.

• Carefully instruct patient who will give subcutaneous injection about proper administration technique, and advise him to use only syringes provided by manufacturer.

• Advise patient that if another syringe must be substituted, a low-dose insulin syringe (U-100, 0.5 ml) is acceptable.

• Advise patient to store drug at room temperature, protected from light and heat.

• Reassure patient with a history of undesirable effects from other endocrine therapies that this drug is much easier to tolerate. Tell patient that adverse effects are transient and will disappear after about 1 week.

• Warn patient that worsening of prostate cancer symptoms may occur when therapy starts.

• Instruct woman to have a bone-density evaluation before and after therapy. Recommend supplemental calcium to minimize bone loss.

☑ Evaluation

• Patient exhibits improvement in underlying condition.

• Patient demonstrates pretherapy thought processes.

• Patient and family state understanding of drug therapy.

levalbuterol hydrochloride
(leev-al-BYOO-teh-rohl high-droh-KLOR-ighd)
Xopenex, Xopenex HFA

Pharmacologic class: beta$_2$ agonist
Therapeutic class: bronchodilator
Pregnancy risk category: C

Indications and dosages

▶ **To prevent or treat bronchospasm in patients with reversible obstructive airway disease.** *Adults and children age 12 and older:* 0.63 mg (3 ml) solution for inhalation by nebulizer t.i.d. q 6 to 8 hours. Patients with more severe asthma who don't respond adequately to 0.63-mg doses may benefit from 1.25 mg t.i.d. *Children ages 6 to 11:* 0.31 mg given t.i.d. by nebulizer. Maximum dosage 0.63 mg t.i.d.

▶ **Treatment of acute episode of bronchospasm or prevention of asthmatic symptoms.** *Adults and children 4 and older:* 2 inhalations (90 mcg) q 4 to 6 hours. In some patients, 1 inhalation q 4 hours is sufficient.

Contraindications and cautions

• Contraindicated in patients hypersensitive to the drug or any of its components, or racemic albuterol.

• Use cautiously in patients with CV disorders, especially coronary insufficiency, hypertension, and arrhythmias. Also use cautiously in patients with seizure disorders, hyperthyroidism, or diabetes mellitus and in patients who are unusually responsive to sympathomimetic amines.

⚙ **Lifespan:** In pregnant women, use only when benefits outweigh risks to fetus. In breast-feeding women, use cautiously. In children younger than age 6 and patients age 65 and older, safety and effectiveness are unknown.

Adverse reactions

CNS: dizziness, migraine, nervousness, tremor, anxiety, pain, *headache.*
CV: tachycardia.
EENT: *rhinitis,* sinusitis, turbinate edema.
GI: dyspepsia.
Musculoskeletal: leg cramps.
Respiratory: increased cough, ***bronchospasm, asthma exacerbation.***
Other: flulike syndrome, accidental injury, *viral infection.*

Interactions

Drug-drug. *Beta blockers:* Blocks pulmonary effect of the drug and, possibly, causes severe bronchospasm. Don't use together. If drug is needed, a cardioselective beta blocker may be considered, but give it with caution.
Digoxin: Decreases digoxin levels up to 22%. Monitor digoxin level and monitor for loss of therapeutic effect.
Epinephrine, short-acting sympathomimetic aerosol bronchodilators: Increases adverse adrenergic effects. To avoid serious CV effects, use additional adrenergics with caution.
Loop and thiazide diuretics: Increases risk of ECG changes and hypokalemia. Use together cautiously; monitor cardiac condition and potassium level.
MAO inhibitors, tricyclic antidepressants: May increase levalbuterol action on the vascular system. Use caution when giving these drugs within 2 weeks of each other.

Effects on lab test results

None reported.

Pharmacokinetics

Absorption: Some.
Distribution: Unknown.
Metabolism: Unknown.
Excretion: Unknown. *Half-life:* 3¼ to 4 hours.

Route	Onset	Peak	Duration
Inhalation			
solution	10–17 min	90 min	5–8 hr
aerosol	Unknown	< 1 hr	Unknown

Action

Chemical effect: Activates beta$_2$ receptors on airway smooth muscle, which causes smooth muscle from trachea to terminal bronchioles to relax, relieving bronchospasm and reducing airway resistance. Inhibits the release of mediators from mast cells in the airway.
Therapeutic effect: Improves ventilation.

Available forms

Inhalation aerosol: 15 g containing 200 actuations
Solution for inhalation: 0.31 mg, 0.63 mg, or 1.25 mg in 3-ml vials

NURSING PROCESS

℞ Assessment
• Obtain history of patient's underlying condition before starting therapy, and reassess regularly thereafter to monitor the drug's effectiveness.
• Make sure that patient has a thorough physical examination before starting drug therapy.
• Be alert for adverse reactions and drug interactions.
• Assess patient's and family's knowledge of drug therapy.

🗲 Nursing diagnoses
• Impaired gas exchange related to underlying respiratory condition
• Risk for injury related to drug-induced adverse reactions
• Deficient knowledge related to drug therapy

❯ Planning and implementation
Ⓢ **ALERT:** Drug may produce life-threatening paradoxical bronchospasm. If this reaction occurs, immediately stop giving the drug and start alternative therapy.
• Rarely, drug may produce significant CV effects. If they occur, stop the drug.
• Compatibility, effectiveness, and safety of levalbuterol when mixed with other drugs in a nebulizer haven't been established.
Patient teaching
• Warn patient to stop taking the drug and notify prescriber if drug worsens breathing.
• Tell patient to call prescriber immediately if drug becomes less effective, if signs and symptoms worsen, or if drug is needed more often than usual.

L

• Urge patient not to increase the dose or frequency without consulting prescriber.
• Tell patient to prime the inhaler before first use or if it has not been used for more than 3 days. To prime inhaler, release 4 test sprays into the air away from the face.
• Tell patient to breathe as calmly, deeply, and evenly as possible until no more mist is formed in the nebulizer reservoir (5 to 15 minutes).
• Teach patient to correctly use and clean nebulizer unit.
• Tell patient that the drug's effects may last up to 8 hours.
• Urge patient to use other inhalations and anti-asthma drugs only as directed while taking this drug.
• Tell woman to notify prescriber if she becomes pregnant or intends to breast-feed.
• Tell patient to keep unopened vials in foil pouch. Once the foil pouch is opened, use vials within 2 weeks. Inform patient that vials removed from the pouch should be protected from light and heat and used within 1 week.

☑ **Evaluation**
• Patient's respiration improves.
• Patient doesn't experience injury from adverse reactions caused by drug.
• Patient and family state understanding of drug therapy.

levetiracetam
(leev-ah-tah-RACE-ah-tam)
Keppra

Pharmacologic class: pyrrolidine derivative
Therapeutic class: anticonvulsant
Pregnancy risk category: C

Indications and dosages

▶ **Adjunctive treatment of partial-onset seizures in epilepsy.** *Adults and adolescents 16 years and older:* Initially, 500 mg b.i.d. Increase dosage 500 mg b.i.d., p.r.n., for seizure control at 2-week intervals to maximum, 1,500 mg b.i.d.
Children age 4 to 16 years: 10 mg/kg P.O. b.i.d. Increase dose by 10 mg/kg b.i.d. at 2-week intervals to recommended dose of 30 mg/kg b.i.d. If patient can't tolerate this dose, it may be re-

duced. Patients who weigh 20 kg or less should use the oral solution.
◩ **Adjust-a-dose:** For adult patients with renal impairment, if creatinine clearance is greater than 80 ml/minute, give 500 to 1,500 mg q 12 hours; if clearance is 50 to 80 ml/minute, give 500 to 1,000 mg q 12 hours; if clearance is 30 to 50 ml/minute, give 250 to 750 mg q 12 hours; if clearance is less than 30 ml/minute, give 250 to 500 mg q 12 hours. For dialysis patients, give 500 to 1,000 mg q 24 hours. Give one dose of 250 to 500 mg after dialysis.

Contraindications and cautions

• Contraindicated in patients hypersensitive to the drug or any of its components.
• Use cautiously in immunocompromised patients and in those with poor renal function.
❦ **Lifespan:** In breast-feeding women, use cautiously; it isn't known if the drug appears in breast milk. In children younger than age 4, drug isn't indicated. In elderly patients, use cautiously because of their greater risk of falls.

Adverse reactions

CNS: *asthenia, headache, somnolence,* dizziness, depression, vertigo, paresthesia, nervousness, hostility, emotional lability, ataxia, amnesia, anxiety.
EENT: diplopia, pharyngitis, rhinitis, sinusitis.
GI: anorexia.
Hematologic: *leukopenia, neutropenia.*
Musculoskeletal: pain.
Respiratory: cough.
Other: infection.

Interactions

Drug-drug. *Antihistamines, benzodiazepines, opioids, tricyclic antidepressants, other drugs that cause drowsiness:* May lead to severe sedation. Avoid using together.
Carbamazepine, clozapine, and other drugs known to cause leukopenia or neutropenia: May increase the risk of infection. Monitor patient closely; monitor hematologic studies.
Drug-lifestyle. *Alcohol use:* Increases risk of severe sedation. Discourage using together.

Effects on lab test results

• May decrease WBC and neutrophil counts.

Pharmacokinetics

Absorption: Rapid. Level peaks in about 1 hour. When given with food, peak level is delayed by about 1½ hours and level will be slightly lower. Level reaches steady-state in about 2 days.
Distribution: Protein binding is minimal.
Metabolism: No active metabolites.
Excretion: About 66% of drug is unchanged by glomerular filtration and tubular reabsorption.
Half-life: About 7 hours in patients with normal renal function.

Route	Onset	Peak	Duration
P.O.	1 hr	1 hr	12 hr

Action

Chemical effect: May inhibit kindling in hippocampus, preventing simultaneous neuronal firing that leads to seizures.
Therapeutic effect: Prevents seizures.

Available forms

Oral solution: 100 mg/ml
Tablets: 250 mg, 500 mg, 750 mg

NURSING PROCESS

⚕ Assessment
● Obtain history of patient's underlying condition before starting therapy, and reassess regularly thereafter to monitor the drug's effectiveness.
● Assess renal function before starting therapy.
● Monitor patient closely for dizziness, which may lead to falls.
● Assess patient's and family's knowledge of drug therapy.

Nursing diagnoses
● Risk for trauma related to seizures.
● Risk for infection related to drug-induced leukopenia and neutropenia.
● Deficient knowledge related to drug therapy.

Planning and implementation
● Drug can be taken with or without food.
● Use drug only with other anticonvulsants. It isn't recommended for monotherapy.
● Taper drug to reduce the risk of seizures.
● **ALERT:** Don't confuse Keppra with Kaletra.

Patient teaching
● Tell patient to use a calibrated device for measuring a dose of oral solution; a household spoon is inadequate.
● Warn patient that drug may cause dizziness and somnolence and to use extra care when rising to a sitting or standing position to avoid becoming dizzy or falling; also to avoid driving, bike riding or other activities that may be hazardous until drugs effects are known.
● Advise patient to call prescriber, but not to abruptly stop taking drug, if an adverse reaction occurs.
● Tell patient to take drug with other prescribed seizure drugs.
● Inform patient that drug can be taken with or without food.

☑ Evaluation
● Patient is free from seizures.
● Patient doesn't develop infection.
● Patient and family state understanding of drug therapy.

levodopa
(lee-voh-DOH-puh)
Larodopa

Pharmacologic class: precursor of dopamine
Therapeutic class: antiparkinsonian
Pregnancy risk category: C

Indications and dosages

▶ **Idiopathic parkinsonism, postencephalitic parkinsonism, and symptomatic parkinsonism after carbon monoxide or manganese intoxication or with cerebral arteriosclerosis.**
Adults and children older than age 12: Initially, 0.5 to 1 g P.O. daily divided into two or more doses with food; increase by no more than 0.75 g daily q 3 to 7 days until daily dosage of 3 to 6 g is reached. Maximum, 8 g daily. Adjust dosage carefully to patient requirements, tolerance, and response. Closely supervise higher dosages.

Contraindications and cautions
● Contraindicated in patients hypersensitive to the drug or any of its components, in those who have taken an MAO inhibitor within 14 days,

and in those with acute angle-closure glaucoma, melanoma, or undiagnosed skin lesions.
• Use cautiously in patients with severe CV, renal, hepatic, or pulmonary disorders; peptic ulcer; psychiatric illness; MI with residual arrhythmias; bronchial asthma; emphysema; or endocrine disease.

⚙ **Lifespan:** In pregnant women, use cautiously; safety hasn't been established. In breastfeeding women, drug is contraindicated. In children age 12 and younger, safety and effectiveness haven't been established.

Adverse reactions

CNS: *aggressive behavior, abnormal movements (choreiform, dystonic, dyskinetic), involuntary grimacing and head movements, myoclonic body jerks,* **seizures,** *ataxia, tremor, muscle twitching, bradykinetic episodes, psychiatric disturbance, memory loss, mood changes, nervousness, anxiety, disturbing dreams, euphoria, malaise, fatigue, severe depression,* **suicidal tendencies,** *dementia, delirium, hallucinations.*
CV: *orthostatic hypotension,* cardiac irregularities, flushing, hypertension, phlebitis.
EENT: *blepharospasm,* blurred vision, diplopia, mydriasis or miosis, widening of palpebral fissures, activation of latent Horner's syndrome, oculogyric crises, nasal discharge.
GI: dry mouth, excessive salivation, bitter taste, *nausea, vomiting, anorexia,* constipation, flatulence, diarrhea, epigastric pain.
GU: urinary frequency, urine retention, incontinence, darkened urine, priapism.
Hematologic: hemolytic anemia, *leukopenia, agranulocytosis.*
Hepatic: *hepatotoxicity.*
Metabolic: weight loss.
Respiratory: hyperventilation, hiccups.
Other: dark perspiration, excessive and inappropriate sexual behavior.

Interactions

Drug-drug. *Antacids:* May increase levodopa absorption. Give antacids 1 hour after levodopa.
Anticholinergics: May increase gastric deactivation and decrease intestinal absorption of levodopa. Avoid using together.
Benzodiazepines: Levodopa's therapeutic value may be lessened. Monitor patient closely.
Furazolidone, procarbazine: May increase risk of severe hypertension. Avoid using together.

Inhaled halogen anesthetics, sympathomimetics: May increase risk of arrhythmias. Monitor ECG and vital signs closely.
MAO inhibitors (phenelzine, tranylcypromine): May cause a hypertensive reaction. Don't use together.
Metoclopramide: May accelerate gastric emptying of levodopa. Give metoclopramide 1 hour after levodopa.
Papaverine, phenothiazines and other antipsychotics, phenytoin, rauwolfia alkaloids: May decrease levodopa effect. Use together cautiously.
Pyridoxine (vitamin B₆): May decrease the effectiveness of levodopa. Avoid using together. (Pyridoxine has little to no effect on the combination drug levodopa and carbidopa.)
Tricyclic antidepressants: May delay absorption and decrease bioavailability of levodopa. Hypertensive episodes have occurred. Monitor patient closely.
Drug-herb. *Kava:* May interfere with drug and with natural dopamine, worsening symptoms of Parkinson's disease. Discourage using together.
Rauwolfia: May decrease effectiveness of levodopa. Discourage using together.
Drug-food. *Foods high in protein:* May decrease levodopa absorption. Don't give with high-protein foods.
Drug-lifestyle. *Cocaine:* May increase risk of arrhythmias. Inform patient of this interaction.

Effects on lab test results

• May increase BUN, ALT, AST, alkaline phosphatase, LDH, bilirubin, and uric acid levels. May decrease hemoglobin level and hematocrit.
• May decrease WBC and granulocyte counts.
• May falsely increase urine catecholamine level. May falsely decrease urine vanillylmandelic acid level. May cause false-positive Coombs' test or tests for urine glucose with reagents that use copper sulfate. May cause false-negative results with tests that use glucose enzymatic methods. May cause false-positive or false-negative tests for urine ketones and urine phenylketonuria.

Pharmacokinetics

Absorption: Rapid, by active amino acid transport system, with 30% to 50% reaching general circulation.

Distribution: Wide to most body tissues but not CNS, which receives less than 1% of dose because of extensive metabolism in periphery.
Metabolism: 95% of levodopa is converted to dopamine.
Excretion: Primarily in urine. *Half-life:* 1 to 3 hours.

Route	Onset	Peak	Duration
P.O.	Unknown	1–3 hr	About 5 hr but varies greatly

Action

Chemical effect: May be decarboxylated to dopamine, countering dopamine depletion in extrapyramidal centers.
Therapeutic effect: Improves voluntary movement.

Available forms

Capsules: 100 mg, 250 mg, 500 mg
Tablets: 100 mg, 250 mg, 500 mg

NURSING PROCESS

⚕ Assessment
• Assess patient's condition before starting therapy and regularly thereafter to monitor the drug's effectiveness.
• Observe and monitor vital signs, especially during dosage adjustments.
• Test patient receiving long-term therapy regularly for diabetes and acromegaly; periodically monitor kidney, liver, and hematopoietic function.
• Assess mental status before initiation of treatment and periodically thereafter.
• Be alert for adverse reactions and drug interactions.
• Assess patient's and family's knowledge of drug therapy.

⊕ Nursing diagnoses
• Impaired physical mobility related to presence of parkinsonism
• Disturbed thought processes related to drug-induced adverse reactions
• Deficient knowledge related to drug therapy

⊳ Planning and implementation
• To minimize GI upset, give drug with food but not a high-protein meal, which can impair absorption and reduce effectiveness.
• In a patient undergoing surgery, continue drug as long as oral intake is permitted, usually until 6 to 24 hours before surgery. Resume drug as soon as patient can take oral drug.
• Protect drug from heat, light, and moisture. If preparation darkens, discard because it has lost potency.
⊛ **ALERT:** Muscle twitching and eyelid twitching may be early signs of drug overdose. Report signs immediately.
• Reestablish effectiveness of lower dose by not giving the drug for a period of time (called a drug holiday). Because the drug holiday may cause symptoms that resemble neuroleptic malignant syndrome, observe patient when drug is abruptly stopped or the dose is abruptly lowered.

Patient teaching
• Advise patient to take drug with food, but not with high-protein meals. If patient has trouble swallowing pills, tell him or family member to crush tablets and mix with applesauce or baby food.
• Teach patient and family that behavioral or thought changes may occur and to report symptoms promptly for evaluation.
• Warn patient and family not to increase dose without prescriber's orders.
• Warn patient about dizziness and lightheadedness, especially at start of therapy. Tell patient to change positions slowly and dangle legs before getting out of bed. Elastic stockings may help control this reaction.
• Advise patient and family that multivitamin preparations, fortified cereals, and certain OTC drugs may contain pyridoxine (vitamin B_6), which can block effects of levodopa.
• Warn patient about risk of arrhythmias if he uses cocaine while taking drug.

☑ Evaluation
• Patient has improved physical mobility.
• Patient maintains normal thought process.
• Patient and family state understanding of drug therapy.

L

levodopa and carbidopa
(LEE-vuh-doh-puh and kar-bih-DOH-puh)
Sinemet, Sinemet CR

Pharmacologic class: dopamine precursor and decarboxylase inhibitor combination
Therapeutic class: antiparkinsonian
Pregnancy risk category: C

Indications and dosages

▶ **Idiopathic Parkinson's disease, postencephalitic parkinsonism, and symptomatic parkinsonism resulting from carbon monoxide or manganese intoxication.** *Adults:* 1 tablet of 100 mg levodopa and 25 mg carbidopa or 1 tablet of 100 mg levodopa and 10 mg carbidopa P.O. t.i.d. followed by increase of 1 tablet daily or q other day p.r.n.; maximum daily, 8 tablets. Substitute 250 mg levodopa and 25 mg carbidopa or 100 mg levodopa and 10 mg carbidopa tablets as required. Determine optimum daily dosage by carefully adjusting dosage for each patient. Patients taking conventional tablets may receive extended-release tablets; dosage is calculated on current levodopa intake. Initially, give extended-release tablets equal to 10% more levodopa per day, increase as needed and tolerated to 30% more levodopa per day. Give in divided doses at intervals of 4 to 8 hours.

Contraindications and cautions

• Contraindicated in patients hypersensitive to drugs or any of its components; in patients with acute angle-closure glaucoma, melanoma, or undiagnosed skin lesions; and within 14 days of MAO inhibitor therapy.
• Use cautiously in patients with severe CV, renal, hepatic, endocrine, or pulmonary disorders; history of peptic ulcer; psychiatric illness; MI with residual arrhythmias; bronchial asthma; emphysema; or well-controlled, chronic, open-angle glaucoma.
❀ **Lifespan:** In pregnant women, use cautiously. In breast-feeding women, drug combination is contraindicated. In children, safety and effectiveness haven't been established.

Adverse reactions

CNS: *abnormal movements (choreiform, dystonic, dyskinetic), involuntary grimacing, head movements, myoclonic body jerks, ataxia,* tremors, muscle twitching, bradykinetic episodes, psychiatric disturbances, memory loss, nervousness, anxiety, disturbing dreams, euphoria, malaise, fatigue, *severe depression, suicidal tendencies,* dementia, delirium, hallucinations.
CV: orthostatic hypotension, *cardiac irregularities,* flushing, hypertension.
EENT: *blepharospasm,* blurred vision, diplopia, mydriasis or miosis, widening of palpebral fissures, activation of latent Horner's syndrome, oculogyric crises, nasal discharge, excessive salivation.
GI: dry mouth, bitter taste, nausea, vomiting, anorexia, and weight loss at start of therapy; constipation; flatulence; diarrhea; epigastric pain.
GU: urinary frequency, urine retention, urinary incontinence, darkened urine, priapism.
Hematologic: hemolytic anemia.
Hepatic: *hepatotoxicity.*
Respiratory: hyperventilation, hiccups.
Skin: dark perspiration, phlebitis.
Other: excessive and inappropriate sexual behavior.

Interactions

Drug-drug. *Antacids:* May increase absorption of levodopa components. Monitor patient closely.
Antihypertensives: May have additive hypotensive effects. Use together cautiously; monitor blood pressure.
Iron salts: May decrease bioavailability of levodopa and carbidopa. Give iron 1 hour before or 2 hours after giving levodopa and carbidopa.
MAO inhibitors: May increase risk of severe hypertension. Don't use together.
Papaverine, phenytoin: May antagonize antiparkinsonian. Avoid using together.
Phenothiazines, other antipsychotics: May antagonize antiparkinsonian. Use together cautiously; monitor for decreased effect.
Drug-herb. *Kava:* May interfere with action of levodopa and natural dopamine, worsening Parkinson's symptoms. Discourage using together.
Octacosanol: May worsen dyskinesia. Discourage using together.
Drug-food. *Foods high in protein:* May decrease absorption of levodopa. Warn against taking drug with high-protein foods.

Reactions may be *common*, uncommon, *life-threatening*, or COMMON AND LIFE-THREATENING.

Effects on lab test results

• May decrease hemoglobin level and hematocrit.
• May decrease platelet, granulocyte, and WBC counts.
• May falsely increase levels of uric acid, urine ketones, urine catecholamines, and urine vanillylmandelic acid, depending on reagent and test method used.

Pharmacokinetics

Absorption: 40% to 70%.
Distribution: Wide to most body tissues, except CNS.
Metabolism: For carbidopa, not extensive. It inhibits levodopa, increasing its own absorption.
Excretion: 30% unchanged in urine within 24 hours. When given with carbidopa, amount of levodopa unchanged in urine is increased by about 6%. *Half-life:* 1 to 2 hours.

Route	Onset	Peak	Duration
P.O.			
regular-release	Unknown	40 min	Unknown
extended-release	Unknown	2½ hr	Unknown

Action

Chemical effect: Unknown for levodopa. May be decarboxylated to dopamine, countering depletion of striatal dopamine in extrapyramidal centers. Carbidopa inhibits peripheral decarboxylation of levodopa without affecting levodopa's metabolism within CNS, making more levodopa available to be decarboxylated to dopamine in brain.
Therapeutic effect: Improves voluntary movement.

Available forms

Tablets: carbidopa 10 mg with levodopa 100 mg (Sinemet 10-100), carbidopa 25 mg with levodopa 100 mg (Sinemet 25-100), carbidopa 25 mg with levodopa 250 mg (Sinemet 25-250)
Tablets (extended-release): carbidopa 25 mg with levodopa 100 mg, carbidopa 50 mg with levodopa 200 mg (Sinemet CR)
Tablets (orally disintegrating): carbidopa 10 mg with levodopa 100 mg, carbidopa 25 mg with levodopa 100 mg, carbidopa 25 mg with levodopa 250 mg

NURSING PROCESS

⚕ Assessment

• Assess patient's underlying condition before therapy and regularly thereafter. Therapeutic response usually follows each dose, disappears within 5 hours, and may vary considerably.
• Be alert for adverse reactions and drug interactions.
⚠ **ALERT:** Immediately report muscle twitching and blepharospasm, which may be early signs of drug overdose.
• Test patients receiving long-term therapy regularly for diabetes and acromegaly and perform periodic tests of liver, renal, and hematopoietic function.
• Assess patient's and family's knowledge of drug therapy.

⊕ Nursing diagnoses

• Impaired physical mobility related to underlying parkinsonian syndrome
• Disturbed thought processes related to drug-induced CNS adverse reactions
• Deficient knowledge related to drug therapy

▶ Planning and implementation

• If patient is being treated with levodopa only, stop that drug at least 8 hours before starting levodopa and carbidopa combination.
• Give drug with food to minimize adverse GI reactions.
• Adjust dosage according to patient's response and tolerance.
• If vital signs or mental condition change significantly, don't give drug. Notify the prescriber, and then lower the dose or stop giving the drug.
• Treat patient with open-angle glaucoma with caution. Monitor patient closely. Watch for change in intraocular pressure and arrange for periodic eye exams.
Patient teaching
• Caution patient and family not to increase dose without consulting the prescriber.
• Warn patient of dizziness and orthostatic hypotension, especially at start of therapy. Tell patient to change positions slowly and to dangle legs before getting out of bed. Elastic stockings may control this adverse reaction.
• Teach patient and family that behavioral or thought changes may occur and to report symptoms promptly for evaluation.

L

Rapid onset   *Liquid form contains alcohol.   ♦ Canada   ◇ Australia   †OTC   ✐Photoguide   ‡Off-label use

• Instruct patient to report adverse reactions and therapeutic effects.

• Inform patient that pyridoxine (vitamin B₆) doesn't reverse beneficial effects of levodopa and carbidopa. Multivitamins can be taken without decreased drug effectiveness.

☑ Evaluation

• Patient exhibits improved mobility with reduction of muscular rigidity and tremor.

• Patient remains mentally alert.

• Patient and family state understanding of drug therapy.

levodopa, carbidopa, and entacapone
(LEE-vuh-doh-puh, kar-bih-DOH-puh, and en-TAH-kah-pohn)
Stalevo 50, Stalevo 100, Stalevo 150

Pharmacologic class: dopamine precursor, decarboxylase inhibitor, and catechol-O-methyltransferase (COMT) inhibitor
Therapeutic class: antiparkinsonian
Pregnancy risk category: C

Indications and dosages

▶ **Idiopathic parkinsonism.** *Adults:* Individualize and carefully adjust the optimum daily dosage according to response. For maintenance therapy, reduce the total daily dosage by either decreasing the strength of this drug or by decreasing the frequency by extending the time between doses. When more levodopa is required, give the next higher strength of this drug or increase the frequency to maximum, eight doses daily without exceeding the maximum daily dosage.

Contraindications and cautions

• Contraindicated in patients hypersensitive to drug or any of its components, and in patients with angle-closure glaucoma, suspicious undiagnosed skin lesions, or a history of melanoma. Also contraindicated within 14 days of MAO inhibitor therapy. If the intraocular pressure is well controlled, patients with chronic open-angle glaucoma may use drug.

• Use cautiously in patients with liver, renal, or endocrine disease or biliary obstruction. Also

use cautiously in patients with past or current psychosis, severe CV or pulmonary disease, bronchial asthma, or history of MI with residual arrhythmias.

⚖ **Lifespan:** In pregnant women, use only if benefits outweigh risks to the fetus. In breastfeeding women, use cautiously. In children, safety and effectiveness haven't been established.

Adverse reactions

CNS: hallucinations, agitation, anxiety, asthenia, dizziness, *dyskinesia*, fatigue, *hyperkinesia*, hypokinesia, ***neuroleptic malignant syndrome***, somnolence, syncope.
CV: hypotension, chest pain.
GI: *nausea, diarrhea*, abdominal pain, constipation, vomiting, dry mouth, dyspepsia, flatulence, gastritis, gastrointestinal disorder, taste disorder.
GU: urine discoloration, ***nephrotoxicity***.
Hematologic: anemia, ***agranulocytosis, thrombocytopenia, leukopenia***.
Musculoskeletal: back pain.
Respiratory: dyspnea.
Skin: sweating.
Other: bacterial infection.

Interactions

Drug-drug. *Antihypertensives:* May cause postural hypotension. Adjust antihypertensive dose, p.r.n.
Dopamine D₂-receptor antagonists (such as butyrophenones, isoniazid, metoclopramide, phenothiazines, and risperidone): May reduce therapeutic effects of levodopa. Avoid using together.
Drugs metabolized by COMT, such as alphamethyldopa, apomorphine, bitolterol, dobutamine, dopamine, epinephrine, isoetharine, isoproterenol, and norepinephrine: May increase heart rate, arrhythmias, and excessive changes in blood pressure. Use together cautiously.
Drugs that interfere with biliary excretion, glucuronidation, and intestinal beta-glucuronidase, including probenecid, cholestyramine, and some antibiotics (ampicillin, chloramphenicol, erythromycin, rifampicin): May interfere with entacapone excretion. Use together cautiously.
Hydantoin, papaverine: May reduce the effects of levodopa. Avoid using together.

Iron salts: May reduce the bioavailability of drug. Adjust dose p.r.n.

Metoclopramide: May increase bioavailability of carbidopa and levodopa by increasing gastric emptying. Adjust dose p.r.n.

Nonselective MAO inhibitors: May cause a hypertensive reaction. Don't use within 14 days of each other.

Selegiline: May cause severe hypotension. Avoid using together.

Tricyclic antidepressants: May cause hypertension and dyskinesia. Use together cautiously.

Drug-food. *Foods high in protein, such as legumes, red meat, and liquid protein shakes:* May delay and reduce the absorption of levodopa. Give drug on an empty stomach.

Effects on lab test results

• May increase growth hormone level. May decrease prolactin level. May increase or decrease BUN and bilirubin levels.

• May increase liver function test values.

• May cause a false-positive Coombs' test. May cause a false-positive reaction for urinary ketone bodies when using a test tape.

Pharmacokinetics

Absorption: Varies. Carbidopa level peaks within 2½ to 3½ hours. Levodopa level peaks in 1 to 1½ hours. Entacapone level peaks within 1½ hours.

Distribution: Levodopa and carbidopa are minimally bound to protein. Entacapone is 98% bound to albumin.

Metabolism: Carbidopa is metabolized to two main metabolites. Levodopa is extensively metabolized to various metabolites. Entacapone is almost completely metabolized.

Excretion: Carbidopa, primarily in urine unchanged; entacapone, 10% in urine, 90% in feces; levodopa, unknown. *Half-life:* 1½ to 2 hours carbidopa, 1 to 5 hours levodopa, and 1 to 4 hours entacapone.

Route	Onset	Peak	Duration
P.O.	< 1 hr	1–1½ hr	Unknown

Action

Chemical effect: Levodopa, a dopamine precursor, converts to dopamine in the brain. Carbidopa inhibits the decarboxylation of peripheral levodopa. When given with levodopa, carbidopa permits more intact levodopa to be transported into the brain. Entacapone is a selective and reversible inhibitor of COMT.

Therapeutic effect: Decreases symptoms of Parkinson's disease.

Available forms

Tablets: 12.5 mg carbidopa, 50 mg levodopa, and 200 mg entacapone (Stalevo 50); 25 mg carbidopa, 100 mg levodopa, and 200 mg entacapone Stalevo 100); 37.5 mg carbidopa, 150 mg levodopa, and 200 mg entacapone (Stalevo 150)

NURSING PROCESS

✍ Assessment

• Periodically evaluate hepatic, hematopoietic, CV, and renal function.

• Monitor patient for mental disturbances such as hallucinations or depression with suicidal tendencies.

• Be alert for adverse reactions and interactions.

• Assess patient's and family's knowledge of drug therapy.

📋 Nursing diagnoses

• Impaired physical mobility related to underlying parkinsonism

• Risk for injury related to drug-induced adverse reactions

• Deficient knowledge related to drug therapy

▶ Planning and implementation

• Patients taking 200-mg entacapone tablet with each dose of standard-release levodopa and carbidopa can be switched to the corresponding strength of this drug containing the same amount of levodopa and carbidopa.

• Patients who experience signs and symptoms of end-of-dose "wearing off" on standard-release levodopa and carbidopa and have a history of moderate or severe dyskinesia, or take more than 600 mg of levodopa per day are likely to require a reduction in daily levodopa dose when entacapone is added. Adjust dose with levodopa and carbidopa (1:4 ratio) and entacapone, then transfer to a corresponding dose of this drug once the patient is stabilized.

• Don't cut or break tablets.

• If dyskinesia occurs, reduce dose.

⚠ ALERT: If abruptly reducing or stopping drug, especially in a patient also taking an antipsychotic, observe him carefully for a syndrome resembling neuroleptic malignant syndrome: elevated temperature, muscle rigidity, involuntary movements, altered consciousness, confusion, tachycardia, tachypnea, sweating, hypertension or hypotension, leukocytosis, myoglobinuria, and increased myoglobin level.

⚠ **ALERT:** Check for overdose by monitoring respiratory, renal, and CV functions. Use supportive measures along with repeated doses of charcoal over time. Also give I.V. fluids and ensure adequate airway.

Patient teaching

• Advise patient to take drug on an empty stomach preferably, or at least not with high-protein meals or drinks.

• Tell patient to take drug exactly as prescribed.

• Tell patient not to cut or break tablets.

• Warn patient of adverse reactions, such as hallucinations, diarrhea, nausea, and discolored urine, and instruct him to notify prescriber if they occur.

• Instruct patient to notify prescriber of any and all drugs taken to prevent any drug interactions.

☑ Evaluation

• Patient has improved physical mobility.

• Patient doesn't suffer any injury from adverse reactions.

• Patient and family state understanding of drug therapy.

levofloxacin
(lee-voh-FLOCKS-uh-sihn)
Levaquin◆

Pharmacologic class: fluorinated carboxyquinolone
Therapeutic class: broad-spectrum antibiotic
Pregnancy risk category: C

Indications and dosages

▶ **Acute bacterial sinusitis caused by susceptible strains of** *Streptococcus pneumoniae, Moraxella catarrhalis,* **or** *Haemophilus influenzae. Adults:* 500 mg P.O. or I.V. daily for 10 to 14 days; or, 750 mg P.O. or I.V. daily for 5 days.

▶ **Acute bacterial exacerbation of chronic bronchitis caused by** *Staphylococcus aureus, S. pneumoniae, M. catarrhalis,* **or** *H. influen-*

zae **or** *parainfluenzae. Adults:* 500 mg P.O. or I.V. daily for 7 days.

▶ **Community-acquired pneumonia caused by** *S. pneumoniae* **resistant to two or more of the following antibiotics: penicillin, second-generation cephalosporins, macrolides, tetracyclines, trimethoprim, and sulfamethoxazole; or by** *S. aureus, M. catarrhalis, H. influenzae, H. parainfluenzae, Klebsiella pneumoniae, Chlamydia pneumoniae, Legionella pneumophila, Mycoplasma pneumoniae,* **or** *S. pneumoniae. Adults:* 500 mg P.O. or I.V. daily for 7 to 14 days. Or, 750 mg P.O. or I.V. once daily for 5 days (not for multidrug-resistant *S. pneumoniae*).

▶ **Mild to moderate skin and skin-structure infections caused by** *S. aureus* **or** *Streptococcus pyogenes. Adults:* 500 mg P.O. or I.V. daily for 7 to 10 days.

▶ **Chronic bacterial prostatitis caused by** *E. coli, E. faecalis,* **or** *Staphylococcus epidermidis. Adults:* 500 mg P.O. or I.V. daily for 28 days.

▶ **Prevention of inhalation anthrax following confirmed or suspected exposure to** *Bacillus anthracis. Adults:* 500 mg I.V. or P.O. q 24 hours for 60 days.

☒ **Adjust-a-dose:** For patients with renal impairment, if creatinine clearance is 20 to 49 ml/minute, give initial dose of 500 mg and then 250 mg once daily; or (if not treating multidrug-resistant *S. pneumoniae*), give 750 mg initially and then 750 mg q 48 hours. If clearance is 10 to 19 ml/minute, initial dose is 500 mg and then 250 mg q 48 hours; or give 750 mg initially and then 500 mg q 48 hours. For patients on hemodialysis or chronic ambulatory peritoneal dialysis, give initial dose of 500 mg and then 250 mg q 48 hours; or give 750 mg initially and then 500 mg q 48 hours.

▶ **Complicated skin and skin structure infections caused by methicillin-sensitive** *S. aureus, E. faecalis, S. pyogenes, P. mirabilis;* **nosocomial pneumonia caused by methicillin-susceptible** *S. aureus, P. aeruginosa, Serratia marcescens, E. coli, K. pneumoniae, H. influenzae,* **or** *S. pneumoniae. Adults:* 750 mg P.O or I.V. daily for 7 to 14 days.

☒ **Adjust-a-dose:** For patients with renal impairment, if creatinine clearance is 20 to 49 ml/minute, give 750 mg initially and then 750 mg q 48 hours, If clearance is 10 to 19 ml/minute or patient is on hemodialysis or chronic ambulatory peritoneal dialysis, give 750 mg initially and then 500 mg q 48 hours.

► **Mild to moderate UTI caused by** *Enterococcus faecalis, Enterobacter cloacae, E. coli, K. pneumoniae, Proteus mirabilis,* **or** *Pseudomonas aeruginosa. Adults:* 250 mg P.O. or I.V. daily for 10 days.

► **Mild to moderate acute pyelonephritis caused by** *E. coli. Adults:* 250 mg P.O. or I.V. daily for 10 days.

🔲 **Adjust-a-dose:** For patients with renal impairment, if creatinine clearance is 10 to 19 ml/minute, give 250 mg initially and then 250 mg q 48 hours.

► **Mild to moderate uncomplicated UTI caused by** *Escherichia coli, K. pneumoniae,* **or** *Staphylococcus saprophyticus. Adults:* 250 mg P.O. daily for 3 days.

► **Traveler's diarrhea‡.** *Adults:* 500 mg P.O. as a single dose with loperamide hydrochloride.

► **To prevent traveler's diarrhea‡.** *Adults:* 500 mg P.O. daily during period of risk, for up to 3 weeks.

► **Uncomplicated cervical, urethral, or rectal gonorrhea‡.** *Adults and adolescents:* 250 mg P.O. as a single dose.

► **Disseminated gonococcal infection‡.** *Adults and adolescents:* 250 mg I.V. daily and continue for 24 to 48 hours after improvement begins. Switch to 500 mg P.O. daily to complete at least 1 week of therapy.

► **Nongonococcal urethritis; urogenital chlamydial infections‡.** *Adults and adolescents:* 500 mg P.O. daily for 7 days.

► **Acute pelvic inflammatory disease‡.** *Adults and adolescents:* 500 mg I.V. daily with or without metronidazole 500 mg q 8 hours. Stop parenteral drug 24 hours after improvement; then begin 100 mg P.O. b.i.d. of doxycycline to complete 14 days of therapy. Or give 500 mg P.O. levofloxacin daily for 14 days with or without metronidazole 500 mg b.i.d. for 14 days.

▽ I.V. administration

• Dilute in single-use vials with D_5W or normal saline solution for injection to a final concentration of 5 mg/ml.

• Make sure reconstituted solution is clear, slightly yellow, and free of particulates.

• Give only by I.V. infusion over 60 minutes for 500 mg or 90 minutes for 750 mg.

• Diluted solution is stable for 72 hours at room temperature, 14 days when refrigerated in plastic containers, and 6 months when frozen. Thaw at room temperature or in refrigerator.

⊗ **Incompatibilities**
Mannitol 20%, multivalent cations (such as magnesium), sodium bicarbonate 5%. Don't mix drug with other drugs.

Contraindications and cautions

• Contraindicated in patients hypersensitive to the drug or any of its components, or other fluoroquinolones.

⚘ **Lifespan:** In pregnant women, use only when benefits outweigh risks to the fetus. Breast-feeding women should either stop breast-feeding or use another drug. In children, safety and effectiveness haven't been established. In elderly patients with renal impairment, adjust dose.

Adverse reactions

CNS: headache, insomnia, dizziness, *encephalopathy,* paresthesia, pain, *seizures.*
CV: chest pain, palpitations, vasodilation, abnormal ECG.
GI: nausea, diarrhea, constipation, vomiting, abdominal pain, dyspepsia, flatulence, *pseudomembranous colitis.*
GU: vaginitis.
Hematologic: eosinophilia, hemolytic anemia, *lymphocytopenia.*
Metabolic: *hypoglycemia.*
Musculoskeletal: back pain, tendon rupture.
Respiratory: allergic pneumonitis.
Skin: rash, photosensitivity reactions, pruritus, *erythema multiforme, Stevens-Johnson syndrome.*
Other: hypersensitivity reactions, *anaphylaxis, multisystem organ failure.*

Interactions

Drug-drug. *Aluminum hydroxide, aluminum-magnesium hydroxide, calcium carbonate, magnesium hydroxide:* May decrease effects of levofloxacin. Give antacid at least 6 hours before or 2 hours after levofloxacin.
Antidiabetics: May alter glucose levels. Monitor them closely.
Iron salts: May decrease absorption of levofloxacin, reducing anti-infective response. Give at least 2 hours apart.
NSAIDs: May increase CNS stimulation. Monitor patient for seizures.

L

Sucralfate, zinc-containing products: May interfere with GI absorption of levofloxacin. Give at least 2 hours apart.
Theophylline: May decrease theophylline clearance with some fluoroquinolones. Monitor theophylline levels.
Warfarin: May enhance anticoagulant effects. Monitor PT and INR closely.
Drug-lifestyle. *Sun exposure:* May cause photosensitivity reactions. Urge patient to avoid unprotected or prolonged exposure to sunlight.

Effects on lab test results

- May decrease glucose and hemoglobin levels and hematocrit.
- May increase eosinophil count. May decrease WBC and lymphocyte counts.
- May cause false-positive opiate assay results.

Pharmacokinetics

Absorption: Rapid and complete.
Distribution: Wide.
Metabolism: Limited.
Excretion: Primarily unchanged in the urine. *Half-life:* About 6 to 8 hours.

Route	Onset	Peak	Duration
P.O.	Unknown	1–2 hr	30–36 hr
I.V.	immediate	1–1½ hr	30–36 hr

Action

Chemical effect: Inhibits bacterial DNA gyrase and prevents DNA replication, transcription, repair, and recombination in susceptible bacteria.
Therapeutic effect: Kills susceptible bacteria.

Available forms

Infusion (premixed): 250 mg in 50 ml D_5W, 500 mg in 100 ml D_5W, 750 mg in 150 ml D_5W (5 mg/ml)
Single-use vials: 500 mg, 750 mg (25 mg/ml)
Tablets: 250 mg, 500 mg, 750 mg
Oral solution: 25 mg/ml

NURSING PROCESS

Assessment

- Obtain specimen for culture and sensitivity tests before starting therapy and as needed to detect bacterial resistance. Therapy may begin pending results.
- Obtain history of seizure disorders or other CNS diseases, such as cerebral arteriosclerosis, before starting therapy.
- Monitor glucose level and renal, hepatic, and hematopoietic blood studies.
- Assess patient's and family's knowledge of drug therapy.

Nursing diagnoses

- Risk for infection related to presence of bacteria susceptible to drug
- Risk for deficient fluid volume related to drug-induced adverse GI reactions
- Deficient knowledge related to drug therapy

Planning and implementation

- Give oral drugs with plenty of fluids.
- Oral solution should be taken 1 hour before or 2 hours after eating.
- P.O. and I.V. dosages are interchangeable. The oral solution has the same effectiveness as the tablet formulation and provides flexible form needed by patients with renal impairment.

ALERT: If *P. aeruginosa* is or is suspected to be the cause, give combination therapy with an antipseudomonal beta-lactam.

- Treat acute hypersensitivity reactions with epinephrine, oxygen, I.V. fluids, antihistamines, corticosteroids, pressor amines, and airway management.
- If patient has symptoms of excessive CNS stimulation (restlessness, tremor, confusion, hallucinations), stop drug and notify prescriber. Take seizure precautions.
- Most antibacterials can cause pseudomembranous colitis. If diarrhea occurs, notify prescriber. If symptoms are severe or unrelieved by appropriate treatment, stop giving the drug.

Patient teaching

- Tell patient to take drug as prescribed, even if symptoms resolve.
- Advise patient to take drug with plenty of fluids and to avoid antacids, sucralfate, and products containing iron or zinc for at least 2 hours before and after each dose.
- Warn patient to avoid hazardous tasks until the drug's CNS effects are known.
- Advise patient to avoid excessive sunlight, use sunblock, and wear protective clothing when outdoors.
- Instruct patient to stop taking the drug and notify prescriber if rash or other signs or symptoms of hypersensitivity develop.

• Tell patient to notify prescriber if he experiences pain or inflammation; tendon rupture can occur with drug.
• Instruct diabetic patient to monitor glucose level and notify prescriber if a hypoglycemic reaction occurs; may need to stop drug.
• Instruct patient to notify prescriber about loose stools or diarrhea.

☑ Evaluation
• Patient is free from infection after drug therapy.
• Patient maintains adequate hydration throughout drug therapy.
• Patient and family state understanding of drug therapy.

levothyroxine sodium (T₄, L-thyroxine sodium)

levothyroxine sodium (T_4, L-thyroxine sodium)
(lee-voh-thigh-ROKS-een SOH-dee-um)
Eltroxin ◆, Levo-T, Levothroid, Levoxine, Levoxyl◊, Oroxine◇, Synthroid, Thyro-Tabs, Unithroid

Pharmacologic class: thyroid hormone
Therapeutic class: thyroid hormone replacement
Pregnancy risk category: A

Indications and dosages

▶ Myxedema coma. *Adults:* 300 to 500 mcg I.V., followed by parenteral maintenance dosage of 75 to 100 mcg I.V. daily. Switch patient to oral maintenance as soon as possible.
▶ Thyroid hormone replacement. *Adults:* Initially, 25 to 50 mcg P.O. daily; increase by 25 mcg P.O. q 4 to 8 weeks until desired response occurs. Maintenance dosage is 75 to 200 mcg P.O. daily.
Children older than age 12: More than 150 mcg or 2 to 3 mcg/kg P.O. daily.
Children ages 6 to 12: 100 to 150 mcg or 4 to 5 mcg/kg P.O. daily.
Children ages 1 to 5: 75 to 100 mcg or 5 to 6 mcg/kg P.O. daily.
Children ages 6 months to 1 year: 50 to 75 mcg or 6 to 8 mcg/kg P.O. daily.
Children younger than age 6 months: 25 to 50 mcg or 8 to 10 mcg/kg P.O. daily.

Patients older than age 65: 12.5 to 50 mcg P.O. daily; increase by 12.5 to 25 mcg q 6 to 8 weeks, depending on response.

▼ I.V. administration
• Don't confuse mg with mcg dosage (1 mg = 1,000 mcg).
• Initial I.V. dose is about half the previously established oral dose of tablets when used for maintenance of euthyroid state.
• Prepare dose immediately before injection. Dilute powder for injection with 5 ml of normal saline solution for injection or bacteriostatic saline solution injection with benzyl alcohol to 200- or 500-mcg vial; don't use other diluents. Resulting solutions contain 40 or 100 mcg/ml, respectively.
• Inject into vein over 1 to 2 minutes.
• Monitor blood pressure and heart rate closely. High initial dosage is usually tolerated by patients in myxedema coma. Normal levels of T_4 occur within 24 hours, followed by a threefold increase in T_3 in 3 days.
⊗ Incompatibilities
Other I.V. solutions.

Contraindications and cautions

• Contraindicated in patients hypersensitive to the drug or any of its components, and in patients with acute MI uncomplicated by hypothyroidism, untreated thyrotoxicosis, or uncorrected adrenal insufficiency.
• Use cautiously in patients with angina pectoris, hypertension, other CV disorders, renal insufficiency, or ischemia. Also use cautiously in patients with diabetes mellitus, diabetes insipidus, myxedema, or dysphagia.
• Use cautiously in patients with arteriosclerosis. Rapid replacement in these patients may precipitate angina, coronary occlusion, or stroke.
⚖ Lifespan: In breast-feeding women, use cautiously; it's unknown if the drug appears in breast milk. Children typically need a higher dose than adults. Adults older than age 60 typically need a lower dose than younger adults.

Adverse reactions

CNS: fever, headache, *nervousness, insomnia, tremor.*
CV: tachycardia, palpitations, *arrhythmias,* angina pectoris, hypertension, *cardiac arrest.*

GI: appetite change, nausea, diarrhea; choking, gagging, or dysphagia, particularly when not taken with fluids.
GU: menstrual irregularities.
Metabolic: weight loss.
Musculoskeletal: leg cramps.
Skin: diaphoresis.
Other: heat intolerance.

Interactions

Drug-drug. *Cholestyramine, colestipol:* May impair levothyroxine absorption. Separate doses by 4 to 5 hours.
Insulin, oral antidiabetics: May increase glucose level. Monitor glucose level when starting or changing dosage and adjust dosage p.r.n.
I.V. phenytoin: May release free thyroid. Monitor patient for tachycardia.
Oral anticoagulants: May increase PT. Decrease anticoagulants by about one-third when initiating thyroid replacement therapy, monitor PT and INR, and adjust dosage to desired range, if needed.
Sympathomimetics (such as epinephrine): May increase risk of coronary insufficiency. Monitor patient closely.

Effects on lab test results

None reported.

Pharmacokinetics

Absorption: Good.
Distribution: Wide; 99% protein-bound.
Metabolism: Primarily in liver, kidneys, and intestines.
Excretion: 20% to 40% in feces. *Half-life:* 3 to 4 days in hyperthyroidism, 9 to 10 days in hypothyroidism.

Route	Onset	Peak	Duration
P.O. I.V., I.M.	24 hr	Unknown	Unknown

Action

Chemical effect: Not fully defined; stimulates metabolism by accelerating cellular oxidation.
Therapeutic effect: Raises thyroid hormone levels in body.

Available forms

Powder for injection: 200 mcg/vial, 500 mcg/vial

Tablets: 0.025 mg, 0.05 mg, 0.075 mg, 0.088 mg, 0.1 mg, 0.112 mg, 0.125 mg, 0.137 mg, 0.15 mg, 0.175 mg, 0.2 mg, 0.3 mg

NURSING PROCESS

🝖 Assessment

• Assess patient's condition before starting therapy, and regularly thereafter to monitor the drug's effectiveness. Monitor TSH monthly until stable, then yearly if asymptomatic.
• Be alert for adverse reactions and drug interactions.
• In patient with coronary artery disease who must receive thyroid hormone, monitor carefully for coronary insufficiency.
• Assess patient for swallowing difficulties before giving the drug. Advise all patients to take tablet with water.
• Assess patient's and family's knowledge of drug therapy.

🔷 Nursing diagnoses

• Ineffective health maintenance related to presence of hypothyroidism
• Risk for injury related to drug-induced adverse reactions
• Deficient knowledge related to drug therapy

▶ Planning and implementation

ⓢ **ALERT:** Doses of alternative brands of thyroid replacement drugs may not be equivalent, particularly between levothyroxine sodium (synthetic T_4), liothyronine (synthetic T_3), and thyroid hormone from animals (Armour thyroid, desiccated thyroid).
• Thyroid hormone replacement requirements are about 25% lower in patients older than age 60 than in younger adults.
• I.M. use is generally not recommended because of variable absorption and difficulty regulating dose.
• Patients with adult hypothyroidism are unusually sensitive to thyroid hormone. Start patient at lowest dose and adjust to higher dose until reaching a euthyroid state based on symptoms and laboratory data.
• When changing from levothyroxine to liothyronine, stop levothyroxine then begin liothyronine at a low dose. Increase liothyronine dose in small increments after residual effects of levothyroxine disappear. When changing from liothyronine to levothyroxine, to avoid relapse

---

start levothyroxine several days before stopping liothyronine.

• Thyroid hormones alter thyroid non-serum test results. Stop drug 4 weeks before test.

• In patient taking a prescribed anticoagulant with thyroid hormones, lower the dose of anticoagulant if needed.

⑨ **ALERT:** Don't confuse levothyroxine sodium with liothyronine sodium or liotrix.

Patient teaching

• Stress importance of compliance. Tell patient to take thyroid hormones at same time each day, preferably 30 to 60 minutes before breakfast, to maintain constant hormone levels, prevent insomnia, and increase absorption.

• Instruct patient (especially an elderly patient) to immediately notify prescriber if he experiences chest pain, palpitations, sweating, nervousness, shortness of breath, or other signs of overdose or aggravated CV disease.

• Advise patient who has achieved stable response not to change brands without physician advice.

• Advise female patient to alert prescriber if she becomes pregnant.

• Tell patient to report unusual bleeding and bruising.

✓ **Evaluation**

• Patient's thyroid hormone levels are normal.

• Patient doesn't experience any adverse reactions.

• Patient and family state understanding of drug therapy.

lidocaine hydrochloride (lignocaine hydrochloride)

(LIGH-doh-kayn high-droh-KLOR-ighd)
LidoPen Auto-Injector, Xylocaine, Xylocard ♦ ◊

Pharmacologic class: amide derivative
Therapeutic class: ventricular antiarrhythmic
Pregnancy risk category: B

Indications and dosages

▶ **Ventricular arrhythmias resulting from MI, cardiac manipulation, or digoxin toxicity.** *Adults:* 50 to 100 mg (1 to 1.5 mg/kg) by I.V. bolus at 25 to 50 mg/minute. Repeat bolus dose

q 3 to 5 minutes until arrhythmias subside or adverse reactions develop. Don't exceed 300-mg total bolus during 1-hour period. Simultaneously, constant infusion of 20 to 50 mcg/kg/minute (or 1 to 4 mg/minute) is begun. If single bolus has been given, smaller bolus dose may be repeated 5 to 10 minutes after start of infusion to maintain therapeutic level. After 24 hours of continuous infusion, decrease rate by one-half. Or 200 to 300 mg I.M., followed by second I.M. dose 60 to 90 minutes later, if needed. Change to I.V. form as soon as possible.

Children: 1 mg/kg by I.V. bolus, followed by infusion of 20 to 50 mcg/kg/minute.

⊠ **Adjust-a-dose:** For elderly patients, patients who weigh less than 50 kg (110 lb), and patients with heart failure or hepatic disease, give half the normal adult dose.

▶ **Status epilepticus‡.** *Adults:* 1 mg/kg I.V. bolus; then, if seizures continue, give 0.5 mg/kg 2 minutes after first dose. May use an infusion of 30 mcg/kg/minute.

▼ I.V. administration

L

• Only use drug without preservatives. Read label carefully.

• Injections (additive syringes and single-use vials) containing 40, 100, or 200 mg/ml are for the preparation of I.V. infusion solutions only and must be diluted before use.

• Add 1 g of drug (using 25 ml of 4% or 5 ml of 20% injection) to 1 L of D_5W injection to provide a solution containing 1 mg/ml.

• If patient is fluid restricted, use a more concentrated solution of up to 8 mg/ml.

• Patients receiving infusion must be on a cardiac monitor and must be attended at all times. Use infusion-control device to give infusion precisely. Don't exceed 4 mg/minute because doing so greatly increases the risk of toxicity.

⊗ **Incompatibilities**
Fentanyl citrate (higher pH formulations), methohexital sodium, phenytoin sodium.

Contraindications and cautions

• Contraindicated in patients hypersensitive to amide-type local anesthetics and in those with Adams-Stokes syndrome, Wolff-Parkinson-White syndrome, or severe degrees of SA, AV, or intraventricular block in absence of artificial pacemaker.

• Use cautiously and reduce dosage in patients with complete or second-degree heart block or sinus bradycardia, in those with heart failure or renal or hepatic disease, and in those who weigh less than 50 kg.

⚹ **Lifespan:** In pregnant women, use only when benefits outweigh risks to the fetus. In breast-feeding women and in children, safety and effectiveness haven't been established. In elderly patients, use cautiously.

Adverse reactions

CNS: *confusion, tremor,* lethargy, somnolence, *stupor, restlessness,* slurred speech, euphoria, depression, *light-headedness,* paresthesia, muscle twitching, *seizures.*
CV: hypotension, *bradycardia, new or worsened arrhythmias, cardiac arrest.*
EENT: *tinnitus, blurred or double vision.*
Respiratory: *respiratory arrest, status asthmaticus.*
Skin: diaphoresis.
Other: *anaphylaxis,* soreness at injection site, cold sensation.

Interactions

Drug-drug. *Atenolol, metoprolol, nadolol, pindolol, propranolol:* May reduce hepatic metabolism of lidocaine, thus increasing risk of lidocaine toxicity. Give bolus doses of lidocaine at a slower rate and monitor lidocaine level closely.
Cimetidine: May decrease clearance of lidocaine, increasing the risk of lidocaine toxicity. Use a different H_2-antagonist. Monitor lidocaine level closely.
Phenytoin, procainamide, propranolol, quinidine: May have additive cardiac depressant effects. Monitor patient.
Succinylcholine: May prolong neuromuscular blockage. Monitor patient for increased effects.
Tocainide: May increase risk of adverse reactions. Avoid using together.
Drug-herb. *Pareira:* May increase neuromuscular blockage. Avoid using together.
Drug-lifestyle. *Smoking:* May increase lidocaine metabolism. Monitor patient closely; discourage patient from smoking.

Effects on lab test results

• May increase CK level.

Pharmacokinetics

Absorption: Nearly complete.
Distribution: Wide, especially to adipose tissue.

Metabolism: Most of drug in liver to two active metabolites.
Excretion: 90% as metabolites; less than 10% in urine unchanged. *Half-life:* 1½ to 2 hours (may be prolonged in patients with heart failure or hepatic disease).

Route	Onset	Peak	Duration
I.V.	Immediate	30–60 min	10–20 min
I.M.	5–15 min	10 min	2 hr

Action

Chemical effect: Decreases depolarization, automaticity, and excitability in ventricles during diastolic phase by direct action on tissues.
Therapeutic effect: Abolishes ventricular arrhythmias.

Available forms

Infusion (premixed): 0.2% (2 mg/ml), 0.4% (4 mg/ml), 0.8% (8 mg/ml)
Injection for direct I.V. use: 1% (10 mg/ml), 2% (20 mg/ml)
Injection for I.M. use: 300 mg/3 ml automatic injection device
Injection for I.V. admixtures: 4% (40 mg/ml), 10% (100 mg/ml), 20% (200 mg/ml)

NURSING PROCESS

☲ Assessment

• Assess patient's condition before starting therapy and regularly thereafter to monitor the drug's effectiveness.
⊛ **ALERT:** Patient receiving infusion must be on cardiac monitor and attended to at all times.
• Monitor patient's response, especially ECG, blood pressure, and electrolytes, BUN, and creatinine levels.
• Check for therapeutic level (2 to 5 mcg/ml).
• Be alert for adverse reactions and drug interactions.
⊛ **ALERT:** Monitor patient for toxicity. Seizures may be first clinical sign. Severe reactions usually are preceded by somnolence, confusion, and paresthesia.
• Assess patient's and family's knowledge of drug therapy.

⊞ Nursing diagnoses

• Decreased cardiac output related to presence of ventricular arrhythmia

---

Reactions may be *common,* uncommon, *life-threatening*, or COMMON AND LIFE-THREATENING.

• Disturbed thought processes related to adverse CNS reactions
• Deficient knowledge related to drug therapy

Planning and implementation
ALERT: If using I.M. drug in patient with suspected MI, test isoenzymes before starting therapy because patients receiving I.M. drug show sevenfold increase in CK level. Such an increase originates in skeletal muscle, not cardiac muscle.
ALERT: Give I.M. injections only in deltoid muscle.
• Use only the 10% solution for I.M. injection. Read label carefully.
• If signs of toxicity (such as dizziness) occur, immediately stop giving the drug and notify prescriber. Continued infusion could lead to seizures and coma. Give oxygen by way of nasal cannula. Keep oxygen and cardiopulmonary resuscitation equipment available.
• If arrhythmias worsen or if ECG changes, such as with a widening QRS complex or substantially prolonged PR interval, stop drug and notify prescriber.
Patient teaching
• Explain purpose of drug to patient.
• Tell patient or caregiver to report any adverse reactions.
• Instruct patient to avoid smoking during drug therapy.

Evaluation
• Patient's cardiac output returns to normal with abolishment of ventricular arrhythmia.
• Patient maintains normal thought processes throughout therapy.
• Patient and family state understanding of drug therapy.

linezolid
(linn-AYE-zoe-lid)
Zyvox

Pharmacologic class: oxazolidinone
Therapeutic class: antibiotic
Pregnancy risk category: C

Indications and dosages
▶ **Vancomycin-resistant** *Enterococcus faecium* **infections, including those with**

bacteremia. *Adults and children age 12 and older:* 600 mg I.V. or P.O. q 12 hours for 14 to 28 days.
Neonates 7 days or older, infants, and children age 11 and younger: 10 mg/kg I.V. or P.O. q 8 hours for 14 to 28 days.
Neonates younger than 7 days old: 10 mg/kg I.V. or P.O. q 12 hours for 14 to 28 days. If neonate doesn't respond or when he is 7 days old, increase to 10 mg/kg q 8 hours.
▶ **Nosocomial pneumonia caused by** *Staphylococcus aureus* **(methicillin-susceptible [MSSA] and methicillin-resistant [MRSA] strains) or** *Streptococcus pneumonia* **(multidrug-resistant strains [MDRSP] only); complicated skin and skin-structure infections, including diabetic foot infections without osteomyelitis, caused by** *S. aureus* **(MSSA and MRSA),** *Streptococcus pyogenes,* **or** *Streptococcus agalactiae;* **community-acquired pneumonia caused by** *S. pneumoniae* **(including MDRSP), including those with bacteremia, or** *S. aureus* **(MSSA only).** *Adults and children age 12 and older:* 600 mg I.V. or P.O. q 12 hours for 10 to 14 days.
Neonates 7 days or older, infants, and children age 11 and younger: 10 mg/kg I.V. or P.O. q 8 hours for 10 to 14 days.
Preterm neonates younger than 7 days old: 10 mg/kg I.V. or P.O. q 12 hours for 10 to 14 days. Increase to 10 mg/kg q 8 hours if neonate doesn't respond or when he is 7 days old.
▶ **Uncomplicated skin and skin-structure infections caused by** *S. aureus* **(MSSA only) or** *S. pyogenes.* *Adults:* 400 mg P.O. q 12 hours for 10 to 14 days.
Children ages 12 to 18: 600 mg P.O. q 12 hours for 10 to 14 days.
Children ages 5 to 11: 10 mg/kg P.O. q 12 hours for 10 to 14 days.
Neonates 7 days or older, infants, and children younger than age 5: 10 mg/kg P.O. q 8 hours for 10 to 14 days.
Neonates younger than 7 days old: 10 mg/kg I.V. or P.O. q 12 hours for 10 to 14 days. Increase to 10 mg/kg q 8 hours if neonate doesn't respond or when he is 7 days old.

I.V. administration
• Drug is compatible with D_5W, normal saline solution for injection, and lactated Ringer's injection.

• Infuse over 30 to 120 minutes. Don't infuse in a series connection.
• Store drug at room temperature in its protective overwrap. The solution may turn yellow over time, but potency isn't affected. Use within 21 days.

⊗ **Incompatibilities**

Amphotericin B, ceftriaxone sodium, chlorpromazine hydrochloride, diazepam, erythromycin lactobionate, pentamidine isethionate, phenytoin sodium, trimethoprim-sulfamethoxazole. Don't mix with other I.V. drugs.

Contraindications and cautions

• Contraindicated in patients hypersensitive to the drug or any of its components.
• Safety and effectiveness of therapy for longer than 28 days haven't been studied.
 Lifespan: In pregnant women, use only if benefits outweigh risks to the fetus. In breastfeeding women, use cautiously. In children, safety and effectiveness haven't been established.

Adverse reactions

CNS: *headache,* insomnia, dizziness, fever.
GI: *diarrhea, nausea,* constipation, vomiting, altered taste, tongue discoloration, oral candidiasis, *pseudomembranous colitis.*
GU: vaginal candidiasis.
Hematologic: anemia, *leukopenia, neutropenia, thrombocytopenia.*
Skin: rash.
Other: fungal infection.

Interactions

Drug-drug. *Adrenergics (such as dopamine, epinephrine, pseudoephedrine):* Increases risk of hypertension. Monitor blood pressure and heart rate. Start continuous infusions of dopamine and epinephrine at lower doses, and adjust to response.
Serotoninergics: Increases risk of serotonin syndrome (confusion, delirium, restlessness, tremor, blushing, diaphoresis, hyperpyrexia). If these symptoms occur, stop serotoninergic.
Drug-food. *Foods and beverages high in tyramine (such as aged cheese, draft beer, red wine, air-dried meat, soy sauce, sauerkraut):* May increase blood pressure. Advise patient to avoid these foods; tell him that tyramine content of meals shouldn't exceed 100 mg.

Effects on lab test results

• May increase ALT, AST, bilirubin, alkaline phosphatase, creatinine, BUN, amylase, and lipase levels. May decrease hemoglobin level and hematocrit.
• May decrease WBC, neutrophil, and platelet counts.

Pharmacokinetics

Absorption: Rapid and complete. Bioavailability is about 100%.
Distribution: Good. Protein-binding is about 31%.
Metabolism: Undergoes oxidative metabolism to two inactive metabolites.
Excretion: At steady-state, about 30% unchanged in urine and about 50% as metabolites.
Half-life: 6¼ hours.

Route	Onset	Peak	Duration
P.O.			
tablet	Unknown	1 hr	4¾–5½ hr
suspension	Unknown	1 hr	4½ hr
I.V.	Unknown	½ hr	4¾ hr

Action

Chemical effect: Bacteriostatic against enterococci and staphylococci. Bactericidal against most strains of streptococci. Interferes with bacterial protein synthesis.
Therapeutic effect: Hinders or kills susceptible bacteria.

Available forms

Injection: 2 mg/ml
Powder for oral suspension: 100 mg/5 ml when reconstituted
Tablets: 400 mg, 600 mg

NURSING PROCESS

 Assessment

• Obtain history of patient's underlying condition before starting therapy, and reassess regularly thereafter to monitor the drug's effectiveness.
• Obtain specimen for culture and sensitivity tests before starting therapy. Use sensitivity results to guide subsequent therapy.
• Monitor platelet count in patient with increased risk of bleeding, patient with thrombocytopenia, patient taking drugs that may cause

thrombocytopenia, or patient taking linezolid for more than 14 days.

- Monitor patient for persistent diarrhea; if it occurs, consider the possibility of pseudomembranous colitis.
- Assess patient's and family's knowledge of drug therapy.

Nursing diagnoses

- Infection related to presence of susceptible bacteria
- Risk for injury related to drug-induced adverse reactions
- Deficient knowledge related to drug therapy

Planning and implementation

- Because inappropriate use of antibiotics may lead to resistant organisms, carefully consider other drugs before starting therapy, especially in an outpatient setting.
- No dosage adjustment is needed when switching from I.V. to P.O. dosage forms.

ALERT: Don't confuse Zyvox with Zovirax. They both come in a 400-mg tablet.

Patient teaching

- Inform patient that tablets and oral suspension may be taken with or without meals.
- Stress to patient the importance of completing the entire course of therapy, even if he feels better.
- Tell patient to alert prescriber if he has hypertension, is taking cough or cold preparations, or is taking a selective serotonin reuptake inhibitor or another antidepressant.
- Inform patient with phenylketonuria that each 5 ml of oral suspension contains 20 mg of phenylalanine. Tablets and injection don't contain phenylalanine.

Evaluation

- Patient is free from infection.
- Patient doesn't experience injury as a result of drug-induced adverse reactions.
- Patient and family state understanding of drug therapy.

lisinopril

(ligh-SIN-uh-pril)

Prinivil, Zestril

Pharmacologic class: ACE inhibitor
Therapeutic class: antihypertensive
Pregnancy risk category: C (D in second and third trimesters)

Indications and dosages

▶ **Hypertension.** *Adults:* Initially, 10 mg P.O. daily. If patient also takes a diuretic, reduce initial dosage to 5 mg P.O. daily. Usual effective dosage is 20 to 40 mg daily. Maximum dosage, 80 mg daily.
Children ages 6 to 16: Initially 0.07 mg/kg P.O. once daily (up to 5 mg total). Adjust dosage by blood pressure response. Doses above 0.61 mg/kg (or in excess of 40 mg) haven't been tested in children.

▶ **Adjunct therapy in heart failure (with diuretics and digoxin).** *Adults:* Initially, 5 mg P.O. daily. Usual effective dosage range is 5 to 20 mg daily. In patients with hyponatremia (sodium level below 130 mEq/L) or creatinine above 3 mg/dl, start with 2.5 mg P.O. once daily.

▶ **Hemodynamically stable patients within 24 hours of acute MI to improve survival.** *Adults:* Initially, 5 mg P.O. Then 5 mg P.O. after 24 hours, 10 mg P.O. after 48 hours, and 10 mg P.O. once daily for 6 weeks. In patients with systolic blood pressure of 120 mm Hg or less at start of therapy or during first 3 days after an MI, reduce dosage to 2.5 mg.

Contraindications and cautions

- Contraindicated in patients hypersensitive to ACE inhibitors and in those with a history of angioedema from previous therapy with an ACE inhibitor.
- Use cautiously in patients with impaired kidney function; adjust dosage as directed. Also use cautiously in patients at risk for hyperkalemia (those with renal insufficiency or diabetes or who use drugs that raise potassium level).

Lifespan: In pregnant women, use in first trimester when benefits to woman exceed risks to fetus. In last two trimesters, drug is contraindicated. In breast-feeding women, use cautiously. In children younger than age 6 and in children with glomerular filtration rate of less than

30 ml/min/1.73 m², safety and effectiveness haven't been established.

Adverse reactions

CNS: *dizziness, headache, fatigue,* depression, somnolence, paresthesia.
CV: hypotension, *orthostatic hypotension,* chest pain.
EENT: *nasal congestion.*
GI: *diarrhea,* nausea, dyspepsia, dysgeusia.
GU: impotence.
Metabolic: *hyperkalemia.*
Musculoskeletal: *muscle cramps.*
Respiratory: *dry, persistent, tickling, nonproductive cough.*
Skin: rash.
Other: *angioedema, anaphylaxis,* decreased libido.

Interactions

Drug-drug. *Capsaicin:* May cause or worsen coughing caused by ACE inhibitors. Monitor patient closely.
Digoxin: May increase digoxin levels. Monitor levels.
Diuretics: May cause excessive hypotension. Stop diuretics for 2 to 3 days or increase salt intake before lisinopril therapy or reduce lisinopril dosage to 5 mg P.O. once daily. Monitor blood pressure closely until stabilized.
Indomethacin: May lessen hypotensive effect. Monitor blood pressure.
Insulin, oral antidiabetics: May increase risk of hypoglycemia, especially when starting lisinopril. Monitor glucose closely.
Lithium: May increase lithium level. Monitor patient for toxicity.
Phenothiazines: May increase effects of drug. Monitor blood pressure.
Potassium-sparing diuretics, potassium supplements: May increase risk of hyperkalemia. Monitor potassium level.
Thiazide diuretics: May lessen potassium loss caused by thiazide diuretics. Monitor potassium level.
Tizanidine: May cause severe hypotension. Monitor patient closely.
Drug-herb. *Licorice:* May cause sodium retention and increase blood pressure, interfering with the therapeutic effects of ACE inhibitors. Discourage using together.
Drug-food. *Salt substitutes with potassium:* May increase risk of hyperkalemia. Monitor pa-

tient closely; discourage patient from using unless directed by prescriber.

Effects on lab test results

- May increase BUN, creatinine, potassium, and bilirubin levels.
- May increase liver function test values.

Pharmacokinetics

Absorption: Variable.
Distribution: Wide, although minimally to brain. Protein-binding appears insignificant.
Metabolism: None.
Excretion: Unchanged in urine. *Half-life:* 12 hours.

Route	Onset	Peak	Duration
P.O.	1 hr	7 hr	24 hr

Action

Chemical effect: Unknown; may result primarily from suppression of renin-angiotensin-aldosterone system.
Therapeutic effect: Lowers blood pressure.

Available forms

Tablets: 2.5 mg, 5 mg, 10 mg, 20 mg, 40 mg

NURSING PROCESS

Assessment
- Assess patient's condition before starting therapy and regularly thereafter to monitor the drug's effectiveness. The drug's beneficial effects may require several weeks to appear.
- Monitor WBC with differential counts before therapy, q 2 weeks for first 3 months of therapy, and periodically thereafter.
- Be alert for adverse reactions and drug interactions.
- Assess patient's and family's knowledge of drug therapy.

Nursing diagnoses
- Risk for injury related to presence of hypertension
- Decreased cardiac output related to drug-induced hypotension
- Deficient knowledge related to drug therapy

Planning and implementation
- If drug doesn't control blood pressure, add diuretics.

⊛ **ALERT:** Don't confuse lisinopril with fosinopril or Lioresal.

⊛ **ALERT:** Don't confuse Prinivil with Proventil or Prilosec.

⊛ **ALERT:** Don't confuse Zestril with Zostrix, Zetia, Zebeta, or Zyrtec.

Patient teaching

• Advise patient to report signs or symptoms of angioedema (including laryngeal edema), such as breathing difficulty or swelling of face, eyes, lips, or tongue.

• Tell patient that light-headedness may occur, especially during first few days of therapy. Tell him to rise slowly to avoid this effect and to report symptoms to prescriber. If syncope occurs, tell patient to stop taking drug and call prescriber immediately.

• Tell patient not to abruptly stop taking the drug but to call the prescriber if an adverse reaction occurs.

• Advise patient to report signs of infection, such as fever and sore throat.

• Tell patient to notify prescriber and stop taking the drug if she becomes pregnant.

☑ **Evaluation**

• Patient's blood pressure is within normal limits.

• Patient maintains adequate cardiac output throughout therapy.

• Patient and family state understanding of drug therapy.

lithium carbonate
(LITH-ee-um KAR-buh-nayt)
Carbolith♦, Duralith♦, Eskalith, Eskalith CR, Lithane, Lithicarb◇, Lithizine♦, Lithobid, Lithonate, Lithotabs

lithium citrate
Lithium Citrate Syrup*

Pharmacologic class: alkali metal
Therapeutic class: antipsychotic
Pregnancy risk category: D

Indications and dosages

▶ **To prevent or control acute manic or mixed episodes in patients with bipolar disorder.** *Adults:* 300 to 600 mg P.O. up to q.i.d., increasing on basis of drug level to achieve thera-

peutic dosage, usually 1,800 mg P.O. daily. Therapeutic drug level: 1 to 1.5 mEq/L for acute mania; 0.6 to 1.2 mEq/L for maintenance therapy; and 2 mEq/L as maximum level.

▶ **Major depression, schizoaffective disorder, schizophrenic disorder, alcohol dependence**‡ *Adults:* 300 mg lithium carbonate P.O. t.i.d. or q.i.d.

▶ **Apparent mixed bipolar disorder in children**‡ *Children:* Initially, 15 to 60 mg/kg or 0.5 to 1.5 g/m² lithium carbonate P.O. daily in three divided doses. Don't exceed usual adult dosage. Adjust dosage based on patient's response and lithium level. Usual range, 150 to 300 mg daily in divided doses to maintain lithium level of 0.5 to 1.2 mEq/L.

▶ **Chemotherapy-induced neutropenia in children and patients with AIDS receiving zidovudine.**‡ *Adults and children:* 300 to 1,000 mg P.O. daily.

Contraindications and cautions

• Contraindicated if therapy can't be closely monitored.

• Use cautiously in patients receiving neuroleptics, neuromuscular blockers, or diuretics; in debilitated patients; and in patients with thyroid disease, seizure disorder, renal or CV disease, severe debilitation or dehydration, or sodium depletion.

⚘ **Lifespan:** In pregnant and breast-feeding women, drug is contraindicated. In children younger than age 12, safety and effectiveness haven't been established. In elderly patients, use cautiously because of possible decreased rate of excretion.

Adverse reactions

CNS: tremor, drowsiness, headache, confusion, restlessness, dizziness, psychomotor retardation, stupor, lethargy, *coma,* syncope, *epileptiform seizures,* EEG changes, worsened organic mental syndrome, impaired speech, ataxia, weakness, incoordination.

CV: *reversible ECG changes, arrhythmias,* hypotension, ankle and wrist edema.

EENT: tinnitus, blurred vision.

GI: dry mouth, metallic taste, nausea, vomiting, anorexia, diarrhea, thirst, abdominal pain, flatulence, indigestion.

GU: polyuria, glycosuria, *renal toxicity,* albuminuria.

Hematologic: *reversible leukocytosis.*

L

Metabolic: goiter, hypothyroidism, hyponatremia, transient hyperglycemia.
Skin: pruritus, rash, diminished or absent sensation, drying and thinning of hair, psoriasis, acne, alopecia.

Interactions

Drug-drug. *Acetazolamide, aminophylline, sodium bicarbonate, urine alkalinizers:* May increase lithium excretion. Avoid salt loads; monitor lithium levels for increase.
Carbamazepine, indomethacin, methyldopa, NSAIDS, piroxicam, probenecid: May increase effect of lithium. Monitor patient for lithium toxicity.
Diuretics: May increase reabsorption of lithium by kidneys with a toxic effect. Use cautiously and monitor lithium and electrolyte levels (especially sodium).
Fluoxetine: May increase lithium level. Monitor patient for toxicity.
Neuroleptics: May cause encephalopathy. Watch for signs and symptoms (lethargy, tremor, extrapyramidal symptoms), and stop drug if they occur.
Neuromuscular blockers: May cause prolonged paralysis or weakness. Monitor patient closely.
Thyroid hormones: Lithium may induce hypothyroidism. Monitor thyroid function and treat with thyroid hormones as needed.

Effects on lab test results

• May increase glucose level. May decrease sodium, T_3, T_4, and protein-bound iodine levels.
• May increase ^{131}I uptake and WBC and neutrophil counts.

Pharmacokinetics

Absorption: Complete within 8 hours.
Distribution: Wide; levels in thyroid gland, bone, and brain exceed serum levels.
Metabolism: Not metabolized.
Excretion: 95% unchanged in urine. *Half-life:* 18 hours (adolescents) to 36 hours (elderly).

Route	Onset	Peak	Duration
P.O.	Unknown	½–3 hr	Unknown

Action

Chemical effect: Unknown; probably alters chemical transmitters in CNS, possibly by interfering with ionic pump mechanisms in brain cells, and may compete with sodium ions.
Therapeutic effect: Stabilizes mood.

Available forms

lithium carbonate
Capsules: 150 mg, 300 mg, 600 mg
Tablets: 300 mg (300 mg = 8.12 mEq lithium)
Tablets (controlled-release): 300 mg, 450 mg
lithium citrate
Syrup (sugarless)*: 8 mEq of lithium per 5 ml (8 mEq lithium = 300 mg of lithium carbonate)

NURSING PROCESS

☞ Assessment
• Assess patient's condition before starting therapy and regularly thereafter to monitor the drug's effectiveness. Expect delay of 1 to 3 weeks before drug's beneficial effects are noticed.
• Monitor baseline ECG, thyroid and kidney studies, and electrolyte levels.
• Monitor lithium blood levels 8 to 12 hours after first dose, usually before morning dose, two or three times weekly in first month, and then weekly to monthly during maintenance therapy. With blood levels below 1.5 mEq/L, adverse reactions usually remain mild, although toxicity may occur even at therapeutic levels.
• Check urine-specific gravity, and report level below 1.005, which may indicate diabetes insipidus.
• Monitor glucose level closely. Lithium may alter glucose tolerance in diabetic patient.
• Be alert for adverse reactions and drug interactions.
• Assess patient's and family's knowledge of drug therapy.

⊕ Nursing diagnoses
• Disturbed thought processes related to presence of bipolar disorder
• Ineffective health maintenance related to drug-induced endocrine dysfunction
• Deficient knowledge related to drug therapy

▷ Planning and implementation
⑤ ALERT: Don't confuse Lithobid with Levbid, Lithonate with Lithostat, or Lithotabs with Lithobid or Lithostat.

Reactions may be *common,* uncommon, *life-threatening*, or COMMON AND LIFE-THREATENING.

• Monitoring lithium level is crucial to safe use of drug. Don't use in patient who can't have level checked regularly.
• Give with plenty of water and after meals to minimize GI reactions.
• Before leaving bedside, make sure patient has swallowed drug.
• Notify prescriber if patient's behavior hasn't improved in 3 weeks or if it worsens.
• Perform outpatient follow-up of thyroid and kidney function q 6 to 12 months. Palpate thyroid to check for enlargement.
Patient teaching
• Tell patient to take drug with plenty of water and after meals to minimize GI upset.
• Explain that lithium has narrow therapeutic margin of safety. A blood level that is even slightly high can be dangerous.
• Warn patient and family to watch for signs of toxicity (diarrhea, vomiting, tremor, drowsiness, muscle weakness, ataxia) and to expect transient nausea, polyuria, thirst, and discomfort during the first few days. Tell patient not to abruptly stop taking the drug unless he has symptoms of toxicity. If he does, he should call his prescriber and not take the next dose.
• Warn patient to avoid activities that require alertness and good psychomotor coordination until the drug's CNS effects are known.
• Tell patient not to switch brands or take other prescription or OTC drugs without prescriber's approval.
• Advise patient to wear or carry medical identification.

☑ **Evaluation**
• Patient exhibits improved behavior and thought processes.
• Patient maintains normal endocrine function throughout therapy.
• Patient and family state understanding of drug therapy.

lomustine (CCNU)
(loh-MUH-steen)
CeeNU

Pharmacologic class: alkylating drug, nitrosourea
Therapeutic class: antineoplastic
Pregnancy risk category: D

Indications and dosages

► **Brain tumor, Hodgkin's disease, lymphomas.** *Adults and children:* 100 to 130 mg/m² P.O. as single dose q 6 weeks. Reduce dosage according to degree of bone marrow suppression. Don't repeat doses until WBC count is more than 4,000/mm³ and platelet count is more than 100,000/mm³.

Contraindications and cautions

• Contraindicated in patients hypersensitive to the drug or any of its components.
• Use cautiously in patients with lowered platelet, WBC, or RBC count and in those receiving other myelosuppressant drugs.
☀ **Lifespan:** In pregnant and breast-feeding women, drug is contraindicated.

Adverse reactions

GI: *nausea, vomiting,* stomatitis.
GU: *nephrotoxicity,* progressive azotemia, *renal impairment.*
Hematologic: anemia, *leukopenia, thrombocytopenia, bone marrow suppression.*
Hepatic: *hepatotoxicity.*
Respiratory: *pulmonary fibrosis.*
Other: *secondary malignant disease.*

Interactions

Drug-drug. *Anticoagulants, aspirin:* Increases bleeding risk. Avoid using together.

Effects on lab test results

• May increase urine urea, liver enzyme, BUN, and creatinine levels. May decrease hemoglobin level and hematocrit.
• May decrease WBC, RBC, and platelet counts.

Pharmacokinetics

Absorption: Rapid and good.
Distribution: Wide; crosses blood-brain barrier to significant extent.
Metabolism: Rapid and extensive in liver.
Excretion: Metabolites primarily in urine. *Half-life:* 1 to 2 days.

Route	Onset	Peak	Duration
P.O.	Unknown	Unknown	Unknown

L

Action

Chemical effect: Cross-links strands of cellular DNA and interferes with RNA transcription.
Therapeutic effect: Kills selected cancer cells.

Available forms

Capsules: 10 mg, 40 mg, 100 mg, dose pack (two 10-mg, two 40-mg, two 100-mg capsules)

⚷ Assessment

• Assess patient's condition before starting therapy and regularly thereafter to monitor the drug's effectiveness.
• Monitor CBC weekly because bone marrow toxicity is delayed by 4 to 6 weeks post treatment.
• Periodically monitor liver function test results.
• Be alert for adverse reactions and drug interactions.
• Assess patient's and family's knowledge of drug therapy.

⊕ Nursing diagnoses

• Ineffective health maintenance related to presence of neoplastic disease
• Ineffective protection related to adverse hematologic reactions
• Deficient knowledge related to drug therapy

⊠ Planning and implementation

• Give antiemetic before giving drug to help patient avoid nausea.
• Give 2 to 4 hours after meals because drug is better absorbed on an empty stomach.
• Repeat dose only when CBC results reveal safe blood counts.
• Institute infection control and bleeding precautions.

Patient teaching

• Warn patient to watch for signs of infection (fever, sore throat, fatigue) and bleeding (easy bruising, nosebleeds, bleeding gums, melena) and to take temperature daily.
• Instruct patient to avoid OTC products containing aspirin.
• Advise woman of childbearing age to avoid pregnancy during therapy and to consult with prescriber before becoming pregnant.

☑ Evaluation

• Patient responds well to therapy.

• Patient regains normal hematologic function.
• Patient and family state understanding of drug therapy.

loperamide
(loh-PEH-ruh-mighd)
Imodium, Imodium A-D†, Kaopectate II Caplets†, Maalox Anti-Diarrheal Caplets†, Neo-Diaral†, Pepto Diarrhea Control†

Pharmacologic class: piperidine derivative
Therapeutic class: antidiarrheal
Pregnancy risk category: B

Indications and dosages

▶ **Acute diarrhea.** *Adults and children age 12 and older:* Initially, 4 mg P.O.; then 2 mg after each unformed stool. Maximum dosage, 16 mg daily.
Children ages 8 to 12 who weigh more than 30 kg (66 lb): 2 mg P.O. t.i.d. on first day. On subsequent days, doses of 1 mg/10 kg of body weight may be given after each unformed stool. Maximum dosage, 6 mg daily.
Children ages 6 to 8 who weigh 20 to 30 kg (44 to 66 lb): 2 mg P.O. b.i.d. on first day. On subsequent days, doses of 1 mg/10 kg of body weight may be given after each unformed stool. Maximum dosage, 4 mg daily.
Children ages 2 to 5 who weigh 13 to 20 kg (29 to 44 lb): 1 mg P.O. t.i.d. on first day. On subsequent days, give doses of 1 mg/10 kg of body weight after each unformed stool. Maximum dosage, 3 mg daily.
▶ **Chronic diarrhea.** *Adults:* Initially, 4 mg P.O.; then 2 mg after each unformed stool until diarrhea subsides. Adjust dosage to individual response. Maximum dosage, 16 mg daily. If patient doesn't improve in 10 days, consider different therapy.
Children‡: 0.08 to 0.24 mg/kg P.O. daily in two to three divided doses. Report persistent diarrhea to prescriber.
▶ **Self-medication of acute diarrhea including traveler's diarrhea.** *Adults:* 4 mg† after first loose bowel movement followed by 2 mg† after each subsequent loose bowel movement; maximum, 8 mg P.O. daily for 2 days.

Contraindications and cautions

• Contraindicated in patients hypersensitive to the drug or any of its components; in patients in whom constipation must be avoided; in patients with pseudomembranous colitis from antibiotic use; and patients with *Shigella, Salmonella,* or enteroinvasive *Escherichia coli* infection. OTC form is contraindicated in patients with bloody diarrhea and those with temperature over 101° F (38° C). Contraindicated in children less than 2 years old.

• Use cautiously in patients with hepatic disease because of risk of encephalopathy.

※ **Lifespan:** In pregnant women, use cautiously. In breast-feeding women, use cautiously; it's unknown if the drug appears in breast milk. In children younger than age 2, drug is contraindicated.

Adverse reactions

CNS: drowsiness, fatigue, dizziness.
GI: dry mouth; abdominal pain, distention, or discomfort; *constipation;* nausea; vomiting.
Skin: rash.
Other: hypersensitivity reactions.

Interactions

Saquinavir: May increase levels of loperamide while decreasing saquinavir levels. Avoid use together.

Effects on lab test results

None reported.

Pharmacokinetics

Absorption: Poor.
Distribution: Unknown.
Metabolism: In liver.
Excretion: Primarily in feces; less than 2% in urine. *Half-life:* 9 to 14½ hours.

Route	Onset	Peak	Duration
P.O.	Unknown	2½–5 hr	24 hr

Action

Chemical effect: Inhibits peristalsis, prolonging passage of intestinal contents.
Therapeutic effect: Relieves diarrhea.

Available forms

Capsules: 2 mg
Oral liquid*: 1 mg/5 ml†, 1 mg/ml†
Tablets: 2 mg†

NURSING PROCESS

🔲 Assessment

• Assess patient's diarrhea before starting therapy and regularly thereafter to monitor the drug's effectiveness.
• Be alert for adverse reactions.
Ⓢ **ALERT:** Monitor children closely for CNS effects because they may be more sensitive than adults.
• Monitor patient's hydration.
• Assess patient's and family's knowledge of drug therapy.

🔲 Nursing diagnoses

• Diarrhea related to underlying condition
• Risk for deficient fluid volume related to drug-induced adverse GI reactions
• Deficient knowledge related to drug therapy

🔲 Planning and implementation

• If patient doesn't improve in 48 hours, stop use.
• If patient has severe abdominal pain, bloating, or firmness or if drug is ineffective, notify prescriber.
• If drug is given by NG tube, flush tube to clear it and ensure drug's passage to stomach.
Ⓢ **ALERT:** Oral liquids are available in different concentrations. Check dose carefully. For children, consider an oral liquid product that doesn't contain alcohol.
Ⓢ **ALERT:** Don't confuse Imodium with Ionamin.
Patient teaching
• Advise patient not to exceed recommended dosage.
• Tell patient with acute diarrhea to contact prescriber if patient doesn't improve within 48 hours. For chronic diarrhea, tell patient to notify prescriber and stop taking the drug if no improvement occurs after taking 16 mg daily for at least 10 days.
• Advise patient to stop taking drug and to notify prescriber immediately if abdominal pain, bloating, or firmness develop because of risk of toxic megacolon.

🔲 Evaluation

• Patient's diarrhea is relieved.
• Patient is adequately hydrated throughout therapy.
• Patient and family state understanding of drug therapy.

Rapid onset   *Liquid form contains alcohol.   ◆ Canada   ◇ Australia   †OTC   ✐Photoguide   ‡Off-label use

lopinavir and ritonavir
(loe-PIN-a-veer and rih-TOH-nuh-veer)
Kaletra&

Pharmacologic class: protease inhibitor
Therapeutic class: antiretroviral
Pregnancy risk category: C

Indications and dosages

▶ **HIV infection, with other antiretrovirals in treatment-naive adults.** *Adults:* 800 mg lopinavir and 200 mg ritonavir (4 tablets or 10 ml) P.O. once daily or divided evenly b.i.d.
▶ **HIV infection, with other antiretrovirals in treatment-experienced patients.** *Adults and children older than age 12:* 400 mg lopinavir and 100 mg ritonavir (2 tablets or 5 ml) P.O. b.i.d.
Children ages 6 months to 12 years who weigh 15 to 40 kg (33 to 88 lb): 10 mg/kg (lopinavir content) P.O. b.i.d. with food up to a maximum of 400 mg lopinavir and 100 mg ritonavir in children weighing more than 40 kg.
Children ages 6 months to 12 years who weigh 7 to 15 kg (15 to 33 lb): 12 mg/kg (lopinavir content) P.O. b.i.d. with food.
❚ Adjust-a-dose: In treatment-experienced patients older than age 12 also taking efavirenz, nevirapine, fosamprenavir without ritonavir, or nelfinavir, consider dosage of 600 mg lopinavir and 150 mg ritonavir (3 tablets) P.O. b.i.d. For patients using oral solution and also taking efavirenz, nevirapine, amprenavir, or nelfinavir, 533 mg lopinavir and 133 mg ritonavir (6.5 ml) b.i.d. with food is recommended. In treatment-experienced patients ages 6 months to 12 years also taking amprevavir, efavirenz or nevirapine and weighing 7 to 15 kg, give 13 mg/kg (lopinavir content) P.O. b.i.d. with food. For these patients weighing 15 to 45 kg, give 11 mg/kg (lopinavir content) P.O. b.i.d. with food up to a maximum dose of 533 mg lopinavir and 133 mg ritonavir b.i.d. in children weighing more than 45 kg.

Contraindications and cautions

• Contraindicated in patients hypersensitive to the drug or any of its components.
• Use cautiously in patients with a history of pancreatitis or with hepatic impairment, hepati-tis B or C, marked elevations in liver enzyme levels, or hemophilia.
⚕ Lifespan: In breast-feeding women, either stop breast-feeding or use another drug. In infants younger than age 6 months, safety and effectiveness haven't been established. In elderly patients, use cautiously because of possible decreased rate of excretion.

Adverse reactions

CNS: pain, asthenia, headache, fever, insomnia, malaise, abnormal dreams, agitation, amnesia, anxiety, ataxia, confusion, depression, dizziness, dyskinesia, emotional lability, *encephalopathy,* hypertonia, nervousness, neuropathy, paresthesia, peripheral neuritis, somnolence, abnormal thinking, tremor.
CV: chest pain, *deep vein thrombosis,* hypertension, palpitations, peripheral edema, thrombophlebitis, vasculitis, facial edema, edema.
EENT: sinusitis, abnormal vision, eye disorder, otitis media, tinnitus, sialadenitis, stomatitis, taste perversion, ulcerative stomatitis.
GI: abdominal pain, abnormal stools, *diarrhea, nausea,* vomiting, anorexia, cholecystitis, constipation, dry mouth, dyspepsia, dysphagia, enterocolitis, eructation, esophagitis, fecal incontinence, flatulence, gastritis, gastroenteritis, GI disorder, *hemorrhagic colitis,* increased appetite, *pancreatitis.*
GU: abnormal ejaculation, decreased libido, gynecomastia, hypogonadism, renal calculus, urine abnormality.
Hematologic: anemia, *leukopenia, neutropenia,* lymphadenopathy; *thrombocytopenia* in children.
Hepatic: hyperbilirubinemia in children.
Metabolic: Cushing's syndrome, hypothyroidism, dehydration, decreased glucose tolerance, *lactic acidosis,* weight loss, hyperglycemia, hyperuricemia, *hypercholesterolemia,* hyponatremia in children.
Musculoskeletal: back pain, arthralgia, arthrosis, myalgia.
Respiratory: bronchitis, dyspnea, *lung edema.*
Skin: rash, acne, alopecia, dry skin, exfoliative dermatitis, furunculosis, nail disorder, pruritus, benign skin neoplasm, skin discoloration, sweating.
Other: chills, flulike syndrome, viral infection.

Interactions

Drug-drug. *Amiodarone, bepridil, lidocaine, quinidine:* May increase antiarrhythmic levels. Use cautiously. Monitor levels of these drugs; adjust dosage, if needed.

Amprenavir, efavirenz, nelfinavir, nevirapine: May decrease lopinavir level. Consider increasing lopinavir and ritonavir dose. Don't use a once-daily Kaletra regimen with these drugs.

Antiarrhythmics (flecainide, propafenone), pimozide: May increase risk of cardiac arrhythmias. Don't use together.

Atovaquone, methadone: May decrease levels of these drugs. Consider increasing doses of these drugs.

Carbamazepine, corticosteroids, phenobarbital, phenytoin: May decrease lopinavir level. Use cautiously.

Clarithromycin: May increase clarithromycin levels in patients with renal impairment. Adjust clarithromycin dose.

Cyclosporine, rapamycin, tacrolimus: May increase levels of these drugs. Monitor therapeutic levels.

Delavirdine: May increase lopinavir level. May be prescribed together for this effect.

Didanosine: May decrease absorption of didanosine because lopinavir and ritonavir dose is taken with food. Give didanosine 1 hour before or 2 hours after lopinavir and ritonavir.

Dihydroergotamine, ergonovine, ergotamine, methylergonovine: May increase risk of ergot toxicity characterized by peripheral vasospasm and ischemia. Don't use together.

Disulfiram, metronidazole: May increase risk of disulfiram-like reaction. Avoid using together.

Felodipine, nicardipine, nifedipine: May increase levels of these drugs. Use cautiously. Monitor patient.

Fluticasone: Significantly increases fluticasone exposure leading to significantly decreased serum cortisol concentrations which may lead to systemic corticosteroid effects (including Cushing syndrome). Don't use together, if possible.

HMG-CoA reductase inhibitors: May increase risk of adverse reactions, such as myopathy and rhabdomyolysis. Atorvastatin, fluvastatin, and pravastatin may be used with careful monitoring; Avoid using lovastatin or simvastatin.

Hormonal contraceptives (ethinyl estradiol): May decrease effectiveness of contraceptives. Recommend nonhormonal contraception.

Indinavir, saquinavir: May increase level of these drugs. May be prescribed together for this effect.

Itraconazole, ketoconazole: May increase levels of these drugs. Don't give more than 200 mg/day of these drugs.

Methadone: May decrease methadone absorption. May need to increase dose. Monitor patient closely.

Midazolam, triazolam: May prolong or increase sedation or respiratory depression. Don't use together.

Rifabutin: May increase rifabutin level. Decrease rifabutin dose by 75%; monitor patient for adverse effects.

Rifampin: May decrease effectiveness of lopinavir and ritonavir. Avoid using together.

Sildenafil, tadalafil, vardenafil: May increase levels and risk of adverse effects of these drugs, such as hypotension and prolonged erection. Don't exceed 25 mg of sildenafil in a 48 hours, 10 mg of tadalafil in 72 hours, or 2.5 mg of vardenafil in 72 hours. Use cautiously, and monitor patient for adverse reactions.

Trazodone: may increase trazodone level causing nausea, dizziness, hypotension and syncope. Avoid use together. If unavoidable, use cautiously with a lower dose of trazodone.

Warfarin: May affect warfarin level. Monitor PT and INR.

Drug-herb. *St. John's wort:* May cause loss of virologic response and resistance to drug. Discourage using together.

Drug-food. *Any food:* May increase absorption of oral solution. Give drug with food.

Effects on lab test results

• May increase amylase, liver enzyme, glucose, uric acid, cholesterol, and triglyceride levels. May decrease hemoglobin level and hematocrit. In children, may increase bilirubin level and decrease sodium level.

• May decrease WBC, neutrophil, and platelet counts.

Pharmacokinetics

Absorption: Peak levels are achieved in 4 hours. Drug better absorbed when taken with food.

Distribution: Lopinavir is 98% or 99% protein-bound.

Metabolism: Lopinavir is extensively metabolized by the CYP 3A isoenzyme. Ritonavir is a

potent inhibitor of CYP 3A, which inhibits the metabolism of lopinavir and increases lopinavir level.
Excretion: In urine and feces. Less than 3% of the drug is excreted unchanged. *Half-life:* About 6 hours.

Route	Onset	Peak	Duration
P.O.	Unknown	4 hr	6 hr

Action

Chemical effects: Inhibits the HIV protease. Ritonavir inhibits the metabolism of lopinavir, increasing lopinavir level.
Therapeutic effect: Prevents the cleavage of the Gag-Pol polyprotein, resulting in the production of immature, noninfectious viral particles.

Available forms

Tablets: 200 mg lopinavir and 50 mg ritonavir
Solution: lopinavir 400 mg and ritonavir 100 mg per 5 ml (80 mg and 20 mg per ml)

NURSING PROCESS

Assessment
• Assess underlying condition before starting therapy, and reassess regularly to monitor the drug's effectiveness.
• Monitor total cholesterol and triglycerides before starting therapy and periodically thereafter.
• To monitor maternal-fetal outcomes of pregnant women exposed to lopinavir and ritonavir, an Antiretroviral Pregnancy Registry has been established. Enroll patients by calling 1-800-258-4263, or register online at www.apregistry.com.
⑤ **ALERT:** This drug interacts with many other drugs. Review current drugs that patient is taking.
• Assess patient's and family's knowledge of drug therapy.

Nursing diagnoses
• Risk for falls related to drug-induced adverse CNS effects
• Risk for powerlessness related to chronic disease and need for aggressive medical management
• Deficient knowledge related to drug therapy

Planning and implementation
• Tablets may be taken without regard to meals. Oral solution must be taken with food.
⑤ **ALERT:** Tablets must be swallowed whole. Don't crush, divide, or let patient chew.
• Refrigerated drug remains stable until expiration date on package. If stored at room temperature, use drug within 2 months.
• Monitor patient for signs of fat redistribution, including central obesity, buffalo hump, peripheral wasting, breast enlargement, and cushingoid appearance.
• Monitor patient for signs of pancreatitis: nausea, vomiting, abdominal pain, and increased lipase and amylase values.
• Monitor patient for signs of bleeding.
• For an overdose, induce emesis or perform gastric lavage. Activated charcoal may be used to aid in removing unabsorbed drug. Dialysis is unlikely to help remove drug.
⑤ **ALERT:** Don't confuse Kaletra with Keppra.
Patient teaching
• Tell patient to take oral solution with food.
• Tell patient also taking didanosine to take it 1 hour before or 2 hours after lopinavir and ritonavir.
• Advise patient to report side effects to prescriber.
• Tell patient to immediately report severe nausea, vomiting, or abdominal pain.
• Warn patient to tell prescriber about any other prescription or nonprescription drug he is taking, including herbal supplements.
• Tell patient that drug isn't a cure for HIV.
• If patient takes a drug for erectile dysfunction, caution about an increased risk of adverse events, including hypotension, visual changes, and priapism, and the need to promptly report any symptoms. Tell him not to take more than directed.
• Advise HIV-infected mothers not to breast-feed because breast-feeding may transmit HIV to their infants.

Evaluation
• Patient doesn't experience falls.
• Patient has adequate support, personal and professional, to deal with emotional aspects of having HIV disease.
• Patient and family state understanding of drug therapy.

loracarbef
(loh-ruh-KAR-bef)
Lorabid

Pharmacologic class: synthetic beta-lactam antibiotic of carbacephem class
Therapeutic class: cephalosporin
Pregnancy risk category: B

Indications and dosages

▶ **Secondary bacterial infections of acute bronchitis.** *Adults:* 200 to 400 g P.O. q 12 hours for 7 days.
▶ **Acute bacterial exacerbations of chronic bronchitis.** *Adults:* 400 mg P.O. q 12 hours for 7 days.
▶ **Pneumonia.** *Adults:* 400 mg P.O. q 12 hours for 14 days.
▶ **Pharyngitis and tonsillitis.** *Adults:* 200 mg P.O. q 12 hours for 10 days. *Children:* 15 mg/kg P.O. daily in divided doses q 12 hours for 10 days.
▶ **Sinusitis:** *Adults:* 400 mg P.O. q 12 hours for 10 days. *Children:* 15 mg/kg P.O. daily in divided doses q 12 hours for 10 days.
▶ **Acute otitis media.** *Children:* 30 mg/kg (oral suspension) P.O. daily in divided doses q 12 hours for 10 days.
▶ **Uncomplicated skin and skin-structure infections.** *Adults:* 200 mg P.O. q 12 hours for 7 days.
▶ **Impetigo.** *Children:* 15 mg/kg P.O. daily in divided doses q 12 hours for 7 days.
▶ **Uncomplicated cystitis.** *Adults:* 200 mg P.O. daily for 7 days.
▶ **Uncomplicated pyelonephritis.** *Adults:* 400 mg P.O. q 12 hours for 14 days.
🕲 **Adjust-a-dose:** For patients with renal impairment, if creatinine clearance is 10 to 49 ml/minute, give half of usual dose at same intervals. If clearance is below 10 ml/minute, give usual dose q 3 to 5 days. Give hemodialysis patients another dose after dialysis.

Contraindications and cautions

• Contraindicated in patients hypersensitive to drug, other cephalosporins, or related antibiotics, and in patients with diarrhea caused by pseudomembranous colitis.

☀ **Lifespan:** In pregnant women, use cautiously. In breast-feeding women, use cautiously; it's unknown if the drug appears in breast milk. In infants younger than age 6 months, safety and effectiveness haven't been established.

Adverse reactions

CNS: headache, somnolence, nervousness, insomnia, dizziness, *seizures.*
CV: vasodilation.
GI: diarrhea, nausea, vomiting, abdominal pain, anorexia, *pseudomembranous colitis.*
GU: vaginal candidiasis.
Hematologic: *transient thrombocytopenia, leukopenia,* eosinophilia.
Skin: rash, urticaria, pruritus, *erythema multiforme.*
Other: hypersensitivity reactions, *anaphylaxis.*

Interactions

Drug-drug. *Aminoglycosides, loop diuretics:* May increase risk of nephrotoxicity. Use together cautiously.
Probenecid: May decrease loracarbef excretion, increasing level. Monitor patient for toxicity.
Drug-food. *Any food:* May decrease absorption. Give drug 1 hour before or 2 hours after meals.

Effects on lab test results

• May increase BUN, creatinine, ALT, AST, and alkaline phosphatase levels.
• May increase PT, INR, and eosinophil count. May decrease platelet, WBC, RBC, and neutrophil counts.
• May cause false-positive direct Coombs' test.

Pharmacokinetics

Absorption: About 90%.
Distribution: About 25% of circulating drug is bound to proteins.
Metabolism: None.
Excretion: Primarily in urine. *Half-life:* About 1 hour.

Route	Onset	Peak	Duration
P.O.	Unknown	30–60 min	Unknown

Action

Chemical effect: Inhibits cell-wall synthesis, promoting osmotic instability; usually bactericidal.
Therapeutic effect: Kills susceptible bacteria.

Available forms

Powder for oral suspension: 100 mg/5 ml, 200 mg/5 ml
Pulvules: 200 mg, 400 mg

NURSING PROCESS

⚕ Assessment
• Assess patient's infection before starting therapy and regularly thereafter to monitor the drug's effectiveness.
• Obtain specimen for culture and sensitivity tests before starting therapy. Begin therapy pending test results.
• Be alert for adverse reactions and drug interactions.
⚙ ALERT: Watch for seizures. Beta-lactam antibiotics may trigger seizures in a susceptible patient, especially when given without dosage modification to a patient with renal impairment.
• If patient has an adverse GI reaction, monitor his hydration.
• Assess patient's and family's knowledge of drug therapy.

⚙ Nursing diagnoses
• Infection related to presence of susceptible bacteria
• Risk for deficient fluid volume related to drug-induced adverse GI reactions
• Deficient knowledge related to drug therapy

❱ Planning and implementation
• To reconstitute powder for oral suspension, add 30 ml of water in two portions to 50-ml bottle, or add 60 ml of water in two portions to 100-ml bottle. Shake after each addition.
• After reconstitution, store oral suspension for 14 days at constant room temperature (59° to 86° F [15° to 30° C]).
• If seizure occurs, stop giving the drug and tell prescriber. Give anticonvulsants.
⚙ ALERT: Don't confuse Lorabid with Lortab.
Patient teaching
• Tell patient to take drug on an empty stomach, at least 1 hour before or 2 hours after meals.
• Tell patient to shake suspension well before measuring dose and to take drug exactly as prescribed.
• Instruct patient to discard unused portion after 14 days.

☑ Evaluation
• Patient is free from infection.
• Patient maintains adequate hydration throughout therapy.
• Patient and family state understanding of drug therapy.

loratadine
(loo-RAH-tuh-deen)
Alavert†, Claritin†, Claritin Reditabs†, Claritin Syrup†, Claritin-D 12 Hour†, Claritin-D 24 Hour†, Claratyne◇, Tavist ND Allergy†

Pharmacologic class: peripherally selective piperidine
Therapeutic class: antihistamine
Pregnancy risk category: B

Indications and dosages

▶ **Allergic rhinitis, chronic idiopathic urticaria.** *Adults and children age 6 and older:* 10 mg P.O. daily.
Children ages 2 to 5: 5 mg P.O. daily.
⊠ Adjust-a-dose: For patients with renal or hepatic impairment, adjust dosage as follows: in adults and children age 6 and older with liver impairment or creatinine clearance less than 30 ml/minute, give 10 mg q other day. In children ages 2 to 5 with liver impairment or renal insufficiency, give 5 mg q other day.

Contraindications and cautions

• Contraindicated in patients hypersensitive to the drug or any of its components.
• Use cautiously in patients with hepatic impairment.
☀ Lifespan: In pregnant women, use only when benefits outweigh risks to the fetus. In breast-feeding women, use cautiously because it isn't known if drug appears in breast milk. In children younger than age 2, safety and effectiveness haven't been established.

Adverse reactions

CNS: *headache,* drowsiness, fatigue, insomnia, nervousness.
EENT: *dry mouth.*

Interactions

Drug-drug. *Erythromycin, ketoconazole:* Increases loratadine levels. Monitor patient closely.
Drug-lifestyle. *Alcohol use:* Increases CNS depression. Discourage using together.

Effects on lab test results

None reported.

Pharmacokinetics

Absorption: Good. Food may delay peak levels by 1 hour.
Distribution: Doesn't readily cross blood-brain barrier; about 97% bound to protein.
Metabolism: Extensive, although specific enzyme system hasn't been identified.
Excretion: About 80%, distributed equally between urine and feces. *Half-life:* 8½ hours.

Route	Onset	Peak	Duration
P.O.	1 hr	4–6 hr	24 hr

Action

Chemical effect: Blocks effects of histamine at H_1-receptor sites. Drug's chemical structure prevents entry into CNS, preventing sedation.
Therapeutic effect: Relieves allergy symptoms.

Available forms

Syrup: 1 mg/ml†
Tablets: 10 mg†
Tablets (rapidly disintegrating): 10 mg†

NURSING PROCESS

✎ Assessment

• Assess patient's condition before starting therapy and regularly thereafter to monitor the drug's effectiveness.
• Be alert for adverse reactions and drug interactions.
• Assess patient's and family's knowledge of drug therapy.

⊕ Nursing diagnoses

• Ineffective health maintenance related to underlying allergy condition
• Fatigue related to drug's adverse effect
• Deficient knowledge related to drug therapy

❯ Planning and implementation

• Give drug on an empty stomach.

• If drug is ineffective, notify prescriber.
Patient teaching
• Tell patient to take drug at least 2 hours after a meal, to avoid eating for at least 1 hour after taking drug, and to take drug only once daily.
• Advise patient taking rapidly disintegrating tablets to place tablet on the tongue, where it disintegrates within a few seconds. It can be swallowed with or without water.
• Tell patient to contact prescriber if symptoms persist or worsen.
• Advise patient to stop taking drug 4 days before allergy skin tests to preserve accuracy of tests.
• Tell patient not to drink alcohol and not to drive or engage in other activities that require alertness until the drug's CNS effects are known.

☑ Evaluation

• Patient states that allergy symptoms are relieved.
• Patient describes coping strategies for fatigue.
• Patient and family state understanding of drug therapy.

lorazepam

(loo-RAZ-eh-pam)
Apo-Lorazepam ♦ , Ativan, Lorazepam
Intensol, Novo-Lorazem ♦ , Nu-Loraz ♦

Pharmacologic class: benzodiazepine
Therapeutic class: anxiolytic, sedative-hypnotic
Pregnancy risk category: D
Controlled substance schedule: IV

Indications and dosages

❯ **Anxiety.** *Adults:* 2 to 6 mg P.O. daily in divided doses. Maximum, 10 mg daily.
❯ **Insomnia caused by anxiety.** *Adults:* 2 to 4 mg P.O. h.s.
▧ **Adjust-a-dose:** For elderly patients, initially, 1 to 2 mg P.O. daily in divided doses. Adjust as needed and as tolerated.
❯ **Status epilepticus.** *Adults:* 4 mg I.V. If seizures continue or recur after 10 to 15 minutes, another 4 mg may be given. *Children‡:* 0.05 to 0.1 mg/kg I.V.
❯ **Premedication before operative procedure.** *Adults:* 0.05 mg/kg I.M. 2 hours before proce-

dure. Maximum dosage, 4 mg. Or 2 mg total or 0.044 mg/kg I.V., whichever is smaller.
► **Nausea and vomiting caused by emetogenic cancer chemotherapy‡.** *Adults:* 2.5 mg P.O. the evening before chemotherapy; repeat just after the initiation of chemotherapy. Or 1.5 mg/m^2 (maximum, 3 mg) I.V. over 5 minutes, 45 minutes before chemotherapy.

▼ I.V. administration

• Have emergency resuscitation equipment and oxygen available.
• Dilute with equal volume of sterile water for injection, normal saline solution for injection, or D$_5$W injection.
• Don't exceed 2-mg dose preoperatively in patients older than age 50.
• Check respirations before each dose and q 5 to 15 minutes thereafter until respiratory condition is stable.
• Give drug slowly, at no more than 2 mg/minute.
⊗ **Incompatibilities**
Aldesleukin, aztreonam, buprenorphine, foscarnet, idarubicin, imipenem-cilastatin sodium, ondansetron hydrochloride, sargramostim, sufentanil citrate, thiopental.

Contraindications and cautions

• Contraindicated in patients hypersensitive to the drug or any of its components or other benzodiazepines. Contraindicated in patients with acute angle-closure glaucoma or acute alcohol intoxication. I.M. and I.V. forms contraindicated in patients with renal or hepatic impairment.
• Use cautiously in patients with pulmonary impairment. Use oral forms cautiously in patients with renal or hepatic impairment. Also use cautiously and at a reduced dosage in acutely ill or debilitated patients.
⚖ **Lifespan:** In pregnant and breast-feeding women, drug is contraindicated. In children, safety and effectiveness haven't been established. In elderly patients, use cautiously and at a lower dose.

Adverse reactions

CNS: *drowsiness, lethargy, hangover,* fainting, anterograde amnesia, restlessness, psychosis.
CV: transient hypotension.
EENT: visual disturbances.
GI: dry mouth, abdominal discomfort.

GU: incontinence, urine retention.
Other: *acute withdrawal syndrome.*

Interactions

Drug-drug. *CNS depressants:* May increase CNS depression. Avoid using together.
Digoxin: May increase digoxin level, increasing toxicity. Monitor level.
Levodopa: May decrease antiparkinson effect. Monitor patient.
Scopolamine: May increase the incidence of sedation, hallucinations, and irrational behavior. Monitor patient.
Drug-herb. *Catnip, kava, lady's slipper, lemon balm, passion flower, sassafras, skullcap, valerian:* May enhance sedative effects. Discourage using together.
Drug-lifestyle. *Alcohol use:* May cause additive CNS effects. Strongly discourage using together.
Smoking: May decrease drug effectiveness. Monitor patient closely; discourage patient from smoking.

Effects on lab test results

• May increase liver function test values.

Pharmacokinetics

Absorption: Good with P.O. use; unknown with I.M. use.
Distribution: Wide; 85% protein-bound.
Metabolism: In liver.
Excretion: In urine. *Half-life:* 10 to 20 hours.

Route	Onset	Peak	Duration
P.O.	1 hr	2 hr	12–24 hr
I.V.	1–5 min	1–1½ hr	6–8 hr
I.M.	15–30 min	1–1½ hr	6–8 hr

Action

Chemical effect: May stimulate gamma-aminobutyric receptors in ascending reticular activating system.
Therapeutic effect: Relieves anxiety and promotes calmness and sleep.

Available forms

Injection: 2 mg/ml, 4 mg/ml
Oral solution (concentrated): 2 mg/ml
S.L. tablets: 0.5 mg ♦, 1 mg ♦, 2 mg ♦
Tablets: 0.5 mg, 1 mg, 2 mg

Reactions may be *common,* uncommon, *life-threatening*, or COMMON AND LIFE-THREATENING.

NURSING PROCESS

⚕ Assessment
- Assess patient's condition before starting therapy and regularly thereafter to monitor drug's effectiveness.
- Monitor liver, kidney, and hematopoietic function studies periodically in patient receiving repeated or prolonged therapy.
- Be alert for adverse reactions and drug interactions.
- Assess patient's and family's knowledge of drug therapy.

⊕ Nursing diagnoses
- Anxiety related to underlying condition
- Risk for injury related to drug-induced adverse CNS effects
- Deficient knowledge related to drug therapy

⧉ Planning and implementation
- For I.M. injection, inject drug deep into muscle mass. Don't dilute.
- Refrigerate parenteral form to prolong shelf life.
- ⊗ ALERT: Possibility of abuse and addiction exists. Don't abruptly stop giving the drug after long-term use. Withdrawal symptoms may occur.
- ⊗ ALERT: Don't confuse lorazepam with alprazolam.

Patient teaching
- Warn patient to avoid hazardous activities until the drug's CNS effects are known.
- Tell patient not to drink alcohol or smoke during therapy.
- Explain the risks of dependence and addiction with prolonged use of drug.
- Teach patient not to stop drug abruptly after prolonged use because of risk of seizures or other withdrawal symptoms.

☑ Evaluation
- Patient is less anxious.
- Patient doesn't experience injury as result of adverse CNS reactions.
- Patient and family state understanding of drug therapy.

losartan potassium
(loh-SAR-tan poh-TAH-see-um)
Cozaar◊

Pharmacologic class: angiotensin II receptor antagonist
Therapeutic class: antihypertensive
Pregnancy risk category: C (D in second and third trimesters)

Indications and dosages
▶ **Nephropathy in type 2 diabetes mellitus.**
Adults: 50 mg P.O. daily. Increase dose to 100 mg daily based on blood pressure response.
▶ **Hypertension.** *Adults:* Initially, 25 to 50 mg P.O. daily. Maximum daily dosage, 100 mg in one or two divided doses.
▶ **To reduce risk of stroke in patients with hypertension and left ventricular hypertrophy.** *Adults:* Initially, 50 mg P.O. once daily. Adjust dosage based on blood pressure response, adding hydrochlorothiazide 12.5 mg once daily, increasing losartan to 100 mg daily, or both. If further adjustments are required, may increase the daily dosage of hydrochlorothiazide to 25 mg.

Contraindications and cautions
- Contraindicated in patients hypersensitive to the drug or any of its components.
- Use cautiously in patients with impaired kidney or liver function and in volume-depleted, hypotensive patients.
- ☀ Lifespan: In pregnant women, drug is contraindicated in second and third trimesters; use very cautiously in first trimester. If pregnancy occurs, stop drug as soon as possible. Breast-feeding women should stop breast-feeding or use another drug. In children, safety and effectiveness haven't been established.

Adverse reactions
For hypertension and left ventricular hypertrophy
CNS: dizziness, asthenia, fatigue, headache, insomnia.
CV: edema, chest pain.
EENT: nasal congestion, sinusitis, pharyngitis, sinus disorder.
GI: abdominal pain, nausea, diarrhea, dyspepsia.

Rapid onset   *Liquid form contains alcohol.   ◆ Canada   ◇ Australia   †OTC   ◊Photoguide   ‡Off-label use

Musculoskeletal: muscle cramps, myalgia, back or leg pain.
Respiratory: cough, upper respiratory tract infection.
Other: *anaphylaxis, angioedema.*
For nephropathy
CNS: *asthenia, fatigue,* fever, hypoesthesia, diabetic neuropathy.
CV: *chest pain,* hypotension, orthostatic hypotension, *diabetic vascular disease.*
EENT: sinusitis, cataract.
GI: *diarrhea,* dyspepsia, gastritis.
GU: UTI.
Hematologic: *anemia.*
Metabolic: *hyperkalemia,* HYPOGLYCEMIA, weight gain.
Musculoskeletal: *back pain,* leg or knee pain, muscle weakness.
Respiratory: *cough, bronchitis.*
Skin: cellulitis.
Other: infection, *flulike syndrome,* trauma, *anaphylaxis, angioedema.*

Interactions

Drug-drug. *Fluconazole:* May increase antihypertensive effects and adverse reactions. Monitor patient.
Indomethacin: May decrease hypotensive effect. Monitor blood pressure.
Phenobarbital: May decrease absorption of losartan. Monitor patient.
Potassium-sparing diuretics, potassium supplements: May cause hyperkalemia. Monitor potassium level.
Rifamycins: May decrease antihypertensive effects. Monitor blood pressure.
Drug-herb. *Red yeast rice:* May increase the risk of adverse events or toxicity because herb contains components similar to those of statin drugs. Discourage using together.
Drug-food. *Salt substitutes containing potassium:* May increase risk of hyperkalemia. Monitor patient closely; advise patient to use only under prescriber's guidance.

Effects on lab test results

None reported.

Pharmacokinetics

Absorption: Good with extensive first-pass metabolism; systemic bioavailability of drug is 33%.
Distribution: Highly bound to proteins.

Metabolism: Involves CYP 2C9 and 3A4.
Excretion: Primarily in feces with smaller amount in urine. *Half-life:* 2 hours.

Route	Onset	Peak	Duration
P.O.	Unknown	1–4 hr	Unknown

Action

Chemical effect: Inhibits vasoconstricting and aldosterone-secreting effects of angiotensin II by selectively blocking binding of angiotensin II to receptor sites in many tissues, including vascular smooth muscle and adrenal glands.
Therapeutic effect: Lowers blood pressure.

Available forms

Tablets: 25 mg, 50 mg, 100 mg

NURSING PROCESS

⚗ Assessment
● Assess patient's blood pressure before starting therapy and regularly thereafter to monitor drug's effectiveness. When drug is used alone, its effect on blood pressure is notably less in black patients than in patients of other races.
● Regularly assess creatinine and BUN levels to check kidney function. Patients with severe heart failure whose kidney function depends on angiotensin-aldosterone system may experience acute renal impairment during therapy. Closely monitor patient, especially during first few weeks of therapy.
● Be alert for adverse reactions.
● If patient is taking a diuretic, monitor him for symptomatic hypotension.
● Assess patient's and family's knowledge of drug therapy.

⊕ Nursing diagnoses
● Risk for injury related to presence of hypertension
● Disturbed sleep pattern related to drug-induced insomnia
● Deficient knowledge related to drug therapy

▷ Planning and implementation
● In patient with impaired liver function, or patient with volume depletion (such as patient taking diuretic), use initial dose of 25 mg.
● Black patients with hypertension and left ventricular hypertrophy have a lower risk of stroke

---

on atenolol than on this drug, but the cause is unknown.

• Drug can be used alone or with other antihypertensives.

• Determine trough level to measure effect. If giving once daily isn't effective, divide same total daily into two daily doses or increase dose.

• Give once-daily dose in the morning to prevent insomnia.

• If pregnancy is suspected, stop giving the drug and immediately notify prescriber.

⑤ **ALERT:** Don't confuse Cozaar with Zocor.

Patient teaching

• Tell patient to avoid sodium substitutes because they may contain potassium, which can cause hyperkalemia in patients taking drug.

• Tell woman of childbearing age to notify prescriber immediately if she suspects she is pregnant.

☑ **Evaluation**

• Patient's blood pressure is normal.

• Patient states that insomnia hasn't occurred.

• Patient and family state understanding of drug therapy.

lovastatin (mevinolin)
(loh-vuh-STAH-tin)
Altoprev, Mevacor⌀

Pharmacologic class: HMG-CoA reductase inhibitor
Therapeutic class: cholesterol-lowering drug
Pregnancy risk category: X

Indications and dosages

▶ **Primary prevention of coronary artery disease; coronary artery disease; hyperlipidemia.** *Adults:* Initially, 20 mg immediate release tablets P.O. once daily with evening meal. Recommended range is 10 to 80 mg in single or two divided doses; maximum dosage, 80 mg daily. Or 20 to 60 mg extended-release P.O. h.s. Starting dose of 10 mg can be used for patients requiring smaller reductions. Usual dosage range is 10 to 60 mg daily for the extended-release tablets.

▶ **Heterozygous familial hypercholesterolemia.** *Children ages 10 to 17:* 10 to 40 mg P.O. (immediate-release) daily with evening meal. In

patients requiring reductions in LDL level of 20% or more, start with 20 mg daily.

⑤ **Adjust-a-dose:** For patients also taking cyclosporine, give 10 mg P.O. daily, not to exceed 20 mg daily. Avoid use of drug with fibrates or niacin; if used with either, don't give more than 20 mg of lovastatin daily. If using with amiodarone or verapamil (immediate-release), don't exceed 40 mg/day.

For patients with renal impairment, if creatinine clearance is less than 30 ml/minute, take care when considering dosage increase above 20 mg daily.

Contraindications and cautions

• Contraindicated in patients hypersensitive to the drug or any of its components, and in those with active liver disease or conditions linked to unexplained persistent elevations of transaminase levels.

• Use cautiously in patients who consume substantial quantities of alcohol or have history of liver disease.

⚘ **Lifespan:** In pregnant and breast-feeding women, drug is contraindicated. In women of childbearing age, drug is contraindicated unless they have no risk of pregnancy. In children younger than age 10, safety and effectiveness haven't been established.

Adverse reactions

CNS: headache, dizziness, peripheral neuropathy.
EENT: blurred vision.
GI: constipation, diarrhea, dyspepsia, flatulence, abdominal pain or cramps, heartburn, dysgeusia, nausea.
Musculoskeletal: muscle cramps, myalgia, myositis, *rhabdomyolysis.*
Skin: rash, pruritus.

Interactions

Drug-drug. *Bile acid sequestrants:* Decreases lovastatin bioavailability. Administer separately.
Cyclosporine or other immunosuppressants, erythromycin, gemfibrozil, niacin: Increases risk of polymyositis and rhabdomyolysis. Monitor patient closely.
Digoxin: May slightly elevate digoxin levels. Monitor patient.
Fluconazole, itraconazole, ketoconazole: May increase level and adverse effects of lovastatin.

L

Avoid this combination. If drugs must be given together, reduce dose of lovastatin.

Isradipine: May increase clearance of lovastatin and its metabolites by increasing hepatic blood flow. Monitor patient for loss of therapeutic effect.

Nicotinic acid: May increase risk of severe myopathy or rhabdomyolysis. Monitor patient closely.

Oral anticoagulants: May enhance oral anticoagulant effects. Monitor PT and INR.

Drug-herb. *Red yeast rice:* May increase the risk of adverse events or toxicity because herb contains components similar to those of drug. Discourage using together.

Drug-lifestyle. *Alcohol use:* May increase risk of hepatotoxicity. Discourage using together.

Sun exposure: May cause photosensitivity reactions. Tell patient to avoid unprotected or prolonged exposure to sunlight.

Effects on lab test results

• May increase ALT, AST, and CK levels. May decrease lipid level.

Pharmacokinetics

Absorption: About 30%. Giving with food improves levels of total inhibitors by about 30%. Extended-release tablets have greater bioavailability than immediate-release tablets.

Distribution: Less than 5% because of extensive first-pass hepatic extraction. More than 95% bound to proteins.

Metabolism: In liver.

Excretion: About 80% in feces, about 10% in urine. *Half-life:* 3 hours.

Route	Onset	Peak	Duration
P.O.	Unknown	2–6 hr	4–6 wk
P.O. extended-release	Unknown	14 hr	Unknown

Action

Chemical effect: Inhibits HMG-CoA reductase. This enzyme is an early and rate-limiting step in synthetic pathway of cholesterol.

Therapeutic effect: Lowers LDL and total cholesterol levels.

Available forms

Tablets: 10 mg, 20 mg, 40 mg

Tablets (extended-release): 10 mg, 20 mg, 40 mg, 60 mg

NURSING PROCESS

⚡ Assessment

• Obtain history of patient's lipoprotein and cholesterol levels before starting therapy, and reassess regularly to monitor the drug's effectiveness.

• Use for heterozygous familial hypercholesterolemia in girls who are at least 1 year postmenarche and boys (ages 10 to 17) who have the following findings after an adequate trial of diet therapy: LDL level higher than 189 mg/dl or LDL level higher than 160 mg/dl with a family history of premature CV disease or two or more other CV disease risk factors.

• Perform liver function tests before starting therapy and periodically thereafter.

• Be alert for adverse reactions and drug interactions.

• Assess patient's and family's knowledge of drug therapy.

⊕ Nursing diagnoses

• Risk for injury related to underlying condition
• Pain related to drug-induced adverse musculoskeletal reactions
• Deficient knowledge related to drug therapy

⟩ Planning and implementation

• Begin drug therapy only after diet and other nonpharmacologic therapies have proven ineffective. Make sure patient is following a standard low-cholesterol diet.

• Give drug with evening meal; absorption is enhanced and cholesterol biosynthesis is greater in evening.

⊛ **ALERT:** Don't confuse lovastatin with Lotensin, Leustatin, or Livostin. Don't confuse Mevacor with Mivacron.

Patient teaching

• Instruct patient to take drug with evening meal.

• Advise patient not to crush or chew extended-release tablets.

• Teach patient to manage lipid level by restricting total fat and cholesterol intake. If appropriate, recommend weight control, exercise, and smoking cessation programs to control other cardiac disease risk factors.

• Advise patient to have periodic eye examinations.

Reactions may be *common*, uncommon, *life-threatening*, or COMMON AND LIFE-THREATENING.

• Tell patient to store drug at room temperature in light-resistant container.
• Instruct patient to avoid alcohol consumption during drug therapy.
⑤ ALERT: Inform patient that drug is contraindicated during pregnancy. Tell her to notify prescriber immediately if she becomes pregnant.

☑ Evaluation
• Patient's LDL and cholesterol levels are within normal limits.
• Patient doesn't experience musculoskeletal pain.
• Patient and family state understanding of drug therapy.

lymphocyte immune globulin (LIG) (antithymocyte globulin [equine], ATG),
(LIM-foh-sight ih-MYOON GLOH-byoo-lin)
Atgam

Pharmacologic class: immunoglobulin
Therapeutic class: immunosuppressant
Pregnancy risk category: C

Indications and dosages
▶ **To prevent acute renal allograft rejection.** *Adults and children:* 15 mg/kg I.V. daily for 14 days, followed by alternate-day doses for 14 days. Give first dose within 24 hours of transplantation.
▶ **Acute renal allograft rejection.** *Adults and children:* 10 to 15 mg/kg I.V. daily for 14 days, followed by alternate-day doses for 14 days. Start therapy when rejection is diagnosed.
▶ **Aplastic anemia.** *Adults:* 10 to 20 mg/kg I.V. daily for 8 to 14 days. Additional alternate-day therapy up to total of 21 doses can be given.
▶ **Skin allotransplantation‡.** *Adults:* 10 mg/ kg I.V. 24 hours before allograft; then 10 to 15 mg/kg q other day. Maintenance dosage ranges from 5 to 40 mg/kg daily based on response. Therapy usually continues until allograft covers less than 20% of total body surface area, usually 40 to 60 days.

▼ I.V. administration
• Dilute dose in 250 to 1,000 ml of half-normal or normal saline solution for injection. Don't

exceed final concentration of 4 mg/ml. When adding drug to solution, make sure container is inverted so drug doesn't contact air inside container. The proteins in drug can be denatured by air. Gently rotate or swirl container to mix contents; don't shake because this may cause excessive foaming and may alter drug.
• Allow diluted drug to reach room temperature before infusion.
• Infuse with in-line filter with pore size of 0.2 to 1 micron over no less than 4 hours (most facilities specify 4 to 8 hours) into a vascular shunt, arterial venous fistula, or high-flow central vein.
• Don't use solutions that are more than 12 hours old, including actual infusion time.
• Refrigerate drug at 35° to 47° F (2° to 8° C). Don't freeze. Drug is heat sensitive.
⊗ **Incompatibilities**
Dextrose solutions, solutions with low salt concentration, acidic solutions.

Contraindications and cautions
• Contraindicated in patients hypersensitive to the drug or any of its components.
• Use cautiously in patients receiving additional immunosuppressive therapy (such as corticosteroids and azathioprine) because of increased risk of infection.
⚕ **Lifespan:** In pregnant women, use cautiously. In breast-feeding women, drug isn't recommended because it is unknown if drug is excreted in breast milk.

Adverse reactions
CNS: malaise, *seizures,* headache.
CV: *hypotension, chest pain,* thrombophlebitis, tachycardia, edema, *iliac vein obstruction,* renal artery stenosis.
EENT: *laryngospasm.*
GI: *nausea, vomiting,* diarrhea, epigastric pain, abdominal distention, stomatitis.
Hematologic: *leukopenia, thrombocytopenia,* hemolysis, *aplastic anemia,* lymphadenopathy.
Metabolic: hyperglycemia.
Musculoskeletal: arthralgia.
Respiratory: *dyspnea,* hiccups, *pulmonary edema.*
Skin: rash.
Other: febrile reactions, serum sickness, *anaphylaxis,* infection, night sweats.

Interactions

Drug-drug. *Muromonab-CD3, immunosuppressants:* May increase risk of infection. Monitor patient closely.

Effects on lab test results

• May increase liver enzyme and glucose levels. May decrease hemoglobin level and hematocrit.
• May decrease WBC and platelet counts.

Pharmacokinetics

Absorption: Administered I.V.
Distribution: Unknown.
Metabolism: Unknown.
Excretion: About 1% in urine, mainly as unchanged drug. *Half-life:* About 6 days.

Route	Onset	Peak	Duration
I.V.	Unknown	5 days	Unknown

Action

Chemical effect: Inhibits cell-mediated immune responses by either altering T-cell function or eliminating antigen-reactive T cells.
Therapeutic effect: Prevents or relieves signs and symptoms of renal allograft rejection; also relieves signs and symptoms of aplastic anemia.

Available forms

Injection: 50 mg of equine immunoglobulin/ml

NURSING PROCESS

🔁 Assessment

• Assess patient's condition before starting therapy and regularly thereafter to monitor the drug's effectiveness.
• Be alert for adverse reactions and drug interactions.
• Assess patient's and family's knowledge of drug therapy.

⊕ Nursing diagnoses

• Ineffective health maintenance related to underlying condition
• Ineffective immune protection related to adverse hematologic reactions
• Deficient knowledge related to drug therapy

▷ Planning and implementation

• Perform an intradermal skin test at least 1 hour before giving the first dose. Marked local swelling or erythema larger than 10 mm indicates increased risk of severe systemic reaction, such as anaphylaxis. Severe reactions to skin test, such as hypotension, tachycardia, dyspnea, generalized rash, or anaphylaxis, rule out further use.

⊛ **ALERT:** Keep airway adjuncts and anaphylaxis drugs at bedside while giving the drug.

Patient teaching

• Warn patient that he is likely to develop a fever. Instruct him to report adverse drug effects.
• Instruct patient to take infection-control and bleeding precautions.

☑ Evaluation

• Patient responds well to therapy.
• Patient doesn't experience serious adverse hematologic reactions.
• Patient and family state understanding of drug therapy.

magnesium chloride (MgCl₂)
(mag-NEE-see-um KLOR-ighd)
Slow-Mag

magnesium sulfate (MgSO₄)

Pharmacologic class: magnesium salts
Therapeutic class: anticonvulsant, mineral, antiarrhythmic
Pregnancy risk category: A

Indications and dosages

▶ **Mild hypomagnesemia.** *Adults:* 1 g I.M. q 6 hours for four doses, depending on magnesium level.
▶ **Severe hypomagnesemia (magnesium level 0.8 mEq/L or less with symptoms).** *Adults:* Up to 2 mEq (0.5 ml of 50% solution)/kg I.M. within a 4- hour period may be given, or 5 g (about 40 mEq) I.V. in 1 L of solution over 3 hours. Subsequent doses depend on magnesium level.
▶ **Magnesium supplementation.** *Adults:* 54 to 483 mg P.O. daily in divided doses (MgCl₂ only).

▶ **Magnesium supplementation in total parenteral nutrition (TPN).** *Adults:* 8 to 24 mEq I.V. daily added to TPN solution.
Infants: 2 to 10 mEq I.V. daily added to TPN solution. Each 2 ml of 50% solution contains 1 g, or 8.12 mEq, magnesium sulfate.

▶ **Hypomagnesemic seizures.** *Adults:* 1 to 2 g of 10% solution I.V. over 15 minutes; then 1 g I.M. q 4 to 6 hours, based on patient's response and magnesium level.

▶ **Seizures caused by hypomagnesemia in acute nephritis.** *Children:* 20 to 40 mg/kg I.M. p.r.n. to control seizures. Dilute the 50% concentration to a 20% solution and give 0.1 to 0.2 ml/kg of the 20% solution. Or, 100 to 200 mg/kg as a 1% to 3% solution I.V. slowly over one hour with 50% of dose given in first 15 to 20 minutes. Adjust dosage according to magnesium level and seizure response.

▶ **Paroxysmal atrial tachycardia in patients unresponsive to other therapies‡.** *Adults:* 3 to 4 g I.V. of 10% solution over 30 seconds with close monitoring of ECG.

▶ **To reduce CV morbidity and mortality from acute MI‡.** *Adults:* 2 g I.V. over 5 to 15 minutes, followed by infusion of 18 g over 24 hours (12.5 mg/minute). Initiate therapy as soon as possible, but no longer than 6 hours after MI.

▶ **To manage preterm labor‡.** *Adults:* 4 to 6 g I.V. over 20 minutes as a loading dose, followed by maintenance infusions of 2 to 4 g/hour for 12 to 24 hours, as tolerated, after contractions subside.

▶ **Severe acute asthma unresponsive to conventional therapy‡.** *Children:* 25 to 50 mg/kg (up to 2 g) I.V. over 10 to 20 minutes.

▼ **I.V. administration**

● Solutions must be diluted to a concentration of 20% (200 mg/ml) or less prior to administration.
● Inject I.V. bolus dose slowly. Use infusion pump for continuous infusion to avoid respiratory or cardiac arrest. Don't exceed 150 mg/ minute (1.5 ml of a 10% solution). Rapid drip causes heat sensation.
● When giving I.V. for severe hypomagnesemia, watch for respiratory depression and signs and symptoms of heart block. Give dose only when respirations are more than 16 breaths/minute.
● Monitor vital signs q 15 minutes when giving drug I.V.

● For preterm labor, monitor I.V. fluids and rates carefully to avoid circulatory overload. Monitor patient for pulmonary edema.

⊗ **Incompatibilities**
Alcohol in high concentrations, alkali carbonates and bicarbonates, amiodarone, amphotericin B, arsenates, barium, calcium gluconate, cefepime, ciprofloxacin, clindamycin, cyclosporine, dobutamine, ethanol, heavy metals, hydrocortisone sodium succinate, I.V. fat emulsion 10%, polymyxin B, procaine, salicylates, sodium bicarbonate, soluble phosphates, tartrates.

Contraindications and cautions

● Contraindicated in patients with myocardial damage, marked myocardial disease, or heart block. I.V. form is contraindicated in patients with preeclampsia during the 2 hours preceding delivery. Magnesium chloride is contraindicated in patients with renal impairment.
● Use magnesium sulfate cautiously in patients with impaired kidney function.

⚘ **Lifespan:** Use during all trimesters of pregnancy if clearly needed except during active labor when drug is contraindicated. Continuous I.V. infusion longer than 24 hours in toxemic mothers may cause neonatal magnesium toxicity. In breast-feeding women small amount of drug is excreted in breast milk but use if clearly needed. Elderly patients may need a lower dose because of renal insufficiency. If patient is severely renally impaired, don't exceed 20 g in 48 hours.

Adverse reactions

CNS: *depressed deep tendon reflexes,* flaccid paralysis, hypothermia, drowsiness, perioral paresthesia, twitching carpopedal spasm, tetany, *seizures.*
CV: *slow, weak pulse; arrhythmias; hypotension;* circulatory collapse; depressed cardiac function; *heart block.*
Metabolic: hypocalcemia.
Respiratory: *respiratory paralysis.*
Other: diaphoresis, flushing.

Interactions

Drug-drug. *Anesthetics, CNS depressants:* May cause additive CNS depression. Use together cautiously.
Digoxin: May cause serious cardiac conduction changes. Give cautiously.

M

Neuromuscular blockers: May increase neuro-muscular blockage. Use cautiously; monitor patient for increased effects.
Nitrofurantoin, penicillamine, tetracyclines: Decreases bioavailability with oral magnesium supplements. Separate administration times by 2 to 3 hours.

Effects on lab test results

• May increase magnesium level. May decrease calcium and potassium levels.

Pharmacokinetics

Absorption: 35% to 40% of P.O. dose. High-fat diets may interfere.
Distribution: About 30% is bound intracellularly to proteins and energy-rich phosphates.
Metabolism: None.
Excretion: Parenteral dose primarily in urine, P.O. dose in urine and feces. *Half-life:* Unknown.

Route	Onset	Peak	Duration
P.O.	Unknown	4 hr	4–6 hr
I.V.	Immediate	Unknown	30 min
I.M.	1 hr	Unknown	3–4 hr

Action

Chemical effect: Replaces and maintains magnesium levels; as anticonvulsant, reduces muscle contractions by interfering with release of acetylcholine at myoneural junction.
Therapeutic effect: Raises magnesium levels, alleviates seizures, and restores normal sinus rhythm.

Available forms

magnesium chloride
Injectable solutions: 20% (1.97 mEq/ml)
Tablets (delayed-release): 64 mg elemental magnesium
magnesium sulfate
Injectable solutions: 4% (0.325 mEq/ml), 8% (0.65 mEq/ml), 10% (0.8 mEq/ml), 12.5% (1 mEq/ml), 50% (4 mEq/ml)

NURSING PROCESS

🗓 Assessment

• Assess patient's condition before therapy and regularly thereafter to monitor the drug's effectiveness.
• Check magnesium level after repeated doses.

⚠ **ALERT:** Watch for respiratory depression and signs of heart block. Make sure respirations are 16 breaths/minute before each dose.
• Monitor patient's fluid intake and output. Make sure output is 100 ml or more during the 4 hours before giving.
• Be alert for adverse reactions and drug interactions.
• Assess patient's and family's knowledge of drug therapy.

🔄 Nursing diagnoses

• Ineffective health maintenance related to underlying condition
• Risk for injury related to drug-induced adverse reactions
• Deficient knowledge related to drug therapy

❯ Planning and implementation

• Keep I.V. calcium gluconate available at bedside to reverse magnesium intoxication.
• For cases of severe hypermagnesemia, peritoneal dialysis or hemodialysis may be needed.
• Undiluted 50% solutions may be given to adults by deep I.M. injection. When giving to children, dilute solutions to 20% or less.
⚠ **ALERT:** Test knee-jerk (patellar) reflexes before each additional dose. If no reflex, notify prescriber and withhold magnesium until reflexes return. Check magnesium level because it may be toxic. Signs of hypermagnesemia begin to appear at a level of 4 mEq/L.
• If used to treat seizures, institute appropriate seizure precautions.
Patient teaching
• Instruct patient taking parenteral drug to immediately report any adverse reactions.
• Review oral administration schedule with patient. Tell him not to take more than prescribed.

✓ Evaluation

• Patient has positive response to drug administration.
• Patient sustains no injury from adverse reactions.
• Patient and family state understanding of drug therapy.

magnesium citrate
(citrate of magnesia)
(mag-NEE-see-um SIH-trayt)
Citro-Mag ♦, Evac-Q-Mag†

magnesium hydroxide (Mg(OH)$_2$)
Milk of Magnesia†, Milk of Magnesia
Concentrated†, Phillips' Milk of Magnesia†,
Phillips' Milk of Magnesia Concentrated†

magnesium sulfate (MgSO$_4$)
Epsom salts†

Pharmacologic class: magnesium salts
Therapeutic class: saline laxatives
Pregnancy risk category: NR

Indications and dosages

▶ **Constipation, to evacuate bowel before surgery.** *Adults and children age 12 and older:* 11 to 25 g magnesium citrate P.O. daily as single dose or divided. Or 2 to 4 tbs Mg(OH)$_2$ at h.s. or on rising, followed by 240 ml (8 oz) of liquid. Or 10 to 30 g MgSO$_4$ P.O. daily as single dose or divided.
Children ages 6 to 11: 5.5 to 12.5 g magnesium citrate P.O. daily as single dose or divided. Or 1 to 2 tbs Mg(OH) $_2$ followed by 240 ml (8 oz) of liquid. Don't use dosage cup. Or 5 to 10 g MgSO$_4$ P.O. daily as single dose or divided.
Children ages 2 to 5: 2.7 to 6.25 g magnesium citrate P.O. daily as single dose or divided. Or 1 to 3 tsp Mg(OH)$_2$ followed by 240 ml (8 oz) of liquid. Don't use dosage cup. Or 2.5 to 5 g MgSO$_4$ P.O. daily as single dose or divided.
▶ **Acid indigestion, gastroesophageal reflux disease, peptic ulcer disease, heartburn.**
Adults and children age 12 and older: Don't use dosage cup. 1 to 3 tsp Mg(OH)$_2$ with a little water, up to four times a day, or as directed by prescriber. Or, for adults, 5 to 15 ml Mg citrate P.O. t.i.d. or q.i.d.

Contraindications and cautions

● Contraindicated in patients with abdominal pain, nausea, vomiting, other symptoms of appendicitis or acute surgical abdomen, myocardial damage, heart block, fecal impaction, rectal fissures, intestinal obstruction or perforation, or renal disease.

● Use cautiously in patients with rectal bleeding.
⚙ **Lifespan:** In pregnant women, use cautiously. During labor and delivery, drug is contraindicated. In breast-feeding women, use cautiously; small amounts of the drug appears in breast milk. In children, use cautiously.

Adverse reactions

GI: *abdominal cramping, nausea, diarrhea,* laxative dependence with long-term or excessive use.
Metabolic: fluid and electrolyte disturbances.

Interactions

Drug-drug. *Benzodiazepines, chloroquine, corticosteroids, digoxin, H$_2$-antagonists, hydantoins, iron, nitrofurantoin, penicillamine, phenothiazines, tetracyclines:* May decrease pharmacologic effects of these drugs. Monitor patient.
Ciprofloxacin, gatifloxacin, levofloxacin, lomefloxacin, moxifloxacin, norfloxacin, ofloxacin: Magnesium hydroxide may decrease effects of quinolones. Give drug at least 6 hours before or 2 hours after quinolones.
Dicumarol, quinidine, sulfonylureas: May increase pharmacologic effects of these drugs. Monitor patient.
Oral drugs: Impairs absorption. Separate administration times.

Effects on lab test results

● May increase or decrease fluid and electrolyte levels with prolonged use.

Pharmacokinetics

Absorption: About 15% to 30% may be systemic (posing risk to patients with renal impairment).
Distribution: Unknown.
Metabolism: Unknown.
Excretion: Unabsorbed drug in feces; absorbed drug rapidly in urine. *Half-life:* Unknown.

Route	Onset	Peak	Duration
P.O.	30 min–3 hr	Varies	Varies

Action

Chemical effect: Reduces total acid load in GI tract, elevates gastric pH to inhibit pepsin, strengthens gastric mucosal barrier, and increases esophageal sphincter tone.

M

Therapeutic effect: Soothes stomach upset, relieves constipation, and raises magnesium level.

Available forms

magnesium citrate
Oral solution: about 3.85 to 4.71 mEq Mg/5 ml†
magnesium hydroxide
Oral suspension: 7% to 8.5% (about 80 mEq Mg/30 ml)†
magnesium sulfate
Granules: about 40 mEq Mg/5 g†

NURSING PROCESS

⚕ Assessment
• Assess patient's condition before therapy and regularly thereafter to monitor the drug's effectiveness.
• Before giving for constipation, determine whether patient has adequate fluid intake, exercise, and diet.
⚠ **ALERT:** Monitor electrolyte levels during prolonged use. Magnesium may accumulate in patients with renal insufficiency.
• Be alert for adverse reactions and drug interactions.
• Assess patient's and family's knowledge of drug therapy.

⚕ Nursing diagnoses
• Constipation related to underlying condition
• Diarrhea related to therapy
• Deficient knowledge related to drug therapy

▶ Planning and implementation
• Give the drug at a time that doesn't interfere with scheduled activities or sleep.
• Chill magnesium citrate before use to improve its palatability.
• Shake suspension well. Give with large amount of water when used as laxative. When giving through NG tube, make sure tube is placed properly and is patent. After instilling drug, flush tube with water to ensure passage to stomach and to maintain tube patency.
⚠ **ALERT:** Drug is for short-term therapy only.
• Magnesium sulfate is more potent than other saline laxatives.
Patient teaching
• Teach patient about dietary sources of bulk, such as bran, other high-fiber cereals, and fresh fruit and vegetables.

• Warn patient that frequent or prolonged use may cause dependence.

☑ Evaluation
• Patient's constipation is relieved.
• Diarrhea doesn't develop.
• Patient and family state understanding of drug therapy.

magnesium oxide
(mag-NEE-see-um OKS-ighd)
Mag-Ox 400†, Maox 420†, Uro-Mag†

Pharmacologic class: magnesium salt
Therapeutic class: antacid, mineral
Pregnancy risk category: NR

Indications and dosages
▶ **Antacid.** *Adults:* 140 mg (capsules) P.O. 3 to 4 times daily, or 400 to 800 mg (tablets) daily.
▶ **Mild hypomagnesemia.** *Adults:* 400 to 840 mg P.O. daily based on magnesium level.

Contraindications and cautions
• In patients with renal disease, use cautiously and under the supervision of a physician.
⚘ **Lifespan:** In pregnant women, use cautiously. In breast-feeding women, use cautiously; it's unknown if the drug appears in breast milk.

Adverse reactions
GI: *diarrhea,* nausea, abdominal pain.
Metabolic: hypermagnesemia.

Interactions
Drug-drug. *Allopurinol, antibiotics (including fluoroquinolones and tetracyclines), diflunisal, digoxin, iron, isoniazid, penicillamine, phenothiazines, quinidine:* Decreases pharmacologic effect, possibly because of impaired absorption. Separate administration times.
Enteric-coated drugs: May release prematurely in stomach. Separate doses by at least 1 hour.

Effects on lab test results
• May increase magnesium level.

Pharmacokinetics
Absorption: Small.
Distribution: Unknown.
Metabolism: None.

Reactions may be *common,* uncommon, *life-threatening*, or COMMON AND LIFE-THREATENING.

Excretion: Unabsorbed drug in feces; absorbed drug in urine. *Half-life:* Unknown.

Route	Onset	Peak	Duration
P.O.			
fasting	20 min	Unknown	20–60 min
non-fasting	20 min	Unknown	20–60 min

Action

Chemical effect: Reduces total acid load in GI tract, elevates gastric pH to inhibit pepsin, strengthens gastric mucosal barrier, and increases esophageal sphincter tone.
Therapeutic effect: Soothes stomach upset, relieves constipation, and raises magnesium level.

Available forms

Capsules: 140 mg (84.5 mg elemental magnesium)†
Tablets: 400 mg (241.3 mg elemental magnesium)†, 420 mg†, 500 mg†

NURSING PROCESS

⚄ Assessment
• Assess patient's condition before therapy and regularly thereafter to monitor the drug's effectiveness.
⊛ ALERT: Monitor magnesium level. In a patient with renal impairment on long-term therapy, watch for signs and symptoms of hypermagnesemia (hypotension, nausea, vomiting, depressed reflexes, respiratory depression, and coma).
• Be alert for adverse reactions and drug interactions.
• Assess patient's and family's knowledge of drug therapy.

⊞ Nursing diagnoses
• Ineffective health maintenance related to underlying condition
• Risk for injury related to potential for hypermagnesemia
• Deficient knowledge related to drug therapy

▷ Planning and implementation
• Don't give other oral drugs 1 to 2 hours before or after therapy.
• If patient has diarrhea, use a different drug.
Patient teaching
• Advise patient not to take drug indiscriminately or to switch antacids without prescriber's advice.

☑ Evaluation
• Patient responds well to therapy.
• Patient maintains normal magnesium level throughout therapy.
• Patient and family state understanding of drug therapy.

mannitol
(MAN-ih-tol)
Osmitrol

Pharmacologic class: osmotic diuretic
Therapeutic class: diuretic
Pregnancy risk category: C

Indications and dosages

▶ **Test dose for marked oliguria or suspected inadequate kidney function.** *Adults and children older than age 12:* 200 mg/kg or 12.5 g as 15% or 20% I.V. solution over 3 to 5 minutes. Response is adequate if 30 to 50 ml of urine/ hour is excreted over 2 to 3 hours. If response is inadequate, give second test dose. If still no response after second dose, stop drug.
Children age 12 and younger‡: 200 mg/kg or 6 g/m^2 I.V. as a 15 or 20% solution over 3 to 5 minutes. Measure response adequacy as above.
▶ **Oliguria.** *Adults and children older than age 12:* 50 to 100 g I.V. of a 15% to 25% solution. *Children age 12 and younger‡:* 2 g/kg or 60 g/ m^2 I.V. as a 15 or 20% solution.
▶ **To prevent oliguria or acute renal impairment.** *Adults and children older than age 12:* 50 to 100 g I.V. of concentrated solution, followed by 5% to 10% solution. Exact concentration determined by fluid requirements.
▶ **Edema; ascites caused by renal, hepatic, or cardiac failure.** *Adults and children older than age 12:* 100 g I.V. as 10% to 20% solution over 2 to 6 hours.
Children age 12 and younger‡: 2 g/kg or 60 g/m^2 I.V. as a 15% or 20% solution over 2 to 6 hours.
▶ **To reduce intraocular or intracranial pressure.** *Adults and children older than age 12:* 1.5 to 2 g/kg as 15% to 25% I.V. solution over 30 to 60 minutes.
Children age 12 and younger‡: 2 g/kg or 60 g/m^2 I.V. as a 15% or 20% solution over 30 to 60 minutes.

M

▶ **Diuresis in drug intoxication.** *Adults and children older than age 12:* Concentration depends on fluid requirement and urine output. If benefit not seen after 200 mg, discontinue infusion.
Children age 12 and younger‡: 2 g/kg or 60 g/m² I.V. as a 5% or 10% solution, p.r.n.
▶ **Irrigating solution during transurethral resection of prostate.** *Adults:* 2.5% solution, p.r.n.

▼ I.V. administration

● Crystals may form in solution at low temperatures or in concentrations greater than 15%. To dissolve, warm bottle in hot water bath and shake vigorously. Cool to body temperature before giving. Don't use solution with undissolved crystals.
● Give as intermittent or continuous infusion, using in-line filter and infusion pump. Direct injection isn't recommended. Check I.V. line patency at infusion site before and during administration.
● Watch for signs of infiltration, including inflammation, edema, and necrosis.
⊗ **Incompatibilities**
Blood products, cefepime, doxorubicin liposomal, filgrastim, imipenem-cilastatin, meropenem, potassium chloride, sodium chloride, strongly acidic or alkaline solutions.

Contraindications and cautions

● Contraindicated in patients hypersensitive to the drug or any of its components, and in those with anuria, severe pulmonary congestion, frank pulmonary edema, severe heart failure, severe dehydration, metabolic edema, progressive renal disease or dysfunction, or active intracranial bleeding except during craniotomy.
⚵ **Lifespan:** In pregnant women, use cautiously. In breast-feeding women, use cautiously; it's unknown if drug appears in breast milk. In children age 12 and younger, safety and effectiveness haven't been established.

Adverse reactions

CNS: headache, confusion, *seizures.*
CV: circulatory overload, heart failure, tachycardia; chest pain.
EENT: blurred vision, rhinitis.
GI: thirst, nausea, vomiting, *diarrhea.*
GU: urine retention.

Metabolic: *water intoxication,* cellular dehydration, electrolyte imbalances.

Interactions

Drug-drug. *Lithium:* Increases urinary excretion of lithium. Monitor patient closely; monitor lithium level.

Effects on lab test results

● May cause electrolyte imbalance.

Pharmacokinetics

Absorption: Administered I.V.
Distribution: Remains in extracellular compartment; doesn't cross blood-brain barrier.
Metabolism: Minimal.
Excretion: In urine. *Half-life:* About 1½ hours.

Route	Onset	Peak	Duration
I.V.	30–60 min	≤ 1 hr	6–8 hr

Action

Chemical effect: Increases osmotic pressure of glomerular filtrate, inhibiting tubular reabsorption of water and electrolytes. This elevates blood osmolality, enhancing water and sodium flow into extracellular fluid.
Therapeutic effect: Increases water excretion, decreases intracranial or intraocular pressure, prevents or treats kidney dysfunction, and promotes excretion of drug overdosage.

Available forms

Injection: 5%, 10%, 15%, 20%, 25%

NURSING PROCESS

⚗ **Assessment**
● Assess patient's condition before therapy and regularly thereafter to monitor the drug's effectiveness.
● Monitor vital signs, central venous pressure, and fluid intake and output hourly. Insert urethral catheter in comatose or incontinent patient because therapy is based on strict evaluation of fluid intake and output. In patient with urethral catheter, use hourly urometer collection bag for accurate evaluation.
● Monitor weight and kidney function, as well as serum and urine sodium and potassium levels, daily.
● Be alert for adverse reactions and drug interactions.

• Assess patient's and family's knowledge of drug therapy.

⊞ Nursing diagnoses
• Ineffective health maintenance related to underlying condition
• Risk for deficient fluid volume related to drug-induced adverse GI reactions
• Deficient knowledge related to drug therapy

⊅ Planning and implementation
• For maximum intraocular pressure reduction before surgery, give 1 to 1½ hours before surgery.
• When used as irrigating solution for prostate surgery, a concentration of 3.5% or greater is needed to avoid hemolysis.
• If patient's oliguria increases or he has adverse reactions, notify prescriber immediately.
Patient teaching
• Tell patient he may feel thirsty or have a dry mouth, and emphasize the importance of drinking only the amount of fluid provided.
• Instruct patient to immediately report pain in chest, back, or legs, or shortness of breath.

☑ Evaluation
• Patient responds well to mannitol.
• Patient maintains adequate hydration throughout therapy.
• Patient and family state understanding of drug therapy.

mebendazole
(meh-BEN-duh-zohl)
Vermox

Pharmacologic class: benzimidazole
Therapeutic class: anthelmintic
Pregnancy risk category: C

Indications and dosages
▶ **Pinworm.** *Adults and children older than age 2:* 100 mg P.O. as single dose. If infection persists for 3 weeks, repeat therapy.
▶ **Roundworm, whipworm, hookworm.** *Adults and children older than age 2:* 100 mg P.O. b.i.d. for 3 days. If infection persists for 3 weeks, repeat therapy.

▶ **Trichinosis‡.** *Adults and children older than age 2:* 200 to 400 mg P.O. t.i.d. for 3 days, then 400 to 500 mg t.i.d. for 10 days.
▶ **Capillariasis‡.** *Adults and children older than age 2:* 200 mg P.O. b.i.d. for 20 days.
▶ **Toxocariasis‡.** *Adults and children:* 100 to 200 mg P.O. b.i.d. for 5 days.
▶ **Dracunculiasis‡.** *Adults and children older than age 2:* 400 to 800 mg P.O. daily for 6 days.

Contraindications and cautions
• Contraindicated in patients hypersensitive to the drug or any of its components.
▩ **Lifespan:** In pregnant women, use cautiously. In breast-feeding women, safety and effectiveness haven't been established. In children younger than 2 years, safety and effectiveness haven't been established.

Adverse reactions
GI: transient abdominal pain, diarrhea.

Interactions
Drug-drug. *Carbamazepine, hydantoins:* May reduce level of mebendazole, possibly decreasing its therapeutic effect. Monitor patient for effect.
Cimetidine: Increases mebendazole levels. Monitor patient for toxicity.

Effects on lab test results
None reported.

Pharmacokinetics
Absorption: About 5% to 10%; varies widely among patients.
Distribution: Highly bound to proteins.
Metabolism: To inactive metabolites.
Excretion: Mostly in feces; 2% to 10% in urine. *Half-life:* 3 to 9 hours.

Route	Onset	Peak	Duration
P.O.	Unknown	2–5 hr	Varies

Action
Chemical effect: Selectively and irreversibly inhibits uptake of glucose and other nutrients in susceptible helminths.
Therapeutic effect: Kills helminth infestation.

Available forms
Tablets (chewable): 100 mg

Assessment
• Assess patient's condition before therapy and regularly thereafter to monitor the drug's effectiveness.
• Be alert for adverse reactions and drug interactions.
• Assess patient's and family's knowledge of drug therapy.

Nursing diagnoses
• Infection related to presence of helminths
• Diarrhea related to drug-induced adverse GI reactions
• Deficient knowledge related to drug therapy

Planning and implementation
• Tablets may be chewed, swallowed whole, or crushed and mixed with food.
• Give drug to all family members to decrease risk of spreading infection.
• No dietary restrictions, laxatives, or enemas are needed.

Patient teaching
• Teach patient about personal hygiene, especially good hand-washing technique. To avoid reinfection, teach patient to wash perianal area daily, to change undergarments and bedclothes daily, and to wash hands and clean fingernails before meals and after bowel movements.
• Advise patient not to prepare food for others.

Evaluation
• Patient is free from infestation.
• Patient's bowel pattern returns to normal after therapy is stopped.
• Patient and family state understanding of drug therapy.

mechlorethamine hydrochloride (nitrogen mustard)
(meh-klor-ETH-uh-meen high-droh-KLOR-ighd)
Mustargen

Pharmacologic class: alkylating drug
Therapeutic class: antineoplastic
Pregnancy risk category: D

Indications and dosages

▶ **Hodgkin's disease.** *Adults and children:* 6 mg/m² I.V. daily on days 1 and 8 of 28-day cycle given with other antineoplastics, such as mechlorethamine-vincristine-procarbazine-prednisone (MOPP). Repeat dosage for six cycles.
▷ **Adjust-a-dose:** Reduce subsequent doses by 50% during MOPP therapy when WBC count is between 3,000 and 3,999/mm³, and by 75% when WBC count is between 1,000 and 2,999/mm³; or when platelet count is between 50,000 and 100,000/mm³.
▶ **Polycythemia vera, chronic lymphocytic leukemia, chronic myelocytic leukemia, bronchogenic cancer, lymphosarcoma, mycosis fungoides.** *Adults and children:* 0.4 mg/kg I.V. daily as a single dose or divided into 2 doses of 0.2 mg/kg or 4 doses of 0.1 mg/kg. Base dosage on ideal dry body weight without edema or ascites. Subsequent courses can't be given until patient has recovered hematologically, usually within 3 weeks.

I.V. administration

• Follow facility personal protection policy to reduce risks. Preparation and administration of parenteral form are linked to carcinogenic, mutagenic, and teratogenic risks.
• Prepare solution immediately before infusion because it's unstable. Use within 15 minutes, and discard unused solution.
• Reconstitute drug using 10 ml of sterile water for injection. Resulting solution contains 1 mg/ml of drug. Give by direct injection into I.V. line containing free-flowing compatible solution.
• Don't use solutions that are discolored or contain particulates. Don't use vials that appear to contain droplets of water.
• Make sure I.V. solution doesn't extravasate because drug is a potent vesicant. If it does, infiltrate area with sterile (1/6 molar) isotonic sodium thiosulfate and apply cold compresses for 6 to 12 hours.
• Dispose of used equipment properly and according to facility policy. Neutralize unused solution with equal volume of 5% sodium bicarbonate and 5% sodium thiosulfate for 45 minutes.
⊗ **Incompatibilities**
Allopurinol, cefepime, methohexital.

Reactions may be *common,* uncommon, *life-threatening*, or COMMON AND LIFE-THREATENING.

Contraindications and cautions

- Contraindicated in patients with infectious disease or previous anaphylactic reactions to the drug.
- Use cautiously in patients with chronic lymphatic lymphoma caused by increased drug toxicity.
- Use cautiously in patients with widely disseminated neoplasms. In patients with inoperable neoplasms or in the terminal stage of the disease, weigh risks and discomfort from use against limited potential gain.

Lifespan: Women of childbearing age shouldn't become pregnant while taking drug. In pregnant women, use cautiously because of risks to the fetus. Breast-feeding women should stop breast-feeding or not take the drug. In children, safety and effectiveness of drug haven't been established.

Adverse reactions

CNS: headache, weakness, drowsiness, vertigo.
CV: thrombophlebitis.
EENT: tinnitus, hearing loss.
GI: metallic taste, nausea, vomiting, anorexia.
Hematologic: ***thrombocytopenia, agranulocytosis,*** lymphocytopenia, ***myelosuppression,*** anemia.
Skin: *alopecia,* rash, sloughing, severe irritation if drug extravasates or touches skin.
Other: herpes zoster, ***anaphylaxis, secondary malignant disease.***

Interactions

Drug-drug. *Anticoagulants, aspirin:* Increases risk of bleeding. Monitor PT and INR and monitor patient for bleeding; adjust dosage, if needed.

Effects on lab test results

- May increase PT, INR, and urine urea level. May decrease hemoglobin level and hematocrit.
- May decrease platelet, granulocyte, lymphocyte, WBC, and RBC counts.

Pharmacokinetics

Absorption: Incomplete, probably from deactivation by body fluids in cavity.
Distribution: Doesn't cross blood-brain barrier.
Metabolism: Converted rapidly to its active form, which reacts quickly with various cellular components before being deactivated.
Excretion: Metabolites in urine.

Route	Onset	Peak	Duration
I.V., intracavitary	Rapid	Unknown	Unknown

Action

Chemical effect: Cross-links strands of cellular DNA and interferes with RNA transcription, causing imbalance of growth that leads to cell death.
Therapeutic effect: Kills certain cancer cells.

Available forms

Injection: 10-mg vials

NURSING PROCESS

Assessment

- Assess patient's condition before therapy and regularly thereafter to monitor the drug's effectiveness.
- Monitor CBC and platelet counts regularly. Mild anemia begins in 2 to 3 weeks.
- Monitor uric acid level.
- Be alert for adverse reactions and drug interactions.
- Monitor patient for signs and symptoms of infection caused by immunosuppression. Myelosuppression peaks in 4 to 10 days and lasts 10 to 21 days per cycle.
- Neurotoxicity and ototoxicity increases with dose and patient age.
- Assess patient's and family's knowledge of drug therapy.

Nursing diagnoses

- Ineffective health maintenance related to presence of neoplastic disease
- Ineffective immune protection related to adverse hematologic reactions
- Deficient knowledge related to drug therapy

Planning and implementation

ALERT: Drug is highly toxic. Avoid inhalation of dust or vapors. Also avoid contact with skin or mucous membranes. Use personal protection equipment, clean drug equipment, and neutralize unused drug according to manufacturer's instructions.

- To prevent hyperuricemia with resulting uric acid nephropathy, make sure patient is adequately hydrated.

M

• If patient develops the acute phase of herpes zoster, stop giving the drug to avoid progression to generalized herpes zoster.

Patient teaching
• Warn patient to watch for signs of infection (fever, sore throat, fatigue) and bleeding (easy bruising, nosebleeds, bleeding gums, melena). Have patient take temperature daily.
• Instruct patient to avoid OTC products that contain aspirin.
• Advise woman of childbearing age to avoid becoming pregnant during therapy and to consult with prescriber before attempting to become pregnant.

☑ Evaluation
• Patient responds positively to drug.
• Patient regains normal hematologic parameters.
• Patient and family state understanding of drug therapy.

meclizine hydrochloride (meclozine hydrochloride)
(MEK-lih-zeen high-droh-KLOR-ighd)
Ancolan◇, Antivert†, Antivert/25, Antivert/50, Antrizine, Bonamine♦, Bonine†, Dramamine Less Drowsy Formula†, Meni-D, Vergon†

Pharmacologic class: piperazine-derivative antihistamine; anticholinergic
Therapeutic class: antiemetic, antivertigo drug
Pregnancy risk category: B

Indications and dosages
▶ **Vertigo, dizziness.** *Adults:* 25 to 100 mg P.O. daily in divided doses. Dosage varies with patient response.
▶ **Motion sickness.** *Adults:* 25 to 50 mg P.O. 1 hour before travel, repeat daily for duration of journey.

Contraindications and cautions
• Contraindicated in patients hypersensitive to the drug or any of its components.
• Use cautiously in patients with asthma, glaucoma, or prostatic hyperplasia.
⚘ **Lifespan:** In pregnant women, safety and effectiveness haven't been established. In breast-

feeding women, use cautiously; it's unknown if drug appears in breast milk. In children, safety and effectiveness haven't been established.

Adverse reactions
CNS: *drowsiness,* fatigue, nervousness, excitation.
CV: hypotension, palpitations, *tachycardia.*
EENT: blurred vision.
GI: dry mouth, anorexia, nausea, vomiting, diarrhea.
GU: urinary frequency.
Skin: rash, urticaria.

Interactions
Drug-drug. *CNS depressants:* May increase drowsiness. Use together cautiously; monitor patient for safety.

Effects on lab test results
None reported.

Pharmacokinetics
Absorption: Unknown.
Distribution: Good.
Metabolism: May be in liver.
Excretion: Unchanged in feces; metabolites in urine. *Half-life:* About 6 hours.

Route	Onset	Peak	Duration
P.O.	1 hr	Unknown	8–24 hr

Action
Chemical effect: May affect neural pathways originating in labyrinth to inhibit nausea and vomiting.
Therapeutic effect: Relieves vertigo and nausea.

Available forms
Capsules: 25 mg, 30 mg†
Tablets: 12.5 mg, 25 mg†, 50 mg
Tablets (chewable): 25 mg†

NURSING PROCESS

☲ Assessment
• Assess patient's condition before therapy and regularly thereafter to monitor the drug's success.
• Be alert for adverse reactions and drug interactions.

• Assess patient's and family's knowledge of drug therapy.

⊕ Nursing diagnoses
• Risk for injury related to vertigo
• Risk for deficient fluid volume related to motion sickness
• Deficient knowledge related to drug therapy

⟫ Planning and implementation
• Don't abruptly stop giving the drug after long-term therapy. Paradoxical reactions or sudden reversal of improved state may occur.
⑨ ALERT: Don't confuse Antivert with Axert.
Patient teaching
• Advise patient to refrain from driving and performing other hazardous activities that require alertness until the drug's CNS effects are known.
• If drug is to be used long term, stress the importance of not abruptly stopping it.
• Advise patient not to use alcohol while taking this drug and to consult prescriber before taking this drug if he's already taking sedatives or tranquilizers.

✔ Evaluation
• Patient states that vertigo is relieved.
• Patient states that motion sickness doesn't occur.
• Patient and family state understanding of drug therapy.

---

medroxyprogesterone acetate
(med-roks-ee-proh-JES-ter-ohn AS-ih-tayt)
Amen, Cycrin, Depo-Provera, Provera◊

Pharmacologic class: synthetic hormone
Therapeutic class: progestin, antineoplastic
Pregnancy risk category: X

Indications and dosages
▶ **Abnormal uterine bleeding caused by hormonal imbalance.** *Women:* 5 to 10 mg P.O. daily for 5 to 10 days beginning on day 16 or 21 of menstrual cycle. If patient also has received estrogen, 10 mg P.O. daily for 10 days beginning on day 16 of cycle.
▶ **Secondary amenorrhea.** *Women:* 5 to 10 mg P.O. daily for 5 to 10 days.

▶ **Endometrial or renal carcinoma.** *Adults:* 400 to 1,000 mg I.M. weekly. If disease improves within a few weeks to months and seems stable, it may be possible to maintain response with 400 mg monthly.
▶ **Contraception.** *Women:* 150 mg I.M. once q 3 months.
▶ **Paraphilia‡.** *Men:* Initially, 200 mg I.M. b.i.d. or t.i.d. or 500 mg I.M. weekly. Base dosage on response.

Contraindications and cautions
• Contraindicated in patients hypersensitive to the drug or any of its components, and in those with active thromboembolic disorders, breast cancer, undiagnosed abnormal vaginal bleeding, missed abortion, hepatic dysfunction, or a history of thromboembolic disorders, cerebrovascular disease, or stroke. Tablets are contraindicated in patients with liver dysfunction or known or suspected genital cancer.
• Use cautiously in patients with diabetes mellitus, seizure disorder, migraine, cardiac or renal disease, asthma, or depression.
⚕ **Lifespan:** In pregnant women, drug is contraindicated. In breast-feeding women, drug has no adverse effects on infants; it may increase milk production and duration of lactation.

Adverse reactions
CNS: dizziness, migraine, lethargy, depression, nervousness, asthenia, *stroke.*
CV: hypertension, thrombophlebitis, edema, *thromboembolism.*
EENT: intolerance to contact lenses.
GI: nausea, vomiting, abdominal cramps.
GU: breakthrough bleeding, dysmenorrhea, amenorrhea, cervical erosion, abnormal secretions, uterine fibromas, vaginal candidiasis.
Hepatic: *cholestatic jaundice, tumors,* gallbladder disease.
Metabolic: hyperglycemia, *weight gain.*
Respiratory: *pulmonary embolism.*
Skin: melasma, rash, pain, induration, sterile abscesses, acne, alopecia.
Other: breast tenderness, enlargement, or secretion; decreased libido, hypersensitivity reactions.

Interactions
Drug-drug. *Aminoglutethimide, rifampin:* May decrease progestin effects. Monitor patient for diminished therapeutic response. Tell patient to

M

---

use nonhormonal contraceptive during therapy with these drugs.

Bromocriptine: May cause amenorrhea, interfering with bromocriptine's effects. Avoid using together.

Drug-food. *Caffeine:* May increase caffeine levels. Monitor patient for effect.

Drug-lifestyle. *Smoking:* Increases risk of adverse CV effects. If smoking continues, may need alternative therapy. Discourage patient from smoking.

Effects on lab test results

• May increase thyroxin-binding globulin and T_4 levels.
• May increase liver function test values.

Pharmacokinetics

Absorption: Rapid.
Distribution: Extensively protein bound, mainly albumin and corticosteroid binding globulin.
Metabolism: Rapid, primarily in the liver.
Excretion: Primarily in urine. *Half-life:* 2¼ to 9 hours orally, 10 weeks I.M.

Route	Onset	Peak	Duration
P.O.	Rapid	1–2 hr	3–5 days
I.M.	Rapid	24 hr	3–4 mo

Action

Chemical effect: Acts as progestin: suppresses ovulation, possibly by inhibiting pituitary gonadotropin secretion.
Therapeutic effect: Regulates menses or acts as a contraceptive depending on dose; promotes anti-androgenic effects in men; and slows growth of some cancer cells.

Available forms

Injection (suspension): 150 mg/ml, 400 mg/ml
Tablets: 2.5 mg, 5 mg, 10 mg

NURSING PROCESS

🔲 Assessment
• Assess patient's condition before therapy and regularly thereafter to monitor the drug's effectiveness.
• Be alert for adverse reactions and drug interactions.
• Monitor injection sites for evidence of sterile abscess.

• Assess patient's and family's knowledge of drug therapy.

🔵 Nursing diagnoses
• Ineffective health maintenance related to underlying condition
• Excessive fluid volume related to drug-induced edema
• Deficient knowledge related to drug therapy

🔷 Planning and implementation
• Rotate injection sites to prevent muscle atrophy.
Patient teaching
• Explain to patient adverse effects of progestins before giving the first dose.
• Instruct patient not to smoke or use caffeine during therapy.
🔸 **ALERT:** Tell patient to immediately report unusual symptoms and to stop taking drug and notify prescriber about disturbed vision or migraine.
• Teach woman how to perform routine monthly breast self-examination.
• Warn patient that I.M. injection may be painful.

✅ Evaluation
• Patient responds well to drug therapy.
• Patient doesn't develop fluid excess throughout drug therapy.
• Patient and family state understanding of drug therapy.

mefloquine hydrochloride
(MEF-loh-kwin high-droh-KLOR-ighd)
Lariam

Pharmacologic class: quinine derivative
Therapeutic class: antimalarial
Pregnancy risk category: C

Indications and dosages

▶ **Acute malaria infections caused by mefloquine-sensitive strains of** *Plasmodium falciparum* **and** *P. vivax. Adults age 17 and older:* 1,250 mg P.O. as single dose, with 240 ml (8 oz) water. Give patients with *P. vivax* infections primaquine or other 8-aminoquinoline to avoid relapse of initial infection after therapy.

Children age 6 months to 16 years: 20 to 25 mg/kg in 2 divided doses given 6 to 8 hours apart, with ample water.
► **To prevent malaria.** *Adults:* 250 mg P.O. once weekly. Give 1 week before patient enters endemic area and continue for 4 weeks after return. Can begin prophylaxis 2 to 3 weeks before departure when taken with other drugs.

Contraindications and cautions

• Contraindicated in patients hypersensitive to the drug or related compounds. Don't give preventively to patients with active depression, a recent history of depression, generalized anxiety disorder, psychosis, schizophrenia, or other major psychiatric disorders; or with a history of convulsions.
• Use cautiously in patients with a previous history of depression and in patients with cardiac disease or seizure disorders.
⚠ **Lifespan:** In pregnant women, use cautiously. In breast-feeding women, use cautiously; it's unknown if the drug appears in breast milk. In infants less than 6 months, safety and effectiveness haven't been established.

Adverse reactions

CNS: dizziness, fever, fatigue, syncope, headache, *seizures,* tremor, ataxia, mood changes, panic attacks, *suicide.*
CV: extrasystoles, chest pain, edema.
EENT: tinnitus.
GI: loss of appetite, vomiting, *nausea,* loose stools, diarrhea, GI discomfort, dyspepsia.
Skin: rash.
Other: chills.

Interactions

Drug-drug. *Beta blockers, quinidine, quinine:* ECG abnormalities and cardiac arrest may occur. Avoid using together.
Chloroquine, quinine: May increase risk of seizures. Do not use together.
Halofantrine: May increase risk of fatal prolongation of QTc interval. Don't use together.
Oral live typhoid vaccine: May reduce effectiveness of immunization. Complete immunization at least 3 days before giving drug.
Valproic acid, other anticonvulsants: May cause loss of seizure control by lowering drug levels. Check anticonvulsant level.

Effects on lab test results

• May increase transaminase levels. May decrease hemoglobin level and hematocrit.
• May decrease WBC and platelet counts.

Pharmacokinetics

Absorption: Good.
Distribution: Concentrated in RBCs; about 98% protein-bound.
Metabolism: By liver.
Excretion: Primarily by liver; small amounts in urine. *Half-life:* About 21 days.

Route	Onset	Peak	Duration
P.O.	Unknown	7–24 hr	Unknown

Action

Chemical effect: May be related to its ability to form complexes with hemin.
Therapeutic effect: Inhibits or kills malaria-causing organisms.

Available forms

Tablets: 250 mg

NURSING PROCESS

☑ Assessment

• Assess patient's condition before therapy and regularly thereafter to monitor the drug's effectiveness.
• Periodically monitor liver function.
• Be alert for adverse reactions and drug interactions.
• If patient has an adverse GI reaction, monitor his hydration.
• Assess patient's and family's knowledge of drug therapy.

⊞ Nursing diagnoses

• Infection related to presence of malaria organisms
• Risk of deficient fluid volume related to drug-induced adverse reactions
• Deficient knowledge related to drug therapy

▷ Planning and implementation

Ⓢ **ALERT:** During preventive use, psychiatric symptoms may precede a more serious reaction. Stop giving the drug and use an alternative.
• If *P. falciparum* infection is life-threatening or overwhelming, start with an I.V. antimalarial drug, and complete therapy with mefloquine.

• Because health risks from simultaneous administration of quinine and mefloquine are great, don't begin therapy within 12 hours of last dose of quinine or quinidine.
• Patients with infections caused by *P. vivax* are at high risk for relapse because drug doesn't eliminate hepatic phase (exoerythrocytic parasites). Follow-up therapy with primaquine or an 8-aminoquinoline is advisable.
• Give drug with food and full glass of water to minimize adverse GI reactions.

Patient teaching
• Advise patient to take drug on the same day each week when using it for prevention.
• Advise patient to use caution when performing hazardous activities that require alertness and coordination because dizziness, disturbed sense of balance, and neuropsychiatric reactions may occur.
• Instruct patient taking drug as prevention to stop taking the drug and notify prescriber if he notices signs or symptoms of impending toxicity, such as unexplained anxiety, depression, confusion, or restlessness.
• For patient undergoing long-term therapy, recommend that he have periodic ophthalmologic examinations.

☑ Evaluation
• Patient is free from infection.
• Patient maintains adequate hydration throughout therapy.
• Patient and family state understanding of drug therapy.

megestrol acetate
(meh-JES-trol AS-ih-tayt)
Megace, Megace ES, Megostat ◊

Pharmacologic class: synthetic progestin
Therapeutic class: antineoplastic
Pregnancy risk category: X

Indications and dosages

▶ **Breast cancer.** *Adults:* 40 mg P.O. q.i.d.
▶ **Endometrial cancer.** *Women:* 40 to 320 mg P.O. daily in divided doses.
▶ **Anorexia, cachexia, or unexplained significant weight loss in patients with AIDS.** *Adults:* 800 mg P.O. (20 ml regular oral suspen-

sion) or 625 mg P.O. (5 ml concentrated ES oral suspension) once daily.
▶ **Anorexia or cachexia in patients with neoplastic disease‡.** *Adults:* 480 to 600 mg P.O. daily.

Contraindications and cautions

• Contraindicated in patients hypersensitive to the drug or any of its components.
• Use cautiously in patients with history of thrombophlebitis.
☀ Lifespan: In pregnant women, drug is contraindicated in the first 4 months of pregnancy. In breast-feeding women, use cautiously; it's unknown if drug appears in breast milk. In children, safety and effectiveness haven't been established.

Adverse reactions

CV: hypertension, thrombophlebitis, *heart failure, thromboembolism.*
GI: nausea, vomiting, abdominal pain.
GU: breakthrough menstrual bleeding.
Metabolic: weight gain, increased appetite.
Musculoskeletal: carpal tunnel syndrome, back pain.
Respiratory: *pulmonary embolism.*
Skin: alopecia, hirsutism.
Other: breast tenderness.

Interactions

Drug-drug. *Dofetilide:* May increase risk of cardiotoxicity. Monitor QT level.

Effects on lab test results

• May increase glucose level.

Pharmacokinetics

Absorption: Good.
Distribution: May be stored in fatty tissue; highly bound to proteins.
Metabolism: Complete.
Excretion: In urine. *Half-life:* 2¼ to 9 hours.

Route	Onset	Peak	Duration
P.O.	Rapid	1–2 hr	3–5 days

Action

Chemical effect: Changes tumor's hormonal environment and alters neoplastic process. Mechanism of appetite stimulation is unknown.
Therapeutic effect: Hinders cancer cell growth and increases appetite.

Available forms

Oral suspension: 40 mg/ml
Oral suspension (concentrated): 125 mg/ml
Tablets: 20 mg, 40 mg

NURSING PROCESS

Assessment
• Assess patient's condition before therapy and regularly thereafter to monitor the drug's effectiveness.
• Be alert for adverse reactions.
• If patient has an adverse GI reaction, monitor his hydration.
• Assess patient's and family's knowledge of drug therapy.

Nursing diagnoses
• Ineffective health maintenance related to underlying condition
• Risk for deficient fluid volume related to drug-induced adverse GI reactions
• Deficient knowledge related to drug therapy

Planning and implementation
• Two months is adequate trial when treating cancer.
• If patient develops pronounced back pain, abdominal pain, headache, or nausea and vomiting, notify prescriber.
Patient teaching
• Inform patient that therapeutic response isn't immediate.
ALERT: Tell patient the ES oral suspension is more concentrated than the regular oral suspension so a smaller amount is needed for the proper dose.
• Advise breast-feeding woman to stop breast-feeding during therapy because of infant toxicity.
• Encourage women to use nonhormonal contraceptives during therapy.

Evaluation
• Patient responds well to therapy.
• Patient maintains adequate hydration throughout therapy.
• Patient and family state understanding of drug therapy.

meloxicam
(mell-OX-ih-kam)
Mobic

Pharmacologic class: NSAID
Therapeutic class: anti-inflammatory, analgesic
Pregnancy risk category: C

Indications and dosages

▶ **Osteoarthritis or rheumatoid arthritis.**
Adults: 7.5 mg P.O. once daily. May increase to maximum of 15 mg daily, p.r.n.
▶ **Pauciarticular or polyarticular course juvenile rheumatoid arthritis.** *Children ages 2 to 17:* 0.125 mg/kg P.O. once daily. Maximum dose 7.5 mg.

Contraindications and cautions

• Contraindicated in patients hypersensitive to the drug or any of its components and in those who have experienced asthma, urticaria, or allergic-type reactions after taking aspirin or other NSAIDs. Contraindicated in patients with severe renal impairment and for the treatment of perioperative pain following CABG surgery.
• Use cautiously in patients with a history of ulcers or GI bleeding and in patients with dehydration, anemia, hepatic disease, renal disease, hypertension, fluid retention, heart failure, or asthma.
Lifespan: In pregnant women, avoid use especially during the third trimester. In breast-feeding women, do not use. In children younger that age 2, safety and effectiveness haven't been established. In elderly and debilitated patients, use cautiously because of greater risk of fatal GI bleeding.

Adverse reactions

CNS: dizziness, headache, insomnia, fatigue, *seizures,* paresthesia, fever, tremor, vertigo, anxiety, confusion, depression, nervousness, somnolence, malaise, syncope.
CV: *arrhythmias,* palpitations, tachycardia, angina, *heart failure,* hypertension, hypotension, *MI,* edema.
EENT: pharyngitis, abnormal vision, conjunctivitis, tinnitus.
GI: abdominal pain, diarrhea, dyspepsia, flatulence, nausea, constipation, colitis, dry mouth,

M

duodenal ulcer, esophagitis, gastric ulcer, gastritis, GI reflux, ***hemorrhage, pancreatitis,*** vomiting, increased appetite, taste perversion.
GU: albuminuria, hematuria, urinary frequency, ***renal impairment,*** UTI.
Hematologic: anemia, ***leukopenia, thrombocytopenia,*** purpura, ***agranulocytosis.***
Hepatic: bilirubinemia, jaundice, ***hepatitis, liver failure.***
Metabolic: dehydration, weight changes.
Musculoskeletal: arthralgia, back pain.
Respiratory: upper respiratory tract infection, ***asthma, bronchospasm,*** dyspnea, cough.
Skin: rash, pruritus, alopecia, bullous eruption, photosensitivity reactions, sweating, urticaria, ***erythema multiforme, exfoliative dermatitis, Stevens-Johnson syndrome, toxic epidermal necrolysis.***
Other: accidental injury, allergic reaction, ***angioedema,*** flulike symptoms, ***anaphylactoid reactions, shock.***

Interactions

Drug-drug. *ACE inhibitors:* May diminish antihypertensive effects. Monitor patient's blood pressure.
Aspirin: May increase risk of adverse effects. Avoid using together.
Bile acid sequestrants: May increase clearance of meloxicam. Monitor patient's pain level.
Cyclosporine: May increase risk of nephrotoxicity. Monitor patient.
Lithium: May increase lithium level. Monitor lithium level closely for toxicity.
Methotrexate: May increase the toxicity of methotrexate. Use cautiously together.
Thiazide and loop diuretics: May reduce sodium excretion linked to diuretics, leading to sodium retention. Monitor patient for edema and increased blood pressure.
Warfarin: May increase PT or INR. Monitor PT and INR, and check for signs and symptoms of bleeding.
Drug-herb. *Dong quai, feverfew, garlic, ginger, horse chestnut, ma huang, meadowsweet, red clover:* May increase risk of bleeding. Discourage using together.
St. John's wort: May increase risk of photosensitivity reactions. Advise patient to avoid unprotected or prolonged exposure to sunlight.
Drug-lifestyle. *Alcohol use:* May increase risk of GI irritation and bleeding. Monitor patient for bleeding; discourage using together.
Smoking: May increase risk of GI irritation and bleeding. Monitor patient for bleeding; discourage patient from smoking.

Effects on lab test results

- May increase BUN, creatinine, ALT, AST, and bilirubin levels. May decrease hemoglobin level and hematocrit.
- May decrease WBC and platelet counts.

Pharmacokinetics

Absorption: Bioavailability is 89% and doesn't appear to be affected by food or antacids. Steady-state conditions are reached after 5 days of daily administration.
Distribution: 99.4% bound to proteins.
Metabolism: Almost complete, to pharmacologically inactive metabolites.
Excretion: In both urine and feces, primarily as metabolites. *Half-life:* 15 to 20 hours.

Route	Onset	Peak	Duration
P.O.	Unknown	Unknown	Unknown

Action

Chemical effect: May be related to prostaglandin (cyclooxygenase) synthetase inhibition.
Therapeutic effect: Relief of signs and symptoms of osteoarthritis.

Available forms

Tablets: 7.5 mg, 15 mg
Oral suspension: 7.5 mg/5 ml

NURSING PROCESS

Assessment

- Obtain accurate history of drug allergies. Drug can produce allergic-like reactions in patients hypersensitive to aspirin and other NSAIDs.
- Assess patient for increased risk of GI bleeding. Risk factors include history of ulcers or GI bleeding, therapy with corticosteroids or anticoagulants, long duration of NSAID therapy, smoking, alcoholism, old age, and poor overall health.
- Monitor patient for signs and symptoms of overt and occult bleeding.

ALERT: NSAIDs may increase the risk of serious thrombotic events, MI, or stroke. The risk may increase with duration of use and be higher in patients with CV disease or risk factors for CV disease.

• Monitor children for abdominal pain, vomiting, diarrhea, headache, and pyrexia, which may occur more frequently than in adults.
• Monitor patient for fluid retention; closely monitor patient who has hypertension, edema, or heart failure.
• Monitor liver function.
• Assess patient's and family's knowledge of drug therapy.

⊕ Nursing diagnoses
• Chronic pain related to underlying condition
• Risk for injury related to drug-induced adverse reactions
• Deficient knowledge related to drug therapy

▶ Planning and implementation
• Drug may be taken with food to prevent GI upset.
• Rehydrate dehydrated patient before therapy.
• If patient develops evidence of liver disease (eosinophilia, rash), stop giving the drug.
Patient teaching
• Tell patient to notify prescriber about history of allergic reactions to aspirin or other NSAIDs before therapy.
• Oral solution may be substituted on a milligram-per-milligram basis for tablets. Shake suspension gently before use.
• Tell patient to report signs and symptoms of GI ulcerations and bleeding, such as vomiting blood, blood in stool, and black, tarry stools.
• Instruct patient to report skin rash, weight gain, or edema.
• Advise patient to report warning signs of hepatotoxicity (nausea, fatigue, lethargy, pruritus, jaundice, right upper quadrant tenderness, and flulike symptoms).
• Warn patient with a history of asthma that it may recur during therapy and that he should stop taking the drug and notify prescriber if it does.
• Tell woman to notify prescriber if she becomes pregnant or is planning to become pregnant during therapy.
• Inform patient that it may take several days before consistent pain relief is achieved.

✓ Evaluation
• Patient is free from pain.
• Patient sustains no injury as a result of drug-induced adverse reactions.

• Patient and family state understanding of drug therapy.

melphalan
(L-phenylalanine mustard)
(MEL-feh-len)
Alkeran

Pharmacologic class: nitrogen mustard; alkylating drug
Therapeutic class: antineoplastic
Pregnancy risk category: D

Indications and dosages
▶ **Multiple myeloma.** *Adults:* 6 mg P.O. daily for 2 to 3 weeks; then stop drug for up to 4 weeks or until WBC and platelet counts begin to rise again; then give maintenance dosage of 2 mg daily.
▶ **Alternative therapy for multiple myeloma.** *Adults:* 0.15 mg/kg P.O. daily for 7 days at 2- to 6-week intervals, then begin maintenance therapy at or less than 0.05 mg/kg/day when WBC and platelet counts increase. Or 0.25 mg/kg P.O. daily for 4 days, repeat q 4 to 6 weeks. Or 10 mg/day for 7 to 10 days, maintenance therapy at 2 mg/day, adjust dosage within 1- to 3-mg range daily based on hematological response. Or for patients who can't tolerate oral therapy, give 16 mg/m^2 by I.V. infusion over 15 to 20 minutes q 2 weeks for four doses. After patient has recovered from toxicity, give drug q 4 weeks.
◪ **Adjust-a-dose:** For patients with renal impairment, reduce I.V. dosage by 50% to reduce risk of severe leukopenia and drug-related death.
▶ **Nonresectable advanced ovarian cancer.** *Women:* 0.2 mg/kg P.O. daily for 5 days. Repeat q 4 to 6 weeks, depending on bone marrow recovery.

▼ I.V. administration
• Follow facility policy to reduce risks. Preparation and administration of parenteral form are linked to carcinogenic, mutagenic, and teratogenic risks for personnel.
• Because drug isn't stable in solution, reconstitute immediately before giving, using 10 ml of sterile diluent supplied by manufacturer. Shake vigorously until solution is clear. Resulting solution contains 5 mg/ml. Immediately dilute re-

M

quired dose in normal saline solution for injection. Don't exceed a final concentration of 0.45 mg/ml.
• Give promptly after diluting because reconstituted product begins to degrade within 30 minutes. After final dilution, nearly 1% of drug degrades q 10 minutes. Administration must be completed within 60 minutes of reconstitution.
• Give by I.V. infusion over 15 to 20 minutes.
• Don't refrigerate reconstituted product because precipitate will form.
⊗ **Incompatibilities**
Amphotericin B, chlorpromazine, D₅W, lactated Ringer's injection. Compatibility with normal saline injection depends on the concentration.

Contraindications and cautions

• Contraindicated in patients hypersensitive to the drug or any of its components, and in those whose disease is resistant to drug. Patients hypersensitive to chlorambucil may have cross-sensitivity to drug.
• Drug isn't recommended for patients with severe leukopenia, thrombocytopenia, anemia, or chronic lymphocytic leukemia.
⚹ **Lifespan:** In pregnant and breast-feeding women, drug isn't recommended. In children, safety and effectiveness haven't been established.

Adverse reactions

Hematologic: *thrombocytopenia, leukopenia, bone marrow suppression.*
Hepatic: *hepatotoxicity.*
Respiratory: pneumonitis, *pulmonary fibrosis.*
Skin: dermatitis, pruritus, rash, alopecia.
Other: *anaphylaxis,* hypersensitivity reactions.

Interactions

Drug-drug. *Anticoagulants, aspirin:* May increase risk of bleeding. Use cautiously together.
Antigout drugs: May decrease effectiveness. Dosage adjustments may be needed.
Bone marrow suppressants: May have additive toxicity. Monitor patient closely.
Carmustine: May reduce carmustine lung toxicity threshold. Monitor patient closely for signs of toxicity.
Cisplatin: May affect melphalan's pharmacokinetics by inducing renal dysfunction and altering melphalan clearance. Monitor patient for toxicity.

Cyclosporine: May increase toxicity of cyclosporine, particularly nephrotoxicity. Monitor cyclosporine level and renal function tests.
Interferon alfa: May decrease melphalan level. Monitor level closely.
Nalidixic acid: May increase risk of severe hemorrhagic necrotic enterocolitis in children. Monitor patient closely.
Vaccines: May decrease effectiveness of killed-virus vaccines and increase risk of toxicity from live-virus vaccines. Postpone routine immunization for at least 3 months after last dose of melphalan.
Drug-food. *Any food:* May decrease absorption of oral drug. Separate administration times; give drug on an empty stomach.

Effects on lab test results

• May increase urine urea level. May decrease hemoglobin level and hematocrit.
• May decrease RBC, WBC, and platelet counts.

Pharmacokinetics

Absorption: Incomplete and variable.
Distribution: Rapid and wide in total body water; initially 50% to 60% bound to proteins and increases to 80% to 90% over time.
Metabolism: Extensively deactivated by hydrolysis.
Excretion: Primarily in urine. *Half-life:* 2 hours.

Route	Onset	Peak	Duration
P.O., I.V.	Unknown	Unknown	Unknown

Action

Chemical effect: Cross-links strands of cellular DNA and interferes with RNA transcription.
Therapeutic effect: Kills certain cancer cells.

Available forms

Injection: 50 mg
Tablets (scored): 2 mg

NURSING PROCESS

⚕ **Assessment**
• Assess patient's condition before therapy and regularly thereafter to monitor the drug's effectiveness.
• Monitor uric acid level and CBC.
• Be alert for adverse reactions and drug interactions.

Reactions may be *common,* uncommon, *life-threatening,* or COMMON AND LIFE-THREATENING.

- Assess patient's and family's knowledge of drug therapy.

🔲 Nursing diagnoses
- Ineffective health maintenance related to presence of neoplastic disease
- Ineffective immune protection related to adverse hematologic reactions
- Deficient knowledge related to drug therapy

▶ Planning and implementation
- Dosage may need to be reduced in patient with renal impairment.
- Melphalan is drug of choice with prednisone in patients with multiple myeloma.
- Give drug on empty stomach.
- Anaphylaxis may occur. Keep antihistamines and steroids readily available.

⚠ **ALERT:** Don't confuse melphalan with Mephyton.

Patient teaching
- Tell patient to take oral drug on empty stomach.
- Warn patient to watch for signs of infection (fever, sore throat, fatigue) and bleeding (easy bruising, nosebleed, bleeding gums, melena). Have patient take temperature daily.
- Instruct patient to avoid OTC products that contain aspirin.
- Advise woman of childbearing age not to become pregnant during therapy and to consult with prescriber before becoming pregnant.

✓ Evaluation
- Patient responds well to therapy.
- Patient regains normal hematologic function when therapy is completed.
- Patient and family state understanding of drug therapy.

memantine hydrochloride
(MEHM-en-tyn high-droh-KLOR-ighd)
Namenda

Pharmacologic class: N-methyl-D-aspartate (NMDA) receptor antagonist
Therapeutic class: Alzheimer's disease drug
Pregnancy risk category: B

Indications and dosages
▶ **Moderate to severe Alzheimer's type dementia.** *Adults:* Initially, 5 mg P.O. once daily. Increase by 5 mg/day each week up to the target dosage. Maximum, 10 mg P.O. b.i.d. Divide doses larger than 5 mg b.i.d.
🔲 **Adjust-a-dose:** If the patient has moderate renal impairment, reduce dosage.

Contraindications and cautions
- Contraindicated in patients allergic to the drug or any of its components. In patients with severe renal impairment, drug isn't recommended.
- Use cautiously in patients with seizures, hepatic impairment, or moderate renal impairment. Also use cautiously in patients who may have an increased urine pH (from drugs, diet, renal tubular acidosis, or severe UTI).
⚖ **Lifespan:** In pregnant women, use only if benefits outweigh risks to the fetus. In breast-feeding women, use cautiously; it's unknown if the drug appears in breast milk. In children, safety and effectiveness haven't been established. In elderly patients, use cautiously.

Adverse reactions
CNS: abnormal gait, aggressiveness, agitation, anxiety, ataxia, confusion, *stroke*, depression, dizziness, fatigue, hallucinations, headache, hypokinesia, insomnia, pain, somnolence, syncope, transient ischemic attack, vertigo.
CV: edema, *heart failure,* hypertension.
EENT: cataracts, conjunctivitis.
GI: anorexia, constipation, diarrhea, nausea, vomiting.
GU: incontinence, urinary frequency, UTI.
Hematologic: anemia.
Metabolic: weight loss.
Musculoskeletal: arthralgia, back pain.
Respiratory: bronchitis, coughing, dyspnea, pneumonia, upper respiratory tract infection.
Skin: rash.
Other: falls, flulike symptoms, inflicted injury.

Interactions
Drug-drug. *Cimetidine, hydrochlorothiazide, quinidine, ranitidine, triamterene:* May alter drug levels. Monitor patient.
NMDA antagonists (amantadine, ketamine, dextromethorphan): May interact. Use together cautiously.
Urine alkalinizers (carbonic anhydrase inhibitors, sodium bicarbonate): May decrease

memantine clearance. Monitor patient for adverse effects.

Drug-herb. *Herbs that alkalinize urine:* May increase drug level and adverse effects. Discourage using together.

Drug-food. *Foods that alkalinize urine:* May increase drug level and adverse effects. Discourage using together.

Drug-lifestyle. *Alcohol use:* May decrease drug's effectiveness or increase adverse effects. Discourage using together.
Smoking: May alter levels of drug and nicotine. Discourage using together.

Effects on lab test results

• May increase alkaline phosphatase level. May decrease hemoglobin level and hematocrit.

Pharmacokinetics

Absorption: Good.
Distribution: About 45% bound to proteins.
Metabolism: Little.
Excretion: Unchanged, primarily in the urine.
Half-life: 60 to 80 hours.

Route	Onset	Peak	Duration
P.O.	Unknown	3–7 hr	Unknown

Action

Chemical effect: Antagonizes NMDA receptors, the persistent activation of which seems to increase Alzheimer's symptoms.
Therapeutic effect: Decreases dementia.

Available forms

Tablets: 5 mg, 10 mg
Oral solution: 2mg/ml

NURSING PROCESS

≈ Assessment
• Assess patient's condition before therapy and regularly thereafter to monitor the drug's effectiveness.
• Assess patient's and family's knowledge of drug therapy.

⊕ Nursing diagnoses
• Acute or chronic confusion related to underlying disease
• Risk for imbalanced fluid volume related to drug-induced GI effects
• Deficient knowledge related to drug therapy

⊵ Planning and implementation
• Drug isn't indicated for mild Alzheimer's disease or other types of dementia.
• Give drug with or without food.
Patient teaching
• Explain that drug doesn't cure Alzheimer's disease but may improve the symptoms.
• Tell patient to report adverse effects.
• Urge patient not to drink alcohol during therapy.
• Advise patient not to take herbal or OTC cold and cough or GI products without consulting the prescriber.

☑ Evaluation
• Patient's cognition improves, and he experiences less confusion.
• Patient and family state that adverse GI effects haven't occurred or have been managed effectively.
• Patient and family state understanding of drug therapy.

menotropins
(meh-noh-TROH-pins)
Pergonal, Repronex

Pharmacologic class: gonadotropin
Therapeutic class: ovulation stimulant, spermatogenesis stimulant
Pregnancy risk category: X

Indications and dosages

▶ **Anovulation.** *Women:* 75 international units each of follicle-stimulating hormone (FSH) and luteinizing hormone (LH) I.M. daily for 7 to 12 days; follow by 5,000 to 10,000 units of human chorionic gonadotropin (HCG) I.M. 1 day after last dose of drug. Repeat for one to three menstrual cycles or until ovulation occurs.
▶ **Infertility with ovulation.** *Women:* 75 international units each of FSH and LH I.M. daily for 7 to 12 days; follow by 5,000 to 10,000 units of HCG I.M. 1 day after last dose of menotropins. Repeat for two menstrual cycles; then increase to 150 international units each of FSH and LH daily for 7 to 12 days; follow by 5,000 to 10,000 units of HCG I.M. 1 day after last dose of drug. Repeat for two menstrual cycles.
▶ **Infertility.** *Men:* Give 5,000 units HCG three times a week for 4 to 6 months; then 75 interna-

---

tional units each of FSH and LH I.M. three times weekly (with 2,000 units HCG two times weekly) for at least 4 months. If spermatogenesis doesn't increase, increase dosage to 150 international units each of FSH and LH three times weekly (keep HCG dosage the same).

Contraindications and cautions

• Contraindicated in patients hypersensitive to the drug or any of its components; in women with primary ovarian failure, uncontrolled thyroid or adrenal dysfunction, pituitary tumor, abnormal uterine bleeding, uterine fibromas, or ovarian cysts or enlargement; and in men with normal pituitary function, primary testicular failure, or infertility disorders other than hypogonadotropic hypogonadism.
⚕ **Lifespan:** In pregnant women, breastfeeding women, and children, drug is contraindicated.

Adverse reactions

CNS: *stroke.*
CV: fever, tachycardia, *arterial occlusion.*
GI: nausea, vomiting, diarrhea.
GU: *ovarian enlargement,* multiple births, ovarian hyperstimulation syndrome.
Hematologic: hemoconcentration with fluid loss into abdomen.
Respiratory: atelectasis, *acute respiratory distress syndrome; pulmonary embolism, pulmonary infarction.*
Other: *gynecomastia,* hypersensitivity reactions, *anaphylaxis.*

Interactions

None significant.

Effects on lab test results

None reported.

Pharmacokinetics

Absorption: Unknown.
Distribution: Unknown.
Metabolism: Unknown.
Excretion: In urine. *Half-life:* I.M., 60 hours.

Route	Onset	Peak	Duration
I.M.	9–12 days	Unknown	Unknown

Action

Chemical effect: When given to women who haven't had primary ovarian failure, mimics

FSH in inducing follicular growth and LH in aiding follicular maturation. In men with hypogonadotrophic hypogonadism, stimulates testosterone production and virilization.
Therapeutic effect: Stimulates ovulation and spermatogenesis.

Available forms

Injection: 75 international units of LH and 75 international units of FSH activity/ampule; 150 international units of LH and 150 international units of FSH activity/ampule

NURSING PROCESS

🗓 **Assessment**
• Assess patient's condition before therapy and regularly thereafter to monitor the drug's effectiveness.
• Be alert for adverse reactions.
⑤ **ALERT:** Monitor women for rare ovarian hyperstimulation syndrome (ovarian enlargement with possible pain and abdominal distension, ascites, and possible pleural effusion with hemoconcentration). Stop drug immediately and hospitalize patient for symptomatic treatment.
• Assess patient's and family's knowledge of drug therapy.

🔲 **Nursing diagnoses**
• Sexual dysfunction related to underlying disorder
• Risk for deficient fluid volume related to drug-induced adverse reactions
• Deficient knowledge related to drug therapy

▷ **Planning and implementation**
• Monitor patient closely to ensure adequate hormonal stimulation.
• Reconstitute with 1 to 2 ml of sterile normal saline solution. Use immediately.
• Rotate injection sites.
Patient teaching
• Discuss risk of multiple births.
• For infertility in women, encourage patient to have intercourse daily from the day before HCG is given until ovulation occurs.
• Tell patient that pregnancy usually occurs 4 to 6 weeks after therapy.
• Instruct patient to immediately report severe abdominal pain, bloating, swelling of hands or feet, nausea, vomiting, diarrhea, substantial weight gain, or shortness of breath.

M

Rapid onset   *Liquid form contains alcohol.   ◆ Canada   ◇ Australia   †OTC   ⌀Photoguide   ‡Off-label use

☑ Evaluation
- Patient or partner becomes pregnant.
- Patient maintains adequate hydration throughout therapy.
- Patient and family state understanding of drug therapy.

meperidine hydrochloride (pethidine hydrochloride)
(meh-PER-uh-deen high-droh-KLOR-ighd)
Demerol

Pharmacologic class: opioid
Therapeutic class: analgesic, adjunct to anesthesia
Pregnancy risk category: C
Controlled substance schedule: II

Indications and dosages
▶ **Moderate to severe pain.** *Adults:* 50 to 150 mg P.O., I.M., or subcutaneously q 3 to 4 hours, p.r.n. Or 15 to 35 mg/hour by continuous I.V. infusion.
Children: 1.1 to 1.76 mg/kg P.O., I.M., or subcutaneously q 3 to 4 hours. Maximum dosage is 100 mg q 4 hours, p.r.n.
▶ **Preoperatively.** *Adults:* 50 to 100 mg I.M., I.V., or subcutaneously 30 to 90 minutes before surgery.
Children: 1 to 2.2 mg/kg I.M., I.V., or subcutaneously up to adult dose 30 to 90 minutes before surgery.
▶ **Adjunct to anesthesia.** *Adults:* Repeat slow I.V. injections of fractional doses (such as 10 mg/ml). Or continuous I.V. infusion of more dilute solution (1 mg/ml); adjust to needs of patient.
▶ **Obstetric analgesia.** *Adults:* 50 to 100 mg I.M. or subcutaneously when pain becomes regular; repeat at 1- to 3-hour intervals.

▽ I.V. administration
- Drug is compatible with most I.V. solutions, including D_5W, normal saline solution, and Ringer's or lactated Ringer's solutions.
- Keep resuscitation equipment and naloxone available.
- Give slowly by direct I.V. injection or slow continuous I.V. infusion.

⊗ Incompatibilities
Acyclovir, allopurinol, aminophylline, amobarbital, amphotericin B, cefepime, cefoperazone, doxorubicin liposomal, ephedrine, furosemide, heparin, hydrocortisone sodium succinate, idarubicin, imipenem-cilastatin sodium, methylprednisolone sodium succinate, morphine, pentobarbital, phenobarbital sodium, phenytoin, sodium bicarbonate, sodium iodide, sulfonamides, thiopental.

Contraindications and cautions
- Contraindicated in patients hypersensitive to the drug or any of its components and in those who have received MAO inhibitors within 14 days.
- Use cautiously in debilitated patients and in patients with increased intracranial pressure, head injury, asthma, other respiratory conditions, supraventricular tachycardias, seizures, acute abdominal conditions, hepatic or renal disease, hypothyroidism, Addison's disease, urethral stricture, or prostatic hyperplasia.
※ **Lifespan:** In pregnant women, use cautiously. In breast-feeding women, use cautiously because it's unknown if drug appears in breast milk. In the elderly, use cautiously because of increased risk of renal insufficiency.

Adverse reactions
CNS: *sedation, somnolence, clouded sensorium, euphoria,* paradoxical excitement, tremors, dizziness, *seizures.*
CV: hypotension, *bradycardia,* tachycardia, *cardiac arrest, shock.*
GI: nausea, vomiting, constipation, ileus.
GU: urine retention.
Musculoskeletal: muscle twitching.
Respiratory: *respiratory depression, respiratory arrest.*
Skin: local tissue irritation and induration, phlebitis.
Other: pain at injection site, physical dependence.

Interactions
Drug-drug. *Chlorpromazine:* May cause excessive sedation and hypotension. Don't use together.
CNS depressants, general anesthetics, hypnotics, other opioid analgesics, phenothiazines, sedatives, tricyclic antidepressants: May cause respiratory depression, hypotension, profound

---

sedation, or coma. Use together cautiously. Reduce meperidine dosage as directed.
MAO inhibitors: May increase CNS excitation or depression that can be severe or fatal. Don't use together.
Phenytoin: May decrease level of meperidine. Monitor patient for decreased analgesia.
Drug-lifestyle. *Alcohol use:* May have additive CNS effects. Discourage using together.

Effects on lab test results

• May increase amylase and lipase levels.

Pharmacokinetics

Absorption: Unknown.
Distribution: Wide.
Metabolism: Primarily by hydrolysis in liver.
Excretion: Primarily in urine, enhanced by acidifying urine. *Half-life:* 2½ to 4 hours.

Route	Onset	Peak	Duration
P.O.	15 min	60–90 min	2–4 hr
I.V.	1 min	5–7 min	2–4 hr
I.M., SubQ	10–15 min	30–50 min	2–4 hr

Action

Chemical effect: Binds with opioid receptors in CNS, altering both perception of and emotional response to pain through unknown mechanism.
Therapeutic effect: Relieves pain.

Available forms

Injection: 25 mg/ml, 50 mg/ml, 75 mg/ml, 100 mg/ml
Injection (for infusion only): 10 mg/ml
Syrup: 50 mg/5 ml
Tablets: 50 mg, 100 mg

NURSING PROCESS

⚏ Assessment

• Assess patient's pain before therapy and regularly thereafter to monitor the drug's effectiveness.
• Be alert for adverse reactions and drug interactions.
• Meperidine and its active metabolite normeperidine accumulate in the body. Monitor patient for increased toxic effect, especially in patient with renal impairment.
• Monitor respirations of neonate exposed to drug during labor.

• Do not stop drug abruptly after long-term use, may cause withdrawal symptoms.
• Assess patient's and family's knowledge of drug therapy.

⊕ Nursing diagnoses

• Acute pain related to underlying condition
• Risk for injury related to drug-induced adverse reactions
• Deficient knowledge related to drug therapy

⊠ Planning and implementation

• Drug may be used in patients with pain who are allergic to morphine.
• Because drug toxicity often appears after several days of therapy, it isn't recommended for chronic pain.
• **ALERT:** If respiratory rate is less than 12 breaths/minute, if respiratory depth decreases, or if pupil size decreases, don't give drug.
• **ALERT:** Oral dose is less than half as effective as parenteral dose. Give I.M., if possible. When changing from parenteral to oral route, increase dose.
• Syrup has local anesthetic effect. Give with full glass of water.
• Subcutaneous injection is painful; avoid if possible.
• **ALERT:** Don't confuse Demerol with Demulen, Dymelor, or Temaril.
Patient teaching
• Warn outpatient to avoid hazardous activities until the drug's CNS effects are known.
• Instruct patient not to use alcohol during therapy.
• Teach patient to manage adverse reactions, such as constipation.
• Tell family members not to give the drug and to notify the prescriber if patient's respiratory rate decreases.

☑ Evaluation

• Patient is free from pain.
• Patient doesn't experience injury.
• Patient and family state understanding of drug therapy.

M

mercaptopurine
(6-mercaptopurine, 6-MP)
(mer-cap-toh-PYOO-reen)
Purinethol

Pharmacologic class: antimetabolite
Therapeutic class: antineoplastic
Pregnancy risk category: D

Indications and dosages

▶ **Acute lymphatic leukemia (lymphocytic, lymphoblastic), acute myelogenous and acute myelomonocytic leukemia.** *Adults:* 2.5 mg/kg P.O. daily as single dose, up to 5 mg/kg P.O. daily. Maintenance dosage is 1.5 to 2.5 mg/kg P.O. daily.
Children age 5 and older: 2.5 mg/kg P.O. daily. Maintenance dosage is 1.5 to 2.5 mg/kg P.O. daily.
▶ **Intractable Crohn's disease‡.** *Adults:* 1 to 1.5 mg/kg P.O. daily (maximum 125 mg/day) with other therapies. *Children:* 1 to 1.5 mg/kg P.O. daily (maximum 75 mg/day) with other therapies.

Contraindications and cautions

• Contraindicated in patients whose disease has resisted drug.
※ **Lifespan:** In pregnant and breast-feeding women, drug is contraindicated.

Adverse reactions

GI: nausea, vomiting, anorexia, stomatitis, *pancreatitis.*
Hematologic: *leukopenia, thrombocytopenia,* anemia.
Hepatic: biliary stasis, jaundice, *hepatotoxicity.*
Metabolic: hyperuricemia.
Skin: rash, hyperpigmentation.

Interactions

Drug-drug. *Allopurinol:* May slow inactivation of mercaptopurine. Decrease mercaptopurine to one-fourth or one-third normal dose.
Hepatotoxic drugs: May enhance hepatotoxicity of mercaptopurine. Monitor patient closely; monitor liver function test results.
Warfarin: May antagonize anticoagulant effect. Monitor PT and INR.

Effects on lab test results

• May increase alkaline phosphatase, bilirubin, and liver enzyme levels. May decrease hemoglobin level and hematocrit.
• May decrease WBC, RBC, and platelet counts.
• May falsely increase glucose and uric acid levels.

Pharmacokinetics

Absorption: Incomplete and variable; about 50%.
Distribution: Wide in total body water.
Metabolism: Extensive.
Excretion: In urine. *Half-life:* Unknown.

Route	Onset	Peak	Duration
P.O.	Unknown	Unknown	Unknown

Action

Chemical effect: Inhibits RNA and DNA synthesis. Strongly inhibits primary immune response by suppressing humoral immunity.
Therapeutic effect: Inhibits growth of certain cancer cells.

Available forms

Tablets (scored): 50 mg

NURSING PROCESS

☞ Assessment

• Assess patient's condition before therapy and regularly thereafter to monitor the drug's effectiveness.
• Monitor blood count and transaminase, alkaline phosphatase, and bilirubin levels weekly during initiation of treatment until remission is achieved and monthly during maintenance.
• Observe for signs of bleeding and infection.
• Monitor fluid intake and output and uric acid level.
• Be alert for adverse reactions and drug interactions. Adverse GI reactions are less common in children.
Ⓢ **ALERT:** Watch for jaundice, clay-colored stools, and frothy, dark urine. Hepatic dysfunction is reversible when drug is stopped. If hepatic tenderness occurs, stop giving the drug and notify prescriber.
• Assess patient's and family's knowledge of drug therapy.

Photoguide to tablets and capsules

This photoguide provides full-color photographs of some of the most commonly prescribed tablets and capsules. These drugs, organized by generic name, are shown in actual size and color with page references to corresponding drug information. Each drug is labeled with its trade name and its strength.

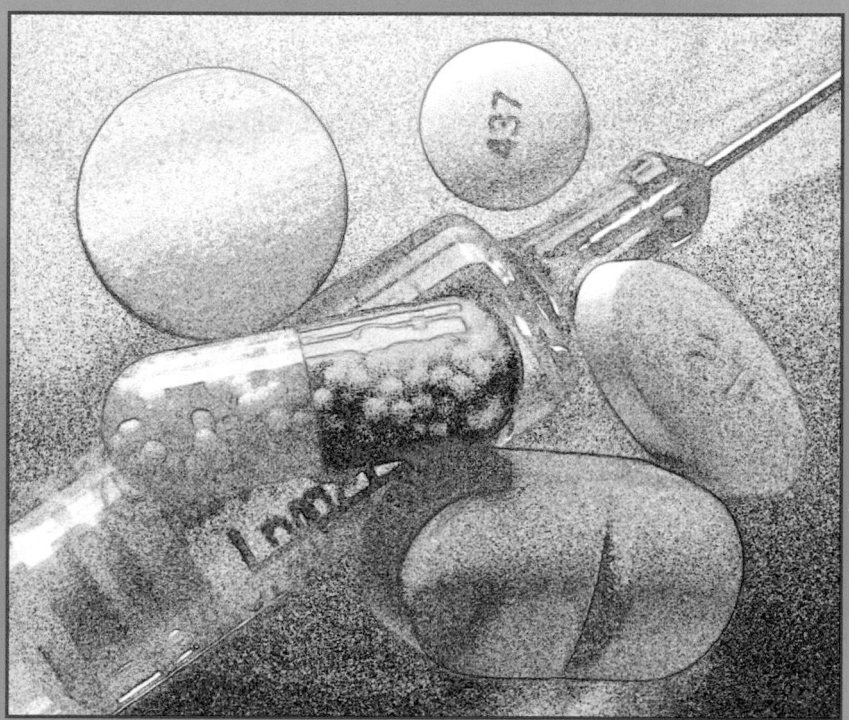

Adapted from Facts & Comparisons, St. Louis, Mo.

For the list of companies permitting the use of these photographs, see pages 1406–1407.

ACAMPROSATE CALCIUM

Campral
(page 94)

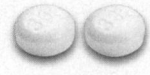

333 mg

ALENDRONATE SODIUM

Fosamax
(page 119)

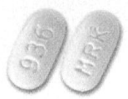

10 mg   40 mg   70 mg

ALPRAZOLAM

Xanax
(page 127)

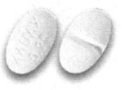   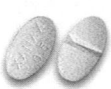   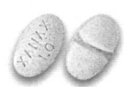

0.25 mg   0.5 mg   1 mg

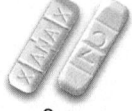

2 mg

AMLODIPINE BESYLATE

Norvasc
(page 144)

    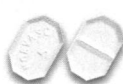   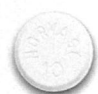

2.5 mg   5 mg   10 mg

ANASTROZOLE

Arimidex
(page 165)

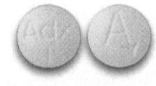

1 mg

ARIPIPRAZOLE

Abilify
(page 172)

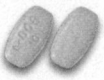   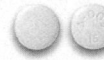   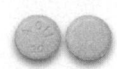

10 mg   15 mg   30 mg

ATENOLOL
Tenormin
(page 183)

 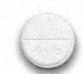 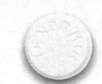

25 mg   50 mg   100 mg

ATOMOXETINE HYDROCHLORIDE
Strattera
(page 185)

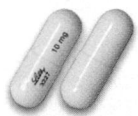 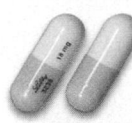 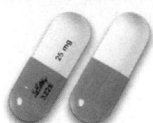

10 mg   18 mg   25 mg

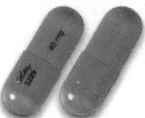 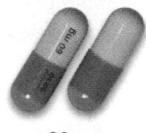

40 mg   60 mg

ATORVASTATIN CALCIUM
Lipitor
(page 187)

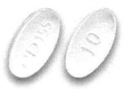 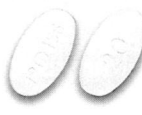 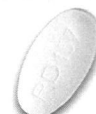

10 mg   20 mg   40 mg

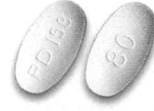

80 mg

AZITHROMYCIN
Zithromax
(page 200)

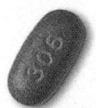 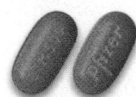 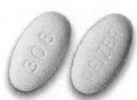

250 mg   500 mg   600 mg

BUPROPION HYDROCHLORIDE
Wellbutrin SR
(page 243)

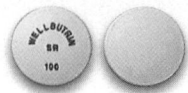 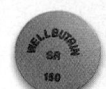 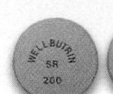

100 mg   150 mg   200 mg

CAPTOPRIL

Capoten
(page 263)

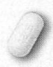

12.5 mg   25 mg

CEFADROXIL MONOHYDRATE

Duricef
(page 277)

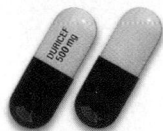 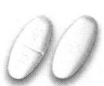

500 mg   1,000 mg

CELECOXIB

Celebrex
(page 302)

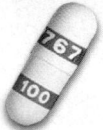 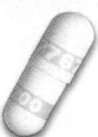

100 mg   200 mg

CIPROFLOXACIN HYDROCHLORIDE

Cipro
(page 330)

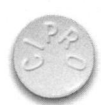 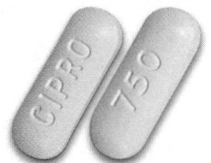

250 mg   500 mg   750 mg

CITALOPRAM HYDROBROMIDE

Celexa
(page 335)

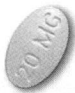 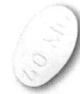

20 mg   40 mg

DARIFENACIN HYDROBROMIDE

Enablex
(page 389)

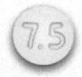

7.5 mg   15 mg

DESLORATADINE

Clarinex
(page 398)

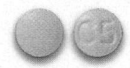

5 mg

DIAZEPAM

Valium
(page 413)

2 mg   5 mg   10 mg

DIGOXIN

Lanoxin
(page 424)

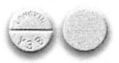   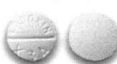

0.125 mg   0.25 mg

DILTIAZEM HYDROCHLORIDE

Cardizem
(page 429)

        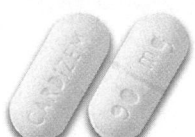

30 mg   90 mg

Cardizem CD
(page 429)

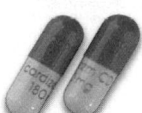   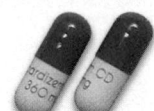

180 mg   360 mg

Cardizem LA
(page 429)

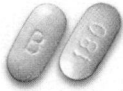   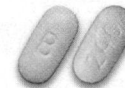   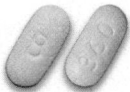

180 mg   240 mg   360 mg

DIVALPROEX SODIUM

Depakote

(page 1295)

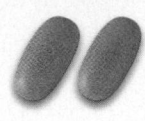 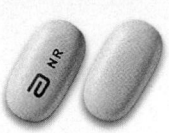 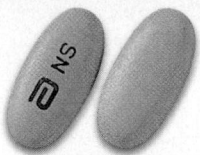

125 mg   250 mg   500 mg

DULOXETINE HYDROCHLORIDE

Cymbalta

(page 471)

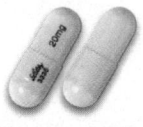 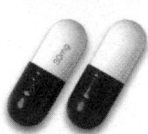 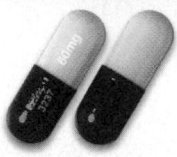

20 mg   30 mg   60 mg

ENALAPRIL MALEATE

Vasotec

(page 483)

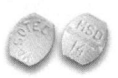 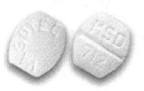 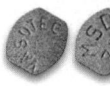

2.5 mg   5 mg   10 mg

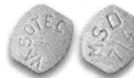

20 mg

ERYTHROMYCIN BASE

Eryc

(page 511)

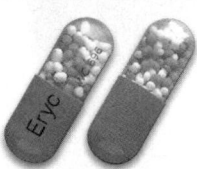

250 mg

ESCITALOPRAM OXALATE

Lexapro

(page 514)

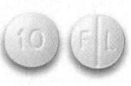 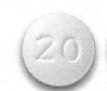 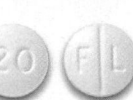

10 mg   20 mg

ESTRADIOL
Estrace
(page 521)

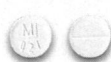 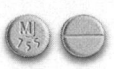 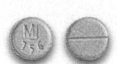

| 0.5 mg | 1 mg | 2 mg |

ESZOPICLONE
Lunesta
(page 533)

| 1 mg | 2 mg | 3 mg |

EZETIMBE
Zetia
(page 559)

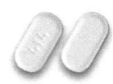

10 mg

FAMOTIDINE
Pepcid
(page 561)

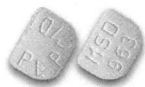 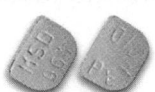

| 20 mg | 40 mg |

FLUCONAZOLE
Diflucan
(page 577)

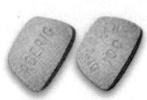 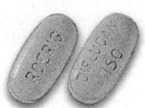 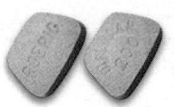

| 100 mg | 150 mg | 200 mg |

FLUOXETINE HYDROCHLORIDE
Prozac
(page 587)

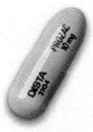 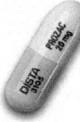 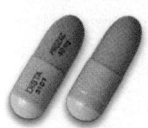

| 10 mg | 20 mg | 40 mg |

90 mg

FOSINOPRIL SODIUM

Monopril
(page 612)

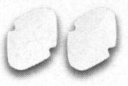

10 mg   20 mg   40 mg

FROVATRIPTAN SUCCINATE

Frova
(page 615)

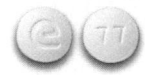

2.5 mg

FUROSEMIDE

Lasix
(page 618)

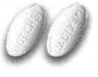   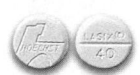   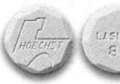

20 mg   40 mg   80 mg

GABAPENTIN

Neurontin
(page 620)

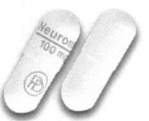   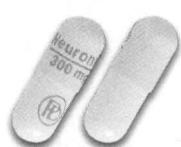   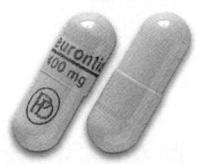

100 mg   300 mg   400 mg

GLIPIZIDE

Glucotrol
(page 638)

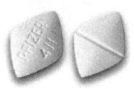   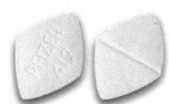

5 mg   10 mg

Glucotrol XL
(page 638)

5 mg   10 mg

GLYBURIDE

DiaBeta
(page 644)

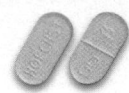   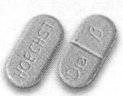   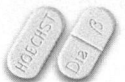

| 1.25 mg | 2.5 mg | 5 mg |

Micronase
(page 644)

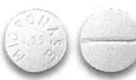

| 1.25 mg | 2.5 mg | 5 mg |

LANSOPRAZOLE

Prevacid
(page 751)

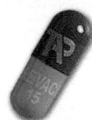   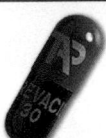

| 15 mg | 30 mg |

LEVOFLOXACIN

Levaquin
(page 768)

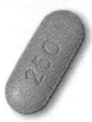   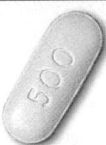

| 250 mg | 500 mg |

LEVOTHYROXINE SODIUM

Levoxyl
(page 771)

   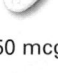

| 25 mcg | 50 mcg | 75 mcg |

| 88 mcg | 100 mcg | 112 mcg |

| 125 mcg | 137 mcg | 150 mcg |

   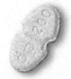   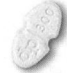

| 175 mcg | 200 mcg | 300 mcg |

LISINOPRIL

Prinivil
(page 777)

2.5 mg   5 mg   10 mg

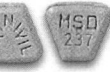

20 mg   40 mg

LOPINAVIR AND RITONAVIR

Kaletra
(page 784)

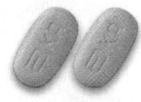

200mg/50 mg

LOSARTAN POTASSIUM

Cozaar
(page 791)

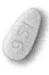

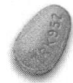

25 mg   50 mg

LOVASTATIN

Mevacor
(page 793)

10 mg   20 mg   40 mg

MEDROXYPROGESTERONE ACETATE

Provera
(page 807)

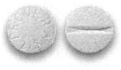

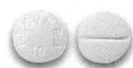

2.5 mg   5 mg   10 mg

METFORMIN HYDROCHLORIDE
Glucophage
(page 827)

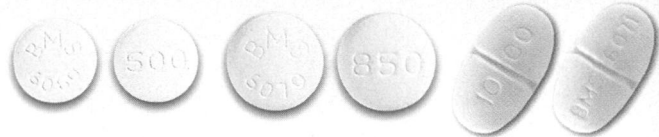

| 500 mg | 850 mg | 1,000 mg |

Glucophage XR
(page 827)

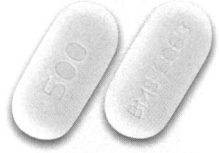

500 mg

METHYLPHENIDATE HYDROCHLORIDE
Ritalin
(page 839)

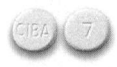 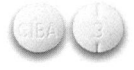 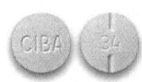

| 5 mg | 10 mg | 20 mg |

METOPROLOL SUCCINATE
Toprol-XL
(page 848)

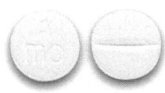  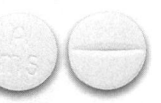

| 50 mg | 100 mg | 200 mg |

MONTELUKAST SODIUM
Singulair
(page 876)

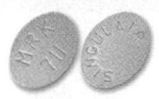

| 4 mg | 5 mg | 10 mg |

NIFEDIPINE
Procardia XL
(page 914)

  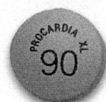

| 30 mg | 60 mg | 90 mg |

NORTRIPTYLINE HYDROCHLORIDE

Pamelor
(page 930)

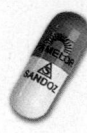   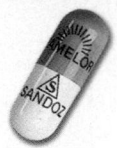   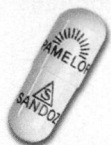

10 mg   25 mg   50 mg

OMEPRAZOLE

Prilosec
(page 944)

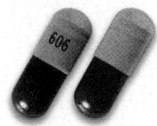   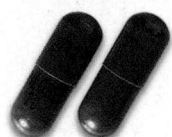   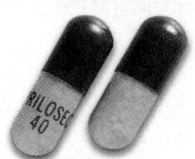

10 mg   20 mg   40 mg

OXYCODONE HYDROCHLORIDE

OxyContin
(page 960)

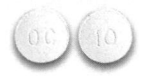   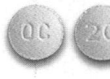   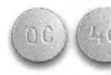

10 mg   20 mg   40 mg

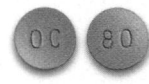

80 mg

PHENYTOIN SODIUM

Dilantin Kapseals
(page 1020)

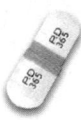   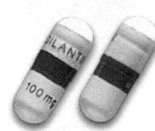

30 mg   100 mg

POTASSIUM CHLORIDE

K-Dur 20
(page 1036)

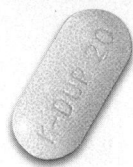

20 mEq

PRAVASTATIN SODIUM

Pravachol
(page 1046)

 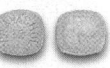   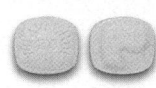   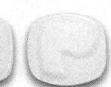

10 mg   20 mg   40 mg

PROMETHAZINE HYDROCHLORIDE

Phenergan
(page 1064)

    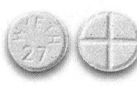   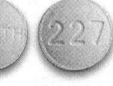

12.5 mg   25 mg   50 mg

QUINAPRIL HYDROCHLORIDE

Accupril
(page 1083)

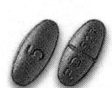

5 mg   10 mg   20 mg

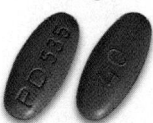

40 mg

RISEDRONATE SODIUM

Actonel
(page 1112)

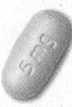   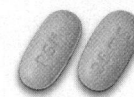

5 mg   35 mg

RISPERIDONE

Risperdal
(page 1114)

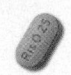 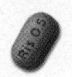

0.25 mg   0.5 mg   1 mg

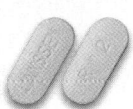 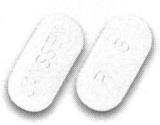

2 mg   3 mg   4 mg

Risperdal M-Tab
(page 1114)

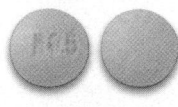

0.5 mg

ROSIGLITAZONE MALEATE

Avandia
(page 1125)

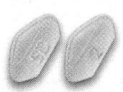 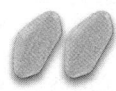 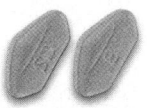

2 mg   4 mg   8 mg

ROSUVASTATIN CALCIUM

Crestor
(page 1129)

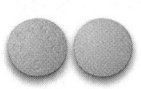 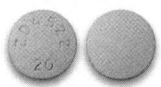

5 mg   10 mg   20 mg

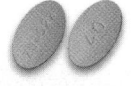

40 mg

SERTRALINE HYDROCHLORIDE

Zoloft
(page 1142)

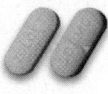 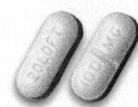

50 mg   100 mg

SILDENAFIL CITRATE

Viagra
(page 1149)

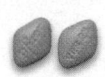 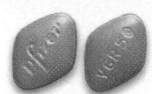 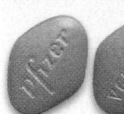

| 25 mg | 50 mg | 100 mg |

SIMVASTATIN

Zocor
(page 1151)

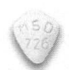 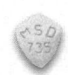 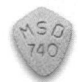

| 5 mg | 10 mg | 20 mg |

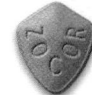

40 mg

TERAZOSIN HYDROCHLORIDE

Hytrin
(page 1211)

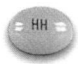

| 1 mg | 5 mg | 10 mg |

VARDENAFIL HYDROCHLORIDE

Levitra
(page 1298)

     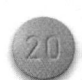

| 5 mg | 10 mg | 20 mg |

VENLAFAXINE HYDROCHLORIDE

Effexor XR
(page 1303)

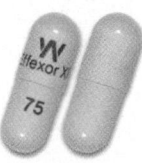 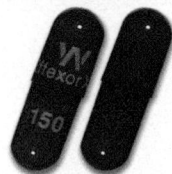

| 75 mg | 150 mg |

VERAPAMIL HYDROCHLORIDE

Calan
(page 1304)

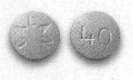 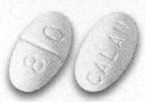 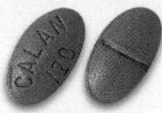

40 mg   80 mg   120 mg

WARFARIN SODIUM

Coumadin
(page 1321)

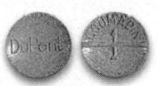 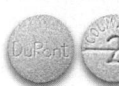 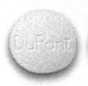

1 mg   2 mg   2.5 mg

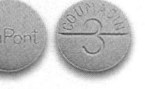 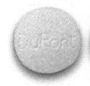

3 mg   4 mg   5 mg

 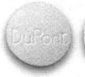 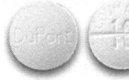

6 mg   7.5 mg   10 mg

ZOLPIDEM TARTRATE

Ambien
(page 1337)

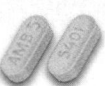 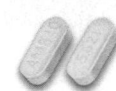

5 mg   10 mg

🖵 Nursing diagnoses

- Ineffective health maintenance related to presence of leukemia
- Ineffective immune protection related to drug-induced adverse hematologic reactions
- Deficient knowledge related to drug therapy

▷ Planning and implementation

- Adjust dosage after chemotherapy or radiation therapy and in a patient with depressed neutrophil or platelet count, or impaired liver or kidney function.
- Be aware that drug is usually used with other antineoplastics as response is poor with monotherapy.
- ⊛ **ALERT:** Sometimes drug is ordered as 6-mercaptopurine or 6-MP. The numeral 6 is part of drug name and doesn't signify number of dosage units. To prevent confusion, avoid these designations.
- Therapy must continue despite nausea and vomiting. If patient has an adverse GI reaction, notify prescriber and give an antiemetic.
- Encourage adequate fluid intake (3 L daily).
- Give allopurinol cautiously.
- If hepatic tenderness occurs, stop giving the drug and notify prescriber.
- ⊛ **ALERT:** Don't confuse Purinethol with propylthiouracil.

Patient teaching

- Tell patient to notify prescriber if vomiting occurs shortly after taking dose because antiemetic will be needed so drug therapy can continue.
- Instruct patient to watch for signs of infection (fever, sore throat, fatigue) and bleeding (easy bruising, nosebleed, bleeding gums, melena). Have patient take his temperature daily.
- Advise woman of childbearing age not to become pregnant during therapy and to consult with prescriber before becoming pregnant after therapy.

☑ Evaluation

- Patient responds well to therapy.
- Patient doesn't develop serious ill effects when hematologic studies are abnormal.
- Patient and family state understanding of drug therapy.

meropenem
(mer-oh-PEN-em)
Merrem I.V.

Pharmacologic class: synthetic broad-spectrum carbapenem
Therapeutic class: antibiotic
Pregnancy risk category: B

Indications and dosages

▶ **Complicated skin and skin structure infections caused by** *Staphylococcus aureus* **(beta-lactamase and non-beta-lactamase producing, methicillin-susceptible isolates only),** *Streptococcus pyogenes, S. agalactiae, viridans group streptococci, Enterococcus faecalis* **(excluding vancomycin-resistant isolates),** *Pseudomonas aeruginosa, Escherichia coli, Proteus mirabilis, Bacteroides fragilis* **and** *Peptostreptococcus* **species.** *Adults and children weighing more than 50 kg (110 lb):* 500 mg I.V. q 8 hours over 15 to 30 minutes as I.V. infusion.
Children ages 3 months and older weighing 50 kg or less: 10 mg/kg I.V. q 8 hours over 15 to 30 minutes as I.V. infusion or over 3 to 5 minutes as I.V. bolus injection (5 to 20 ml); maximum dose is 500 mg I.V. q 8 hours.
▶ **Complicated appendicitis and peritonitis caused by viridans group streptococci,** *Escherichia coli, Klebsiella pneumoniae, Pseudomonas aeruginosa, Bacteroides fragilis, B. thetaiotaomicron,* **and** *Peptostreptococcus* **species.** *Adults and children weighing more than 50 kg:* 1 g I.V. q 8 hours over 15 to 30 minutes as I.V. infusion or over 3 to 5 minutes as I.V. bolus injection (5 to 20 ml).
Children ages 3 months and older, weighing 50 kg or less: 20 mg/kg I.V. q 8 hours over 15 to 30 minutes as I.V. infusion or over 3 to 5 minutes as I.V. bolus injection (5 to 20 ml); maximum dose is 1 g I.V. q 8 hours.
▤ **Adjust-a-dose:** For adults with creatinine clearance of 26 to 50 ml/minute, give usual dose q 12 hours. If clearance is 10 to 25 ml/minute, give half usual dose q 12 hours; if clearance is less than 10 ml/minute, give half usual dose q 24 hours.
▶ **Bacterial meningitis caused by** *Streptococcus pneumoniae, Haemophilus influenzae,* **and** *Neisseria meningitides. Children weighing more than 50 kg:* 2 g I.V. q 8 hours.

M

Children ages 3 months and older weighing 50 kg or less: 40 mg/kg I.V. q 8 hours; maximum dose, 2 g I.V. q 8 hours.

▽ I.V. administration

• For I.V. bolus administration, add 10 ml of sterile water for injection to 500-mg/20-ml vial or add 20 ml to 1-g/30-ml vial. Shake to dissolve, and let stand until clear.
• For I.V. infusion, infusion vials (500 mg/100 ml and 1 g/100 ml) may be directly reconstituted with compatible infusion fluid. Or an injection vial may be reconstituted, then the resulting solution added to an I.V. container, and further diluted with appropriate infusion fluid. Don't use ADD-Vantage vials for this purpose.
• Follow manufacturer's guidelines closely when using ADD-Vantage vials.
• Use freshly prepared solutions of drug immediately.
• Stability of drug varies with form of drug used (injection vial, infusion vial, or ADD-Vantage container).
⊗ **Incompatibilities**
Other I.V. drugs.

Contraindications and cautions

• Contraindicated in patients hypersensitive to the drug or any of its components or other drugs in the same class. Also contraindicated in those who have had anaphylactic reactions to beta-lactams.
• Use cautiously and at a reduced dosage in patients with renal impairment.
⚕ **Lifespan:** In pregnant women, use only when benefits outweigh risks to the fetus. In breast-feeding women, use cautiously because it's unknown if the drug appears in breast milk. In infants younger than age 3 months, safety and effectiveness haven't been established.

Adverse reactions

CNS: headache, insomnia, somnolence, confusion, nervousness, agitation.
CV: thrombophlebitis at injection site, *heart failure, cardiac arrest,* tachycardia, hypertension, *MI, pulmonary embolism, bradycardia,* hypotension.
GI: diarrhea, nausea, vomiting, constipation, oral candidiasis, *pseudomembranous colitis,* glossitis, anorexia, cholestatic jaundice.
GU: dysuria, *renal failure.*
Hematologic: eosinophilia, anemia.

Respiratory: *apnea.*
Skin: rash, pruritus, urticaria.
Other: hypersensitivity reactions, *anaphylaxis,* inflammation at injection site, pain.

Interactions

Drug-drug. *Probenecid:* Inhibits renal excretion of meropenem. Don't give together.

Effects on lab test results

• May increase ALT, AST, bilirubin, alkaline phosphatase, LDH, creatinine, and BUN levels. May decrease hemoglobin level and hematocrit.
• May increase eosinophil count. May decrease WBC count. May increase or decrease platelet count and PT.

Pharmacokinetics

Absorption: Administered I.V.
Distribution: Protein-binding is 2%. Penetrates into most body fluids and tissues, including CSF.
Metabolism: In kidneys.
Excretion: In urine. *Half-life:* 1 hour.

Route	Onset	Peak	Duration
I.V.	Unknown	< 1 hr	Unknown

Action

Chemical effect: Readily penetrates the cell wall of most gram-positive and gram-negative bacteria to reach penicillin-binding protein targets, where it inhibits cell wall synthesis.
Therapeutic effect: Bactericidal.

Available forms

Powder for injection: 500 mg/15 ml, 500 mg/20 ml, 500 mg/100 ml, 1 g/15 ml, 1 g/30 ml, 1 g/100 ml

NURSING PROCESS

▥ **Assessment**
• Obtain specimen for culture and sensitivity tests before giving first dose. Therapy may begin pending test results.
🖐 **ALERT:** Serious and occasionally fatal hypersensitivity reactions may occur. Before therapy, determine whether patient has ever had a hypersensitivity reaction to penicillins, cephalosporins, other beta-lactams, or other allergens.
• Monitor patient for signs and symptoms of superinfection.

Reactions may be *common*, uncommon, *life-threatening*, or COMMON AND LIFE-THREATENING.

• Periodically assess organ-system functions during prolonged therapy.
• Assess patient's and family's knowledge of drug therapy.

Nursing diagnoses
• Infection related to bacteria
• Risk for deficient fluid volume related to effect on kidneys
• Deficient knowledge related to drug therapy

Planning and implementation
• Drug isn't used to treat methicillin-resistant staphylococci.
• If patient develops diarrhea, suspect pseudomembranous colitis. If confirmed, stop giving the drug, begin fluid and electrolyte management, and give an antibacterial effective against *Clostridium difficile.*
• If overdose occurs (usually in patients with renal impairment), stop giving the drug and provide general supportive therapy until renal elimination occurs. Drug is removable by hemodialysis, if needed.
Patient teaching
• Instruct patient to report adverse reactions.

Evaluation
• Patient is free from infection.
• Patient maintains adequate hydration.
• Patient and family state understanding of drug therapy.

mesalamine
(mez-AL-uh-meen)
Asacol, Canasa, Mesasal ♦, Novo-5 ASA ♦, Pentasa, Rowasa, Salofalk ♦

Pharmacologic class: salicylate
Therapeutic class: anti-inflammatory
Pregnancy risk category: B

Indications and dosages
▶ **Active mild to moderate distal ulcerative colitis, proctitis, proctosigmoiditis.** *Adults:*
800 mg P.O. (tablets) t.i.d. for total dose of 2.4 g daily for 6 weeks, or 1 g P.O. (capsules) q.i.d. for total dose of 4 g daily up to 8 weeks. Or 500 mg P.R. (suppository) b.i.d. Increase to t.i.d. after 2 weeks. Have patient retain for 1 to 3 hours or longer. Or 4 g as retention enema

once daily (preferably h.s.) retained for about 8 hours. Usual course of therapy for P.R. form is 3 to 6 weeks.
▶ **Maintenance of remission of ulcerative colitis.** *Adults:* 1.6 g P.O. daily in divided doses for 6 months. Or, 60 ml (4 g) rectal suspension q 2 to 3 nights or 1 to 3 g rectal suspension daily; retain for approximately 8 hours.

Contraindications and cautions
• Contraindicated in patients hypersensitive to the drug, any of its components, or salicylates.
• Use cautiously in patients with renal impairment; absorbed drug may cause nephrotoxicity.
Lifespan: In pregnant women, use cautiously. In breast-feeding women, rectal form of drug is contraindicated. Oral form may be used with caution. It's unknown if the drug appears in breast milk. In children, drug is contraindicated. In the elderly, use cautiously.

Adverse reactions
CNS: headache, dizziness, fatigue, fever, malaise.
GI: abdominal pain, cramps, or discomfort; flatulence; diarrhea; rectal pain; bloating; *nausea, vomiting, belching; pancolitis; pancreatitis.*
Respiratory: wheezing, URI.
Skin: pruritus, rash, urticaria, hair loss, acne.
Other: pain, *anaphylaxis.*

Interactions
None significant.

Effects on lab test results
• May increase BUN, creatinine, AST, ALT, alkaline phosphatase, LDH, amylase, and lipase levels.

Pharmacokinetics
Absorption: Poor with P.R. use.
Distribution: Not clearly defined.
Metabolism: Undergoes acetylation, but whether this takes place at colonic or systemic sites is unknown.
Excretion: P.O. form primarily in urine; most of P.R. form in feces. *Half-life:* about 5 to 10 hours.

Route	Onset	Peak	Duration
P.O., P.R.	Unknown	3–12 hr	Unknown

M

Action

Chemical effect: May act topically by inhibiting prostaglandin production in colon.
Therapeutic effect: Relieves inflammation in lower GI tract.

Available forms

Capsules (controlled-release): 250 mg, 500 mg
Rectal suspension: 4 g/60 ml
Suppositories: 500 mg, 1,000 mg
Tablets (delayed-release): 400 mg

NURSING PROCESS

Assessment

● Assess patient's condition before therapy and regularly thereafter to monitor the drug's effectiveness.
● Periodically monitor kidney function in patient on long-term therapy.
● Because it contains potassium metabisulfite, drug may cause hypersensitivity reactions in patient sensitive to sulfites.
● Be alert for adverse reactions.
● Assess patient's and family's knowledge of drug therapy.

Nursing diagnoses

● Impaired tissue integrity related to underlying condition
● Acute pain related to drug-induced adverse GI reactions
● Deficient knowledge related to drug therapy

Planning and implementation

● Have patient swallow tablets and capsules whole; don't crush or let him chew them.
● For maximum effectiveness, have patient retain suppository as long as possible. When giving rectal suspension, shake bottle before application.
● **ALERT:** Don't confuse Asacol with Os-Cal or mesalamine with mecamylamine.
Patient teaching
● Teach patient how to take oral and rectal form, and instruct him to carefully follow instructions supplied with drug.
● Instruct patient to stop taking drug if he experiences fever or rash. Patient intolerant of sulfasalazine or aminosalicylic acid may also be hypersensitive to this drug.

Evaluation

● Patient reports relief from GI symptoms.
● Patient states that no new pain is experienced during therapy.
● Patient and family state understanding of drug therapy.

mesna
(MEZ-nah)
Mesnex, Uromitexan ◆

Pharmacologic class: thiol derivative
Therapeutic class: uroprotectant
Pregnancy risk category: B

Indications and dosages

▶ **To prevent hemorrhagic cystitis in patients taking ifosfamide.** *Adults:* Dosage varies with amount of ifosfamide given. If using 1.2-g/m^2 ifosfamide, give 240 mg/m^2 as I.V. bolus with ifosfamide dose. Repeat dose at 4 hours and 8 hours to a total of 60% of the ifosfamide dose. Or, give 20% as a single bolus injection followed by two oral doses (40% each). If using 1.2-g/m^2 ifosfamide, give 240 mg/m^2 I.V. mesna with ifosfamide, then 480 mg/m^2 P.O. at 2 and 6 hours.
▶ **To prevent hemorrhagic cystitis in bone marrow recipients taking cyclophosphamide‡.** *Adults:* Give 60% to 160% of the cyclophosphamide daily dose I.V. in three to five divided doses or by continuous infusion. Or, in patients receiving 50 to 60 mg/kg cyclophosphamide I.V. daily for 2 to 4 days, give 10 mg/kg I.V. loading dose followed by 60 mg/kg by continuous infusion over 24 hours. Give with each cyclophosphamide dose and continue for 24 hours after last dose of cyclophosphamide.

▼ I.V. administration

● Dilute drug in D_5W, dextrose 5% combined with normal saline solution for injection, normal saline solution for injection, or lactated Ringer's solution to obtain final solution of 20 mg/ml.
● After mixing, inspect drug for particulate matter and discoloration before administering.
● Drug and ifosfamide are compatible in same I.V. infusion.
● Although diluted solution is stable for 24 hours at room temperature, refrigerate after preparation and use within 6 hours. After open-

ing ampule, discard any unused drug because it decomposes quickly into inactive compound.
⊗ **Incompatibilities**
Amphotericin B, carboplatin, cisplatin.

Contraindications and cautions

• Contraindicated in patients hypersensitive to the drug or other compounds containing thiol.
⚘ **Lifespan:** In pregnant women, use cautiously. In breast-feeding women and in children, safety and effectiveness haven't been established.

Adverse reactions

CNS: *fatigue, fever, asthenia,* dizziness, headache, somnolence, anxiety, confusion, insomnia, pain.
CV: chest pain, edema, hypotension, tachycardia, flushing.
GI: nausea, vomiting, diarrhea, constipation, anorexia, abdominal pain, dyspepsia.
GU: hematuria.
Hematologic: *leukopenia, thrombocytopenia, anemia, granulocytopenia.*
Metabolic: hypokalemia, dehydration.
Musculoskeletal: back pain.
Respiratory: dyspnea, coughing, pneumonia.
Skin: alopecia, increased sweating, pallor.
Other: *allergy,* injection site reaction.

Interactions

None significant.

Effects on lab test results

• Drug may interfere with diagnostic tests for urine ketones.

Pharmacokinetics

Absorption: Food doesn't affect it.
Distribution: Remains in vascular compartment.
Metabolism: Rapid, to one metabolite.
Excretion: In urine. *Half-life:* 4 to 8 hours.

Route	Onset	Peak	Duration
P.O., I.V.	Unknown	Unknown	Unknown

Action

Chemical effect: Detoxifies urotoxic ifosfamide metabolites.
Therapeutic effect: Prevents ifosfamide from adversely affecting bladder tissue.

Available forms

Injection: 100 mg/ml in 2- and 10-ml vials (contains benzyl alcohol)
Tablets: 400 mg

NURSING PROCESS

ᗅ Assessment

• Assess patient's condition before therapy and regularly thereafter to monitor the drug's effectiveness.
• Up to 6% of patients may not respond to drug's protective effects.
• Monitor urine samples for hematuria daily in patient taking mesna.
• Be alert for adverse reactions.
• If patient has an adverse GI reaction, monitor his hydration.
• Assess patient's and family's knowledge of drug therapy.

⊕ Nursing diagnoses

• Risk for deficient fluid volume related to drug-induced adverse GI reactions
• Deficient knowledge related to drug therapy

▷ Planning and implementation

• If patient vomits within 2 hours of taking drug P.O., repeat the dose or give I.V.
• Because drug is used with ifosfamide and other chemotherapeutics, it's difficult to determine adverse reactions attributable solely to this drug.
• Drug isn't effective in preventing hematuria from other causes (such as thrombocytopenia).
• Although formulated to prevent hemorrhagic cystitis from ifosfamide, drug won't protect against other toxicities linked to ifosfamide.
Patient teaching
• Instruct patient to report hematuria immediately and to notify prescriber about adverse GI reactions.

☑ Evaluation

• Patient maintains adequate hydration throughout therapy.
• Patient and family state understanding of drug therapy.

M

metaproterenol sulfate
(met-uh-proh-TER-eh-nul SUL-fayt)
Alupent

Pharmacologic class: beta agonist
Therapeutic class: bronchodilator
Pregnancy risk category: C

Indications and dosages

▶ **Asthma; bronchospasm.** *Oral. Adults and children age 9 and older or weighing more than 27.3 kg (60 lb):* 20 mg P.O. t.i.d. to q.i.d.
Adults and children younger than age 9 or weighing less 27.3 kg (60 lb): 10 mg P.O. t.i.d. to q.i.d.
Children younger than age 6: 1.3 to 2.6 mg/kg/day P.O. in divided doses.
Aerosol inhalation
Adults and children older than age 12: 2 to 3 inhalations with at least 2 minutes between inhalations. Don't repeat inhalations more often than q 3 to 4 hours. Maximum, 12 inhalations daily.
Intermittent positive pressure breathing (IPPB) or nebulizer
Adults and children age 12 and older: 0.2 to 0.3 ml of 5% solution diluted in 2.5 ml of normal saline solution or 2.5 ml of commercially available 0.4% or 0.6% solution q 4 hours, p.r.n.
Hand-bulb nebulizer
Adults and children age 12 and older: 10 inhalations of an undiluted 5% solution.
▶ **Acute asthma attacks.** *Children age 6 and older:* Use 5% solution for inhalation only. Give 0.1 to 0.2 ml in saline to a total volume of 3 ml given by nebulizer at time of attack.

Contraindications and cautions

• Contraindicated in patients hypersensitive to the drug or any of its components, in those receiving cyclopropane or halogenated hydrocarbon general anesthetics, and in those with tachycardia or arrhythmias caused by tachycardia, peripheral or mesenteric vascular thrombosis, or profound hypoxia or hypercapnia.
• Use cautiously in patients with hypertension, hyperthyroidism, heart disease, diabetes, or cirrhosis and in those receiving digoxin.
🌸 **Lifespan:** In pregnant women, use cautiously. In breast-feeding women, use cautiously. It's unknown if the drug appears in breast milk.

Adverse reactions

CNS: *nervousness, weakness,* drowsiness, tremors.
CV: tachycardia, hypertension, ECG changes, palpitations, *cardiac arrest.*
GI: vomiting, nausea, heartburn, taste perversion.
Respiratory: *paradoxical bronchoconstriction.*

Interactions

Drug-drug. *Other sympathomimetics:* May have additive effects and toxicity. Separate administration times.
Propranolol, other beta blockers: Blocks bronchodilating effect of metaproterenol. Monitor patient.
Theophylline, aminophylline: May increase risk of cardiotoxicity. Monitor ECG and vital signs closely.

Effects on lab test results

None reported.

Pharmacokinetics

Absorption: Good in GI tract. Minimally through the lungs.
Distribution: Wide.
Metabolism: Extensive on first pass through liver.
Excretion: In urine. *Half-life:* Unknown.

Route	Onset	Peak	Duration
P.O.	15 min	1 hr	1–4 hr
Inhalation	1 min	1 hr	2–6 hr
Nebulization	5–30 min	1 hr	2–6 hr

Action

Chemical effect: Relaxes bronchial smooth muscle by acting on beta$_2$-adrenergic receptors.
Therapeutic effect: Improves breathing.

Available forms

Aerosol inhaler: 0.65 mg/metered spray
Solution for nebulizer inhalation: 0.4%, 0.6%, 5% solution
Syrup: 10 mg/5 ml
Tablets: 10 mg, 20 mg

NURSING PROCESS

📝 Assessment
• Assess patient's condition before therapy and regularly thereafter to monitor the drug's effectiveness.

Reactions may be *common,* uncommon, *life-threatening*, or COMMON AND LIFE-THREATENING.

• Be alert for adverse reactions and drug interactions.
• If patient has an adverse GI reaction, monitor his hydration.
• Assess patient's and family's knowledge of drug therapy.

◙ Nursing diagnoses
• Impaired gas exchange related to underlying respiratory condition
• Risk for deficient fluid volume related to drug-induced adverse GI reactions
• Deficient knowledge related to drug therapy

▶ Planning and implementation
• Aerosol nebulization solution can be given by IPPB with drug diluted in normal saline solution or by hand-bulb nebulizer at full strength.
③ ALERT: Don't use solution if discolored or precipitated.
③ ALERT: Don't confuse metaproterenol with metoprolol or metipranolol.
③ ALERT: Don't confuse Alupent with Atrovent.
Patient teaching
• Give patient the following instructions for using metered-dose inhaler: clear nasal passages and throat. Breathe out, expelling as much air from lungs as possible. Place mouthpiece well into mouth and inhale deeply as you release a dose from inhaler. Hold breath for several seconds, remove mouthpiece, and exhale slowly. Allow 2 minutes between inhalations.
• Instruct patient to store drug in light-resistant container.
• Tell patient using corticosteroid inhaler to use bronchodilator first and then to wait 5 to 15 minutes before using corticosteroid. This allows bronchodilator to open air passages for maximum effectiveness of corticosteroid.
• Warn patient to immediately stop taking the drug and notify the prescriber if he has paradoxical bronchospasm.
• Tell patient that if dose doesn't work, he should notify his prescriber for an increase.

▨ Evaluation
• Patient's respiratory status improves.
• Patient maintains adequate hydration.
• Patient and family state understanding of drug therapy.

metformin hydrochloride
(met-FOR-min high-droh-KLOR-ighd)
Apo-Metformin♦, Fortamet, Gen-Metformin♦, Glucophage⌀, Glucophage XR⌀, Glumetza, Nu-Metformin♦, PMS-Metformin♦, Rhoxal-metformin♦, Riomet

Pharmacologic class: biguanide
Therapeutic class: antidiabetic
Pregnancy risk category: B

Indications and dosages

▶ **Adjunct to diet and exercise to lower glucose level in patients with type 2 (non–insulin-dependent) diabetes mellitus.** *Adults:* Initially, 500 mg P.O. b.i.d. with morning and evening meals. Increase by 500 mg q week or to 850 mg b.i.d. Maximum daily, 2,500. Or 850 mg P.O. once daily with morning meal; increase by 850 mg q other week to daily maximum, 2,550 mg. Doses greater than 2,000 mg may be better tolerated if divided t.i.d. If using extended-release form, give 500 mg P.O. daily with the evening meal; increase by 500 mg q week to daily maximum, 2,000 mg. If higher daily dose is needed, change to the regular release form.
Children ages 10 to 16: 500 mg P.O. b.i.d. using the regular-release form only. Increase dosage in increments of 500 mg weekly up to a maximum of 2,000 mg daily in divided doses. Don't use extended-release form in children.
▶ **Adjunct to diet and exercise in type 2 diabetes, as monotherapy or with a sulfonylurea or insulin.** *Adults and adolescents age 17 and older:* Initially, 500 to 1,000 mg of Fortamet P.O. with evening meal. Increase dosage based on glucose level in increments of 500 mg/week to a maximum of 2,500 mg daily. When used with a sulfonylurea or insulin, base dosage on blood glucose level, and adjust slowly until desired therapeutic effect occurs. Decrease insulin dosage by 10% to 25% when fasting blood glucose level is less than 120 mg/dl.
▶ **Adjunct to diet and exercise in type 2 diabetes as monotherapy or with a sulfonylurea or insulin (Glumetza).** *Adults:* Initially, 1,000 mg P.O. once daily in the evening with food. Increase as needed by 500 mg in weekly increments up to a maximum of 2,000 mg daily.

M

If glycemic control not attained at this dose, give 1,000 mg b.i.d.

When used with a sulfonylurea or insulin, base dosage on glucose level and adjust slowly until desired therapeutic effect occurs. Decrease insulin dose by 10% to 25% when fasting blood glucose level is less than 120 mg/dl.

🔲 **Adjust-a-dose:** For malnourished or debilitated patients, don't adjust to maximum dosage.

Contraindications and cautions

• Contraindicated in patients hypersensitive to the drug or any of its components; in those with hepatic disease, renal disease or renal dysfunction, acute or chronic metabolic acidosis; and in heart failure patients who require other drugs. Temporarily withhold drug in patients undergoing radiologic studies involving parenteral administration of iodinated contrast materials; using such products may result in acute renal dysfunction. If patient enters hypoxic state, stop drug.

• Use cautiously in debilitated or malnourished patients and in those with adrenal or pituitary insufficiency because of increased risk of hypoglycemia.

⚜ **Lifespan:** In pregnant women, safety and effectiveness haven't been established. In breastfeeding women, use cautiously; it's unknown if drug appears in breast milk. In children younger than age 10, safety and effectiveness of regular form haven't been established. In children younger than age 17, safety and effectiveness of extended-release form haven't been established. In elderly patients, use cautiously.

Adverse reactions

CNS: headache, dizziness, asthenia.
GI: *diarrhea, nausea, vomiting,* abdominal discomfort, *flatulence,* indigestion, unpleasant or metallic taste.
Hematologic: megaloblastic anemia.
Metabolic: *lactic acidosis.*

Interactions

Drug-drug. *Calcium channel blockers, corticosteroids, estrogens, hormonal contraceptives, isoniazid, nicotinic acid, phenothiazines, phenytoin, sympathomimetics, thiazide and other diuretics, thyroid drugs:* May cause hyperglycemia. Monitor patient's glycemic control. Increase metformin dosage.

Cationic drugs (such as amiloride, cimetidine, digoxin, morphine, procainamide, quinidine, quinine, ranitidine, triamterene, trimethoprim, vancomycin): May reduce metformin clearance and increase metformin level. Monitor patient's glucose level. Adjust dosages, if needed.
Furosemide, nifedipine: May increase metformin levels. Monitor patient and decrease dosage.
Iodinated contrast material: May cause lactic acidosis, leading to acute renal impairment. Withhold metformin on or before the day of the study, and resume after 48 hours, if renal function is normal.
Drug-herb. *Aloe, bilberry leaf, bitter melon, burdock, dandelion, fenugreek, garlic, ginseng:* May improve glucose control and allow reduction of antidiabetic. Tell patient to discuss use of herbal remedies with prescriber before therapy.
Drug-lifestyle. *Alcohol use:* May increase drug effects. Discourage using together.

Effects on lab test results

• May decrease pH, bicarbonate, triglyceride, total cholesterol, LDL, glucose, hemoglobin, and glycosylated hemoglobin levels and hematocrit.
• May decrease RBC count.

Pharmacokinetics

Absorption: Food decreases rate and extent for tablets, but increases extent for oral solution.
Distribution: Negligible.
Metabolism: None.
Excretion: Unchanged in urine. *Half-life:* About 6 hours.

Route	Onset	Peak	Duration
P.O.			
regular	Unknown	2–4 hr	Unknown
solution	Unknown	2½ hr	Unknown
extended-release	Unknown	4–8 hr	24–48 hr

Action

Chemical effect: Decreases hepatic glucose production and intestinal absorption of glucose and improves insulin sensitivity (increases peripheral glucose uptake and utilization).
Therapeutic effect: Lowers blood glucose level.

Available forms

Oral solution: 500 mg/5 ml

Tablets: 500 mg, 850 mg, 1,000 mg
Tablets (extended-release): 500 mg, 750 mg, 1000 mg

NURSING PROCESS

🔬 Assessment

• Assess patient's glucose level before therapy and regularly thereafter to monitor the drug's effectiveness.
• Assess patient's kidney function before therapy and reassess at least annually. If renal impairment is detected, expect prescriber to switch to different antidiabetic.
• Monitor patient's hematologic lab test results for megaloblastic anemia. Patients with low vitamin B_{12} or calcium intake or absorption may be more likely to develop a below-normal vitamin B_{12} level. Check their vitamin B_{12} level every 2 to 3 years.
• Be alert for adverse reactions and drug interactions.
• Monitor patient closely during times of stress, such as infection, fever, surgery, or trauma. Insulin therapy may be needed.
• The risk of drug-induced lactic acidosis is very low but may occur in diabetics with significant renal or hepatic insufficiency, other medical or surgical problems, and multiple drug therapies. The risk of lactic acidosis increases with the degree of renal impairment and patient's age. Don't give drug to patient age 80 or older unless measurement of creatinine clearance shows renal function is normal.
• Assess patient's and family's knowledge of drug therapy.

⊕ Nursing diagnoses

• Ineffective health maintenance related to presence of hyperglycemia
• Risk for deficient fluid volume related to drug-induced adverse GI reactions
• Deficient knowledge related to drug therapy

▷ Planning and implementation

• When switching from standard oral antidiabetic (except chlorpropamide) to metformin, usually no transition period is needed. When switching from chlorpropamide to metformin, use care during first 2 weeks of metformin therapy because prolonged retention of chlorpropamide increases risk of hypoglycemia during this time.

🚫 **Adjust-a-dose:** Don't use extended-release formulation in children.
⚠ **ALERT:** Don't cut, crush or chew extended-release tablets; swallow whole.
• If glucose level rises despite therapy, notify prescriber.
• If patient hasn't responded to 4 weeks of therapy using maximum dosage, add oral sulfonylurea while continuing metformin at maximum dosage. If patient still doesn't respond after several months, stop both drugs and start insulin therapy.
⚠ **ALERT:** If patient develops conditions linked to hypoxemia or dehydration, stop giving the drug immediately and notify prescriber because of risk of lactic acidosis.
• Stop therapy temporarily for a surgical procedure (except minor procedures not related to restricted intake of food and fluids), and don't restart until patient's oral intake and kidney function are normal.
Patient teaching
• Tell patient to take once-daily dose with breakfast (except Fortamet, which is to be taken with dinner) and twice-daily dose with breakfast and dinner.
• Tell patient not to crush or chew extended-release tablets.
• Instruct patient to stop drug and tell prescriber about unexplained hyperventilation, myalgia, malaise, unusual somnolence, or other symptoms of early lactic acidosis.
• Warn patient to avoid alcohol consumption while taking drug.
⚠ **ALERT:** Teach patient about diabetes and the importance of complying with therapy; adhering to diet, weight reduction, exercise, and hygiene programs; and avoiding infection. Explain how and when to monitor glucose level and how to differentiate between hypoglycemia and hyperglycemia.
• Tell patient not to change dose without prescriber's consent. Encourage patient to report abnormal glucose test results.
• Advise patient not to take other drugs, including OTC drugs, without checking with prescriber.
• Instruct patient to wear or carry medical identification.

✓ Evaluation

• Patient's glucose level is normal.

M

Rapid onset   *Liquid form contains alcohol.   ◆ Canada   ◇ Australia   †OTC   ⌀ Photoguide   ‡Off-label use

• Patient maintains adequate hydration throughout therapy.
• Patient and family state understanding of drug therapy.

methadone hydrochloride
(METH-eh-dohn high-droh-KLOR-ighd)
Dolophine, Methadose, Physeptone◊

Pharmacologic class: opioid
Therapeutic class: analgesic, opioid detoxification adjunct
Pregnancy risk category: C
Controlled substance schedule: II

Indications and dosages

▶ **Severe pain.** *Adults:* 2.5 to 10 mg P.O., I.M., or subcutaneously q 3 to 4 hours, p.r.n. unless patient is opiate naïve, then give q 8 to 12 hours. *Children‡:* 0.7 mg/kg P.O. q 4 to 6 hours.
▶ **Opiate withdrawal syndrome.** *Adults:* 15 to 40 mg P.O. daily initially based on previous opiate exposure (highly individualized). Maintenance dosage is 20 to 120 mg P.O. daily. Adjust dosage p.r.n. Daily doses greater than 120 mg require state and federal approval.

Contraindications and cautions

• Contraindicated in patients hypersensitive to the drug or any of its components.
• Use cautiously in debilitated patients and in patients with acute abdominal conditions, severe hepatic or renal impairment, hypothyroidism, Addison's disease, prostatic hyperplasia, urethral stricture, head injury, increased intracranial pressure, asthma, or other respiratory conditions.
❧ **Lifespan:** In pregnant women, use cautiously. In breast-feeding women, don't use. It's unknown if the drug appears in breast milk. In children, safety and effectiveness haven't been established. In elderly patients, use cautiously.

Adverse reactions

CNS: headache, agitation, lightheadedness, syncope, insomnia, *sedation, somnolence, clouded sensorium, euphoria,* dizziness, chorea, *seizures.*
CV: hypotension, *bradycardia, shock, cardiac arrest, arrhythmias.*
EENT: visual disturbances.

GI: nausea, vomiting, constipation, ileus.
GU: urine retention.
Respiratory: *respiratory depression, respiratory arrest.*
Skin: diaphoresis.
Other: decreased libido, *physical dependence,* pain at injection site, tissue irritation, induration after subcutaneous injection.

Interactions

Drug-drug. *Ammonium chloride and other urine acidifiers, phenytoin:* May reduce methadone effect. Monitor patient for decreased pain control.
Cimetidine: may increase methadone levels. Monitor patient for increased CNS and respiratory depression.
CNS depressants, general anesthetics, hypnotics, MAO inhibitors, sedatives, tranquilizers, tricyclic antidepressants: May cause respiratory depression, hypotension, profound sedation, or coma. Use together cautiously and monitor patient.
Rifampin: May cause withdrawal symptoms; reduces blood levels of methadone. Use together cautiously.
Drug-lifestyle. *Alcohol use:* May have additive effects. Discourage patient from using together.

Effects on lab test results

• May increase amylase or lipase levels.

Pharmacokinetics

Absorption: Good in P.O. use; unknown in I.M. use.
Distribution: Highly bound to tissue protein.
Metabolism: Primarily in liver.
Excretion: Primarily in urine; metabolites in feces. *Half-life:* 15 to 25 hours.

Route	Onset	Peak	Duration
P.O.	30–60 min	1–2 hr	4–7 hr
I.M.	10–30 min	½–1 hr	4–7 hr
SubQ	Unknown	1–1½ hr	4–7 hr

Action

Chemical effect: Binds to opioid receptors at many sites in CNS, altering both perception of and emotional response to pain through unknown mechanism.
Therapeutic effect: Relieves pain and symptoms of opioid withdrawal.

Reactions may be *common,* uncommon, *life-threatening,* or COMMON AND LIFE-THREATENING.

Available forms

Dispersible tablets (for maintenance therapy): 40 mg
Injection: 10 mg/ml
Oral solution (contains 8% alcohol): 5 mg/ 5 ml, 10 mg/5 ml, 10 mg/ml (concentrate)
Tablets: 5 mg, 10 mg

NURSING PROCESS

Assessment
• Assess patient's pain or opioid dependence before and during therapy.
• Monitor patient closely because drug has cumulative effect. Marked sedation can occur after repeated doses.
• Be alert for adverse reactions and drug interactions.
• Assess patient's and family's knowledge of drug therapy.

Nursing diagnoses
• Chronic pain related to underlying condition
• Ineffective individual coping related to opioid dependence
• Deficient knowledge related to drug therapy

Planning and implementation
• Liquid form is legally required in maintenance programs. Dissolve tablets in 120 ml of orange juice or powdered citrus drink.
• P.O. dose is one-half as potent as injected dose.
• For parenteral use, I.M. injection is preferred. Rotate injection sites.
• Around-the-clock therapy is needed to manage severe, chronic pain.
• Duration of action is prolonged to 22 to 48 hours with repeated doses of drug. Depressant effects from overdosage can also last 36 to 48 hours.
❸ ALERT: Very high doses of methadone may cause QT interval prolongation and torsades de pointes.
❸ ALERT: Don't confuse methadone with Metadate.
Patient teaching
• Warn patient about getting out of bed or walking. Warn outpatient to avoid hazardous activities until drug's CNS effects are known.
• Instruct patient to avoid alcohol consumption during drug therapy.

Evaluation
• Patient is free from pain.
• Patient doesn't exhibit opioid withdrawal symptoms.
• Patient and family state understanding of drug therapy.

methamphetamine hydrochloride
(meth-am-FET-uh-meen high-droh-KLOR-ighd)
Desoxyn

Pharmacologic class: amphetamine
Therapeutic class: CNS stimulant, short-term adjunct anorexigenic, sympathomimetic amine
Pregnancy risk category: C.
Controlled substance schedule: II

Indications and dosages

▶ **Attention deficit hyperactivity disorder.**
Children age 6 and older: Initially, 5 mg P.O. once daily or b.i.d., increase by 5-mg increments weekly p.r.n. Usual effective dosage is 20 to 25 mg daily.
▶ **Short-term adjunct in exogenous obesity.**
Adults and children older than age 12: 5 mg P.O. 30 minutes before each meal. Treatment should not exceed a few weeks.

Contraindications and cautions

• Contraindicated in patients hypersensitive to sympathomimetic amines; patients with idiosyncratic reactions to sympathomimetic amines; patients with moderate to severe hypertension, hyperthyroidism, symptomatic CV disease, advanced arteriosclerosis, glaucoma, or history of drug abuse; patients who have taken an MAO inhibitor within 14 days; and agitated patients.
• Use cautiously in patients who are debilitated, asthenic, psychopathic, or patients who have a history of suicidal or homicidal tendencies.
⚘ Lifespan: In pregnant and breast-feeding women, drug is contraindicated. In children younger than age 6, safety and effectiveness haven't been established. In elderly patients, use cautiously.

Adverse reactions

CNS: *nervousness, insomnia,* irritability, *talkativeness,* dizziness, headache, hyperexcitability, euphoria, tremors, exacerbation of Tourette syndrome, tics, psychotic episodes.

M

CV: hypertension, *reflex bradycardia*, tachycardia, *palpitations, arrhythmias, cardiomyopathy.*
EENT: blurred vision, mydriasis.
GI: metallic taste, dry mouth, nausea, vomiting, abdominal cramps, diarrhea, constipation, *anorexia.*
GU: impotence.
Skin: urticaria.
Other: altered libido; growth suppression in children.

Interactions

Drug-drug. *Acetazolamide, antacids, sodium bicarbonate:* May increase renal reabsorption. Monitor patient for enhanced effects.
Ammonium chloride, ascorbic acid: May decrease levels and increase renal excretion of methamphetamine. Monitor patient for decreased methamphetamine effects.
Furazolidone: increased sensitivity to amphetamines. Monitor patient for toxicity and adjust dose as needed.
Guanethidine: May decrease the antihypertensive effectiveness of guanethidine. Monitor blood pressure.
Haloperidol, phenothiazines, tricyclic antidepressants: May increase CNS effects. Avoid using together.
Insulin, oral antidiabetics: May decrease antidiabetic requirement. Monitor glucose level.
MAO inhibitors: May cause severe hypertension; possible hypertensive crisis. Don't use within 14 days of MAO inhibitor therapy.
SSRIs: increased sensitivity to sympathomimetics; risk of serotonin syndrome. Monitor and adjust dose as needed.
Drug-herb. *Melatonin:* May enhance monoaminergic effects of drug; may worsen insomnia. Discourage using together.
Drug-food. *Caffeinated beverages:* May increase drug effects. Discourage using together.

Effects on lab test results
• May increase corticosteroid level.

Pharmacokinetics
Absorption: Rapid.
Distribution: Wide.
Metabolism: In liver to at least seven metabolites.
Excretion: In urine. *Half-life:* 4 to 5 hours.

Route	Onset	Peak	Duration
P.O.	Unknown	Unknown	24 hr

Action
Chemical effect: Probably promotes nerve impulse transmission by releasing stored norepinephrine from nerve terminals in brain. Main sites appear to be cerebral cortex and reticular activating system. In hyperkinetic children, drug has paradoxical calming effect.
Therapeutic effect: Promotes calmness in children with attention deficit disorder and causes weight loss.

Available forms
Tablets: 5 mg

NURSING PROCESS

Assessment
• Assess patient's condition before therapy, and regularly thereafter to monitor the drug's effectiveness.
• Be alert for adverse reactions and drug interactions particularly growth suppression in children and cardiomyopathy with prolonged use.
• Assess patient's and family's knowledge of drug therapy.

Nursing diagnoses
• Ineffective health maintenance related to underlying condition
• Disturbed sleep pattern related to drug-induced insomnia
• Deficient knowledge related to drug therapy

Planning and implementation
ALERT: Don't confuse Desoxyn with digitoxin or digoxin.
• Drug isn't the first-line therapy for obesity. Use as anorexigenic is prohibited in some states.
• When used for obesity, make sure patient is on weight-reduction program.
• If tolerance to anorexigenic effect develops, notify prescriber and stop giving the drug.
Patient teaching
• Warn patient of high risk of abuse. Advise him that drug shouldn't be used to prevent fatigue.
• Advise patient to take last dose of drug at least 6 hours before bedtime.
• Warn patient to avoid activities that require alertness or good coordination until the drug's CNS effects are known.

- Tell patient not to use caffeine during therapy.
- Instruct patient to report signs of excessive stimulation.
- Instruct patient not to crush long-acting tablets.

☑ Evaluation
- Patient has positive response to drug therapy.
- Patient doesn't experience insomnia.
- Patient and family state understanding of drug therapy.

methimazole
(meth-IH-muh-zohl)
Tapazole

Pharmacologic class: thyroid hormone antagonist
Therapeutic class: antithyroid drug
Pregnancy risk category: D

Indications and dosages

▶ **Hyperthyroidism.** *Adults:* If mild, 15 mg P.O. daily. If moderately severe, 30 to 40 mg daily. If severe, 60 mg daily. Daily dosage divided into three doses at 8-hour intervals. Maintenance dosage is 5 to 15 mg daily.
Children: 0.4 mg/kg P.O. daily in divided doses q 8 hours. Maintenance dosage is 0.2 mg/kg P.O. daily in divided doses q 8 hours. Or 0.5 to 0.7 mg/kg P.O. daily in three divided doses. Maintenance dosage is one-third to two-thirds of initial dose. Maximum dosage 30 mg/24 hours.

Contraindications and cautions

- Contraindicated in patients hypersensitive to the drug or any of its components.
- ❊ **Lifespan:** In pregnant women, use cautiously. In breast-feeding women, use cautiously; it's unknown if drug appears in breast milk.

Adverse reactions

CNS: headache, drowsiness, vertigo, neuropathies, neuritis, paresthesias, CNS stimulation, depression.
GI: diarrhea, nausea, vomiting, epigastric distress, salivary gland enlargement, loss of taste.
Hematologic: *agranulocytosis, leukopenia, thrombocytopenia, aplastic anemia,* lymphadenopathy.

Hepatic: jaundice.
Metabolic: hypothyroidism.
Musculoskeletal: arthralgia, myalgia.
Skin: alopecia, rash, urticaria, skin discoloration.
Other: drug-induced fever.

Interactions

Drug-drug. *Anticoagulants:* May enhance anti–vitamin K effects. Monitor PT and INR.
Beta blockers, digoxin, theophylline: May increase levels of these drugs when a hyperthyroid patient becomes euthyroid. Reduce dosage of these drugs, if needed.

Effects on lab test results
- May decrease hemoglobin level and hematocrit.
- May decrease granulocyte, WBC, RBC, and platelet counts.

Pharmacokinetics
Absorption: Rapid.
Distribution: Concentrated in thyroid and isn't protein-bound.
Metabolism: Hepatic.
Excretion: Primarily in urine. *Half-life:* 5 to 13 hours.

Route	Onset	Peak	Duration
P.O.	Unknown	30 min–1 hr	Unknown

Action

Chemical effect: Inhibits oxidation of iodine in thyroid gland, blocking iodine's ability to combine with tyrosine to form T_4. Also may prevent coupling of monoiodotyrosine and diiodotyrosine to form T_4 and T_3.
Therapeutic effect: Reduces thyroid hormone level.

Available forms

Tablets: 5 mg, 10 mg

NURSING PROCESS

☒ Assessment
- Assess patient's thyroid condition before therapy and regularly thereafter to monitor the drug's effectiveness.
- Monitor thyroid function studies.
- Monitor CBC and liver function periodically.

M

⊛ **ALERT:** Dosages higher than 30 mg daily increase risk of agranulocytosis, especially in patients older than age 40.
• Be alert for adverse reactions.
• Assess patient's and family's knowledge of drug therapy.

⊞ **Nursing diagnoses**
• Ineffective health maintenance related to presence of hyperthyroidism
• Ineffective immune protection related to drug-induced adverse hematologic reactions
• Deficient knowledge related to drug therapy

▷ **Planning and implementation**
• Pregnant women may need a lower dosage as pregnancy progresses. Thyroid hormone may be added. Drug may be stopped during last weeks of pregnancy.
• Notify prescriber about signs and symptoms of hypothyroidism and adjust dosage.
⊛ **ALERT:** If severe rash occurs or cervical lymph nodes become enlarged, stop giving the drug and notify prescriber.
⊛ **ALERT:** Don't confuse methimazole with mebendazole, methazolamide, or rabeprazole.
Patient teaching
• Tell patient to take drug with meals.
• Warn patient to immediately report fever, sore throat, or mouth sores (signs of agranulocytosis); skin eruptions (sign of hypersensitivity); or anorexia, pruritus, right upper quadrant pain, and yellow skin or sclera (signs of hepatic dysfunction).
• Tell patient to ask prescriber about using iodized salt and eating shellfish.
• Warn patient against taking OTC cough products, because many contain iodine.
• Instruct patient to store drug in light-resistant container.

⛊ **Evaluation**
• Patient has normal thyroid hormone level.
• Patient maintains normal hematologic parameters throughout therapy.
• Patient and family state understanding of drug therapy.

methotrexate
(amethopterin, MTX)
(meth-oh-TRECKS-ayt)
Trexall

methotrexate sodium
Methotrexate LPF, Rheumatrex Dose Pack

Pharmacologic class: antimetabolite
Therapeutic class: antineoplastic, immunosuppressant, antirheumatic
Pregnancy risk category: X

Indications and dosages
▶ **Trophoblastic tumors (choriocarcinoma, hydatidiform mole).** *Adults:* 15 to 30 mg P.O. or I.M. daily for 5 days. May repeat course after 1 or more weeks, based on response or toxicity. Three to five courses usually are used.
▶ **Acute lymphoblastic and lymphatic leukemia.** *Adults and children:* 3.3 mg/m^2 P.O. or I.M. daily for 4 to 6 weeks or until remission occurs; then 20 to 30 mg/m^2 P.O. or I.M. twice weekly. Or, 2.5 mg/kg I.V. q 14 days.
▶ **Meningeal leukemia.** *Adults and children:* 12 mg/m^2 intrathecally (maximum of 15 mg) q 2 to 5 days and repeat until cell count of CSF returns to normal, then give one additional dose. Or, 12 mg/m^2 once weekly for 2 weeks, then once monthly thereafter. Or intrathecal dose based on age in years, *younger than 1 year,* 6 mg; *1 year,* 8 mg; *2 years,* 10 mg; *3 years or older,* 12 mg.
▶ **Burkitt's lymphoma (stage I or stage II).** *Adults:* 10 to 25 mg P.O. daily for 4 to 8 days with 7- to 10-day rest intervals.
▶ **Lymphosarcoma (stage III).** *Adults:* 0.625 to 2.5 mg/kg P.O., I.M., or I.V. daily.
▶ **Osteosarcoma.** *Adults:* 12 g/m^2 I.V. as a 4-hour infusion. May increase to 15 g/m^2 in subsequent treatments if peak serum concentration at the end of infusion does not reach 1,000 micromolar (10^{-3} mol/L).
▶ **Mycosis fungoides.** *Adults:* 2.5 to 10 mg P.O. daily, or 50 mg I.M. weekly, or 25 mg I.M. twice weekly.
▶ **Psoriasis.** *Adults:* 10 to 25 mg P.O., I.M., or I.V. as single weekly dose. Do not exceed 30 mg/week. Or, 2.5 mg q. 12 hours for 3 doses each week. Do not exceed 30 mg/week. A 5- to

10-mg test dose should be tried the week before therapy starts.

▶ **Rheumatoid arthritis.** *Adults:* Initially, 7.5 mg P.O. once weekly, or divided as 2.5 mg P.O. q 12 hours for three doses once a week. Gradually increase dosage to maximum, 20 mg weekly.
Adults‡: 7.5 to 15 mg I.M. once weekly.
▶ **Head and neck carcinoma‡.** *Adults:* 40 to 60 mg/m² I.V. once weekly. Response to therapy is limited to 4 months.

▼ I.V. administration

• Follow facility policy to reduce risks. Preparation and administration of parenteral forms are linked to carcinogenic, mutagenic, and teratogenic risks.
• Liquid methotrexate sodium injection with preservatives may be given undiluted except intrathecally or in high I.V. doses.
• Preservative-free liquid methotrexate sodium injection may be given undiluted or may be further diluted with normal saline solution.
• For reconstitution of lyophilized powders, reconstitute immediately before use, and discard unused drug. Dilute with D₅W or normal saline solution. Dilute the 20-mg vial to a concentration no greater than 25 mg/ml. Reconstitute 1-g vial with 19.4 ml of diluent for a maximum concentration of 50 mg/ml.
• For intrathecal use, only use 20-mg vials of powder with no preservatives. Reconstitute immediately before using, with preservative-free normal saline solution injection. Dilute to maximum of 1 mg/ml. Use only new vials of drug and diluent.
• Drug may be given daily or weekly, depending on the disease.
• Storage for 24 hours at 70° to 77° F (21° to 25° C) results in a product that is within 90% of label potency. Protect from light.
⊗ **Incompatibilities**
Bleomycin, chlorpromazine, dexamethasone sodium phosphate, droperidol, fluorouracil, gemcitabine, idarubicin, ifosfamide, metoclopramide, midazolam, nalbuphine, prednisolone, promethazine, propofol, sodium phosphate, vancomycin.

Contraindications and cautions

• Contraindicated in patients hypersensitive to the drug or any of its components and in those with psoriasis or rheumatoid arthritis who also have alcoholism, alcoholic liver, chronic liver disease, immunodeficiency syndromes, or blood dyscrasias.
• Use cautiously and at modified dosage in patients with impaired liver or kidney function, bone marrow suppression, aplasia, leukopenia, thrombocytopenia, or anemia. Also use cautiously in patients with infection, peptic ulceration, or ulcerative colitis and in debilitated patients.
⚖ **Lifespan:** In pregnant and breast-feeding women, drug is contraindicated. In children younger than age 2, safety and effectiveness haven't been established for uses other than cancer. In elderly patients, use cautiously.

Adverse reactions

CNS: *seizures,* malaise, dizziness, headache, *arachnoiditis,* subacute neurotoxicity, demyelination, *leukoencephalopathy.*
EENT: pharyngitis, blurred vision, gingivitis.
GI: stomatitis, diarrhea, enteritis, *intestinal perforation,* nausea, vomiting.
GU: nephropathy, TUBULAR NECROSIS, *renal impairment, renal failure.*
Hematologic: *anemia, leukopenia, thrombocytopenia.*
Hepatic: *acute toxicity, chronic toxicity, cirrhosis, hepatic fibrosis.*
Metabolic: hyperuricemia.
Musculoskeletal: osteoporosis in children with long-term use.
Respiratory: *pulmonary fibrosis, pulmonary interstitial infiltrates,* pneumonitis.
Skin: *urticaria,* pruritus, alopecia, hyperpigmentation, psoriatic lesions, rash, photosensitivity reactions.
Other: *severe infections, sudden death.*

Interactions

Drug-drug. *Digoxin:* May decrease digoxin level. Monitor digoxin level.
Folic acid derivatives: May antagonize methotrexate effect. Monitor patient.
NSAIDs, phenylbutazone, salicylates, sulfonamides: May increase methotrexate toxicity. Use together cautiously; monitor methotrexate levels.
Phenytoin: May decrease phenytoin level. Monitor phenytoin level.
Probenecid: May impair excretion of methotrexate, causing increased levels, effects, and toxicity. Monitor level closely, and decrease dosage accordingly.

Procarbazine: May increase nephrotoxicity of methotrexate. Monitor renal function closely.
Vaccines: May inactivate vaccine; may increase risk of disseminated infection with live-virus vaccines. Consult with prescriber about safe time to give vaccine.
Drug-food. *Food:* May delay drug absorption and reduce peak levels of methotrexate. Take on empty stomach.
Drug-lifestyle. *Alcohol use:* May increase hepatotoxicity. Discourage using together.
Sun exposure: May cause photosensitivity reactions. Urge patient to avoid unprotected or prolonged exposure to sunlight.

Effects on lab test results

• May increase uric acid, BUN, creatinine, and liver enzyme levels. May decrease hemoglobin level and hematocrit.
• May decrease WBC, RBC, and platelet counts.

Pharmacokinetics

Absorption: For small P.O. doses, almost complete, but for large doses, incomplete and variable. For I.M. use, complete.
Distribution: Wide, with highest levels in kidneys, gallbladder, spleen, liver, and skin; about 50% bound to protein.
Metabolism: Only slight.
Excretion: Primarily in urine. *Half-life for doses below 30 mg/m^2:* About 3 to 10 hours. *For doses of 30 mg/m^2 and above:* 8 to 15 hours.

Route	Onset	Peak	Duration
P.O.	Unknown	1–2 hr	Unknown
I.V., intrathecal	Unknown	Immediate	24 hr
I.M.	Unknown	30 min–1 hr	Unknown

Action

Chemical effect: Prevents reduction of folic acid to tetrahydrofolate by binding to dihydrofolate reductase.
Therapeutic effect: Kills certain cancer cells and reduces inflammation.

Available forms

methotrexate
Tablets: 2.5 mg, 5 mg, 7.5 mg, 10 mg, 15 mg
methotrexate sodium
Injection (lyophilized powder, preservative free): 20 mg (as base); 1-g (as base) vials

Injection (preservative free): 25 mg/ml in 2-, 4-, 8-, and 10-ml vials
Injection (with preservatives): 25 mg/ml in 2- and 10-ml vials
Tablets: 2.5 mg

NURSING PROCESS

☒ Assessment

• Assess patient's condition before therapy and regularly thereafter to monitor the drug's effectiveness.
• Perform baseline pulmonary function tests before therapy, and repeat periodically.
• Monitor fluid intake and output daily.
• Monitor uric acid level.
• Watch for increases in AST, ALT, and alkaline phosphatase levels, which are signs of hepatic dysfunction.
• Regularly monitor CBC.
• Be alert for adverse reactions and drug interactions.
• Assess patient's and family's knowledge of drug therapy.

⊕ Nursing diagnoses

• Ineffective health maintenance related to underlying condition
• Ineffective immune protection related to drug-induced adverse hematologic reactions
• Deficient knowledge related to drug therapy

⊠ Planning and implementation

• CSF volume depends on age, not body surface area (BSA). Basing dose on BSA for meningeal leukemia may cause low CSF methotrexate level in children and high level and neurotoxicity in adults. Instead, base dose on patient's age. Elderly patients may need a reduced dosage because CSF volume and turnover may decrease with age.
• Arachnoiditis can develop within hours of intrathecal use but subacute neurotoxicity may begin a few weeks later.
• Have patient drink 2 to 3 L of fluids daily.
• **⊛ ALERT:** Alkalinize urine by giving sodium bicarbonate tablets to prevent precipitation of drug, especially with high doses. Maintain urine pH at more than 6.5. If BUN level reaches 20 to 30 mg/dl or creatinine level reaches 1.2 to 2 mg/dl, reduce dosage. Report BUN level over 30 mg/dl or creatinine level over 2 mg/dl, and stop drug.

• Rash, redness, ulcerations in mouth, or adverse pulmonary reactions may signal serious complications. If ulcerative stomatitis or other severe adverse GI reaction occurs, or if pulmonary toxicity is detected, stop giving the drug.
• Leucovorin rescue is used with high-dose (greater than 100 mg) protocols. This technique works against systemic toxicity but doesn't interfere with tumor cells' absorption of methotrexate.

Patient teaching
• Teach and encourage diligent mouth care to reduce risk of superinfection in mouth.
• Tell patient to take oral form on empty stomach.
• Advise patient to avoid prolonged exposure to sunlight, wear protective clothing, and use highly protective sunblock.
• Tell patient to continue leucovorin rescue despite severe nausea and vomiting and to tell prescriber. Parenteral leucovorin therapy may be needed.
• Warn patient not to become pregnant during or immediately after therapy, because of risk of spontaneous abortion or congenital anomalies.
• Instruct patient not to use alcohol during therapy.

☑ **Evaluation**
• Patient exhibits positive response to drug therapy.
• Patient doesn't experience serious complications when hematologic parameters are depressed during therapy.
• Patient and family state understanding of drug therapy.

methyldopa
(meth-il-DOH-puh)
Aldomet, Apo-Methyldopa ♦, Dopamet ♦, Hydopa ◊, Novomedopa ♦, Nu-Medopa ♦

methyldopate hydrochloride
Aldomet

Pharmacologic class: centrally acting antiadrenergic
Therapeutic class: antihypertensive
Pregnancy risk category: B (P.O.), C (I.V.)

Indications and dosages

▶ **Hypertension, hypertensive crisis.** *Adults:* Initially, 250 mg P.O. b.i.d. to t.i.d. in first 48 hours. Then increase p.r.n. q 2 days. Entire daily dosage may be given in evening or h.s. If other antihypertensives are added to or removed from therapy, adjust dosages p.r.n. Maintenance dosage, 500 mg to 2 g daily divided b.i.d. or q.i.d. Maximum daily dosage, 3 g. Or, 250 to 500 mg I.V. q 6 hours. Maximum dosage, 1 g q 6 hours. Switch to P.O. antihypertensives as soon as possible.
Children: Initially, 10 mg/kg P.O. daily in two to four divided doses. Or, 20 to 40 mg/kg I.V. daily in four divided doses. Increase dosage at least q 2 days until desired response occurs. Maximum, 65 mg/kg, 2 g/m², or 3 g daily, whichever is least.

▼ **I.V. administration**
• Dilute appropriate dose in 100 ml D₅W. Alternatively, the required dose may be administered in 5% dextrose injection in a concentration of 10 mg/ml.
• Infuse slowly over 30 to 60 minutes.
• When control has been obtained, substitute oral therapy starting with the same parenteral dosage schedule.

⊗ **Incompatibilities**
Amphotericin B; drugs with poor solubility in acidic media, such as barbiturates and sulfonamides; methohexital; some total parenteral nutrition solutions.

Contraindications and cautions
• Contraindicated in patients hypersensitive to drug or any of its components (including sulfites) and in those with active hepatic disease (such as acute hepatitis) or active cirrhosis. Also contraindicated if previous methyldopa therapy has been linked to liver disorders. Coadministration with MAO inhibitors is contraindicated.
• Use cautiously in patients with renal impairment or a history of impaired liver function.
⚠ **Lifespan:** Drug has been used effectively in pregnant women without apparent harm to the fetus. In breast-feeding women, use cautiously; it's unknown if the drug appears in breast milk. In elderly patients, use cautiously because they may experience syncope from increased sensitivity.

M

Adverse reactions

CNS: *sedation,* headache, asthenia, weakness, dizziness, *decreased mental acuity,* involuntary choreoathetoid movements, psychic disturbances, depression, nightmares.
CV: *bradycardia, heart failure,* orthostatic hypotension, aggravated angina, *myocarditis,* edema.
EENT: nasal congestion.
GI: nausea, vomiting, diarrhea, constipation, *pancreatitis, dry mouth.*
GU: decreased libido, impotence.
Hematologic: hemolytic anemia, *thrombocytopenia.*
Hepatic: *hepatic necrosis.*
Metabolic: weight gain.
Skin: rash.
Other: gynecomastia, galactorrhea, *drug-induced fever.*

Interactions

Drug-drug. *Amphetamines, norepinephrine, phenothiazines, tricyclic antidepressants:* May decrease hypotensive effects. Monitor blood pressure carefully.
Antihypertensives, diuretics: May increase hypotensive effects. Decrease the methyldopa dosage.
Barbiturates: May increase likelihood of orthostatic hypotension. Monitor patient and blood pressure.
Haloperidol: May produce dementia and sedation. Use together cautiously.
Levodopa: May have additive hypotensive effects and may increase adverse CNS reactions. Monitor patient closely.
Lithium: May increase lithium level. Monitor lithium level and toxicity.
MAO inhibitors: May increase sympathetic stimulation, which may result in hypertensive crisis. Don't use together.
Oral iron therapy: May increase hypotensive effects. Use together cautiously; monitor blood pressure.
Drug-herb. *Capsicum:* May reduce antihypertensive effectiveness. Discourage using together.
Yohimbe: May interfere with blood pressure. Discourage using together.

Effects on lab test results

• May increase creatinine level. May decrease hemoglobin level and hematocrit.

• May decrease liver function test values and granulocyte, platelet, RBC, and WBC counts.
• May cause positive direct Coombs' test.

Pharmacokinetics

Absorption: Partial.
Distribution: Wide; bound weakly to proteins.
Metabolism: Extensive in liver and intestinal cells.
Excretion: Absorbed drug in urine; unabsorbed drug in feces. *Half-life:* About 2 hours.

Route	Onset	Peak	Duration
P.O.	Unknown	4–6 hr	12–48 hr
I.V.	Unknown	4–6 hr	10–16 hr

Action

Chemical effect: May involve inhibition of central vasomotor centers, decreasing sympathetic outflow to heart, kidneys, and peripheral vasculature.
Therapeutic effect: Lowers blood pressure.

Available forms

methyldopa
Tablets: 250 mg, 500 mg
methyldopate hydrochloride
Injection: 50 mg/ml in 5- and 10-mg vials

NURSING PROCESS

Assessment
• Assess patient's blood pressure before therapy and regularly thereafter to monitor the drug's effectiveness.
• Monitor CBC with differential counts before therapy, every 2 weeks for first 3 months of therapy, and periodically thereafter.
• Monitor patient's Coombs' test results. In patient who has received this drug for several months, positive reaction to direct Coombs' test indicates hemolytic anemia.
• Be alert for adverse reactions and drug interactions.
• Assess patient's and family's knowledge of drug therapy.

Nursing diagnoses
• Ineffective health maintenance related to presence of hypertension
• Risk for injury related to drug-induced adverse CNS reactions
• Deficient knowledge related to drug therapy

▷ Planning and implementation

• Report involuntary choreoathetoid movements. Drug may be stopped.

• Tolerance may occur, usually between the second and third months of therapy, and addition of a diuretic or a dosage adjustment may be needed. If patient's response changes significantly, notify prescriber.

• If hypertension occurs after dialysis, notify prescriber. Patient may need extra dose of drug.

• In a patient who needs blood transfusions, perform direct and indirect Coombs' tests to prevent crossmatching problems.

Ⓢ **ALERT:** Don't confuse Aldomet with Aldoril or Anzemet.

Patient teaching

• Advise patient to report signs of infection, such as fever and sore throat.

• Tell patient to report adverse reactions but not to stop taking drug.

• Tell patient to check his weight daily and to report weight gain of more than 5 lb (2.27 kg). Diuretics can relieve sodium and water retention.

• Warn patient that drug may impair mental alertness, particularly at start of therapy. Once-daily dose h.s. minimizes daytime drowsiness.

• Tell patient to rise slowly and avoid sudden position changes.

• Tell patient that dry mouth can be relieved with ice chips, sugarless gum, or hard candy.

• Advise patient that urine may turn dark in bleached toilet bowls.

ⓜ Evaluation

• Patient's blood pressure is normal.

• Patient doesn't experience injury as result of drug-induced adverse CNS reactions.

• Patient and family state understanding of drug therapy.

---

methylphenidate hydrochloride
(meth-il-FEN-ih-dayt high-droh-KLOR-ighd)
Concerta, Metadate CD, Metadate ER, Methylin, Methylin ER, Ritalin◈, Ritalin LA, Ritalin SR

Pharmacologic class: piperidine derivative
Therapeutic class: CNS stimulant

Pregnancy risk category: NR (Metadate ER, Methylin, Methylin ER, Ritalin, Ritalin SR); C (Concerta, Metadate CD, Ritalin LA)
Controlled substance schedule: II

Indications and dosages

▶ **Attention deficit hyperactivity disorder (ADHD).** *Children age 6 and older:* Initially 5 mg, Methylin or Ritalin P.O. b.i.d. before breakfast and lunch. Increase in 5- to 10-mg increments weekly, p.r.n., until an optimum daily dosage of 2 mg/kg is reached, not to exceed 60 mg/day. Ritalin SR, Metadate ER, Methylin ER, Metadate CD, or Ritalin LA may be used in place of above tablets by calculating the dose of methylphenidate in 8 hours, and giving the total dosage P.O. once daily before breakfast. Or, initially, 20 mg Metadate CD or Ritalin LA P.O. daily before breakfast; increase in 10-mg increments weekly to maximum, 60 mg daily.

Adolescents ages 13 to 17 not on methylphenidate, or for patients on other stimulants: 18 mg P.O. extended-release Concerta once daily in the morning. Adjust dosage by 18 mg at weekly intervals to a maximum of 72 mg P.O. (not to exceed 2 mg/kg) once daily in the morning.

Children ages 6 to 12 not on methylphenidate, or for patients on other stimulants: 18 mg P.O. extended-release Concerta once daily in the morning. Adjust dosage by 18 mg at weekly intervals to a maximum of 54 mg P.O. once daily in the morning.

Children age 6 and older on methylphenidate: If the previous methylphenidate daily dosage is 5 mg b.i.d. or t.i.d. or 20 mg of sustained-release, the recommended dose of Concerta is 18 mg P.O. q morning. If the previous methylphenidate daily dose is 10 mg b.i.d. or t.i.d. or 40 mg sustained-release, the recommended dosage of Concerta is 36 mg P.O. q morning. If the previous methylphenidate daily dosage is 15 mg b.i.d. or t.i.d. or 60 mg of sustained release, the recommended dose of Concerta is 54 mg P.O. q morning. Maximum conversion daily dose is 54 mg. After conversion is complete, adjust adolescents ages 13 to 17 to maximum, 72 mg once daily (not to exceed 2 mg/kg).

▶ **Narcolepsy.** *Adults:* 10 mg Methylin or Ritalin P.O. b.i.d. or t.i.d. 30 to 45 minutes before meals. Dosage varies with patient needs; average dose is 40 to 60 mg P.O. daily. Ritalin SR, Metadate ER, and Methylin ER tablets may be used in place of methylphenidate tablets by cal-

M

culating the dosage of methylphenidate in 8 hours and administering the total dosage P.O. once daily before breakfast.

Contraindications and cautions

• Contraindicated in patients hypersensitive to the drug or any of its components, and in those with glaucoma, motor tics, family history or diagnosis of Tourette syndrome, or history of marked anxiety, tension, or agitation. Ritalin, Ritalin SR, and Ritalin LA are contraindicated during therapy with MAO inhibitors and within 14 days of MAO inhibitor therapy.
• Use cautiously in patients with hypertension, history of drug abuse, GI stricture or narrowing, seizures, or EEG abnormalities.
⚜ **Lifespan:** In pregnant women, use cautiously. In breast-feeding women, use cautiously. It's unknown if the drug appears in breast milk. In children younger than age 6, safety and effectiveness haven't been established.

Adverse reactions

CNS: *nervousness, insomnia,* Tourette syndrome, dizziness, headache, akathisia, dyskinesia, *seizures.*
CV: *palpitations,* angina, *tachycardia,* changes in blood pressure and pulse rate.
EENT: dry throat, pharyngitis, sinusitis.
GI: vomiting; nausea, abdominal pain, anorexia.
Hematologic: *thrombocytopenia, thrombocytopenic purpura, leukopenia.*
Metabolic: weight loss, delayed growth.
Respiratory: upper respiratory tract infection, cough.
Skin: rash, urticaria, exfoliative dermatitis, *erythema multiforme.*

Interactions

Drug-drug. *Anticonvulsants (phenobarbital, phenytoin, primidone):* Increases level of anticonvulsants. Patient may need dosage adjustment.
Centrally acting antihypertensives: Decreases antihypertensive effect. Monitor blood pressure.
Clonidine: May cause serious adverse events. Avoid using together.
Coumadin: May increase levels. Monitor PT and INR and monitor patient for bleeding.
Drugs that increase gastric pH (antacids, proton pump inhibitors, H₂-receptor antagonists):

May alter the release of Ritalin LA extended-release capsules. Separate administration times.
MAO inhibitors: May cause severe hypertension or hypertensive crisis. Don't use together or within 14 days of each other.
Tricyclic antidepressants: Increases levels of these drugs. Avoid using together.
Drug-food. *Caffeine:* May increase amphetamine and related amine effects. Discourage using together.

Effects on lab test results

• May decrease hemoglobin level and hematocrit.
• May decrease WBC and platelet counts.

Pharmacokinetics

Absorption: Rapid and complete. Ritalin LA and Metadate CD have two distinct peaks.
Distribution: Unknown. Ritalin LA is 10% to 33% protein-bound.
Metabolism: By the liver.
Excretion: In urine. *Half-life:* 12 hours.

Route	Onset	Peak	Duration
P.O.			
Methylin, Ritalin	Unknown	2 hr	3–6 hr
Concerta	Unknown	6–8 hr	8–12 hr
Methylin ER, Ritalin SR	Unknown	4¾ hr	3–8 hr
Metadate CD	Unknown	1st peak, 1½ hr; 2nd peak, 4½ hr	8–12 hr
Ritalin LA	Unknown	1st peak, 1–3 hr; 2nd peak, 4–7 hr	8–12 hr

Action

Chemical effect: Probably promotes nerve impulse transmission by releasing stored norepinephrine from nerve terminals in brain. Main site appears to be cerebral cortex and reticular activating system.
Therapeutic effect: Promotes calmness in hyperkinesis, and prevents sleep.

Available forms

Capsules (extended-release) (Metadate CD, Ritalin LA): 10 mg, 20 mg, 30 mg, 40 mg
Tablets (chewable) (Methylin): 2.5 mg, 5 mg, 10 mg
Tablets (immediate-release) (Methylin, methylphenidate, Ritalin): 5 mg, 10 mg, 20 mg

---

Tablets (extended-release) (Metadate ER, Methylin ER, Ritalin SR): 10 mg, 20 mg
Tablets (extended-release core) (Concerta): 18 mg, 27 mg, 36 mg, 54 mg
Oral solution: 5 mg/5 ml, 10 mg/5 ml

NURSING PROCESS

⚕ Assessment
• Assess patient's condition before therapy and regularly thereafter to monitor the drug's effectiveness.
• Drug may precipitate Tourette syndrome in children. Monitor effects, especially at start of therapy.
• Observe patient for signs of excessive stimulation. Monitor blood pressure.
• When using long term, periodically monitor CBC, differential, and platelet counts.
• Monitor height and weight in child receiving long-term therapy. Drug may delay growth, but child will attain normal height when drug is stopped.
⧄ ALERT: Chronic abuse can lead to marked tolerance and psychological dependence. Careful supervision is needed. Monitor patient for tolerance or psychological dependence.
• Be alert for adverse reactions and drug interactions.
• Assess patient's and family's knowledge of drug therapy.

⧉ Nursing diagnoses
• Ineffective health maintenance related to underlying condition
• Disturbed sleep pattern related to drug-induced insomnia
• Deficient knowledge related to drug therapy

⧁ Planning and implementation
⧄ ALERT: This is drug of choice for ADHD and is usually stopped after puberty.
• Don't use to prevent fatigue.
• Metadate CD and Ritalin-LA may be swallowed whole, or the contents of the capsule may be sprinkled onto a small amount of applesauce and given immediately with a full glass of water.
• Give at least 6 hours before bedtime to prevent insomnia. Give after meals to reduce appetite suppression.
• Methylin ER and Ritalin SR tablets have a duration of about 8 hours and may be used in

place of regular tablets when 8-hour dosage of sustained release tablets corresponds to the adjusted dosage of the regular tablets.
⧄ ALERT: Don't confuse Ritalin with Rifadin or Metadate with methadone.

Patient teaching
• Tell patient to swallow Ritalin SR and Concerta tablets whole and not to chew or crush them. Metadate CD may be swallowed whole, or the contents of the capsule may be sprinkled onto a small amount of applesauce and given immediately.
• Warn patient to avoid activities that require alertness until the drug's CNS effects are known.
• Tell patient to avoid caffeine.
• Advise patient with seizure disorder to notify prescriber.
• Inform patient that he will need more rest as drug effects wear off.
• Warn patient that the shell of the Concerta tablet may appear in the stool.

⧉ Evaluation
• Patient responds positively to drug therapy.
• Patient doesn't experience insomnia during therapy.
• Patient and family state understanding of drug therapy.

methylprednisolone
(meth-il-pred-NIS-uh-lohn)
Medrol, Meprolone

methylprednisolone acetate
depMedalone 40, depMedalone 80, Depo-Medrol, Depopred-40, Depopred-80

methylprednisolone sodium succinate
A-MethaPred, Solu-Medrol

Pharmacologic class: glucocorticoid
Therapeutic class: anti-inflammatory, immunosuppressant
Pregnancy risk category: NR

Indications and dosages
▶ **Severe inflammation or immunosuppression.** *Adults:* 2 to 60 mg methylprednisolone

M

P.O. daily in four divided doses. Or 10 to 80 mg methylprednisolone acetate I.M. daily, or 4 to 80 mg into joint or soft tissue, p.r.n. May repeat q 1 to 5 weeks p.r.n. Or 10 to 250 mg methylprednisolone succinate I.M. or I.V. q 4 hours. *Children:* 0.03 to 0.2 mg/kg or 1 to 6.25 mg/m² methylprednisolone succinate I.M. once or twice daily. Although dosage may be reduced in infants and children, give dose based more on severity of condition and response than by age or size. Don't give less than 0.5 mg/kg daily.

▶ **Shock.** *Adults:* 100 to 250 mg methylprednisolone succinate I.V. at 2- to 6-hour intervals. Or 30 mg/kg I.V. initially, repeat q 4 to 6 hours, p.r.n. Continue therapy for 2 to 3 days or until patient is stable.

▶ **Acute exacerbations of multiple sclerosis.** *Adults:* Give 200 mg I.M. prednisolone daily for 1 week, followed by 80 mg I.M. q other day for 1 month. (Note that 5 mg of prednisolone is equivalent to 4 mg of methylprednisolone.)

▶ **Severe lupus nephritis‡.** *Adults:* 1 g methylprednisolone succinate I.V. over 1 hour for 3 days. Continue orally at 0.5 mg/kg daily using prednisone or prednisolone. *Children:* 30 mg/kg methylprednisolone succinate I.V. q other day for 6 doses.

▶ **To minimize motor and sensory defects caused by acute spinal cord injury‡.** *Adults:* Initially, 30 mg/kg I.V. over 15 minutes, followed in 45 minutes by 5.4 mg/kg/hour I.V. infusion for 23 hours.

▶ **Adjunct treatment for moderate to severe** *Pneumocystis jiroveci (carinii)* **pneumonia‡.** *Adults and children older than age 13:* 30 mg I.V. b.i.d. for 5 days; then 30 mg I.V. daily for 5 days; then 15 mg I.V. daily for 11 days (or until completion of anti-infective therapy).

▽ I.V. administration

• Compatible solutions include D₅W, normal saline solution, and D₅W in normal saline solution.
• Use within 48 hours after mixing.
• Give only methylprednisolone sodium succinate I.V., never the acetate form. Reconstitute according to manufacturer's directions using supplied diluent or bacteriostatic water for injection with benzyl alcohol.
• For direct injection, inject diluted drug into vein or I.V. line containing free-flowing compatible solution over at least 1 minute. For shock,

give massive doses over at least 10 minutes to prevent arrhythmias and circulatory collapse.
• For intermittent or continuous infusion, dilute solution according to manufacturer's instructions and give over prescribed duration. In continuous infusion, change solution q 24 hours.
• Rapid administration of large I.V. doses (0.5 to 1 g in less than 10 to 120 minutes) may result in circulatory collapse, cardiac arrhythmias, or fatal cardiac arrest.

⊗ **Incompatibilities**
Allopurinol, aminophylline, calcium gluconate, cephalothin, ciprofloxacin, cytarabine, diltiazem, docetaxel, doxapram, etoposide, gemcitabine, filgrastim, glycopyrrolate, metaraminol, nafcillin, ondansetron, paclitaxel, penicillin G sodium, potassium chloride, propofol, sargramostim, vinorelbine, vitamin B complex with C.

Contraindications and cautions

• Contraindicated in patients hypersensitive to drug or any of its components, and in those with systemic fungal infections.
• Use cautiously in patients with GI ulceration or renal disease, hypertension, osteoporosis, diabetes mellitus, hypothyroidism, cirrhosis, diverticulitis, nonspecific ulcerative colitis, recent intestinal anastomoses, thromboembolic disorders, seizures, myasthenia gravis, heart failure, tuberculosis, ocular herpes simplex, emotional instability, or psychotic tendencies.
⚹ **Lifespan:** In pregnant women, use cautiously. In breast-feeding women, don't use because it's unknown if drug appears in breast milk. In premature infants, methylprednisolone acetate and methylprednisolone succinate are contraindicated because they contain benzyl alcohol.

Adverse reactions

CNS: *euphoria, insomnia,* psychotic behavior, pseudotumor cerebri.
CV: *heart failure,* hypertension, edema, *thromboembolism, fatal arrest, circulatory collapse, arrhythmias.*
EENT: cataracts, glaucoma.
GI: peptic ulceration, GI irritation, increased appetite, *pancreatitis.*
Metabolic: hypokalemia, hyperglycemia, carbohydrate intolerance, growth suppression in children.
Musculoskeletal: muscle weakness, osteoporosis.

Skin: hirsutism, delayed wound healing, acne, various skin eruptions.
Other: susceptibility to infections, *acute adrenal insufficiency.*

Interactions

Drug-drug. *Anticholinesterases:* May cause profound weakness. Use together cautiously.
Aspirin, indomethacin, other NSAIDs: Increases risk of GI distress and bleeding. Give together cautiously.
Cyclosporins: May increase risk of adverse events and convulsions. May need to increase methylprednisolone dose.
CYP 3A4 inducers (barbiturates, ephedrine, phenytoin, rifampin): Decreases corticosteroid effect. Increase corticosteroid dosage.
CYP 3A4 inhibitors (ketoconazole, macrolides): May decrease glucocorticoid clearance. Adjust dosage, if needed.
Hormonal contraceptives: Reduces metabolism of corticosteroids. Dose of steroid may need to be reduced.
Oral anticoagulants: Alters dosage requirements. Monitor PT and INR closely.
Potassium-depleting drugs (such as thiazide and loop diuretics): Enhances potassium-wasting effects. Monitor potassium level.
Skin-test antigens: Decreases response. Defer skin testing until therapy is completed.
Toxoids, live-virus vaccines: Decreases antibody response and increases risk of neurologic complications. Avoid using together.

Effects on lab test results

• May increase glucose and cholesterol levels. May decrease potassium and calcium levels.

Pharmacokinetics

Absorption: Good after P.O. use; sodium succinate is rapid while acetate is much slower.
Distribution: Rapid to muscle, liver, skin, intestines, and kidneys.
Metabolism: In liver.
Excretion: Primarily in urine. *Half-life:* 18 to 36 hours.

Route	Onset	Peak	Duration
P.O.	Rapid	1–2 hr	30–36 hr
I.V.	Immediate	Immediate	Unknown
I.M.	6–48 hr	Unknown	4–8 days

Action

Chemical effect: Not clear; decreases inflammation, mainly by stabilizing leukocyte lysosomal membranes. Drug also suppresses immune response, stimulates bone marrow, and influences protein, fat, and carbohydrate metabolism.
Therapeutic effect: Relieves inflammation and suppresses immune system function.

Available forms

methylprednisolone
Tablets: 2 mg, 4 mg, 8 mg, 16 mg, 24 mg, 32 mg
methylprednisolone acetate
Injection (suspension): 20 mg/ml, 40 mg/ml, 80 mg/ml
methylprednisolone sodium succinate (contains benzyl alcohol)
Injection: 40-, 125-, 500-, 1,000-, and 2,000-mg vials

NURSING PROCESS

Assessment

• Assess patient's condition before therapy and regularly thereafter to monitor the drug's effectiveness.
• Watch for enhanced response in patient with hypothyroidism or cirrhosis.
• Monitor patient's weight, blood pressure, electrolyte levels (especially glucose), and sleep patterns. Euphoria may initially interfere with sleep, but patient typically adjusts to drug after 1 to 3 weeks.
• Be alert for adverse reactions and drug interactions.
• Assess patient's and family's knowledge of drug therapy.

Nursing diagnoses

• Ineffective health maintenance related to underlying condition
• Risk for injury related to drug-induced adverse reactions
• Deficient knowledge related to drug therapy

Planning and implementation

ALERT: Salt formulations are not interchangeable.
• Drug may be used for alternate-day therapy.
• For better results and less risk of toxicity, give once-daily dose in morning.

Rapid onset   *Liquid form contains alcohol.   ♦ Canada   ◊ Australia   †OTC   ✐ Photoguide   ‡ Off-label use

• Don't inject subcutaneously. Atrophy and sterile abscesses may occur.

• Give with food whenever possible. Critically ill patients may also need antacid or H_2-receptor antagonist therapy.

• Give I.M. injection deep into gluteal muscle.

• Dermal atrophy may occur with large dose of acetate salt. Use multiple small injections rather than single large dose, and rotate injection sites.

⊛ ALERT: Don't give intrathecally because severe adverse reactions may occur.

• Don't use acetate salt when immediate onset of action is needed.

⊛ ALERT: Acute adrenal insufficiency may occur in patients on long term therapy who are under stress (infection, surgery, or trauma).

• Always adjust to lowest effective dose.

• Give potassium supplements, p.r.n.

• Gradually stop giving the drug after long-term therapy. Abruptly stopping drug may be fatal or cause inflammation, fatigue, weakness, arthralgia, fever, dizziness, lethargy, depression, fainting, orthostatic hypotension, dyspnea, anorexia, or hypoglycemia.

⊛ ALERT: Don't confuse Solu-Medrol with Solu-Cortef.

⊛ ALERT: Don't confuse methylprednisolone with medroxyprogesterone.

Patient teaching

• Tell patient most adverse reactions are dose or duration dependent.

• Tell patient not to abruptly stop taking the drug without prescriber's consent.

• Teach patient signs of early adrenal insufficiency: fatigue, muscle weakness, joint pain, fever, anorexia, nausea, dyspnea, dizziness, and fainting.

• Instruct patient to wear or carry medical identification.

• Warn patient receiving long-term therapy about cushingoid symptoms, and tell him to report sudden weight gain or swelling. Suggest exercise or physical therapy, and advise him to ask prescriber about vitamin D or calcium supplements.

☑ Evaluation

• Patient responds positively to drug therapy.

• Patient sustains no injury from adverse reactions.

• Patient and family state understanding of drug therapy.

metoclopramide hydrochloride
(met-oh-KLOH-preh-mighd high-droh-KLOR-ighd)
Apo-Metoclop ♦ , Clopra, Maxeran ♦ ,
Maxolon, Octamide, Octamide PFS,
Pramin ◇ , Reclomide, Reglan

Pharmacologic class: para-aminobenzoic acid derivative; dopamine-receptor agonist
Therapeutic class: antiemetic, GI stimulant
Pregnancy risk category: B

Indications and dosages

▶ **To prevent or reduce nausea and vomiting induced by cisplatin alone or with other chemotherapeutics.** *Adults:* 1 to 2 mg/kg I.V. 30 minutes before chemotherapy; then repeat q 2 hours for two doses; then q 3 hours for three doses.

▶ **To prevent or reduce postoperative nausea and vomiting.** *Adults:* 10 to 20 mg I.M. near end of surgical procedure, repeat q 4 to 6 hours, p.r.n.

▶ **To facilitate small-bowel or upper G.I. intubation and aid in radiologic examinations.** *Adults and children older than age 14:* 10 mg (2 ml) I.V. as single dose over 1 to 2 minutes.
Children ages 6 to 14: 2.5 to 5 mg I.V. (0.5 to 1 ml).
Children younger than age 6: 0.1 mg/kg I.V.

▶ **Delayed gastric emptying caused by diabetic gastroparesis.** *Adults:* 10 mg P.O. for mild symptoms; slow I.V. infusion for severe symptoms 30 minutes before meals and h.s. for 2 to 8 weeks, depending on response.

▶ **Gastroesophageal reflux disease.** *Adults:* 10 to 15 mg P.O. q.i.d., p.r.n., 30 minutes before meals and h.s.

⊠ Adjust-a-dose: For patients with renal impairment, if creatinine clearance is less than 40 ml/minute, reduce initial dose by 50% and adjust dose, as tolerated.

▼ I.V. administration

• Drug is compatible with D_5W, normal saline solution for injection, dextrose 5% in half-normal saline solution, Ringer's solution, and lactated Ringer's solution. Normal saline is the preferred diluent because drug is most stable in this solution.

• Dilute doses larger than 10 mg in 50 ml of compatible diluent, and infuse over at least 15 minutes.

• Give doses of 10 mg or less by direct injection over 1 to 2 minutes.

• Closely monitor blood pressure.

• If giving infusion mixture within 24 hours, protection from light is unnecessary. If protected from light and refrigerated, it's stable for 48 hours.

⊗ **Incompatibilities**
Allopurinol, ampicillin, amphotericin B, calcium gluconate, cefepime, chloramphenicol sodium succinate, cisplatin, doxorubicin liposomal, erythromycin lactobionate, fluorouracil, furosemide, methotrexate sodium, penicillin G potassium, propofol, sodium bicarbonate.

Contraindications and cautions

• Contraindicated in patients hypersensitive to the drug or any of its components; patients allergic to procainamide may also be allergic to metoclopramide. Also contraindicated in patients taking drugs that are likely to cause extrapyramidal reactions (phenothiazines, butyrophenones), in those for whom stimulation of GI motility might be dangerous (such as those with hemorrhage), and in those with pheochromocytoma or seizure disorder.

• Use cautiously in patients with a history of depression, Parkinson's disease, hypertension, or renal impairment.

• Safety and effectiveness haven't been established for therapy that lasts longer than 12 weeks.

⚘ **Lifespan:** In pregnant women, use cautiously. In breast-feeding women, use cautiously; It's unknown if the drug appears in breast milk. In elderly patients, use cautiously and at a reduced dose.

Adverse reactions

CNS: *restlessness, anxiety, drowsiness,* fatigue, fever, *lassitude,* insomnia, **suicidal ideation, seizures,** headache, dizziness, extrapyramidal symptoms, tardive dyskinesia, dystonic reactions, sedation.
CV: transient hypertension, **bradycardia, AV block,** hypotension, **heart failure, arrhythmias.**
GI: nausea, bowel disturbances, diarrhea.
Hematologic: **agranulocytosis, neutropenia, leukopenia, neonatal methemoglobinemia.**

Skin: rash.
Other: prolactin secretion, loss of libido.

Interactions

Drug-drug. *Acetaminophen, aspirin, cyclosporine, diazepam, levodopa, lithium, tetracycline:* May increase absorption of these drugs. Monitor patient for adverse effects.
Anticholinergics, opioid analgesics: May antagonize GI motility effects of metoclopramide. Use together cautiously.
CNS depressants: May cause additive CNS depression. Avoid using together.
Digoxin: May decrease absorption of digoxin. Monitor digoxin levels.
Insulin: May influence the rate of food absorption. Adjust insulin dosage, if needed.
Drug-lifestyle. *Alcohol use:* May cause additive CNS depression. Discourage using together.

Effects on lab test results

• May increase aldosterone and prolactin levels.
• May decrease neutrophil and granulocyte counts.

Pharmacokinetics

Absorption: After P.O. use, rapid and complete. After I.M. use, about 74% to 96% bioavailable.
Distribution: To most body tissues and fluids, including brain.
Metabolism: Not extensive.
Excretion: In urine and feces. *Half-life:* 4 to 6 hours.

Route	Onset	Peak	Duration
P.O.	30–60 min	1–2 hr	1–2 hr
I.V.	1–3 min	Unknown	1–2 hr
I.M.	10–15 min	Unknown	1–2 hr

Action

Chemical effect: Stimulates motility of upper GI tract by increasing lower esophageal sphincter tone. Blocks dopamine receptors at chemoreceptor trigger zone.
Therapeutic effect: Prevents or minimizes nausea and vomiting. Also reduces gag reflex, improves gastric emptying, and reduces gastric reflux.

Available forms

Injection: 5 mg/ml

Syrup: 5 mg/5 ml (sugar-free), 10 mg/ml
Tablets: 5 mg, 10 mg

NURSING PROCESS

☰ Assessment
• Assess patient's condition before therapy and regularly thereafter to monitor the drug's effectiveness.
• Frequently monitor blood pressure in patient taking I.V. form of drug.
• Be alert for adverse reactions and drug interactions.
• Assess patient's and family's knowledge of drug therapy.

⊞ Nursing diagnoses
• Risk for deficient fluid volume related to nausea and vomiting
• Risk for injury related to drug-induced adverse CNS reactions
• Deficient knowledge related to drug therapy

❯ Planning and implementation
• Dilute oral concentrate just before administration using water, juice, or carbonated beverage. Semisolid food, such as applesauce or pudding, also may be used.
• Commercially available I.M. preparations may be used without further dilution.
Ⓢ ALERT: Extrapyramidal effects caused by high drug doses are counteracted by 25 mg diphenhydramine I.V.
Ⓢ ALERT: Don't confuse Reglan with Relafen.
Patient teaching
• Instruct patient not to drink alcohol during therapy.
• Advise patient to avoid activities requiring alertness for 2 hours after taking each dose.

☑ Evaluation
• Patient responds positively to drug and doesn't develop fluid volume deficit.
• Patient doesn't experience injury from adverse reactions.
• Patient and family state understanding of drug therapy.

metolazone
(meh-TOH-luh-zohn)
Mykrox, Zaroxolyn

Pharmacologic class: quinazoline derivative
Therapeutic class: diuretic, antihypertensive
Pregnancy risk category: B

Indications and dosages
❯ **Edema in heart failure or renal disease.**
Adults: 5 to 10 mg P.O. daily; may increase to 20 mg daily.
❯ **Mild to moderate essential hypertension.**
Adults: Initially, 1.25 to 2.5 mg P.O. daily; increase gradually until desired therapeutic response has been achieved. Usual maintenance dose is 2.5 to 5 mg daily. Maintenance dosage determined by patient's blood pressure. If response is inadequate, add another antihypertensive. If Mykrox is used, initial dose is 0.5 mg P.O. daily in the a.m. If response is inadequate, increase to maximum of 1 mg daily. If response is inadequate, add another antihypertensive.

Contraindications and cautions
• Contraindicated in patients hypersensitive to thiazides or other sulfonamide-derived drugs and in patients with anuria, hepatic coma, or precoma.
• Use cautiously in patients with impaired kidney or liver function.
⚖ Lifespan: In pregnant women, use only when benefits outweigh risks to the fetus. In breast-feeding women and in children, safety and effectiveness haven't been established.

Adverse reactions
CNS: *dizziness,* headache, fatigue.
CV: volume depletion, orthostatic hypotension, palpitations, chest pain.
GI: anorexia, nausea, *pancreatitis.*
GU: nocturia, polyuria, frequent urination.
Hematologic: *aplastic anemia, agranulocytosis, leukopenia, thrombocytopenia,* hyperlipidemia.
Hepatic: *hepatic encephalopathy.*
Metabolic: hyperglycemia, glucose tolerance impairment, hyperuricemia, hypokalemia, *metabolic alkalosis,* hypercalcemia, dilutional hyponatremia, hypochloremia, dehydration.

Musculoskeletal: acute gouty attacks, muscle cramps, swelling.
Skin: dermatitis, photosensitivity reactions, rash.
Other: hypersensitivity reactions.

Interactions

Drug-drug. *Amphotericin B, corticosteroids:* May cause hypokalemia. Monitor potassium level.
Barbiturates, opioids: May increase orthostatic hypotensive effect. Monitor blood pressure closely.
Bumetanide, ethacrynic acid, furosemide, torsemide: May cause excessive diuretic response resulting in serious electrolyte abnormalities or dehydration. Adjust doses carefully while monitoring patient closely.
Cholestyramine, colestipol: May decrease intestinal absorption of thiazides. Separate doses by 1 hour.
Diazoxide: May increase antihypertensive, hyperglycemic, and hyperuricemic effects. Use together cautiously.
Digoxin: May increase risk of digoxin toxicity from metolazone-induced hypokalemia. Monitor potassium and digitalis levels.
Insulin, sulfonylureas: May increase requirements in diabetic patients. Adjust dosages.
Lithium: May decrease lithium clearance, increasing risk of lithium toxicity. Avoid giving together.
NSAIDs: May increase risk of NSAID-induced renal impairment. Monitor patient for signs of renal impairment.
Drug-lifestyle. *Alcohol use:* May increase orthostatic hypotensive effect. Discourage using together.
Sun exposure: May cause photosensitivity reactions. Urge patient to avoid unprotected or prolonged exposure to sunlight.

Effects on lab test results

• May increase glucose, calcium, cholesterol, pH, bicarbonate, uric acid, and triglyceride levels. May decrease potassium, sodium, magnesium, chloride, and hemoglobin levels and hematocrit.
• May decrease granulocyte, platelet, and WBC counts.

Pharmacokinetics

Absorption: About 65% in healthy adults; in cardiac patients, falls to 40%. Mykrox formulation has more rapid absorption.
Distribution: 50% to 70% erythrocyte-bound; 33% protein-bound. Mykrox formulation more bioavailable than standard formulations.
Metabolism: Insignificant.
Excretion: 70% to 95% unchanged in urine.
Half-life: About 14 hours.

Route	Onset	Peak	Duration
P.O.	≤ 1 hr	2–8 hr	12–24 hr

Action

Chemical effect: Increases sodium and water excretion by inhibiting sodium reabsorption in cortical diluting site of ascending loop of Henle.
Therapeutic effect: Promotes water and sodium elimination and lowers blood pressure.

Available forms

Tablets: 2.5 mg, 5 mg, 10 mg
Tablets (Mykrox): 0.5 mg

NURSING PROCESS

M

🗲 Assessment
• Assess patient's condition before therapy and regularly thereafter to monitor the drug's effectiveness. In hypertensive patients, therapeutic response may be delayed several days.
• Unlike thiazide diuretics, drug is effective in patients with decreased kidney function.
• Monitor fluid intake and output, weight, blood pressure, and electrolyte level.
• Monitor uric acid level, especially in patient with a history of gout.
• Be alert for adverse reactions and drug interactions.
• Assess patient's and family's knowledge of drug therapy.

Nursing diagnoses
• Excessive fluid volume related to presence of edema
• Risk for injury related to presence of hypertension
• Deficient knowledge related to drug therapy

Planning and implementation
• Drug may be used with potassium-sparing diuretic to prevent potassium loss.

Rapid onset   *Liquid form contains alcohol.   ♦Canada   ◇ Australia   †OTC   ✐Photoguide   ‡Off-label use

• Give drug in morning to prevent nocturia.

• Drug is used as adjunct in furosemide-resistant edema.

⑤ ALERT: The metolazone formulations are not bioequivalent or therapeutically equivalent at the same doses. Do not interchange brands.

⑤ ALERT: Don't confuse Zaroxolyn with Zarontin or metolazone with metoprolol.

Patient teaching

• Advise patient to not change position suddenly and to rise slowly, to avoid orthostatic hypotension.

• Advise patient to wear protective clothing, avoid prolonged exposure to sunlight, and use sunblock to prevent photosensitivity reactions.

• Instruct patient to avoid alcohol consumption during drug therapy.

✓ Evaluation

• Patient doesn't have edema.

• Patient's blood pressure is normal.

• Patient and family state understanding of drug therapy.

metoprolol succinate
(meh-TOH-pruh-lol SUHK-seh-nayt)
Toprol-XL◊

metoprolol tartrate
(meh-TOH-pruh-lol TAR-trayt)
Apo-Metoprolol ◆, Apo-Metoprolol
(Type L) ◆, Betaloc ◆ ◊, Betaloc
Durules ◆, Lopresor ◆, Lopressor,
Minax ◊, Novometoprol ◆, Nu-Metop ◆

Pharmacologic class: selective beta$_1$ blocker
Therapeutic class: antihypertensive, adjunct therapy of acute MI
Pregnancy risk category: C

Indications and dosages

▶ **Hypertension.** *Adults:* Initially, 50 to 100 mg succinate P.O. once daily. Adjust dosage as needed and tolerated at intervals of no less than 1 week to maximum, 400 mg daily. For metoprolol tartrate, initially, 100 mg P.O. daily in single or divided doses; usual maintenance dosage is 100 to 450 mg daily.

▶ **Early intervention in acute MI.** *Adults:* 5 mg tartrate I.V. push q 2 to 5 minutes up to a total of 15 mg based on hemodynamic status.

Then, 15 minutes after last dose, 25 to 50 mg P.O. q 6 hours for 48 hours. Maintenance dosage is 100 mg P.O. b.i.d. In patients who do not tolerate full 15 mg dose in 10 to 15 minutes, may decrease oral dose to 25 mg initially. If severe intolerance, discontinue drug.

▶ **Angina pectoris.** *Adults:* Initially, 100 mg succinate P.O. daily as single dose. Increase at weekly intervals until adequate response or pronounced decrease in heart rate is seen. Safety and effectiveness of daily dose higher than 400 mg aren't known. Or, 100 mg metoprolol tartrate P.O. in two divided doses. Increase at weekly intervals until adequate response or pronounced decrease in heart rate is seen. Maintenance dosage, 100 to 400 mg P.O. daily.

▶ **Stable, symptomatic heart failure (New York Heart Association class II) resulting from ischemia, hypertension, or cardiomyopathy.** *Adults:* 25 mg succinate P.O. once daily for 2 weeks. In patients with more severe heart failure, start with 12.5 mg P.O. once daily for 2 weeks. Double the dose q 2 weeks as tolerated to a maximum of 200 mg daily.

▶ **Atrial tachyarrhythmias after acute MI‡.** *Adults:* 2.5 to 5 mg I.V. q 2 to 5 minutes to control rate up to 15 mg over a 10- to 15-minute period. Once heart rate is controlled or normal sinus rhythm is restored, therapy may continue with 50 mg P.O. b.i.d. for 24 hours starting 15 minutes after the last I.V. dose. Increase dosage to 100 mg P.O. b.i.d. as tolerated. When therapeutic response is achieved or if systolic blood pressure is less than 100 mm Hg or heart rate is less than 50 beats/minute, stop drug.

▶ **Unstable angina or non–ST-segment elevation MI at high risk for ischemic events‡.** *Adults:* 5 mg I.V. bolus q 5 minutes for 3 doses. May continue therapy with P.O. drug.

▽ I.V. administration

• Give drug undiluted and by direct injection.

• Drug is only compatible with meperidine hydrochloride or morphine sulfate, or with alteplase infusions at Y-site connection.

• Store drug at room temperature and protect from light. If solution is discolored or contains particulates, discard.

⊗ **Incompatibilities**
Amphotericin B, other I.V. drugs.

Contraindications and cautions

• Contraindicated in patients hypersensitive to the drug or other beta blockers, and in those with sinus bradycardia, heart block greater than first-degree, cardiogenic shock, or overt cardiac failure when used to treat hypertension or angina. When used to treat MI, drug is also contraindicated in patients with heart rate below 45 beats/minute, second- or third-degree heart block, PR interval of 0.24 second or more with first-degree heart block, systolic blood pressure lower than 100 mm Hg, or moderate-to-severe cardiac failure.

• Use cautiously in patients with heart failure, diabetes, or respiratory or hepatic disease.

⚖ **Lifespan:** In pregnant women, use cautiously. In breast-feeding women, don't use. It's unknown if drug appears in breast milk. In children, safety and effectiveness haven't been established.

Adverse reactions

CNS: fatigue, lethargy, dizziness, fever.
CV: *bradycardia,* hypotension, *heart failure, AV block,* peripheral vascular disease.
GI: nausea, vomiting, diarrhea.
GU: decreased libido.
Musculoskeletal: arthralgia.
Respiratory: dyspnea, *bronchospasm.*
Skin: rash.

Interactions

Drug-drug. *Amobarbital, aprobarbital, butabarbital, butalbital, mephobarbital, pentobarbital, phenobarbital, primidone, secobarbital:* May reduce the effects of metoprolol. Increase beta blocker dose.
Antihypertensives: May produce additive effects. Monitor blood pressure.
Chlorpromazine: May decrease hepatic clearance. Monitor patient for increased beta blockade.
Cimetidine: May increase the pharmacologic effects of beta blocker. Consider another H₂ agonist or decrease the dose of beta blocker.
CYP 2D6 inhibitors, such as amiodarone, fluoxetine, paroxetine, propafenone, quinidine: May increase metoprolol level. Monitor patient for increased adverse effects.
Digoxin, diltiazem: May cause excessive bradycardia and increase depressant effect on myocardium. Use together cautiously.

Hydralazine: May increase levels and effects of both drugs. Monitor patient closely. Adjust dosage of either drug, if needed.
Indomethacin: May decrease antihypertensive effect. Monitor blood pressure and adjust dosage.
Insulin, oral antidiabetics: May alter dosage requirements in previously stabilized diabetic patient. Observe patient carefully.
I.V. lidocaine: May reduce metabolism of lidocaine, increasing the risk of toxicity. Give bolus doses of lidocaine at a slower rate, and monitor lidocaine levels closely.
MAO inhibitors: May cause bradycardia during use with MAO inhibitors. Monitor ECG and patient closely.
Prazosin: May increase the risk of orthostatic hypotension in the early phases of use together. Assist patient to stand slowly until effects are known.
Rifampin: May increase metabolism of metoprolol. Monitor patient for decreased effect.
Thioamine: May alter pharmacokinetics of metoprolol, increasing the effects of metoprolol. Monitor patient.
Thyroid hormones: May impair actions of metoprolol when patient is converted to euthyroid state. Monitor patient.
Verapamil: May increase the effects of both drugs. Monitor cardiac function closely and decrease dosages p.r.n.
Drug-food. *Any food:* May increase absorption. Give together.

Effects on lab test results

• May increase transaminase, alkaline phosphatase, LDH, and uric acid levels.

Pharmacokinetics

Absorption: Rapid and almost complete; food enhances absorption of metoprolol tartrate.
Distribution: Wide; about 12% protein-bound.
Metabolism: In liver.
Excretion: About 95% in urine. *Half-life:* 3 to 7 hours.

Route	Onset	Peak	Duration
P.O.	≤ 15 min	1–12 hr	6–24 hr
I.V.	≤ 5 min	20 min	5–8 hr

Action

Chemical effect: Unknown. Known to depress renin secretion.

Therapeutic effect: Reduces blood pressure; decreases myocardial contractility, heart rate, and cardiac output; reduces myocardial oxygen consumption; and helps to prevent myocardial tissue damage.

Available forms

metoprolol succinate
Tablets (extended-release): 25 mg, 50 mg, 100 mg, 200 mg
metoprolol tartrate
Injection: 1 mg/ml in 5-ml ampules
Tablets: 50 mg, 100 mg
Tablets (extended-release): 100 mg ♦, 200 mg ♦

NURSING PROCESS

⚙ Assessment
● Assess patient's condition before therapy and regularly thereafter to monitor the drug's effectiveness.
● Frequently monitor blood pressure. Drug masks common signs of shock.
● Be alert for adverse reactions and drug interactions.
● Assess patient's and family's knowledge of drug therapy.

⚙ Nursing diagnoses
● Ineffective health maintenance related to underlying disorder
● Risk for injury related to drug-induced adverse CNS reactions
● Deficient knowledge related to drug therapy

⚙ Planning and implementation
⚕ **ALERT:** Always check patient's apical pulse rate before giving drug. If it's slower than 60 beats/minute, don't give the drug and immediately call the prescriber.
● Give drug with meals because food may increase absorption.
⚕ **ALERT:** Don't confuse metoprolol with metaproterenol or metolazone or Toprol XL with Topamax, Tegretol, or Tegretol-XR.
Patient teaching
● Tell patient that abruptly stopping therapy can worsen angina and precipitate MI. He should stop taking the drug gradually over 1 to 2 weeks.
● Instruct patient to take oral form with meals to enhance absorption.

● Advise patient to report adverse reactions to prescriber.
● Warn patient to avoid performing hazardous activities until the drug's CNS effects are known.

☑ Evaluation
● Patient responds well to therapy.
● Patient doesn't experience injury from adverse CNS reactions.
● Patient and family state understanding of drug therapy.

metronidazole
(met-roh-NIGH-duh-zohl)
Apo-Metronidazole ♦, Flagyl, Flagyl ER, Flagyl 375, Metric 21, MetroCream, MetroGel, MetroGel-vaginal, MetroLotion, Metrogyl ◇, Metrozine ◇, NidaGel ♦, Noritate, Novonidazol ♦, Protostat, Trikacide ♦

metronidazole hydrochloride
Flagyl I.V. RTU, Metro I.V., Novonidazol ♦

Pharmacologic class: nitroimidazole
Therapeutic class: antibacterial, antiprotozoal, amebicide
Pregnancy risk category: B

Indications and dosages

▶ **Amebic hepatic abscess.** *Adults:* 500 to 750 mg P.O. t.i.d. for 5 to 10 days.
Children: 35 to 50 mg/kg daily (in three doses) for 10 days.
▶ **Intestinal amebiasis.** *Adults:* 750 mg P.O. t.i.d. for 5 to 10 days.
Children: 35 to 50 mg/kg daily (in three doses) for 10 days; maximum of 750 mg/dose. Therapy is followed by P.O. iodoquinol.
▶ **Trichomoniasis.** *Adults:* 250 mg P.O. t.i.d. for 7 days, or 500 mg b.i.d. for 7 days or 2 g P.O. in single dose (may give 2-g dose as two 1-g doses on same day); allow 4 to 6 weeks between courses of therapy. Both partners should be treated.
Children: 5 mg/kg dose P.O. t.i.d. for 7 days. Maximum dosage, 2 g daily.
▶ **Refractory trichomoniasis.** *Adults:* 500 mg P.O. b.i.d. for 7 days. For repeated failures, 2 g P.O. daily for 3 to 5 days.

Reactions may be *common*, uncommon, *life-threatening*, or COMMON AND LIFE-THREATENING.

▶ **Bacterial infections caused by anaerobic microorganisms.** *Adults:* Loading dose, 15 mg/kg I.V. infused over 1 hour (about 1 g for 70-kg [154-lb] adult). Maintenance dosage, 7.5 mg/kg I.V. or P.O. q 6 hours (about 500 mg for 70-kg adult). Give first maintenance dose 6 hours after loading dose. Maximum, 4 g daily.

▶ **To prevent postoperative infection in contaminated or potentially contaminated colorectal surgery.** *Adults:* 15 mg/kg I.V. infused over 30 to 60 minutes and completed about 1 hour before surgery. Then, 7.5 mg/kg I.V. infused over 30 to 60 minutes at 6 and 12 hours after initial dose.

▶ **Inflammatory papules and pustules of acne rosacea.** *Adults:* If using a 0.75% preparation, apply thin film to affected area b.i.d., morning and evening. If using a 1% preparation, apply thin film to affected area once daily. Frequency and duration of therapy are adjusted after response is seen. Results are usually noticed within 3 weeks.

▶ **Pelvic inflammatory disease‡.** *Adults:* 500 mg I.V. q 8 hours with other drugs. Or, 500 mg P.O. b.i.d. for 14 days given with ofloxacin, 400 mg P.O. b.i.d.

▶ **Bacterial vaginosis‡.** *Adults:* 500 mg P.O. b.i.d. for 7 days. Or, 2 g P.O. as a single dose. Or, 250 mg P.O. t.i.d. for 7 days.

▶ **Active Crohn's disease‡.** *Adults:* 400 mg P.O. b.i.d. For refractory perineal disease, 20 mg/kg (1 to 1.5 g) P.O. daily in three to five divided doses.

▶ **To prevent sexually transmitted diseases in sexual assault victims‡.** *Adults:* 2 g P.O. given with other drugs.

▶ *Helicobacter pylori* **with peptic ulcer disease‡.** *Adults:* 250 to 500 mg P.O. t.i.d. to q.i.d. given with other drugs. Continue for 7 to 14 days depending on the regimen used. *Children:* 15 to 20 mg/kg P.O. daily, divided in two doses for 4 weeks given with other drugs.

▶ **Giardiasis‡.** *Adults:* 250 mg P.O. t.i.d. for 7 days.

▼ I.V. administration

● No preparation is needed for Flagyl I.V. RTU form.

● Add 4.4 ml of sterile water for injection, bacteriostatic water for injection, sterile normal saline solution injection, or bacteriostatic normal saline solution injection. Reconstituted drug contains 100 mg/ml.

● Add contents of vial to 100 ml of D_5W, lactated Ringer's injection, or normal saline solution for final concentration of 5 mg/ml. Do not exceed a concentration of 8 mg/ml.

● The resulting highly acidic solution must be neutralized before giving. Carefully add 5 mEq of sodium bicarbonate for each 500 mg of metronidazole. Carbon dioxide will form and may need to be vented.

● Don't use equipment (needles, hubs) containing aluminum to reconstitute the drug or to transfer reconstituted drug. Equipment that contains aluminum will turn the solution orange; the potency isn't affected.

● Infuse drug over at least 1 hour. Don't give I.V. push.

● Don't refrigerate neutralized diluted solution. Precipitation may occur. If Flagyl I.V. RTU is refrigerated, crystals may form. These will disappear after solution is gently warmed to room temperature.

⊗ **Incompatibilities**
Aluminum, amino acid 10%, amphotericin B, aztreonam, ceftriaxone, dopamine, filgrastim, meropenem, warfarin; other I.V. drugs.

Contraindications and cautions

● Contraindicated in patients hypersensitive to the drug or other nitroimidazole derivatives.

● Use cautiously in patients receiving hepatotoxic drugs and in patients with history of blood dyscrasia or CNS disorder, retinal or visual field changes, hepatic disease, or alcoholism.

⚠ **Lifespan:** In pregnant women, don't use during first trimester unless benefits outweigh risks to the fetus. In breast-feeding women, use cautiously. It isn't known if drug appears in breast milk.

Adverse reactions

CNS: vertigo, headache, ataxia, fever, incoordination, confusion, irritability, depression, restlessness, weakness, fatigue, drowsiness, insomnia, sensory neuropathy, paresthesia of limbs, psychic stimulation, *seizures,* neuropathy.
CV: flattened T wave, edema, flushing, thrombophlebitis.
EENT: eye tearing.
GI: abdominal cramping, stomatitis, *nausea, vomiting, anorexia,* diarrhea, constipation, proctitis, dry mouth, metallic taste.

M

GU: darkened urine, polyuria, dysuria, pyuria, incontinence, cystitis, dyspareunia, dry vagina and vulva, sense of pelvic pressure.
Hematologic: *transient leukopenia, neutropenia, thrombocytopenia.*
Skin: burning and stinging, contact dermatitis, dry skin, local allergic reaction or irritation, pruritus, rash, worsening of rosacea.
Other: decreased libido, gynecomastia, overgrowth of nonsusceptible organisms, glossitis.

Interactions

Drug-drug. *Azathioprine, fluorouracil:* May increase risk of transient neutropenia. Use cautiously.
Barbiturates, phenobarbital, phenytoin: May decrease metronidazole effectiveness because of increased hepatic clearance. Monitor patient closely for effect.
Cimetidine: Increases risk of metronidazole toxicity because of inhibited hepatic metabolism. Monitor patient.
Disulfiram: May cause acute psychoses and confusional states. Don't use together.
Lithium: May increase lithium level, resulting in toxicity. Monitor lithium level closely.
Oral anticoagulants: May increase anticoagulant effects. Monitor patient for bleeding; monitor PT and INR.
Drug-lifestyle. *Alcohol use:* May cause disulfiram-like reaction (nausea, vomiting, headache, cramps, flushing). Discourage using together.

Effects on lab test results

• May decrease WBC and neutrophil counts.

Pharmacokinetics

Absorption: About 80%; food delays peak levels to about 2 hours.
Distribution: To most body tissues and fluids; less than 20% bound to proteins.
Metabolism: To active metabolite and to other metabolites.
Excretion: Primarily in urine; 6% to 15% in feces. *Half-life:* 6 to 8 hours.

Route	Onset	Peak	Duration
P.O.	Unknown	1–2 hr	Unknown
I.V.	Immediate	Immediate	Unknown
Topical	Unknown	6-10 hr	Unknown

Action

Chemical effect: Direct-acting trichomonacide and amebicide that works at both intestinal and extraintestinal sites.
Therapeutic effect: Hinders growth of selected organisms, including most anaerobic bacteria and protozoa.

Available forms

Capsules: 375 mg
Injection: 5 mg/ml
Oral suspension (benzoyl metronidazole): 200 mg/5 ml ◊
Tablets: 200 mg ◊, 250 mg, 400 mg ◊, 500 mg
Tablets (extended-release): 750 mg
Topical gel: 0.75%; 1%

NURSING PROCESS

Assessment

• Assess patient's infection before therapy and regularly thereafter to monitor the drug's effectiveness.
• Watch carefully for edema, especially in patients also receiving corticosteroids, because Flagyl I.V. RTU may cause sodium retention.
• Record number and character of stools when used in amebiasis.
• Be alert for adverse reactions and drug interactions.
• I.V. infusion may cause thrombophlebitis at site; observe closely.
• Assess skin for severity, areas of rosacea before and after therapy, and any local adverse reactions
• Assess patient's and family's knowledge of drug therapy.

Nursing diagnoses

• Infection related to presence of susceptible organisms
• Risk for deficient fluid volume related to drug-induced adverse GI reactions
• Deficient knowledge related to drug therapy

Planning and implementation

• Give drug (except Flagyl ER) with meals to minimize GI distress. Give Flagyl ER at least 1 hour before or 2 hours after meals.
• Use only after *T. vaginalis* has been confirmed by wet smear or culture or *E. histolytica* has been identified; simultaneously treat asymptomatic sexual partners to avoid reinfection.

Reactions may be *common*, uncommon, *life-threatening*, or COMMON AND LIFE-THREATENING.

• To treat trichomoniasis during pregnancy, give drug for 7 days instead of 2-g single dose.
Patient teaching
• Tell patient not to use alcohol or drugs that contain alcohol during therapy and for at least 48 hours after therapy is completed.
• Tell patient that metallic taste and dark or red-brown urine may occur.
• Instruct patient to take oral form with meals to minimize reactions.
• Urge patient to complete full course of therapy even if he feels better.
• Instruct patient in proper hygiene.
• Teach patient to cleanse affected skin areas twice daily before applying MetroLotion
• Instruct users of topical drug to report worsening of rosacea promptly to prescriber.

☑ Evaluation
• Patient is free from infection.
• Patient maintains adequate hydration throughout therapy.
• Patient and family state understanding of drug therapy.

mexiletine hydrochloride
(MEKS-il-eh-teen high-droh-KLOR-ighd)
Mexitil

Pharmacologic class: lidocaine analogue, sodium channel antagonist
Therapeutic class: class IB ventricular antiarrhythmic
Pregnancy risk category: C

Indications and dosages

▶ **Refractory life-threatening ventricular arrhythmias, including ventricular tachycardia and PVCs.** *Adults:* 200 mg (if rapid control of arrhythmia is not necessary) to 400 mg (for rapid arrhythmia control) P.O., followed by 200 mg q 8 hours. If satisfactory control isn't obtained, increase dosage in 2 to 3 days to 400 mg q 8 hours. Patients who respond well to a 12-hour schedule may be given up to 450 mg q 12 hours. Maximum daily dose is 1,200 mg.
▶ **Diabetic neuropathy‡.** *Adults:* 150 mg P.O. daily for 3 days; then give 300 mg P.O. daily for 3 days followed by 10 mg/kg P.O. daily.

Contraindications and cautions

• Contraindicated in patients with cardiogenic shock or second- or third-degree AV block in absence of artificial pacemaker.
• Use cautiously in patients with first-degree heart block, ventricular pacemaker, sinus node dysfunction, intraventricular conduction disturbances, hypotension, severe heart failure, or seizure disorder.
☀ Lifespan: In pregnant women, use cautiously. In breast-feeding women, use cautiously; it's unknown if drug appears in breast milk. In children, safety and effectiveness haven't been established.

Adverse reactions

CNS: *tremor, dizziness,* blurred vision, ataxia, diplopia, confusion, nystagmus, nervousness, headache.
CV: *hypotension, bradycardia, widened QRS complex, arrhythmias,* palpitations, chest pain.
GI: *heartburn,* nausea, vomiting, diarrhea, constipation.
Skin: rash.

Interactions

Drug-drug. *Antacids, atropine, opioids:* May slow mexiletine absorption. Monitor patient; separate administration times.
Cimetidine: May increase or decrease mexiletine level. Monitor patient for effect or toxicities.
Methylxanthines (such as theophylline): May reduce clearance of methylxanthines, possibly resulting in toxicity. Monitor levels.
Metoclopramide: May accelerate absorption. Monitor patient for toxicity.
Phenobarbital, phenytoin, rifampin, urine acidifiers: May decrease mexiletine level. Monitor patient.
Urine alkalinizers: May increase mexiletine level. Monitor patient.
Drug-food. *Caffeine:* May reduce clearance of methylxanthines, resulting in toxicity. Monitor patient.

Effects on lab test results

• May increase AST level.

Pharmacokinetics

Absorption: About 90%.
Distribution: Wide. Volume declines in patients with liver disease, resulting in toxic levels with

M

usual doses. About 50% to 60% of circulating drug is bound to proteins.
Metabolism: Almost complete, in liver.
Excretion: In urine. *Half-life:* 10 to 12 hours.

Route	Onset	Peak	Duration
P.O.	½–2 hr	2–3 hr	Unknown

Action

Chemical effect: Blocks fast sodium channel in cardiac tissues without involvement of autonomic nervous system. Reduces acceleration and amplitude of action potential and decreases automaticity in Purkinje fibers. It also shortens action potential and, to a lesser extent, decreases the effective refractory period in Purkinje fibers.
Therapeutic effect: Abolishes ventricular arrhythmias.

Available forms

Capsules: 100 mg ◆, 150 mg, 200 mg, 250 mg

NURSING PROCESS

Assessment
• Assess patient's condition until arrhythmia is abolished.
• Monitor drug levels. Therapeutic levels are 0.75 to 2 mcg/ml.
• Be alert for adverse reactions and drug interactions.
• Monitor patient for toxicity. Early signs include tremors–usually fine tremor of hands. As drug's blood level increases, additional signs of toxicity such as dizziness, ataxia and nystagmus may develop. Ask patient about these symptoms.
• If patient has an adverse GI reaction, monitor his hydration.
• Assess patient's and family's knowledge of drug therapy.

Nursing diagnoses
• Decreased cardiac output related to presence of ventricular arrhythmia
• Risk for deficient fluid volume related to drug-induced adverse GI reactions
• Deficient knowledge related to drug therapy

Planning and implementation
• Give with meals or antacids to lessen GI distress.

• If patient appears to be good candidate for b.i.d. therapy, notify prescriber. This dose enhances compliance.
• Notify prescriber of any significant changes in blood pressure, heart rate, and heart rhythm.
Patient teaching
• Instruct patient taking oral form of drug to take it with food.
• Instruct patient to report adverse reactions.

Evaluation
• Patient regains normal cardiac output.
• Patient maintains adequate hydration throughout therapy.
• Patient and family state understanding of drug therapy.

micafungin sodium
(my-kah-FUN-jin SOE-dee-um)
Mycamine

Pharmacologic class: echinocandin antifungal
Therapeutic class: antifungal
Pregnancy risk category: C

Indications and dosages

► **Esophageal candidiasis.** *Adults:* 150 mg I.V. daily for 10 to 30 days.
► **Prevention of candidal infection in hematopoietic stem cell transplant recipients.** *Adults:* 50 mg I.V. daily for 6 to 51 days.

I.V. administration

• Use aseptic technique when preparing micafungin.
• Reconstitute each 50-mg vial with 5 ml of normal saline solution for injection or D_5W.
• To minimize foaming, dissolve powder by swirling the vial; don't shake it.
• Dilute dose in 100 ml of normal saline solution for injection.
• Flush I.V. line with normal saline solution for injection before infusing drug.
• Infuse drug over 1 hour.
• Reconstituted product and diluted infusion may be stored for up to 24 hours at room temperature.
• Protect diluted solution from light.
⊗ **Incompatibilities**
Other I.V. drugs.

Contraindications and cautions

• Contraindicated in patients hypersensitive to drug.
• Use cautiously in patients with severe hepatic disease.
🕯 **Lifespan:** In pregnant women, only use if clearly needed. Use cautiously in breast-feeding women; it isn't known whether micafungin appears in breast milk. In children, safety hasn't been established.

Adverse reactions

CNS: headache, delirium.
GI: abdominal pain, diarrhea, nausea, vomiting.
Hematologic: anemia, *leukopenia, neutropenia, thrombocytopenia.*
Hepatic: hyperbilirubinemia, hepatocellular damage.
Metabolic: hypocalcemia, hypokalemia, *hypomagnesemia,* hypophosphatemia, hemolytic anemia.
Skin: infusion site inflammation, phlebitis, pruritus, rash.
Other: pyrexia, rigors, *shock.*

Interactions

Drug-drug. *Nifedipine:* May increase nifedipine level. Monitor blood pressure, and decrease nifedipine dose if needed.
Sirolimus: May increase sirolimus level. Monitor patient for evidence of toxicity, and decrease the sirolimus dose if needed.

Effects on lab test results

• May increase alkaline phosphatase, ALT, AST, bilirubin, BUN, creatinine, and LDH levels. May decrease calcium, magnesium, phosphorous, potassium, and hemoglobin levels and hematocrit.
• May decrease neutrophil and platelet counts.

Pharmacokinetics

Absorption: Administered I.V.
Distribution: More than 99% protein-bound, mainly to albumin.
Metabolism: By several pathways in the liver.
Excretion: Mainly fecal.

Route	Onset	Peak	Duration
I.V.	Unknown	Unknown	Unknown

Action

Chemical effect: Inhibits synthesis of 1,3-β-D-glucan, which is an essential component of fungal cell walls that isn't found in mammal cells.
Therapeutic effect: Hinders fungal growth, including *Candida albicans, C. glabrata, C. krusei, C. parapsilosis,* and *C. tropicalis.*

Available forms

Lyophilized powder for injection: 50 mg single-use vial

NURSING PROCESS

🏵 Assessment
• Assess patient's fungal infection prior to treatment, and regularly thereafter.
• Be alert for adverse reactions and drug interactions.
• Monitor hepatic and renal function during therapy.
• Monitor patient for hemolysis and hemolytic anemia.
• Assess patient's and family's knowledge of drug therapy.

🏵 Nursing diagnoses
• Infection related to presence of susceptible fungi
• Risk for injury related to potential for drug-induced hypersensitivity reaction
• Deficient knowledge related to drug therapy

▷ Planning and implementation
• Be aware that injection site reactions occur more often in patients receiving drug by peripheral I.V. route.
• Histamine-mediated reactions may occur more often if drug is infused over less than 1 hour.
• Discontinue infusion if patient develops signs of serious hypersensitivity reaction, including shock.
• Be aware that in the case of overdose, dialysis doesn't remove micafungin.
Patient teaching
• Advise patient to report pain or redness at infusion site.
• Tell patient to expect to undergo laboratory tests during treatment to monitor hematologic, renal, and hepatic function.

M

☑ Evaluation

• Patient responds to drug therapy and is free from infection.
• Patient does not experience hypersensitivity reaction.
• Patient and family state understanding of drug therapy.

midazolam hydrochloride
(MID-ayz-oh-lam high-droh-KLOR-ighd)
Hypnovel ◊

Pharmacologic class: benzodiazepine
Therapeutic class: sedative
Pregnancy risk category: D
Controlled substance schedule: IV

Indications and dosages

▶ **Preoperative sedation (to induce sleepiness or drowsiness and relieve apprehension).**
Adults younger than age 60: 0.07 mg to 0.08 mg/kg I.M. about 1 hour before surgery.
▶ **Conscious sedation before short diagnostic or endoscopic procedures.** *Adults younger than age 60:* Initially, up to 2.5 mg slow I.V.; repeat in 2 minutes if needed, in small increments of initial dose over at least 2 minutes. Total dose that exceeds 5 mg usually isn't needed.
Adults age 60 and older: 1.5 mg or less over at least 2 minutes. If additional adjustment is needed, give at no more than 1 mg over 2 minutes. Total doses exceeding 3.5 mg aren't usually needed.
▶ **Induction of general anesthesia.** *Adults younger than age 55:* If patient hasn't received preanesthesia drug, 0.3 to 0.35 mg/kg I.V. over 20 to 30 seconds. If patient has received preanesthesia drug, 0.15 to 0.35 mg/kg I.V. over 20 to 30 seconds. To complete induction, give additional increments of 25% of initial dose p.r.n. Total dose that exceeds 0.6 mg/kg usually isn't needed.
Adults age 55 and older: If patient hasn't been premedicated, 0.3 mg/kg I.V. over 20 to 30 seconds. If patient has received sedation or opioid, 0.2 mg/kg I.V. over 20 to 30 seconds. To complete induction, give additional increments of 25% of initial dose p.r.n.
▶ **To induce sleepiness and amnesia and to relieve apprehension before anesthesia or before or during procedures in children.**

Children: 0.1 to 0.15 mg/kg I.M. Doses up to 0.5 mg/kg can be used for more anxious patients. Total dose usually doesn't exceed 10 mg. I.M. depending on age of child.
Children ages 12 to 16: Initially, give dose of 2.5 mg or less I.V. slowly; repeat in 2 minutes, if needed, in small increments of initial dose over at least 2 minutes to achieve desired effect. Slowly titrate additional doses to maintain desired level of sedation in increments of 25% of dose used to first reach the sedative endpoint. Total dose that exceeds 5 mg usually isn't needed.
Children ages 6 to 12: 0.025 to 0.05 mg/kg I.V. over 2 to 3 minutes. Additional doses may be given in small increments after 2 to 3 minutes. Total dose that exceeds 0.4 mg/kg usually isn't needed.
Children ages 6 months to 5 years: Initially, 0.05 to 0.1 mg/kg I.V. over 2 to 3 minutes. Additional doses may be given in small increments after 2 to 3 minutes. Total dose that exceeds 0.6 mg/kg usually isn't needed.
▶ **Continuous infusion for sedation of intubated patients in the critical care setting.**
Adults: Initially, 0.01 to 0.05 mg/kg I.V. over several minutes, repeat at 10- to 15-minute intervals, until adequate sedation is achieved. To maintain sedation, infuse initially at 0.02 to 0.1 mg/kg/hour. Some patients may need higher loading doses or infusion rates. Use the lowest effective rate.
Children: Initially, 0.05 to 0.2 mg/kg I.V. over at least 2 to 3 minutes; then continuous infusion at 0.06 to 0.12 mg/kg/hour. Increase or decrease infusion to maintain desired effect.
Neonates born at 32 weeks' gestation or later: Initially 0.06 mg/kg/hour. Adjust rate, p.r.n., using lowest possible rate.
Neonates born earlier than 32 weeks' gestation: Initially 0.03 mg/kg/hour. Adjust rate, p.r.n., using lowest possible rate.

▽▼ I.V. administration

• When mixing infusion, use 5-mg/ml vial, dilute to 0.5 mg/ml with D_5W or normal saline solution.
• Give slowly over at least 2 minutes, and wait at least 2 minutes when adjusting doses to desired effect.
• Watch for irritation and infiltration. Extravasation can cause tissue damage and necrosis.

Reactions may be *common*, uncommon, *life-threatening*, or COMMON AND LIFE-THREATENING.

⊗ **Incompatibilities**
Albumin, amphotericin B, ampicillin sodium, bumetanide, butorphanol, ceftazidime, cefuroxime, clonidine, dexamethasone sodium phosphate, dimenhydrinate, dobutamine, foscarnet, fosphenytoin, furosemide, hydrocortisone, imipenem-cilastatin sodium, methotrexate sodium, nafcillin, pentobarbital sodium, perphenazine, prochlorperazine edisylate, ranitidine hydrochloride, sodium bicarbonate, thiopental, some total parenteral nutrition formulations, trimethoprim-sulfamethoxazole.

Contraindications and cautions

• Contraindicated in patients hypersensitive to the drug or any of its components and in those with acute angle-closure glaucoma, shock, coma, or acute alcohol intoxication.
• Use cautiously in patients with uncompensated acute illness and in debilitated patients.
⚡ **Lifespan:** In pregnant women, drug is contraindicated. In breast-feeding women, use cautiously; it's unknown if the drug appears in breast milk. In elderly patients, use drug cautiously.

Adverse reactions

CNS: headache, oversedation, involuntary movements, combativeness, amnesia.
CV: variations in blood pressure and pulse rate, *hypotension, cardiac arrest.*
GI: nausea, vomiting, hiccups.
Respiratory: decreased respiratory rate, APNEA.
Other: pain, tenderness at injection site.

Interactions

Drug-drug. *Cimetidine, verapamil:* May increase effects of benzodiazepine. Monitor patient closely.
CNS depressants: May increase risk of apnea. Monitor vital signs and respiratory condition closely.
CYP 3A4 inducers (rifampin, carbamazepine, phenytoin, phenobarbital): May decrease midazolam concentration. Monitor patient for effect; adjust dosage if needed.
Diltiazem: May increase CNS depression and prolonged effects of midazolam. Use lower dose of midazolam.
Fluconazole, itraconazole, ketoconazole, miconazole: May increase and prolong levels, and may increase CNS depression and psychomotor impairment. Don't use together.

Hormonal contraceptives: May prolong benzodiazepine half-life. Monitor patient closely.
Indinavir, ritonavir: May cause prolonged or severe sedation and respiratory depression. Monitor patient closely.
Opioid analgesics: May increase midazolam's hypnotic effect and increase risk of hypotension. Monitor patient closely; adjust dosage as needed.
Rifamycin: May decrease midazolam levels. Monitor patient for effect.
Drug-food. *Grapefruit juice:* May increase bioavailability of oral midazolam. Discourage using together.
Drug-lifestyle. *Alcohol use:* May cause additive CNS effects. Strongly discourage using together.

Effects on lab test results

None reported.

Pharmacokinetics

Absorption: 80% to 100%.
Distribution: Large volume; about 97% protein-bound.
Metabolism: In liver by CYP 3A4 isoenzyme.
Excretion: In urine. *Half-life:* 2 to 6 hours.

Route	Onset	Peak	Duration
P.O.	10–20 min	45–60 min	2–6 hr
I.V.	1½–5 min	Rapid	2–6 hr
I.M.	≤ 15 min	15–60 min	2–6 hr

Action

Chemical effect: May depress CNS at limbic and subcortical levels of brain by potentiating effects of GABA.
Therapeutic effect: Promotes calmness and sleep.

Available forms

Injection: 1 mg/ml, 5 mg/ml
Syrup: 2 mg/ml

NURSING PROCESS

⚗ **Assessment**
• Assess patient's condition before therapy and regularly thereafter to monitor the drug's effectiveness.

• Monitor blood pressure, heart rate and rhythm, respirations, airway integrity, and arterial oxygen saturation during procedure, especially in patients premedicated with opioids.
• Assess patient's and family's knowledge of drug therapy.

⊕ Nursing diagnoses
• Anxiety related to surgery
• Ineffective breathing pattern related to drug's effect on respiratory system
• Deficient knowledge related to drug therapy

▶ Planning and implementation
• Have oxygen and resuscitation equipment available in case of severe respiratory depression. Excessive dose or too rapid infusion may cause respiratory arrest, particularly in an elderly or debilitated patient.
• Abrupt withdrawal of drug can cause seizures.
• For I.M. dose, give deep into large muscle mass.
Patient teaching
• Use extra caution when teaching patient because drug will diminish predrug memory. Provide written information, family member instruction, and follow-up contact to ensure that patient has adequate information.
• Instruct patient not to use alcohol during therapy.

☑ Evaluation
• Patient exhibits calmness.
• Patient maintains adequate breathing pattern throughout therapy.
• Patient and family state understanding of drug therapy.

miglitol
(MIG-lih-tall)
Glyset

Pharmacologic class: alpha-glucosidase inhibitor
Therapeutic class: antidiabetic
Pregnancy risk category: B

Indications and dosages

▶ **Type 2 diabetes mellitus where hyperglycemia can't be managed with diet alone; with a sulfonylurea when diet plus either miglitol**

or sulfonylurea alone yield inadequate glycemic control. *Adults:* 25 mg P.O. t.i.d. with the first bite of each main meal; some patients may start at 25 mg P.O. daily to minimize GI side effects. Increase dosage after 4 to 8 weeks to maintenance dosage of 50 mg P.O. t.i.d. Further increase dosage after 3 months, based on glycosylated hemoglobin level, to maximum of 100 mg P.O. t.i.d.

Contraindications and cautions

• Contraindicated in patients hypersensitive to the drug or any of its components. Also contraindicated in patients with diabetic ketoacidosis, inflammatory bowel disease, colonic ulceration, or partial intestinal obstruction; patients predisposed to intestinal obstruction or those with chronic intestinal diseases related to disorders of digestion or absorption; and patients with conditions that may deteriorate as a result of increased gas formation in the intestine.
• Use cautiously in patients with serum creatinine more than 2 mg/dl.
• Use cautiously in patients also receiving insulin or oral sulfonylureas.
⚕ **Lifespan:** In pregnant women, use cautiously when benefits outweigh risks to the fetus. In breast-feeding women, don't use. In children, safety and effectiveness haven't been established.

Adverse reactions

GI: abdominal pain, diarrhea, flatulence.
Skin: rash.

Interactions

Drug-drug. *Digestive enzyme preparations (such as amylase, pancreatin), intestinal absorbents (such as charcoal):* May reduce the effectiveness of miglitol. Avoid using together.
Digoxin, propranolol, ranitidine: May decrease the bioavailability of these drugs. Monitor patient for loss of effectiveness and adjust dosages.
Insulin, oral sulfonylureas: May increase the effect of these drugs. Adjust dosage of these drugs if needed. Monitor these patients for hypoglycemia.
Drug-herb. *Aloe, bilberry leaf, bitter melon, burdock, dandelion, fenugreek, garlic, ginseng, stinging nettle:* May improve glucose level control, allowing for a reduced antidiabetic dosage.

Reactions may be *common*, uncommon, *life-threatening*, or COMMON AND LIFE-THREATENING.

Advise patient to discuss the use of herbal remedies with prescriber before therapy.

Effects on lab test results

• May decrease iron and glucose levels.

Pharmacokinetics

Absorption: A 25-mg dose is completely absorbed, whereas a 100-mg dose is only 50% to 70% absorbed.
Distribution: Primarily into the extracellular fluid. Protein-binding is less than 4%.
Metabolism: None.
Excretion: Primarily renal. More than 95% of a dose in urine as unchanged drug. *Half-life:* About 2 hours.

Route	Onset	Peak	Duration
P.O.	Unknown	2–3 hr	Unknown

Action

Chemical effect: Lowers glucose level through reversible inhibition of alpha glucosidases in the small intestine; they convert oligosaccharides and disaccharides to glucose. Inhibiting these enzymes delays glucose absorption. Drug has no effect on insulin secretion.
Therapeutic effect: Lowers glucose level.

Available forms

Tablets: 25 mg, 50 mg, 100 mg

NURSING PROCESS

Assessment

• Obtain history of patient's condition before therapy, and reassess regularly to monitor the drug's effectiveness.
• Regularly monitor glucose level, especially during increased stress, such as infection, fever, surgery, and trauma.
• Check glycosylated hemoglobin level every 3 months to monitor long-term glycemic control.
• Assess patient's and family's knowledge of drug therapy.

Nursing diagnoses

• Ineffective health maintenance related to hyperglycemia
• Risk for injury related to drug-induced hypoglycemia
• Deficient knowledge related to drug therapy

Planning and implementation

• Give with the first bite of each main meal.
• Manage type 2 diabetes with diet control, exercise program, and regular testing of urine and glucose levels.
• Treat mild to moderate hypoglycemia with dextrose, such as glucose tablets or gel, or orange juice with sugar packets. Severe hypoglycemia may require I.V. glucose or glucagon.
• GI adverse effects decrease with continued treatment.

Patient teaching

• Tell patient about the importance of adhering to prescriber's diet, weight reduction, and exercise instructions and to have glucose and glycosylated hemoglobin level tested regularly.
• Inform patient that drug therapy relieves symptoms but doesn't cure diabetes.
• Teach patient the signs and symptoms of hyperglycemia and hypoglycemia.
• Instruct patient to treat hypoglycemia with glucose tablets and to have a source of glucose readily available when miglitol is taken with a sulfonylurea or insulin.
• Advise patient to promptly seek medical advice during periods of stress such as fever, trauma, infection, or surgery, because drug requirements may change.
• Instruct patient to take drug t.i.d. with the first bite of each main meal.
• Show patient how and when to monitor glucose level.
• Advise patient that adverse GI effects are most common during the first few weeks of therapy and should improve over time.
• Urge patient to always carry medical identification.

Evaluation

• Patient's glucose level is normal.
• Patient sustains no injury from drug-induced hypoglycemia.
• Patient and family state understanding of drug therapy.

milrinone lactate
(MIL-rih-nohn LAK-tayt)
Primacor

Pharmacologic class: bipyridine phosphodiesterase inhibitor
Therapeutic class: inotropic vasodilator
Pregnancy risk category: C

Indications and dosages

▶ **Short-term therapy for acute decompensated heart failure.** *Adults:* Loading dose is 50 mcg/kg I.V., given slowly over 10 minutes, followed by continuous I.V. infusion of 0.375 to 0.75 mcg/kg/minute. Adjust infusion dose based on response. Maximum dose is 1.13 mg/kg/day.
⊟ Adjust-a-dose: For patients with renal impairment, if creatinine clearance is 50 ml/minute or less, decrease dosage to achieve maximum effect, not to exceed 1.13 mg/kg I.V. daily.

▼ I.V. administration

• Dilute with half-normal or normal saline solution or D₅W. Prepare 100-mcg/ml solution by adding 180 ml of diluent per 20-mg (20-ml) vial, 150-mcg/ml solution by adding 113 ml of diluent per 20-mg (20-ml) vial, and 200-mcg/ml solution by adding 80 ml of diluent per 20-mg (20-ml) vial.
• Decreased blood pressure requires stopping or slowing infusion.
• Drug hasn't been shown to be safe or effective for more than 48 hours. Avoid using longer.
⊗ **Incompatibilities**
Bumetanide, furosemide, procainamide.

Contraindications and cautions

• Contraindicated in patients hypersensitive to the drug, or any of its components.
• Use cautiously in patients with severe aortic or pulmonic valvular disease in place of surgical correction of obstruction, or for patients in acute phase of MI.
• Use cautiously in patients with atrial flutter or fibrillation because drug slightly shortens AV node conduction time and may increase ventricular response rate.
❈ **Lifespan:** In pregnant women, use cautiously. In breast-feeding women, use cautiously; it's unknown if the drug appears in breast milk. In children, safety and effectiveness haven't been established.

Adverse reactions

CNS: headache.
CV: chest pain, hypotension, VENTRICULAR ARRHYTHMIAS, *ventricular ectopic activity, ventricular tachycardia, ventricular fibrillation.*

Interactions

Drug-drug. *Nesiritide:* May increase hypotensive effect. Avoid using together.

Effects on lab test results

None reported.

Pharmacokinetics

Absorption: Administered I.V.
Distribution: About 70% bound to protein.
Metabolism: About 12% to glucuronide metabolite.
Excretion: About 83% unchanged in urine.
Half-life: 2½ to 2¾ hours.

Route	Onset	Peak	Duration
I.V.	5–15 min	1–2 hr	3–6 hr

Action

Chemical effect: Produces inotropic action by increasing cellular levels of cAMP; produces vasodilation by relaxing vascular smooth muscle.
Therapeutic effect: Relieves acute signs and symptoms of heart failure.

Available forms

Injection: 1 mg/ml
Premixed injection: 200 mcg/ml in 100 ml D₅W injection; 200 mcg/ml in 200 ml D₅W injection

NURSING PROCESS

⚏ Assessment
• Assess patient's heart failure before therapy and regularly thereafter to monitor the drug's effectiveness.
• Monitor fluid and electrolyte levels, blood pressure, heart rate, and kidney function during therapy.
• Continuously monitor patient's ECG.
• Be alert for adverse reactions.
• Assess patient's and family's knowledge of drug therapy.

⊕ **Nursing diagnoses**
• Impaired gas exchange related to presence of heart failure
• Decreased cardiac output related to drug-induced cardiac arrhythmias
• Deficient knowledge related to drug therapy

▶ **Planning and implementation**
• Drug is typically given with digoxin and diuretics.
• Inotropics may aggravate outflow tract obstruction in hypertrophic subaortic stenosis.
Ⓢ **ALERT:** Improvement of cardiac output may result in enhanced urine output. Reduce diuretic dose as heart failure improves. Potassium loss may predispose patient to digitalis toxicity.
Ⓢ **ALERT:** Don't confuse milrinone with inamrinone.
Patient teaching
• Tell patient to report headache. Mild analgesic can be given for relief.

☑ **Evaluation**
• Patient exhibits adequate gas exchange as heart failure is resolved.
• Drug-induced arrhythmias don't develop during therapy.
• Patient and family state understanding of drug therapy.

minocycline hydrochloride
(migh-noh-SIGH-kleen high-droh-KLOR-ighd)
Akamin◇, Alti-Minocycline♦, Apo-Minocycline♦, Dynacin, Minocin, Minomycin◇, Novo-Minocycline♦, PMS-Minocycline♦, Vectrin

Pharmacologic class: tetracycline
Therapeutic class: antibiotic
Pregnancy risk category: D

Indications and dosages
▶ **Infections caused by sensitive gram-negative and gram-positive organisms, trachoma, amebiasis.** *Adults:* 200 mg I.V.; then 100 mg I.V. q 12 hours. Maximum 400 mg I.V. daily. Or 200 mg P.O. initially; then 100 mg P.O. q 12 hours. Some clinicians use 100 or 200 mg P.O. initially, followed by 50 mg q.i.d. *Children older than age 8:* Initially, 4 mg/kg P.O. or I.V., followed by 2 mg/kg P.O. q

12 hours. Give I.V. in 500- to 1,000-ml solution without calcium over 6 hours.
▶ **Gonorrhea in patients sensitive to penicillin.** *Adults:* Initially, 200 mg P.O.; then 100 mg q 12 hours for at least 4 days.
▶ **Syphilis in patients sensitive to penicillin.** *Adults:* Initially, 200 mg P.O.; then 100 mg q 12 hours for 10 to 15 days.
▶ **Meningococcal carrier state.** *Adults:* 100 mg P.O. q 12 hours for 5 days.
▶ **Uncomplicated urethral, endocervical, or rectal infection caused by** *Chlamydia trachomatis* **or** *Ureaplasma urealyticum.* *Adults:* 100 mg P.O. b.i.d. for at least 7 days.
▶ **Uncomplicated gonococcal urethritis in men.** *Adults:* 100 mg P.O. b.i.d. for 5 days.
▶ **Cholera.** *Adults:* Initially, 200 mg P.O., then 100 mg P.O. q. 12 hours for 2 to 3 days.
▶ **Multibacillary leprosy‡.** *Adults:* 100 mg P.O. daily with clofazimine and ofloxacin for 6 months, followed by 100 mg P.O. daily for an additional 18 months in conjunction with clofazimine.
▶ **Nongonococcal urethritis caused by** *C. trachomatis* **or** *mycoplasma‡.* *Adults:* 100 mg P.O. daily in one or two divided doses for 1 to 3 weeks.

▼ **I.V. administration**
• Reconstitute 100 mg of powder with 5 ml of sterile water for injection, with further dilution of 500 to 1,000 ml for I.V. infusion.
• Infusions are usually given over 6 hours.
• Thrombophlebitis may develop. Watch for irritation and infiltration; extravasation can cause tissue damage and necrosis.
• Switch to P.O. form as soon as possible.
• Solution is stable for 24 hours at room temperature.
⊗ **Incompatibilities**
Adrenocorticotropic hormone (ACTH), allopurinol, amifostine, aminophylline, amobarbital sodium, amphotericin B, bicarbonate infusion mixtures, calcium gluconate or calcium chloride, carbenicillin, cephalothin sodium, cefazolin sodium, chloramphenicol succinate, colistin sulfate, doxapram, heparin sodium, hydrocortisone sodium succinate, hydromorphone, iodine sodium, meperidine, morphine, penicillin, pentobarbital, phenytoin sodium, piperacillin sodium-tazobactam sodium, polymyxin, prochlorperazine, propofol, rifampin, sodium ascorbate, sulfadiazine, sulfisoxazole,

thiopental sodium, thiotepa, vitamin K (sodium bisulfate or sodium salt), whole blood.

Contraindications and cautions

• Contraindicated in patients hypersensitive to the drug or other tetracyclines.

• Use cautiously in patients with impaired kidney or liver function.

🔆 **Lifespan:** In breast-feeding women, don't use because it's unknown if drug appears in breast milk. In children younger than age 8, don't use. Drug may cause permanent discoloration of teeth, enamel defects, and bone growth retardation. In pregnant women, don't use in the last trimester because of these same effects on the fetus.

Adverse reactions

CNS: light-headedness or dizziness from vestibular toxicity, *intracranial hypertension (pseudotumor cerebri).*
CV: pericarditis, *thrombophlebitis.*
EENT: dysphagia, glossitis.
GI: *anorexia,* epigastric distress, oral candidiasis, *nausea,* vomiting, *diarrhea,* enterocolitis, inflammatory anogenital lesions.
Hematologic: eosinophilia, *neutropenia, thrombocytopenia.*
Musculoskeletal: bone growth retardation.
Skin: maculopapular and erythematous rashes, photosensitivity reactions, increased pigmentation, urticaria.
Other: permanent discoloration of teeth, enamel defects, *hypersensitivity reactions, anaphylaxis,* superinfection.

Interactions

Drug-drug. *Antacids (including sodium bicarbonate) and laxatives containing aluminum, magnesium, or calcium; antidiarrheals:* May decrease antibiotic absorption. Give antibiotic 1 hour before or 2 hours after these drugs.
Cimetidine: May decrease absorption of minocycline. Monitor patient.
Digoxin: May increase digoxin level. Decrease digoxin dose, if needed.
Ferrous sulfate, other iron products, zinc: May decrease antibiotic absorption. Give drug 3 hours after or 2 hours before iron.
Hormonal contraceptives: May decrease contraceptive effectiveness and increase risk of breakthrough bleeding. Recommend a nonhormonal contraceptive.

Methoxyflurane: May cause nephrotoxicity with tetracyclines. Avoid using together; monitor patient carefully.
Oral anticoagulants: May increase anticoagulant effect. Monitor PT and INR. Adjust dosage if needed.
Penicillins: May interfere with bactericidal action of penicillins. Avoid using together.
Drug-herb. *St. John's wort:* May increase photosensitivity reactions. Urge patient to avoid unprotected or prolonged exposure to sunlight.
Drug-lifestyle. *Sun exposure:* May cause photosensitivity reaction. Urge patient to avoid unprotected or prolonged exposure to sunlight.

Effects on lab test results

• May increase BUN and liver enzyme levels. May decrease hemoglobin level and hematocrit.
• May increase eosinophil count. May decrease platelet and neutrophil counts.
• Parenteral form may cause false-positive reading of copper sulfate tests (Clinitest). All forms may cause false-negative reading of glucose enzymatic tests (Diastix).

Pharmacokinetics

Absorption: 90% to 100%.
Distribution: Wide, including into synovial, pleural, prostatic, and seminal fluids; bronchial secretions; saliva; and aqueous humor. CSF penetration is poor. Drug is 70% to 80% protein-bound.
Metabolism: Partial.
Excretion: In bile salts, urine, and feces. *Half-life:* 11 to 26 hours.

Route	Onset	Peak	Duration
P.O.	Unknown	1–4 hr	Unknown
I.V.	Immediate	Immediate	Unknown

Action

Chemical effect: May exert bacteriostatic effect by binding to ribosomal subunit of microorganisms, inhibiting protein synthesis.
Therapeutic effect: Hinders bacterial cell growth.

Available forms

Akamin ◊, *Minomycin* ◊
Capsules: 100 mg
Tablets: 50 mg

Reactions may be *common,* uncommon, *life-threatening,* or COMMON AND LIFE-THREATENING.

Alti-Minocycline ♦, *Apo-Minocycline* ♦,
Novo-Minocycline ♦, *PMS-Minocycline* ♦
Capsules: 50 mg, 100 mg
Dynacin
Capsules: 50 mg, 75 mg, 100 mg
Tablets: 50 mg, 75 mg, 100 mg
Minocin
Capsules (pellet-filled): 50 mg, 100 mg
Injection: 100 mg/vial

NURSING PROCESS

▓ Assessment
• Assess patient's infection before therapy and
regularly thereafter to monitor the drug's effectiveness.
• Obtain specimen for culture and sensitivity
tests before giving first dose. Begin therapy
pending results.
• Be alert for adverse reactions and drug interactions.
• If patient has an adverse GI reaction, monitor
patient's hydration.
• Assess patient's and family's knowledge of
drug therapy.

▓ Nursing diagnoses
• Infection related to presence of susceptible
bacteria
• Risk for deficient fluid volume related to
drug-induced adverse reactions
• Deficient knowledge related to drug therapy

▓ Planning and implementation
⊛ **ALERT:** Check expiration date. Outdated or de-
teriorated tetracyclines have been linked to re-
versible nephrotoxicity (Fanconi's syndrome).
• Don't expose these drugs to light or heat.
Keep cap tightly closed.
• Drug may cause tooth discoloration in chil-
dren and young adults. If it occurs, inform pre-
scriber.
⊛ **ALERT:** Don't confuse Minocin with niacin
and Mithracin.
⊛ **ALERT:** Don't confuse Dynacin with Dyna-
Circ.
Patient teaching
• Inform patient that drug may be taken with
food, and instruct him to take drug exactly as
prescribed.
• Instruct patient to take oral form with full
glass of water and to avoid taking it within 1
hour of bedtime to avoid esophagitis.

• Warn patient to avoid hazardous tasks until
the drug's CNS effects are known.
• Instruct patient to avoid direct sunlight and ultraviolet light, to use sunblock, and to wear protective clothing in order to avoid photosensitivity reaction.
• Advise patient who uses hormonal contraceptives that barrier method of contraception
should also be used. Also inform her that she
may experience breakthrough bleeding.

▓ Evaluation
• Patient is free from infection.
• Patient maintains adequate hydration through-
out therapy.
• Patient and family state understanding of drug
therapy.

mirtazapine
(mir-TAH-zuh-peen)
Remeron, Remeron SolTab

Pharmacologic class: piperazinoazepine
Therapeutic class: antidepressant
Pregnancy risk category: C

Indications and dosages

▶ **Depression.** *Adults:* Initially, 15 mg P.O. h.s.
Maintenance dosage is 15 to 45 mg daily. Adjust dosage at intervals of at least 1 to 2 weeks.

Contraindications and cautions

• Contraindicated in patients hypersensitive to
the drug or any of its components and in those
taking MAO inhibitors.
• Use cautiously in patients with CV or cerebrovascular disease, seizure disorders, suicidal
ideation, impaired hepatic or renal function, or
history of mania or hypomania.
⚖ **Lifespan:** In pregnant women, use only if
benefits outweigh risks to the fetus. In breast-
feeding women, use cautiously; it's unknown if
the drug appears in breast milk. In children,
safety and effectiveness haven't been established, and drug shouldn't be used to treat major
depressive disorder. Increased risk of suicidal
behavior has been noted in this population, although not proven to be attributable to drug.

M

Adverse reactions

CNS: *somnolence,* dizziness, asthenia, abnormal dreams, abnormal thinking, tremor, confusion, neurosis, neuropathy.
CV: edema, peripheral edema.
GI: nausea, increased appetite, dry mouth, constipation.
GU: urinary frequency.
Hematologic: *neutropenia, agranulocytosis.*
Metabolic: *weight gain.*
Musculoskeletal: back pain, myalgia.
Respiratory: dyspnea.
Other: flulike syndrome.

Interactions

Drug-drug. *Diazepam, other CNS depressants:* May have additive CNS effects. Avoid using together.
MAO inhibitors: May cause serious and sometimes fatal reactions. Don't use drug within 14 days of an MAO inhibitor.
Drug-lifestyle. *Alcohol use:* May have additive CNS effects. Discourage using together.

Effects on lab test results

• May increase ALT level.
• May decrease neutrophil and granulocyte counts.

Pharmacokinetics

Absorption: Rapid.
Distribution: 85% bound to proteins.
Metabolism: Extensive.
Excretion: Mainly in urine; some in feces.
Half-life: About 20 to 40 hours.

Route	Onset	Peak	Duration
P.O.	Unknown	< 2 hr	Unknown

Action

Chemical effect: Enhances central noradrenergic and serotonergic action; potent antagonist of histamine receptors.
Therapeutic effect: Relieves depression.

Available forms

Orally disintegrating tablets: 15 mg, 30 mg, 45 mg
Tablets: 15 mg, 30 mg, 45 mg

NURSING PROCESS

Assessment
• Assess mental status before initiating drug and regularly throughout treatment.
• Monitor for signs of infection and other adverse reactions.
• Assess patient's and family's knowledge of drug therapy.

Nursing diagnoses
• Disturbed thought processes related to adverse effects
• Risk for injury related to sedation and orthostatic hypotension
• Deficient knowledge related to drug therapy

Planning and implementation
• If patient develops a sore throat, fever, stomatitis, or other signs of infection with a low WBC count, stop giving the drug and monitor him closely.
• Don't abruptly stop giving the drug because doing so increases the risk of suicidal behavior. Monitor patient and take suicide precautions.
Patient teaching
• Instruct patient to remove orally disintegrating tablet from blister pack and immediately place on the tongue. Tell him he won't need water to swallow the tablet because drug dissolves rapidly.
• Tell patient not to break or split tablet.
• Warn patient to avoid hazardous activities if somnolence occurs.
• Tell patient to report signs and symptoms of infection or flulike symptoms.
• Advise patient not to use alcohol or take other CNS depressants.
• Stress importance of compliance with therapy.
• Instruct patient not to take other drugs without prescriber's approval.
• Tell woman to notify prescriber if she suspects pregnancy or if she is breast-feeding.

Evaluation
• Patient regains normal thought processes.
• Patient sustains no injury from adverse reactions.
• Patient and family state understanding of drug therapy.

Reactions may be *common,* uncommon, *life-threatening,* or COMMON AND LIFE-THREATENING.

misoprostol
(mee-SOH-pruh-stol)
Cytotec

Pharmacologic class: prostaglandin E₁ analogue
Therapeutic class: gastric mucosal protectant
Pregnancy risk category: X

Indications and dosages

▶ **Prevention of NSAID-induced gastric ulcer in elderly or debilitated patients at high risk for complications from gastric ulcer and in patients with history of NSAID-induced ulcer.** *Adults:* 200 mcg P.O. q.i.d. with food. If dosage isn't tolerated, decrease to 100 mcg P.O. q.i.d.
▶ **Duodenal or gastric ulcer‡.** *Adults:* 100 to 200 mcg P.O. q.i.d. with meals and h.s. for 4 to 8 weeks.

Contraindications and cautions

• Contraindicated in patients with a known allergy to prostaglandins.
✱ **Lifespan:** In pregnant women, don't use because of risk of uterine rupture and fetal death. In breast-feeding women, don't use because significant diarrhea in infants has been reported. In children, safety and effectiveness haven't been established.

Adverse reactions

CNS: headache, lethargy, vertigo.
GI: *diarrhea, abdominal pain,* nausea, flatulence, dyspepsia, vomiting, constipation, *pancreatitis.*
GU: hypermenorrhea, dysmenorrhea, spotting, cramps, menstrual disorders, UTI, hematuria.
Other: *anaphylaxis.*

Interactions

Drug-drug. *Antacids:* Reduces misoprostol level insignificantly. Monitor patient.

Effects on lab test results

• May increase alkaline phosphatase, aminotransferase, and cardiac enzyme levels. May decrease hemoglobin level and hematocrit.
• May increase erythrocyte sedimentation rate. May decrease platelet count.

Pharmacokinetics

Absorption: Rapid.
Distribution: Highly bound to proteins.
Metabolism: Rapidly de-esterified to misoprostol acid, the biologically active metabolite.
Excretion: About 15% in feces; rest in urine.
Half-life: 20 to 40 minutes.

Route	Onset	Peak	Duration
P.O.	30 min	60–90 min	3 hr

Action

Chemical effect: Replaces gastric prostaglandins depleted by NSAID therapy. Decreases basal and stimulated gastric acid secretion and may increase gastric mucus and bicarbonate production.
Therapeutic effect: Protects gastric mucosa from ulcerating.

Available forms

Tablets: 100 mcg, 200 mcg

NURSING PROCESS

⚕ Assessment

• Obtain history of patient's GI condition before therapy.
• In woman of childbearing age, make sure that negative pregnancy test is obtained within 2 weeks before therapy begins.
• Be alert for adverse reactions and drug interactions.
• Assess patient's and family's knowledge of drug therapy.

⚕ Nursing diagnoses

• Risk for injury related to potential for gastric ulceration
• Acute pain related to headache
• Deficient knowledge related to drug therapy

▶ Planning and implementation

⚕ ALERT: Take special precautions not to use drug in a pregnant woman. Make sure she is fully aware of dangers of drug to fetus and that she receives both verbal and written warnings regarding these dangers. Also make sure she can comply with effective contraceptive use.
• Uterine rupture is linked to certain risk factors, including later trimester pregnancies, higher doses of the drug, prior cesarean delivery or

M

uterine surgery, or five or more previous pregnancies.

⊛ **ALERT:** Don't confuse misoprostol with mifepristone.

Patient teaching
● Instruct patient to report to prescriber headache, diarrhea that doesn't resolve within three weeks or is severe, or severe abdominal pain.
● Instruct patient not to share drug as drug may cause miscarriage, usually with life-threatening bleeding, in women of child-bearing age.
● Advise her not to begin therapy until second or third day of next normal menstrual period.

☑ Evaluation
● Patient remains free from signs and symptoms of gastric ulceration.
● Patient states that drug-induced headache doesn't occur.
● Patient and family state understanding of drug therapy.

mitomycin (mitomycin-C)
(might-oh-MIGH-sin)
Mutamycin

Pharmacologic class: antibiotic
Therapeutic class: antineoplastic
Pregnancy risk category: NR

Indications and dosages

▶ **Disseminated adenocarcinomas of the pancreas and stomach.** *Adults:* 20 mg/m^2 I.V. as single dose. Repeat cycle after 6 to 8 weeks when WBC and platelet counts have returned to normal.
⬗ **Adjust-a-dose:** If WBC count at nadir after last dose is 2,000 to 2,999 mm^3 and platelet count is 25,000 to 74,999 mm^3, give 70% of regular dose. If WBC count is less than 2,000 mm^3 and platelet count is less than 25,000 mm^3, give 50% of regular dose.
▶ **Bladder cancer‡.** *Adults:* 20 to 60 mg intravesically once per week for 8 weeks.

▼ I.V. administration

● Follow facility policy to reduce risks. Preparation and administration are related to mutagenic, teratogenic, and carcinogenic risks to personnel.
● To reconstitute 5-mg vial use 10 ml sterile water for injection; to reconstitute 20-mg vial,

use 40 ml of sterile water for injection; to reconstitute a 40-mg vial, use 80 ml sterile water for injection, to give a concentration of 0.5 mg/ml. Allow to stand at room temperature until complete dissolution occurs.
● Give drug into the Y-connector of a freeflowing I.V. line.
● Watch for irritation and infiltration. Extravasation can cause tissue damage and necrosis. If extravasation occurs, stop infusion immediately and notify prescriber because of risk of severe ulceration and necrosis.
● When reconstituted with sterile water for injection to a concentration of 0.5 mg/ml, drug is stable for 14 days refrigerated or 7 days at room temperature. When diluted to a concentration of 20 to 40 mcg/ml, stable in D$_5$W for 3 hours, normal saline solution for 12 hours, sodium lactate for 24 hours.
● The combination of 5 to 15 mg mitomycin and 1,000 to 10,000 units heparin in 30 ml of normal saline solution for injection is stable at room temperature for 48 hours.

⊗ **Incompatibilities**
Aztreonam, bleomycin, cefepime, etoposide, filgrastim, gemcitabine, piperacillin sodium-tazobactam sodium, sargramostim, vinorelbine.

Contraindications and cautions

● Contraindicated in patients hypersensitive to the drug or any of its components and in those with thrombocytopenia, coagulation disorder, or increased bleeding tendency from other causes.
⚹ **Lifespan:** In pregnant and breast-feeding women, use only when benefits outweigh risks to the fetus and infant. In children, safety and effectiveness haven't been established.

Adverse reactions

CNS: headache, neurologic abnormalities, confusion, drowsiness, fatigue, *fever.*
GI: *nausea, vomiting,* anorexia, stomatitis.
GU: *renal toxicity, hemolytic uremic syndrome.*
Hematologic: THROMBOCYTOPENIA, LEUKOPENIA, *microangiopathic hemolytic anemia.*
Respiratory: *pulmonary edema,* dyspnea, nonproductive cough, *acute respiratory distress syndrome, interstitial pneumonitis.*
Skin: desquamation, induration, pruritus, and *pain* at injection site; *septicemia;* cellulitis, ulceration, and sloughing with extravasation; *re-*

versible alopecia; purple coloration of nail beds.

Interactions

Drug-drug. *Vinca alkaloids:* May cause acute respiratory distress. Avoid using together.

Effects on lab test results

• May decrease hemoglobin level and hematocrit.
• May decrease platelet and WBC counts.

Pharmacokinetics

Absorption: Administered I.V.
Distribution: Wide; doesn't cross blood-brain barrier.
Metabolism: By hepatic microsomal enzymes and deactivated in kidneys, spleen, brain, and heart.
Excretion: Primarily in urine; small portion in bile and feces. *Half-life:* About 50 minutes.

Route	Onset	Peak	Duration
I.V.	Unknown	Unknown	Unknown

Action

Chemical effect: Acts like alkylating drug, cross-linking strands of DNA. This causes imbalance of cell growth, leading to cell death.
Therapeutic effect: Kills certain cancer cells.

Available forms

Injection: 5-, 20-, and 40-mg vials

NURSING PROCESS

🗓 Assessment

• Assess patient's condition before therapy and regularly thereafter to monitor the drug's effectiveness.
• Obtain CBC and blood studies.
• Monitor kidney function tests.
• Be alert for adverse reactions and drug interactions.
• Assess patient's and family's knowledge of drug therapy.

🔲 Nursing diagnoses

• Ineffective health maintenance related to presence of neoplastic disease
• Ineffective protection related to adverse hematologic reactions
• Deficient knowledge related to drug therapy

▶ Planning and implementation

• Never give drug I.M. or subcutaneously.
• Base dosage adjustments on nadir of leukocyte and platelet counts after previous dose.
• Hemolytic uremic syndrome is characterized by microangiopathic hemolytic anemia, thrombocytopenia, and renal impairment.
• Watch for leukopenia up to 8 weeks post infusion; also can be cumulative with successive doses.
🄯 **ALERT:** Don't confuse mitomycin with mithramycin.

Patient teaching
• Instruct patient to watch for signs of infection and bleeding and to take temperature daily.
• Warn patient that alopecia may occur, but assure him that it's reversible.
• Tell patient to promptly report to prescriber any adverse reaction.

✅ Evaluation

• Patient responds well to therapy.
• Patient doesn't develop serious complications.
• Patient and family state understanding of drug therapy.

mitoxantrone hydrochloride
(migh-toh-ZAN-trohn high-droh-KLOR-ighd)
Novantrone

Pharmacologic class: antibiotic
Therapeutic class: antineoplastic
Pregnancy risk category: D

Indications and dosages

▶ **Combination initial therapy for acute non-lymphocytic leukemia.** *Adults:* Induction begins with 12 mg/m² I.V. daily on days 1 through 3, given with 100 mg/m² daily of cytarabine on days 1 through 7. If response isn't adequate, give second induction. Maintenance therapy: 12 mg/m² on days 1 and 2, given with cytarabine on days 1 through 5.
▶ **To reduce neurologic disability and frequency of relapse in chronic progressive, progressive relapsing, or worsening relapsing-remitting multiple sclerosis.** *Adults:* 12 mg/m² I.V. over 5 to 15 minutes q 3 months.
▶ **Pain from advanced hormone-refractory prostate cancer.** *Adults:* 12 to 14 mg/m² I.V. in-

fusion over 15 to 30 minutes q 21 days with corticosteroids.

▽ I.V. administration

• Preparation and administration of parenteral
form carries mutagenic, teratogenic, and carcinogenic risks. Check facility policy.
• Dilute dose (available as aqueous solution of
2 mg/ml in volumes of 10, 12.5, and 15 ml) in at
least 50 ml of normal saline solution injection
or D₅W injection. Give drug by direct injection
into free-flowing I.V. line of normal saline solution or D₅W injection over at least 3 minutes,
usually 15 to 30 minutes.
• Although drug isn't a vesicant, if dose extravasates, stop infusion immediately and notify
prescriber.
• Store undiluted solution at room temperature.
Once vial is penetrated, undiluted solution may
be stored at room temperature for 7 days, or
14 days in refrigerator. Don't freeze.
⊗ **Incompatibilities**
Amphotericin B, aztreonam, cefepime, doxorubicin liposomal, heparin sodium, hydrocortisone, other I.V. drugs, paclitaxel, piperacillin
sodium and tazobactam sodium, propofol, sargramostim.

Contraindications and cautions

• Contraindicated in patients hypersensitive to
the drug or any of its components.
• Use cautiously in patients previously exposed
to anthracyclines or other cardiotoxic drugs.
▒ **Lifespan:** In pregnant and breast-feeding
women, drug is contraindicated. In children,
safety and effectiveness haven't been established.

Adverse reactions

CNS: *seizures,* headache.
CV: *heart failure, arrhythmias,* tachycardia,
fatal myocardial toxicity.
EENT: conjunctivitis.
GI: BLEEDING, abdominal pain, diarrhea, nau-
sea, mucositis, vomiting, stomatitis.
GU: uric acid nephropathy, *renal impairment.*
Hematologic: *myelosuppression, secondary
acute myelogenous leukemia.*
Hepatic: *jaundice.*
Metabolic: hyperuricemia.
Respiratory: dyspnea, cough.
Skin: petechiae, ecchymoses, alopecia.

Interactions

None significant.

Effects on lab test results

• May increase ALT, AST, bilirubin, BUN, creatinine, and uric acid levels. May decrease hemoglobin level and hematocrit.
• May decrease WBC, RBC, and platelet
counts.

Pharmacokinetics

Absorption: Administered I.V.
Distribution: 78% protein-bound.
Metabolism: In liver.
Excretion: By renal and hepatobiliary systems.
Half-life: 5¼ days.

Route	Onset	Peak	Duration
I.V.	Unknown	Unknown	Unknown

Action

Chemical effect: Not fully understood; may be
cell cycle–nonspecific. Drug reacts with DNA,
producing cytotoxic effect.
Therapeutic effect: Hinders susceptible cancer
cell growth.

Available forms

Injection: 2 mg/ml in 10-, 12.5-, and 15-ml
vials

NURSING PROCESS

▣ Assessment

• Assess patient's condition before therapy and
regularly thereafter to monitor the drug's effectiveness.
• Monitor CBC and other lab test results regularly.
• Monitor left ventricular ejection fraction and
signs of heart failure or cardiac toxicity with
each dose.
• Be alert for adverse reactions and drug interactions.
• Assess patient's and family's knowledge of
drug therapy.

▣ Nursing diagnoses

• Ineffective health maintenance related to presence of leukemia
• Ineffective immune protection related to drug-
induced myelosuppression
• Deficient knowledge related to drug therapy

⊠ Planning and implementation
• Don't give to patient with neutrophil count below 1,500 cells/mm³ or to patient with LVEF < 50% unless benefits outweigh risks.
• Cardiotoxicity is linked to a cumulative dose > 140 mg/m².
• Give allopurinol, if needed. Uric acid nephropathy can be avoided by adequately hydrating patient before and during therapy.
• If severe nonhematologic toxicity occurs during first course of therapy, delay second course until patient recovers.

Patient teaching
• Inform patient that urine may appear blue-green within 24 hours after administration, and that some bluish discoloration of sclera may occur. These effects aren't harmful.
• Teach patient infection control and bleeding precautions. Tell him to watch for and report signs of bleeding and infection.
• Tell patient to report sudden weight gain, peripheral edema, shortness of breath, or chest discomfort to prescriber immediately.
• Advise woman of childbearing age not to become pregnant during therapy and to consult prescriber before becoming pregnant.

✅ Evaluation
• Patient responds well to therapy.
• Patient develops no serious complications from drug-induced myelosuppression.
• Patient and family state understanding of drug therapy.

mivacurium chloride
(migh-vuh-KYOO-ree-um KLOR-ighd)
Mivacron

Pharmacologic class: nondepolarizing neuromuscular blocker
Therapeutic class: skeletal muscle relaxant
Pregnancy risk category: C

Indications and dosages
▶ **Adjunct to general anesthesia, to facilitate endotracheal intubation, and to relax skeletal muscles during surgery or mechanical ventilation.** *Adults:* Dosage is highly individualized. Usually, 0.15 mg/kg I.V. push over 5 to 15 seconds provides adequate muscle relaxation within 135 seconds for endotracheal intubation. Sup-

plemental doses of 0.1 mg/kg I.V. q 15 minutes is usually sufficient to maintain muscle relaxation. Or maintain neuromuscular blockade with continuous infusion of 4 mcg/kg/minute begun simultaneously with initial dose, or 9 to 10 mcg/kg/minute started after evidence of spontaneous recovery caused by initial dose. When used with isoflurane or enflurane anesthesia, reduce dosage about 35% to 40%.
Children ages 2 to 12: 0.2 mg/kg I.V. push given over 5 to 15 seconds. Neuromuscular blockade is usually evident in less than 2 minutes. Maintenance doses are generally needed more frequently in children. Or maintain neuromuscular blockade with continuous I.V. infusion, adjusted to effect. Most children respond to 5 to 31 mcg/kg/minute.
⊠ **Adjust-a-dose:** For patients with end-stage renal or hepatic disease, decrease infusion rates by as much as 50%.

▼ I.V. administration
• Give only under direct medical supervision of clinician skilled in use of neuromuscular blockers and techniques for maintaining airway. Don't use unless emergency equipment for respiratory support and antagonist are within reach.
• To avoid patient distress, don't give until patient is unconscious by general anesthetic because drug has no effect on consciousness or pain threshold.
• Use with D₅W, normal saline solution injection, D₅W in normal saline solution injection, lactated Ringer's injection, or D₅W in lactated Ringer's injection.
• Drug is compatible with alfentanil, fentanyl, sufentanil, droperidol, and midazolam.
• For premixed infusion in D₅W, remove protective outer wrap and check container for minor leaks by squeezing bag before giving. Don't use container in series connections.
• Drug may be given by direct injection over 5 to 15 seconds.
• Diluted solutions are stable for 24 hours at room temperature.
⊗ **Incompatibilities**
Alkaline solutions such as barbiturate solutions, other I.V. drugs.

Contraindications and cautions
• Contraindicated in patients hypersensitive to the drug, any of its components, or other drugs containing benzylisoquinolinium. Also contrain-

dicated in patients with allergy to benzyl alcohol.

• Use very cautiously in patients who are homozygous for atypical pseudocholinesterase gene. Drug is metabolized to inactive compounds by pseudocholinesterase.

• Use cautiously in patients with significant CV disease and in those who may be adversely affected by release of histamine (such as asthmatic patients).

• Also use cautiously, possibly at reduced dosage, in debilitated patients; in patients with metastatic cancer, severe electrolyte disturbances, or neuromuscular diseases; and in those in whom potentiation or difficulty in reversal of neuromuscular blockade is anticipated. Patients with myasthenia gravis or myasthenic syndrome (Eaton-Lambert syndrome) are particularly sensitive to effects of nondepolarizing relaxants.

⚠ Lifespan: In pregnant women, use cautiously. In breast-feeding women, use cautiously. It's unknown if the drug appears in breast milk. In children younger than age 2, safety and effectiveness of drug haven't been established.

Adverse reactions

CNS: dizziness.
CV: *flushing,* hypotension, tachycardia, ***bradycardia, arrhythmias,*** phlebitis.
Musculoskeletal: prolonged muscle weakness, muscle spasms.
Respiratory: *bronchospasm,* wheezing, ***respiratory insufficiency, apnea.***
Skin: rash, urticaria, erythema.

Interactions

Drug-drug. *Amikacin, gentamicin, neomycin, streptomycin, tobramycin:* May increase the effects of mivacurium, including prolonged respiratory depression. Use together only when necessary. Reduce mivacurium dose if needed.
Bacitracin, clindamycin, colistimethate, colistin, ketamine, parenteral verapamil, polymyxin B sulfate, tetracycline: May increase neuromuscular blockade, leading to increased skeletal muscle relaxation and prolonged effect. Use together cautiously.
Carbamazepine, phenytoin: May decrease the effects of mivacurium. Increase dose, if needed.
Inhaled anesthetics (especially enflurane, isoflurane), magnesium salts, quinidine: May enhance or prolong action of nondepolarizing neu-

romuscular blockers. Monitor patient for excessive weakness.

Effects on lab test results

None reported.

Pharmacokinetics

Absorption: Administered I.V.
Distribution: Not extensive.
Metabolism: Rapidly hydrolyzed by pseudocholinesterase to inactive components.
Excretion: Metabolites in urine and bile. *Half-life:* 2 minutes for two main metabolites; 55 minutes for minor metabolite.

Route	Onset	Peak	Duration
I.V.	1–2 min	2–5 min	20–35 min

Action

Chemical effect: Competes with acetylcholine for receptor sites at motor end plate. Because cholinesterase inhibitors may antagonize this action, drug is considered a competitive antagonist. Drug is mixture of three stereoisomers, each with neuromuscular blocking action.
Therapeutic effect: Relaxes skeletal muscles.

Available forms

Infusion: 0.5 mg/ml in 50 ml of D_5W
Injection: 2 mg/ml in 5- and 10-ml vials

NURSING PROCESS

⚖ Assessment
• Assess patient's need for drug before therapy and regularly thereafter.
• Closely monitor respiratory rate until patient is fully recovered from neuromuscular blockade, as evidenced by tests of muscle strength (hand grip, head lift, and ability to cough).
• Be alert for adverse reactions and drug interactions.
• Assess patient's and family's knowledge of drug therapy.

⊕ Nursing diagnoses
• Ineffective breathing pattern related to drug's effect on respiratory muscles
• Deficient knowledge related to drug therapy

▷ Planning and implementation
⊛ ALERT: Give test dose to assess burn patient's sensitivity to drug. Patients with severe burns

---

develop resistance to nondepolarizing neuro-muscular blockers; however, they also may have reduced pseudocholinesterase activity, drug's mechanism of action.

• Monitor nerve stimulator and train-of-four to document antagonism of neuromuscular block-ade and recovery of muscle strength. Before attempting reversal with neostigmine or edrophonium, wait for some signs of spontaneous recovery.

• Experimental evidence suggests that acid-base and electrolyte balances may influence actions of nondepolarizing neuromuscular blockers. Alkalosis may counteract paralysis; acidosis may enhance it.

• In patients 30% or more above their ideal weight, adjust the dose to ideal body weight to avoid prolonged neuromuscular blockade.

• Effect lasts about 150% longer in patients with end-stage renal disease and 300% longer in patients with hepatic dysfunction.

• Like other neuromuscular blockers, dose requirements for children are higher on mg/kg basis than those for adults. Onset and recovery of neuromuscular blockade occur more rapidly in children.

⊛ ALERT: Don't confuse Mivacron with Mazicon or Mevacor.

Patient teaching

• Instruct patient and family in drug use during surgery and side effects of intubation.

☑ **Evaluation**

• Patient maintains adequate ventilation with or without assistance.

• Patient and family state understanding of drug therapy.

modafinil
(moh-DAFF-ih-nil)
Provigil

Pharmacologic class: CNS stimulant
Therapeutic class: analeptic
Pregnancy risk category: C
Controlled substance schedule: IV

Indications and dosages

▶ **Narcolepsy, obstructive sleep apnea/hypopnea syndrome.** *Adults:* 200 mg P.O. daily, given as a single dose in the morning.

▶ **Shift-work sleep disorder.** *Adults:* 200 mg P.O. once daily one hour before start of shift work.

☒ **Adjust-a-dose:** For patients with severe hepatic impairment, reduce dosage by 50%.

Contraindications and cautions

• Contraindicated in patients hypersensitive to the drug or any of its components. Don't use in patients with a history of left ventricular hypertrophy or ischemic ECG changes, chest pain, arrhythmias, or other signs or symptoms of mitral valve prolapse caused by CNS stimulant use.

• Use cautiously in patients with recent MI or unstable angina, in those with history of psychosis, and in those receiving therapy with MAO inhibitors.

• Use cautiously and at reduced dosage in patients with severe hepatic impairment, with or without cirrhosis.

• Safety and effectiveness of drug in patients with severe renal impairment hasn't been established.

⚛ **Lifespan:** In pregnant women, use only when benefits outweigh risks to the fetus. In breast-feeding women, use cautiously because it's unknown if the drug appears in breast milk. In children younger than age 16, safety and effectiveness haven't been established. In elderly patients with renal or hepatic impairment, use cautiously and at a low dose.

Adverse reactions

CNS: *headache,* nervousness, dizziness, depression, anxiety, fever, cataplexy, insomnia, paresthesia, dyskinesia, hypertonia, confusion, amnesia, emotional lability, ataxia, syncope, tremor.
CV: hypotension, hypertension, vasodilation, *arrhythmias,* chest pain.
EENT: *rhinitis,* pharyngitis, epistaxis, amblyopia, abnormal vision.
GI: *nausea,* diarrhea, dry mouth, mouth ulcer, gingivitis, thirst, anorexia, vomiting.
GU: abnormal urine, urine retention, abnormal ejaculation.
Hematologic: eosinophilia.
Metabolic: hyperglycemia.
Musculoskeletal: neck pain, rigid neck, joint disorder.
Respiratory: lung disorders, dyspnea, *asthma.*
Skin: herpes simplex, dry skin.
Other: chills, infection.

M

Interactions

Drug-drug. *Cyclosporine, theophylline:* Reduces levels of these drugs. Use together cautiously.
Drugs that induce CYP 3A4 (carbamazepine, phenobarbital, rifampin), drugs that inhibit CYP 3A4 (itraconazole, ketoconazole): Alters modafinil levels. Monitor patient closely.
Drugs metabolized by CYP 2C9 (diazepam, phenytoin, propranolol): May increase levels of these drugs. Use together cautiously. Adjust dosage p.r.n.
Hormonal contraceptives: Reduces levels of these drugs, resulting in reduced contraceptive effectiveness. Recommend additional or alternative contraceptive method during modafinil therapy and for 1 month afterward.
Methylphenidate: Delays modafinil absorption. Separate administration times.
Phenytoin, warfarin: May inhibit CYP 2C9 and increase levels of phenytoin and warfarin. Monitor patient closely for signs of toxicity.
Tricyclic antidepressants (clomipramine, desipramine): May increase tricyclic antidepressant levels. Reduce dosage of these drugs.

Effects on lab test results

• May increase glucose, GGT, and AST levels.
• May increase eosinophil count.

Pharmacokinetics

Absorption: Rapid, with levels peaking in 2 to 4 hours.
Distribution: Good. About 60% binds to protein, primarily albumin.
Metabolism: About 90% in the liver.
Excretion: Less than 10% from the kidneys as unchanged drug. *Half-life:* 15 hours.

Route	Onset	Peak	Duration
P.O.	Unknown	2–4 hr	Unknown

Action

Chemical effect: Unknown. It has wake-promoting actions similar to those of sympathomimetics, including amphetamines, but it's structurally distinct from amphetamines and doesn't appear to alter the release of either dopamine or norepinephrine to produce CNS stimulation.
Therapeutic effect: Improves daytime wakefulness.

Available forms

Tablets: 100 mg, 200 mg

NURSING PROCESS

⚗ Assessment
• Obtain history of patient's condition before therapy, and reassess regularly thereafter to monitor the drug's effectiveness.
• Assess patient's renal function before therapy.
• Closely monitor hypertensive patient.
• Assess patient's and family's knowledge of drug therapy.

⊕ Nursing diagnoses
• Disturbed sleep pattern related to drug-induced insomnia
• Risk for injury related to drug-induced CNS adverse effects
• Deficient knowledge related to drug therapy

❯ Planning and implementation
• Food has no effect on overall bioavailability, but it may delay modafinil absorption by 1 hour.
• Although single, daily, 400-mg dose is usually well tolerated, no consistent evidence exists that this dosage provides additional benefit beyond daily 200-mg doses.
Patient teaching
• Drug may impair judgment. Advise patient to be careful while driving or performing other activities that require alertness until the drug's CNS effects are known.
• Instruct patient not to take other prescription or OTC drugs without consulting prescriber because of possible drug interactions.
• Advise patient not to drink alcohol during therapy.
• Tell patient to notify prescriber if he develops a rash, hives, or a related allergic reaction.
• Caution woman that use of hormonal contraceptives (including depot or implantable contraceptives) with modafinil tablets may increase the risk of pregnancy. Recommend barrier method as alternative or additional contraception during therapy and for 1 month after therapy ends.
• Advise woman to notify prescriber if she becomes pregnant or intends to become pregnant during therapy.
• Tell woman to notify prescriber if she's breast-feeding.

Reactions may be *common*, uncommon, *life-threatening*, or COMMON AND LIFE-THREATENING.

☑ **Evaluation**
• Patient develops and maintains normal sleep-wake patterns.
• Patient has no adverse CNS effects.
• Patient and family state understanding of drug therapy.

moexipril hydrochloride
(moh-EKS-eh-pril high-droh-KLOR-ighd)
Univasc

Pharmacologic class: ACE inhibitor
Therapeutic class: antihypertensive
Pregnancy risk category: C (D in second and third trimesters)

Indications and dosages
▶ **Hypertension.** *Adults:* Initially, 7.5 mg P.O. daily in patients not receiving a diuretic, given 1 hour before meals. If inadequate response, increase or divide dose. Maintenance dosage, 7.5 to 30 mg daily in one or two divided doses 1 hour before meals.
❊ **Adjust-a-dose:** For patients with renal impairment, if creatinine clearance is 40 ml/minute/1.73 m² or less, start dosage at 3.75 mg P.O. daily. Maximum, 15 mg P.O. daily. For patients taking diuretics, if diuretic can't be discontinued, start dosage at 3.75 mg P.O. daily.

Contraindications and cautions
• Contraindicated in patients hypersensitive to the drug or any of its components, and in those with history of angioedema with previous ACE inhibitor therapy.
• Use cautiously in patients with impaired kidney function, heart failure, or renal artery stenosis.
❊ **Lifespan:** In pregnant women, use cautiously during first trimester; contraindicated in second and third trimesters. In breast-feeding women, use cautiously; it's unknown if the drug appears in breast milk. In children, safety and effectiveness haven't been established.

Adverse reactions
CNS: *dizziness,* headache, fatigue, pain.
CV: peripheral edema, hypotension, orthostatic hypotension, chest pain, flushing.
EENT: pharyngitis, rhinitis, sinusitis.
GI: diarrhea, dyspepsia, nausea.

GU: urinary frequency.
Hematologic: *neutropenia.*
Metabolic: *hyperkalemia.*
Musculoskeletal: myalgia.
Respiratory: *persistent, nonproductive cough;* upper respiratory tract infection.
Skin: rash.
Other: *anaphylaxis, angioedema,* flulike syndrome.

Interactions
Drug-drug. *Antacids:* May decrease bioavailability of ACE inhibitors. Give drug on an empty stomach.
Digoxin: May increase or decrease digoxin level. Monitor digoxin level and patient closely.
Diuretics: May increase risk of excessive hypotension. Monitor blood pressure closely.
Indomethacin: May reduce hypotensive effects of ACE inhibitors. Avoid using together; monitor blood pressure.
Lithium: May increase lithium level and lithium toxicity. Use together cautiously. Monitor lithium level frequently.
Potassium-sparing diuretics, potassium supplements: May increases risk of hyperkalemia. Monitor potassium level closely.
Drug-herb. *Capsaicin:* May cause or worsen coughing from ACE inhibitor therapy. Discourage using together.
Drug-food. *Salt substitutes that contain potassium:* May increase risk of hyperkalemia. Monitor potassium level closely; urge patient to avoid salt substitutes containing potassium.

Effects on lab test results
• May increase potassium level.
• May decrease neutrophil and granulocyte counts.

Pharmacokinetics
Absorption: Incomplete, with bioavailability of about 13%. Food significantly decreases bioavailability.
Distribution: About 50% protein-bound.
Metabolism: Extensive, to the active metabolite moexiprilat.
Excretion: Primarily in feces, with small amount in urine. *Half-life:* 2 to 9 hours.

Route	Onset	Peak	Duration
P.O.	1 hr	3–6 hr	24 hr

Action

Chemical effect: May suppress renin-angiotensin-aldosterone system. Inhibits ACE, inhibiting production of angiotensin II (a potent vasoconstrictor and stimulator of aldosterone secretion).
Therapeutic effect: Lowers blood pressure.

Available forms

Tablets: 7.5 mg, 15 mg

NURSING PROCESS

Assessment
• Assess patient's blood pressure before therapy.
• Measure blood pressure at lowest point just before dose to verify adequate control. Drug is less effective in reducing trough blood pressure in blacks than in others.
• Monitor patient for hypotension.
• Assess kidney function before therapy and periodically thereafter. Monitor potassium level.
• Monitor CBC with differential counts before therapy, especially in patient who has collagen-vascular disease with impaired kidney function.
• Be alert for adverse reactions and interactions.
• Assess patient's and family's knowledge of drug therapy.

Nursing diagnoses
• Risk for injury related to presence of hypertension
• Disturbed sleep pattern related to cough
• Deficient knowledge related to drug therapy

Planning and implementation
⊛ ALERT: Excessive hypotension can occur when drug is given with diuretics. If possible, stop giving diuretics 2 to 3 days before giving this drug to decrease risk of reaction. If drug doesn't adequately control blood pressure, restart diuretic with care.
⊛ ALERT: Angioedema involving tongue, glottis, or larynx may be fatal because of airway obstruction. Give epinephrine and ensure a patent airway.
• If cough interferes with patient's ability to sleep, notify prescriber.
Patient teaching
• Instruct patient to take drug on an empty stomach; high-fat meals can impair absorption.

• Tell patient to avoid salt substitutes. These products may contain potassium, which can cause hyperkalemia.
• Advise patient to rise slowly to minimize light-headedness. If syncope occurs, tell him to stop taking the drug and immediately call the prescriber.
• Urge patient to use caution in hot weather and during exercise. Inadequate fluid intake, vomiting, diarrhea, and excessive perspiration can lead to light-headedness and syncope.
• Advise patient to report signs of infection, such as fever and sore throat; easy bruising or bleeding; swelling of tongue, lips, face, eyes, mucous membranes, or limbs; difficulty swallowing or breathing; and hoarseness.
• Tell woman to notify prescriber if she becomes pregnant.

Evaluation
• Patient's blood pressure is normal.
• Patient states that sleep disturbance doesn't occur.
• Patient and family state understanding of drug therapy.

---

mometasone furoate
(moe-MEH-tah-zone fuhr-OH-eight)
Asmanex Twisthaler

Pharmacologic class: corticosteroid
Therapeutic class: anti-inflammatory, antiasthmatic
Pregnancy risk category: C

Indications and dosages

▶ **Maintenance therapy for asthma; asthma in patients who need oral corticosteroids.**
Adults and children age 12 and older who use a bronchodilator or inhaled corticosteroids: Initially, 220 mcg by oral inhalation q day in the evening. Maximum, 440 mcg/day.
Adults and children age 12 and older who take oral corticosteroids: 440 mcg b.i.d. by oral inhalation. Maximum, 880 mcg/day. Reduce oral corticosteroid dosage by no more than 2.5 mg/day at weekly intervals starting at least 1 week after starting mometasone. After stopping oral corticosteroids, reduce mometasone dose to the lowest effective amount.

Contraindications and cautions

• Contraindicated in patients hypersensitive to drug or its ingredients and as primary treatment of status asthmaticus or other acute episodes of asthma or bronchospasm.

• Use cautiously in patients at high risk for decreased bone mineral content (those with a family history of osteoporosis, prolonged immobilization, long-term use of drugs that reduce bone mass), patients switching from systemic to inhaled corticosteroids, and patients with active or quiescent tuberculosis, untreated systemic infections, ocular herpes simplex, or immunosuppression.

⚖ **Lifespan:** In pregnant women, use only if benefits outweigh risks to the fetus. In breast-feeding women; use cautiously; it isn't known if drug appears in breast milk. In children younger than age 12, safety hasn't been established.

Adverse reactions

CNS: depression, fatigue, *headache,* insomnia.
EENT: *allergic rhinitis,* dry throat, dysphonia, earache, epistaxis, nasal irritation, *pharyngitis,* sinus congestion, sinusitis.
GI: abdominal pain, anorexia, dyspepsia, flatulence, gastroenteritis, nausea, oral candidiasis, vomiting.
GU: dysmenorrhea, menstrual disorder, UTI.
Musculoskeletal: arthralgia, back pain, myalgia, pain.
Respiratory: respiratory disorder, *upper respiratory tract infection.*
Other: accidental injury, flulike symptoms, infection.

Interactions

Drug-drug. *Ketoconazole:* May increase mometasone level. Use together cautiously.

Effects on lab test results

None reported.

Pharmacokinetics

Absorption: Low in plasma.
Distribution: None in RBCs.
Metabolism: Extensive in the liver by CYP 3A4 to multiple metabolites.
Excretion: Mainly in feces; some in urine.

Route	Onset	Peak	Duration
Inhalation	Unknown	Unknown	Unknown

Action

Chemical effect: Unknown, although corticosteroids inhibit many cells and mediators involved in inflammation and the asthmatic response.
Therapeutic effect: Reduces inflammation in the lungs and airways to improve pulmonary function.

Available forms

Inhalation powder: 220 mcg per inhalation

NURSING PROCESS

⚗ Assessment

• Obtain patient's medical history including current treatments for asthma prior to initiating drug.

⊛ **ALERT:** If patient is switching from an oral corticosteroid to an inhaled form, watch closely for evidence of adrenal insufficiency, such as fatigue, lethargy, weakness, nausea, vomiting, and hypotension.

• Because inhaled corticosteroids can be systemically absorbed, watch for cushingoid effects.

• If a woman takes corticosteroids during pregnancy, monitor newborn for hypoadrenalism.

• Assess patient for bone loss during long-term use.

• Watch for evidence of localized mouth infections, glaucoma, and immunosuppression.

• Monitor elderly patients for increased sensitivity to drug effects.

• Assess patient's and family's knowledge of drug therapy.

🔲 Nursing diagnoses

• Impaired gas exchange related to underlying condition and poor pulmonary function
• Activity intolerance related to underlying asthmatic condition
• Deficient knowledge related to drug therapy

▷ Planning and implementation

⊛ **ALERT:** Don't use this drug to treat acute bronchospasm.

• Wean patient slowly from systemic corticosteroids once he switches to mometasone. Monitor lung function tests, beta-agonist use, and asthma symptoms.

• After oral corticosteroids are withdrawn, it may take months for hypothalamic-pituitary-

M

adrenal (HPA) function to recover. Patients are particularly vulnerable to adrenal insufficiency or adrenal crisis during this period of HPA recovery if they experience trauma, stress, infection, or surgery.
• Maximum benefits may not occur for 1 to 2 weeks or longer after mometasone therapy is initiated.

Patient teaching
• Tell patient to use thc mometasone inhaler regularly and at the same time each day. If he uses it only once daily, tell him to do so in the evening.
• Caution patient not to use drug for immediate relief of an asthmatic attack or bronchospasm.
• Inform patient that maximum benefits may not occur for 1 to 2 weeks or longer after mometasone therapy starts; instruct him to notify the prescriber if his condition fails to improve or if it worsens.
• Explain that, if bronchospasm develops after taking mometasone, he should immediately use a fast-acting bronchodilator. Urge him to contact the prescriber immediately if bronchospasm doesn't respond to the fast-acting bronchodilator.
ALERT: If patient has been weaned from oral corticosteroids, urge him to resume them during severe asthmatic attack or periods of stress and to contact the prescriber for instructions.
• Warn patient to avoid exposure to chickenpox or measles and to notify the prescriber if such exposure occurs.
• Tell patient to report vision changes; long-term use of an inhaled corticosteroid may increase the risk of cataracts or glaucoma.
• Advise patient to write the date on a new inhaler on the day he opens it and to discard the unit after 45 days or when the dose counter reads "00".
• Instruct patient on the proper use and routine care of the inhaler.

☑ Evaluation
• Patient has normal respiratory rate and optimal air exchange.
• Patient experiences improved exercise and activity tolerance.
• Patient and family state understanding of drug therapy.

montelukast sodium
(mon-tih-LOO-kist SOH-dee-um)
Singulair

Pharmacologic class: leukotriene receptor antagonist
Therapeutic class: antiasthmatic
Pregnancy risk category: B

Indications and dosages
▶ **Asthma, seasonal allergic rhinitis.** *Adults and children age 15 and older:* one 10 mg tablet P.O. daily in evening.
Children ages 6 to 14: 5 mg chewable tablet P.O. daily in the evening.
Children ages 2 to 5: 4 mg chewable tablet P.O. or one packet of 4-mg oral granules daily in the evening.
▶ **Asthma.** *Children ages 12 to 23 months:* One packet of 4-mg granules P.O. daily in the evening.
▶ **Perennial allergic rhinitis in children.** *Children 6 to 23 months:* One packet of 4-mg granules P.O. daily in the evening.
▶ **Prevention of exercise-induced bronchospasm‡.** *Adults and children age 15 and older:* 10 mg P.O. daily.
Children ages 6 to 14: 5 mg P.O. daily.

Contraindications and cautions
• Contraindicated in patients hypersensitive to the drug or any of its components and in patients with acute asthmatic attacks or status asthmaticus.
• Use cautiously and with appropriate monitoring when systemic corticosteroid dosages are reduced.
Lifespan: In children younger than age 6 months, safety and effectiveness haven't been established.

Adverse reactions
CNS: *headache,* dizziness, fatigue, fever, asthenia.
EENT: nasal congestion.
GI: dyspepsia, infectious gastroenteritis, abdominal pain.
GU: pyuria.
Respiratory: cough.
Skin: rash.
Other: trauma, influenza, dental pain.

Interactions

Drug-drug. *Phenobarbital, rifampin:* May decrease bioavailability of montelukast by inducing hepatic metabolism. Monitor patient closely for decreased effects.

Effects on lab test results

• May increase ALT and AST levels.

Pharmacokinetics

Absorption: Rapid with an oral bioavailability of 64% in adults without regard to meals.
Distribution: More than 99% bound to plasma proteins.
Metabolism: Extensive, by cytochrome P isoenzymes in GI tract.
Excretion: About 86% in the feces. *Half-life:* 2¾ to 5½ hours.

Route	Onset	Peak	Duration
P.O.			
chewable	Unknown	2–2½ hr	24 hr
coated	Unknown	3–4 hr	24 hr
granules	Unknown	2 hr	24 hr

Action

Chemical effect: Inhibits action of cysteinyl leukotriene₁ (CysLT₁) receptor by binding with CysLT₁. This reduces early- and late-phase bronchoconstriction caused by antigen challenge.
Therapeutic effect: Improves breathing.

Available forms

Granules: 4-mg packet
Tablets (chewable): 4 mg, 5 mg
Tablets (film-coated): 10 mg

NURSING PROCESS

Assessment
• Assess patient's underlying condition before therapy and regularly thereafter to monitor the drug's effectiveness.
• Monitor patient for adverse reactions and drug interactions.
• Assess patient's and family's knowledge of drug therapy.

Nursing diagnoses
• Impaired gas exchange related to asthma
• Activity intolerance related to asthma
• Deficient knowledge related to drug therapy

Planning and implementation
• Don't abruptly substitute drug for inhaled or oral corticosteroids.
• Drug isn't indicated for patients with acute asthmatic attacks or status asthmaticus. It's also not indicated as monotherapy for managing exercise-induced bronchospasm. Continue rescue drug for acute exacerbations.
• Give oral granules directly in mouth or mixed with a teaspoonful of cold or room-temperature applesauce, carrots, rice, or ice cream. After opening packet, give within 15 minutes. If mixed with food, don't store excess for future use; discard any unused portion.
• Don't dissolve oral granules in liquid, but liquids may be given afterwards.
• Don't give oral granules with high-fat meals.
• Give drug daily in the evening for asthma or asthma with allergic rhinitis; in the morning, give only for allergic rhinitis.
Patient teaching
• Advise patient not to use drug on an as-needed basis but to take drug daily, even if asymptomatic, and to contact prescriber if asthma isn't well controlled.
• Warn patient not to reduce or stop taking other prescribed antiasthma drugs without prescriber's approval.
• Tell parent the oral granules may be given directly into the child's mouth, dissolved in 1 tsp of cold or room temperature baby formula or breast milk, or mixed in a spoonful of applesauce, carrots, rice, or ice cream.
• Warn patient that drug isn't beneficial in acute asthma attacks or in exercise-induced bronchospasm, and advise him to keep appropriate rescue drugs available.
• Advise patient with known aspirin sensitivity to continue not to use aspirin or other NSAIDs.
• Advise patient with phenylketonuria that chewable tablet contains phenylalanine.

Evaluation
• Patient's respiratory signs and symptoms improve.
• Patient can perform normal activities of daily living.
• Patient and family state understanding of drug therapy.

moricizine hydrochloride
(MOR-ih-sigh-zeen high-droh-KLOR-ighd)
Ethmozine

Pharmacologic class: sodium channel blocker
Therapeutic class: antiarrhythmic
Pregnancy risk category: B

Indications and dosages

▶ **Life-threatening ventricular arrhythmias.**
Adults: Individualized dosage is based on response and patient tolerance. Begin therapy in hospital. Most patients respond to 600 to 900 mg P.O. daily in divided doses q 8 hours. Increase daily dosage within this range q 3 days by 150 mg until desired effect is achieved.
◙ **Adjust-a-dose:** For patients with hepatic or renal impairment, give 600 mg or less P.O. daily. Monitor ECG before increasing dosage.

Contraindications and cautions

• Contraindicated in patients hypersensitive to the drug or any of its components, in patients with second- or third-degree AV block or right bundle-branch heart block when linked to left hemiblock (bifascicular block) unless artificial pacemaker is present, and in patients with cardiogenic shock.
• Use cautiously in patients with sick sinus syndrome because drug may cause sinus bradycardia or sinus arrest. Also use cautiously in patients with coronary artery disease and left ventricular dysfunction because these patients may be at risk for sudden death when treated with drug.
• Give cautiously to patients with hepatic or renal impairment.
⚜ **Lifespan:** In pregnant and breast-feeding women use only if benefits outweigh risks to fetus and infant; drug does appear in breast milk. In children, safety and effectiveness haven't been established.

Adverse reactions

CNS: *dizziness, headache, fatigue,* anxiety, hypoesthesia, asthenia, nervousness, paresthesia, sleep disorders.
CV: *ventricular tachycardia, PVCs, supraventricular arrhythmias,* ECG abnormalities, AV block, *heart failure,* palpitations, *cardiac death,* chest pain.

EENT: blurred vision.
GI: nausea, vomiting, abdominal pain, dyspepsia, diarrhea, dry mouth.
GU: urine retention, urinary frequency, dysuria.
Musculoskeletal: muscle pain.
Respiratory: dyspnea.
Skin: diaphoresis, rash.
Other: drug-induced fever.

Interactions

Drug-drug. *Cimetidine:* Increases levels and decreases clearance of moricizine. Begin moricizine therapy at low dosage (not more than 600 mg daily) and monitor therapeutic effect and signs of toxicity closely.
Digoxin, propranolol: May cause additive prolongation of PR interval, but does not increase incidence of second or third degree heart block. Monitor patient closely; monitor ECG.
Theophylline: Increases clearance and reduces levels of theophylline. Monitor levels and therapeutic response; adjust theophylline dosage.

Effects on lab test results

None reported.

Pharmacokinetics

Absorption: Using within 30 minutes of a meal delays absorption and lowers peak levels but has no effect on extent.
Distribution: 95% protein-bound.
Metabolism: Significant in first-pass.
Excretion: 50% in feces; 39% excreted in urine. *Half-life:* 1½ to 3½ hours.

Route	Onset	Peak	Duration
P.O.	≤ 2 hr	30 min–2 hr	10–24 hr

Action

Chemical effect: Reduces fast inward current carried by sodium ions across myocardial cell membranes. Stabilizes membranes.
Therapeutic effect: Reduces risk of recurrence of ventricular arrhythmias.

Available forms

Tablets: 200 mg, 250 mg, 300 mg

Reactions may be *common,* uncommon, *life-threatening,* or COMMON AND LIFE-THREATENING.

NURSING PROCESS

⚖ Assessment
• Assess patient's condition before therapy and regularly thereafter to monitor the drug's effectiveness.
• Be alert for adverse reactions and drug interactions.
• Assess patient's and family's knowledge of drug therapy.

⊞ Nursing diagnoses
• Decreased cardiac output related to presence of ventricular arrhythmia
• Risk for injury related to drug-induced adverse reactions
• Deficient knowledge related to drug therapy

⊠ Planning and implementation
• When substituting this drug for another antiarrhythmic, stop giving previous drug for one or two of drug's half-lives before giving this drug. When stopping or adjusting drug, hospitalize patient with tendency to develop life-threatening arrhythmias after stopping the drug. Start this drug as follows: 6 to 12 hours after last dose of disopyramide; 8 to 12 hours after last dose of mexiletine; 3 to 6 hours after last dose of procainamide; 8 to 12 hours after last dose of propafenone; 6 to 12 hours after last dose of quinidine; 8 to 12 hours after last dose of tocainide.
• Obtain electrolyte levels and correct imbalances before therapy. Hypokalemia, hyperkalemia, and hypomagnesemia may alter effects of drug.
ⓈALERT: Don't confuse Ethmozine with Erythrocin.
Patient teaching
• Tell patient to promptly report adverse reactions.

☑ Evaluation
• Patient regains normal cardiac output with alleviation of ventricular arrhythmia.
• Patient sustains no injury from adverse reactions.
• Patient and family state understanding of drug therapy.

morphine hydrochloride
(MOR-feen high-droh-KLOR-ighd)
M.O.S. ♦, M.O.S.-SR ♦

morphine sulfate
Astramorph PF, Avinza, DepoDur, DMS Concentrate, Duramorph PF, Infumorph 200, Infumorph 500, Kadian, Morphine H.P. ♦, MS Contin, MSIR, MS/L, MS/L Concentrate, OMS Concentrate, Oramorph SR, RMS Uniserts, Roxanol, Roxanol 100, Roxanol T, Statex ♦

morphine tartrate ◊

Pharmacologic class: opioid agonist
Therapeutic class: analgesic
Pregnancy risk category: C
Controlled substance schedule: II

Indications and dosages

▶ **Severe pain.** *Adults:* 5 to 20 mg/70 kg subcutaneously or I.M. q 4 hours, p.r.n. Or 2 to 10 mg/70 kg I.V. q 4 hours, p.r.n. Or 10 to 30 mg P.O. q 4 hours, p.r.n. Or, 10 to 20 mg P.R. q 4 hours, p.r.n. Or 15 to 30 mg of controlled-release tablets P.O. q 8 to 12 hours. Or 5 mg of epidural injection by epidural catheter. Maximum total epidural dose, 10 mg. If adequate pain relief not obtained within 1 hour, give additional doses of 1 to 2 mg at intervals sufficient to assess effectiveness.
Children: 0.1 to 0.2 mg/kg I.M. or subcutaneously q 4 hours, p.r.n. Maximum single dose is 15 mg. Or, 0.05 to 0.1 mg/kg by slow I.V. injection.
▶ **Moderate to severe pain requiring continuous, around-the-clock opioid.** *Adults:* Give loading dose of 15 mg or more by continuous I.V. infusion; then continuous infusion (concentration of 1 mg/ml) of 0.8 to 80 mg/hour. Or individualize dosage of Avinza according to patient's previous drug schedule.
Children: Give 0.025 to 2.6 mg/kg/hour by I.V. infusion.
▶ **Pain following major surgery.** *Adults:* Inject 10 to 15 mg DepoDur (maximum 20 mg) by lumbar epidural administration into lumbar epidural space before surgery or after clamping of umbilical cord during cesarean delivery. Inject undiluted or dilute up to 5 ml total volume

M

with preservative-free normal saline solution. Don't mix with other drugs. Don't give other drugs into epidural space for at least 48 hours.

▼ I.V. administration

• Drug is compatible with most common I.V. solutions.
• For direct injection, dilute 2.5 to 15 mg in 4 or 5 ml of sterile water for injection and give over 4 to 5 minutes.
• For continuous infusion, mix with D_5W to yield 0.1 to 1 mg/ml.
⊗ **Incompatibilities**
Aminophylline, amobarbital, cefepime, chlorothiazide, fluorouracil, haloperidol, heparin sodium, meperidine, pentobarbital, phenobarbital sodium, phenytoin sodium, prochlorperazine, promethazine hydrochloride, sodium bicarbonate, thiopental.

Contraindications and cautions

• Contraindicated in patients hypersensitive to the drug or any of its components and in those with conditions that preclude I.V. administration of opioids (acute bronchial asthma or upper airway obstruction).
• Use cautiously in debilitated patients and in patients with head injury, increased intracranial pressure, seizures, chronic pulmonary disease, prostatic hyperplasia, severe hepatic or renal disease, acute abdominal conditions, hypothyroidism, Addison's disease, or urethral stricture.
❧ **Lifespan:** In pregnant women, use cautiously. In breast-feeding women, wait 2 to 3 hours after last dose before breast-feeding to avoid sedation in infant. In elderly patients, use cautiously.

Adverse reactions

CNS: *sedation, somnolence, clouded sensorium, euphoria, **seizures,** dizziness, nightmares.*
CV: *hypotension, flushing, **bradycardia, shock, cardiac arrest.***
GI: *nausea, vomiting, constipation, ileus.*
GU: *urine retention.*
Hematologic: *thrombocytopenia.*
Respiratory: *respiratory depression, respiratory arrest.*
Skin: *pruritus and flushing.*
Other: *physical dependence.*

Interactions

Drug-drug. *Antihistamines, chloral hydrate, CNS depressants, general anesthetics,*

glutethimide, hypnotics, MAO inhibitors, methocarbamol, other opioid analgesics, sedatives, tranquilizers, tricyclic antidepressants: May cause respiratory depression, hypotension, profound sedation, or coma. Use cautiously. Reduce morphine dosage, and monitor patient.
Drug-lifestyle. *Alcohol use:* May have additive CNS effects. Also, use with Avinza and Kadian may compromise the extended-release capsule characteristics and cause a life-threatening dose of morphine to be released. Urge patient to avoid using alcohol during drug therapy.

Effects on lab test results

• May increase amylase level.
• May decrease platelet count.

Pharmacokinetics

Absorption: Variable when given P.O.; unknown for other routes.
Distribution: Wide.
Metabolism: Primarily in liver.
Excretion: In urine and bile. *Half-life:* 2 to 3 hours.

Route	Onset	Peak	Duration
P.O.	1 hr	1–2 hr	4–12 hr
I.V.	< 5 min	20 min	4–5 hr
I.M.	10–30 min	30–60 min	4–5 hr
SubQ	10–30 min	50–90 min	4–5 hr
P.R.	20–60 min	20–60 min	4–5 hr
Epidural	15–60 min	15–60 min	24 hr
Intrathecal	15–60 min	Unknown	24 hr

Action

Chemical effect: Binds with opioid receptors in CNS, altering both perception of and emotional response to pain through unknown mechanism.
Therapeutic effect: Relieves pain.

Available forms

morphine hydrochloride ◆
Oral solution ◆ : 1 mg/ml, 5 mg/ml, 10 mg/ml, 20 mg/ml, 50 mg/ml
Suppositories ◆ : 10 mg, 20 mg, 30 mg
Syrup ◆ : 1 mg/ml, 5 mg/ml, 10 mg/ml, 20 mg/ml, 50 mg/ml
Tablets ◆ : 10 mg, 20 mg, 40 mg, 60 mg
Tablets (extended-release) ◆ : 30 mg, 60 mg
morphine sulfate
Capsules: 15 mg, 30 mg

Capsules (extended-release beads) (Avinza): 30 mg, 60 mg, 90 mg, 120 mg
Capsules (sustained-release pellets) (Kadian): 20 mg, 30 mg, 50 mg, 60 mg, 100 mg
Injection (with preservative): 1 mg/ml, 2 mg/ml, 4 mg/ml, 5 mg/ml, 8 mg/ml, 10 mg/ml, 15 mg/ml, 25 mg/ml, 50 mg/ml
Injection (without preservative): 0.5 mg/ml, 1 mg/ml, 10 mg/ml, 15 mg/ml, 25 mg/ml, 50 mg/ml
Liposomal injection (preservative-free): 10 mg/ml, 15 mg/1.5 ml, 20 mg/2 ml
Oral solution: 10 mg/5 ml, 20 mg/5 ml
Oral solution (concentrated): 20 mg/ml, 100 mg/5 ml
Soluble tablets: 10 mg, 15 mg, 30 mg
Suppositories: 5 mg, 10 mg, 20 mg, 30 mg
Tablets: 15 mg, 30 mg.
Tablets (extended-release): 15 mg, 30 mg, 60 mg, 100 mg, 200 mg
Tablets (sustained-release): 15 mg, 30 mg, 60 mg, 100 mg, 200 mg
morphine tartrate ◊
Injection: 80 mg/ml ◊

NURSING PROCESS

🔬 Assessment

• Assess patient's pain before therapy and regularly thereafter to monitor drug's effectiveness.
• Drug may worsen or mask gallbladder pain.
• Monitor patient for respiratory depression after administration. When given epidurally, monitor patient for up to 24 hours after injection. Check respiratory rate and depth q 30 to 60 minutes for 24 hours.
• Frequently assess for constipation; adjust GI drugs as needed when increasing morphine dose.
• Be alert for adverse reactions and drug interactions.
• Assess patient's and family's knowledge of drug therapy.

🔲 Nursing diagnoses

• Acute pain related to underlying condition
• Ineffective breathing pattern related to drug's depressive effect on respiratory system
• Deficient knowledge related to drug therapy

▷ Planning and implementation

• Preservative-free preparations are available for giving by epidural or intrathecal route.

🟢 **ALERT:** Highly concentrated injections containing 10 or 25 mg/ml are meant for continuous, controlled microinfusion devices. Don't use for I.M., subcutaneous, I.V epidural, or intrathecal individual doses because of the risk of substantial overdose.
• Solutions of various strengths are available as well as concentrated P.O. solutions (20 mg/ml, 100 mg/5 ml). Double-check the orders written against the strength you are giving carefully. Serious events and fatalities may occur from dispensing and using wrong concentrations.
• Don't crush or break extended- or sustained-release tablets.
• For use with gastrostomy tube, immediately give opened Kadian capsule pellets in 10 ml water, swirling them into prewetted gastrostomy tube. Flush with additional water to clear all pellets; don't use in NG tube and don't crush pellets.
• May open controlled-release capsules and sprinkle beads or pellets onto small amount of applesauce for immediate use P.O. Follow with 4 to 8 oz water.
• Store DepoDur in refrigerator. Unopened vials can be stored at room temperature for up to 7 days. After withdrawn from vial, drug can be stored at room temperature for up to 4 hours before use.
• No need to refrigerate rectal suppositories.
• If using S.L., measure solution with tuberculin syringe. Give dose a few drops at a time to maximize S.L. absorption and minimize swallowing.
• In some patients, P.R. and P.O. absorption may not be equivalent.
• Morphine is drug of choice in relieving pain of MI. It may cause transient decrease in blood pressure.
• Keep opioid antagonist and resuscitation equipment available.
• Around-the-clock therapy best manages severe, chronic pain.

🟢 **ALERT:** If respiratory rate is below 12 breaths/minute except in terminal conditions, don't give the dose. Notify prescriber.
• Because constipation is often severe with maintenance dose, give stool softener or other laxative.

🟢 **ALERT:** Don't confuse morphine with hydromorphone. Don't confuse Avinza with Invanz.
🟢 **ALERT:** Dose of Kadian is not bioequivalent to other controlled-release formulations. Therefore, observe patient carefully for oversedation

M

or inadequate analgesia, and adjust dosage or time interval accordingly.

Patient teaching

• Teach patient use of standardized pain-rating scale to facilitate communication about analgesic effectiveness.

③ **ALERT:** Consuming alcoholic beverages or drugs containing alcohol while taking Avinza may cause extended-release coating to fail, releasing a potentially fatal dose of morphine. Warn patient against the use of alcohol in any form, and stress need to read labels on OTC products carefully.

• Warn patient about getting out of bed or walking without assistance. Warn outpatient not to drive or perform other hazardous activities until the drug's CNS effects are known.

• Tell patient to report continued pain and not to increase dose independently.

• Instruct patient to keep opioids locked safely out of reach of children or cognitively impaired individuals.

• Instruct patient not to use alcohol during therapy.

☒ **Evaluation**

• Patient states that pain is relieved.

• Patient maintains adequate breathing patterns throughout therapy.

• Patient and family state understanding of drug therapy.

---

moxifloxacin hydrochloride
(mox-ih-FLOX-uh-sin high-droh-CLOR-ighd)
Avelox, Avelox I.V.

Pharmacologic class: fluoroquinolone
Therapeutic class: antibiotic
Pregnancy risk category: C

Indications and dosages

▶ **Acute bacterial sinusitis caused by** *Streptococcus pneumoniae, Haemophilus influenzae,* or *Moraxella catarrhalis. Adults:* 400 mg P.O. or I.V. once daily for 10 days.

▶ **Acute bacterial exacerbation of chronic bronchitis caused by** *S. pneumoniae, H. influenzae, H. parainfluenzae, Klebsiella pneumoniae, Staphylococcus aureus,* or *M. catarrhalis. Adults:* 400 mg P.O. or I.V. once daily for 5 days.

▶ **Community-acquired pneumonia caused by multidrug resistant** *Streptococcus pneumoniae* **(resistance to two or more of the following antibiotics: penicillin, second-generation cephalosporins, macrolides, tetracyclines, trimethoprim and sulfamethoxazole),** *Chlamydia pneumoniae, Haemophilus influenzae, Klebsiella pneumoniae, Mycoplasma pneumoniae, Moraxella catarrhalis,* or *Staphylococcus aureus. Adults:* 400 mg P.O. or I.V. once daily for 7 to 14 days.

▶ **Uncomplicated skin and skin-structure infections caused by** *S. aureus* **and** *Streptococcus pyogenes. Adults:* 400 mg P.O daily for 7 days.

▶ **Complicated skin and skin structure infections caused by methicillin-susceptible** *Staphylococcus aureus, Escherichia coli, Klebsiella pneumoniae,* or *Enterobacter cloacae. Adults:* 400 mg P.O. or I.V. q 24 hours for 7 to 21 days.

▶ **Complicated intra-abdominal infections caused by** *Escherichia coli, Bacteroides fragilis, Streptococcus anginosis, S. constellatus, Enterococcus faecalis, Proteus mirabilis, Clostridium perfringens, Bacteroides thetaiotaomicrom,* or *Peptostreptococcus* **species.** *Adults:* 400 mg P.O. or I.V. q 24 hours for 5 to 14 days. Therapy usually begins with the I.V. formulation.

▼ I.V. administration

• If particulate matter is visible, don't use.

• Flush I.V. line with a compatible solution such as D_5W, normal saline solution, or Ringer's lactate solution before and after use.

• Infuse over 60 minutes by direct infusion or through a Y-type IV infusion set. Avoid rapid infusion or bolus injection.

• Switch from I.V. to P.O. form when warranted.

⊗ **Incompatibilities**
Other I.V. drugs or additives.

Contraindications and cautions

• Contraindicated in patients hypersensitive to drug, any of its components, or other fluoroquinolones.

• Use cautiously in patients with known or suspected CNS disorders and in patients with risk factors that may predispose them to seizures or lower the seizure threshold. Use cautiously in patients with prolonged QT interval or uncorrected hypokalemia.

Reactions may be *common*, uncommon, **life-threatening**, or COMMON AND LIFE-THREATENING.

🜲 **Lifespan:** In pregnant women, breast-feeding women, and children, safety and effectiveness haven't been established. In elderly patients, monitor cardiac function carefully, especially with I.V. form.

Adverse reactions

CNS: dizziness, headache, asthenia, pain, malaise, insomnia, nervousness, anxiety, confusion, somnolence, tremor, vertigo, paresthesia.
CV: *prolonged QT interval,* chest pain, palpitations, tachycardia, hypertension, peripheral edema.
GI: *pseudomembranous colitis,* nausea, diarrhea, abdominal pain, vomiting, dyspepsia, dry mouth, constipation, oral candidiasis, anorexia, stomatitis, glossitis, flatulence, gastrointestinal disorder, taste perversion.
GU: vaginitis, vaginal candidiasis.
Hematologic: *thrombocytosis, thrombocytopenia, leukopenia,* eosinophilia.
Hepatic: liver dysfunction, cholestatic jaundice.
Musculoskeletal: leg pain, back pain, arthralgia, myalgia, tendon rupture.
Respiratory: dyspnea.
Skin: rash (maculopapular, purpuric, pustular), pruritus, sweating, phototoxicity.
Other: candidiasis, *allergic reaction,* injection site reaction.

Interactions

Drug-drug. *Aluminum hydroxide, aluminum-magnesium hydroxide, calcium carbonate, magnesium hydroxide:* May decrease effects of moxifloxacin. Give antacid at least 4 hours before or 8 hours after.
Class IA (quinidine, procainamide) or Class III (amiodarone, sotalol) antiarrhythmics: May enhance adverse CV effects. Avoid using together.
Didanosine, metal cations (such as aluminum, magnesium, iron, zinc), multivitamins: May decrease absorption and lower levels. Give moxifloxacin at least 4 hours before or 8 hours after these drugs.
Drugs known to prolong the QT interval, such as antipsychotics, erythromycin, tricyclic antidepressants: May have an additive effect when combined with these drugs. Avoid using together.
NSAIDs: May increase risk of CNS stimulation and seizures. Don't use together.
Sucralfate: May decrease absorption of moxifloxacin, reducing anti-infective effect. If use together can't be avoided, give at least 6 hours apart.
Warfarin: May enhance anticoagulant effects. Monitor PT and INR closely.
Drug-lifestyle. *Sun exposure:* May cause photosensitivity reactions. Discourage prolonged or unprotected exposure to sunlight or tanning bed use.

Effects on lab test results

• May increase GGT, glucose, amylase, lipid, and LDH levels.
• May increase eosinophil count. May decrease WBC count. May increase or decrease platelet count, PT, and INR.

Pharmacokinetics

Absorption: Good.
Distribution: Wide, about 50% protein-bound.
Metabolism: About 50% to inactive conjugates.
Excretion: About 45% of dose unchanged in urine and feces. *Half-life:* About 12 hours.

Route	Onset	Peak	Duration
P.O., I.V.	Unknown	1–3 hr	24 hr

Action

Chemical effect: Inhibits the enzymes needed for bacterial DNA replication, transcription, repair, and recombination.
Therapeutic effect: Kills susceptible bacteria.

Available forms

Injection (premixed solution): 400 mg
Tablets (film-coated): 400 mg

NURSING PROCESS

🗈 Assessment

• Obtain history of patient's condition before therapy, and reassess regularly to monitor the drug's effectiveness.
• Obtain specimen for culture and sensitivity tests before first dose. Begin therapy pending culture results.
• Monitor patient for hypersensitivity reactions and symptoms of CNS toxicity, including seizures, prolonged QT interval, pseudomembranous colitis, phototoxicity, and tendon rupture.
• Assess patient's and family's knowledge of drug therapy.

M

⊞ Nursing diagnoses

• Infection related to presence of bacteria susceptible to drug
• Risk for injury related to drug-induced adverse reactions
• Deficient knowledge related to drug therapy

⊠ Planning and implementation

• Correct hypokalemia before therapy.
• Give with or without food. Give at same time each day to provide consistent absorption.
• Provide plenty of fluids.
• The most common adverse reactions are nausea, vomiting, stomach pain, diarrhea, dizziness, and headache.
• Store drug at controlled room temperature.
Patient teaching
• Instruct patient to take drug once daily, at the same time each day.
• Tell patient to finish the entire course of therapy, even if symptoms resolve.
• Advise the patient to drink plenty of fluids and to take moxifloxacin 6 hours before or 2 hours after antacids, sucralfate, or products containing iron and zinc.
• Tell patient to avoid hazardous activities, such as driving or operating machinery, until the drug's CNS effects are known.
• Instruct patient to contact prescriber if he experiences adverse effects.

⊠ Evaluation

• Patient is free from infection after drug therapy.
• Patient sustains no injury as a result of drug-induced adverse reactions.
• Patient and family state understanding of drug therapy.

---

moxifloxacin hydrochloride ophthalmic solution

(mocks-ih-FLOCKS-ah-sin high-droe-KLOR-ighd off-THAL-mick suh-LOO-shun)
Vigamox

Pharmacologic class: fluoroquinolone
Therapeutic class: antibiotic
Pregnancy risk category: C

Indications and dosages

▶ **Bacterial conjunctivitis.** *Adults and children age 1 and older:* 1 drop into affected eye t.i.d. for 7 days.

Contraindications and cautions

• Contraindicated in patients hypersensitive to the drug, any of its components, or other fluoroquinolones. Contraindicated in patients with epithelial herpes simplex keratitis, vaccinia, varicella, mycobacterial infections of the eye, fungal diseases of the ocular structure, or use of steroid combinations after uncomplicated removal of a corneal foreign body.
⚕ **Lifespan:** In pregnant women, use only when benefits of therapy outweigh risks to the fetus. In breast-feeding women, use cautiously because it's unknown if the drug appears in breast milk. In children younger than age 1, don't use drug.

Adverse reactions

EENT: conjunctivitis; dry eyes; increased lacrimation; keratitis; ocular hyperemia; ocular discomfort, pain, and pruritus; otitis media; pharyngitis; reduced visual acuity; rhinitis; subconjunctival hemorrhage.
Respiratory: increased cough.
Skin: rash.
Other: infection, fever.

Interactions

None reported.

Effects on lab test results

None reported.

Pharmacokinetics

Absorption: Local.
Distribution: Local tissues and plasma 1,000 to 1,600 times less than oral doses.
Metabolism: Unknown.
Excretion: In urine and bile. *Half-life:* 13 hours.

Route	Onset	Peak	Duration
Ocular	Immediate	Unknown	Unknown

Action

Chemical effect: Inhibits DNA gyrase and topoisomerase IV, preventing cell replication, transcription, repair of bacterial DNA, and cell division.

Reactions may be *common,* uncommon, *life-threatening*, or COMMON AND LIFE-THREATENING.

Therapeutic effect: Kills susceptible bacteria causing infection.

Available forms

Solution: 0.5%

NURSING PROCESS

⚕ Assessment

• Assess patient's allergy history before therapy.
• Monitor patient for superinfection, particularly with repeated use.
• Monitor patient for adverse reactions.
• Assess patient's and family's knowledge of drug therapy.

⊕ Nursing diagnoses

• Infection related to presence of bacteria susceptible to drug
• Disturbed visual sensory perception related to adverse effects of the drug
• Deficient knowledge related to drug therapy

▶ Planning and implementation

• Don't inject solution subconjunctivally, or into the eye's anterior chamber.
• Drug has caused serious hypersensitivity reactions; if patient has an allergic reaction, stop giving the drug and treat symptoms.
Patient teaching
• Tell patient to stop taking the drug and immediately seek medical treatment if he develops an allergic reaction (itching, rash, swelling of the face or throat, or difficulty breathing).
• Tell patient not to wear contact lenses during therapy.
• Instruct patient not to touch dropper tip to anything, including eyes and fingers.

☑ Evaluation

• Patient is free from infection after drug therapy.
• Patient doesn't experience adverse drug effects.
• Patient and family state understanding of drug therapy.

muromonab-CD3
(myoo-roh-MOH-nab see dee three)
Orthoclone OKT*3

Pharmacologic class: monoclonal antibody
Therapeutic class: immunosuppressive
Pregnancy risk category: C

Indications and dosages

▶ **Acute allograft rejection in heart, liver, or kidney transplant.** *Adults:* 5 mg I.V. daily for 10 to 14 days.
Children: Initially, 2.5 mg/day (if 30 kg or less) or 5 mg/day (if more than 30 kg) I.V. as a single bolus over less than 1 minute for 10 to 14 days. Increase daily dosage in 2.5 mg increments to decrease CD3-positive cells.

▽ I.V. administration

• Don't give by infusion.
• Draw solution into syringe through low–protein-binding 0.2- or 0.22-micron filter. Discard filter and attach needle for bolus injection.
• Give bolus over less than 1 minute.
• Store drug in the refrigerator at 2° to 8° C (36° to 46° F). Do not freeze.
⊗ **Incompatibilities**
Other I.V. drugs.

Contraindications and cautions

• Contraindicated in patients hypersensitive to the drug or to other products of murine origin. Also contraindicated in patients who have anti-mouse antibody titers of 1:1,000 or more; who have fluid overload, as evidenced by chest X-ray or weight gain greater than 3% in the week before therapy; and who have history of or predisposition to seizures.
⚞ **Lifespan:** In pregnant and breast-feeding women, drug is contraindicated. In children, safety and effectiveness haven't been established.

Adverse reactions

CNS: *asthenia,* fatigue, lethargy, malaise, *fever, seizures,* dizziness, *headache,* **meningitis,** *tremor,* confusion, depression, nervousness, somnolence.
CV: vasodilation, **arrhythmia, bradycardia,** hypertension, hypotension, chest pain, tachycardia, **vascular occlusion,** edema.

M

EENT: photophobia, tinnitus.
GI: anorexia, *diarrhea, nausea,* abdominal pain, GI pain, *vomiting.*
GU: *renal dysfunction.*
Hematologic: anemia, *leukocytosis, leukopenia, thrombocytopenia.*
Musculoskeletal: arthralgia, myalgia.
Respiratory: *dyspnea,* hyperventilation, *hypoxia,* pneumonia, *pulmonary edema,* respiratory congestion, wheezing, *acute respiratory distress syndrome.*
Skin: diaphoresis, pruritus, *rash.*
Other: chills, pain in trunk area, *cytokine release syndrome, hypersensitivity reactions.*

Interactions

Drug-drug. *Immunosuppressants:* Increases risk of infection. Monitor patient closely.
Indomethacin: May increase muromonab-CD3 levels with CNS effects, including encephalopathy. Monitor patient closely.
Live-virus vaccines: May increase replication and effects of vaccine. Postpone vaccination when possible and consult prescriber.

Effects on lab test results

• May increase BUN and creatinine levels. May decrease hemoglobin level and hematocrit.
• May decrease platelet count. May may increase or decrease WBC count.

Pharmacokinetics

Absorption: Administered I.V.
Distribution: Unknown.
Metabolism: Unknown.
Excretion: Unknown. *Half-life:* Unknown.

Route	Onset	Peak	Duration
I.V.	Immediately	Unknown	1 wk after therapy

Action

Chemical effect: Reacts in T-lymphocyte membrane with CD3 needed for antigen recognition and depletes blood of CD3-positive T cells.
Therapeutic effect: Halts acute allograft rejection in kidney transplantation.

Available forms

Injection: 1 mg/ml in 5-ml ampules

NURSING PROCESS

🜚 Assessment
• Assess patient's condition before therapy and regularly thereafter to monitor the drug's effectiveness.
• Obtain chest X-ray within 24 hours before drug therapy.
• Assess patient for signs of fluid overload before therapy.
• Be alert for adverse reactions and drug interactions.
• If patient has an adverse GI reaction, monitor his hydration.
• Assess patient's and family's knowledge of drug therapy.

🜚 Nursing diagnoses
• Risk for injury related to presence of acute allograft rejection
• Risk for deficient fluid volume related to drug-induced adverse GI reactions
• Deficient knowledge related to drug therapy

⟫ Planning and implementation
• Begin therapy in facility equipped and staffed for cardiopulmonary resuscitation where patient can be closely monitored.
• Most adverse reactions develop within 30 minutes to 6 hours after first dose.
• **ALERT:** Give antipyretic before giving drug to lower risk of expected pyrexia and chills. It is recommended that methylprednisolone sodium succinate 8 mg/kg be administered I.V. 1 to 4 hours before initial dose of muromonab-CD3 to reduce the risk for and severity of cytokine release syndrome.
• If second course of therapy is attempted, patient may develop antibodies to drug that can lead to loss of effectiveness and more severe adverse reactions; use for one course of therapy only.

Patient teaching
• Inform patient of expected adverse reactions, and reassure him that they will lessen as therapy progresses.

☑ Evaluation
• Patient shows no signs of organ rejection.
• Patient maintains adequate hydration.
• Patient and family state understanding of drug therapy.

---

mycophenolate mofetil
(migh-koh-FEN-oh-layt MOH-feh-til)
CellCept

mycophenolate mofetil hydrochloride
CellCept Intravenous

Pharmacologic class: mycophenolic acid derivative
Therapeutic class: immunosuppressant
Pregnancy risk category: C

Indications and dosages

▶ **Prevention of organ rejection in patients receiving allogenic renal transplant.** *Adults:* 1 g I.V. infused over 2 hours b.i.d. with cyclosporine and corticosteroids. Begin I.V. infusion within 24 hours after transplantation. For oral use, give 1 g P.O. b.i.d. as soon as possible after surgery.
Children age 1 and older: 600 mg/m² oral suspension P.O. b.i.d. up to a maximum daily dosage of 2 g/10 ml. Or give child with 1.25 m² to 1.5 m² body surface area 750 mg capsules P.O. b.i.d. Give child with a greater than 1.5 m² body surface area 1 g P.O. tablets or capsules b.i.d. For oral use, give as soon as possible after surgery.
🛇 **Adjust-a-dose:** For patients with renal impairment, if GFR is less than 25 ml/minute/1.73 m² outside the immediate post-transplant period, avoid doses above 1 g b.i.d. If neutropenia develops, interrupt or reduce dose.
▶ **Prevention of organ rejection in patients receiving allogenic cardiac transplant.** *Adults:* 1.5 g P.O. or I.V. b.i.d. with cyclosporine and corticosteroids.
▶ **Prevention of organ rejection in patients receiving allogenic hepatic transplants.** *Adults:* 1 g I.V. b.i.d. over no less than 2 hours or 1.5 g P.O. b.i.d., with cyclosporine and corticosteroids.
🛇 **Adjust-a-dose:** If neutropenia develops, interrupt or reduce dose.

▼ I.V. administration

• Avoid direct contact with solution.
• Reconstitute under aseptic conditions.
• Reconstitute the contents of each CellCept Intravenous vial with 14 ml of D₅W. Use two vials to prepare a 1-g dose and 3 vials for a 1.5-g dose. Gently shake the vial to dissolve drug.

• For a 1-g dose, dilute 2 vials further into 140 ml of D₅W; for a 1.5-g dose, dilute 3 vials further into 210 ml of 5% dextrose injection. The final concentration of both solutions is 6 mg/ml.
• Never give drug by rapid or bolus I.V. injection. Give infusion over at least 2 hours.
• Use within 4 hours of reconstitution and dilution.
⊗ **Incompatibilities**
• Other I.V. solutions.

Contraindications and cautions

• Contraindicated in patients hypersensitive to the drug or any of its components.
• Use cautiously in patients with GI disorders.
⚖ **Lifespan:** In pregnant and breast-feeding women, use only when benefits outweigh risks to fetus and infant. In children, safety and effectiveness for cardiac and hepatic transplantation haven't been established.

Adverse reactions

CNS: tremor, insomnia, dizziness, headache, pain, fever, asthenia.
CV: *chest pain, hypertension, edema,* tachycardia, peripheral edema.
EENT: pharyngitis.
GI: diarrhea, constipation, nausea, dyspepsia, vomiting, oral candidiasis, abdominal pain, HEMORRHAGE.
GU: UTI, hematuria, kidney tubular necrosis.
Hematologic: anemia, *leukopenia,* THROMBO-CYTOPENIA, hypochromic anemia, leukocytosis.
Metabolic: *hypercholesteremia, hypophosphatemia, hypokalemia, hyperkalemia, hyperglycemia.*
Musculoskeletal: *back pain.*
Respiratory: *dyspnea, cough,* infection, bronchitis, pneumonia.
Skin: *acne,* rash.
Other: infection, *sepsis.*

Interactions

Drug-drug. *Acyclovir, ganciclovir, other drugs known to undergo tubular secretion:* Increases risk of toxicity for both drugs. Monitor patient closely.
Antacids with magnesium and aluminum hydroxides: Decreases absorption of mycophenolate mofetil. Separate administration times.
Azathioprine: Hasn't been studied. Avoid using together.

M

Cholestyramine: May interfere with enterohepatic recirculation, reducing mycophenolate bioavailability. Don't give together.
Hormonal contraceptives: May reduce effectiveness of hormonal contraceptives. Advise patient to use barrier birth control methods.

Effects on lab test results

• May increase cholesterol and glucose levels. May decrease phosphorous and hemoglobin levels and hematocrit. May increase or decrease potassium level.
• May decrease platelet count. May increase or decrease WBC count.

Pharmacokinetics

Absorption: Good.
Distribution: 97% bound to proteins.
Metabolism: Complete, to mycophenolic acid.
Excretion: Primarily in urine, with small amount in feces. *Half-life:* About 18 hours.

Route	Onset	Peak	Duration
P.O.	Unknown	Unknown	Unknown
I.V.	Unknown	Unknown	10–17 hr

Action

Chemical effect: Inhibits proliferative responses of T- and B-lymphocytes, suppresses antibody formation by B-lymphocytes, and may inhibit recruitment of leukocytes into sites of inflammation and graft rejection.
Therapeutic effect: Prevents organ rejection.

Available forms

mycophenolate mofetil
Capsules: 250 mg
Powder for oral suspension (contains aspartame): 200 mg/ml
Tablets: 500 mg
mycophenolate mofetil hydrochloride
Injection: 500 mg/vial

NURSING PROCESS

⚏ Assessment
• Obtain history of patient's kidney transplant.
• Monitor CBC regularly.
• Be alert for adverse reactions and drug interactions.
• Assess patient's and family's knowledge of drug therapy.

⚏ Nursing diagnoses
• Ineffective health maintenance related to need for kidney transplant
• Ineffective immune protection related to drug-induced immunosuppression
• Deficient knowledge related to drug therapy

⚏ Planning and implementation
• Give drug on an empty stomach.
• **⚠ ALERT:** Because of risk of teratogenic effects, don't open or crush capsules. Avoid inhaling powder in capsules or letting it contact skin or mucous membranes. If it does, wash skin thoroughly with soap and water and rinse eyes with plain water.
• If patient develops neutropenia, notify prescriber.
Patient teaching
• Warn patient not to open or crush capsule but to swallow it whole on an empty stomach.
• Stress importance of not interrupting therapy without consulting prescriber.
• Tell woman to do a pregnancy test 1 week before therapy. Tell her to use two forms of contraception simultaneously unless abstinent and to use effective contraception until at least 6 weeks after therapy ends, even if she has a history of infertility (unless she has had a hysterectomy). If patient becomes pregnant, tell her to immediately contact her prescriber.

⚏ Evaluation
• Patient shows no signs and symptoms of organ rejection.
• Neutropenia doesn't develop.
• Patient and family state understanding of drug therapy.

nabumetone
(nuh-BYOO-meh-tohn)
Apo-Nabumetone ♦ , Relafen

Pharmacologic class: NSAID
Therapeutic class: anti-inflammatory, analgesic, antipyretic
Pregnancy risk category: C

Indications and dosages

▶ **Rheumatoid arthritis, osteoarthritis.**
Adults: Initially, 1,000 mg P.O. daily as single dose or in divided doses b.i.d. Maximum dosage, 2,000 mg daily.

Contraindications and cautions

• Contraindicated in patients hypersensitive to the drug or any of its components and in patients with history of aspirin- or NSAID-induced asthma, urticaria, or other allergic reactions.
• Use cautiously in patients with renal or hepatic impairment, peptic ulcer disease, heart failure, hypertension, or other conditions that may predispose patient to fluid retention.
⚠ **Lifespan:** In pregnant and breast-feeding women, only use when benefits outweigh risks to fetus and infant. In children, safety and effectiveness haven't been established. In the elderly, use cautiously because of possible impaired excretion.

Adverse reactions

CNS: *dizziness, headache,* fatigue, insomnia, nervousness, somnolence.
CV: vasculitis, *edema.*
EENT: tinnitus.
GI: diarrhea, dyspepsia, abdominal pain, constipation, flatulence, nausea, dry mouth, gastritis, stomatitis, vomiting, *bleeding,* ulceration.
Respiratory: dyspnea, pneumonitis.
Skin: *pruritus, rash,* increased sweating.

Interactions

Drug-drug. *Diuretics:* NSAIDs may decrease diuretic effectiveness. Monitor patient for effect.
Drugs highly bound to proteins (such as warfarin): Increases risk of adverse effects from displacement of drug by nabumetone. Use together cautiously; monitor patient for adverse effects.
Drug-herb. *Dong quai, feverfew, garlic, ginger, horse chestnut, red clover:* Increases risk of bleeding. Discourage using together.
St. John's wort: Increases risk of photosensitivity. Advise patient to avoid unprotected or prolonged exposure to sunlight.
Drug-food. *Any food:* Increases the rate of absorption. Give together.
Drug-lifestyle. *Alcohol use:* Increases risk of additive GI toxicity. Discourage using together.

Effects on lab test results

None reported.

Pharmacokinetics

Absorption: Good. Use with food increases absorption rate and peak levels of principal metabolite but doesn't change total amount absorbed.
Distribution: More than 99% of metabolite is bound to proteins.
Metabolism: To inactive metabolites in liver.
Excretion: Metabolites primarily in urine; about 9% in feces. *Half-life:* About 24 hours.

Route	Onset	Peak	Duration
P.O.	Unknown	2–4 hr	Unknown

Action

Chemical effect: Unknown; may inhibit prostaglandin synthesis.
Therapeutic effect: Relieves pain.

Available forms

Tablets: 500 mg, 750 mg

NURSING PROCESS

⚚ Assessment

• Assess patient's arthritis before starting therapy and regularly thereafter to monitor the drug's effectiveness.
• During long-term therapy, periodically monitor renal and liver function, CBC, and hematocrit; assess patient for evidence of GI bleeding.
• Watch for fluid retention, especially in a patient with heart failure and hypertension.
• Be alert for adverse reactions and drug interactions.
• Assess patient's and family's knowledge of drug therapy.

⊞ Nursing diagnoses

• Chronic pain related to arthritic condition
• Impaired tissue integrity related to adverse drug effect on GI mucosa
• Deficient knowledge related to drug therapy

▶ Planning and implementation

• Give drug with food to increase absorption rate.
• Notify prescriber about adverse reactions.
⊛ **ALERT:** Don't confuse Relafen with Rifadin.

N

Patient teaching
• Instruct patient to take drug with food, milk, or antacids for best absorption.
• Advise patient to limit alcohol intake because of additive GI toxicity.
• Teach patient to recognize and report signs and symptoms of GI bleeding.

☑ **Evaluation**
• Patient is free from pain.
• Patient's GI tissue integrity is maintained throughout drug therapy.
• Patient and family state understanding of drug therapy.

nadolol
(nay-DOH-lol)
Apo-Nadol ♦ , Corgard

Pharmacologic class: nonselective beta blocker
Therapeutic class: antihypertensive, antianginal
Pregnancy risk category: C

Indications and dosages

▶ **Angina pectoris.** *Adults:* Initially, 40 mg P.O. once daily. Increase in 40- to 80-mg increments q 3 to 7 days until optimum response occurs. Usual maintenance dosage is 40 to 80 mg daily; a maximum dose of 160 or 240 mg may be needed.
▶ **Hypertension.** *Adults:* Initially, 20 to 40 mg P.O. once daily. Increase by 40- to 80-mg increments q 2 to 14 days until optimum response occurs. Usual maintenance dosage is 40 to 80 mg daily; doses up to 240 or 320 mg may be needed.
🔲 **Adjust-a-dose:** In patients with renal impairment, if creatinine clearance is 31 to 50 ml/minute, give q 24 to 36 hours; if 10 to 30 ml/minute, give q 24 to 48 hours; if less than 10 ml/minute, give q 40 to 60 hours.
▶ **Arrhythmias‡.** *Adults:* 60 to 160 mg P.O. daily or in divided doses.
▶ **To prevent vascular headaches‡.** *Adults:* 20 to 40 mg P.O. daily; gradually increase to 120 mg daily, if needed.

Contraindications and cautions

• Contraindicated in patients with bronchial asthma, sinus bradycardia, greater than first-degree heart block, and cardiogenic shock.

• Use cautiously in patients undergoing major surgery involving general anesthesia and in those with heart failure, chronic bronchitis, emphysema, renal or hepatic impairment, or diabetes.
🔥 **Lifespan:** In pregnant women, use only if benefits outweigh risks to the fetus. In breast-feeding women, don't use because it's unknown if drug appears in breast milk. In children, safety and effectiveness haven't been established.

Adverse reactions

CNS: fatigue, lethargy, dizziness, fever.
CV: *bradycardia, hypotension, heart failure,* peripheral vascular disease.
GI: nausea, vomiting, diarrhea, constipation.
Respiratory: *increased airway resistance.*

Interactions

Drug-drug. *Antihypertensives:* May enhance antihypertensive effect. Monitor patient's blood pressure closely.
Digoxin, diltiazem: May cause excessive bradycardia and affect AV conduction. Use together cautiously; monitor ECG.
Epinephrine: May cause an initial hypertensive episode followed by bradycardia. Stop beta blocker 3 days before anticipated epinephrine use. Monitor patient closely.
Insulin: May mask symptoms of hypoglycemia as a result of beta blockade (such as tachycardia). Use cautiously in patients with diabetes.
I.V. lidocaine: May reduce hepatic metabolism of lidocaine increasing the risk of toxicity. Give bolus doses of lidocaine at a slower rate and monitor lidocaine level closely.
NSAIDs: May decrease antihypertensive effect. Monitor blood pressure and adjust dosage.
Oral antidiabetics: May alter dosage requirements in diabetic patients. Monitor glucose level.
Prazosin: May increase the risk of orthostatic hypotension in the early phases of use together. Teach patient to stand slowly until effects are known.
Verapamil: May increase the effects of both drugs. Monitor cardiac function closely for excessive bradycardia and decrease dosage.

Effects on lab test results

None reported.

Pharmacokinetics

Absorption: 30% to 40% without regard to meals.
Distribution: Distributed throughout body; about 30% protein-bound.
Metabolism: None.
Excretion: Most excreted unchanged in urine; remainder in feces. *Half-life:* About 10 to 24 hours.

Route	Onset	Peak	Duration
P.O.	Unknown	2–4 hr	24 hr

Action

Chemical effect: Reduces cardiac oxygen demand by blocking catecholamine-induced increases in heart rate, blood pressure, and myocardial contraction. Depresses renin secretion.
Therapeutic effect: Lowers blood pressure, relieves and prevents recurrence of angina.

Available forms

Tablets: 20 mg, 40 mg, 80 mg, 120 mg, 160 mg

NURSING PROCESS

⏲ Assessment

• Assess patient's condition before starting therapy and regularly thereafter to monitor the drug's effectiveness.
• Drug masks common signs of shock, hyperthyroidism, and hypoglycemia.
• Be alert for adverse reactions and drug interactions.
• Assess patient's and family's knowledge of drug therapy.

⊕ Nursing diagnoses

• Risk for injury related to presence of hypertension
• Acute pain related to angina
• Deficient knowledge related to drug therapy

▷ Planning and implementation

⊛ **ALERT:** Always check apical pulse before giving drug. If slower than 60 beats/minute, don't give the dose. Notify prescriber.
• If patient develops severe hypotension, give vasopressor.
⊛ **ALERT:** Reduce dosage gradually over 1 to 2 weeks. Abruptly stopping the drug can worsen angina and MI.
⊛ **ALERT:** Don't confuse Corgard with Coreg.

Patient teaching

• Explain importance of taking drug as prescribed, even when feeling well.
• Warn patient not to abruptly stop taking the drug.

☑ Evaluation

• Patient's blood pressure is normal.
• Patient reports reduced angina.
• Patient and family state understanding of drug therapy.

nafcillin sodium
(naf-SIL-in SOH-dee-um)

Pharmacologic class: penicillinase-resistant penicillin
Therapeutic class: antibiotic
Pregnancy risk category: B

Indications and dosages

▶ **Systemic infections caused by susceptible organisms (including methicillin-sensitive *Staphylococcus aureus*).** *Adults:* 500 mg to 1 g I.V. q 4 hours depending on severity of the infection.
Infants and children older than age 1 month: 50 to 200 mg/kg I.V. daily in equally divided doses q 4 to 6 hours depending on the severity of the infection.
Neonates age 7 days or younger who weigh less than 2 kg (4.4 lb): 25 mg/kg I.V. q 12 hours.
Neonates age 7 days or younger who weigh more than 2 kg: 25 mg/kg I.V. q 8 hours.
Neonates older than 7 days who weigh less than 2 kg: 25 mg/kg I.V. q 8 hours.
Neonates older than 7 days who weigh more than 2 kg: 25 mg/kg I.V. q 6 hours.
▶ **Meningitis.** *Adults:* 100 to 200 mg/kg I.V. daily in divided doses q 4 to 6 hours.
Neonates age 7 days or younger who weigh less than 2 kg: 50 mg/kg I.V. q 12 hours.
Neonates age 7 days or younger who weigh more than 2 kg: 50 mg/kg I.V. q 8 hours.
Neonates older than 7 days who weigh less than 2 kg: 50 mg/kg I.V. q 8 hours.
Neonates older than 7 days who weigh more than 2 kg: 50 mg/kg I.V. q 6 hours.
▶ **Acute or chronic osteomyelitis caused by susceptible organism.** *Adults:* 1 to 2 g I.V. ⌐ 4 hours for 4 to 8 weeks.

N

Children older than age 1 month: 100 to
200 mg/kg daily in equally divided doses q 4 to
6 hours for 4 to 8 weeks.
▶ **Native valve endocarditis caused by susceptible organisms.** *Adults:* 2 g I.V. q 4 hours
for 4 to 6 weeks with gentamicin.
Children older than age 1 month: 100 to
200 mg/kg daily in equally divided doses q 4 to
6 hours for 4 to 8 weeks with gentamicin.

▽ I.V. administration

• After thawing at room temperature or under
refrigeration, check and discard container with
leaks, cloudiness, or precipitate.
• Give by intermittent I.V. infusion over 30 to
60 minutes.
• Avoid continuous I.V. infusion to avoid vein
irritation.
• Change I.V. site q 48 hours to reduce the risk
of vein irritation.
⊗ **Incompatibilities**
Aminoglycosides, aminophylline, ascorbic acid,
aztreonam, bleomycin, cytarabine, diltiazem,
droperidol, gentamicin, hydrocortisone sodium
succinate, insulin, labetalol, meperidine,
methylprednisolone sodium succinate, midazolam, nalbuphine, pentazocine lactate, promazine, vancomycin, verapamil hydrochloride,
vitamin B complex with C.

Contraindications and cautions

• Contraindicated in patients hypersensitive to
the drug or other penicillins.
• Use cautiously in patients with GI distress and
those with other drug allergies, especially to
cephalosporins.
⚜ **Lifespan:** In pregnant women, use cautiously. In breast-feeding women, use cautiously; it's
unknown if the drug appears in breast milk.

Adverse reactions

CV: thrombophlebitis.
GI: *nausea,* vomiting, diarrhea.
Hematologic: *transient leukopenia, neutrope-
nia, granulocytopenia, thrombocytopenia.*
Other: hypersensitivity reactions, *anaphylaxis,*
vein irritation.

Interactions

Drug-drug. *Aminoglycosides:* May have synergistic effect; may use together for this effect.
Monitor patient closely.

Cyclosporine: May cause subtherapeutic cyclosporine level. Monitor level.
Probenecid: May increase level of nafcillin.
Probenecid may be used for this purpose.
Rifampin: May cause dose-dependent antagonism. Monitor patient closely.
Warfarin: May increase risk of bleeding when
used with I.V. nafcillin. Monitor patient for
bleeding.

Effects on lab test results

• May decrease neutrophil, granulocyte, WBC,
and platelet counts.
• May falsely elevate urine or serum proteins or
cause false-positive results in certain tests for
them.

Pharmacokinetics

Absorption: Administered I.V.
Distribution: Wide. CSF penetration is poor
but enhanced by meningeal inflammation. Drug
is 70% to 90% protein-bound.
Metabolism: Metabolized primarily in liver;
undergoes enterohepatic circulation.
Excretion: Excreted primarily in bile; 25% to
30% is excreted in urine unchanged. *Half-life:*
30 to 90 minutes.

Route	Onset	Peak	Duration
I.V.	Immediate	Immediate	Unknown

Action

Chemical effect: Inhibits cell wall synthesis
during microorganism multiplication; resists
bacteria-produced penicillinases.
Therapeutic effect: Kills susceptible bacteria,
such as penicillinase-producing staphylococci,
and some gram-positive aerobic and anaerobic
bacilli.

Available forms

Injection: 1 g, 2 g

NURSING PROCESS

🗷 Assessment

• Assess patient's infection before starting therapy and regularly thereafter to monitor the
drug's effectiveness.
• Before giving drug, ask patient about allergic
reactions to penicillins and cephalosporins. Remember that allergic reactions may occur even
in patients with no history of penicillin allergy.

• Obtain specimen for culture and sensitivity tests before giving first dose. Begin therapy pending results.

⑤ ALERT: Monitor WBC counts twice weekly in patients receiving nafcillin for longer than 2 weeks. Neutropenia commonly occurs in the third week.

• Be alert for adverse reactions and drug interactions.

• If patient has an adverse GI reaction, monitor his hydration.

• Assess patient's and family's knowledge of drug therapy.

⊕ Nursing diagnoses
• Infection related to susceptible bacteria
• Risk for deficient fluid volume related to drug-induced adverse GI reactions
• Deficient knowledge related to drug therapy

⫸ Planning and implementation
• Give drug at least 1 hour before bacteriostatic antibiotics.
• If urinalysis is abnormal, notify prescriber because this may indicate drug-induced interstitial nephritis.
Patient teaching
• Tell patient to notify prescriber if rash, fever, or chills develop.
• Instruct patient to report pain, burning, edema, or redness at I.V. site.

☑ Evaluation
• Patient is free from infection.
• Patient maintains adequate hydration throughout drug therapy.
• Patient and family state understanding of drug therapy.

nalbuphine hydrochloride
(NAL-byoo-feen high-droh-KLOR-ighd)
Nubain

Pharmacologic class: synthetic opioid partial agonist/antagonist
Therapeutic class: analgesic, adjunct to anesthesia
Pregnancy risk category: B

Indications and dosages
▶ Moderate to severe pain. *Adults:* For patient who weighs about 70 kg (154 lb), give 10 to 20 mg I.V., I.M., or subcutaneously q 3 to 6 hours, p.r.n. Maximum daily dosage is 160 mg.
▶ Adjunct in balanced anesthesia. *Adults:* 0.3 mg/kg to 3 mg/kg I.V. over 10 to 15 minutes, followed by maintenance doses of 0.25 to 0.5 mg/kg in single I.V. doses p.r.n.

▼ I.V. administration
• Keep resuscitation equipment available.
• Inject slowly over at least 2 minutes into vein or into line containing compatible, free-flowing solution, such as D_5W, normal saline solution, or lactated Ringer's solution.
• Respiratory depression can be reversed with naloxone.
⊗ Incompatibilities
Allopurinol, amphotericin B, cefepime, diazepam, docetaxel, ketorolac, methotrexate sodium, nafcillin, pentobarbital sodium, piperacillin and tazobactam sodium, promethazine, sargramostim, sodium bicarbonate, thiethylperazine.

Contraindications and cautions
• Contraindicated in patients hypersensitive to the drug or sulfites present in some preparations of drug.
• Use cautiously in substance abusers and in those with emotional instability, head injury, increased intracranial pressure, impaired ventilation, MI accompanied by nausea and vomiting, upcoming biliary surgery, and hepatic or renal disease.
⚘ Lifespan: In pregnant women, use cautiously. In breast-feeding women, use cautiously because it's unknown if drug appears in breast milk. In children, safety and effectiveness haven't been established.

Adverse reactions
CNS: headache, *sedation,* dizziness, vertigo, nervousness, depression, restlessness, crying, euphoria, hostility, unusual dreams, confusion, hallucinations, speech difficulty, delusions.
CV: hypertension, hypotension, tachycardia, *bradycardia.*
EENT: blurred vision.
GI: cramps, dyspepsia, bitter taste, dry mouth, nausea, vomiting, constipation.

N

GU: urinary urgency.
Respiratory: *respiratory depression, pulmonary edema.*
Skin: itching; burning; urticaria; sweaty, clammy feeling.

Interactions

Drug-drug. *CNS depressants, hypnotics, MAO inhibitors, sedatives, tranquilizers, tricyclic antidepressants:* May cause respiratory depression, hypertension, profound sedation, or coma. The dose of one or both drugs may need to be decreased.
General anesthetics: May increase respiratory depression, sedation and coma; may cause hypertension or hypotension.
Opioid analgesics: May decrease analgesic effect and increase withdrawal symptoms. Avoid using together.
Drug-lifestyle. *Alcohol use:* May cause respiratory depression, hypertension, profound sedation, or coma. Discourage using together.

Effects on lab test results

None reported.

Pharmacokinetics

Absorption: Unknown.
Distribution: Not measurably bound to proteins.
Metabolism: In liver.
Excretion: In urine and bile. *Half-life:* 5 hours.

Route	Onset	Peak	Duration
I.V.	2–3 min	≤ 30 min	3–4 hr
I.M.	≤ 15 min	≤ 60 min	3–6 hr
SubQ	≤ 15 min	30–60 min	3–6 hr

Action

Chemical effect: Binds with opioid receptors in CNS, altering pain perception and response to pain by unknown mechanism.
Therapeutic effect: Relieves pain and enhances anesthesia.

Available forms

Injection: 10 mg/ml, 20 mg/ml

NURSING PROCESS

⚖ Assessment
● Assess patient's pain or anesthetic requirement before starting therapy and regularly thereafter to monitor the drug's effectiveness.
● Observe for signs of withdrawal in patient receiving long-term opioid therapy.
● Monitor patient closely for respiratory depression.
● Monitor patient for signs and symptoms of constipation.
● Be alert for adverse reactions and drug interactions.
● Assess patient's and family's knowledge of drug therapy.

⊕ Nursing diagnoses
● Acute pain related to underlying condition
● Disturbed thought processes related to drug's effect on CNS
● Deficient knowledge related to drug therapy

❯ Planning and implementation
● Psychological and physical dependence may occur with prolonged use.
● Drug acts as an opioid antagonist and may precipitate withdrawal syndrome. For patients receiving long-term opioid therapy, start with 25% of usual dose.
● Give stool softener or other laxative to prevent constipation. Encourage patient to drink fluids and eat fiber.
● **ALERT:** If patient's respirations are shallow or rate is below 12 breaths/minute, withhold dose and notify prescriber.
● **ALERT:** Don't confuse Nubain with Navane.
Patient teaching
● Warn ambulatory patient about getting out of bed or walking.
● Instruct outpatient to avoid hazardous activities until the drug's CNS effects are known.

☑ Evaluation
● Patient is free from pain.
● Patient maintains normal thought processes throughout therapy.
● Patient and family state understanding of drug therapy.

naloxone hydrochloride
(nal-OKS-ohn high-droh-KLOR-ighd)
Narcan

Pharmacologic class: opioid antagonist
Therapeutic class: adjunct to opiate cessation
Pregnancy risk category: B

Indications and dosages

▶ **Known or suspected opioid-induced respiratory depression, including that caused by pentazocine and propoxyphene.** *Adults:* 0.4 to 2 mg I.V. May be given I.M. or subcutaneously if I.V. route unavailable. Repeat q 2 to 3 minutes, p.r.n. If no response is observed after 10 mg has been given, reevaluate diagnosis.
▶ **Postoperative reversal of opioid effects.**
Adults: 0.1 to 0.2 mg I.V. q 2 to 3 minutes, p.r.n.
Children: 0.005 to 0.01 mg/kg dose I.V. Repeat q 2 to 3 minutes, p.r.n.
Neonates (asphyxia neonatorum): 0.01 mg/kg I.V. into umbilical vein. May repeat q 2 to 3 minutes until response is obtained.
▶ **Naloxone challenge for diagnosing opiate dependence‡** *Adults:* 0.16 mg I.M. naloxone; if no signs of withdrawal after 20 to 30 minutes, give second dose of 0.24 mg. Test is negative if no withdrawal symptoms within 30 minutes.

▼ I.V. administration

• If 0.02 mg/ml isn't available for neonatal concentration, adult concentration (0.4 mg) may be diluted by mixing 0.5 ml with 9.5 ml of sterile water or saline solution for injection.
• Give continuous I.V. infusion to control adverse effects of epidural morphine.
⊗ **Incompatibilities**
All other I.V. drugs, especially preparations containing bisulfite, sulfite, long-chain or high-molecular-weight anions, or alkaline solutions.

Contraindications and cautions

• Contraindicated in patients hypersensitive to the drug or any of its components.
• Use cautiously in patients with cardiac irritability and opioid addiction. Abrupt reversal of opioid-induced CNS depression may cause nausea, vomiting, diaphoresis, tachycardia, CNS excitement, and increased blood pressure.

⚠ **Lifespan:** In pregnant women, use cautiously. In breast-feeding women, safety and effectiveness haven't been established.

Adverse reactions

CNS: tremors, *seizures.*
CV: tachycardia and hypertension with high doses, *ventricular fibrillation.*
GI: nausea and vomiting with high doses.
Respiratory: *pulmonary edema.*
Other: *withdrawal symptoms.*

Interactions

None significant.

Effects on lab test results

None reported.

Pharmacokinetics

Absorption: Unknown.
Distribution: Rapid.
Metabolism: Rapid.
Excretion: In urine. *Half-life:* 60 to 90 minutes in adults, 3 hours in neonates.

Route	Onset	Peak	Duration
I.V.	1–2 min	Unknown	Varies
I.M., SubQ	2–5 min	Unknown	Varies

Action

Chemical effect: Unknown; may displace opioid analgesics from their receptors (competitive antagonism). Has no pharmacologic activity.
Therapeutic effect: Reverses opioid effects.

Available forms

Injection: 0.02 mg/ml, 0.4 mg/ml, 1 mg/ml

NURSING PROCESS

✐ Assessment
• Assess patient's opioid use before starting therapy, and reassess regularly to monitor the drug's effectiveness.
• Duration of opioid may exceed that of naloxone, causing relapse into respiratory depression. Monitor patient's respiratory depth and rate.
• Patients who receive naloxone to reverse opioid-induced respiratory depression may develop tachypnea.
• If patient has an adverse GI reaction, monitor his hydration.

N

• Assess patient's and family's knowledge of drug therapy.

🔄 Nursing diagnoses
• Ineffective health maintenance related to opioid use
• Risk for deficient fluid volume related to drug-induced adverse GI reactions
• Deficient knowledge related to drug therapy

▷ Planning and implementation
• High doses of drug may cause withdrawal symptoms in opioid dependent patients.
🔵 **ALERT:** Drug is effective only in reversing respiratory depression caused by opioids. Use flumazenil to treat respiratory depression caused by diazepam or other benzodiazepines.
🔵 **ALERT:** Provide oxygen, ventilation, and other resuscitation measures to patient with severe respiratory depression from acute opioid overdose.
🔵 **ALERT:** Don't confuse naloxone with naltrexone.
Patient teaching
• Instruct patient and family to report adverse reactions.

☑ Evaluation
• Patient responds well to drug.
• Patient maintains adequate hydration.
• Patient and family state understanding of drug therapy.

naltrexone hydrochloride
(nal-TREKS-ohn high-droh-KLOR-ighd)
Depade, ReVia

Pharmacologic class: opioid antagonist
Therapeutic class: adjunct in opioid detoxification/cessation
Pregnancy risk category: C

Indications and dosages

▶ **Adjunct in maintaining opioid-free state in detoxified patients.** *Adults:* Initially, 25 mg P.O. If no withdrawal signs occur within 1 hour, additional 25 mg is given. Once patient takes 50 mg q 24 hours, flexible maintenance schedule may be used.
▶ **Alcohol dependence.** *Adults:* 50 mg P.O. once daily for up to 12 weeks.

Contraindications and cautions
• Contraindicated in patients hypersensitive to the drug or any of its components; in those who are receiving opioid analgesics, have a positive urine screen for opioids, or are opioid dependent; in those who have acute opioid withdrawal; and in those with acute hepatitis or liver failure.
• Use cautiously in patients with mild hepatic disease or history of recent hepatic disease.
≋ **Lifespan:** In pregnant women, use cautiously. In breast-feeding women and in children, safety and effectiveness haven't been established.

Adverse reactions
CNS: *insomnia, anxiety, nervousness, headache,* depression, **suicidal ideation.**
GI: *nausea, vomiting,* anorexia, *abdominal pain.*
Hematologic: lymphocytosis.
Hepatic: *hepatotoxicity.*
Musculoskeletal: *muscle and joint pain.*

Interactions
Drug-drug. *Products containing opioids (such as cough and cold and antidiarrheal products):* Decreases response to these products. Recommend using a nonopioid product.
Thioridazine: Increases somnolence and lethargy. Monitor patient closely.

Effects on lab test results
• May increase AST, ALT, and LDH levels.
• May increase lymphocyte count.

Pharmacokinetics
Absorption: Good.
Distribution: Wide but variable. Drug is about 21% to 28% protein-bound.
Metabolism: Extensive. Its major metabolite may be pure antagonist and contribute to its effectiveness. Drug and metabolites may undergo enterohepatic recirculation.
Excretion: Mainly by kidneys. *Half-life:* About 4 hours.

Route	Onset	Peak	Duration
P.O.	15–30 min	1-2 hr	24 hr

Action
Chemical effect: May reversibly block subjective effects of I.V. opioids by occupying opioid receptors in brain.

Reactions may be *common,* uncommon, *life-threatening*, or COMMON AND LIFE-THREATENING.

Therapeutic effect: Helps prevent opioid dependence and treats alcohol dependence.

Available forms

Tablets: 25 mg, 50 mg, 100 mg

NURSING PROCESS

⚕ Assessment

• Assess patient's opioid or alcohol dependence before starting therapy and regularly thereafter to monitor the drug's effectiveness.
• Assess patient's and family's knowledge of drug therapy.

⊕ Nursing diagnoses

• Health-seeking behavior related to desire to remain free from opioid dependence
• Disturbed sleep pattern related to drug-induced insomnia
• Deficient knowledge related to drug therapy

▷ Planning and implementation

⊛ ALERT: Begin therapy for opioid dependency after giving naloxone challenge, a provocative test of opioid dependency. If signs of opioid withdrawal persist after challenge, don't give the drug.

⊛ ALERT: Patient must be completely free from opioids before taking the drug or severe withdrawal symptoms may occur. Wait at least 7 days in patient addicted to short-acting opioids, such as heroin and meperidine. Wait at least 10 days in patient addicted to longer-acting opioids, such as methadone.

• Use a nonopioid analgesic for analgesia. If an opioid analgesic is needed in an emergency, give an opioid analgesic in a higher dose than usual to surmount naltrexone's effect. Respiratory depression caused by opioid analgesic may be longer and deeper.
• For patient with opioid dependence who isn't expected to comply, use flexible maintenance regimen: 100 mg on Monday and Wednesday, 150 mg on Friday.
• Use naltrexone only as part of comprehensive rehabilitation program.

⊛ ALERT: Don't confuse naltrexone with naloxone.

Patient teaching

• Advise patient to wear or carry medical identification. Warn him to tell medical personnel that he takes naltrexone.

• Give patient names of nonopioid drugs he can take for pain, diarrhea, or cough.

☑ Evaluation

• Patient maintains opioid-free state.
• Patient reports no insomnia.
• Patient and family state understanding of drug therapy.

naproxen
(nuh-PROK-sin)
Apo-Naproxen ♦ , EC-Naprosyn, Naprosyn, Naprosyn SR ♦ ◇ , Naxen ♦ ◇ , Novo-Naprox ♦ , Nu-Naprox ♦

naproxen sodium
Aleve† , Anaprox, Anaprox DS, Apo-Napro-Na ♦ , Apo-Napro-Na DS ♦ , Naprelan, Novo-Naprox Sodium ♦ , Synflex ♦ , Synflex DS ♦

Pharmacologic class: NSAID
Therapeutic class: analgesic, antipyretic, anti-inflammatory
Pregnancy risk category: B

Indications and dosages

▶ **Rheumatoid arthritis, osteoarthritis, ankylosing spondylitis.** *Adults:* 250 to 500 mg naproxen P.O. b.i.d. Or 375 mg to 500 mg EC Naprosyn P.O. b.i.d. Or, 275 to 550 mg naproxen sodium P.O. b.i.d. Or 750 mg or 1,000 mg Naprelan P.O. daily. Or where suppository is available, 500 mg P.R. h.s. with naproxen P.O. during day.
▶ **Juvenile arthritis.** *Children age 2 and older:* 10 mg/kg naproxen P.O. in two divided doses.
▶ **Acute gout.** *Adults:* 750 mg naproxen P.O., followed by 250 mg q 8 hours until attack subsides. Or 825 mg naproxen sodium initially; then 275 mg q 8 hours until attack subsides. Or 1,000 mg to 1,500 mg Naprelan P.O. on the first day, then 1,000 mg daily until attack subsides.
▶ **Mild to moderate pain, primary dysmenorrhea, acute tendinitis and bursitis.** *Adults:* 500 mg naproxen P.O., followed by 250 mg q 6 to 8 hours p.r.n. Or 550 mg naproxen sodium P.O. initially; then 275 mg P.O. q 6 to 8 hours p.r.n. Or 1,000 mg Naprelan P.O. daily; use 1,500 mg P.O. daily for limited period.

N

Contraindications and cautions

• Contraindicated in patients hypersensitive to the drug or any of its components, and in patients with asthma, rhinitis, or nasal polyps.

• Use cautiously in those with renal disease, CV disease, GI disorders, hepatic disease, or peptic ulcer disease.

⚠ Lifespan: In women in the last trimester of pregnancy and in breast-feeding women, drug is contraindicated. In children younger than age 2, safety and effectiveness haven't been established. In elderly patients, use cautiously because of possible delayed excretion.

Adverse reactions

CNS: *headache, drowsiness, dizziness,* cognitive dysfunction, aseptic meningitis.
CV: *peripheral edema,* palpitations, digital vasculitis.
EENT: visual disturbances, *tinnitus.*
GI: *epigastric distress, occult blood loss,* nausea, peptic ulceration.
GU: *nephrotoxicity.*
Hematologic: *agranulocytosis, thrombocytopenia, neutropenia.*
Metabolic: *hyperkalemia.*
Respiratory: dyspnea.
Skin: *pruritus, rash,* urticaria.

Interactions

Drug-drug. *ACE inhibitors:* May increase risk of renal disease. Don't use together.
Aspirin, corticosteroids: May increase risk of adverse GI reactions. Use cautiously and monitor patient for abdominal pain, bleeding.
Cyclosporine: May increase nephrotoxicity of both drugs. Monitor renal function tests.
Diuretics: May decrease effect of these drugs. Monitor patient.
Drugs that are highly protein-bound, oral anticoagulants, sulfonylureas: May increase risk of toxicity. Monitor patient closely.
Methotrexate: May increase risk of toxicity. Monitor levels.
Probenecid: May decrease elimination of naproxen. Monitor patient for toxicity.
Drug-herb. *Dong quai, feverfew, garlic, ginger, horse chestnut, red clover:* May increase risk of bleeding. Discourage using together.
St. John's wort: May increase risk of photosensitivity. Advise patient to avoid unprotected or prolonged exposure to sunlight.

Drug-lifestyle. *Alcohol use:* May increase risk of adverse GI reactions. Discourage using together.

Effects on lab test results

• May increase BUN, creatinine, ALT, AST, and potassium levels.
• May increase bleeding time. May decrease granulocyte, platelet, and neutrophil counts.
• May interfere with urinary assays of 5-hydroxyindoleacetic acid and may falsely elevate urine 17-ketosteroid concentrations.

Pharmacokinetics

Absorption: Rapid and complete.
Distribution: Highly protein-bound.
Metabolism: In liver.
Excretion: In urine. *Half-life:* 10-20 hours.

Route	Onset	Peak	Duration
P.O.	≤ 1 hr	1–6 hr	7–12 hr
P.R.	Unknown	Unknown	Unknown

Action

Chemical effect: Unknown; produces anti-inflammatory, analgesic, and antipyretic effects, possibly by inhibiting prostaglandin synthesis.
Therapeutic effect: Relieves pain, fever, and inflammation.

Available forms

naproxen
Oral suspension: 125 mg/5 ml
Suppositories: 500 mg ◊
Tablets: 250 mg, 375 mg, 500 mg
Tablets (delayed-release, enteric-coated): 375 mg, 500 mg
Tablets (extended-release) ♦ : 750 mg, 1,000 mg
naproxen sodium
275 mg naproxen sodium equals 250 mg naproxen.
Tablets (controlled-release): 375 mg, 500 mg
Tablets: 220 mg†, 275 mg, 550 mg

NURSING PROCESS

⚗ Assessment

• Assess patient's condition before starting therapy and regularly thereafter to monitor the drug's effectiveness,

• Monitor CBC, electrolytes, and renal and hepatic function q 4 to 6 months during long-term therapy.
• NSAIDs may mask signs and symptoms of infection.
• If patient has an adverse GI reaction, monitor his hydration.
• Assess patient's and family's knowledge of drug therapy.

⊞ **Nursing diagnoses**
• Acute pain related to underlying condition
• Risk for deficient fluid volume related to drug-induced adverse GI reactions
• Deficient knowledge related to drug therapy

❯ **Planning and implementation**
⊗ **ALERT:** Don't exceed 1.25 g of naproxen or 1.375 of naproxen sodium daily.
• Give drug with food or milk to minimize GI upset.
• Suppository isn't available in the United States.
• Don't use in patients with inflammatory lesion of the rectum or anus.
Patient teaching
• Tell patient taking prescription doses of naproxen for arthritis that full therapeutic effect may take 2 to 4 weeks.
• Tell patient to take a full glass of water or other liquid with each dose.
• Tell patient not to break, crush or chew delayed-release tablets.
⊗ **ALERT:** Warn patient against taking naproxen and naproxen sodium at the same time.
• Teach patient to recognize and report evidence of GI bleeding. Serious GI toxicity, including peptic ulceration and bleeding, can occur in patients taking NSAIDs, despite absence of GI symptoms.
• Warn patient that use with aspirin, alcohol, or corticosteroids may increase risk of adverse GI reactions.
• Advise patient to have periodic eye examinations.

☑ **Evaluation**
• Patient is free from pain.
• Patient maintains adequate hydration.
• Patient and family state understanding of drug therapy.

naratriptan hydrochloride
(nah-rah-TRIP-tin high-droh-KLOR-ighd)
Amerge, Naramig ◊

Pharmacologic class: selective agonist of serotonin
Therapeutic class: antimigraine drug
Pregnancy risk category: C

Indications and dosages

❯ **Acute migraine headaches with or without aura.** *Adults:* 1 or 2.5 mg P.O. as a single dose. If headache returns or responds only partially, dose may be repeated after 4 hours, for maximum dosage of 5 mg in 24 hours.
⊠ **Adjust-a-dose:** For patients with mild or moderate renal or hepatic impairment, don't use more than 2.5 mg P.O. in 24 hours. If creatinine clearance is less than 15 ml/minute or if patient has severe hepatic impairment, don't use drug.

Contraindications and cautions

• Contraindicated in patients hypersensitive to the drug or any of its components, and in those who have received ergot-containing, ergot-type, or other 5-HT$_1$ agonists in the previous 24 hours. Also contraindicated in patients with a history of, or signs and symptoms of, cardiac ischemia, cerebrovascular disease, peripheral vascular disease, significant underlying CV disease, uncontrolled hypertension, creatinine clearance below 15 ml/minute, or severe hepatic impairment (Child-Pugh grade C).
• Unless a CV evaluation determines that patient is free from cardiac disease, use cautiously in patient with risk factors for coronary artery disease, such as hypertension, hypercholesterolemia, obesity, diabetes, a strong family history of coronary artery disease, surgical or physiologic menopause (women), age older than 40 (men), and smoking. For patients with cardiac risk factors but a satisfactory CV evaluation, give first dose in a medical facility and consider ECG monitoring.
• Safety and effectiveness haven't been established for cluster headaches or for treating more than four migraine headaches in a 30-day period.
⚕ **Lifespan:** In pregnant women, drug is contraindicated. In breast-feeding women, small amounts of drug may appear in breast milk. In

N

children, safety and effectiveness haven't been established. In elderly patients, drug is contraindicated.

Adverse reactions

CNS: paresthesias, dizziness, drowsiness, malaise, fatigue, vertigo, syncope.
CV: palpitations, increased blood pressure, *tachyarrhythmias, PR and QT interval prolongation, ST/T wave abnormalities, PVCs, atrial flutter, fibrillation, coronary artery vasospasm,* transient myocardial ischemia, *MI, ventricular tachycardia, ventricular fibrillation.*
EENT: ear, nose, and throat infections; photophobia.
GI: nausea, hyposalivation, vomiting.
Other: warm or cold temperature sensations; pressure, tightness, and heaviness sensations.

Interactions

Drug-drug. *Ergot-containing or ergot-type drugs (dihydroergotamine, methysergide), other 5-HT₁ agonists:* Prolong vasospastic reactions. Don't give within 24 hours of naratriptan.
Hormonal contraceptives: May cause slightly higher naratriptan levels. Monitor patient.
Sibutramine: Signs of serotonin syndrome, including CNS irritability, motor weakness, shivering, myoclonus may occur. Use together cautiously.
SSRIs, such as fluoxetine, fluvoxamine, paroxetine, sertraline: May cause weakness, hyperreflexia, and incoordination. Monitor patient.
Drug-lifestyle. *Smoking:* Increases naratriptan clearance. Discourage using together; urge patient to stop smoking.

Effects on lab test results

None reported.

Pharmacokinetics

Absorption: Good. Bioavailability of 70%.
Distribution: About 28% to 31% protein-bound.
Metabolism: To a number of inactive metabolites by wide range of cytochrome P isoenzymes.
Excretion: Primarily in urine with 50% of dose recovered unchanged and 30% as metabolites.
Half-life: 6 hours.

Route	Onset	Peak	Duration
P.O.	Unknown	2–3 hr	Unknown

Action

Chemical effect: May activate receptors in intracranial blood vessels, leading to vasoconstriction and relief of migraine headache; activation of receptors on sensory nerve endings in trigeminal system may inhibit proinflammatory neuropeptide release.
Therapeutic effect: Relieves migraine pain.

Available forms

Tablets: 1 mg, 2.5 mg

NURSING PROCESS

℞ Assessment

● Assess baseline cardiac function before starting therapy. Perform periodic cardiac reevaluation in patients who develop risk factors for coronary artery disease.
● Assess renal and liver function test results before starting drug therapy, and report abnormalities.
● Assess patient's and family's knowledge of drug therapy.

⊕ Nursing diagnoses

● Acute pain related to presence of migraine headache
● Risk for injury related to drug-induced adverse CV reactions
● Deficient knowledge related to drug therapy

❯ Planning and implementation

● Give drug only for a definite diagnosis of migraine. Drug isn't intended for preventing migraine headaches or treating hemiplegic headaches, basilar migraines, or cluster headaches.
● If patient has pain or tightness in chest or throat, arrhythmias, or increased blood pressure, withhold the drug and notify prescriber.
● Don't give the drug to a patient with history of coronary artery disease, hypertension, arrhythmias, or risk factors for coronary artery disease because drug may cause coronary vasospasm and hypertension.
● For patients with cardiac risk factors who have had a satisfactory cardiac evaluation, give first dose while monitoring ECG. Keep emergency equipment readily available.
Patient teaching
● Instruct patient to take drug only as prescribed.

• Tell patient that drug is intended to relieve migraine headaches, not to prevent them.
• Instruct patient to take dose soon after headache starts. If no response occurs to first tablet, tell patient to seek prescriber approval before taking second tablet. If prescriber approves a second dose, patient may take a second tablet, but no sooner than 4 hours after first tablet. Warn patient not to exceed two tablets in 24 hours.
• Teach patient to alert prescriber about risk factors for coronary artery disease or bothersome adverse effects.

☑ **Evaluation**
• Patient has relief of migraine headache.
• Patient has no pain or tightness in chest or throat, arrhythmias, or increase in blood pressure.
• Patient and family state understanding of drug therapy.

nateglinide
(na-TEG-li-nide)
Starlix

Pharmacologic class: amino acid derivative
Therapeutic class: antidiabetic
Pregnancy risk category: C

Indications and dosages

▶ **Alone or with metformin or a thiazolidinedione to lower glucose levels in patients with type 2 diabetes whose hyperglycemia isn't adequately controlled by diet and exercise and who haven't received long-term therapy with other antidiabetics.** *Adults:* 120 mg P.O. t.i.d., taken 1 to 30 minutes before meals. If patient's glycosylated hemoglobin level is near normal when therapy starts, he may receive 60 mg P.O. t.i.d.

Contraindications and cautions

• Contraindicated in patients hypersensitive to the drug or any of its components and in patients with type 1 diabetes or diabetic ketoacidosis.
• Use cautiously in malnourished patients and patients with moderate to severe liver dysfunction or adrenal or pituitary insufficiency.

⚝ **Lifespan:** In pregnant women, don't use. In breast-feeding women, use cautiously; it's unknown if the drug appears in breast milk. In children, safety and effectiveness haven't been established. In elderly patients, use cautiously because some elderly patients have greater sensitivity to the glucose-lowering effects than others.

Adverse reactions

CNS: dizziness.
GI: diarrhea.
Metabolic: *hypoglycemia.*
Musculoskeletal: back pain, arthropathy.
Respiratory: upper respiratory tract infection, bronchitis, coughing.
Other: flulike symptoms, accidental trauma.

Interactions

Drug-drug. *Corticosteroids, sympathomimetics, thiazides, thyroid drugs:* May reduce the hypoglycemic action of nateglinide. Monitor patient for hyperglycemia, and monitor glucose levels closely.
MAO inhibitors, nonselective beta blockers, NSAIDs, salicylates: May increase the hypoglycemic action of nateglinide. Monitor patient for hypoglycemia and monitor glucose levels closely.

Effects on lab test results

• May decrease glucose level.

Pharmacokinetics

Absorption: Rapid when taken immediately before a meal.
Distribution: 98% bound to proteins, primarily albumin.
Metabolism: In the liver.
Excretion: Rapid and complete. *Half-life:* About 1½ hours.

Route	Onset	Peak	Duration
P.O.	20 min	1 hr	4 hr

Action

Chemical effect: Stimulates insulin secretion from the pancreas.
Therapeutic effect: Lowers glucose level.

Available forms

Tablets: 60 mg, 120 mg

NURSING PROCESS

⚖ Assessment
• Assess underlying condition before starting therapy, and reassess regularly to monitor the drug's effectiveness.
• Monitor glucose level regularly to evaluate drug's effectiveness.
• When other drugs are started or stopped, monitor glucose level closely to detect drug interactions.
• Periodically monitor HbA1c levels.
• Assess patient's and family's knowledge of drug therapy.

⊕ Nursing diagnoses
• Ineffective health maintenance related to hyperglycemia
• Risk for injury related to adverse drug effect of hypoglycemia
• Deficient knowledge related to nateglinide therapy

❯ Planning and implementation
• Don't use with or instead of glyburide or other oral antidiabetics. Drug may be used with metformin.
• Give drug 1 to 30 minutes before a meal. If patient misses a meal, skip the scheduled dose.
⊛ ALERT: Risk of hypoglycemia rises with strenuous exercise, alcohol ingestion, insufficient caloric intake, and use with other oral antidiabetics.
• Symptoms of hypoglycemia may be masked in patients with autonomic neuropathy and in those who use beta blockers.
• Insulin may be needed for glycemic control in patients with fever, infection, trauma, or impending surgery.
• Effectiveness may decline over time.
⊛ ALERT: Observe patient for evidence of hypoglycemia, including sweating, rapid pulse, trembling, confusion, headache, irritability, and nausea. To minimize the risk of hypoglycemia, follow dose immediately with a meal. If hypoglycemia occurs and the patient remains conscious, give an oral form of glucose. If unconscious, give I.V. glucose.

Patient teaching
• Tell patient to take nateglinide 1 to 30 minutes before a meal.

• To reduce the risk of hypoglycemia, advise patient to skip the scheduled dose if he misses a meal.
• Educate patient about the risk of hypoglycemia and its signs and symptoms (sweating, rapid pulse, trembling, confusion, headache, irritability, and nausea). Advise patient to treat these symptoms by eating or drinking something containing sugar.
• Teach patient how to monitor and log glucose levels to evaluate diabetes control.
• Instruct patient to adhere to the prescribed diet and exercise regimen.
• Explain the long-term complications of diabetes and the importance of regular preventive therapy.
• Encourage patient to wear or carry medical identification that shows he has diabetes.

☑ Evaluation
• Patient's glucose level is normal.
• Patient doesn't become hypoglycemic and sustains no injury.
• Patient and family state understanding of drug therapy.

nefazodone hydrochloride
(nef-AZ-oh-dohn high-droh-KLOR-ighd)

Pharmacologic class: serotonin modulator
Therapeutic class: antidepressant
Pregnancy risk category: C

Indications and dosages
▶ **Depression.** *Adults:* Initially, 200 mg P.O. daily in two divided doses. Increase dosage in increments of 100 to 200 mg daily at intervals of no less than 1 week. Usual daily dosage range, 300 to 600 mg. Maximum dosage is 600 mg.

Contraindications and cautions
• Contraindicated in patients hypersensitive to the drug or any of its components, other phenylpiperazine antidepressants, or in patients who are withdrawn from drug because of liver injury. Also contraindicated within 14 days of MAO inhibitor therapy.
• Use cautiously in patients with CV or cerebrovascular disease that could be worsened by hypotension (such as history of MI, angina, or

stroke) and conditions that predispose to hypotension (such as dehydration, hypovolemia, and therapy with antihypertensives).
• Also use cautiously in patients with history of mania.
≉ **Lifespan:** In pregnant women, use cautiously. In breast-feeding women, use cautiously; it's unknown if drug appears in breast milk. In children, drug isn't approved for use because children may have an increased risk of suicidal behavior.

Adverse reactions

CNS: headache, fever, *somnolence, dizziness, asthenia,* insomnia, *light-headedness, confusion,* memory impairment, paresthesia, abnormal dreams, decreased concentration, ataxia, incoordination, psychomotor retardation, tremor, hypertonia, *suicidal ideation.*
CV: vasodilation, orthostatic hypotension, hypotension, peripheral edema.
EENT: *blurred vision, abnormal vision,* pharyngitis, tinnitus, visual field defect.
GI: *dry mouth, nausea, constipation,* dyspepsia, diarrhea, increased appetite, vomiting, taste perversion.
GU: urinary frequency, UTI, urine retention, vaginitis.
Hepatic: *liver failure.*
Metabolic: hyponatremia.
Musculoskeletal: neck rigidity, arthralgia.
Respiratory: cough.
Skin: pruritus, rash.
Other: infection, flulike syndrome, chills, thirst, breast pain.

Interactions

Drug-drug. *Alprazolam, triazolam:* May increase effects of these drugs. Avoid using together or substantially reduce dosage of alprazolam and triazolam.
Calcium channel blockers, HMG-CoA reductase inhibitors: May increase levels of these drugs. Adjust dosage if needed.
CNS-active drugs: May alter CNS activity. Use together cautiously.
Digoxin: May increase digoxin level. Use together cautiously and monitor digoxin levels.
MAO inhibitors (phenelzine, selegiline, tranylcypromine): May cause serotonin syndrome (CNS irritability, shivering, and altered consciousness). Don't give together. Wait at least 2 weeks after stopping an MAO inhibitor before

giving any selective serotonin reuptake inhibitors.
Other drugs highly bound to proteins: May increase adverse reactions. Monitor patient closely.
Sibutramine, sumatriptan: May cause severe excitation, hyperpyrexia, seizures, delirium, coma, or a fatal reaction. Avoid using together.
Drug-herb. *St. John's wort:* May cause additive effects and serotonin syndrome (CNS irritability, shivering, and altered consciousness). Discourage using together.
Drug-lifestyle. *Alcohol use:* Enhances CNS depression. Discourage using together.

Effects on lab test results

• May decrease sodium level.

Pharmacokinetics

Absorption: Rapid and complete.
Distribution: Wide. Drug is extensively bound to proteins.
Metabolism: Extensive.
Excretion: In urine. *Half-life:* 2 to 4 hours.

Route	Onset	Peak	Duration
P.O.	Unknown	1 hr	Unknown

Action

Chemical effect: Not precisely defined. Drug inhibits neuronal uptake of serotonin ($5\text{-}HT_2$) and norepinephrine; it also occupies serotonin and alpha$_1$-adrenergic receptors in CNS.
Therapeutic effect: Relieves depression.

Available forms

Tablets: 50 mg, 100 mg, 150 mg, 200 mg, 250 mg

NURSING PROCESS

☏ Assessment
• Assess patient's depression before starting therapy and regularly thereafter to monitor the drug's effectiveness.
🕲 **ALERT:** Calculate a risk-benefit ratio before using drug for depression because of the risk for hepatic failure and emergence of suicidal ideation and attempts.
• Record mood changes. Monitor patient for suicidal tendencies.
• Be alert for adverse reactions and drug interactions.

N

• Assess patient's and family's knowledge of drug therapy.

⊕ Nursing diagnoses
• Disturbed thought processes related to depression
• Risk for injury related to drug-induced adverse CNS reactions
• Deficient knowledge related to drug therapy

▶ Planning and implementation
⊛ **ALERT:** Allow at least 7 days after stopping drug before starting patient on an MAO inhibitor. Allow at least 14 days after stopping an MAO inhibitor before starting patient on the drug.
⊛ **ALERT:** Don't initiate therapy in patients with active liver disease or with elevated baseline transaminase levels. Preexisting liver disease doesn't appear to increase the likelihood of developing liver failure, but baseline abnormalities can complicate patient monitoring.
⊛ **ALERT:** If patient has signs and symptoms of liver dysfunction, such as AST or ALT levels greater than or equal to 3 times upper limit of normal, stop giving the drug and don't restart.
Patient teaching
• Warn patient not to engage in hazardous activity until the drug's CNS effects of drug are known.
⊛ **ALERT:** Instruct man with prolonged or inappropriate erections to stop drug at once and call prescriber.
• Instruct woman to call prescriber if she becomes pregnant or intends to become pregnant during therapy.
• Teach patient the signs and symptoms of liver dysfunction (jaundice, anorexia, GI complaints, and malaise), and tell him to immediately report them to prescriber.
• Instruct patient not to drink alcohol during therapy.
• Tell patient who develops rash, hives, or related allergic reaction to notify prescriber.
• Inform patient that several weeks of therapy may be needed to obtain full antidepressant effect. Once improvement occurs, tell patient not to stop drug until directed by prescriber.
⊛ **ALERT:** Inform family members to be particularly vigilant for suicidal tendencies during therapy with nefazodone.
• Urge patient to notify prescriber before taking any OTC drugs.

☑ Evaluation
• Patient exhibits improved thought processes.
• Patient sustains no injuries from drug-induced adverse CNS reactions.
• Patient and family state understanding of drug therapy.

nelfinavir mesylate
(nel-FIN-uh-veer MES-ih-layt)
Viracept

Pharmacologic class: HIV protease inhibitor
Therapeutic class: antiretroviral
Pregnancy risk category: B

Indications and dosages

▶ **HIV infection when antiretroviral therapy is warranted.** *Adults and children older than age 13:* 750 mg P.O. t.i.d., or 1,250 mg P.O. b.i.d. with meal.
Children ages 2 to 13: 45 to 55 mg/kg b.i.d. or 25 to 35 mg/kg t.i.d. with meal. Maximum dose 2,500 mg/day.
▶ **Prophylaxis after occupational exposure to HIV‡.** *Adults:* 750 mg P.O. t.i.d. with two other antiretrovirals for 4 weeks.

Contraindications and cautions

• Contraindicated in patients hypersensitive to the drug or any of its components and in patients receiving amiodarone, ergot derivatives, lovastatin, midazolam, pimozide, quinidine, simvastatin, or triazolam.
• Use cautiously in patients with hepatic dysfunction or hemophilia type A and B.
⚕ **Lifespan:** In pregnant women, use only when clearly needed. Women shouldn't breast-feed to avoid transmitting HIV to infant.

Adverse reactions

CNS: asthenia, anxiety, depression, dizziness, emotional lability, headache, malaise, paresthesia, *seizures,* sleep disorders, *suicidal ideation.*
EENT: conjunctivitis, iritis, pharyngitis, rhinitis, sinusitis.
GI: *diarrhea,* flatulence, mouth ulceration, nausea, *pancreatitis.*
GU: renal calculus, sexual dysfunction.
Hematologic: anemia, *leukopenia, thrombocytopenia.*
Hepatic: *hepatitis.*

Reactions may be *common*, uncommon, *life-threatening*, or COMMON AND LIFE-THREATENING.

Metabolic: dehydration, *diabetes mellitus,* hyperlipidemia, hyperuricemia, *hypoglycemia.*
Musculoskeletal: arthralgia, myalgia, myasthenia, myopathy.
Respiratory: diaphoresis, dyspnea
Skin: dermatitis, pruritus, rash, urticaria.
Other: allergic reactions, fever, redistribution or accumulation of body fat.

Interactions

Drug-drug. *Amiodarone, ergot derivatives, lovastatin, midazolam, pimozide, quinidine, simvastatin, triazolam:* May increase levels of these drugs, causing increased risk of serious or life-threatening adverse reactions. Avoid using together.
Atorvastatin, lovastatin, simvastatin: May increase level of atorvastatin. Use lowest dose or consider using pravastatin or fluvastatin instead.
Azithromycin: May increase azithromycin levels. Monitor patient for liver impairment.
Carbamazepine, phenobarbital: May reduce the effectiveness of nelfinavir. Use together cautiously; monitor drug levels and virologic response.
Cyclosporine, sirolimus, tacrolimus: May increase levels of these immunosuppressants. Use together cautiously.
Delavirdine, HIV protease inhibitors (indinavir or saquinavir), nevirapine: May increase levels of protease inhibitors. Use together cautiously.
Didanosine: May decrease didanosine absorption. Take nelfinavir with food at least 2 hours before or 1 hour after didanosine.
Ethinyl estradiol: May decrease level of contraceptive. Advise patient to use alternative contraceptive measures during therapy.
Methadone, phenytoin: May decrease levels of these drugs. Adjust dosage of these drugs accordingly.
Rifabutin: Increases rifabutin level and decreases level of nelfinavir. Reduce dose of rifabutin to one-half the usual dose, and increase nelfinavir to 1,250 mg b.i.d.
Sildenafi, tadalafil, vardenafil: May increase adverse effects of these drugs. Use together cautiously. Don't exceed 25 mg of sildenafil in a 48-hour period, 10 mg of tadalafil in a 72-hour period, or 2.5 mg of vardenafil in a 72-hour period.
Drug-herb. *St. John's wort:* Decreases nelfinavir level. Discourage using together.

Effects on lab test results
● May increase ALT, AST, alkaline phosphatase, bilirubin, GGT, amylase, CK, and uric acid levels. May decrease hemoglobin level and hematocrit. May increase or decrease glucose level.
● May decrease WBC and platelet counts.

Pharmacokinetics
Absorption: Level peaks higher when drug is taken with food.
Distribution: More than 98% bound to protein.
Metabolism: Primarily by CYP 3A and CYP 2C19.
Excretion: Mainly in feces. *Half-life:* 3½ to 5 hours.

Route	Onset	Peak	Duration
P.O.	Unknown	2–4 hr	Unknown

Action
Chemical effect: Inhibits protease enzyme and prevents splitting of the viral polyprotein.
Therapeutic effect: Produces immature, noninfectious virus; prevention of AIDS progression.

Available forms
Powder (for suspension): 50 mg/g powder
Tablets (film-coated): 250 mg, 625 mg

NURSING PROCESS

⟐ Assessment
● Obtain baseline assessment of patient's condition before starting therapy, and reassess regularly to monitor drug the drug's effectiveness.
● Monitor liver function test results.
● Assess patient for increased bleeding tendencies, especially if he has hemophilia type A or B.
● Monitor patient for excessive diarrhea, and treat as directed.
● Assess patient's and family's knowledge of drug therapy.

⟐ Nursing diagnoses
● Risk for injury related to adverse GI effects of drug
● Risk for impaired skin integrity secondary to drug-induced adverse effects
● Deficient knowledge related to drug therapy

N

▶ Planning and implementation

• Give oral powder to children unable to take tablets. Mix powder with small amount of water, milk, formula, soy formula, soy milk, or dietary supplements. Tell patient to consume entire contents.

• Don't reconstitute drug with water in its original container.

• Use reconstituted powder within 6 hours.

• Mixing with acidic foods or juice isn't recommended because of the bitter taste.

• Enroll pregnant women with the Antiretroviral Pregnancy Registry by calling 1-800-258-4263 or visiting www.apregistry.com.

⑨ **ALERT:** Don't confuse nelfinavir with nevirapine.

Patient teaching

• Advise patient to take drug with food.

• Explain that drug doesn't cure HIV infection or reduce the risk of transmitting HIV to others.

• Tell patient that the drug's long-term effects are unknown.

• Instruct patient to take drug daily as prescribed and not to alter dose or stop drug without medical approval.

• Tell patient that diarrhea is the most common adverse effect and that it can be controlled with loperamide.

• If patient misses a dose, tell him to take it immediately and then return to his normal schedule, but do not double the dose.

• Instruct patient taking hormonal contraceptives to use an additional (or different) contraceptive measure while taking drug.

⑨ **ALERT:** Warn patient with phenylketonuria that powder contains 11.2 mg phenylalanine per gram.

• Instruct patient to report use of other prescribed or OTC drugs because of interactions.

• Advise patient taking sildenafi, tadalafil, or vardenafil of an increased risk of adverse events, including hypotension, visual changes, and priapism; tell him to promptly report any symptoms to prescriber. Tell him not to exceed 25 mg of sildenafil in a 48-hour period, 10 mg of tadalafil in a 72-hour period, or 2.5 mg of vardenafil in a 72-hour period.

✓ Evaluation

• Patient has no adverse GI reactions.

• Patient and family state understanding of drug therapy.

• Skin integrity remains intact.

neomycin sulfate
(nee-oh-MIGH-sin SUL-fayt)
Mycifradin, Neo-Fradin, Neo-Tabs

Pharmacologic class: aminoglycoside
Therapeutic class: antibiotic
Pregnancy risk category: D

Indications and dosages

▶ **Infectious diarrhea caused by enteropathogenic *Escherichia coli*.** *Adults:* 50 mg/kg daily P.O. in four divided doses for 2 to 3 days. *Children:* 50 to 100 mg/kg daily P.O. divided q 4 to 6 hours for 2 to 3 days.

▶ **Preoperative suppression of intestinal bacteria.** *Adults:* 1 g P.O. q hour for four doses; then 1 g q 4 hours for balance of 24 hours. For the 2- to 3-day regimen, 88 mg/kg/day in 6 equally divided doses at 4-hour intervals. Give a saline cathartic before first dose. *Children:* 40 to 100 mg/kg daily P.O. divided q 4 to 6 hours. Give a saline cathartic before first dose.

▶ **Adjunct in hepatic coma.** *Adults:* 1 to 3 g P.O. q.i.d. for 5 to 6 days. Or 200 ml of 1% solution or 100 ml of 2% solution as enema retained for 20 to 60 minutes q 6 hours.

▶ **Hypercholesterolemia‡** *Adults:* 500 mg to 2 g P.O. daily in 2 to 3 divided doses with or immediately after meals.

Contraindications and cautions

• Contraindicated in patients hypersensitive to other aminoglycosides and in those with intestinal obstruction.

• Use cautiously in patients with renal impairment, neuromuscular disorders, or ulcerative bowel lesions.

⚕ **Lifespan:** In pregnant women, only use drug when clearly needed because of the potential for harm. In breast-feeding women, safety and effectiveness haven't been established. In elderly patients, use cautiously.

Adverse reactions

CNS: headache, lethargy.
EENT: *ototoxicity.*
GI: nausea, vomiting.
GU: *nephrotoxicity.*
Skin: rash, urticaria.
Other: *hypersensitivity reactions.*

Reactions may be *common,* uncommon, ***life-threatening***, or COMMON AND LIFE-THREATENING.

Interactions

Drug-drug. *Acyclovir, amphotericin B, cisplatin, methoxyflurane, other aminoglycosides, vancomycin:* Increases risk of nephrotoxicity. Use together cautiously.
Atracurium, doxacurium, mivacurium, pancuronium, rocuronium, tubocurarine, vecuronium: May increase the effects of nondepolarizing muscle relaxant, such as prolonged respiratory depression. Use together only when needed. Reduce dose.
Cephalothin: Increases risk of nephrotoxicity. Use together cautiously; monitor renal function.
Digoxin: Decreases digoxin absorption. Monitor patient for loss of therapeutic effect.
Dimenhydrinate: May mask symptoms of ototoxicity. Use cautiously.
I.V. loop diuretics (such as furosemide): Increases risk of ototoxicity. Use cautiously; monitor hearing function.
Methotrexate: Decreases effects of methotrexate. Monitor patient for decreased effect.
Oral anticoagulants: Inhibits vitamin K–producing bacteria; may increase anticoagulant effect. Monitor patient for bleeding; monitor PT and INR.

Effects on lab test results

• May increase BUN, creatinine, and nonprotein nitrogen levels.

Pharmacokinetics

Absorption: About 3%. Enhanced in patients with impaired GI motility or mucosal intestinal ulcerations.
Distribution: Local.
Metabolism: None.
Excretion: Primarily unchanged in feces. *Half-life:* 2 to 3 hours.

Route	Onset	Peak	Duration
P.O.	Unknown	1–4 hr	8 hr

Action

Chemical effect: Inhibits protein synthesis by binding directly to 30S ribosomal subunit.
Therapeutic effect: Kills susceptible bacteria, such as many aerobic gram-negative organisms and some aerobic gram-positive organisms. Inhibits ammonia-forming bacteria in GI tract, reducing ammonia and improving neurologic status of patients with hepatic encephalopathy.

Available forms

Oral solution: 125 mg/5 ml
Tablets: 500 mg

NURSING PROCESS

⚕ Assessment

• Assess patient's condition before starting therapy and regularly thereafter to monitor the drug's effectiveness.
• Evaluate patient's hearing before starting therapy and regularly thereafter.
• Monitor renal function (output, specific gravity, urinalysis, BUN and creatinine levels, and creatinine clearance).
• Be alert for adverse reactions and drug interactions.
• If patient has adverse GI reactions, monitor his hydration.
• Assess patient's and family's knowledge of drug therapy.

⊞ Nursing diagnoses

• Infection related to organisms
• Risk for deficient fluid volume related to drug-induced adverse GI reactions
• Deficient knowledge related to drug therapy

▶ Planning and implementation

⚠ ALERT: Never give drug parenterally.
• Drug is nonabsorbable at recommended dosage. More than 4 g daily may be systemically absorbed and lead to nephrotoxicity.
• Make sure patient is well hydrated while taking drug to minimize chemical irritation of renal tubules.
• For preoperative disinfection, provide low-residue diet and cathartic immediately before giving the drug orally.
• In adjunct therapy of hepatic coma, decrease patient's dietary protein and assess neurologic status frequently during therapy.
• The ototoxic and nephrotoxic properties of neomycin limit its usefulness.
• Drug is available with polymyxin B as urinary bladder irrigant.
• Notify prescriber about signs of decreasing renal function or complaints of tinnitus, vertigo, or hearing loss. Deafness may begin several weeks after drug is stopped.

Patient teaching
• Instruct patient to report adverse reactions, especially hearing loss or change in urinary elimination.
• Emphasize the need to drink 2 L of fluid each day.
• Tell patient to alert prescriber if infection worsens or doesn't improve.

☑ Evaluation
• Patient is free from infection.
• Patient maintains adequate hydration throughout drug therapy.
• Patient and family state understanding of drug therapy.

neostigmine bromide
(nee-oh-STIG-meen BROH-mighd)
Prostigmin

neostigmine methylsulfate
Prostigmin

Pharmacologic class: cholinesterase inhibitor
Therapeutic class: muscle stimulant
Pregnancy risk category: C

Indications and dosages
▶ **Myasthenia gravis.** *Adults:* 15 to 30 mg P.O. t.i.d. (range, 15 to 375 mg daily). Or, 0.5 mg (1:2,000 solution) subcutaneously, I.M., or I.V. as needed.
Children: 7.5 to 15 mg P.O. t.i.d. or q.i.d. or 2 mg/kg/day P.O. divided q 3 to 4 hours. Or, 0.01 to 0.04 mg/kg/dose I.M., I.V., or subcutaneously q 2 to 3 hours p.r.n. Subsequent dosages must be highly individualized, depending on response and tolerance of adverse effects. Therapy may be required day and night.
▶ **To diagnose myasthenia gravis.** *Adults:* 0.022 mg/kg I.M. 30 minutes after 0.011 mg/kg I.M. of atropine sulfate.
Children: 0.025 to 0.04 mg/kg. I.M. after 0.011 mg/kg atropine sulfate subcutaneously.
▶ **Postoperative abdominal distention and bladder atony.** *Adults:* 0.25 to 0.5 mg (1:4,000 solution) I.M. or subcutaneously q 4 to 6 hours for 2 to 3 days.
▶ **Antidote for nondepolarizing neuromuscular blockers.** *Adults:* 0.5 to 2.5 mg I.V. slowly.

Repeat p.r.n. to total of 5 mg. Before antidote dose, give 0.6 to 1.2 mg I.V. atropine sulfate.
Children age 12 months and older: 0.025 to 0.08 mg/kg/dose I.V. given with atropine or glycopyrrolate.
Infants up to age 12 months: 0.025 to 0.1 mg/kg/dose I.V. given with atropine or glycopyrrolate.
▶ **Supraventricular tachycardia from tricyclic antidepressant overdose‡.** *Children:* 0.5 to 1 mg I.V. slowly, followed by 0.25 to 0.5 mg I.V. q 1 to 3 hours, p.r.n.
▶ **Decrease small bowel transit time during radiography‡.** *Adults:* 0.5 to 0.75 mg subcutaneously.

▼ I.V. administration
• A 1:1,000 solution of injectable solution contains 1 mg/ml; a 1:2,000 solution contains 0.5 mg/ml.
• Give drug at slow, controlled rate of no more than 1 mg/minute in adults and 0.5 mg/minute in children.
⊗ **Incompatibilities**
None reported.

Contraindications and cautions
• Contraindicated in patients hypersensitive to cholinergics or bromide and in those with peritonitis or mechanical obstruction of intestine or urinary tract.
• Use cautiously in patients with bronchial asthma, bradycardia, seizure disorders, recent coronary occlusion, vagotonia, hyperthyroidism, arrhythmias, or peptic ulcer.
⚘ **Lifespan:** In pregnant women, safety and effectiveness haven't been established.

Adverse reactions
CNS: dizziness, headache, mental confusion, jitters.
CV: *bradycardia,* hypotension, *cardiac arrest.*
EENT: blurred vision, lacrimation, miosis.
GI: *nausea, vomiting, diarrhea, abdominal cramps,* excessive salivation.
GU: urinary frequency.
Musculoskeletal: *muscle cramps,* muscle weakness, muscle fasciculations.
Respiratory: *depressed respiratory drive, bronchospasm, bronchoconstriction, respiratory arrest.*
Skin: rash (with bromide), diaphoresis.
Other: *hypersensitivity reactions, anaphylaxis.*

Reactions may be *common,* uncommon, *life-threatening,* or COMMON AND LIFE-THREATENING.

Interactions

Drug-drug. Aminoglycosides, anticholinergics, atropine, corticosteroids, magnesium sulfate, procainamide, quinidine: May reverse cholinergic effects. Observe patient for lack of drug effect.

Effects on lab test results

None reported.

Pharmacokinetics

Absorption: 1% to 2% after P.O. use. Unknown after subcutaneous. or I.M. use.
Distribution: About 15% to 25% of dose binds to serum albumin.
Metabolism: Hydrolyzed by cholinesterases and metabolized by microsomal liver enzymes.
Excretion: About 80% of drug in urine. *Half-life:* 52 to 53 minutes.

Route	Onset	Peak	Duration
P.O.	45–75 min	1–2 hr	2–4 hr
I.V.	4–8 min	1–2 hr	2–4 hr
I.M.	20–30 min	1–2 hr	2–4 hr
SubQ	Unknown	1–2 hr	2–4 hr

Action

Chemical effect: Inhibits destruction of acetylcholine released from parasympathetic and somatic efferent nerves. Acetylcholine accumulates, increasing stimulation of receptor.
Therapeutic effect: Stimulates muscle contraction.

Available forms

neostigmine bromide
Tablets: 15 mg
neostigmine methylsulfate
Injection: 0.25 mg/ml, 0.5 mg/ml, 1 mg/ml

NURSING PROCESS

Assessment
• Assess patient's condition before starting therapy.
• Monitor patient's response after each dose. Watch closely for improvement in strength, vision, and ptosis 45 to 60 minutes after each dose. Show patient how to record variations in muscle strength.
• Monitor vital signs frequently.
• Assess patient's and family's knowledge of drug therapy.

Nursing diagnoses
• Impaired physical mobility related to condition
• Diarrhea related to drug's adverse effect on GI tract
• Deficient knowledge related to drug therapy

Planning and implementation
ALERT: For diagnosis of myasthenia gravis, stop any anticholinesterases for at least 8 hours before giving drug.
• For myasthenia gravis, schedule doses before fatigue. For example, if patient has dysphagia, schedule dose 30 minutes before each meal.
• Give atropine injection and provide respiratory support p.r.n.
• When drug is used to prevent abdominal distention and GI distress, use a rectal tube to help passage of gas.
ALERT: Although drug is commonly used to reverse effects of nondepolarizing neuromuscular blockers in patients who have undergone surgery, it may worsen blockade produced by succinylcholine.
• Patient may develop resistance to drug.
• Give oral drug with food or milk.
ALERT: Use I.M. drug instead of edrophonium to diagnose myasthenia gravis when lengthy procedures involving testing of limb strength are used.
ALERT: Don't confuse neostigmine with etomidate (Amidate) vials. They may look alike.
Patient teaching
• Tell patient to take drug with food or milk to reduce GI distress.
• When using for myasthenia gravis, explain that drug will relieve ptosis, double vision, difficulty chewing and swallowing, and trunk and limb weakness. Stress need to take drug exactly as ordered. Explain that it may have to be taken for life.
• Advise patient to wear or carry medical identification indicating that he has myasthenia gravis.

Evaluation
• Patient performs activities of daily living without assistance.
• Patient has normal bowel patterns.
• Patient and family state understanding of drug therapy.

N

nesiritide
(ne-SIR-I-tide)
Natrecor

Pharmacologic class: human B-type natriuretic peptide
Therapeutic class: inotropic vasodilator
Pregnancy risk category: C

Indications and dosages

▶ **Acutely decompensated heart failure in patients with dyspnea at rest or with minimal activity.** *Adults:* 2 mcg/kg by I.V. bolus over 60 seconds followed by continuous infusion of 0.01 mcg/kg/minute.

▽ I.V. administration

• Use these formulas to calculate bolus volume (2 mcg/kg) and infusion flow rate (0.01 mcg/kg/minute):

$$\frac{\text{Bolus volume}}{\text{(ml)}} = 0.33 \times \frac{\text{patient weight}}{\text{(kg)}}$$

$$\frac{\text{Infusion flow rate}}{\text{(ml/hr)}} = 0.1 \times \frac{\text{patient weight}}{\text{(kg)}}$$

• Reconstitute one 1.5-mg vial with 5 ml of diluent (such as D_5W, normal saline solution, 5% dextrose and 0.2% saline solution injection, or 5% dextrose and half-normal saline solution) from a prefilled 250-ml I.V. bag.
• Don't shake vial. Gently rock until solution is clear and colorless.
• Withdraw contents of vial and add back to the 250-ml bag to yield 6 mcg/ml. Invert the bag several times to ensure complete mixing, and use the solution within 24 hours.
• Drug binds heparin and could bind the heparin lining of a heparin-coated catheter, decreasing the amount of nesiritide delivered. Don't give nesiritide through a central heparin-coated catheter.
• Before starting bolus dose, prime the tubing. Give the bolus over 60 seconds through a port in the tubing.
• Immediately after giving bolus, infuse drug at 0.1 ml/kg/hour to deliver 0.01 mcg/kg/minute.
• Store drug at a controlled room temperature.

⊗ **Incompatibilities**
Bumetanide, enalaprilat, ethacrynate sodium, furosemide, heparin, hydralazine, insulin, sodium metabisulfite preservative.

Contraindications and cautions

• Contraindicated in patients hypersensitive to the drug or any of its components.
• Avoid using drug as primary therapy in patients with cardiogenic shock, systolic blood pressure below 90 mm Hg, low cardiac filling pressures, conditions in which cardiac output is dependent on venous return, or conditions that make vasodilators inappropriate, such as valvular stenosis, restrictive or obstructive cardiomyopathy, constrictive pericarditis, or pericardial tamponade.
⚞ **Lifespan:** In pregnant women, use cautiously. In breast-feeding women, use cautiously; it's unknown if the drug appears in breast milk. In children, safety and effectiveness haven't been established. Some older patients are more sensitive to drug effects than younger patients, but no overall difference in effectiveness has been noted.

Adverse reactions

CNS: headache, confusion, somnolence, insomnia, dizziness, anxiety, paresthesia, tremor, fever.
CV: *hypotension, ventricular tachycardia,* ventricular extrasystoles, angina, *bradycardia,* atrial fibrillation, AV node conduction abnormalities.
GI: nausea, vomiting, abdominal pain.
Hematologic: anemia.
Musculoskeletal: back pain, leg cramps.
Respiratory: *apnea,* cough.
Skin: rash, sweating, pruritus.
Other: injection-site reactions, pain at the site.

Interactions

Drug-drug. *ACE inhibitors:* Increases hypotension symptoms. Monitor blood pressure closely.

Effects on lab test results

• May increase creatinine level more than 0.5 mg/dl above baseline. May decrease hemoglobin level and hematocrit.

Pharmacokinetics

Absorption: Administered I.V.
Distribution: Unknown.

Metabolism: Unknown.
Excretion: Three independent paths: lysosomal proteolysis after drug binds to cell surface receptors, proteolytic cleavage by endopeptidases in the vascular lumen, and renal filtration. *Half-life:* 18 minutes.

Route	Onset	Peak	Duration
I.V.	15 min	1 hr	3 hr

Action

Chemical effect: Binds to receptors on vascular smooth muscle and endothelial cells, which leads to relaxation of smooth muscles and dilation of veins and arteries.
Therapeutic effect: Produces a dose-dependent reduction in pulmonary capillary wedge pressure and systemic arterial pressure in patients with heart failure.

Available forms

Injection: Single-dose vials of 1.5-mg sterile, lyophilized powder

NURSING PROCESS

Assessment
• Assess underlying condition before starting therapy, and reassess regularly to monitor the drug's effectiveness.
• **ALERT:** Drug may cause hypotension. Monitor patient's blood pressure closely, particularly if patient also takes an ACE inhibitor.
• Evaluate patient's renal function because drug affects renal function in some people. In patients with severe heart failure whose renal function depends on the renin-angiotensin-aldosterone system, therapy may lead to azotemia.
• Monitor patient's cardiac status before, during, and after drug administration.
• Assess patient's and family's knowledge of drug therapy.

Nursing diagnoses
• Ineffective tissue perfusion (cardiopulmonary) related to drug-induced hypotension
• Excess fluid volume related to heart failure
• Deficient knowledge related to nesiritide therapy

Planning and implementation
• Because of hypotension, don't start drug at dose higher than recommended. If hypotension develops during administration, reduce dose or stop giving the drug, then restart at a lower dose.
• Limited data exist about giving this drug for longer than 48 hours.

Patient teaching
• Tell patient to report discomfort at I.V. site.
• Urge patient to report symptoms of hypotension, such as dizziness, light-headedness, blurred vision, or sweating.
• Tell patient to report other adverse effects promptly.

Evaluation
• Patient's blood pressure remains normal during therapy.
• Patient's volume status improves.
• Patient and family state understanding of drug therapy.

nevirapine
(neh-VEER-uh-peen)
Viramune

Pharmacologic class: nonnucleoside reverse transcriptase inhibitor
Therapeutic class: antiretroviral
Pregnancy risk category: C

Indications and dosages

▶ **Adjunct for deteriorating patients with HIV-1 infection.** *Adults:* 200 mg P.O. daily for first 14 days, followed by 200 mg P.O. b.i.d. with nucleoside analogue antiretroviral drugs.
▶ **Adjunct therapy in children infected with HIV-1.** *Children age 8 and older:* 4 mg/kg P.O. once daily for first 14 days, followed by 4 mg/kg P.O. b.i.d. thereafter. Maximum, 400 mg daily.
Children ages 2 months to 7 years: 4 mg/kg P.O. once daily for first 14 days, followed by 7 mg/kg P.O. b.i.d. thereafter. Maximum dosage is 400 mg daily.
▶ **Prevention of maternal-fetal transmission of HIV‡.** *Mother:* Give 200 mg P.O. as a single dose at the onset of labor.
Neonate: Give 2 mg/kg P.O. as a single dose 48 to 72 hours after birth. Usually given with a three-part zidovudine regimen.

Contraindications and cautions

• Contraindicated in patients hypersensitive to the drug or any of its components and in those with severe hepatic impairment.

• Use cautiously in patients with impaired renal and hepatic function or coinfection with hepatitis B or C. Use extreme caution in women and patients with CD4 counts greater than 250 cells/mm^3.

☀ **Lifespan:** In pregnant women, use only if benefits outweigh risks to the fetus. Women shouldn't breast-feed to reduce risk of giving HIV to infant. In the elderly, choose dose cautiously.

Adverse reactions

CNS: *headache,* paresthesia, *fever.*
GI: *nausea,* diarrhea, abdominal pain, ulcerative stomatitis.
Hepatic: *hepatitis, hepatotoxicity.*
Musculoskeletal: myalgia.
Skin: rash, blistering, *Stevens-Johnson syndrome, toxic epidermal necrolysis.*
Other: *severe hypersensitivity reactions,* fat redistribution.

Interactions

Drug-drug. *CYP 3A4 inhibitors (cimetidine, macrolides):* May increase nevirapine levels. Monitor patient for adverse effects.
Drugs extensively metabolized by CYP 3A4 (rifabutin, rifampin): May decrease nevirapine levels of these drugs. Adjust dosages of these drugs if needed.
Ketoconazole: Decreases ketoconazole levels and increase nevirapine levels. Avoid using together.
Hormonal contraceptives, protease inhibitors: Decreases levels of these drugs. Monitor patient for effect; advise patient to use nonhormonal contraception.
Drug-herb. *St. John's wort:* Decreases nevirapine levels. Discourage using together.

Effects on lab test results

• May increase ALT, AST, GGT, and bilirubin levels. May decrease hemoglobin level and hematocrit.
• May decrease neutrophil count.

Pharmacokinetics

Absorption: Good, > 90%.
Distribution: Wide.

Metabolism: By liver.
Excretion: In urine and feces. *Terminal-phase half-life:* 45 hours (single dose); 25 to 30 hours (multiple dosing).

Route	Onset	Peak	Duration
P.O.	Unknown	4 hr	Unknown

Action

Chemical effect: Binds to reverse transcriptase and blocks RNA-dependent and DNA-dependent DNA polymerase activities.
Therapeutic effect: May inhibit replication of HIV-1.

Available forms

Oral suspension: 50 mg/5 ml
Tablets: 200 mg

NURSING PROCESS

⚖ Assessment

• Obtain lab tests, including liver and renal function tests, before and during therapy.
• Monitor patient for blistering, oral lesions, conjunctivitis, muscle or joint aches, or general malaise. Be especially alert for severe rash, rash accompanied by fever, or rash accompanied by elevated AST and ALT. Requires drug cessation. Report such signs and symptoms immediately to prescriber.

⊕ Nursing diagnoses

• Infection related to presence of virus
• Deficient knowledge related to drug therapy

⟩ Planning and implementation

• If clinical hepatitis occurs, stop giving the drug permanently.
• Use drug with at least one other antiretroviral.
• Notify the Antiretroviral Pregnancy Registry if woman is or becomes pregnant while taking drug by calling 1-800-258-4263 or visiting www.apregistry.com.
⚠ **ALERT:** Don't confuse nelfinavir with nevirapine.

Patient teaching

• Inform patient that drug doesn't cure HIV infection, that he can still develop illnesses linked to advanced HIV infection, and can still transmit HIV to others.
• Instruct patient to report rash at once and to stop taking the drug if one develops.

Reactions may be *common*, uncommon, *life-threatening*, or COMMON AND LIFE-THREATENING.

• Instruct women to use at least two barrier methods of contraception as hormonal contraceptive's effectiveness is reduced.

• Tell patient not to use other drugs unless approved by prescriber.

• If therapy is interrupted for more than 7 days, instruct patient to resume it as if for the first time.

• Tell patient with signs or symptoms of hepatitis (such as fatigue, malaise, anorexia, nausea, jaundice, liver tenderness or hepatomegaly, with or without initially abnormal transaminase levels) to stop taking the drug and immediately seek medical evaluation.

☑ **Evaluation**

• Patient shows no signs of worsening condition.

• Patient and family state understanding of drug therapy.

niacin (vitamin B3, nicotinic acid)
(NIGH-uh-sin)
Niacin TR Tablets, Niacor, Niaspan, Nicolar, Nicotinex*, Slo Niacin

niacinamide (nicotinamide)†

Pharmacologic class: B-complex vitamin
Therapeutic class: vitamin B_3, antilipemic, peripheral vasodilator
Pregnancy risk category: A (C in dosages that exceed the RDA)

Indications and dosages

▶ **RDA.** *Neonates and infants younger than 6 months:* 2 mg.
Infants ages 6 months to 1 year: 4 mg.
Children ages 1 to 3: 6 mg.
Children ages 4 to 8: 8 mg.
Children ages 9 to 13: 12 mg.
Males age14 and older: 16 mg.
Females age 14 and older: 14 mg.
Pregnant women: 18 mg.
Breast-feeding women: 17 mg.

▶ **Pellagra.** *Adults:* 300 to 500 mg P.O. daily in divided doses, depending on severity of niacin deficiency.
Children: Up to 300 mg P.O. daily, depending on severity of niacin deficiency. After symptoms

subside, advise adequate nutrition and RDA supplements to prevent recurrence.

▶ **Hartnup disease.** *Adults:* 50 to 200 mg P.O. daily.

▶ **Niacin deficiency.** *Adults:* up to 100 mg P.O. daily.

▶ **Hyperlipidemias, especially with hypercholesterolemia.** *Adults:* Initially, 250 mg P.O. as a single dose following evening meal. Then increase q 4 to 7 days to 1 to 2 g P.O. b.i.d. or t.i.d. with meals until desired LDL level is achieved. Maximum, 6 g daily. Or, for extended-release tablets, initially start at 500 mg P.O. daily h.s. for 1 to 4 weeks; then increase to 1,000 mg h.s. during weeks 5 to 8. After week 8, increase dose by 500 mg q 4 weeks. Maximum, 2 g daily.

Contraindications and cautions

• Contraindicated in patients hypersensitive to the drug or any of its components and in those with hepatic dysfunction, active peptic ulcers, severe hypotension, or arterial hemorrhage.

• Use cautiously in patients with gallbladder disease, diabetes mellitus, or coronary artery disease and in patients with history of liver disease, peptic ulcer, allergy, or gout.

⚖ **Lifespan:** In pregnant women, use above the RDA hasn't been studied. In breast-feeding women, use above the RDA is not recommended. In children, safety of doses that exceed the RDA hasn't been established.

Adverse reactions

CNS: dizziness, transient headache.
CV: *flushing, excessive peripheral vasodilation, arrhythmias.*
GI: *nausea, vomiting, diarrhea,* activation of peptic ulceration, epigastric or substernal pain.
Hepatic: *hepatic dysfunction.*
Metabolic: hyperglycemia, hyperuricemia.
Skin: pruritus, dryness, tingling.

Interactions

Drug-drug. *Antihypertensives:* May increase risk of orthostatic hypotension. Use together cautiously; also warn patient about orthostatic hypotension.
HMG-CoA reductase inhibitors, such as lovastatin: Coadministration may result in myopathy and rhabdomyolysis. Avoid using together.

N

Effects on lab test results

• May increase glucose, AST, ALT, and uric acid levels.

Pharmacokinetics

Absorption: Rapid after P.O. use. Unknown after subcutaneous or I.M. use.
Distribution: Wide.
Metabolism: By liver to active metabolites.
Excretion: In urine. *Half-life:* About 45 minutes.

Route	Onset	Peak	Duration
P.O.	Unknown	45 min	Unknown

Action

Chemical effect: Niacin and niacinamide stimulate lipid metabolism, tissue respiration, and glycogenolysis; niacin decreases synthesis of low-density lipoproteins and inhibits lipolysis in adipose tissue.
Therapeutic effect: Restores normal level of vitamin B_3, lowers triglyceride and cholesterol levels, and dilates peripheral blood vessels.

Available forms

niacin
Capsules (timed-release): 125 mg†, 250 mg†, 400 mg†, 500 mg
Elixir: 50 mg/5 ml*†
Tablets: 50 mg†, 100 mg†, 250 mg†, 500 mg
Tablets (extended-release): 500 mg, 750 mg, 1000 mg
Tablets (timed-release): 250 mg†, 500 mg†, 750 mg†
niacinamide
Tablets: 50 mg†, 100 mg†, 500 mg†

NURSING PROCESS

⏱ Assessment

• Assess patient's condition before starting therapy and regularly thereafter to monitor the drug's effectiveness.
• Monitor hepatic function and glucose levels.
• Be alert for adverse reactions and drug interactions.
• If patient has an adverse GI reactions, monitor his hydration.
• Assess patient's and family's knowledge of drug therapy.

⊞ Nursing diagnoses

• Imbalanced nutrition: less than body requirements related to decreased intake of vitamin B_3
• Risk for deficient fluid volume related to drug-induced adverse GI reactions
• Deficient knowledge related to drug therapy

⊠ Planning and implementation

⊛ ALERT: Give aspirin (325 mg P.O. 30 minutes before niacin dose) to help reduce persistent or distressing flushing.
• Timed-release niacin or niacinamide may prevent excessive flushing that occurs with large doses, but this drug form also has been linked to hepatic dysfunction, even at doses as low as 1 g daily.
• Give drug with meals to minimize GI adverse effects.
⊛ ALERT: Don't confuse Nicobid and Nicotinex with Nicoderm, Nicotrol, or Nicorette.
Patient teaching
• Explain that skin flushing or warm sensation is usually harmless and will usually subside with continued use.
• Advise patient to decrease flushing by taking drug with a low-fat snack and not taking it after alcohol, hot beverages, hot or spicy foods, a hot shower, or exercise.
• Stress that drug is a potent drug that may cause serious adverse effects. Explain importance of adhering to therapy.
• Advise patient against self-medicating for hyperlipidemia.

✓ Evaluation

• Patient's vitamin B_3 levels are normal.
• Patient maintains adequate hydration throughout drug therapy.
• Patient and family state understanding of drug therapy.

nifedipine
(nigh-FEH-duh-peen)
**Adalat, Adalat CC, Adalat P.A. ♦,
Adalat XL ♦ , Nifedical XL, Nu-Nifed ♦ ,
Procardia, Procardia XL⌀**

Pharmacologic class: calcium channel blocker
Therapeutic class: antianginal
Pregnancy risk category: C

Indications and dosages

▶ **Vasospastic angina (also called Prinzmetal's [variant] angina) and classic chronic stable angina pectoris.** *Adults:* Initially, 10 mg P.O. (capsules) t.i.d. Usual effective dosage range is 10 to 20 mg t.i.d. Some patients may need up to 30 mg q.i.d. Maximum daily dose is 180 mg.

▶ **Hypertension.** *Adults:* 30 or 60 mg P.O. (extended-release tablets) once daily. Adjust over 7- to 14-day period. Maximum, 120 mg daily.

Contraindications and cautions

• Contraindicated in patients hypersensitive to the drug or any of its components.
• Use cautiously in those with heart failure or hypotension.
• Use extended-release tablets cautiously in patients with severe GI narrowing because obstructive symptoms may occur.
✠ **Lifespan:** In pregnant and breast-feeding women, drug is contraindicated. In children, safety and effectiveness haven't been established. In geriatric patients, use cautiously.

Adverse reactions

CNS: *dizziness, light-headedness, headache,* weakness, **syncope.**
CV: *flushing,* peripheral edema, hypotension, palpitations, **heart failure, MI.**
EENT: nasal congestion.
GI: nausea, heartburn, diarrhea.
Metabolic: *hypokalemia.*
Musculoskeletal: muscle cramps.
Respiratory: dyspnea, **pulmonary edema.**
Skin: rash, pruritus.

Interactions

Drug-drug. *Beta blockers, such as propranolol:* May cause hypotension and heart failure. Use together cautiously; monitor vital signs.
Cimetidine, ranitidine: May decrease nifedipine metabolism. Monitor patient closely for increased adverse effects.
I.V. magnesium sulfate: May cause neuromuscular blockade and hypotension. Don't use together. Monitor patient.
Quinidine: May cause hypotension, bradycardia, ventricular tachycardia, AV block, and pulmonary edema. Reduce quinidine dosage and monitor level. Monitor ECG and vital signs.

Drug-food. *Grapefruit juice:* Increases drug bioavailability. Discourage using together because effects vary.

Effects on lab test results

• May increase ALT, AST, alkaline phosphatase, and LDH levels. May decrease potassium level.

Pharmacokinetics

Absorption: Rapid and about 90%, but only about 45% to 75% reaches circulation because of significant first-pass effect in liver.
Distribution: About 92% to 98% is bound to proteins.
Metabolism: In liver.
Excretion: In urine and feces as inactive metabolites. *Half-life:* 2 to 5 hours.

Route	Onset	Peak	Duration
P.O.	20 min	30 min–2 hr	Unknown

Action

Chemical effect: Unknown; may inhibit calcium ion influx across cardiac and smooth-muscle cells, decreasing myocardial contractility and oxygen demand. Also may dilate coronary arteries and arterioles.
Therapeutic effect: Reduces blood pressure and prevents angina.

Available forms

Capsules: 10 mg, 20 mg
Tablets (extended-release): 30 mg, 60 mg, 90 mg

NURSING PROCESS

✐ Assessment
• Assess patient's condition before starting therapy and regularly thereafter to monitor the drug's effectiveness.
• Monitor blood pressure regularly, especially if patient also takes a beta blocker or an antihypertensive.
• Monitor potassium level regularly.
• Be alert for adverse reactions and drug interactions.
• Assess patient's and family's knowledge of drug therapy.

🔟 Nursing diagnoses
• Risk for injury related to presence of hypertension

- Pain related to angina
- Deficient knowledge related to drug therapy

> **Planning and implementation**

⑤ **ALERT:** When rapid response to drug is desired, instruct patient to bite and swallow capsule. When using this method, continuously monitor blood pressure and ECG.

⑤ **ALERT:** Don't use S.L. route for nifedipine capsules despite previous widespread use. Peak level may be lower and take longer to peak than when capsule is bitten and swallowed.

⑤ **ALERT:** Procardia XL and Adalat CC aren't equivalent.

- S.L. nitroglycerin may be prescribed for acute angina.
- Although rebound effect hasn't been observed when drug is stopped, reduce dosage slowly.

⑤ **ALERT:** Don't confuse nifedipine with nicardipine or nisoldipine.

Patient teaching

- If patient is kept on nitrate therapy while adjusting nifedipine dose, urge continued compliance with both drugs.
- Warn patient that angina may worsen when therapy starts or dose increases. Reassure him that this is temporary.
- Instruct patient to swallow extended-release tablets without breaking, crushing, or chewing them.
- Advise patient who takes extended-release form of drug that he may pass the tablet's wax-matrix "ghost" in stool.

⑤ **ALERT:** Warn patient not to switch brands of this drug. Procardia XL and Adalat CC aren't equivalent because they have differing pharmacokinetics.

- Tell patient to protect capsules from direct light and moisture and to store them at room temperature.

☑ **Evaluation**

- Patient's blood pressure is normal.
- Patient's angina is less frequent and severe.
- Patient and family state understanding of drug therapy.

nisoldipine
(nigh-SOHL-dih-peen)
Sular

Pharmacologic class: calcium channel blocker
Therapeutic class: antihypertensive
Pregnancy risk category: C

Indications and dosages

▶ **Hypertension.** *Adults:* Initially, 20 mg P.O. once daily; then increase by 10 mg weekly or at longer intervals, as indicated. Usual maintenance dosage is 20 to 40 mg once daily. Dosages above 60 mg daily aren't recommended.

⊠ **Adjust-a-dose:** For patients older than age 65 and those who have liver dysfunction, initial dosage is 10 mg P.O. daily.

Contraindications and cautions

- Contraindicated in patients hypersensitive to dihydropyridine calcium channel blockers.
- Use cautiously in patients with severe hepatic impairment, heart failure, or compromised ventricular function, and particularly in those taking beta blockers.

⚓ **Lifespan:** In pregnant women, use cautiously. In breast-feeding women, don't use drug. In children, safety and effectiveness haven't been established.

Adverse reactions

CNS: *headache,* dizziness.
CV: vasodilation, palpitations, chest pain, *peripheral edema.*
EENT: sinusitis, pharyngitis.
GI: nausea.
Skin: rash.

Interactions

Drug-drug. *Cimetidine:* Increases bioavailability and peak levels of nisoldipine. Monitor patient for increased adverse effects.
Quinidine: May decrease bioavailability, but not peak levels, of nisoldipine. Monitor patient.
Drug-food. *Grapefruit juice:* May increase peak concentration of drug, increasing therapeutic and adverse effects. Give drug 1 hour before or after patient eats or drinks grapefruit.
High-fat meal: May increase peak drug level. Don't give drug with a high-fat meal.

Effects on lab test results

None reported.

Pharmacokinetics

Absorption: Good; high-fat foods significantly affect rate of release of drug.
Distribution: About 99% protein-bound.
Metabolism: Extensive.
Excretion: In urine. *Half-life:* 7 to 12 hours.

Route	Onset	Peak	Duration
P.O.	Unknown	6–12 hr	24 hr

Action

Chemical effect: Prevents entry of calcium ions into vascular smooth-muscle cells, causing dilation of arterioles, which decreases peripheral vascular resistance.
Therapeutic effect: Lowers blood pressure.

Available forms

Extended-release tablets: 10 mg, 20 mg, 30 mg, 40 mg

NURSING PROCESS

Assessment

• Assess patient's blood pressure before starting therapy, and monitor regularly, especially during dose adjustment.
• Monitor patient carefully. Some patients, especially those with severe obstructive coronary artery disease, may develop increased frequency, duration, or severity of angina or acute MI when starting calcium channel blocker therapy or increasing dose.
• Be alert for adverse reactions and interactions.
• Assess patient's and family's knowledge of drug therapy.

Nursing diagnoses

• Risk for injury related to hypertension
• Excessive fluid volume related to edema
• Deficient knowledge related to drug therapy

Planning and implementation

• Don't give drug with a high-fat meal or grapefruit products.
⊛ **ALERT:** Don't confuse nisoldipine with nifedipine or nicardipine.
Patient teaching
• Tell patient to take drug as prescribed.

• Instruct patient to swallow tablet whole and not to chew, divide, or crush it.

Evaluation

• Patient's blood pressure is normal.
• Patient doesn't exhibit signs of edema.
• Patient and family state understanding of drug therapy.

nitrofurantoin macrocrystals
(nigh-troh-fyoo-RAN-toyn MAH-kroh-kris-tuls)
Macrobid, Macrodantin

nitrofurantoin microcrystals
Apo-Nitrofurantoin ◆, Furadantin, Furalan, Macrodantin

Pharmacologic class: nitrofuran
Therapeutic class: urinary tract anti-infective
Pregnancy risk category: B

Indications and dosages

▶ **UTI caused by susceptible *Escherichia coli*, *Staphylococcus aureus*, enterococci, and certain strains of *Klebsiella* and *Enterobacter*.**
Adults and children older than age 12: 50 to 100 mg P.O. q.i.d. with milk or meals. Or 100 mg Macrobid PO q 12 hours for 7 days.
Children ages 1 month to 12 years: 5 to 7 mg/kg P.O. daily, divided q.i.d.
▶ **Long-term suppression therapy.** *Adults:* 50 to 100 mg P.O. q h.s.
Children age 1 month and older: 1 to 2 mg/kg P.O. q h.s.

Contraindications and cautions

• Contraindicated in patients who are hypersensitive to the drug or any of its components. Contraindicated in patients with moderate to severe renal impairment (creatinine clearance less than 60 ml/minute), anuria, or oliguria.
• Use cautiously in patients with renal impairment, anemia, diabetes mellitus, electrolyte abnormalities, vitamin B deficiency, debilitating disease, or G6PD deficiency.
⚹ **Lifespan:** In pregnant women, use cautiously. In breast-feeding women, use cautiously; it's unknown if the drug appears in breast milk. In infants age 1 month and younger, drug is contraindicated.

Adverse reactions

CNS: *peripheral neuropathy,* headache, dizziness, drowsiness, *ascending polyneuropathy.*
GI: anorexia, nausea, vomiting, abdominal pain, diarrhea.
Hematologic: *hemolysis in patients with G6PD deficiency, agranulocytosis, thrombocytopenia, leukopenia.*
Hepatic: *hepatitis, hepatic necrosis.*
Respiratory: *asthma,* pulmonary sensitivity.
Skin: maculopapular, erythematous, or eczematous eruption; pruritus; urticaria; exfoliative dermatitis; *Stevens-Johnson syndrome.*
Other: hypersensitivity reactions, *anaphylaxis,* transient alopecia, drug fever, overgrowth of nonsusceptible organisms in urinary tract.

Interactions

Drug-drug. *Magnesium-containing antacids:* Decreases nitrofurantoin absorption. Separate ingestion by 1 hour.
Probenecid, sulfinpyrazone: Increases blood level and decreases urine level. May result in increased toxicity and lack of therapeutic effect. Don't use together.
Quinolones (such as nalidixic acid, norfloxacin): May decrease effectiveness of quinolone derivatives. Avoid using together.
Drug-food. *Any food:* Increases drug absorption. Give drug with food.

Effects on lab test results

• May increase phosphorous, bilirubin, and alkaline phosphatase levels. May decrease glucose and hemoglobin levels and hematocrit.
• May decrease granulocyte and platelet counts.
• May cause false-positive results with urine glucose test using copper sulfate reduction method (Clinitest), Benedict's solution, or Fehling's solution, but not with glucose enzymatic test.

Pharmacokinetics

Absorption: Good. Food aids drug's dissolution and speeds absorption. Macrocrystal form has slower dissolution and absorption.
Distribution: Into bile; 60% binds to proteins.
Metabolism: Partially in liver.
Excretion: About 30% to 50% in urine. *Half-life:* 15 minutes to 1 hour.

Route	Onset	Peak	Duration
P.O.	Unknown	Unknown	Unknown

Action

Chemical effect: Unknown; may interfere with bacterial enzyme systems and cell wall formation.
Therapeutic effect: Hinders growth of many common gram-positive and gram-negative urinary pathogens.

Available forms

nitrofurantoin macrocrystals
Capsules: 25 mg, 50 mg, 100 mg
Capsules (dual-release): 100 mg
nitrofurantoin microcrystals
Capsules: 50 mg, 100 mg
Oral suspension: 25 mg/5 ml
Tablets: 50 mg, 100 mg

NURSING PROCESS

Assessment
• Assess patient's infection before starting therapy and regularly thereafter to monitor the drug's effectiveness.
• Obtain urine specimen for culture and sensitivity tests before starting therapy, and repeat p.r.n. Start therapy pending results.
• Monitor fluid intake and output. May turn urine darker or even brown.
• Monitor CBC and pulmonary status regularly.
• Assess for renal impairment before and during therapy especially with high doses as increased risk of ascending polyneuropathy.
• Be alert for adverse reactions and drug interactions.
• If patient has adverse GI reactions, monitor his hydration.
• Assess patient's and family's knowledge of drug therapy.

Nursing diagnoses
• Infection related to susceptible bacteria
• Risk for deficient fluid volume related to drug-induced adverse GI reactions
• Deficient knowledge related to drug therapy

Planning and implementation
• Drug has no effect on blood or tissue outside urinary tract.

• Notify prescriber if patient develops cough, chest pains, fever, chills, and dyspnea (signs of pulmonary sensitivity).
• Be aware that patients with G6PD deficiency who develop hemolysis during therapy will recover when drug is stopped.
⑨ **ALERT:** Hypersensitivity may develop during long-term therapy.
• Dual-release capsules (25-mg nitrofurantoin macrocrystals combined with 75-mg nitrofurantoin monohydrate) enable twice-daily dosing.
• Continue therapy for 3 days after urine specimens become sterile.
• Patient may experience fewer adverse GI effects with nitrofurantoin macrocrystals.
• Store drug in amber container. Avoid metals other than stainless steel or aluminum to avoid precipitate formation.

Patient teaching
• Tell patient to take drug with food or milk to minimize GI distress.
• Teach patient how to measure intake and output. Warn him that drug will turn urine darker or even brown.
• Instruct patient how to store drug.

☑ Evaluation
• Patient is free from infection.
• Patient maintains adequate hydration throughout drug therapy.
• Patient and family state understanding of drug therapy.

nitroglycerin (glyceryl trinitrate)
(nigh-troh-GLIH-suh-rin)
Anginine◇, Deponit, Minitran, Nitradisc◇, Nitro-Bid, Nitro-Bid IV, Nitrodisc, Nitro-Dur, Nitrogard, Nitroglyn, Nitrolingual, NitroQuick, Nitrostat, Nitro-Time, Transderm-Nitro, Transiderm-Nitro◇, Tridil

Pharmacologic class: nitrate
Therapeutic class: antianginal, vasodilator
Pregnancy risk category: C

Indications and dosages
▶ **Prevention of chronic anginal attacks.**
Adults: 2.5 mg or 2.6 mg sustained-release capsule q 8 to 12 hours. Or 2% ointment: Start with ½ inch of ointment and increase by ½-inch increments until headache occurs; then decrease

to previous dose. Range of dosage with ointment is ½ to 5 inches. Usual dose is 1 to 2 inches. Or Nitrodisc, Nitro-Dur, or Transderm-Nitro transdermal disk or pad, 0.2 to 0.4 mg/hour once daily.
▶ **Acute angina pectoris; to prevent or minimize anginal attacks when taken immediately before stressful events.** *Adults:* 1 S.L. tablet (grain [gr] ½₀₀, ⅟₁₅₀, ⅟₁₀₀) dissolved under tongue or in buccal pouch as soon as angina begins. Repeat q 5 minutes for up to 15 minutes if symptoms persist. Or, using Nitrolingual spray, 1 or 2 sprays into mouth, preferably onto or under tongue. Repeat q 3 to 5 minutes if symptoms persist, to maximum of three doses in 15-minute period. Or, 1 to 3 mg transmucosally q 3 to 5 hours during waking hours.
▶ **Hypertension related to surgery; heart failure linked to MI; angina pectoris in acute situations; to produce controlled hypotension during surgery.** *Adults:* Initial infusion rate is 5 mcg/minute. Increase p.r.n. by 5 mcg/minute q 3 to 5 minutes until response occurs. If 20-mcg/minute rate doesn't produce response, increase dosage by as much as 20 mcg/minute q 3 to 5 minutes. Up to 100 mcg/minute I.V. may be needed.
▶ **Hypertensive crisis‡.** *Adults:* Infuse at 5 to 100 mcg/minute I.V.

▼ I.V. administration
• Mix in glass bottles and avoid I.V. filters because drug binds to plastic. Regular polyvinyl chloride tubing can bind up to 80% of drug, requiring higher doses. Special nonabsorbent, nonpolyvinyl chloride tubing is available from manufacturer.
• Dilute drug with D₅W or normal saline solution for injection to a concentration no stronger than 400 mcg/ml.
• Always use same type of infusion set when changing I.V. lines.
• When changing concentration of nitroglycerin infusion, flush I.V. administration set with 15 to 20 ml of new concentration before use. This will clear line of old drug solution.
• Give with infusion control device and titrate to desired response.
⊗ **Incompatibilities**
Alteplase, bretylium, hydralazine, levofloxacin, phenytoin sodium, other I.V. drugs.

Contraindications and cautions

• Contraindicated in patients hypersensitive to nitrates and in those with early MI (S.L. form), severe anemia, increased intracranial pressure, angle-closure glaucoma, orthostatic hypotension, and allergy to adhesives (transdermal form). I.V. nitroglycerin is contraindicated in patients with hypovolemia, hypotension, cardiac tamponade, restrictive cardiomyopathy, constrictive pericarditis, or hypersensitivity to I.V. form.

• Use cautiously in patients with hypotension or volume depletion.

⚥ **Lifespan:** In pregnant women, use cautiously. In breast-feeding women, use cautiously; it's unknown if the drug appears in breast milk. In children, safety and effectiveness haven't been established.

Adverse reactions

CNS: *headache, throbbing, dizziness,* weakness.
CV: *orthostatic hypotension, tachycardia, flushing,* palpitations, fainting.
EENT: sublingual burning.
GI: nausea, vomiting.
Skin: cutaneous vasodilation, contact dermatitis (patch), rash.
Other: hypersensitivity reactions.

Interactions

Drug-drug. *Alteplase:* Decreases t-PA antigen concentrations. Avoid using together. If use together is unavoidable, use the lowest effective dose of nitroglycerin.
Antihypertensives: May enhance hypotensive effect. Monitor patient closely.
Dihydroergotamine: May decrease antianginal effect or increase mean standing systolic blood pressure. Avoid use together.
Sildenafil, tadalafil, vardenafil: May cause severe hypotension. Use of nitrates in any form with erectile dysfunction drugs is contraindicated.
Drug-lifestyle. *Alcohol use:* May increase hypotension. Urge patient to avoid alcohol during therapy.

Effects on lab test results

• May interfere with Zlatkis-Zak color reaction, causing false report of decreased cholesterol level.

Pharmacokinetics

Absorption: For P.O. use, good but incomplete. For S.L. use, relatively complete. For topical or transdermal use, good.
Distribution: Wide; about 60% bound to proteins.
Metabolism: In liver.
Excretion: Metabolites in urine. *Half-life:* About 1 to 4 minutes.

Route	Onset	Peak	Duration
P.O.	20–45 min	Unknown	3–8 hr
I.V.	Immediate	Immediate	3–5 min
Topical	30 min	Unknown	2–12 hr
Transdermal	30 min	Unknown	≤ 24 hr
S.L.	1–3 min	Unknown	30–60 min
Buccal	3 min	Unknown	5 hr
Translingual	2–4 min	Unknown	30–60 min

Action

Chemical effect: Reduces cardiac oxygen demand by decreasing left ventricular end-diastolic pressure (preload) and, to a lesser extent, systemic vascular resistance (afterload). Also increases blood flow through collateral coronary vessels.
Therapeutic effect: Prevents or relieves acute angina, lowers blood pressure, and helps minimize heart failure caused by MI.

Available forms

Aerosol (translingual): 0.4 mg metered spray
Capsules (sustained-release): 2.5 mg, 6.5 mg, 9 mg
I.V.: 0.5 mg/ml, 0.8 mg/ml, 5 mg/ml
I.V. premixed solutions in dextrose: 100 mcg/ml, 200 mcg/ml, 400 mcg/ml
Tablets (buccal): 2 mg, 3 mg
Tablets (S.L.): 0.3 mg (gr 1/200) 0.4 mg (gr 1/150), 0.6 mg (gr 1/100)
Topical: 2% ointment
Transdermal: 2.5 mg/24 hours, 5 mg/24 hours, 7.5 mg/24 hours, 10 mg/24 hours, 15 mg/24 hours, 20 mg/24 hours

NURSING PROCESS

Assessment
• Assess patient's condition before starting therapy and regularly thereafter to monitor the drug's effectiveness.

• Monitor vital signs and drug response. Be particularly aware of blood pressure. Excessive hypotension may worsen MI.
• Be alert for adverse reactions and drug interactions.
• Assess patient's and family's knowledge of drug therapy.

Nursing diagnoses
• Pain related to angina
• Risk for injury related to drug-induced adverse reactions
• Deficient knowledge related to drug therapy

Planning and implementation
• Give P.O. tablets on empty stomach, either 30 minutes before or 1 to 2 hours after meals.
• Don't allow patient to swallow or chew S.L. tablets.
• Give S.L. tablet at first sign of attack. Wet tablet with patient's saliva, then place under patient's tongue until completely absorbed. Have patient sit down and rest until pain subsides.
• Repeat dose q 5 minutes for up to three doses. If drug doesn't provide relief, immediately notify prescriber.
• If patient complains of tingling sensation with S.L. form, place tablet in buccal pouch.
• When giving translingual aerosol form, make sure patient doesn't inhale spray. Release it onto or under tongue, and have patient wait about 10 seconds or so before swallowing.
• To apply ointment, measure prescribed amount on application paper, then place paper on any nonhairy area. Don't rub in. Cover with plastic film to aid absorption and protect clothing.
• If using Tape-Surrounded Appli-Ruler (TSAR) system, keep TSAR on skin to protect patient's clothing and to make sure that ointment remains in place.
• Remove excess ointment from previous site before applying next dose. Avoid getting ointment on fingers.
• Apply transdermal forms to any nonhairy area, except lower parts of arms or legs, to promote maximum absorption.
ALERT: Remove transdermal patch before defibrillation. Electric current may cause patch to arc, causing burn to patient or damage to paddles.
• When stopping transdermal therapy for angina, gradually reduce dose and frequency of application over 4 to 6 weeks.
• If drug is ineffective, immediately notify prescriber, keep patient at rest.
• Drug may cause headache, especially at start of therapy. Lower the dose temporarily. Tolerance to drug without headache response may develop. Treat headache with aspirin or acetaminophen.
• Minimize drug tolerance with 10- to 12-hour daily nitrate-free interval. For example, remove transdermal system in early evening and apply a new system the next morning. Or omit the last daily dose of buccal, sustained-release, or ointment form. If tolerance is suspected, alter dosage.
ALERT: Don't confuse Nitro-Bid with Nicobid.
ALERT: Don't confuse nitroglycerin with nitroprusside.

Patient teaching
• Teach patient how to use the form of drug prescribed.
• Tell patient to place transmucosal tablet between lip and gum above incisors, or between cheek and gum.
• Tell patient to swallow oral tablets whole and not to chew them.
• Instruct patient to take drug regularly, as prescribed, and to have it accessible at all times.
• Tell patient that abruptly stopping the drug causes coronary vasospasm.
• Inform patient that an additional dose may be taken before anticipated stress or h.s. if angina is nocturnal.
• Instruct patient to use caution when wearing transdermal patch near microwave oven. Leaking radiation may heat metallic backing of patch and cause burns.
• Advise patient not to drink alcohol during therapy.
• Tell patient to change to upright position slowly. Advise him to go up and down stairs carefully and to lie down at first sign of dizziness.
• Urge patient to store drug in cool, dark place in tightly closed container. To ensure potency, tell him to replace S.L. tablets 6 months after opening (mark bottle with date opened), and to remove cotton because it absorbs drug.
• Tell patient to store S.L. tablets in original container or other container specifically approved for this use and to carry container in jacket pocket or purse, not in a pocket close to body.

Evaluation
• Patient reports pain relief.

N

• Patient doesn't experience injury from adverse reactions.
• Patient and family state understanding of drug therapy.

nitroprusside sodium
(nigh-troh-PRUHS-ighd SOH-dee-um)
Nipride ◆, Nitropress

Pharmacologic class: vasodilator
Therapeutic class: antihypertensive
Pregnancy risk category: C

Indications and dosages

▶ **To lower blood pressure quickly in hypertensive emergencies; to produce controlled hypotension during anesthesia; to reduce preload and afterload in cardiac pump failure or cardiogenic shock (may be used with or without dopamine).** *Adults:* Begin infusion at 0.25 to 0.3 mcg/kg/minute I.V. and gradually titrate q few minutes to a maximum infusion rate of 10 mcg/kg/minute. Average dose is 3 mcg/kg/minute. Patients taking other antihypertensives are extremely sensitive to nitroprusside. Adjust dosage.

▼ I.V. administration

• Dissolve 50 mg in 2 to 3 ml of D_5W injection. Further dilute concentration in 250, 500, or 1,000 ml of D_5W to provide solutions with 200, 100, or 50 mcg/ml, respectively. Reconstitute ADD-Vantage vials labeled as containing 50 mg of drug according to manufacturer's directions.
• Because drug is sensitive to light, wrap infusion bag in foil; wrapping the tubing isn't needed.
• Infuse with infusion pump. Drug is best given by piggyback through peripheral line with no other drug. Don't adjust rate of main line while drug is being infused. Even small bolus of nitroprusside can cause severe hypotension.
• Check blood pressure every 5 minutes at start of infusion and every 15 minutes thereafter.
• If severe hypotension occurs, stop infusion. Effects of drug reverse quickly. Notify prescriber.
• Start arterial pressure line. Adjust flow to specified level.
• If cyanide toxicity occurs, stop drug immediately and notify prescriber.

• Fresh solution will have faint brownish tint. Discard drug after 24 hours.
⊗ **Incompatibilities**
Bacteriostatic water for injection, other I.V. drug, or preservative.

Contraindications and cautions

• Contraindicated in patients hypersensitive to the drug or any of its components, and in those with compensatory hypertension (as in arteriovenous shunt or coarctation of aorta), inadequate cerebral circulation, congenital optic atrophy, or tobacco-induced amblyopia.
• Use cautiously in patients with increased intracranial pressure and in those with hypothyroidism, hepatic or renal disease, hyponatremia, or low vitamin B_{12} level.
⁂ **Lifespan:** In pregnant women, use cautiously. In breast-feeding women and in children, safety and effectiveness haven't been established.

Adverse reactions

CNS: *headache, dizziness,* ataxia, loss of consciousness, *coma, increased intracranial pressure,* weak pulse, absent reflexes, dilated pupils, *restlessness, muscle twitching.*
CV: distant heart sounds, palpitations, *bradycardia,* tachycardia, *hypotension.*
GI: vomiting, nausea, abdominal pain.
Hematologic: *methemoglobinemia.*
Metabolic: *acidosis.*
Respiratory: dyspnea, shallow breathing.
Skin: pink color, *diaphoresis.*
Other: *thiocyanate toxicity, cyanide toxicity.*

Interactions

Drug-drug. *Antihypertensives:* May cause sensitivity to nitroprusside. Adjust dosage.
Ganglionic blockers, general anesthetics, negative inotropics, other antihypertensives: May have additive effects. Monitor blood pressure closely.
Sildenafil, tadalafil, vardenafil: May increase hypotensive effects. Don't use together.
Tricyclic antidepressants: May increase the pressor response and cause arrhythmias. Use with caution.

Effects on lab test results

• May increase creatinine, thiocyanide, and methemoglobin levels.

Pharmacokinetics

Absorption: Administered I.V.
Distribution: Unknown.
Metabolism: Rapid in erythrocytes and tissues to cyanide radical and then converted to thiocyanate in liver.
Excretion: Primarily as metabolites in urine. *Half-life:* 2 minutes.

Route	Onset	Peak	Duration
I.V.	Immediate	1–2 min	10 min

Action

Chemical effect: Relaxes arteriolar and venous smooth muscle.
Therapeutic effect: Lowers blood pressure and reduces preload and afterload.

Available forms

Injection: 50 mg/vial in 2-ml, 5-ml vials

NURSING PROCESS

Assessment

- Assess patient's condition before starting therapy.
- Obtain baseline vital signs before giving drug, and find out what parameters prescriber wants to achieve.

ALERT: Excessive doses or rapid infusion (more than 15 mcg/kg/minute) can cause cyanide toxicity; check thiocyanate levels q 72 hours. Levels above 100 mcg/ml may cause toxicity. Watch for profound hypotension, metabolic acidosis, dyspnea, headache, loss of consciousness, ataxia, and vomiting.

- Be alert for adverse reactions and drug interactions.
- Assess patient's (if appropriate) and family's knowledge of drug therapy.

Nursing diagnoses

- Risk for injury related to hypertension
- Decreased cardiac output related to heart failure
- Deficient knowledge related to drug therapy

Planning and implementation

- Keep patient in supine position when starting therapy or adjusting dose.

ALERT: Don't confuse nitroprusside with nitroglycerin.

Patient teaching

- Advise patient, if alert, to report adverse reactions or discomfort at the I.V. site immediately.

Evaluation

- Patient's blood pressure is normal.
- Patient has normal cardiac output.
- Patient and family state understanding of drug therapy.

nizatidine

(nigh-ZAT-ih-deen)
Axid, Axid AR†, Tazac ♦

Pharmacologic class: histamine$_2$ (H_2)-receptor antagonist
Therapeutic class: gastric antisecretory
Pregnancy risk category: B

Indications and dosages

▶ **Active duodenal ulcer.** *Adults:* 300 mg P.O. daily h.s. Or 150 mg P.O. b.i.d.
▶ **Maintenance therapy for duodenal ulcer.** *Adults:* 150 mg P.O. daily h.s.
▶ **Benign gastric ulcer.** *Adults:* 150 mg P.O. b.i.d. or 300 mg P.O. h.s. for 8 weeks.
▶ **Gastroesophageal reflux disease.** *Adults:* 150 mg P.O. b.i.d.
▶ **Relief or prevention of heartburn†.** *Adults:* 75 mg tablet 1 to 2 times daily.

Adjust-a-dose: For patients with renal impairment, if creatinine clearance is 20 to 50 ml/minute, give 150 mg P.O. daily for active duodenal ulcer or 150 mg q other day for maintenance therapy. If creatinine clearance is less than 20 ml/minute, give 150 mg P.O. q other day for active ulcer or 150 mg q third day for maintenance.

Contraindications and cautions

- Contraindicated in patients hypersensitive to H_2-receptor antagonists.
- Use cautiously in patients with renal impairment.

Lifespan: In pregnant women, use cautiously. In breast-feeding women, use cautiously; it's unknown if the drug appears in breast milk. In children, safety and effectiveness haven't been established.

N

Adverse reactions

CNS: *somnolence,* fever.
CV: *arrhythmias.*
Hematologic: *thrombocytopenia.*
Hepatic: liver damage.
Metabolic: hyperuricemia.
Skin: *diaphoresis,* rash, urticaria, exfoliative
dermatitis.

Interactions

Drug-drug. *Aspirin:* May elevate salicylate levels (with high doses). Monitor patient for salicylate toxicity.
Drug-lifestyle. *Alcohol use:* May increase alcohol level. Discourage using together.

Effects on lab test results

• May increase liver enzyme and uric acid levels.
• May decrease platelet count.
• May cause false-positive test results for uro-
bilinogen.

Pharmacokinetics

Absorption: Greater than 90%. May be slightly
enhanced by food and slightly impaired by
antacids.
Distribution: About 35% of drug is bound to
proteins.
Metabolism: Unknown, but may undergo hepatic metabolism.
Excretion: More than 90% excreted in urine;
less than 6% in feces. *Half-life:* 1 to 2 hours.

Route	Onset	Peak	Duration
P.O.	≤ 30 min	30 min–3 hr	≤ 12 hr

Action

Chemical effect: Competitively inhibits action
of H_2 at receptor sites of parietal cells.
Therapeutic effect: Decreases gastric acid secretion.

Available forms

Capsules: 75 mg†, 150 mg, 300 mg

NURSING PROCESS

⚚ Assessment

• Assess patient's condition before starting therapy and regularly thereafter to monitor the
drug's effectiveness.

• Be alert for adverse reactions and drug interactions.
• Assess patient for abdominal pain. Note presence of blood in emesis, stool, or gastric aspirate.
• Assess patient's and family's knowledge of
drug therapy.

⊕ Nursing diagnoses

• Impaired tissue integrity related to ulceration
of GI mucosa
• Decreased cardiac output related to drug-
induced arrhythmias
• Deficient knowledge related to drug therapy

❯ Planning and implementation

• If needed, open capsules and mix contents
with apple juice.
Patient teaching
• Urge patient not to smoke cigarettes because
they may increase gastric acid secretion and
worsen disease.
• Have patient report blood in stool or emesis.
• Warn patient to take drug as directed, even after pain subsides, to allow for adequate healing.
• Instruct users of OTC dose to report worsening symptoms to provider and not to exceed recommended dose without provider instruction.

✔ Evaluation

• Patient reports pain relief.
• Patient maintains normal cardiac output
throughout drug therapy.
• Patient and family state understanding of drug
therapy.

norepinephrine bitartrate (levarterenol bitartrate, noradrenaline acid tartrate)

(nor-ep-ih-NEF-rin bigh-TAR-trayt)
Levophed

Pharmacologic class: adrenergic
Therapeutic class: vasopressor
Pregnancy risk category: C

Indications and dosages

▶ **To restore blood pressure in severe hypotension, shock, and during cardiac arrest.**
Adults: Initially, 8 to 12 mcg/minute by I.V. in-

fusion, adjust to maintain low normal blood pressure (systolic blood pressure 80 to 100 mm Hg). Or 0.5 to 1 mcg/minute I.V. infusion, titrate to effect. Average maintenance dosage is 2 to 4 mcg/minute.

Children: 2 mcg/m²/minute by I.V. infusion; adjust dosage based on patient response. Or, initial I.V. infusion rate of 0.1 mcg/kg/minute, titrate to effect.

▶ **GI bleeding‡.** *Adults:* Give 8 mg in 250 ml normal saline solution intraperitoneally. Or give 8 mg in 100 ml of normal saline solution by NG tube q 1 hour for 6 to 8 hours and then q 2 hours for 4 to 6 hours.

▽ I.V. administration

• Prepare by adding 4 mg of norepinephrine to 1 L of 5% dextrose injection to equal a concentration of 4 mcg/ml.

• Never leave patient unattended during infusion.

• Use central venous catheter or large vein, such as in antecubital fossa, to minimize risk of extravasation. Dilute in dextrose 5% in normal saline solution for injection. Use continuous infusion pump to regulate flow rate and piggyback setup so I.V. line remains open if drug is stopped.

• Titrate infusion rate according to assessment findings and prescriber's guidelines. In previously hypertensive patients, don't raise blood pressure higher than 30 to 40 mm Hg below previous systolic pressure.

• Check site frequently for blanching and other signs of extravasation. If it occurs, change infusion site immediately and call prescriber. Counteract effect by infiltrating area with 5 to 10 mg phentolamine and 10 to 15 ml of normal saline solution. Untreated extravasation can lead to tissue necrosis.

• If prolonged I.V. therapy is needed, change injection site frequently.

• Protect drug from light. Discard discolored solutions or solutions that contain precipitate. Drug solutions deteriorate after 24 hours.

⊗ **Incompatibilities**

Alkaline solutions, aminophylline, amobarbital, chlorothiazide, chlorpheniramine, iron salts, lidocaine, normal saline solution, oxidizing drugs, pentobarbital sodium, phenobarbital sodium, phenytoin sodium, ranitidine hydrochloride, sodium bicarbonate, streptomycin, thiopental, whole blood.

Contraindications and cautions

• Contraindicated in patients receiving cyclopropane or halothane anesthesia and in patients with mesenteric or peripheral vascular thrombosis, profound hypoxia, hypercapnia, or hypotension caused by blood volume deficits.

• Use cautiously in patients receiving MAO inhibitors, tricyclic antidepressants, or certain antihistamines and in patients with sulfite sensitivity.

⚖ **Lifespan:** In pregnant and breast-feeding women, drug is contraindicated. In children, safety and effectiveness haven't been established. Use cautiously in elderly patients because of increased risk of vasoconstrictive adverse reactions.

Adverse reactions

CNS: *headache,* anxiety, fever, weakness, dizziness, tremor, restlessness, insomnia.

CV: *bradycardia, severe hypertension,* marked increase in peripheral resistance, *decreased cardiac output, arrhythmias.*

GU: decreased urine output.

Metabolic: *metabolic acidosis,* hyperglycemia, increased glycogenolysis.

Respiratory: *respiratory difficulties, asthmatic episodes.*

Other: tissue sloughing with extravasation, swelling and enlargement of thyroid, *anaphylaxis.*

Interactions

Drug-drug. *Alpha blockers:* May antagonize drug effects. Monitor patient.

Antihistamines, ergot alkaloids, guanethidine, methyldopa: Use with sympathomimetics may cause severe hypertension. Don't give together.

Bretylium: May cause arrhythmias. Monitor ECG closely.

Inhaled anesthetics: Increases risk of arrhythmias. Monitor ECG closely.

MAO inhibitors: Increases risk of hypertensive crisis. Monitor patient closely.

Tricyclic antidepressants: May increase the pressor response and cause arrhythmias. Use with caution.

Effects on lab test results

• May increase glucose level.

Pharmacokinetics

Absorption: Administered I.V.

Distribution: Drug localizes in sympathetic nerve tissues.
Metabolism: Metabolized in liver and other tissues to inactive compounds.
Excretion: Excreted in urine. *Half-life:* About 1 minute.

Route	Onset	Peak	Duration
I.V.	Immediate	Immediate	1–2 min

Action

Chemical effect: Stimulates alpha- and beta$_1$-adrenergic receptors in sympathetic nervous system.
Therapeutic effect: Raises blood pressure.

Available forms

Injection: 1 mg/ml in 4-ml ampules

NURSING PROCESS

Assessment
• Assess patient's condition before starting therapy.
• During infusion, frequently monitor ECG, cardiac output, central venous pressure, pulmonary capillary wedge pressure, pulse rate, urine output, and color and temperature of limbs. Also, check blood pressure q 2 minutes until stabilized; then check q 5 minutes.
• Be alert for adverse reactions and drug interactions.
• Monitor vital signs closely when therapy ends. Watch for sudden drop in blood pressure.
• Assess patient's and family's knowledge of drug therapy.

Nursing diagnoses
• Decreased cardiac output related to hypotension
• Risk for injury related to drug-induced adverse reactions
• Deficient knowledge related to drug therapy

Planning and implementation
• Drug isn't a substitute for blood or fluid volume deficit. If deficit exists, replace fluid before giving vasopressors.
• Keep emergency drugs on hand to reverse effects of norepinephrine: atropine for reflex bradycardia, phentolamine for vasopressor effects, and propranolol for arrhythmias.

• Immediately report to prescriber any decrease in urine output.
• When stopping drug, gradually slow infusion rate and report sudden drop in blood pressure.

Patient teaching
• Tell patient to immediately report discomfort at infusion site or difficulty breathing.

Evaluation
• Patient has normal cardiac output.
• Patient sustains no injuries from drug-induced adverse reactions.
• Patient and family state understanding of drug therapy.

norethindrone
(nor-ETH-in-drohn)
Camila, Errin, Jolivette, Micronor, Nora-BE, Nor-QD

norethindrone acetate
Aygestin, Norlutate ◆

Pharmacologic class: progestin
Therapeutic class: contraceptive
Pregnancy risk category: X

Indications and dosages

▶ **Amenorrhea, abnormal uterine bleeding.** *Women:* 2.5 to 10 mg norethindrone acetate P.O. daily for 5 to 10 days during second half of the theoretical menstrual cycle.
▶ **Endometriosis.** *Women:* 5 mg norethindrone acetate P.O. daily for 14 days; then increase by 2.5 mg daily q 2 weeks up to 15 mg daily.
▶ **To prevent pregnancy.** *Women:* Initially, 0.35 mg norethindrone P.O. on first day of menstruation; then 0.35 mg daily.

Contraindications and cautions

• Contraindicated in patients hypersensitive to the drug or any of its components; in patients with thromboembolic disorders, cerebrovascular insufficiency, or a history of these conditions; and patients with breast cancer, undiagnosed abnormal vaginal bleeding, severe hepatic disease, or missed abortion.
• Use cautiously in patients with diabetes mellitus, seizure disorder, migraine, cardiac or renal disease, asthma, or depression.

Reactions may be *common*, uncommon, *life-threatening*, or COMMON AND LIFE-THREATENING.

🤰 **Lifespan:** In pregnant women, drug is contraindicated. Breast-feeding woman may start taking progestin-only pills (POPs) 6 weeks after delivery. A woman who is partially breast-feeding (supplementing with formula) can start taking drug by 3 weeks after delivery. In children, safety and effectiveness haven't been established.

Adverse reactions

CNS: ***stroke,*** dizziness, migraine, lethargy, depression.
CV: hypertension, thrombophlebitis, ***pulmonary embolism, thromboembolism,*** *edema.*
GI: nausea, vomiting, abdominal cramps.
GU: breakthrough bleeding, dysmenorrhea, amenorrhea, cervical erosion, abnormal secretions, uterine fibromas, vaginal candidiasis.
Hepatic: cholestatic jaundice.
Metabolic: hyperglycemia, weight changes.
Skin: melasma, rash, hirsutism.
Other: decreased libido; breast tenderness, enlargement, or secretion.

Interactions

Drug-drug. *Barbiturates, carbamazepine, rifampin:* Decreases progestin effects. Monitor patient for lack of effect.
Bromocriptine: May cause amenorrhea, thus interfering with bromocriptine effects. Avoid using together.
Drug-food. *Caffeine:* May increase caffeine level. Monitor patient for caffeine effects.
Drug-lifestyle. *Smoking:* Increases risk of CV effects. If smoking continues, may need alternative therapy.

Effects on lab test results

- May increase glucose level.
- May increase liver function test values. May decrease T_3 uptake and glucose tolerance.

Pharmacokinetics

Absorption: Well absorbed from GI tract.
Distribution: Distributed widely; about 80% protein-bound.
Metabolism: Metabolized primarily in liver; it undergoes extensive first-pass metabolism.
Excretion: Excreted primarily in feces. *Half-life:* 5 to 14 hours.

Route	Onset	Peak	Duration
P.O.	Unknown	1–2 hr	Unknown

Action

Chemical effect: Suppresses ovulation, possibly by inhibiting pituitary gonadotropin secretion, and forms thick cervical mucus.
Therapeutic effect: Prevents pregnancy and relieves symptoms of endometriosis, amenorrhea, and abnormal uterine bleeding.

Available forms

norethindrone
Tablets: 0.35 mg, 0.5 mg
norethindrone acetate
Tablets: 5 mg

NURSING PROCESS

Assessment

- Assess patient's condition before starting therapy and regularly thereafter to monitor the drug's effectiveness.
- Be alert for adverse reactions and drug interactions.
- Assess patient's and family's knowledge of drug therapy.
- Monitor blood pressure and edema.

Nursing diagnoses

- Ineffective health maintenance related to underlying condition
- Excessive fluid volume related to drug-induced edema
- Deficient knowledge related to drug therapy

Planning and implementation

ALERT: Norethindrone acetate is twice as potent as norethindrone. Don't use as contraception.
- Preliminary estrogen therapy is usually needed by patients with menstrual disorders.

ALERT: If visual disturbance, migraine, or headache occurs or if pulmonary emboli are suspected, withhold drug, notify prescriber, and provide supportive care.
ALERT: Don't confuse Micronor with Micro-K or Micronase.

Patient teaching
- If switching from combined hormonal contraceptives to progestin-only pill (POP), tell patient to take the first POP the day after the last active combined pill.

N

• If switching from POPs to combined pills, tell patient to take the first active combined pill on the first day of menstruation, even if the POPs pack isn't finished.

• Explain adverse effects of progestin and have patient read package insert before taking first dose.

• Tell patient to take drug at same time each day when used as a contraceptive. If she is more than 3 hours late or has missed a pill, tell her to take pill as soon as she remembers, to continue with her normal schedule, and to use backup contraception for the next 48 hours.

• Instruct patient to immediately report unusual symptoms. Tell her to stop taking the drug and call prescriber if visual disturbance or migraine occurs.

• Teach patient how to perform routine monthly breast self-examination.

• Warn patient that edema and weight gain are likely. Advise her to restrict sodium intake.

◪ Evaluation

• Patient responds well to therapy.

• Patient's drug-induced edema is minimized with sodium restriction.

• Patient and family state understanding of drug therapy.

norfloxacin

(nor-FLOKS-uh-sin)
Noroxin

Pharmacologic class: fluoroquinolone
Therapeutic class: broad-spectrum antibiotic
Pregnancy risk category: C

Indications and dosages

▶ **UTI caused by susceptible strains of _Escherichia coli, Klebsiella, Enterobacter, Proteus, Pseudomonas aeruginosa, Citrobacter, Staphylococcus aureus, Staphylococcus epidermidis,_ and group D streptococci.** _Adults:_ For uncomplicated infections, 400 mg P.O. b.i.d. for 7 to 10 days. For complicated infections, 400 mg b.i.d. for 10 to 21 days.

▶ **UTI caused by _E. coli, K. pneumoniae,_ or _Proteus mirabilis._** _Adults:_ 400 mg P.O. b.i.d. for 3 days.

▶ **Acute, uncomplicated gonorrhea.** _Adults:_ 800 mg P.O. as single dose, followed by doxy-cycline therapy to treat coexisting chlamydial infection.

▶ **Prostatitis from _E. coli._** _Men:_ 400 mg P.O. q 12 hours for 28 days.

▶ **Gastroenteritis‡.** _Adults:_ 400 mg P.O. b.i.d. for 5 days.

▶ **Traveler's diarrhea‡.** _Adults:_ 400 mg P.O. b.i.d. for 3 days.

◪ Adjust-a-dose: For patients with renal impairment, if creatinine clearance is less than 30 ml/minute, give 400 mg once daily.

Contraindications and cautions

• Contraindicated in patients hypersensitive to fluoroquinolones. Contraindicated in patients with a history of tendonitis or tendon rupture associated with fluoroquinolones.

• Use cautiously in patients with conditions that may predispose them to seizure disorders, such as cerebral arteriosclerosis and epilepsy.

⚖ Lifespan: In pregnant women, breast-feeding women, adolescents, and children, safety and effectiveness haven't been established.

Adverse reactions

CNS: fatigue, somnolence, headache, fever, dizziness, _seizures._
GI: nausea, constipation, flatulence, heartburn, dry mouth.
GU: crystalluria.
Hematologic: eosinophilia.
Musculoskeletal: arthralgia, arthritis, myalgia, joint swelling.
Skin: rash, photosensitivity reaction.
Other: hypersensitivity reaction, rash, _anaphylactoid reactions._

Interactions

Drug-drug. _Aluminum hydroxide, aluminum-magnesium hydroxide, calcium carbonate, magnesium hydroxide:_ May decrease effects of norfloxacin. Give antacid at least 6 hours before or 2 hours after norfloxacin.
Cimetidine: May interfere with norfloxacin elimination. Use cautiously.
Cyclosporine: May increase cyclosporine level. Monitor level.
Didanosine: Decrease absorption of norfloxacin. Avoid use together.
Iron salts: May decrease absorption of norfloxacin, reducing anti-infective response. Give at least 2 hours apart.

Nitrofurantoin: Decreases norfloxacin's effectiveness. Don't use together.

NSAIDs: May increase risk of CNS stimulation and seizures. Monitor patient closely.

Oral anticoagulants: Increases anticoagulant effect. Monitor patient closely for bleeding; monitor PT and INR.

Probenecid: May increase levels of norfloxacin by decreasing its excretion. Monitor patient for toxicity.

Sucralfate: May decrease absorption of norfloxacin, reducing anti-infective response. If use together can't be avoided, give at least 6 hours apart.

Theophylline: May impair theophylline metabolism, resulting in increased theophylline level and risk of toxicity. Monitor theophylline level closely.

Warfarin: May increase anticoagulant effect. Monitor patient and INR closely.

Drug-food. *Any food:* Decreases absorption of drug. Give drug 1 hour before or 2 hours after meals.

Caffeine: May increase pharmacologic effects of caffeine. Discourage caffeine use.

Drug-lifestyle. *Sunlight:* May cause photosensitivity reaction. Urge patient to avoid unprotected or prolonged sun exposure.

Effects on lab test results

• May increase BUN, creatinine, ALT, AST, and alkaline phosphatase levels. May decrease hemoglobin level and hematocrit.

• May increase eosinophil count. May decrease neutrophil count.

Pharmacokinetics

Absorption: About 30% to 40%. As dose increases, percentage absorbed decreases. Food may reduce absorption.

Distribution: Into renal tissue, liver, gallbladder, prostatic fluid, testicles, seminal fluid, bile, and sputum. About 10% to 15% binds to proteins.

Metabolism: Unknown.

Excretion: Mostly excreted by kidneys with about 30% appearing in bile. *Half-life:* 3 to 4 hours.

Route	Onset	Peak	Duration
P.O.	Unknown	1–2 hr	Unknown

Action

Chemical effect: Inhibits bacterial DNA synthesis, mainly by blocking DNA gyrase.

Therapeutic effect: Kills certain bacteria.

Available forms

Tablets: 400 mg

NURSING PROCESS

☑ Assessment

• Assess patient's infection before starting therapy and regularly thereafter to monitor the drug's effectiveness.

• Obtain a sample for culture and sensitivity tests before starting therapy, and repeat p.r.n. throughout therapy. May begin therapy pending test results.

• Be alert for adverse reactions and drug interactions.

• Assess patient's and family's knowledge of drug therapy.

⊞ Nursing diagnoses

• Infection related to bacteria

• Risk for injury related to drug-induced adverse CNS reactions

• Deficient knowledge related to drug therapy

▷ Planning and implementation

• Give drug on empty stomach.

• Make sure patient is well hydrated before and during therapy to avoid crystalluria.

⑤ **ALERT:** Don't confuse Noroxin with Neurontin or Floxin.

Patient teaching

• Urge patient to take drug 1 hour before or 2 hours after meals to promote absorption.

• Warn patient not to exceed recommended dosage.

• Encourage patient to drink several glasses of water throughout the day to maintain hydration and adequate urine output.

• Warn patient to avoid hazardous activities until the drug's CNS effects are known.

☑ Evaluation

• Patient is free from infection.

• Patient has no injuries from drug-induced adverse CNS reactions.

• Patient and family state understanding of drug therapy.

nortriptyline hydrochloride
(nor-TRIP-teh-leen high-droh-KLOR-ighd)
Allegron◇, Aventyl*, Pamelor*℘

Pharmacologic class: tricyclic antidepressant
Therapeutic class: antidepressant
Pregnancy risk category: D

Indications and dosages

▶ **Depression.** *Adults:* 25 mg P.O. t.i.d. or
q.i.d.; gradually increase to maximum of 150 mg
daily. Or entire dosage may be given h.s.
▶ **Premenstrual symptoms‡.** *Adults:* 50 to
125 mg/day.
▶ **Dermatologic disorders (chronic urticaria,
angioedema, nocturnal pruritus in atopic
eczema)‡.** *Adults:* 20 to 75 mg/day.
❏ **Adjust-a-dose:** For elderly and debilitated patients, give 30 mg to 50 mg P.O. once daily or in
divided doses.

Contraindications and cautions

• Contraindicated in patients hypersensitive to
the drug or any of its components, patients in
acute recovery phase after MI, and patients who
have taken an MAO inhibitor within 14 days.
• Use cautiously in patients taking thyroid drugs
and patients with glaucoma, suicidal tendency,
history of urine retention or seizures, CV disease, or hyperthyroidism.
❧ **Lifespan:** In pregnant women, breast-
feeding women, and children, don't use unless
benefits outweigh potential risks. In elderly patients, use cautiously and at a lower dose.

Adverse reactions

CNS: *drowsiness, dizziness,* excitation,
seizures, tremor, weakness, confusion, headache, nervousness, EEG changes, extrapyramidal reactions, **suicidal ideation, stroke.**
CV: *tachycardia,* ECG changes, hypertension,
heart block, MI.
EENT: *blurred vision,* tinnitus, mydriasis.
GI: *dry mouth, constipation,* nausea, vomiting,
anorexia, paralytic ileus.
GU: urine retention.
Hematologic: **bone marrow depression,** eosinophilia, **agranulocytosis, thrombocytopenia.**
Skin: diaphoresis, rash, urticaria, photosensitiv-
ity.
Other: hypersensitivity reaction.

Interactions

Drug-drug. *Anticholinergics:* Increases anticholinergic effect. Paralytic ileus may occur.
Monitor patient.
Barbiturates, CNS depressants: Enhances CNS
depression. Avoid using together.
*Bupropion, cimetidine, methylphenidate, SSRIs,
valproic acid:* May increase nortriptyline levels.
Monitor patient for adverse reactions.
Carbamazepine: May increase levels of nortriptyline and carbamazepine, leading to toxicity. Use with caution.
Clonidine: May cause loss of blood pressure
control with potentially life-threatening eleva-
tions in blood pressure. Don't use together.
Epinephrine, norepinephrine: Increases hypertensive effect. Use together cautiously; monitor
blood pressure.
MAO inhibitors: May cause severe excitation,
hyperpyrexia, or seizures. Do not use together.
Quinolones: Increases risk of life-threatening
arrhythmias, including torsades de pointes.
Don't use together.
Rifamycin: Decreases nortriptyline levels. Monitor levels for decreased effect.
Drug-herb. *SAMe, St. John's wort, yohimbe:*
Use with some tricyclic antidepressants may increase serotonin levels. Discourage using together.
Drug-lifestyle. *Alcohol use:* Enhances CNS depression. Discourage using together.
Smoking: May lower nortriptyline level. Monitor patient for lack of drug effect.
Sun exposure: Increases risk of photosensitivity
reaction. Urge patient to avoid unprotected or
prolonged exposure to sunlight.

Effects on lab test results

• May increase or decrease glucose level.
• May increase liver function test values and
eosinophil count. May decrease RBC, WBC,
granulocyte, and platelet counts.

Pharmacokinetics

Absorption: Rapid.
Distribution: Distributed widely into body, including CNS. Drug is 95% protein-bound.
Metabolism: Metabolized by liver; significant
first-pass effect may account for variability of
levels in different patients taking same dosage.
Excretion: Most excreted in urine; some in feces. *Half-life:* 18 to 24 hours.

Route	Onset	Peak	Duration
P.O.	Unknown	7–8½ hr	16–90 hr

Action

Chemical effect: Unknown; increases amount of norepinephrine, serotonin, or both in CNS by blocking their reuptake by presynaptic neurons. **Therapeutic effect:** Relieves depression.

Available forms

Capsules: 10 mg, 25 mg, 50 mg, 75 mg
Oral solution: 10 mg/5 ml*
Tablets: 10 mg ◇, 25 mg ◇

NURSING PROCESS

Assessment

• Assess patient's depression before starting therapy and regularly thereafter to monitor the drug's effectiveness.
• Be alert for adverse reactions and drug interactions.
• If dosage is greater than 100 mg/day, monitor levels and maintain in the range of 50 to 150 nanograms/ml.
• Assess patient's and family's knowledge of drug therapy.

Nursing diagnoses

• Disturbed thought processes related to depression
• Risk for injury related to drug-induced adverse CNS reactions
• Deficient knowledge related to drug therapy

Planning and implementation

• Lower the dosage in geriatric or debilitated patient.
⊗ **ALERT:** Abruptly stopping long-term therapy may cause the patient to experience nausea, headache, and malaise.
⊗ **ALERT:** Because hypertensive episodes may occur during surgery in patients receiving tricyclic antidepressants, gradually stop giving the drug beginning several days before surgery.
• If signs of psychosis occur or increase, reduce dosage.
⊗ **ALERT:** Don't confuse nortriptyline with amitriptyline.
Patient teaching
• Advise patient to take full dose h.s. to reduce risk of orthostatic hypotension.

• Warn patient to avoid hazardous activities until CNS effects of drug are known. Drowsiness and dizziness usually subside after a few weeks.
• Tell patient to avoid alcohol during drug therapy.
• Warn patient not to stop drug suddenly.
• Advise patient to consult prescriber before taking other prescription or OTC drugs.
• Advise patient to use sunblock, wear protective clothing, and avoid prolonged exposure to sunlight to avoid photosensitivity.

Evaluation

• Patient's depression improves.
• Patient experiences no injuries from drug-induced adverse CNS reactions.
• Patient and family state understanding of drug therapy.

nystatin
(nigh-STAT-in)
Mycostatin*, Nilstat, Nystex*, Nystop

Pharmacologic class: polyene macrolide
Therapeutic class: antifungal
Pregnancy risk category: C

Indications and dosages

▶ **GI tract infections.** *Adults:* 500,000 to 1 million units as oral tablets P.O. t.i.d.
▶ **Oral infections caused by** *Candida albicans* **and other** *Candida* **sp.** *Adults and children:* 400,000 to 600,000 units suspension P.O. q.i.d. Or 200,000 or 400,000 units (1 or 2 lozenges) 4 or 5 times daily.
Infants: 200,000 units suspension P.O. q.i.d.
▶ **Vaginal infections.** *Adults:* 100,000 units, as vaginal tablets, inserted high into vagina, daily for 14 days.
▶ **Cutaneous or mucocutaneous yeast infections.** *Adults:* Apply topical products to affected areas 2 to 3 times daily.
▶ **Candidal diaper dermatitis‡** 100,000 units suspension P.O. q.i.d. as an adjunct to topical nystatin therapy.

Contraindications and cautions

• Contraindicated in patients hypersensitive to the drug or any of its components.
⚖ **Lifespan:** In pregnant women, use only when benefits outweigh risks to the fetus. In

N

breast-feeding women, safety and effectiveness haven't been established.

Adverse reactions

GI: transient nausea, vomiting, diarrhea.
Skin: rash.

Interactions

None significant.

Effects on lab test results

None reported.

Pharmacokinetics

Absorption: Not absorbed from GI tract, intact skin, or mucous membranes.
Distribution: None.
Metabolism: None.
Excretion: Oral form excreted almost entirely unchanged in feces. *Half-life:* Unknown.

Route	Onset	Peak	Duration
P.O., topical, vaginal	Unknown	Unknown	Unknown

Action

Chemical effect: Unknown; probably acts by binding to sterols in fungal cell membrane, altering cell permeability and allowing leakage of intracellular components.
Therapeutic effect: Kills susceptible yeasts and fungi.

Available forms

Cream/ointment/powder: 100,000 units/g
Oral suspension: 100,000 units/ml*
Tablets: 500,000 units
Lozenges: 200,000 units
Vaginal tablets: 100,000 units

NURSING PROCESS

Assessment
• Assess patient's infection before starting therapy and regularly thereafter to monitor the drug's effectiveness.
• Be alert for adverse reactions.
• If patient has adverse GI reactions, monitor his hydration.
• Assess patient's and family's knowledge of drug therapy.

Nursing diagnoses
• Infection related to organisms
• Risk for deficient fluid volume related to drug-induced adverse GI reactions
• Deficient knowledge related to drug therapy

Planning and implementation
• Drug isn't effective against systemic infections.
• When treating oral candidiasis (thrush), clean food debris from patient's mouth and have patient hold suspension in mouth for several minutes before swallowing.
• When treating an infant, swab drug on oral mucosa.
• Immunosuppressed patients with oral candidiasis are sometimes instructed by prescriber to suck on vaginal tablets (100,000 units) because doing so provides prolonged contact with oral mucosa.
• Pregnant patients can use vaginal tablets up to 6 weeks before term to treat infection that may cause thrush in neonates.
Patient teaching
• Advise patient to take drug for at least 2 days after symptoms disappear to prevent reinfection. Consult prescriber for duration of therapy.
• Tell patient not to chew or swallow lozenge (troche) but to allow it to dissolve slowly in the mouth.
• Tell patient to premoisten oral mucosa and maintain adequate hydration when using lozenge (troche) formulation.
• Instruct patient to continue therapy during menstruation.
• Instruct patient in oral hygiene techniques. Poorly fitting dentures and overuse of mouthwash may alter oral flora and promote infection.
• Explain that predisposing factors for vaginal infection include use of antibiotics, hormonal contraceptives, and corticosteroids; diabetes; reinfection by sexual partner; and tight-fitting undergarments. Encourage patient to wear cotton (not synthetic) underpants.
• Teach patient about hygiene for affected areas, including wiping perineal area from front to back.
• Advise patient to report redness, swelling, or irritation.

Evaluation
• Patient is free from infection.

- Patient maintains adequate hydration throughout drug therapy.
- Patient and family state understanding of drug therapy.

octreotide acetate
(ok-TREE-oh-tighd AS-ih-tayt)
Sandostatin, Sandostatin LAR Depot

Pharmacologic class: synthetic polypeptide
Therapeutic class: somatotropic hormone
Pregnancy risk category: B

Indications and dosages

▶ **Flushing and diarrhea caused by carcinoid tumors.** *Adults:* 100 to 600 mcg daily subcutaneously in two to four divided doses for first 2 weeks (usual daily dosage 300 mcg). Subsequent dosage based on patient's response. Patients currently on Sandostatin can switch to Sandostatin LAR Depot 20 mg I.M. to gluteal area q 4 weeks for 2 months. Octreotide immediate-release injection should be continued at the previous dosage during at least the first 2 weeks of therapy with the long-acting formulation.
▶ **Watery diarrhea caused by vasoactive intestinal polypeptide secreting tumors (VIPomas).** *Adults:* 200 to 300 mcg daily subcutaneously in two to four divided doses for first 2 weeks of therapy. Subsequent dosage based on individual response; typically doesn't exceed 450 mcg daily. Patients currently on Sandostatin can switch to Sandostatin LAR Depot 20 mg I.M. to gluteal area q 4 weeks for 2 months.
▶ **Acromegaly.** *Adults:* Initially, 50 mcg subcutaneously t.i.d.; then adjust by somatomedin C (IGF-1) or growth hormone (GH) levels q 2 weeks. Usual effective dosage, 100 mcg subcutaneously t.i.d. Some patients may need up to 500 mcg subcutaneously t.i.d., but doses higher than 300 mg t.i.d. often add no benefits. Switch patients on Sandostatin to 20 mg Sandostatin LAR Depot I.M. to gluteal area q 4 weeks for 3 months.

▶ **GI fistula**‡. *Adults:* 0.05 to 0.2 mg subcutaneously q 8 hours.
▶ **Variceal bleeding**‡. *Adults:* 0.025 to 0.05 mg/hour continuous I.V. infusion. Duration is from 18 hours to 5 days.
▶ **AIDS-related diarrhea**‡. *Adults:* 0.1 to 0.5 mg subcutaneously t.i.d.
▶ **Short bowel (ileostomy) syndrome**‡. *Adults:* 0.025 mg/hour continuous I.V. infusion or 0.05 mg subcutaneously b.i.d.
▶ **Chemotherapy- and radiation-induced diarrhea**‡. *Adults:* 0.05 to 0.1 mg subcutaneously t.i.d. for 1 to 3 days.
▶ **Pancreatic fistula**‡. *Adults:* 0.05 to 0.2 mg subcutaneously q 8 hours.
▶ **Irritable bowel syndrome**‡. *Adults:* 0.1 mg single dose to 0.125 mg subcutaneously b.i.d.
▶ **Dumping syndrome**‡. *Adults:* 0.05 to 0.15 mg subcutaneously daily.

Contraindications and cautions

- Contraindicated in patients hypersensitive to the drug or any of its components.
☀ **Lifespan:** In pregnant women, use cautiously. In breast-feeding women and in children, safety and effectiveness haven't been established.

Adverse reactions

CNS: pain, dizziness, headache, lightheadedness, fatigue.
CV: flushing, *arrhythmias, bradycardia.*
GI: *nausea, diarrhea, abdominal pain or discomfort,* loose stools, vomiting, fat malabsorption, gallbladder abnormalities.
Metabolic: *hyperglycemia, hypoglycemia,* hypothyroidism.
Skin: edema, wheal, erythema and pain at injection site.
Other: burning at subcutaneous injection site.

Interactions

Drug-drug. *Cyclosporine:* May decrease cyclosporine level. Monitor patient.
Drug-food. *Dietary fats:* Drug may alter the absorption of dietary fats.
Vitamin B$_{12}$: May decrease vitamin B$_{12}$ level; monitor level.

Effects on lab test results

- May decrease T$_4$ and thyroid-stimulating hormone levels. May increase or decrease glucose level.

Pharmacokinetics

Absorption: Rapid and complete after subcutaneous use.
Distribution: To plasma, where it binds to lipoprotein and albumin.
Metabolism: Not clearly defined.
Excretion: About 35% unchanged in urine.
Half-life: About 1½ hours.

Route	Onset	Peak	Duration
I.M., SubQ	≤ 30 min	30–60 min	12 hr–6 wk

Action

Chemical effect: Mimics action of naturally occurring somatostatin.
Therapeutic effect: Relieves flushing and diarrhea caused by certain tumors and treats acromegaly.

Available forms

Depot: 10 mg/5 ml, 20 mg/5 ml, 30 mg/5 ml
Injection: 0.05-mg, 0.1-mg, 0.5-mg ampules; 0.2-mg/ml, 1-mg/ml multidose vials

NURSING PROCESS

☜ Assessment
• Assess patient's condition before starting therapy, and regularly thereafter to monitor the drug's effectiveness.
• Monitor IGF-1 or GH levels every 2 weeks. Base dose on this level.
• Monitor laboratory tests, such as thyroid function tests, urine 5-hydroxyindoleacetic acid, serotonin, substance P (for carcinoid tumors), and vasoactive intestinal peptide levels (for VIPomas), at baseline and then periodically.
• Monitor fluid and electrolyte levels.
• Be alert for adverse reactions and drug interactions.
• Assess patient's and family's knowledge of drug therapy.

⊞ Nursing diagnoses
• Diarrhea related to condition
• Fatigue related to drug-induced adverse CNS reaction
• Deficient knowledge related to drug therapy

▷ Planning and implementation
• Give drug in divided doses for first 2 weeks of therapy; subsequent daily dose depends on patient's response.

• Read drug labels carefully, and check dosage and strength.
⑤ ALERT: For LAR Depot injection, give drug I.M. only. Avoid deltoid muscle because of discomfort at site.
• Drug therapy may alter fluid and electrolyte balance and may require adjustment of other drugs.
• Adjust LAR Depot dosing q 3 months based on GH level; range for depot dosing, 10 to 40 mg at intervals no sooner than 4 weeks.

Patient teaching
• Tell patient to report signs of gallbladder disease such as abdominal discomfort. Drug may be linked to cholelithiasis.
• Inform patient that laboratory tests are needed during therapy.
• Advise diabetic patient to monitor glucose level closely. Antidiabetics may need dosage adjustment.

☑ Evaluation
• Patient's bowel pattern is normal.
• Patient uses energy-saving measures to combat fatigue.
• Patient and family state understanding of drug therapy.

ofloxacin
(oh-FLOKS-eh-sin)
Apo-Oflox ◆ , Floxin, Floxin Otic, Ocuflox

Pharmacologic class: fluoroquinolone
Therapeutic class: antibiotic
Pregnancy risk category: C

Indications and dosages

▶ **Lower respiratory tract infections caused by susceptible strains of *Haemophilus influenzae* or *Streptococcus pneumoniae*.** *Adults:* 400 mg P.O. q 12 hours for 10 days.
▶ **Cervicitis or urethritis caused by *Chlamydia trachomatis* or *Neisseria gonorrhoeae*.** *Adults:* 300 mg P.O. q 12 hours for 7 days.
▶ **Acute pelvic inflammatory disease.** *Adults:* 400 mg P.O. q 12 hours for 10 to 14 days.
▶ **Acute uncomplicated gonorrhea.** *Adults:* 400 mg P.O. as single dose.
▶ **Mild to moderate skin and skin-structure infections caused by susceptible strains of *Staphylococcus aureus, Staphylococcus epi-***

dermidis, Streptococcus pyogenes, **or** *Proteus mirabilis. Adults:* 400 mg P.O. q 12 hours for 10 days.

▶**Cystitis caused by** *Escherichia coli* **or** *Klebsiella pneumoniae. Adults:* 200 mg P.O. q 12 hours for 3 days.

▶**UTIs caused by susceptible strains of** *Citrobacter diversus, Enterobacter aerogenes, E. coli, P. mirabilis,* **or** *Pseudomonas aeruginosa. Adults:* 200 mg P.O. q 12 hours for 7 days. Complicated infections may need 10 days of therapy.

▶**Prostatitis caused by** *E. coli. Adults:* 300 mg P.O. q 12 hours for 6 weeks.

▶**Bacterial conjunctivitis.** *Adults and children age 1 year and older:* 1 or 2 drops every 2 to 4 hours in the affected eye on days 1 and 2, then 1 or 2 drops q.i.d. on days 3 through 7.

▶**Otitis externa (swimmer's ear).** *Adults and children age 13 and older:* 10 drops (or 2 single-dispensing containers) into affected ear twice daily for 10 days.
Children 1 to 12 years old: 5 drops (or 1 single-dispensing container) into affected ear twice daily for 10 days.

▶**Otitis media with tympanostomy tubes.** *Children ages 1 to 12:* 1 single-dispensing container into affected ear twice daily for 10 days.

▶**Chronic suppurative otitis media with perforated tympanic membranes.** *Adults and children age 12 and older:* 2 dispensing-containers in affected ear twice daily for 14 days.

▶**Adjunct for** *Brucella* **infections** ‡. *Adults:* 400 mg P.O. daily for 6 weeks.

▶**Typhoid fever** ‡. *Adults:* 200 to 400 mg P.O. q 12 hours for 7 to 14 days.

▶**Tuberculosis adjunct** ‡. *Adults:* 300 mg P.O. daily.

▶**Postoperative sternotomy or soft tissue wounds caused by** *Mycobacterium fortuitum* ‡. *Adults:* 300 or 600 mg P.O. daily for 3 to 6 months.

▶**Acute Q fever pneumonia** ‡. *Adults:* 600 mg P.O. daily for up to 16 days.

▶**Mediterranean spotted fever** ‡. *Adults:* 200 mg P.O. q 12 hours for 7 days.

▶**Traveler's diarrhea** ‡. *Adults:* 300 mg P.O. b.i.d. for 3 days.

▶**Inhalational anthrax post-exposure prophylaxis/treatment** ‡. *Adults:* 400 mg P.O. b.i.d. for 60 days.

▶**Legionnaire's disease** ‡. *Adults:* 400 mg P.O. q 12 hours for 2 to 3 weeks.

◘ **Adjust-a-dose:** For patients with renal impairment, if creatinine clearance is 20 to 50 ml/minute, give usual recommended dose q 24 hours; if creatinine clearance is less than 20 ml/minute, give one-half of recommended dose q 24 hours.

For patients with hepatic impairment, maximum daily dose is 400 mg.

Contraindications and cautions

● Contraindicated in patients hypersensitive to the drug or other fluoroquinolones.

● Use cautiously in patients with renal impairment, history of seizures, or other CNS diseases such as cerebral arteriosclerosis.

▧ **Lifespan:** In pregnant women, use cautiously. In breast-feeding women and in infants younger than age 1, safety and effectiveness haven't been established.

Adverse reactions

CNS: *headache,* dizziness, fever, fatigue, lethargy, malaise, drowsiness, sleep disorders, nervousness, light-headedness, insomnia, *seizures.*
CV: chest pain.
EENT: visual disturbances.
GI: *nausea,* anorexia, abdominal pain or discomfort, diarrhea, vomiting, dry mouth, flatulence, dysgeusia.
GU: vaginitis, vaginal discharge, genital pruritus.
Hematologic: eosinophilia, anemia, leukocytosis, *neutropenia, lymphocytopenia, leukopenia.*
Metabolic: *hypoglycemia,* hyperglycemia.
Musculoskeletal: trunk pain, transient arthralgia, myalgia.
Skin: rash, pruritus, photosensitivity reaction.
Other: hypersensitivity reactions, *anaphylaxis.*

Interactions

Drug-drug. *Aluminum hydroxide, aluminum-magnesium hydroxide, calcium carbonate, magnesium hydroxide:* May decrease effects of ofloxacin. Give antacid at least 6 hours before or 2 hours after oral ofloxacin.
Cimetidine: May interfere with the elimination of ofloxacin. Monitor patient for toxicity.
Divalent or trivalent cations (such as zinc), or didanosine (chewable or buffered tablets or pediatric powder for oral solution): May interfere with GI absorption of ofloxacin. Give these

drugs at least 2 hours before or 2 hours after taking oral ofloxacin.

Iron salts: May decrease absorption of ofloxacin, reducing anti-infective response. Give at least 2 hours apart.

NSAIDs: May increase risk of CNS stimulation and convulsive seizures. Avoid using together. Monitor patient for tremors and seizures if used together.

Oral anticoagulants: May increase anticoagulant effect. Monitor patient for bleeding and altered PT and INR.

Procainamide: May increase procainamide concentration. Monitor procainamide concentration; adjust dose accordingly.

Sucralfate: May decrease absorption of oral ofloxacin, reducing anti-infective response. If use together can't be avoided, give at least 2 hours apart.

Theophylline: Some fluoroquinolones may decrease theophylline clearance. Monitor theophylline level.

Drug-food. *Any food:* May decrease oral drug absorption. Give drug on an empty stomach.

Drug-lifestyle. *Sun exposure:* May cause photosensitivity reactions. Urge patient to avoid unprotected or prolonged sun exposure.

Effects on lab test results

● May increase ALT, AST, and alkaline phosphatase levels. May decrease hemoglobin level and hematocrit. May increase or decrease glucose level.

● May increase eosinophil count. May decrease neutrophil and lymphocyte counts. May increase or decrease WBC count.

● May produce false-positive opiate assay results.

Pharmacokinetics

Absorption: Good.
Distribution: Wide.
Metabolism: Pyridobenzoxazine ring decreases extent.
Excretion: 68% to 90% unchanged in urine; less than 5% in feces. *Half-life:* 4 to 7½ hours.

Route	Onset	Peak	Duration
P.O.	Unknown	1–2 hr	Unknown
Topical	Unknown	Unknown	Unknown

Action

Chemical effect: May inhibit bacterial DNA gyrase and prevent DNA replication in susceptible bacteria.

Therapeutic effect: Kills susceptible aerobic gram-positive and gram-negative organisms.

Available forms

Tablets: 200 mg, 300 mg, 400 mg
Ophthalmic solution: 0.3% in 1ml, 5 ml, 10 ml
Otic solution: 0.3% in 0.25-ml single-dispensing containers, 5 ml, 10 ml

NURSING PROCESS

▨ Assessment

● Assess patient's infection before starting therapy, and regularly thereafter to monitor the drug's effectiveness.

● Monitor regular blood studies and hepatic and renal function tests during long-term therapy.

● Give serologic test for syphilis to patient treated for gonorrhea. Drug isn't effective against syphilis, and treating gonorrhea may mask or delay symptoms of syphilis.

● Be alert for adverse reactions and drug interactions.

● If patient has an adverse GI reaction, monitor his hydration.

● Assess patient's and family's knowledge of drug therapy.

⊞ Nursing diagnoses

● Infection related to presence of bacteria
● Risk for deficient fluid volume related to drug-induced adverse GI reactions
● Deficient knowledge related to drug therapy

➤ Planning and implementation

● Give oral drug on empty stomach.

⊛ ALERT: If patient experiences restlessness, tremor, confusion, or hallucinations, stop giving the drug and notify prescriber. Take seizure precautions.

⊛ ALERT: The ophthalmic and otic forms both come in 3% strengths. Don't confuse them; they're not interchangeable.

Patient teaching

● Advise patient to take oral drug with plenty of fluids but not with meals. Also, tell patient to avoid antacids, sucralfate, and products containing iron or zinc for at least 2 hours before and after each dose.

Reactions may be *common*, uncommon, *life-threatening*, or COMMON AND LIFE-THREATENING.

• Advise patient to complete full course of antibiotics, as directed.

• Warn patient to avoid hazardous tasks until the drug's CNS effects are known.

• Advise patient to use sunblock and protective clothing to avoid photosensitivity reactions.

• Tell patient to stop taking the drug and notify prescriber if rash or other signs of hypersensitivity reactions develop.

• Tell patient to warm ear drops before instilling by holding the bottle in his hands for 1 or 2 minutes; this will avoid dizziness that may occur following instillation of cold solution.

• Give the patient these instructions for using eardrops: lie down with the affected ear upward and drop in the prescribed amount of drops. Remain lying down for 5 minutes to allow the drug to reach the ear canal. If treating middle ear infections, press the cartilage by the opening of the ear four times to help drug get to the middle ear.

• Advise patient using ear drops or eye drops to avoid contaminating the tip of the multidose container with his fingers, infectious material or other sources.

🛚 **Evaluation**

• Patient is free from infection.

• Patient maintains adequate hydration throughout drug therapy.

• Patient and family state understanding of drug therapy.

olanzapine
(oh-LAN-za-peen)
Zyprexa, Zyprexa Intramuscular, Zyprexa Zydis

Pharmacologic class: thienobenzodiazepine derivative
Therapeutic class: atypical antipsychotic
Pregnancy risk category: C

Indications and dosages

▶ **Short-term therapy for acute manic episodes related to bipolar I disorder.** *Adults:* Initially, 10 or 15 mg P.O. daily. Adjust dosage p.r.n. by increments of 5 mg daily at intervals of 24 hours or more. Maximum, 20 mg P.O. daily. Therapy lasts 3 or 4 weeks.

▶ **Short-term therapy for acute manic episodes of bipolar I disorder, given with lithium or valproate.** *Adults:* 10 mg P.O. once daily. Dosage range, 5 to 20 mg daily. Therapy lasts for 6 weeks.

▶ **Long-term therapy for bipolar I disorder.** *Adults:* 5 to 20 mg P.O. daily.

▶ **Agitation from schizophrenia and bipolar I mania.** *Adults:* 2.5 to 10 mg I.M. Maximum daily dose, 30 mg I.M., in no more than 3 divided doses.

▶ **Long-term therapy for schizophrenia.** *Adults:* Initially, 5 to 10 mg P.O. daily. Goal, 10 mg P.O. daily within several days of starting therapy. Increase dosage weekly in increments of 5 mg daily to a maximum of 20 mg daily.

🛚 **Adjust-a-dose:** For patients who are debilitated, have a predisposition to hypotensive reactions, have risk factors for slower metabolism of drug (nonsmoking women older than age 65), or may be more pharmacodynamically sensitive to drug, the recommended starting dosage is 5 mg P.O. or 2.5 to 5 mg I.M. daily. In these patients, increase dose with caution.

Contraindications and cautions

• Contraindicated in patients hypersensitive to the drug or any of its components.

• Use cautiously in patients with heart disease, cerebrovascular disease, conditions that predispose patient to hypotension, history of seizures or conditions that might lower the seizure threshold, or hepatic impairment. Also use cautiously in patients with a history of paralytic ileus and in those at risk for aspiration pneumonia, prostatic hyperplasia, or angle-closure glaucoma.

Ⓢ **ALERT:** Hyperglycemia may occur in patients taking drug. Monitor patients with diabetes regularly. Test patients with risk factors for diabetes with a fasting blood glucose test for baseline and periodically thereafter. In some cases, hyperglycemia is reversible when antipsychotic is stopped.

🔥 **Lifespan:** In pregnant women, use drug only if benefits outweigh potential risks to the fetus. Breast-feeding women should stop breast-feeding or use another drug. Safety and effectiveness haven't been established in children younger than age 18. In elderly people with dementia, don't use; such patients may have an increased risk of stroke while using this drug.

Adverse reactions

CNS: *dizziness, somnolence, asthenia, parkinsonism, insomnia,* akathisia, extrapyramidal events, personality disorder, fever, abnormal gait, speech impairment, tardive dyskinesia, *neuroleptic malignant syndrome, suicide attempt* (P.O.).
CV: orthostatic hypotension, chest pain, tachycardia, hypertension, peripheral edema.
EENT: rhinitis, pharyngitis, amblyopia, conjunctivitis.
GI: *constipation, dry mouth, dyspepsia,* increased appetite, vomiting, increased salivation and thirst.
GU: urinary incontinence, UTI, amenorrhea, hematuria, metrorrhagia, vaginitis.
Hematologic: *leukopenia.*
Metabolic: weight gain, *hyperglycemia.*
Musculoskeletal: joint pain, joint stiffness and twitching, extremity pain, back pain, hypertonia.
Respiratory: increased cough, dyspnea.
Skin: ecchymosis, sweating, injection site pain.
Other: dental pain, flulike syndrome, injury.

Interactions

Drug-drug. *Antihypertensives:* May increase hypotensive effects. Monitor blood pressure closely.
Carbamazepine, omeprazole, rifampin: May increase olanzapine clearance. Monitor patient.
Diazepam: May increase CNS effects. Monitor patient closely.
Dopamine agonists, levodopa: May antagonize these drugs. Monitor patient.
Fluvoxamine: May decrease the clearance of olanzapine. Consider lower dose of olanzapine.
Drug-herb. *Nutmeg:* May reduce effectiveness of or interfere with drug therapy. Discourage using together.
Drug-lifestyle. *Alcohol use:* May increase CNS effects. Discourage using together.

Effects on lab test results

• May increase AST, ALT, GGT, CK, and prolactin levels.

Pharmacokinetics

Absorption: Food doesn't affect rate or extent. About 40% of dose is limited by first-pass metabolism.

Distribution: Extensive, with a volume of distribution of about 1,000 L. About 93% protein-bound, primarily to albumin and alpha$_1$-acid glycoprotein.
Metabolism: By direct glucuronidation and CYP-mediated oxidation.
Excretion: About 57% in urine and 30% in feces as metabolites. Only 7% of dose is recovered in urine unchanged. *Half-life:* 21 to 54 hours.

Route	Onset	Peak	Duration
P.O.	Unknown	6 hr	Unknown
I.M.	Rapid	15–45 min	Unknown

Action

Chemical effect: Binds to dopamine and serotonin receptors; may antagonize adrenergic, cholinergic, and histaminergic receptors.
Therapeutic effect: Relieves signs and symptoms of psychosis.

Available forms

Powder for injection: 10 mg
Tablets: 2.5 mg, 5 mg, 7.5 mg, 10 mg, 15 mg, 20 mg
Tablets (orally disintegrating): 5 mg, 10 mg, 15 mg, 20 mg

NURSING PROCESS

ℤ Assessment

• Obtain history of patient's underlying condition before starting therapy, and reassess regularly thereafter to monitor the drug's effectiveness.
• Obtain baseline and periodic glucose levels and liver function tests.
• Monitor patient for signs of neuroleptic malignant syndrome (hyperpyrexia, muscle rigidity, altered mental condition, autonomic instability), which is rare but fatal. If patient has symptoms, stop drug immediately, notify prescriber, and treat symptoms.
• Monitor patient for tardive dyskinesia, which may occur after prolonged use. It may not appear until months or years later, and it may disappear spontaneously or persist for life despite stopping therapy.
• Monitor patient for abnormal body temperature regulation, especially if patient is exercising strenuously, exposed to extreme heat, receiving anticholinergics, or at risk for dehydration.

• Monitor patient for symptoms of hyperglycemia, including polydipsia, polyuria, polyphagia, and weakness; if symptoms develop, test fasting glucose level.
• Regularly re-evaluate the drug's long-term effectiveness, especially in patients taking more than 20 mg daily.
• Assess patient's and family's knowledge of drug therapy.

⊕ Nursing diagnoses
• Disturbed thought processes related to underlying condition
• Risk for injury related to drug-induced adverse CNS reactions
• Deficient knowledge related to drug therapy

▶ Planning and implementation
• Start with a 5-mg dose in a patient who is debilitated, predisposed to hypotension, sensitive to drug, or affected by altered metabolism caused by smoking, gender, or age.
• Orally disintegrating tablets contain phenylalanine.
• Inspect I.M. solution for particulate matter and discoloration before administration.
• Store vials at 68 to 77° F (20 to 25° C). Protect from light and don't freeze. To reconstitute I.M. injection, dissolve contents of 1 vial with 2.1 ml of sterile water for injection to yield a 5 mg/ml solution that is clear and yellow in appearance. Store at room temperature and administer within 1 hour of reconstitution. Discard any unused solution.
• Postural hypotension and bradycardia may be lessened after I.M. injection by keeping patient recumbent.
⊛ ALERT: Don't confuse olanzapine with olsalazine or ondansetron.
⊛ ALERT: Don't confuse Zyprexa with Zyrtec or Celexa.
Patient teaching
• Drug can be taken with or without food.
• Tell patient to avoid hazardous tasks until the drug's CNS effects are known.
• Warn patient against exposure to extreme heat; drug may impair body's ability to reduce core temperature.
• Tell patient not to drink alcohol during therapy.
• Tell patient to rise slowly to avoid effects of orthostatic hypotension.

• Instruct patient to relieve dry mouth with ice chips or sugarless candy or gum.
• Advise woman to notify prescriber if she becomes pregnant or intends to become pregnant during drug therapy. Advise her not to breast-feed during therapy.

☑ Evaluation
• Patient's behavior and communication show improved thought processes.
• Patient sustains no injury from adverse CNS reactions.
• Patient and family state understanding of drug therapy.

olmesartan medoxomil
(ol-meh-SAHR-tan me-DOKS-oh-mil)
Benicar

Pharmacologic class: angiotensin II receptor antagonist
Therapeutic class: antihypertensive
Pregnancy risk category: C (first trimester) and D (second and third trimesters)

Indications and dosages

▶ **Hypertension.** *Adults:* 20 mg P.O. daily in patients who aren't volume-contracted. If blood pressure isn't reduced after 2 weeks of therapy, increase dosage to 40 mg P.O. once daily.
⧅ **Adjust-a-dose:** In patients whose intravascular volume may be depleted, consider lower starting dose.

Contraindications and cautions

• Contraindicated in patients hypersensitive to the drug or any of its components.
• Use cautiously in patients who are volume- or salt-depleted, in those whose renal function depends on the renin-angiotensin-aldosterone system (such as patients with severe heart failure), and in those with renal artery stenosis.
≋ **Lifespan:** In pregnant women, drug isn't recommended. If woman becomes pregnant, stop drug immediately. Breast-feeding women should either stop breast-feeding or use another drug. In children, safety and effectiveness haven't been established. In elderly patients, use cautiously because they may have greater sensitivity to drug.

Adverse reactions

CNS: headache.
EENT: pharyngitis, rhinitis, sinusitis.
GI: diarrhea.
GU: hematuria.
Metabolic: hyperglycemia, hypertriglyceridemia, hypercholesterolemia.
Musculoskeletal: back pain.
Respiratory: bronchitis, cough, upper respiratory tract infection.
Other: flulike symptoms, accidental injury.

Interactions

None reported.

Effects on lab test results

• May increase glucose, triglyceride, uric acid, liver enzyme, bilirubin, cholesterol, potassium, and CK levels. May decrease hemoglobin level and hematocrit.

Pharmacokinetics

Absorption: Rapid and complete. Steady-state level is achieved within 3 to 5 days.
Distribution: 99% bound to proteins.
Metabolism: None.
Excretion: In the urine and feces. *Half-life:* 13 hours.

Route	Onset	Peak	Duration
P.O.	Rapid	1–2 hr	24 hr

Action

Chemical effect: Blocks the vasoconstrictor and aldosterone-secreting effects of angiotensin II by selectively blocking the binding of angiotensin II to the angiotensin receptor in the vascular smooth muscle.
Therapeutic effect: Lowers blood pressure.

Available forms

Tablets: 5 mg, 20 mg, 40 mg

NURSING PROCESS

⚚ Assessment

• Monitor patients with heart failure closely for oliguria, azotemia, and acute renal impairment.
• Monitor BUN and creatinine levels in patients with renal artery stenosis.
• Be alert for adverse reactions.
• Assess patient's and family's knowledge of drug therapy.

⊕ Nursing diagnoses

• Risk for injury related to presence of hypertension
• Disturbed sleep pattern related to drug-induced cough
• Deficient knowledge related to drug therapy

⊠ Planning and implementation

• Symptomatic hypotension may occur in patients who are volume- or salt-depleted, especially those being treated with high doses of a diuretic. If hypotension occurs, place patient supine and treat supportively. When blood pressure is stabilized, therapy can continue.
• If blood pressure isn't adequately controlled, a diuretic or other antihypertensive may be added.
Patient teaching
• Tell patient to take drug exactly as prescribed and not to stop even if he feels better.
• Tell patient that drug may be taken with or without food.
• Tell patient to immediately report adverse reactions, especially light-headedness and syncope, to prescriber.
• Advise a woman of childbearing age to immediately report pregnancy to prescriber.
• Inform diabetic patient that glucose readings may become higher, and the dosage of their antidiabetics may need adjustment.
• Warn patient that reduced fluid volume from inadequate fluid intake, excessive perspiration, diarrhea, or vomiting may cause a drop in blood pressure, leading to light-headedness and fainting.
• Inform patient that other antihypertensives can have additive or synergistic effects. Patient should inform prescriber of all drugs (including OTC) that he's taking.

☑ Evaluation

• Patient's blood pressure is normal.
• Patient's sleep patterns are undisturbed throughout therapy.
• Patient and family state understanding of drug therapy.

---

olsalazine sodium
(olh-SAL-uh-zeen SOH-dee-um)
Dipentum

Pharmacologic class: salicylate
Therapeutic class: anti-inflammatory
Pregnancy risk category: C

Indications and dosages

▶ Maintenance of remission of ulcerative colitis in patients intolerant of sulfasalazine.
Adults: 500 mg P.O. b.i.d. with meals.

Contraindications and cautions

• Contraindicated in patients hypersensitive to salicylates.
• Use cautiously in patients with renal disease. Renal tubular damage may result from absorbed drug or its metabolites.
⚞ Lifespan: In pregnant women, use cautiously. In breast-feeding women, use cautiously; it's unknown if the drug appears in breast milk. In children, safety and effectiveness haven't been established.

Adverse reactions

CNS: headache, depression, vertigo, dizziness.
GI: *diarrhea,* nausea, abdominal pain, heartburn.
Musculoskeletal: arthralgia.
Skin: rash, itching.

Interactions

Drug-drug. *Anticoagulants, coumarin derivatives:* May increase anticoagulant effects. Monitor patient closely for bleeding.

Effects on lab test results

• May increase AST and ALT levels.

Pharmacokinetics

Absorption: About 2%.
Distribution: Liberated mesalamine is absorbed slowly from colon, resulting in very high local levels.
Metabolism: 0.1% in liver; remainder reaches colon, where it's rapidly converted to mesalamine by colonic bacteria.
Excretion: About 80% in feces; less than 1% in urine. *Half-life:* About 1 hour.

Route	Onset	Peak	Duration
P.O.	Unknown	1 hr	Unknown

Action

Chemical effect: May convert to 5-aminosalicylic acid (5-ASA or mesalamine) in colon, where it has local anti-inflammatory effect.
Therapeutic effect: Prevents flare-up of ulcerative colitis.

Available forms

Capsules: 250 mg

NURSING PROCESS

⬛ Assessment
• Assess patient's condition before starting therapy, and regularly thereafter to monitor the drug's effectiveness.
• Monitor BUN and creatinine levels and urinalysis in patient with renal disease.
• Be alert for adverse reactions.
• Assess patient's and family's knowledge of drug therapy.

⬛ Nursing diagnoses
• Impaired tissue integrity related to ulcerative colitis
• Diarrhea related to drug's adverse effect on GI tract
• Deficient knowledge related to drug therapy

⬛ Planning and implementation
• Give drug in evenly divided doses with food to decrease GI irritation.
• Report diarrhea to prescriber. Although diarrhea appears dose-related, it's difficult to distinguish from worsening of disease symptoms. Worsening of disease has been noted with similar drugs.
⚞ ALERT: Don't confuse olsalazine with olanzapine.
Patient teaching
• Tell patient to take drug in evenly divided doses, with food, to minimize GI irritation.
• Urge patient to notify prescriber about adverse reactions, especially diarrhea or increased pain.

⬛ Evaluation
• Patient has no evidence of ulcerative colitis.
• Patient is free from diarrhea.

0

• Patient and family state understanding of drug therapy.

omalizumab
(oh-mah-LIZZ-uh-mahb)
Xolair

Pharmacologic class: monoclonal antibody
Therapeutic class: antiasthmatic
Pregnancy risk category: B

Indications and dosages

▶ **Moderate to severe persistent asthma in patients who have positive skin test or in vitro reactivity to a seasonal allergen and whose symptoms are inadequately controlled with inhaled corticosteroids.** *Adults and children age 12 and older:* Dosage is determined by total immunoglobulin E (IgE) level (international unit/ml) measured before the start of therapy and by body weight (kg). See tables on next page. Divide doses greater than 150 mg and use more than one injection site. Inject subcutaneously q 2 or 4 weeks.

Contraindications and cautions

• Contraindicated in patients hypersensitive to the drug or any of its components.
⚱ **Lifespan:** In pregnant women, use only when potential benefits outweigh risks to the fetus. In breast-feeding women, use cautiously; it's unclear if the drug appears in breast milk. In children younger than age 12, safety and effectiveness of drug haven't been established.

Adverse reactions

CNS: *headache,* pain, fatigue, dizziness.
EENT: *sinusitis,* pharyngitis, earache.
Musculoskeletal: arthralgia, fracture, leg pain, arm pain.
Respiratory: *upper respiratory tract infection.*
Skin: pruritus, dermatitis.
Other: *injection site reaction, viral infections, anaphylaxis,* hypersensitivity reaction, malignancy.

Interactions

None reported.

Effects on lab test results

• May increase IgE levels for up to 1 year after therapy.

Pharmacokinetics

Absorption: Slow, with a bioavailability of about 62%.
Distribution: None specified.
Metabolism: Unknown.
Excretion: In liver and bile. *Half-life:* About 26 days.

Route	Onset	Peak	Duration
SubQ	Unknown	7–8 days	Unknown

Action

Chemical effect: Inhibits binding of IgE to a high-affinity receptor on the surface of mast cells and basophils. Reducing IgE limits the release of mediators of the allergic response and reduces the number of receptors on basophils.
Therapeutic effect: Treats asthma symptoms.

Available forms

Powder for injection: 150 mg in 5-ml vial

NURSING PROCESS

🔍 **Assessment**
• Assess patient's respiratory condition before starting therapy, and regularly thereafter to monitor the drug's effectiveness.
• Be alert for adverse reactions.
⑤ **ALERT:** Observe patient after injection and have drugs available to treat severe hypersensitivity reactions. If a severe hypersensitivity reaction occurs, stop therapy.
• Assess patient's and family's knowledge of drug therapy.

📋 **Nursing diagnoses**
• Impaired gas exchange related to presence of bronchospasms
• Acute pain related to drug-induced headache
• Deficient knowledge related to drug therapy

▷ **Planning and implementation**
⑤ **ALERT:** Don't use for acute bronchospasm or status asthmaticus.
• Don't abruptly stop giving systemic or inhaled corticosteroids when starting this drug. Gradually decrease corticosteroids with prescriber nearby.

Reactions may be *common,* uncommon, *life-threatening*, or COMMON AND LIFE-THREATENING.

DOSE EVERY 4 WEEKS

Pretreatment IgE (international unit/ml)	Body weight (kg)			
	30–60	> 60–70	> 70–90	> 90–150
≥ 30–100	150 mg	150 mg	150 mg	300 mg
> 100–200	300 mg	300 mg	300 mg	See table below.
> 200–300	300 mg	See table below.	See table below.	See table below.

DOSE EVERY 2 WEEKS

Pretreatment IgE (international unit/ml)	Body weight (kg)			
	30–60	> 60–70	> 70–90	> 90–150
> 100–200	See table above.	See table above.	See table above.	225 mg
> 200–300	See table above.	225 mg	225 mg	300 mg
> 300–400	225 mg	225 mg	300 mg	Don't give.
> 400–500	300 mg	300 mg	375 mg	Don't give.
> 500–600	300 mg	375 mg	Don't give.	Don't give.
> 600–700	375 mg	Don't give.	Don't give.	Don't give.

• Because the solution is slightly viscous, it may take 5 to 10 seconds to inject.
• Patient may have injection site reactions, including bruising, redness, warmth, burning, stinging, itching, hives, pain, induration, and inflammation. Most reactions occur within 1 hour of injection, last less than 8 days, and decrease in frequency with subsequent injections.
• Total IgE levels may elevate during therapy and remain elevated for up to 1 year after therapy stops; testing IgE levels during therapy can't be used as a guide to determine dose. If therapy has been stopped for less than 1 year, use IgE levels from the original dose determination. If therapy has been stopped for 1 year or more, retest total IgE levels.

Patient teaching
• Tell patient not to decrease the dose or stop taking his other antiasthmatics unless directed by prescriber.
• Tell patient not to expect immediate improvement in his asthma after starting therapy.

☑ Evaluation
• Patient exhibits normal breathing pattern.
• Patient states that drug-induced headache is relieved by analgesic.
• Patient and family state understanding of drug therapy.

omega-3 acid ethyl esters
(oh-MAY-gah THREE ASS-id ETH-ill ESS-turs)
Omacor

Pharmacologic class: ethyl ester
Therapeutic class: lipid regulator
Pregnancy risk category: C

Indications and dosages
▶ **Adjunct to diet to reduce triglyceride level of 500 mg/dl or more.** *Adults:* 4 g P.O. once daily or divided equally b.i.d.

Contraindications and cautions
• Contraindicated in patients hypersensitive to drug or any of its components.
• Use cautiously in patients sensitive to fish.
※ **Lifespan:** In pregnant women, use only if benefits outweigh risks to the fetus. In breast-feeding women, use cautiously. Safety and effectiveness in children haven't been established.

Adverse reactions
CNS: pain.
CV: angina pectoris.
GI: altered taste, belching, dyspepsia.
Musculoskeletal: back pain.
Skin: rash.
Other: flulike syndrome, infection.

Interactions

Drug-drug. *Anticoagulants:* May prolong bleeding time. Monitor patient.

Effects on lab test results

• May increase ALT and LDL levels.

Pharmacokinetics

Absorption: Good.
Distribution: Unknown.
Metabolism: Unknown.
Excretion: Unknown.

Route	Onset	Peak	Duration
P.O.	Unknown	Unknown	Unknown

Action

Chemical effect: May be a poor substrate for the enzymes needed for triglyceride synthesis. Blocks formation of other fatty acids.
Therapeutic effect: Decreases triglyceride levels.

Available forms

Capsules: 1 g

NURSING PROCESS

☼ Assessment

• Assess patient for conditions that increase triglyceride level, such as diabetes and hypothyroidism, before therapy.
• Assess patient's current history for drugs known to sharply increase triglyceride levels, including estrogen therapy, thiazide diuretics, and beta blockers. Drug made not be needed after stopping these drugs.
• Monitor patient for adverse drug effects.
• Assess patient's and family's knowledge of drug therapy.

⊞ Nursing diagnoses

• Ineffective health maintenance related to elevated triglyceride levels
• Risk for injury related to very high triglyceride levels
• Deficient knowledge related to drug therapy

▷ Planning and implementation

• Start therapy only after diet and lifestyle modifications have proven unsuccessful.
• Obtain baseline triglyceride levels to confirm that they're consistently abnormal before ther-

apy; then recheck periodically during therapy. If patient has an inadequate response after 2 months, stop drug.
• Monitor LDL level to make sure it doesn't increase excessively during therapy.

Patient teaching
• Explain that drug doesn't reduce the importance of following the recommended diet and exercise plan.
• Remind patient of the need for follow-up blood work to evaluate progress.
• Advise patient to notify prescriber about bothersome side effects.
• Tell patient to report planned or suspected pregnancy.

☑ Evaluation

• Patient reduces triglyceride level with diet, exercise, lifestyle modifications, and drug therapy.
• Patient has reduced triglyceride level.
• Patient and family state understanding of drug therapy.

omeprazole

(oh-MEH-pruh-zohl)
Losec ◆ ◇ , Prilosec⊘ , Prilosec OTC† ,
Zegerid

Pharmacologic class: substituted benzimidazole
Therapeutic class: proton pump inhibitor
Pregnancy risk category: C

Indications and dosages

▶ **Erosive esophagitis; symptomatic, poorly responsive gastroesophageal reflux disease (GERD).** *Adults with GERD who are unresponsive to H₂-receptor antagonist:* 20 mg P.O. daily for 4 to 8 weeks. May increase dose to 40 mg daily if needed and extend therapy up to 12 weeks.
Children 2 to 16 years weighing less than 20 kg: 10 mg P.O. daily.
Children 2 to 16 years weighing 20 kg or more: 20 mg P.O. daily.
▶ **GERD without erosive esophagitis.** *Adults:* 20 mg P.O. daily for 4 weeks.
▶ **Pathologic hypersecretory conditions (such as Zollinger-Ellison syndrome).** *Adults:* Initially, 60 mg P.O. daily; adjust to patient's response. If daily amount exceeds 80 mg, give in divided doses. Dosages up to 120 mg t.i.d. may be given.

▶ **Duodenal ulcer (short-term therapy).**
Adults: 20 mg P.O. daily for 2 to 8 weeks.
▶ **Gastric ulcer.** *Adults:* 40 mg P.O. daily for 4 to 8 weeks.
▶ *Helicobacter pylori* **eradication to reduce risk of duodenal ulcer recurrence as part of triple therapy with clarithromycin and amoxicillin.** *Adults:* 20 mg P.O. with 500 mg clarithromycin P.O. and 1,000 mg amoxicillin P.O., each given b.i.d. for 10 days. For patients with ulcers when therapy starts, another 18 days of 20 mg omeprazole P.O. once daily is recommended.
▶ *Helicobacter pylori* **eradication to reduce risk of duodenal ulcer recurrence as part of dual therapy with clarithromycin.** *Adults:* 40 mg P.O. once daily with clarithromycin 500 mg, P.O., t.i.d. for 14 days. For patients with ulcers present at the start of therapy, give 20 mg omeprazole P.O. once daily for 14 more days.
▶ **Heartburn on 2 or more days per week.**
Adults: 20 mg P.O. (Prilosec OTC) daily before breakfast for 14 days. May repeat the 14-day course q 4 months.
▶ **Posterior laryngitis‡.** *Adults:* 40 mg q h.s. for 6 to 24 weeks.

Contraindications and cautions

• Contraindicated in patients hypersensitive to the drug or any of its components.
⚕ **Lifespan:** In pregnant women, use cautiously. In breast-feeding women, use cautiously; it's unknown if the drug appears in breast milk. In children ages 2 to 16 years, drug may be used to treat GERD, erosive esophagitis, and for maintenance of healing in erosive esophagitis (tablets and capsules only).

Adverse reactions

CNS: headache, dizziness.
GI: diarrhea, abdominal pain, nausea, vomiting, constipation, flatulence.
Musculoskeletal: back pain.
Respiratory: cough.
Skin: rash.

Interactions

Drug-drug. *Ampicillin esters, iron derivatives, ketoconazole:* May decrease absorption. Give separately.
Clarithromycin: May increase levels of either drug. Monitor patient for drug toxicity.

Diazepam, phenytoin, warfarin: May decrease hepatic clearance of these drugs, possibly leading to increased levels. Monitor patient closely.
Sucralfate: May delay absorption and reduce omeprazole bioavailability. Separate administration times by 30 minutes or more.
Drug-herb. *Male fern:* May inactivate herb. Discourage using together.
Pennyroyal: May change the rate at which toxic metabolites of herb form. Discourage using together.

Effects on lab test results

None reported.

Pharmacokinetics

Absorption: Rapid, but bioavailability is about 40% because of instability in gastric acid as well as substantial first-pass effect. Bioavailability increases slightly with repeated dosing.
Distribution: Protein-binding is about 95%.
Metabolism: Primarily in liver.
Excretion: Primarily in urine. *Half-life:* 30 to 60 minutes.

Route	Onset	Peak	Duration
P.O.	≤ 1 hr	30 min-2 hr	< 3 days

Action

Chemical effect: Inhibits acid (proton) pump and binds to hydrogen-potassium adenosine triphosphatase on secretory surface of gastric parietal cells to block formation of gastric acid.
Therapeutic effect: Relieves symptoms caused by excessive gastric acid.

Available forms

Capsules (delayed-release): 10 mg, 20 mg, 40 mg
Tablets (delayed-release): 20 mg
Powder for oral suspension: 20 mg

NURSING PROCESS

⚕ Assessment
• Assess patient's condition before starting therapy, and regularly thereafter to monitor the drug's effectiveness.
• Be alert for adverse reactions and drug interactions.
• If adverse GI reaction occurs, monitor patient's hydration.

• Assess patient's and family's knowledge of drug therapy.

🖳 **Nursing diagnoses**
• Impaired tissue integrity related to upper gastric disorder
• Risk for deficient fluid volume related to drug-induced adverse GI reactions
• Deficient knowledge related to drug therapy

▷ **Planning and implementation**
• Give tablets or capsules 30 minutes before meals; powder for oral suspension 1 hour before meals.
• Zegerid powder for oral suspension may be used for short-term treatment of duodenal ulcers, GERD, and maintenance of healing of erosive esophagitis; don't use in children younger than age 18.
• Use 2 tbs of water to mix 1 packet of powder for oral suspension; don't use any other liquids or food.
• Powder for oral suspension contains 460 mg of sodium per dose and 20 mEq of sodium bicarbonate.
• Lower doses aren't needed for patients with renal or hepatic impairment.
⑤ **ALERT:** Don't confuse Prilosec with Prozac, prilocaine, or Prinivil.
⑤ **ALERT:** Don't confuse Losec with Lasix.
Patient teaching
• Explain importance of taking drug exactly as prescribed.
• Warn patient not to crush or chew tablets or capsules.
• Explain to patient how to reconstitute powder for oral suspension: Empty packet contents into a small cup containing 2 tbs of water; stir well and drink immediately. Refill cup with water and drink.
• Advise patient that OTC drug isn't intended for immediate relief of heartburn or to treat occasional heartburn (one episode of heartburn a week or less).
• Inform patient that OTC drug may require 1 to 4 days for full effect, although some patients may get complete relief of symptoms within 24 hours.

☑ **Evaluation**
• Patient responds well to therapy.
• Patient maintains adequate hydration throughout drug therapy.

• Patient and family state understanding of drug therapy.

ondansetron hydrochloride
(on-DAN-seh-tron high-droh-KLOR-ighd)
Zofran, Zofran ODT

Pharmacologic class: serotonin receptor antagonist
Therapeutic class: antiemetic
Pregnancy risk category: B

Indications and dosages

▶ **To prevent nausea and vomiting caused by moderately emetogenic chemotherapy.**
Adults and children age 12 and older: 8 mg P.O. 30 minutes before start of chemotherapy. Follow with 8 mg P.O. 8 hours after first dose. Then follow with 8 mg q 12 hours for 1 to 2 days. Or, three doses of 0.15 mg/kg I.V. Give first dose 30 minutes before chemotherapy; give subsequent doses 4 and 8 hours after first dose. Infuse drug over 15 minutes. Or, adults may receive a single dose of 32 mg I.V. infused over 15 minutes, 30 minutes before chemotherapy. Don't repeat this dose.
Children ages 4 to 11: 4 mg P.O. 30 minutes before start of chemotherapy. Follow with 4 mg P.O. 4 and 8 hours after first dose. Then follow with 4 mg q 8 hours for 1 to 2 days.
Children ages 6 months to 11 years: Three doses of 0.15 mg/kg I.V. Give first dose 30 minutes before chemotherapy; give subsequent doses 4 and 8 hours after first dose. Infuse drug over 15 minutes.
▶ **To prevent nausea and vomiting caused by highly emetogenic chemotherapy.** *Adults:* 24 mg P.O. 30 minutes before start of chemotherapy.
▶ **To prevent postoperative nausea and vomiting.** *Adults:* 4 mg I.V. (undiluted) over 2 to 5 minutes immediately before induction of anesthesia or postoperatively. Or, 4 mg I.M. as a single injection immediately before induction of anesthesia or postoperatively. Or, 16 mg P.O. 1 hour before induction of anesthesia.
Children ages 1 month to 12 years who weigh 40 kg (88 lb) or less: 0.1 mg/kg I.V. Give dose over 2 to 5 minutes as a single dose.

Children ages 1 month to 12 years who weigh more than 40 kg: Give 4 mg I.V. over 2 to 5 minutes as a single dose.

▶ **To prevent nausea and vomiting from radiation therapy—total body irradiation, a single high-dose fraction, or daily fractions to the abdomen.** *Adults:* 8 mg P.O. t.i.d.

❑ **Adjust-a-dose:** For patients with severe liver impairment, don't exceed total daily dose of 8 mg P.O. or a single maximum dose of 8 mg I.V. over 15 minutes.

▼ I.V. administration

• Dilute drug in 50 ml of D_5W injection or normal saline solution for injection before giving.
• Infuse drug over 15 minutes.
• Drug is stable for up to 48 hours after dilution in 5% dextrose and normal saline injection, 5% dextrose in half-normal saline injection, and 3% saline injection.
⊗ **Incompatibilities**
Acyclovir sodium, allopurinol, aminophylline, amphotericin B, ampicillin sodium, ampicillin sodium and sulbactam sodium, cefepime, cefoperazone, dexamethasone sodium phosphate, droperidol, fluorouracil, furosemide, ganciclovir, lorazepam, meropenem, methylprednisolone sodium succinate, piperacillin sodium, sargramostim, sodium bicarbonate.

Contraindications and cautions

• Contraindicated in patients hypersensitive to the drug or any of its components.
• Use cautiously and at a lower dose in patients with liver failure.
⚘ **Lifespan:** In pregnant women, use cautiously. In breast-feeding women, use cautiously; it's unknown if the drug appears in breast milk. In children, safety and effectiveness of the 24-mg tablet or the use of oral forms of drug for postoperative nausea and vomiting or radiation-induced nausea and vomiting haven't been established. In children younger than age 2, information on safety and effectiveness of injection forms of drug is limited.

Adverse reactions

CNS: *headache,* extrapyramidal syndrome.
CV: hypotension, chest pain, *bradycardia, arrhythmias.*
GI: diarrhea, constipation.
Skin: rash, pruritus.

Interactions

Drug-drug. *Drugs that alter hepatic drug-metabolizing enzymes (such as cimetidine, phenobarbital):* May alter pharmacokinetics of ondansetron. No dosage adjustment is needed.
Rifampin: May reduce ondansetron levels, decreasing antiemetic effect. Monitor patient for adequate antiemetic effect; adjust dosage.

Effects on lab test results

• May increase ALT and AST levels.

Pharmacokinetics

Absorption: Variable; bioavailability is 50% to 60%.
Distribution: 70% to 76% is protein-bound.
Metabolism: Extensive.
Excretion: Primarily in urine. *Half-life:* 4 hours.

Route	Onset	Peak	Duration
P.O., I.V.	Unknown	Unknown	Unknown

Action

Chemical effect: Blocking action may take place in CNS at chemoreceptor trigger zone and in peripheral nervous system on terminals of vagus nerve.
Therapeutic effect: Prevents nausea and vomiting from emetogenic chemotherapy or surgery.

Available forms

Injection: 2 mg/ml
Oral solution: 4 mg/5 ml
Tablets: 4 mg, 8 mg, 24 mg
Tablets (orally disintegrating): 4 mg, 8 mg

NURSING PROCESS

▨ **Assessment**
• Assess patient's condition before starting therapy, and regularly thereafter to monitor the drug's effectiveness.
• Be alert for adverse reactions and drug interactions.
• Assess patient's and family's knowledge of drug therapy.

⊞ **Nursing diagnoses**
• Risk for deficient fluid volume related to nausea and vomiting
• Pain related to drug-induced headache
• Deficient knowledge related to drug therapy

⟫ Planning and implementation
⊛ **ALERT:** Don't confuse Zofran with Zantac or Zosyn.
⊛ **ALERT:** Don't confuse Zofran with Precedex. These vials appear very similar.
⊛ **ALERT:** Don't confuse ondansetron with olanzapine
Patient teaching
● Instruct patient when to take drug.
● Tell patient to report adverse reactions.
● Advise patient to report any discomfort at I.V. site.

☑ Evaluation
● Patient maintains adequate hydration.
● Patient does not experience any drug-induced headaches.
● Patient and family state understanding of drug therapy.

orlistat
(OR-lih-stat)
Xenical

Pharmacologic class: lipase inhibitor
Therapeutic class: antiobesity drug
Pregnancy risk category: B

Indications and dosages
▶ **Management of obesity, including weight loss and weight maintenance, given with a reduced-calorie diet; reduction of risk of weight regain after weight loss.** *Adults:* 120 mg P.O. t.i.d. with each main meal containing fat (during or up to 1 hour after the meal).

Contraindications and cautions
● Contraindicated in patients hypersensitive to the drug or any of its components and in patients with chronic malabsorption syndrome or cholestasis.
● Use cautiously in patients with a history of hyperoxaluria or calcium oxalate nephrolithiasis, patients who are at risk for anorexia nervosa or bulimia, and patients who are receiving cyclosporine therapy because of changes in cyclosporine absorption related to variations in diet.
≋ **Lifespan:** In pregnant and breast-feeding women, drug isn't recommended. In children, safety and effectiveness haven't been established.

Adverse reactions
CNS: *headache*, dizziness, fatigue, sleep disorder, anxiety, depression.
CV: pedal edema.
EENT: otitis.
GI: *oily spotting, flatus with discharge, fecal urgency, fatty or oily stool, oily evacuation, increased defecation, abdominal pain,* fecal incontinence, nausea, infectious diarrhea, rectal pain, vomiting.
GU: menstrual irregularity, vaginitis, UTI.
Musculoskeletal: *back pain,* leg pain, arthritis, myalgia, joint disorder, tendinitis.
Respiratory: *influenza, upper respiratory tract infection,* lower respiratory tract infection.
Skin: rash, dry skin.
Other: tooth and gingival disorders.

Interactions
Drug-drug. *Cyclosporine:* May alter cyclosporine absorption. Monitor cyclosporine levels.
Fat-soluble vitamins such as vitamin E, beta-carotene: May decrease vitamin absorption. Separate administration times by 2 hours.
Pravastatin: May slightly increase pravastatin levels and lipid-lowering effects. Monitor patient.
Warfarin: May change coagulation parameters. Monitor INR.

Effects on lab test results
● May decrease vitamin D, beta-carotene, LDL, and total cholesterol levels.

Pharmacokinetics
Absorption: Only a small amount.
Distribution: More than 99% binds to proteins. Lipoproteins and albumin are major binding proteins.
Metabolism: Primarily in GI wall.
Excretion: Mostly unchanged in feces. *Half-life:* 1 to 2 hours.

Route	Onset	Peak	Duration
P.O.	Unknown	Unknown	Unknown

Action
Chemical effect: Binds with the active site of gastric and pancreatic lipases. These inactivated enzymes are thus unavailable to hydrolyze dietary fat, in the form of triglycerides, into absorbable free fatty acids and monoglycerides. Because the undigested triglycerides aren't ab-

sorbed, the resulting caloric deficit may help with weight control. The recommended dosage of 120 mg t.i.d. inhibits dietary fat absorption by about 30%.
Therapeutic effect: Weight loss and weight maintenance.

Available forms

Capsules: 120 mg

NURSING PROCESS

Assessment

• Obtain history of patient's underlying condition before starting therapy, and reassess regularly thereafter to monitor the drug's effectiveness.
• Screen patient for anorexia nervosa or bulimia; as with any weight-loss drug, drug can be misused.
• Organic causes of obesity, such as hypothyroidism, must be ruled out before patient starts orlistat therapy.
• In diabetic patient, monitor glucose level frequently during weight loss. Dose of oral antidiabetic or insulin may need to be reduced.
• Assess patient's and family's knowledge of drug therapy.

Nursing diagnoses

• Imbalanced nutrition: More than body requirements related to obesity
• Disturbed body image related to obesity
• Deficient knowledge related to drug therapy

Planning and implementation

• Use drug for a patient with an initial body mass index of 30 kg/m^2 or more (27 kg/m^2 or more if patient has other risk factors, such as hypertension, diabetes, or dyslipidemia).
• It's unknown whether drug is safe and effective to use longer than 2 years.
• Tell patient to follow dietary guidelines. GI effects may increase when patient takes drug with high-fat foods—specifically, when more than 30% of total daily calories come from fat.
• Drug reduces absorption of some fat-soluble vitamins and beta-carotene.
ALERT: Don't confuse Xenical with Xeloda.

Patient teaching

• Advise patient to follow a nutritionally balanced, reduced-calorie diet that derives only 30% of its calories from fat. Daily intake of fat, carbohydrate, and protein should be distributed over three main meals. If a meal is occasionally missed or contains no fat, tell patient that dose can be skipped.
• To ensure adequate nutrition, advise patient to take a daily multivitamin supplement that contains fat-soluble vitamins no sooner than within 2 hours of taking drug, such as h.s.
• Tell patient with diabetes that weight loss may improve glycemic control, so the dose of his oral antidiabetic or insulin may need to be reduced.
• Tell woman to inform prescriber if she is pregnant, plans to become pregnant, or is breast-feeding.

Evaluation

• Patient's nutritional intake is adequate according to proper dietary guidelines.
• Patient reaches and maintains a stable weight.
• Patient and family state understanding of drug therapy.

oseltamivir phosphate

(ah-sul-TAM-ih-veer FOS-fayt)
Tamiflu

Pharmacologic class: neuraminidase inhibitor
Therapeutic class: antiviral
Pregnancy risk category: C

Indications and dosages

▶ **Uncomplicated, acute illness from influenza in patients who have been symptomatic for 2 days or less.** *Adults, children age 13 and older, and children who weigh more than 40 kg (88 lb):* 75 mg P.O. b.i.d. for 5 days.
Children age 1 and older who weigh 23 to 40 kg (51 to 88 lb): 60 mg oral suspension P.O. b.i.d.
Children age 1 and older who weigh 15 to 23 kg (33 to 51 lb): 45 mg oral suspension P.O. b.i.d.
Children age 1 and older who weigh 15 kg (33 lb) or less: 30 mg oral suspension P.O. b.i.d.
Adjust-a-dose: For patients with renal impairment, if creatinine clearance is 10 to 30 ml/minute, give 75 mg P.O. once daily for 5 days.
▶ **Prevention of influenza after close contact with infected person.** *Adults and children age 13 and older:* 75 mg P.O. once daily beginning within 2 days of exposure and lasting at least 7 days.

Σ **Adjust-a-dose:** For patients with renal impairment, if creatinine clearance is 10 to 30 ml/minute, give 75 mg once q other day or 30 mg of oral suspension daily.

▶ **Prevention of influenza during a community outbreak.** *Adults and children age 13 and older:* 75 mg P.O. daily for up to 6 weeks.

Σ **Adjust-a-dose:** For patients with renal impairment, if creatinine clearance is 10 to 30 ml/minute, give 75 mg once q other day or 30 mg of oral suspension daily.

Contraindications and cautions

• Contraindicated in patients hypersensitive to the drug or any of its components.

▓ **Lifespan:** In breast-feeding women, use only if benefits outweigh potential risks to the infant. In children younger than age 1, use for treatment of influenza hasn't been established. In children younger than age 13, use for prevention of influenza hasn't been established.

Adverse reactions

CNS: dizziness, insomnia, headache, vertigo, fatigue.
GI: abdominal pain, diarrhea, nausea, vomiting.
Respiratory: bronchitis, cough.

Interactions

None significant.

Effects on lab test results

None reported.

Pharmacokinetics

Absorption: Good. More than 75% reaches systemic circulation as oseltamivir carboxylate.
Distribution: Protein-binding is 3 to 42%.
Metabolism: Extensive.
Excretion: Mostly in urine by glomerular filtration and tubular secretion. Less than 20% is eliminated in feces. *Half-life:* 1 to 10 hours.

Route	Onset	Peak	Duration
P.O.	Unknown	Unknown	Unknown

Action

Chemical effect: Inhibits the enzyme neuraminidase in influenza virus particles. This action may inhibit viral replication, possibly by interfering with viral particle aggregation and release from the host cell.

Therapeutic effect: Lessens the symptoms of influenza.

Available forms

Capsules: 75 mg
Oral suspension: 12 mg/ml after reconstitution

NURSING PROCESS

Ӿ **Assessment**
• Obtain complete medical history before starting therapy.
• Assess renal function before giving drug, as directed.
• Assess patient's and family's knowledge of drug therapy.

▣ **Nursing diagnoses**
• Infection related to influenza virus
• Imbalanced nutrition: Less than body requirements related to drug's adverse GI effects
• Deficient knowledge related to drug therapy

▷ **Planning and implementation**
• Drug is used primarily to treat symptoms and isn't a replacement for an annual influenza vaccination.
• No evidence supports use in treating other viral infections.
• Drug may be given with meals to decrease adverse GI effects.
• Safety and effectiveness of repeated courses of therapy haven't been established.
Patient teaching
• Tell patient to start drug within 2 days of start of symptoms.
• Inform patient that receiving this drug isn't a substitute for receiving the flu vaccination. Urge patient to continue receiving an annual vaccination.

▨ **Evaluation**
• Patient recovers from influenza.
• Patient has no adverse GI effects and maintains adequate hydration.
• Patient and family state understanding of drug therapy.

oxaliplatin
(ox-ah-leh-PLA-tin)
Eloxatin

Pharmacologic class: alkylating drug
Therapeutic class: antineoplastic
Pregnancy risk category: D

Indications and dosages

▶ **Advanced colorectal cancer when given
with 5-fluorouracil (5-FU) and leucovorin.**
Adults: On day one, 85 mg/m² oxaliplatin I.V.
in 250 to 500 ml D₅W and 200 mg/m² leucovorin I.V. in D₅W, given simultaneously over
120 minutes in separate bags using a Y-line.
Then, 400 mg/m² 5-FU I.V. bolus given over
2 to 4 minutes, followed by 600 mg/m² 5-FU
I.V. infusion in 500 ml D₅W over 22 hours. On
day two, 200 mg/m² leucovorin I.V. infusion
over 120 minutes. Then, 400 mg/m² 5-FU I.V.
bolus given over 2 to 4 minutes, followed by
600 mg/m² 5-FU I.V. infusion in 500 ml D₅W
over 22 hours. Repeat cycle q 2 weeks.
◙ **Adjust-a-dose:** In patients with unresolved
and persistent grade 2 neurosensory events
(events that interfere with function, but not daily
activities), reduce dose to 65 mg/m². In patients
with persistent grade 3 neurosensory events
(pain and functional impairment that affect daily
activity), consider stopping drug. In patients recovering from grade 3/4 GI (despite prophylaxis) or hematologic (neutrophil count less than
1.5 × 10⁹/L and platelet count less than 100 ×
10⁹/L) events, reduce dose to 65 mg/m². Also
reduce dose of 5-FU by 20%.
▶ **With 5-FU and leucovorin for the adjuvant treatment of stage III colon cancer in
patients who have undergone complete resection of the primary tumor.** *Adults:* On day
one, give oxaliplatin, 85 mg/m² I.V. in 250 to
500 ml D₅W and leucovorin 200 mg/m² I.V. infusion in D₅W, both over 120 minutes at the
same time, in separate bags, using a Y-line. Follow with 5-FU 400 mg/m² I.V. bolus over 2 to
4 minutes, then 600 mg/m² 5-FU in 500 ml
D₅W as a 22-hour continuous infusion. On day
two, give leucovorin, 200 mg/m² I.V. infused
over 120 minutes followed by 5-FU 400 mg/m²
as an I.V. bolus over 2 to 4 minutes, then,
600 mg/m² 5-FU infusion in 500 ml D₅W over
22 hours. Repeat cycle q 2 weeks for a total of

6 months. Premedicate with antiemetics, with or
without dexamethasone.
◙ **Adjust-a-dose:** For patients with persistent
grade 2 neurotoxicity, consider an oxaliplatin
dose reduction to 75 mg/m². For patients with
persistent Grade 3 neurosensory events, consider discontinuing oxaliplatin therapy. For patients
who recovered from a grade 3/4 GI events
(despite prophylaxis) or grade 3/4 hematologic
toxicity, reduce oxaliplatin to 75 mg/m² and
5-FU to a 300 mg/m² bolus and 500 mg/m²
22-hour infusion. Delay dose until neutrophils
are ≥ 1.5 x 10⁹/L and platelets are ≥ 75 x 10⁹/L.

▼ I.V. administration

● Preparing and giving drug may have carcinogenic, mutagenic, and teratogenic risks. Follow
facility policy to reduce risks.
● Reconstitute powder using sterile water for injection or D₅W. Add 10 ml to a 50-mg vial or
20 ml to a 100-mg vial for a final concentration
of 5 mg/ml. Never reconstitute with sodium
chloride solution or other solution containing
chloride.
● Further dilute reconstituted solutions in an infusion solution of 250 to 500 ml of D₅W.
● Inspect bag for particulate matter and discoloration before giving; discard if present.
● Don't use needles or I.V. administration sets
that contain aluminum because they will react
with platinum in drug, causing loss of potency
and formation of a black precipitate.
● Drug doesn't require prehydration.
● Premedicate with antiemetics with or without
dexamethasone.
● Flush infusion line with D₅W before giving
any other drugs simultaneously.
● Give drug and leucovorin over 2 hours at the
same time in separate bags, using a Y-line. May
extend the infusion time of the oxaliplatin to
6 hours to decrease acute toxicities.
● Avoid ice and cold exposure during infusion
of drug because cold temperatures can exacerbate acute neurologic symptoms. Cover patient
with a blanket during infusion.
● Store unopened vials at room temperature.
Reconstituted solutions are stable if refrigerated
(36° to 46° F [2° to 8° C]) for up to 24 hours.
After final dilution, solutions are stable for
6 hours at room temperature and up to 24 hours
under refrigeration.

O

⊗ **Incompatibilities**
Alkaline solutions, solutions containing chloride, or drugs such as 5-FU.

Contraindications and cautions

• Contraindicated in patients allergic to the drug or other compounds containing platinum.
• Use cautiously in patients with preexisting renal impairment or peripheral sensory neuropathy.
⚄ **Lifespan:** In pregnant women, drug is contraindicated. In breast-feeding women and in children, safety and effectiveness haven't been established. In the elderly, use cautiously because diarrhea, dehydration, hypokalemia, and fatigue may occur more frequently in these patients.

Adverse reactions

CNS: *pain, peripheral neuropathy, fatigue, headache, dizziness, insomnia, fever.*
CV: chest pain, ***thromboembolism,*** edema, flushing, peripheral edema.
EENT: *rhinitis,* pharyngitis, epistaxis, abnormal lacrimation.
GI: *nausea, vomiting, diarrhea, stomatitis, abdominal pain, anorexia, constipation, dyspepsia, taste perversion,* gastroesophageal reflux, flatulence, mucositis.
GU: dysuria, hematuria.
Hematologic: FEBRILE NEUTROPENIA, *anemia,* LEUKOPENIA, THROMBOCYTOPENIA.
Metabolic: hypokalemia, dehydration.
Musculoskeletal: *back pain, arthralgia.*
Respiratory: *dyspnea, cough, upper respiratory tract infection,* hiccups, ***pulmonary toxicity.***
Skin: rash, alopecia.
Other: *injection site reaction, **anaphylaxis,** hand-foot syndrome,* allergic reaction, rigors.

Interactions

Drug-drug. *Nephrotoxic drugs (such as gentamicin):* May decrease oxaliplatin elimination and increase level. Monitor patient for signs and symptoms of toxicity.

Effects on lab test results

• May increase creatinine, bilirubin, AST, and ALT levels. May decrease potassium and hemoglobin levels and hematocrit.
• May decrease neutrophil, WBC, and platelet counts.

Pharmacokinetics

Absorption: Administered I.V.
Distribution: Wide. More than 90% protein-bound.
Metabolism: Undergoes non-enzymatic biotransformation.
Excretion: Primarily renal. *Half-life:* Unknown.

Route	Onset	Peak	Duration
I.V.	Unknown	Unknown	Unknown

Action

Chemical effect: May inhibit cell replication and transcription by forming platinum complexes that cross-link with DNA molecules.
Therapeutic effect: Inhibits cancer cell formation.

Available forms

Powder for injection: 50- or 100-mg vials
Injection: 5 mg/ml

NURSING PROCESS

⚗ Assessment
• Monitor CBC, platelet count, and liver and kidney function before each chemotherapy cycle.
• Monitor patient for hypersensitivity reactions, which may occur within minutes of giving drug.
• Monitor patient for injection site reaction. Extravasation may occur.
• Monitor patient for neuropathy and pulmonary toxicity. Peripheral neuropathy may be acute or persistent. Acute neuropathy is reversible; it occurs within 2 days of therapy and resolves within 14 days. Persistent peripheral neuropathy occurs more than 14 days after therapy and causes paresthesias, dysesthesias, hypoesthesias, and decrease in sensation that can interfere with daily activities, such as walking or swallowing.
• Assess patient's and family's knowledge of drug therapy.

⊞ Nursing diagnoses
• Ineffective health maintenance related to cancer
• Ineffective protection related to drug-induced adverse hematologic reactions
• Deficient knowledge related to drug therapy

> **Planning and implementation**
- Drug clearance is reduced in patients with renal impairment. Dose adjustment for patients with renal impairment hasn't been established.

Patient teaching
- Inform patient of potential adverse reactions.
- Tell patient to avoid exposure to cold or cold objects (such as cold drinks or ice cubes), which can bring on or worsen acute symptoms of peripheral neuropathy. Advise patient to have warm drinks, wear warm clothing, and cover any exposed skin. Have patient warm the air going into his lungs by wearing a scarf or ski mask. Have him wear gloves when touching cold objects (such as foods in the freezer, outside door handles, and mailbox).
- Tell patient to immediately notify prescriber if he has trouble breathing or experiences signs and symptoms of an allergic reaction (rash, hives, swelling of lips or tongue, sudden cough).
- Tell patient to contact prescriber if fever, signs and symptoms of an infection, persistent vomiting, diarrhea, or signs and symptoms of dehydration (thirst, dry mouth, light-headedness, and decreased urination) occur.

☑ **Evaluation**
- Patient responds well to therapy.
- Patient develops no serious complications from drug-induced adverse hematologic reactions.
- Patient and family state understanding of drug therapy.

---

oxaprozin potassium
(oks-uh-PROH-zin puh-TAH-see-um)
Apo-Oxaprozin ♦, Daypro, Daypro ALTA, Rhoxal-Oxaprozin ♦

Pharmacologic class: NSAID
Therapeutic class: analgesic, anti-inflammatory
Pregnancy risk category: C

Indications and dosages
▶ **Osteoarthritis, rheumatoid arthritis.**
Adults: 1,200 mg P.O. once daily. Divide doses in patients unable to tolerate single doses. For osteoarthritis patients with low body weight and milder disease, give an initial dose of 600 mg once daily. Maximum daily dose, 1,800 mg.

⧨ **Adjust-a-dose:** For patients with renal impairment and those undergoing hemodialysis, initial dose is 600 mg P.O. daily.

Contraindications and cautions
- Contraindicated in patients hypersensitive to the drug or any of its components and in those with syndrome of nasal polyps, angioedema, and bronchospastic reactions to aspirin or other NSAIDs.
- Use cautiously in patients with history of peptic ulcer disease, hepatic or renal dysfunction, hypertension, CV disease, or conditions that predispose to fluid retention.
- ☀ **Lifespan:** In pregnant women, use cautiously. In breast-feeding women, use cautiously; it's unknown if the drug appears in breast milk. In children, safety and effectiveness haven't been established.

Adverse reactions
CNS: depression, sedation, somnolence, confusion, sleep disturbances.
EENT: tinnitus, visual disturbances.
GI: *nausea, dyspepsia, diarrhea, constipation,* abdominal pain or distress, anorexia, flatulence, vomiting, *GI hemorrhage.*
GU: dysuria, renal insufficiency, urinary frequency.
Skin: *rash,* photosensitivity.

Interactions
Drug-drug. *Antihypertensives, diuretics:* May decrease effect. Monitor patient closely and adjust dosage.
Aspirin: May displace salicylates from protein-binding sites, increasing risk of salicylate toxicity. Avoid using together.
Aspirin, corticosteroids: May increase risk of adverse GI reactions. Avoid using together.
Cyclosporine: May increase risk of nephrotoxicity by both drugs. Monitor renal function tests.
Methotrexate: Increases risk of methotrexate toxicity. Avoid using together.
Oral anticoagulants: May increase risk of bleeding. Use together cautiously; monitor patient for bleeding.
Drug-herb. *Dong quai, feverfew, garlic, ginger, horse chestnut, red clover:* May increase risk of bleeding. Discourage using together.
St. John's wort: May increase risk of photosensitivity. Advise patient to avoid unprotected or prolonged exposure to sunlight.

Drug-lifestyle. *Alcohol use:* May increase risk of adverse GI reactions. Discourage using together.
Sun exposure: May cause photosensitivity reactions. Urge patient to avoid unprotected or prolonged exposure to sunlight.

Effects on lab test results

• May increase ALT, AST, BUN, and creatinine levels. May decrease hemoglobin level and hematocrit.
• May increase bleeding time.

Pharmacokinetics

Absorption: Bioavailability is 95%; food may reduce rate but not extent.
Distribution: About 99.9% protein-bound.
Metabolism: In liver.
Excretion: In urine (65%) and feces (35%).
Half-life: 42 to 50 hours.

Route	Onset	Peak	Duration
P.O.	Unknown	2 hr	Unknown

Action

Chemical effect: May inhibit prostaglandin synthesis.
Therapeutic effect: Relieves pain, fever, and inflammation.

Available forms

Caplets: 600 mg
Tablets: 600 mg

NURSING PROCESS

⧉ Assessment
• Assess patient's condition before starting therapy, and regularly thereafter to monitor the drug's effectiveness.
• Monitor liver function test results periodically during long-term therapy, and closely monitor patient with abnormal test results. Liver function values may be elevated. These abnormal findings may persist, worsen, or resolve with continued therapy. Rarely, patient may progress to severe hepatic dysfunction.
• Be alert for adverse reactions and drug interactions.
• Assess patient's and family's knowledge of drug therapy.

⧉ Nursing diagnoses
• Chronic pain related to condition
• Impaired tissue integrity related to adverse GI effects of drug
• Deficient knowledge related to drug therapy

⧉ Planning and implementation
• Give drug on empty stomach unless adverse GI reactions occur.
• Notify prescriber immediately about adverse reactions, especially GI symptoms.
⊛ **ALERT:** Don't confuse oxaprozin with oxazepam.
Patient teaching
• Tell patient experiencing adverse GI effects, to take drug with milk or meals.
• Explain that full therapeutic effects may be delayed for 2 to 4 weeks.
• Tell patient to report adverse visual or auditory reactions immediately.
• Teach patient to recognize and promptly report signs and symptoms of GI bleeding.
• Advise patient to use sunscreen, wear protective clothing, and avoid prolonged exposure to sunlight.
• Warn patient to avoid hazardous activities until CNS effects of drug are known.

⧉ Evaluation
• Patient is free from pain.
• Patient maintains GI tissue integrity.
• Patient and family state understanding of drug therapy.

oxazepam

(oks-AZ-ih-pam)
Alepam◇, **Apo-Oxazepam**♦, **Murelax**◇, **Novoxapam**♦, **Serax, Serepax**◇

Pharmacologic class: benzodiazepine
Therapeutic class: anxiolytic
Pregnancy risk category: D
Controlled substance schedule: IV

Indications and dosages

▶ **Alcohol withdrawal.** *Adults:* 15 to 30 mg P.O. t.i.d. or q.i.d.
▶ **Severe anxiety.** *Adults:* 15 to 30 mg P.O. t.i.d. or q.i.d.
▶ **Mild to moderate anxiety.** *Adults:* 10 to 15 mg P.O. t.i.d. or q.i.d.

▶ **Older patients with anxiety, tension, irritability, and agitation.** *Adults:* 10 mg P.O. t.i.d. May increase cautiously to 15 mg P.O. t.i.d. to q.i.d.

Contraindications and cautions

- Contraindicated in patients hypersensitive to the drug or any of its components.
- Use cautiously in patients with history of drug abuse and in those for whom a drop in blood pressure could lead to cardiac problems.

Lifespan: In pregnant and breast-feeding women, don't use. In children, safety and effectiveness haven't been established. In the elderly, use cautiously.

Adverse reactions

CNS: drowsiness, lethargy, hangover, fainting, *mental changes.*
CV: transient hypotension.
GI: nausea, vomiting, abdominal discomfort.
Hepatic: ***hepatic dysfunction.***
Other: increased risk for falls.

Interactions

Drug-drug. *CNS depressants:* May increase CNS depression. Avoid using together.
Digoxin: May increase digoxin levels, increasing toxicity. Monitor levels closely.
Hormonal contraceptives: May increase clearance of oxazepam. Monitor patient for decreased effect.
Lamotrigine: May decrease lamotrigine levels. Adjust lamotrigine dose as needed.
Phenytoin: May increase oxazepam clearance and increase phenytoin concentration. Monitor patient closely for phenytoin toxicity.
Drug-herb. *Catnip, kava, lady's slipper, lemon balm, passionflower, sassafras, skullcap, valerian:* May enhance sedative effects. Discourage using together.
Drug-lifestyle. *Alcohol use:* May increase CNS depression. Discourage using together.
Smoking: May increase benzodiazepine clearance. Monitor patient for lack of drug effect.

Effects on lab test results

- May increase liver function test values.

Pharmacokinetics

Absorption: Good.
Distribution: Wide. Drug is 85% to 95% protein-bound.
Metabolism: In liver.
Excretion: In urine. *Half-life:* 5 to 13 hours.

Route	Onset	Peak	Duration
P.O.	Unknown	3 hr	Unknown

Action

Chemical effect: May stimulate GABA receptors in ascending reticular activating system.
Therapeutic effect: Relieves anxiety and promotes calmness.

Available forms

Capsules: 10 mg, 15 mg, 30 mg
Tablets: 10 mg, 15 mg, 30 mg

NURSING PROCESS

Assessment

- Assess patient's condition before starting therapy, and regularly thereafter to monitor the drug's effectiveness.
- Monitor liver, renal, and hematopoietic function studies periodically in patient receiving repeated or prolonged therapy.
- Be alert for adverse reactions and drug interactions.
- Assess patient's and family's knowledge of drug therapy.

Nursing diagnoses

- Disturbed thought processes related to condition
- Risk for injury related to drug-induced adverse CNS reactions
- Deficient knowledge related to drug therapy

Planning and implementation

- Lower the dose in an elderly or debilitated patient.
- Possibility of abuse and addiction exists. Don't abruptly stop giving the drug; withdrawal symptoms may occur.

ALERT: Don't confuse oxazepam with oxaprozin.

Patient teaching

- Warn patient to avoid hazardous activities until CNS effects of drug are known.
- Tell patient to avoid alcohol during therapy.
- Warn patient not to stop drug abruptly; withdrawal signs may occur.

O

☑ Evaluation
• Patient has less anxiety.
• Patient sustains no injury as result of drug therapy.
• Patient and family state understanding of drug therapy.

oxcarbazepine
(ox-car-BAY-zah-peen)
Trileptal

Pharmacologic class: carboxamide derivative
Therapeutic class: antiepileptic
Pregnancy risk category: C

Indications and dosages

▶ **Adjunctive therapy for partial seizures in patients with epilepsy.** *Adults:* Initially, 300 mg P.O. b.i.d. Increase by maximum of 600 mg daily (300 mg P.O. b.i.d.) at weekly intervals. Recommended daily dosage is 600 mg P.O. b.i.d.
Children ages 4 to 16: Initially, 4 to 5 mg/kg P.O. b.i.d., not to exceed 600 mg P.O. daily. Target maintenance dosage depends on patient weight. If patient weighs 20 to 29 kg (44 to 64 lb), target maintenance dosage is 900 mg daily. If 29.1 to 39 kg (64 to 86 lb), target maintenance dosage is 1,200 mg daily. If more than 39 kg (86 lb), target maintenance dosage is 1,800 mg daily. Achieve target dosage over 2 weeks.
▶ **Conversion to monotherapy for partial seizures in patients with epilepsy.** *Adults:* Initially, 300 mg P.O. b.i.d. with simultaneous reduction in dosage of other antiepileptics. Increase by a maximum of 600 mg daily at weekly intervals over 2 to 4 weeks. Recommended daily dose is 2,400 mg P.O., divided b.i.d. Withdraw other antiepileptics completely over 3 to 6 weeks.
Children ages 4 to 16: Initially 8 to 10 mg/kg P.O. daily divided b.i.d., with simultaneous reduction in dose of other antiepileptics. Increase by a maximum of 10 mg/kg daily at weekly intervals. Withdraw other antiepileptics completely over 3 to 6 weeks.
▶ **Initial monotherapy for partial seizures in patients with epilepsy.** *Adults:* Initially, 300 mg P.O. b.i.d. Increase by 300 mg daily q third day to a total daily dose of 1,200 mg.

Children ages 4 to 16: Initially, 8 to 10 mg/kg P.O. daily divided b.i.d., increasing the dosage by 5 mg/kg daily q third day to the recommended daily dosage:
20 to 24 kg (44 to 54 lb)–600 to 900 mg
25 to 34 kg (55 to 76 lb)–900 to 1,200 mg
35 to 44 kg (77 to 98 lb)–900 to 1,500 mg
45 to 49 kg (99 to 109 lb)–1,200 to 1,500 mg
50 to 59 kg (110 to 131 lb)–1,200 to 1,800 mg
60 to 69 kg (132 to 153 lb)–1,200 to 2,100 mg
70 kg (154 lb)–1,500 to 2,100 mg.
☒ **Adjust-a-dose:** For patients with renal impairment, if creatinine clearance is less than 30 ml/minute, therapy starts at 150 mg P.O. b.i.d. (one-half the usual starting dose) and increases slowly to achieve desired clinical response.

Contraindications and cautions

• Contraindicated in patients hypersensitive to the drug or any of its components.
• Use cautiously in patients who have had hypersensitivity reactions to carbamazepine.
⚠ Lifespan: Effects during pregnancy are unknown. Breast-feeding women should either stop breast-feeding or use another drug.

Adverse reactions

CNS: *fatigue,* fever, asthenia, feeling abnormal, *headache, dizziness, somnolence, ataxia, abnormal gait,* insomnia, *tremor,* nervousness, agitation, abnormal coordination, speech disorder, confusion, anxiety, amnesia, **aggravated seizures,** hypoesthesia, emotional lability, impaired concentration, *vertigo.*
CV: hypotension, edema, chest pain.
EENT: *nystagmus, diplopia, abnormal vision,* abnormal accommodation, rhinitis, sinusitis, pharyngitis, epistaxis.
GI: *nausea, vomiting, abdominal pain,* diarrhea, dyspepsia, constipation, gastritis, anorexia, dry mouth, rectal hemorrhage, taste perversion, thirst.
GU: UTI, urinary frequency, vaginitis.
Metabolic: hyponatremia, weight gain.
Musculoskeletal: muscle weakness, back pain.
Respiratory: *upper respiratory tract infection,* coughing, bronchitis, chest infection.
Skin: *Stevens–Johnson syndrome, toxic epidermal necrosis,* acne, purpura, rash, bruising, increased sweating.
Other: allergic reaction, hot flushes, toothache.

Interactions

Drug-drug. *Carbamazepine, valproic acid, verapamil:* May decrease levels of the active metabolite of oxcarbazepine. Monitor patient and levels closely.
Felodipine: May decrease felodipine level. Monitor patient closely.
Hormonal contraceptives: May decrease levels of ethinyl estradiol and levonorgestrel, which reduces contraceptive effect. Women of child-bearing age should use other forms of contraception.
Lamotrigine: May decrease levels of lamotrigine. Adjust lamotrigine dose as needed.
Phenobarbital: May decrease levels of the active metabolite of oxcarbazepine and increase phenobarbital level. Monitor patient closely.
Phenytoin: May decrease levels of the active metabolite of oxcarbazepine. Watch for reduced effect. May increase phenytoin level in adults receiving high doses of oxcarbazepine. Monitor phenytoin levels closely when starting therapy in these patients.
Drug-lifestyle. *Alcohol use:* Increases CNS depression. Discourage using together.

Effects on lab test results

• May decrease sodium and T_4 levels.

Pharmacokinetics

Absorption: Complete.
Distribution: About 40% of active metabolite is bound to proteins, mostly to albumin.
Metabolism: Rapid; 4% of dose is oxidized to inactive metabolite.
Excretion: Mainly by the kidneys. *Half-life:* About 2 hours for drug, about 9 hours for active metabolite. Children younger than age 8 have about 30% to 40% increased clearance of drug.

Route	Onset	Peak	Duration
P.O.	Unknown	Variable	Unknown

Action

Chemical effect: May result from blockade of voltage-sensitive sodium channels, which causes stabilized hyperexcited neural membranes, inhibited repetitive neuronal firing, and reduced synaptic impulses. May stem from increased potassium conductance and modulation of high-voltage activated calcium channels.
Therapeutic effect: Controls partial seizures.

Available forms

Oral suspension: 60 mg/ml, 300 mg/5 ml*
Tablets (film-coated): 150 mg, 300 mg, 600 mg

NURSING PROCESS

⚗ Assessment
⑤ ALERT: Ask patient about history of hypersensitivity reaction to carbamazepine because 25% to 30% of affected patients may develop hypersensitivity to this drug. If signs or symptoms of hypersensitivity occur, stop drug immediately.
• Obtain history of patient's underlying condition before starting therapy, and reassess regularly thereafter to monitor the drug's effectiveness.
⑤ ALERT: Drug is linked to several adverse neurologic events, including psychomotor slowing, difficulty with concentration, speech or language problems, somnolence, fatigue, and abnormal coordination (including ataxia and gait disturbances). Monitor patient closely.
• Monitor patient for evidence of hyponatremia, including nausea, malaise, headache, lethargy, confusion, and decreased sensation.
• Assess patient's and family's knowledge of drug therapy.

⬡ Nursing diagnoses
• Risk for trauma related to seizures
• Risk for injury related to drug-induced adverse reactions
• Deficient knowledge related to drug therapy

⬢ Planning and implementation
⑤ ALERT: Gradually stop giving the drug to minimize risk of increased seizure frequency.
• Correct hyponatremia p.r.n.
• Shake oral suspension well before giving. Suspension can be mixed with water or may be swallowed directly from the syringe. Oral suspension and tablets may be interchanged at equal doses. Suspension can be taken without regard to food.
• Serious skin reactions including Stevens-Johnson syndrome and toxic epidermal necrosis can occur.
Patient teaching
• Advise patient to tell prescriber if he has ever had a hypersensitivity reaction to carbamazepine.

• Tell patient that drug may be taken with or without food.

• Warn patient to avoid hazardous activities until the drug's CNS effects are known.

• Tell patient not to drink alcohol while taking drug.

• Advise patient not to interrupt therapy without consulting prescriber.

• Advise patient to immediately report skin rashes to his prescriber.

• Advise patient to report fever and swollen lymph nodes to his prescriber; multi-organ hypersensitivity reactions may occur, with diverse signs and symptoms.

• Advise patient to report signs and symptoms of hyponatremia, such as nausea, malaise, headache, lethargy, or confusion.

• Advise women using hormonal contraceptives to use a barrier method of birth control while taking drug.

☑ Evaluation

• Patient experiences no or fewer seizures during drug therapy.

• Patient sustains no injury from drug-induced adverse reactions.

• Patient and family state understanding of drug therapy.

oxybutynin chloride
(oks-ee-BYOO-tih-nin KLOR-ighd)
Apo-Oxybutynin ◆ , Ditropan, Ditropan XL, Oxytrol

Pharmacologic class: synthetic tertiary amine
Therapeutic class: urinary antispasmodic
Pregnancy risk category: B

Indications and dosages

▶ **Uninhibited or reflex neurogenic bladder.**
Adults: 5 mg P.O. b.i.d. to t.i.d., up to 5 mg q.i.d.
Children older than age 5: 5 mg P.O. b.i.d., up to 5 mg t.i.d.

▶ **Overactive bladder.** *Adults:* Initially, 5 mg Ditropan XL P.O. once daily. Adjust dosage weekly in 5-mg increments, p.r.n., to a maximum of 30 mg P.O. daily. Or, 1 transdermal patch (Oxytrol) twice weekly applied to dry, intact skin on abdomen, hip, or buttocks.

Contraindications and cautions

• Contraindicated in patients hypersensitive to the drug or any of its components, in debilitated patients with intestinal atony, in hemorrhaging patients with unstable CV condition, and in patients with myasthenia gravis, GI obstruction, glaucoma, adynamic ileus, megacolon, severe colitis, ulcerative colitis with megacolon, or obstructive uropathy.

• Use cautiously in patients with autonomic neuropathy, reflux esophagitis, or hepatic or renal disease. Use transdermal patch cautiously in patients with bladder outflow obstruction, gastroesophageal reflux, intestinal atony, and in those taking bisphosphonates.

※ **Lifespan:** In pregnant women, use cautiously. In breast-feeding women, use cautiously; it's unknown if the drug appears in breast milk. In the elderly, use cautiously. In the elderly who have intestinal atony, drug is contraindicated.

Adverse reactions

Oral form
CNS: *drowsiness,* fever, dizziness, insomnia, restlessness, impaired alertness.
CV: flushing, palpitations, tachycardia.
EENT: *transient blurred vision,* mydriasis, cycloplegia.
GI: nausea, vomiting, *constipation,* bloated feeling, *dry mouth.*
GU: impotence, urinary hesitancy, urine retention.
Skin: decreased diaphoresis, rash, urticaria.
Other: suppressed lactation, allergic reactions.
Transdermal form
CNS: fatigue, somnolence, headache.
CV: flushing.
EENT: abnormal vision.
GI: *dry mouth,* diarrhea, abdominal pain, flatulence, nausea.
GU: dysuria.
Musculoskeletal: back pain.
Skin: *pruritus,* erythema, vesicles, macules, rash, burns.

Interactions

Drug-drug. *Amantadine, anticholinergics:* May increase anticholinergic effects. Use together cautiously.
Atenolol, digoxin: May increase levels of these drugs. Monitor patient closely. Use of digoxin elixir or capsules may avoid the interaction.

CNS depressants: May increase CNS effects. Use cautiously.

Drug-lifestyle. *Alcohol use:* May increase CNS effects. Discourage using together.

Exercise, hot weather: May precipitate heatstroke. Urge patient to avoid exercise or increased activity during hot and humid weather and to stay hydrated.

Effects on lab test results

None reported.

Pharmacokinetics

Absorption: Rapid.

Distribution: Unknown. Transdermal system is widely distributed.

Metabolism: By liver. Transdermal system is metabolized by liver and gut wall by CYP 3A4; bypasses first-pass metabolism.

Excretion: Primarily in urine. *Transdermal half-life:* 2 hours.

Route	Onset	Peak	Duration
P.O.	30–60 min	3–4 hr	6–10 hr
Transdermal	24–48 hr	Varies	96 hr

Action

Chemical effect: Produces direct spasmolytic effect and antimuscarinic (atropine-like) effect on smooth muscles of urinary tract, increasing bladder capacity and providing some local anesthesia and mild analgesia.

Therapeutic effect: Relieves bladder spasms.

Available forms

Syrup: 5 mg/5 ml
Tablets: 5 mg
Tablets (extended-release): 5 mg, 10 mg, 15 mg
Transdermal patch: 36-mg patch (delivers 3.9 mg/day)

NURSING PROCESS

Assessment

• Assess patient's bladder condition before starting therapy.

• Before giving drug, confirm neurogenic bladder by cystometry and rule out partial intestinal obstruction in patients with diarrhea, especially those with colostomy or ileostomy.

• Prepare patient for periodic cystometry to evaluate response to therapy.

• Watch geriatric patients for confusion and mental changes.

• Be alert for adverse reactions.

• Drug may aggravate symptoms of hyperthyroidism, coronary artery disease, heart failure, arrhythmias, tachycardia, hypertension, or prostatic hyperplasia.

• Assess patient's and family's knowledge of drug therapy.

Nursing diagnoses

• Acute pain related to bladder spasms

• Risk for injury related to drug-induced adverse CNS reactions

• Deficient knowledge related to drug therapy

Planning and implementation

• If patient has a UTI, give antibiotics.

• To minimize tendency toward tolerance, periodically stop therapy to determine whether patient can be weaned off drug.

ALERT: Don't confuse Ditropan with diazepam or Dithranol.

Patient teaching

• Warn patient to avoid hazardous activities until the drug's CNS effects are known.

• Tell patient not to drink alcohol during therapy.

• Advise patient that taking drug in hot weather raises the risk of fever or heatstroke, and urge patient to take precautions to avoid excessive heat and maintain adequate hydration.

• Instruct patient to change transdermal patch two times per week and avoid using the same site within 7 days. Also warn patient to wear only one patch at a time and to properly dispose of old patches to prevent accidental application or ingestion.

• Advise patient to store drug in tightly closed containers at room temperature.

Evaluation

• Patient is free from bladder pain.

• Patient sustains no injuries from drug-induced adverse CNS reactions.

• Patient and family state understanding of drug therapy.

oxycodone hydrochloride
(oks-ee-KOH-dohn high-droh-KLOR-ighd)
Endocodone, Endone◇, M-Oxy,
OxyContin✍, Oxydose, OxyFAST, OxyIR,
OxyNorm◇, Percolone, Roxicodone*,
Roxicodone Intensol, Supeudol

oxycodone pectinate
Proladone◇

Pharmacologic class: opioid
Therapeutic class: analgesic
Pregnancy risk category: B
Controlled substance schedule: II

Indications and dosages

▶ **Moderate to severe pain.** *Adults:* 5 mg P.O.
q 6 hours, p.r.n. Or, 1 to 3 suppositories P.R.
daily, p.r.n.
Adults not taking opioids who need a continu-
ous around-the-clock analgesic for an extended
period: 10 mg extended-release tablets P.O. q
12 hours. May increase dose q 1 to 2 days, p.r.n.
The 80-mg form is for opioid-tolerant patients
only.
Adjust-a-dose: For patients with impaired hepatic function, start extended-release tablets at
⅓ to ½ of usual dosage and adjust carefully. In
patients with impaired renal function, if creatinine clearance is less than 60 ml/minute, reduce
initial extended-release dose and adjust carefully.

Contraindications and cautions

• Contraindicated in patients hypersensitive to
the drug or any of its components.
• Oxycodone extended-release tablets are contraindicated in patients with known or suspected
paralytic ileus.
• Use cautiously in debilitated patients and in
those with head injury, increased intracranial
pressure, seizures, asthma, COPD, prostatic hyperplasia, severe hepatic or renal disease, acute
abdominal conditions, urethral stricture, hypothyroidism, Addison's disease, or arrhythmias.
✿ **Lifespan:** In pregnant women, use cautiously. In breast-feeding women, use cautiously; it's
unknown if the drug appears in breast milk. In
children, drug isn't recommended. In the elderly, use cautiously due to increased risk of delayed renal excretion and of CNS effects.

Adverse reactions

CNS: *sedation, somnolence, clouded sensori-*
um, euphoria, dizziness.
CV: *hypotension,* **bradycardia.**
GI: nausea, vomiting, constipation, ileus.
GU: urine retention.
Respiratory: *respiratory depression.*
Other: physical dependence.

Interactions

Drug-drug. *Anticoagulants:* May increase anticoagulant effect if combination product with aspirin is used. Monitor PT and INR. Use together
cautiously; monitor patient for bleeding.
CNS depressants, general anesthetics, hyp-
notics, MAO inhibitors, other opioid analgesics,
protease inhibitors, sedatives, tranquilizers, tri-
cyclic antidepressants: May have additive effects. Use together cautiously. Reduce oxycodone dose as directed, and monitor patient
response.
Drug-lifestyle. *Alcohol use:* May increase CNS
depression. Discourage using together.

Effects on lab test results

• May increase amylase and lipase levels.

Pharmacokinetics

Absorption: Unknown.
Distribution: Unknown.
Metabolism: In liver.
Excretion: Primarily in urine. *Half-life:* 2 to
3 hours.

Route	Onset	Peak	Duration
P.O.	10–15 min	≤ 1 hr	3–6 hr
P.R.	Unknown	Unknown	Unknown

Action

Chemical effect: Binds with opioid receptors in
CNS, altering response to pain by an unknown
mechanism.
Therapeutic effect: Relieves pain.

Available forms

oxycodone hydrochloride
Capsules: 5 mg
Oral solution: 5 mg/5 ml, 20 mg/ml
Tablets: 5 mg, 15 mg, 30 mg
Tablets (extended-release): 10 mg, 20 mg,
40 mg, 80 mg
oxycodone pectinate
Suppositories: 10 mg♦, 30 mg◇

Reactions may be *common,* uncommon, *life-threatening*, or COMMON AND LIFE-THREATENING.

NURSING PROCESS

❧ Assessment
• Assess patient's pain before and after giving drug.
• Monitor circulation and respirations.
• Be alert for adverse reactions and drug interactions.
• Monitor patient for development of constipation.
• Assess patient's and family's knowledge of drug therapy.

🔲 Nursing diagnoses
• Acute pain related to condition
• Ineffective breathing pattern related to drug-induced respiratory depression
• Deficient knowledge related to drug therapy

⊠ Planning and implementation
• Give drug with food or milk to avoid GI upset.
⊛ ALERT: Drug isn't intended for p.r.n. use or for immediate postoperative pain. Drug is only indicated for postoperative use if patient was receiving it before surgery or if pain is expected to persist for an extended period of time.
• For best results, give drug before patient has intense pain.
• Single-agent oxycodone solution or tablet is especially useful for patient who can't take aspirin or acetaminophen.
⊛ ALERT: If respirations are shallow or rate falls below 12 breaths/minute, withhold dose and notify prescriber.
⊛ ALERT: Don't confuse oxycodone immediate-release tablets with OxyContin extended-release tablets.
⊛ ALERT: Drug is addictive and abused as much as morphine. Chewing, crushing, snorting, or injecting it can lead to overdose and death.
⊛ ALERT: Don't confuse Roxicodone Intensol with other Intensol products manufactured by Roxane.
Patient teaching
• Instruct patient to take drug with food or milk to minimize GI upset.
• Tell patient to ask for drug before pain becomes intense.
• Tell patient not to chew or crush OxyIR or extended-release forms.
• Warn ambulatory patient about getting out of bed or walking. Warn outpatient to avoid hazardous activities until CNS effects of drug are known.

☑ Evaluation
• Patient is free from pain.
• Patient's respiratory rate and pattern remain within normal limits.
• Patient and family state understanding of drug therapy.

oxymorphone hydrochloride
(oks-ee-MOR-fohn high-droh-KLOR-ighd)
Numorphan

Pharmacologic class: opioid
Therapeutic class: analgesic
Pregnancy risk category: C
Controlled substance schedule: II

Indications and dosages
▶ **Moderate to severe pain.** *Adults:* 1 to 1.5 mg I.M. or subcutaneously q 4 to 6 hours, p.r.n. Or, 0.5 mg I.V. q 4 to 6 hours, p.r.n. Or, 5 mg P.R. q 4 to 6 hours, p.r.n.

▽ I.V. administration
• Give drug by direct I.V. injection. If needed, dilute in normal saline solution.
• To minimize hypotension, keep patient supine while giving drug.
⊗ **Incompatibilities**
None reported.

Contraindications and cautions
• Contraindicated in patients hypersensitive to the drug or any of its components.
• Use cautiously in debilitated patients and in those with head injury, increased intracranial pressure, seizures, asthma, COPD, acute abdominal conditions, prostatic hyperplasia, severe hepatic or renal disease, urethral stricture, respiratory depression, hypothyroidism, Addison's disease, or arrhythmias.
⚘ **Lifespan:** In pregnant women, use cautiously. In breast-feeding women, use cautiously; it's unknown if the drug appears in breast milk. In the elderly, use cautiously due to increased risk of delayed renal excretion and of CNS effects. In children, drug is contraindicated.

Adverse reactions

CNS: *sedation, somnolence, clouded sensorium, euphoria,* dizziness, ***seizures*** with large doses.
CV: *hypotension,* ***bradycardia.***
GI: *nausea, vomiting, constipation,* ileus.
GU: urine retention.
Respiratory: ***respiratory depression.***
Other: physical dependence.

Interactions

Drug-drug. *CNS depressants, general anesthetics, MAO inhibitors, tricyclic antidepressants:* May have additive effects. Use together cautiously.
Drug-lifestyle. *Alcohol use:* May have additive effects. Discourage using together.

Effects on lab test results

- May increase amylase level.

Pharmacokinetics

Absorption: Good.
Distribution: Wide.
Metabolism: Primarily in liver.
Excretion: Primarily in urine. *Half-life:* Unknown.

Route	Onset	Peak	Duration
I.V.	5–10 min	15–30 min	3–6 hr
I.M.	10–15 min	30–90 min	3–6 hr
SubQ	10–15 min	60–90 min	3–6 hr
P.R.	15–30 min	2 hr	3–6 hr

Action

Chemical effect: Binds with opioid receptors in CNS, altering response to pain by an unknown mechanism.
Therapeutic effect: Relieves pain.

Available forms

Injection: 1 mg/ml, 1.5 mg/ml
Suppositories: 5 mg

NURSING PROCESS

Assessment

- Assess patient's pain before and after giving drug.
- Be alert for adverse reactions and drug interactions.
- Assess patient's and family's knowledge of drug therapy.

Nursing diagnoses

- Acute pain related to condition
- Ineffective breathing pattern related to drug-induced respiratory depression
- Deficient knowledge related to drug therapy

Planning and implementation

- Keep opioid antagonist (naloxone) and resuscitation equipment available.
- Don't give drug for mild to moderate pain.
- Drug may worsen gallbladder pain.
- Give drug before patient's pain becomes too intense.

ALERT: If respirations decrease or rate is below 12 breaths/minute, withhold dose and notify prescriber.

- Dependence can develop with long-term use.
- Giving laxatives or stool softeners may help prevent or relieve constipation.

ALERT: Don't confuse oxymorphone with oxymetholone.

Patient teaching

- Instruct patient to take drug before pain becomes intense.
- Warn ambulatory patient about getting out of bed or walking. Warn outpatient to avoid hazardous activities until the drug's CNS effects are known.
- Tell patient to refrigerate suppositories.
- Advise patient or family to report a decreased respiratory rate.
- Teach patient about increasing fluid and fiber intake to prevent constipation.

Evaluation

- Patient is free from pain.
- Patient's respiration is normal.
- Patient and family state understanding of drug therapy.

oxytocin, synthetic injection

(oks-ih-TOH-sin, sin-THET-ik in-JEK-shun)
Pitocin, Syntocinon

Pharmacologic class: exogenous hormone
Therapeutic class: oxytocic, lactation stimulant
Pregnancy risk category: NR

Indications and dosages

▶ **To induce or stimulate labor.** *Adults:* Initially, 1-ml ampule (10 units) I.V. in 1,000 ml of

D₅W, lactated Ringer's, or normal saline solution infused at 0.5 to 2 milliunits/minute. Increase rate in increments of no more than 1 to 2 milliunits/minute at 30- to 60-minute intervals until normal contraction pattern is established. Decrease rate when labor is firmly established. Rates exceeding 9 to 10 milliunits/minute rarely are required; maximum dose 20 milliunits/minute.

▶ **To reduce postpartum bleeding after expulsion of placenta.** *Adults:* 10 to 40 units I.V. in 1,000 ml of D₅W or normal saline solution infused at rate that controls bleeding, usually 20 to 40 milliunits/minute. Give 10 units I.M. after delivery of placenta.

▶ **Incomplete or inevitable abortion.** *Adults:* 10 units I.V. in 500 ml of normal saline solution or dextrose 5% in normal saline solution or D₅W. Infuse at 10 to 20 milliunits/minute (20 to 40 gtt/minute).

▶ **Oxytocin challenge test to assess fetal distress in high-risk pregnancies greater than 31 weeks' gestation‡.** *Adults:* 5 to 10 units I.V. in 1 L of D₅W injection, yielding a solution of 5 to 10 milliunits per ml. Infuse 0.5 milliunits/minute, gradually increasing at 15-minute intervals to a maximum infusion of 20 milliunits/minute. Stop infusion when three moderate uterine contractions occur within a 10-minute period. Response of fetal heart rate may be used to evaluate prognosis.

▽ I.V. administration
• Give only by infusion.
• Give by piggyback infusion so drug can be stopped without interrupting I.V. line.
• Use an infusion pump.
⊗ **Incompatibilities**
Plasmin, norepinephrine bitartrate, Normosol-M with dextrose 5%, prochlorperazine, warfarin sodium.

Contraindications and cautions
• Contraindicated in patients hypersensitive to the drug or any of its components. Also contraindicated in cephalopelvic disproportion or delivery that requires conversion, as in transverse lie; in fetal distress when delivery isn't imminent; in prematurity; in other obstetric emergencies; and in severe toxemia, hypertonic uterine patterns, total placenta previa, or vasa previa.
• During first and second stages of labor, use cautiously because cervical laceration, uterine

rupture, and maternal and fetal death may occur. In patients with grand multiparity, uterine sepsis, traumatic delivery, or overdistended uterus, use cautiously.
• Use cautiously in patients with invasive cervical carcinoma and in patients with history of cervical or uterine surgery.
≜ **Lifespan:** Drug is only indicated for pregnant and postpartum women.

Adverse reactions
Maternal
CNS: *subarachnoid hemorrhage from hypertension, seizures, coma from water intoxication.*
CV: *hypertension;* increased heart rate, systemic venous return, and cardiac output; *arrhythmias.*
GI: nausea, vomiting.
GU: *tetanic uterine contractions, abruptio placentae, impaired uterine blood flow, pelvic hematoma, increased uterine motility, uterine rupture.*
Hematologic: afibrinogenemia (may be related to postpartum bleeding).
Other: hypersensitivity reactions, *anaphylaxis.*
Fetal
CV: *bradycardia,* tachycardia, PVCs.
Hematologic: hyperbilirubinemia.
Respiratory: *anoxia, asphyxia.*

Interactions
Drug-drug. *Cyclopropane anesthetics:* May cause less pronounced tachycardia but more severe hypotension. May cause maternal sinus bradycardia with abnormal atrioventricular arrhythmias. Use together cautiously.
Thiopental anesthetics: May delay induction. Use together cautiously.
Vasoconstrictors: May cause severe hypertension in patients receiving caudal block anesthetic. Avoid using together.

Effects on lab test results
None reported.

Pharmacokinetics
Absorption: Unknown.
Distribution: Through extracellular fluid.
Metabolism: Rapid, in kidneys and liver. In early pregnancy, a circulating enzyme, oxytocinase, can inactivate drug.

O

Excretion: Small amounts in urine. *Half-life:* 3 to 5 minutes.

Route	Onset	Peak	Duration
I.V.	Immediate	Unknown	1 hr
I.M.	3–5 min	Unknown	2–3 hr

Action

Chemical effect: Causes potent and selective stimulation of uterine and mammary gland smooth muscle.

Therapeutic effect: Induces labor and milk ejection and reduces postpartum bleeding.

Available forms

Injection: 10 units/ml in ampule, vial, or syringe

NURSING PROCESS

Assessment

- Assess patient's condition before starting therapy and regularly thereafter.
- Monitor and record uterine contractions, heart rate, blood pressure, intrauterine pressure, fetal heart rate, and blood loss q 15 minutes.
- Be alert for adverse reactions and drug interactions.
- Monitor fluid intake and output. Antidiuretic effect may lead to fluid overload, seizures, and coma.
- Assess patient's and family's knowledge of drug therapy.

Nursing diagnoses

- Risk for deficient fluid volume related to postpartum bleeding
- Excessive fluid volume related to drug-induced antidiuretic effect
- Deficient knowledge related to drug therapy

Planning and implementation

- Drug is used to induce or reinforce labor only when pelvis is known to be adequate, vaginal delivery is indicated, fetal maturity is ensured, and fetal position is favorable. Use only in hospital where critical care facilities and experienced clinician are immediately available.
- Drug isn't recommended for routine I.M. use, but 10 units may be given I.M. after delivery of placenta to control postpartum uterine bleeding.
- Never give oxytocin simultaneously by more than one route.
- Have 20% solution of magnesium sulfate available for relaxation of myometrium.

ALERT: If contractions are less than 2 minutes apart, if they're above 50 mm Hg, or if they last 90 seconds or longer, stop infusion, turn patient on her side, and notify prescriber.

ALERT: Don't confuse Pitocin with Pitressin.

ALERT: Don't confuse oxytocin with OxyContin.

Patient teaching

- Instruct patient to report unusual feelings or adverse effects at once.
- Instruct patient to remain lying down during administration.

Evaluation

- Patient maintains adequate fluid balance with drug therapy.
- Patient doesn't develop edema.
- Patient and family state understanding of drug therapy.

P

paclitaxel

(pak-lih-TAK-sil)

Onxol, Taxol

Pharmacologic class: antimitotic
Therapeutic class: antineoplastic
Pregnancy risk category: D

Indications and dosages

▶ **First-line and subsequent therapy for advanced ovarian cancer.** *Previously untreated adults:* 175 mg/m² over 3 hours q 3 weeks followed by cisplatin 75 mg/m² or 135 mg/m² over 24 hours followed by cisplatin 75 mg/m² q 3 weeks.

Previously treated adults: 135 or 175 mg/m² I.V. over 3 hours q 3 weeks.

▶ **Breast cancer that doesn't respond to combination chemotherapy for metastatic disease or relapse within 6 months of chemotherapy that included an anthracycline; node-positive breast cancer (after combination chemotherapy that includes doxoru-**

bicin). *Adults:* 175 mg/m² I.V. over 3 hours q 3 weeks.

► **Initial therapy for advanced non–small-cell lung cancer in patients who aren't candidates for curative surgery or radiation.** *Adults:* 135 mg/m² I.V. infusion over 24 hours; follow with cisplatin 75 mg/m². Repeat cycle q 3 weeks.

⊠ **Adjust-a-dose:** For all indications, give subsequent courses when neutrophil count is at least 1,500/mm³ and platelet count is at least 100,000/mm³. For patients who experience severe neutropenia (neutrophil count less than 500/mm³ for at least 7 days) or severe peripheral neuropathy, reduce dose by 20% for subsequent courses.

► **AIDS-related Kaposi's sarcoma.** *Adults:* 135 mg/m² I.V. over 3 hours q 3 weeks, or 100 mg/m² I.V. over 3 hours q 2 weeks. Don't give if baseline or subsequent neutrophil counts are less than 1,000/mm³.

⊠ **Adjust-a-dose:** In patients who experience severe neutropenia (neutrophil count less than 500/mm³ for a week or longer) or severe peripheral neuropathy, reduce dosage by 20% for subsequent courses. In patients with elevated liver enzymes, toxicity increases. Adjust dosage.

▼ I.V. administration

• Preparing and giving drug are linked to carcinogenic, mutagenic, and teratogenic risks. Follow facility policy for safe handling.
• Dilute concentrate to 0.3 to 1.2 mg/ml before infusion. Compatible solutions include normal saline solution for injection, D₅W, dextrose 5% in normal saline for injection, and dextrose 5% in lactated Ringer's injection.
• Don't allow undiluted concentrate to come in contact with polyvinyl chloride I.V. bags or tubing. Prepare and store infusion solutions in glass containers. Store diluted solution in glass or polypropylene bottles, or use polypropylene or polyolefin bags. Administer through polyethylene-lined administration sets, and use in-line 0.22-micron filter.
• If extravasation occurs, stop infusion and notify prescriber.
• Diluted solutions are stable for 27 hours at room temperature. Prepared solution may appear hazy.

⊗ **Incompatibilities**
Amphotericin B, chlorpromazine, cisplatin, doxorubicin liposomal, hydroxyzine hydrochloride, methylprednisolone sodium succinate, mitoxantrone.

Contraindications and cautions

• Contraindicated in patients hypersensitive to the drug or to polyoxyethylated castor oil, a vehicle used in drug solution, and in patients with solid tumors with baseline neutrophil counts below 1,500/mm³. When used to treat AIDS-related Kaposi's sarcoma, contraindicated in patients with baseline neutrophil counts below 1,000/mm³.
• Use cautiously in patients who have received radiation therapy; they may have more frequent or severe myelosuppression.
⚘ **Lifespan:** In pregnant and breast-feeding women, drug isn't recommended. In children, safety and effectiveness haven't been established.

Adverse reactions

CNS: fever, peripheral neuropathy.
CV: *bradycardia,* hypotension, abnormal ECG.
GI: nausea, vomiting, diarrhea, mucositis.
Hematologic: *neutropenia, leukopenia, thrombocytopenia,* anemia, *bleeding.*
Musculoskeletal: myalgia, arthralgia.
Skin: *alopecia,* phlebitis, cellulitis at injection site.
Other: hypersensitivity reactions, *anaphylaxis.*

Interactions

Drug-drug. *Cisplatin:* May have additive myelosuppressive effects. Use together cautiously.
Cyclosporine, dexamethasone, diazepam, estradiol, etoposide, ketoconazole, quinidine, retinoic acid, teniposide, testosterone, verapamil, vincristine: May inhibit paclitaxel metabolism. Use together cautiously.
Doxorubicin: May increase levels of doxorubicin and its metabolites. Dose adjustments may be needed.
Phenobarbital, carbamazepine: May increase the metabolism of paclitaxel. Monitor patient for effectiveness.

Effects on lab test results

• May increase alkaline phosphatase, AST, and triglyceride levels. May decrease hemoglobin level and hematocrit.
• May decrease neutrophil, WBC, and platelet counts.

Pharmacokinetics

Absorption: Administered I.V.
Distribution: About 89% to 98% of drug is bound to proteins.
Metabolism: May be metabolized in liver by CYP 2C8 and CYP 3A4.
Excretion: Unknown. *Half-life:* 2¼ to 5¾ hours.

Route	Onset	Peak	Duration
I.V.	Unknown	Unknown	Unknown

Action

Chemical effect: Inhibits normal reorganization of microtubule network needed for mitosis and other vital cellular functions.
Therapeutic effect: Stops ovarian and breast cancer cell activity.

Available forms

Injection: 6 mg/ml

NURSING PROCESS

Assessment

• Assess patient's condition before starting therapy, and regularly thereafter to monitor the drug's effectiveness.
• Continuously monitor patient for first 30 minutes of infusion. Monitor patient closely throughout infusion.
• Monitor blood counts and liver function test results frequently during therapy.
• Be alert for adverse reactions and drug interactions.
• Assess patient's and family's knowledge of drug therapy.

Nursing diagnoses

• Ineffective health maintenance related to cancer
• Ineffective protection related to drug-induced adverse hematologic reactions
• Deficient knowledge related to drug therapy

Planning and implementation

• To reduce severe hypersensitivity, pretreat patient with corticosteroids, such as dexamethasone, and antihistamines. H₁-receptor antagonists, such as diphenhydramine, and H₂-receptor antagonists, such as cimetidine or ranitidine, may be used.

Ⓢ **ALERT:** Don't confuse paclitaxel with paroxetine. Don't confuse Taxol with Paxil or Taxotere.
Ⓢ **ALERT:** Severe hypersensitivity reactions occur in about 4% of patients, usually within 2 or 3 minutes and almost always within 10 minutes.

Patient teaching
• Warn patient to watch for signs of bleeding and infection.
• Teach patient symptoms of peripheral neuropathy, such as tingling, burning, or numbness in limbs, and urge him to report them immediately to prescriber. Dose reduction may be needed.
• Warn patient that alopecia occurs in up to 82% of patients.
• Advise woman of childbearing age not to become pregnant during therapy. Recommend consulting prescriber before becoming pregnant.

☑ Evaluation

• Patient responds well to therapy.
• Patient develops no serious complications from drug-induced adverse hematologic reactions.
• Patient and family state understanding of drug therapy.

paclitaxel protein-bound particles
(pack-lih-TAK-sil)
Abraxane

Pharmacologic class: antimicrotubule drug
Therapeutic class: antineoplastic
Pregnancy risk category: D

Indications and dosages

▶ **Metastatic breast cancer after failure of combination chemotherapy or relapse within 6 months of adjuvant chemotherapy.** Previous therapy should have included an anthracycline unless clinically contraindicated. *Adults:* 260 mg/m² I.V. over 30 minutes q 3 weeks.
Ⓢ **Adjust-a-dose:** For patients with severe sensory neuropathy or a neutrophil count less than 500 cells/mm³ for a week or longer, reduce dose to 220 mg/m². For recurrence of severe sensory neuropathy or severe neutropenia, reduce dose to 180 mg/m². For grade 3 sensory neuropathy, hold drug until condition improves to a grade 1

or 2; then resume drug at a reduced dose for the duration of treatment.

▼ I.V. administration

• Because of the drug's cytotoxicity, handle it cautiously and wear gloves. If the drug contacts your skin, wash thoroughly with soap and water. If it contacts mucous membranes, flush them thoroughly with water.
• Reconstitute the vial with 20 ml of normal saline solution. Direct the stream slowly, over at least 1 minute, onto the inside wall of the vial to avoid foaming.
• Let the vial sit for 5 minutes to ensure proper wetting of the powder.
• Gently swirl or invert the vial for at least 2 minutes until completely dissolved. If foaming occurs, let the solution stand for 15 minutes for the foam to subside.
• If particles are visible, gently invert the vial again to ensure complete resuspension. The solution should be milky and uniform in appearance.
• Each reconstituted vial contains 5 mg/ml paclitaxel. Inject the dose into an empty polyvinyl chloride I.V. bag.
• Give the drug I.V. over 30 minutes.
• Store unopened vials at room temperature in the original package. Use the contents of reconstituted vials immediately, or, if needed, refrigerate at 36° to 46° F (2° to 8° C) for a maximum of 8 hours. If not used immediately, the vial should be protected from light.
• The suspension for infusion prepared as recommended in an infusion bag is stable at room temperature and ambient lighting for up to 8 hours.

⊗ **Incompatibilities**
None known.

Contraindications and cautions

• Contraindicated in patients with baseline neutrophil counts of less than 1,500/mm³.
• Use hasn't been studied in patients with serum creatinine level more than 2 mg/dl or bilirubin level more than 1.5 mg/dl.
⚘ **Lifespan:** Women of childbearing age should avoid becoming pregnant during treatment. Women shouldn't breast-feed during treatment. In children, safety and effectiveness haven't been established.

Adverse reactions

CNS: *asthenia, sensory neuropathy.*
CV: *abnormal ECG, **cardiac arrest, chest pain,** edema,* hypertension, hypotension, ***PE, supraventricular tachycardia, thromboembolism, thrombosis.***
EENT: visual disturbances.
GI: *diarrhea, **intestinal obstruction, ischemic colitis,** mucositis, nausea, oral candidiasis, **pancreatitis, perforation,** vomiting.*
Hematologic: *anemia,* bleeding, NEUTROPE-NIA, ***thrombocytopenia.***
Hepatic: ***hepatic encephalopathy, hepatic necrosis.***
Musculoskeletal: *arthralgia, myalgia.*
Respiratory: cough, *dyspnea, pneumonia, respiratory tract infection.*
Skin: *alopecia,* injection site reactions.
Other: *hypersensitivity reactions, infections, **angioedema, anaphylaxis.***

Interactions

Cytochrome P450 inhibitors: May decrease Abraxane metabolism. Use together cautiously.

Effects on lab test results

• May increase alkaline phosphatase, AST, bilirubin, creatinine, and GGT levels. May decrease hemoglobin level.
• May decrease neutrophil and platelet counts.

Pharmacokinetics

Absorption: Given I.V.
Distribution: Serum protein–binding is 89% to 98%.
Metabolism: Heavily metabolized by several isoenzymes in the cytochrome P450 pathway.
Excretion: 4% of drug recovered in urine unchanged. Less than 1% recovered in urine as metabolites. Fecal excretion 20% of the dose. *Half life:* 27 hours.

Route	Onset	Peak	Duration
I.V.	Unknown	Unknown	Unknown

Action

Chemical effect: Prevents depolymerization of cellular microtubules, inhibiting reorganization of the microtubule network and disrupting mitosis and other vital cell functions.
Therapeutic effect: Inhibits breast cancer cell growth.

P

Available forms

Lyophilized powder for injection: 100 mg in single-use vial

NURSING PROCESS

⚕ Assessment

• Assess patient's condition before starting therapy, and regularly thereafter to monitor the drug's effectiveness.
• Assess the patient for symptoms of sensory neuropathy and severe neutropenia.
• Monitor liver and kidney function tests.
• Monitor infusion site closely.
• Assess patient's and family's knowledge of drug therapy.

⊕ Nursing diagnoses

• Risk for injury related to drug-induced hematologic reactions
• Ineffective health maintenance related to presence of neoplastic disease
• Deficient knowledge related to drug therapy

❯ Planning and implementation

• Give only under the supervision of a practitioner experienced in using chemotherapy in a facility that can manage its complications.
• ⊛ **ALERT:** Don't substitute this drug for other forms of paclitaxel.
• Because Abraxane contains human albumin, there's a remote risk of transmitting viral disease and Creutzfeldt-Jakob disease.
• Complications of overdose may include bone marrow suppression, sensory neurotoxicity, and mucositis; there's no known antidote for overdose.

Patient teaching

• Advise male patients to avoid fathering children while taking this drug.
• Warn the patient that alopecia is common, but is reversible when treatment ends.
• Teach the patient to recognize signs of neuropathy, such as tingling, burning, and numbness in limbs.
• Tell the patient to report fever or other signs of infection, severe abdominal pain, or severe diarrhea.
• Advise the patient to contact her health care provider if nausea and vomiting persist or interfere with her ability to maintain nutrition. Reassure her that a drug can be prescribed that may help.

• Explain that many patients experience weakness and fatigue, so it's important to rest. Tiredness, paleness, and shortness of breath may result from low blood counts, and the patient may need a transfusion.
• To reduce or prevent mouth sores, remind the patient to perform proper oral hygiene.

☑ Evaluation

• Patient does not develop serious adverse hematologic reactions.
• Patient responds to pharmacologic therapy.
• Patient and family state understanding of drug therapy.

palifermin
(pahl-ee-FUR-mihn)
Kepivance

Pharmacologic class: human keratinocyte growth factor
Therapeutic class: growth factor
Pregnancy risk category: C

Indications and dosages

❯ **To decrease the occurrence and duration of severe oral mucositis in patients with hematologic malignancies who are receiving myelotoxic therapy that requires hematopoietic stem cell support.** *Adults:* 60 mcg/kg/day by I.V. bolus for 3 consecutive days before myelotoxic therapy, with the third dose 24 to 48 hours before myelotoxic therapy starts. Repeat dose for 3 consecutive days after myelotoxic therapy, for a total of six doses. The first dose after myelotoxic therapy should be given after, but on the same day of, hematopoietic stem cell infusion and at least 4 days after the most recent palifermin dose.

▼ I.V. administration

• To reconstitute powder, slowly add 1.2 ml sterile water for injection to the vial.
• Swirl the vial gently; don't shake or agitate.
• The final concentration will be 5 mg/ml, and the solution should be clear and colorless.
• Use drug immediately after preparing it or refrigerate it for up to 24 hours.
• Discard any drug that sits at room temperature for more than 1 hour.
• Don't filter drug while preparing or giving it.

Reactions may be *common*, uncommon, *life-threatening*, or COMMON AND LIFE-THREATENING.

- Give palifermin by I.V. bolus; if the I.V. line has been flushed with heparin, flush it with normal saline solution before and after giving palifermin.
- Protect drug from light.

⊗ **Incompatibilities**
Heparin.

Contraindications and cautions

- Contraindicated in patients hypersensitive to *Escherichia coli*–derived proteins, palifermin, or any other component of the product.
- Use cautiously in patients with nonhematologic malignancies.
- **Lifespan:** In pregnant women, use drug only if benefits outweigh potential risk to the fetus. Use cautiously in breast-feeding women; it's unknown if drug appears in breast milk. In children, safety and effectiveness haven't been established.

Adverse reactions

CNS: *dysesthesia, fever, hyperesthesia, hypoesthesia, paresthesia.*
CV: hypertension.
GI: *mouth or tongue thickness or discoloration, taste alteration.*
Musculoskeletal: *arthralgia.*
Skin: *erythema, pruritus, rash.*
Other: *edema, pain.*

Interactions

Drug-drug. *Heparin:* May bind to palifermin and alter dose. Flush I.V. line with normal saline solution before and after giving palifermin.
Myelotoxic chemotherapy: May increase severity and duration of oral mucositis. Don't give palifermin within 24 hours before, during, or within 24 hours after chemotherapy.

Effects on lab test results

- May increase amylase and lipase levels.

Pharmacokinetics

Absorption: Unknown.
Distribution: Extravascular.
Metabolism: Unknown.
Excretion: Unknown. *Half-life:* 3.3 to 5.7 hours.

Route	Onset	Peak	Duration
I.V.	Immediate	1–4 hr	Unknown

Action

Chemical effect: Increases proliferation of epithelial cells, increasing the thickness of tongue tissue, buccal mucosa, and GI tract.
Therapeutic effect: Prevents the development of mouth sores (oral mucositis) caused by chemotherapy or radiation therapy; expedites the healing of the sores if they develop.

Available forms

Lyophilized powder for injection: 6.25-mg vials

NURSING PROCESS

⊞ Assessment
- Assess patient's condition before starting therapy, and regularly thereafter to monitor drug's effectiveness
- Monitor patient for fever, arthralgia, and adverse mucocutaneous effects
- Assess patient's and family's knowledge of drug therapy

⊞ Nursing diagnoses
- Impaired oral mucous membrane related to myelotoxic therapy
- Risk for injury related to drug-induced growth of tumor cells
- Deficient knowledge related to drug therapy

⊠ Planning and implementation
- **⊛ ALERT:** To avoid increasing the severity and duration of oral mucositis, don't give palifermin within 24 hours of myelotoxic chemotherapy.
- Skin-related toxicities are most likely to occur 6 days after the first three consecutive doses.
- Drug may enhance growth of tumor cells.

Patient teaching
- Tell patient to report rash, reddening of the skin, swelling, itching, an unpleasant sensation around the mouth, tongue discoloration or thickening, altered taste, fever, and joint pain.
- Explain that palifermin may stimulate the growth of other types of cancer cells.
- Urge patient to keep all scheduled appointments for treatment.

⊠ Evaluation
- Patient responds to palifermin therapy.
- Patient does not experience increased growth of tumor cells.

P

• Patient and family state understanding of drug therapy.

palivizumab
(pal-ih-VYE-zoo-mab)
Synagis

Pharmacologic class: monoclonal antibody
Therapeutic class: antiviral
Pregnancy risk category: C

Indications and dosages

▶ **To prevent serious lower respiratory tract disease caused by RSV in children at high risk.** *Infants and children:* 15 mg/kg I.M. monthly throughout RSV season, with first dose before RSV season.

Contraindications and cautions

• Contraindicated in children hypersensitive to the drug or any of its components.
• Use cautiously in children with thrombocytopenia or other coagulation disorders.
⚖ **Lifespan:** Drug is only indicated in children.

Adverse reactions

CNS: nervousness, pain.
EENT: *otitis media, rhinitis,* pharyngitis, sinusitis, conjunctivitis.
GI: diarrhea, vomiting, gastroenteritis, oral candidiasis.
Hematologic: anemia.
Respiratory: *upper respiratory tract infection,* cough, wheeze, bronchiolitis, *apnea,* pneumonia, bronchitis, *asthma,* croup, dyspnea.
Skin: *rash,* fungal dermatitis, eczema, seborrhea.
Other: hernia, *failure to thrive,* injection site reaction, viral infection, flulike syndrome, hypersensitivity, *anaphylaxis.*

Interactions

None significant.

Effects on lab test results

• May increase ALT and AST levels. May decrease hemoglobin level and hematocrit.

Pharmacokinetics

Absorption: Absorbed well.

Distribution: Unknown.
Metabolism: Unknown.
Excretion: Unknown. *Half-life:* About 18 days.

Route	Onset	Peak	Duration
I.M.	Unknown	Unknown	Unknown

Action

Chemical effect: Inhibits RSV replication.
Therapeutic effect: Prevents RSV infection in high-risk children.

Available forms

Injection (single-use vial): 50 mg, 100 mg

NURSING PROCESS

ᴙ Assessment
• Obtain accurate medical history before giving drug; ask if child has any coagulation disorders or liver dysfunction.
• Be alert for adverse reactions.
• Assess patient's and family's knowledge of drug therapy.

🔟 Nursing diagnoses
• Risk for infection related to RSV infection
• Risk for injury related to drug-induced adverse reactions
• Deficient knowledge related to drug therapy

⟩ Planning and implementation
• Very rarely, nonfatal cases of anaphylaxis may occur following re-exposure to drug. Rare severe acute hypersensitivity reactions may occur on initial exposure or re-exposure to drug. If a severe hypersensitivity reaction occurs, permanently stop drug. If milder hypersensitivity reactions occur, restart drug cautiously. If anaphylaxis or severe allergic reactions occur, give drug such as epinephrine and provide supportive care as needed.
• To reconstitute, slowly add 0.6 ml of sterile water for injection to the 50-mg vial or 1 ml of sterile water for injection into a 100-mg vial. Gently swirl vial for 30 seconds to avoid foaming; don't shake. Let reconstituted solution stand at room temperature for 20 minutes. Give within 6 hours of reconstitution.
• Give drug in front thigh muscle, off to one side. Don't use gluteal muscle routinely as an injection site because of risk of damage to sciatic nerve. Divide injections larger than 1 ml.

Reactions may be *common,* uncommon, *life-threatening*, or COMMON AND LIFE-THREATENING.

• Give monthly doses throughout RSV season, even if RSV infection develops. In the northern hemisphere, RSV season typically lasts from November to April.

• For patients undergoing cardiopulmonary bypass, give dose immediately after the bypass, even if it's been less than a month since the last dose.

Patient teaching
• Explain to parent or caregiver that drug is used to prevent RSV and not to treat it.
• Advise parent that monthly injections are recommended throughout RSV season.
• Tell parent to immediately report adverse reactions or unusual bruising, bleeding, or weakness.

☑ Evaluation
• Patient doesn't develop RSV infection.
• Patient sustains no injury from drug-induced adverse reactions.
• Patient and family state understanding of drug therapy.

palonosetron hydrochloride
(pa-LOW-no-suh-tron high-droh-KLOHR-ighd)
Aloxi

Pharmacologic class: selective serotonin receptor antagonist
Therapeutic class: antiemetic
Pregnancy risk category: B

Indications and dosages

▶ **To prevent acute nausea and vomiting caused by moderately or highly emetogenic chemotherapy or delayed nausea and vomiting caused by moderately emetogenic chemotherapy.** *Adults:* 0.25 mg I.V. over 30 seconds; give 30 minutes before the start of chemotherapy. Give once per cycle, not more than q 7 days.

▽ I.V. administration

• Don't mix with other drugs.
• Give by either peripheral or central I.V. access.
• Give by rapid I.V. injection over 30 seconds. Flush I.V. line before and after with normal saline solution.

⊗ Incompatibilities
Don't mix (Y-site or otherwise) with other I.V. drugs.

Contraindications and cautions

• Contraindicated in patients hypersensitive to the drug or any of its components.
• Use cautiously in patients hypersensitive to other selective serotonin receptor antagonists; cross-sensitivity may occur. Also use cautiously in patients with cardiac conduction abnormalities, hypokalemia, or hypomagnesemia and in patients taking drugs that affect cardiac conduction.
⚥ Lifespan: In pregnant women, use only if benefits outweigh potential risks to fetus. Breast-feeding women should stop breast-feeding or use a different antiemetic; it's unknown if drug appears in breast milk. In children, safety and effectiveness haven't been established.

Adverse reactions

CNS: anxiety, dizziness, headache, weakness.
CV: *bradycardia*, hypotension, *nonsustained ventricular tachycardia.*
GI: constipation, diarrhea.
Metabolic: *hyperkalemia.*

Interactions

Drug-drug. *Antiarrhythmics or other drugs that may prolong the QT interval, diuretics with potential for inducing electrolyte abnormalities, high doses of anthracycline:* May increase risk of prolonged QT interval. Use together cautiously.

Effects on lab test results

• May increase potassium level.

Pharmacokinetics

Absorption: Administered I.V.
Distribution: Distributes well into tissues. Drug is 60% bound to proteins.
Metabolism: 50% is metabolized to inactive metabolites by CYP 2D6 and, to a lesser extent, CYP 3A4 and 1A2.
Excretion: 80% of drug and inactive metabolites is eliminated in the urine. *Half-life:* 40 hours.

Route	Onset	Peak	Duration
I.V.	30 min	Unknown	5 days

Action

Chemical effect: Binds to the 5-HT$_3$ receptor, which inhibits emesis caused by cytotoxic chemotherapy.
Therapeutic effect: Prevents vomiting from chemotherapy.

Available forms

Injection: 0.25 mg/5 ml (single-use vial).

NURSING PROCESS

⚗ Assessment

• Assess patient's condition before starting therapy, and regularly thereafter to monitor the drug's effectiveness.
• Obtain baseline potassium level.
• In patients with known cardiac conduction abnormalities, obtain baseline ECG.
• Be alert for adverse reactions and drug interactions.
• Assess patient's and family's knowledge of drug therapy.

⊞ Nursing diagnoses

• Risk for deficient fluid volume related to nausea and vomiting
• Pain related to drug-induced headache
• Deficient knowledge related to drug therapy

⧉ Planning and implementation

• Give 30 minutes before chemotherapy on day 1 of each cycle.
• Consider giving with corticosteroids as part of the antiemetic therapy, particularly for patients receiving highly emetogenic chemotherapy.
• Give additional antiemetics for breakthrough nausea and vomiting.
Patient teaching
• Advise patients to take a different antiemetic for breakthrough nausea and vomiting, and tell patient to take it at the first sign of nausea and not to wait until symptoms are severe.
• Tell patients with a history of cardiac conduction abnormalities to report any changes in their drug regimen, such as the adding or stopping of antiarrhythmics.

☑ Evaluation

• Patient maintains adequate hydration.
• Patient doesn't experience drug-induced headaches.

• Patient and family state understanding of drug therapy.

pamidronate disodium
(pam-ih-DROH-nayt digh-SOH-dee-um)
Aredia

Pharmacologic class: bisphosphonate, pyrophosphate analogue
Therapeutic class: bone resorption inhibitor
Pregnancy risk category: D

Indications and dosages

▶ **Moderate to severe hypercalcemia related to malignancy (with or without metastases).**
Adults: Dosage depends on severity of hypercalcemia. Calcium levels are corrected for serum albumin as follows:

Corrected serum calcium (cCa) (in mg/dl)	=	serum calcium (in mg/dl)	+	0.8 (4 – serum albumin) (in g/dl)

Patients with moderate hypercalcemia (cCa levels of 12 to 13.5 mg/dl) may receive 60 to 90 mg I.V. infusion as a single dose over 2 to 24 hours. Patients with severe hypercalcemia (cCa levels higher than 13.5 mg/dl) may receive 90 mg over 2 to 24 hours. Wait at least 7 days to give repeat dose to allow for full response to initial dose.
▶ **Osteolytic bone lesions of multiple myeloma.** *Adults:* 90 mg I.V. over 4 hours once monthly.
▶ **Osteolytic bone lesions of breast cancer.** *Adults:* 90 mg I.V. over 2 hours q 3 to 4 weeks.
▶ **Moderate to severe Paget's disease.** *Adults:* 30 mg I.V. as 4-hour infusion on 3 consecutive days for total dose of 90 mg. Cycle repeated, p.r.n.

▽ I.V. administration

• Reconstitute vial with 10 ml sterile water for injection. Once drug is completely dissolved, add to 250-ml (2-hour infusion), 500-ml (4-hour infusion), or 1,000-ml (up to 24-hour infusion) bag of half-normal or normal saline solution injection or D$_5$W. Inspect for precipitate before administering.
• Give drug only by I.V. infusion. Nephropathy may occur with rapid bolus injections.

• Infusions of more than 2 hours may reduce the risk of renal toxicity, particularly in patients with renal insufficiency.
• Solution is stable for 24 hours at room temperature.

⊗ **Incompatibilities**
Calcium-containing infusion solutions, such as Ringer's injection or lactated Ringer's solution.

Contraindications and cautions

• Contraindicated in patients hypersensitive to the drug or to other bisphosphonates, such as etidronate.
• Use cautiously in patients with renal impairment.
⚖ **Lifespan:** In pregnant women, drug is contraindicated. In breast-feeding women, use cautiously; it's unknown if the drug appears in breast milk. In children, safety and effectiveness haven't been established.

Adverse reactions

CNS: *pain, fever, fatigue, headache, insomnia, anxiety, seizures.*
CV: hypertension, atrial fibrillation.
GI: *abdominal pain, anorexia, constipation, nausea, vomiting, diarrhea, dyspepsia, GI hemorrhage.*
GU: *UTI, renal failure.*
Hematologic: *leukopenia,* THROMBOCYTOPENIA, GRANULOCYTOPENIA, *anemia.*
Metabolism: hypophosphatemia, *hypokalemia, hypomagnesemia,* hypocalcemia.
Musculoskeletal: *bone pain, arthralgia, myalgia.*
Other: METASTASES.

Interactions

None significant.

Effects on lab test results

• May increase creatinine level. May decrease phosphate, potassium, magnesium, calcium, and hemoglobin levels and hematocrit.
• May decrease WBC and platelet counts.

Pharmacokinetics

Absorption: Administered I.V.
Distribution: About 50% to 60% of dose is rapidly taken up by bone; drug is also taken up by kidneys, liver, spleen, teeth, and tracheal cartilage.
Metabolism: None.

Excretion: By kidneys. *Half-life:* Alpha, 1½ hours; beta, 27¼ hours.

Route	Onset	Peak	Duration
I.V.	Unknown	Unknown	Unknown

Action

Chemical effect: Inhibits bone resorption. Adsorbs to hydroxyapatite crystals in bone and may directly block calcium phosphate dissolution.
Therapeutic effect: Lowers calcium levels.

Available forms

Powder for injection: 30 mg/vial, 90 mg/vial
Solution for injection: 3 mg/ml, 6 mg/ml, 9 mg/ml in 10-ml vials

NURSING PROCESS

🏥 Assessment
• Assess patient's condition before starting therapy, and regularly thereafter to monitor the drug's effectiveness.
• Assess hydration before therapy.
• Closely monitor electrolyte levels, CBC and differential. Check creatinine level before each dose.
• Carefully monitor patient with anemia, leukopenia, or thrombocytopenia during first 2 weeks of therapy.
• Monitor patient's temperature. Fever is most likely 24 to 48 hours after therapy.
• Be alert for adverse reactions and drug interactions. Patients with renal impairment are at a greater risk for adverse reactions.
• Assess patient's and family's knowledge of drug therapy.

🔲 Nursing diagnoses
• Ineffective health maintenance related to hypercalcemia
• Risk for injury related to drug-induced hypocalcemia
• Deficient knowledge related to drug therapy

▶ Planning and implementation
• Use drug only after patient has been vigorously hydrated with saline solution. In patients with mild to moderate hypercalcemia, hydration alone may be sufficient.
• If patient has severe hypocalcemia, short-term administration of calcium may be needed.

P

• For a patient with multiple myeloma, limited information is available on those with creatinine level greater than 3 mg/dl. Before infusion, adequately hydrate patient with marked Bence Jones proteinuria and dehydration. Optimal duration of therapy is unknown, but may be 21 months.

⧆ **ALERT:** Because of the risk of renal dysfunction leading to renal failure, don't give single doses of more than 90 mg.

• In patient treated for bone metastases who has renal dysfunction, don't give the dose until renal function returns to baseline. Use in patient with severe renal impairment isn't recommended.

• In patient with breast cancer, optimal duration of therapy isn't known; may be 24 months for overall benefit.

⧆ **ALERT:** Don't confuse Aredia with Meridia.

Patient teaching
• Instruct patient to report unusual signs or symptoms at once.
• Inform patient of need for frequent tests to monitor effectiveness of drug and detect adverse reactions.

☒ **Evaluation**
• Patient's calcium level returns to normal.
• Patient doesn't develop hypocalcemia during drug therapy.
• Patient and family state understanding of drug therapy.

pancuronium bromide
(pan-kyoo-ROH-nee-um BROH-mighd)

Pharmacologic class: nondepolarizing neuromuscular blocker
Therapeutic class: skeletal muscle relaxant
Pregnancy risk category: C

Indications and dosages

▶ **Adjunct to anesthesia to induce skeletal muscle relaxation; to facilitate intubation; to lessen muscle contractions in pharmacologically or electrically induced seizures; to assist with mechanical ventilation.** Dosage depends on anesthetic used, individual needs, and response. Dosages shown are representative; individualize dosage.

Adults and children age 1 month and older: Initially, 0.04 to 0.1 mg/kg I.V.; then 0.01 mg/kg q 25 to 60 minutes.

Neonates younger than age 1 month: Individualize dosages. Give a test dose of 0.02 mg/kg to assess response.

▼ **I.V. administration**
• Mix drug only with fresh solutions.
• Store drug in refrigerator. Don't store in plastic containers or syringes, although plastic syringes may be used for administration.
⊗ **Incompatibilities**
Barbiturates, diazepam, other alkaline solutions.

Contraindications and cautions

• Contraindicated in patients hypersensitive to bromides, in those with tachycardia, and in those for whom even a minor increase in heart rate is undesirable.
• Use cautiously in debilitated patients and in those with respiratory depression, myasthenia gravis, myasthenic syndrome of lung cancer, bronchogenic carcinoma, dehydration, thyroid disorders, collagen diseases, porphyria, electrolyte disturbances, hyperthermia, toxemic states, or renal, hepatic, or pulmonary impairment.
⚕ **Lifespan:** In pregnant women undergoing cesarean section and in breast-feeding women, use large doses cautiously. In the elderly, use cautiously.

Adverse reactions

CV: tachycardia, increased blood pressure.
EENT: excessive salivation.
Musculoskeletal: residual muscle weakness.
Respiratory: *prolonged, dose-related respiratory insufficiency or apnea;* wheezing.
Skin: transient rashes, excessive diaphoresis.
Other: burning sensation, *allergic or idiosyncratic hypersensitivity reactions.*

Interactions

Drug-drug. *Amikacin, gentamicin, neomycin, streptomycin, tobramycin:* May increase the effects of nondepolarizing muscle relaxant, including prolonged respiratory depression. Use together only when needed. Dose of nondepolarizing muscle relaxant may need to be reduced.
Carbamazepine, phenytoin: May decrease the effects of pancuronium causing it to be less ef-

fective. May need to increase the dose of pancuronium.

Clindamycin; general anesthetics; kanamycin; ketamine; polymyxin antibiotics, such as polymyxin B sulfate and colistin; quinidine: May increase neuromuscular blockade, leading to an increase in skeletal muscle relaxation and prolonged effect. Use cautiously during surgical and postoperative periods.

Lithium, opioid analgesics, verapamil: May increase neuromuscular blockade, leading to an increase in skeletal muscle relaxation and respiratory paralysis. Use cautiously, and reduce pancuronium dosage, as directed.

Succinylcholine: May increase intensity and duration of blockade. Allow succinylcholine effects to subside before giving pancuronium.

Theophylline: May reverse the neuromuscular blocking effects of pancuronium.

Effects on lab test results

None reported.

Pharmacokinetics

Absorption: Administered I.V.
Distribution: About 87% plasma protein-binding.
Metabolism: Unknown.
Excretion: Excreted mainly in urine; some biliary excretion. *Half-life:* About 2 hours.

Route	Onset	Peak	Duration
I.V.	30–45 sec	3–4½ min	35–45 min

Action

Chemical effect: Prevents acetylcholine from binding to receptors on muscle end plate, thus blocking depolarization.
Therapeutic effect: Relaxes skeletal muscles.

Available forms

Injection: 1 mg/ml, 2 mg/ml

NURSING PROCESS

▚ Assessment

• Assess patient's condition before starting therapy, and regularly thereafter to monitor the drug's effectiveness.
• Monitor baseline electrolyte determinations (electrolyte imbalance can increase neuromuscular effects) and vital signs.

• Measure fluid intake and output; renal dysfunction may prolong duration of action because 25% of drug is unchanged before excretion.
• Monitor nerve stimulator and train-of-four to avoid overdosage and to confirm antagonism of neuromuscular blockade and recovery of muscle strength. Don't attempt reversal with neostigmine until you see signs of spontaneous recovery.
• Monitor respirations closely until patient fully recovers from neuromuscular blockade, as evidenced by tests of muscle strength (hand grip, head lift, and ability to cough).
• Be alert for adverse reactions and drug interactions.
• Assess patient's and family's knowledge of drug therapy.

⬙ Nursing diagnoses

• Ineffective health maintenance related to condition
• Ineffective breathing pattern related to drug's effect on respiratory muscles
• Deficient knowledge related to drug therapy

▷ Planning and implementation

• Administer sedatives or general anesthetics before neuromuscular blockers. Neuromuscular blockers don't reduce consciousness or alter pain threshold. Give analgesics for pain.
• Give drug only if skilled in airway management.
• Have emergency respiratory support equipment (endotracheal equipment, ventilator, oxygen, atropine, edrophonium, epinephrine, and neostigmine) immediately available.
• If giving with succinylcholine, allow succinylcholine effects to subside before giving this drug.
• Once spontaneous recovery starts, drug-induced neuromuscular blockade may be reversed with an anticholinesterase (such as neostigmine or edrophonium). Usually given with an anticholinergic such as atropine.
• **ALERT:** Don't confuse pancuronium with pipecuronium.
Patient teaching
• Explain all events to patient because he can still hear.
• Reassure patient that he'll be monitored at all times and that pain drug will be provided, if appropriate.

P

• Tell patient that he may feel burning sensation at injection site.

☑ Evaluation
• Patient's condition improves.
• Patient maintains adequate ventilation with mechanical assistance.
• Patient and family state understanding of drug therapy.

pantoprazole sodium
(pan-TOE-pra-zole SOH-dee-um)
Protonix, Protonix IV

Pharmacologic class: proton pump inhibitor
Therapeutic class: gastric acid suppressant
Pregnancy risk category: B

Indications and dosages

▶ **Short-term therapy for erosive esophagitis related to gastroesophageal reflux disease (GERD).** *Adults:* 40 mg P.O. once daily for up to 8 weeks. For those patients who haven't healed after 8 weeks of therapy, an additional 8-week course may be considered.
▶ **Patients with GERD who are unable to continue pantoprazole sodium delayed-release tablets.** *Adults:* 40 mg I.V. daily for 7 to 10 days. Switch to oral form as soon as patient is able to take oral drugs.
▶ **Long-term maintenance of healing erosive esophagitis and reduction in relapse rates of daytime and nighttime heartburn symptoms in patients with GERD.** *Adults:* 40 mg P.O. once daily.
▶ **Pathological hypersecretion conditions related to Zollinger-Ellison syndrome or other neoplastic conditions.** *Adults:* Individualize dosage. Usual starting dose is 40 mg P.O. b.i.d. Adjust dose to a maximum of 240 mg daily. Or, 80 mg I.V. q 12 hours for no more than 6 days. For those needing a higher dose, 80 mg q 8 hours is expected to maintain acid output below 10 mEq/h. Maximum daily dose, 240 mg.

▼ I.V. administration
• Reconstitute each vial with 10 ml of normal saline solution.
• Compatible diluents for infusion include 5% dextrose, normal saline solution, or lactated Ringer's injection.

• For GERD, further dilute with 100 ml of diluent to a final concentration of 0.4 mg/ml.
• For hypersecretion conditions, combine two reconstituted vials and further dilute with 80 ml of diluent to a total volume of 100 ml, with a final concentration of 0.8 mg/ml.
• Infuse diluted solutions I.V. over 15 minutes at a rate not greater than 3 mg/min (7 ml/min) for GERD and 6 mg/min (7 ml/min) for pathological hypersecretory conditions.
• Don't give another infusion simultaneously through the same line.
• The reconstituted solution may be stored for up to 2 hours at room temperature, and the diluted solutions may be stored for up to 12 hours at room temperature.
• Stop I.V. drug as soon as P.O. use is possible.
⊗ **Incompatibilities**
Midazolam (Y-site), zinc-containing products or solutions.

Contraindications and cautions
• Contraindicated in patients hypersensitive to the drug or any of its components.
🕭 **Lifespan:** Use in pregnancy only when clearly needed. In breast-feeding women, use cautiously. In children, safety and effectiveness haven't been established.

Adverse reactions
CNS: headache, insomnia, asthenia, migraine, anxiety, dizziness, pain.
CV: chest pain.
EENT: pharyngitis, rhinitis, sinusitis.
GI: diarrhea, flatulence, abdominal pain, eructation, constipation, dyspepsia, gastroenteritis, gastrointestinal disorder, nausea, vomiting.
GU: rectal disorder, urinary frequency, UTI.
Metabolic: hyperglycemia, hyperlipidemia.
Musculoskeletal: back pain, neck pain, arthralgia, hypertonia.
Respiratory: bronchitis, increased cough, dyspnea, upper respiratory tract infection.
Skin: rash.
Other: flulike syndrome, infection.

Interactions
Drug-drug. *Ampicillin esters, iron salts, ketoconazole:* May decrease absorption of these drugs. Monitor patient closely, and try to separate doses.
Drug-herb. *St. John's wort:* May increase risk of sunburn. Discourage use together.

Reactions may be *common*, uncommon, *life-threatening*, or COMMON AND LIFE-THREATENING.

Drug-food. *Food:* May delay absorption of pantoprazole for up to 2 hours, but the extent of absorption isn't affected. Give with or without meals.

Effects on lab test results

• May increase glucose, uric acid, and lipid levels.
• May increase or decrease liver function test values.
• May cause false-positive urine screen for tetrahydrocannabinol.

Pharmacokinetics

Absorption: Good, with an absolute bioavailability of 77%. Peak level occurs at 2½ hours. Food may delay absorption up to 2 hours, but the extent of absorption isn't affected.
Distribution: Mainly in the extracellular fluid. Protein binding is about 98%, mainly to albumin.
Metabolism: Extensive.
Excretion: About 71% in urine and 18% in feces through bile. *Half-life:* 1 hour.

Route	Onset	Peak	Duration
P.O.	Unknown	2½	24 hr
I.V.	15–30 min	Unknown	24 hr

Action

Chemical effect: Inhibits the activity of the proton pump by binding to hydrogen-potassium adenosine triphosphatase, located at secretory surface of the gastric parietal cells.
Therapeutic effect: Suppresses gastric acid secretion.

Available forms

Injection: 40-mg vial
Tablets (delayed-release): 20 mg, 40 mg

NURSING PROCESS

⚗ Assessment

• Assess underlying condition before starting therapy, and regularly thereafter to monitor the drug's effectiveness.
• Assess patient for complaints of epigastric or abdominal pain and for bleeding (such as blood in stool or emesis).
• Be alert for adverse reactions and interactions.
• Assess patient's and family's knowledge of drug therapy.

⊞ Nursing diagnoses

• Risk for imbalanced fluid volume related to drug-induced adverse reactions
• Risk for aspiration related to underlying gastrointestinal disorder
• Deficient knowledge related to pantoprazole therapy

⊠ Planning and implementation

• Symptomatic response to therapy doesn't rule out gastric malignancy.
⊛ **ALERT:** Don't confuse Protonix with Lotronex, Prilosec, Prozac, or Prevacid.
Patient teaching
• Instruct patient to take exactly as prescribed and at approximately the same time every day.
• Tell patient that drug can be taken with or without food.
• Inform patient that tablet is to be swallowed whole and not crushed, split, or chewed.
• Tell patient that antacids don't affect the absorption of pantoprazole.
• Instruct patient to report abdominal pain or signs of bleeding, such as tarry stool.
• Advise patient not to drink alcohol, eat food, or take other drugs (such as aspirin, NSAIDs) that could cause gastric irritation.

⊠ Evaluation

• Patient maintains adequate hydration throughout therapy.
• Patient responds well to therapy and doesn't aspirate.
• Patient and family state understanding of pantoprazole therapy.

paroxetine hydrochloride
(par-OKS-eh-teen high-droh-KLOR-ighd)
Paxil, Paxil CR

Pharmacologic class: SSRI
Therapeutic class: antidepressant
Pregnancy risk category: D

Indications and dosages

▶ **Major depressive disorder.** *Adults:* Initially, 20 mg P.O. daily, preferably in morning, as directed. Increase by 10 mg daily at weekly intervals, to maximum of 50 mg daily, if needed. Or, initially, 25 mg Paxil CR P.O. as a single daily dose, usually in the morning, with or without food. May increase dose at intervals of at least 1 week by 12.5 mg daily increments, up to a maximum of 62.5 mg daily.

▶ **Obsessive-compulsive disorder.** *Adults:* Initially, 20 mg P.O. daily, preferably in morning, as directed. Increase by 10 mg daily at weekly intervals to target dose of 40 mg daily. Maximum daily dose, 60 mg.

▶ **Panic disorder.** *Adults:* Initially, 10 mg P.O. daily. Increase by 10-mg increments at no less than weekly intervals to target dose of 40 mg daily. Maximum daily dose is 60 mg. Or, initially, 12.5 mg Paxil CR P.O. as a single daily dose, usually in the morning, with or without food. May increase dose at intervals of at least 1 week by 12.5 mg daily increments, up to a maximum of 75 mg. Daily.

▶ **Generalized anxiety disorder.** *Adults:* Initially, 20 mg P.O. daily. Increase dose by 10 mg daily at increments of at least 1 week. Maximum daily dose, 50 mg.

▶ **Posttraumatic stress disorder.** *Adults:* Initially, 20 mg P.O. daily. Increase dose by 10 mg daily at intervals of at least 1 week. Maximum daily dose, 50 mg.

▶ **Premenstrual dysphoric disorder (PMDD).** *Adults:* Initially, 12.5 mg P.O. (Paxil CR) once daily as a single daily dose, usually in the morning, with or without food. May increase to 25 mg daily after at least 1 week. May be given either daily or limited to the luteal phase of the menstrual cycle.

▶ **Social anxiety disorder.** *Adults:* 20 mg P.O. (Paxil) once daily in the morning. Or, initially, 12.5 mg P.O (Paxil CR) once daily in the morning. Increase dosage at weekly intervals in increments of 12.5 mg/day, up to a maximum of 37.5 mg. daily.

▷ **Adjust-a-dose:** For geriatric or debilitated patients and patients with severe hepatic or renal disease, initially, give 10 mg P.O. (immediate-release) daily, preferably in morning. If patient doesn't respond, increase by 10-mg increments at weekly intervals to maximum daily dose of 40 mg. The recommended initial dosage of Paxil CR is 12.5 mg daily. Don't exceed 50 mg daily.

▶ **Diabetic neuropathy‡.** *Adults:* 40 mg P.O. daily.

▶ **Headache‡.** *Adults:* 10 to 50 mg P.O daily for 3 to 9 months.

▶ **Premature ejaculation‡.** *Adults:* 20 mg P.O. 3 to 4 hours before planned intercourse or 10 to 40 mg daily to increase ejaculatory latency time.

Contraindications and cautions

● Contraindicated in patients taking MAO inhibitors or thioridazine. Don't give drug within 14 days of an MAO inhibitor. Also, contraindicated in patients hypersensitive to the drug or any ingredient in the formulation.

● Use cautiously in patients with a history of seizures or mania; patients with severe, concomitant systemic illness; and patients at risk for volume depletion.

● Adults and children with major depressive disorders may experience suicidal ideation and behavior even while taking an antidepressant. Monitor patients for worsening depression or suicidal ideation, especially at the beginning of therapy and during dosage changes.

※ **Lifespan:** In pregnant women, use cautiously in first trimester because of risk of congenital malformations in the fetus. Neonates of women taking drug in the latter part of the third trimester may require prolonged hospitalization due to respiratory problems and feeding difficulties. In breast-feeding women, use cautiously; drug is distributed in breast milk. Not approved for use in children.

Adverse reactions

CNS: *asthenia,* blurred vision, *somnolence, dizziness, insomnia, tremor, headache,* nervousness, anxiety, paresthesia, confusion.

CV: palpitations, vasodilation, orthostatic hypotension.

EENT: lump or tightness in throat, dysgeusia.

GI: *dry mouth, nausea, constipation, diarrhea,* taste perversion, increased or decreased appetite, flatulence, vomiting, dyspepsia, *bleeding.*

GU: abnormal ejaculation, *male genital disorders (including anorgasmy, erectile difficulties, delayed ejaculation or orgasm, impotence, and sexual dysfunction),* urinary frequency, other urinary disorder, *female genital disorder (including anorgasmy, difficulty with orgasm).*

Metabolic: hyponatremia.

Musculoskeletal: myopathy, myalgia, myasthenia.

Skin: excessive sweating, rash.

Other: decreased libido, yawning.

Interactions

Drug-drug. *Buspirone, dextromethorphan, dihydroergotamine, isoniazid, lithium, meperidine, sumatriptan, tramadol, trazodone, tri-*

Reactions may be *common,* uncommon, *life-threatening,* or COMMON AND LIFE-THREATENING.

cyclic antidepressants: May cause serotonin syndrome. Avoid use together.
Cimetidine: May decrease hepatic metabolism of paroxetine, leading to risk of toxicity. Dosage adjustments may be needed.
Digoxin: May decrease digoxin level. Monitor level closely.
NSAIDs, warfarin: May increase risk of bleeding. Use with caution; monitor patient closely for bleeding.
Phenelzine, selegiline, tranylcypromine: May cause serotonin syndrome, including CNS irritability, shivering, and altered consciousness. Don't give together. Wait at least 2 weeks after stopping an MAO inhibitor before giving any SSRI.
Phenobarbital, phenytoin: May alter pharmacokinetics of both drugs. Dosage adjustments may be needed.
Procyclidine: May increase procyclidine levels. Monitor patient for excessive anticholinergic effects.
Sumatriptan: May cause weakness, hyperreflexia, and incoordination. Monitor patient.
Theophylline: Theophylline clearance may decrease threefold. Dosage reduction may be needed.
Thioridazine: May prolong QT interval and increase risk of serious ventricular arrhythmias, such as torsades de pointes and sudden death. Avoid use together.
Tricyclic antidepressants: May inhibit tricyclic antidepressant metabolism. Dose of tricyclic antidepressant may need to be reduced. Monitor patient closely.
Tryptophan: May increase risk of adverse reactions, such as nausea and dizziness. Avoid using together.
Drug-herb. *St. John's wort:* May result in sedative-hypnotic intoxication. Discourage using together.
Drug-lifestyle. *Alcohol use:* May alter psychomotor function. Discourage using together.

Effects on lab test results

• May decrease sodium level.
• May alter platelet count.

Pharmacokinetics

Absorption: Complete.
Distribution: Throughout body, including CNS; only 1% remains in plasma. About 93% to 95% bound to protein.

Metabolism: About 36%.
Excretion: About 64% in urine. *Half-life:* About 24 hours.

Route	Onset	Peak	Duration
P.O.			
immediate-release	1–4 wk	2–8 hr	Unknown
controlled-release	Unknown	6–10 hr	Unknown

Action

Chemical effect: May inhibit CNS neuronal uptake of serotonin.
Therapeutic effect: Relieves depression.

Available forms

Suspension: 10 mg/5ml
Tablets: 10 mg, 20 mg, 30 mg, 40 mg
Tablets (controlled-release): 12.5 mg, 25 mg, 37.5 mg

NURSING PROCESS

✐ Assessment

• Assess patient's depression before starting therapy, and regularly thereafter to monitor the drug's effectiveness.
• Be alert for adverse reactions and drug interactions.
• Assess patient's and family's knowledge of drug therapy.
• For PMDD, the effectiveness of Paxil CR for longer than 3 menstrual cycles hasn't been established.
• Periodically reassess the need for continuing therapy.

✐ Nursing diagnoses

• Disturbed thought processes related to depression
• Risk for injury related to drug-induced adverse CNS reactions
• Deficient knowledge related to drug therapy

✐ Planning and implementation

• Don't give drug within 14 days of MAO inhibitor therapy.
• Don't crush CR tablet. If patient can't swallow a CR tablet whole, give a regular-release form.
• If signs of psychosis occur or increase, reduce dosage.

P

Rapid onset   *Liquid form contains alcohol.   ♦Canada   ◇Australia   †OTC   ✐Photoguide   ‡Off-label use*

• Gradually reduce dosage to prevent withdrawal symptoms.

⑤ **ALERT:** Don't confuse paroxetine with paclitaxel.

⑤ **ALERT:** Don't confuse Paxil with Doxil, Taxol, or Plavix.

Patient teaching

• Warn patient to avoid hazardous activities until the drug's CNS effects are known.

• Warn patient not to chew or crush Paxil CR tablet but to swallow it whole.

• Tell patient that he may notice improvement in 1 to 4 weeks but that he must continue with prescribed regimen to continue feeling benefits.

• Tell patient to abstain from alcohol during drug therapy.

⑤ **ALERT:** If patient wishes to switch from an SSRI to St. John's wort, tell him to wait a few weeks for the SSRI to fully leave his system before starting the herb. The exact time required will depend on which SSRI he takes.

⚕ Evaluation

• Patient's depression improves.

• Patient sustains no injuries because of drug-induced adverse CNS reactions.

• Patient and family state understanding of drug therapy.

pegaspargase (PEG-L-asparaginase)

(peg-AHS-per-jays)
Oncaspar

Pharmacologic class: modified version of enzyme L-asparaginase
Therapeutic class: antineoplastic
Pregnancy risk category: C

Indications and dosages

▶ **Acute lymphoblastic leukemia (ALL) in patients who need L-asparaginase but have developed hypersensitivity to native forms of L-asparaginase.** *Adults and children with body surface area of at least 0.6 m²:* 2,500 international units/m² I.M. or I.V. q 14 days.
Children with body surface area less than 0.6 m²: 82.5 international units/kg I.M. or I.V. q 14 days.

▼ I.V. administration

• Handle and give solution with care; wear gloves. Avoid inhaling vapors and contact with skin or mucous membranes, especially in eyes. If contact occurs, wash with plenty of water for at least 15 minutes.

• Avoid excessive agitation; don't shake. Keep refrigerated at 36° to 46° F (2° to 8° C). If cloudy, precipitated, or stored at room temperature for more than 48 hours, don't use.

• Give drug over 1 to 2 hours in 100 ml of normal saline solution or D₅W through infusion that is already running.

• Keep patient under observation for 1 hour after use and keep resuscitation equipment (such as epinephrine, oxygen, and I.V. steroids) within reach to treat anaphylaxis. If moderate to life-threatening hypersensitivity reactions occur, stop drug.

• Increased risk of hepatotoxicity, coagulopathy, and GI and renal disorders when compared to the I.M. route. Use only when clearly needed.

• Discard unused portions. Use only one dose per vial; don't reenter vial. Don't save unused drug for later use.

⊗ **Incompatibilities**
Other I.V. drugs.

Contraindications and cautions

• Contraindicated in patients with pancreatitis or history of pancreatitis; in those who have had significant hemorrhagic events with previous L-asparaginase therapy; and in those with previous serious allergic reactions, such as generalized urticaria, bronchospasm, laryngeal edema, hypotension, or other unacceptable adverse reactions to pegaspargase.

• Use cautiously in patients with liver dysfunction.

⚕ **Lifespan:** In pregnant and breast-feeding women, use only when benefits outweigh risks.

Adverse reactions

CNS: *seizures,* headache, paresthesia, *status epilepticus,* somnolence, *coma,* mental status changes, dizziness, emotional lability, mood changes, parkinsonism, confusion, disorientation, fatigue, malaise.
CV: hypotension, tachycardia, chest pain, subacute bacterial endocarditis, hypertension, edema.
EENT: epistaxis.

Reactions may be *common*, uncommon, *life-threatening*, or COMMON AND LIFE-THREATENING.

GI: nausea, vomiting, abdominal pain, anorexia, diarrhea, constipation, indigestion, flatulence, GI pain, mucositis, *pancreatitis,* colitis, mouth tenderness.

GU: increased urinary frequency, hematuria, severe hemorrhagic cystitis, renal dysfunction, *renal failure.*

Hematologic: *thrombosis, leukopenia, pancytopenia, agranulocytosis, thrombocytopenia, disseminated intravascular coagulation,* hemolytic anemia, easy bruising, *hemorrhage.*

Hepatic: jaundice, bilirubinemia, ascites, hypoalbuminemia, fatty changes in liver, *liver failure.*

Metabolic: hyperuricemia, hyponatremia, uric acid nephropathy, hypoproteinemia, proteinuria, weight loss, *metabolic acidosis,* hyperglycemia, *hypoglycemia.*

Musculoskeletal: arthralgia, myalgia, musculoskeletal pain, joint stiffness, cramps.

Respiratory: cough, *severe bronchospasm,* upper respiratory tract infection.

Skin: ecchymosis, itching, alopecia, fever blister, purpura, white hands, urticaria, fungal changes, nail whiteness and ridging, erythema simplex, petechial rash, nighttime sweating.

Other: *hypersensitivity reactions (including anaphylaxis,* pain, fever, chills, peripheral edema; infection); *sepsis; septic shock;* injection pain or reaction; localized edema.

Interactions

Drug-drug. *Aspirin, dipyridamole, heparin, NSAIDs, warfarin:* Imbalances in coagulation factors may occur, predisposing patient to bleeding or thrombosis. Use together cautiously.

Methotrexate: May interfere with action of methotrexate, which requires cell replication for its lethal effect. Monitor patient for decreased effectiveness.

Protein-bound drugs: Protein depletion may increase toxicity of other drugs that bind to proteins. Monitor patient for toxicity. May interfere with enzymatic detoxification of other drugs, particularly in liver. Give together cautiously.

Effects on lab test results

• May increase antithrombin III, fibrinogen, BUN, creatinine, amylase, lipase, bilirubin, ALT, AST, uric acid, and ammonia levels. May decrease sodium, protein, and hemoglobin levels and hematocrit. May increase or decrease glucose level.

• May increase PT, INR, and PTT. May decrease WBC, RBC, platelet, and granulocyte counts.

Pharmacokinetics

Absorption: Unknown.
Distribution: Unknown.
Metabolism: Unknown.
Excretion: Unknown. *Half-life:* 2 to 6 days.

Route	Onset	Peak	Duration
I.M.,I.V.	Unknown	Unknown	Unknown

Action

Chemical effect: Destroys cancer cells by inactivating the amino acid asparagine. Asparagine is required by tumor cells to synthesize proteins. Because tumor cells can't synthesize their own asparagine, protein synthesis and, eventually, synthesis of DNA and RNA are inhibited.

Therapeutic effect: Kills selected leukemic cells.

Available forms

Injection: 750 international units/ml

NURSING PROCESS

⚏ Assessment

• Assess patient's condition before starting therapy, and regularly thereafter to monitor the drug's effectiveness.

• Closely monitor patient for hypersensitivity reactions, including life-threatening anaphylaxis, which may occur during therapy, especially in patient hypersensitive to other forms of L-asparaginase.

• Monitor patient's peripheral blood count and bone marrow. A drop in circulating lymphoblasts may occur with a marked rise in uric acid levels.

• Monitor amylase levels to detect early evidence of pancreatitis. Monitor patient's glucose levels during therapy because hyperglycemia may occur.

• Monitor patient for liver dysfunction when used with hepatotoxic chemotherapeutics.

• Drug may affect a number of plasma proteins; monitor fibrinogen, PT, and PTT.

• Be alert for adverse reactions and drug interactions.

• Assess patient's and family's knowledge of drug therapy.

P

⌬ **Nursing diagnoses**
• Ineffective health maintenance related to leukemia
• Ineffective protection related to drug-induced adverse hematologic reactions
• Deficient knowledge related to drug therapy

⬙ **Planning and implementation**
• Use as monotherapy only in unusual situation when combined regimen that uses other chemotherapeutic drugs is inappropriate because of toxicity, because patient is refractory to other therapy, or because of other specific patient-related factors.
• Don't use thawed drug. Although drug may look unchanged, freezing destroys its activity. Obtain new dose from pharmacist.
• Hydrate patient before therapy. Hyperuricemia may result from rapid lysis of leukemic cells. Allopurinol may be ordered.
• Limit volume administered at single injection site to 2 ml. If volume is larger than 2 ml, use multiple injection sites.
Patient teaching
• Inform patient about hypersensitivity reactions and importance of alerting staff at once.
• Instruct patient to ask prescriber before taking other drugs, including OTC preparations. Using together may increase risk of bleeding, or may increase toxicity of other drugs.
• Instruct patient to report signs and symptoms of infection (fever, chills, and malaise) to prescriber because drug may suppress immune system.

☑ **Evaluation**
• Patient responds well to therapy.
• Patient develops no serious complications caused by drug-induced adverse hematologic reactions.
• Patient and family state understanding of drug therapy.

pegfilgrastim
(peg-FILL-grass-tihm)
Neulasta

Pharmacologic class: colony-stimulating factor
Therapeutic class: neutrophil-growth stimulator
Pregnancy risk category: C

Indications and dosages
▶ **To reduce frequency of infection in patients with nonmyeloid malignancies taking myelosuppressive anticancer drugs that may cause febrile neutropenia.** *Adults:* 6 mg subcutaneously once per chemotherapy cycle. Don't give in the period between 14 days before and 24 hours after administration of cytotoxic chemotherapy.

Contraindications and cautions
• Contraindicated in patients hypersensitive to *Escherichia coli*–derived proteins, filgrastim, or any component of the drug.
• Don't use for peripheral blood progenitor cell mobilization.
• Use cautiously in patients with sickle cell disease, those receiving chemotherapy causing delayed myelosuppression, and those receiving radiation therapy.
⚘ **Lifespan:** In pregnant women, use drug only if benefits outweigh potential risks to the fetus. In breast-feeding women, use cautiously; it's unknown if the drug appears in breast milk. In infants, children, and adolescents who weigh less than 45 kg (99 lb), don't use the 6-mg single-use syringe dose. In children, safety and effectiveness haven't been established.

Adverse reactions
CNS: *dizziness, headache, fatigue, insomnia, fever.*
CV: *peripheral edema.*
GI: *nausea, diarrhea, vomiting, constipation, anorexia, taste perversion, dyspepsia, abdominal pain, stomatitis, mucositis.*
Hematologic: GRANULOCYTOPENIA, NEUTROPENIC FEVER, *splenic rupture.*
Musculoskeletal: skeletal pain, generalized weakness, arthralgia, myalgia, bone pain.
Respiratory: *acute respiratory distress syndrome (ARDS).*
Skin: alopecia.

Interactions
Drug-drug. *Lithium:* May increase the release of neutrophils. Monitor neutrophil counts closely.

Effects on lab test results
• May increase LDH, alkaline phosphatase, and uric acid levels.

Reactions may be *common,* uncommon, *life-threatening*, or COMMON AND LIFE-THREATENING.

• May increase WBC, granulocyte, and neutrophil counts.

Pharmacokinetics
Absorption: Unknown.
Distribution: Unknown.
Metabolism: Unknown.
Excretion: Unknown. *Half-life:* 15 to 80 hours.

Route	Onset	Peak	Duration
SubQ	Unknown	Unknown	Unknown

Action
Chemical effect: Binds cell receptors to stimulate proliferation, differentiation, commitment, and end-cell function of neutrophils. Pegfilgrastim and filgrastim have the same mechanism of action. Pegfilgrastim has a reduced renal clearance and therefore a longer half-life than filgrastim.
Therapeutic effect: Increases WBC count.

Available forms
Injection: 6 mg/0.6 ml single-use, preservative-free, prefilled syringes

NURSING PROCESS

⚏ Assessment
• Assess patient's underlying condition before starting therapy, and regularly thereafter to monitor the drug's effectiveness.
• Obtain CBC and platelet count before starting therapy.
• Monitor patient's hemoglobin level, hematocrit, and CBC and platelet count; as well as LDH, alkaline phosphatase, and uric acid levels during therapy.
• Assess patient's and family's knowledge of drug therapy.

⚎ Nursing diagnoses
• Acute pain related to adverse musculoskeletal effects of drug
• Risk for infection related to underlying condition and treatment
• Deficient knowledge related to pegfilgrastim therapy

⚏ Planning and implementation
• The maximum amount of filgrastim that can be given is unknown. Treat patient having symptomatic leukocytosis with leukapheresis.

⚠ **ALERT:** Splenic rupture may occur rarely with filgrastim use. Evaluate patient who experiences signs or symptoms of left upper abdominal or shoulder pain for an enlarged spleen or splenic rupture.
• Monitor patient for allergic reactions, including anaphylaxis, skin rash, and urticaria.
• Evaluate patient who develops fever, lung infiltrates, or respiratory distress for ARDS. If ARDS occurs, stop drug.
• Keep patient with sickle cell disease well hydrated, and monitor patient for symptoms of sickle cell crisis.
• Pegfilgrastim may act as a growth factor for tumors.
Patient teaching
• Inform patient of the drug's potential side effects.
• Advise patient to immediately report upper left abdominal or shoulder tip pain.
• Tell patient to report signs and symptoms of allergic reactions, fever, or breathing problems.
• Tell patient with sickle cell disease to maintain hydration and report signs or symptoms of sickle cell crisis.
• Instruct patient or caregiver how to give drug if it is to be given at home.
• Instruct patient or caregiver not to freeze drug. If accidentally frozen, thaw in refrigerator before administration. Tell them to discard if frozen twice.

⚏ Evaluation
• Patient states that pain management is adequate.
• Patient's WBC count is normal.
• Patient and family state understanding of drug therapy.

peginterferon alfa-2a
(peg-inter-FEAR-on AL-fah TOO AY)
Pegasys

Pharmacologic class: biological response modifier
Therapeutic class: antiviral
Pregnancy risk category: C (X if used with ribavirin)

Indications and dosages

▶ **Chronic hepatitis C in patients with compensated liver disease and not previously treated with interferon alfa.** *Adults:* 180 mcg subcutaneously in abdomen or thigh, once weekly for 48 weeks, on the same day each week.

▶ **Chronic hepatitis C (regardless of genotype) in HIV infected patients not previously treated with interferon.** *Adults:* 180 mcg subcutaneously weekly along with ribavirin (Copegus) 800 mg P.O. daily given in 2 divided doses for 48 weeks.

☒ **Adjust-a-dose:** For patients who experience moderate to severe adverse reactions, decrease dose to 135 mcg subcutaneously once a week; in some cases, decrease to 90 mcg subcutaneously once a week.

For patients who experience hematologic reactions, if absolute neutrophil count (ANC) is less than 750/mm³, reduce dose to 135 mcg subcutaneously once a week; if ANC is less than 500/mm³, stop drug until ANC exceeds 1,000/mm³ and restart at 90 mcg subcutaneously once a week. If platelet count is less than 50,000/mm³, reduce dose to 90 mcg subcutaneously once a week; stop drug if platelet count drops below 25,000/mm³.

In patients on hemodialysis, decrease dose to 135 mcg subcutaneously once a week.

In patients with ALT level increases above baseline, decrease dose to 135 mcg subcutaneously once a week; if hepatic impairment worsens or bilirubin level increases, stop therapy.

If patient develops mild depression, continue drug, but evaluate weekly. For moderate depression, reduce dose to 135 mcg for 4 to 8 weeks and evaluate patient q week; in some cases, reduce to 90 mcg. If symptoms improve and remain stable for 4 weeks, continue at present dose or resume previous dose. If severe depression occurs, discontinue drug permanently.

Contraindications and cautions

• Contraindicated in patients hypersensitive to interferon alfa-2a or its components and in patients with autoimmune hepatitis or decompensated liver disease before or during therapy.
• Use cautiously in patients with a history of depression, drug addiction, suicidal ideation, or suicide attempts. Also use cautiously in patients with baseline ANC less than 1,500/mm³, base-line platelet counts less than 90,000/mm³, or baseline hemoglobin level less than 10 g/dl. Use cautiously in patients with cardiac disease or hypertension, thyroid disease, autoimmune disorders, pulmonary disorders, colitis, pancreatitis, or ophthalmologic disorders. Also use cautiously in patients with creatinine clearance less than 50 ml/minute.

• Safety and effectiveness of drug haven't been established for hepatitis C in organ-transplant recipients, for patients with hepatitis C infected with hepatitis B, or in patients who haven't responded to other alpha interferon therapy.

⚖ **Lifespan:** In pregnant women, use only if benefits outweigh potential risks to the fetus; women of childbearing age must use effective contraception. In breast-feeding women, use cautiously; it's unknown whether drug appears in breast milk. In neonates and premature infants, don't use the drug because it contains benzyl alcohol. In children, safety and effectiveness of drug haven't been established. In the elderly, use cautiously because risk for adverse reactions increases.

Adverse reactions

CNS: *pain, insomnia, dizziness, cerebral hemorrhage, coma,* aggressive behavior, anxiety, bipolar disorder, concentration and memory impairment, *depression, irritability, drug overdose* and relapse of drug addiction, *suicide.*
CV: *pulmonary embolism, myocardial infarction,* hypotension, arrhythmias.
GI: *nausea, diarrhea, abdominal pain,* vomiting, dry mouth, anorexia, *pancreatitis, ulcerative colitis, hemorrhagic or ischemic colitis.*
Hematologic: *anemia, lymphopenia,* NEUTROPENIA, *thrombocytopenia.*
Metabolic: diabetes mellitus, *hypoglycemia,* hyper- or hypothyroidism.
Musculoskeletal: *myalgia, arthralgia,* back pain.
Respiratory: *pneumonia, interstitial pneumonitis.*
Skin: *alopecia, pruritus,* increased sweating, dermatitis, rash.
Other: *flulike symptoms, injection site reaction, infection.*

Interactions

Drug-drug. *Ribavirin:* May increase risk of hematologic toxicity (neutropenia, anemia). The two drugs are commonly given together for additive therapeutic benefit, but laboratory values and symptoms must be monitored closely. *Theophylline:* May increase theophylline level. Monitor theophylline level and adjust dosage, p.r.n.

Effects on lab test results

• May increase ALT and triglyceride levels. May decrease hemoglobin level and hematocrit. May increase or decrease glucose level.
• May decrease ANC, WBC, and platelet counts. May increase or decrease thyroid function test values.

Pharmacokinetics

Absorption: Unknown.
Distribution: Unknown.
Metabolism: Possibly in liver and kidney.
Excretion: Unknown, about 30% is excreted by the kidneys. *Half-life:* 80 hours.

Route	Onset	Peak	Duration
SubQ	Unknown	3–4 days	≤ 1 wk

Action

Chemical effect: Binds to specific receptors on the cell surface, which causes rapid gene transcription that starts complex intracellular events and immunomodulation.
Therapeutic effect: Inhibits viral replication in infected cells and decreases cell proliferation.

Available forms

Injection: 180-mcg/ml single-dose vials, 180-mcg/0.5 ml prefilled syringes

NURSING PROCESS

Assessment

• Monitor patient weekly for psychiatric reactions, such as depression and thoughts of suicide, during the first 8 weeks of therapy. These symptoms may occur in a patient without earlier psychiatric illness. If moderate depression occurs and doesn't go away after decreasing dose, refer patient for psychiatric consultation. If severe depression occurs, immediately stop the drug and start psychiatric therapy.
• Obtain CBC and differential before starting therapy, and monitor it routinely thereafter. Stop giving the drug in the case of a large decrease in neutrophil or platelet counts.

• Obtain baseline eye examination and repeat periodically thereafter during therapy. If patient has a new or worsening eye disorder, stop the drug.
• Monitor lab values for kidney or liver impairment and for thyroid or glucose level changes that require therapy.

Nursing diagnoses

• Ineffective health maintenance related to underlying condition
• Risk for suicide related to adverse CNS effects of drug
• Deficient knowledge related to peginterferon alfa-2a therapy

Planning and implementation

• If uncontrollable thyroid disease, hyperglycemia, hypoglycemia, or diabetes mellitus occurs, stop giving the drug. Thyroid dysfunction may persist after drug is stopped.
• If persistent or unexplained pulmonary infiltrates or pulmonary dysfunction occur, stop giving the drug.
• If signs and symptoms of colitis (abdominal pain, bloody diarrhea, and fever) occur, stop giving the drug. Symptoms will resolve within 3 weeks.
• If signs and symptoms of pancreatitis or autoimmune hepatitis occur, stop giving the drug.
Patient teaching
• Teach patient proper technique for giving himself the drug and for properly disposing of needles and syringes.
• Tell patient to immediately report depression, mood or sleep changes, or thoughts of suicide.
• Tell patient to report signs and symptoms of pancreatitis, GI upset, eye disorders, flulike symptoms, or respiratory disorders.
• Instruct women of childbearing age who are taking drug or who are sexual partners of men taking drug to use two forms of effective contraception during therapy and for 6 months following the end of therapy.
• Inform patient, or partner of patient, who becomes pregnant during or for 6 months posttreatment, to notify prescriber immediately or call the Pregnancy Registry at 1-800-526-6367.
• Advise patient to avoid driving or operating machinery if dizziness, fatigue, confusion, or somnolence occur.

P

☑ **Evaluation**

• Patient has improved health.
• Patient denies suicidal ideation.
• Patient and family state understanding of drug therapy.

peginterferon alfa-2b
(pehg-in-ter-FEAR-ahn AL-fah TOO BEE)
PEG-Intron

Pharmacologic class: biological response modifier
Therapeutic class: antiviral
Pregnancy risk category: C (X if used with ribavirin)

Indications and dosages

▶ **Chronic hepatitis C in patients with compensated liver disease not previously treated with interferon alfa therapy.** *Adults:* Recommended regimen is about 1 mcg/kg subcutaneously once weekly for 48 weeks on the same day each week. Recommended doses are as follows:
37 to 45 kg (81 to 99 lb): 40 mcg (0.4 ml) of 100-mcg/ml strength
46 to 56 kg (100 to 123 lb): 50 mcg (0.5 ml) of 100-mcg/ml strength
57 to 72 kg (124 to 158 lb): 64 mcg (0.4 ml) of 160-mcg/ml strength
73 to 88 kg (159 to 194 lb): 80 mcg (0.5 ml) of 160-mcg/ml strength
89 to 106 kg (195 to 233 lb): 96 mcg (0.4 ml) of 240-mcg/ml strength
107 to 136 kg (234 to 299 lb): 120 mcg (0.5 ml) of 240-mcg/ml strength
137 to 160 kg (300 to 352 lb): 150 mcg (0.5 ml) of 300-mcg/ml strength
▶ **Chronic hepatitis C in patients not previously treated with interferon alpha, given with ribavirin.** *Adults:* Recommended regimen is about 1.5 mcg/kg subcutaneously once weekly for 48 weeks on same day each week. Specific doses are as follows:
Less than 40 kg (< 88 lb): 50 mcg (0.5 ml) of 100-mcg/ml strength
40 to 50 kg (88 to 110 lb): 64 mcg (0.4 ml) of 160-mcg/ml strength
51 to 60 kg (111 to 132 lb): 80 mcg (0.5 ml) of 160-mcg/ml strength

61 to 75 kg (133 to 165 lb): 96 mcg (0.4 ml) of 240-mcg-mcg/ml strength
76 to 85 kg (166 to 187 lb): 120 mcg (0.5 ml) of 240-mcg-mcg/ml strength
More than 85 kg (187 lb): 150 mcg (0.5 ml) of 300-mcg/ml strength
⧉ **Adjust-a-dose:** In patients with WBC counts less than 1,500/mm³, neutrophil counts less than 750/mm³, or platelet counts less than 80,000/mm³, decrease dose by one-half. Oral ribavirin dose can be continued. If hemoglobin level is less than 10 g/dl, reduce oral ribavirin dose by 200 mg daily. If hemoglobin level is less than 8.5 g/dl, WBC counts less than 1000/mm³, neutrophil counts less than 500/mm³, or platelet counts less than 50,000/mm³, stop both drugs.

If patient develops mild depression, continue drug, but evaluate weekly. For moderate depression, reduce dose by one-half for 4 to 8 weeks and evaluate patient q week. If symptoms improve and remain stable for 4 weeks, continue at present dose or resume previous dose. If severe depression occurs, stop drug.

For patients with stable CV disease whose hemoglobin level decreases more than 2 g/dl in any 4-week period, decrease peginterferon alfa-2b dosage by one-half and ribavirin dosage by 200 mg daily. If hemoglobin level is less than 12 g/dl after 4 weeks of reduced dosages, stop both drugs.

Contraindications and cautions

• Contraindicated in patients hypersensitive to the drug or any of its components, and in patients with renal impairment (creatinine clearance below 50 ml/minute), pulmonary infiltrates, autoimmune hepatitis, or decompensated liver disease (Child-Pugh class B and C).
• Don't use drug in organ transplant recipients, patients who haven't responded to other alpha interferon therapy, or those with HIV or hepatitis B virus.
• Use cautiously in patients with psychiatric disorders; diabetes mellitus; cardiovascular disease; pulmonary function impairment; or autoimmune, ischemic, and infectious disorders.
⚖ **Lifespan:** In pregnant women and men whose sexual partners are pregnant, drug is contraindicated. Breast-feeding women should either stop breast-feeding or drug. In neonates and infants, drug is contraindicated because it contains benzyl alcohol. In children, safety and effectiveness haven't been established.

Reactions may be *common*, uncommon, *life-threatening*, or COMMON AND LIFE-THREATENING.

Adverse reactions

CNS: dizziness, hypertonia, fever, depression, insomnia, anxiety, emotional lability, irritability, headache, fatigue, malaise, *suicidal behavior.*
CV: flushing.
EENT: pharyngitis, sinusitis.
GI: nausea, anorexia, diarrhea, abdominal pain, vomiting, dyspepsia, right upper quadrant pain, colitis.
Hematologic: *neutropenia, thrombocytopenia.*
Hepatic: hepatomegaly.
Metabolic: hypothyroidism, hyperthyroidism, weight decrease.
Musculoskeletal: musculoskeletal pain.
Respiratory: cough.
Skin: alopecia, pruritus, dry skin, rash, increased sweating.
Other: injection site reaction (inflammation), injection site pain, viral infection, flulike symptoms, rigors.

Interactions

None reported.

Effects on lab test results

• May increase ALT, bilirubin, and uric acid levels. May increase or decrease TSH levels.
• May decrease neutrophil and platelet counts.

Pharmacokinetics

Absorption: Slowed to mean of 4.6 hours by pegylation of interferon alfa-2b.
Distribution: Unknown.
Metabolism: Unknown.
Excretion: Unknown, about 30% is excreted by the kidneys. *Half-life:* 40 hours.

Route	Onset	Peak	Duration
SubQ	Unknown	15–44 hr	48–72 hr

Action

Chemical effect: Binds to specific receptors on the cell surface, which causes rapid gene transcription that initiates complex intracellular events and various immunomodulating activities.
Therapeutic effect: Inhibits viral replication in infected cells, and decreases cell proliferation.

Available forms

Injection: 100 mcg/ml, 160 mcg/ml, 240 mcg/ml, 300 mcg/ml

NURSING PROCESS

Assessment
• Assess underlying condition before starting therapy, and regularly thereafter to monitor the drug's effectiveness.
• Assess patient for preexisting uncontrolled diabetes or thyroid disorder. Drug may cause or aggravate hypothyroidism, hyperthyroidism, or diabetes.
• If patient has cardiac history, obtain ECG before starting therapy.
• Evaluate patient's volume and make sure patient is hydrated before starting therapy.
• Obtain eye examination in patients with diabetes or hypertension before starting therapy. Retinal hemorrhages, cotton wool spots, and retinal artery or vein obstruction may occur.
• Monitor CBC, platelet count, and AST, ALT, bilirubin, and TSH levels before starting therapy and periodically during therapy.
• Assess patient's and family's knowledge of drug therapy.

Nursing diagnoses
• Ineffective health maintenance related to underlying condition
• Risk for suicide related to adverse CNS effects of drug
• Deficient knowledge related to peginterferon alfa-2b therapy

Planning and implementation
• Drug may be used alone or with ribavirin for chronic hepatitis B.
• If patient has history of MI or arrhythmias, watch closely for hypotension, arrhythmias, tachycardia, cardiomyopathy, and MI.
ALERT: Alpha interferons may cause or aggravate life-threatening neuropsychiatric, autoimmune, ischemic, and infectious disorders. Monitor patient closely and periodically assess for them. Stop therapy in patient with persistently severe or worsening signs or symptoms of these disorders. In many cases, they resolve after stopping therapy.
• Monitor patient for depression and other psychiatric illness. If symptoms are severe, stop giving the drug and refer patient for psychiatric care.
• Monitor patient for signs and symptoms of colitis, such as abdominal pain, bloody diarrhea, and fever. If colitis occurs, stop giving the drug.

Symptoms will resolve 1 to 3 weeks after stopping drug.

• Monitor patient for signs and symptoms of pancreatitis or hypersensitivity reactions. If these occur, stop giving the drug.

• Monitor patient with pulmonary disease for dyspnea, pulmonary infiltrates, pneumonitis, and pneumonia.

• If patient has renal disease, watch for signs and symptoms of toxicity.

• If patient has severe neutropenia or thrombocytopenia, stop giving the drug.

Patient teaching

• Explain appropriate use of the drug and its benefits and risks. Tell patient that adverse reactions may continue for several months after therapy is stopped.

• Advise patient that laboratory tests are required before therapy starts and periodically thereafter.

• Tell patient to take drug h.s. and to use antipyretics to decrease the effect of flulike symptoms.

• Emphasize the importance of properly disposing of needles and syringes, and warn against reusing old needles and syringes.

• Tell patient that drug isn't known to prevent transmission of hepatitis C. It also isn't known whether drug cures hepatitis C or prevents cirrhosis, liver failure, or liver cancer that may result from hepatitis C.

• Advise patient to immediately report symptoms of depression or thoughts of suicide.

☑ Evaluation

• Patient has improved health.

• Patient reports no suicidal ideation.

• Patient and family state understanding of drug therapy.

pemetrexed
(peh-meh-TREK-sed)
Alimta

Pharmacologic class: folate antagonist
Therapeutic class: antineoplastic
Pregnancy risk category: D

Indications and dosages

▶ **With cisplatin, malignant pleural mesothelioma in patients whose disease is unresect-** able or who aren't candidates for surgery. *Adults:* 500 mg/m^2 I.V. over 10 minutes on day 1 of each 21-day cycle. 30 minutes after infusion ends, give 75 mg/m^2 cisplatin I.V. over 2 hours.

▶ **Locally advanced or metastatic non–small-cell lung cancer after chemotherapy.** *Adults:* 500 mg/m^2 I.V. over 10 minutes on day 1 of each 21-day cycle.

⧅ Adjust-a-dose: For patients who develop toxic reactions, see table on next page.

▼ I.V. administration

• Reconstitute 500-mg vial with 20 ml of preservative-free normal saline solution to yield 25 mg/ml.

• Swirl the vial gently until powder is completely dissolved. The solution will be clear and colorless to yellow or yellow-green.

• Calculate the appropriate dose, and further dilute with 100 ml normal saline solution.

• Give I.V. over 10 minutes.

• Reconstituted solution and dilution are stable for 24 hours refrigerated or at room temperature under ambient lighting.

⊗ **Incompatibilities**
Calcium-containing diluents including Ringer's or lactated Ringer's for injection; other drugs or diluents.

Contraindications and cautions

• Contraindicated in patients with a history of severe hypersensitivity reaction to drug or its components. Don't use in patients with creatinine clearance less than 45 ml/minute.

⚖ **Lifespan:** In pregnant women, use only when benefits outweigh potential risks to the fetus. Breast-feeding women should stop breast-feeding or stop drug. In children, drug hasn't been adequately studied.

Adverse reactions

CNS: *depression, fatigue, fever, neuropathy.*
CV: cardiac ischemia, *chest pain, edema, emboli,* thrombosis.
EENT: *pharyngitis*
GI: *anorexia, constipation, diarrhea, esophagitis, nausea,* painful difficult swallowing, *stomatitis, vomiting.*
GU: *renal failure.*
Hematologic: ANEMIA, LEUKOPENIA, NEUTROPENIA, THROMBOCYTOPENIA.
Metabolic: dehydration.
Musculoskeletal: arthralgia, *myalgia.*

Reactions may be *common,* uncommon, *life-threatening*, or COMMON AND LIFE-THREATENING.

Toxic reaction	Dosage adjustment
Grade 3 (severe or undesirable) or 4 (life-threatening or disabling) diarrhea Diarrhea that calls for hospitalization Grade 3 toxicity (except mucositis and increased transaminase levels) Grade 4 toxicity (except mucositis) Platelet count ≥ 50,000/mm^3 and absolute neutrophil count < 500/mm^3	Give 75% of previous pemetrexed and cisplatin doses.
Platelet count < 50,000/mm^3	Give 50% of previous pemetrexed and cisplatin doses.
Grade 3 or 4 mucositis	Give 50% of previous pemetrexed dose and 100% of previous cisplatin dose.
Grade 2 neurotoxicity	Give 100% of previous pemetrexed dose and 50% of previous cisplatin dose.
Grade 3 or 4 neurotoxicity Any grade 3 or 4 toxicity (except increased transaminase levels) after two dose reductions	Stop therapy.

Respiratory: *dyspnea.*
Skin: *alopecia, rash.*
Other: allergic reaction, *infection.*

Interactions

Drug-drug. *Ibuprofen:* May decrease pemetrexed clearance in patients with mild to moderate renal insufficiency (creatinine clearance 45-79 ml/minute). Use together cautiously.
Nephrotoxic drugs, probenecid: May delay pemetrexed clearance. Monitor patient.
NSAIDs: May decrease pemetrexed clearance in patients with mild to moderate renal insufficiency. For NSAIDs with short half-lives, avoid use for 2 days before, during, and 2 days after pemetrexed therapy. For NSAIDs with long half-lives, avoid use for 5 days before, during, and 2 days after pemetrexed therapy.

Effects on lab test results

• May increase ALT, AST, and creatinine levels. May decrease hemoglobin level and hematocrit.
• May decrease absolute neutrophil, platelet, and WBC counts.

Pharmacokinetics

Absorption: Administered I.V.
Distribution: 81% bound to plasma proteins.
Metabolism: None significant.
Excretion: 70% to 90% is unchanged in urine.
Half life: 3½ hours.

Route	Onset	Peak	Duration
I.V.	Unknown	Unknown	Unknown

Action

Chemical effect: Disturbs cell replication by inhibiting several folate-dependent enzymes involved in nucleotide synthesis. When given with other antineoplastics, drug inhibits growth of certain mesothelioma cell lines.
Therapeutic effect: Inhibits replication of certain cancer cells.

Available forms

Injection: 500 mg in single-use vials

NURSING PROCESS

P

Assessment
• Assess patient's condition before therapy and regularly thereafter to monitor the drug's effectiveness.
• Monitor renal function, CBC, platelet count, hemoglobin level, hematocrit, and liver function test values.
• Assess patient for neurotoxicity, mucositis, and diarrhea. Severe symptoms may warrant dose reduction.
• If the patient has an adverse GI reaction, monitor his hydration.
• Assess patient's and family's knowledge of drug therapy.

Nursing diagnoses
• Ineffective protection related to drug-induced adverse hematologic reactions

• Risk for deficient fluid volume related to drug-induced adverse GI reactions
• Deficient knowledge related to drug therapy

▷ **Planning and implementation**
• For a patient with pleural effusion and ascites, drain effusion before therapy.
• Don't start a new cycle of therapy unless absolute neutrophil count is 1,500/mm³ or more, platelet count is 100,000/mm³ or more, and creatinine clearance is 45 ml/minute or more.
⚡ **ALERT:** To reduce the occurrence and severity of cutaneous reactions, give a corticosteroid, such as dexamethasone 4 mg P.O. b.i.d., the day before, the day of, and the day after giving drug.
⚡ **ALERT:** To reduce toxicity, give 350 to 1,000 mcg of folic acid starting 5 days before the first drug dose and ending 21 days after therapy.
⚡ **ALERT:** Give 1,000 mcg vitamin B$_{12}$ I.M. once during the week before the first dose and q three cycles thereafter. After the first cycle, vitamin injections may be given on the first day of the cycle.
Patient teaching
• Inform patient that he may receive corticosteroids and vitamins before pemetrexed to help minimize its adverse effects.
• Tell patient to avoid NSAIDs for several days before, during, and after therapy.
• Urge patient to report adverse reactions, especially fever, sore throat, infection, diarrhea, fatigue, limb pain, unusual bleeding or bruising, black tarry stools, blood in urine or stools, and pinpoint red spots on skin.

☑ **Evaluation**
• Patient doesn't develop serious complications from adverse hematologic reactions.
• Patient maintains adequate hydration.
• Patient and family state understanding of drug therapy.

penicillamine
(pen-ih-SIL-uh-meen)
Cuprimine, Depen

Pharmacologic class: chelating agent
Therapeutic class: heavy metal antagonist, antirheumatic
Pregnancy risk category: D

Indications and dosages
▷ **Wilson's disease.** *Adults and children:* 0.75 to 1.5 g P.O. in divided doses 60 minutes before meals. Initially, adjust dosage to achieve urinary copper excretion of greater than 2 mg daily. After 3 months, base dosage on maintaining a serum free copper level of less than 10 mcg/dL.
▷ **Cystinuria.** *Adults:* 250 mg to 1 g P.O. q.i.d. 60 minutes before meals. Adjust dosage to achieve urinary cystine excretion of less than 100 mg daily when renal calculi are present or 100 to 200 mg daily when no calculi are present. Maximum, 4 g daily.
Children: 30 mg/kg P.O. daily divided q.i.d. 60 minutes before meals. Adjust dosage to achieve urinary cystine excretion of less than 100 mg daily when renal calculi are present or 100 to 200 mg daily when no calculi are present.
▷ **Severe, active rheumatoid arthritis unresponsive to conventional therapy.** *Adults:* Initially, 125 to 250 mg P.O. daily, with increases of 125 to 250 mg q 1 to 3 months, if needed. Maximum, 1.5 g daily.
▷ **Adjunct in heavy metal poisoning‡.** *Adults:* 500 to 1,500 mg P.O. daily for 1 to 2 months.
▷ **Primary biliary cirrhosis‡.** *Adults:* Initially, 250 mg P.O. daily with increases of 250 mg P.O. q 2 weeks. Maximum, 1 g daily in divided doses.
◩ **Adjust-a-dose:** Reduce dose to 250 mg daily if elective surgery is necessary during penicillamine therapy.

Contraindications and cautions
• Contraindicated in patients with previous penicillamine-related aplastic anemia or agranulocytosis; patients with rheumatoid arthritis and history or other evidence of renal insufficiency.
• Use cautiously, in patients hypersensitive to penicillin.
✾ **Lifespan:** In pregnant women, except those with Wilson's disease or certain patients with cystinuria, drug is contraindicated. Breast-feeding women should stop breast-feeding or use another drug. In children with rheumatoid arthritis, safety and effectiveness haven't been established. In elderly patients, use cautiously due to possible increase in adverse reactions.

Adverse reactions
CNS: tinnitus, optic neuritis, peripheral sensory and motor neuropathies, visual and psychic disturbances, mental disorders, agitation, anxiety.

Reactions may be *common,* uncommon, ***life-threatening***, or COMMON AND LIFE-THREATENING.

GI: *anorexia, epigastric pain, nausea, vomiting, diarrhea, loss of taste or altered taste perception,* stomatitis, oral ulcerations, reactivated peptic ulcer, *pancreatitis.*
GU: *nephrotic syndrome, glomerulonephritis, renal failure,* proteinuria, hematuria, *renal vasculitis.*
Hematologic: *leukopenia,* eosinophilia, *thrombocytopenia,* monocytosis, *agranulocytopenia, aplastic anemia,* sideroblastic anemia, *lymphadenopathy.*
Hepatic: *hepatotoxicity, hepatic failure.*
Metabolic: thyroiditis, *hypoglycemia.*
Musculoskeletal: migratory polyarthralgia, synovitis.
Respiratory: *interstitial pneumonitis, obliterative bronchiolitis, pulmonary fibrosis* in patients with severe rheumatoid arthritis, *bronchial asthma.*
Skin: alopecia; friability, especially at pressure spots; wrinkling; erythema; urticaria; ecchymoses, early and late rashes, exfoliative dermatitis, pemphigus.
Other: lupus-like syndrome, myasthenia gravis syndrome with long-term use, drug fever, *allergic reactions, Goodpasture's syndrome,* vasculitis.

Interactions

Drug-drug. *Antacids, oral iron:* May decrease effectiveness of penicillamine. Give at least 2 hours apart.
Antimalaria drugs, cytotoxic drugs, gold therapy, oxyphenbutazone, phenylbutazone: May increase risk of toxicity. Avoid giving together.
Digoxin: May decrease digoxin effect. Adjust dosage if needed.
Drug-food. *Any food:* May delay absorption of drug. Give drug 1 hour before or 2 hours after meals.

Effects on lab test results

• May increase liver enzyme and urinary protein levels. May decrease glucose and hemoglobin levels and hematocrit.
• May increase eosinophil count, antinuclear antibody titer, and sedimentation rate. May decrease platelet, WBC, and granulocyte counts.

Pharmacokinetics

Absorption: Readily absorbed from the GI tract.
Distribution: Highly protein bound.

Metabolism: In liver to inactive disulfides.
Excretion: Slow, mainly renal. *Half-life:* 1½ to 3 hours.

Route	Onset	Peak	Duration
P.O.	Unknown	1–3 hr	4–6 days

Action

Chemical effect: Chelates heavy metals, binds cystine into more soluble form, dissociates macroglobulins like rheumatoid factor without causing overall immunoglobulin suppression, depresses T-cell activity, and interferes with cross-links between tropocollagen molecules.
Therapeutic effect: Binds copper for renal excretion in Wilson's disease, enhances excretion of cystine, and relieves symptoms of rheumatoid arthritis.

Available forms

Capsules: 125 mg, 250 mg
Tablets (scored): 250 mg

NURSING PROCESS

Assessment
• Obtain history of patient's underlying condition before starting therapy.
• Obtain baseline 24-hour urinary copper excretion before giving the drug for Wilson's disease. Goal is more than 2 mg copper excreted daily.
• Monitor CBC with differential and urinalysis two times a week for one month, then q 2 weeks for 5 months, then monthly throughout therapy; observing for hematologic and GU adverse effects. Assess patient's skin, lymph nodes, and body temperature on same schedule.
• Monitor liver function tests q 3 months for first year of therapy for Wilson's disease, and q 6 months thereafter. For patient taking drug for other diagnoses, monitor liver function tests q 6 months.
• If patient has rheumatoid arthritis, check 24-hour urinary protein q 1 to 2 weeks.
• In patient with rheumatoid arthritis, check joint mobility and range of motion, pain, and swelling to evaluate the drug's effectiveness.
• Monitor yearly X-ray for renal calculi in patients with cystinuria.
• Be alert for adverse reactions and drug interactions.
• Assess patient's and family's knowledge of drug therapy.

⊕ Nursing diagnoses
- Impaired physical mobility related to Wilson's disease
- Impaired urinary elimination related to drug-induced renal dysfunction
- Deficient knowledge related to drug therapy

⊠ Planning and implementation
- Give dose on an empty stomach to facilitate absorption, preferably 1 hour before or 2 hours after meals. Don't give drug within 1 hour of any other drug, milk, antacid, or preparation that contains zinc or iron due to risk of metal binding in GI tract.
- Penicillamine therapy should be continued on daily basis. Sensitivity reactions may occur when therapy is reinstituted following interruptions.
- Give 25 mg supplemental pyridoxine daily to patients with Wilson's disease or cystinuria.
- If annoying GI symptoms or rash don't resolve within 6 weeks of starting therapy, reduce dose to minimum of 250 mg daily and then increase more slowly.
- If patient has mild skin reaction, give antihistamines. Handle patient carefully to avoid skin damage.
- **⊛ ALERT:** Immediately report rash and fever (important signs of toxicity to prescriber). If pemphigus, unexplained gross hematuria or persistent microscopic hematuria is noted, stop the drug.
- If WBC count falls below 3,500/mm³ or platelet count falls below 100,000/mm³, don't give the drug and notify prescriber. A progressive decline in platelet or WBC count in three successive blood tests may require a temporary stop, even if the counts are within normal limits.
- If 24-hour urinary protein is greater than 1 g or is progressively increasing, reduce or stop drug.
- **⊛ ALERT:** Don't confuse penicillamine with penicillin.
Patient teaching
- Tell patient with rheumatoid arthritis or Wilson's disease that drug may not take effect for up to 3 months.
- Tell patient with cystinuria to drink 1 L (1 qt) of water throughout the night.
- Teach patient with Wilson's disease to follow low-copper diet: no chocolate, nuts, shellfish, mushrooms, liver, molasses, broccoli, and cereals or products containing added copper such as multivitamins.
- Advise patient to report early signs of granulocytopenia or thrombocytopenia: fever, sore throat, chills, bruising, and bleeding.
- Reassure patient that taste impairment usually resolves in 6 weeks without change in dosage.

☑ Evaluation
- Patient reports increase in physical mobility.
- Patient maintains normal urinary elimination pattern.
- Patient and family state understanding of drug therapy.

penicillin G benzathine (benzylpenicillin benzathine)
(pen-ih-SIL-in gee BENZ-uh-theen)
Bicillin L-A, Permapen

Pharmacologic class: natural penicillin
Therapeutic class: long-acting antibiotic
Pregnancy risk category: B

Indications and dosages
▶ **Congenital syphilis.** *Children younger than age 2:* 50,000 units/kg I.M. as single dose.
▶ **Group A streptococcal upper respiratory tract infections.** *Adults:* 1.2 million units I.M. as single injection.
Children who weigh 27 kg (60 lb) or more: 900,000 units I.M. as single injection.
Children who weigh less than 27 kg (60 lb): 300,000 to 600,000 units I.M. as single injection.
▶ **To prevent poststreptococcal rheumatic fever and glomerulonephritis.** *Adults and children:* 1.2 million units I.M. once monthly or 600,000 units twice monthly.
▶ **Syphilis of less than 1 year's duration.** *Adults:* 2.4 million units I.M. as single dose.
Children: 50,000 units/kg I.M. up to adult dosage as a single dose.
▶ **Syphilis of more than 1 year's duration.** *Adults:* 2.4 million units I.M. weekly for 3 successive weeks.
Children: 50,000 units/kg I.M. up to adult dosage weekly for 3 successive weeks.
▶ **Yaws, bejel, and pinta.** *Adults:* 1.2 million units I.M. as a single dose.

▶ **To prevent diphtheria‡.** *Adults and children older than age 6 or weighing 30 kg (66 lb) or more:* 1.2 million units I.M. as a single injection.

Children younger than age 6 or weighing less than 30 kg (66 lb): 600,000 units I.M. as a single dose.

⊠ **Adjust-a-dose:** Decrease dosage in patients with severe renal or hepatic disease.

Contraindications and cautions

● Contraindicated in patients hypersensitive to drug or other penicillins.
● Use cautiously in patients with other drug allergies, especially to cephalosporins.
❀ **Lifespan:** In pregnant women, use cautiously. In breast-feeding women, don't use; drug appears in breast milk and may sensitize infant to drug, causing an adverse reaction.

Adverse reactions

CNS: pain, neuropathy, *seizures.*
Hematologic: eosinophilia, hemolytic anemia, *thrombocytopenia, leukopenia.*
Other: hypersensitivity reactions (maculopapular and exfoliative dermatitis, chills, fever, edema, *anaphylaxis*), sterile abscess at injection site.

Interactions

Drug-drug. *Aspirin, ethacrynic acid, furosemide, indomethacin, phenylbutazone, sulfonamides, thiazide diuretics:* May compete with penicillin G for renal tubular secretion and prolong penicillin half-life.
Heparin, oral anticoagulants: May increase risk of bleeding. Monitor PT, PTT, and INR. Monitor patient for bleeding.
Hormonal contraceptives: May decrease effectiveness of hormonal contraceptives and increase breakthrough bleeding. Advise patient to use another method during therapy.
Probenecid: May increase levels of penicillin. Probenecid may be used for this purpose.

Effects on lab test results

● May decrease hemoglobin level and hematocrit.
● May increase eosinophil count. May decrease platelet, WBC, and granulocyte counts.
● May cause false-positive urine glucose test results.

Pharmacokinetics

Absorption: Slow.
Distribution: Wide. CSF penetration is poor but enhanced in patients with inflamed meninges. 45% to 68% protein-bound.
Metabolism: At injection site. 16% to 30% to inactive compounds.
Excretion: Primarily in urine. *Half-life:* 30 to 60 minutes.

Route	Onset	Peak	Duration
I.M.	Unknown	13–24 hr	1–4 wk

Action

Chemical effect: Inhibits cell wall synthesis during microorganism multiplication.
Therapeutic effect: Kills susceptible bacteria.

Available forms

Injection: 300,000 units/ml, 600,000 units/ml

NURSING PROCESS

☷ Assessment
● Assess patient's infection before starting therapy, and regularly thereafter to monitor the drug's effectiveness.
● Before giving drug, ask the patient about allergic reactions to penicillin, cephalosporins, and cephamycins. Absence of past reactions is no guarantee against future allergic reactions.
● Obtain specimen for culture and sensitivity tests before giving first dose. If a sexually transmitted disease (STD) is suspected, obtain baseline venereal disease research laboratory, or VDRL, and rapid plasma reagin, or RPR, tests. Start therapy pending test results.
● Be alert for adverse reactions and drug interactions.
● Observe patient closely. Large doses and prolonged therapy raise the risk of bacterial or fungal superinfection, especially in an elderly, debilitated, or immunosuppressed patient.
● Assess patient's and family's knowledge of drug therapy.

⊞ Nursing diagnoses
● Infection related to presence of bacteria
● Ineffective protection related to risk of hypersensitivity reactions to drug
● Deficient knowledge related to drug therapy

▧ Planning and implementation

• Shake drug well before injection.
• Inject at a slow, steady rate to prevent needle from becoming blocked by suspended material in product.
⚡ **ALERT:** Never give drug I.V.; doing so has caused cardiac arrest and death.
• Inject deep into upper outer quadrant of buttocks in adult; in midlateral thigh in infant and young child. Avoid injection into or near major nerves or blood vessels to prevent severe neurovascular damage.
• If a high dose of penicillin is required for several days, change to an I.V. formulation (penicillin G potassium or penicillin G sodium) to avoid muscle fibrosis and atrophy from repeated I.M. injections (particularly in neonates and infants).
• Drug's extremely slow absorption makes allergic reactions difficult to treat. If patient develops signs of anaphylactic shock, such as rapidly developing dyspnea and hypotension, immediately stop giving the drug. Notify prescriber and immediately administer epinephrine, corticosteroids, antihistamines, or other resuscitative measures.
⚡ **ALERT:** Be aware of the various preparations of penicillin. They aren't interchangeable.
• Periodically monitor renal and hematopoietic function in patient receiving long-term therapy.
⚡ **ALERT:** Don't confuse penicillin with penicillamine. Don't confuse penicillin G potassium with penicillin G sodium, penicillin G procaine, or penicillin G benzathine.
⚡ **ALERT:** Bicillin L-A is the only penicillin G benzathine product indicated for the treatment of sexually transmitted infections, including syphilis. Don't substitute Bicillin C-R in its place as this may cause ineffective treatment.
Patient teaching
• Tell patient to call prescriber if rash, fever, or chills develop.
• Tell patient taking drug for active STD to take safe sex precautions, to reduce risks to fetus and neonate of syphilis during pregnancy, and to complete full drug course and follow-up testing.
• Instruct patient treated for active STD to bring partners in for therapy as well.
• Warn patient that injection may be painful but that ice applied to site may ease discomfort.

☑ Evaluation

• Patient is free from infection.
• Patient shows no signs of allergy.
• Patient and family state understanding of drug therapy.

penicillin G potassium (benzylpenicillin potassium)
(pen-ih-SIL-in gee poh-TAH-see-um)
Pfizerpen

Pharmacologic class: natural penicillin
Therapeutic class: rapid-acting antibiotic
Pregnancy risk category: B

Indications and dosages

▶ **Moderate to severe systemic infection.**
Adults and children age 12 and older: Individualize dose. 1 to 24 million units I.M. or I.V. daily in divided doses q 4 to 6 hours.
Children younger than age 12: Highly individualized; 25,000 to 400,000 units/kg I.M. or I.V. daily in divided doses q 4 to 6 hours.
▶ **Anthrax.** *Adults:* 5 to 20 million units I.V. daily in divided doses q 4 to 6 hours for at least 14 days after symptoms subside. Or, 80,000 units/kg in the first hour followed by a maintenance dose of 320,000 units/kg/day. Average adult dosage, 4 million units q 4 hours or 2 million units q 2 hours.
Children: 100,000 to 150,000 units/kg/day I.V. in divided doses q 4 to 6 hours for at least 14 days after symptoms subside.
▶ **Necrotizing ulcerative gingivitis.** *Adults:* 5 to 10 million units I.M. or I.V. daily.
▶ **To eliminate the diphtheria carrier-state:** *Adults:* 2 to 3 million units per day I.M. in divided doses q 4 to 6 hours for 10 to 12 days.
⬕ **Adjust-a-dose:** For patients with renal impairment, if creatinine clearance is less than 10 ml/min, give full loading dose and then one-half of usual dose q 8 to 10 hours or usual dose q 12 to 18 hours; if creatinine clearance is more than 10 ml/minute, give full loading dose and then give one-half dose q 4 to 6 hours for additional doses.

▼ I.V. administration

• Use continuous I.V. infusion when large doses are required (10 million units or more). Otherwise, give by intermittent I.V. infusion over 1 to 2 hours.

⊗ **Incompatibilities**

Alcohol 5%, amikacin, aminoglycosides, aminophylline, amphotericin B sodium, chlorpromazine, dextran, dopamine, heparin sodium, hydroxyzine hydrochloride, lincomycin, metoclopramide, pentobarbital sodium, phenytoin sodium, prochlorperazine mesylate, promethazine hydrochloride, sodium bicarbonate, thiopental, vancomycin, vitamin B complex with C.

Contraindications and cautions

• Contraindicated in patients hypersensitive to the drug or other penicillins.

• Use cautiously in patients with other drug allergies, especially to cephalosporins and cephamycins.

⚠ **Lifespan:** In pregnant women, use cautiously. In breast-feeding women, don't use; drug appears in breast milk and may sensitize infant to penicillin and cause an adverse reaction.

Adverse reactions

CNS: neuropathy, *coma, seizures.*
CV: thrombophlebitis.
Hematologic: hemolytic anemia, *thrombocytopenia, leukopenia.*
Metabolic: *severe potassium poisoning.*
Other: hypersensitivity reactions (rash, urticaria, maculopapular eruptions, exfoliative dermatitis, chills, fever, edema, *anaphylaxis*), overgrowth of nonsusceptible organisms, pain at injection site.

Interactions

Drug-drug. *Aminoglycoside antibiotics:* May be synergistic with some penicillins but can deactivate some beta-lactam penicillins if mixed in same syringe or I.V. solution and administration set. May reduce oral aminoglycoside levels when given with parenteral penicillins to renally impaired patients.

Aspirin, ethacrynic acid, furosemide, indomethacin, phenylbutazone, sulfonamides, thiazide diuretics: May compete with penicillin G for renal tubular secretion and prolong penicillin half-life.

Heparin, oral anticoagulants: May increase risk of bleeding. Monitor PT, PTT, and INR. Monitor patient for bleeding.

Hormonal contraceptives: May decrease effectiveness of hormonal contraceptives and increase breakthrough bleeding. Advise patient to use another contraceptive during therapy.

Potassium-sparing diuretics: May increase risk of hyperkalemia. Don't use together.

Probenecid: May increase levels of penicillin. Probenecid may be used for this purpose.

Effects on lab test results

• May increase potassium level. May decrease hemoglobin level and hematocrit.

• May increase eosinophil count. May decrease platelet, WBC, and granulocyte counts.

Pharmacokinetics

Absorption: Rapid from I.M. injection site.
Distribution: Wide. CSF penetration is poor but is enhanced in patients with inflamed meninges. Drug is 45% to 68% protein-bound.
Metabolism: At injection site.
Excretion: Primarily in urine. *Half-life:* 30 to 60 minutes.

Route	Onset	Peak	Duration
I.V.	Immediate	Immediate	4 hr
I.M.	Unknown	15–30 min	4 hr

Action

Chemical effect: Inhibits cell wall synthesis during microorganism multiplication.
Therapeutic effect: Kills susceptible bacteria.

Available forms

Injection (powder): 5 million units, 20 million units
Injection (premixed in dextrose): 1 million units, 2 million units, 3 million units

NURSING PROCESS

⚕ Assessment

• Assess patient's infection before starting therapy, and regularly thereafter to monitor the drug's effectiveness.

• Before giving, ask the patient about any allergic reactions to penicillin, cephalosporins, and cephamycins. Negative history of penicillin allergy is no guarantee against future allergic reactions.

• Obtain specimen for culture and sensitivity tests before first dose. Start therapy pending test results.

• Assess renal, cardiac, and vascular conditions with physical exams and laboratory testing before start of therapy. Drug contains 1.7 mEq potassium and 0.3 mEq sodium per 1 million units. If risk of fluid overload or electrolyte imbalance, decrease dose and monitor electrolytes and renal tests frequently during therapy.
• Be alert for adverse reactions and drug interactions.
• Observe patient closely. Large doses and prolonged therapy raise the risk of neutropenia and bacterial or fungal superinfection especially in an elderly, debilitated, or immunosuppressed patient.
• Assess patient's and family's knowledge of drug therapy.

Nursing diagnoses
• Infection related to presence of bacteria
• Ineffective protection related to risk of hypersensitivity reactions to drug
• Deficient knowledge related to drug therapy

Planning and implementation
• Reconstitute vials with sterile water for injection, D_5W, or normal saline solution for injection. Volume of diluent varies with manufacturer.
• Inject deep into upper outer quadrant of buttocks in adult and in midlateral thigh in infant and young child. Avoid injection into or near major nerves or blood vessels to prevent severe neurovascular damage.
• ALERT: The various preparations of penicillin aren't interchangeable.
• Monitor level in patients taking large doses. A high level may lead to seizures. Take precautions and periodically monitor renal and hematopoietic function in patient receiving long-term therapy.
• Give drug I.M. deep into large muscle; warn patient that injection may be painful.
• ALERT: Don't confuse penicillamine with penicillin. Don't confuse penicillin G potassium with penicillin G sodium, penicillin G procaine, or penicillin G benzathine.
Patient teaching
• Tell patient to call prescriber if rash, fever, or chills develop.
• Warn patient that I.M. injection may be painful but that ice applied to site may ease discomfort.

Evaluation
• Patient is free from infection.
• Patient shows no signs of allergy.
• Patient and family state understanding of drug therapy.

penicillin G procaine
(benzylpenicillin procaine)
(pen-ih-SIL-in gee PROH-kayn)
Wycillin

Pharmacologic class: natural penicillin
Therapeutic class: long-acting antibiotic
Pregnancy risk category: B

Indications and dosages
▶ **Moderately severe infections of upper respiratory tract including pneumococcal pneumonia; tonsils; pharynx; and skin and soft tissues.** *Adults and children who weigh 27 kg (60 lb) or more:* 600,000 to 1.2 million units I.M. daily in 1 or 2 doses for at least 10 days. *Children who weigh less than 27 kg (60 lb):* 300,000 units I.M. daily in single dose for at least 10 days.
▶ **Anthrax caused by** *Bacillus anthracis,* **including prophylaxis after exposure to inhalation anthrax.** *Adults:* 1.2 million units I.M. q 12 hours for up to 60 days.
Children: 25,000 units/kg I.M. (maximum, 1.2 million units) q 12 hours for up to 60 days.
▶ **Cutaneous anthrax.** *Adults:* 600,000 to 1 million units I.M. daily for 5 to 60 days depending on source of exposure.
▶ **Necrotizing ulcerative gingivitis.** *Adults:* 600,000 to 1 million units I.M. daily.
▶ **Syphilis with negative CSF test.** *Adults and children older than age 12:* 600,000 units I.M. daily for 8 days.
▶ **Syphilis with no CSF test or positive CSF test.** *Adults and children older than age 12:* 600,000 units I.M. daily for 10 to 15 days.
▶ **Neurosyphilis.** *Adults and children older than age 12:* 2.4 million units I.M. daily with probenecid 500 mg P.O. q.i.d. for 10 to 14 days.
▶ **Congenital syphilis.** *Children less than 32 kg (70 lb):* 50,000 units/kg/day I.M. for 10 to 14 days.

Contraindications and cautions

• Contraindicated in patients hypersensitive to drug, other penicillins, or procaine.
• Use cautiously in patients with other drug allergies, especially to cephalosporins, and cephamycins.
⚕ **Lifespan:** In pregnant women, use cautiously. In breast-feeding women, don't use; drug appears in breast milk and drug use may sensitize infant to penicillin and cause adverse effects. Avoid use in newborns due to concern of sterile abscesses and procaine toxicity.

Adverse reactions

CNS: *seizures.*
Hematologic: *thrombocytopenia,* hemolytic anemia, *leukopenia.*
Musculoskeletal: arthralgia.
Other: hypersensitivity reactions (rash, urticaria, chills, fever, edema, prostration, *anaphylaxis*), overgrowth of nonsusceptible organisms.

Interactions

Drug-drug. *Aspirin, ethacrynic acid, furosemide, indomethacin, phenylbutazone, sulfonamides, thiazide diuretics:* May compete with penicillin G for renal tubular secretion and prolong penicillin half-life.
Heparin, oral anticoagulants: May increase risk of bleeding. Monitor PT, PTT, and INR. Monitor patient for bleeding.
Hormonal contraceptives: May decrease effectiveness of hormonal contraceptives and increase breakthrough bleeding. Advise patient to use alternative method during therapy.
Probenecid: May increase levels of penicillin. Probenecid may be used for this purpose.

Effects on lab test results

• May decrease hemoglobin level and hematocrit.
• May increase eosinophil count. May decrease platelet, WBC, and granulocyte counts.

Pharmacokinetics

Absorption: Slow.
Distribution: Distributed widely. CSF penetration poor. Drug is 45% to 68% protein-bound.
Metabolism: Occurs at injection site. From 16% to 30% metabolized to inactive compounds.

Excretion: Excreted primarily in urine. *Half-life:* 30 to 60 minutes.

Route	Onset	Peak	Duration
I.M.	Unknown	1–4 hr	1–2 days

Action

Chemical effect: Inhibits cell wall synthesis during microorganism multiplication.
Therapeutic effect: Kills susceptible bacteria.

Available forms

Injection: 600,000 units/ml

NURSING PROCESS

🔬 Assessment

• Assess patient's infection before starting therapy, and regularly thereafter to monitor the drug's effectiveness.
• Before giving, ask patient about allergic reactions to penicillin, cephalosporins, and cephamycins. Negative history of penicillin allergy is no guarantee against future allergic reaction.
• Assess for allergy to drug. Give test dose of 0.1 ml of 1% or 2% intradermally and observe for erythema, wheal, flare, or eruption. If positive for sensitivity, drug is contraindicated.
• Obtain specimen for culture and sensitivity tests before giving first dose. Start therapy pending test results.
• Be alert for adverse reactions and drug interactions.
• Observe patient closely. Large doses and prolonged therapy raise the risk of neutropenia and bacterial or fungal superinfection, especially in a geriatric, debilitated, or immunosuppressed patient.
• Assess patient's and family's knowledge of drug therapy.

🔆 Nursing diagnoses

• Infection related to presence of bacteria
• Ineffective protection related to risk of hypersensitivity reactions to drug
• Deficient knowledge related to drug therapy

▷ Planning and implementation

• Shake drug well before injection.
• Inject at a slow, steady rate to prevent needle from becoming blocked by suspended material in product.

P

• Inject deep into upper outer quadrant of buttocks in adults; in midlateral thigh in infants and small children. Avoid injection into or near major nerves or blood vessels to prevent severe neurovascular damage.
⊛ **ALERT:** Never give I.V.; doing so has caused cardiac arrest and death.
• If high dose is required for several days, consider change to I.V. penicillin G potassium or penicillin G sodium to avoid muscle fibrosis and atrophy from repeated I.M. injections.
• In patients with renal insufficiency or those taking high doses of I.M. drug, give penicillin G procaine at least 1 hour before bacteriostatic oral antibiotics such as aminoglycosides because it may inactivate such oral drugs.
⊛ **ALERT:** Don't confuse penicillin G procaine, with penicillin G sodium, penicillin G potassium, or penicillin G benzathine.
• The drug's extremely slow absorption makes allergic reactions difficult to treat. If patient develops signs of anaphylactic shock, such as rapidly developing dyspnea and hypotension, immediately stop giving the drug. Notify prescriber and immediately administer epinephrine, corticosteroids, antihistamines, or other resuscitative measures.
• For a patient receiving long-term therapy, periodically monitor renal and hematopoietic function.
⊛ **ALERT:** Be aware of the various preparations of penicillin. They aren't interchangeable.
Patient teaching
• Tell patient to call prescriber if rash, fever, or chills develop.
• Warn patient that injection may be painful but that ice applied to site may ease discomfort.
• Teach patient taking drug for active STD about safe sex practices, and address the risks of syphilis to fetus and neonate during pregnancy and the need to complete full drug course and follow-up testing.
• Instruct patient treated for active STD to bring partners in for treatment as well.

☑ **Evaluation**
• Patient is free from infection.
• Patient shows no signs of allergy.
• Patient and family state understanding of drug therapy.

penicillin G sodium (benzylpenicillin sodium)
(pen-ih-SIL-in gee SOH-dee-um)
Crystapen ◆

Pharmacologic class: natural penicillin
Therapeutic class: rapid-acting antibiotic
Pregnancy risk category: B

Indications and dosages

▶ **Moderate to severe systemic infections.**
Adults and children age 12 and older: Highly individualized; 1 to 24 million units daily I.M. or I.V. in divided doses q 4 to 6 hours.
Children: Highly individualized; 25,000 to 400,000 units/kg daily I.M. or I.V. in divided doses q 4 to 6 hours.
▶ **Bacterial endocarditis.** *Adults and children age 12 and older:* 5 to 30 million units daily I.V. in divided doses q 4 to 6 hours for 2 to 6 weeks depending on bacterial strain and severity of infection.
Children younger than age 12: 150,000 to 250,000 units/kg daily I.M. or I.V. in divided doses q 4 weeks.
▶ **Anthrax.** *Adults:* 5 to 20 million units I.V. daily in divided doses q 4 to 6 hours, for at least 14 days after symptoms abate. Or, 80,000 units/kg in the first hour, followed by a maintenance dose of 320,000 units/kg/day. The average adult dosage is 4 million units q 4 hours or 2 million units q 2 hours.
Children: 100,000 to 150,000 units/kg/day I.V. in divided doses q 4 to 6 hours for at least 14 days after symptoms lessen.
▶ **Neurosyphilis.** *Adults:* 18 to 24 million units I.V. daily in divided doses q 4 hours for 10 to 14 days.
▶ **Necrotizing ulcerative gingivitis.** *Adults:* 5 to 10 million units I.M. or I.V. daily.
Ⓢ **Adjust-a-dose:** For patients with renal impairment, if creatinine clearance is less than 10 ml/min, give full loading dose and then half of usual dose q 8 to 10 hours or usual dose q 12 to 18 hours; if creatinine clearance is more than 10 ml/minute, give full loading dose and then give half dose q 4 to 6 hours.

▼ **I.V. administration**

• Reconstitute vials with sterile water for injection, normal saline solution for injection, or

D_5W. Volume of diluent varies with manufacturer and concentration needed.

• For patient receiving 10 million units of drug or more daily, dilute in 1 to 2 liters of compatible solution and administer over 24 hours. Otherwise, give by intermittent I.V. infusion: Dilute drug in 50 to 100 ml and give over 1 to 2 hours every 4 to 6 hours.

• In a neonate or child, give divided doses, usually over 15 to 30 minutes.

⊗ **Incompatibilities**

Aminoglycosides, amphotericin B, bleomycin, chlorpromazine, cytarabine, fat emulsions 10%, heparin sodium, hydroxyzine hydrochloride, invert sugar 10%, lincomycin, methylprednisolone sodium succinate, potassium chloride, prochlorperazine mesylate, promethazine hydrochloride.

Contraindications and cautions

• Contraindicated in patients hypersensitive to the drug or other penicillins.

• Use cautiously in patients with other drug allergies, especially to cephalosporins, and cephamycins.

⚫ **Lifespan:** In pregnant women, use cautiously. In breast-feeding women, don't use; drug appears in breast milk and may sensitize infant to penicillin and cause adverse effects.

Adverse reactions

CNS: neuropathy, *seizures.*
CV: thrombophlebitis.
Hematologic: hemolytic anemia, *leukopenia, thrombocytopenia.*
Musculoskeletal: arthralgia.
Other: hypersensitivity reactions (exfoliative dermatitis, urticaria, *anaphylaxis*), overgrowth of nonsusceptible organisms, vein irritation, pain at injection site.

Interactions

Drug-drug. *Aminoglycoside antibiotics:* May deactivate some beta-lactam penicillins if mixed in same syringe or I.V. solution and administration set. Oral aminoglycoside level may be reduced when given with parenteral penicillins to a renally compromised patient.
Aspirin, ethacrynic acid, furosemide, indomethacin, phenylbutazone, sulfonamides, thiazide diuretics: May compete with penicillin G for renal tubular secretion and prolong penicillin half-life. Monitor patient.

Heparin, oral anticoagulants: May increase risk of bleeding. Monitor PT, PTT, and INR. Monitor patient for bleeding.
Hormonal contraceptives: May decrease effectiveness of hormonal contraceptives and increase breakthrough bleeding. Advise patient to use alternative contraception during therapy.
Probenecid: May increase levels of penicillin. Probenecid may be used for this purpose.

Effects on lab test results

• May decrease hemoglobin level and hematocrit.

• May increase eosinophil count. May decrease platelet, WBC, and granulocyte counts.

Pharmacokinetics

Absorption: Rapid.
Distribution: Wide. CSF penetration is poor but is enhanced in patients with inflamed meninges. 45% to 68% protein-bound.
Metabolism: At injection site. 16% to 30% to inactive compounds.
Excretion: Primarily in urine. *Half-life:* 30 to 60 minutes.

Route	Onset	Peak	Duration
I.V.	Immediate	Immediate	4 hr
I.M.	Unknown	15–30 min	4 hr

Action

Chemical effect: Inhibits cell wall synthesis during microorganism multiplication.
Therapeutic effect: Kills susceptible bacteria.

Available forms

Injection: 5-million-unit vial

NURSING PROCESS

Assessment

• Assess patient's infection before starting therapy, and regularly thereafter to monitor the drug's effectiveness.

• Before giving, ask patient about allergic reactions to penicillin, cephalosporins, and cephamycins. Negative history of penicillin allergy is no guarantee against future allergic reaction.

• Obtain specimen for culture and sensitivity tests before first dose. Start therapy pending test results.

• Assess renal, cardiac, and vascular conditions with physical exams and laboratory testing be-

fore the start of therapy. Drug contains 2 mEq sodium per 1 million units. Assess risk of fluid overload or electrolyte imbalance; decrease dose and monitor electrolytes and renal tests frequently during therapy.
- Be alert for adverse reactions and drug interactions.
- Observe patient closely. Large doses and prolonged therapy raise the risk of neutropenia and bacterial or fungal superinfection, especially in geriatric, debilitated, or immunosuppressed patients.
- Assess patient's and family's knowledge of drug therapy.

Nursing diagnoses
- Infection related to presence of bacteria
- Ineffective protection related to risk of hypersensitivity reactions to drug
- Deficient knowledge related to drug therapy

Planning and implementation
- Give drug I.M. deep in upper outer quadrant of buttocks in adult; in midlateral thigh in young child. Don't massage injection site. Avoid injection near major nerves or blood vessels to prevent severe neurovascular damage.
- Give penicillin G sodium at least 1 hour before bacteriostatic antibiotics, and if given I.M., at different sites.
- Periodically monitor renal and hematopoietic function in patient receiving long-term therapy.

ALERT: Be aware of the various preparations of penicillin. They aren't interchangeable.
- Monitor level in patient taking large doses. A high level may lead to seizures. Take precautions.

ALERT: Don't confuse penicillamine with penicillin. Don't confuse penicillin G sodium with penicillin G potassium, penicillin G procaine, or penicillin G benzathine.

Patient teaching
- Tell patient to report discomfort at I.V. site
- Warn patient that I.M. injection may be painful but that ice applied to site may ease discomfort.

Evaluation
- Patient is free from infection.
- Patient shows no signs of allergy.
- Patient and family state understanding of drug therapy.

penicillin V (phenoxymethylpenicillin)
(pen-ih-SIL-in VEE)

penicillin V potassium (phenoxymethylpenicillin potassium)
Abbocillin VK◇, Apo-Pen-VK♦, Beepen-VK, Cilicaine VK◇, Nadopen-V♦, Nadopen-V-200♦, Nadopen-V-400♦, Novo-Pen-VK♦, Nu-Pen-VK, Pen-Vee K, PVF K♦, PVK◇, V-Cillin K, Veetids

Pharmacologic class: natural penicillin
Therapeutic class: antibiotic
Pregnancy risk category: B

Indications and dosages
▶ **Mild to moderately severe infections of upper respiratory tract (including pneumococcal pneumonia), oropharynx, sinuses, and skin and soft tissues; necrotizing ulcerative gingivitis.** *Adults and children older than age 12:* 125 to 500 mg (200,000 to 800,000 units) P.O. q 6 to 8 hours.
Children age 1 month to 12 years: 15 to 62.5 mg/kg (25,000 to 100,000 units/kg) P.O. daily, in divided doses q 4 to 8 hours.
▶ **Prophylaxis for rheumatic fever.** *Adults and children older than age 12:* 125 to 250 mg P.O. b.i.d.
▶ **Prophylaxis for pneumococcal infections‡.** *Children age 5 and older:* 250 mg P.O. b.i.d.
Children 3 months to younger than age 5: 125 mg P.O. b.i.d.
▶ **Lyme disease‡.** *Adults:* 250 to 500 mg P.O. q.i.d. for 10 to 20 days.

Contraindications and cautions
- Contraindicated in patients hypersensitive to the drug or other penicillins.
- Use cautiously in patients with other drug allergies, especially to cephalosporins and cephamycins and in patients with hyperacidity of the GI tract since decreased pH can inactivate drug.

Lifespan: In pregnant women, use cautiously. In breast-feeding women, don't use; drug appears in breast milk and use of drug may sensitize infant to penicillin and cause adverse effects.

Adverse reactions

CNS: neuropathy, *seizures.*
GI: *epigastric distress,* vomiting, diarrhea, *nausea.*
Hematologic: eosinophilia, hemolytic anemia, *leukopenia, thrombocytopenia.*
Other: hypersensitivity reactions (rash, urticaria, chills, fever, edema, *anaphylaxis*), overgrowth of nonsusceptible organisms.

Interactions

Drug-drug. *Beta blockers:* May increase risk of anaphylactic reactions to oral penicillins.
Hormonal contraceptives containing estrogen: May decrease effectiveness of hormonal contraceptive. Monitor patient for breakthrough bleeding. Advise patient to use alternative forms of birth control.
Oral neomycin: May reduce oral penicillin level. Monitor patient.
Probenecid: May increase level of penicillin. Probenecid may be used for this purpose.

Effects on lab test results

- May decrease hemoglobin level and hematocrit.
- May increase eosinophil count. May decrease platelet, WBC, and granulocyte counts.

Pharmacokinetics

Absorption: About 60% to 75%.
Distribution: Distributed widely. CSF penetration is poor. Drug is 75% to 89% protein-bound.
Metabolism: Primarily in small intestine.
Excretion: Excreted primarily in urine. *Half-life:* 30 minutes.

Route	Onset	Peak	Duration
P.O.	Unknown	30–60 min	6–8 hr

Action

Chemical effect: Inhibits cell wall synthesis during microorganism multiplication.
Therapeutic effect: Kills susceptible bacteria.

Available forms

penicillin V
Oral suspension: 125 mg/5 ml, 250 mg/5 ml (after reconstitution)
Tablets: 250 mg, 500 mg
penicillin V potassium
Capsules: 250 mg ◊

Oral suspension: 125 mg/5 ml, 250 mg/5 ml (after reconstitution)
Tablets: 125 mg, 250 mg, 500 mg
Tablets (film-coated): 250 mg, 500 mg

NURSING PROCESS

🖉 Assessment

- Assess patient's infection before starting therapy, and regularly thereafter to monitor the drug's effectiveness.
- Before giving drug, ask patient about any allergic reactions to penicillin, cephalosporins, and cephamycins. Negative history of penicillin allergy is no guarantee against future allergic reaction.
- Obtain specimen for culture and sensitivity tests before giving first dose. Start therapy pending test results.
- Periodically assess renal and hematopoietic function in patient receiving long-term therapy.
- Be alert for adverse reactions and drug interactions.
- Observe patient closely. Large doses and prolonged therapy raise the risk of bacterial or fungal superinfection, especially in geriatric, debilitated, or immunosuppressed patients.
- Assess patient's and family's knowledge of drug therapy.

📋 Nursing diagnoses

- Infection related to presence of bacteria
- Ineffective protection related to risk of hypersensitivity reactions to drug
- Deficient knowledge related to drug therapy

🔼 Planning and implementation

- Give drug at least 1 hour before bacteriostatic antibiotics.
- Ⓢ **ALERT:** Don't confuse penicillamine with penicillin.
Patient teaching
- Tell patient to take drug exactly as prescribed, even after he feels better.
- Tell patient that drug may be taken without regard to meals. If GI disturbances occur, drug may be taken with meals.
- Warn patient never to use leftover penicillin V for new illness or to share penicillin with family and friends.
- Inform patients using oral solution that any remaining solution must be discarded after 14 days.

P

• Drug of choice for endocarditis prophylaxis is amoxicillin
• Tell patient to call prescriber if rash, fever, or chills develop.

🗹 Evaluation
• Patient is free from infection.
• Patient shows no signs of allergy.
• Patient and family state understanding of drug therapy.

pentamidine isethionate
(pen-TAM-eh-deen ighs-eh-THIGH-oh-nayt)
NebuPent, Pentacarinat ♦, Pentam 300

Pharmacologic class: diamidine derivative
Therapeutic class: antiprotozoal
Pregnancy risk category: C

Indications and dosages
▶ **Pneumocystis jiroveci (carinii) pneumonia.**
Adults and children: 4 mg/kg I.V. or I.M. once daily for 14 to 21 days.
▶ **Prevention of *P. jiroveci (carinii)* pneumonia in high-risk patients.** *Adults:* 300 mg by inhalation (using Respirgard II jet nebulizer) once q 4 weeks.

▼ I.V. administration
• Reconstitute drug with 3 ml of sterile water for injection; then dilute in 50 to 250 ml of D_5W. Inject over 1 to 2 hours.
• To minimize hypotension, infuse drug slowly with patient lying down.
⊗ **Incompatibilities**
Aldesleukin, cephalosporins, fluconazole, foscarnet.

Contraindications and cautions
• Contraindicated in patients with history of anaphylactic reaction to drug.
• Use cautiously in patients with hypertension, hypotension, hypoglycemia, hypocalcemia, leukopenia, thrombocytopenia, anemia, pancreatitis, hepatic or renal dysfunction or history of ventricular tachycardia or Stevens-Johnson syndrome.
❄ **Lifespan:** In pregnant women, use cautiously. In breast-feeding women, drug isn't recommended.

Adverse reactions
Parenteral form
CNS: confusion, fever, hallucinations, dizziness, neuralgia.
CV: *hypotension,* facial flushing, *ventricular tachycardia,* cardiac arrhythmias.
GI: *pancreatitis,* metallic taste, anorexia, nausea, vomiting, diarrhea, abdominal discomfort.
GU: *renal toxicity, acute renal failure.*
Hematologic: *leukopenia, thrombocytopenia, anemia.*
Metabolic: *hypoglycemia,* hyperglycemia, *hypocalcemia, hyperkalemia.*
Respiratory: cough, *bronchospasm.*
Skin: pruritus, rash, *Stevens-Johnson syndrome.*
Other: *sterile abscess, pain and induration at injection site* with I.M. route; phlebitis, tissue necrosis or sloughing from extravasation with I.V. route; *anaphylactoid reactions.*
Aerosol form
CNS: *fatigue, dizziness,* decreased taste or smell, fever, confusion, headache, tremors.
CV: *chest pain,* hypertension, hypotension.
GI: abdominal discomfort, anorexia, *metallic taste,* nausea, vomiting, diarrhea, *pancreatitis, pharyngitis.*
Hematologic: *leukopenia, thrombocytopenia, anemia.*
Metabolic: hyperglycemia, *hypocalcemia, hypoglycemia.*
Respiratory: *shortness of breath, chest congestion, cough,* BRONCHOSPASM.
Skin: *rash.*
Other: *night sweats, chills.*

Interactions
Drug-drug. Aminoglycosides, amphotericin B, capreomycin, cisplatin, colistin, methoxyflurane, polymyxin B, vancomycin: Increases risk of nephrotoxicity. Monitor patient closely.

Effects on lab test results
• May increase BUN, creatinine, potassium, and liver enzyme levels. May decrease calcium and hemoglobin levels and hematocrit. May increase or severely decrease glucose levels.
• May decrease WBC and platelet counts.

Pharmacokinetics
Absorption: Limited after aerosol administration. Well absorbed after I.M. administration.

Reactions may be *common,* uncommon, *life-threatening,* or COMMON AND LIFE-THREATENING.

Distribution: Drug appears to be extensively tissue-bound. CNS penetration is poor. Extent of protein-binding is unknown.
Metabolism: Unknown.
Excretion: Excreted unchanged in urine. *Half-life:* Varies according to route of administration: 9 to 13¼ hours for I.M., about 6½ hours for I.V., and unknown for aerosol.

Route	Onset	Peak	Duration
I.V.	Unknown	Immediate	Unknown
I.M.	Unknown	30 min–1 hr	Unknown
Aerosol	Unknown	Unknown	Unknown

Action

Chemical effect: Interferes with infectious organism's biosynthesis of DNA, RNA, phospholipids, and proteins.
Therapeutic effect: Hinders growth of susceptible organisms.

Available forms

Aerosol: 300-mg vial
Injection: 300-mg vial

NURSING PROCESS

Assessment
• Assess patient's infection before starting therapy and regularly thereafter to monitor the drug's effectiveness.
⊛ **ALERT:** Monitor glucose level before therapy, daily during parenteral administration, and regularly afterwards. Glucose level may decrease initially, and hypoglycemia may be severe. Hyperglycemia and insulin-dependent diabetes mellitus may follow months after therapy ends and may be permanent.
• Monitor CBC, platelet count, calcium, liver function tests, potassium, and renal function tests before, during, and after therapy. Monitor BUN, creatinine, calcium, and potassium levels daily during parenteral therapy due to risks of acute renal failure, hypocalcemia, and hyperkalemia.
• Closely monitor blood pressure during I.V. administration.
⊛ **ALERT:** Screen and treat patient for tuberculosis (TB) before using inhaled form. The risk of spreading TB to health care personnel and family members increases with high-pressure nebulizer use due to cough and droplet spread. If you're pregnant or plan to become pregnant,

have another staff member care for this patient. Standard personal protection equipment is ineffective. Use care in choosing a room for patient using inhaled form.
• Be alert for adverse reactions and drug interactions.
• Assess patient's and family's knowledge of drug therapy.

Nursing diagnoses
• Infection related to presence of organisms
• Risk for injury related to drug-induced adverse CNS reactions
• Deficient knowledge related to drug therapy

Planning and implementation
• For I.M. use, reconstitute drug with 3 ml of sterile water to make solution containing 100 mg/ml; administer deeply, preferably using Z-track technique. Expect pain and induration at site.
• In patient with AIDS, this drug may produce less severe adverse reactions than cotrimoxazole and may be drug of choice.
• Give aerosol form only by Respirgard II jet nebulizer manufactured by Marquest (flow rate of 5 to 7 liters/minute from 40 to 50 pounds per square inch [psi] compressor). Dosage is based on particle size and delivery rate of this device; don't change to low-pressure (below 20 psi) compressors.
• To use aerosol, mix contents of one vial in 6 ml of sterile water for injection. Don't use normal saline solution; it will cause precipitation.
• Don't mix with other drugs.
• Inhaling drug may induce bronchospasm or cough, especially in patients with a history of smoking or asthma.
Patient teaching
• Instruct patient to use aerosol device until chamber is empty, which may take up to 45 minutes.
• Advise patient with significant cough and bronchospasm to report effects to prescriber. Aerosol bronchodilator may be prescribed for use just before therapy.
• Warn patient that I.M. injection is painful. Application of warm soaks is helpful.
• Tell patient to report light-headedness or signs and symptoms of hypoglycemia immediately.

☑ **Evaluation**
• Patient is free from infection.
• Patient sustains no injuries because of drug-induced adverse CNS reactions.
• Patient and family state understanding of drug therapy.

pentazocine hydrochloride
(pen-TAZ-oh-seen high-droh-KLOR-ighd)
Talwin

pentazocine hydrochloride and acetaminophen
Talacen

pentazocine and naloxone hydrochlorides
Talwin NX

pentazocine lactate
Talwin

Pharmacologic class: opioid agonist-antagonist, opioid partial agonist
Therapeutic class: analgesic, adjunct to anesthesia
Pregnancy risk category: C
Controlled substance schedule: IV

Indications and dosages
▶ **Moderate to severe pain.** *Adults:* 50 to 100 mg Talwin NX P.O. q 3 to 4 hours, p.r.n. Maximum oral dosage, 600 mg daily. Or, 1 tablet Talacen P.O. q 4 hours, up to 6 tablets daily. Or, 30 mg I.M., I.V., or subcutaneously q 3 to 4 hours, p.r.n. Maximum total parenteral dosage is 360 mg in 24 hours. Single doses above 30 mg I.V. or 60 mg I.M. or subcutaneously aren't recommended.
▶ **Labor.** *Women:* 30 mg I.M. as a single dose or 20 mg I.V. q 2 to 3 hours when contractions become regular.

▼ I.V. administration
• Give drug by direct I.V. injection.
• Administer slowly.
⊗ **Incompatibilities**
Aminophylline, amobarbital, glycopyrrolate, heparin sodium, nafcillin sodium, pentobarbital

sodium, phenobarbital sodium, sodium bicarbonate.

Contraindications and cautions
• Contraindicated in patients hypersensitive to the drug or any of its components.
• Use cautiously in patients with hepatic or renal disease, acute MI, head injury, increased intracranial pressure, or respiratory depression.
⚘ **Lifespan:** In pregnant women, use cautiously. In breast-feeding women, use cautiously; it's unknown if the drug appears in breast milk. In children younger than age 12, drug isn't recommended. In the elderly, use cautiously because they may be more sensitive to the drug's CNS effects.

Adverse reactions
CNS: *sedation,* visual disturbances, hallucinations, drowsiness, *dizziness, light-headedness,* confusion, *euphoria,* headache, psychotomimetic effects.
CV: hypotension, *shock.*
EENT: dry mouth, dysgeusia.
GI: nausea, vomiting, constipation.
GU: urine retention.
Respiratory: *respiratory depression.*
Skin: induration, nodules, sloughing, and sclerosis of injection site.
Other: hypersensitivity reactions *(anaphylaxis),* physical and psychological dependence.

Interactions
Drug-drug. *CNS depressants:* May have additive effects. Use together cautiously.
Fluoxetine: May cause diaphoresis, ataxia, flushing, and tremor suggestive of serotonin syndrome. Use together cautiously.
Opioid analgesics: May decrease analgesic effect. Avoid using together.
Drug-lifestyle. *Alcohol use:* May have additive effects. Discourage using together.
Smoking: May increase requirements for pentazocine. Monitor drug's effectiveness; urge patient to stop smoking.

Effects on lab test results
• May interfere with laboratory tests for urinary 17-hydroxycorticosteroids.

Pharmacokinetics
Absorption: Well absorbed after P.O. or parenteral administration, although P.O. form un-

dergoes first-pass metabolism in liver and less than 20% of dose reaches systemic circulation unchanged. Bioavailability is increased in patients with hepatic dysfunction; patients with cirrhosis absorb 60% to 70% of drug.
Distribution: Appears to be widely distributed throughout body.
Metabolism: Metabolized in liver. Metabolism may be prolonged in patients with impaired hepatic function.
Excretion: Excreted primarily in urine, with very small amounts excreted in feces. *Half-life:* 2 to 3 hours.

Route	Onset	Peak	Duration
P.O.	15–30 min	60–90 min	2–3 hr
I.V.	2–3 min	15–30 min	2–3 hr
I.M., SubQ	15–20 min	15–60 min	4–6 hr

Action

Chemical effect: Binds with opioid receptors at many sites in CNS, altering pain response by unknown mechanism.
Therapeutic effect: Relieves pain.

Available forms

pentazocine hydrochloride
Tablets: 50 mg ◊
pentazocine hydrochloride and acetaminophen
Tablets: 25 mg pentazocine hydrochloride and 650 mg acetaminophen
pentazocine and naloxone hydrochlorides
Tablets: 50 mg pentazocine hydrochloride and 0.5 mg naloxone hydrochloride
pentazocine lactate
Injection: 30 mg/ml

NURSING PROCESS

Assessment
• Assess patient's pain before and after giving the drug.
• Monitor vital signs closely, especially respirations.
• Be alert for adverse reactions and drug interactions.
• Assess patient's and family's knowledge of drug therapy.

Nursing diagnoses
• Acute pain related to condition
• Ineffective breathing pattern related to drug-induced respiratory depression

• Deficient knowledge related to drug therapy

Planning and implementation
• Talwin NX, the oral pentazocine available in the U.S., contains the opioid antagonist naloxone, which prevents illicit use.
ALERT: Talwin NX is for P.O. use only. Severe, potentially fatal reaction may occur if given by injection.
• When giving I.M. or subcutaneously, rotate injection sites to minimize tissue irritation. If possible, avoid giving subcutaneously.
• Drug has opioid antagonist properties. May precipitate withdrawal syndrome in an opioid-dependent patient.
• Dependence may occur with prolonged use.
ALERT: If respiratory rate drops significantly, hold drug and notify prescriber. Have naloxone readily available to reverse respiratory depression.
Patient teaching
• Warn ambulatory patient about getting out of bed or walking. Warn outpatient to avoid hazardous activities until the drug's CNS effects are known.
• Inform patient about the risk of dependence.

Evaluation
• Patient is free from pain.
• Patient maintains respiratory rate and pattern within normal limits.
• Patient and family state understanding of drug therapy.

pentetate calcium trisodium (Ca-DTPA)
(PEN-tuh-tayt KAL-see-um try-SOE-dee-um)

pentetate zinc trisodium (Zn-DTPA)

Pharmacologic class: chelating drug
Therapeutic class: radiation emergency drug
Pregnancy risk category: C (Ca-DTPA); B (Zn-DTPA)

Indications and dosages

▶ **To increase the rate of plutonium, americium, or curium elimination in patients with internal contamination.** *Adults and children* *age 12 and older:* Initially, 1 g Ca-DTPA by slow I.V. push over 3 to 4 minutes (or dilute in 100 to 250 ml D_5W, Ringer's lactate, or normal saline solution and infuse over 30 minutes) within the first 24 hours of exposure. Then, 1 g once daily of Zn-DTPA by slow I.V. push over 3 to 4 minutes (or dilute in 100 to 250 ml D_5W, Ringer's lactate, or normal saline solution and infuse over 30 minutes) until radioactive substances are removed. If patient was exposed by inhalation, give solution by nebulizer at a ratio of 1:1 with sterile water or saline.

Children younger than age 12: Initially, 14 mg/kg Ca-DTPA (maximum dose, 1 g) by slow I.V. push over 3 to 4 minutes within the first 24 hours of exposure. Then, 14 mg/kg once daily of Zn-DTPA by slow I.V. push over 3 to 4 minutes (maximum dose, 1 g) until radioactive substances are removed.

▽ I.V. administration

• Use a sterile filter if particles appear after ampule is opened.
• Give by slow I.V. push over 3 to 4 minutes or dilute in 100 to 250 ml of D_5W, lactated Ringer's solution, or normal saline solution and infuse over 30 minutes.
• Store at room temperature.
⊗ **Incompatibilities**
None reported.

Contraindications and cautions

• Use cautiously in patients with severe hemochromatosis. Use inhalation route cautiously in patients with asthma.
⚞ **Lifespan:** In pregnant women, start and continue with Zn-DTPA unless patient has a high level of internal radioactive contamination. If the level of contamination is high, start with a single dose of Ca-DTPA and vitamin or mineral supplements containing zinc. Breast-feeding women should stop breast-feeding or use a different drug; it's unknown if drug appears in breast milk, but radiocontaminants do. Patient shouldn't breast-feed during therapy and should take precautions when discarding breast milk. In children, safety and effectiveness of inhaled form haven't been established.

Adverse reactions

CNS: headache, light-headedness.
CV: chest pain.
GI: diarrhea, metallic taste, nausea.

Skin: dermatitis, injection site reactions.
Other: allergic reaction.

Interactions

None known.

Effects on lab test results

• May decrease manganese, magnesium, and zinc levels with prolonged therapy.

Pharmacokinetics

Absorption: Unknown, not in GI system, organs, erythrocytes; 20% in lungs with inhalational route.
Distribution: Rapid, throughout extracellular space after I.V. use.
Metabolism: Minimal.
Excretion: Almost exclusively in urine by glomerular filtration. *Half-life:* About 7 hours.

Route	Onset	Peak	Duration
I.V., inhalation	1½ min	Unknown	< 24 hr

Action

Chemical effect: Forms stable complexes with metal ions by exchanging calcium or zinc ions for radioactive plutonium, americium, or curium ions. The complexes are excreted into urine faster than the unbound radioactive contaminants, thus speeding removal from the body.
Therapeutic effect: Reduces the effects of exposure to radioactive plutonium, americium, or curium.

Available forms

Injection: 200 mg/ml in 5-ml single-use vials

NURSING PROCESS

⚗ Assessment

• Obtain history of patient's radiation exposure before therapy.
• Obtain baseline CBC, zinc, BUN, and electrolyte levels, urinalysis, and blood and urine radioassays before starting therapy.
• During therapy, measure the radioactivity of blood, urine, and feces weekly.
• Regularly monitor urinalysis, CBC, BUN, and electrolyte levels during therapy.
• Assess patient's and family's knowledge of drug therapy.

⊞ Nursing diagnoses
- Potential for injury related to internal radioactive contamination
- Ineffective protection related to drug-induced depletion of endogenous trace metals
- Deficient knowledge related to drug therapy

⊠ Planning and implementation
- The binding capacity of Ca-DTPA is greatest in the first 24 hours after exposure.
- **⑤ ALERT:** If patient needs further therapy after Ca-DTPA, switch to Zn-DTPA to avoid mineral depletion. If Zn-DTPA isn't available, continue Ca-DTPA as long as the patient receives supplemental zinc, magnesium, and manganese.
- When the route of contamination is unknown or if contamination occurs by multiple routes, use I.V. drug.
- If contamination occurs only by inhalation and within 24 hours, use nebulizer. Dilute drug 1:1 with sterile water or saline solution.
- The elimination rate is based on the quantity of radioactivity taken in.

Patient teaching
- Instruct patient to drink plenty of fluids so that he urinates frequently.
- Remind patient that drug eliminates radioactivity through urine, which may make urine highly radioactive and dangerous to others.
- Instruct patient to flush the toilet several times after each use and to wash hands thoroughly after urinating.
- If the patient is coughing, tell him to dispose of phlegm carefully and not to swallow it, if possible.
- Tell parents of a young child to dispose of dirty diapers properly and to avoid handling urine, feces, or phlegm.

☑ Evaluation
- The effects of radiation contamination are reduced.
- Patient experiences minimal loss of trace metals or receives mineral supplements as appropriate.
- Patient and family state understanding of drug therapy.

pentobarbital (pentobarbitone)
(pen-toh-BAR-beh-tol)
Nembutal

pentobarbital sodium
Nembutal Sodium, Novo-Pentobarb ◊

Pharmacologic class: barbiturate
Therapeutic class: anticonvulsant, sedative-hypnotic
Pregnancy risk category: D
Controlled substance schedule: II (oral and parenteral); III (rectal)

Indications and dosages

▶ **Sedation.** *Adults:* 20 to 40 mg P.O. b.i.d., t.i.d., or q.i.d.
Children: 2 to 6 mg/kg daily P.O. or P.R. t.i.d. Maximum daily dosage, 100 mg.
▶ **Short-term therapy for insomnia.** *Adults:* 100 to 200 mg P.O. h.s. or 150 to 200 mg I.M. Or, 120 to 200 mg P.R. Or, initially, 100 mg I.V. with additional small doses, to a total of 500 mg.
Children: 2 to 6 mg/kg I.M. Maximum dose is 100 mg. Or, for children ages 2 months to 1 year, give 30 mg P.R.; for children ages 1 to 4 years, give 30 or 60 mg P.R.; for children ages 5 to 12 years, give 60 mg P.R.; for children ages 12 to 14 years, give 60 or 120 mg P.R.
▶ **Preoperative sedation.** *Adults:* 150 to 200 mg I.M.
Children: 5 mg/kg P.O. or I.M. In children younger than age 10, the dose is usually given rectally.

▼ I.V. administration

- I.V. use of barbiturates may cause severe respiratory depression, laryngospasm, or hypotension. Have emergency resuscitation equipment available.
- To minimize deterioration, use I.V injection solution within 30 minutes after opening container. Don't use cloudy solution.
- Reserve I.V. injection for emergencies and give under close supervision. Give slowly (50 mg/minute or less).
- Parenteral solution is alkaline. Local tissue reactions and injection site pain may result. Monitor site for irritation and infiltration; extravasation can lead to tissue damage and necrosis.

P

Assess patency of I.V. site before and during administration.

⊗ **Incompatibilities**
Other I.V. drugs or solutions.

Contraindications and cautions

• Contraindicated in patients with porphyria or hypersensitivity to barbiturates.
• Use cautiously in debilitated patients and in those with acute or chronic pain, depression, suicidal tendencies, history of drug abuse, or renal or hepatic impairment.
⚠ **Lifespan:** In pregnant and breast-feeding women, drug isn't recommended. In the elderly, use cautiously because of possible delayed renal excretion.

Adverse reactions

CNS: *drowsiness, lethargy, hangover,* paradoxical excitement in elderly patients.
GI: nausea, vomiting.
Hematologic: worsening of porphyria.
Respiratory: *respiratory depression.*
Skin: rash, urticaria, *Stevens-Johnson syndrome.*
Other: *angioedema.*

Interactions

Drug-drug. *CNS depressants, including opioid analgesics:* May cause excessive CNS and respiratory depression. Use together cautiously.
Corticosteroids, doxycycline, estrogens and hormonal contraceptives, oral anticoagulants quinidine, theophylline, verapamil: May enhance metabolism of these drugs. Monitor patient for decreased effect.
MAO inhibitors: May inhibit barbiturate metabolism and prolong CNS depression. Reduce barbiturate dosage.
Metoprolol, propranolol: May reduce the effects of these drugs. Increase beta blocker dose.
Rifampin: May decrease barbiturate levels. Monitor patient for decreased effect.
Drug-lifestyle. *Alcohol use:* May impair coordination, increase CNS effects, and cause death. Strongly discourage use together.

Effects on lab test results

None reported.

Pharmacokinetics

Absorption: Rapid after P.O. use. Unknown after I.M. use.

Distribution: Wide. About 35% to 45% of drug is protein-bound.
Metabolism: In liver.
Excretion: 99% of drug is in urine. *Half-life:* 35 to 50 hours.

Route	Onset	Peak	Duration
P.O.	≤ 15 min	30–60 min	1–4 hr
I.V.	Immediate	Immediate	15 min
I.M.	10–25 min	Unknown	Unknown

Action

Chemical effect: May interfere with transmission of impulses from thalamus to cortex of brain.
Therapeutic effect: Promotes sleep and calmness.

Available forms

Capsules: 50 mg, 100 mg
Injection: 50 mg/ml
Suppositories: 30 mg, 60 mg, 120 mg, 200 mg

NURSING PROCESS

Assessment
• Assess patient's condition before starting therapy, and regularly thereafter to monitor the drug's effectiveness.
• An elderly patient may be more sensitive to the drug's CNS effects.
• Inspect patient's skin. Skin eruptions may precede life-threatening reactions to barbiturate therapy.
• Be alert for adverse reactions and drug interactions.
• Assess patient's and family's knowledge of drug therapy.

Nursing diagnoses
• Disturbed sleep pattern related to condition
• Risk for injury related to drug-induced adverse CNS reactions
• Deficient knowledge related to drug therapy

Planning and implementation
• Give I.M. injection deeply. Superficial injection may cause pain, sterile abscess, and sloughing.
⊛ **ALERT:** If skin reactions occur, stop drug and notify prescriber. In some patients, high fever, stomatitis, headache, or rhinitis may precede skin reactions.

• Drug has no analgesic effect and may cause restlessness or delirium in a patient with pain.
⑤ **ALERT:** Long-term use isn't recommended; drug loses its effectiveness in promoting sleep after 14 days of continued use. Long-term high doses may cause dependence and may lead to withdrawal symptoms if drug is suddenly stopped. Gradually stop giving barbiturates.
⑤ **ALERT:** Don't confuse pentobarbital with phenobarbital.

Patient teaching
• Warn patient about performing activities that require alertness or physical coordination. For an acute care inpatient, particularly an elderly patient, supervise walking and raise bed rails.
• Inform patient that morning hangover is common after hypnotic dose, which suppresses REM sleep. Patient's dreams may increase after therapy stops.
• Tell woman who uses hormonal contraceptives to use barrier-method birth control because drug may decrease contraceptive effect.

☑ Evaluation
• Patient reports satisfactory sleep.
• Patient sustains no injuries from drug-induced adverse CNS reactions.
• Patient and family state understanding of drug therapy.

pentoxifylline
(pen-tok-SIH-fi-lin)
Trental

Pharmacologic class: xanthine derivative
Therapeutic class: hemorheologic
Pregnancy risk category: C

Indications and dosages
▶ **Intermittent claudication caused by chronic occlusive vascular disease.** *Adults:* 400 mg P.O. t.i.d. with meals for at least 8 weeks.

Contraindications and cautions
• Contraindicated in patients who are intolerant of methylxanthines, such as caffeine and theophylline, and in those with recent cerebral or retinal hemorrhage.
※ **Lifespan:** In pregnant women, use cautiously. In breast-feeding women, drug isn't recom-

mended. In children, safety and effectiveness haven't been established.

Adverse reactions
CNS: headache, dizziness.
GI: dyspepsia, nausea, vomiting.

Interactions
Drug-drug. *Anticoagulants:* May increase anticoagulant effect. Monitor PT and INR, and adjust anticoagulant dosage as needed.
Antihypertensives: May increase hypotensive effect. Adjust dosage; monitor patient's blood pressure closely.
Theophylline: May increase theophylline level. Monitor level; adjust theophylline dosage.
Drug-lifestyle. *Smoking:* May cause vasoconstriction. Advise patient to avoid smoking because it may worsen his condition.

Effects on lab test results
None reported.

Pharmacokinetics
Absorption: Rapid and almost completely absorbed by the GI tract.
Distribution: Bound by erythrocyte membrane.
Metabolism: Extensively by erythrocytes and liver.
Excretion: Primarily in urine. *Half-life:* About 30 to 45 minutes.

Route	Onset	Peak	Duration
P.O.	Unknown	1 hr	Unknown

Action
Chemical effect: May increase RBC flexibility and lower blood viscosity.
Therapeutic effect: Improves capillary blood flow.

Available forms
Tablets (controlled-release): 400 mg
Tablets (extended-release): 400 mg

NURSING PROCESS

☞ Assessment
• Assess patient's condition before starting therapy, and regularly thereafter to monitor the drug's effectiveness.
• Be alert for adverse reactions and drug interactions.

- In an elderly patient, watch for increased CNS effects.
- If adverse GI reaction occurs, monitor patient's hydration.
- Assess patient's and family's knowledge of drug therapy.

🔵 Nursing diagnoses
- Ineffective peripheral tissue perfusion related to condition
- Risk for deficient fluid volume related to drug-induced adverse GI reactions
- Deficient knowledge related to drug therapy

▷ Planning and implementation
- Drug is useful in patient who isn't a good surgical candidate.
- Report adverse reactions to prescriber; dose may need to be lowered.
- Monitor blood pressure for hypotension, particularly in patients also on antihypertensive therapy.

⚠ ALERT: Don't confuse Trental with Trendar or Trandate.

Patient teaching
- Advise patient to take drug with meals to minimize GI upset.
- Instruct patient to swallow drug whole, without breaking, crushing, or chewing.
- Tell patient to report adverse GI or CNS reactions.
- Advise patient not to smoke because nicotine causes vasoconstriction that can worsen his condition.
- Advise patient that effects of drug may not be seen for 2 to 4 weeks.
- Tell patient not to stop taking the drug during first 8 weeks of therapy unless directed by prescriber.

✅ Evaluation
- Patient has adequate peripheral tissue perfusion.
- Patient maintains adequate hydration throughout therapy.
- Patient and family state understanding of drug therapy.

pergolide mesylate
(PER-goh-lighd MES-ih-layt)
Permax

Pharmacologic class: dopaminergic agonist
Therapeutic class: antiparkinsonian
Pregnancy risk category: B

Indications and dosages

▶ **Adjunct therapy with levodopa and carbidopa in management of symptoms caused by Parkinson's disease.** *Adults:* Initially, 0.05 mg P.O. daily for first 2 days; increase dose by 0.1 to 0.15 mg q third day over 12 days. Increase later doses by 0.25 mg q third day until optimum response is seen. Drug usually is given in divided doses t.i.d. Gradual reductions in levodopa and carbidopa dosage may be made during dosage adjustment. Usual total daily dosage, 3 mg.

Contraindications and cautions

- Contraindicated in patients hypersensitive to the drug or ergot alkaloids.
- Use cautiously in patients prone to arrhythmias and in patients with a history of pleuritis, pleural effusion, pleural fibrosis, pericarditis, pericardial effusion, cardiac valvulopathy or retroperitoneal fibrosis.
- Because of the risk of increased sedative effects, use caution when patient is also taking other CNS depressants.
- Hypotension may occur, especially during initial therapy.
- Symptoms similar to neuroleptic malignant syndrome may occur with rapid dose reduction.

⚘ Lifespan: In pregnant women, use cautiously. In breast-feeding women and in children, safety and effectiveness haven't been established.

Adverse reactions

CNS: headache, asthenia, *dyskinesia, dizziness, hallucinations,* dystonia, confusion, *somnolence,* syncope, insomnia, anxiety, depression, tremor, abnormal dreams, personality disorder, psychosis, abnormal gait, akathisia, extrapyramidal syndrome, incoordination, akinesia, hypertonia, neuralgia, speech disorder, twitching, paresthesia.

CV: chest pain; *orthostatic hypotension;* vasodilation; palpitations; hypotension; hypertension; *arrhythmias; MI;* facial, peripheral, or generalized edema; *valvulopathy, fibrosis.*
EENT: *rhinitis,* epistaxis, abnormal vision, diplopia, eye disorder.
GI: dry mouth, dysgeusia, abdominal pain, *nausea, constipation,* diarrhea; dyspepsia, anorexia, vomiting.
GU: urinary frequency, UTI, hematuria.
Metabolic: weight gain.
Musculoskeletal: neck and back pain, arthralgia, bursitis, myalgia.
Skin: diaphoresis, rash.
Other: flulike syndrome, chills, infection.

Interactions

Drug-drug. *Butyrophenones, metoclopramide, other dopamine antagonists, phenothiazines, thioxanthenes:* May antagonize effects of pergolide. Avoid using together.
CNS depressants: May cause additive CNS effects. Monitor patient closely.
Levodopa: May cause additive neurologic effects, such as hallucinations. Monitor patient closely.

Effects on lab test results

None reported.

Pharmacokinetics

Absorption: Well absorbed.
Distribution: About 90% protein-bound.
Metabolism: To at least 10 different compounds, some of which retain pharmacologic activity.
Excretion: Mainly by kidneys. *Half-life:* Unknown.

Route	Onset	Peak	Duration
P.O.	Unknown	Unknown	Unknown

Action

Chemical effect: Directly stimulates dopamine receptors in nigrostriatal system.
Therapeutic effect: Helps to relieve signs and symptoms of Parkinson's disease.

Available forms

Tablets: 0.05 mg, 0.25 mg, 1 mg

NURSING PROCESS

✍ Assessment

• Assess patient's condition before starting therapy. Monitor drug effectiveness by regularly checking patient's body movements for improvement.
• Monitor blood pressure and heart rate and rhythm. Symptomatic orthostatic or sustained hypotension may occur, especially at start of therapy. Drug also may induce arrhythmias.
• Evaluate patient for underlying valvular disease, including echocardiogram, before beginning therapy with pergolide.
• Be alert for adverse reactions and drug interactions.
• Assess patient's and family's knowledge of drug therapy.
• Periodically evaluate patient for somnolence. If a patient develops significant daytime sleepiness or episodes of falling asleep during activities that require participation (such as conversations or eating), stop the drug. If patient continues therapy, advise patient not to drive and to avoid other potentially dangerous activities. Dose reduction may reduce the degree of somnolence, but not enough information is available to establish that dose reduction will stop it.

⊕ Nursing diagnoses

• Impaired physical mobility related to Parkinson's disease
• Decreased cardiac output related to drug-induced adverse CV reactions
• Deficient knowledge related to drug therapy

▶ Planning and implementation

• Gradually increase dosage by patient's response and tolerance.
• Perform regular cardiovascular follow-up during the course of the drug therapy.
• Stop therapy if patient develops a fibrotic condition or cardiac valvular disease during treatment.
• If patient has significant changes in vital signs or mental status, notify prescriber.
• When stopping drug, taper slowly to avoid malignant neuroleptic syndrome, confusion, and hallucinations.
Patient teaching
• Inform patient of potential adverse reactions, especially hallucinations and confusion.

P

• Warn patient to avoid activities that could result in injury from orthostatic hypotension and syncope.

• Advise patient of the possibility of suddenly falling asleep while performing daily activities, including driving a car. Many patients who fall asleep have no warning of somnolence. Advise patient with increased somnolence or new episodes of falling asleep during daily living not to drive or participate in potentially dangerous activities until he has contacted his prescriber.

☑ **Evaluation**
• Patient has improved mobility.
• Patient maintains cardiac output.
• Patient and family state understanding of drug therapy.

perphenazine
(per-FEN-uh-zeen)
Apo-Perphenazine ◆, Trilafon, Trilafon Concentrate*

Pharmacologic class: phenothiazine (piperazine derivative)
Therapeutic class: antipsychotic, antiemetic
Pregnancy risk category: C

Indications and dosages

▶ **Psychosis in nonhospitalized patients.**
Adults: Initially, 4 to 8 mg P.O. t.i.d. Reduce to minimum effective dosage as soon as possible.
Children older than age 12: Lowest adult dose.
▶ **Psychosis in hospitalized patients.** *Adults:* Initially, 8 to 16 mg P.O. b.i.d., t.i.d., or q.i.d., increase to 64 mg daily, p.r.n. Or, 5 to 10 mg I.M. q 6 hours, p.r.n. Maximum daily I.M. dose, 30 mg.
Children older than age 12: Lowest limit of adult dosage.
▶ **Severe nausea and vomiting.** *Adults:* 5 to 10 mg I.M., p.r.n.

Contraindications and cautions

• Contraindicated in patients hypersensitive to the drug or any of its components; in comatose patients; in patients with CNS depression, blood dyscrasia, bone marrow depression, liver damage, or subcortical damage; and in those taking large doses of CNS depressants and itraconazole.

• Use cautiously with other CNS depressants or anticholinergics. Also use cautiously in debilitated patients and patients with alcohol withdrawal, depression, suicidal tendency, severe adverse reactions to other phenothiazines, impaired renal function, or respiratory disorders.
⚖ **Lifespan:** In pregnant women, use cautiously; a neonate whose mother uses drug during pregnancy may have prolonged jaundice, extrapyramidal signs, hyperreflexia or hyporeflexia. In breast-feeding women, drug appears in breast milk; avoid using unless the benefit outweighs the risk to the infant. In children age 12 and younger, safety and effectiveness haven't been established. In the elderly, use cautiously because of risk of increased effects.

Adverse reactions

CNS: *extrapyramidal reaction, tardive dyskinesia,* sedation, pseudoparkinsonism, EEG changes, dizziness, *seizures, neuroleptic malignant syndrome.*
CV: *orthostatic hypotension,* tachycardia, ECG changes, *cardiac arrest.*
EENT: ocular changes, blurred vision.
GI: dry mouth, constipation.
GU: *urine retention,* dark urine, menstrual irregularities, inhibited ejaculation.
Hematologic: *transient leukopenia,* hyperprolactinemia, *agranulocytosis, hemolytic anemia, thrombocytopenia.*
Hepatic: cholestatic jaundice.
Metabolic: weight gain, increased appetite.
Skin: *mild photosensitivity reaction,* sterile abscess.
Other: allergic reactions, pain at I.M. injection site, gynecomastia.

Interactions

Drug-drug. *Antacids:* May inhibit oral phenothiazine absorption. Administer drugs separately.
Anticonvulsants: May lower the seizure threshold. Monitor patient.
Barbiturates: May decrease phenothiazine effect. Observe patient closely.
Bromocriptine: May decrease bromocriptine effectiveness. Monitor patient for effect.
CNS depressants: May increase CNS depression. Avoid using together.
Lithium: May cause severe neurological toxicity with encephalitis-like syndrome; decreased ther-

apeutic response to perphenazine. Don't use together.
Drug-herb. *Dong quai, St. John's wort:* May increase photosensitivity. Discourage using together.
Evening primrose oil: May increase risk of seizures. Discourage using together.
Kava: May increase risk of dystonic reactions. Discourage using together.
Milk thistle: May decrease liver toxicity caused by phenothiazines. Monitor liver enzyme levels.
Yohimbe: May increase risk of yohimbe toxicity. Discourage using together.
Drug-lifestyle. *Alcohol use:* May increase CNS depression, particularly psychomotor skills. Strongly discourage use together.
Sun exposure: May increase photosensitivity reaction. Urge patient to avoid unprotected or prolonged exposure to sunlight.

Effects on lab test results

• May increase prolactin levels. May decrease hemoglobin level and hematocrit.
• May increase liver function test values and eosinophil count. May decrease WBC, granulocyte, and platelet counts.
• May produce false-positive phenylketonuria or pregnancy test results.

Pharmacokinetics

Absorption: Rate and extent vary. Erratic and variable for P.O. tablet; much more predictable for P.O. concentrate. Rapid from I.M. injection.
Distribution: Distributed widely; 91% to 99% of drug is protein-bound.
Metabolism: Metabolized extensively by liver.
Excretion: Most of drug excreted in urine; some in feces. *Half-life:* 9 to 12 hours.

Route	Onset	Peak	Duration
P.O., I.M.	Varies	1–3 hr	Unknown

Action

Chemical effect: Probably blocks postsynaptic dopamine receptors in brain and inhibits medullary chemoreceptor trigger zone.
Therapeutic effect: Relieves signs and symptoms of psychosis; also relieves nausea and vomiting.

Available forms

Injection: 5 mg/ml
Oral concentrate: 16 mg/5 ml*

Syrup: 2 mg/5 ml ◆
Tablets: 2 mg, 4 mg, 8 mg, 16 mg

NURSING PROCESS

Assessment
• Assess patient's condition before starting therapy, and regularly thereafter to monitor the drug's effectiveness.
• Obtain baseline blood pressure before starting therapy, and monitor it regularly. Watch for orthostatic hypotension, especially with I.M. administration.
• Test bilirubin level weekly during first month, and obtain periodic blood tests (CBC and liver function) and ophthalmic tests (long-term use).
• Be alert for adverse reactions and drug interactions.
• Monitor patient for tardive dyskinesia, which may occur after prolonged use. It may not appear until months or years later and may disappear spontaneously or persist for life despite no longer using the drug.
• If drug is used for nausea and vomiting, monitor patient's hydration.
• Assess patient's and family's knowledge of drug therapy.

Nursing diagnoses
• Disturbed thought processes related to psychosis
• Risk for deficient fluid volume related to nausea or vomiting
• Deficient knowledge related to drug therapy

Planning and implementation
• When giving liquid form, dilute with fruit juice, milk, carbonated beverage, or semisolid food just before giving.
• Concentrate causes turbidity or precipitation in colas, black coffee, grape or apple juice, or tea. Don't mix with them.
• When given I.M., inject drug deep in upper outer quadrant of buttocks. Injection may sting.
• Massage slowly after injection to prevent sterile abscess.
• Keep patient supine for 1 hour after injection because of risk of hypotension.
• Prevent contact dermatitis by keeping drug away from skin and clothes. Wear gloves when preparing liquid forms.

P

• Protect drug from light. Slight yellowing of injection or concentrate doesn't affect potency. Discard markedly discolored solutions.
• Don't abruptly stop giving the drug unless severe adverse reaction occurs. After abruptly stopping long-term therapy, patient may experience gastritis, nausea, vomiting, dizziness, tremors, feeling of warmth or cold, diaphoresis, tachycardia, headache, or insomnia.
• If patient develops jaundice, symptoms of blood dyscrasia (fever, sore throat, infection, cellulitis, weakness), or extrapyramidal reactions that last longer than a few hours, withhold dose and notify prescriber.
• Acute dystonic reactions may be treated with diphenhydramine.
⊛ **ALERT:** Don't confuse perphenazine with prochlorperazine.
Patient teaching
• Advise patient to change positions slowly to minimize orthostatic hypotension.
• Teach patient which fluids are appropriate for diluting concentrate.
• Warn patient to avoid hazardous activities until the drug's CNS effects are known. Drowsiness and dizziness usually subside after a few weeks.
• Tell patient to avoid alcohol during drug therapy.
• Advise patient to report urine retention or constipation.
• Tell patient to use sunblock and to wear protective clothing to avoid photosensitivity reactions.
• Tell patient to relieve dry mouth with sugarless gum or hard candy.

☑ **Evaluation**
• Patient's thought processes are normal.
• Patient maintains adequate hydration throughout drug therapy.
• Patient and family state understanding of drug therapy.

phenazopyridine hydrochloride (phenylazo diamino pyridine hydrochloride)
(fen-eh-soh-PEER-eh-deen high-droh-KLOR-ighd)
Azo-Dine, Azo-Gesic, Azo-Standard†, Baridium†, Geridium, Phenazo◆, Prodium†, Pyridiate, Pyridium, Pyridium Plus, RE-Azo, Urodine†, Urogesic, UTI Relief

Pharmacologic class: azo dye
Therapeutic class: urinary analgesic
Pregnancy risk category: B

Indications and dosages
▶ **Relief of symptoms of urinary tract irritation or infection.** *Adults:* 200 mg P.O. t.i.d. *Children:* 12 mg/kg P.O. daily divided into three equal doses.

Contraindications and cautions
• Contraindicated in patients with glomerulonephritis, severe hepatitis, uremia, or renal insufficiency.
⚖ **Lifespan:** In pyelonephritis during pregnancy, drug is contraindicated. In breast-feeding women, safety and effectiveness haven't been established. In children younger than age 12, don't use.

Adverse reactions
CNS: headache, vertigo.
EENT: staining of contact lenses.
GI: nausea, mild GI disturbance.
Skin: rash, pruritus.

Interactions
None significant.

Effects on lab test results
• May alter urine glucose results when Diastix is used. May interfere with urinalysis based on spectrometry or color reactions.

Pharmacokinetics
Absorption: Unknown.
Distribution: Unknown.
Metabolism: In liver.
Excretion: 65% excreted in urine unchanged.
Half-life: Unknown.

Reactions may be *common,* uncommon, *life-threatening*, or COMMON AND LIFE-THREATENING.

Route	Onset	Peak	Duration
P.O.	Unknown	Unknown	Unknown

Action

Chemical effect: Unknown; has local anesthetic effect on urinary mucosa.
Therapeutic effect: Relieves urinary tract pain.

Available forms

Tablets: 95 mg†, 97.2 mg, 100 mg†, 200 mg

NURSING PROCESS

Assessment
• Assess patient's pain before and after giving drug.
• Be alert for adverse reactions.
• If nausea occurs, monitor patient's hydration.
• Assess patient's and family's knowledge of drug therapy.

Nursing diagnoses
• Acute pain related to underlying urinary tract condition
• Risk for deficient fluid volume related to drug-induced nausea
• Deficient knowledge related to drug therapy

Planning and implementation
• Administer drug with food to minimize nausea.
• **ALERT:** Don't confuse Pyridium with pyridoxine, pyrimethamine, or pyridine.
Patient teaching
• Advise patient that taking drug with meals may minimize nausea.
• Tell patient to stop taking drug and notify prescriber if skin or sclera becomes yellow-tinged.
• Warn patient that drug colors urine red or orange. Drug may stain fabrics and contact lenses.
• Tell patient to notify prescriber if urinary tract pain persists after 2 days and the patient isn't also taking an antibiotic. If using drug with an antibiotic, stop drug after 2 days because it has no additional effectiveness. Drug isn't for long-term use.

Evaluation
• Patient is free from pain.
• Patient maintains adequate hydration.
• Patient and family state understanding of drug therapy.

phenobarbital (phenobarbitone)
(feen-oh-BAR-bih-tol)
Solfoton

phenobarbital sodium (phenobarbitone sodium)
Luminal Sodium

Pharmacologic class: barbiturate
Therapeutic class: anticonvulsant, sedative-hypnotic
Pregnancy risk category: D
Controlled substance schedule: IV

Indications and dosages

▶ **All forms of epilepsy except absence seizures; febrile seizures in children.** *Adults:* 60 to 250 mg P.O. daily, in divided doses t.i.d. or as single dose h.s.
Children: 1 to 6 mg/kg P.O. daily, divided q 12 hours for total of 100 mg; can be given once daily, usually h.s.
▶ **Status epilepticus.** *Adults:* 200 to 600 mg by slow I.V. injection; may repeat in 6 hours, if needed.
Children: 15 to 20 mg/kg by slow I.V. injection.
▶ **Sedation.** *Adults:* 30 to 120 mg P.O. daily in two or three divided doses.
Children: 8 to 32 mg P.O. daily in divided doses t.i.d.
▶ **Insomnia.** *Adults:* 100 to 200 mg P.O. or I.M. h.s.
▶ **Preoperative sedation.** *Adults:* 100 to 200 mg I.M. 60 to 90 minutes before surgery.
Children: 1 to 3 mg/kg I.V. or I.M. 60 to 90 minutes before surgery.

I.V. administration

• Injection is reserved for emergencies because patients respond differently.
• Have resuscitation equipment available.
• If injectable solution contains precipitate, don't use.
• Observe patient with status epilepticus for decrease of seizures; stop drug when convulsions cease.
• Don't give more than 60 mg/minute because respiratory depression may occur. Monitor respirations closely.

P

⊗ **Incompatibilities**
Acidic solutions, amphotericin B, chlorpromazine, dimenhydrinate, diphenhydramine, ephedrine, hydralazine, hydrocortisone sodium succinate, hydromorphone, insulin, kanamycin, levorphanol, meperidine, morphine, norepinephrine, pentazocine lactate, phenytoin, prochlorperazine mesylate, promethazine hydrochloride, ranitidine hydrochloride, streptomycin, vancomycin.

Contraindications and cautions

• Contraindicated in patients hypersensitive to barbiturates and in those with hepatic dysfunction, respiratory disease with dyspnea or obstruction, nephritis, or a history of manifest or latent porphyria.
• Use cautiously in debilitated patients and in patients with acute or chronic pain, depression, suicidal tendencies, history of drug abuse, altered blood pressure, CV disease, shock, or uremia.
⚕ Lifespan: In pregnant and breast-feeding women, drug isn't recommended. In the elderly, use cautiously; drug causes paradoxical excitement in these patients.

Adverse reactions

CNS: drowsiness, lethargy, hangover.
CV: *bradycardia,* hypotension.
GI: nausea, vomiting.
Hematologic: exacerbation of porphyria.
Respiratory: *respiratory depression, apnea.*
Skin: rash; *erythema multiforme, Stevens-Johnson syndrome,* urticaria.
Other: *angioedema;* pain, swelling, thrombophlebitis, necrosis, nerve injury at injection site.

Interactions

Drug-drug. *Chloramphenicol, MAO inhibitors, valproic acid:* May increase barbiturate effect. Monitor patient for increased CNS and respiratory depression.
CNS depressants, including opioid analgesics: May increase CNS depression. Use together cautiously.
Carbamazepine, corticosteroids, digitoxin, doxorubicin, doxycycline, estrogens and hormonal contraceptives, oral anticoagulants, quinidine, theophylline, tricyclic antidepressants, verapamil: May enhance metabolism of these drugs. Monitor patient for decreased effect.
Diazepam: May increase effects of both drugs. Use together cautiously.

Griseofulvin: May decrease griseofulvin absorption. Administer drug separately.
Mephobarbital, primidone: May increase phenobarbital levels. Monitor patient closely.
Metoprolol, propranolol: May reduce the effects of these drugs. Increase beta blocker dose.
Rifampin: May decrease barbiturate levels. Monitor patient for decreased effect.
Drug-lifestyle. *Alcohol use:* May impair coordination, increase CNS effects, and cause death. Strongly discourage use together.

Effects on lab test results

• May decrease bilirubin level.

Pharmacokinetics

Absorption: Good after P.O. use. 100% from I.M. injection.
Distribution: Wide. About 25% to 30% protein-bound.
Metabolism: In liver.
Excretion: In urine. *Half-life:* 5 to 7 days.

Route	Onset	Peak	Duration
P.O.	20–60 min	Unknown	10–12 hr
I.V.	5 min	≥ 15 min	10–12 hr
I.M.	> 60 min	Unknown	10–12 hr

Action

Chemical effect: Unknown; may depress CNS synaptic transmission and increase seizure activity threshold in motor cortex. As sedative, may interfere with transmission of impulses from thalamus to brain cortex.
Therapeutic effect: Prevents and stops seizure activity; promotes calmness and sleep.

Available forms

Capsules: 16 mg
Elixir*: 20 mg/5 ml
Injection: 30 mg/ml, 60 mg/ml, 65 mg/ml, 130 mg/ml
Tablets: 15 mg, 16 mg, 30 mg, 60 mg, 100 mg

NURSING PROCESS

⚕ **Assessment**
• Assess patient's condition before starting therapy, and regularly thereafter to monitor the drug's effectiveness.
• Monitor drug level closely. Therapeutic level is 15 to 40 mcg/ml.

Reactions may be *common,* uncommon, *life-threatening*, or COMMON AND LIFE-THREATENING.

• Be alert for adverse reactions and drug interactions.
• Assess patient's and family's knowledge of drug therapy.

🔆 **Nursing diagnoses**
• Risk for trauma related to seizures
• Risk for injury related to drug-induced adverse CNS reactions
• Deficient knowledge related to drug therapy

▶ **Planning and implementation**
• Don't abruptly stop giving the drug; seizures may worsen. If adverse reaction occurs, immediately notify prescriber.
• Give drug by deep I.M. injection. Superficial injection may cause pain, sterile abscess, and tissue sloughing.
⚠ **ALERT:** Don't confuse phenobarbital with pentobarbital.
Patient teaching
• Tell patient that phenobarbital is available in different strengths and sizes. Advise him to check prescription and refills closely.
• Inform patient that full effects don't occur for 2 to 3 weeks except when loading dose is used.
• Advise patient to avoid hazardous activities until the drug's CNS effects are known.
• Warn patient and parents not to abruptly stop taking the drug.
• Tell patient using hormonal contraceptives to use barrier-method birth control.

✅ **Evaluation**
• Patient is free from seizure activity.
• Patient has no injury from drug-induced adverse CNS reactions.
• Patient and family state understanding of drug therapy.

phentermine hydrochloride
(FEN-ter-meen high-droh-KLOR-ighd)
Adipex-P, Duromine ◇ **, Ionamin, Ona Mast, Pro-Fast HS, Pro-Fast SA, Pro-Fast SR**

Pharmacologic class: indirect-acting sympathomimetic amine
Therapeutic class: anorexigenic
Pregnancy risk category: C
Controlled substance schedule: IV

Indications and dosages
▶ **Short-term adjunct in exogenous obesity.**
Adults: 8 mg P.O. t.i.d. 30 minutes before meals. Or, 15 to 37.5 mg daily before breakfast or 10 to 14 hours before bed time. Give Pro-Fast HS or Pro-Fast SR capsules 2 hours after breakfast. Give Adipex-P before breakfast or 1 to 2 hours after breakfast.

Contraindications and cautions
• Contraindicated in agitated patients, patients hypersensitive to sympathomimetic amines, patients who have idiosyncratic reactions to them, patients who have taken an MAO inhibitor within 14 days, and patients with hyperthyroidism, moderate to severe hypertension, advanced arteriosclerosis, symptomatic CV disease, or glaucoma.
• Use cautiously in patients with mild hypertension.
🌺 **Lifespan:** In pregnant and breast-feeding women, drug isn't recommended. Use in children younger than 16 years of age isn't recommended.

Adverse reactions
CNS: overstimulation, headache, euphoria, dysphoria, dizziness, *insomnia.*
CV: palpitations, tachycardia, increased blood pressure, *pulmonary hypertension.*
EENT: mydriasis, eye irritation, blurred vision.
GI: dry mouth, dysgeusia, constipation, diarrhea, other GI disturbances.
GU: impotence.
Skin: urticaria.
Other: altered libido.

Interactions
Drug-drug. *Acetazolamide, antacids, sodium bicarbonate:* May increase renal reabsorption. Monitor patient.
Ammonium chloride, ascorbic acid: May decrease levels and increase renal excretion of phentermine. Monitor patient for decreased effects.
Furazolidone, MAO inhibitors: May cause severe hypertension and hypertensive crisis. Don't use within 14 days of an MAO inhibitor.
Guanethidine: May decrease hypotensive effect. Monitor blood pressure closely.
Haloperidol, phenothiazines, tricyclic antidepressants: May increase CNS effects. Avoid using together.

P

Insulin, oral antidiabetics: May alter antidiabetic requirements. Monitor glucose levels.
SSRIs: May increase sensitivity to phentermine with risk of serotonin syndrome.
Drug-food. *Caffeine:* May increase CNS stimulation. Discourage using together.

Effects on lab test results

None reported.

Pharmacokinetics

Absorption: Absorbed readily from GI tract.
Distribution: Distributed throughout body.
Metabolism: Unknown.
Excretion: Excreted in urine. *Half-life:* 19 to 24 hours.

Route	Onset	Peak	Duration
P.O.	Unknown	Unknown	12–14 hr

Action

Chemical effect: Unknown; probably works by releasing stored norepinephrine from nerve terminals in the brain (primarily in the cerebral cortex and reticular activating system), thus promoting nerve impulse transmission.
Therapeutic effect: Depresses appetite.

Available forms

Capsules: 15 mg, 18.75 mg, 30 mg, 37.5 mg
Capsules (extended-release): 15 mg, 30 mg
Tablets: 8 mg, 15 mg, 18.75 mg, 30 mg, 37.5 mg

NURSING PROCESS

Assessment
• Weigh patient before starting therapy, and regularly thereafter to monitor the drug's effectiveness.
• Be alert for adverse reactions and drug interactions.
• Monitor patient for habituation and tolerance.
• Assess patient's and family's knowledge of drug therapy.

Nursing diagnoses
• Imbalanced nutrition: more than body requirements related to food intake
• Disturbed sleep pattern related to drug-induced insomnia
• Deficient knowledge related to drug therapy

Planning and implementation
• Give drug at least 6 hours before bedtime to avoid insomnia.
• Make sure patient is following a weight-reduction program.
⑤ ALERT: Don't confuse phentermine with phentolamine.

Patient teaching
• Instruct patient to take drug at least 6 hours before bedtime to avoid sleep interference.
• Warn patient to avoid hazardous activities until the drug's CNS effects are known.
• Instruct patient that drug is to meant to suppress appetite while patient maintains a reducing diet and that he shouldn't use the drug for more than 3 to 4 weeks.
• Tell patient to avoid caffeine because it increases the effects of amphetamines and related amines.
• Tell patient to report signs of excessive stimulation.
• Inform patient that fatigue may result as drug effects wear off.

Evaluation
• Patient loses weight.
• Patient doesn't have insomnia.
• Patient and family state understanding of drug therapy.

phenylephrine hydrochloride
(fen-il-EF-rin high-droh-KLOR-ighd)
Neo-Synephrine

Pharmacologic class: adrenergic
Therapeutic class: vasoconstrictor
Pregnancy risk category: C

Indications and dosages

▶ **Hypotensive emergencies during spinal anesthesia.** *Adults:* Initially, 0.1 to 0.2 mg I.V., followed by 0.1 to 0.2 mg, p.r.n.
▶ **Maintenance of blood pressure during spinal or inhalation anesthesia.** *Adults:* 2 to 3 mg subcutaneously or I.M. 3 or 4 minutes before anesthesia.
Children: 0.044 to 0.088 mg/kg subcutaneously or I.M.
▶ **Prolongation of spinal anesthesia.** *Adults:* 2 to 5 mg added to anesthetic solution.

▶ **Vasoconstrictor for regional anesthesia.** *Adults:* 1 mg phenylephrine added to 20 ml local anesthetic.

▶ **Mild to moderate hypotension.** *Adults:* 2 to 5 mg subcutaneously or I.M.; repeated in 1 to 2 hours as needed and tolerated. Maximum first dose, 5 mg. Or, 0.1 to 0.5 mg slow I.V., no more than q 10 to 15 minutes.
Children: 0.1 mg/kg I.M. or subcutaneously; repeated in 1 to 2 hours as needed and tolerated.

▶ **Severe hypotension and shock (including drug-induced).** *Adults:* 0.1 to 0.18 mg/minute I.V. infusion. After blood pressure stabilizes, maintain at 0.04 to 0.06 mg/minute and adjust to patient response.

▶ **Paroxysmal supraventricular tachycardia.** *Adults:* Initially, 0.5 mg rapid I.V. Increase later doses by 0.1 to 0.2 mg. Maximum dose, 1 mg.

▽ **I.V. administration**

• For direct injection, dilute 10 mg (1 ml) with 9 ml sterile water for injection to provide solution containing 1 mg/ml.
• Prepare I.V. infusions by adding 10 mg of drug to 500 ml of D₅W or normal saline solution for injection.
• Initial infusion rate is usually 100 to 180 mcg/minute; maintenance rate is usually 40 to 60 mcg/minute.
• Use central venous catheter or large vein, as in antecubital fossa, to minimize risk of extravasation.
• Use continuous infusion pump to regulate flow rate.
• During infusion, frequently monitor ECG, blood pressure, cardiac output, central venous pressure, pulmonary capillary wedge pressure, pulse rate, urine output, and color and temperature of limbs. Titrate infusion rate according to findings and prescriber's guidelines.
• To treat extravasation, infiltrate site promptly with 10 to 15 ml of normal saline solution for injection that contains 5 to 10 mg phentolamine. Use a fine needle.
• After prolonged I.V. infusion, avoid abrupt withdrawal.
• Store at room temperature and protect from light.

⊗ **Incompatibilities**
Alkaline solutions, butacaine sulfate, iron salts, other metals, phenytoin sodium, thiopental sodium.

Contraindications and cautions

• Contraindicated in patients hypersensitive to the drug or any of its components, and in patients with severe hypertension or ventricular tachycardia.
• Use cautiously in patients with heart disease, hyperthyroidism, severe atherosclerosis, bradycardia, partial heart block, myocardial disease, or sulfite sensitivity.
• Correct blood volume depletion before using phenylephrine.
⚘ **Lifespan:** In pregnant women, use cautiously. In breast-feeding women, use cautiously; it's unknown if the drug appears in breast milk. In the elderly, use cautiously.

Adverse reactions

CNS: *headache, restlessness, light-headedness, weakness.*
CV: palpitations, *bradycardia, arrhythmias,* hypertension, angina, decreased cardiac output.
EENT: blurred vision.
GI: vomiting.
Respiratory: *asthma attacks.*
Skin: pilomotor response, feeling of coolness.
Other: tachyphylaxis, *decreased organ perfusion with prolonged use,* tissue sloughing with extravasation, *anaphylaxis.*

Interactions

Drug-drug. *Alpha blockers, phenothiazines:* May decrease vasopressor response. Monitor patient closely.
Bretylium: May increase risk of arrhythmias. Monitor ECG.
Guanethidine, oxytocics: May increase pressor response and cause severe, persistent hypertension. Monitor patient and blood pressure closely.
Halogenated hydrocarbon anesthetics: May lead to serious arrhythmias. Use with caution.
MAO inhibitors: May potentiate cardiac and pressor effects. Avoid use together.
Phenelzine, tranylcypromine: May cause severe headache, hypertension, fever, and hypertensive crisis. Avoid using together.
Tricyclic antidepressants: May increase the pressor response and cause arrhythmias. Use cautiously.

Effects on lab test results

None reported.

P

Pharmacokinetics

Absorption: Unknown.
Distribution: Unknown.
Metabolism: Metabolized in liver and intestine.
Excretion: Unknown. *Half-life:* Unknown.

Route	Onset	Peak	Duration
I.V.	Immediate	Unknown	15–20 min
I.M.	10–15 min	Unknown	½–2 hr
SubQ	10–15 min	Unknown	50–60 min

Action

Chemical effect: Mainly stimulates alpha-adrenergic receptors in sympathetic nervous system.
Therapeutic effect: Raises blood pressure and stops paroxysmal supraventricular tachycardia.

Available forms

Injection: 10 mg/ml (1%)

NURSING PROCESS

☒ Assessment
● Assess patient's condition before starting therapy, and regularly thereafter to monitor the drug's effectiveness.
● Monitor blood pressure frequently; avoid severe increase.
● Monitor ECG throughout therapy.
● Be alert for adverse reactions and drug interactions.
● Assess patient's and family's knowledge of drug therapy.

▦ Nursing diagnoses
● Ineffective tissue perfusion (cerebral, cardiopulmonary, peripheral, GI, renal) related to underlying condition
● Decreased cardiac output related to drug-induced adverse reaction
● Deficient knowledge related to drug therapy

▷ Planning and implementation
● Maintain blood pressure slightly below patient's normal level. In previously normotensive patient, maintain systolic pressure at 80 to 100 mm Hg; in previously hypertensive patient, maintain systolic pressure at 30 to 40 mm Hg below usual level.
Patient teaching
● Tell patient to immediately report discomfort at infusion site.

☑ Evaluation
● Patient maintains tissue perfusion and cellular oxygenation.
● Patient maintains adequate cardiac output.
● Patient and family state understanding of drug therapy.

phenytoin (diphenylhydantoin)
(FEN-uh-toyn)
Dilantin-125, Dilantin Infatabs

phenytoin sodium (extended)
Dilantin Kapseals⬦, Phenytek

phenytoin sodium (prompt)
Dilantin

Pharmacologic class: hydantoin derivative
Therapeutic class: anticonvulsant
Pregnancy risk category: D

Indications and dosages

▶ **Control of tonic-clonic (grand mal) and complex partial (temporal lobe) seizures.**
Adults: Highly individualized. Initially, 100 mg P.O. t.i.d. Increase in increments of 100 mg P.O. q 2 to 4 weeks until desired response is obtained. Usual range is 300 to 600 mg daily. If patient is stabilized with extended-release capsules, may give once-daily dosing with 300-mg extended-release capsules.
Children: 5 mg/kg or 250 mg/m² P.O. extended-release capsules divided b.i.d. or t.i.d. Maximum daily dose is 300 mg.
▶ **For patient requiring a loading dose.**
Adults: Initially, 1 g P.O. daily divided into three doses and administered at 2-hour intervals. Or, 10 to 15 mg/kg I.V. at a rate not exceeding 50 mg/minute. Normal maintenance dose is started 24 hours later with frequent level determinations.
Children: Initially, 5 mg/kg P.O. daily in two or three equally divided doses with subsequent dose individualized to maximum of 300 mg daily. Usual dosage is 4 to 8 mg/kg P.O. daily. Children older than age 6 may require the minimum adult dosage (300 mg daily).
▶ **To prevent and treat seizures during neurosurgery.** *Adults:* 100 to 200 mg I.M or I.V. q 4 hours during surgery and continued in the immediate postoperative period.

Reactions may be *common*, uncommon, *life-threatening*, or COMMON AND LIFE-THREATENING.

▶ **Status epilepticus.** *Adults:* Loading dose of
10 to 15 mg/kg I.V. (1 to 1.5 g may be needed)
at a rate not exceeding 50 mg/minute; then
maintenance dosage of 100 mg P.O. or I.V. q
6 to 8 hours.
Children: Loading dose of 15 to 20 mg/kg I.V.,
at a rate not exceeding 1 to 3 mg/kg/minute;
then highly individualized maintenance doses.
▶ **Alternative to magnesium sulfate for
severe preeclampsia.** 15 mg/kg I.V. given as
10 mg/kg initially and 5 mg/kg 2 hours later.
▶ **Cardiac glycoside–induced arrhythmias‡.**
50 mg I.V. q 5 minutes to a total of 1 g or oral
loading dose of 14 mg/kg followed by maintenance dose of 200 to 400 mg/day I.V. or P.O.
Adjust-a-dose: Elderly patients may need
lower dosages.

▼ I.V. administration

• Check patency of I.V. catheter before administering. Extravasation may cause severe local tissue damage.
• Never use cloudy solution.
• Avoid giving phenytoin by I.V. push into veins
on back of hand to avoid discoloration known as
purple glove syndrome. Inject into larger veins
or central venous catheter.
• Administer drug slowly (50 mg/minute) as an
I.V. bolus.
• If giving as infusion, don't mix drug with
D₅W because it will precipitate. Clear I.V. tubing first with normal saline solution. May mix
with normal saline solution if needed and infuse
over 30 to 60 minutes when possible.
• Infusion must begin within 1 hour after preparation and run through in-line filter.
• Discard 4 hours after preparation.
⊗ **Incompatibilities**
Amikacin, aminophylline, amphotericin B,
bretylium, cephapirin, ciprofloxacin, D₅W, diltiazem, dobutamine, enalaprilat, fat emulsions,
hydromorphone, insulin (regular), levorphanol,
lidocaine, lincomycin, meperidine, morphine
sulfate, nitroglycerin, norepinephrine, other I.V.
drugs or infusion solutions, pentobarbital sodium, potassium chloride, procaine, propofol,
streptomycin, sufentanil citrate, theophylline,
vitamin B complex with C.

Contraindications and cautions

• Contraindicated in patients hypersensitive to
hydantoin and in patients with sinus bradycar-

dia, SA block, second- or third-degree AV
block, or Adams-Stokes syndrome.
• Use cautiously in debilitated patients, patients
taking other hydantoin derivatives, and patients
with hepatic dysfunction, hypotension, myocardial insufficiency, diabetes, or respiratory depression.
• Don't stop drug in pregnant women using the
drug to prevent major seizures. An increase in
seizure activity may occur in pregnant woman
due to changes in drug absorption or metabolism, so monitor levels carefully.
Lifespan: In pregnant women, drug isn't recommended; infants born to mothers taking
phenytoin may have bleeding defects. Give vitamin K to the mother 1 month before and during
delivery and to the neonate immediately after
birth. In breast-feeding women, drug isn't recommended. In the elderly, use cautiously; they
tend to metabolize drug slowly and may need
lower dosages.

Adverse reactions

CNS: *ataxia, slurred speech, confusion,* dizzi-
ness, insomnia, nervousness, twitching, head-
ache.
CV: hypotension.
EENT: nystagmus, diplopia, blurred vision,
gingival hyperplasia.
GI: nausea, vomiting.
Hematologic: *thrombocytopenia, leukopenia,
agranulocytosis, pancytopenia,* macrocythemia,
megaloblastic anemia, lymphadenopathy.
Hepatic: *toxic hepatitis.*
Metabolic: hyperglycemia.
Musculoskeletal: osteomalacia.
Skin: scarlatiniform or morbilliform rash;
bullous, exfoliative, or purpuric dermatitis;
*Stevens-Johnson syndrome; hirsutism; toxic
epidermal necrolysis;* photosensitivity reaction,
hypertrichosis.
Other: periarteritis nodosa; lupus erythematosus; pain, necrosis, or inflammation at injection
site.

Interactions

Drug-drug. *Amiodarone, allopurinol, antihistamines, chloramphenicol, cimetidine, clonazepam, cycloserine, diazepam, disulfiram,
fluconazole, influenza vaccine, isoniazid,
phenylbutazone, phenothiazines, salicylates,
sulfamethizole, tricyclic antidepressants, val-*

proate: May increase therapeutic effects of phenytoin. Monitor patient for toxicity.
Antacids, carbamazepine, dexamethasone, diazoxide, folic acid, phenobarbital, rifampin, theophylline: May decrease phenytoin activity. Monitor patient closely.
Atracurium, cisatracurium, doxacurium, mivacurium, pancuronium, rocuronium, vecuronium: May decrease the effects of nondepolarizing muscle relaxant causing it to be less effective. May need to increase the dose of the nondepolarizing muscle relaxant.
Lithium: May increase toxicity. Monitor lithium levels.
Meperidine: May increase toxic effects of meperidine while decreasing analgesic effect. Monitor patient for decreased effect and toxicity.
Warfarin: May displace warfarin. Monitor patient for bleeding complications.
Drug-herb. *Milk thistle:* May decrease risk of liver toxicity. Monitor patient.
Drug-food. *Enteral nutrition therapy:* May reduce orally administered phenytoin concentrations. Consider giving phenytoin 2 hours before starting enteral feeding, or wait 2 hours after stopping enteral feeding to administer phenytoin.
Drug-lifestyle. *Alcohol use:* May decrease phenytoin activity. Discourage using together.

Effects on lab test results

• May increase alkaline phosphatase, GGT, and glucose levels. May decrease protein-bound iodine, free thyroxine, urinary 17-hydroxysteroid, 17-ketosteroid, and hemoglobin levels and hematocrit.
• May increase urine 6-hydroxycortisol excretion. May decrease platelet, WBC, RBC, and granulocyte counts.
• May decrease dexamethasone suppression and metyrapone test values.

Pharmacokinetics

Absorption: Slow after P.O. administration. Formulation-dependent; bioavailability may differ among products. Erratic from I.M. site.
Distribution: Distributed widely throughout body. Drug is about 90% protein-bound.
Metabolism: Metabolized by liver.
Excretion: Excreted in urine; exhibits dose-dependent (zero-order) elimination kinetics. Above certain dosage level, small increases in

dosage disproportionately increase levels. *Half-life:* Varies with dose and concentration changes.

Route	Onset	Peak	Duration
P.O.	Unknown	½–2 hr	Unknown
P.O. extended-release	Unknown	4–12 hr	Unknown
I.V.	Immediate	1–2 hr	Unknown
I.M.	Unknown	Unknown	Unknown

Action

Chemical effect: Unknown; probably limits seizure activity by either increasing efflux or decreasing influx of sodium ions across cell membranes in motor cortex during generation of nerve impulses.
Therapeutic effect: Prevents and stops seizure activity.

Available forms

phenytoin
Oral suspension: 125 mg/5 ml
Tablets (chewable): 50 mg
phenytoin sodium (extended)
Capsules: 30 mg (27.6-mg base), 100 mg (92-mg base), 200 mg (184-mg base), 300 mg (276-mg base)
phenytoin sodium (prompt)
Capsules: 100 mg (92-mg base)
Injection: 50 mg/ml (46-mg base)

NURSING PROCESS

Assessment
• Assess patient's condition before starting therapy, and regularly thereafter to monitor the drug's effectiveness.
• Monitor phenytoin level; therapeutic level is 10 to 20 mcg/ml.
• Monitor CBC and calcium level q 6 months, and periodically monitor hepatic function.
• Check vital signs, blood pressure, and ECG during I.V. administration.
• Be alert for adverse reactions and drug interactions.
• Mononucleosis may decrease phenytoin level. Monitor patient for increased seizure activity.
• Assess patient's and family's knowledge of drug therapy.

Reactions may be *common*, uncommon, *life-threatening*, or COMMON AND LIFE-THREATENING.

Nursing diagnoses
- Risk for trauma related to seizures
- Impaired oral mucous membrane related to gingival hyperplasia
- Deficient knowledge related to drug therapy

Planning and implementation
- Use only clear or slightly yellow solution for injection. Don't refrigerate.
- Divided doses given with or after meals may decrease adverse GI reactions.
- Dilantin capsule is only P.O. form that can be given once daily. If any other brand or form is given once daily, toxic levels may result.
- Don't give drug I.M. unless dosage adjustments are made. Drug may precipitate at site, cause pain, and be erratically absorbed.
- If rash appears, stop giving the drug. If rash is scarlatiniform or morbilliform, drug may be resumed after rash clears. If rash reappears, stop giving the drug. If rash is exfoliative, purpuric, or bullous, don't resume.
- Don't abruptly stop giving the drug; seizures may worsen. If adverse reaction occurs, immediately notify prescriber.
- If patient has megaloblastic anemia, prescriber may order folic acid and vitamin B_{12}.

ALERT: Don't confuse phenytoin with Mephyton or fosphenytoin.

ALERT: Don't confuse Dilantin with Dilaudid.

Patient teaching
- Advise patient to avoid hazardous activities until the drug's CNS effects are known.
- Advise patient not to change brand, dose, or form.
- Warn patient and parents not to abruptly stop taking the drug.
- Promote oral hygiene and regular dental examinations. Gingivectomy may be needed periodically if dental hygiene is poor.
- Inform patient that drug may color urine pink, red, or red-brown.
- Tell patient that heavy alcohol use may diminish drug's benefits.

Evaluation
- Patient is free from seizure activity.
- Patient expresses importance of good oral hygiene and regular dental examinations.
- Patient and family state understanding of drug therapy.

physostigmine salicylate (eserine salicylate)
(fiz-oh-STIG-meen sa-LIS-il-ayt)

Antilirium

Pharmacologic class: cholinesterase inhibitor
Therapeutic class: antimuscarinic antidote
Pregnancy risk category: C

Indications and dosages
▶ **To reverse CNS toxicity caused by anticholinergics.** *Adults:* 0.5 to 2 mg I.M. or slow I.V. injection (1 mg/minute or slower). If coma, seizures, or arrhythmias recur, repeat q 10 minutes p.r.n.

Children: 0.02 mg/kg I.M. or slow I.V. injection (0.5 mg/min or slower). Repeat q 5 to 10 minutes until patient responds. Maximum dosage, 2 mg. Drug is only for life-threatening situations.

I.V. administration
- Use only clear solution. Darkening of solution may indicate loss of potency.
- Give drug I.V. at controlled rate; use direct injection at no more than 1 mg/minute. Rapid administration may cause bradycardia and hypersalivation, leading to respiratory difficulties and seizures.

⊗ **Incompatibilities**

None reported.

Contraindications and cautions
- Contraindicated in patients taking choline esters or depolarizing neuromuscular blockers and in patients with mechanical obstruction of intestine or urogenital tract, asthma, gangrene, diabetes, CV disease, or vagotonia.
- Use cautiously in patients with sensitivity or allergy to sulfites.

Lifespan: In pregnant women, use cautiously. In breast-feeding women, safety and effectiveness haven't been established. In children, use only in life-threatening situations.

Adverse reactions
CNS: ***seizures,*** hallucinations, muscle twitching, muscle weakness, ataxia, *restlessness, excitability, sweating.*
CV: irregular pulse, palpitations, ***bradycardia,*** hypotension.

P

EENT: miosis.
GI: nausea, vomiting, epigastric pain, *diarrhea, excessive salivation.*
GU: urinary urgency.
Respiratory: *bronchospasm,* bronchial constriction, dyspnea.

Interactions

Drug-drug. *Anticholinergics, atropine, procainamide, quinidine:* May reverse cholinergic effects. Observe patient for lack of drug effect.
Ganglionic blockers: May decrease blood pressure. Avoid using together.
Drug-herb. *Jaborandi tree, pill-bearing spurge:* May have additive effects and increase risk of toxicity. Discourage using together.

Effects on lab test results

None reported.

Pharmacokinetics

Absorption: Absorbed well from injection site.
Distribution: Distributed widely and crosses blood-brain barrier.
Metabolism: Cholinesterase hydrolyzes physostigmine relatively quickly.
Excretion: Primary mode of excretion unknown; small amount excreted in urine. *Half-life:* 1 to 2 hours.

Route	Onset	Peak	Duration
I.V.	3–5 min	≤ 5 min	30–60 min
I.M.	3–5 min	20–30 min	30–60 min

Action

Chemical effect: Inhibits destruction of acetylcholine released from parasympathetic and somatic efferent nerves. Acetylcholine accumulates, promoting increased stimulation of receptor.
Therapeutic effect: Reverses anticholinergic signs and symptoms.

Available forms

Injection: 1 mg/ml

NURSING PROCESS

☡ Assessment

• Assess patient's condition before starting therapy and regularly thereafter. Effect is often immediate and dramatic, but may be transient and require repeated doses.

• Frequently monitor vital signs, especially respirations.
• Be alert for adverse reactions and drug interactions.
• Assess patient's and family's knowledge of drug therapy.

⊞ Nursing diagnoses

• Ineffective health maintenance related to underlying condition
• Risk for injury related to drug-induced adverse CNS reactions
• Deficient knowledge related to drug therapy

⧐ Planning and implementation

• Position patient to ease breathing. If hypersensitivity or cholinergic crisis occurs, have atropine injection readily available and give 0.5 mg subcutaneously or slow I.V. push. Provide respiratory support p.r.n. Best administered in presence of prescriber.
• If patient becomes restless or hallucinates, raise side rails of bed. Adverse reaction may indicate drug toxicity. Notify prescriber.
• If patient has excessive salivation or emesis, frequent urination, or diarrhea, stop the drug.
• If patient has excessive sweating or nausea, lower dose.
Patient teaching
• Tell patient to report adverse reactions, especially pain at the I.V. site.

☑ Evaluation

• Patient responds well to therapy.
• Patient doesn't experience injury from adverse CNS reactions.
• Patient and family state understanding of drug therapy.

phytonadione (vitamin K₁)

(figh-toh-neh-DIGH-ohn)
AquaMEPHYTON, Mephyton

Pharmacologic class: synthetic analog of vitamin K
Therapeutic class: blood coagulation modifier
Pregnancy risk category: C

Indications and dosages

▶ **RDA.** *Infants age 6 months and younger:* 5 mcg.

Infants ages 6 months to 1 year: 10 mcg.
Children ages 1 to 3: 15 mcg.
Children ages 4 to 6: 20 mcg.
Children ages 7 to 10: 30 mcg.
Children ages 11 to 14: 45 mcg.
Men ages 15 to 18: 65 mcg.
Men ages 19 to 24: 70 mcg.
Men age 25 and older: 80 mcg.
Women ages 15 to 18: 55 mcg.
Women ages 19 to 24: 60 mcg.
Women age 25 and older, pregnant or breast-feeding women: 65 mcg.
► **Hypoprothrombinemia secondary to vitamin K malabsorption, drug therapy, or excessive vitamin A.** *Adults:* Depending on severity, 2.5 to 25 mg P.O., subcutaneously, or I.M.; repeat and increase up to 50 mg, if needed.
► **Hypoprothrombinemia secondary to effect of oral anticoagulants.** *Adults:* 2.5 to 10 mg P.O., subcutaneously, or I.M. based on PT; repeat if needed within 12 to 48 hours after P.O. dose or within 6 to 8 hours after parenteral dose.
► **To prevent hemorrhagic disease of newborns.** *Neonates:* 0.5 to 1 mg I.M. or subcutaneously within 1 hour after birth.
► **Hemorrhagic disease of newborns.** *Neonates:* 1 mg subcutaneously or I.M. based on laboratory tests. Higher doses may be needed if mother has been taking anticoagulants P.O.

▼ I.V. administration

⊛ **ALERT:** Severe reactions, including fatalities, have occurred with I.V. injection. Use I.V. route only if other routes are not available and when the benefit outweighs the serious risk.
• Dilute drug with normal saline solution for injection, D_5W, or 5% dextrose in normal saline solution for injection.
• Protect parenteral products from light. Wrap infusion container with aluminum foil.
⊗ **Incompatibilities**
Dobutamine, phenytoin sodium, ranitidine.

Contraindications and cautions

• Contraindicated in patients hypersensitive to the drug or any of its components.
🜲 **Lifespan:** In pregnant women, use cautiously. In breast-feeding women, use cautiously; it's unknown if the drug appears in breast milk. In children, safety and effectiveness haven't been established. In neonates, use cautiously and don't exceed recommended dosage.

Adverse reactions

CNS: dizziness, seizurelike movements.
CV: flushing, transient hypotension after I.V. administration, rapid and weak pulse, cardiac irregularities.
Skin: diaphoresis, erythema.
Other: cramplike pain; *anaphylaxis and anaphylactoid reactions* (usually after rapid I.V. administration); pain, swelling, and hematoma at injection site.

Interactions

Drug-drug. *Anticoagulants:* May cause temporary resistance to prothrombin-depressing anticoagulants, especially when larger doses of phytonadione are used. Monitor patient closely.
Cholestyramine resin, mineral oil: May inhibit GI absorption of oral vitamin K. Administer separately.

Effects on lab test results

• May decrease PT and INR.

Pharmacokinetics

Absorption: Drug requires presence of bile salts for GI tract absorption after P.O. administration. Unknown after I.M. or subcutaneous administration.
Distribution: Concentrates in liver for short time.
Metabolism: Metabolized rapidly by liver.
Excretion: Not clearly defined. *Half-life:* Unknown.

Route	Onset	Peak	Duration
P.O.	6–12 hr	Unknown	12–14 hr
I.V., I.M., SubQ	1–2 hr	Unknown	12–14 hr

Action

Chemical effect: An antihemorrhagic factor that promotes hepatic formation of active prothrombin.
Therapeutic effect: Controls abnormal bleeding.

Available forms

Injection (aqueous colloidal solution): 2 mg/ml, 10 mg/ml
Tablets: 5 mg

⚖ Assessment

• Assess patient's condition before starting therapy and regularly thereafter to monitor the drug's effectiveness.
• Monitor PT to determine dosage effectiveness.
• Failure to respond to vitamin K may indicate coagulation defects.
• Be alert for adverse reactions and drug interactions.
• If adverse GI reactions occur, monitor patient's hydration.
• Assess patient's and family's knowledge of drug therapy.

⊕ Nursing diagnoses

• Ineffective protection related to underlying vitamin K deficiency
• Risk for deficient fluid volume related to adverse GI reactions
• Deficient knowledge related to drug therapy

▶ Planning and implementation

• Check brand name labels for administration route restrictions.
• Subcutaneous is the preferred route of administration.
• Give drug I.M. in upper outer quadrant of buttocks in an adult; inject in infant's outer thigh.
• If severe bleeding occurs, don't delay other therapy, such as fresh frozen plasma or whole blood.
• Does not counteract the anticoagulant effects of heparin or low–molecular-weight heparin.
Patient teaching
• Explain drug's purpose.
• Instruct patient to report adverse reactions.

☑ Evaluation

• Patient achieves normal PT levels with drug therapy.
• Patient maintains adequate hydration throughout drug therapy.
• Patient and family state understanding of drug therapy.

pimecrolimus
(py-meck-roh-LY-muhs)
Elidel

Pharmacologic class: topical immuno-modulator
Therapeutic class: topical skin product
Pregnancy risk category: C

Indications and dosages

▶ **Short-term and intermittent long-term therapy for mild to moderate atopic dermatitis in nonimmunocompromised patients in whom the use of alternative, conventional therapies is deemed inadvisable or for patients who aren't adequately responding to or are intolerant of conventional therapies.** *Adults and children age 2 and older:* Apply a thin layer to the affected skin twice daily and rub in gently and completely.

Contraindications and cautions

• Contraindicated in patients hypersensitive to the drug or any of the cream's components.
• Don't use on areas of active cutaneous viral infections or infected atopic dermatitis.
• Not recommended for use in patients with Netherton's syndrome or in immunocompromised patients.
• Use cautiously in patients with varicella zoster virus infection, herpes simplex virus infection, or eczema herpeticum.
⚠ **Lifespan:** In pregnant women, safety and effectiveness haven't been established. Breast-feeding women should stop breast-feeding or use another drug. In children younger than age 2, drug isn't recommended. In patients age 65 and older, safety and effectiveness haven't been established.

Adverse reactions

CNS: *headache.*
EENT: *nasopharyngitis,* otitis media, sinusitis, pharyngitis, eye infection, nasal congestion, rhinorrhea, sinus congestion, rhinitis, epistaxis, conjunctivitis, earache.
GI: gastroenteritis, abdominal pain, sore throat, tonsillitis, vomiting, diarrhea, nausea, toothache, constipation, loose stools.
GU: dysmenorrhea.
Musculoskeletal: back pain, arthralgias.

Reactions may be *common,* uncommon, *life-threatening*, or COMMON AND LIFE-THREATENING.

Respiratory: *upper respiratory tract infections, pneumonia, bronchitis,* cough, asthma, wheezing, dyspnea.
Skin: skin infections, impetigo, folliculitis, molluscum contagiosum, varicella, skin papilloma, urticaria, acne.
Other: herpes simplex, *application site reaction* (burning, irritation, erythema, pruritus), *influenza, pyrexia,* flulike illness, hypersensitivity reaction, bacterial infection, staphylococcal infection, viral infection.

Interactions

Drug-drug. *CYP 3A family of inhibitors (erythromycin, itraconazole, ketoconazole, fluconazole, calcium channel blockers):* May have an effect on metabolism of pimecrolimus. Use together cautiously.
Drug-lifestyle. *Natural or artificial sunlight:* Drug may shorten the time to skin tumor formation. Avoid or minimize exposure to sunlight.

Effects on lab test results

None reported.

Pharmacokinetics

Absorption: Low systemic absorption.
Distribution: 74% to 87% bound to proteins.
Metabolism: No evidence of skin-mediated drug metabolism exists.
Excretion: Following the administration of a single oral radiolabeled dose, about 81% of the administered radioactivity was recovered, primarily in the feces (78.4%) as metabolites. Less than 1% of the radioactivity found in the feces was because of unchanged drug. *Half-life:* Unknown.

Route	Onset	Peak	Duration
Topical	Unknown	Unknown	Unknown

Action

Chemical effect: Unknown. May inhibit T cell activation by blocking the transcription of early cytokines. May also prevent the release of inflammatory cytokines and mediators from mast cells in vitro after stimulation by antigen/immunoglobulin E.
Therapeutic effect: Improves skin integrity.

Available forms

Cream: 1% in tubes of 15 g, 30 g, and 100 g (Base contains the following alcohols: benzyl alcohol, cetyl alcohol, oleyl alcohol, and stearyl alcohol.)

NURSING PROCESS

Assessment
• Assess underlying skin condition before starting therapy, and regularly thereafter to monitor the drug's effectiveness. Clear up infections at disease sites before use.
• Assess patient's and family's knowledge of drug therapy.

Nursing diagnoses
• Risk for situational low self-esteem related to skin disorder
• Impaired skin integrity related to underlying skin condition
• Deficient knowledge related to pimecrolimus therapy

Planning and implementation
• May be used on all skin surfaces, including the head, neck, and intertriginous areas.
• Use only after other treatments have failed because of risk of cancer with its use.
• If disease resolves, stop giving the drug.
• If symptoms persist beyond 6 weeks, reevaluate patient.
⚠ ALERT: Don't use with occlusive dressing; this may promote systemic exposure.
• May cause local symptoms such as skin burning. Most local reactions start within 1 to 5 days, are mild to moderately severe, and last no more than 5 days.
• Monitor patient for lymphadenopathy. If the cause isn't clear or the patient has acute infectious mononucleosis, consider stopping drug.
• Papillomas or warts may occur. If skin papillomas worsen or don't respond to conventional therapy, consider stopping drug.
Patient teaching
• Instruct patient to use as directed; this drug is for external use on the skin only. Tell patient to report any signs or symptoms of adverse reactions.
• Tell patient not to use drug with an occlusive dressing.
• Instruct patient to wash hands after application if hands aren't being treated.
• Tell patient to stop using the drug after signs and symptoms of atopic dermatitis have re-

P

solved. Tell patient to contact prescriber if symptoms persist beyond 6 weeks.
• Advise patient to resume therapy at the first signs or symptoms of recurrence.
• Instruct patient to minimize or avoid exposure to natural or artificial sunlight (including tanning beds and ultraviolet A and B therapy) while using this drug.
• Tell patient that application site reactions are expected, but to notify prescriber if reaction is severe or persists for more than 1 week.

☑ Evaluation
• Patient has improved self-esteem as skin condition clears.
• Patient has improved skin condition.
• Patient and family state understanding of drug therapy.

pioglitazone hydrochloride
(pigh-oh-GLIH-tah-zohn high-droh-KLOR-ighd)
Actos

Pharmacologic class: thiazolidinedione
Therapeutic class: antidiabetic
Pregnancy risk category: C

Indications and dosages

▶ **Monotherapy adjunct to diet and exercise to improve glycemic control in patients with type 2 diabetes mellitus, or combination therapy with a sulfonylurea, metformin, or insulin when diet, exercise, and the single drug don't yield adequate glycemic control.** *Adults:* Initially, 15 or 30 mg P.O. once daily. For patients who respond inadequately to initial dose, increase in increments; maximum daily dose is 45 mg. If used in combination therapy, don't exceed 30 mg daily.

Contraindications and cautions

• Contraindicated in patients hypersensitive to the drug or any of its components. Not recommended for New York Heart Association Class III and IV cardiac patients.
• Also contraindicated in patients with type 1 diabetes mellitus or diabetic ketoacidosis, patients with evidence of active liver disease, patients with ALT levels more than 2½ times the upper limit of normal, and patients who experienced jaundice while taking troglitazone.

☀ **Lifespan:** In pregnant women, use only if benefits outweigh potential risks to the fetus; insulin is the preferred antidiabetic for use during pregnancy. Potentially excreted in breast milk. Avoid use if breast-feeding. Safety has not been established in children younger than 18.

Adverse reactions

CNS: headache.
CV: edema, *heart failure.*
EENT: sinusitis, pharyngitis.
Hematologic: anemia.
Metabolic: *hypoglycemia with combination therapy,* aggravated diabetes mellitus, weight gain.
Musculoskeletal: myalgia.
Respiratory: upper respiratory tract infection.
Other: tooth disorder.

Interactions

Drug-drug. *Hormonal contraceptives:* May reduce levels of hormonal contraceptives, resulting in less effective contraception. Advise patients taking pioglitazone and hormonal contraceptives to consider additional birth control measures.
Ketoconazole: May inhibit pioglitazone metabolism. Monitor patient's glucose levels more frequently.
Drug-herb. *Aloe, bilberry leaf, bitter melon, burdock, dandelion, fenugreek, garlic, ginseng:* May improve blood glucose control and allow reduction of antidiabetic dosage. Advise patient to discuss herbal remedies with prescriber before using them.

Effects on lab test results

• May increase liver enzyme and HDL levels. May decrease glucose, triglyceride, and hemoglobin levels and hematocrit.

Pharmacokinetics

Absorption: When taken on an empty stomach, rapidly absorbed and measurable in serum within 30 minutes; level peaks within 2 hours. Food slightly delays time to peak levels (to 3 to 4 hours), but doesn't affect the overall extent of absorption.
Distribution: Drug and its metabolites are extensively protein-bound (more than 98%), primarily to albumin.

Metabolism: Extensively metabolized by the liver. Three metabolites, M-II, M-III, and M-IV, are pharmacologically active.
Excretion: About 15% to 30% of dose is recovered in urine, primarily as metabolites and their conjugates. Most of P.O. dose is excreted in bile and eliminated in feces. *Half-life:* 3 to 7 hours.

Route	Onset	Peak	Duration
P.O.	Unknown	< 2 hr	Unknown

Action

Chemical effect: Decreases insulin resistance in the periphery and in the liver, resulting in decreased glucose output by the liver.
Therapeutic effect: Lowers glucose level.

Available forms

Tablets: 15 mg, 30 mg, 45 mg

NURSING PROCESS

Assessment
● Obtain history of patient's underlying condition before starting therapy, and regularly thereafter to monitor the drug's effectiveness.
● Assess patient for excessive fluid volume. Monitor patient with heart failure for increased edema.
● Measure liver enzymes at start of therapy, q 2 months for the first year of therapy, and periodically thereafter. Obtain liver function test results in patients who develop evidence of liver dysfunction, such as nausea, vomiting, abdominal pain, fatigue, anorexia, or dark urine.
● Monitor hemoglobin level and hematocrit, especially during the first 4 to 12 weeks of therapy.
● Monitor glucose level regularly, especially during situations of increased stress, such as infection, fever, surgery, and trauma.
● Check glycosylated hemoglobin level periodically to evaluate therapeutic response to drug.
● Assess patient's and family's knowledge of drug therapy.

Nursing diagnoses
● Ineffective health maintenance related to hyperglycemia
● Risk for injury related to drug-induced hyperglycemia
● Deficient knowledge related to drug therapy

Planning and implementation
● If patient develops jaundice or if results of liver function tests show ALT elevations greater than three times the upper limit of normal, notify prescriber and stop giving the drug.
● Drug alone or with insulin can cause fluid retention that may lead to or exacerbate heart failure. Observe patients for signs or symptoms of heart failure. If cardiac condition deteriorates, stop drug.
● Watch for hypoglycemia in patients taking pioglitazone with insulin or a sulfonylurea. Dosage adjustments of these drugs may be needed.
● Premenopausal, anovulatory women with insulin resistance may need contraception because ovulation may resume.
Patient teaching
● Tell patient to control his diet in order to manage type 2 diabetes because calorie restrictions, weight loss, and exercise improve insulin sensitivity and make drug therapy more effective.
● Instruct patient to adhere to dietary instructions and to have glucose and glycosylated hemoglobin level tested regularly.
● Inform patient taking drug with insulin or an oral antidiabetic about the signs and symptoms of hypoglycemia.
● Tell patient to notify prescriber about periods of stress, such as fever, trauma, infection, or surgery, because drug requirements may change.
● Inform patient that blood tests for liver function will be performed before the start of therapy, every 2 months for the first year, and periodically thereafter.
● Tell patient to report unexplained nausea, vomiting, abdominal pain, fatigue, anorexia, or dark urine immediately because these signs and symptoms may indicate liver problems.
● Advise patient to contact prescriber if he has signs or symptoms of heart failure (unusually rapid increase in weight or edema, shortness of breath).
● Inform patient that pioglitazone can be taken with or without meals.
● If patient misses a dose, warn against doubling the dose the following day.
● Advise premenopausal, anovulatory woman with insulin resistance that drug may restore ovulation; recommend that she consider contraception as needed.

P

Evaluation

• Patient's glucose level is normal with drug therapy.
• Patient doesn't experience hypoglycemia.
• Patient and family state understanding of drug therapy.

piperacillin sodium and tazobactam sodium

(pigh-PER-uh-sil-in SOH-dee-um and taz-oh-BAK-tem SOH-dee-um)
Zosyn

Pharmacologic class: extended-spectrum penicillin, beta-lactamase inhibitor
Therapeutic class: antibiotic
Pregnancy risk category: B

Indications and dosages

▶ **Moderate to severe infections caused by piperacillin-resistant, piperacillin and tazobactam–susceptible, beta-lactamase–producing strains of microorganisms in the following conditions: appendicitis (complicated by rupture or abscess) and peritonitis caused by** *Escherichia coli, Bacteroides fragilis, B. ovatus, B. thetaiotaomicron, B. vulgatus;* **skin and skin-structure infections caused by** *Staphylococcus aureus;* **postpartum endometritis or pelvic inflammatory disease caused by** *E. coli;* **moderately severe community-acquired pneumonia caused by** *Haemophilus influenzae. Adults:* 3.375 g (3 g piperacillin/0.375 g tazobactam) q 6 hours as a 30-minute I.V. infusion for 7 to 10 days.
§ **Adjust-a-dose:** For patients with renal impairment, if creatinine clearance is 20 to 40 ml/minute, give 2.25 g (2 g piperacillin/0.25 g tazobactam) q 6 hours; if clearance is less than 20 ml/minute, give same dose q 8 hours.

In patients undergoing continuous ambulatory peritoneal dialysis (CAPD), give same dose q 12 hours. In hemodialysis patients, give same dose q 12 hours with a supplemental dose of 0.75 g (0.67 g piperacillin/0.08 g tazobactam) after each dialysis period.
▶ **Moderate to severe nosocomial pneumonia caused by piperacillin-resistant, beta-lactamase–producing strains of** *S. aureus* **and by piperacillin and tazobactam–susceptible**

Acinetobacter baumannii, H. influenzae, Klebsiella pneumoniae, **and** *Pseudomonas aeruginosa. Adults:* 4.5 g (4 g piperacillin/0.5 g tazobactam) q 6 hours given with an aminoglycoside for 7 to 14 days. For patients with *P. aeruginosa,* continue aminoglycoside therapy; if *P. aeruginosa* isn't isolated, may stop aminoglycoside therapy.
§ **Adjust-a-dose:** For patients with renal impairment, if creatinine clearance is 20 to 40 ml/minute, give 3.375 g (3 g piperacillin and 0.375 g tazobactam) q 6 hours; if clearance is less than 20 ml/minute, give 2.25 g (2 g piperacillin and 0.25 g tazobactam) q 6 hours. In CAPD patients, give 2.25 g (2 g piperacillin and 0.25 g tazobactam) q 8 hours.

▼ I.V. administration

• Reconstitute each gram of drug with 5 ml of diluent, such as sterile or bacteriostatic water for injection, normal saline solution for injection, bacteriostatic normal saline solution for injection, D_5W, 5% dextrose in normal saline solution for injection, or dextran 6% in normal saline solution for injection. Shake until dissolved. Further dilute to final volume of 50 ml before infusion.
• Infuse drug over at least 30 minutes. Stop other primary infusions during administration if possible. Aminoglycoside antibiotics (such as gentamicin and tobramycin) are chemically incompatible with drug. Don't mix in same I.V. container.
• Use drug immediately after reconstitution. Discard unused drug in single-dose vials after 24 hours if held at room temperature; after 48 hours if refrigerated. Diluted drug is stable in I.V. bags for 24 hours at room temperature or 1 week if refrigerated.
• Change I.V. site every 48 hours.
⊗ **Incompatibilities**
Acyclovir sodium, aminoglycosides, amphotericin B, chlorpromazine, cisatracurium, cisplatin, dacarbazine, daunorubicin, dobutamine, doxorubicin, doxycycline hyclate, droperidol, famotidine, ganciclovir, gemcitabine, haloperidol lactate, hydroxyzine hydrochloride, idarubicin, lactated Ringer's solution, minocycline, mitomycin, mitoxantrone, nalbuphine, prochlorperazine edisylate, promethazine hydrochloride, streptozocin, vancomycin.

Contraindications and cautions

• Contraindicated in patients hypersensitive to the drug or other penicillins.

• Use cautiously in patients with other drug allergies, especially to cephalosporins (risk of cross-sensitivity), and in those with bleeding tendencies, uremia, or hypokalemia.

⚕ Lifespan: In pregnant women, use cautiously. In breast-feeding women, use cautiously; it's unknown if the drug appears in breast milk. In children younger than age 12, safety and effectiveness haven't been established.

Adverse reactions

CNS: pain, *headache, insomnia,* agitation, fever, dizziness, anxiety.
CV: hypertension, tachycardia, chest pain, edema.
EENT: rhinitis.
GI: *diarrhea, nausea, constipation,* vomiting, dyspepsia, stool changes, abdominal pain.
Hematologic: *thrombocytopenia.*
Respiratory: dyspnea.
Skin: rash (including maculopapular, bullous, urticarial, and eczematoid), pruritus.
Other: *anaphylaxis,* candidiasis, inflammation and phlebitis at I.V. site.

Interactions

Drug-drug. *Anticoagulants:* May increase risk of bleeding. Monitor PT, PTT, and INR, and monitor patient for bleeding.
Hormonal contraceptives: May decrease effectiveness of hormonal contraceptives. Advise alternative barrier method during therapy.
Probenecid: May increase levels of piperacillin. Probenecid may be used for this purpose.
Vecuronium: May prolong neuromuscular blockage. Monitor patient closely.

Effects on lab test results

• May decrease hemoglobin level and hematocrit.
• May increase eosinophil count. May decrease WBC and platelet counts.

Pharmacokinetics

Absorption: Administered I.V.
Distribution: Both drugs are about 30% protein-bound.
Metabolism: Piperacillin is metabolized to a minor, microbiologically active desethyl metabolite. Tazobactam is metabolized to a

single metabolite that lacks pharmacologic and antibacterial activities.
Excretion: Excreted in urine and bile. *Half-life:* piperacillin, 40 minutes; tazobactam, 70 minutes.

Route	Onset	Peak	Duration
I.V.	Immediate	Immediate	Unknown

Action

Chemical effect: Piperacillin inhibits cell wall synthesis during microorganism multiplication; tazobactam increases piperacillin effectiveness by inactivating beta-lactamases, which destroy penicillins.
Therapeutic effect: Kills susceptible bacteria.

Available forms

Powder for injection: 2 g piperacillin and 0.25 g tazobactam per vial, 3 g piperacillin and 0.375 g tazobactam per vial, 4 g piperacillin and 0.5 g tazobactam per vial

NURSING PROCESS

☞ Assessment
• Before giving drug, ask patient about previous allergic reactions to this drug or other penicillins. Negative history of penicillin allergy doesn't guarantee future safety.
• Assess patient's infection before starting therapy, and regularly thereafter to monitor the drug's effectiveness.
• Obtain specimen for culture and sensitivity tests before first dose. Start therapy pending test results.
• Be alert for adverse reactions and drug interactions.
• If adverse GI reaction occurs, monitor patient's hydration.
• Assess patient's and family's knowledge of drug therapy.

⊕ Nursing diagnoses
• Infection related to presence of bacteria
• Risk of deficient fluid volume related to adverse GI reactions
• Deficient knowledge related to drug therapy

▷ Planning and implementation
• Because hemodialysis removes 6% of piperacillin dose and 21% of tazobactam dose, supplemental doses may be needed after hemodialysis.

P

Patient teaching
• Tell patient to report pain or discomfort at I.V. site.
• Advise patient to limit salt intake while taking drug because piperacillin contains 1.98 mEq of sodium per gram.
• Tell patient to report adverse reactions.

☑ **Evaluation**
• Patient is free from infection.
• Patient maintains adequate hydration.
• Patient and family state understanding of drug therapy.

polyethylene glycol and electrolyte solution

(pol-ee-ETH-ih-leen GLIGH-kohl and ee-LEK-troh-light soh-LOO-shun)
CoLyte, GoLYTELY, NuLYTELY, OCL, TriLyte

Pharmacologic class: polyethylene glycol (PEG) 3350 nonabsorbable solution
Therapeutic class: laxative and bowel evacuant
Pregnancy risk category: C

Indications and dosages

▶ **Bowel preparation before GI examination.**
Adults: 240 ml P.O. q 10 minutes until 4 L are consumed. Typically, give 4 hours before examination, allowing 3 hours for drinking and 1 hour for bowel evacuation.
▶ **Management of acute iron overdose‡.**
Children older than age 3: 2,953 ml/kg over 5 days.

Contraindications and cautions

• Contraindicated in patients with GI obstruction or perforation, gastric retention, toxic colitis, or megacolon.
⚜ **Lifespan:** In pregnant women, use cautiously. In breast-feeding women, use cautiously; it's unknown if the drug appears in breast milk.

Adverse reactions

GI: nausea, bloating, cramps, vomiting.

Interactions

Drug-drug. *Oral drugs:* May decrease absorption if given within 1 hour of starting therapy. Don't give with other oral drugs.

Effects on lab test results

None reported.

Pharmacokinetics

Absorption: None.
Distribution: Not applicable because drug isn't absorbed.
Metabolism: Not applicable because drug isn't absorbed.
Excretion: In GI tract. *Half-life:* None.

Route	Onset	Peak	Duration
P.O.	≤ 1 hr	Varies	Varies

Action

Chemical effect: Acts as an osmotic agent. Sodium sulfate greatly reduces sodium absorption. The electrolyte concentration causes virtually no net absorption or secretion of ions.
Therapeutic effect: Cleanses bowel.

Available forms

Oral solution: PEG 3350 (6 g), sodium sulfate decahydrate (1.29 g), sodium chloride (146 mg), potassium chloride (75 mg), sodium bicarbonate (168 mg), polysorbate 80 (30 mg) per 100 ml (OCL)
Powder for oral solution: PEG 3350 (240 g), sodium sulfate (22.72 g), sodium chloride (5.84 g), potassium chloride (2.98 g), sodium bicarbonate (6.72 g) per 4 L (CoLyte); PEG 3350 (236 g), sodium sulfate (22.74 g), sodium bicarbonate (6.74 g), sodium chloride (5.86 g), potassium chloride (2.97 g) per 4 L (GoLYTELY); PEG 3350 (420 g), sodium bicarbonate (5.72 g), sodium chloride (11.2 g), potassium chloride (1.48 g) per 4 L (NuLYTELY)

NURSING PROCESS

🗷 **Assessment**
• Assess patient's condition before starting therapy, and regularly thereafter to monitor the drug's effectiveness.
• Be alert for adverse reactions and drug interactions.
• Assess patient's and family's knowledge of drug therapy.

🔠 **Nursing diagnoses**
• Health-seeking behavior (testing) related to need to determine cause of underlying GI problem

• Risk for deficient fluid volume related to adverse GI reactions
• Deficient knowledge related to drug therapy

Planning and implementation
• Use tap water to reconstitute powder. Shake vigorously to make sure all powder is dissolved. Refrigerate solution but use within 48 hours.
ALERT: Don't add flavoring or additional ingredients to solution or administer chilled solution. Hypothermia has developed after ingestion of large amounts of chilled solution.
• If patient is scheduled for midmorning examination, give solution early in morning. Oral solution induces diarrhea in 30 to 60 minutes that rapidly cleans bowel, usually within 4 hours.
• When used as preparation for barium enema, give solution the evening before examination, to avoid interfering with barium coating of colonic mucosa.
• If giving to adult via NG tube infuse at 20 to 30 ml/minute.
• If given to semiconscious patient or to patient with impaired gag reflex, take care to prevent aspiration.
• No major shifts in fluid or electrolyte balance have been reported.
Patient teaching
• Tell patient to fast for 4 hours before taking solution and to ingest only clear fluids until examination is complete.
• Warn patient about adverse GI reactions to drug.
• Advise patient that rapid drinking of each portion is preferred to drinking small amounts continuously.

Evaluation
• Patient is able to have examination.
• Patient maintains adequate fluid volume.
• Patient and family state understanding of drug therapy.

---

potassium acetate
(poh-TAS-ee-um AS-ih-tayt)

Pharmacologic class: potassium supplement
Therapeutic class: electrolyte
Pregnancy risk category: C

Indications and dosages
▶ **Hypokalemia.** *Adults:* No more than 20 mEq I.V. hourly at concentration of 40 mEq/L or less. Maximum daily dose, 150 mEq. Monitor ECG and perform frequent potassium tests with potassium replacement. Use I.V. route only for life-threatening hypokalemia or when oral replacement isn't feasible.
▶ **To prevent hypokalemia.** *Adults:* Dosage is individualized to patient's needs, not to exceed 150 mEq daily. Give as an additive to I.V. infusions. Usual dosage is 20 mEq/L infused at no more than 20 mEq/hour.
Children: Individualized dosage not to exceed 3 mEq/kg daily. Give as an additive to I.V. infusions.

I.V. administration
• Give drug only by I.V. infusion, never by I.V. push or I.M. route.
• Dilute drug before administration and give slowly; life-threatening hyperkalemia may result from a rapid infusion.
• Watch for pain and redness at infusion site. Large-bore needle reduces local irritation.
⊗ **Incompatibilities**
Calcium, phosphate, and sulfate solutions.

Contraindications and cautions
• Contraindicated in patients with severe renal impairment with oliguria, anuria, or azotemia; those with untreated Addison's disease or adrenocortical insufficiency; and those with acute dehydration, heat cramps, hyperkalemia, hyperkalemic form of familial periodic paralysis, and conditions related to extensive tissue breakdown.
• Use cautiously in patients with cardiac disease or renal impairment.
Lifespan: In pregnant women, use cautiously. In breast-feeding women, use cautiously; it's unknown if the drug appears in breast milk.

Adverse reactions
CNS: paresthesia of limbs, listlessness, mental confusion, weakness or heaviness of legs, flaccid paralysis.
CV: *arrhythmias, cardiac arrest, heart block,* ECG changes.
GI: nausea, vomiting, abdominal pain, diarrhea.
GU: oliguria.

P

Respiratory: *respiratory paralysis.*
Skin: cold skin, gray pallor.
Other: pain, redness at infusion site.

Interactions

Drug-drug. *ACE inhibitors, potassium-sparing diuretics:* May increase risk of hyperkalemia. Use cautiously.
Drug-herb. *Cascara, licorice:* May antagonize effects of potassium supplements. Discourage using together.
Drug-food. *Salt substitutes:* May increase risk of hyperkalemia. Don't use together.

Effects on lab test results

● May increase potassium level.

Pharmacokinetics

Absorption: Administered I.V.
Distribution: Distributed throughout body.
Metabolism: None significant.
Excretion: Largely by kidneys. *Half-life:* Unknown.

Route	Onset	Peak	Duration
I.V.	Immediate	Immediate	Unknown

Action

Chemical effect: Aids in transmitting nerve impulses, contracting cardiac and skeletal muscle, and maintaining intracellular tonicity, cellular metabolism, acid-base balance, and normal renal function.
Therapeutic effect: Replaces and maintains potassium level.

Available forms

Injection: 2 mEq/ml in 20-ml, 50-ml, 100-ml vials; 4 mEq/ml in 50-ml vial

NURSING PROCESS

Assessment
● Assess patient's condition before starting therapy, and regularly thereafter to monitor the drug's effectiveness.
● During therapy, monitor ECG, renal function, fluid intake and output, and potassium, creatinine, and BUN levels.
● Be alert for adverse reactions and drug interactions.

● Assess patient's and family's knowledge of drug therapy.

Nursing diagnoses
● Ineffective health maintenance related to presence of hypokalemia
● Risk for injury related to drug-induced hyperkalemia
● Deficient knowledge related to drug therapy

Planning and implementation
● Don't give potassium postoperatively until urine flow is established.
⊛ ALERT: Potassium preparations aren't interchangeable. Verify preparation before giving.
Patient teaching
● Inform patient of need for potassium supplementation.
● Tell patient that drug will be given through an I.V. line.
● Instruct patient to report adverse reactions.

Evaluation
● Patient's potassium level returns to normal with drug therapy.
● Patient doesn't develop hyperkalemia as result of drug therapy.
● Patient and family state understanding of drug therapy.

potassium bicarbonate
(poh-TAS-ee-um bigh-KAR-buh-nayt)
K+ Care ET

Pharmacologic class: potassium supplement
Therapeutic class: mineral
Pregnancy risk category: C

Indications and dosages

▶ **Hypokalemia.** *Adults:* 25 to 50 mEq dissolved in 4 to 8 oz (120 to 240 ml) of water and given P.O. once daily to b.i.d.

Contraindications and cautions

● Contraindicated in patients with untreated Addison's disease, acute dehydration, heat cramps, hyperkalemia, hyperkalemic form of familial periodic paralysis, other conditions linked to extensive tissue breakdown, or severe renal impairment with oliguria, anuria, or azotemia.

• Use cautiously in patients with cardiac disease or renal impairment.
Lifespan: In pregnant women, use cautiously. In breast-feeding women, use cautiously; it's unknown if the drug appears in breast milk. In children, safety and effectiveness haven't been established.

Adverse reactions

CNS: paresthesia of limbs, listlessness, mental confusion, weakness or heaviness of legs, flaccid paralysis.
CV: ***arrhythmias, cardiac arrest, heart block,*** ECG changes (prolonged PR interval, widened QRS complex, ST-segment depression, and tall, tented T waves).
GI: *nausea, vomiting, abdominal pain,* diarrhea, ulcerations, ***hemorrhage, obstruction, perforation.***

Interactions

Drug-drug. *ACE inhibitors, potassium-sparing diuretics:* May increase risk of hyperkalemia. Use cautiously.
Drug-food. *Salt substitutes:* May increase risk of hyperkalemia. Don't use together.

Effects on lab test results

• May increase potassium level.

Pharmacokinetics

Absorption: Well absorbed from GI tract.
Distribution: Distributed throughout body.
Metabolism: None significant.
Excretion: Excreted largely by kidneys. *Half-life:* Unknown.

Route	Onset	Peak	Duration
P.O.	Unknown	≤ 4 hr	Unknown

Action

Chemical effect: Aids in transmitting nerve impulses, contracting cardiac and skeletal muscle, and maintaining intracellular tonicity, cellular metabolism, acid-base balance, and normal renal function.
Therapeutic effect: Replaces and maintains potassium level.

Available forms

Effervescent tablets: 6.5 mEq, 25 mEq

NURSING PROCESS

Assessment

• Assess patient's condition before starting therapy, and regularly thereafter to monitor the drug's effectiveness.
• During therapy, monitor ECG, renal function, fluid intake and output, and potassium, creatinine, and BUN levels.
• Be alert for adverse reactions and drug interactions.
• Assess patient's and family's knowledge of drug therapy.

Nursing diagnoses

• Ineffective health maintenance related to presence of hypokalemia
• Risk for injury related to potassium-induced hyperkalemia
• Deficient knowledge related to drug therapy

Planning and implementation

• Dissolve potassium bicarbonate tablets completely in 6 to 8 oz of cold water to minimize GI irritation.
• Ask patient's flavor preference. Available in lime, fruit punch, and orange flavors.
• Have patient take with meals and sip slowly over 5 to 10 minutes.
• Don't give potassium supplements postoperatively until urine flow has been established.
ALERT: Potassium preparations aren't interchangeable. Verify preparation before giving.

Patient teaching

• Inform patient about need for potassium supplementation.
• Teach patient how to prepare and take drug.
• Instruct patient to report adverse reactions.

Evaluation

• Patient's potassium level returns to normal.
• Patient doesn't develop hyperkalemia as result of drug therapy.
• Patient and family state understanding of drug therapy.

potassium chloride

(poh-TAS-ee-um KLOR-ighd)

Apo-K*, Cena-K, Gen-K, K-8, K-10*, K+10, Kaochlor, Kaochlor S-F*, Kaon-Cl, Kaon-Cl-10, Kaon-Cl 20%*, Kay Ciel*, K+ Care, K-Dur 10, K-Dur 20◆, K-Lease, K-Lor, Klor-Con, Klor-Con 8, Klor-Con 10, Klor-Con/25, Klorvess, Klotrix, K·Lyte/Cl, K-Norm, K-Tab, K-Vescent, Micro-K Extencaps, Micro-K 10 Extencaps, Micro-K LS, Potasalan, Slow-K, Ten-K

Pharmacologic class: potassium supplement
Therapeutic class: mineral
Pregnancy risk category: C

Indications and dosages

▶ **Prevention of hypokalemia.** *Adults and children:* Initially, 20 mEq P.O. daily in divided doses. Adjust dosage, p.r.n., based on potassium level.

▶ **Hypokalemia.** *Adults and children:* 40 to 100 mEq P.O. daily divided into two to four doses. Use I.V. potassium chloride when oral replacement isn't feasible. Maximum dose of diluted I.V. potassium chloride is 20 mEq/hour of 40 mEq/L solution. Further dose based on potassium level. Don't exceed 150 mEq P.O. daily in adults and 3 mEq/kg P.O. daily in children. Further doses are based on potassium level and blood pH. Monitor ECG and obtain potassium level frequently when giving I.V. potassium replacement.

▶ **Severe hypokalemia.** *Adults and children:* Dilute potassium chloride in a suitable I.V. solution to 80 mEq/L or less and give at no more than 40 mEq/hour. Base next dose on potassium level. Don't exceed 150 mEq I.V. daily in adults and 3 mEq/kg I.V. daily or 40 mEq/m² daily for children.

▶ **Acute MI‡.** *Adults:* High dose—80 mEq/L at 1.5 ml/kg/hour for 24 hours with an I.V. infusion of 25% dextrose and 50 units/L regular insulin. Low dose—40 mEq/L at 1 ml/kg/hour for 24 hours, with an I.V. infusion of 10% dextrose and 20 units/L regular insulin.

▼ I.V. administration

● Give parenteral drug only by infusion, never by I.V. push or I.M. route.

● Give slowly as dilute solution; life-threatening hyperkalemia may result from a rapid infusion.

⊗ **Incompatibilities**
Amikacin, amphotericin B, diazepam, dobutamine, ergotamine, fat emulsion 10%, methylprednisolone sodium succinate, penicillin G sodium, phenytoin sodium, promethazine hydrochloride.

Contraindications and cautions

● Contraindicated in patients with untreated Addison's disease, adrenocortical insufficiency, acute dehydration, heat cramps, hyperkalemia, hyperkalemic form of familial periodic paralysis, other conditions linked to extensive tissue breakdown, or severe renal impairment with oliguria, anuria, or azotemia.

● Use cautiously in patients with cardiac disease or renal impairment.

❀ **Lifespan:** In pregnant women, use cautiously. In breast-feeding women, use cautiously; it's unknown if the drug appears in breast milk.

Adverse reactions

CNS: paresthesia of limbs, listlessness, mental confusion, weakness or heaviness of limbs, flaccid paralysis.
CV: *arrhythmias, heart block, cardiac arrest,* ECG changes (prolonged PR interval, widened QRS complex, ST-segment depression, and tall, tented T waves).
GI: nausea, vomiting, abdominal pain, diarrhea, *GI ulcerations (stenosis, hemorrhage, obstruction, perforation).*
GU: oliguria.
Respiratory: *respiratory paralysis.*
Skin: cold skin, gray pallor, phlebitis.

Interactions

Drug-drug. *ACE inhibitors, potassium-sparing diuretics:* May increase risk of hyperkalemia. Use cautiously.
Drug-herb. *Cascara, licorice:* May antagonize effects of potassium supplements. Discourage using together.
Drug-food. *Salt substitutes:* May increase risk of hyperkalemia. Don't use together.

Effects on lab test results

● May increase potassium level.

Pharmacokinetics

Absorption: Well absorbed.

Distribution: Distributed throughout body.
Metabolism: None significant.
Excretion: Excreted largely by kidneys; small amounts may be excreted by skin and intestinal tract, but intestinal potassium is usually reabsorbed. *Half-life:* Unknown.

Route	Onset	Peak	Duration
P.O.	Unknown	≤ 4 hr	Unknown
I.V.	Immediate	Immediate	Unknown

Action

Chemical effect: Aids in transmitting nerve impulses, contracting cardiac and skeletal muscle, and maintaining intracellular tonicity, cellular metabolism, acid-base balance, and normal renal function.
Therapeutic effect: Replaces and maintains potassium level.

Available forms

Capsules (controlled-release): 8 mEq, 10 mEq
Injection concentrate: 1.5 mEq/ml, 2 mEq/ml
Injection for I.V. infusion: 0.1mEq/ml, 0.2 mEq/ml, 0.3 mEq/ml, 0.4 mEq/ml
Oral liquid: 20 mEq/15 ml*, 30 mEq/15 ml, 40 mEq/15 ml*
Powder for oral administration: 15 mEq/packet, 20 mEq/packet, 25 mEq/packet
Tablets (controlled-release): 6.7 mEq, 8 mEq, 10 mEq, 20 mEq
Tablets (extended-release): 8 mEq, 10 mEq

NURSING PROCESS

Assessment

- Assess patient's condition before starting therapy, and regularly thereafter to monitor the drug's effectiveness.
- During therapy, monitor ECG, renal function, fluid intake and output, and potassium, creatinine, and BUN levels.
- Be alert for adverse reactions and drug interactions.
- Assess patient's and family's knowledge of drug therapy.

Nursing diagnoses

- Ineffective health maintenance related to presence of hypokalemia
- Risk for injury related to drug-induced hyperkalemia
- Deficient knowledge related to drug therapy

Planning and implementation

- When giving I.V. potassium replacement, monitor ECG and take potassium level frequently.
- Give cautiously because different potassium supplements deliver varying amounts of potassium. Never switch products without prescriber's order.
- Make sure powders are completely dissolved before giving.
- Don't crush sustained-release potassium products.
- Give potassium with or after meals with full glass of water or fruit juice to lessen GI distress.
- If tablet or capsule passage is likely to be delayed, as in GI obstruction, use sugar-free liquid (Kaochlor S-F 10%). Have patient sip slowly to minimize GI irritation.
- Enteric-coated tablets increase risk of GI bleeding and small-bowel ulcerations; use cautiously.
- Tablets in wax matrix sometimes lodge in esophagus and cause ulceration in cardiac patients who have esophageal compression from enlarged left atrium. Use liquid form in such patients and in those with esophageal stasis or obstruction.
- Drug is commonly given with potassium-wasting diuretics to maintain potassium levels.

ALERT: Potassium preparations aren't interchangeable. Verify preparation before giving.
ALERT: Don't give potassium postoperatively until urine flow is established.

Patient teaching

- Tell patient that controlled-release tablets may appear in stool but that the drug has already been absorbed.
- Instruct patient to report adverse reactions and pain at the I.V. site.

Evaluation

- Patient's potassium level returns to normal.
- Patient doesn't develop hyperkalemia.
- Patient and family state understanding of drug therapy.

P

potassium gluconate
(poh-TAS-ee-um GLOO-kuh-nayt)
Kaon, Kaylixir*, K-G Elixir*

Pharmacologic class: potassium supplement
Therapeutic class: mineral
Pregnancy risk category: C

Indications and dosages

▶ **Hypokalemia.** *Adults:* 40 to 100 mEq P.O.
daily in three or four divided doses; 20 mEq
P.O. daily for prevention. Further dosage based
on potassium level determinations.

Contraindications and cautions

• Contraindicated in patients with untreated Addison's disease, acute dehydration, heat cramps, hyperkalemia, hyperkalemic form of familial periodic paralysis, other conditions related to extensive tissue breakdown, or severe renal impairment with oliguria, anuria, or azotemia.
• Use cautiously in patients with cardiac disease or renal impairment.
⚠ Lifespan: In pregnant women, use cautiously. In breast-feeding women, use cautiously; it's unknown if the drug appears in breast milk. In children, safety and effectiveness haven't been established.

Adverse reactions

CNS: paresthesia of limbs, listlessness, mental confusion, weakness or heaviness of legs, flaccid paralysis.
CV: *arrhythmias,* ECG changes (prolonged PR interval, widened QRS complex, ST-segment depression, and tall, tented T waves).
GI: *nausea and vomiting; abdominal pain;* diarrhea; *GI ulcerations* that may be accompanied by stenosis, *hemorrhage, obstruction or perforation* (with oral products, especially enteric-coated tablets).

Interactions

Drug-drug. *ACE inhibitors, potassium-sparing diuretics:* May increase risk of hyperkalemia. Use cautiously.
Drug-food. *Salt substitutes:* May increase risk of hyperkalemia. Don't use together.

Effects on lab test results

• May increase potassium level.

Pharmacokinetics

Absorption: Well absorbed from GI tract.
Distribution: Distributed throughout body.
Metabolism: None significant.
Excretion: Excreted largely by kidneys; small amounts may be excreted by skin and intestinal tract, but intestinal potassium is usually reabsorbed. *Half-life:* Unknown.

Route	Onset	Peak	Duration
P.O.	Unknown	≤ 4 hr	Unknown

Action

Chemical effect: Aids in transmitting nerve impulses, contracting cardiac and skeletal muscle, and maintaining intracellular tonicity, cellular metabolism, acid-base balance, and normal renal function.
Therapeutic effect: Replaces and maintains potassium level.

Available forms

Liquid: 20 mEq/15 ml*
Tablets: 500 mg†, 595 mg† (83.45 mg and 99 mg potassium, respectively)

NURSING PROCESS

⚕ Assessment
• Assess patient's condition before starting therapy, and regularly thereafter to monitor the drug's effectiveness.
• During therapy, monitor ECG, renal function, fluid intake and output, and potassium, creatinine, and BUN levels.
• Be alert for adverse reactions and drug interactions.
• Assess patient's and family's knowledge of drug therapy.

⚕ Nursing diagnoses
• Ineffective health maintenance related to presence of hypokalemia
• Risk for injury related to potassium-induced hyperkalemia
• Deficient knowledge related to drug therapy

▷ Planning and implementation
• Give cautiously because different potassium supplements deliver varying amounts of potassium. Never switch products without prescriber's order.

• Give drug with or after meals with glass of water or fruit juice.
• Have patient sip liquid potassium slowly to minimize GI irritation.
• Enteric-coated tablets aren't recommended because of increased risk of GI bleeding and small-bowel ulcerations.
⊛ **ALERT:** Potassium preparations aren't interchangeable. Verify preparation before giving.
⊛ **ALERT:** Don't give potassium supplements postoperatively until urine flow is established.
Patient teaching
• Inform patient of need for potassium supplementation.
• Teach patient how to take drug.
• Instruct patient to report adverse reactions.

☑ **Evaluation**
• Patient's potassium level returns to normal.
• Patient doesn't develop hyperkalemia as result of drug therapy.
• Patient and family state understanding of drug therapy.

potassium iodide
(poh-TAS-ee-um IGH-uh-dighd)
Iosat, Pima, Thyro-Block

potassium iodide, saturated solution (SSKI)

strong iodine solution (Lugol's solution)

Pharmacologic class: antithyroid
Therapeutic class: radiation protectant
Pregnancy risk category: D

Indications and dosages

▶ **Preparation for thyroidectomy.** *Adults and children:* 0.1 to 0.3 ml (2 to 6 drops) strong iodine solution P.O. t.i.d. for 10 days before surgery.
▶ **Thyrotoxic crisis.** *Adults and children:* 500 mg P.O. q 4 hours (about 10 drops of 1 g/ml solution).
▶ **Radiation protectant for thyroid gland.** *Adults:* 130 mg P.O. daily for 10 days after radiation exposure. Start no later than 3 to 4 hours

after acute exposure. Or, 3 ml Pima P.O. daily 24 hours before and for 10 days after exposure. *Children older than age 3:* 65 mg P.O. daily for 10 days after exposure. Start no later than 3 to 4 hours after acute exposure. *Children older than age 1:* 2 ml Pima P.O. once daily 24 hours before and for 10 days after exposure. *Infants and children younger than age 1:* 1 ml Pima P.O. daily 24 hours before and for 10 days after exposure to radioactive isotopes of iodine.
▶ **Hyperthyroidism.** *Adults and children:* 50 to 250 mg (1 to 5 drops of 1 g/ml solution) potassium iodide t.i.d. for 10 to 14 days before surgery. Or, 0.1 to 0.3 strong iodine solution (3 to 5 drops) t.i.d.

Contraindications and cautions
• Contraindicated in patients with tuberculosis, acute bronchitis, iodide hypersensitivity, impaired renal function, or hyperkalemia. Some forms contain sulfites, which may cause allergic reactions in hypersensitive people.
• Use cautiously in patients with hypocomplementemic vasculitis, goiter, or autoimmune thyroid disease.
⚖ **Lifespan:** In pregnant and breast-feeding women, drug isn't recommended.

Adverse reactions
CNS: fever, frontal headache.
EENT: acute rhinitis, inflammation of salivary glands, periorbital edema, conjunctivitis, hyperemia.
GI: burning, irritation, *nausea*, vomiting, diarrhea (sometimes bloody), *metallic taste*.
Metabolic: *potassium toxicity* (confusion, irregular heart beat, numbness, tingling, pain or weakness in hands and feet, tiredness).
Skin: acneiform rash, mucous membrane ulceration.
Other: hypersensitivity reactions, tooth discoloration.

Interactions
Drug-drug. *ACE inhibitors, potassium-sparing diuretics:* May increase risk of hyperkalemia. Avoid using together.
Antithyroid drugs: May increase hypothyroid or goitrogenic effects. Monitor effects closely.
Lithium carbonate: May cause hypothyroidism. Use together cautiously.

Drug-food. *Salt substitutes:* May increase risk of hyperkalemia. Don't use together.

Effects on lab test results

• May increase potassium level.
• May increase or decrease thyroid function test results.

Pharmacokinetics

Absorption: Unknown.
Distribution: Unknown.
Metabolism: Unknown.
Excretion: Unknown. *Half-life:* Unknown.

Route	Onset	Peak	Duration
P.O.	≤ 24 hr	10–15 days	Unknown

Action

Chemical effect: Inhibits thyroid hormone formation by blocking iodotyrosine and iodothyronine synthesis, limits iodide transport into thyroid gland, and blocks thyroid hormone release.
Therapeutic effect: Lowers thyroid hormone levels.

Available forms

potassium iodide
Oral solution: 500 mg/15 ml
Scored tablets: 130 mg
Syrup: 325 mg/5 ml
potassium iodide, saturated solution
Oral solution: 1 g/ml
strong iodine solution
Oral solution: iodine 50 mg/ml and potassium iodide 100 mg/ml

NURSING PROCESS

⁜ Assessment
• Assess patient's condition before starting therapy, and regularly thereafter to monitor the drug's effectiveness.
• Be alert for adverse reactions and drug interactions.
• Earliest signs of delayed hypersensitivity reactions caused by iodides are irritation and swelling of eyelids.
• Assess patient's and family's knowledge of drug therapy.

⊞ Nursing diagnoses
• Ineffective health maintenance related to underlying thyroid condition

• Ineffective protection related to hypersensitivity reactions
• Deficient knowledge related to drug therapy

⟩ Planning and implementation
• Potassium iodide is usually given with other antithyroid drugs.
• Dilute oral doses in water, milk, or fruit juice to hydrate patient and mask salty taste; give drug after meals to prevent gastric irritation.
• Give iodide through straw to prevent tooth discoloration.
• Store drug in light-resistant container.
Patient teaching
• Warn patient that suddenly stopping the drug may cause thyroid crisis.
• Tell patient to ask prescriber whether he can use iodized salt or eat shellfish.
• Tell patient to report adverse reactions.

☑ Evaluation
• Patient's thyroid hormone level is lower with potassium iodide therapy.
• Patient doesn't experience hypersensitivity reactions.
• Patient and family state understanding of drug therapy.

pralidoxime chloride (pyridine-2-aldoxime methochloride; 2-PAM chloride)
(pral-ih-DOKS-eem KLOR-ighd)
Protopam Chloride

Pharmacologic class: quaternary ammonium oxime
Therapeutic class: antidote
Pregnancy risk category: C

Indications and dosages

▶ **Antidote for organophosphate poisoning.**
Adults: 1 to 2 g in 100 ml of saline solution by I.V. infusion over 15 to 30 minutes. If patient has pulmonary edema, give by slow I.V. push over at least 5 minutes. Repeat in 1 hour if muscle weakness persists; may give further doses cautiously. Use I.M. or subcutaneous injection if I.V. route isn't feasible.
▶ **Anticholinesterase overdose.** *Adults:* 1 to 2 g I.V., followed by 250 mg I.V. q 5 minutes.

▼ I.V. administration

• Give I.V. preparation slowly as diluted solution. Dilute with unpreserved sterile water.
• To lessen muscarinic effects and block accumulation of acetylcholine from organophosphate poisoning, give atropine 2 to 6 mg I.V. along with pralidoxime unless patient has cyanosis. (If he is cyanotic, give atropine I.M.) Give atropine q 5 to 60 minutes in adults until muscarinic signs and symptoms disappear; if they reappear, repeat the dose. Maintain atropinization for at least 48 hours.
• Infuse slowly since tachycardia, laryngospasm, muscle rigidity, and worsening of cholinergic symptoms may occur with rapid administration. Maximum injection rate is 200 mg/minute.

⊗ **Incompatibilities**
None reported.

Contraindications and cautions

• Use cautiously in patients with myasthenia gravis; overdose may cause myasthenic crisis.
⚖ **Lifespan:** In pregnant women, use cautiously. In breast-feeding women and in children, safety and effectiveness haven't been established.

Adverse reactions

CNS: dizziness, headache, drowsiness, excitement, manic behavior after recovery of consciousness.
CV: tachycardia, increased blood pressure.
EENT: blurred vision, diplopia, impaired accommodation.
GI: nausea.
Musculoskeletal: muscle weakness, muscle rigidity.
Respiratory: hyperventilation.
Other: pain at injection site.

Interactions

Drug-drug. *Atropine:* May cause flushing, tachycardia, dry mouth. Monitor patient.
Barbiturates: May increase the effects of barbiturates. Use together cautiously.

Effects on lab test results

• May increase AST, ALT, and CK levels.

Pharmacokinetics

Absorption: Unknown after I.M. or subcutaneous use.

Distribution: Distributed throughout extracellular fluid; it isn't appreciably bound to protein. It doesn't readily pass into CNS.
Metabolism: Unknown but hepatic metabolism is considered likely.
Excretion: Excreted rapidly in urine. *Half-life:* 1½ hours.

Route	Onset	Peak	Duration
I.V.	Unknown	5–15 min	Unknown
I.M.	Unknown	10–20 min	Unknown
SubQ	Unknown	Unknown	Unknown

Action

Chemical effect: Reactivates cholinesterase that has been inactivated by organophosphorus pesticides and related compounds, permitting degradation of accumulated acetylcholine and facilitating normal functioning of neuromuscular junctions.
Therapeutic effect: Alleviates signs and symptoms of organophosphate poisoning and cholinergic crisis in myasthenia gravis.

Available forms

Injection: 1 g/20 ml in 20-ml vial without diluent or syringe; 1 g/20 ml in 20-ml vial with diluent, syringe, needle, and alcohol swab (emergency kit); 600 mg/2 ml autoinjector (may contain benzyl alcohol), parenteral

NURSING PROCESS

▓ Assessment
• Assess patient's condition before starting therapy and regularly thereafter. Drug relieves paralysis of respiratory muscles but is less effective in relieving depression of respiratory center.
• Drug isn't effective against poisoning caused by phosphorus, inorganic phosphates, or organophosphates that have no anticholinesterase activity.
• If poison was ingested, observe patient for 48 to 72 hours. Absorption from lower bowel may be delayed. It's difficult to distinguish between toxic effects produced by atropine or organophosphate compounds and those resulting from this drug.
• Watch for signs of rapid weakening in patient with myasthenia gravis who was treated for overdose of cholinergics. Patient can pass quickly from cholinergic crisis to myasthenic crisis and may need more cholinergic drugs to

treat myasthenia. Keep edrophonium (Tensilon) available in such situations for establishing differential diagnosis.
• Be alert for adverse reactions.
• Assess patient's and family's knowledge of drug therapy.

🔅 **Nursing diagnoses**
• Ineffective health maintenance related to underlying condition
• Risk for injury related to adverse CNS reactions
• Deficient knowledge related to drug therapy

▷ **Planning and implementation**
• Use drug only in hospitalized patients; have respiratory and other supportive measures available. If possible, obtain accurate medical history and chronology of poisoning. Give drug as soon as possible; it's most effective when started within 24 hours.
• Remove secretions, maintain patent airway, and start artificial ventilation if needed. After dermal exposure to organophosphate, remove patient's clothing and wash his skin and hair with sodium bicarbonate, soap, water, and alcohol immediately. A second washing may be needed. When washing patient, wear protective gloves and clothes to avoid exposure.
• Draw blood for cholinesterase levels before giving drug.
⊛ **ALERT:** Don't confuse pralidoxime with pramoxine or pyridoxine.
Patient teaching
• Tell patient to report adverse reactions immediately.
• Advise patient treated for organophosphate poisoning to avoid contact with insecticides for several weeks.

✅ **Evaluation**
• Patient responds well to therapy.
• Patient sustains no injury from adverse CNS reactions.
• Patient and family state understanding of drug therapy.

pramipexole dihydrochloride
(pram-ih-PEKS-ohl digh-high-droh-KLOR-ighd)
Mirapex

Pharmacologic class: dopamine agonist
Therapeutic class: antiparkinsonian
Pregnancy risk category: C

Indications and dosages

▶ **Signs and symptoms of idiopathic Parkinson's disease.** *Adults:* Initially, 0.375 mg P.O. daily in three divided doses; don't increase more often than q 5 to 7 days. Maintenance daily dosage range is 1.5 to 4.5 mg in three divided doses.
⧄ **Adjust-a-dose:** For patients with renal impairment, if creatinine clearance is greater than 60 ml/minute, initial dose is 0.125 mg P.O. t.i.d., up to 1.5 mg t.i.d. If creatinine clearance is 35 to 59 ml/minute, initial dose is 0.125 mg P.O. b.i.d. up to 1.5 mg b.i.d. If creatinine clearance is 15 to 34 ml/minute, initial dose is 0.125 mg P.O. daily, up to 1.5 mg daily.

Contraindications and cautions

• Contraindicated in patients hypersensitive to the drug or any of its components.
• Use cautiously in patients with renal impairment; adjust dosage if needed.
⚛ **Lifespan:** Use during pregnancy only if benefits outweigh potential risks to the fetus. In breast-feeding women, use cautiously. In children, safety and effectiveness haven't been established. In the elderly, use cautiously.

Adverse reactions

CNS: malaise, akathisia, amnesia, *asthenia, confusion,* delusions, *dizziness, dream abnormalities, dyskinesia,* dystonia, *extrapyramidal syndrome,* gait abnormalities, *hallucinations,* hypoesthesia, hypertonia, *insomnia,* myoclonus, paranoid reaction, *somnolence,* sleep disorders, thought abnormalities, fever.
CV: chest pain, peripheral edema, general edema, *orthostatic hypotension.*
EENT: accommodation abnormalities, diplopia, rhinitis, vision abnormalities.
GI: dry mouth, anorexia, *constipation,* dysphagia, *nausea.*
GU: impotence, urinary frequency, UTI, urinary incontinence.

Reactions may be *common,* uncommon, *life-threatening,* or COMMON AND LIFE-THREATENING.

Metabolic: weight loss.
Musculoskeletal: arthritis, bursitis, twitching, myasthenia.
Respiratory: dyspnea, pneumonia.
Skin: skin disorders.
Other: decreased libido, *accidental injury.*

Interactions

Drug-drug. *Butyrophenones, metoclopramide, phenothiazines, thiothixenes:* May diminish pramipexole effectiveness. Monitor patient closely.
Cimetidine, diltiazem, quinidine, quinine, ranitidine, triamterene, verapamil: May decrease pramipexole clearance. Adjust dosage.
Levodopa: May increase adverse effects of levodopa. Decrease levodopa dosage, as directed.
Drug-herb. *Black horehound:* May have additive dopaminergic effects. Discourage using together.
Kava: May decrease dopaminergic effects. Discourage use together.

Effects on lab test results

None reported.

Pharmacokinetics

Absorption: Rapid. Absolute bioavailability exceeds 90%.
Distribution: Extensively distributed throughout body.
Metabolism: 90% of dose is excreted unchanged in urine.
Excretion: Primary route of elimination is urinary. *Half-life:* 8 to 12 hours.

Route	Onset	Peak	Duration
P.O.	Rapid	2 hr	8–12 hr

Action

Chemical effect: Precise mechanism is unknown, but drug probably stimulates dopamine receptors in striatum.
Therapeutic effect: Relieves symptoms of idiopathic Parkinson's disease.

Available forms

Tablets: 0.125 mg, 0.25 mg, 0.5 mg, 1 mg, 1.5 mg

NURSING PROCESS

Assessment

- Monitor vital signs carefully because drug may cause orthostatic hypotension, especially during dose escalation.
- Assess patient's risk for physical injury from adverse CNS effects of drug (dyskinesia, dizziness, hallucinations, and somnolence).
- Assess patient's response to drug therapy and adjust dose.
- Assess patient's and family's knowledge of drug therapy.

Nursing diagnoses

- Impaired physical mobility related to underlying Parkinson's disease
- Disturbed thought processes related to drug-induced CNS adverse reactions
- Deficient knowledge related to drug therapy

Planning and implementation

- Institute safety precautions.

ALERT: Don't abruptly stop giving the drug. Adjust dose gradually according to patient's response and tolerance.

- Provide ice chips, drinks, or hard, sugarless candy to relieve dry mouth. Increase fluid and fiber intake to prevent constipation.

Patient teaching

- Instruct patient not to rise rapidly after sitting or lying down because of risk of orthostatic hypotension.
- Warn patient to avoid hazardous activities until the drug's CNS effects are known.
- Tell patient to contact prescriber before taking this drug with other drugs.
- Tell patient—especially geriatric patient—that hallucinations may occur.
- If nausea develops, advise patient to take drug with food.
- If woman is breast-feeding or intends to do so, tell her to notify prescriber.

Evaluation

- Patient has improved mobility and reduced muscle rigidity and tremor.
- Patient remains mentally alert.
- Patient and family state understanding of drug therapy.

pramlintide acetate
(PRAM-lihn-tighd As-ih-tayt)
Symlin

Pharmacologic class: human amylin analogue
Therapeutic class: antidiabetic
Pregnancy risk category: C

Indications and dosages

▶ **Adjunct to insulin in patients with type 1 diabetes who haven't achieved the desired glucose control.** *Adults:* Initially, 15 mcg subcutaneously immediately before major meals (more than 250 calories or 30 g of carbohydrates). Reduce preprandial rapid-acting or short-acting insulin dose, including fixed-mix insulin such as 70/30, by 50%. Increase pramlintide dose by 15-mcg increments every 3 days as long as no nausea has occurred, to a maintenance dose of 30 to 60 mcg. Adjust insulin dose as needed.

▶ **Adjunct to insulin in patients with type 2 diabetes who haven't achieved the desired glucose control, with or without a sulfonylurea or metformin.** *Adults:* Initially, 60 mcg subcutaneously immediately before major meals. Reduce preprandial rapid-acting or short-acting insulin dose, including fixed-mix insulin, by 50%. Increase pramlintide dose to 120 mcg when no significant nausea has occurred for 3 to 7 days. Adjust insulin dose as needed.

Contraindications and cautions

• Contraindicated in patients hypersensitive to drug or its components, including metacresol, and in patients with gastroparesis or hypoglycemia unawareness. Don't use drug in patients noncompliant with current insulin and glucose monitoring regimen, patients with a glycosylated hemoglobin (HbA$_{1c}$) level greater than 9%, patients with severe hypoglycemia during the previous 6 months, and patients who take drugs that stimulate GI motility.
≋ **Lifespan:** Use during pregnancy only if benefits outweigh potential risks to the fetus. Use cautiously in breast-feeding women; it isn't known whether drug appears in breast milk. Safety and effectiveness haven't been established in children. Use cautiously in elderly patients; drug seems to have similar effects on eld-

erly and younger adults, but some older adults may have greater sensitivity to it.

Adverse reactions

CNS: dizziness, fatigue, *headache.*
EENT: pharyngitis.
GI: abdominal pain, *anorexia, nausea, vomiting.*
Metabolic: *hypoglycemia.*
Musculoskeletal: arthralgia.
Respiratory: cough.
Skin: injection site reaction.
Other: allergic reaction, *inflicted injury.*

Interactions

Drug-drug. *ACE inhibitors, disopyramide, fibrates, fluoxetine, MAO inhibitors, oral antidiabetics, pentoxifylline, propoxyphene, salicylates, sulfonamide antibiotics:* May increase the risk of hypoglycemia. Monitor blood glucose level closely.
Alpha glucosidase inhibitors (such as acarbose) and anticholinergics (such as atropine, tricyclic antidepressants, benztropine): May alter GI motility. Avoid using together.
Beta blockers, clonidine, guanethidine, reserpine: May mask signs of hypoglycemia. Monitor blood glucose level closely.
Oral drugs dependent on rapid onset of action (such as analgesics): May delay absorption because of slowed gastric emptying. If rapid effect is needed, give oral drug 1 hour before or 2 hours after pramlintide.

Effects on lab test results

None reported.

Pharmacokinetics

Absorption: 30% to 40% bioavailable.
Distribution: Not extensively bound to blood cells or albumin.
Metabolism: Mainly by the kidneys.
Excretion: *Half-life of parent drug and active metabolite:* About 48 minutes each.

Route	Onset	Peak	Duration
SubQ	Unknown	19–21 min	Unknown

Action

Chemical effect: Slows the rate at which food leaves the stomach, reducing the initial postprandial increase in plasma glucose level. Drug also reduces postprandial glucagon concentra-

---

Reactions may be *common,* uncommon, ***life-threatening***, or COMMON AND LIFE-THREATENING.

tions, which decreases hyperglycemia, and reduces total caloric intake by modulating appetite.
Therapeutic effect: Lowers glucose level.

Available forms

Injection: 0.6 mg/ml in 50-ml vials

NURSING PROCESS

Assessment
• Before starting drug, review patient's HbA$_{1c}$ level, recent blood glucose monitoring data, history of insulin-induced hypoglycemia, current insulin regimen, and body weight.
• Monitor patient's blood glucose level.
• Assess patient for signs of hypoglycemia including dizziness, restlessness, diaphoresis, tremor, nausea, irritability, and poor concentration.
• Monitor patient for severe nausea and vomiting. Dosage reduction may be needed.
• Assess patient's and family's knowledge of drug therapy.

Nursing diagnoses
• Risk for injury related to drug-induced hypoglycemia
• Ineffective health maintenance related to hyperglycemia
• Deficient knowledge related to drug therapy

Planning and implementation
• To give drug, use a U-100 insulin syringe, preferably a 0.3-ml size.
• Don't mix drug with any type of insulin, and give it as a separate injection.
• Give each dose subcutaneously into the abdomen or thigh. Rotate injection sites, and use a site separate from the insulin site used at the same time.
• **ALERT:** Pramlintide may increase the risk of insulin-induced severe hypoglycemia, particularly in patients with type 1 diabetes.
• The risk of severe, drug-related hypoglycemia is highest within the first 3 hours after an injection.
• Symptoms of hypoglycemia may be masked in patients with a long history of diabetes, diabetic nerve disease, or intensified diabetes control.
• Stop drug if patient has persistent nausea or recurrent, unexplained hypoglycemia that requires medical assistance. Also stop drug if patient doesn't comply with blood glucose monitoring or drug dosage adjustments.

Patient teaching
• Teach patient how to take drug exactly as prescribed, immediately before mealtimes. Explain that it doesn't replace daily insulin but may lower the amount of insulin needed, especially before meals.
• Explain that a major meal contains more than 250 calories or 30 g of carbohydrates.
• Caution patient not to mix drug with insulin; instruct him to give the injections at separate sites.
• Instruct patient not to change doses of pramlintide or insulin without consulting the prescriber.
• Tell patient to refrain from driving, operating heavy machinery, or performing other risky activities where he could hurt himself or others, until drug affects his blood glucose are known.
• Caution patient about the possibility of severe hypoglycemia, particularly within 3 hours of injection.
• Teach patient and family members the signs and symptoms of hypoglycemia, including hunger, headache, sweating, tremor, irritability, and trouble concentrating.
• Instruct patient and family members what to do if hypoglycemia occurs.
• Tell patient to report severe nausea and vomiting.
• Advise woman of child-bearing potential to tell the prescriber if she is, could be, or is planning to become pregnant.
• Teach patient how to handle unusual situations, such as illness or stress, an inadequate or omitted insulin dose, inadvertent use of too much insulin or pramlintide, inadequate food intake, or missed meals.
• Tell patient to refrigerate vials. Contents of open vials should be used within 28 days and unopened vials before expiration date.

Evaluation
• Patient does not experience hypoglycemia and sustains no injury.
• Patient's glucose level is normal with drug therapy.
• Patient and family state understanding of drug therapy.

P

pravastatin sodium (eptastatin)
(PRAH-vuh-stat-in SOH-dee-um)
Pravachol⬧

Pharmacologic class: HMG-CoA reductase inhibitor
Therapeutic class: antilipemic
Pregnancy risk category: X

Indications and dosages

▶ **Primary hypercholesterolemia and mixed dyslipidemia; primary and secondary prevention of coronary events; hyperlipidemia; homozygous familial hypercholesterolemia.**
Adults: Initially, 40 mg P.O. once daily at the same time each day, with or without food. Adjust dosage q 4 weeks based on patient tolerance and response; maximum daily dose, 80 mg.
▶ **Heterozygous familial hypercholesterolemia.** *Children ages 14 to 18:* 40 mg P.O. once daily.
Children ages 8 to 13: 20 mg P.O. once daily.
⬧ **Adjust-a-dose:** For patients with renal or hepatic impairment, start with 10 mg P.O. daily.
For patients also taking immunosuppressants, begin therapy with 10 mg P.O. h.s. and adjust to higher doses cautiously. Most patients given combination will receive maximum daily dose of 20 mg.

Contraindications and cautions

• Contraindicated in patients hypersensitive to the drug or any of its components, and in patients with active liver disease or unexplained persistent elevations of transaminase levels.
• Use cautiously in patients who consume large quantities of alcohol or have a history of liver disease.
⚘ **Lifespan:** In pregnant women, breastfeeding women, and women of childbearing age (unless they have no risk of pregnancy), drug is contraindicated. In children younger than age 8, safety and effectiveness haven't been established.

Adverse reactions

CNS: headache, fatigue, dizziness.
CV: chest pain.
EENT: rhinitis.
GI: vomiting, diarrhea, heartburn, nausea.
GU: *renal failure* secondary to myoglobinuria.

Musculoskeletal: myositis, myopathy, localized muscle pain, myalgia, *rhabdomyolysis.*
Respiratory: cough.
Skin: rash.
Other: flulike symptoms.

Interactions

Drug-drug. *Cholestyramine, colestipol:* May decrease pravastatin levels. Give pravastatin 1 hour before or 4 hours after these drugs.
Drugs that decrease levels or activity of endogenous steroids (such as cimetidine, spironolactone): May increase risk of endocrine dysfunction. No intervention needed. Take complete drug history in patients who develop endocrine dysfunction.
Erythromycin, fibric acid derivatives (such as clofibrate, gemfibrozil), high doses of niacin, immunosuppressants: May increase risk of rhabdomyolysis. Don't use together.
Fluconazole, itraconazole, ketoconazole: May increase level and adverse effects of pravastatin. Avoid this combination. If they must be given together, reduce dose of pravastatin.
Gemfibrozil: May decrease protein-binding and urinary clearance of pravastatin. Avoid using together.
Hepatotoxic drugs: May increase risk of hepatotoxicity. Avoid using together.
Drug-herb. *Kava:* May increase risk of hepatotoxicity. Discourage using together.
Red yeast rice: May increase the risk of adverse events or toxicity because herb contains components similar to those of statin drugs. Discourage using together.
Drug-lifestyle. *Alcohol use:* May increase risk of hepatotoxicity. Discourage using together.

Effects on lab test results

• May increase ALT, AST, CK, alkaline phosphatase, and bilirubin levels.
• May alter thyroid function test values.

Pharmacokinetics

Absorption: Rapidly absorbed. Although food reduces bioavailability, drug effects are the same if drug is taken with or 1 hour before meals.
Distribution: About 50% bound to proteins. Drug undergoes extensive first-pass extraction, possibly because of active transport system into hepatocytes.

Reactions may be *common*, uncommon, *life-threatening*, or COMMON AND LIFE-THREATENING.

Metabolism: Metabolized in liver; at least six metabolites have been identified. Some are active.
Excretion: Excreted by liver and kidneys. *Half-life:* 1¼ to 2¼ hours.

Route	Onset	Peak	Duration
P.O.	Unknown	1 hr	Unknown

Action
Chemical effect: Inhibits HMG-CoA reductase, which is an early and rate-limiting step in the synthesis of cholesterol.
Therapeutic effect: Lowers LDL and total cholesterol levels in some patients.

Available forms
Tablets: 10 mg, 20 mg, 40 mg, 80 mg

NURSING PROCESS

☞ Assessment
• Assess patient's condition before starting therapy, and regularly thereafter to monitor the drug's effectiveness.
• Obtain liver function tests at start of therapy and periodically thereafter. If elevations persist, arrange for patient to have a liver biopsy.
• Be alert for adverse reactions and drug interactions.
• Monitor patient for signs of rhabdomyolysis, such as muscle aches and weakness.
• If adverse GI reaction occurs, monitor patient's hydration.
• Assess patient's and family's knowledge of drug therapy.

▦ Nursing diagnoses
• Risk for injury related to elevated cholesterol levels
• Risk for deficient fluid volume related to adverse GI reactions
• Deficient knowledge related to drug therapy

▧ Planning and implementation
• Begin only after diet and other nondrug therapies have proved ineffective.
Patient teaching
• Instruct patient to take recommended dosage in evening, preferably h.s.
• Teach patient about proper cholesterol-lowering diet (restricting total fat and cholesterol), and how to control other cardiac disease

risk factors. Recommend weight control, exercise, and smoking cessation programs.
• Inform woman that drug is contraindicated during pregnancy. Advise her to notify prescriber immediately if she becomes pregnant.

☑ Evaluation
• Patient's LDL and total cholesterol levels are within normal range.
• Patient maintains adequate hydration.
• Patient and family state understanding of drug therapy.

prazosin hydrochloride
(PRAH-zoh-sin high-droh-KLOR-ighd)
Minipress

Pharmacologic class: alpha blocker
Therapeutic class: antihypertensive
Pregnancy risk category: C

Indications and dosages
▶ **Mild to moderate hypertension, alone or with diuretic or other antihypertensive.**
Adults: Initial dosage is 1 mg P.O. b.i.d. to t.i.d. Increase slowly; maximum daily dosage is 20 mg. Maintenance dosage is 6 to 15 mg daily in three divided doses. Some patients need larger dosages (up to 40 mg daily). If other antihypertensives or diuretics are added, decrease to 1 to 2 mg t.i.d. and readjust.
Children: 0.5 to 7 mg P.O. t.i.d.
▶ **BPH‡.** *Adults:* Initially, 2 mg P.O. b.i.d. Daily dose may range from 1 to 9 mg.

Contraindications and cautions
• Use cautiously in patients taking other antihypertensives.
❋ **Lifespan:** In pregnant women, use cautiously. In breast-feeding women, drug isn't recommended. In children, safety and effectiveness haven't been established.

Adverse reactions
CNS: *dizziness,* headache, drowsiness, weakness, *first-dose syncope,* depression.
CV: orthostatic hypotension, *palpitations.*
EENT: blurred vision.
GI: vomiting, diarrhea, abdominal cramps, constipation, *nausea,* dry mouth.
GU: priapism, impotence.

Interactions

Drug-drug. *Acebutolol, atenolol, betaxolol, carteolol, esmolol, metoprolol, nadolol, pindolol, propranolol, sotalol, timolol:* May increase risk of orthostatic hypotension in the early phases of use together. Assist patient to stand slowly until effects of drug are known.
Clonidine: May decrease antihypertensive effect of clonidine. Monitor blood pressure.
Diuretics: May increase frequency of syncope with loss of consciousness.
Indomethacin: May decrease antihypertensive action of prazosin. Monitor blood pressure.
Verapamil: May increase prazosin level and increase risk of postural hypotension. Advise patient to sit or lie down if dizziness occurs.
Drug-herb. *Saw palmetto.* May have additive effect when used together for BPH.
Yohimbe: May antagonize antihypertensive effects. Discourage using together.

Effects on lab test results

• May increase BUN and uric acid levels.
• May increase liver function test values.

Pharmacokinetics

Absorption: Variable.
Distribution: Distributed throughout body; highly protein-bound (about 97%).
Metabolism: Extensive in liver.
Excretion: More than 90% excreted in feces by bile; remainder excreted in urine. *Half-life:* 2 to 4 hours.

Route	Onset	Peak	Duration
P.O.	30–90 min	2–4 hr	7–10 hr

Action

Chemical effect: Unknown; effects probably stem from alpha blocking activity.
Therapeutic effect: Lowers blood pressure.

Available forms

Capsules: 1 mg, 2 mg, 5 mg

NURSING PROCESS

Assessment
• Assess patient's condition before starting therapy, and regularly thereafter to monitor the drug's effectiveness.

• Frequently monitor patient's blood pressure and pulse rate.
• An elderly patient may be more sensitive to hypotensive effects of drug.
• Be alert for adverse reactions and drug interactions.
• Assess patient's and family's knowledge of drug therapy.

Nursing diagnoses
• Risk for injury related to presence of hypertension
• Sexual dysfunction related to drug-induced impotence
• Deficient knowledge related to drug therapy

Planning and implementation
• If first dose is larger than 1 mg, severe syncope with loss of consciousness may occur (first-dose syncope).
ALERT: Don't stop therapy abruptly.
• If you suspect compliance problems, discuss twice-daily dosing with prescriber.
Patient teaching
• Tell patient not to abruptly stop taking drug, but to call prescriber if unpleasant adverse reactions occur.
• Advise patient to minimize effects of orthostatic hypotension by rising slowly and avoiding sudden position changes.
• Dry mouth can be relieved with sugarless chewing gum, sour hard candy, or ice chips.
• Inform male patient of the possibility of impotence, and advise him to seek counseling to learn how to cope with this adverse effect.

Evaluation
• Patient's blood pressure is normal.
• Patient seeks counseling for alternative methods of sexual gratification because of drug-induced impotence.
• Patient and family state understanding of drug therapy.

prednisolone (systemic)
(pred-NIS-uh-lohn)
Delta-Cortef, Prelone

prednisolone acetate
Cotolone, Key-Pred-25, Predalone 50,
Predcor-50

prednisolone sodium phosphate
Hydeltrasol, Key-Pred SP, Orapred,
Pediapred

prednisolone tebutate
Nor-Pred TBA, Predate TBA, Predcor-TBA,
Prednisol TBA

Pharmacologic class: glucocorticoid, mineralocorticoid
Therapeutic class: anti-inflammatory, immunosuppressant
Pregnancy risk category: C

Indications and dosages

▶ **Severe inflammation, modification of body's immune response to disease.** *Adults:* 2.5 to 15 mg prednisolone P.O. b.i.d., t.i.d., or q.i.d. Or, 2 to 30 mg prednisolone acetate I.M. q 12 hours. Or, 5 to 60 mg prednisolone sodium phosphate I.M., I.V., or P.O. daily. Or, 4 to 40 mg prednisolone tebutate injected into joints and lesions, p.r.n.
Children: Initially, 0.14 to 2 mg/kg prednisolone P.O. or 4 to 60 mg/m² prednisolone P.O. daily in four divided doses. Or, 0.04 to 0.25 mg/kg prednisolone acetate or 1.5 to 7.5 mg/m² prednisolone acetate I.M. once or twice daily. Or, initially, 0.14 to 2 mg/kg prednisolone sodium phosphate or 4 to 60 mg/m² prednisolone sodium phosphate I.M., I.V., or P.O. daily in three or four divided doses.
▶ **Acute exacerbations of multiple sclerosis.** *Adults:* 200 mg prednisolone sodium phosphate P.O. daily for 1 week, followed by 80 mg q other day.
▶ **Nephrotic syndrome.** *Children:* 60 mg/m² prednisolone sodium phosphate P.O. daily in three divided doses for 4 weeks, followed by 4 weeks of single-dose, alternate-day therapy at 40 mg/m².
▶ **Uncontrolled asthma in patients taking inhaled corticosteroids and long-acting bron-** chodilators. *Children:* 1 to 2 mg/kg prednisolone sodium phosphate P.O. daily in single or divided doses. Short course or "burst" therapy should continue until a child achieves a peak expiratory flow rate of 80% of his personal best or symptoms resolve. This usually requires 3 to 10 days of therapy, although it can take longer. No evidence shows that tapering the dose after improvement will prevent a relapse.

▼ I.V. administration

● Give only prednisolone sodium phosphate I.V. Never give acetate or tebutate form I.V.
● When giving drug as direct injection, inject undiluted over at least 1 minute.
● When giving drug as intermittent or continuous infusion, dilute solution according to manufacturer's instructions and give over prescribed duration.
● D₅W and normal saline solution are recommended as diluents for I.V. infusions.
⊗ **Incompatibilities**
Calcium gluconate, dimenhydrinate, methotrexate sodium, polymyxin B, prochlorperazine edisylate, promazine, promethazine hydrochloride.

Contraindications and cautions

● Contraindicated in patients hypersensitive to the drug or any of its components, and in those with fungal infections.
● Use cautiously in patients with recent MI, GI ulcer, renal disease, hypertension, osteoporosis, diabetes mellitus, hypothyroidism, cirrhosis, diverticulitis, nonspecific ulcerative colitis, recent intestinal anastomoses, thromboembolic disorders, seizures, myasthenia gravis, heart failure, tuberculosis, ocular herpes simplex, emotional instability, or psychotic tendencies.
⚖ **Lifespan:** In pregnant women, use cautiously. In breast-feeding women, high doses aren't recommended.

Adverse reactions

Most reactions to corticosteroids are dose- or duration-dependent.
CNS: *euphoria, insomnia,* psychotic behavior, pseudotumor cerebri, *seizures.*
CV: *heart failure, thromboembolism,* hypertension, edema.
EENT: cataracts, glaucoma.
GI: *peptic ulceration,* GI irritation, increased appetite, *pancreatitis.*

P

Metabolic: hypokalemia, hyperglycemia, carbohydrate intolerance, growth suppression in children.
Musculoskeletal: muscle weakness, osteoporosis.
Skin: hirsutism, delayed wound healing, acne, various skin eruptions.
Other: susceptibility to infections, *acute adrenal insufficiency with increased stress (infection, surgery, or trauma) or abrupt withdrawal after long-term therapy.*

Interactions

Drug-drug. *Antihypertensives:* May counteract effect of antihypertensives. Adjust dose of antihypertensive as needed.
Aspirin, indomethacin, other NSAIDs: Increases risk of GI distress and bleeding. Avoid using together.
Barbiturates, phenytoin, rifampin: May decrease corticosteroid effect. Increase corticosteroid dosage.
Oral anticoagulants: May alter dosage requirements. Monitor PT and INR closely.
Potassium-depleting drugs (such as thiazide diuretics): May enhance potassium-wasting effects of prednisolone. Monitor potassium levels.
Skin-test antigens: May decrease skin-test response. Defer skin testing until therapy is completed.
Toxoids, vaccines: May decrease antibody response and increase risk of neurologic complications. Check with prescriber about when to reschedule vaccine, if possible.

Effects on lab test results

● May increase glucose and cholesterol levels. May decrease potassium and calcium levels.

Pharmacokinetics

Absorption: Absorbed readily after P.O. use; variable with other routes.
Distribution: Distributed to muscle, liver, skin, intestine, and kidneys. Drug is extensively bound to proteins. Only unbound portion is active.
Metabolism: Metabolized in liver.
Excretion: Inactive metabolites and small amounts of unmetabolized drug are excreted in urine; insignificant amount excreted in feces.
Half-life: 18 to 36 hours.

Route	Onset	Peak	Duration
P.O.	Rapid	1–2 hr	30–36 hr
I.V.	Rapid	< 1 hr	Unknown
I.M.	Rapid	< 1 hr	< 4 wk
P.R.	Unknown	Unknown	Unknown
Intra-articular, intralesional	1–2 days	Unknown	3 days–4 wk

Action

Chemical effect: Not clearly defined; decreases inflammation, mainly by stabilizing leukocyte lysosomal membranes; suppresses immune response; stimulates bone marrow; and influences protein, fat, and carbohydrate metabolism.
Therapeutic effect: Relieves inflammation and induces immunosuppression.

Available forms

prednisolone
Syrup: 5 mg/ml, 15 mg/5 ml
Tablets: 5 mg
prednisolone acetate
Injection: 25 mg/ml, 50 mg/ml suspension
prednisolone sodium phosphate
Injection: 20 mg/ml solution
Oral liquid: 5 mg/5 ml, 15 mg/5 ml
prednisolone tebutate
Injection: 20 mg/ml suspension

NURSING PROCESS

℞ Assessment

● Assess patient's condition before starting therapy, and regularly thereafter to monitor the drug's effectiveness.
● Monitor patient's weight, blood pressure, and electrolyte levels.
● Watch for depression or psychotic episodes, especially with high dose.
● Monitor glucose levels in a diabetic patient; he may need increase in insulin.
● Monitor patient's stress level; a dose adjustment may be needed.
● Assess for adequate calcium supplementation.
● Be alert for adverse reactions and drug interactions.
● Assess patient's and family's knowledge of drug therapy.

Nursing diagnoses

● Ineffective health maintenance related to underlying condition

• Ineffective protection related to drug-induced adverse reactions
• Deficient knowledge related to drug therapy

Planning and implementation
• Always adjust to lowest effective dose, which may need to be increased during times of physiologic stress (such as surgery, trauma, or infection).
• Prednisolone salts (acetate, sodium phosphate, and tebutate) are used parenterally less often than other corticosteroids that have more potent anti-inflammatory action.
• Drug may be used for alternate-day therapy.
• Give dose with food when possible to reduce GI irritation.
• Refrigerate Orapred at 36° to 46° F (2° to 8° C).
• Inject drug I.M. deep into gluteal muscle.
• Alternate injection sites to prevent muscle atrophy.
• Avoid subcutaneous injection because atrophy and sterile abscesses may occur.
• Unless contraindicated, give low-sodium diet high in potassium and protein. Give potassium supplements, p.r.n.
• Notify prescriber immediately if serious adverse reactions occur, and give supportive care.
• After long-term therapy, reduce dose gradually. Abrupt withdrawal may cause rebound inflammation, fatigue, weakness, arthralgia, fever, dizziness, lethargy, depression, fainting, orthostatic hypotension, dyspnea, anorexia, or hypoglycemia. Sudden withdrawal after prolonged use may be fatal.
ALERT: Don't confuse prednisolone with prednisone.

Patient teaching
• Tell patient not to stop drug without prescriber's knowledge.
• Tell patient that if he misses a dose, he should take it as soon as possible unless it is near the time for his next dose. Tell him not to attempt to make up missed doses that are long overdue.
• Advise patient to take oral form with meals to minimize GI reactions.
• Warn patient receiving long-term therapy about cushingoid symptoms.
• Teach signs of early adrenal insufficiency: fatigue, muscle weakness, joint pain, fever, anorexia, nausea, dyspnea, dizziness, and fainting.
• Instruct patient to wear or carry medical identification that indicates his need for systemic glucocorticoids during stress.
• Tell patient to report slow healing, sudden weight gain, or swelling.
• Advise patient receiving long-term therapy to exercise or have physical therapy and to ask prescriber about vitamin D or calcium supplements.

Evaluation
• Patient responds well to therapy.
• Patient has no serious adverse reactions.
• Patient and family state understanding of drug therapy.

prednisone
(PRED-nih-sohn)
Apo-Prednisone ♦, Deltasone, Liquid Pred*, Meticorten, Novo-Prednisone ♦, Orasone, Panafcort ♦, Panasol-S, Prednicen-M, Prednisone Intensol*, Sone ♦, Sterapred, Winpred ♦

Pharmacologic class: adrenocorticoid
Therapeutic class: anti-inflammatory, immunosuppressant
Pregnancy risk category: C

Indications and dosages
▶ **Severe inflammation or immunosuppression.** *Adults:* 5 to 60 mg P.O. daily in single or divided doses. Maximum, 250 mg daily. Maintenance dosage given once daily or q other day. Dosage must be individualized.
▶ **Acute exacerbations of multiple sclerosis.** *Adults:* 200 mg P.O. daily for 1 week; then 80 mg P.O. q other day for 1 month.

Contraindications and cautions
• Contraindicated in patients hypersensitive to the drug or any of its components, and in those with systemic fungal infections.
• Use cautiously in patients with GI ulcer, renal disease, hypertension, osteoporosis, diabetes mellitus, hypothyroidism, cirrhosis, diverticulitis, nonspecific ulcerative colitis, recent intestinal anastomoses, thromboembolic disorders, seizures, myasthenia gravis, heart failure, tuberculosis, ocular herpes simplex, emotional instability, or psychotic tendencies.

P

⚜ Lifespan: In pregnant women, use cautiously. In breast-feeding women, high doses aren't recommended.

Adverse reactions

Most reactions are dose- or duration-dependent.
CNS: *euphoria, insomnia,* psychotic behavior, pseudotumor cerebri, *seizures.*
CV: *heart failure, thromboembolism,* hypertension, edema.
EENT: cataracts, glaucoma.
GI: *peptic ulceration,* GI irritation, increased appetite, *pancreatitis.*
Metabolic: hypokalemia, hyperglycemia, carbohydrate intolerance, growth suppression in children.
Musculoskeletal: muscle weakness, osteoporosis.
Skin: hirsutism, delayed wound healing, acne, various skin eruptions.
Other: susceptibility to infections.

Interactions

Drug-drug. *Antihypertensives:* May counteract effect of antihypertensives. Adjust dose of antihypertensive as needed.
Aspirin, indomethacin, other NSAIDs: May increase risk of GI distress and bleeding. Give together cautiously.
Barbiturates, phenytoin, rifampin: May decrease corticosteroid effect. Increase corticosteroid dosage.
Oral anticoagulants: May alter dosage requirements. Monitor PT and INR closely.
Potassium-depleting drugs (such as thiazide diuretics): May enhance potassium-wasting effects of prednisone. Monitor potassium levels.
Skin-test antigens: May decrease skin test response. Defer skin testing until therapy is completed.
Toxoids, vaccines: May decrease antibody response and increases risk of neurologic complications. Don't give together.

Effects on lab test results

• May increase glucose and cholesterol levels. May decrease potassium and calcium levels.

Pharmacokinetics

Absorption: Absorbed readily after P.O. use.
Distribution: Distributed to muscle, liver, skin, intestine, and kidneys. Drug is extensively bound to proteins. Only unbound portion is active.
Metabolism: Metabolized in liver.
Excretion: Inactive metabolites and small amounts of unmetabolized drug are excreted in urine; insignificant amounts excreted in feces. *Half-life:* 18 to 36 hours.

Route	Onset	Peak	Duration
P.O.	Varies	Varies	Varies

Action

Chemical effect: Not clearly defined; decreases inflammation; suppresses immune response; stimulates bone marrow; and influences protein, fat, and carbohydrate metabolism.
Therapeutic effect: Relieves inflammation and induces immunosuppression.

Available forms

Oral solution: 5 mg/5 ml*, 5 mg/ml (concentrate)*
Syrup: 5 mg/5 ml*
Tablets: 1 mg, 2.5 mg, 5 mg, 10 mg, 20 mg, 25 mg, 50 mg

NURSING PROCESS

☞ Assessment

• Assess patient's condition before starting therapy, and regularly thereafter to monitor the drug's effectiveness.
• Monitor patient's weight, blood pressure, and electrolyte levels.
• Watch for depression or psychotic episodes, especially when given in high doses.
• Monitor glucose level in a diabetic patient; he may need an increase in insulin.
• Monitor patient's stress level; dose adjustment may be needed.
• Be alert for adverse reactions and drug interactions.
• Assess patient's and family's knowledge of drug therapy.

🔲 Nursing diagnoses

• Ineffective health maintenance related to underlying condition
• Ineffective protection related to drug-induced adverse reactions
• Deficient knowledge related to drug therapy

◼ Planning and implementation

• Always adjust to lowest effective dose, which may need to be increased during times of physiologic stress (such as surgery, trauma, or infection).

• Drug may be used for alternate-day therapy.

• For better results and less toxicity, give once-daily dose in morning.

• Give oral dose with food to reduce GI irritation.

• After long-term therapy, reduce dose gradually. Abruptly stopping the drug may cause rebound inflammation, fatigue, weakness, arthralgia, fever, dizziness, lethargy, depression, fainting, orthostatic hypotension, dyspnea, anorexia, or hypoglycemia. After long-term therapy, increased stress or abrupt withdrawal may cause acute adrenal insufficiency. Sudden withdrawal after prolonged use may be fatal.

• Unless contraindicated, give low-sodium diet high in potassium and protein. Give potassium supplements, p.r.n.

• If serious adverse reactions occur, notify prescriber immediately and give supportive care.

⊛ **ALERT:** Don't confuse prednisone with prednisolone.

Patient teaching

• Tell patient not to stop taking the drug without prescriber's knowledge.

• Advise patient to take oral form with meals to minimize GI reactions.

• Tell patient to report sudden weight gain, swelling, or slow healing.

• Advise patient receiving long-term therapy to exercise or have physical therapy, to ask prescriber about vitamin D or calcium supplements, and to have periodic eye examinations.

• Instruct patient to wear or carry medical identification that indicates his need for systemic glucocorticoids during stress.

• Warn patient receiving long-term therapy about cushingoid symptoms.

• Teach signs of early adrenal insufficiency: fatigue, muscular weakness, joint pain, fever, anorexia, nausea, dyspnea, dizziness, and fainting.

▨ Evaluation

• Patient responds well to therapy.

• Patient doesn't experience serious adverse reactions.

• Patient and family state understanding of drug therapy.

pregabalin
(preh-GAH-bah-linn)
Lyrica

Pharmacologic class: CNS drug
Therapeutic class: analgesic, anticonvulsant
Pregnancy risk category: C
Controlled substance schedule: V

Indications and dosages

▶ **Diabetic peripheral neuropathy.** *Adults:* Initially, 50 mg P.O. t.i.d. May increase to 100 mg P.O. t.i.d. within 1 week.

▶ **Postherpetic neuralgia.** *Adults:* Initially, 75 mg P.O. b.i.d. or 50 mg P.O. t.i.d. May increase to 300 mg/day in two or three equally divided doses within 1 week. If pain relief is insufficient after 2 to 4 weeks, may increase to 300 mg b.i.d. or 200 mg t.i.d.

▶ **Adjunctive treatment of partial onset seizures.** *Adults:* Initially, 75 mg P.O. b.i.d. or 50 mg P.O. t.i.d. Range, 150 to 600 mg/day.

⧄ **Adjust-a-dose:** If creatinine clearance is 30 to 60 ml/minute, give 75 to 300 mg/day in two to three divided doses. If clearance is 15 to 30 ml/minute, give 25 to 150 mg/day in one dose or divided into two doses. If clearance is less than 15 ml/minute, give 25 to 75 mg/day in one dose.

If patient undergoes hemodialysis, give one supplemental dose according to these guidelines. If patient takes 25 mg daily, give 25 or 50 mg. If patient takes 25 to 50 mg daily, give 50 or 75 mg. If patient takes 75 mg daily, give 100 or 150 mg.

Contraindications and cautions

• Contraindicated in patients hypersensitive to pregabalin or any of its components.

• Use cautiously in patients with New York Heart Association class III or class IV heart failure.

⚖ **Lifespan:** Use drug in pregnancy only if benefits outweigh potential risks to the fetus. It isn't known whether drug appears in breast milk. Patient should either stop breast-feeding or stop drug. Safety and effectiveness haven't been established in pediatric patients. Older adults may be more sensitive to side effects.

P

Adverse reactions

CNS: abnormal gait, abnormal thinking, amnesia, anxiety, asthenia, *ataxia,* confusion, depersonalization, *dizziness,* euphoria, headache, hypesthesia, hypertonia, incoordination, myoclonus, nervousness, nystagmus, paresthesia, *somnolence,* stupor, *tremor,* twitching, vertigo.
CV: *edema,* **PR interval prolongation.**
EENT: blurred or abnormal vision, conjunctivitis, diplopia, eye disorder, otitis media, tinnitus.
GI: abdominal pain, constipation, *dry mouth,* flatulence, gastroenteritis, vomiting.
GU: anorgasmia, impotence, urinary incontinence, urinary frequency
Metabolic: HYPOGLYCEMIA, increased or decreased appetite, *weight gain.*
Musculoskeletal: arthralgia, back and chest pain, leg cramps, myalgia, myasthenia, neuropathy.
Respiratory: bronchitis, dyspnea.
Skin: ecchymosis, pruritus.
Other: *accidental injury, allergic reaction,* decreased libido, flu syndrome, *infection,* pain.

Interactions

Drug-drug. *CNS depressants:* May have additive effects on cognitive and gross motor function. Monitor patient for increased dizziness and somnolence.
Pioglitazone, rosiglitazone: May cause additive fluid retention and weight gain. Monitor patient closely.
Drug-lifestyle. *Alcohol use:* May have additive depressant effects on cognitive and gross motor function. Discourage alcohol use.

Effects on lab test results

• May increase CK level.
• May decrease platelet count.

Pharmacokinetics

Absorption: Well absorbed. Bioavailability exceeds 90%. Rate but not extent of absorption is decreased when drug is taken with food.
Distribution: Steady state is achieved in 24 to 48 hours. Doesn't bind to plasma proteins.
Metabolism: Negligible.
Excretion: Nearly proportional to creatinine clearance. About 90% eliminated via the kidneys as unchanged drug. *Half-life:* 6½ hours.

Route	Onset	Peak	Duration
P.O.	Unknown	1½–3 hr	Unknown

Action

Chemical effect: Drug may contribute to analgesic and anticonvulsant effects by binding to sites in CNS.
Therapeutic effect: Prevents seizure activity; relieves nerve pain caused by diabetic peripheral neuropathy or postherpetic neuralgia.

Available forms

Capsules: 25 mg, 50 mg, 75 mg, 100 mg, 150 mg, 200 mg, 225 mg, 300 mg

NURSING PROCESS

⚕ Assessment
• Assess patient's seizure disorder or diabetic peripheral neuropathy or postherpetic neuralgia prior to therapy and regularly thereafter.
• Monitor patient's weight and fluid status, especially if he has heart failure.
• Check for changes in vision.
• Watch for signs of rhabdomyolysis, such as dark, red, or cola-colored urine; muscle tenderness; generalized weakness; or muscle stiffness or aching.
• Evaluate patient's and family's knowledge of drug therapy.

⊕ Nursing diagnoses
• Risk for injury related to seizure disorder
• Acute pain related to diabetic peripheral neuropathy or postherpetic neuralgia
• Deficient knowledge related to drug therapy

⧁ Planning and implementation
• Taper drug gradually over at least 1 week. Stopping abruptly may result in increased seizure frequency, insomnia, headache, nausea, and diarrhea.
• In the case of overdose, treatment is supportive. Four hours of hemodialysis removes about 50% of drug. Contact poison control center.
Patient teaching
• Explain that drug may be taken with or without food.
• Warn patient not to stop drug abruptly.
• Caution patient to avoid hazardous activities until drug's effects are known.
• Instruct patient to watch for weight changes and water retention.
• Advise patient to report vision changes and malaise or fever accompanied by muscle pain, tenderness, or weakness.

Reactions may be *common,* uncommon, *life-threatening,* or COMMON AND LIFE-THREATENING.

• Inform a woman of childbearing age to immediately report planned or suspected pregnancy to prescriber.
• Tell a man who plans to father a child to consult prescriber about risks to fetus.
• If patient has diabetes, urge him to inspect his skin closely for ulcer formation.

☑ Evaluation
• Patient does not experience seizures while taking drug.
• Patient reports pain relief.
• Patient and family state understanding of drug therapy.

primidone
(PRIH-mih-dohn)
Apo-Primidone ◆ , Mysoline,
PMS Primidone, Sertan ◆

Pharmacologic class: barbiturate analogue
Therapeutic class: anticonvulsant
Pregnancy risk category: D

Indications and dosages

▶ **Generalized tonic-clonic, focal, and complex-partial (psychomotor) seizures.**
Adults and children age 8 and older: Initially, 100 to 125 mg P.O. h.s. on days 1 to 3; then 100 to 125 mg P.O. b.i.d. on days 4 to 6; then 100 to 125 mg P.O. t.i.d. on days 7 to 9; followed by maintenance dosage of 250 mg P.O. t.i.d. to q.i.d.; maximum dosage, 2 g daily.
Children younger than age 8: Initially, 50 mg P.O. h.s. for 3 days; then 50 mg P.O. b.i.d. for 4 to 6 days; then 100 mg P.O. b.i.d. for 7 to 9 days; followed by maintenance dosage of 125 to 250 mg P.O. t.i.d., or 10 to 25 mg/kg daily in divided doses.
▶ **Benign familial tremor (essential tremor).**
Adults: 750 mg P.O. daily.

Contraindications and cautions

• Contraindicated in patients with phenobarbital hypersensitivity or porphyria.
⚡ **Lifespan:** In pregnant and breast-feeding women, drug is contraindicated.

Adverse reactions

CNS: *drowsiness, ataxia,* emotional disturbances, vertigo, hyperirritability, fatigue.

CV: edema.
EENT: *diplopia,* nystagmus, edema of eyelids.
GI: anorexia, nausea, vomiting, thirst.
GU: impotence, polyuria.
Hematologic: *leukopenia,* eosinophilia, *thrombocytopenia.*
Skin: morbilliform rash, alopecia.

Interactions

Drug-drug. *Acetazolamide:* May decrease primidone level. Monitor patient for effect.
Carbamazepine: May decrease primidone level and increase carbamazepine level. Observe patient for lack of effect or carbamazepine toxicity.
Isoniazid, nicotinamide: May increase primidone level. Monitor patient for toxicity.
Metoprolol, propranolol: May reduce the effects of these drugs. Consider an increased beta blocker dose.
Phenytoin: May increase conversion of primidone to phenobarbital. Observe patient for increased phenobarbital effect.
Drug-herb. *Glutamate:* May antagonize anticonvulsant effects of drug. Discourage using together.
Drug-lifestyle. *Alcohol use:* May impair coordination, increase CNS effects, and cause death. Strongly discourage use together.

Effects on lab test results

• May decrease hemoglobin level and hematocrit.
• May increase eosinophil count. May decrease WBC and platelet counts.

Pharmacokinetics

Absorption: Absorbed readily.
Distribution: Wide.
Metabolism: Metabolized slowly by liver to phenylethylmalonamide (PEMA) and phenobarbital; PEMA is the major metabolite.
Excretion: Excreted in urine. *Half-life:* 5 to 15 hours.

Route	Onset	Peak	Duration
P.O.	Unknown	3–4 hr	Unknown

Action

Chemical effect: Unknown; some activity may be caused by PEMA and phenobarbital.
Therapeutic effect: Prevents seizures.

Available forms

Oral suspension: 250 mg/5 ml
Tablets: 50 mg, 250 mg

NURSING PROCESS

⏱ Assessment
• Assess patient's condition before starting therapy, and regularly thereafter to monitor the drug's effectiveness.
• Monitor blood levels. Therapeutic primidone level is 5 to 12 mcg/ml. Therapeutic phenobarbital level is 15 to 40 mcg/ml.
• Monitor CBC and routine blood chemistry q 6 months.
• Monitor patient's hydration throughout drug therapy.
• Assess patient's and family's knowledge of drug therapy.

⊕ Nursing diagnoses
• Risk for trauma related to seizures
• Risk for deficient fluid volume related to adverse reactions
• Deficient knowledge related to drug therapy

▷ Planning and implementation
• Shake liquid suspension well.
• Don't abruptly stop giving the drug, because seizures may worsen.
• Call prescriber immediately if adverse reactions develop.
• **③ ALERT:** Don't confuse primidone with prednisone.
Patient teaching
• Advise patient to avoid hazardous activities until the drug's CNS effects are known.
• Warn patient and parents not to stop drug suddenly.
• Tell patient that full therapeutic response may take 2 weeks or more.

☑ Evaluation
• Patient is free from seizure activity.
• Patient maintains adequate hydration throughout drug therapy.
• Patient and family state understanding of drug therapy.

probenecid
(proh-BEN-uh-sid)
Benuryl ◇ , Probalan

Pharmacologic class: sulfonamide derivative
Therapeutic class: uricosuric
Pregnancy risk category: B

Indications and dosages

▶ **Adjunct to penicillin therapy.** *Adults and children older than age 14 or who weigh more than 50 kg (110 lb):* 500 mg P.O. q.i.d.
Children ages 2 to 14 or who weigh 50 kg or less: Initially, 25 mg/kg P.O.; then 40 mg/kg in divided doses q.i.d.
▶ **Gonorrhea.** *Adults:* 3.5 g ampicillin P.O. with 1 g probenecid P.O. given together. Or, 1 g probenecid P.O. 30 minutes before 4.8 million units of aqueous penicillin G procaine I.M., injected at two different sites.
▶ **Hyperuricemia of gout, gouty arthritis.** *Adults:* 250 mg P.O. b.i.d. for first week; then 500 mg b.i.d., to maximum of 3 g daily. Reevaluate maintenance dosage q 6 months and reduce in increments of 500 mg.
▶ **To diagnose parkinsonian syndrome or mental depression‡.** *Adults:* 500 mg P.O. q 12 hours for 5 doses.
◻ Adjust-a-dose: For patients with renal impairment with a GFR of 30 ml/minute or greater, dose may need to be increased. Increases can be made in 0.5 g increments q 4 weeks. Usual daily dose is 2 g or less.

Contraindications and cautions

• Contraindicated in patients hypersensitive to the drug or any of its components, and in patients with uric acid kidney stones, blood dyscrasias, or acute gout attack.
• Use cautiously in patients with history of allergy to sulfa drugs; peptic ulcer or renal impairment.
※ Lifespan: In pregnant women, use cautiously. In breast-feeding women, use cautiously; it's unknown if the drug appears in breast milk. In children younger than age 2, drug is contraindicated.

Adverse reactions

CNS: *headache,* fever, dizziness.
CV: flushing, hypotension.

Reactions may be *common,* uncommon, *life-threatening*, or COMMON AND LIFE-THREATENING.

GI: anorexia, nausea, vomiting, sore gums, *gastric distress.*
GU: urinary frequency, renal colic.
Hematologic: hemolytic anemia, *aplastic anemia.*
Hepatic: *hepatic necrosis.*
Skin: alopecia, dermatitis, pruritus.
Other: hypersensitivity reaction, *anaphylaxis.*

Interactions

Drug-drug. *Methotrexate:* May impair excretion of methotrexate, causing increased level, effects, and toxicity. Monitor level closely and adjust dosage accordingly.
NSAIDs: May increase NSAID levels and increase risk of toxicity. Adjust dosage, p.r.n.
Oral antidiabetics: May enhance hypoglycemic effect. Monitor glucose levels closely. Dosage adjustment may be needed.
Rifampin: May decrease rifampin levels. Monitor patient for lack of effect.
Salicylates: May inhibit uricosuric effect of probenecid, causing urate retention. Don't use together.
Sulfonamides: May decrease sulfonamide excretion. Monitor patient for signs of toxicity.
Sulfonylureas: May increase half-life of these drugs. Monitor blood glucose.
Zidovudine: May increase absorption of zidovudine. Monitor patient for cutaneous drug eruption, malaise, myalgia, and fever.
Drug-lifestyle. *Alcohol use:* May increase urate levels. Discourage using together.

Effects on lab test results

● May decrease hemoglobin level and hematocrit.
● May cause false-positive glucose test results with Benedict's solution or Clinitest.

Pharmacokinetics

Absorption: Complete.
Distribution: Distributed throughout body; about 75% protein-bound.
Metabolism: Metabolized in liver to active metabolites, with some uricosuric effect.
Excretion: Drug and metabolites excreted in urine; probenecid is actively reabsorbed but metabolites aren't. *Half-life:* 3 to 8 hours after 500-mg dose, 6 to 12 hours after larger doses.

Route	Onset	Peak	Duration
P.O.	Unknown	2–4 hr	8 hr

Action

Chemical effect: Blocks renal tubular reabsorption of uric acid, increasing excretion, and inhibits active renal tubular secretion of many weak organic acids, such as penicillins and cephalosporins.
Therapeutic effect: Lowers uric acid and prolongs penicillin action.

Available forms

Tablets: 500 mg

NURSING PROCESS

⚕ Assessment
● Assess patient's condition before starting therapy, and regularly thereafter to monitor the drug's effectiveness.
● Periodically monitor BUN and renal function tests in patient on long-term therapy.
● Be alert for adverse reactions and drug interactions.
● If adverse GI reactions occur, monitor patient's hydration.
● Assess patient's and family's knowledge of drug therapy.

⊕ Nursing diagnoses
● Ineffective health maintenance related to underlying condition
● Risk for deficient fluid volume related to adverse GI reactions
● Deficient knowledge related to drug therapy

▶ Planning and implementation
● Drug is ineffective in patients with chronic renal insufficiency and a GFR less than 30 ml/minute.
● Give drug with milk, food, or antacids to minimize GI distress. Continued disturbances may indicate need to lower dose.
● Encourage patient to drink to maintain minimum daily output of 2 L of water a day. Alkalinize urine with sodium bicarbonate or potassium citrate. These measures will prevent hematuria, renal colic, urate stone development, and costovertebral pain.
● Therapy doesn't start until acute attack subsides. Drug contains no analgesic or anti-inflammatory drug and isn't useful during acute gout attacks.
● Drug may increase frequency, severity, and duration of acute gout attacks during first 6 to

P

12 months of therapy. Prophylactic colchicine or another anti-inflammatory is given during first 3 to 6 months.

ALERT: Don't confuse probenecid with Procanbid.

Patient teaching

- Instruct patient to take drug with food or milk to minimize GI distress.
- Advise patient with gout to avoid all drugs that contain aspirin, which may precipitate gout. Acetaminophen may be used for pain.
- Tell patient with gout to avoid alcohol during drug therapy; it increases urate level.
- Tell patient with gout to limit intake of foods high in purine, such as anchovies, liver, sardines, kidneys, sweetbreads, peas, and lentils.
- Instruct patient and family that drug must be taken regularly or gout attacks may result. Tell patient to visit prescriber regularly so uric acid can be monitored and dosage adjusted, if needed. Lifelong therapy may be required in patients with hyperuricemia.

Evaluation

- Patient responds positively to therapy.
- Patient maintains adequate hydration.
- Patient and family state understanding of drug therapy.

procainamide hydrochloride

(proh-KAYN-uh-mighd high-droh-KLOR-ighd)

Procainamide Durules ♦, Procan SR, Procanbid, Promine, Pronestyl, Pronestyl-SR

Pharmacologic class: procaine derivative
Therapeutic class: antiarrhythmic
Pregnancy risk category: C

Indications and dosages

▶ **Symptomatic PVCs; life-threatening ventricular tachycardia.** *Adults:* 100 mg q 5 minutes by slow I.V. push, no faster than 25 to 50 mg/minute, until arrhythmias disappear, adverse effects develop, or 500 mg have been given. Usual effective loading dose is 500 to 600 mg. Alternatively, give a loading dose of 500 to 600 mg I.V. infusion over 25 to 30 minutes. Maximum total dose is 1 g. When arrhythmias disappear, give continuous infusion of 2 to 6 mg/minute. If arrhythmias recur, repeat bolus as above and increase infusion rate. For I.M. administration, give 50 mg/kg/day divided q 3 to 6 hours; for arrhythmias during surgery, 100 to 500 mg I.M. For oral therapy, initiate dosage at 50 mg/kg P.O. of conventional tablets or capsules in divided doses q 3 hours until therapeutic levels are reached. For the maintenance dosage, substitute sustained-release form q 6 hours or extended-release form (Procanbid) at dosage of 50 mg/kg P.O. in two divided doses q 12 hours.

Children‡: Dosage not established. Recommendations include 2 to 5 mg/kg, not exceeding 100 mg, repeated, p.r.n., at 5- to 10-minute intervals not exceeding 15 mg/kg in 24 hours or 500 mg in a 30-minute period; or 15 mg/kg infused over 30 to 60 minutes, followed by maintenance infusion of 0.02 to 0.08 mg/kg/minute.

Adjust-a-dose: For patients with renal or hepatic dysfunction, decrease dosage or give at longer intervals.

▶ **To maintain normal sinus rhythm after conversion of atrial flutter‡.** *Adults:* 0.5 to 1 g P.O. of conventional tablets or capsules q 4 to 6 hours.

▶ **Loading dose to prevent atrial fibrillation or paroxysmal atrial tachycardia‡.** *Adults:* 1.25 g P.O. of conventional tablets or capsules. If arrhythmias persist after 1 hour, give additional 750 mg. If no change occurs, give 500 mg to 1 g P.O. q 2 hours until arrhythmias disappear or adverse effects occur. Maintenance dose is 1 g extended release q 6 hours.

▶ **Malignant hyperthermia‡.** *Adults:* 200 to 900 mg I.V., followed by an infusion.

I.V. administration

- Vials for I.V. injection contain 1 g of drug: 100 mg/ml (10 ml) or 500 mg/ml (2 ml).
- Use infusion control device to give infusion precisely.
- Keep patient in supine position during I.V. use. If drug is given too rapidly, hypotension can occur. Watch closely for adverse reactions during infusion, and notify prescriber if they occur.
- Patient receiving infusions must be monitored at all times.
- If solution becomes discolored, check with pharmacy and expect to discard.

⊗ **Incompatibilities**
Bretylium, esmolol, ethacrynate, milrinone, phenytoin sodium.

Contraindications and cautions

• Contraindicated in patients hypersensitive to procaine and related drugs; in those with complete, second-, or third-degree heart block in absence of artificial pacemaker; and in those with myasthenia gravis or systemic lupus erythematosus. Also contraindicated in patients with atypical ventricular tachycardia (torsades de pointes) because procainamide may aggravate this condition.
• Use cautiously when giving drug to treat ventricular tachycardia during coronary occlusion.
• Use cautiously in patients with hepatic or renal insufficiency, blood dyscrasias, bone marrow suppression, heart failure, or other conduction disturbances, such as bundle-branch heart block, sinus bradycardia, or digoxin intoxication.
⚡ **Lifespan:** In pregnant women, use cautiously. In breast-feeding women, drug isn't recommended. In children, safety and effectiveness haven't been established.

Adverse reactions

CNS: hallucinations, fever, confusion, depression, dizziness.
CV: hypotension, *ventricular asystole,* bradycardia, AV block, *ventricular fibrillation* after parenteral use, *heart failure.*
GI: nausea, vomiting, anorexia, diarrhea, bitter taste with large doses.
Hematologic: *thrombocytopenia, neutropenia* (especially with sustained-release forms), *agranulocytosis,* hemolytic anemia.
Musculoskeletal: *myalgia.*
Skin: maculopapular rash.
Other: *lupuslike syndrome* (especially after prolonged use).

Interactions

Drug-drug. *Amiodarone:* May increase procainamide level and toxicity with additive effects on QT interval and QRS complex. Avoid using together.
Anticholinergics: May have additive anticholinergic effects. Monitor patient closely.

Anticholinesterases: May decrease anticholinesterase effect. Anticholinesterase dosage may need to be increased.
Cimetidine: May increase procainamide level. Avoid this combination if possible. Monitor procainamide level closely and adjust the dose p.r.n.
Lidocaine: May have additive cardiodepressant effects. Monitor ECG.
Neuromuscular skeletal muscle relaxants: May increase skeletal muscle relaxant effects. Monitor patient.
Propranolol, ranitidine: May increase procainamide level. Monitor patient for toxicity.
Quinidine, trimethoprim: May elevate procainamide and N-acetylprocainamide (NAPA) levels. Monitor patient for toxicity.
Drug-herb. *Jimson weed:* May adversely affect CV function. Discourage using together.
Licorice: May prolong QT interval and be additive. Discourage using together.

Effects on lab test results

• May increase ALT, AST, alkaline phosphatase, LDH, and bilirubin levels. May decrease hemoglobin level and hematocrit.
• May increase antinuclear antibody titer. May decrease neutrophil, granulocyte, and platelet counts.

Pharmacokinetics

Absorption: Usually 75% to 95% of P.O. dose. Unknown after I.M. use.
Distribution: Distributed widely in most body tissues, including CSF, liver, spleen, kidneys, lungs, muscles, brain, and heart. About 15% binds to proteins.
Metabolism: Metabolized in liver.
Excretion: Excreted in urine. *Half-life:* About 2½ to 4¾ hours.

Route	Onset	Peak	Duration
P.O.	Unknown	1–2 hr	Unknown
I.V.	Immediate	Immediate	Unknown
I.M.	10–30 min	15–60 min	Unknown

Action

Chemical effect: Class IA antiarrhythmic that decreases excitability, conduction velocity, automaticity, and membrane responsiveness with prolonged refractory period. Larger doses may induce AV block.

Therapeutic effect: Restores normal sinus rhythm.

Available forms

Capsules: 250 mg, 375 mg, 500 mg
Injection: 100 mg/ml, 500 mg/ml
Tablets: 250 mg, 375 mg, 500 mg
Tablets (extended-release): 500 mg, 1000 mg
Tablets (sustained-release): 250 mg, 500 mg, 750 mg

NURSING PROCESS

⚕ Assessment
• Assess patient's condition before starting therapy, and regularly thereafter to monitor the drug's effectiveness.
• Monitor levels of procainamide and its active metabolite, NAPA. To suppress ventricular arrhythmias, therapeutic level of procainamide is 4 to 8 mcg/ml; therapeutic level of NAPA is 10 to 30 mcg/ml.
• Monitor QT interval closely in patient with renal impairment.
• Hypokalemia predisposes patient to arrhythmias; monitor electrolytes, especially potassium level.
• Monitor blood pressure and ECG continuously during I.V. use. Watch for prolonged QT intervals and QRS complexes, heart block, or increased arrhythmias.
• Monitor CBC frequently during first 3 months, particularly in patient taking sustained-release form.
• Be alert for adverse reactions and drug interactions.
• Assess patient's and family's knowledge of drug therapy.

🖥 Nursing diagnoses
• Decreased cardiac output related to presence of arrhythmia
• Ineffective protection related to adverse hematologic reactions
• Deficient knowledge related to drug therapy

▷ Planning and implementation
Ⓢ **ALERT:** Some drug products contain tartrazine and sulfites. Ask if patient is allergic to these agents.
Ⓢ **ALERT:** If blood pressure changes significantly or ECG changes occur, withhold drug, obtain rhythm strip, and notify prescriber immediately.

Ⓢ **ALERT:** Don't confuse procainamide with probenecid.
• Positive antinuclear antibody titer occurs in about 60% of patients without lupuslike symptoms. This response seems to be related to prolonged use, not to dosage. May progress to systemic lupus erythematosus if drug isn't stopped.
Patient teaching
• Instruct patient to report fever, rash, muscle pain, diarrhea, bleeding, bruises, or pleuritic chest pain.
• Stress importance of taking drug exactly as prescribed. This may require use of alarm clock for nighttime doses.
• Inform patient taking extended-release form that wax-matrix "ghost" from tablet may be passed in stool. Assure patient that drug is completely absorbed before this occurs.
• Tell patient not to crush or break sustained-release or extended-release tablets.

☑ Evaluation
• Patient regains normal cardiac output after drug stops abnormal heart rhythm.
• Patient maintains normal CBC.
• Patient and family state understanding of drug therapy.

procarbazine hydrochloride
(proh-KAR-buh-zeen high-droh-KLOR-ighd)
Matulane, Natulan ◆

Pharmacologic class: antibiotic
Therapeutic class: antineoplastic
Pregnancy risk category: D

Indications and dosages
▶ **Hodgkin's disease, lymphoma, brain and lung cancer.** *Adults:* 2 to 4 mg/kg P.O. daily in single dose or divided doses for first week. Then, 4 to 6 mg/kg daily until WBC count decreases to below 4,000/mm³ or platelet count decreases to below 100,000/mm³. If hematologic toxicity occurs, resume at 1 to 2 mg/kg daily.
Children: 50 mg/m² P.O. daily for first week; then 100 mg/m² until response or toxicity occurs. Maintenance dosage is 50 mg/m² P.O. daily after bone marrow recovery.

Contraindications and cautions

• Contraindicated in patients hypersensitive to the drug or any of its components and in those with inadequate bone marrow reserve as shown by bone marrow aspiration.

• Use cautiously in patients with impaired hepatic or renal function.

Lifespan: In pregnant and breast-feeding women, drug isn't recommended.

Adverse reactions

CNS: nervousness, depression, insomnia, nightmares, paresthesia, neuropathy, *hallucinations,* confusion, ***seizures, coma.***
EENT: retinal hemorrhage, nystagmus, photophobia.
GI: *nausea, vomiting,* anorexia, stomatitis, dry mouth, dysphagia, diarrhea, constipation.
Hematologic: ***bleeding tendency, thrombocytopenia, leukopenia,*** anemia.
Hepatic: ***hepatotoxicity.***
Respiratory: *pleural effusion,* pneumonitis.
Skin: dermatitis, reversible alopecia.

Interactions

Drug-drug. *CNS depressants:* May have additive depressant effects. Avoid using together.
Digoxin: May decrease digoxin level. Monitor level closely.
Levodopa: May cause flushing and a significant rise in blood pressure within 1 hour of levodopa use. Separate administration times; monitor patient's blood pressure closely.
Local anesthetics, sympathomimetics, tricyclic antidepressants: May cause tremors, palpitations, and increased blood pressure. Monitor patient closely.
Opioids: May cause severe hypotension and death. Don't give together.
Drug-food. *Caffeine:* May result in arrhythmias, severe hypertension. Discourage caffeine intake.
Foods high in tyramine (cheese, red wine): May cause tremors, palpitations, and increased blood pressure. Monitor patient closely.
Drug-lifestyle. *Alcohol use:* May cause mild disulfiram-like reaction. Warn patient to avoid alcohol.

Effects on lab test results

• May increase liver enzyme levels. May decrease hemoglobin level and hematocrit.

• May increase eosinophil count. May decrease platelet, WBC, and RBC counts.

Pharmacokinetics

Absorption: Rapid and complete.
Distribution: Distributes widely into body tissues, with highest levels in liver, kidneys, intestinal wall, and skin. Drug crosses blood-brain barrier.
Metabolism: Extensively metabolized in liver; some metabolites have cytotoxic activity.
Excretion: Drug and metabolites excreted primarily in urine. *Half-life:* About 10 minutes.

Route	Onset	Peak	Duration
P.O.	Unknown	Unknown	Unknown

Action

Chemical effect: Unknown; thought to inhibit DNA, RNA, and protein synthesis.
Therapeutic effect: Kills selected cancer cells.

Available forms

Capsules: 50 mg

NURSING PROCESS

Assessment

• Assess patient's condition before starting therapy, and regularly thereafter to monitor the drug's effectiveness.

• Monitor CBC and platelet counts.

• Be alert for adverse reactions and drug interactions.

• Assess patient's and family's knowledge of drug therapy.

Nursing diagnoses

• Ineffective health maintenance related to presence of neoplastic disease

• Ineffective protection related to adverse hematologic reactions

• Deficient knowledge related to drug therapy

Planning and implementation

• Give drug h.s. to lessen nausea.

ALERT: If patient becomes confused or if paresthesia or other neuropathies develop, stop giving the drug and notify prescriber.

Patient teaching

• Advise patient to take drug h.s. and in divided doses.

P

• Warn patient to watch for signs of infection (fever, sore throat, fatigue) and bleeding (easy bruising, nosebleeds, bleeding gums, melena). Tell him to take his temperature daily.

• Warn patient not to drink alcohol during therapy.

• Tell patient to stop taking the drug and immediately notify the prescriber if disulfiram-like reaction occurs (chest pains, rapid or irregular heartbeat, severe headache, stiff neck).

• Tell patient to avoid foods high in tyramine, such as cheese, yogurt, and bananas.

• Warn patient to avoid hazardous activities until the drug's CNS effects are known.

• Advise woman of childbearing age not to become pregnant during therapy, and to consult with prescriber before becoming pregnant.

✓ Evaluation

• Patient responds well to therapy.

• Patient develops no serious adverse hematologic reactions.

• Patient and family state understanding of drug therapy.

prochlorperazine
(proh-klor-PER-ah-zeen)
Compazine, PMS Prochlorperazine ♦,
Prorazin ♦, Stemetil

prochlorperazine edisylate
Compa-Z, Compazine Syrup, Cotranzine,
Ultrazine-10

prochlorperazine maleate
Compazine Spansule, PMS
Prochlorperazine ♦, Prorazin ♦, Stemetil ♦

Pharmacologic class: phenothiazine (piperazine derivative)
Therapeutic class: antipsychotic, antiemetic, anxiolytic
Pregnancy risk category: C

Indications and dosages

▶ **Preoperative nausea control.** *Adults:* 5 to 10 mg I.M. 1 to 2 hours before induction of anesthesia; repeat once in 30 minutes, if needed. Or, 5 to 10 mg I.V. 15 to 30 minutes before induction of anesthesia; repeat once if needed. Or, 20 mg/L D₅W or normal saline solution by I.V.

infusion. Begin infusion 15 to 30 minutes before induction of anesthesia.

▶ **Severe nausea and vomiting.** *Adults:* 5 to 10 mg P.O., t.i.d. or q.i.d. Or, 15 mg P.O. (sustained-release) on arising. Or, 10-mg sustained-release form P.O. q 12 hours. Or, 25 mg P.R., b.i.d. Or, 5 to 10 mg I.M. repeated q 3 to 4 hours, p.r.n. Or, 5 to 10 mg may be given I.V. Maximum parenteral dosage is 40 mg daily.
Children who weigh 18 to 39 kg (39 to 86 lb): 2.5 mg P.O. or P.R., t.i.d. Or, 5 mg P.O. or P.R., b.i.d. Maximum dosage is 15 mg daily. Or, give 0.132 mg/kg by deep I.M. injection. Control usually is obtained with one dose.
Children who weigh 14 to 17 kg (31 to 38 lb): 2.5 mg P.O. or P.R., b.i.d. or t.i.d. Maximum dosage, 10 mg daily. Or give 0.132 mg/kg by deep I.M. injection. Control usually is obtained with one dose.
Children who weigh 9 to 14 kg (20 to 30 lb): 2.5 mg P.O. or P.R. once daily or b.i.d. Maximum dosage is 7.5 mg daily. Or give 0.132 mg/kg by deep I.M. injection. Control usually is obtained with one dose.

▶ **To manage symptoms of psychotic disorders.** *Adults and children age 12 and older:* 5 to 10 mg P.O., t.i.d. or q.i.d.
Children ages 2 to 12: 2.5 mg P.O. or P.R., b.i.d. or t.i.d. Don't exceed 10 mg on day 1. Increase dosage gradually to recommended maximum, if needed. In children ages 2 to 5, maximum daily dosage is 20 mg. In children ages 6 to 12, maximum daily dosage is 25 mg.

▶ **To manage symptoms of severe psychoses.** *Adults and children age 12 and older:* 10 to 20 mg I.M. repeated in 1 to 4 hours, if needed. Rarely, patients may require 10 to 20 mg q 4 to 6 hours. Institute P.O. therapy after symptoms are controlled.
Children ages 2 to 12: 0.13 mg/kg I.M. then switch to oral dosage.

▶ **Nonpsychotic anxiety.** *Adults:* 5 to 10 mg by deep I.M. injection q 3 to 4 hours, not to exceed 40 mg daily; or 5 to 10 mg P.O., t.i.d., or q.i.d. Or, give 15-mg extended-release capsule once daily or 10-mg extended-release capsule q 12 hours.

▼ I.V. administration

• Drug may be given undiluted or diluted in an isotonic solution.

• Don't give faster than 5 mg/minute. Don't give by bolus injection.

⊗ Incompatibilities

Aldesleukin, allopurinol, amifostine, aminophylline, amphotericin B, ampicillin sodium, aztreonam, calcium gluconate, chloramphenicol sodium succinate, chlorothiazide, dexamethasone sodium phosphate, dimenhydrinate, etoposide, filgrastim, fludarabine, foscarnet, furosemide, gemcitabine, heparin sodium, hydrocortisone sodium succinate, hydromorphone, ketorolac, solutions containing methylparabens, midazolam hydrochloride, morphine, penicillin G potassium, penicillin G sodium, pentobarbital, phenobarbital sodium, phenytoin sodium, piperacillin sodium and tazobactam sodium, solutions containing propylparabens, thiopental, vitamin B complex with C.

Contraindications and cautions

• Contraindicated in patients hypersensitive to phenothiazines, patients with CNS depression (including coma), patients undergoing pediatric surgery, patients taking adrenergic blockers, and patients under the influence of alcohol.
• Use cautiously in patients who have been exposed to extreme heat and patients with impaired CV function, glaucoma, or seizure disorders.
⚕ Lifespan: In pregnant women, drug is contraindicated except in cases of continuous nausea and vomiting when benefits outweigh risk to the fetus. In breast-feeding women, use cautiously; it's unknown if the drug appears in breast milk. In acutely ill children, use cautiously. In children younger than age 2 who weigh less than 9 kg (20 lb), drug is contraindicated. In the elderly, use cautiously, and gradually increase the dose.

Adverse reactions

CNS: *extrapyramidal reactions,* sedation, pseudoparkinsonism, EEG changes, dizziness.
CV: *orthostatic hypotension,* tachycardia, ECG changes.
EENT: ocular changes, blurred vision.
GI: dry mouth, constipation.
GU: *urine retention,* dark urine, menstrual irregularities, inhibited ejaculation.
Hematologic: hyperprolactinemia, *transient leukopenia, agranulocytosis.*
Hepatic: cholestatic jaundice.
Metabolic: weight gain, increased appetite.
Skin: *mild photosensitivity,* exfoliative dermatitis.
Other: allergic reactions, gynecomastia.

Interactions

Drug-drug. *Antacids:* May inhibit absorption of oral phenothiazines. Separate antacid doses by at least 2 hours.
Anticholinergics, including antidepressants and antiparkinsonian drugs: May increase anticholinergic activity and aggravated parkinsonian symptoms. Use together cautiously.
Barbiturates: May decrease phenothiazine effect. Monitor patient for decreased effect.
Lithium: May cause disorientation, unconsciousness, and extrapyramidal symptoms. Monitor patient closely.
Drug-herb. *Dong quai, St. John's wort:* May increase photosensitivity reactions. Discourage using together.
Ginkgo: May decrease effects of phenothiazines. Monitor patient.
Kava: May increase risk of dystonic reactions. Discourage using together.
Milk thistle: May decrease liver toxicity caused by phenothiazines. Monitor liver enzyme levels if used together.
Yohimbe: May increase risk for yohimbe toxicity when used together. Discourage using together.
Drug-lifestyle. *Alcohol use:* May increase CNS depression, particularly decreasing psychomotor skills. Strongly discourage alcohol use.
Sun exposure: May cause photosensitivity reaction. Urge patient to avoid unprotected or prolonged sun exposure.

Effects on lab test results

• May decrease WBC and granulocyte counts. May alter liver function test values.

Pharmacokinetics

Absorption: Erratic and variable with P.O. tablet; more predictable with P.O. concentrate. Unknown for P.R. use. Rapid for I.M. use.
Distribution: Distributed widely into body; 91% to 99% protein-bound.
Metabolism: Metabolized extensively by liver, but no active metabolites are formed.
Excretion: Excreted primarily in urine; some excreted in feces. *Half-life:* Unknown.

Route	Onset	Peak	Duration
P.O.	30–40 min	Unknown	3–12 hr
I.V.	Immediate	Immediate	Unknown
I.M.	10–20 min	Unknown	3–4 hr
P.R.	60 min	Unknown	3–4 hr

P

Action

Chemical effect: Acts on chemoreceptor trigger zone to inhibit nausea and vomiting; in larger doses, partially depresses vomiting center.
Therapeutic effect: Relieves nausea and vomiting, signs and symptoms of psychosis, and anxiety.

Available forms

prochlorperazine
Injection: 5 mg/ml
Suppositories: 2.5 mg, 5 mg, 25 mg
Tablets: 5 mg, 10 mg
prochlorperazine edisylate
Syrup: 1 mg/ml
prochlorperazine maleate
Capsules (sustained-release): 10 mg, 15 mg, 30 mg
Tablets: 5 mg, 10 mg, 25 mg

NURSING PROCESS

⚒ Assessment
• Assess patient's condition before starting therapy, and regularly thereafter to monitor the drug's effectiveness.
• Watch for orthostatic hypotension, especially when giving drug I.V.
• Monitor CBC and liver function test results during long-term therapy.
• Be alert for adverse reactions and drug interactions.
• Assess patient's and family's knowledge of drug therapy.

⊞ Nursing diagnoses
• Risk for deficient fluid volume related to nausea and vomiting
• Disturbed thought processes related to presence of psychosis
• Deficient knowledge related to drug therapy

▷ Planning and implementation
• Dilute solution with tomato or fruit juice, milk, coffee, carbonated beverage, tea, water, or soup; or mix with pudding.
• Inject I.M. deep into upper outer quadrant of gluteal region.
• Don't give subcutaneously or mix in syringe with another drug.
• Avoid getting concentrate or injection solution on hands or clothing.

• Drug is used only if vomiting can't be otherwise controlled or if only a few doses are needed. If more than four doses are needed in 24 hours, notify prescriber.
• Store drug in light-resistant container. Slight yellowing doesn't affect potency; discard extremely discolored solutions.

Patient teaching
• Tell patient to mix oral solution with flavored liquid to mask taste.
• Advise patient to wear protective clothing when exposed to sunlight.
• Tell patient to notify prescriber about adverse reactions.

☑ Evaluation
• Patient's nausea and vomiting are relieved.
• Patient's behavior and communication show better thought processes.
• Patient and family state understanding of drug therapy.

promethazine hydrochloride
(proh-METH-uh-zeen high-droh-KLOR-ighd)
Anergan 50, Phenergan*✦

promethazine theoclate
Avomine ◊

Pharmacologic class: phenothiazine derivative
Therapeutic class: antiemetic, antihistamine, sedative
Pregnancy risk category: C

Indications and dosages

▶ **Motion sickness.** *Adults:* Give 25 mg P.O. or P.R. b.i.d. Take initial dose 30 to 60 minutes before anticipated travel, and repeat in 8 to 12 hours, if needed.
Children older than age 2: Give 12.5 to 25 mg P.O. or P.R. b.i.d.
▶ **Nausea and vomiting.** *Adults:* Give 12.5 to 25 mg P.O., I.M., or P.R. q 4 to 6 hours, p.r.n.
Children older than age 2: Give 12.5 to 25 mg P.O. or P.R. q 4 to 6 hours, p.r.n. Or, 6.25 to 12.5 mg I.M. q 4 to 6 hours, p.r.n.
▶ **Rhinitis, allergy symptoms.** *Adults:* Give 12.5 mg P.O. or P.R. q.i.d. (before meals and h.s.). Or, 25 mg P.O. or P.R. h.s.
Children older than age 2: Give 6.25 to 12.5 mg P.O. or P.R. t.i.d. Or, 25 mg P.O. or P.R. h.s.

Reactions may be *common*, uncommon, *life-threatening*, or COMMON AND LIFE-THREATENING.

▶ **Sedation.** *Adults:* Give 25 to 50 mg P.O., P.R., or I.M. h.s. or p.r.n.
Children older than age 2: Give 12.5 to 25 mg P.O., I.M., or P.R. h.s.
▶ **Routine preoperative or postoperative sedation or adjunct to analgesics.** *Adults:* Give 25 to 50 mg I.M., I.V., P.R., or P.O.
Children older than age 2: Give 0.5 to 1.1 mg/kg I.M., P.R., or P.O.

▼ I.V. administration

• Don't give in concentration greater than 25 mg/ml or at rate exceeding 25 mg/minute.
• Shield I.V. solution from direct light.
⊗ **Incompatibilities**
Aldesleukin, allopurinol, aminophylline, amphotericin B, cephalosporins, chloramphenicol sodium succinate, chloroquine phosphate, chlorothiazide, diatrizoate meglumine (34.3%) and diatrizoate sodium (35%), diatrizoate meglumine (52%) and diatrizoate sodium (8%), diatrizoate sodium (75%), dimenhydrinate, doxorubicin liposomal, foscarnet, furosemide, heparin sodium, hydrocortisone sodium succinate, iodipamide meglumine (52%), iothalamate meglumine (60%), iothalamate sodium (80%), ketorolac, methohexital, morphine, nalbuphine, penicillin G potassium and sodium, pentobarbital sodium, phenobarbital sodium, phenytoin sodium, thiopental, vitamin B complex.

Contraindications and cautions

• Contraindicated in patients hypersensitive to the drug or any of its components, and in those with intestinal obstruction, prostatic hyperplasia, bladder-neck obstruction, seizure disorders, coma, CNS depression, or stenosing peptic ulcerations.
• Use cautiously in patients with pulmonary, hepatic, or CV disease or asthma.
• Avoid combining drug with other respiratory depressants.
▲ **Lifespan:** In pregnant women, safety and effectiveness haven't been established. In breast-feeding women, neonates, premature neonates, and acutely ill or dehydrated children, drug is contraindicated. Don't use in children for nausea and vomiting when the cause of the vomiting is unknown. In children younger than age 2, drug is contraindicated. Use with caution in children ages 2 and older, using the lowest effective dose and watch for respiratory depressant effects. In the elderly, use cautiously.

Adverse reactions

CNS: *sedation,* confusion, restlessness, tremors, *drowsiness* (especially geriatric patients), extrapyramidal reactions.
CV: hypotension, ECG changes.
EENT: transient myopia, nasal congestion.
GI: anorexia, nausea, vomiting, constipation, *dry mouth.*
GU: urine retention.
Hematologic: *leukopenia, agranulocytosis, thrombocytopenia.*
Skin: photosensitivity, venous thrombosis at injection site.

Interactions

Drug-drug. *CNS depressants:* May increase sedation. Use together cautiously.
Epinephrine: May block or reverse effects of epinephrine. Use another vasopressor.
Levodopa: May decrease antiparkinsonian action of levodopa. Avoid using together.
Lithium: May reduce GI absorption or enhance renal elimination of lithium. Avoid using together.
MAO inhibitors: May increase extrapyramidal effects. Don't use together.
Protease inhibitors, SSRIs: May increase levels of these drugs and cause serious adverse cardiac effects. Don't use together.
Drug-herb. *Dong quai, St. John's wort:* May increase photosensitivity reactions. Discourage using together.
Kava: May increase risk of dystonic reactions. Discourage using together.
Yohimbe: May increase risk of yohimbe toxicity when used together. Discourage using together.
Drug-lifestyle. *Alcohol use:* May increase sedation. Discourage using together.
Sun exposure: May cause photosensitivity reaction. Urge patient to avoid unprotected or prolonged sun exposure.

Effects on lab test results

• May increase glucose and hemoglobin levels and hematocrit.
• May decrease WBC, platelet, and granulocyte counts.
• May cause false-positive immunologic urine pregnancy test using Gravindex and false-negative results using Prepurex or Dap tests. May interfere with blood typing of ABO group.

P

Rapid onset   *Liquid form contains alcohol.   ◆ Canada   ◇ Australia   †OTC   ✐Photoguide   ‡Off-label use

Pharmacokinetics

Absorption: Well absorbed after P.O. use; fairly rapid after P.R. or I.M. use.
Distribution: Distributed widely throughout body.
Metabolism: Metabolized in liver.
Excretion: Excreted in urine and feces. *Half-life:* Unknown.

Route	Onset	Peak	Duration
P.O.	15–60 min	Unknown	≤ 12 hr
I.V.	3–5 min	Unknown	≤ 12 hr
I.M., P.R.	20 min	Unknown	≤ 12 hr

Action

Chemical effect: Competes with histamine for H_1-receptor sites on effector cells. Prevents, but doesn't reverse, histamine-mediated responses.
Therapeutic effect: Prevents motion sickness and relieves nausea, nasal congestion, and allergy symptoms. Also promotes calmness.

Available forms

promethazine hydrochloride
Injection: 25 mg/ml, 50 mg/ml (I.M. use only)
Suppositories: 12.5 mg, 25 mg, 50 mg
Syrup: 6.25 mg/5 ml*
Tablets: 12.5 mg, 25 mg, 50 mg
promethazine theoclate
Tablets: 25 mg†

NURSING PROCESS

⚖ Assessment
• Assess patient's condition before starting therapy, and regularly thereafter to monitor the drug's effectiveness.
• Be alert for adverse reactions and drug interactions.
• Assess patient's and family's knowledge of drug therapy.

✥ Nursing diagnoses
• Ineffective health maintenance related to underlying condition
• Risk for injury related to drug's sedating effects
• Deficient knowledge related to drug therapy

▶ Planning and implementation
• Pronounced sedative effect limits use in many ambulatory patients.

• Drug is used as adjunct to analgesics (usually to increase sedation); it has no analgesic activity.
• Give drug with food or milk to reduce GI distress.
⚠ **ALERT:** Phenergan brand ampules contain sulfite. Check patient for sulfite allergy before administering Phenergan I.M.
• Inject I.M. deep into large muscle mass. Rotate injection sites.
• Don't give subcutaneously.
• Drug may be safely mixed with meperidine (Demerol) in same syringe.
• In patient scheduled for myelogram, stop drug 48 hours before procedure and don't resume giving the drug until 24 hours after the procedure, because of risk of seizures.
⚠ **ALERT:** Caution should be used in children 2 years of age and older. This includes using the lowest effective dose, monitoring for respiratory depressant effects and avoiding combining promethazine hydrochloride with other drugs that are known to depress the respiratory system.

Patient teaching
• When treating for motion sickness, tell patient to take first dose 30 to 60 minutes before travel. Tell him to take dose after rising and with evening meal on next days of travel.
• Warn patient not to drink alcohol or engage in hazardous activities until the drug's CNS effects are known.
• Tell patient that coffee or tea may reduce drowsiness. Sugarless gum, sugarless sour hard candy, or ice chips may relieve dry mouth.
• Warn patient about photosensitivity and precautions to avoid it.
• Advise patient to stop drug 4 days before allergy skin tests.

☑ Evaluation
• Patient responds well to therapy.
• Patient doesn't experience injury from adverse reactions.
• Patient and family state understanding of drug therapy.

---

propafenone hydrochloride
(proh-puh-FEE-nohn high-droh-KLOR-ighd)
Rythmol, Rythmol SR

Pharmacologic class: sodium channel antagonist
Therapeutic class: antiarrhythmic (class IC)
Pregnancy risk category: C

Indications and dosages

▶ **Suppression of life-threatening ventricular arrhythmias, such as sustained ventricular tachycardia; prevention of supraventricular tachycardia associated with disabling symptoms and for disabling paroxysmal atrial fibrillation/flutter.** *Adults:* Initially, 150 mg P.O. q 8 hours. May increase dosage at 3- to 4-day intervals to 225 mg q 8 hours. If needed, increase dosage to 300 mg q 8 hours. Maximum daily dosage is 900 mg.
🅽 **Adjust-a-dose:** For patients with hepatic failure, manufacturer recommends dosage reduction of 20% to 30%.

Contraindications and cautions

• Contraindicated in patients hypersensitive to the drug or any of its components, and in those with severe or uncontrolled heart failure, cardiogenic shock, bradycardia, marked hypotension, bronchospastic disorders, electrolyte imbalance, or SA, AV, or intraventricular disorders of impulse conduction in absence of pacemaker.
• Use cautiously in patients with heart failure because propafenone can have negative inotropic effect. Also use cautiously in patients taking other cardiac depressant drugs and in those with hepatic or renal impairment.
🔆 **Lifespan:** In pregnant women, safety and effectiveness haven't been established. In breastfeeding women, drug isn't recommended. In children, safety and effectiveness haven't been established.

Adverse reactions

CNS: anxiety, ataxia, dizziness, drowsiness, fatigue, headache, insomnia, syncope, tremor, weakness.
CV: atrial fibrillation, *bradycardia,* bundle branch block, *heart failure,* chest pain, edema, first-degree AV block, hypotension, increased QRS duration, intraventricular conduction de-

lay, palpitations, *proarrhythmic events (ventricular tachycardia, PVCs).*
EENT: blurred vision.
GI: abdominal pain or cramps, constipation, diarrhea, dyspepsia, flatulence, nausea, vomiting, dry mouth, unusual taste, anorexia.
Musculoskeletal: joint pain.
Respiratory: dyspnea.
Skin: rash, diaphoresis.

Interactions

Drug-drug. *Antiarrhythmics:* May increase risk of heart failure. Monitor patient closely.
Cimetidine: May decrease metabolism of propafenone. Monitor patient for toxicity.
Digoxin, oral anticoagulants: May increase levels of these drugs by about 35% to 85%, resulting in toxicity. Monitor patient's PT, INR, and digoxin level closely.
Local anesthetics: May increase risk of CNS toxicity. Monitor patient closely.
Metoprolol, propranolol: May slow metabolism of these drugs. Monitor patient for toxicity.
Quinidine: May slow propafenone metabolism. Avoid using together.
Rifampin: May increase propafenone clearance. Monitor patient for lack of effect.

Effects on lab test results

None reported.

Pharmacokinetics

Absorption: Good. Because of significant first-pass effect, bioavailability is limited, but it increases with dosage.
Distribution: 97% protein-bound.
Metabolism: Metabolized in liver.
Excretion: Excreted mainly in feces; some in urine. *Half-life:* 2 to 32 hours.

Route	Onset	Peak	Duration
P.O.	Unknown	≤ 3½ hr	Unknown

Action

Chemical effect: Reduces inward sodium current in Purkinje and myocardial cells. Decreases excitability, conduction velocity, and automaticity in AV nodal, His-Purkinje, and intraventricular tissue; causes slight but significant prolongation of refractory period in AV nodal tissue.
Therapeutic effect: Restores normal sinus rhythm.

Available forms

Capsules (extended-release): 225 mg, 325 mg, 425 mg
Tablets: 150 mg, 225 mg, 300 mg

NURSING PROCESS

☡ Assessment

• Assess patient's condition before starting therapy, and regularly thereafter to monitor the drug's effectiveness.
• Continuous cardiac monitoring is recommended at start of therapy and during dose adjustments.
• Be alert for adverse reactions and drug interactions.
• Assess patient's and family's knowledge of drug therapy.

⊞ Nursing diagnoses

• Decreased cardiac output related to presence of arrhythmia
• Ineffective protection related to drug-induced proarrhythmias
• Deficient knowledge related to drug therapy

▷ Planning and implementation

• Give drug with food to minimize adverse GI reactions.
⊛ ALERT: If PR interval or QRS complex increases by more than 25%, notify prescriber because reduction in dose may be needed.
• During use with digoxin, monitor ECG and digoxin level frequently.
Patient teaching
• Tell patient to take drug with food.
• Stress importance of taking drug exactly as ordered.
• Warn patient to avoid hazardous activities if adverse CNS disturbances occur.

☑ Evaluation

• Patient regains adequate cardiac output when arrhythmia is corrected.
• Patient doesn't develop any proarrhythmic events.
• Patient and family state understanding of drug therapy.

propoxyphene hydrochloride (dextropropoxyphene hydrochloride)
(proh-POK-sih-feen high-droh-KLOR-ighd)
Darvon, 642 ♦

propoxyphene napsylate (dextropropoxyphene napsylate)
Darvon-N

Pharmacologic class: opioid
Therapeutic class: analgesic
Pregnancy risk category: C
Controlled substance schedule: IV

Indications and dosages

▶ Mild to moderate pain. *Adults:* 65 mg propoxyphene hydrochloride P.O. q 4 hours p.r.n. Maximum, 390 mg P.O. daily. Or, 100 mg propoxyphene napsylate P.O. q 4 hours p.r.n. Maximum, 600 mg P.O. daily.

Contraindications and cautions

• Contraindicated in patients hypersensitive to the drug or any of its components, and in patients who are suicidal or addiction-prone.
• Use cautiously in patients with hepatic or renal disease, emotional instability, or history of drug or alcohol abuse.
⚶ Lifespan: In pregnant women, use cautiously. In breast-feeding women, use cautiously; it's unknown if the drug appears in breast milk. In children, safety and effectiveness haven't been established.

Adverse reactions

CNS: *dizziness*, headache, *sedation*, euphoria, paradoxical excitement, insomnia.
GI: nausea, vomiting, *constipation*.
Respiratory: respiratory depression.
Other: psychological and physical dependence.

Interactions

Drug-drug. *Barbiturate anesthetics:* May increase respiratory and CNS depression. Use together cautiously.
Carbamazepine: May increase carbamazepine levels. Monitor levels closely.
CNS depressants: May have additive effects. Use together cautiously.

Reactions may be *common*, uncommon, *life-threatening*, or COMMON AND LIFE-THREATENING.

Protease inhibitors: May increase CNS and respiratory depression. Monitor patient.
Warfarin: May increase anticoagulant effect. Monitor PT and INR and patient for bleeding.
Drug-lifestyle. *Alcohol use:* May have additive effects. Discourage using together.

Effects on lab test results

• May increase or decrease liver function test values.
• May cause false decreases in urinary steroid excretion tests.

Pharmacokinetics

Absorption: Absorbed primarily in upper small intestine.
Distribution: Drug enters CSF.
Metabolism: Metabolized in liver; about one-quarter of dose is metabolized to norpropoxyphene, an active metabolite.
Excretion: Excreted in urine. *Half-life:* 6 to 12 hours.

Route	Onset	Peak	Duration
P.O.	¼–1 hr	2–2½ hr	4–6 hr

Action

Chemical effect: Binds with opioid receptors in CNS, altering both perception of and emotional response to pain through unknown mechanism.
Therapeutic effect: Relieves pain.

Available forms

propoxyphene hydrochloride
Capsules: 65 mg
propoxyphene napsylate
Tablets: 50 mg, 100 mg

NURSING PROCESS

Assessment

• Assess patient's pain before and after giving drug.
• Be alert for adverse reactions and drug interactions.
• If adverse GI reaction occurs, monitor patient's hydration.
• Assess patient's and family's knowledge of drug therapy.

Nursing diagnoses

• Acute pain related to underlying condition

• Risk for deficient fluid volume related to GI upset
• Deficient knowledge related to drug therapy

Planning and implementation

• Give with food to minimize adverse GI reactions.
• Consider giving laxative to prevent constipation.
• Drug can be considered a mild opioid analgesic, but pain relief is equivalent to that provided by aspirin. Tolerance and physical dependence have been observed. Typically used with aspirin or acetaminophen to maximize analgesia.
⑤ ALERT: A dose of 65 mg of propoxyphene hydrochloride equals 100 mg of propoxyphene napsylate.
Patient teaching
• Advise patient to take drug with food or milk to minimize GI upset.
• Warn patient not to exceed recommended dosage. Respiratory depression, hypotension, profound sedation, and coma may result if used in excess or with other CNS depressants. Products that contain propoxyphene alone or with other drugs are major cause of drug-related overdose and death.
• Advise patient not to drink alcohol during therapy.
• Warn ambulatory patient about getting out of bed or walking. Warn outpatient to avoid driving and other hazardous activities until drug's CNS effects are known.

Evaluation

• Patient is free from pain.
• Patient maintains adequate hydration.
• Patient and family state understanding of drug therapy.

propranolol hydrochloride
(proh-PRAH-nuh-lohl high-droh-KLOR-ighd)
Apo-Propranolol ♦, Detensol ♦, Inderal, Inderal LA, InnoPran XL, Novopranol ♦, PMS Propranolol ♦

Pharmacologic class: beta blocker
Therapeutic class: antihypertensive, antianginal, antiarrhythmic
Pregnancy risk category: C

Indications and dosages

▶ **Angina pectoris.** *Adults:* Total daily dosages of 80 to 320 mg P.O. when given b.i.d., t.i.d., or q.i.d. Or, one 80-mg extended-release capsule daily. Increase dosage at 7- to 10-day intervals.
▶ **Mortality reduction after MI.** *Adults:* 180 to 240 mg P.O. daily in divided doses beginning 5 to 21 days after MI. Usually given t.i.d. or q.i.d.
▶ **Supraventricular, ventricular, and atrial arrhythmias; tachyarrhythmias caused by excessive catecholamine action during anesthesia.** *Adults:* 0.5 to 3 mg by slow I.V. push, not to exceed 1 mg/minute. After 3 mg have been given, another dose may be given in 2 minutes; subsequent doses, no sooner than q 4 hours. May be diluted and infused slowly. Usual maintenance dosage is 10 to 30 mg P.O. t.i.d. to q.i.d.
Children‡: 0.01 to 0.1 mg/kg I.V. to a maximum of 1 mg/dose by slow infusion over 5 minutes.
▶ **Hypertension.** *Adults:* Initially, 80 mg P.O. daily in two to four divided doses or extended-release form once daily. Increase at 3- to 7-day intervals to maximum daily dosage of 640 mg. Usual maintenance dosage is 120 to 240 mg daily in two or three divided doses or 120 to 160 mg sustained-release once daily. Or, 80 mg InnoPran XL P.O. once daily h.s. Take consistently with or without food. Adjust to maximum of 120 mg daily if needed.
Children‡: 1 mg/kg P.O. daily, up to a maximum daily dose of 16 mg/kg.
▶ **Prevention of frequent, severe, uncontrollable, or disabling migraine or vascular headache.** *Adults:* Initially, 80 mg P.O. daily in divided doses or one extended-release capsule daily. Usual maintenance dosage is 160 to 240 mg daily.
▶ **Essential tremor.** *Adults:* 40 mg (tablets, solution) P.O. b.i.d. Usual maintenance dosage is 120 to 320 mg daily in three divided doses.
▶ **Hypertrophic subaortic stenosis.** *Adults:* 10 to 20 mg P.O. t.i.d. or q.i.d. before meals and at bedtime or 80 to 160 mg extended-release capsule daily.
▶ **Adjunct therapy in pheochromocytoma.** *Adults:* 60 mg P.O. daily in divided doses with alpha blocker 3 days before surgery.
▶ **Adjunctive therapy in anxiety‡.** *Adults:* 10 to 80 mg P.O. 1 hour before anxiety-provoking activity.

▼ I.V. administration

● Drug is compatible with D_5W, half-normal and normal saline solutions, and lactated Ringer's solution.
● Give drug by direct injection into large vessel or I.V. line containing free-flowing, compatible solution; continuous I.V. infusion generally isn't recommended.
● Or dilute drug with normal saline solution and give by intermittent infusion over 10 to 15 minutes in 0.1- to 0.2-mg increments.
⊗ **Incompatibilities**
Amphotericin B, diazoxide.

Contraindications and cautions

● Contraindicated in patients with bronchial asthma, sinus bradycardia, heart block greater than first-degree, cardiogenic shock, or overt cardiac failure (unless failure is secondary to tachyarrhythmia that can be treated with propranolol).
● Use cautiously in patients taking other antihypertensives and in those with renal impairment, nonallergic bronchospastic diseases, Wolff-Parkinson-White syndrome, hepatic disease, diabetes mellitus (drug blocks some symptoms of hypoglycemia), or thyrotoxicosis (drug may mask some signs of that disorder).
⚘ **Lifespan:** In pregnant women, use cautiously. In breast-feeding women, drug isn't recommended. In children, safety and effectiveness haven't been established.

Adverse reactions

CNS: *fatigue, lethargy,* vivid dreams, fever, hallucinations, mental depression, dizziness (InnoPran XL).
CV: *bradycardia,* hypotension, *heart failure,* intermittent claudication.
GI: nausea, vomiting, diarrhea, constipation (InnoPran XL).
Hematologic: *agranulocytosis.*
Musculoskeletal: arthralgia.
Respiratory: increased airway resistance.
Skin: rash.

Interactions

Drug-drug. *Aminophylline, theophylline:* May act antagonistically reducing the effects of one or both drugs. May reduce elimination of theophylline. Monitor theophylline level and patient closely.

Amobarbital, aprobarbital, butabarbital, butalbital, mephobarbital, pentobarbital, phenobarbital, primidone, secobarbital: May reduce the effects of propranolol. Increase beta blocker dose.

Cimetidine: May increase the pharmacologic effects of beta blocker. Consider a different H₂-agonist or decrease the dose of beta blocker.

Digoxin, diltiazem, verapamil: May cause hypotension, bradycardia, and increased depressant effect on myocardium. Use together cautiously.

Epinephrine: May cause an initial hypertensive episode followed by bradycardia. Stop the beta blocker 3 days before anticipated epinephrine use. Monitor patient closely.

Glucagon, isoproterenol: May antagonize propranolol effect. May be used therapeutically and in emergencies.

Hydralazine: May increase levels and pharmacologic effects of both drugs. Monitor patient closely. Dosage adjustment of either drug may be needed.

Insulin: May mask symptoms of hypoglycemia (such as tachycardia) as a result of beta blockade. Use cautiously in patients with diabetes.

Lidocaine I.V.: May reduce hepatic metabolism of lidocaine, increasing the risk of toxicity. Give bolus doses of lidocaine at a slower rate and monitor lidocaine levels closely.

Oral antidiabetics: May alter requirements for these drugs in previously stabilized diabetic patients. Monitor patient for hypoglycemia.

Prazosin: May increase the risk of orthostatic hypotension in the early phases of use together. Assist patient to stand slowly until effects are known.

Verapamil: May increase the effects of both drugs. Monitor cardiac function closely and decrease dosages p.r.n.

Drug-herb. *Ginkgo:* May alter drug level. Discourage use of herb.

Melatonin: May reverse the negative effects of drug on nocturnal sleep. Advise patient to discuss use with prescriber.

Drug-lifestyle. *Cocaine use:* May increase angina-inducing potential of cocaine. Inform patient of this potentially dangerous combination.

Effects on lab test results

• May increase BUN, transaminase, alkaline phosphatase, and LDH levels.
• May decrease granulocyte count.

Pharmacokinetics

Absorption: Almost complete. Absorption is enhanced when given with food. Food increases the lag time and the time to maximum concentration of InnoPran XL.

Distribution: Distributed widely throughout body. Drug is more than 90% protein-bound.

Metabolism: Metabolized almost totally in liver. P.O. form undergoes extensive first-pass metabolism.

Excretion: About 96% to 99% excreted in urine as metabolites; remainder excreted in feces as unchanged drug and metabolites. *Half-life:* About 4 hours; 8 hours for InnoPran XL.

Route	Onset	Peak	Duration
P.O.	30 min	60–90 min	12 hr
P.O. InnoPran XL	Unknown	12–14 hr	24 hr
I.V.	≤ 1 min	≤1 min	< 5 min

Action

Chemical effect: Reduces cardiac oxygen demand by blocking catecholamine-induced increases in heart rate, blood pressure, and force of myocardial contraction. Depresses renin secretion and prevents vasodilation of cerebral arteries.

Therapeutic effect: Relieves anginal and migraine pain, lowers blood pressure, restores normal sinus rhythm, and helps limit MI damage.

Available forms

Capsules (extended-release): 60 mg, 80 mg, 120 mg, 160 mg
Injection: 1 mg/ml
Oral solution: 4 mg/ml, 8 mg/ml, 80 mg/ml (concentrate)
Tablets: 10 mg, 20 mg, 40 mg, 60 mg, 80 mg, 90 mg

NURSING PROCESS

⚕ Assessment

• Assess patient's condition before starting therapy, and regularly thereafter to monitor the drug's effectiveness.
• Frequently monitor blood pressure, ECG, and heart rate and rhythm, especially when giving I.V.
• Be alert for adverse reactions and drug interactions.

- Assess patient's and family's knowledge of drug therapy.

🔁 **Nursing diagnoses**
- Ineffective health maintenance related to underlying condition
- Impaired gas exchange related to airway resistance
- Deficient knowledge related to drug therapy

⊠ **Planning and implementation**
- Check patient's apical pulse before therapy. If extremes in pulse rate occur, don't give the drug and immediately call the prescriber.
- ⊛ **ALERT:** Don't confuse Inderal with Inderide or Isordil.
- Double-check dose and route. I.V. doses are much smaller than oral doses.
- Give oral drug with meals. Food may increase absorption.
- Don't stop giving the drug before surgery for pheochromocytoma. Before any surgical procedure, notify anesthesiologist that patient is taking propranolol.
- If patient develops severe hypotension, notify prescriber; vasopressor may be prescribed.
- In an elderly patient, adverse reactions may increase and he may need an adjusted dose.
- Don't abruptly stop giving the drug.
- For overdose, give I.V. isoproterenol, I.V. atropine, or glucagon; refractory cases may require pacemaker.

Patient teaching
- Teach patient how to check pulse rate, and tell him to do so before each dose. Tell him to notify prescriber if rate changes significantly.
- Tell patient that taking drug twice a day or as extended-release capsule may improve compliance. Advise him to check with prescriber.
- Advise patient to continue taking drug as prescribed, even when he's feeling well. Tell him not to stop drug suddenly because doing so can worsen angina and MI.

✓ **Evaluation**
- Patient responds well to therapy.
- Patient maintains adequate gas exchange.
- Patient and family state understanding of drug therapy.

propylthiouracil (PTU)
(proh-pil-thigh-oh-YOOR-uh-sil)
Propyl-Thyracil ◆

Pharmacologic class: thyroid hormone antagonist
Therapeutic class: antihyperthyroid drug
Pregnancy risk category: D

Indications and dosages

▶ **Hyperthyroidism.** *Adults:* 300 to 450 mg P.O. daily in divided doses. Patients with severe hyperthyroidism or very large goiters may need initial doses of 600 to 1,200 mg daily. Continue until patient is euthyroid; then start maintenance dose of 100 mg to 150 mg P.O. daily.
Children age 10 and older: Initially, 150 to 300 mg P.O. daily in divided doses. Continue until patient is euthyroid. Individualize maintenance dose.
Children ages 6 to 10: Initially, 50 to 150 mg P.O. daily in divided doses q 8 hours. Continue until patient is euthyroid. Individualize maintenance dose.
Neonates and children: 5 to 7 mg/kg P.O. daily in divided doses q 8 hours, or give according to age as above.
▶ **Thyrotoxic crisis.** *Adults and children:* 200 to 400 mg P.O. q 4 to 6 hours on first day; after symptoms are under control, gradually reduce dosage to usual maintenance levels.

Contraindications and cautions

- Contraindicated in patients hypersensitive to the drug or any of its components.
- ⚕ **Lifespan:** In pregnant women, use cautiously. Pregnant women may need a lower dose as pregnancy progresses; monitor thyroid function studies closely. In breast-feeding women, drug is contraindicated.

Adverse reactions

CNS: headache, drowsiness, vertigo.
CV: vasculitis.
EENT: visual disturbances.
GI: diarrhea, *nausea, vomiting* (may be dose-related), salivary gland enlargement, loss of taste.
Hematologic: *agranulocytosis, thrombocytopenia, aplastic anemia, leukopenia,* lymphadenopathy.

Reactions may be *common*, uncommon, *life-threatening*, or COMMON AND LIFE-THREATENING.

Hepatic: jaundice, *hepatotoxicity.*
Metabolic: dose-related hypothyroidism (mental depression; cold intolerance; hard, nonpitting edema).
Musculoskeletal: arthralgia, myalgia.
Skin: rash, urticaria, skin discoloration, pruritus.
Other: drug-induced fever.

Interactions

Drug-drug. *Aminophylline, oxtriphylline, theophylline:* May decrease drug clearance. Dosage may need adjustment.
Anticoagulants: May increase anticoagulant effects. Monitor PT, PTT, and INR and monitor patient for bleeding.
Digoxin: May increase glycoside levels. May need to decrease dose.
Potassium iodide: May decrease response to drug. May need to increase dose of antithyroid drug.

Effects on lab test results

• May increase liver enzyme levels. May decrease hemoglobin level and hematocrit.
• May decrease granulocyte, WBC, and platelet counts.

Pharmacokinetics

Absorption: About 80% of drug is absorbed rapidly and readily from GI tract.
Distribution: Drug appears to be concentrated in thyroid gland. About 75% to 80% of drug is protein-bound.
Metabolism: Metabolized rapidly in the liver.
Excretion: About 35% excreted in urine. *Half-life:* 1 to 2 hours.

Route	Onset	Peak	Duration
P.O.	Unknown	1–1½ hr	Unknown

Action

Chemical effect: Inhibits oxidation of iodine in thyroid gland, blocking iodine's ability to combine with tyrosine to form T_4, and may prevent coupling of monoiodotyrosine and diiodotyrosine to form T_4 and T_3.
Therapeutic effect: Lowers thyroid hormone level.

Available forms

Tablets: 50 mg, 100 mg ◆

NURSING PROCESS

☲ Assessment

• Assess patient's condition before starting therapy, and regularly thereafter to monitor the drug's effectiveness.
• Watch for signs of hypothyroidism (depression; cold intolerance; hard, nonpitting edema); adjust dose as directed.
• Monitor CBC to detect impending leukopenia, thrombocytopenia, and agranulocytosis.
• Be alert for adverse reactions.
• If adverse GI reaction occurs, monitor patient's hydration.
• Assess patient's and family's knowledge of drug therapy.

⊞ Nursing diagnoses

• Ineffective health maintenance related to thyroid condition
• Risk for deficient fluid volume related to adverse GI reaction
• Deficient knowledge related to drug therapy

⊠ Planning and implementation

• Give drug with meals to reduce adverse GI reaction.
• If patient develops severe rash or enlarged cervical lymph nodes, stop giving the drug and notify prescriber.
• Maintenance daily dose is about ⅓ to ⅔ of initial daily dose.
• Store drug in light-resistant container.
⑤ **ALERT:** Don't confuse propylthiouracil with Purinethol.
Patient teaching
• Tell patient to report skin eruptions (sign of hypersensitivity), fever, sore throat, or mouth sores (early signs of agranulocytosis).
• Instruct patient to ask prescriber whether he can use iodized salt and eat shellfish.
• Warn patient against OTC cough medicines because many contain iodine.

☑ Evaluation

• Patient's thyroid hormone level is normal.
• Patient maintains adequate hydration.
• Patient and family state understanding of drug therapy.

P

protamine sulfate
(PROH-tuh-meen SUL-fayt)

Pharmacologic class: antidote
Therapeutic class: heparin antagonist
Pregnancy risk category: C

Indications and dosages

▶ **Heparin overdose.** *Adults:* Dosage based on venous blood coagulation studies, usually 1 mg for each 90 to 115 units of heparin. Give by slow I.V. injection over 10 minutes, not to exceed 50 mg.

I.V. administration

- May be given without further dilution or diluted in D_5W or normal saline solution.
- Give by slow injection over 10 minutes.
- Refrigerate at 36° to 46° F (2° to 8° C).
- Don't store diluted solutions; they contain no preservatives.

⊗ **Incompatibilities**
Cephalosporins, diatrizoate meglumine 52% and diatrizoate sodium 8%, diatrizoate sodium 60%, ioxaglate meglumine 39.3% and ioxaglate sodium 19.6%, penicillins.

Contraindications and cautions

- Contraindicated in patients hypersensitive to the drug or any of its components.
- Use cautiously after cardiac surgery.

Lifespan: In pregnant women, use cautiously. In breast-feeding women, use cautiously; it's unknown if the drug appears in breast milk. In children, safety and effectiveness haven't been established.

Adverse reactions

CV: transitory flushing, drop in blood pressure, ***bradycardia, circulatory collapse.***
Respiratory: dyspnea, ***pulmonary edema, acute pulmonary hypertension.***
Other: feeling of warmth, ***anaphylaxis, anaphylactoid reactions.***

Interactions

None significant.

Effects on lab test results

None reported.

Pharmacokinetics

Absorption: Administered I.V.
Distribution: Unknown.
Metabolism: Unknown, although it appears to be partially degraded, with release of some heparin.
Excretion: Unknown. *Half-life:* Shorter than heparin.

Route	Onset	Peak	Duration
I.V.	30–60 sec	Unknown	2 hr

Action

Chemical effect: Forms inert complex with heparin sodium.
Therapeutic effect: Blocks heparin's effects.

Available forms

Injection: 10 mg/ml

NURSING PROCESS

Assessment

- Assess patient's heparin overdose before therapy.
- Continually monitor patient; frequently check vital signs.
- Watch for spontaneous bleeding (heparin rebound), especially in patients undergoing dialysis and in those who have undergone cardiac surgery. Protamine sulfate may act as anticoagulant in very high doses.
- Assess patient's and family's knowledge of drug therapy.

Nursing diagnoses

- Ineffective protection related to heparin overdose
- Risk for injury related to anaphylaxis
- Deficient knowledge related to drug therapy

Planning and implementation

- Calculate dose carefully. One milligram of drug neutralizes 90 to 115 units of heparin depending on salt (heparin calcium or heparin sodium) and source of heparin (beef or pork).
- Give drug slowly by direct injection. Treat shock.

ALERT: Don't confuse protamine with Protopam.

Patient teaching

- Instruct patient to report adverse reactions immediately.

☑ Evaluation
• Patient doesn't experience injury.
• Patient and family state understanding of drug therapy.

pseudoephedrine hydrochloride
(soo-doh-eh-FED-rin high-droh-KLOR-ighd)
Cenafed, Children's Sudafed Liquid†, Decofed†, DeFed-60†, Dimetapp†, Dorcol Children's Decongestant†, Drixoral Non-Drowsy Formula ♦ †, Eltor 120 ♦ †, Genaphed†, Halofed†, Halofed Adult Strength†, Maxenal ♦ †, Myfedrine†, Novafed†, PediaCare Infants' Oral Decongestant Drops†, Pseudo 60†, Pseudofrin ♦, Pseudogest†, Robidrine ♦ †, Sudafed†, Sudafed 12 Hour†, Sudafed 60†, Sufedrin†, Triaminic†

pseudoephedrine sulfate
Afrin†, Drixoral†, Drixoral 12 Hour Non-Drowsy Formula ♦ †

Pharmacologic class: sympathomimetic
Therapeutic class: decongestant
Pregnancy risk category: C

Indications and dosages
▶ **Nasal and eustachian tube decongestion.**
Adults and children age 12 and older: 60 mg P.O. q 4 to 6 hours; or 120 mg P.O. extended-release tablet q 12 hours; or 240 mg P.O. controlled-release tablet daily. Maximum dosage is 240 mg daily.
Children ages 6 to 11: 30 mg P.O. q 4 to 6 hours. Maximum dosage, 120 mg daily.
Children ages 2 to 5: 15 mg P.O. q 4 to 6 hours. Maximum dosage is 60 mg daily, or 4 mg/kg or 125 mg/m² P.O. divided q.i.d.
Children younger than age 2: Consult a prescriber for specific dosage.

Contraindications and cautions
• Contraindicated in patients taking MAO inhibitors and in patients with severe hypertension or severe coronary artery disease.
• Use cautiously in patients with hypertension, cardiac disease, diabetes, glaucoma, hyperthyroidism, or prostatic hyperplasia.

☀ Lifespan: Use cautiously during pregnancy and breast-feeding. In children younger than age 12, extended-release forms are contraindicated.

Adverse reactions
CNS: *anxiety,* transient stimulation, tremor, dizziness, headache, *insomnia, nervousness.*
CV: *arrhythmias, palpitations,* tachycardia, hypertension.
GI: anorexia, nausea, vomiting, dry mouth.
GU: difficulty urinating.
Respiratory: *respiratory difficulty,* stinging, burning, drying of nasal mucosa, sneezing, excessive nasal discharge with topical drug forms.
Skin: pallor.

Interactions
Drug-drug. *Antihypertensives:* May attenuate hypotensive effect. Monitor blood pressure.
Phenelzine, tranylcypromine: May cause severe headache, hypertension, fever, and hypertensive crisis. Avoid using together.
Drug-herb. *Bitter orange:* May increase risk of hypertension and adverse CV effects. Discourage using together.

Effects on lab test results
None reported.

Pharmacokinetics
Absorption: Unknown.
Distribution: Widely distributed throughout body.
Metabolism: Incompletely metabolized in liver to inactive compounds.
Excretion: Excreted in urine; rate is accelerated with acidic urine. *Half-life:* 3 to 16 hours, depending on urine pH.

Route	Onset	Peak	Duration
P.O.	15–30 min	30–60 min	3–12 hr

Action
Chemical effect: Stimulates alpha-adrenergic receptors in upper respiratory tract, resulting in vasoconstriction.
Therapeutic effect: Relieves congestion of nasal passages and eustachian tube.

Available forms
pseudoephedrine hydrochloride
Capsules†: 60 mg
Capsules (liquid gel)†: 30 mg

Liquid†: 7.5 mg/0.8 ml, 15 mg/5 ml, 30 mg/ 5 ml
Tablets†: 30 mg, 60 mg
Tablets (chewable)†: 15 mg
Tablets (controlled-release)†: 240 mg (60-mg immediate, 180-mg delayed release)
Tablets (extended-release)†: 120 mg
pseudoephedrine sulfate
Tablets (extended-release)†: 120 mg (60-mg immediate, 60-mg delayed release)

NURSING PROCESS

⚗ Assessment
• Assess patient's condition before starting therapy, and regularly thereafter to monitor the drug's effectiveness.
• Be alert for adverse reactions and drug interactions.
• Elderly patients are more sensitive to drug's effects.
• Some OTC topical preparations contain sulfites. Determine patient allergy to sulfites before therapy.
• Assess patient's and family's knowledge of drug therapy.

⊕ Nursing diagnoses
• Ineffective health maintenance related to congestion
• Disturbed sleep pattern related to drug-induced insomnia
• Deficient knowledge related to drug therapy

⨺ Planning and implementation
• Don't crush or break extended-release forms.
• Give last dose at least 2 hours before bedtime to minimize insomnia.
Patient teaching
• Teach patient to read OTC drug labels so he can avoid using products containing other sympathomimetics or sulfites (if allergic).
• Tell patient not to take immediate-release drug within 2 hours of bedtime because it can cause insomnia.
• Tell patient to relieve dry mouth with sugarless gum or hard candy.
• Instruct patient to stop drug if he becomes unusually restless and to notify prescriber promptly.
• Inform patient about risk of overuse of nasal sprays and consequent rebound congestion. Warn against exceeding recommended dosage

and use longer than 3 days unless instructed to do so by a physician.
• Instruct patient to stop drug and call prescriber if no improvement with oral dosage within 7 days.
• Inform patient of risks of overdosage if he exceeds recommended daily dosing.
• Teach patient proper administration of sprays, drops and inhalers, as needed.

☑ Evaluation
• Patient's congestion is relieved.
• Patient has no insomnia.
• Patient and family state understanding of drug therapy.

pyridostigmine bromide
(peer-ih-doh-STIG-meen BROH-mighd)
Mestinon*, Mestinon SR ♦ , Mestinon Timespans, Regonol

Pharmacologic class: cholinesterase inhibitor
Therapeutic class: muscle stimulant
Pregnancy risk category: NR

Indications and dosages
▶ **Antidote for nondepolarizing neuromuscular blockers.** *Adults:* 10 to 20 mg I.V. preceded by atropine sulfate 0.6 to 1.2 mg I.V.
▶ **Myasthenia gravis.** *Adults:* 60 to 120 mg P.O. t.i.d. Usual dosage is 600 mg daily, but a higher dosage may be needed (up to 1,500 mg daily). For I.M. or I.V. use, give ⅟₃₀ of oral dosage. Adjust dosage for each patient, depending on response and tolerance. Or, 180 to 540 mg sustained-release tablets (1 to 3 tablets) P.O. daily to b.i.d., with at least 6 hours between doses. *Children:* 7 mg/kg or 200 mg/m^2 P.O. daily in five or six divided doses. Or, 0.05 to 0.15 mg/ kg/dose I.V. or I.M.
▶ **To increase survival after exposure to the nerve agent Soman.** *Adults in the military:* 30 mg P.O. q 8 hours starting about 8 hours before Soman exposure.

▽ I.V. administration
• Give I.V. injection no faster than 1 mg/minute. If administration is too rapid, bradycardia and seizures may result.
⊗ **Incompatibilities**
Alkaline solutions.

Reactions may be *common,* uncommon, *life-threatening,* or COMMON AND LIFE-THREATENING.

Contraindications and cautions

• Contraindicated in patients hypersensitive to anticholinesterases, in those with mechanical obstruction of the intestine or urinary tract, and in those with history of a reaction to bromides.
• Use cautiously in patients with bronchial asthma, bradycardia, or arrhythmias.
⚜ **Lifespan:** In pregnant and breast-feeding women, safety and effectiveness haven't been established. In neonates, Regonol is contraindicated because it contains benzyl alcohol.

Adverse reactions

CNS: headache with large doses, weakness, sweating, *seizures.*
CV: *bradycardia,* hypotension, thrombophlebitis.
EENT: miosis.
GI: abdominal cramps, nausea, vomiting, diarrhea, excessive salivation.
Musculoskeletal: muscle cramps, muscle fasciculations.
Respiratory: *bronchospasm, bronchoconstriction,* increased bronchial secretions.
Skin: rash.

Interactions

Drug-drug. *Aminoglycosides:* May increase response to drug. Use together cautiously.
Anesthetics, anticholinergics, atropine, corticosteroids, magnesium, procainamide, quinidine: May antagonize cholinergic effects. Observe patient for lack of drug effect.
Ganglionic blockers: May increase risk of hypotension. Monitor patient closely.

Effects on lab test results

None reported.

Pharmacokinetics

Absorption: Poor.
Distribution: Unknown.
Metabolism: Unknown.
Excretion: Excreted in urine. *Half-life:* 1 to 3 hours, depending on route.

Route	Onset	Peak	Duration
P.O.	20–60 min	1–2 hr	3–12 hr
I.V.	2–5 min	Unknown	2–3 hr
I.M.	15 min	Unknown	2–3 hr

Action

Chemical effect: Inhibits destruction of acetylcholine released from parasympathetic and somatic efferent nerves. This allows acetylcholine to accumulate.
Therapeutic effect: Reverses effect of nondepolarizing neuromuscular blockers and myasthenia gravis.

Available forms

Injection: 5 mg/ml in 2-ml ampules or 5-ml vials
Syrup: 60 mg/5 ml
Tablets: 60 mg
Tablets (military use only): 30 mg
Tablets (sustained-release): 180 mg

NURSING PROCESS

⚗ Assessment

• Assess patient's condition before starting therapy, and regularly thereafter to monitor the drug's effectiveness.
• Monitor and document patient's response after each dose; optimum dosage is difficult to judge.
• Monitor patient's vital signs, especially respirations.
• Be alert for adverse reactions and drug interactions.
• Assess patient's and family's knowledge of drug therapy.

⊕ Nursing diagnoses

• Impaired physical mobility related to underlying condition
• Ineffective breathing pattern related to adverse respiratory reactions
• Deficient knowledge related to drug therapy

▶ Planning and implementation

• Stop all other cholinergics before giving drug.
• Don't crush extended-release tablets.
• When using sweet syrup for patient who has difficulty swallowing, pour over ice chips if he can't tolerate flavor.
• Position patient to ease breathing. Have atropine injection readily available, and provide respiratory support as needed.
• If patient's muscle weakness is severe, prescriber will determine if it's caused by drug-induced toxicity or worsening of myasthenia gravis. Test dose of edrophonium I.V. will ag-

P

gravate drug-induced weakness but will temporarily relieve weakness caused by disease.

• The U.S. formulation of Regonol contains benzyl alcohol preservative, which may cause toxicity in neonates if given in large doses. The Canadian formulation of this drug doesn't contain benzyl ethanol.

• If appropriate, obtain prescriber's order for hospitalized patient to have bedside supply of tablets. Patients with long-standing disease often insist on self-administration.

⊛ **ALERT:** If drug is taken immediately before or during Soman exposure, drug may be ineffective against Soman, and may worsen the effects of Soman.

⊛ **ALERT:** Don't confuse Mestinon with Mesantoin or Metatensin.

Patient teaching

• When giving drug for myasthenia gravis, stress the importance of taking it exactly as ordered, on time, in evenly spaced doses. If prescriber has ordered extended-release tablets, tell patient to take tablets at same time each day, at least 6 hours apart. Tell him that he may have to take drug for life.

• Advise patient to wear or carry medical identification at all times.

☑ Evaluation

• Patient has improved physical mobility.
• Patient maintains adequate respiratory pattern.
• Patient and family state understanding of drug therapy.

pyridoxine hydrochloride (vitamin B₆)

(peer-ih-DOKS-een high-droh-KLOR-ighd)
Aminoxin, Beesix, Nestrex†, Rodex

Pharmacologic class: water-soluble vitamin
Therapeutic class: nutritional supplement
Pregnancy risk category: A

Indications and dosages

▶ **RDA.** *Men age 15 and older:* 2 mg.
Men ages 11 to 14: 1.7 mg.
Women age 19 and older: 1.6 mg.
Women ages 15 to 18: 1.5 mg.
Women ages 11 to 14: 1.4 mg.
Pregnant women: 2.2 mg.

Breast-feeding women: 2.1 mg.
Children ages 7 to 10: 1.4 mg.
Children ages 4 to 6: 1.1 mg.
Children ages 1 to 3: 1 mg.
Infants ages 6 months to 1 year: 0.6 mg.
Neonates and infants up to age 6 months: 0.3 mg.

▶ **Dietary vitamin B₆ deficiency.** *Adults:* 2.5 to 10 mg P.O. daily for 3 weeks; then 2 to 5 mg daily as supplement to proper diet.

▶ **Seizures related to vitamin B₆ deficiency or dependency.** *Adults and children:* 10 to 100 mg I.M. or I.V. in single dose.

▶ **Vitamin B₆-responsive anemias or dependency syndrome (inborn errors of metabolism).** *Adults:* up to 600 mg I.M., P.O., or I.V. daily until symptoms subside; then 30 mg daily for life.

▶ **Prevention of vitamin B₆ deficiency during drug therapy.** *Adults:* 6 to 100 mg P.O. daily for isoniazid therapy.

▶ **Drug-induced vitamin B₆ deficiency.** *Adults:* 100 to 200 mg P.O. daily for 3 weeks, followed by 25 to 100 mg P.O. daily to prevent relapse.

▶ **Antidote for isoniazid poisoning.** *Adults:* 1 to 4 g I.V., followed by 1 g I.M. q 30 minutes until amount of pyridoxine given equals amount of isoniazid ingested.

▶ **Premenstrual syndrome‡.** *Adults:* 40 to 500 mg P.O., I.M., or I.V. daily.

▶ **Carpal tunnel syndrome‡.** *Adults:* 100 to 200 mg P.O. daily for 12 weeks or longer.

▶ **Hyperoxaluria type I‡.** *Adults:* 25 to 300 mg P.O. daily.

▼ I.V. administration

• Protect drug from light. Don't use solution if it contains precipitate, although slight darkening is acceptable.

• Inject undiluted drug into I.V. line containing free-flowing compatible solution. Or, infuse diluted drug over prescribed duration for intermittent infusions. Don't use for continuous infusion.

⊗ **Incompatibilities**
Alkaline solutions, erythromycin estolate, iron salts, kanamycin, oxidizers, riboflavin phosphate sodium, streptomycin.

Contraindications and cautions

• Contraindicated in patients hypersensitive to the drug or any of its components, and in patients with heart disease.

⚖ **Lifespan:** No considerations reported.

Adverse reactions

CNS: drowsiness, paresthesia, unstable gait.

Interactions

Drug-drug. *Levodopa:* May decrease the effectiveness of levodopa. Avoid using pyridoxine with levodopa. Pyridoxine has little to no effect on the combination drug levodopa and carbidopa.
Phenobarbital, phenytoin: May decrease anticonvulsant level, increasing risk of seizures. Monitor level closely; institute seizure precautions.
Drug-lifestyle. *Alcohol use:* May increase risk of delirium and lactic acidosis. Discourage using together.

Effects on lab test results

• May increase AST level. May decrease folic acid level.

Pharmacokinetics

Absorption: Drug and its substituents are absorbed readily from GI tract. May be diminished in patients with malabsorption syndromes or following gastric resection.
Distribution: Drug is stored mainly in liver.
Metabolism: Metabolized in liver.
Excretion: In erythrocytes, pyridoxine is converted to pyridoxal phosphate and pyridoxamine is converted to pyridoxamine phosphate. The phosphorylated form of pyridoxine is transaminated to pyridoxal and pyridoxamine, which is phosphorylated rapidly. Conversion of pyridoxine phosphate to pyridoxal phosphate requires riboflavin. *Half-life:* 15 to 20 days.

Route	Onset	Peak	Duration
P.O., I.V., I.M.	Unknown	Unknown	Unknown

Action

Chemical effect: Vitamin B_6 stimulates various metabolic functions, including amino acid metabolism.
Therapeutic effect: Raises pyridoxine levels, prevents and relieves seizure activity related to pyridoxine deficiency or dependency, and blocks effects of isoniazid poisoning.

Available forms

Injection: 100 mg/ml

Tablets: 10 mg†, 25 mg†, 50 mg†, 100 mg†, 200 mg†, 250 mg†, 500 mg†
Tablets (enteric-coated): 20 mg†
Tablets (extended-release): 200 mg

NURSING PROCESS

⚖ Assessment
• Assess patient before starting therapy, and regularly thereafter to monitor the drug's effectiveness.
• Be alert for adverse CNS reactions and drug interactions. Patient taking high dose (2 to 6 g daily) may have difficulty walking because of reduced proprioceptive and sensory function.
• Monitor patient's diet. Excessive protein intake increases daily drug requirements.
• Assess patient's and family's knowledge of drug therapy.

⊞ Nursing diagnoses
• Ineffective health maintenance related to underlying condition
• Risk for injury related to drug-induced adverse CNS reactions
• Deficient knowledge related to drug therapy

▷ Planning and implementation
• When using drug to treat isoniazid toxicity, give anticonvulsants.
• If sodium bicarbonate is required to control acidosis in isoniazid toxicity, don't mix in same syringe with pyridoxine.
⊛ ALERT: Don't confuse pyridoxine with pralidoxime, pyrimethamine, or Pyridium.
Patient teaching
• Advise patient taking levodopa alone to avoid multivitamins containing pyridoxine because of decreased levodopa effect.
• If prescribed for maintenance therapy to prevent recurrence of deficiency, stress importance of compliance and good nutrition. Explain that pyridoxine with isoniazid has specific therapeutic purpose and isn't just a vitamin.

☑ Evaluation
• Patient responds well to therapy.
• Patient doesn't experience injury from adverse CNS reactions.
• Patient and family state understanding of drug therapy.

P

pyrimethamine
(peer-ih-METH-uh-meen)
Daraprim

pyrimethamine with sulfadoxine
Fansidar

Pharmacologic class: folic acid antagonist
Therapeutic class: antimalarial
Pregnancy risk category: C

Indications and dosages

▶ **Malaria prophylaxis and transmission control.** *Adults and children older than age 10:* 25 mg pyrimethamine P.O. weekly.
Children ages 4 to 10: 12.5 mg pyrimethamine P.O. weekly.
Children younger than age 4: 6.25 mg pyrimethamine P.O. weekly.
Continued in all age groups at least 10 weeks after leaving endemic area.
▶ **Acute attacks of malaria.** *Adults and children older than age 10:* 25 mg pyrimethamine P.O. daily for 2 days when used with faster-acting antimalarials; when used alone, 50 mg P.O. daily for 2 days.
Children ages 4 to 10: 25 mg pyrimethamine P.O. daily for 2 days.
▶ **Acute attacks of malaria.** *Adults:* 2 to 3 tablets pyrimethamine with sulfadoxine as single dose, either alone or in sequence with quinine.
Children ages 9 to 14: 2 tablets pyrimethamine with sulfadoxine.
Children ages 4 to 8: 1 tablet pyrimethamine with sulfadoxine.
Children younger than age 4: ½ tablet pyrimethamine with sulfadoxine.
▶ **Malaria prophylaxis.** *Adults:* 1 tablet pyrimethamine with sulfadoxine weekly, or 2 tablets q 2 weeks.
Children ages 9 to 14: ¾ tablet pyrimethamine with sulfadoxine weekly, or 1½ tablets q 2 weeks.
Children ages 4 to 8: ½ tablet pyrimethamine with sulfadoxine weekly, or 1 tablet q 2 weeks.
Children younger than age 4: ¼ tablet pyrimethamine with sulfadoxine weekly, or ½ tablet q 2 weeks.
▶ **Toxoplasmosis.** *Adults:* Initially, 50 to 75 mg pyrimethamine P.O. daily for 1 to 3 weeks; then 25 mg P.O. daily for 4 to 5 weeks along with 1 g sulfadiazine P.O. q 6 hours.

Children: Initially, 1 mg/kg pyrimethamine P.O. daily (not to exceed 100 mg) in two equally divided doses for 2 to 4 days; then 0.5 mg/kg daily for 4 weeks along with 100 mg sulfadiazine/kg P.O. daily, divided q 6 hours.
▶ **Isosporiasis‡.** *Adults:* 50 to 75 mg pyrimethamine P.O. daily.

Contraindications and cautions

• Contraindicated in patients hypersensitive to the drug or any of its components, and in those with megaloblastic anemia caused by folic acid deficiency. Pyrimethamine with sulfadoxine is contraindicated in patients with porphyria because it contains sulfadoxine, a sulfonamide.
• Repeated use of pyrimethamine with sulfadoxine is contraindicated in patients hypersensitive to pyrimethamine or sulfonamides, and in patients with severe renal insufficiency, marked liver parenchymal damage or blood dyscrasias, or megaloblastic anemia caused by folate deficiency.
• Use cautiously in patients with impaired hepatic or renal function, severe allergy or bronchial asthma, or G6PD deficiency; in those with seizure disorders (smaller doses may be needed); and in those treated with chloroquine.
⚇ **Lifespan:** In pregnant women at term, infants younger than age 2 months, and breast-feeding women, repeated use of pyrimethamine with sulfadoxine is contraindicated.

Adverse reactions

CNS: stimulation, *seizures.*
GI: anorexia, vomiting, diarrhea, atrophic glossitis.
Hematologic: *agranulocytosis, aplastic anemia,* megaloblastic anemia, *bone marrow suppression, leukopenia, thrombocytopenia, pancytopenia.*
Skin: rash, *erythema multiforme, Stevens-Johnson syndrome, toxic epidermal necrolysis.*

Interactions

Drug-drug. *Co-trimoxazole, methotrexate, sulfonamides:* May increase risk of bone marrow suppression. Don't use together.
Folic acid, PABA: May decrease antitoxoplasmic effects. May require dosage adjustment.
Lorazepam: May cause mild hepatotoxicity. Monitor liver enzymes.

Effects on lab test results

• May decrease hemoglobin level and hematocrit.

• May decrease granulocyte, WBC, platelet, and RBC counts.

Pharmacokinetics

Absorption: Well absorbed from intestinal tract.
Distribution: Distributed to kidneys, liver, spleen, and lungs. About 80% bound to proteins.
Metabolism: Metabolized to several unidentified compounds.
Excretion: Excreted in urine. *Half-life:* 4 days.

Route	Onset	Peak	Duration
P.O.	Unknown	1½–8 hr	Unknown

Action

Chemical effect: Inhibits enzyme dihydrofolate reductase, impeding reduction of this enzyme to tetrahydrofolic acid. Sulfadoxine competitively inhibits use of PABA.
Therapeutic effect: Prevents malaria and treats malaria and toxoplasmosis infections. Spectrum of activity includes asexual erythrocytic forms of susceptible plasmodia and *Toxoplasma gondii.*

Available forms

pyrimethamine
Tablets: 25 mg
pyrimethamine with sulfadoxine
Tablets: pyrimethamine 25 mg, sulfadoxine 500 mg

NURSING PROCESS

Assessment
• Assess patient's condition before starting therapy, and regularly thereafter to monitor the drug's effectiveness.
• Obtain twice-weekly blood counts, including platelets, for patients with toxoplasmosis because dosages used approach toxic levels.
• Be alert for adverse reactions and drug interactions.
• Assess patient's and family's knowledge of drug therapy.

Nursing diagnoses
• Infection related to presence of susceptible organism
• Ineffective protection related to adverse hematologic reactions
• Deficient knowledge related to drug therapy

Planning and implementation
• Give drug with meals to minimize GI distress.
• If signs of folic acid or folinic acid deficiency develop, reduce dosage or stop drug while patient receives parenteral folinic acid (leucovorin) until blood counts become normal.
• For toxoplasmosis, patients with AIDS may need lifelong drug therapy and suppressive therapy.
• Leucovorin should be administered concomitantly when drug is used for the treatment of toxoplasmosis.
⊗ **ALERT:** Because of possibly severe skin reactions, use pyrimethamine with sulfadoxine only in regions where chloroquine-resistant malaria is prevalent and only when traveler plans to stay in region longer than 3 weeks.
Patient teaching
• Advise patient to take drug with food.
• Teach patient to watch for and immediately report signs of folic or folinic acid deficiency and acute toxicity.
• Warn patient taking pyrimethamine with sulfadoxine to stop drug and notify prescriber at first sign of rash.
• Instruct patient to take first prophylactic dose of pyrimethamine with sulfadoxine 1 to 2 days before traveling to endemic area.

Evaluation
• Patient is free from infection.
• Patient maintains normal hematologic parameters.
• Patient and family state understanding of drug therapy.

quetiapine fumarate
(KWET-ee-uh-peen FYOO-muh-rayt)
Seroquel

Pharmacologic class: dibenzothiazepine derivative
Therapeutic class: antipsychotic
Pregnancy risk category: C

Indications and dosages

▶ **Schizophrenia.** *Adults:* Initially, 25 mg P.O. b.i.d.; increase in increments of 25 to 50 mg b.i.d. or t.i.d. on days 2 and 3, as tolerated. Target dosage range is 300 to 400 mg daily, divided into two or three daily doses by day 4. Make further dosage adjustments at intervals of not less than 2 days. Dosages can be increased or decreased by 25 to 50 mg b.i.d. based on response. Safety of doses above 800 mg daily hasn't been evaluated.

▶ **Monotherapy and adjunct therapy with lithium or divalproex for the short-term treatment of acute manic episodes associated with bipolar I disorder.** *Adults:* Initially, 50 mg P.O. b.i.d. Increase dosage in increments of 100 mg/day in 2 divided doses, to 200 mg P.O. b.i.d. on day 4. May increase dosage in increments not greater than 200 mg/day, up to 800 mg/day by day 6. Usual dose, 400 to 800 mg daily.

🆂 **Adjust-a-dose:** For patients with hepatic impairment, initially give 25 mg P.O. daily. Increase in increments of 25 to 50 mg daily to an effective dose, depending on the patient's response and tolerance.

Contraindications and cautions

• Contraindicated in patients hypersensitive to the drug or any of its ingredients.

• Use cautiously in patients with CV or cerebrovascular disease or conditions that predispose them to hypotension; in those with history of seizures or conditions that lower seizure threshold; in those at risk for aspiration pneumonia; and in those who could experience conditions in which core body temperature may be elevated. Also use cautiously in patients who are debilitated.

⚕ **Lifespan:** In pregnant women, use only if benefits outweigh potential risks to the fetus. In breast-feeding women, stop breast-feeding or use a different drug. In children, safety and effectiveness haven't been established. In the elderly, use cautiously and at a lower dose.

Adverse reactions

CNS: fever, asthenia, *dizziness, headache, seizures, somnolence,* hypertonia, dysarthria, *neuroleptic malignant syndrome,* tardive dyskinesia, extrapyramidal symptoms.
CV: orthostatic hypotension, tachycardia, palpitations, peripheral edema.

EENT: pharyngitis, rhinitis, ear pain, cataracts, sinusitis, nasal congestion.
GI: dry mouth, dyspepsia, abdominal pain, constipation, anorexia.
GU: urine retention.
Hematologic: *leukopenia.*
Metabolic: *weight gain,* hypothyroidism, *hyperglycemia.*
Musculoskeletal: back pain.
Respiratory: increased cough, dyspnea.
Skin: rash, sweating.
Other: flulike syndrome.

Interactions

Drug-drug. *Antihypertensives:* May increase drug effects. Monitor blood pressure.
Carbamazepine, glucocorticoids, phenobarbital, phenytoin, rifampin, thioridazine: May increase quetiapine clearance. Increase quetiapine dose, p.r.n.
Cimetidine, erythromycin, fluconazole, itraconazole, ketoconazole: May decrease quetiapine clearance. Use together cautiously.
CNS depressants: May increase CNS effects. Use together cautiously.
Dopamine agonists, levodopa: May antagonize effects of these drugs. Monitor patient for effects.
Lorazepam: May reduce lorazepam clearance. Monitor patient.
Drug-lifestyle. *Alcohol use:* May increase CNS effects. Discourage use together.

Effects on lab test results

• May increase glucose, liver enzyme, cholesterol, and triglyceride levels.
• May decrease T_4 and thyroid-stimulating hormone levels.
• May decrease WBC count.

Pharmacokinetics

Absorption: Rapid; 100% bioavailability.
Distribution: Wide; 83% bound to protein.
Metabolism: Extensive.
Excretion: About 73% in urine, 20% in feces.
Half-life: 6 hours.

Route	Onset	Peak	Duration
P.O.	Unknown	1½ hr	Unknown

Action

Chemical effect: May block dopamine D_2 receptors and serotonin $5\text{-}HT_2$ receptors in the

---

Reactions may be *common*, uncommon, *life-threatening*, or COMMON AND LIFE-THREATENING.

brain. It also may act at histamine H_1 receptors and alpha$_1$-adrenergic receptors.
Therapeutic effect: Reduces symptoms of psychotic disorders.

Available forms

Tablets: 25 mg, 100 mg, 200 mg, 300 mg

NURSING PROCESS

Assessment
• Monitor patient for tardive dyskinesia. Condition may not appear until months or years after starting drug and may disappear spontaneously or persist for life, despite stopping the drug.
• Monitor patient's vital signs carefully, especially during the 3- to 5-day period of initial use and when restarting or increasing the dose.
• Assess patient's risk of physical injury from adverse CNS effects.
• Be alert for adverse reactions and drug interactions.
• Assess patient's and family's knowledge of drug therapy.

Nursing diagnoses
• Risk for imbalanced body temperature related to drug-induced hyperpyrexia
• Impaired physical mobility related to drug-induced adverse CNS effects
• Deficient knowledge related to drug therapy

Planning and implementation
• An elderly or debilitated patient or patient with hepatic impairment or tendency for hypotensive reactions usually requires a lower initial dose and more gradual dose adjustment.
• Effectiveness for more than 3 weeks hasn't been thoroughly studied. Periodically reevaluate the long-term usefulness of drug.
• **ALERT:** If symptoms of neuroleptic malignant syndrome (hyperpyrexia, muscle rigidity, altered mental status, or autonomic instability) occur, stop the drug and notify prescriber.
• Provide ice chips, drinks, or sugarless hard candy to help relieve dry mouth.
• **ALERT:** Drug may cause hyperglycemia. Monitor patient with diabetes regularly. For patients with risk factors for diabetes, test fasting glucose level at baseline and periodically during therapy. Monitor all patients for symptoms of hyperglycemia, including excessive hunger or thirst, frequent urinating, and weakness; if

symptoms develop, test fasting glucose level. Hyperglycemia may reverse once drug is stopped.

Patient teaching
• Warn patient about risk of orthostatic hypotension, especially during initial use or after a dose increase.
• Tell patient to avoid becoming overheated or dehydrated during therapy.
• Advise patient to avoid activities that require mental alertness until the drug's CNS effects are known.
• Remind patient to have eye examination before starting drug therapy and every 6 months during therapy to check for cataract formation.
• Tell patient to notify prescriber of other prescription or OTC drugs he is taking or plans to take.
• Tell woman to notify prescriber if she becomes pregnant or intends to become pregnant during therapy. Advise her not to breast-feed during therapy.
• Advise patient not to drink alcohol during therapy.
• Tell patient that drug may be taken with or without food.

Evaluation
• Patient maintains normal body temperature.
• Patient maintains physical mobility and doesn't experience extrapyramidal effects of drug.
• Patient and family state understanding of drug therapy.

quinapril hydrochloride
(KWIN-eh-pril high-droh-KLOR-ighd)
Accupril◊, Asig ◊

Pharmacologic class: ACE inhibitor
Therapeutic class: antihypertensive
Pregnancy risk category: C (D in second and third trimesters)

Indications and dosages
▶ **Hypertension.** *Adults younger than age 65:* Initially, 10 to 20 mg P.O. daily. Adjust dosage based on patient response at intervals of about 2 weeks. Most patients are controlled at 20, 40, or 80 mg daily as a single dose or in two divided doses.

Adults age 65 and older: Initially 10 mg P.O. once daily. Adjust dose based on patient's response and tolerance.

⊠ **Adjust-a-dose:** For patients with renal impairment, if creatinine clearance exceeds 60 ml/minute, maximum initial dose is 10 mg P.O.; if clearance is 30 to 60 ml/minute, 5 mg; and if clearance is 10 to 30 ml/minute, 2.5 mg. No dose recommendations are available for creatinine clearance less than 10 ml/minute.

▶ **Heart failure.** *Adults:* Initially, 5 mg P.O. b.i.d. if patient is taking a diuretic and 10 mg P.O. b.i.d. if patient isn't taking a diuretic. Increase dosage at weekly intervals. Usual effective dosage is 20 to 40 mg daily in equally divided doses.

⊠ **Adjust-a-dose:** For patients with renal impairment, if creatinine clearance exceeds 30 ml/minute, the recommended initial dose is 5 mg P.O.; if clearance is 10 to 30 ml/minute, 2.5 mg. No dose recommendations are available for creatinine clearance less than 10 ml/minute.

Contraindications and cautions

• Contraindicated in patients hypersensitive to ACE inhibitors, in those with a history of angioedema during previous ACE inhibitor therapy, and in those with renal artery stenosis.
• Use cautiously in patients with impaired kidney function and increased potassium levels.
※ **Lifespan:** In pregnant women in the second or third trimester, drug isn't recommended. In breast-feeding women, use cautiously; it's unknown if the drug appears in breast milk. In children, safety and effectiveness haven't been established.

Adverse reactions

CNS: somnolence, vertigo, light-headedness, syncope, malaise, nervousness, depression.
CV: palpitations, vasodilation, tachycardia, *hypertensive crisis,* angina, orthostatic hypotension, *arrhythmias.*
EENT: dry throat.
GI: dry mouth, abdominal pain, constipation, *GI hemorrhage.*
Metabolic: hyperkalemia.
Musculoskeletal: back pain.
Respiratory: dry, persistent, tickling, nonproductive cough.
Skin: pruritus, exfoliative dermatitis, *photosensitivity reaction,* diaphoresis.
Other: *angioedema.*

Interactions

Drug-drug. *Digoxin:* May increase digoxin level. Monitor level.
Diuretics, other antihypertensives: May increase the risk of excessive hypotension. Expect to stop diuretic or lower dosage.
Lithium: May increase lithium levels and lithium toxicity. Avoid using together.
Potassium-sparing diuretics: May increase risk of hyperkalemia. Monitor patient, ECG, and potassium levels closely.
Drug-herb. *Licorice:* May cause sodium retention and increase blood pressure, interfering with the therapeutic effects of ACE inhibitors. Discourage using together.
Drug-food. *High-fat foods:* May impair absorption. Discourage using together.
Sodium substitutes containing potassium: May increase risk of hyperkalemia. Discourage using together; monitor patient closely.

Effects on lab test results

• May increase potassium level.
• May decrease liver function test values.

Pharmacokinetics

Absorption: At least 60%; rate and extent drop by 25% to 30% when given with high-fat meal.
Distribution: About 97% of drug and active metabolite are bound to proteins.
Metabolism: 38% of dose de-esterified in liver to active metabolite.
Excretion: Primarily in urine. *Elimination half-life:* 2 hours; *terminal half-life:* 25 hours.

Route	Onset	Peak	Duration
P.O.	≤ 1 hr	2–4 hr	24 hr

Action

Chemical effect: Inhibits conversion of angiotensin I to angiotensin II, which lowers peripheral arterial resistance and decreases aldosterone secretion.
Therapeutic effect: Lowers blood pressure.

Available forms

Tablets: 5 mg, 10 mg, 20 mg, 40 mg

NURSING PROCESS

☞ **Assessment**
• Assess patient's blood pressure before therapy and regularly thereafter. Take blood pressure

---

just before giving a dose and then again 2 to 6 hours after dose to make sure blood pressure is controlled.
• Assess kidney and liver function before starting therapy and regularly thereafter.
• Monitor potassium levels.
• Other ACE inhibitors have been linked to agranulocytosis and neutropenia. Monitor CBC with differential before therapy, q 2 weeks for first 3 months of therapy, and periodically thereafter.
• Be alert for adverse reactions and drug interactions.
• Assess patient's and family's knowledge of drug therapy.

🕮 **Nursing diagnoses**
• Risk for injury related to presence of hypertension
• Disturbed sleep pattern related to drug-induced cough
• Deficient knowledge related to drug therapy

▷ **Planning and implementation**
• If patient has renal impairment, give a lower dose.
• Give drug on empty stomach. High-fat meals can impair absorption.
Patient teaching
• Advise patient to report signs of infection, such as fever and sore throat.
• Tell patient to immediately report signs of angioedema (breathing difficulty and swelling of face, eyes, lips, or tongue), especially after first dose.
• Warn patient that light-headedness can occur, especially at start of drug therapy. Tell him to rise slowly and to stop taking the drug and notify prescriber if he experiences blackouts.
• Inadequate fluid intake, vomiting, diarrhea, and excessive perspiration can lead to light-headedness and syncope. Tell patient to maintain adequate hydration/fluid intake and to use caution in hot weather and during exercise.
• Warn patient not to take potassium supplements or use sodium substitutes that contain potassium during therapy.
• Tell women to notify prescriber about suspected or confirmed pregnancy. Drug will need to be stopped.

🗹 **Evaluation**
• Patient's blood pressure is normal.

• Patient's sleep patterns are undisturbed throughout therapy.
• Patient and family state understanding of drug therapy.

quinidine bisulfate
(KWIN-eh-deen bigh-SUL-fayt)
(66.4% quinidine base)
Biquin Durules ◆ , Kinidin Durules ◇

quinidine gluconate
(62% quinidine base)
Quinaglute Dura-Tabs, Quinalan, Quinate ◆

quinidine sulfate
(83% quinidine base)
Apo-Quinidine ◆ , Cin-Quin, Quinidex Extentabs ◆ , Quinora

Pharmacologic class: cinchona alkaloid
Therapeutic class: antiarrhythmic, antimalarial
Pregnancy risk category: C

Indications and dosages
▶ **Atrial flutter or fibrillation.** *Adults:* 200 mg quinidine sulfate or equivalent base P.O. q 2 to 3 hours for five to eight doses, with subsequent daily increases until sinus rhythm is restored or toxic effects develop. Drug is given only after digitalization to avoid increasing AV conduction. Maximum dosage, 3 to 4 g daily. Or 300 mg Quinidex Extentabs P.O. (extended-release) q 8 to 12 hours.
▶ **Paroxysmal supraventricular tachycardia.** *Adults:* 400 to 600 mg quinidine sulfate P.O. q 2 to 3 hours until toxic adverse reactions develop or arrhythmia subsides.
▶ **Premature atrial and ventricular contractions; paroxysmal AV junctional rhythm; paroxysmal atrial tachycardia; paroxysmal ventricular tachycardia; maintenance after cardioversion of atrial fibrillation or flutter.** *Adults:* Test dose: 200 mg quinidine sulfate or equivalent base P.O., then 200 to 300 mg P.O. q 4 to 6 hours. Or give a test dose of 200 mg quinidine gluconate I.M., then give initial dose of 600 mg I.M., followed by 400 mg I.M. q 2 hours, p.r.n. Adjust each dose by the effect of the previous. Or 300 to 600 mg quinidine sulfate or gluconate sustained-release tablets P.O. q 8 or 12 hours. Or, 800 mg quinidine gluconate

I.V. diluted in 40 ml of D_5W and infused at 1 ml/minute.
Children: Test dose is 2 mg/kg; then 30 mg/kg P.O. daily or 900 mg/m² P.O. daily in five divided doses.

► Severe *Plasmodium falciparum* malaria.
Adults: 10 mg/kg quinidine gluconate I.V. Dilute in 250 ml of normal saline solution and infuse over 1 to 2 hours; then give continuous maintenance infusion of 0.02 mg/kg/minute for 72 hours or until parasitemia is less than 1%. Or dilute 15 mg/kg quinidine gluconate I.V. in 250 ml of normal saline solution and infuse over 4 hours. Begin maintenance therapy 24 hours after the start of the loading dose, at 7.5 mg/kg infused over 4 hours, q 8 hours for 7 days, or until oral therapy can be instituted.

▽ I.V. administration

• Use drug I.V. only for malaria or acute arrhythmias.
• Mix 10 ml (800 mg) of quinidine gluconate with 40 ml of D_5W and infuse at a slow rate of 1 ml/minute for maximum safety.
• Never use discolored (brownish) quinidine solution.

⊗ **Incompatibilities**
Alkalies, amiodarone, atracurium besylate, furosemide, heparin sodium, iodides.

Contraindications and cautions

• Contraindicated in patients hypersensitive to quinidine or related cinchona derivatives; in patients with idiosyncratic reactions to them; and in patients with intraventricular conduction defects, complete heart block, left bundle branch block, history of drug-induced torsades de pointes or prolonged QT interval, digitalis toxicity with grossly impaired AV conduction, or abnormal rhythms caused by escape mechanisms.
• Use cautiously in patients with asthma, muscle weakness, or infection with fever (hypersensitivity reactions to drug may be masked). Also use cautiously in patients with hepatic, renal, or cardiac impairment.
❧ **Lifespan:** In pregnant women, use cautiously. In breast-feeding women, drug isn't recommended. In children, safety and effectiveness haven't been established.

Adverse reactions

CNS: *vertigo, headache, light-headedness,* confusion, restlessness, cold sweats, pallor, fainting, fever, dementia.
CV: *PVCs, ventricular tachycardia, torsades de pointes, severe hypotension, SA and AV block, ventricular fibrillation, cardiotoxicity,* tachycardia, *aggravated heart failure, ECG changes (widening of QRS complex, notched P waves, widened QT interval, ST-segment depression),* hypotension.
EENT: *tinnitus,* blurred vision.
GI: *diarrhea, nausea, vomiting,* excessive salivation, anorexia, petechial hemorrhage of buccal mucosa, abdominal pain.
Hematologic: hemolytic anemia, *thrombocytopenia, agranulocytosis.*
Hepatic: *hepatotoxicity.*
Respiratory: *acute asthma attack, respiratory arrest.*
Skin: rash, pruritus.
Other: *angioedema,* cinchonism, hypersensitivity reaction, lupus erythematosus.

Interactions

Drug-drug. *Acetazolamide, antacids, sodium bicarbonate, thiazide diuretics:* May increase quinidine levels because of alkaline urine. Monitor patient for increased effect.
Amiodarone: May increase quinidine level, producing potentially fatal cardiac arrhythmias. If use together can't be avoided, monitor quinidine level closely. Adjust quinidine p.r.n.
Anticoagulants: May increase anticoagulant effect. Monitor patient closely for bleeding.
Barbiturates, nifedipine, phenytoin, rifampin: May decrease level of quinidine. Monitor patient for decreased quinidine effect.
Cimetidine: May increase quinidine levels. Monitor patient for increased effect.
Digoxin: May increase digoxin level after quinidine therapy starts. Monitor patient closely for digitalis toxicity.
Other antiarrhythmics (such as lidocaine, procainamide, propranolol): May increase risk of toxicity. Use together cautiously.
Propafenone: May increase propafenone levels and its effects. Use together cautiously.
Succinylcholine and nondepolarizing neuromuscular blockades: May increase neuromuscular blockade. Avoid using together.
Sucralfate: May decrease quinidine levels. Adjust dose, p.r.n.

Verapamil: May result in hypotension, bradycardia, or AV block. Monitor blood pressure and heart rate.
Drug-herb. *Jimson weed:* May adversely affect CV function. Discourage using together.
Licorice: May prolong the QT interval. Discourage using together.
Drug-food. *Grapefruit:* May delay absorption and onset of action of drug. Advise patient to avoid eating or drinking grapefruit.

Effects on lab test results

- May increase liver enzyme levels. May decrease hemoglobin level and hematocrit.
- May decrease platelet and granulocyte counts.

Pharmacokinetics

Absorption: Although all salts are well absorbed, levels vary greatly among individuals.
Distribution: Well distributed in all tissues except brain; about 80% bound to proteins.
Metabolism: About 60% to 80% metabolized in liver to two metabolites.
Excretion: 10% to 30% excreted in urine. Urine acidification increases excretion; alkalinization decreases it. *Half-life:* 5 to 12 hours.

Route	Onset	Peak	Duration
P.O.	1–3 hr	1–2 hr	6–8 hr
I.V.	Immediate	Immediate	Unknown
I.M.	Unknown	Unknown	Unknown

Action

Chemical effect: Has direct and indirect (anticholinergic) effects on cardiac tissue. Automaticity, conduction velocity, and membrane responsiveness are decreased. The effective refractory period is prolonged. Anticholinergic action reduces vagal tone.
Therapeutic effect: Restores normal sinus rhythm and relieves signs and symptoms of malaria infection.

Available forms

quinidine bisulfate
Tablets (sustained-release): 250 mg ♦ ◇
quinidine gluconate
Injection: 80 mg/ml
Tablets (sustained-release): 324 mg, 325 mg, 330 mg
quinidine sulfate
Tablets: 200 mg, 300 mg
Tablets (sustained-release): 300 mg

NURSING PROCESS

Assessment

- Assess patient's arrhythmia before starting therapy and regularly thereafter to monitor the drug's effectiveness.
- Monitor drug level. Therapeutic level for arrhythmias is 2 to 5 mcg/ml.
- Check apical pulse rate and blood pressure before starting therapy. Hypotension may occur, usually with parenteral use.
- Monitor liver function test results during first 4 to 8 weeks of therapy.
- Be alert for adverse reactions and drug interactions.
- Assess patient's and family's knowledge of drug therapy.

Nursing diagnoses

- Decreased cardiac output related to presence of arrhythmia
- Risk for deficient fluid volume related to drug-induced adverse GI reactions
- Deficient knowledge related to drug therapy

Planning and implementation

- Give anticoagulant before starting therapy in a patient with long-standing atrial fibrillation because restoration of normal sinus rhythm may dislodge thrombi from atrial wall, causing thromboembolism.
- If patient develops unexplained fever or elevated hepatic enzyme level, monitor him for hepatotoxicity.
- If patient develops symptoms of cardiotoxicity, such as increased PR and QT intervals, 50% widening of the QRS complex, ventricular tachyarrhythmias, frequent ventricular ectopic beats, or tachycardia, stop drug immediately.
- Don't crush sustained-release tablets.

ALERT: Sustained-release preparations aren't interchangeable.
ALERT: Don't confuse quinidine with clonidine.

Patient teaching

- Tell patient to take drug with meals.
- Tell patient to report signs of toxicity, including ringing in ears, visual disturbances, dizziness, headache, nausea, rash, or shortness of breath.
- Stress importance of follow-up care.

☑ Evaluation
• Patient regains normal cardiac output with resolution of arrhythmia.
• Patient maintains adequate hydration throughout therapy.
• Patient and family state understanding of drug therapy.

quinupristin and dalfopristin
(QUIN-uh-pris-tin and DALF-oh-pris-tin)
Synercid

Pharmacologic class: streptogramin
Therapeutic class: antibiotic
Pregnancy risk category: B

Indications and dosages

▶ **Serious or life-threatening infections linked to vancomycin-resistant** *Enterococcus faecium* **bacteremia.** *Adults and children age 16 and older:* 7.5 mg/kg I.V. infusion over 1 hour q 8 hours. Length of therapy determined by site and severity of infection.
▶ **Complicated skin and skin-structure infections caused by** *Staphylococcus aureus* **(methicillin susceptible) or** *Streptococcus pyogenes.* *Adults and children age 16 and older:* 7.5 mg/kg by I.V. infusion over 1 hour q 12 hours for at least 7 days.

▼ I.V. administration
• Flush line with D_5W before and after each dose.
• Reconstitute powder for injection by adding 5 ml of sterile water for injection or D_5W. Gently swirl vial to dissolve powder completely; to limit foaming, don't shake the vial. Reconstituted solutions must be further diluted within 30 minutes.
• Add dose of reconstituted solution to 250 ml of D_5W; maximum concentration, 2 mg/ml. Diluted solution is stable for 5 hours at room temperature or 54 hours when refrigerated.
• Fluid-restricted patient with a central venous catheter may receive dose in 100 ml of D_5W. This concentration isn't recommended for peripheral venous administration.
• Give all doses by I.V. infusion over 1 hour. Use an infusion pump or device to control rate of infusion.

• If moderate to severe peripheral venous irritation occurs, consider increasing infusion volume to 500 or 750 ml, changing injection site, or infusing by central venous catheter.
⊗ Incompatibilities
Saline and heparin solutions.

Contraindications and cautions

• Contraindicated in patients hypersensitive to the drug or other streptogramin antibiotics.
⚘ Lifespan: In pregnant women, use only if benefits outweigh potential risks to the fetus. In breast-feeding women, use cautiously; it's unknown if the drug appears in breast milk. In children younger than age 16, safety and effectiveness haven't been established.

Adverse reactions

CNS: headache, pain.
CV: thrombophlebitis.
GI: nausea, diarrhea, vomiting.
Musculoskeletal: arthralgia, myalgia.
Skin: *inflammation, pain, and edema at infusion site;* rash; pruritus.

Interactions

Drug-drug. *Cyclosporine:* May decrease metabolism of cyclosporine and increase level. Monitor cyclosporine levels.
Drugs metabolized by CYP 3A4 (carbamazepine, delavirdine, diazepam, diltiazem, disopyramide, docetaxel, indinavir, lidocaine, lovastatin, methylprednisolone, midazolam, nevirapine, nifedipine, paclitaxel, ritonavir, tacrolimus, verapamil, vinblastine, and others): May increase levels, therapeutic effects, and adverse reactions of these drugs. Use together cautiously.
Drugs metabolized by CYP 3A4 that may prolong the QT interval (such as quinidine): May decrease metabolism of these drugs and prolong QT interval. Avoid using together.

Effects on lab test results

• May increase AST, ALT, and bilirubin levels.

Pharmacokinetics

Absorption: Administered I.V.
Distribution: Protein-binding is moderate.
Metabolism: Quinupristin and dalfopristin are converted to several active major metabolites by nonenzymatic reactions.

Excretion: About 75% of both drugs and their metabolites excreted in feces. About 15% of quinupristin and 19% of dalfopristin excreted in urine. *Half-life:* About 1 hour for quinupristin; about ¾ hours for dalfopristin.

Route	Onset	Peak	Duration
I.V.	Unknown	Unknown	Unknown

Action

Chemical effect: Inhibit or destroy susceptible bacteria through combined inhibition of protein synthesis in bacterial cells. Dalfopristin inhibits the early phase of protein synthesis in the bacterial ribosome, and quinupristin inhibits the late phase of protein synthesis.
Therapeutic effect: Inactivation or death of bacterial cells.

Available forms

Injection: 500 mg/10 ml (150 mg quinupristin and 350 mg dalfopristin)

NURSING PROCESS

🔖 Assessment
• Obtain history of patient's underlying condition before starting therapy, and reassess regularly thereafter to monitor the drug's effectiveness.
• Overgrowth of nonsusceptible organisms may occur. Monitor patient closely for signs and symptoms of superinfection.
• Monitor liver function during therapy.
• Assess patient's and family's knowledge of drug therapy.

🔵 Nursing diagnoses
• Risk for infection related to presence of bacteria
• Diarrhea related to drug-induced adverse effect
• Deficient knowledge related to drug therapy

➤ Planning and implementation
⚠ ALERT: Drug isn't active against *Enterococcus faecalis*. Make sure cultures are drawn to avoid misidentifying *E. faecalis* as *E. faecium*.
• To reduce adverse reactions, such as arthralgia and myalgia, decrease dose interval to q 12 hours.
• If patient develops diarrhea during or following therapy, notify prescriber because mild to life-threatening pseudomembranous colitis may occur.

Patient teaching
• Advise patient to immediately report irritation at I.V. site, pain in joints or muscles, and diarrhea.
• Tell patient to report persistent or worsening signs and symptoms of infection, such as pain and erythema.

☑ Evaluation
• Patient is free from infection.
• Patient doesn't experience diarrhea.
• Patient and family state understanding of drug therapy.

rabeprazole sodium
(rah-BEH-pruh-zohl SOH-dee-um)
AcipHex

Pharmacologic class: proton pump inhibitor
Therapeutic class: antiulcerative
Pregnancy risk category: B

Indications and dosages
➤ **Erosive or ulcerative gastroesophageal reflux disease (GERD).** *Adults:* 20 mg P.O. daily for 4 to 8 weeks. Additional 8-week course may be considered, if needed.
➤ **To maintain healing of erosive or ulcerative GERD.** *Adults:* 20 mg P.O. daily.
➤ **Duodenal ulcers.** *Adults:* 20 mg P.O. daily after morning meal for up to 4 weeks.
➤ **Pathological hypersecretory conditions, including Zollinger-Ellison syndrome.** *Adults:* 60 mg P.O. daily; increase p.r.n. to 100 mg P.O. daily or 60 mg P.O. twice daily.
➤ **Symptomatic GERD, including daytime and nighttime heartburn.** *Adults:* 20 mg P.O. daily for 4 weeks. Additional 4-week course may be considered, if needed.
➤ *Helicobacter pylori* **eradication to reduce the risk of duodenal ulcer recurrence.** *Adults:* Three drug regimen: rabeprazole 20 mg P.O. b.i.d. given with amoxicillin 1,000 mg P.O.

b.i.d. and clarithromycin 500 mg P.O. b.i.d. for a total of 7 days.

Contraindications and cautions

• Contraindicated in patients hypersensitive to drug, other benzimidazoles (such as lansoprazole or omeprazole), or components in these formulations. For *H. pylori* eradication, clarithromycin is contraindicated in patients hypersensitive to any macrolide antibiotic and in those taking pimozide. Amoxicillin is contraindicated in patients hypersensitive to any penicillin.

• Use cautiously in patients with severe hepatic impairment.

⚛ **Lifespan:** In pregnant women, clarithromycin is contraindicated for *H. pylori* eradication. In children, safety and effectiveness haven't been established.

Adverse reactions

CNS: headache.

Interactions

Drug-drug. *Clarithromycin:* May increase levels of rabeprazole. Monitor patient closely.
Cyclosporine: May inhibit cyclosporine metabolism. Use together cautiously.
Digoxin, ketoconazole, other gastric pH–dependent drugs: May decrease or increase drug absorption at increased pH values. Monitor patient closely.
Drug-herb. *St. John's wort:* May increase risk of sunburn. Discourage using together; urge patient to avoid unprotected or prolonged sun exposure.

Effects on lab test results

None reported.

Pharmacokinetics

Absorption: Acid labile; enteric coating allows drug to pass through the stomach relatively intact. Level peaks over a period of 2 to 5 hours.
Distribution: 96.3% protein-bound.
Metabolism: Extensively metabolized by the liver to inactive compounds.
Excretion: 90% eliminated in urine as metabolites. Remaining 10% of metabolites eliminated in feces. *Half-life:* 1 to 2 hours.

Route	Onset	Peak	Duration
P.O.	< 1 hr	2–5 hr	> 24 hr

Action

Chemical effect: Blocks activity of the acid (proton) pump by inhibiting gastric hydrogen-potassium adenosine triphosphatase at the secretory surface of gastric parietal cells, thereby blocking gastric acid secretion.
Therapeutic effect: Promotes healing of gastric erosion or ulceration by stopping gastric acid secretion.

Available forms

Tablets (delayed-release): 20 mg

NURSING PROCESS

⚖ Assessment

• Obtain history of patient's underlying condition before starting therapy, and reassess regularly thereafter to monitor the drug's effectiveness.
• Determine if patient is hypersensitive to penicillin because anaphylaxis may occur.
• Be alert for adverse reactions and drug interactions.
• Assess patient's and family's knowledge of drug therapy.

⊞ Nursing diagnoses

• Acute pain related to underlying condition
• Risk for injury related to drug-induced adverse reactions
• Deficient knowledge related to drug therapy

⟩ Planning and implementation

• Don't crush, split, or allow patient to chew tablets.
• If duodenal ulcer or GERD isn't healed after first course of therapy, additional courses of therapy may be needed.
⑤ ALERT: Symptomatic response to therapy doesn't rule out presence of gastric malignancy.
• In patient who doesn't respond to therapy for *H. pylori*, test for susceptibility. If resistance to clarithromycin occurs or susceptibility testing isn't possible, give a different antimicrobial.
⑤ ALERT: For *H. pylori* eradication, pseudomembranous colitis may occur with nearly all antibacterials, including clarithromycin and amoxicillin. Monitor patient closely.
Patient teaching
• Explain importance of taking drug exactly as prescribed.

Reactions may be *common*, uncommon, *life-threatening*, or COMMON AND LIFE-THREATENING.

• Tell patient to swallow delayed-release tablets whole and not crush, chew, or split them.
• Tell patient that drug may be taken without regard to meals, unless patient is being treated for *H. pylori*; then all three drugs should be taken twice daily with the morning and evening meals.

🗹 Evaluation
• Patient experiences decreased pain with drug therapy.
• Patient sustains no injury as a result of drug-induced adverse reactions.
• Patient and family state understanding of drug therapy.

---

rabies immune globulin, human
(RAY-bees ih-MYOON GLOH-byoo-lin, HYOO-mun)
BayRab, Imogam Rabies-HT

Pharmacologic class: immune serum
Therapeutic class: rabies prophylaxis drug
Pregnancy risk category: C

Indications and dosages
▶ **Rabies exposure.** *Adults and children:* 20 international units/kg at time of first dose of rabies vaccine. If feasible, infiltrate the full dose in the area around and in the wounds. Give remainder, if any, I.M. separate from rabies vaccine injection site.

Contraindications and cautions
• Give only one dose to prevent interference with effectiveness of vaccine.
• Use cautiously in patients hypersensitive to thimerosal, in patients with a history of systemic allergic reactions after using human immunoglobulin, and in patients with immunoglobulin A deficiency.
※ Lifespan: In pregnant women, use cautiously. In breast-feeding women, safety and effectiveness haven't been established.

Adverse reactions
CV: slight fever, slight headache, malaise.
GU: nephrotic syndrome.
Skin: *rash,* pain, redness, induration at injection site.
Other: *anaphylaxis, angioedema.*

Interactions
Drug-drug. *Corticosteroids, immunosuppressive drugs:* May interfere with the active antibody response, predisposing patient to rabies. Avoid these drugs during postexposure immunization period.
Live-virus vaccines: May interfere with response to vaccine. Delay immunization.
Rabies vaccine: May partially suppress the antibody response to rabies immune globulin. Give full dose of immune globulin into wound, if feasible.

Effects on lab test results
None reported.

Pharmacokinetics
Absorption: Slow.
Distribution: Unknown.
Metabolism: Unknown.
Excretion: Unknown. *Half-life:* About 24 days.

Route	Onset	Peak	Duration
I.M.	Unknown	2–13 days	Unknown

Action
Chemical effect: Provides passive immunity to rabies.
Therapeutic effect: Prevents rabies.

Available forms
Injection: 150 international units/ml in 2-ml, 10-ml vials

NURSING PROCESS

R

🗺 Assessment
• Obtain history of animal bites, allergies, and immunization reactions.
• Ask patient when he last received a tetanus immunization. Prescriber may order booster.
• Be alert for adverse reactions and drug interactions.
• Assess patient's and family's knowledge of drug therapy.

⊞ Nursing diagnoses
• Risk for injury related to rabies exposure
• Ineffective protection related to drug-induced hypersensitivity reaction
• Deficient knowledge related to drug therapy

▶ Planning and implementation

• Use only with rabies vaccine and immediate local treatment of wound. Don't give in same syringe or at same site as rabies vaccine. Give drug regardless of interval between exposure and start of therapy.

• Don't give live-virus vaccines within 3 months of this drug.

⊛ **ALERT:** Drug provides passive immunity. Don't confuse with rabies vaccine, which is suspension of attenuated or killed microorganisms used to give active immunity. The two drugs usually are given together for prophylaxis after exposure to known or suspected rabid animals.

⊛ **ALERT:** Have epinephrine 1:1,000 immediately available to treat any acute anaphylactic reactions.

⊛ **ALERT:** Don't give more than 5 ml at one I.M. injection site; instead, divide I.M. doses larger than 5 ml and give at different sites. Use a large muscle, such as the gluteus.

Patient teaching

• Tell patient he may develop a slight fever and pain and redness at injection site.

• Explain that tetanus booster may be needed.

• Instruct patient to report signs of hypersensitivity immediately.

☑ Evaluation

• Patient has passive immunity to rabies.

• Patient shows no signs of hypersensitivity after receiving drug.

• Patient and family state understanding of drug therapy.

raloxifene hydrochloride
(rah-LOKS-ih-feen high-droh-KLOR-ighd)
Evista

Pharmacologic class: selective estrogen receptor modulator (SERM)
Therapeutic class: antiosteoporotic
Pregnancy risk category: X

Indications and dosages

▶ **To prevent and treat osteoporosis.** *Postmenopausal women:* 60 mg P.O. daily.

Contraindications and cautions

• Contraindicated in women hypersensitive to the drug or any of its components, and in those with current or past venous thromboembolic events, including deep vein thrombosis (DVT), pulmonary embolism, or retinal vein thrombosis.

• Use cautiously in women with severe hepatic impairment.

• Use with hormone replacement therapy or systemic estrogen isn't recommended.

⚘ **Lifespan:** In women who are pregnant or planning to become pregnant, in breast-feeding women, and in children, drug is contraindicated. In men, safety and effectiveness haven't been evaluated.

Adverse reactions

CNS: depression, insomnia, migraine, fever.
CV: chest pain, peripheral edema.
EENT: *sinusitis,* pharyngitis, laryngitis.
GI: nausea, dyspepsia, vomiting, flatulence, GI disorder, gastroenteritis, abdominal pain.
GU: vaginitis, UTI, cystitis, leukorrhea, endometrial disorder, vaginal bleeding.
Metabolic: weight gain.
Musculoskeletal: *arthralgia,* myalgia, arthritis, leg cramps.
Respiratory: increased cough, pneumonia.
Skin: rash, sweating.
Other: hot flushes, infection, flulike syndrome, breast pain.

Interactions

Drug-drug. *Cholestyramine:* May significantly reduce raloxifene absorption. Don't give these drugs together.
Highly protein-bound drugs (such as clofibrate, diazepam, diazoxide, ibuprofen, indomethacin, naproxen): May interfere with binding sites. Use together cautiously.
Warfarin: May decrease PT. Monitor PT and INR closely.

Effects on lab test results

• May increase calcium, inorganic phosphate, total protein, albumin, hormone-binding globulin, and apolipoprotein A levels. May decrease total and low-density lipoprotein cholesterol levels and apolipoprotein B levels.

Pharmacokinetics

Absorption: Rapid, with about 60% of dose absorbed after P.O. administration.
Distribution: Widely distributed and highly bound to proteins.

Metabolism: Extensive first-pass metabolism to glucuronide conjugates.
Excretion: Primarily excreted in feces, with less than 0.2% excreted unchanged in urine. *Half-life:* 27½ hours.

Route	Onset	Peak	Duration
P.O.	Unknown	Unknown	24 hr

Action

Chemical effect: Reduces resorption of bone and decreases overall bone turnover by selectively activating and blocking estrogen receptors, resulting in increased bone mineral density.
Therapeutic effect: Prevents bone breakdown in postmenopausal women.

Available forms

Tablets: 60 mg

NURSING PROCESS

Assessment

- Obtain history of patient's condition before starting therapy, and reassess regularly thereafter to monitor the drug's effectiveness.
- Monitor patient for signs of blood clots. The greatest risk of thromboembolic events is during the first 4 months of therapy.
- Monitor patient for breast abnormalities.
- Monitor lipid levels, blood pressure, body weight, and liver function.
- Assess patient's and family's knowledge of drug therapy.

Nursing diagnoses

- Ineffective peripheral tissue perfusion related to potential DVT formation
- Imbalanced nutrition: less than body requirements related to drug-induced adverse GI reactions
- Deficient knowledge related to drug therapy

Planning and implementation

ALERT: Stop drug at least 72 hours before prolonged immobilization, and resume only after patient is fully mobile.
- If you suspect thromboembolic event, stop giving the drug and notify prescriber.
- Report unexplained uterine bleeding immediately to prescriber.
- Effect on bone mineral density with more than 2 years of drug therapy isn't known.

Patient teaching

- Advise patient to avoid long periods of restricted movement (such as during traveling) because it increases the risk of venous thromboembolic events.
- Inform patient that hot flashes or flushing may occur and that drug doesn't aid in reducing them.
- Instruct patient to take other bone-loss prevention measures, including taking supplemental calcium and vitamin D if dietary intake is inadequate, performing weight-bearing exercises, and stopping alcohol consumption and smoking.
- Tell patient that drug may be taken with or without food.
- Advise patient to report any unexplained uterine bleeding or breast abnormalities.
- Explain drug's adverse effects; instruct patient to read package insert before starting therapy and to read it again each time prescription is renewed.

Evaluation

- Patient doesn't develop pain, redness, or swelling in legs.
- Patient maintains normal dietary intake.
- Patient and family state understanding of drug therapy.

ramelteon
(rah-MEHL-tee-on)
Rozerem

Pharmacologic class: melatonin receptor agonist
Therapeutic class: hypnotic
Pregnancy risk category: C

Indications and dosages

▶ **Insomnia characterized by trouble falling asleep.** *Adults:* 8 mg P.O. within 30 minutes h.s. Don't give with or immediately after a high-fat meal.

Contraindications and cautions

- Contraindicated in those hypersensitive to the drug or any of its components. Don't use in patients taking fluvoxamine or in patients with severe hepatic impairment, severe sleep apnea, or severe COPD.

R

• Use cautiously in patients with depression or moderate hepatic impairment.

⚞ **Lifespan:** Use drug in pregnancy only if benefits outweigh potential risks to the fetus. In breast-feeding women, avoid use. In children, safety and effectiveness haven't been established.

Adverse reactions

CNS: depression, dizziness, fatigue, headache, somnolence, worsened insomnia.
GI: diarrhea, impaired taste, nausea.
Musculoskeletal: arthralgia, myalgia.
Respiratory: upper respiratory tract infection.
Other: flulike symptoms.

Interactions

Drug-drug. *CNS depressants:* May cause excessive CNS depression. Use together cautiously.
Fluconazole (strong CYP 2C9 inhibitor), keto-conazole (strong CYP 3A4 inhibitor), weak CYP 1A2 inhibitors: May increase ramelteon level. Use together cautiously.
Fluvoxamine (strong CYP 1A2 inhibitor): May increase ramelteon level. Avoid use together.
Rifampin (strong CYP enzyme inducer): May decrease ramelteon level. Monitor patient for lack of effect.
Drug-food. *Food (especially high-fat meals):* May delay time to peak drug effect. Tell patient to take drug on an empty stomach.
Drug-lifestyle. *Alcohol use:* May cause excessive CNS depression. Discourage alcohol use.

Effects on lab test results

• May increase prolactin level. May alter blood cortisol and testosterone levels.

Pharmacokinetics

Absorption: Rapid. Oral bioavailability is 1.8%. Food consumption decreases and delays peak level by 45 minutes.
Distribution: 82% bound to protein; 70% to serum albumin. Tissue distribution is substantial.
Metabolism: Rapid, first pass metabolism. Metabolized mainly by CYP 1A2 (also by CYP 2C and CYP 3A4), with four active metabolites formed.
Excretion: 84% in urine, 4% in feces. Less than 0.1% is excreted as the parent compound. Elimination complete 96 hours after dose. *Half-life:*

Parent compound, 1 to 2½ hours; metabolite M-II, 2 to 5 hours.

Route	Onset	Peak	Duration
P.O.	Rapid	½–1½ hr	Unknown

Action

Chemical effect: Acts on receptors believed to maintain the circadian rhythm underlying the normal sleep-wake cycle.
Therapeutic effect: Promotes sleep.

Available forms

Tablets: 8 mg

NURSING PROCESS

⚖ Assessment

• Thoroughly evaluate the cause of insomnia before starting drug.
• Assess patient for behavioral or cognitive disorders.
• Evaluate patient's and family's knowledge of drug therapy.

⬢ Nursing diagnoses

• Disturbed sleep pattern related to presence of insomnia
• Risk for injury related to drug-induced adverse CNS effects
• Deficient knowledge related to drug therapy

▶ Planning and implementation

• Administer drug on an empty stomach to prevent delays in peak effect.
• Drug doesn't cause physical dependence.
• In cases of overdose, consider the possibility of multiple drug ingestion, and contact a poison control center. Treat symptomatically.
Patient teaching
• Instruct patient to take dose within 30 minutes of bedtime.
• Tell patient not to take drug with or after a heavy meal.
• Caution against performing activities that require mental alertness or physical coordination after taking drug.
• Caution patient to avoid alcohol while taking ramelteon.
• Tell patient to consult prescriber if insomnia worsens or behavior changes.

Reactions may be *common*, uncommon, ***life-threatening***, or COMMON AND LIFE-THREATENING.

• Urge woman to consult prescriber if menses stops, libido decreases, or breast discharge or fertility problems develop.

☑ Evaluation

• Patient reports that drug effectively promotes sleep.

• Patient does not experience injury from adverse CNS effects.

• Patient and family state understanding of drug therapy.

ramipril
(reh-MIH-pril)
Altace, Ramace ◊ , Tritace ◊

Pharmacologic class: ACE inhibitor
Therapeutic class: antihypertensive
Pregnancy risk category: C (D in second and third trimesters)

Indications and dosages

▶ **Hypertension (either alone or with thiazide diuretics).** *Adults:* Initially, 2.5 mg P.O. daily in patients not receiving diuretic therapy. Adjust dose based on blood pressure response. Usual maintenance dosage is 2.5 to 20 mg daily as a single dose or in two equal doses.
⊠ Adjust-a-dose: For patients with renal impairment, if creatinine clearance is less than 40 ml/minute (creatinine higher than 2.5 mg/dl), recommended initial dose is 1.25 mg daily, adjusted upward to maximum dose of 5 mg based on blood pressure response.

In patients receiving diuretic therapy, symptomatic hypotension may occur. To minimize this, stop diuretic, if possible, 2 to 3 days before starting ramipril. When this isn't possible, give initial dose of 1.25 mg.
▶ **Heart failure post-MI.** *Adults:* Initially, 2.5 mg P.O. b.i.d. Adjust to target dose of 5 mg P.O. b.i.d.
⊠ Adjust-a-dose: For patients with renal impairment, start therapy with 1.25 mg P.O. once daily, and increase to 1.25 mg b.i.d. Maximum dosage is 2.5 mg b.i.d.
▶ **Reduction in risk of MI, stroke, and death from CV causes.** *Adults age 55 and older:* 2.5 mg P.O. once daily for 1 week, then 5 mg P.O. once daily for 3 weeks. Increase as tolerat-

ed to a maintenance dosage of 10 mg P.O. once daily.
⊠ Adjust-a-dose: For patients with renal impairment, if creatinine clearance is less than 40 ml/minute, give one-quarter of recommended dose.

Contraindications and cautions

• Contraindicated in patients hypersensitive to ACE inhibitors, in those with history of angioedema during previous therapy with ACE inhibitor, and in those with renal artery stenosis.

• Use cautiously in patients with renal impairment.

⚘ Lifespan: In pregnant and breast-feeding women, drug isn't recommended. In children, safety and effectiveness haven't been established.

Adverse reactions

CNS: headache, dizziness, fatigue, syncope, asthenia, malaise, light-headedness, anxiety, amnesia, *seizures,* depression, insomnia, nervousness, neuralgia, neuropathy, paresthesia, somnolence, tremors, vertigo.
CV: orthostatic hypotension, angina, *arrhythmias,* chest pain, palpitations, *MI,* edema.
EENT: epistaxis, tinnitus.
GI: nausea, vomiting, abdominal pain, anorexia, constipation, diarrhea, dyspepsia, dry mouth, gastroenteritis.
GU: impotence.
Metabolic: *hyperkalemia,* weight gain.
Musculoskeletal: arthralgia, arthritis, myalgia.
Respiratory: dry, persistent, tickling, nonproductive cough; dyspnea.
Skin: rash, dermatitis, pruritus, photosensitivity reaction, increased diaphoresis.
Other: hypersensitivity reactions, *angioedema.*

Interactions

Drug-drug. *Diuretics:* May cause excessive hypotension, especially at start of therapy. Stop diuretic at least 3 days before starting ramipril, increase sodium intake, or reduce starting dose of ramipril.
Insulin, oral antidiabetics: May increase risk of hypoglycemia, especially at start of ramipril therapy. Monitor patient closely.
Lithium: May increase lithium levels. Use together cautiously, and monitor lithium levels for toxicity.
Potassium-sparing diuretics, potassium supplements: May increase risk of hyperkalemia be-

R

cause ramipril attenuates potassium loss. Monitor potassium level closely.

Drug-herb. *Capsaicin:* May increase risk of cough. Discourage using together.

Licorice: May cause sodium retention and increase blood pressure, interfering with therapeutic effects of ACE inhibitors. Discourage using together.

Drug-food. *Salt substitutes containing potassium:* May increase risk of hyperkalemia because ramipril attenuates potassium loss. Monitor potassium level closely.

Effects on lab test results

• May increase BUN, creatinine, bilirubin, liver enzyme, glucose, and potassium levels. May decrease hemoglobin level and hematocrit.

Pharmacokinetics

Absorption: 50% to 60%.
Distribution: 73% protein-bound; ramiprilat (metabolite), 58%.
Metabolism: Almost completely converted to ramiprilat, which is six times more potent than parent drug.
Excretion: 60% in urine; 40% in feces. *Half-life:* 13 to 17 hours.

Route	Onset	Peak	Duration
P.O.	1–2 hr	< 1 hr	24 hr

Action

Chemical effect: May inhibit conversion from angiotensin I to angiotensin II, a potent vasoconstrictor. This decreases peripheral arterial resistance, thus decreasing aldosterone secretion.
Therapeutic effect: Lowers blood pressure.

Available forms

Capsules: 1.25 mg, 2.5 mg, 5 mg, 10 mg

NURSING PROCESS

Assessment

• Assess patient's blood pressure before starting therapy and regularly thereafter to monitor the drug's effectiveness.
• Closely assess kidney function during first few weeks of therapy. Regularly assess creatinine and BUN levels. Patient with severe heart failure whose kidney function depends on angiotensin-aldosterone system may experience acute renal impairment during therapy. Hyper-

tensive patient with renal artery stenosis also may show signs of worsening kidney function at start of therapy.
• Monitor CBC before therapy, q 2 weeks for first 3 months of therapy, and periodically thereafter.
• Monitor potassium level. Risk factors for hyperkalemia include renal insufficiency, diabetes, and use of drugs that raise potassium levels.
• Be alert for adverse reactions and drug interactions.
• Assess patient's and family's knowledge of drug therapy.

Nursing diagnoses

• Risk for injury related to presence of hypertension
• Disturbed sleep pattern related to drug-induced cough
• Deficient knowledge related to drug therapy

Planning and implementation

• Stop diuretic 2 to 3 days before starting therapy, if possible.
• If patient has trouble swallowing pills whole, capsule may be opened and the contents sprinkled onto 4 ounces of applesauce or mixed in 4 ounces (118 ml) of water or apple juice. These mixtures may be stored at room temperature for up to 24 hours, or refrigerated for up to 48 hours.

Patient teaching
• Instruct patient not to use salt substitutes or potassium supplements during therapy.
• If patient has trouble swallowing, tell him to open capsules and sprinkle contents on food.
• Tell patient to rise slowly to avoid initial lightheadedness. If syncope occurs, tell him to stop taking the drug and notify the prescriber.
• Tell patient not to abruptly stop therapy.
• Advise patient to report signs of angioedema and laryngeal edema, which may occur after first dose.
• Tell patient to report signs of infection.
• Tell woman to report pregnancy. Drug will need to be stopped.

Evaluation

• Patient's blood pressure is normal.
• Patient's sleep patterns are undisturbed throughout therapy.
• Patient and family state understanding of drug therapy.

ranitidine hydrochloride

(ruh-NIH-tuh-deen high-droh-KLOR-ighd)

Zantac*, Zantac-C ♦, Zantac EFFERdose, Zantac GELdose, Zantac 75†

Pharmacologic class: H_2-receptor antagonist
Therapeutic class: antiulcerative
Pregnancy risk category: B

Indications and dosages

▶ **Intractable duodenal ulcer; pathologic hypersecretory conditions, such as Zollinger-Ellison syndrome; short-term therapy for patients unable to tolerate oral forms (I.V. only).** *Adults:* 150 mg P.O. b.i.d. or 300 mg q h.s. Or, 50 mg I.V. or I.M. q 6 to 8 hours. Patients with Zollinger-Ellison syndrome may need up to 6 g P.O. daily. Or, for Zollinger-Ellison syndrome, 1 mg/kg/hour for 4 hours, then increase in increments of 0.5 mg/kg/hr if needed, to a maximum of 2.5 mg/kg/hour.

▶ **Duodenal and gastric ulcer.** *Children ages 1 month to 16 years:* 2 to 4 mg/kg P.O. twice daily to a maximum of 300 mg/day. Maintenance dosage is 2 to 4 mg/kg P.O. once daily to a maximum of 150 mg daily.

▶ **Maintenance therapy for duodenal ulcer.** *Adults:* 150 mg P.O. h.s.

▶ **Gastroesophageal reflux disease.** *Adults:* 150 mg P.O. b.i.d.
Children age 1 month and older: 5 to 10 mg/kg P.O. daily in 2 divided doses.

▶ **Erosive esophagitis.** *Adults:* 150 mg P.O. q.i.d.; maintenance dosage, 150 mg P.O. b.i.d.
Children age 1 month and older: 5 to 10 mg/kg P.O. daily in 2 divided doses.

▶ **Self-medication for occasional heartburn, acid indigestion, and sour stomach.** *Adults and children age 12 and older:* 75 mg† once or twice daily; maximum daily dosage, 150 mg.

Adjust-a-dose: For patients with renal impairment, if creatinine clearance is less than 50 ml/min, give 150 mg P.O. q 24 hours or 50 mg I.M. or I.V. q 18 to 24 hours.

I.V. administration

• To prepare I.V. injection, dilute 2 ml (50 mg) with compatible I.V. solution to a total volume of 20 ml, and inject over at least 5 minutes. Compatible solutions include sterile water for injection, normal saline solution for injection, D_5W, and lactated Ringer's injection.
• To give drug by intermittent I.V. infusion, dilute 50 mg (2 ml) in 100 ml compatible solution and infuse at a rate of 5 to 7 ml/minute. The premixed solution is 50 ml and doesn't need further dilution. Infuse over 15 to 20 minutes. After dilution, solution is stable for 48 hours at room temperature.
• For premixed I.V. infusion, give by slow I.V. drip (over 15 to 20 minutes). Don't add other drugs to solution. If used with primary I.V. fluid system, stop primary solution during infusion.
• Store I.V. vial at 39° to 86° F (4° to 30° C). Store premixed containers at 36° F to 77° F (2° C to 25° C).

⊗ **Incompatibilities**
Amphotericin B, atracurium, cefazolin, cefoxitin, ceftazidime, cefuroxime, chlorpromazine, clindamycin phosphate, diazepam, ethacrynate sodium, hetastarch, hydroxyzine, insulin, methotrimeprazine, midazolam, norepinephrine, pentobarbital sodium, phenobarbital, phytonadione.

Contraindications and cautions

• Contraindicated in patients hypersensitive to the drug or any of its components.
• Use cautiously in patients with hepatic dysfunction. Adjust dosage in patients with impaired kidney function.

Lifespan: In pregnant women, use cautiously. In breast-feeding women, use cautiously; it's unknown if the drug appears in breast milk. In children, safety and effectiveness haven't been established for pathological hypersecretory conditions or the maintenance of healing duodenal ulcer. In neonates younger than 1 month, safety and effectiveness haven't been established. Safety and effectiveness have been established in children age 1 month to 16 years for treatment of gastroesophageal reflux disease. In the elderly, use cautiously.

Adverse reactions

CNS: vertigo, malaise.
EENT: blurred vision.
Hematologic: ***reversible leukopenia, pancytopenia, thrombocytopenia.***
Hepatic: jaundice.
Other: burning and itching at injection site, ***anaphylaxis, angioedema.***

R

Interactions

Drug-drug. *Antacids:* May interfere with ranitidine absorption. Stagger doses.
Diazepam: May decrease diazepam absorption. Monitor patient for decreased effectiveness; adjust dose.
Glipizide: May increase hypoglycemic effect. Adjust glipizide dosage.
Procainamide: May decrease renal clearance of procainamide. Monitor patient for procainamide toxicity.
Warfarin: May interfere with warfarin clearance. Monitor patient closely for bleeding.
Drug-lifestyle. *Smoking:* May increase gastric acid secretion and worsen disease. Discourage using together.

Effects on lab test results

• May increase creatinine and ALT levels.
• May decrease RBC, WBC, and platelet counts.
• May cause false-positive test for urine protein using Multistix.

Pharmacokinetics

Absorption: About 50% to 60% of P.O. dose; rapid from parenteral sites after I.M. dose.
Distribution: Distributed to many body tissues and appears in CSF; about 10% to 19% protein-bound.
Metabolism: Metabolized in liver.
Excretion: Excreted in urine and feces. *Half-life:* 2 to 3 hours.

Route	Onset	Peak	Duration
P.O.	≤ 1 hr	1–3 hr	≤ 13 hr
I.V., I.M.	Unknown	Unknown	≤ 13 hr

Action

Chemical effect: Competitively inhibits action of H_2 at receptor sites of parietal cells, decreasing gastric acid secretion.
Therapeutic effect: Relieves GI discomfort.

Available forms

Capsules: 150 mg, 300 mg
Granules (effervescent): 150 mg
Infusion: 0.5 mg/ml in 100-ml containers
Injection: 25 mg/ml
Syrup: 15 mg/ml*
Tablets: 75 mg†, 150 mg, 300 mg
Tablets (dispersible): 150 mg†
Tablets (effervescent): 25 mg, 150 mg

NURSING PROCESS

⚖ Assessment

• Assess patient's GI condition before starting therapy and regularly thereafter to monitor the drug's effectiveness.
• Zantac EFFERdose contains phenylalanine.
• Be alert for adverse reactions and drug interactions.
• Assess patient's and family's knowledge of drug therapy.

⊞ Nursing diagnoses

• Impaired tissue integrity related to underlying GI condition
• Risk for injury related to drug-induced adverse CNS reactions
• Deficient knowledge related to drug therapy

▶ Planning and implementation

• Don't use aluminum-based needles or equipment when mixing or giving drug parenterally because drug is incompatible with aluminum.
• No dilution is needed when giving drug I.M.
• The effervescent tablet may be dissolved in 5 ml of water and given with an oral syringe or in a medicine cup.
⊛ ALERT: Don't confuse ranitidine with rimantadine.
⊛ ALERT: Don't confuse Zantac with Xanax or Zyrtec.
Patient teaching
• Remind patient taking drug once daily to take it h.s.
• Instruct patient to take drug with or without food.
• Urge patient not to smoke cigarettes; smoking may increase gastric acid secretion and worsen disease.

☑ Evaluation

• Patient states that GI discomfort is relieved.
• Patient sustains no injury as result of drug-induced adverse CNS reactions.
• Patient and family state understanding of drug therapy.

Reactions may be *common*, uncommon, *life-threatening*, or COMMON AND LIFE-THREATENING.

repaglinide
(reh-PAG-lih-nighd)
Prandin

Pharmacologic class: meglitinide
Therapeutic class: antidiabetic
Pregnancy risk category: C

Indications and dosages

▶ **Adjunct to diet and exercise to lower glucose levels in patients with type 2 diabetes mellitus (non–insulin-dependent diabetes mellitus) whose hyperglycemia can't be controlled satisfactorily by diet and exercise alone; adjunct to diet, exercise, and metformin, rosiglitazone, or pioglitazone.** *Adults:* For patients not previously treated or whose glycosylated hemoglobin (HbA$_{1c}$) is below 8%, start dose at 0.5 mg P.O. given 15 minutes before meal; however, time may vary from immediately before to as long as 30 minutes before meal. For patients previously treated with glucose-lowering drugs and whose HbA$_{1c}$ is 8% or more, initial dose is 1 to 2 mg P.O. with each meal. Recommended dosage range is 0.5 to 4 mg with meals b.i.d., t.i.d., or q.i.d. Maximum, 16 mg daily. Base dosage on glucose-level response. May double dosage up to 4 mg with each meal until satisfactory glucose-level response is achieved. Allow at least 1 week between dosage adjustments to assess response to each dose.
⊠ Adjust-a-dose: For patients with severe renal impairment, starting dose is 0.5 mg P.O. with meals.

Contraindications and cautions

• Contraindicated in patients hypersensitive to the drug or any of its components and in those with insulin-dependent diabetes mellitus or diabetic ketoacidosis with or without coma.
• Use cautiously in patients with hepatic insufficiency. Reduced metabolism may increase drug level and cause hypoglycemia. Also use cautiously in debilitated and malnourished patients and in those with adrenal or pituitary insufficiency because they're more susceptible to the hypoglycemic effect of glucose-lowering drugs.
⚘ Lifespan: In pregnant women and breastfeeding women, don't use. In children, safety

and effectiveness haven't been established. In the elderly, use cautiously.

Adverse reactions

CNS: *headache,* paresthesia.
CV: angina, chest pain.
EENT: rhinitis, sinusitis.
GI: constipation, diarrhea, dyspepsia, nausea, vomiting.
GU: UTI.
Metabolic: HYPOGLYCEMIA, hyperglycemia.
Musculoskeletal: arthralgia, back pain.
Respiratory: bronchitis, upper respiratory infection.
Other: tooth disorder.

Interactions

Drug-drug. *Barbiturates, carbamazepine, rifampin:* May increase repaglinide metabolism. Monitor glucose level.
Beta blockers, chloramphenicol, coumarins, MAO inhibitors, NSAIDs, other drugs that are highly protein-bound, probenecid, salicylates, sulfonamides: May increase hypoglycemic action of repaglinide. Monitor glucose level.
Calcium channel blockers, corticosteroids, estrogens, hormonal contraceptives, isoniazid, nicotinic acid, phenothiazines, phenytoin, sympathomimetics, thiazides and other diuretics, thyroid products: May produce hyperglycemia and loss of glycemic control. Monitor glucose level.
Erythromycin, gemfibrozil, inhibitors of CYP 3A4, ketoconazole, miconazole: May inhibit repaglinide metabolism. Monitor glucose levels and avoid using gemfibrozil and repaglinide together.
Levonorgestrel and ethinyl estradiol, simvastatin: May increase repaglinide levels. Monitor glucose level.
Drug-herb. *Aloe, bilberry leaf, bitter melon, burdock, dandelion, fenugreek, garlic, ginseng:* May improve glucose control so that antidiabetic dosage needs to be reduced. Advise patient to discuss the use of herbal remedies before taking drug.

Effects on lab test results

• May increase or decrease glucose level.

Pharmacokinetics

Absorption: Rapid and complete. Absolute bioavailability is 56%.

R

Distribution: More than 98% bound to proteins.
Metabolism: Completely metabolized by oxidative biotransformation and direct conjugation with glucuronic acid.
Excretion: About 90% is recovered in feces and 8% in urine. *Half-life:* 1 hour.

Route	Onset	Peak	Duration
P.O.	Rapid	1 hr	Unknown

Action

Chemical effect: Stimulates the release of insulin from beta cells in the pancreas.
Therapeutic effect: Lowers glucose level.

Available forms

Tablets: 0.5 mg, 1 mg, 2 mg

NURSING PROCESS

Assessment
• Monitor glucose level before starting therapy, and regularly thereafter to monitor the drug's effectiveness.
• Be alert for adverse reactions and drug interactions.
• Monitor elderly patients and patients taking beta blockers carefully because hypoglycemia may be difficult to recognize in these patients.
• Assess patient's and family's knowledge of drug therapy.

Nursing diagnoses
• Imbalanced nutrition: more than body requirements related to patient's underlying condition
• Risk for injury related to drug-induced hypoglycemic episode
• Deficient knowledge related to drug therapy

Planning and implementation
• Increase dose carefully in a patient with renal impairment who needs dialysis.
• If repaglinide alone is inadequate, metformin may be added.
• Loss of glycemic control can occur during stress, such as fever, trauma, infection, or surgery. Stop giving the drug and give insulin.
• Oral antidiabetics have been linked to increased CV mortality compared to changing diet alone.
• Give drug immediately or up to 30 minutes before meals.

Patient teaching
• Teach patient about importance of diet and exercise along with drug therapy.
• Discuss symptoms of hypoglycemia with patient and family.
• Advise patient to monitor glucose level periodically to determine minimum effective dose.
• Encourage patient to keep regular medical appointments and have glucose level checked to monitor long-term glucose control.
• Tell patient to take drug before meals, usually 15 minutes before start of meal; however, time can vary from immediately to up to 30 minutes before meal.
• Tell patient to skip dose if he skips a meal and to add dose if he adds a meal.
• Teach patient how to monitor glucose levels carefully and what to do when he is ill, undergoing surgery, or under added stress.

Evaluation
• Patient's glucose level is controlled and an adequate nutritional balance is maintained.
• Patient doesn't experience severe decreases in glucose level.
• Patient and family state understanding of drug therapy.

reteplase, recombinant
(REE-teh-plays, ree-KUHM-buh-nent)
Retavase

Pharmacologic class: recombinant plasminogen activator
Therapeutic class: thrombolytic enzyme
Pregnancy risk category: C

Indications and dosages

▶ **Acute MI.** *Adults:* Double-bolus injection of 10 + 10 units. Give each bolus I.V. over 2 minutes. If complications don't occur after first bolus, give second bolus 30 minutes after start of first.

I.V. administration
• Reconstitute drug according to manufacturer's instructions.
⊗ **Incompatibilities**
Other I.V. drugs.

Contraindications and cautions

• Contraindicated in patients with active internal bleeding, bleeding diathesis, history of stroke, recent intracranial or intraspinal surgery or trauma, severe uncontrolled hypertension, intracranial neoplasm, arteriovenous malformation, or aneurysm.

• Use cautiously in patients who've had major surgery, obstetric delivery, organ biopsy, or trauma within 10 days and in those with previous puncture of noncompressible vessel, cerebrovascular disease, recent GI or GU bleeding, or heart disease.

⚸ Lifespan: Use in pregnancy only if benefits outweigh potential risks to the fetus. In breast-feeding women, use cautiously; it's unknown if the drug appears in breast milk. In children, safety and effectiveness haven't been established.

Adverse reactions

CNS: *intracranial hemorrhage.*
CV: *arrhythmias, cholesterol embolization, hemorrhage.*
GI: *hemorrhage.*
GU: hematuria.
Hematologic: anemia, *bleeding tendency.*
Other: bleeding at puncture sites.

Interactions

Drug-drug. Heparin, oral anticoagulants, platelet inhibitors (abciximab, aspirin, dipyridamole): May increase risk of bleeding. Use together cautiously.

Effects on lab test results

• May decrease plasminogen, fibrinogen, and hemoglobin levels and hematocrit.
• May cause unreliable results of coagulation tests or measurements of fibrinolytic activity.

Pharmacokinetics

Absorption: Administered I.V.
Distribution: Rapid distribution.
Metabolism: Unknown.
Excretion: In urine and feces. *Half-life:* 13 to 16 minutes.

Route	Onset	Peak	Duration
I.V.	Unknown	Unknown	Unknown

Action

Chemical effect: Enhances cleavage of plasminogen to generate plasmin.
Therapeutic effect: Dissolves and breaks up clots.

Available forms

Injection: 10.8 international units (18.8 mg)/vial. Supplied in kit with components for reconstitution for 2 single-use vials. Also available in half kits with 1 single use vial.

NURSING PROCESS

⮐ Assessment
• Monitor ECG.
• Monitor patient for bleeding. Avoid I.M. injections, invasive procedures, and unneeded handling of patient.
• Assess patient's and family's knowledge of drug therapy.

⮐ Nursing diagnoses
• Ineffective cardiopulmonary tissue perfusion related to underlying condition
• Risk for injury related to adverse effects of drug
• Deficient knowledge related to drug therapy

⮐ Planning and implementation
• Reteplase is administered I.V. as double-bolus injection. If bleeding or allergic reaction occurs after first bolus, notify prescriber.
• Avoid noncompressible pressure sites during therapy. If an arterial puncture is needed, use a vessel in the arm that can be compressed manually. Apply pressure for at least 30 minutes; then apply a pressure dressing. Check site often for bleeding.
Patient teaching
• Teach patient and family about drug.
• Tell patient to report adverse reactions immediately.

⮐ Evaluation
• Patient's cardiopulmonary assessment findings show improved perfusion.
• Patient is free from serious adverse reactions caused by therapy.
• Patient and family state understanding of drug therapy.

R

Rho(D) immune globulin, human
(ARR AITCH OH DEE ih-MYOON GLOH-byoo-lin, HYOO-mun)

Rho(D) immune globulin, human (Rho[D] IGIM)
BayRho-D Full Dose, RhoGAM

Rho(D) immune globulin, human (Rho[D] IGIV)
WinRho SDF, Rhophylac

Rho(D) immune globulin, human, microdose (Rho[D] IG microdose)
BayRho-D Mini-Dose, MICRhoGAM

Pharmacologic class: immune serum
Therapeutic class: anti-Rh_0(D)-positive prophylaxis drug
Pregnancy risk category: C

Indications and dosages

▶ **Rh exposure (postabortion, postmiscarriage, ectopic pregnancy, postpartum, or threatened abortion 13 weeks or later).**
Women: Transfusion unit or blood bank determines fetal packed RBC volume entering patient's blood. Give one vial I.M. if fetal packed RBC volume is below 15 ml. More than one vial I.M. may be required if large fetomaternal hemorrhage occurs. Must be given within 72 hours after delivery or miscarriage.
▶ **Transfusion accident.** *Adults and children:* Usually, 600 mcg I.V. q 8 hours or 1,200 mcg I.M. q 12 hours until total dose given. Total dose depends on volume of packed RBCs or whole blood infused. Consult blood bank or transfusion unit at once. Must be given within 72 hours.
▶ **Postabortion or postmiscarriage to prevent Rh antibody formation up to and including 12 weeks' gestation.** *Women:* Consult transfusion unit or blood bank. One microdose vial suppresses immune reaction to 2.5 ml Rh_0(D)-positive RBCs. Should be given within 3 hours but may be given up to 72 hours after abortion or miscarriage.

▶ **Amniocentesis or abdominal trauma during pregnancy.** *Women:* Base dose on extent of fetomaternal hemorrhage.
▶ **Idiopathic thrombocytopenia purpura.**
Adults and children: 250 units/kg (50 mcg/kg) I.V. as single dose or in two divided doses given on separate days. If patient responded to initial dose, maintenance dose is 125 to 300 units/kg (25 to 60 mcg/kg) based on platelet count and hemoglobin level. If patient had inadequate response to initial dose and hemoglobin level is more than 10 g/dl, maintenance dose is 250 to 300 units/kg (50 to 60 mcg/kg); for those with hemoglobin level of 8 to 10 g/dl maintenance dose is 125 to 200 units/kg (25 to 40 mcg/kg).

▼ I.V. administration

• Reconstitute only with normal saline solution: 2.5 ml for the 120-mcg and 300-mcg vials and 8.5 ml for the 1,000-mcg vial. Slowly inject diluent into vial and gently swirl vial until dissolved. Don't shake vial.
• Give injection over 3 to 5 minutes.
• Refrigerate drug at 36° to 46° F (2° to 8° C).
⊗ **Incompatibilities**
Other I.V. drugs.

Contraindications and cautions

• Contraindicated in Rh_0(D)-positive or D^u-positive patients, those previously immunized to Rh_0(D) blood factor, those with anaphylactic or severe systemic reaction to human globulin, and those with immunoglobulin A deficiency.
• Use cautiously in patients with thrombocytopenia or bleeding disorders.
⚹ **Lifespan:** In pregnant women, use cautiously. In breast-feeding women, use cautiously; it's unknown if the drug appears in breast milk. Microdose must not be used for any indication with continuation of pregnancy.

Adverse reactions

CNS: slight fever.
Other: *anaphylaxis*, discomfort at injection site.

Interactions

Drug-drug. *Live-virus vaccines:* May interfere with response to Rh_0(D) immune globulin. Delay immunization for 3 months.

Effects on lab test results

None reported.

Pharmacokinetics
Absorption: Unknown.
Distribution: Unknown.
Metabolism: Unknown.
Excretion: Unknown. *Half-life:* 24 to 30 days.

Route	Onset	Peak	Duration
I.V., I.M.	Unknown	Unknown	Unknown

Action
Chemical effect: Suppresses active antibody response and formation of anti-Rh$_o$(D) in Rh$_o$(D)-negative, D^u-negative people exposed to Rh-positive blood.
Therapeutic effect: Blocks adverse effects of Rh-positive exposure.

Available forms
I.M. injection: 300 mcg of Rh$_o$(D) immune globulin/vial (standard dose); 50 mcg of Rh$_o$(D) immune globulin/vial (microdose)
I.V. infusion: 120 mcg, 300 mcg, 1,000 mcg

NURSING PROCESS

Assessment
• Obtain history of Rh-negative patient's Rh-positive exposure, allergies, and reactions to immunizations.
• Assess patient's and family's knowledge of drug therapy.

Nursing diagnoses
• Risk for injury related to Rh-positive exposure
• Ineffective protection related to drug-induced anaphylaxis
• Deficient knowledge related to drug therapy

Planning and implementation
• Inject I.M. into the anterolateral aspect of the upper thigh or deltoid muscle.
• If administering 1,000 mcg, don't give entire dose in one muscle; divide dose between several different sites.
• Make sure epinephrine 1:1,000 is available in case of anaphylaxis.
• After delivery, have neonate's cord blood typed and crossmatched; confirm if mother is Rh$_o$(D)-negative and D^u-negative. Give to mother only if infant is Rh$_o$(D)-positive or D^u-positive.
• Drug gives passive immunity to woman exposed to Rh$_o$(D)-positive fetal blood during pregnancy and prevents formation of maternal antibodies, which would endanger future Rh$_o$(D)-positive pregnancies.
• Defer vaccination with live-virus vaccines for 3 months after giving drug.
• MICRhoGAM is recommended for every woman having an abortion or miscarriage up to 12 weeks' gestation unless she is Rh$_o$(D)-positive or D^u-positive, she has Rh antibodies, or father or fetus is Rh-negative.
Patient teaching
• Explain how drug protects future Rh$_o$(D)-positive fetuses.

Evaluation
• Patient shows evidence of passive immunity to exposure to Rh$_o$(D)-positive blood.
• Patient doesn't develop anaphylaxis after drug administration.
• Patient and family state understanding of drug therapy.

ribavirin
(righ-beh-VIGH-rin)
Copegus, Rebetol, Virazole

Pharmacologic class: synthetic nucleoside
Therapeutic class: antiviral
Pregnancy risk category: X

Indications and dosages
▶ **Hospitalized patients infected by RSV.** *Infants and young children:* 20-mg/ml solution delivered by small particle aerosol generator (SPAG-2) and mechanical ventilator or oxygen hood, face mask, or oxygen tent at about 12.5 L of mist per minute. Therapy lasts 12 to 18 hours daily for 3 to 7 days.
▶ **Chronic hepatitis C.** *Adults weighing 75 kg (165 lb) or less:* 1,000 mg Rebetol P.O. daily in divided doses (400 mg in morning, 600 mg in evening) with interferon alfa-2b 3 million units subcutaneously three times weekly. Or, 1,000 mg Copegus with 180 mcg of Pegasys (peginterferon alfa-2a).
Adults weighing more than 75 kg: 1,200 mg Rebetol P.O. divided b.i.d. (600 mg in morning, 600 mg in evening) with interferon alfa-2b, 3 million units subcutaneously three times weekly. Or, 1,200 mg Copegus with 180 mcg of Pegasys.

R

▶ **Chronic hepatitis C (regardless of geno-type) in HIV-infected patients who have not previously been treated with interferon.**
Adults: 800 mg (Copegus) P.O. daily given in two divided doses with peginterferon alfa-2a (Pegasys) 180 mcg subcutaneously weekly for 48 weeks.

Contraindications and cautions

• Contraindicated in patients hypersensitive to the drug or any of its components, and in those with creatinine clearance less than 50 ml/minute, history of significant or unstable cardiac disease, Child-Pugh class B or C, or hemoglobinopathies, such as sickle cell anemia and thalassemia.
• Use cautiously in patients with renal impairment.
⚠ **Lifespan:** In women who are or may become pregnant and in men whose sexual partners are pregnant, drug is contraindicated. Breast-feeding women should stop breast-feeding or use another drug, taking into consideration the importance of the drug. In children, capsules and tablets are contraindicated. In the elderly, use cautiously.

Adverse reactions

CNS: headache, dizziness, *seizures,* asthenia, *depression, suicide,* fatigue, anxiety, insomnia.
CV: *cardiac arrest,* hypotension, chest pains.
EENT: conjunctivitis, rhinitis, pharyngitis, lacrimation, rash or erythema of eyelids.
GI: nausea.
Hematologic: reticulocytosis, *severe anemia,* hemolytic anemia, *thrombocytopenia, neutropenia.*
Musculoskeletal: arthralgia, myalgia.
Respiratory: *worsening of respiratory state, bronchospasms, apnea,* bacterial pneumonia, *pneumothorax.*
Skin: rash.
Other: weight decrease, *flulike syndrome.*

Interactions

Drug-drug. *Acetaminophen; antacids containing magnesium, aluminum, or simethicone; aspirin; cimetidine:* May affect drug level. Monitor patient.
Didanosine: May increase toxicity. Avoid using together.
Stavudine, zidovudine: May decrease antiretroviral activity. Use together cautiously.

Effects on lab test results

• May increase bilirubin, AST, and ALT levels. May decrease hemoglobin level and hematocrit.
• May increase reticulocyte count. May decrease platelet and WBC counts.

Pharmacokinetics

Absorption: Some ribavirin is absorbed systemically.
Distribution: Concentrates in bronchial secretions.
Metabolism: Metabolized to 1,2,4-triazole-3-carboxamide (deribosylated ribavirin).
Excretion: Most of drug excreted in urine.
Half-life: First phase, 9¼ hours; second phase, 40 hours.

Route	Onset	Peak	Duration
Inhalation	Immediate	Immediate	Unknown

Action

Chemical effect: Inhibits viral activity by unknown mechanism, possibly by inhibiting RNA and DNA synthesis by depleting intracellular nucleotide pools.
Therapeutic effect: Inhibits RSV activity.

Available forms

Capsules: 200 mg
Powder to be reconstituted for inhalation: 6 g in 100-ml glass vial
Tablets: 200 mg, 400 mg
Oral solution: 40 mg/ml

NURSING PROCESS

⚐ Assessment
• Assess patient's respiratory infection before starting therapy, and regularly thereafter to monitor the drug's effectiveness.
• Monitor ventilator function. Drug may precipitate in ventilator apparatus, causing equipment malfunction with serious consequences.
• Watch for anemia in patient taking drug longer than 1 to 2 weeks.
• Be alert for adverse reactions.
• Assess patient's and family's knowledge of drug therapy.

⚐ Nursing diagnoses
• Infection related to presence of RSV

Reactions may be *common,* uncommon, *life-threatening*, or COMMON AND LIFE-THREATENING.

- Risk for injury related to drug-induced adverse CV reactions
- Deficient knowledge related to drug therapy

Planning and implementation

- Aerosol form is indicated only for severe lower respiratory tract infection caused by RSV. Start therapy pending test results, but existence of RSV infection must be documented.
- Most infants and children with RSV infection don't need treatment. Infants with underlying conditions, such as prematurity or cardiopulmonary disease, benefit most from using aerosol form of drug.
- Give drug by SPAG-2 only. Don't use any other aerosol generator.
- For reconstitution, use sterile USP water for injection, not bacteriostatic water. Water used to reconstitute this drug must not contain an antimicrobial.
- Discard solutions placed in SPAG-2 unit at least every 24 hours before adding newly reconstituted solution.
- Avoid unneeded occupational exposure to drug. Adverse effects reported in health care personnel exposed to aerosolized drug include eye irritation and headache.
- Capsules and tablets aren't effective as monotherapy for chronic hepatitis C.
- Store reconstituted solutions at room temperature for 24 hours.
- Stop drug at first sign of pancreatitis.

ALERT: Don't confuse ribavirin with riboflavin.

Patient teaching

- Inform parents of children with RSV infection of need for drug therapy, and answer their questions.
- Advise patient to use correct device.
- Explain to women of childbearing age and men with sexual partners of childbearing age the effects of drug on a fetus and the need to inform the prescriber immediately if pregnancy occurs.

Evaluation

- Patient is free from infection.
- Patient doesn't develop adverse CV reactions after drug administration.
- Parents state understanding of drug therapy.

rifabutin
(rif-uh-BYOO-tin)
Mycobutin

Pharmacologic class: semisynthetic ansamycin
Therapeutic class: antimycobacterial
Pregnancy risk category: B

Indications and dosages

▶ To prevent disseminated *Mycobacterium avium* complex (MAC) in patients with advanced HIV infection. *Adults:* 300 mg P.O. daily as single dose or divided b.i.d.

Contraindications and cautions

- Contraindicated in patients hypersensitive to drug or other rifamycin derivatives (such as rifampin).
- Use cautiously in patients with neutropenia and thrombocytopenia.

Lifespan: Use during pregnancy only when clearly needed. In breast-feeding women, drug isn't recommended. In children, safety and effectiveness haven't been established.

Adverse reactions

CNS: fever, headache.
CV: ECG changes.
GI: dyspepsia, eructation, flatulence, diarrhea, nausea, vomiting, abdominal pain.
GU: discolored urine.
Hematologic: anemia, eosinophilia, LEUKOPENIA, NEUTROPENIA, *thrombocytopenia.*
Musculoskeletal: myalgia.
Skin: *rash,* uveitis.

Interactions

Drug-drug. *Corticosteroids:* May decrease corticosteroid effects. Double dose of corticosteroids, if needed.
Cyclosporine: May reduce immunosuppressive effects. Don't use together.
Drugs metabolized by the liver, benzodiazepines, beta blockers, buspirone, doxycycline, hydantoins, indinavir, losartan, macrolides, methadone, morphine, nelfinavir, quinidine, theophylline, tricyclic antidepressants, zidovudine: May decrease level of these drugs. Because rifabutin, like rifampin, induces liver enzymes, it may lower levels of many other drugs as well. Monitor patient for effect.

R

Hormonal contraceptives: May decrease effectiveness. Instruct patient to use nonhormonal forms of birth control.
Warfarin: May decrease anticoagulation effect. Increase dose of anticoagulant.
Drug-food. *High-fat foods:* May slow absorption of drug. Discourage taking drug with high-fat meals.

Effects on lab test results
• May increase alkaline phosphatase, AST, and ALT levels. May decrease hemoglobin level and hematocrit.
• May increase eosinophil count. May decrease neutrophil, WBC, and platelet counts.

Pharmacokinetics
Absorption: Readily absorbed from GI tract.
Distribution: Because of its high lipophilicity, rifabutin demonstrates high propensity for distribution and intracellular tissue uptake. About 85% of drug is bound to proteins.
Metabolism: Metabolized in liver.
Excretion: Excreted primarily in urine; about 30% excreted in feces. *Half-life:* 45 hours.

Route	Onset	Peak	Duration
P.O.	Unknown	1½–4 hr	Unknown

Action
Chemical effect: Blocks bacterial protein synthesis by inhibiting DNA-dependent RNA polymerase in susceptible bacteria.
Therapeutic effect: Prevents disseminated MAC in patients with advanced HIV infection.

Available forms
Capsules: 150 mg

NURSING PROCESS

⚕ Assessment
• Assess patient's condition before starting therapy, and regularly thereafter to monitor the drug's effectiveness.
• Perform baseline hematologic studies and repeat periodically.
• Be alert for adverse reactions and drug interactions.
• Assess patient's and family's knowledge of drug therapy.

⚕ Nursing diagnoses
• Infection related to advanced HIV infection and decreased immune system
• Ineffective protection related to drug-induced adverse hematologic reactions
• Deficient knowledge related to drug therapy

⚕ Planning and implementation
• High-fat meals slow rate but not extent of absorption.
• Give drug with food. Mix with soft foods for patient who has difficulty swallowing.
• No evidence exists that drug will provide effective prophylaxis against *Mycobacterium tuberculosis.* Patients requiring prophylaxis against both *M. tuberculosis* and MAC may require rifampin and rifabutin.
⚕ ALERT: Don't confuse rifabutin, rifampin, and rifapentine.
Patient teaching
• Tell patient that drug may turn urine, feces, sputum, saliva, tears, and skin brownish-orange. Tell him not to wear soft contacts because they may be permanently stained.
• Instruct patient to report photophobia, excessive lacrimation, or eye pain. Drug may rarely cause uveitis.

⚕ Evaluation
• Patient doesn't develop disseminated MAC.
• Patient maintains normal hematologic values throughout therapy.
• Patient and family state understanding of drug therapy.

rifampin (rifampicin)
(rih-FAM-pin)
Rifadin, Rifadin IV, Rimactane, Rimycin◊, Rofact◆

Pharmacologic class: macrocytic antibiotic
Therapeutic class: antituberculotic
Pregnancy risk category: C

Indications and dosages
▶ **Pulmonary tuberculosis.** *Adults:* 10 mg/kg P.O. or I.V. daily in single dose. Maximum, 600 mg daily.
Children older than age 5: 10 to 20 mg/kg P.O. or I.V. daily in single dose. Maximum, 600 mg

daily. Use with other antituberculotics is recommended.

► **Meningococcal carriers.** *Adults:* 600 mg P.O. or I.V. b.i.d. for 2 days or once daily for 4 days.
Children ages 1 month to 12 years: 10 mg/kg P.O. or I.V. b.i.d. for 2 days or once daily for 4 days. Maximum, 600 mg daily.
Neonates: 5 mg/kg P.O. or I.V. b.i.d. for 2 days.

► **Prophylaxis of** *Haemophilus influenzae* **type B.** *Adults and children:* 20 mg/kg P.O. daily for 4 days. Maximum, 600 mg daily.

► **Leprosy‡.** *Adults:* 600 mg P.O. once monthly, usually with other drugs.

▼ I.V. administration

• When dextrose is contraindicated, drug may be diluted with normal saline solution for injection.
• Reconstitute vial with 10 ml of sterile water for injection to make solution containing 60 mg/ml.
• Add to 100 ml of D₅W and infuse over 30 minutes, or add to 500 ml of D₅W and infuse over 3 hours.

⊗ **Incompatibilities**
Diltiazem, minocycline, I.V. solutions other than dextrose or normal saline.

Contraindications and cautions

• Contraindicated in patients hypersensitive to the drug or any of its components.
• Use cautiously and under strict medical supervision in patients with liver disease.
⚖ **Lifespan:** In pregnant women, use only when benefits outweigh potential risks to the fetus. During the last 2 weeks of pregnancy, use of the drug may lead to postnatal hemorrhage in the mother or infant. Monitor clotting factors closely. In breast-feeding women, use cautiously. It's unknown if the drug appears in breast milk.

Adverse reactions

CNS: ataxia, behavioral changes, confusion, dizziness, fatigue, headache, drowsiness, generalized numbness.
CV: *shock.*
EENT: visual disturbances, exudative conjunctivitis.
GI: epigastric distress, anorexia, nausea, vomiting, abdominal pain, diarrhea, flatulence, sore mouth and tongue, *pseudomembranous colitis, pancreatitis.*
GU: hemoglobinuria, hematuria, *acute renal failure,* menstrual disturbances.

Hematologic: eosinophilia, *transient leukopenia, thrombocytopenia,* hemolytic anemia.
Hepatic: *hepatotoxicity,* worsening of porphyria.
Metabolic: hyperuricemia.
Musculoskeletal: osteomalacia.
Respiratory: shortness of breath, wheezing.
Skin: pruritus, urticaria, rash.
Other: flulike syndrome, discoloration of body fluids.

Interactions

Drug-drug. *Analgesics, anticoagulants, anticonvulsants, barbiturates, beta blockers, chloramphenicol, clofibrate, corticosteroids, cyclosporine, dapsone, diazepam, digoxin, disopyramide, doxycycline, hormonal contraceptives, macrolides, methadone, mexiletine, opioids, progestins, protease inhibitors, quinidine, sulfonylureas, theophylline, verapamil:* May reduce effectiveness of these drugs. Avoid using together.
Halothane: May increase risk of hepatotoxicity in both drugs. Monitor liver function closely.
Ketoconazole, para-aminosalicylate sodium: May interfere with absorption of rifampin. Give these drugs 8 to 12 hours apart.
Probenecid: May increase rifampin levels. Use cautiously.
Drug-herb. *Kava:* May increase the risk of hepatotoxicity. Discourage use.
Drug-lifestyle. *Alcohol use:* May increase risk of hepatotoxicity. Discourage using together.

Effects on lab test results

• May increase ALT, AST, alkaline phosphatase, bilirubin, BUN, creatinine, and uric acid levels. May decrease hemoglobin level and hematocrit.
• May increase eosinophil count. May decrease platelet and WBC counts.

Pharmacokinetics

Absorption: Complete. Food delays absorption.
Distribution: Wide. 84% to 91% protein-bound.
Metabolism: Extensive.
Excretion: Primarily in bile; drug, but not metabolite, is reabsorbed. Some in urine. *Half-life:* 1¼ to 5 hours.

Route	Onset	Peak	Duration
P.O.	Unknown	2–4 hr	Unknown
I.V.	Unknown	Unknown	Unknown

Action

Chemical effect: Kills bacteria by inhibiting DNA-dependent RNA polymerase, thus impairing RNA synthesis.
Therapeutic effect: Kills susceptible bacteria.

Available forms

Capsules: 150 mg, 300 mg
Injection: 600 mg

NURSING PROCESS

⚕ Assessment

• Assess patient's infection before starting therapy, and regularly thereafter to monitor the drug's effectiveness.
• Monitor liver function, hematopoiesis, and uric acid levels.
• Be alert for adverse reactions and drug interactions.
• Watch closely for signs of hepatic impairment.
• If adverse GI reaction occurs, monitor hydration.
• Assess patient's and family's knowledge of drug therapy.

Nursing diagnoses

• Infection related to presence of susceptible bacteria
• Risk for deficient fluid volume related to drug-induced adverse reactions
• Deficient knowledge related to drug therapy

Planning and implementation

• Give drug 1 hour before or 2 hours after meals for optimal absorption; if GI irritation occurs, patient may take with meals.
• Drug may inhibit standard assays for folate and vitamin B_{12}. Consider alternative assay method.
• Giving at least one additional antituberculotic is recommended.
• **ALERT:** Don't confuse rifampin, rifabutin, and rifapentine.

Patient teaching

• Warn patient about drowsiness and red-orange discoloration of urine, feces, saliva, sweat, sputum, and tears. Soft contact lenses may be permanently stained.
• Advise patient not to drink alcohol while taking the drug.

✓ Evaluation

• Patient is free from infection.
• Patient maintains adequate hydration throughout therapy.
• Patient and family state understanding of drug therapy.

rifapentine
(rif-ah-PEN-tin)
Priftin

Pharmacologic class: macrocytic antibiotic
Therapeutic class: antituberculotic
Pregnancy risk category: C

Indications and dosages

▶ **Pulmonary tuberculosis, with at least one other antituberculotic to which the isolate is susceptible.** *Adults:* During intensive phase of short-course therapy, 600 mg P.O. twice weekly for 2 months, with an interval between doses of not less than 3 days (72 hours). During the continuation phase of short-course therapy, 600 mg P.O. once weekly for 4 months with isoniazid or another drug to which the isolate is susceptible.

Contraindications and cautions

• Contraindicated in patients hypersensitive to rifamycin (rifapentine, rifampin, or rifabutin).
• Use drug cautiously and with frequent monitoring in patients with liver disease.
• **Lifespan:** During last 2 weeks of pregnancy, drug may lead to postnatal hemorrhage in mother or infant; monitor clotting parameters closely. Use with caution in breast-feeding women. It isn't known if drug is excreted in breast milk.

Adverse reactions

CNS: pain, headache, dizziness.
CV: hypertension.
GI: anorexia, nausea, vomiting, dyspepsia, diarrhea, *pseudomembranous colitis.*
GU: pyuria, proteinuria, hematuria, urinary casts.
Hematologic: *neutropenia, lymphopenia,* anemia, *leukopenia,* thrombocytosis.
Metabolic: *hyperuricemia.*
Musculoskeletal: arthralgia.
Respiratory: hemoptysis.
Skin: rash, pruritus, acne, maculopapular rash.

Interactions

Drug-drug. *Antiarrhythmics, antibiotics, anticonvulsants, antifungals, barbiturates, benzodiazepines, beta blockers, calcium channel blockers, clofibrate, corticosteroids, digoxin, haloperidol, HIV protease inhibitors, hormonal contraceptives, immunosuppressants, levothyroxine, opioid analgesics (methadone), oral anticoagulants, oral hypoglycemics, progestins, quinine, reverse transcriptase inhibitors, sildenafil, theophylline, tricyclic antidepressants:* May induce metabolism of CYP, decreasing the activity of these drugs. Dosage adjustments may be needed.

Effects on lab test results

• May increase uric acid, ALT, and AST levels. May decrease hemoglobin level and hematocrit.
• May increase platelet count. May decrease neutrophil and WBC counts.

Pharmacokinetics

Absorption: Relative bioavailability is 70%.
Distribution: About 98% bound to proteins.
Metabolism: Hydrolyzed by an esterase enzyme to the microbiologically active 25-desacetyl rifapentine. Rifapentine contributes 62% to drug's activity and 25-desacetyl contributes 38%.
Excretion: About 17% is excreted in urine and 70% in feces. *Half-life:* 13 hours.

Route	Onset	Peak	Duration
P.O.	Unknown	5–6 hr	Unknown

Action

Chemical effect: Kills susceptible strains of *Mycobacterium tuberculosis,* both inside and outside cells, by inhibiting DNA-dependent RNA polymerase. Rifapentine and rifampin share similar antimicrobial action.
Therapeutic effect: Kills susceptible bacteria.

Available forms

Tablets (film-coated): 150 mg

NURSING PROCESS

Assessment

• Assess patient's condition before starting therapy, and regularly thereafter to monitor the drug's effectiveness.

• Assess patient's understanding of disease and stress importance of strict compliance with drug and daily companion medications, as well as needed follow-up visits and laboratory tests.
• Monitor liver function, CBC, and uric acid levels.
• Monitor patient for persistent or severe diarrhea and notify prescriber if it occurs.
• Assess patient's and family's knowledge of drug therapy.

Nursing diagnoses

• Infection related to patient's underlying condition
• Noncompliance related to long-term therapeutic regimen
• Deficient knowledge related to drug therapy

Planning and implementation

• Give pyridoxine (vitamin B_6) during rifapentine therapy to a malnourished patient, a patient predisposed to neuropathy (alcoholic, diabetic), or an adolescent.
• Drug must be given with appropriate daily companion drugs. Compliance with all drugs, especially with daily companion drugs on the days when rifapentine isn't given, is crucial for early sputum conversion and protection from tuberculosis relapse.
ALERT: Don't confuse rifampin, rifabutin, and rifapentine.
Patient teaching
• Stress importance of strict compliance with regimen of drug and daily companion drugs, as well as needed follow-up visits and laboratory tests.
• Advise patient to use barrier-method of birth control.
• Tell patient to take drug with food if nausea, vomiting, or GI upset occurs.
• Instruct patient to notify prescriber if any of the following occur: fever, loss of appetite, malaise, nausea, vomiting, darkened urine, yellowish discoloration of skin and eyes, pain or swelling of joints, and excessive loose stools or diarrhea.
• Instruct patient to protect pills from excessive heat.
• Tell patient that drug can turn body fluids red-orange. Contact lenses can become permanently stained.

R

☑ Evaluation
- Patient experiences sputum conversion and recovers from tuberculosis.
- Patient is compliant with therapeutic regimen.
- Patient and family state understanding of drug therapy.

rifaximin
rih-FAX-ih-mehn
Xifaxan

Pharmacologic class: rifamycin antibacterial
Therapeutic class: nonabsorbed antibiotic
Pregnancy risk category: C

Indications and dosages
▶ **Traveler's diarrhea caused by noninvasive strains of** *Escherichia coli. Adults and children age 12 and older:* 200 mg P.O. t.i.d. for 3 days.

Contraindications and cautions
- Contraindicated in patients hypersensitive to rifaximin or any rifamycin antibacterial.
- ⚜ **Lifespan:** In pregnant women, use only if benefits outweigh potential risks to the fetus. In breast-feeding women, use cautiously. It isn't known if drug appears in breast milk. In children younger than age 12, safety and effectiveness haven't been established.

Adverse reactions
CNS: fever, headache.
GI: abdominal pain, constipation, defecation urgency, flatulence, nausea, rectal tenesmus, vomiting.

Interactions
None significant.

Effects on lab test results
None reported.

Pharmacokinetics
Absorption: Poor.
Distribution: In the gut.
Metabolism: Not specified.
Excretion: In feces as unchanged drug.

Route	Onset	Peak	Duration
P.O.	Unknown	Unknown	Unknown

Action
Chemical effect: Drug binds to the beta-subunit of bacterial DNA–dependent RNA polymerase, which inhibits bacterial RNA synthesis and kills the *E. coli.*
Therapeutic effect: Kills susceptible bacteria and resolves traveler's diarrhea.

Available forms
Tablets: 200 mg

NURSING PROCESS

☞ Assessment
- Assess patient's condition before starting therapy, and regularly thereafter to monitor the drug's effectiveness.
- Monitor patient's hydration status.
- Be alert for adverse drug reactions.
- Monitor patient for overgrowth of nonsusceptible organisms.
- Assess patient's and family's knowledge of drug therapy.

☺ Nursing diagnoses
- Diarrhea related to infection with *E. coli*
- Risk for imbalanced fluid volume related to underlying medical condition and drug-induced adverse GI effects
- Deficient knowledge related to drug therapy

▶ Planning and implementation
- Don't use drug in patients whose illness may be caused by *Campylobacter jejuni, Shigella,* or *Salmonella.*
- ⓧ **ALERT:** Don't use drug in patients with blood in the stool, diarrhea with fever, or diarrhea from pathogens other than *E. coli.*
- Stop drug if diarrhea worsens or lasts longer than 24 to 48 hours. The patient may need a different antibiotic.
- Patient who has diarrhea after antibiotic therapy may have pseudomembranous colitis, which may range from mild to life-threatening.
Patient teaching
- Explain that drug may be taken with or without food.
- Tell patient to take all of the prescribed drug, even if he feels better before the drug is finished.
- Advise patient to notify his prescriber if diarrhea worsens or lasts longer than 1 or 2 days af-

ter starting treatment. A different treatment may be needed.

• Tell patient to call the prescriber if he develops a fever or has blood in his stool.

• Explain that this drug is only for treating diarrhea caused by contaminated foods or beverages while traveling and not for any other type of infection.

• Caution patient not to share this drug with others.

☑ Evaluation

• Patient's diarrhea resolves with drug therapy.
• Patient maintains adequate hydration.
• Patient and family state understanding of drug therapy.

riluzole
(RIGH-loo-zohl)
Rilutek

Pharmacologic class: benzothiazole
Therapeutic class: neuroprotector
Pregnancy risk category: C

Indications and dosages

▶ **Amyotrophic lateral sclerosis (ALS).**
Adults: 50 mg P.O. q 12 hours on empty stomach.

Contraindications and cautions

• Contraindicated in patients hypersensitive to the drug or any of its components.

• Use cautiously in patients with hepatic or renal dysfunction. Also use cautiously in women and Japanese patients (who may have a lower metabolic capacity to eliminate riluzole compared with men and white patients, respectively).

⚠ **Lifespan:** In pregnant patients, use only if benefits outweigh potential risks; risks specific to fetus aren't known. In breast-feeding women, drug isn't recommended. In children, safety and effectiveness haven't been established. In the elderly, use cautiously.

Adverse reactions

CNS: headache, aggravation reaction, *asthenia,* hypertonia, depression, dizziness, insomnia, malaise, somnolence, vertigo, circumoral paresthesia.

CV: hypertension, tachycardia, palpitations, orthostatic hypotension, peripheral edema.
EENT: rhinitis, sinusitis.
GI: abdominal pain, *nausea,* vomiting, dyspepsia, anorexia, diarrhea, flatulence, stomatitis, dry mouth, oral candidiasis.
GU: UTI, dysuria.
Hematologic: *neutropenia.*
Metabolic: weight loss.
Musculoskeletal: back pain, arthralgia.
Respiratory: *decreased lung function,* increased cough.
Skin: pruritus, eczema, alopecia, exfoliative dermatitis.
Other: tooth disorder, phlebitis.

Interactions

Drug-drug. *Allopurinol, methyldopa, sulfasalazine:* May increase risk of hepatotoxicity. Monitor patient closely.
Inducers of CYP 1A2 (omeprazole, rifampicin): May increase riluzole elimination. Monitor patient for loss of therapeutic effect.
Potential inhibitors of CYP 1A2 (amitriptyline, phenacetin, quinolones, theophylline): May decrease riluzole elimination. Monitor patient closely for toxicity.
Drug-food. *Any food:* May decrease drug bioavailability. Give 1 hour before or 2 hours after meals.
Caffeine: May decrease riluzole elimination. Monitor patient for adverse reactions.
Charbroiled foods: May increase riluzole elimination. Discourage patient from eating these foods while on drug therapy.
Drug-lifestyle. *Alcohol use:* May increase risk of hepatotoxicity. Discourage using together.
Smoking: May increase riluzole elimination. Urge patient to stop smoking.

Effects on lab test results

• May increase AST, ALT, bilirubin, and GGT levels.
• May decrease neutrophil count.

Pharmacokinetics

Absorption: Well absorbed from GI tract, with average absolute oral bioavailability of about 60%. High-fat meal decreases absorption.
Distribution: 96% protein-bound.
Metabolism: Extensively metabolized in liver.

R

Excretion: Excreted primarily in urine, with small amount in feces. *Half-life:* 12 hours with repeated doses.

Route	Onset	Peak	Duration
P.O.	Unknown	Unknown	Unknown

Action

Chemical effect: Unknown.
Therapeutic effect: Improves signs and symptoms of ALS.

Available forms

Tablets: 50 mg

NURSING PROCESS

Assessment
• Obtain history of patient's ALS.
• Obtain liver and renal function studies and CBC before and during therapy.
• Monitor patient carefully because rare but severe cases of neutropenia have occurred.
• Assess patient's and family's knowledge of drug therapy.

Nursing diagnoses
• Impaired physical mobility related to ALS.
• Risk for deficient fluid volume related to adverse GI reactions
• Deficient knowledge related to drug therapy

Planning and implementation
• If baseline liver function test results (especially bilirubin level) rise, don't use drug. Drug may increase aminotransferase level. If level exceeds 10 times upper limit of normal, or if jaundice develops, notify prescriber.
• Give drug at least 1 hour before or 2 hours after a meal.
Patient teaching
• Tell patient to take drug at same time each day. If he misses a dose, instruct him not to double the dose but to take the next dose as scheduled.
• Instruct patient to report febrile illness; check his WBC count.
• Warn patient to avoid hazardous activities until drug's CNS effects are known.
• Advise patient to limit alcohol intake during therapy.
• Tell patient to store drug at room temperature, protected from bright light and out of children's reach.

Evaluation
• Patient responds well to therapy.
• Patient maintains adequate hydration.
• Patient and family state understanding of drug therapy.

risedronate sodium
(ri-SEH-droe-nate SOE-dee-um)
Actonel

Pharmacologic class: bisphosphonate
Therapeutic class: antiresorptive
Pregnancy risk category: C

Indications and dosages

▶ **To prevent and treat postmenopausal osteoporosis.** *Adults:* 5-mg tablet P.O. once daily, or 35-mg tablet once weekly. Give at least 30 minutes before first food or drink (except water) of the day.
▶ **Glucocorticoid-induced osteoporosis in patients who are either starting or continuing glucocorticoid therapy at 7.5 mg or more of prednisone or equivalent daily.** *Adults:* 5 mg P.O. daily.
▶ **Paget's disease.** *Adults:* 30 mg P.O. daily for 2 months. If relapse occurs or alkaline phosphatase level doesn't normalize, give same dose for 2 months or longer after first course.

Contraindications and cautions

• Contraindicated in patients hypersensitive to the drug or any of its components, and in patients who are hypocalcemic or unable to stand or sit upright for 30 minutes after administration.
• Drug isn't recommended for patients with severe renal impairment (creatinine clearance below 30 ml/minute).
• Use cautiously in patients with upper GI disorders such as dysphagia, esophagitis, and esophageal or gastric ulcers.
⚜ **Lifespan:** In pregnant women, use only when benefits outweigh potential risks to the fetus. In breast-feeding women, use cautiously. It isn't known if drug appears in breast milk. In children, safety and effectiveness of drug haven't been established.

Reactions may be *common,* uncommon, *life-threatening*, or COMMON AND LIFE-THREATENING.

Adverse reactions

CNS: asthenia, *headache,* depression, dizziness, insomnia, anxiety, neuralgia, vertigo, hypertonia, paresthesia, *pain.*
CV: *hypertension,* CV disorder, chest pain, peripheral edema.
EENT: pharyngitis, rhinitis, sinusitis, cataract, conjunctivitis, otitis media, amblyopia, tinnitus.
GI: nausea, diarrhea, abdominal pain, esophageal irritation and ulceration, flatulence, gastritis, rectal disorder, constipation.
GU: *UTI,* cystitis.
Hematologic: anemia.
Musculoskeletal: *arthralgia,* neck pain, *back pain,* myalgia, bone pain, leg cramps, bursitis, tendon disorder.
Respiratory: dyspnea, pneumonia, bronchitis.
Skin: ecchymosis, *rash,* pruritus, *skin carcinoma.*
Other: tooth disorder, *infection.*

Interactions

Drug-drug. *Calcium supplements, antacids that contain calcium, magnesium, or aluminum:* May interfere with risedronate absorption. Advise patient to separate administration times.
Drug-food. *Any food:* May interfere with risedronate absorption. Advise patient to take drug at least 30 minutes before first food or drink of the day (other than water).

Effects on lab test results

• May decrease calcium, phosphorus, and hemoglobin levels and hematocrit.

Pharmacokinetics

Absorption: Absorbed via the GI tract. Steady state occurs in 57 days. Mean absolute oral bioavailability of the 30-mg tablet is 0.63%. Because food alters absorption, give drug at least 30 minutes before breakfast.
Distribution: The mean steady-state volume of distribution is 6.3 L/kg. Protein-binding is about 24%.
Metabolism: No evidence of systemic metabolism.
Excretion: About 50% of a dose is excreted in urine within 24 hours. Unabsorbed drug is eliminated unchanged in feces. *Half-life:* 1½ hours to 20 days. *Half-life:* Unknown.

Route	Onset	Peak	Duration
P.O.	1 hr	Unknown	Unknown

Action

Chemical effect: Reverses the loss of bone mineral density by reducing bone turnover and bone resorption by inhibiting osteoclasts. In patients with Paget's disease, drug causes bone turnover to return to normal.
Therapeutic effect: Reverses the loss of bone mineral density.

Available forms

Tablets: 5 mg, 30 mg, 35 mg

NURSING PROCESS

✍ Assessment

• Assess underlying condition before starting therapy, and regularly thereafter to monitor the drug's effectiveness.
• Evaluate renal function before beginning therapy. Drug isn't recommended for patients with creatinine clearance below 30 ml/minute.
• Assess patient for the following risk factors for the development of osteoporosis: family history, previous fracture, smoking, a decrease in bone mineral density below the premenopausal mean, a thin body frame, white or Asian race, and early menopause.
• Assess patient's and family's knowledge of drug therapy.

⊕ Nursing diagnoses

• Risk for injury related to decreased bone mass
• Ineffective health maintenance related to underlying disease
• Deficient knowledge related to risedronate sodium therapy

❯ Planning and implementation

Ⓢ **ALERT:** Follow dosage instructions carefully because benefits of the drug may be compromised by failure to take it according to instructions. Give drug at least 30 minutes before patient's first food or drink (other than water) of the day.
• Give drug with 6 to 8 oz plain water to facilitate delivery to the stomach. Don't allow patient to lie down for 30 minutes after taking drug.
Ⓢ **ALERT:** Bisphosphonates have been linked to such GI disorders as dysphagia, esophagitis, and esophageal or gastric ulcers. Monitor patient for symptoms of esophageal disease (such as dysphagia, retrosternal pain, or severe persistent or worsening heartburn).

R

Rapid onset   *Liquid form contains alcohol.   ◆ Canada   ◇ Australia   †OTC   ∥Photoguide   ‡Off-label use

• If patient's dietary intake of calcium and vitamin D is inadequate, give supplements. However, because calcium supplements and drugs containing calcium, aluminum, or magnesium may interfere with absorption, separate doses.
• Store drug at 68° to 77° F (20° to 25° C).
• Bisphosphonates can interfere with bone-imaging agents.

Patient teaching
• Explain that risedronate is used to replace bone lost as a result of certain disease processes.
• Instruct patient to adhere to dosage instructions.
• Tell patient to take drug at least 30 minutes before the first food or drink (other than water) of the day. Tell patient to take drug with 6 to 8 oz of water while sitting or standing. Warn against lying down for 30 minutes after taking drug.
• Advise patient not to chew or suck the tablet because doing so could cause mouth irritation.
• Advise patient to notify the prescriber immediately if symptoms of esophageal disease (difficulty or pain when swallowing, retrosternal pain, or severe heartburn) develop.
• Advise patient to take calcium and vitamin D if dietary intake is inadequate, but to take them at a different time than risedronate.
• Advise patient to stop smoking and drinking alcohol, as appropriate. Also, instruct patient to perform weight-bearing exercise.
• Tell patient to store drug in a cool (room temperature), dry place and away from children.
• Urge patient to read the patient information guide before starting therapy.
• Tell patient if he misses a dose of the 35-mg tablet, he should take 1 tablet on the morning after he remembers and return to taking 1 tablet once a week, as originally scheduled on his chosen day. Patients shouldn't take 2 tablets on the same day.

☑ Evaluation
• Patient doesn't suffer any injury related to decreased bone mass.
• Patient shows improvement in underlying condition.
• Patient and family state understanding of drug therapy.

risperidone
(ris-PER-ih-dohn)
Risperdal◆, Risperdal Consta, Risperdal M-Tab◆

Pharmacologic class: benzisoxazole derivative
Therapeutic class: antipsychotic
Pregnancy risk category: C

Indications and dosages

▶ **Short-term therapy for schizophrenia.**
Adults: Initially, 1 mg P.O. b.i.d. Increase in increments of 1 mg b.i.d. on days 2 and 3 to a target dosage of 3 mg b.i.d. Alternatively, 1 mg P.O. on day 1, increase to 2 mg once daily on day 2, and 4 mg once daily on day 3. Wait at least 1 week before adjusting dosage further. Adjust doses by 1 to 2 mg. Maximum, 8 mg daily. Once tolerance to P.O. formulation has been established, patient may be switched to I.M. formulation, if appropriate. Give 25 mg by deep I.M. gluteal injection q 2 weeks; alternating injections between the two buttocks. Adjust dose no sooner than q 4 weeks. Maximum, 50 mg I.M. q 2 weeks. Continue oral antipsychotic for 3 weeks after first I.M. injection. Then stop oral therapy.
▶ **Delaying relapse in long-term therapy for schizophrenia.** *Adults:* Initially, 1 mg P.O. on day 1, increase to 2 mg once daily on day 2, and 4 mg once daily on day 3. Dosage range, 2 to 8 mg daily.
▶ **Monotherapy or combination therapy with lithium or valproate for short-term (3-week) treatment of acute manic or mixed episodes in bipolar I disorder.** *Adults:* 2 to 3 mg P.O. once daily. Adjust dose by 1 mg daily. Dosage range, 1 to 6 mg daily.
☒ **Adjust-a-dose:** For elderly or debilitated patients, hypotensive patients, or patients with severe renal or hepatic impairment, initially give 0.5 mg P.O. b.i.d. Increase dosage in increments of 0.5 mg b.i.d. Increase dosages more than 1.5 mg b.i.d. at intervals of at least 1 week. Subsequent switches to once-daily dosage may be made after patient has received a twice-daily regimen for 2 or 3 days at the target dose.

Contraindications and cautions

• Contraindicated in patients hypersensitive to the drug or any of its components.

• Use cautiously in patients with prolonged QT interval, CV disease, cerebrovascular disease, dehydration, hypovolemia, history of seizures, exposure to extreme heat, or conditions that could affect metabolism or hemodynamic responses. Also use cautiously in patients at risk for aspiration pneumonia.

• Use I.M. injection cautiously in those with hepatic or renal impairment. Stabilize patient on oral drug before switching to I.M. injection.

※ **Lifespan:** In pregnant women, use cautiously. In breast-feeding women, drug is contraindicated. In children, safety and effectiveness haven't been established. In elderly patients with dementia, drug is contraindicated.

Adverse reactions

CNS: *neuroleptic malignant syndrome,* somnolence, extrapyramidal reactions, headache, insomnia, agitation, anxiety, tardive dyskinesia, aggressiveness, dizziness, *suicide attempt,* fever; *transient ischemic attack or stroke in elderly patients with dementia;* hallucination, abnormal thinking and dreaming, akathisia, parkinsonism, tremor, hypoesthesia, fatigue, pain, depression, nervousness (I.M.).

CV: tachycardia, chest pain, orthostatic hypotension, *prolonged QT interval;* peripheral edema, syncope, hypertension (I.M.).

EENT: *rhinitis,* sinusitis, pharyngitis, abnormal vision; ear disorder (I.M.).

GI: *constipation, nausea, vomiting, dyspepsia, abdominal pain, anorexia;* dry mouth, toothache, increased saliva, tooth disorder, diarrhea (I.M.).

Hematologic: anemia.

Metabolic: *weight gain, hyperglycemia;* weight decrease (I.M.).

Musculoskeletal: arthralgia, back pain; leg pain, myalgia (I.M.).

Respiratory: coughing, upper respiratory infection.

Skin: rash, dry skin, photosensitivity; acne, injection site pain (I.M.).

Interactions

Drug-drug. *Antihypertensives:* May enhance hypotensive effects. Monitor blood pressure.

Carbamazepine: May increase risperidone clearance, leading to decreased effectiveness. Monitor patient closely.

Clozapine: May decrease risperidone clearance, increasing toxicity. Monitor patient closely.

CNS depressants: May cause additive CNS depression. Avoid using together.

Dopamine agonists, levodopa: May antagonize the effects of these drugs. Monitor patient closely.

Fluoxetine, paroxetine: May increase risperidone levels, increasing the risk of adverse reactions, including serotonin syndrome. Monitor patient closely and adjust risperidone dose as needed.

Drug-lifestyle. *Alcohol use:* May cause additive CNS depression. Discourage using together.

Sun exposure: May increase photosensitivity reactions. Discourage prolonged or unprotected sun exposure.

Effects on lab test results

• May increase glucose and prolactin levels. May decrease hemoglobin level and hematocrit.

Pharmacokinetics

Absorption: Well absorbed; absolute oral bioavailability is 70%. Slowly absorbed via I.M. injection.

Distribution: Protein-binding is about 90% for risperidone and 77% for its major active metabolite.

Metabolism: Extensively metabolized in liver.

Excretion: Metabolite excreted in urine. *Half-life:* 3 to 20 hours.

Route	Onset	Peak	Duration
P.O.	Unknown	1 hr	Unknown
I.M.	3 wk	4–6 wk	7 wk

Action

Chemical effect: Blocks dopamine and serotonin receptors as well as alpha₁, alpha₂, and H₁ receptors in the CNS.

Therapeutic effect: Relieves signs and symptoms of psychosis.

Available forms

Oral solution: 1 mg/ml
Orally disintegrating tablets: 0.5 mg, 1 mg, 2 mg
Powder for I.M. injection: 25 mg, 37.5 mg, 50 mg
Tablets: 0.25 mg, 0.5 mg, 1 mg, 2 mg, 3 mg, 4 mg

R

NURSING PROCESS

⚖ Assessment
• Assess patient's psychosis before starting therapy, and regularly thereafter to monitor the drug's effectiveness.
• Assess blood pressure before starting therapy, and monitor regularly. Watch for orthostatic hypotension, especially during dose adjustment.
• Monitor CBC, liver functions tests, ECG, serum prolactin, and routine chemistry during prolonged administration.
• Be alert for adverse reactions and drug interactions.
⑤ ALERT: Watch for tardive dyskinesia. It may occur after prolonged use; it may not appear until months or years later and may disappear spontaneously or persist for life despite stopping the drug.
• Assess patient's and family's knowledge of drug therapy.

⊕ Nursing diagnoses
• Disturbed thought processes related to presence of psychosis
• Risk for injury related to drug-induced adverse CNS reactions
• Deficient knowledge related to drug therapy

▷ Planning and implementation
⑤ ALERT: Fatal hyperglycemia may occur in a patient taking atypical antipsychotics. Monitor patient with diabetes regularly. For patients with risk factors for diabetes, perform fasting glucose testing at baseline and periodically. Monitor all patients for symptoms of hyperglycemia, including excessive thirst, hunger, frequent urinating, and weakness; if symptoms develop, perform fasting glucose testing. Hyperglycemia may resolve once therapy is stopped.
• When restarting therapy for patient who has been off drug, follow 3-day dose initiation schedule.
• When switching patient to drug from another antipsychotic, stop other drug immediately when risperidone therapy starts.
• Orally disintegrating tablets contain phenylalanine.
• Give oral antipsychotic for the first 3 weeks of I.M. injection therapy because of injection's prolonged onset of action. Then stop oral therapy.
• To reconstitute I.M. injection, remove dose pack from the refrigerator and allow it to reach

room temperature. Inject premeasured diluent into vial and shake vigorously for at least 10 seconds. Suspension will appear uniform, thick, and milky; particles will be visible, but no dry particles remain. Manufacturer recommends that drug be used immediately; suspension must be used within 6 hours of reconstitution. If more than 2 minutes pass before injection, shake vigorously again. See manufacturer's package insert for more detailed instructions.
• Store I.M. injection kit in refrigerator and protect from light. Drug can be stored at temperatures less than 77° F (25° C) for no more than 7 days before administration.
⑤ ALERT: Fatal cerebrovascular adverse events, such as stroke or transient ischemic attacks, may occur in elderly patients with dementia.
Patient teaching
• Warn patient to rise slowly, avoid hot showers, and use extra caution during first few days of therapy to avoid fainting.
• Warn patient to avoid activities that require alertness until the drug's CNS effects are known. Drowsiness and dizziness usually subside after a few days.
• Tell patient not to drink alcohol and to avoid prolonged exposure to sunlight during therapy.
• Tell patient to use sunblock and to wear protective clothing in sunlight.
• Advise patient to use caution in hot weather to prevent heatstroke; drug may affect the body's ability to regulate temperature.
• Tell woman to notify prescriber if she is or plans to become pregnant during therapy and for at least 12 weeks after last I.M. injection.
• Warn patient not to breast-feed during treatment and for at least 12 weeks after last I.M. injection.
• Inform patient that drug may be taken with or without food.
• Tell patient to dissolve orally disintegrating tablets on tongue. Instruct him not to remove tablets from blister pack until just before use.
• Tell patient not to split or chew orally disintegrating tablets.

☑ Evaluation
• Patient behavior and communication indicate improved thought processes.
• Patient doesn't experience injury as result of drug-induced adverse CNS reactions.
• Patient and family state understanding of drug therapy.

ritonavir
(rih-TOH-nuh-veer)
Norvir

Pharmacologic class: protease inhibitor
Therapeutic class: antiretroviral
Pregnancy risk category: B

Indications and dosages

▶ **HIV infection.** *Adults:* 600 mg P.O. b.i.d.
with meals. If adverse events occur, may give
300 mg b.i.d.; then increase at 2-to 3-day intervals by 100 mg b.i.d. If given with saquinavir,
reduce saquinavir to 400 mg P.O. b.i.d. and ritonavir to 400 or 600 mg P.O. b.i.d.
Children age 1 month and older: Initially,
250 mg/m² P.O. b.i.d. Increase by 50 mg/m²
b.i.d. at 2- to 3-day intervals to target dose of
400 mg/m² b.i.d.

Contraindications and cautions

• Contraindicated in patients hypersensitive to
the drug or any of its components, and in those
who are taking dihydroergotamine or ergotamine drugs. Also contraindicated with alfuzosin,
amiodarone, cisapride, flecainide, propafenone,
quinidine, ergot derivatives, lovastatin, simvastatin, midazolam, triazolam, and voriconazole.
☙ **Lifespan:** Use in pregnancy only if benefits outweigh potential risks to fetus. If used
during pregnancy, contact the antiretroviral
pregnancy registry at 800-258-4263 or
www.APRegistry.com. In breast-feeding
women, use cautiously. It isn't known whether
drug appears in breast milk.

Adverse reactions

CNS: *asthenia,* headache, circumoral paresthesia, dizziness, insomnia, paresthesia, peripheral
paresthesia, somnolence, thinking abnormality,
generalized tonic-clonic seizure, depression,
anxiety, pain, malaise, confusion, fever.
CV: vasodilation, syncope.
EENT: pharyngitis.
GI: abdominal pain, anorexia, constipation, diarrhea, nausea, vomiting, taste perversion, dyspepsia, flatulence, *pancreatitis, pseudomembranous colitis.*
Hematologic: *thrombocytopenia, leukopenia.*
Hepatic: *hepatitis.*
Metabolic: *diabetes mellitus,* weight loss.

Musculoskeletal: myalgia, arthralgia.
Skin: sweating, rash.
Other: fat redistribution/accumulation, *hyper-
sensitivity reactions.*

Interactions

Drug-drug. *Alfuzosin, amiodarone, cisapride,
ergot derivatives, flecainide, midazolam,
propafenone, quinidine, triazolam, voriconazole:* May cause serious and life-threatening adverse reactions. Use together is contraindicated.
*Atovaquone, divalproex, lamotrigine, phenytoin,
warfarin:* May decrease levels of these drugs.
Use together cautiously and monitor drug levels
closely, if appropriate.
*Beta blockers, disopyramide, fluoxetine, mexile-
tine, nefazodone:* May increase levels of these
drugs, causing cardiac and neurologic events.
Use together with caution.
*Bupropion, buspirone, carbamazepine, calcium
channel blockers, clonazepam, clorazepate,
cyclosporine, dexamethasone, diazepam, dronabinol, estazolam, ethosuximide, flurazepam,
lidocaine, methamphetamine, metoprolol, perphenazine, prednisone, propoxyphene, quinine,
risperidone, SSRIs, tacrolimus, tricyclic antidepressants, thioridazine, timolol, tramadol, zolpi-
dem:* May increase levels of these drugs. Use
cautiously together and consider decreasing the
dosage of these drugs by almost 50%.
Clarithromycin: May increase clarithromycin
level. Patients with impaired renal function require 50% reduction in clarithromycin if creatinine clearance is 30 to 60 ml/minute, and a 75%
reduction if it's below 30 ml/minute.
Delavirdine: Increases ritonavir level. Use together cautiously. Dosage recommendations not
established for combined use.
Didanosine: May decrease didanosine absorption. Separate doses by 2½ hours.
Disulfiram, metronidazole: May increase risk of
disulfiram-like reactions since ritonavir formulations contain alcohol. Monitor patient.
Ethinyl estradiol: May decrease ethinyl estradiol plasma concentrations. Use an alternative or
additional method of birth control.
Fluticasone: May increase fluticasone exposure
leading to significantly decreased serum cortisol
concentrations, which may lead to systemic corticosteroid effects (including Cushing's syndrome). Don't use together, if possible.
HMG-CoA reductase inhibitors: May cause a
large increase in statin levels, causing myopa-

R

thy. Avoid use with lovastatin and simvastatin. Use cautiously with atorvastatin. Consider using fluvastatin or pravastatin.

Indinavir: May increase indinavir level. Use together cautiously.

Itraconazole, ketoconazole: May increase levels of these drugs. Don't exceed 200 mg per day of these drugs.

Meperidine: May decrease level of meperidine and its metabolite. Dosage increase and long-term use of meperidine with ritonavir not recommended because of CNS effects. Use cautiously together.

Methadone: May decrease methadone level. Consider increasing methadone dosage.

Phosphodiesterase type 5 (PDE 5) inhibitors (sildenafil, tadalafil, vardenafil): May increase levels of PDE 5 inhibitor causing hypotension, syncope, visual changes, or prolonged erection. Use together cautiously and with increased monitoring for adverse reactions. Tell patient not to exceed 25 mg of sildenafil in a 48-hour period, 10 mg of tadalafil in a 72-hour period, or 2.5 mg of vardenafil in a 72-hour period.

Rifabutin: May increase rifabutin level. Monitor patient and reduce rifabutin daily dosage by at least 75% of usual dose.

Rifampin: May decrease ritonavir level. Consider using rifabutin in place of rifampin.

Saquinavir: May increase saquinavir level. Adjust dose by giving 400 mg saquinavir b.i.d. and 400 mg ritonavir b.i.d.

Theophylline: May decrease theophylline level. Increase dose based on level.

Trazodone: May increase trazodone level causing nausea, dizziness, hypotension and syncope. Avoid use together. If unavoidable, use cautiously with a lower dose of trazodone.

Drug-herb. *St. John's wort:* May substantially reduce drug level. Discourage use together.

Drug-food. *Any food:* May increase drug absorption. Give drug with food.

Drug-lifestyle. *Smoking:* May decrease level of ritonavir. Discourage smoking.

Effects on lab test results

• May increase ALT, AST, GGT, glucose, triglyceride, lipid, CPK, and uric acid levels. May decrease hemoglobin level and hematocrit.
• May decrease WBC, RBC, platelet, and neutrophil counts.

Pharmacokinetics

Absorption: Enhanced by food.
Distribution: Absolute bioavailability unknown; 98% to 100% bound to albumin.
Metabolism: Metabolized in the liver and kidneys.
Excretion: Excreted in the urine and feces.
Half-life: Unknown.

Route	Onset	Peak	Duration
P.O.	Unknown	2–4 hr	Unknown

Action

Chemical effect: HIV protease inhibitor with activity against HIV-1 and HIV-2 proteases; binds to protease-active site and inhibits enzyme activity.

Therapeutic effect: Prevents cleavage of viral polyproteins, resulting in formation of immature noninfectious viral particles.

Available forms

Capsules: 100 mg
Oral solution: 80 mg/ml

NURSING PROCESS

⚗ Assessment
• Use cautiously in patients with hepatic insufficiency.
• Assess patient's and family's knowledge of drug therapy.

⊕ Nursing diagnoses
• Infection related to presence of virus
• Deficient knowledge related to drug therapy

▶ Planning and implementation
⑨ ALERT: Don't confuse Norvir with Norvasc.
Patient teaching
• Inform patient that drug isn't a cure for HIV infection and that illnesses caused by HIV infection may occur. Drug doesn't reduce risk of HIV transmission.
• Tell patient that the taste of oral solution may be improved by mixing with flavored milk within 1 hour of dose.
• Tell patient to take drug with meal.
• If patient misses a dose, instruct him to take next dose at once. He shouldn't take double doses.
• Advise patient to report use of other drugs, including OTC drugs.

Reactions may be *common*, uncommon, **life-threatening**, or COMMON AND LIFE-THREATENING.

• Advise patient taking PDE 5 inhibitors about an increased risk of adverse events, including hypotension, visual changes, and prolonged erection. He should promptly report any symptoms to his prescriber. Tell patient not to exceed 25 mg of sildenafil in a 48-hour period, 10 mg of tadalafil in a 72-hour period, or 2.5 mg of vardenafil in a 72-hour period.

• To prevent transmission of disease, HIV-positive women shouldn't breast-feed.

☑ **Evaluation**
• Patient's infection is controlled.
• Patient and family state understanding of drug therapy.

rivastigmine tartrate
(ri-va-STIG-meen TAR-trayt)
Exelon

Pharmacologic class: cholinesterase inhibitor
Therapeutic class: Alzheimer's disease drug
Pregnancy risk category: B

Indications and dosages

▶ **Symptoms of mild to moderate Alzheimer's disease.** *Adults:* Initially, 1.5 mg P.O. b.i.d. with food. If tolerated, may be increased to 3 mg b.i.d. after 2 weeks. Further increases to 4.5 mg b.i.d. and 6 mg b.i.d. may be given as tolerated after 2 weeks on the previous dose. Effective dosage range is 6 to 12 mg daily, with maximum recommended dosage of 12 mg daily.

Contraindications and cautions

• Contraindicated in patients hypersensitive to the drug, any of its components, or other carbamate derivatives.

• Use cautiously in patients who take NSAIDs and who have a history of ulcers or GI bleeding and in patients with sick sinus syndrome or other supraventricular cardiac conditions, asthma or obstructive pulmonary disease, or seizures.

⚖ **Lifespan:** Use in pregnancy if benefits outweigh potential risks to the fetus. In breast-feeding women, use cautiously because it isn't known if drug appears in breast milk.

Adverse reactions

CNS: syncope, fatigue, asthenia, malaise, *dizziness, headache,* somnolence, tremor, insomnia, confusion, depression, anxiety, hallucination, aggressive reaction, vertigo, agitation, nervousness, delusion, paranoid reaction, pain.
CV: hypertension, chest pain, peripheral edema.
EENT: rhinitis, pharyngitis.
GI: *nausea, vomiting, diarrhea, anorexia, abdominal pain,* dyspepsia, constipation, flatulence, eructation, GI bleeding.
GU: UTI, urinary incontinence, urinary obstruction.
Metabolic: weight loss.
Musculoskeletal: back pain, arthralgia, bone fracture.
Respiratory: upper respiratory tract infection, cough, bronchitis.
Skin: increased sweating, rash.
Other: *accidental trauma,* flulike symptoms.

Interactions

Drug-drug. *Anticholinergics:* May interfere with anticholinergic activity. Monitor patient closely.
Bethanechol, succinylcholine, and other neuromuscular blockers or cholinergic antagonists: May have synergistic effect. Monitor patient closely.
Drug-lifestyle. *Smoking:* May increase rivastigmine clearance. Monitor patient closely.

Effects on lab test results
None reported.

Pharmacokinetics

Absorption: Rapid, with levels peaking in about 1 hour. Although drug is given with food, it delays peak levels by about 1½ hours. Absolute bioavailability is 36%.
Distribution: Widely distributed throughout body; drug crosses the blood-brain barrier. Protein-binding is about 40%.
Metabolism: Rapid and extensive.
Excretion: Elimination is primarily through the kidneys. *Half-life:* About 1½ hours in patients with normal renal function.

Route	Onset	Peak	Duration
P.O.	Unknown	1 hr	12 hr

Action

Chemical effect: Thought to increase acetylcholine levels by reversibly inhibiting its hydrolysis by cholinesterase. Acetylcholine is probably the primary neurotransmitter that is depleted in Alzheimer's disease.
Therapeutic effect: Improves cognitive function.

Available forms

Capsules: 1.5 mg, 3 mg, 4.5 mg, 6 mg
Solution: 2 mg/ml

NURSING PROCESS

⚕ Assessment

• Assess underlying condition before starting therapy and regularly thereafter to monitor drug's effectiveness.
• Perform complete health history, and carefully monitor for adverse effects any patient with a history of GI bleeding, NSAID use, arrhythmias, seizures, or pulmonary conditions.
• Assess patient's and family's knowledge of drug therapy.

⊕ Nursing diagnoses

• Acute or chronic confusion related to underlying disease
• Risk for imbalanced fluid volume related to drug-induced GI effects
• Deficient knowledge related to rivastigmine tartrate therapy

▶ Planning and implementation

• Expect significant GI adverse effects, such as nausea, vomiting, anorexia, and weight loss. They're less common during maintenance doses.
• **ALERT:** Severe vomiting may occur in patient who resumes therapy after an interruption. If therapy is interrupted for more than several days, resume therapy at 1.5 mg b.i.d. to maintenance levels.
• Dramatic memory improvement is unlikely. As disease progresses, the benefits of rivastigmine may decline.
• Monitor patient for symptoms of active or occult GI bleeding.
• Monitor patient for severe nausea, vomiting, and diarrhea, which may lead to dehydration and weight loss.

Patient teaching

• Advise patient to report any episodes of nausea, vomiting, or diarrhea.
• Inform patient and caregiver that memory improvement may be subtle and that a more likely result of therapy is a slower decline in memory loss.
• Tell patient to take rivastigmine with food in the morning and evening.
• Instruct patient to consult prescriber before taking OTC drugs.

☑ Evaluation

• Patient's cognition improves and he experiences less confusion.
• Patient and family state that adverse GI effects haven't occurred or have been managed effectively.
• Patient and family state understanding of drug therapy.

rizatriptan benzoate

(rih-zah-TRIP-tin BEN-zoh-ayt)
Maxalt, Maxalt-MLT

Pharmacologic class: selective 5-hydroxytryptamine (5-HT$_1$) receptor agonist
Therapeutic class: antimigraine drug
Pregnancy risk category: C

Indications and dosages

▶ **Acute migraine headaches with or without aura.** *Adults:* Initially, 5 to 10 mg P.O. If first dose is ineffective, another dose can be given at least 2 hours after first dose. Maximum, 30 mg daily. For patients taking propranolol, 5 mg P.O., up to maximum of three doses (15 mg total) in 24 hours.

Contraindications and cautions

• Contraindicated in patients hypersensitive to the drug or any of its components and in the management of hemiplegic or basilar migraines. Also contraindicated in patients with ischemic heart disease (angina pectoris, history of MI, or documented silent ischemia) or those with evidence of ischemic heart disease, coronary artery vasospasm (Prinzmetal's variant angina), or other significant underlying CV disease. Also contraindicated in patients with uncontrolled hypertension and within 24 hours of another 5-HT$_1$

agonist or with ergotamine-containing or ergot-type drugs, such as dihydroergotamine or methysergide.
• Don't use within 14 days of an MAO inhibitor.
• Use cautiously in patients with hepatic or renal impairment. Also use cautiously in patients with risk factors for coronary artery disease (hypertension, hypercholesterolemia, smoking, obesity, diabetes, strong family history of coronary artery disease, women with surgical or physiologic menopause, or men older than age 40), unless a cardiac evaluation provides evidence that patient is free from cardiac disease.
※ **Lifespan:** Use in pregnancy only if benefits clearly outweigh potential risks to the fetus. In breast-feeding women, don't use drug because the effects on infants are unknown. In children, safety and effectiveness haven't been established.

Adverse reactions

CNS: dizziness, headache, somnolence, paresthesia, asthenia, fatigue, hypesthesia, decreased mental acuity, euphoria, tremor.
CV: flushing, chest pain, pressure or heaviness, palpitations, *coronary artery vasospasm, transient myocardial ischemia, MI, ventricular tachycardia, ventricular fibrillation.*
EENT: neck, throat, and jaw pain, pressure, or heaviness.
GI: dry mouth, nausea, diarrhea, vomiting.
Respiratory: dyspnea.
Other: pain, warm or cold sensations, hot flushes.

Interactions

Drug-drug. *Ergot-containing or ergot-type drugs (dihydroergotamine, methysergide), other 5-HT₁ agonists:* May prolong vasospastic reactions. Don't use within 24 hours of rizatriptan.
MAO inhibitors: May increase rizatriptan level. Don't use together. Allow at least 14 days between stopping an MAO inhibitor and giving rizatriptan.
Propranolol: May increase rizatriptan levels. Reduce rizatriptan dose to 5 mg.
SSRIs: May cause weakness, hyperreflexia, and incoordination. Monitor patient.

Effects on lab test results

None reported.

Pharmacokinetics

Absorption: Complete, with an absolute bioavailability of 45%.
Distribution: Widely distributed, 14% bound to proteins.
Metabolism: Metabolized primarily by oxidative deamination by MAO-A.
Excretion: 82% in urine. *Half-life:* 2 to 3 hours.

Route	Onset	Peak	Duration
P.O.	Unknown	1–1½ hr	Unknown

Action

Chemical effect: Believed to exert its effect by acting as an agonist at serotonin receptors on extracerebral intracranial blood vessels, which results in vasoconstriction of the affected vessels, inhibition of neuropeptide release, and reduction of pain transmission in the trigeminal pathways.
Therapeutic effect: Relieves migraine pain.

Available forms

Tablets: 5 mg, 10 mg
Tablets (disintegrating): 5 mg, 10 mg

NURSING PROCESS

✷ Assessment
• Use drug only after a definite diagnosis of migraine is established.
• Assess patient for history of coronary artery disease, hypertension, arrhythmias, or presence of risk factors for coronary artery disease.
• Perform baseline and periodic CV evaluation in patients who develop risk factors for coronary artery disease.
• Monitor renal and liver function tests before starting therapy, and report abnormalities.
• Assess patient's and family's knowledge of drug therapy.

✤ Nursing diagnoses
• Acute pain related to presence of migraine headache
• Risk for activity intolerance related to adverse drug reactions
• Deficient knowledge related to drug therapy

◩ Planning and implementation
• Don't give to patient with hemiplegic migraine, basilar migraine, or cluster headaches.

R

⊗ **ALERT:** Don't give drug within 24 hours of a drug containing ergot or 5-HT$_1$ agonist or within 14 days of an MAO inhibitor.

• For patient with cardiac risk factors who has had a satisfactory cardiac evaluation, give first dose while monitoring ECG and have emergency equipment readily available.

• If patient develops palpitations or neck, throat, or jaw pain, pressure, or heaviness, stop giving the drug and notify prescriber.

• Safety of treating more than four headaches in a 30-day period, on average, hasn't been established.

• Drug contains phenylalanine.

Patient teaching

• Inform patient that drug doesn't prevent headache.

• For Maxalt-MLT, tell patient to remove blister pack from sachet and to remove drug from blister pack immediately before use. Tell him not to pop tablet out of blister pack but to carefully peel pack away with dry hands, place tablet on tongue, and let it dissolve. Tablet is then swallowed with saliva. No water is needed or recommended. Tell patient that dissolving tablet doesn't provide more rapid headache relief.

• Advise patient that if headache returns after first dose, a second dose may be taken with medical approval at least 2 hours after the first dose. Don't take more than 30 mg in a 24-hour period.

• Tell patient that food may delay onset of drug action.

• Advise patient to notify prescriber if pregnancy occurs or is suspected.

🗹 Evaluation

• Patient has relief from migraine headache.

• Patient maintains baseline activity level.

• Patient and family state understanding of drug therapy.

rocuronium bromide
(roh-kyoo-ROH-nee-um BROH-mighd)
Zemuron

Pharmacologic class: nondepolarizing neuromuscular blocker
Therapeutic class: skeletal muscle relaxant
Pregnancy risk category: C

Indications and dosages

▶ **Adjunct to general anesthesia, to facilitate endotracheal intubation, and to provide skeletal muscle relaxation during surgery or mechanical ventilation.** Dosage depends on anesthetic used, individual needs, and response. Dosages are representative and must be adjusted.

Adults and children age 3 months or older: Initially, 0.6 mg/kg (adults, up to 1.2 mg/kg) I.V. bolus. In most patients, perform tracheal intubation within 2 minutes; muscle paralysis will last about 31 minutes. A maintenance dosage of 0.1 mg/kg will provide additional 12 minutes of muscle relaxation, 0.15 mg/kg will add 17 minutes, and 0.2 mg/kg will add 24 minutes to duration of effect.

⛏ I.V. administration

• Compatible solutions include D$_5$W, normal saline solution for injection, dextrose 5% in normal saline solution for injection, sterile water for injection, and lactated Ringer's injection.

• Give drug by rapid I.V. injection or continuous I.V. infusion. Infusion rates are highly individualized but range from 0.004 to 0.16 mg/kg/minute.

• Store reconstituted solution in refrigerator. Discard after 24 hours.

⊗ **Incompatibilities**

Alkaline solutions such as barbiturates; other I.V. drugs.

Contraindications and cautions

• Contraindicated in patients hypersensitive to the drug or any of its components.

• Use cautiously in patients with hepatic disease, severe obesity, bronchogenic carcinoma, electrolyte disturbances, neuromuscular disease, or altered circulation time caused by CV disease or edema.

⚖ **Lifespan:** In pregnant women, use cautiously. In breast-feeding women, safety and effectiveness haven't been established. In the elderly, use cautiously because of slower circulation.

Adverse reactions

CV: tachycardia, abnormal ECG, *arrhythmias,* transient hypotension, hypertension.
GI: nausea, vomiting.
Respiratory: hiccups, *asthma.*
Skin: rash, pruritus.
Other: injection site edema.

Reactions may be *common,* uncommon, *life-threatening,* or COMMON AND LIFE-THREATENING.

Interactions

Drug-drug. *Amikacin, gentamicin, neomycin, streptomycin, tobramycin:* May increase the effects, including prolonged respiratory depression, of nondepolarizing muscle relaxants. Use together only when needed. Dose of nondepolarizing muscle relaxant may need to be reduced.

Aminoglycoside antibiotics (kanamycin), anticonvulsants, clindamycin, general anesthetics (such as enflurane, halothane, isoflurane), opioid analgesics, polymyxin antibiotics (colistin, polymyxin B sulfate), quinidine, succinylcholine, tetracyclines: May increase neuromuscular blockade, leading to increased skeletal muscle relaxation and increased effect. Use cautiously during surgical and postoperative periods.

Carbamazepine, phenytoin: May decrease the effects of rocuronium. May need to increase the dose of rocuronium.

Effects on lab test results

None reported.

Pharmacokinetics

Absorption: Administered I.V.
Distribution: About 30% bound to proteins.
Metabolism: Unknown, although hepatic clearance may be significant.
Excretion: About 33% excreted in urine. *Half-life:* 14 to 18 minutes in adults; ¾ to 1¼ hours in children.

Route	Onset	Peak	Duration
I.V.	≤ 1 min	≤ 2 min	Varies

Action

Chemical effect: Prevents acetylcholine from binding to receptors on motor end plate, thus blocking depolarization.
Therapeutic effect: Relaxes skeletal muscles.

Available forms

Injection: 10 mg/ml

NURSING PROCESS

🄰 Assessment
● Assess patient's condition before starting therapy, and regularly thereafter to monitor the drug's effectiveness.

● Be alert for adverse reactions and drug interactions.
● Monitor patients with liver disease. They may need higher doses to achieve adequate muscle relaxation and may exhibit prolonged effects from drug.
● Monitor respirations closely until patient is fully recovered from neuromuscular blockade, as evidenced by tests of muscle strength (hand grip, head lift, and ability to cough).
● Assess patient's and family's knowledge of drug therapy.

⊕ Nursing diagnoses
● Ineffective health maintenance related to underlying condition
● Ineffective breathing pattern related to drug's effect on respiratory muscles
● Deficient knowledge related to drug therapy

❯ Planning and implementation
● Give only if skilled in airway management.
● Give sedatives or general anesthetics before neuromuscular blockers because neuromuscular blockers don't affect consciousness or pain perception.
● Give analgesics for pain.
● Keep airway clear. Have emergency respiratory support equipment (endotracheal equipment, ventilator, oxygen, atropine, edrophonium, epinephrine, and neostigmine) on hand.
● Nerve stimulator and train-of-four monitoring are recommended to confirm antagonism of neuromuscular blockade and recovery of muscle strength. Before attempting reversal with neostigmine, note signs of spontaneous recovery.
● Prior administration of succinylcholine may enhance neuromuscular blocking effect and duration of action.
Patient teaching
● Explain all events and happenings to patient because he can still hear.
● Reassure patient that he is being monitored and that muscle use will return when drug has worn off.

☑ Evaluation
● Patient has positive response to drug therapy.
● Patient maintains adequate breathing pattern with mechanical assistance throughout therapy.
● Patient and family state understanding of drug therapy.

R

ropinirole hydrochloride
(roh-PIN-er-ohl high-droh-KLOR-ighd)
Requip

Pharmacologic class: nonergoline dopamine agonist
Therapeutic class: antiparkinsonian
Pregnancy risk category: C

Indications and dosages

▶ **Idiopathic Parkinson's disease.** *Adults:* Initially, 0.25 mg P.O. t.i.d. Dosages can be adjusted weekly. After week 4, dosage may be increased by 1.5 mg daily on a weekly basis up to dosage of 9 mg daily, and then increased weekly by up to 3 mg daily to maximum daily dose of 24 mg.
▶ **Moderate to severe restless leg syndrome.** *Adults:* Initially, 0.25 mg P.O. 1 to 3 hours before bedtime. May increase dose as needed and tolerated after 2 days to 0.5 mg, then to 1 mg by the end of the first week. May further increase dose as needed and tolerated as follows: week 2, give 1 mg once daily. Week 3, give 1.5 mg once daily. Week 4, give 2 mg once daily. Week 5, give 2.5 mg once daily. Week 6, give 3 mg once daily. And week 7, give 4 mg once daily. All doses should be taken 1 to 2 hours before bedtime.

Contraindications and cautions

• Contraindicated in patients hypersensitive to the drug or any of its components.
• Use cautiously in patients with severe hepatic or renal impairment.
⚱ **Lifespan:** Use during pregnancy only if benefits outweigh potential risks to fetus. In nursing mothers, decision should be made whether to stop nursing or to stop drug. In patients older than age 65, clearance is reduced; dose is individually adjusted to response.

Adverse reactions

Early Parkinson's disease (without levodopa)
CNS: pain, asthenia, fatigue, malaise, hallucinations, *dizziness,* aggravated Parkinson's disease, syncope, somnolence, headache, confusion, hyperkinesia, hypesthesia, vertigo, amnesia, impaired concentration.
CV: hypotension, orthostatic symptoms, flushing, hypertension, edema, chest pain, extrasys-

toles, atrial fibrillation, palpitations, tachycardia, peripheral ischemia.
EENT: pharyngitis, abnormal vision, eye abnormality, xerophthalmia, rhinitis, sinusitis.
GI: dry mouth, *nausea, vomiting, dyspepsia,* flatulence, abdominal pain, anorexia, constipation, abdominal pain.
GU: UTI, impotence (male).
Respiratory: bronchitis, dyspnea.
Skin: increased sweating.
Other: viral infection, yawning.
Advanced Parkinson's disease (with levodopa)
CNS: *dizziness,* aggravated parkinsonism, *somnolence, headache,* insomnia, *hallucinations,* abnormal dreaming, confusion, tremor, anxiety, nervousness, amnesia, paresthesia, syncope, pain.
CV: hypotension.
EENT: diplopia, increased saliva.
GI: *nausea,* abdominal pain, dry mouth, vomiting, constipation, diarrhea, dysphagia, flatulence.
GU: UTI, pyuria, urinary incontinence.
Hematologic: anemia.
Metabolic: weight loss.
Musculoskeletal: *dyskinesia,* hypokinesia, paresis, arthralgia, arthritis.
Respiratory: upper respiratory infection, dyspnea.
Skin: increased sweating.
Other: injury, *falls,* viral infection.
Restless leg syndrome
CNS: vertigo, *fatigue, somnolence, dizziness,* paresthesia.
CV: peripheral edema.
EENT: *nasopharyngitis,* nasal congestion.
GI: *nausea, vomiting,* diarrhea, dyspepsia, dry mouth.
Musculoskeletal: arthralgia, muscle cramps, extremity pain.
Respiratory: cough.
Skin: increased sweating.
Other: influenza.

Interactions

Drug-drug. *CNS depressants:* May increase CNS effects. Use together cautiously.
Dopamine antagonists (butyrophenones, metoclopramide, phenothiazines, thioxanthenes): May decrease ropinirole effectiveness. Monitor patient closely.

Estrogens: May decrease ropinirole clearance. If estrogens are started or stopped during therapy, adjust ropinirole dosage.

Inhibitors or substrates of CYP 1A2 (cimetidine, ciprofloxacin, erythromycin, fluvoxamine, diltiazem, tacrine): May decrease ropinirole clearance. If these drugs are started or stopped during therapy, adjust ropinirole dosage.

Drug-lifestyle. *Alcohol use:* May increase sedative effects. Discourage using together.

Smoking: May increase drug clearance. Urge patient to stop smoking, especially during drug therapy.

Effects on lab test results
• May increase BUN and alkaline phosphatase levels. May decrease hemoglobin level and hematocrit.

Pharmacokinetics
Absorption: Rapid, with an absolute bioavailability of 55%.
Distribution: Widely distributed, with about 40% bound to protein.
Metabolism: Extensively metabolized by the liver to inactive metabolites.
Excretion: Less than 10% excreted unchanged in urine. *Half-life:* 6 hours.

Route	Onset	Peak	Duration
P.O.	Unknown	1–2 hr	Unknown

Action
Chemical effect: Unknown. A dopamine agonist thought to stimulate postsynaptic dopamine D₂ receptors in the brain.
Therapeutic effect: Improves physical mobility in patients with parkinsonism.

Available forms
Tablets: 0.25 mg, 0.5 mg, 1 mg, 2 mg, 5 mg

NURSING PROCESS

Assessment
• Assess patient before starting therapy, and frequently thereafter to monitor the drug's effectiveness.
• Monitor patient carefully for orthostatic hypotension, especially during dose escalation.
• Assess patient for adequate nutritional intake.
• Assess patient's and family's knowledge of drug therapy.

Nursing diagnoses
• Impaired physical mobility related to underlying Parkinson's disease
• Disturbed thought processes related to drug-induced CNS adverse reactions
• Deficient knowledge related to drug therapy

Planning and implementation
• Give drug with food to decrease nausea.
• Drug may increase the risk of dopaminergic adverse effects of levodopa and may cause or worsen dyskinesia. Decrease levodopa dosage if needed.
• Don't abruptly stop drug. Withdraw gradually over 7 days to avoid hyperpyrexia and confusion.
• When used for restless leg syndrome, no dose taper is needed when stopping therapy.
Patient teaching
• Tell patient to take drug with food if nausea occurs.
• Explain that hallucinations may occur, particularly in an elderly patient.
• To minimize effects of orthostatic hypotension, instruct patient not to rise rapidly after sitting or lying down, especially when therapy starts or dosage changes.
• Advise patient to avoid hazardous activities until the drug's CNS effects are known.
• Tell patient not to drink alcohol during therapy.
• Tell woman to notify prescriber if pregnancy is suspected or planned, or if she is breastfeeding.

Evaluation
• Patient has improved mobility and reduced muscle rigidity and tremor.
• Patient remains mentally alert.
• Patient and family state understanding of drug therapy.

rosiglitazone maleate
(roh-sih-GLIH-tah-zohn MAL-ee-ayt)
Avandia⊘

Pharmacologic class: thiazolidinedione
Therapeutic class: antidiabetic
Pregnancy risk category: C

Indications and dosages
▶ **Adjunct to diet and exercise (as monotherapy) to improve glycemic control in patients**

with type 2 diabetes mellitus, or (as combination therapy) with sulfonylurea, metformin, or insulin when diet, exercise, and a single drug don't result in adequate glycemic control. *Adults:* Initially, 4 mg P.O. daily in the morning or in divided doses b.i.d. in the morning and evening. If fasting glucose level doesn't improve after 12 weeks, increase to 8 mg P.O. daily or in divided doses b.i.d. Maximum dose is 8 mg daily, except in patients taking insulin. For patients stabilized on insulin, continue insulin dose when therapy starts. Doses greater than 4 mg daily with insulin aren't indicated.

☒ **Adjust-a-dose:** If patient reports hypoglycemia or if fasting glucose levels decrease to less than 100 mg/dL, decrease insulin dose by 10% to 25%. Base further adjustments on response.

Contraindications and cautions

• Contraindicated in patients hypersensitive to the drug or any of its components, and in patients with New York Heart Association Class III or IV cardiac status unless expected benefits outweigh risks. Also contraindicated in patients who developed jaundice while taking troglitazone and in patients with active liver disease, increased baseline liver enzyme levels (ALT level is greater than three times the upper limit of normal), type 1 diabetes, or diabetic ketoacidosis.
• Combination therapy with metformin and rosiglitazone is contraindicated in patients with renal impairment. Rosiglitazone can be used as monotherapy in patients with renal impairment.
• Use cautiously in patients with edema or heart failure.

⚜ **Lifespan:** Drug isn't recommended for pregnant or breast-feeding women.

Adverse reactions

CNS: headache, fatigue.
CV: edema, *heart failure,* peripheral edema.
EENT: sinusitis.
GI: *diarrhea,* weight gain.
Hematologic: anemia.
Metabolic: hyperglycemia, *hypoglycemia.*
Musculoskeletal: back pain.
Respiratory: *upper respiratory tract infection.*
Other: injury.

Interactions

Drug-herb. *Aloe, bilberry leaf, bitter melon, burdock, dandelion, fenugreek, garlic, ginseng:* May improve glucose control. Patient may need

reduced antidiabetic dosage. Discourage using together.

Effects on lab test results

• May increase ALT, HDL, LDL, total cholesterol, and glucose levels. May decrease free fatty acid, glucose, and hemoglobin levels and hematocrit.

Pharmacokinetics

Absorption: Level peaks about 1 hour after a dose. Absolute bioavailability is 99%.
Distribution: About 99.8% of rosiglitazone binds to proteins, primarily albumin.
Metabolism: Extensively metabolized, with no unchanged drug excreted in the urine. Primarily metabolized through N-demethylation and hydroxylation.
Excretion: About 64% and 23% of the dose is eliminated in urine and feces, respectively. *Half-life:* 3 to 4 hours.

Route	Onset	Peak	Duration
P.O.	Unknown	1 hr	Unknown

Action

Chemical effect: Lowers glucose level by improving insulin sensitivity. Highly selective and potent agonist for receptors in key target areas for insulin action, such as adipose tissue, skeletal muscle, and liver.
Therapeutic effect: Lowers glucose level.

Available forms

Tablets: 2 mg, 4 mg, 8 mg

NURSING PROCESS

☞ Assessment

• Obtain history of patient's underlying condition before starting therapy, and reassess regularly thereafter to monitor the drug's effectiveness.
• Check liver enzyme levels before therapy starts. Don't use drug in patients with increased baseline liver enzyme levels. In patients with normal baseline liver enzyme levels, monitor levels q 2 months for the first 12 months and periodically afterward. If ALT level is elevated, recheck levels as soon as possible. If level remains elevated, notify prescriber and stop drug.
• Monitor glucose level regularly and glycosylated hemoglobin level periodically to determine therapeutic response to drug.

• If patient has heart failure, watch for increased edema during rosiglitazone therapy.
• Assess patient's and family's knowledge of drug therapy.

❖ Nursing diagnoses
• Ineffective health maintenance related to hyperglycemia
• Risk for injury related to drug-induced hypoglycemia
• Deficient knowledge related to drug therapy

▷ Planning and implementation
• Before starting drug, treat patient for other causes of poor glycemic control, such as infection.
• Because calorie restriction, weight loss, and exercise help improve insulin sensitivity and make drug therapy effective, these measures are essential.
• For patients inadequately controlled with a maximum dose of a sulfonylurea or metformin, add this drug to current regimen; don't switch therapies.
• This drug alone or with insulin can cause fluid retention that may lead to or exacerbate heart failure. Observe patient for signs or symptoms of heart failure. If cardiac health deteriorates, stop drug.
• Because ovulation may resume in premenopausal, anovulatory woman with insulin resistance, contraceptive measures may need to be considered.
Patient teaching
• Advise patient that rosiglitazone can be taken with or without food.
• Inform patient that blood will be tested to check liver function before therapy starts, every 2 months for the first 12 months, and periodically thereafter.
• Tell patient to immediately report unexplained signs or symptoms—such as nausea, vomiting, abdominal pain, fatigue, anorexia, or dark urine—because they may indicate liver problems.
• Instruct patient to contact prescriber if he has signs or symptoms of heart failure, such as unusually rapid increase in weight, edema, or shortness of breath.
• Inform premenopausal, anovulatory woman with insulin resistance that ovulation may resume and that she may want to consider contraceptive measures.

• Advise patient that diabetes management must include diet control because calorie restriction, weight loss, and exercise improve insulin sensitivity and make drug therapy effective.

☑ Evaluation
• Patient's glucose level is normal with drug therapy.
• Patient doesn't experience hypoglycemia.
• Patient and family state understanding of drug therapy.

rosiglitazone maleate and metformin hydrochloride
(roh-si-GLI-ta-zone and met-FOR-min)
Avandamet

Pharmacologic class: thiazolidinedione and biguanide
Therapeutic class: antidiabetic
Pregnancy risk category: C

Indications and dosages

▶ **Adjunct to diet and exercise to improve glycemic control in patients with type 2 diabetes mellitus who are already treated with rosiglitazone and metformin or who are inadequately controlled on metformin or rosiglitazone alone.** *Adults:* Dosage is based on patient's current doses of rosiglitazone, metformin, or both. Base dose on effectiveness and tolerance and give in two divided doses with meals. For patients inadequately controlled on metformin alone, 2 mg rosiglitazone P.O. b.i.d., plus the dose of metformin already being taken (500 mg or 1,000 mg P.O. b.i.d.). Dosage may be increased after 8 to 12 weeks. For patients inadequately controlled on rosiglitazone alone, 500 mg metformin P.O. b.i.d., plus the dose of rosiglitazone already being taken (2 mg or 4 mg b.i.d.). Dosage may be increased after 1 to 2 weeks. The total daily dose of this drug may be increased in increments of 4 mg rosiglitazone or 500 mg metformin, or both, up to the maximum daily dose of 8 mg rosiglitazone and 2,000 mg metformin in two divided doses.
☒ Adjust-a-dose: In elderly patients, give conservative initial and maintenance doses because these patients' kidney function may be reduced.

Don't give maximum dose to elderly, malnourished, or debilitated patients.

Contraindications and cautions

• Contraindicated in patients hypersensitive to rosiglitazone or metformin and in patients with abnormal creatinine clearance or creatinine levels 1.5 mg/dl or higher in men or 1.4 mg/dl or higher in women; heart failure requiring drug therapy; acute or chronic metabolic acidosis, including diabetic ketoacidosis with or without coma; or evidence of active liver disease or ALT more than 2.5 times the upper limit of normal.

• Don't use with insulin or in patients with type 1 diabetes.

• Use cautiously in patients with edema or those at high risk of heart failure.

⚰ **Lifespan:** In pregnant or breast-feeding women, drug isn't recommended. In children, safety and effectiveness haven't been established. In the elderly, use cautiously because aging often reduces renal function. Don't give an elderly patient the maximum daily dose. Don't give drug to a patient older than age 80 unless renal function is normal.

Adverse reactions

CNS: headache, fatigue.
CV: edema.
EENT: sinusitis.
GI: *diarrhea,* weight loss, weight gain.
Hematologic: anemia.
Metabolic: hyperglycemia, *hypoglycemia.*
Musculoskeletal: back pain, arthralgia.
Respiratory: upper respiratory tract infection.
Other: injury, viral infection.

Interactions

Drug-drug. *Calcium channel blockers, corticosteroids, diuretics, estrogens, hormonal contraceptives, isoniazid, nicotinic acid, phenothiazines, phenytoin, sympathomimetics, thyroid products:* May cause hyperglycemia. Monitor glucose level; adjust dosage, if needed.
Cationic drugs (amiloride, digoxin, morphine, procainamide, quinidine, quinine, ranitidine, triamterene, trimethoprim, vancomycin): May decrease metformin excretion. Monitor glucose level; adjust cationic drugs or metformin, if needed.
Contrast media containing iodine: May increase risk of lactic acidosis and renal failure with met-

formin. Make sure noniodine contrast media is used.
Furosemide: May increase metformin level and decrease furosemide level. Monitor patient closely.
Nifedipine: May increase absorption of metformin. Monitor patient closely.
Drug-herb. *Guar gum:* May decrease hypoglycemic effect. Monitor glucose level.
Drug-lifestyle. *Alcohol use:* May increase effect of metformin on lactate metabolism and increase risk of lactic acidosis. Discourage using together.

Effects on lab test results

• May increase ALT, HDL, LDL, and total cholesterol levels. May decrease vitamin B_{12} and hemoglobin levels and hematocrit. May increase or decrease glucose level.

Pharmacokinetics

Absorption: Absolute bioavailability of rosiglitazone and metformin is 99% and 50% to 60%, respectively.
Distribution: Rosiglitazone is 99.8% bound to proteins, primarily albumin; metformin is negligibly bound to proteins.
Metabolism: Rosiglitazone is extensively metabolized, primarily by N-demethylation and hydroxylation. Rosiglitazone may be predominantly metabolized by CYP 2C8, with CYP 2C9 contributing as a minor pathway. Metformin doesn't undergo hepatic metabolism.
Excretion: 64% and 23% of rosiglitazone is eliminated in the urine and feces, respectively. *Rosiglitazone half-life:* 3 to 4 hours. Metformin is excreted unchanged in the urine. *Metformin half-life:* 6¼ hours to 17½ hours.

Route	Onset	Peak	Duration
P.O.			
rosiglitazone	Unknown	1 hr	Unknown
metformin	Unknown	2½–3 hr	Unknown

Action

Chemical effect: Rosiglitazone improves insulin sensitivity. It's a highly selective and potent agonist for receptors in key target areas for insulin action, such as adipose tissue, skeletal muscle, and the liver. Metformin decreases hepatic glucose production and intestinal absorption of glucose and increases insulin sensitivity.
Therapeutic effect: Lowers glucose level.

Reactions may be *common,* uncommon, *life-threatening*, or COMMON AND LIFE-THREATENING.

Available forms

Tablets: 1 mg rosiglitazone maleate and 500 mg metformin hydrochloride, 2 mg rosiglitazone maleate and 500 mg metformin hydrochloride, 2 mg rosiglitazone maleate and 1,000 mg metformin hydrochloride, 4 mg rosiglitazone maleate and 500 mg metformin hydrochloride, 4 mg rosiglitazone maleate and 1,000 mg metformin hydrochloride

NURSING PROCESS

⏱ Assessment

• Obtain history of patient's underlying condition before starting therapy, and reassess regularly thereafter to monitor the drug's effectiveness.
• Monitor transaminase levels at baseline, q 2 months for the first 12 months, and periodically thereafter. If ALT levels increase to more than three times the upper limit of normal, recheck liver enzymes as soon as possible. If ALT remains more than three times the upper limit of normal, stop drug.
• Monitor CBC and vitamin B_{12} levels.
• Watch for signs and symptoms of heart failure and hepatic dysfunction. If jaundice occurs, stop drug.
• Monitor renal function at baseline and at least annually during therapy.
• Monitor glycosylated hemoglobin level q 3 months.
• Assess patient's and family's knowledge of drug therapy.

⊕ Nursing diagnoses

• Ineffective health maintenance related to hyperglycemia
• Risk for injury related to drug-induced hypoglycemia
• Deficient knowledge related to drug therapy

⧁ Planning and implementation

⑤ **ALERT:** Evaluate patient for ketoacidosis or lactic acidosis. Nonspecific symptoms of lactic acidosis include malaise, myalgias, respiratory distress, abdominal distress, hypotension, and bradyarrhythmias.
• In patient undergoing radiologic studies involving iodinated contrast materials, stop drug before or during the procedure, and withhold for 48 hours after the procedure. Resume drug only after renal function has been re-evaluated and documented to be normal.

• Stop drug temporarily in a patient having surgery. Don't restart until oral intake resumes and renal function is normal.
• If shock, acute heart failure, acute MI, or other conditions linked to hypoxemia occur, stop drug.
⑤ **ALERT:** Don't confuse Avandamet with Anzemet.

Patient teaching

• Stress the importance of dietary instructions, weight loss, and a regular exercise program.
• Tell patient to immediately report unexplained hyperventilation, myalgia, malaise, or unusual somnolence.
• Instruct patient to report a rapid increase in weight, swelling, shortness of breath, or other symptoms of heart failure.
• Tell patient to report unexplained nausea, vomiting, abdominal pain, fatigue, anorexia, or dark urine.
• Explain that it may take 1 to 2 weeks for drug to take effect and up to 2 to 3 months for the full effect to occur.
• Stress the importance of avoiding excessive alcohol intake.
• Discuss the need for contraception with premenopausal women because ovulation may resume.
• Advise patient to take the drug in divided doses with meals to reduce GI side effects.

☑ Evaluation

• Patient's glucose level is normal with drug therapy.
• Patient doesn't experience hypoglycemia.
• Patient and family state understanding of drug therapy.

rosuvastatin calcium
(ro-SOO-va-stat-in KAL-see-uhm)
Crestor◊

Pharmacologic class: HMG-CoA reductase inhibitor
Therapeutic class: antihyperlipidemic
Pregnancy risk category: X

Indications and dosages

▶ **Adjunct to diet to reduce total cholesterol, LDL, apolipoprotein B (ApoB), non-HDL, and triglyceride levels, as well as to increase HDL level in primary hypercholesterolemia** (heterozygous familial and nonfamilial), mixed dyslipidemia (Fredrickson Type IIA and IIB); adjunct to diet to treat elevated triglyceride levels (Fredrickson Type IV). *Adults:* Initially, 10 mg P.O. daily. Increase dosage, p.r.n., to a maximum of 40 mg daily. Increase q 2 to 4 weeks based on lipid levels. If aggressive lipid lowering is needed, drug may be started at 20 mg once daily.

▶ **Adjunct to other lipid-lowering therapies to reduce LDL, ApoB, and total cholesterol levels in homozygous familial hypercholesterolemia.** *Adults:* Initially, 20 mg once daily. Maximum, 40 mg daily.

◩ **Adjust-a-dose:** For patients with renal impairment, if creatinine clearance is less than 30 ml/ minute, start with 5 mg once daily; don't exceed 10 mg once daily. In patients taking 40 mg who develop unexplained persistent proteinuria, reduce dosage. For patients taking gemfibrozil with rosuvastatin, don't exceed 10 mg once daily. For patients requiring less aggressive treatment, those at risk for myopathy, Asian patients, or patients also taking cyclosporine, initial dose is 5 mg.

Contraindications and cautions

• Contraindicated in patients hypersensitive to the drug or any of its components, and in patients with active liver disease or unexplained persistent elevations in transaminases.
• Use cautiously in patients who drink substantial amounts of alcohol and in patients with a history of liver disease. Also use cautiously in patients at increased risk for developing myopathies, such as patients 65 or older or those with renal impairment or hypothyroidism.
• Use with gemfibrozil only when the benefit clearly outweighs the risk. Don't exceed recommended dosage.
⚓ **Lifespan:** In pregnant women, drug is contraindicated. In breast-feeding women, use cautiously; it's unknown if the drug appears in breast milk. In children, safety and effectiveness haven't been established.

Adverse reactions

CNS: headache, asthenia, dizziness, insomnia, paresthesia, depression, anxiety, vertigo, pain, neuralgia, hypertonia.
CV: chest pain, hypertension, palpitation, vasodilation.
EENT: pharyngitis, rhinitis, sinusitis.

GI: diarrhea, dyspepsia, nausea, abdominal pain, vomiting, gastritis, constipation, gastroenteritis, flatulence, periodontal abscess.
GU: UTI, proteinuria.
Hematologic: anemia.
Metabolic: *diabetes mellitus.*
Musculoskeletal: myalgia, back pain, pelvic pain, neck pain, pathological fracture, arthritis, *rhabdomyolysis, myopathy.*
Respiratory: *asthma,* pneumonia, bronchitis, increased cough, dyspnea.
Skin: rash, pruritus, ecchymosis.
Other: flulike syndrome, accidental injury.

Interactions

Drug-drug. *Antacids:* May decrease level of rosuvastatin. Give antacids 2 hours after rosuvastatin.
Cyclosporine: May increase rosuvastatin level and increase risk of myopathy or rhabdomyolysis. Don't exceed 10 mg daily. Monitor patient for signs and symptoms of toxicity.
Gemfibrozil: May increase rosuvastatin level and increase risk of myopathy or rhabdomyolysis. Don't exceed 5 mg daily. Monitor patient for signs and symptoms of toxicity.
Warfarin: May increase warfarin level and increase risk of bleeding. Monitor INR and look for signs of increased bleeding.
Drug-lifestyle. *Alcohol use:* May increase risk of hepatotoxicity. Avoid using together.

Effects on lab test results

• May increase CK, transaminase, glucose, glutamyl transpeptidase, alkaline phosphatase, bilirubin, and thyroid function test levels.
• May cause dipstick-positive proteinuria and microscopic hematuria tests.

Pharmacokinetics

Absorption: About 20%; peak level occurs within 3 to 5 hours. Rate of absorption is decreased by food, but the extent of absorption is unaffected. The drug may be given at any time of day without any change in level.
Distribution: About 88% bound to proteins, primarily albumin.
Metabolism: About 10%.
Excretion: 90% in feces. *Half-life:* About 19 hours.

Route	Onset	Peak	Duration
P.O.	2 wk	Unknown	Unknown

Action

Chemical effect: Inhibits HMG-CoA reductase, which is an early and rate-limiting step in the synthetic pathway of cholesterol.
Therapeutic effect: Lowers total cholesterol, LDL, ApoB, non-HDL, and triglyceride levels.

Available forms

Tablets: 5 mg, 10 mg, 20 mg, 40 mg

NURSING PROCESS

⚗ Assessment

• Assess patient's condition before starting therapy, and regularly thereafter to monitor the drug's effectiveness.
• Perform liver function tests before therapy and again at 12 weeks. Repeat liver function tests 12 weeks following a dosage increase and then twice a year thereafter. If CK levels increase to greater than 10 times the upper limit of normal, stop drug.
• Be alert for adverse reactions and drug interactions.
• If adverse GI reactions occur, monitor hydration.
• Assess patient's and family's knowledge of drug therapy.

⊞ Nursing diagnoses

• Risk for injury related to elevated cholesterol levels
• Risk for deficient fluid volume related to adverse GI reactions
• Deficient knowledge related to drug therapy

⊳ Planning and implementation

• Begin drug only after diet and other nondrug therapies have proven ineffective. Give standard low-cholesterol diet during therapy.
• Withhold drug temporarily in any condition, such as sepsis, hypotension, major surgery, trauma, uncontrolled seizures, and severe metabolic, endocrine, and electrolyte disorders, that may predispose patient to the development of myopathy or rhabdomyolysis.
⊛ **ALERT:** Asian patients are at a greater risk of elevated drug levels.

Patient teaching

• Instruct patient to take drug exactly as prescribed.
• Teach patient about restricting total fat and cholesterol intake, and recommend weight control, exercise, and smoking cessation programs.
• Tell patient to immediately report any signs of unexplained muscle pain, tenderness, or weakness, especially if accompanied by malaise or fever.
• Instruct patient that antacids containing aluminum or magnesium should be taken at least 2 hours after this drug.
• Inform woman that drug is contraindicated during pregnancy. Advise her to notify prescriber immediately if she becomes pregnant.

⊠ Evaluation

• Patient's LDL and total cholesterol levels are within normal range.
• Patient maintains adequate hydration.
• Patient and family state understanding of drug therapy.

salmeterol xinafoate
(sal-MEE-ter-ohl zee-neh-FOH-ayt)
Serevent Diskus

Pharmacologic class: selective beta$_2$ agonist
Therapeutic class: bronchodilator
Pregnancy risk category: C

Indications and dosages

▶ **Long-term maintenance therapy for asthma; to prevent bronchospasm in patients with nocturnal asthma or reversible obstructive airway disease who need regular short-acting beta agonists.** *Adults and children older than age 4:* 1 inhalation (50 mcg) q 12 hours, in the morning and in the evening.
▶ **To prevent exercise-induced bronchospasm.** *Adults and children age 4 and older:* 1 inhalation (50 mcg) at least 30 minutes before exercise.
▶ **Maintenance therapy for bronchospasm with COPD (including emphysema and**

chronic bronchitis). *Adults:* 1 inhalation (50 mcg) q 12 hours, in the morning and in the evening.

Contraindications and cautions

• Contraindicated in patients hypersensitive to the drug or any of its components.
• Use cautiously in patients who are unusually responsive to sympathomimetics and patients with coronary insufficiency, arrhythmias, hypertension or other CV disorders, thyrotoxicosis, or seizure disorders.
⚡ **Lifespan:** In pregnant women, use cautiously. Do not use in breast-feeding women. In children younger than age 4, safety and effectiveness haven't been established.

Adverse reactions

CNS: *headache,* sinus headache, tremor, nervousness, dizziness.
CV: tachycardia, palpitations, *ventricular arrhythmias.*
EENT: *nasopharyngitis,* nasal cavity or sinus disorder, sore throat.
GI: nausea, vomiting, diarrhea, heartburn.
Musculoskeletal: joint and back pain, myalgia.
Respiratory: *upper respiratory tract infection,* cough, lower respiratory tract infection, *bronchospasm.*
Other: *hypersensitivity reactions, anaphylaxis.*

Interactions

Drug-drug. *Beta agonists, methylxanthines, theophylline:* May cause adverse cardiac effects with excessive use. Monitor patient closely.
MAO inhibitors: May cause severe adverse CV effects. Don't use within 14 days of MAO therapy.
Tricyclic antidepressants: May cause moderate to severe adverse CV effects. Use cautiously.

Effects on lab test results

None reported.

Pharmacokinetics

Absorption: Low or undetectable because of low therapeutic dose.
Distribution: Local to lungs; 94% to 99% bound to proteins.
Metabolism: Extensive.
Excretion: Primarily in feces.

Route	Onset	Peak	Duration
Inhalation	10–20 min	3 hr	12 hr

Action

Chemical effect: Unclear; selectively activates beta$_2$-adrenergic receptors, which results in bronchodilation, and blocks release of allergic mediators from mast cells in respiratory tract.
Therapeutic effect: Improves breathing ability.

Available forms

Inhalation powder: 50 mcg/blister

NURSING PROCESS

🗲 Assessment

• Assess patient's respiratory condition before starting therapy, and regularly thereafter to monitor the drug's effectiveness.
• Assess peak flow readings before starting therapy and periodically thereafter.
• Be alert for adverse reactions and drug interactions.
• Assess patient's and family's knowledge of drug therapy.

⊞ Nursing diagnoses

• Ineffective breathing pattern related to respiratory condition
• Acute pain related to drug-induced headache
• Deficient knowledge related to drug therapy

▶ Planning and implementation

• Don't give drug for acute bronchospasm.
• Report insufficient relief or worsening condition.
• If headache occurs, give mild analgesic.
🟢 **ALERT:** A serious asthma episode or asthma-related death may occur, with blacks at greatest risk.
🟢 **ALERT:** Don't confuse Serevent with Serentil.
Patient teaching
• Tell patient to take drug at about 12-hour intervals, even if he is feeling better.
• Tell patient to prevent exercise-induced bronchospasm by taking drug 30 to 60 minutes before exercise.
🟢 **ALERT:** Instruct patient not to use for acute bronchospasm, but to use a short-acting beta agonist (such as albuterol) instead.
• Tell patient to contact prescriber if short-acting beta agonist no longer provides sufficient

relief or if taking more than 4 inhalations daily. Tell patient not to increase the dose.

• If patient is using an inhaled corticosteroid, he should continue. Warn him not to take other drugs without prescriber's consent.

• Instruct patient not to exhale into Diskus, and to only use Diskus in a level, horizontal position.

☑ **Evaluation**

• Patient exhibits normal breathing pattern.

• Patient states that drug-induced headache is relieved after analgesic administration.

• Patient and family state understanding of drug therapy.

saquinavir mesylate
(suh-KWIN-uh-veer MEH-sih-layt)
Invirase

Pharmacologic class: protease inhibitor
Therapeutic class: antiretroviral
Pregnancy risk category: B

Indications and dosages

▶ **Adjunct therapy for advanced HIV infection in selected patients.** *Adults and children older than age 16:* 1,000 mg (five 200 mg capsules) P.O. b.i.d. with 100 mg ritonavir. Or, 400 mg Invirase and 400 mg ritonavir P.O. b.i.d.

Contraindications and cautions

• Contraindicated in patients hypersensitive to the drug and its components, and in patients taking triazolam, midazolam, ergot derivatives, or cisapride.

• Use cautiously in patients with liver impairment.

☀ **Lifespan:** In pregnant women, breast-feeding women, and children younger than age 16, safety and effectiveness haven't been established.

Adverse reactions

CNS: asthenia, paresthesia, headache, dizziness.
CV: chest pain.
GI: diarrhea, mouth ulcers, abdominal pain, nausea, *pancreatitis.*
Hematologic: *pancytopenia, thrombocytopenia.*
Hepatic: *portal hypertension,* cirrhosis, elevated liver enzymes.

Metabolic: *hyperglycemia, new onset diabetes mellitus.*
Musculoskeletal: musculoskeletal pain.
Respiratory: bronchitis, cough.
Skin: rash.
Other: *adipogenic effects.*

Interactions

Drug-drug. *Amprenavir:* May decrease levels of amprenavir. Use together cautiously.
Carbamazepine, phenobarbital, phenytoin: May decrease saquinavir level. Avoid using together.
Delavirdine: May increase saquinavir level. Use cautiously, and monitor hepatic enzymes. Decrease dose when used together.
Dexamethasone: May decrease saquinavir level. Avoid using together.
Efavirenz: May decrease levels of both drugs. Don't use together.
HMG-CoA reductase inhibitors: May increase levels of these drugs, which increases risk of myopathy, including rhabdomyolysis. Avoid using together.
Indinavir, lopinavir and ritonavir, nelfinavir, ritonavir: May increase level of saquinavir. Use together cautiously.
Ketoconazole: May increase saquinavir level. No dosage adjustment needed.
Loperamide: May increase loperamide level while decreasing saquinavir level. Avoid use together.
Macrolide antibiotics such as clarithromycin: May increase levels of both drugs. Use together cautiously.
Nevirapine: May decrease saquinavir level. Monitor patient.
Rifabutin, rifampin: May reduce the steady-state level of saquinavir. Use rifabutin and saquinavir together cautiously. Don't use with rifampin.
Sildenafil: May increase peak level and exposure of sildenafil. Reduce initial dose of sildenafil to 25 mg when given with saquinavir.
Drug-herb. *Garlic supplements:* May decrease drug level by half. Discourage using together.
St. John's wort: May substantially reduce level of drug, causing loss of therapeutic effect. Discourage using together.
Drug-food. *Any food:* May increase drug absorption. Advise patient to take drug with food.
Grapefruit juice: May increase drug level. Give with another liquid.

S

Effects on lab test results

- May increase liver enzyme levels.
- May decrease WBC, RBC, and platelet counts.

Pharmacokinetics

Absorption: Poor.
Distribution: More than 98% bound to proteins.
Metabolism: Rapid.
Excretion: Mainly in feces. *Half-life:* 1 to 2 hours.

Route	Onset	Peak	Duration
P.O.	Unknown	Unknown	7 hr

Action

Chemical effect: Inhibits HIV protease and prevents cleavage of HIV polyproteins, which are essential for HIV maturation.
Therapeutic effect: Hinders HIV activity.

Available forms

Capsules (hard gelatin): 200 mg
Tablets: 500 mg

NURSING PROCESS

Assessment

- Obtain history of patient's HIV infection.
- Monitor CBC and platelet counts and electrolyte, uric acid, liver enzyme, and bilirubin levels before and during therapy.
- Be alert for adverse reactions and drug interactions, including those caused by adjunct therapy (zidovudine or zalcitabine).
- If patient has an adverse GI reaction, monitor his hydration.
- Watch for adipogenic side effects with prolonged therapy (redistribution or accumulation of body fat, dorsocervical fat enlargement, peripheral wasting, breast enlargement, and cushingoid appearance).
- Assess patient's and family's knowledge of drug therapy.

Nursing diagnoses

- Infection related to presence of HIV
- Risk for deficient fluid volume related to adverse GI reactions
- Deficient knowledge related to drug therapy

Planning and implementation

ALERT: If severe toxicity occurs, stop drug until cause is identified or toxicity resolves. Therapy may resume with no dosage change.

- Notify prescriber of adverse reactions, and obtain an order for a mild analgesic, antiemetic, or antidiarrheal, if needed.

Patient teaching

- Tell patient to take drug with meals or within 2 hours after a full meal.
- Urge patient to report adverse reactions.
- Inform patient that drug is usually given with other AIDS-related antiviral drugs.

ALERT: Advise patient taking sildenafil about an increased risk of adverse events, including hypotension, visual changes, and priapism, and the need to report them promptly. Tell patient not to exceed 25 mg of sildenafil in 48 hours.

Evaluation

- Patient responds well to therapy.
- Patient maintains adequate hydration.
- Patient and family state understanding of drug therapy.

sargramostim (granulocyte macrophage colony-stimulating factor, GM-CSF)

(sar-GRAH-moh-stim)
Leukine

Pharmacologic class: biological response modifier
Therapeutic class: hematopoietic growth factor
Pregnancy risk category: C

Indications and dosages

▶ **To accelerate hematopoiesis after autologous bone marrow transplantation (BMT) in patients with malignant lymphoma, acute lymphoblastic leukemia, or chemotherapeutically treated Hodgkin's disease.** *Adults:* 250 mcg/m² daily as 2-hour I.V. infusion beginning 2 to 4 hours after BMT and not less than 24 hours after last dose of chemotherapy or radiation. Patient's post-BMT absolute neutrophil count (ANC) must be at least 500/mm³. Continue until ANC is greater than 1,500/mm³ for 3 consecutive days.

▶ **BMT failure or engraftment delay.** *Adults:* 250 mcg/m^2 as 2-hour I.V. infusion daily for 14 days. May repeat after 7 days off therapy. If engraftment still hasn't occurred, a third course of 500 mcg/m^2 I.V. daily for 14 days may be tried after another 7 days off therapy.

▶ **Neutrophil recovery following chemotherapy in acute myelogenous leukemia.** *Adults:* 250 mcg/m^2 I.V. infusion over 4 hours daily. Start therapy about day 11 or 4 days after end of induction therapy.

▶ **To mobilize hematopoietic progenitor cells into peripheral blood for collection by leukapheresis; to accelerate myeloid engraftment after autologous peripheral blood progenitor cell (PBPC) transplantation.** *Adults:* 250 mcg/m^2 by continuous I.V. infusion over 24 hours or subcutaneously once daily. After PBPC, continue until the ANC is > 1,500/mm^3 for 3 consecutive days.

▼ I.V. administration

• Reconstitute drug with 1 ml of sterile water for injection. Direct stream of sterile water against side of vial and gently swirl contents to minimize foaming. Avoid excessive or vigorous agitation or shaking.

• Dilute in normal saline solution. If final level is less than 10 mcg/ml, add human albumin at final level of 0.1% to saline solution before adding drug to prevent adsorption to components of delivery system. For final level of 0.1% human albumin, add 1 mg human albumin per 1 ml saline solution.

• Give as soon as possible and no later than 6 hours after reconstituting.

• Do not use an in-line membrane filter since adsorption of the drug could occur.

• Vials are for single-dose use and contain no preservatives. Discard unused portion.

• Refrigerate sterile powder, reconstituted solution, and diluted solution for injection. Don't freeze or shake.

⊗ **Incompatibilities**
Other I.V. drugs, unless specific compatibility data are available.

Contraindications and cautions

• Contraindicated in patients hypersensitive to the drug or any of its components or to yeast-derived products. Also contraindicated in patients with excessive leukemic myeloid blasts in bone marrow or peripheral blood.

• Use cautiously in patients with cardiac disease, hypoxia, fluid retention, pulmonary infiltrates, heart failure, or impaired kidney or liver function.

⚖ **Lifespan:** In pregnant women, use cautiously. In breast-feeding women, use cautiously; it's unknown if the drug appears in breast milk. In children, safety and effectiveness haven't been established.

Adverse reactions

CNS: malaise, CNS disorders, asthenia, fever.
CV: edema, *supraventricular arrhythmia,* pericardial effusion.
EENT: mucous membrane disorder.
GI: *nausea, vomiting, diarrhea, anorexia, hemorrhage,* GI disorder, stomatitis.
GU: *urinary tract disorder,* abnormal kidney function.
Hematologic: *blood dyscrasias, hemorrhage.*
Hepatic: *liver damage.*
Respiratory: *dyspnea, lung disorders,* pleural effusion.
Skin: alopecia, rash.
Other: SEPSIS.

Interactions

Drug-drug. *Corticosteroids, lithium:* May increase myeloproliferative effects of sargramostim. Use together cautiously.

Effects on lab test results

• May increase BUN, creatinine, AST, ALT, and bilirubin levels.

Pharmacokinetics

Absorption: Administered I.V.
Distribution: Bound to specific receptors on target cells.
Metabolism: Unknown.
Excretion: Unknown. *Half-life:* About 2 hours.

Route	Onset	Peak	Duration
I.V.	≤ 30 min	2 hr	Unknown
SubQ	Rapid	1–4 hr	Unknown

Action

Chemical effect: Differs from natural human GM-CSF. Induces cellular responses by binding to specific receptors on surfaces of target cells.
Therapeutic effect: Stimulates formation of granulocytes (neutrophils, eosinophils) and macrophages.

Available forms
Liquid: 500 mcg*
Powder for injection: 250 mcg

NURSING PROCESS

⚗ Assessment
• Assess patient's condition before starting therapy, and regularly thereafter to monitor the drug's effectiveness.
• Monitor CBC with differential biweekly, including examination for presence of blast cells.
• Be alert for adverse reactions and drug interactions.
• Monitor patient's hydration throughout drug therapy.
• Assess patient's and family's knowledge of drug therapy.

⊞ Nursing diagnoses
• Ineffective health maintenance related to underlying condition
• Risk for deficient fluid volume related to drug-induced adverse effects
• Deficient knowledge related to drug therapy

▶ Planning and implementation
• Drug's effect may be lessened in patient who has received extensive radiotherapy to hematopoietic sites in abdomen or chest or who has been exposed to multiple drugs (alkylating, anthracycline antibiotics, antimetabolites) before autologous BMT.
• Drug is effective in accelerating myeloid recovery in patients receiving bone marrow purged from monoclonal antibodies.
• Drug can act as growth factor for tumors, particularly myeloid cancers.
• Blood counts return to normal or baseline levels within 3 to 7 days after stopping therapy.
• If severe adverse reaction occurs, notify prescriber. Dose may need to be reduced by half or stopped temporarily. Resume therapy when reaction decreases. Transient rashes and local reactions at injection site may occur; serious allergic or anaphylactic reaction isn't common.
• Stimulation of marrow precursors may result in rapid rise of WBC count. If blast cells appear or increase to 10% or more of WBC count or if underlying disease progresses, stop drug. If ANC is more than 20,000/mm³ or if platelet count is more than 50,000/mm³, temporarily stop drug or reduce dose by half.

Patient teaching
• Inform patient and family about need for therapy.
• Advise patient to report adverse reactions immediately.

☑ Evaluation
• Patient exhibits positive response to drug therapy.
• Patient maintains adequate hydration throughout therapy.
• Patient and family state understanding of drug therapy.

scopolamine (hyoscine)
(skoh-POL-uh-meen)
Scop◇, Transderm Scōp, Scopace

scopolamine butylbromide (hyoscine butylbromide)
Buscopan♦ ◇

scopolamine hydrobromide (hyoscine hydrobromide)

Pharmacologic class: anticholinergic
Therapeutic class: antimuscarinic, antiemetic, antivertigo drug, antiparkinsonian
Pregnancy risk category: C

Indications and dosages
▶ **Spastic states.** *Adults:* 0.4 to 0.8 mg Scopace P.O. daily. Or, 10 to 20 mg scopolamine butylbromide subcutaneously, I.M., or I.V. t.i.d. or q.i.d.
▶ **To reduce secretions preoperatively.** *Adults:* 0.2 to 0.6 mg scopolamine hydrobromide I.M. 30 to 60 minutes before induction of anesthesia. *Children ages 8 to 12:* 0.3 mg scopolamine hydrobromide I.M. 45 minutes before induction of anesthesia. *Children ages 3 to 8:* 0.2 mg scopolamine hydrobromide I.M. 45 minutes before induction of anesthesia. *Children ages 7 months to 3 years:* 0.15 mg scopolamine hydrobromide I.M. 45 minutes before induction of anesthesia. *Infants ages 4 to 7 months:* 0.1 mcg scopolamine hydrobromide I.M. 45 minutes before induction of anesthesia.

▶ **To prevent nausea and vomiting from motion sickness.** *Adults:* 1 Transderm Scōp patch (a circular flat unit), which delivers 1 mg over 3 days (72 hours). Apply to skin behind ear at least 4 hours before antiemetic is needed. Or 0.3 to 0.6 mg scopolamine hydrobromide subcutaneously, I.M., or I.V. Or 0.4 to 0.8 mg P.O.
Children: 0.006 mg/kg or 0.2 mg/m² scopolamine hydrobromide subcutaneously, I.M., or I.V.

▼ I.V. administration

• Intermittent and continuous infusions aren't recommended.
• For direct injection, dilute with sterile water and inject through patent I.V. line.
• Protect I.V. solutions from freezing and light; store at room temperature.
⊗ **Incompatibilities**
Alkalies, anticholinergics, methohexital.

Contraindications and cautions

• Contraindicated in patients with angle-closure glaucoma, obstructive uropathy, obstructive disease of GI tract, asthma, chronic pulmonary disease, myasthenia gravis, paralytic ileus, intestinal atony, unstable CV status in acute hemorrhage, or toxic megacolon.
• Transderm Scōp is contraindicated in patients allergic to scopolamine and other belladonna alkaloids.
• Use cautiously in patients with autonomic neuropathy, hyperthyroidism, coronary artery disease, arrhythmias, heart failure, hypertension, hiatal hernia with reflux esophagitis, hepatic or renal disease, or ulcerative colitis. Also use cautiously in patients in hot or humid environments because of drug-induced heatstroke.
• Use Transderm Scōp cautiously in patients with liver or renal impairment, pyloric obstruction, or urinary bladder and neck obstruction.
⚖ **Lifespan:** In pregnant women and children younger than age 6, use cautiously. In breast-feeding women, don't use. In children, Transderm Scōp is contraindicated. In the elderly, use Transderm Scōp cautiously.

Adverse reactions

CNS: disorientation, restlessness, irritability, dizziness, drowsiness, headache, confusion, hallucinations, delirium, fever.
CV: palpitations, tachycardia, flushing, *paradoxical bradycardia.*

EENT: dilated pupils, blurred vision, photophobia, increased intraocular pressure, difficulty swallowing.
GI: constipation, dry mouth, nausea, vomiting, epigastric distress.
GU: urinary hesitancy, urine retention.
Respiratory: bronchial plugging, *depressed respirations.*
Skin: rash, dryness, contact dermatitis with transdermal patch.

Interactions

Drug-drug. *Centrally acting anticholinergics (antihistamines, phenothiazines, tricyclic antidepressants):* May increase risk of adverse CNS reactions. Monitor patient closely.
CNS depressants: May increase risk of CNS depression. Monitor patient closely.
Digoxin: May increase digoxin level. Monitor patient for cardiac toxicity.
Drug-herb. *Jaborandi tree:* May decrease effects of drug. Discourage using together.
Pill-bearing spurge: May decrease effects of drug. Discourage using together.
Squaw vine: May decrease metabolic breakdown of drug. Discourage using together.
Drug-lifestyle. *Alcohol use:* May increase risk of CNS depression. Discourage using together.

Effects on lab test results

None reported.

Pharmacokinetics

Absorption: Good with P.O., P.R., and transdermal use. Rapidly with I.M. or subcutaneous use.
Distribution: Wide; probably crosses blood-brain barrier.
Metabolism: Probably complete.
Excretion: May be in urine as metabolites.
Half-life: 8 hours.

Route	Onset	Peak	Duration
P.O.	30–60 min	Unknown	4–6 hr
I.V., I.M., SubQ	30 min	Unknown	4 hr
P.R.	Unknown	Unknown	Unknown
Transdermal	3–6 hr	Unknown	≤ 72 hr

Action

Chemical effect: Inhibits muscarinic actions of acetylcholine in the autonomic nervous system. It also may affect neural pathways originating in

S

the labyrinth (inner ear) to inhibit nausea and vomiting.
Therapeutic effect: Relieves spasticity, nausea, and vomiting; reduces secretions; and blocks cardiac vagal reflexes.

Available forms

scopolamine
Transdermal patch: 1.5 mg
scopolamine butylbromide
Capsules: 0.25 mg
Suppositories: 10 mg
Tablets: 10 mg
scopolamine hydrobromide
Injection: 0.3, 0.4, 0.5, 0.6, and 1 mg/ml in 1-ml vials and ampules; 0.86 mg/ml in 0.5-ml ampules

NURSING PROCESS

⬛ Assessment
● Assess patient's condition before starting therapy, and regularly thereafter to monitor the drug's effectiveness.
● Be alert for adverse reactions and drug interactions.
● Assess patient's and family's knowledge of drug therapy.

⊕ Nursing diagnoses
● Risk for deficient fluid volume related to nausea and vomiting
● Risk for injury related to drug-induced adverse CNS reactions
● Deficient knowledge related to drug therapy

▶ Planning and implementation
● In therapeutic doses, drug may produce amnesia, drowsiness, and euphoria; patient may need to be reoriented.
● Raise side rails of bed as a precaution because some patients become temporarily excited or disoriented. Symptoms disappear when sedative effect is complete.
● Tolerance may develop when given for a long time.
● Apply patch the night before patient's expected travel.
⊛ ALERT: Overdose may cause curarelike effects such as respiratory paralysis.
Patient teaching
● Advise patient to apply patch the night before planned trip. Transdermal method releases con-

trolled therapeutic amount of drug. Transderm Scōp is effective if applied 2 or 3 hours before travel but is more effective if applied 12 hours before.
● Advise patient to wash and dry hands thoroughly before applying transdermal patch. After removing patch, he should discard it and wash hands and application site thoroughly, especially before touching eye because pupil may dilate.
● Tell patient that if patch becomes displaced, he should remove it and replace it with another patch on fresh site.
● Alert patient to risk of withdrawal symptoms (nausea, vomiting, headache, dizziness) if transdermal patch is used longer than 72 hours.
● Tell patient to ask pharmacist for the brochure that comes with transdermal patch.
● Tell patient about P.O. or P.R. forms.
● Advise patient to refrain from activities that require alertness until drug's CNS effects are known.
● Instruct patient to report signs of urinary hesitancy or urine retention.
● Recommend use of sugarless gum or hard candy to help minimize dry mouth.

☑ Evaluation
● Patient responds well to therapy.
● Patient doesn't experience injury from adverse CNS reactions.
● Patient and family state understanding of drug therapy.

secobarbital sodium
(sek-oh-BAR-bih-tohl SOH-dee-um)
Novosecobarb ◆ , Seconal Sodium

Pharmacologic class: barbiturate
Therapeutic class: sedative-hypnotic, anticonvulsant
Pregnancy risk category: D
Controlled substance schedule: II

Indications and dosages
▶ **Preoperative sedation.** *Adults:* 200 to 300 mg P.O. 1 to 2 hours before surgery. *Children:* 2 to 6 mg/kg P.O. 1 to 2 hours before surgery. Maximum single dose, 100 mg.
▶ **Insomnia.** *Adults:* 100 mg P.O. h.s.

Reactions may be *common*, uncommon, *life-threatening*, or COMMON AND LIFE-THREATENING.

Contraindications and cautions

• Contraindicated in patients hypersensitive to barbiturates and in patients with marked liver impairment, porphyria, or respiratory disease in which dyspnea or obstruction is evident.

• Use cautiously in patients with acute or chronic pain, depression, suicidal tendencies, history of drug abuse, or hepatic impairment.

❄ **Lifespan:** In pregnant or breast-feeding women, drug isn't recommended.

Adverse reactions

CNS: *drowsiness, lethargy, hangover,* paradoxical excitement in geriatric patients, somnolence.
GI: nausea, vomiting.
Hematologic: exacerbation of porphyria.
Respiratory: *respiratory depression.*
Skin: rash, urticaria, *Stevens-Johnson syndrome.*
Other: *angioedema,* physical or psychological dependence.

Interactions

Drug-drug. *Chloramphenicol, MAO inhibitors, valproic acid:* May inhibit metabolism of barbiturates; may cause prolonged CNS depression. Reduce barbiturate dosage.
CNS depressants, including opioid analgesics: May cause excessive CNS and respiratory depression. Use together cautiously.
Corticosteroids, digitoxin, doxycycline, estrogens, hormonal contraceptives, oral anticoagulants, theophylline, tricyclic antidepressants, verapamil: May enhance metabolism of these drugs, Monitor patient for decreased effect.
Griseofulvin: May decrease absorption of griseofulvin. Monitor patient for decreased griseofulvin effectiveness.
Metoprolol, propranolol: May reduce the effects of these drugs. Consider an increased beta blocker dose
Rifampin: May decrease barbiturate levels. Monitor patient for decreased effect.
Drug-lifestyle. *Alcohol use:* May impair coordination, increase CNS effects, and cause death. Strongly discourage alcohol use with this drug.

Effects on lab test results

• May increase AST and ALT levels.

Pharmacokinetics

Absorption: Rapid; almost complete.

Distribution: Rapid; about 30% to 45% protein-bound.
Metabolism: Oxidized in liver to inactive metabolites.
Excretion: In urine. *Half-life:* About 30 hours.

Route	Onset	Peak	Duration
P.O.	15 min	5–30 min	1–4 hr

Action

Chemical effect: Probably interferes with transmission of impulses from thalamus to cortex of brain.
Therapeutic effect: Promotes pain relief and calmness and relieves acute seizures.

Available forms

Capsules: 50 mg, 100 mg

NURSING PROCESS

Assessment
• Assess patient's condition before starting therapy, and regularly thereafter to monitor the drug's effectiveness.
• Assess mental status before therapy. An elderly patient is more sensitive to the drug's CNS effects.
• Be alert for adverse reactions and drug interactions.
• Assess patient's and family's knowledge of drug therapy.

Nursing diagnoses
• Disturbed sleep pattern related to underlying condition
• Risk for injury related to drug-induced adverse CNS reactions
• Deficient knowledge related to drug therapy

Planning and implementation
• Make sure a patient who is depressed, suicidal, or drug-dependent or who has a history of drug abuse isn't hoarding drug or planning an intentional overdose.
• Skin eruptions may precede a fatal reaction. If skin reactions occur, stop giving the drug and notify the prescriber. In some patients, high fever, stomatitis, headache, or rhinitis may precede skin reactions.
• Long-term use isn't recommended because drug loses its effectiveness after 14 days of continued use.

S

Patient teaching

- Warn patient to avoid activities that require mental alertness or physical coordination. For inpatient, supervise walking and raise bed rails, particularly for an elderly patient.
- Inform patient that morning hangover is common after hypnotic dose, which suppresses REM sleep. Patient may experience increased dreaming after drug is stopped.
- Advise woman who uses a hormonal contraceptive to use a barrier method instead because drug may enhance the metabolism of a hormonal contraceptive and decrease its effect.

☑ Evaluation

- Patient states that drug effectively induces sleep.
- Patient doesn't experience injury from adverse CNS reactions.
- Patient and family state understanding of drug therapy.

selegiline hydrochloride (L-deprenyl hydrochloride)
(seh-LEJ-eh-leen high-droh-KLOR-ighd)
Atapryl, Carbex, Eldepryl, Selpak

Pharmacologic class: MAO inhibitor
Therapeutic class: antiparkinsonian
Pregnancy risk category: C

Indications and dosages

▶ **Adjunct therapy with levodopa and carbidopa for managing symptoms of Parkinson's disease.** *Adults:* 10 mg P.O. daily, taken as 5 mg at breakfast and 5 mg at lunch. After 2 or 3 days of therapy, gradually decrease levodopa-carbidopa dosage.

Contraindications and cautions

- Contraindicated in patients hypersensitive to the drug or any of its components, and in those taking meperidine.
- ☀ **Lifespan:** In pregnant women, use cautiously. In breast-feeding women and in children, safety and effectiveness haven't been established.

Adverse reactions

CNS: *dizziness,* increased tremors, chorea, loss of balance, restlessness, increased bradykinesia, facial grimacing, stiff neck, dyskinesia, involuntary movements, twitching, increased apraxia, behavioral changes, fatigue, headache, confusion, hallucinations, vivid dreams, malaise, syncope.
CV: orthostatic hypotension, hypertension, hypotension, *arrhythmias,* palpitations, angina, tachycardia, peripheral edema.
EENT: blepharospasm.
GI: dry mouth, *nausea,* vomiting, constipation, abdominal pain, anorexia or poor appetite, dysphagia, diarrhea, heartburn.
GU: slow urination, transient nocturia, prostatic hyperplasia, urinary hesitancy, urinary frequency, urine retention, sexual dysfunction.
Metabolic: weight loss.
Skin: rash, hair loss, diaphoresis.

Interactions

Drug-drug. *Adrenergics:* May increase pressor response, particularly in patients who have taken overdose of selegiline. Use together cautiously.
Citalopram, fluoxetine, fluvoxamine, nefazodone, paroxetine, sertraline, venlafaxine: May cause serotonin syndrome involving CNS irritability, shivering, and altered consciousness. Don't give together. Wait at least 2 weeks after stopping an MAO inhibitor before giving any SSRI.
Meperidine: May cause stupor, muscle rigidity, severe agitation, and elevated temperature. Avoid using together.
Drug-herb. *Cacao tree:* May have vasopressor effects. Discourage using together.
Ginseng: May increase risk of adverse reactions, including headache, tremor, and mania. Discourage using together.
Drug-food. *Foods high in tyramine:* May cause hypertensive crisis. Monitor patient's blood pressure; instruct patient to avoid these foods.

Effects on lab test results

None reported.

Pharmacokinetics

Absorption: Rapidly absorbed.
Distribution: Unknown.

Metabolism: Three metabolites include N-desmethyldeprenyl, L-amphetamine, and L-methamphetamine.
Excretion: 45% in urine as metabolite. *Half-life:* selegiline, 2 to 10 hours; N-desmethyldeprenyl, 2 hours; L-amphetamine, 17¾ hours; L-methamphetamine, 20½ hours.

Route	Onset	Peak	Duration
P.O.	Unknown	30 min–2 hr	Unknown

Action

Chemical effect: May act by selectively inhibiting MAO type B (found mostly in brain). It also may directly increase dopaminergic activity by decreasing reuptake of dopamine into nerve cells. Its active metabolites, amphetamine and methamphetamine, may contribute to this effect.
Therapeutic effect: Improves physical mobility.

Available forms

Capsules: 5 mg
Tablets: 5 mg

NURSING PROCESS

Assessment

- Assess patient's condition before starting therapy, and regularly thereafter to monitor the drug's effectiveness.
- Be alert for adverse reactions and drug interactions.
- Assess patient's and family's knowledge of drug therapy.

Nursing diagnoses

- Impaired physical mobility related to underlying condition
- Risk for injury related to drug-induced adverse CNS reactions
- Deficient knowledge related to drug therapy

Planning and implementation

- Some patients experience increased adverse reactions related to levodopa and need a 10% to 30% reduction of levodopa and carbidopa dosage.

ALERT: Don't confuse selegiline with Stelazine or Eldepryl with enalapril.

Patient teaching

- Warn patient to move cautiously at start of therapy because he may experience dizziness.
- Advise patient not to take more than 10 mg daily because greater amount of drug won't improve effectiveness and may increase adverse reactions.
- Tell patient to take drug with food.

Evaluation

- Patient exhibits improved physical mobility.
- Patient doesn't experience injury from adverse CNS reactions.
- Patient and family state understanding of drug therapy.

sertaconazole nitrate

(sir-tah-CON-ah-zole NIGH-trate)
Ertaczo

Pharmacologic class: imidazole derivative
Therapeutic class: topical antifungal
Pregnancy risk category: C

Indications and dosages

▶ **Tinea pedis caused by *Trichophyton mentagrophytes, T. rubrum,* or *Epidermophyton floccosum* in immunocompetent patients.** *Adults and children age 12 and older:* Apply cream twice daily to affected areas between toes and healthy surrounding areas for 4 weeks.

Contraindications and cautions

- Contraindicated in patients hypersensitive to the drug, any of its components, or other imidazoles.

Lifespan: In pregnant women, use cautiously. In breast-feeding women, use cautiously; it's unknown if the drug appears in breast milk. In children younger than age 12, safety and effectiveness haven't been established.

Adverse reactions

Skin: application site reactions, burning skin, contact dermatitis, dry skin, skin tenderness.

Interactions

None known.

Effects on lab test results

- None reported.

Pharmacokinetics

Absorption: Unknown.

S

Distribution: Unknown.
Metabolism: Unknown.
Excretion: Unknown. *Half-life:* Unknown.

Route	Onset	Peak	Duration
Topical	Unknown	Unknown	Unknown

Action

Chemical effect: May inhibit the CYP-dependent synthesis of ergosterol. The lack of ergosterol in the cell membrane alters cell wall permeability and osmotic instability leading to fungal cell injury and death.
Therapeutic effect: Kills susceptible fungus.

Available forms

Topical cream: 2%, in 15- and 30-g tubes

NURSING PROCESS

⚖ Assessment
• Assess area of infection before therapy and regularly thereafter to monitor the drug's effectiveness.
• Monitor patient for adverse effects. Stop giving the drug if skin irritation or sensitivity develops.
• Assess patient's and family's knowledge of drug therapy.

⊞ Nursing diagnoses
• Impaired tissue integrity related to infection with susceptible organisms
• Impaired skin integrity related to adverse effects of drug
• Deficient knowledge related to drug therapy

⊁ Planning and implementation
• Before treatment starts, make sure that diagnosis has been confirmed by direct microscopic examination of infected tissue in potassium hydroxide solution or by culture on an appropriate medium.
• Drug is for use on skin only, not for ophthalmic, oral, or intravaginal use.
• If condition hasn't improved after 2 weeks, review the diagnosis.
Patient teaching
• Warn patient to stop using drug if he develops increased irritation, redness, itching, burning, blistering, swelling, or oozing at the site of application.

• Caution patient that drug is for external use on skin only. Discourage contact with eyes, nose, mouth, and other mucous membranes.
• If cream will be applied after bathing, tell patient to dry the affected area thoroughly before use.
• Tell patient to wash hands after applying cream.
• Urge patient to use the drug for the full duration of treatment, even if symptoms have improved.
• Instruct patient to notify prescriber if condition worsens or fails to improve.
• Caution patient to avoid occlusive coverings unless directed by prescriber.
• Teach patient proper foot hygiene.

☑ Evaluation
• Tissue integrity is restored after treatment.
• Patient doesn't experience adverse drug effects.
• Patient and family state understanding of drug therapy.

sertraline hydrochloride
(SER-truh-leen high-droh-KLOR-ighd)
Zoloft⬦

Pharmacologic class: SSRI
Therapeutic class: antidepressant
Pregnancy risk category: C

Indications and dosages

▶ **Depression.** *Adults:* 50 mg P.O. daily. Adjust dosage as tolerated and needed, at intervals of no less than 1 week. Maximum dosage, 200 mg daily.
▶ **Post-traumatic stress disorder, social anxiety disorder, obsessive compulsive disorder, panic disorder.** *Adults:* Initially, 25 mg P.O. once daily. Increase dosage to 50 mg P.O. once daily after 1 week of therapy. Dosage may be increased at weekly intervals to a maximum of 200 mg daily. Maintain patient on lowest effective dosage.
▶ **Premenstrual dysphoric disorder.** *Women:* Initially, 50 mg daily P.O. continuously, or limited to the luteal phase of the menstrual cycle. Patients not responding may benefit from dose increases at 50-mg increments per menstrual cycle up to 150 mg daily when taken daily

throughout the menstrual cycle, or 100 mg daily when taken during the luteal phase of the menstrual cycle. If a 100-mg daily dose has been established with luteal-phase regimen, a 50-mg daily adjustment step for 3 days should be used at the beginning of each luteal phase.
► **Premature ejaculation‡.** *Adults:* 25 to 50 mg P.O. daily or p.r.n.
⊠ **Adjust-a-dose:** Give lower or less frequent doses with hepatic impairment.

Contraindications and cautions

• Contraindicated in patients hypersensitive to the drug or any of its components, and in patients receiving pimozide.
• Use cautiously in patients at risk for suicide and in those with seizure disorder, major affective disorder, or diseases or conditions that affect metabolism or hemodynamic responses.
• Drug should not be discontinued abruptly.
⚹ **Lifespan:** In pregnant women, use cautiously. In breast-feeding women, use cautiously; it's unknown if the drug appears in breast milk. In children younger than age 18, drug isn't approved for use in treatment of major depressive disorder due to possible increased risk of suicidal behavior.

Adverse reactions

CNS: *headache, tremor, dizziness, insomnia, somnolence,* paresthesia, hypesthesia, hyperesthesia, *fatigue,* twitching, hypertonia, nervousness, anxiety, confusion.
CV: palpitations, chest pain, hot flushes, flushing.
GI: *dry mouth, nausea, diarrhea, loose stools, dyspepsia,* vomiting, constipation, thirst, flatulence, anorexia, abdominal pain, increased appetite.
GU: male sexual dysfunction, decreased libido.
Musculoskeletal: myalgia.
Skin: *diaphoresis,* rash, pruritus.

Interactions

Drug-drug. *Benzodiazepines (except lorazepam and oxazepam), tolbutamide:* May decrease clearance of these drugs. Monitor patient for increased drug effects.
Cimetidine: May decrease sertraline clearance. Monitor patient for toxicity.
Disulfiram: May cause a disulfiram reaction because oral concentrate contains alcohol. Avoid using together.

Phenelzine, selegiline, tranylcypromine: May cause serotonin syndrome, including CNS irritability, shivering, and altered consciousness. Don't give together. Wait at least 2 weeks after stopping an MAO inhibitor before giving any SSRI.
Pimozide: May increase pimozide level and cause bradycardia. Avoid using together.
Sumatriptan: May cause weakness, hyperreflexia, and incoordination. Monitor patient closely.
Tricyclic antidepressants (TCA): May inhibit TCA metabolism. Reduce TCA dose. Monitor patient closely.
Warfarin, other highly protein-bound drugs: May increase levels of warfarin or other highly bound drug. Monitor patient, PT, and INR closely.
Drug-herb. *Ginkgo:* May decrease adverse sexual effects of drug. Advise patient to speak to prescriber before taking any herbal remedy.
St. John's wort: May cause additive effects and serotonin syndrome, including CNS irritability, shivering, and altered consciousness. Discourage use together.
Drug-lifestyle. *Alcohol use:* May enhance CNS effects. Advise patient to avoid alcohol use.

Effects on lab test results

• May increase ALT, AST, cholesterol, and triglyceride levels. May decrease uric acid level.

Pharmacokinetics

Absorption: Well absorbed from GI tract. Rate and extent enhanced when taken with food.
Distribution: Highly protein-bound (greater than 98%).
Metabolism: Metabolism is probably hepatic.
Excretion: Excreted mostly as metabolites in urine and feces. *Half-life:* 26 hours.

Route	Onset	Peak	Duration
P.O.	2–4 wk	4½–8½ hr	Unknown

Action

Chemical effect: Unknown; may be linked to inhibited neuronal uptake of serotonin in CNS.
Therapeutic effect: Relieves depression.

Available forms

Oral concentrate: 20 mg/ml
Tablets: 25 mg, 50 mg, 100 mg

NURSING PROCESS

⚖ Assessment
• Assess patient's condition before starting therapy, and regularly thereafter to monitor the drug's effectiveness.
• Assess patient for risk factors for suicide.
• Be alert for adverse reactions and drug interactions.
• Assess patient's and family's knowledge of drug therapy.

⊕ Nursing diagnoses
• Disturbed thought processes related to presence of depression
• Risk for injury related to drug-induced adverse CNS reactions
• Deficient knowledge related to drug therapy

⟩ Planning and implementation
• Give drug once daily, either morning or evening. Drug may be given with or without food.
• Don't give within 14 days of MAO inhibitor therapy.
• In a patient with a latex allergy, don't use the rubber oral concentrate dropper.
• Don't abruptly discontinue drug. Taper gradually over several weeks, and monitor the patient carefully for serotonin syndrome.

Patient teaching
• Advise patient to use caution when performing hazardous tasks that require alertness and not to drink alcohol or take other drugs that affect CNS while taking this drug.
• Instruct patient to check with prescriber or pharmacist before taking OTC drugs.
• Advise patient to mix the oral concentrate with 4 oz of water, ginger ale, or lemon-lime soda only, and to take the dose right away.

✓ Evaluation
• Patient behavior and communication indicate improved thought processes.
• Patient doesn't experience injury from adverse CNS reactions.
• Patient and family state understanding of drug therapy.

sevelamer hydrochloride
(seh-VEL-ah-mer high-droh-KLOR-ighd)
Renagel

Pharmacologic class: polymeric phosphate binder
Therapeutic class: antihyperphosphatemic
Pregnancy risk category: C

Indications and dosages
▶ **To reduce phosphorus level in patients with end-stage renal disease who are undergoing hemodialysis.** *Adults:* Depends on severity of hyperphosphatemia. Gradually adjust dosage based on phosphorus level, with goal of lowering phosphorus to 6 mg/dl or less. If phosphorus level is 9 mg/dl or more, start with 1.6 g P.O. t.i.d. with meals; if phosphorus level is between 7.5 and 9 mg/dl, 1.2 g P.O. t.i.d. or 1.6 g P.O. t.i.d. with meals; if phosphorus level is between 6 and 7.5 mg/dl, 800 mg P.O. t.i.d. with meals.

Dosage may be increased or decreased by one tablet per meal at 2-week intervals according to the patient's serum phosphorus level. If serum phosphorous level is > 6 mg/dl, increase by 1 tablet per meal. If serum phosphorous level is < 3.5 mg/dl, decrease by 1 tablet per meal.

Contraindications and cautions
• Contraindicated in patients hypersensitive to the drug or any of its components, and in those with hypophosphatemia or bowel obstruction.
• Use cautiously in patients with dysphagia, swallowing disorders, severe GI motility disorders, or major GI tract surgery.
☆ Lifespan: Use in pregnancy only if benefits clearly outweigh potential risks to the fetus. In breast-feeding women, use cautiously; it's unknown if the drug appears in breast milk. In children, safety and effectiveness haven't been established.

Adverse reactions
CNS: headache, pain.
CV: hypertension, hypotension, *thrombosis.*
GI: *vomiting,* nausea, constipation, *diarrhea,* flatulence, *dyspepsia.*
Respiratory: cough.
Other: infection.

Reactions may be *common,* uncommon, *life-threatening*, or COMMON AND LIFE-THREATENING.

Interactions

Drug-drug. *Antiarrhythmics, anticonvulsants:* May interact. Give drug at least 1 hour before or 3 hours after giving these drugs and monitor levels of these drugs.

Effects on lab test results

• May increase alkaline phosphatase level.

Pharmacokinetics

Absorption: Unknown.
Distribution: Binds bile acids in the intestines forming a nonabsorbable complex with phosphorus.
Metabolism: None known systemically.
Excretion: In feces. *Half-life:* Unknown.

Route	Onset	Peak	Duration
P.O.	Unknown	Unknown	Unknown

Action

Chemical effect: Inhibits intestinal phosphate absorption.
Therapeutic effect: Decreases phosphorus level.

Available forms

Capsules: 403 mg
Tablets: 400 mg, 800 mg

NURSING PROCESS

Assessment

• Obtain history of patient's underlying condition before starting therapy, and reassess regularly thereafter to monitor the drug's effectiveness.
• Monitor calcium, bicarbonate, and chloride levels.
• Watch for symptoms of thrombosis (numbness or tingling of limbs, chest pain, shortness of breath), and notify prescriber if they occur.
• Assess patient's and family's knowledge of drug therapy.

Nursing diagnoses

• Ineffective tissue perfusion (cardiopulmonary or peripheral) related to potential drug-induced thrombosis
• Imbalanced nutrition: less than body requirements related to drug-induced adverse GI effects
• Deficient knowledge related to drug therapy

Planning and implementation

• Don't crush or break capsules or tablets, and give only with meals.
• Drug may bind to other drugs given at the same time and decrease their bioavailability. Give other drugs 1 hour before or 3 hours after sevelamer.
ALERT: Drug may reduce vitamins D, E, and K and folic acid. Give a multivitamin supplement.

Patient teaching

• Instruct patient to take with meals and adhere to prescribed diet.
• Inform patient that drug must be taken whole because contents expand in water; tell him not to open or chew capsules.
• Tell patient to take other drugs as directed, but they must be taken either 1 hour before or 3 hours after sevelamer.
• Inform patient about common adverse reactions and instruct him to report them immediately. Teach patient signs and symptoms of thrombosis (numbness, tingling limbs, chest pain, changes in level of consciousness).

Evaluation

• Patient doesn't develop a thrombus.
• Patient maintains adequate nutrition.
• Patient and family state understanding of drug therapy.

sibutramine hydrochloride monohydrate

(sigh-BYOO-truh-meen high-droh-KLOR-ighd mah-noh-HIGH-drayt)
Meridia

Pharmacologic class: serotonin, norepinephrine, and dopamine reuptake inhibitor
Therapeutic class: anorexic
Pregnancy risk category: C
Controlled substance schedule: IV

Indications and dosages

▶ **To manage obesity.** *Adults:* 10 mg P.O. once daily with or without food. If weight loss isn't adequate after 4 weeks, increase dosage to 15 mg P.O. daily. Patients who don't tolerate the 10-mg dose may receive 5 mg P.O. daily. Doses above 15 mg daily aren't recommended.

S

Contraindications and cautions

• Contraindicated in patients hypersensitive to the drug or any of its components, those taking MAO inhibitors or other centrally acting appetite suppressants, and those with anorexia nervosa. Don't use drug in patients with severe renal or hepatic dysfunction, history of hypertension, seizures, coronary artery disease, heart failure, arrhythmias, or stroke.

• Use cautiously in patients with angle-closure glaucoma, and in patients predisposed to bleeding events or taking drugs that affect hemostasis or platelet function.

• Use not recommended for more than 2 years.

⚞ **Lifespan:** In pregnant and breast-feeding women, use isn't recommended. Women of child-bearing age should use adequate contraception and notify prescriber promptly if they become pregnant. In children younger than age 16, safety and effectiveness haven't been established.

Adverse reactions

CNS: asthenia, *headache, insomnia,* dizziness, nervousness, anxiety, depression, paresthesia, somnolence, CNS stimulation, emotional lability, migraine.
CV: tachycardia, vasodilation, hypertension, palpitations, chest pain, generalized edema.
EENT: thirst, *rhinitis, pharyngitis,* sinusitis, ear disorder, ear pain, laryngitis.
GI: *dry mouth,* taste perversion, *anorexia, constipation,* increased appetite, nausea, dyspepsia, gastritis, vomiting, abdominal pain, rectal disorder.
GU: dysmenorrhea, UTI, vaginal candidiasis, metrorrhagia.
Musculoskeletal: arthralgia, myalgia, tenosynovitis, joint disorder, neck or back pain.
Respiratory: cough.
Skin: rash, sweating, acne.
Other: flulike syndrome, injury, herpes simplex, accident, allergic reaction.

Interactions

Drug-drug. *CNS depressants:* May enhance CNS depression. Use cautiously.
Dextromethorphan, dihydroergotamine, fentanyl, fluoxetine, fluvoxamine, lithium, MAO inhibitors, meperidine, paroxetine, pentazocine, sertraline, sumatriptan, tryptophan, venlafaxine: May cause hyperthermia, tachycardia, and loss of consciousness. Don't use together.

Ephedrine, pseudoephedrine: May increase blood pressure or heart rate. Use cautiously.
Erythromycin, cimetidine, ketoconazole: May result in small increases in sibutramine metabolites. Use cautiously together.
Drug-lifestyle. *Alcohol use:* May enhance CNS depression. Discourage using together.

Effects on lab test results

• May increase ALT, AST, GGT, LDH, alkaline phosphatase, and bilirubin levels.

Pharmacokinetics

Absorption: Rapid; about 77% of dose is absorbed.
Distribution: Rapid and extensive. Active metabolites are extensively bound to proteins.
Metabolism: Extensive in the first pass by the liver to two active metabolites, M_1 and M_2.
Excretion: About 77% in urine. *Half-life:* M_1 is 14 hours and M_2 is 16 hours.

Route	Onset	Peak	Duration
P.O.	Unknown	3–4 hr	Unknown

Action

Chemical effect: Inhibits reuptake of norepinephrine, serotonin, and dopamine.
Therapeutic effect: Facilitates weight loss.

Available forms

Capsules: 5 mg, 10 mg, 15 mg

NURSING PROCESS

⯎ Assessment
• Monitor patient for adverse reactions and drug interactions.
• Assess patient for organic causes of obesity before starting therapy.
• Assess patient's dietary intake.
• Measure blood pressure and pulse before starting therapy, with dosage changes, and at regular intervals during therapy.
• Assess patient's and family's knowledge of drug therapy.

⯎ Nursing diagnoses
• Imbalanced nutrition: more than body requirements related to increased caloric intake
• Disturbed sleep pattern related to drug-induced insomnia
• Deficient knowledge related to drug therapy

Reactions may be *common,* uncommon, *life-threatening,* or COMMON AND LIFE-THREATENING.

⧉ Planning and implementation
● Don't give drug within 14 days of MAO inhibitor therapy.
● Give patient ice chips or sugarless hard candy to relieve dry mouth.
● Make sure patient follows appropriate diet regimen.

Patient teaching
● Advise patient to immediately report rash, hives, or other allergic reactions.
● Instruct patient to inform prescriber if he is taking or plans to take other prescription or OTC drugs.
● Advise patient to have blood pressure and pulse monitored at regular intervals. Stress importance of regular follow-up visits with prescriber.
● Advise patient to use drug with reduced calorie diet.
● Tell patient that weight loss can cause gallstones. Teach patient about signs and symptoms and the need to report them to prescriber promptly.

⧉ Evaluation
● Patient achieves nutritional balance with the use of drugs and a reduced-calorie diet.
● Patient experiences normal sleep patterns.
● Patient and family state understanding of drug therapy.

sildenafil citrate
(sil-DEN-ah-fil SIGH-trayt)
Revatio

Pharmacologic class: cyclic guanosine monophosphate (cGMP)–specific phosphodiesterase type 5 (PDE5) inhibitor
Therapeutic class: vasodilator
Pregnancy risk category: B

Indications and dosages
▶ **To improve exercise ability in patients with World Health Organization group I pulmonary arterial hypertension.** *Adults:* 20 mg P.O. t.i.d., 4 to 6 hours apart.

Contraindications and cautions
● Contraindicated in patients hypersensitive to drug or its components and in those taking organic nitrates.

● Don't use in patients with pulmonary venoocclusive disease.
● Use cautiously in patients with resting hypotension, severe left ventricular outflow obstruction, autonomic dysfunction, and volume depletion.
● Use cautiously in patients with hepatic or severe renal impairment, retinitis pigmentosa, bleeding disorders, or active peptic ulcer disease; those who have had an MI, a stroke, or a life-threatening arrhythmia in last 6 months; those with history of coronary artery disease causing unstable angina or uncontrolled high or low blood pressure; those with deformation of the penis and conditions that may cause priapism (such as sickle cell anemia, multiple myeloma, or leukemia); and those taking bosentan.
⚖ **Lifespan:** In pregnant women, use cautiously. Use cautiously in breast-feeding women; it isn't known whether drug appears in breast milk. Safety and effectiveness haven't been established in children. Use cautiously in elderly patients because they have an increased risk of impaired renal, hepatic, and cardiac function and of concurrent disease.

Adverse reactions
CNS: fever, headache, dizziness.
CV: hypotension, flushing.
EENT: epistaxis, rhinitis, sinusitis, photophobia, impaired color discrimination, blurred vision, burning.
GI: dyspepsia, diarrhea, gastritis.
Musculoskeletal: myalgia.
Skin: erythema.

Interactions
Drug-drug. *Alpha blockers:* May cause symptomatic hypotension. Use together cautiously.
Amlodipine: May further reduce blood pressure. Monitor blood pressure closely.
Bosentan: May decrease sildenafil level. Monitor patient.
Cytochrome P450 inducers, rifampin: May reduce sildenafil level. Monitor effect.
Hepatic isoenzyme inhibitors (such as cimetidine, erythromycin, itraconazole, ketoconazole): May increase sildenafil level. Avoid using together.
Isosorbide, nitroglycerin: May cause severe hypotension. Use of nitrates in any form is contraindicated during therapy.

S

Protease inhibitors (ritonavir): May significantly increase sildenafil level. Don't use together.
Vitamin K antagonists: May increase risk of bleeding (primarily epistaxis). Monitor patient.
Drug-food. *Grapefruit:* May increase drug level and delay absorption. Advise patient to avoid using together.

Effects on lab test results

None reported.

Pharmacokinetics

Absorption: Rapid. Absolute bioavailability is 40%.
Distribution: Extensively into body tissues. About 96% bound to proteins.
Metabolism: Mainly in the liver to an active metabolite with properties similar to those of parent drug.
Excretion: About 80% in feces and 13% in urine. *Half-life:* 4 hours.

Route	Onset	Peak	Duration
P.O.	15–30 min	30 min–2 hr	4 hr

Action

Chemical effect: Increases cyclic guanosine monophosphate levels by preventing its breakdown by phosphodiesterase, prolonging smooth muscle relaxation of the pulmonary vasculature, which leads to vasodilation.
Therapeutic effect: Improved exercise tolerance in patients with World Health Organization group I pulmonary arterial hypertension.

Available Forms

Tablets: 20 mg

NURSING PROCESS

Assessment

- Assess patient for underlying conditions that could be adversely affected by vasodilatory effects of the drug including resting hypotension (blood pressure below 90/50 mm Hg), fluid depletion, severe ventricular outflow obstruction, or autonomic dysfunction.
- Monitor patient's vital signs carefully at start of treatment.
- Monitor patient for evidence of pulmonary edema; if it occurs, consider pulmonary veno-occlusive disease.
- Monitor patient for development of visual disturbances such as photophobia, impaired color discrimination, blurred vision, and burning.
- Assess patient's and family's knowledge of drug therapy.

Nursing diagnoses

- Ineffective tissue perfusion (cardiopulmonary) related to underlying condition
- Activity intolerance related to underlying medical condition
- Deficient knowledge related to drug therapy

Planning and implementation

ALERT: Don't substitute Viagra for Revatio because there isn't an equivalent dose.
- Patients with pulmonary arterial hypertension caused by connective tissue disease are more prone to epistaxis during therapy than those with primary pulmonary hypertension.
- The serious CV events linked to this drug's use in erectile dysfunction mainly involve patients with underlying CV disease who are at increased risk for cardiac effects related to sexual activity.

Patient teaching
- Warn patient that drug should never be used with nitrates.
- Advise patient to rise slowly from lying down.
- Inform patient that drug can be taken with or without food.
- Warn patient that discrimination between colors such as blue and green may become impaired during therapy; warn him to avoid hazardous activities that rely on recognizing colors.
- Instruct patient to notify prescriber of visual changes, dizziness, or fainting.
- Caution patient to take drug only as prescribed.

Evaluation

- Patient's pulmonary artery pressure decreases, and patient reaches pulmonary hemodynamic stability.
- Patient experiences improved exercise tolerance with drug therapy.
- Patient and family state understanding of drug therapy.

sildenafil citrate
(sil-DEN-ah-fil SIGH-trayt)
Viagra℘

Pharmacologic class: phosphodiesterase type 5 (PDE 5) inhibitor
Therapeutic class: erectile dysfunction drug
Pregnancy risk category: B

Indications and dosages

▶ **Erectile dysfunction.** *Men younger than age 65:* 50 mg P.O., p.r.n., about 1 hour before sexual activity. Dosage range is 25 to 100 mg, based on effectiveness and tolerance. Maximum, 1 dose daily.
⊠ **Adjust-a-dose:** Men age 65 and older or those with hepatic or severe renal impairment or those taking potent CYP 3A4 inhibitors (erythromycin, ketoconazole, itraconazole, saquinavir) should take 25 mg P.O. about 1 hour before sexual activity. Base dose on patient response. Maximum, 1 dose daily.

Contraindications and cautions

• Contraindicated in patients hypersensitive to the drug or any of its components, those with underlying CV disease, and those using organic nitrates at any frequency and in any form.
• Use cautiously in patients with hepatic or severe renal impairment; those with anatomic deformation of the penis; those with conditions that may predispose them to priapism (such as sickle cell anemia, multiple myeloma, leukemia), retinitis pigmentosa, bleeding disorders, or active peptic ulcer disease; those who have had an MI, stroke, or life-threatening arrhythmia during previous 6 months; and those with history of cardiac failure, coronary artery disease, or uncontrolled high or low blood pressure.
▥ **Lifespan:** In men age 65 and older, use cautiously. Not indicated for use in women or children.

Adverse reactions

CNS: anxiety, *headache,* dizziness, *seizures,* somnolence, vertigo.
CV: *MI, sudden cardiac death, ventricular arrhythmia, cerebrovascular hemorrhage, transient ischemic attack,* hypotension, flushing.
EENT: diplopia, temporary vision loss, decreased vision, ocular redness or bloodshot appearance, increased intraocular pressure, retinal vascular disease, retinal bleeding, vitreous detachment or traction, perimacular edema, abnormal vision (photophobia, color-tinged vision, blurred vision), ocular burning, ocular swelling or pressure.
GI: dyspepsia, diarrhea.
GU: hematuria, priapism, UTI.
Musculoskeletal: arthralgia, back pain.
Respiratory: respiratory tract infection.
Skin: rash.
Other: flulike syndrome.

Interactions

Drug-drug. *Alpha blockers:* May cause hypotension or syncope.Caution patient not to take 50- to 100-mg doses of sildenafil within 4 hours of an alpha blocker. A dose of 25 mg may be taken at any time.
CYP 3A4 inducers, rifampin: May reduce sildenafil level. Monitor drug effect.
Hepatic isoenzyme inhibitors (such as cimetidine, erythromycin, itraconazole, ketoconazole): May reduce clearance of sildenafil. Avoid using together or reduce dosage to 25 mg.
Isosorbide, nitroglycerin, other nitrates: May cause severe hypotension. Use of nitrates in any form with sildenafil is contraindicated.
Protease inhibitors (ritonavir, saquinavir), delavirdine: May increase sildenafil level and may result in an increase in sildenafil-related adverse events, including hypotension, visual changes, and priapism. Tell patient not to exceed 25 mg in a 48-hour period.
Drug-food. *Grapefruit:* May increase levels and delay absorption. Advise patient to avoid consuming grapefruit products.
High-fat meals: Reduces rate of absorption and decreases peak levels. Tell patient to separate dose from meals.

Effects on lab test results

None reported.

Pharmacokinetics

Absorption: Rapid. Absolute bioavailability is 40%.
Distribution: Extensively into body tissues. About 96% bound to proteins.
Metabolism: Mainly in the liver to an active metabolite with properties similar to those of parent drug.

S

Excretion: About 80% in feces and 13% in urine. *Half-life:* 4 hours.

Route	Onset	Peak	Duration
P.O.	30 min	30 min–2 hr	4 hr

Action

Chemical effect: Enhances the effect of nitric oxide (NO) by inhibiting PDE 5. When sexual stimulation causes local release of NO, inhibition of PDE 5 causes increased levels of cyclic guanosine monophosphate in the corpus cavernosum, resulting in smooth muscle relaxation and inflow of blood.
Therapeutic effect: Patient achieves an erection.

Available forms

Tablets: 25 mg, 50 mg, 100 mg

NURSING PROCESS

Assessment
● Discuss patient's history of erectile dysfunction to establish need for drug versus other therapies.
● Assess patient for CV risk factors because serious events have been reported with drug, and report risk factors to prescriber.
● Assess patient's and family's knowledge of drug therapy.

Nursing diagnoses
● Sexual dysfunction related to patient's underlying condition
● Ineffective tissue perfusion (cardiopulmonary) related to drug-induced effects on blood pressure and cardiac output
● Deficient knowledge related to drug therapy

Planning and implementation
⊛ **ALERT:** Serious CV events, including MI, sudden cardiac death, ventricular arrhythmia, cerebrovascular hemorrhage, transient ischemic attack, and hypertension, may occur in patients during or shortly after sexual activity.
⊛ **ALERT:** Drug's systemic vasodilation causes transient decreases in supine blood pressure and cardiac output about 2 hours after use. Together with the cardiac risk of sexual activity, the risk for patients with underlying CV disease is increased.

Patient teaching
● Advise patient that drug is contraindicated with regular or intermittent use of nitrates.
● Warn patient about cardiac risk with sexual activity, especially if he has CV risk factors. If patient has symptoms such as angina pectoris, dizziness, or nausea at the start of sexual activity, instruct him to notify prescriber and refrain from further sexual activity.
● Warn patient that erections lasting more than 4 hours and priapism (painful erections more than 6 hours) may occur and should be reported immediately. If priapism isn't treated immediately, penile tissue damage and permanent loss of potency may result.
● Inform patient that drug doesn't protect against sexually transmitted diseases and that protective measures, such as condoms, should be used.
● Instruct patient to take drug 30 minutes to 4 hours before sexual activity; maximum benefit can be expected less than 2 hours after ingesting drug.
● Advise patient that drug is most rapidly absorbed if taken on an empty stomach.
● Inform patient to avoid potentially hazardous activities that rely on color discrimination because blue and green discrimination may be impaired.
● Instruct patient to notify prescriber if visual changes occur.
● Advise patient that drug is effective only with sexual stimulation.
● Tell patient to take drug only as prescribed.
● Advise patient taking HIV drugs or alpha blockers about an increased risk of sildenafil-related adverse events, including hypotension, visual changes, and priapism, and he should promptly report any symptoms to his prescriber. Tell him not to exceed 25 mg of sildenafil in a 48-hour period.

Evaluation
● Sexual activity improves with drug therapy.
● Patient doesn't experience adverse CV events.
● Patient and family state understanding of drug therapy.

simvastatin (synvinolin)
(sim-vuh-STAT-in)
Lipex ◇ , Zocor◉

Pharmacologic class: HMG-CoA reductase inhibitor
Therapeutic class: antihyperlipemic
Pregnancy risk category: X

Indications and dosages

▶ **To reduce risk of CAD mortality and CV events in patients at high risk.** *Adults:* Initially, 20 to 40 mg P.O. daily in evening. Dosage adjusted q 4 weeks based on patient tolerance and response. Maximum, 80 mg daily.
▶ **To reduce total cholesterol and LDL levels in patients with homozygous familial hypercholesterolemia.** *Adults:* 40 mg daily in evening; or 80 mg daily in three divided doses of 20 mg in morning, 20 mg in afternoon, and 40 mg in evening.
▶ **Heterozygous familial hypercholesterolemia.** *Children ages 10 to 17:* 10 mg P.O. once daily in the evening. Maximum, 40 mg daily.
🔲 **Adjust-a-dose:** For patients taking cyclosporine, initially give 5 mg P.O. daily; don't exceed 10 mg daily. For patients taking fibrates or niacin, maximum is 10 mg P.O. daily. For patients taking amiodarone or verapamil, maximum is 20 mg P.O. daily. For patients with severe renal insufficiency, initially give 5 mg P.O. daily.

Contraindications and cautions

• Contraindicated in patients hypersensitive to the drug or any of its components, and in those with active liver disease or conditions that have unexplained persistent elevations of transaminase levels.
• Use cautiously in patients who consume substantial quantities of alcohol or have a history of liver disease.
⚠ **Lifespan:** In pregnant women, breastfeeding women, and women of childbearing age, drug is contraindicated. In children, safety and effectiveness haven't been established.

Adverse reactions

CNS: headache, asthenia.
GI: abdominal pain, constipation, diarrhea, dyspepsia, flatulence, nausea.
Hepatic: *cirrhosis, hepatitis, hepatic necrosis.*
Musculoskeletal: myalgia.
Respiratory: upper respiratory tract infection.

Interactions

Drug-drug. *Amiodarone, verapamil:* May increase risk of myopathy and rhabdomyolysis. Don't exceed 20 mg simvastatin daily.
Clarithromycin, erythromycin, HIV protease inhibitors, nefazodone: May increase risk of myopathy and rhabdomyolysis. Avoid using together, or suspend therapy during treatment with clarithromycin or erythromycin.
Cyclosporine, fibrates, niacin: May increase risk of myopathy and rhabdomyolysis. Monitor patient closely if use together can't be avoided. Don't exceed 10 mg simvastatin daily.
Digoxin: May elevate digoxin level slightly. Closely monitor at the start of therapy.
Fluconazole, itraconazole, ketoconazole: May increase levels and adverse effects of simvastatin. Avoid this combination. If they must be given together, reduce dose of simvastatin.
Hepatotoxic drugs: May increase risk of hepatotoxicity. Avoid using together.
Warfarin: May enhance anticoagulant effect. Monitor PT and INR at the start of therapy and during dose adjustment.
Drug-herb. *Red yeast rice:* May increase the risk of adverse events or toxicity. Discourage using together.
Drug-food. *Grapefruit juice:* May increase drug level and risk of adverse effects, including myopathy and rhabdomyolysis. Advise patient against drinking a quart or more of juice per day.
Drug-lifestyle. *Alcohol use:* May increase the risk of hepatotoxicity. Discourage using together.

Effects on lab test results

• May increase liver enzyme and CK levels.

Pharmacokinetics

Absorption: Good, but extensive hepatic extraction limits availability of active inhibitors to 5% of dose or less.
Distribution: More than 95% bound to proteins.
Metabolism: Hydrolysis occurs in plasma; at least three major metabolites have been identified.
Excretion: Primarily in bile. *Half-life:* 3 hours.

Route	Onset	Peak	Duration
P.O.	Unknown	1½–2½ hr	Unknown

Action

Chemical effect: Inhibits HMG-CoA reductase. This enzyme is early (and rate-limiting) step in synthetic pathway of cholesterol.
Therapeutic effect: Lowers LDL and total cholesterol levels.

Available forms

Tablets: 5 mg, 10 mg, 20 mg, 40 mg, 80 mg

NURSING PROCESS

⚖ Assessment
● Obtain history of patient's LDL and total cholesterol levels before starting therapy, and reassess regularly thereafter to monitor the drug's effectiveness.
● Obtain liver function test results before starting therapy and periodically thereafter. If enzyme level elevations persist, a liver biopsy may be performed.
● Monitor patient for myalgia—muscular weakness—and for elevated CK level, during treatment. Rhabdomyolysis with and without acute renal insufficiency has been reported.
● Be alert for adverse reactions and drug interactions.
● Assess patient's dietary fat intake.
● Assess patient's and family's knowledge of drug therapy.

⊕ Nursing diagnoses
● Risk for injury related to presence of elevated cholesterol levels
● Constipation related to drug-induced adverse GI reactions
● Deficient knowledge related to drug therapy

▷ Planning and implementation
● Drug therapy starts only after diet and other nondrug therapies have proven ineffective.
● Make sure patient follows a standard low-cholesterol diet during therapy.
● Give drug with evening meal for enhanced effectiveness.
● If cholesterol level falls below target range, dosage may be reduced.
⑤ ALERT: Don't confuse Zocor with Cozaar.
Patient teaching
● Tell patient to take drug with evening meal to enhance absorption and cholesterol biosynthesis.

● Teach patient dietary management of lipids (restricting total fat and cholesterol intake) and measures to control other cardiac disease risk factors. If appropriate, suggest weight control, exercise, and smoking cessation programs.
● Tell patient to inform prescriber about adverse reactions, particularly muscle aches and pains.
⑤ ALERT: Inform woman that drug is contraindicated during pregnancy. Advise her to notify prescriber immediately if pregnancy occurs.

✓ Evaluation
● Patient's LDL and total cholesterol levels are within normal limits.
● Patient regains and maintains normal bowel pattern throughout therapy.
● Patient and family state understanding of drug therapy.

sirolimus
(sir-AH-lih-mus)
Rapamune

Pharmacologic class: macrocyclic lactone
Therapeutic class: immunosuppressant
Pregnancy risk category: C

Indications and dosages

▶ **Prophylaxis of organ rejection in patients receiving renal transplants.** *Adults and children age 13 and older who weigh 40 kg (88 lb) or more:* Initially, 6 mg P.O. as a one-time loading dose as soon as possible after transplantation; then maintenance dose of 2 mg P.O. once daily. Give 4 hours after cyclosporine and corticosteroids.
Children age 13 and older who weigh less than 40 kg: Initially, 3 mg/m² P.O. as a one-time loading dose after transplantation; then maintenance dose of 1 mg/m² P.O. once daily. Maximum daily dose is 40 mg. If a daily dose exceeds 40 mg because of loading dose, give the loading dose over 2 days. Monitor trough levels at least 3 to 4 days after loading dose.
§ Adjust-a-dose: For patients with hepatic impairment, reduce maintenance dose by 33%. Adjusting loading dose isn't needed.

Contraindications and cautions

● Contraindicated in patients hypersensitive to the drug or any of its derivatives or components.

• Use cautiously in patients with hyperlipidemia or impaired liver or renal function.

• The safety and effectiveness of sirolimus haven't been established in liver and lung transplant patients; therefore, such use isn't recommended.

⚱ **Lifespan:** In pregnant women, use only if benefits outweigh potential risks to the fetus. In breast-feeding women, drug is contraindicated. Women of childbearing age should use adequate contraception before starting, during, and for 12 weeks after therapy. In children younger than age 13, safety and effectiveness haven't been established.

Adverse reactions

CNS: *headache, insomnia, tremor, anxiety, depression, asthenia,* malaise, syncope, confusion, dizziness, emotional lability, hypertonia, hypesthesia, hypotonia, neuropathy, paresthesia, somnolence, *fever, pain.*
CV: facial edema, *hypertension, heart failure,* atrial fibrillation, tachycardia, hypotension, *peripheral edema, chest pain, edema, hemorrhage,* palpitations, peripheral vascular disorder, thrombophlebitis, *thrombosis,* vasodilation.
EENT: *pharyngitis,* epistaxis, rhinitis, sinusitis, abnormal vision, cataracts, conjunctivitis, deafness, ear pain, otitis media, tinnitus.
GI: *diarrhea, nausea, vomiting, constipation, abdominal pain, dyspepsia,* enlarged abdomen, hernia, ascites, *peritonitis,* anorexia, dysphagia, eructation, esophagitis, flatulence, gastritis, gastroenteritis, gingivitis, gum hyperplasia, ileus, mouth ulcerations, oral candidiasis, stomatitis.
GU: dysuria, hematuria, albuminuria, *tubular necrosis, UTI,* pelvic pain, glycosuria, bladder pain, hydronephrosis, impotence, kidney pain, nocturia, oliguria, pyuria, scrotal edema, testis disorder, *toxic nephropathy,* urinary frequency, urinary incontinence, urine retention.
Hematologic: *anemia,* THROMBOCYTOPENIA, *leukopenia, thrombotic thrombocytopenic purpura,* leukocytosis, polycythemia, lymphadenopathy.
Hepatic: *hepatic artery thrombosis.*
Metabolic: *hypercholesteremia, hyperlipidemia, hypokalemia, weight gain, hypophosphatemia,* HYPERKALEMIA, hypervolemia, Cushing's syndrome, *diabetes mellitus, acidosis,* dehydration, hypercalcemia, hyperglycemia, hyperphosphatemia, hypocalcemia, *hypoglycemia,* hypomagnesemia, hyponatremia, weight loss.

Musculoskeletal: *back pain, arthralgia,* myalgia, arthrosis, bone necrosis, leg cramps, osteoporosis, tetany.
Respiratory: dyspnea, cough, atelectasis, upper respiratory tract infection, *asthma,* bronchitis, *hypoxia, lung edema,* pleural effusion, pneumonia.
Skin: *rash, acne,* hirsutism, fungal dermatitis, pruritus, skin hypertrophy, skin ulcer, ecchymoses, sweating.
Other: abscess, cellulitis, chills, flulike syndrome, infection, *sepsis,* abnormal healing.

Interactions

Drug-drug. *Aminoglycosides, amphotericin, other nephrotoxic drugs:* May increase risk of nephrotoxicity. Use cautiously.
Bromocriptine, cimetidine, clarithromycin, clotrimazole, danazol, erythromycin, fluconazole, indinavir, itraconazole, metoclopramide, nicardipine, ritonavir, verapamil, other drugs that inhibit CYP 3A4: May decrease sirolimus metabolism, thereby increasing sirolimus level. Monitor patient for toxicity, elevated liver enzymes.
Carbamazepine, phenobarbital, phenytoin, rifabutin, rifapentine, other drugs that induce CYP 3A4: May increase sirolimus metabolism, thereby decreasing sirolimus level. Monitor patient closely.
Cyclosporine: May inhibit sirolimus metabolism, increasing levels and toxicity risk. Give sirolimus 4 hours after cyclosporine to prevent variations in sirolimus concentration.
Diltiazem: May increase sirolimus level. Monitor and reduce dosage of sirolimus as needed.
Ketoconazole: May increase rate and extent of sirolimus absorption. Avoid using together.
Rifampin: May decrease sirolimus level. Consider alternatives to rifampin.
Tacrolimus: May increase risk of hepatic artery thrombosis. Don't use together.
Vaccines: May reduce effectiveness of vaccination. Avoid live vaccines.
Drug-food. *Grapefruit juice:* May decrease drug metabolism if patient drinks a quart or more of grapefruit juice per day. Discourage overuse or dilution of drug with juice.
Drug-lifestyle. *Sun exposure:* May increase risk of skin cancer. Tell patient to take precautions.

S

Rapid onset   *Liquid form contains alcohol.   ◆ Canada   ◇ Australia   †OTC   ∅Photoguide   ‡Off-label use

Effects on lab test results
• May increase BUN, creatinine, liver enzyme, cholesterol, and lipid levels. May decrease sodium, magnesium, and hemoglobin levels and hematocrit. May increase or decrease phosphate, potassium, glucose, and calcium levels.
• May increase RBC count. May decrease platelet count. May increase or decrease WBC count.

Pharmacokinetics
Absorption: Rapid, with mean peak levels occurring in about 1 to 3 hours. Oral bioavailability is about 14%. Food decreases peak levels and increases time to peak level.
Distribution: Extensively partitioned into formed blood elements. Drug is extensively bound to proteins (about 92%).
Metabolism: Extensively metabolized by the mixed function oxidase system, primarily CYP 3A4. Seven major metabolites have been identified in whole blood.
Excretion: 91% in feces and 2.2% in urine.
Half-life: About 62 hours.

Route	Onset	Peak	Duration
P.O.	Unknown	1–3 hr	Unknown

Action
Chemical effect: An immunosuppressant that inhibits T-lymphocyte activation and proliferation that occur in response to antigenic and cytokine stimulation. Also inhibits antibody formation.
Therapeutic effect: Immunosuppression in patients receiving renal transplants.

Available forms
Oral solution: 1 mg/ml
Tablets: 1 mg, 2 mg

NURSING PROCESS

✍ Assessment
• Obtain history of patient's organ transplantation before starting therapy.
• Monitor patient's liver and renal function, and triglyceride level, before starting therapy.
• Monitor drug level in children who weigh less than 40 kg (88 lb), patients with hepatic impairment, patients taking drugs that induce or inhibit CYP 3A4, and patients whose cyclosporine dose has been drastically reduced or stopped.

• Monitor patient for infection and development of lymphoma, which may result from immunosuppression.
• Watch for development of rhabdomyolysis if patient is taking sirolimus and cyclosporine is started as an HMG-CoA reductase inhibitor.
• Assess patient's and family's knowledge of drug therapy.

⊞ Nursing diagnoses
• Risk for injury related to potential for organ rejection
• Ineffective protection related to drug-induced immunosuppression
• Deficient knowledge related to drug therapy

⟫ Planning and implementation
• Give drug consistently with or without food.
⊛ **ALERT:** In patient with mild to moderate hepatic impairment, reduce maintenance dose by about one-third. Loading dose doesn't need to be reduced.
• Dilute oral solution before giving. After dilution, use it immediately.
• When diluting drug, empty correct amount into glass or plastic container filled with at least 2 oz (60 ml) of water or orange juice. Don't use grapefruit juice or any other liquid. Stir vigorously and have patient drink immediately. Refill container with at least 4 oz (120 ml) of water or orange juice, stir again, and have patient drink all contents.
• After opening bottle, use contents within 1 month. If needed, bottles and pouches may be stored at room temperature (up to 77° F [25° C]) for several days. Drug can be kept in oral syringe for 24 hours at room temperature or refrigerated at 36° to 46° F (2° to 8° C).
• A slight haze may develop during refrigeration, but this won't affect quality of drug. If haze develops, bring drug to room temperature and shake gently until haze disappears.
• Use drug in a regimen with cyclosporine and corticosteroids. This drug should be taken 4 hours after cyclosporine dose.
• Two to four months following transplantation, patient with low to moderate risk of graft rejection should be tapered off cyclosporine over 4 to 8 weeks. During the taper, adjust sirolimus dose q 1 to 2 weeks to obtain level between 12 to 24 nanograms/ml. Dosage adjustments should also be based on condition, tissue biopsies, and laboratory findings.

• After transplantation, give antimicrobials for 1 year as directed to prevent *Pneumocystis jiroveci (carinii)* pneumonia and for 3 months as directed to prevent CMV infection.

• If patient has hyperlipidemia, start additional interventions, such as diet, exercise, and lipid-lowering drugs. Use with lipid-lowering drugs is common.

• Don't withdraw cyclosporine in patients with high risk of graft rejection, including patients with Banff grade III acute rejection or vascular rejection before cyclosporine withdrawal, a creatinine level greater than 4.5 mg/dl, or a high panel of reactive antibodies; those who have had retransplants or multi-organ transplants; and those who are dialysis-dependent or African-American.

Patient teaching

• Show patient how to store, dilute, and take drug properly.

• Tell patient to take drug consistently with or without food to minimize absorption variability.

• Advise patient to take drug 4 hours after taking cyclosporine.

• Tell patient to wash area with soap and water if solution touches skin or mucous membranes; tell him to rinse eyes with plain water if solution gets in eyes.

• Inform woman of child-bearing age of risks during pregnancy. Tell her to use effective contraception before and during therapy and for 12 weeks after stopping the drug.

• Advise patient to take precautions against sun exposure.

☑ **Evaluation**

• Patient doesn't experience organ rejection.

• Patient is free from infection and serious bleeding episodes throughout drug therapy.

• Patient and family state understanding of drug therapy.

sodium bicarbonate
(SOH-dee-um bigh-KAR-buh-nayt)
Arm and Hammer Pure Baking Soda†, Bell/ans†, Citrocarbonate†, Soda Mint

Pharmacologic class: alkalinizer
Therapeutic class: ion buffer, oral antacid
Pregnancy risk category: C

Indications and dosages

▶ **Adjunct to advanced cardiovascular life support during cardiopulmonary resuscitation (no longer routinely recommended).**
Adults: Inject either 300 to 500 ml of a 5% solution or 200 to 300 mEq of a 7.5% or 8.4% solution as rapidly as possible. Base further doses on subsequent blood gas values. Alternatively, 1-mEq/kg dose, then repeat 0.5 mEq/kg q 10 minutes.
Children age 2 and younger: 1 mEq/kg I.V. or intraosseous injection of a 4.2 % to 8.4% solution. Give slowly. Don't exceed daily dose of 8 mEq/kg.

▶ **Severe metabolic acidosis.** *Adults:* Dose depends on blood carbon dioxide content, pH, and patient's condition. Generally, give 90 to 180 mEq/L I.V. during first hour, then adjust, p.r.n.

▶ **Less urgent metabolic acidosis.** *Adults and children age 12 and older:* 2 to 5 mEq/kg as a 4- to 8-hour I.V. infusion.

▶ **Urine alkalization.** *Adults:* 48 mEq (4 g) P.O. initially; then 12 to 24 mEq (1 to 2 g) q 4 hours. May need doses of 30 to 48 mEq (2.5 to 4 g) q 4 hours, up to 192 mEq (16 g) daily.
Children: 1 to 10 mEq (84 to 840 mg)/kg P.O. daily.

▶ **Antacid.** *Adults:* 300 mg to 2 g P.O. one to four times daily.

▽ I.V. administration

• Sodium bicarbonate inactivates such catecholamines as norepinephrine and dopamine and forms precipitate with calcium. Don't mix sodium bicarbonate with I.V. solutions of these drugs, and flush I.V. line adequately.

• Drug is usually given by I.V. infusion. When immediate treatment is needed, drug may be given by direct, rapid I.V. injection. However, in neonates and children younger than age 2, slow I.V. administration is preferred to avoid hypernatremia, decreased CSF pressure, and intracranial hemorrhage.

⊗ **Incompatibilities**
Alcohol 5% in dextrose 5%; allopurinol; amiodarone; amphotericin B; amino acids; ascorbic acid injection; bupivacaine; calcium salts; carboplatin; carmustine; cefotaxime; ciprofloxacin; cisatracurium; cisplatin; corticotropin; dextrose 5% in lactated Ringer's injection; diltiazem; dobutamine; dopamine; doxorubicin liposomal;

S

epinephrine hydrochloride; fat emulsion 10%; glycopyrrolate; hydromorphone; idarubicin; imipenem-cilastatin sodium; Ionosol B, D, or G with invert sugar 10%; isoproterenol; labetalol; lactated Ringer's injection; levorphanol; leucovorin calcium; lidocaine; magnesium sulfate; meperidine; meropenem; methylprednisolone sodium succinate; metoclopramide; midazolam; morphine sulfate; nalbuphine; norepinephrine bitartrate; ondansetron; oxacillin; penicillin G potassium; pentazocine lactate; pentobarbital sodium; procaine; Ringer's injection; sargramostim; 1/6 M sodium lactate; streptomycin; succinylcholine; thiopental; ticarcillin disodium and clavulanate potassium; vancomycin; verapamil; vinca alkaloids; vitamin B complex with vitamin C.

Contraindications and cautions

• Contraindicated in patients with metabolic or respiratory alkalosis; patients who are losing chlorides from vomiting or continuous GI suction; patients taking diuretics known to produce hypochloremic alkalosis; and patients with hypocalcemia in which alkalosis may produce tetany, hypertension, seizures, or heart failure. Oral sodium bicarbonate is contraindicated in patients with acute ingestion of strong mineral acids.
• Use cautiously in patients with hypertension, heart failure or other edematous or sodium-retaining conditions or renal insufficiency.
🜲 **Lifespan:** In pregnant women, use cautiously. In breast-feeding women, use cautiously; it's unknown if the drug appears in breast milk.

Adverse reactions

GI: gastric distention, belching, flatulence.
Metabolic: *metabolic alkalosis,* hypernatremia, hypokalemia, hyperosmolarity (with overdose).
Other: pain and irritation at injection site.

Interactions

Drug-drug. *Anorexigenics, flecainide, mecamylamine, quinidine, sympathomimetics:* May increase urine alkalization, decrease renal clearance, and increase pharmacologic or toxic effects. Monitor patient for toxicity.
Chlorpropamide, lithium, methotrexate, salicylates, tetracycline: May increase renal clearance of these drugs, possibly resulting in decreased pharmacologic effects. Monitor patient for lack of effect.

Effects on lab test results

• May increase sodium and lactate levels. May decrease potassium level.

Pharmacokinetics

Absorption: Good.
Distribution: Bicarbonate is confined to systemic circulation.
Metabolism: None.
Excretion: Bicarbonate is filtered and reabsorbed by kidneys; less than 1% of filtered bicarbonate is excreted. *Half-life:* Unknown.

Route	Onset	Peak	Duration
P.O.	Unknown	Unknown	Unknown
I.V.	Immediate	Immediate	Unknown

Action

Chemical effect: Restores body's buffering capacity and neutralizes excess acid.
Therapeutic effect: Restores normal acid-base balance and relieves acid indigestion.

Available forms

Injection: 4% (2.4 mEq/5 ml), 4.2% (5 mEq/10 ml), 5% (297.5 mEq/500 ml), 7.5% (8.92 mEq/10 ml and 44.6 mEq/50 ml), 8.4% (10 mEq/10 ml and 50 mEq/50 ml)
Tablets†: 325 mg, 650 mg

NURSING PROCESS

🜮 Assessment

• Assess patient's condition before starting therapy, and regularly thereafter to monitor the drug's effectiveness.
• To avoid risk of alkalosis, obtain blood pH, Pao_2, $Paco_2$, and electrolyte levels.
• If sodium bicarbonate is being used to produce alkaline urine, monitor urine pH (should be greater than 7) q 4 to 6 hours.
• Be alert for adverse reactions and drug interactions.
• Assess patient's and family's knowledge of drug therapy.

🜛 Nursing diagnoses

• Ineffective health maintenance related to underlying condition
• Risk for injury related to drug-induced adverse reactions
• Deficient knowledge related to drug therapy

▷ Planning and implementation

• Drug isn't routinely recommended for use in cardiac arrest because it may produce paradoxical acidosis from CO_2 production. It shouldn't be routinely given during early stages of resuscitation unless acidosis is clearly present.

• Drug may be used after such interventions as defibrillation, cardiac compression, and administration of first-line drugs.

• Give drug with water, not milk; drug may cause hypercalcemia, alkalosis, or possibly renal calculi.

• Inform prescriber of laboratory results.

Patient teaching

• Tell patient not to take with milk.

• Discourage use as antacid. Offer nonabsorbable alternate antacid if it is to be used repeatedly.

☑ Evaluation

• Patient regains normal acid-base balance.

• Patient doesn't experience injury from drug-induced adverse reactions.

• Patient and family state understanding of drug therapy.

---

sodium chloride
(SOH-dee-um KLOR-ighd)

Pharmacologic class: electrolyte
Therapeutic class: sodium and chloride replacement
Pregnancy risk category: C

Indications and dosages

▶ **Fluid and electrolyte replacement in hyponatremia caused by severe electrolyte loss, severe salt depletion.** *Adults:* Dosage is highly individualized. The 3% and 5% solutions are used only with frequent electrolyte determination and given only by slow I.V. With half-normal saline solution: 3% to 8% of body weight, according to deficiencies, over 18 to 24 hours. With normal saline solution: 2% to 6% of body weight, according to deficiencies, over 18 to 24 hours.

▼ I.V. administration

• Infuse 3% and 5% solutions very slowly and cautiously to avoid pulmonary edema. Use only

for critical situations, and observe patient continually.

⊗ **Incompatibilities**
Amphotericin B, chlordiazepoxide, diazepam, fat emulsion, mannitol, methylprednisolone sodium succinate, phenytoin sodium.

Contraindications and cautions

• Contraindicated in patients with conditions in which giving sodium and chloride is detrimental. The 3% and 5% saline solution injections are contraindicated in patients with increased, normal, or only slightly decreased electrolyte levels.

• Use cautiously in postoperative patients and patients with heart failure, circulatory insufficiency, renal dysfunction, or hypoproteinemia.

≋ **Lifespan:** In pregnant women, use cautiously. In breast-feeding women, use cautiously; it's unknown if the drug appears in breast milk. In the elderly, use cautiously.

Adverse reactions

CV: *aggravation of heart failure,* edema if given too rapidly or in excess, thrombophlebitis.
Metabolic: hypernatremia, *aggravation of existing metabolic acidosis* with excessive infusion, electrolyte disturbances, hypokalemia.
Respiratory: *pulmonary edema* if given too rapidly or in excess.
Skin: local tenderness, abscess, tissue necrosis at injection site.

Interactions

None significant.

Effects on lab test results

• May increase sodium and chloride levels. May decrease potassium and bicarbonate levels.

Pharmacokinetics

Absorption: Absorbed readily.
Distribution: Distributed widely in body.
Metabolism: None significant.
Excretion: Primarily in urine; some excreted in sweat, tears, and saliva. *Half-life:* Unknown.

Route	Onset	Peak	Duration
P.O.	Unknown	Unknown	Unknown
I.V.	Immediate	Immediate	Unknown

Action

Chemical effect: Replaces and maintains sodium and chloride levels.
Therapeutic effect: Restores normal sodium and chloride levels.

Available forms

Injection: *Half-normal saline solution:* 500 ml, 1,000 ml
Normal saline solution: 50 ml, 100 ml, 150 ml, 250 ml, 500 ml, 1,000 ml
3% saline solution: 500 ml
5% saline solution: 500 ml
14.6% saline solution: 20 ml, 40 ml, 200 ml
23.4% saline solution: 30 ml, 50 ml, 200 ml
Tablets (enteric-coated): 650 mg, 1 g, 2.25 g
Tablets (slow-release): 600 mg

NURSING PROCESS

✎ Assessment

• Obtain history of patient's sodium and chloride levels before starting therapy, and reassess regularly thereafter to monitor the drug's effectiveness.
• Monitor other electrolyte levels.
• Assess patient's fluid status.
• Be alert for adverse reactions.
• Assess patient's and family's knowledge of drug therapy.

⊕ Nursing diagnoses

• Imbalanced nutrition: less than body requirements related to subnormal levels of sodium and chloride
• Excess fluid volume related to saline solution's water-drawing power
• Deficient knowledge related to drug therapy

❯ Planning and implementation

• Give tablet with glass of water.
• **ALERT:** Don't confuse concentrates (14.6% and 23.4%) available to add to parenteral nutrient solutions with normal saline solution injection, and never give without diluting. Read label carefully.

Patient teaching
• Tell patient to report adverse reactions promptly.

✓ Evaluation

• Patient's sodium and chloride levels are normal.

• Patient doesn't exhibit signs and symptoms of fluid retention.
• Patient and family state understanding of drug therapy.

sodium ferric gluconate complex
(SOH-dee-um FEH-rik GLOO-kuh-nayt KOM-pleks)
Ferrlecit

Pharmacologic class: macromolecular iron complex
Therapeutic class: hematinic
Pregnancy risk category: B

Indications and dosages

❯ **Iron-deficient anemia in patients undergoing long-term hemodialysis and receiving supplemental erythropoietin therapy.** *Adults and children older than age 15:* Before starting therapeutic doses, a test dose of 2 ml sodium ferric gluconate complex (25 mg elemental iron) diluted in 50 ml normal saline solution may be given I.V. over 1 hour. If test dose is tolerated, give therapeutic dose of 10 ml (125 mg elemental iron) diluted in 100 ml normal saline solution I.V. over 1 hour. May also be given undiluted as a slow I.V. infusion at 12.5 mg/min. Most patients need a minimum cumulative dose of 1 g elemental iron given at more than eight sequential dialysis treatments to achieve a favorable hemoglobin level or hematocrit response. May be given during dialysis session.
Children ages 6 to 15: 0.12 ml/kg (1.5 mg/kg elemental iron) diluted in 25 ml 0.9% sodium chloride I.V. infusion over 1 hour at eight sequential dialysis sessions. Maximum dosage not to exceed 125 mg/dose.

▽ I.V. administration

• Don't add sodium ferric gluconate complex to parenteral nutrition solutions for I.V. infusion.
• Use immediately after dilution in normal saline solution.
• Dilute test dose of sodium ferric gluconate complex in 50 ml normal saline solution and give over 1 hour. Dilute therapeutic doses of drug in 100 ml normal saline solution and give over 1 hour. Don't exceed 2.1 mg/minute.
• Patient may develop profound hypotension with flushing, light-headedness, malaise, fatigue, weakness, or severe chest, back, flank, or

groin pain after rapid I.V. administration of iron. These reactions don't indicate hypersensitivity and may result from rapid administration of drug. Monitor patient closely during infusion.
⊗ **Incompatibilities**
Other I.V. drugs.

Contraindications and cautions

• Contraindicated in patients hypersensitive to the drug or any of its components (such as benzyl alcohol), and in patients with anemias not linked to iron deficiency. Don't give to patients with iron overload.

⁂ **Lifespan:** In breast-feeding women, use cautiously; it's unknown if the drug appears in breast milk. In children younger than age 6, safety and effectiveness haven't been established. In the elderly, begin treatment at lowest dose and observe closely.

Adverse reactions

CNS: asthenia, headache, fatigue, malaise, dizziness, paresthesia, agitation, insomnia, somnolence, syncope, pain, fever.
CV: hypotension, hypertension, tachycardia, *bradycardia,* angina, chest pain, *MI,* edema, flushing.
EENT: conjunctivitis, abnormal vision, rhinitis.
GI: nausea, vomiting, diarrhea, rectal disorder, dyspepsia, eructation, flatulence, melena, abdominal pain.
GU: UTI.
Hematologic: abnormal erythrocytes, anemia, lymphadenopathy.
Metabolic: *hyperkalemia, hypoglycemia,* hypokalemia, hypervolemia.
Musculoskeletal: myalgia, arthralgia, back pain, arm pain, cramps.
Respiratory: dyspnea, coughing, upper respiratory tract infections, pneumonia, *pulmonary edema.*
Skin: pruritus, increased sweating, rash.
Other: infection, injection site reaction, rigors, chills, flulike syndrome, *sepsis, carcinoma, hypersensitivity reactions.*

Interactions

ACE inhibitors (enalapril): May potentiate adverse effects of I.V. iron therapy. Use together cautiously.

Effects on lab test results

• May decrease glucose and hemoglobin levels and hematocrit. May increase or decrease potassium level.

Pharmacokinetics

Absorption: Administered I.V.
Distribution: Unknown.
Metabolism: Unknown.
Excretion: Unknown. *Half-life:* 1 hour in healthy iron-deficient people.

Route	Onset	Peak	Duration
I.V.	Unknown	Unknown	Unknown

Action

Chemical effect: Drug restores total body iron content, which is critical for normal hemoglobin synthesis and oxygen transport.
Therapeutic effect: Restores total body iron content.

Available forms

Injection: 62.5 mg elemental iron (12.5 mg/ml) in 5-ml ampules

NURSING PROCESS

⚗ Assessment

• Obtain history of patient's underlying condition before starting therapy, and reassess regularly to monitor the drug's effectiveness.
• Find out about other sources of iron patient may be taking, such as nonprescription iron preparations and iron-containing multivitamin and mineral supplements.
• Monitor hematocrit and hemoglobin, ferritin, and iron saturation levels during therapy.
• Assess patient's and family's knowledge of drug therapy.

⊕ Nursing diagnoses

• Risk for injury related to drug-induced adverse reactions
• Activity intolerance related to underlying condition
• Deficient knowledge related to drug therapy

⟩ Planning and implementation

• Dose is expressed in milligrams of elemental iron.

S

• Don't give drug to patients with iron overload, which commonly occurs in hemoglobinopathies and other refractory anemias.

⑤ **ALERT:** Life-threatening hypersensitivity reactions (characterized by CV collapse, cardiac arrest, bronchospasm, oral or pharyngeal edema, dyspnea, angioedema, urticaria, or pruritus sometimes linked with pain and muscle spasm of chest or back) may occur during infusion. Have adequate supportive measures readily available. Monitor patient closely.

• Some adverse reactions in hemodialysis patients may be related to dialysis itself or to chronic renal impairment.

⑤ **ALERT:** Drug contains benzyl alcohol and may cause "gasping syndrome" in neonates.

Patient teaching
• Advise to immediately report signs or symptoms of iron poisoning, which include abdominal pain, diarrhea, vomiting, drowsiness, or hyperventilation.

☑ Evaluation
• Patient doesn't experience injury as a result of drug-induced adverse reactions.
• Patient experiences improved activity tolerance.
• Patient and family state understanding of drug therapy.

sodium phosphate
(SOH-dee-um FOS-fayt)
Fleet Enema, Fleet Pediatric Enema, Fleet Phospho-soda†

Pharmacologic class: acid salt
Therapeutic class: saline laxative, mineral
Pregnancy risk category: C (I.V.), NR (P.R.)

Indications and dosages

▶ **Constipation.** *Adults and children age 12 and older:* 20 to 45 ml of solution mixed with 120 ml of cold water P.O. Or, 120 ml P.R. (as enema).
Children ages 10 to 11: 10 to 20 ml of solution mixed with 120 ml of cold water P.O.
Children ages 5 to 9: 5 to 10 ml of solution mixed with 120 ml of cold water P.O.
Children older than age 2: 60 ml P.R.

▶ **Total parenteral nutrition (TPN).** *Adults and children:* Doses are highly individualized.

Usually 10 to 15 millimoles (mM) per liter of TPN solution I.V.; titrate per phosphate levels. Normal range 3 to 4.5 mg/dl for adults, 4 to 7 mg/dl for children.
Infants receiving TPN: Usually 1.5 to 2 mM/kg I.V. daily; titrate per phosphate levels.

▼ I.V. administration
• To avoid errors, drug should be prescribed in terms of millimoles (mM) of phosphorous.
• Dilute and mix with larger volume of fluid.
• To avoid toxicity, infuse slowly.
• Infusions with high concentrations of phosphate may cause hypocalcemia. Monitor calcium levels.

⊗ **Incompatibilities**
None reported.

Contraindications and cautions
• Contraindicated in patients on sodium-restricted diets and in patients with intestinal obstruction or perforation, edema, heart failure, megacolon, impaired renal function, or symptoms of appendicitis or acute surgical abdomen, such as abdominal pain, nausea, and vomiting.
• I.V. sodium phosphate contraindicated in patients with hypernatremia, high phosphate levels, or low calcium levels.
• Use cautiously in patients with large hemorrhoids or anal abrasions.
• Use I.V. sodium phosphate in patients with cardiac disease, renal impairment, adrenal insufficiency, and cirrhosis.

☀ **Lifespan:** In pregnant women, use cautiously. In breast-feeding women, use cautiously because it's unknown if the drug appears in breast milk. In children younger than age 4, use only as directed by prescriber.

Adverse reactions
GI: abdominal cramps.
Metabolic: fluid and electrolyte disturbances (such as hypernatremia, hypocalcemia or hyperphosphatemia) with daily use.
Other: laxative dependence with long-term or excessive use, hypocalcemic tetany.

Interactions
None significant.

Reactions may be *common*, uncommon, *life-threatening*, or COMMON AND LIFE-THREATENING.

Effects on lab test results

● May increase sodium and phosphate levels. May decrease electrolyte levels with prolonged use.

Pharmacokinetics

Absorption: About 1% to 20% of P.O. dose absorbed; unknown after P.R. administration. About 80% of I.V. dose reabsorbed through the renal tubules for homeostasis.
Distribution: Unknown.
Metabolism: Unknown.
Excretion: Renal for I.V. route. *Half-life:* Unknown.

Route	Onset	Peak	Duration
P.O.	30 min–3 hr	Varies	Varies
P.R.	5–10 min	Varies	Ends with evacuation
I.V.	Unknown	Unknown	Unknown

Action

Chemical effect: Oral and rectal use produces osmotic effect in small intestine by drawing water into intestinal lumen. I.V. use maintains body's normal phosphate levels.
Therapeutic effect: Relieves constipation. Prevents hypophosphatemia.

Available forms

Enema: 160 mg/ml sodium phosphate and 60 mg/ml sodium biphosphate
Liquid: 2.4 g/5 ml sodium phosphate and 900 mg/5 ml sodium biphosphate
I.V. infusion: 3 mM phosphate and 4 mEq sodium/L in 10-, 15-, 30-, 50-ml vials

NURSING PROCESS

☑ Assessment

● Assess patient's condition before starting therapy, and regularly thereafter to monitor the drug's effectiveness.
● Before giving drug for constipation, determine whether patient has adequate fluid intake, exercise, and diet.
● Be alert for adverse reactions.
● Assess for signs of overdose during I.V. therapy, including paresthesias of extremities, confusion, paralysis, cardiac arrhythmias.
● **ALERT:** Up to 10% of sodium content of drug may be absorbed.

● Assess patient's and family's knowledge of drug therapy.

☒ Nursing diagnoses

● Constipation related to underlying condition
● Acute pain related to drug-induced abdominal cramping
● Deficient knowledge related to drug therapy

❱ Planning and implementation

● Dilute drug with water before giving. Follow administration with full glass of water.
● Make sure that patient has easy access to bathroom facilities, commode, or bedpan.
● **ALERT:** Severe electrolyte imbalances may occur if recommended dose is exceeded.
Patient teaching
● Teach patient about dietary sources of bulk, which include bran and other cereals, fresh fruit, and vegetables.
● Tell patient to maintain adequate fluid intake of at least 6 to 8 glasses of water or juices daily unless contraindicated.

☑ Evaluation

● Patient's constipation is relieved.
● Patient's abdominal cramping ceases.
● Patient and family state understanding of drug therapy.

sodium phosphate monohydrate
(SOE-dee-um FOS-fate maw-no-HIGH-drate)

sodium phosphate dibasic anhydrous
(SOE-dee-um FOS-fate die-BAY-sick an-HIGH-drus)
Visicol

Pharmacologic class: osmotic laxative
Therapeutic class: bowel evacuant
Pregnancy risk category: C

Indications and dosages

▶ **To cleanse the bowel before colonoscopy.**
Adults: 40 tablets taken in the following manner: The evening before the procedure, 3 tablets P.O. with at least 8 oz of clear liquid q 15 minutes for a total of 20 tablets. The last dose will be only 2 tablets. The day of the procedure, 3 tablets P.O. with at least 8 oz of clear liquid q

15 minutes for a total of 20 tablets, starting 3 to 5 hours before the procedure. The last dose will be only 2 tablets.

Contraindications and cautions

• Contraindicated in patients hypersensitive to the drug or any of its components. Avoid giving drug to patients with heart failure, ascites, unstable angina, gastric retention, ileus, acute intestinal obstruction, pseudo-obstruction, severe chronic constipation, bowel perforation, acute colitis, toxic megacolon, or hypomotility syndrome (hypothyroidism, scleroderma).

• Use cautiously in patients with a history of electrolyte abnormalities, current electrolyte abnormalities, or impaired renal function. Also, use cautiously in patients who take drugs that can induce electrolyte abnormalities or prolong the QT interval.

※ **Lifespan:** In children, safety and effectiveness haven't been established. In the elderly, use cautiously because of greater sensitivity to drug.

Adverse reactions

CNS: headache, dizziness.
GI: nausea, vomiting, abdominal bloating, abdominal pain.

Interactions

Drug-drug. *Oral drugs:* May reduce absorption of these drugs because of rapid peristalsis and diarrhea induced by sodium phosphate monohydrate and sodium phosphate dibasic anhydrous. Separate administration times.

Effects on lab test results

• May increase phosphorus level. May decrease potassium and calcium levels.

Pharmacokinetics

Absorption: Quick. Duration of action is 1 to 3 hours after administration.
Distribution: Unknown.
Metabolism: Not expected to be metabolized by the liver.
Excretion: Eliminated almost entirely via the kidneys. *Half-life:* Unknown.

Route	Onset	Peak	Duration
P.O.	Unknown	3 hr	1–3 hr

Action

Chemical effect: The primary mechanism is thought to be the osmotic action of sodium, which causes large amounts of water to be drawn into the colon.
Therapeutic effect: Cleanses the colon.

Available forms

Tablets: 1.5 g sodium phosphate (1.102 g sodium phosphate monohydrate and 0.398 g sodium phosphate dibasic anhydrous)

NURSING PROCESS

※ Assessment

• Assess underlying condition before starting therapy, and reassess regularly thereafter to monitor the drug's effectiveness.
• Obtain laboratory studies before starting therapy and correct electrolyte imbalances before giving drug.
• Assess patient's and family's knowledge of drug therapy.

⊕ Nursing diagnoses

• Acute pain related to abdominal discomfort
• Risk for deficient fluid volume related to adverse GI effects
• Deficient knowledge related to drug therapy

▷ Planning and implementation

• Undigested or partially digested tablets and other drugs may be seen in the stool or during colonoscopy.
• As with other sodium phosphate cathartic preparations, this drug may induce colonic mucosal ulceration.
• Monitor patient for signs of dehydration.
• Don't repeat administration within 7 days.
• No enema or laxative is needed with drug.
⊛ **ALERT:** Giving other sodium phosphate products may result in death from significant fluid shifts, electrolyte abnormalities, and cardiac arrhythmias. Patient with electrolyte disturbances has an increased risk of prolonged QT interval. Use drug cautiously in patient who is taking other drugs known to prolong the QT interval.
Patient teaching
• Instruct patient to drink at least 8 oz of clear liquid with each dose. Inadequate fluid intake may lead to excessive fluid loss and hypovolemia.

• Tell patient to drink only clear liquids for at least 12 hours before starting the purgative regimen.

• Warn patient against taking an additional enema or laxative, particularly one that contains sodium phosphate.

• Tell patient that undigested or partially digested tablets and other drugs may appear in the stool.

☑ **Evaluation**
• Patient states that pain management methods are effective.
• Patient maintains adequate hydration.
• Patient and family state understanding of therapy.

sodium polystyrene sulfonate
(SOH-dee-um pol-ee-STIGH-reen SUL-fuh-nayt)
Kayexalate, SPS

Pharmacologic class: cation-exchange resin
Therapeutic class: potassium-removing resin
Pregnancy risk category: C

Indications and dosages

▶ **Hyperkalemia.** *Adults:* 15 g P.O. daily to q.i.d. in water or sorbitol (3 to 4 ml/g of resin). Or mix powder with appropriate medium— aqueous suspension or diet appropriate for renal impairment—and instill into NG tube. Or 30 to 50 g q 6 hours as warm emulsion deep into sigmoid colon (20 cm), retained for 30 minutes. In persistent vomiting or paralytic ileus, high-retention enema of sodium polystyrene sulfonate (30 g) suspended in 200 ml of 10% methylcellulose, 10% dextrose, or 25% sorbitol solution may be given.
Children: 1 g of resin P.O. or P.R. for each mEq of potassium to be removed. Or, alternatively, 1 g/kg every 6 hours. P.O. route preferred because drug should stay in intestine for at least 6 hours.

Contraindications and cautions

• Contraindicated in patients hypersensitive to the drug or any of its components, and in those with hypokalemia.
• Use cautiously in patients with severe heart failure, severe hypertension, or marked edema.

❄ **Lifespan:** In pregnant women, use cautiously. In breast-feeding women, use cautiously; it's unknown if the drug appears in breast milk.

Adverse reactions

GI: *constipation,* fecal impaction in elderly patients, anorexia, gastric irritation, nausea, vomiting, *diarrhea* with sorbitol emulsions.
Metabolic: hypokalemia, hypocalcemia, hypomagnesemia, sodium retention.

Interactions

Drug-drug. *Antacids and laxatives (nonabsorbable cation-donating types, including magnesium hydroxide):* May cause systemic alkalosis and reduced potassium exchange capability. Don't use together.

Effects on lab test results

• May increase sodium level. May decrease potassium, calcium, and magnesium levels.

Pharmacokinetics

Absorption: None.
Distribution: None.
Metabolism: None.
Excretion: Unchanged in feces. *Half-life:* Unknown.

Route	Onset	Peak	Duration
P.O., P.R.	2–12 hr	Unknown	Unknown

Action

Chemical effect: Exchanges sodium ions for potassium ions in intestine. Much of exchange capacity is used for cations other than potassium (calcium and magnesium) and, possibly, fats and proteins.
Therapeutic effect: Lowers potassium level.

Available forms

Powder: 1-lb jar (3.5 g/5 ml)
Suspension: 60 ml*, 120 ml*, 200 ml*, 480 ml*, 500 ml*

S

NURSING PROCESS

⚕ **Assessment**
• Obtain history of patient's potassium level before starting therapy.
• Monitor potassium level at least once daily. Treatment may result in potassium deficiency.

Treatment usually stops when potassium level declines to 4 or 5 mEq/L.

⚡ ALERT: Watch for other signs of hypokalemia, such as irritability, confusion, arrhythmias, ECG changes, severe muscle weakness and paralysis, and cardiotoxicity in patient taking digitalis.

• Monitor patient for symptoms of other electrolyte deficiencies (magnesium, calcium) because drug is nonselective. Monitor calcium level in patient receiving sodium polystyrene therapy for more than 3 days. Supplementary calcium may be needed.

• Watch for sodium overload. Drug contains about 100 mg of sodium/g. About one-third of sodium in resin is retained.

• Be alert for adverse reactions and drug interactions.

• Watch for constipation with P.O. or NG use.

• Assess patient's and family's knowledge of drug therapy.

⊞ Nursing diagnoses
• Ineffective health maintenance related to presence of hyperkalemia
• Constipation related to drug-induced adverse GI reactions
• Deficient knowledge related to drug therapy

▷ Planning and implementation
• Don't heat resin because it will impair drug's effectiveness.
• Mix resin only with water or sorbitol for P.O. use. Never mix with orange juice (high potassium content) to disguise taste.
• Chill oral suspension for greater palatability.
• If sorbitol is given, mix with resin suspension.
• Consider solid form. Resin cookie and candy recipes are available. Ask pharmacist or dietitian to supply.
• To prevent constipation, use sorbitol (10 to 20 ml of 70% syrup q 2 hours, p.r.n.) to produce one or two watery stools daily.
• Premixed forms are available (SPS and others) for P.R. use.
• If preparing manually, mix polystyrene resin only with water and sorbitol for P.R. use. Don't use mineral oil for P.R. administration to prevent impaction. Ion exchange requires aqueous medium. Sorbitol content prevents impaction.
• Prepare P.R. dose at room temperature. Stir emulsion gently during administration.
• Use #28 French rubber tube. Insert tube 20 cm into sigmoid colon and tape in place. Or, con-

sider indwelling urinary catheter with 30-ml balloon inflated distal to anal sphincter to aid in retention. This is especially helpful for patients with poor sphincter control (for example, after stroke). Use gravity flow. Drain returns constantly through Y-tube connection. Place patient in knee-chest position or with hips on pillow for a while if back leakage occurs.

• After P.R. administration, flush tubing with 50 to 100 ml of nonsodium fluid to ensure delivery of all drug. Flush rectum to remove resin.

• Prevent fecal impaction in geriatric patient by giving resin P.R. Give cleansing enema before P.R. administration. The patient will need to retain enema, ideally for 6 to 10 hours, but 30 to 60 minutes is acceptable.

• If hyperkalemia is severe, prescriber won't depend solely on polystyrene resin to lower potassium level. Dextrose 50% with regular insulin may be given by I.V. push.

Patient teaching
• Explain importance of following prescribed low-potassium diet.
• Explain need to retain enema, ideally for 6 to 10 hours, but 30 to 60 minutes is acceptable.
• Tell patient to report adverse reactions.

☑ Evaluation
• Patient's potassium level is normal.
• Patient doesn't develop constipation.
• Patient and family state understanding of drug therapy.

solifenacin succinate
(sohl-ih-FEN-ah-sin SUC-sin-eight)
VESIcare

Pharmacologic class: muscarinic receptor antagonist
Therapeutic class: urinary tract antispasmodic
Pregnancy risk category: C

Indications and dosages

▶ **Overactive bladder with urinary urgency, frequency, and urge incontinence.** *Adults:* 5 mg P.O. once daily. May increase to 10 mg once daily if 5-mg dose is well tolerated.
⊠ Adjust-a-dose: If creatinine clearance is less than 30 ml/minute or the patient has moderate liver impairment (Child-Pugh score B), maintain the dose at 5 mg.

Contraindications and cautions

• Contraindicated in patients hypersensitive to drug or any of its components and in patients with urine or gastric retention or uncontrolled narrow-angle glaucoma. Don't use in patients with severe hepatic impairment.

• Use cautiously in patients with a history of prolonged QT interval, those being treated for angle-closure glaucoma, and those with bladder outflow obstruction, decreased GI motility, renal insufficiency, or moderate liver impairment.

⚜ **Lifespan:** In pregnant women, use only if benefits outweigh potential risks to the fetus. Women shouldn't breast-feed while taking drug. Safety and effectiveness in children hasn't been established. In elderly patients, level and half-life may increase though safety and effectiveness are similar to those for younger adults.

Adverse reactions

CNS: depression, dizziness, fatigue.
CV: hypertension, leg swelling.
EENT: blurred vision, dry eyes, pharyngitis.
GI: *constipation, dry mouth,* dyspepsia, nausea, upper abdominal pain, vomiting.
GU: urinary retention, UTI.
Respiratory: cough.
Other: influenza.

Interactions

Drug-drug. *Drugs that prolong the QT interval:* May increase the risk of serious cardiac arrhythmias. Monitor patient and ECG closely.
Potent CYP 3A4 inhibitors (such as ketoconazole): May increase solifenacin levels. Don't exceed solifenacin dose of 5 mg daily when used together.

Effects on lab test results

None reported.

Pharmacokinetics

Absorption: Absolute bioavailability is about 90%.
Distribution: Wide, except in CNS. About 90% bound to plasma proteins.
Metabolism: Extensive, mainly by CYP 3A4.
Excretion: Mainly in urine and, to a lesser extent, feces. *Half-life:* 2 or 3 days.

Route	Onset	Peak	Duration
P.O.	Unknown	3–8 hr	Unknown

Action

Chemical effect: Relaxes smooth muscle of the bladder by competitively antagonizing the muscarinic receptors.
Therapeutic effect: Relieves symptoms of overactive bladder.

Available forms

Tablets (film-coated): 5 mg, 10 mg

NURSING PROCESS

Assessment
• Assess bladder function, and monitor drug effects.
• Monitor patient for decreased gastric motility and constipation.
• Evaluate patient's and family's knowledge of drug therapy.

Nursing diagnoses
• Impaired urinary elimination related to underlying medical condition
• Constipation related to drug-induced adverse effects
• Deficient knowledge related to drug therapy

Planning and implementation
• If patient has bladder outlet obstruction, watch for urine retention.
• If the patient has urinary retention, notify prescriber and prepare for urinary catheterization.
• Dry mouth and constipation are the most frequently reported adverse effects of drug therapy.
• Chronic overdose may result in fixed, dilated pupils, blurred vision, dry skin, tremors, and inability to perform the heel-to-toe exam. These effects should subside when drug is stopped.

Patient teaching
• Explain that drug may blur vision. Tell patient to use caution when performing hazardous activities or tasks that require clear vision until effects of the drug are known.
• Discourage use of other drugs that may cause dry mouth, constipation, urine retention, or blurred vision.
• Urge patient to notify prescriber about abdominal pain or constipation that lasts 3 days or longer.
• Tell patient that drug decreases the ability to sweat normally, and advise cautious use in hot environments or during strenuous activity.

• Tell patient to swallow tablet whole with liquid.
• Inform patient that drug may be taken with or without food.

☑ **Evaluation**
• Patient experiences improved bladder function with drug therapy.
• Patient maintains normal bowel regimen.
• Patient and family state understanding of drug therapy.

somatropin
(soh-muh-TROH-pin)
Genotropin, Genotropin Miniquick, Humatrope, Norditropin, Nutropin, Nutropin AQ, Saizen, Serostim

Pharmacologic class: anterior pituitary hormone
Therapeutic class: human growth hormone (GH)
Pregnancy risk category: C

Indications and dosages

▶ **Long-term therapy for growth failure in patients with inadequate secretion of endogenous GH.** *Children:* 0.18 to 0.3 mg/kg Humatrope subcutaneously or I.M. weekly, divided equally and given either 3 alternate days, six times weekly, or daily. Or, up to 0.3 mg/kg Nutropin or Nutropin AQ subcutaneously weekly in daily divided doses. Or, 0.06 mg/kg Saizen I.M. or subcutaneously three times weekly. Or, 0.024 to 0.034 mg/kg Norditropin subcutaneously, six to seven times weekly. Or 0.16 to 0.24 mg/kg Genotropin subcutaneously weekly, divided into five to seven doses. Or 1.5 mg/kg somatropin depot subcutaneously once monthly or 0.75 mg/kg subcutaneously twice monthly on the same days of each month.
▶ **Growth failure from chronic renal insufficiency up to time of kidney transplant.** *Children:* Weekly dosage of up to 0.35 mg/kg Nutropin or Nutropin AQ subcutaneously divided into daily doses.
▶ **Long-term therapy for short stature related to Turner's syndrome.** *Children:* Up to 0.375 mg/kg Humatrope, Nutropin, or Nutropin AQ subcutaneously weekly, divided into equal doses given three to seven times weekly.

▶ **Long-term therapy for growth failure in children with Prader-Willi syndrome (PWS) diagnosed by genetic testing.** *Children:* 0.24 mg/kg Genotropin subcutaneously weekly, divided into six to seven doses.
▶ **To replace endogenous GH in patients with GH deficiency.** *Adults:* Initially, not more than 0.006 mg/kg Humatrope, Nutropin, or Nutropin AQ subcutaneously daily. Humatrope may be increased to maximum of 0.0125 mg/kg daily. Nutropin and Nutropin AQ may be increased to maximum of 0.025 mg/kg daily in patients younger than age 35 or 0.0125 mg/kg daily in patients older than age 35. With Genotropin, starting dose isn't more than 0.04 mg/kg subcutaneously weekly, divided into six to seven doses. Dose may be increased at 4- to 8-week intervals to a maximum dose of 0.08 mg/kg subcutaneously weekly, divided into six to seven doses. With Saizen, starting dose isn't more than 0.005 mg/kg/day. May increase after 4 weeks to maximum of 0.01 mg/kg/day based on patient tolerance and clinical response.
▶ **AIDS wasting or cachexia.** *Adults and children weighing more than 55 kg (121 lb):* 6 mg Serostim subcutaneously h.s.
Adults and children weighing 45 to 55 kg (99 to 121 lb): 5 mg Serostim subcutaneously h.s.
Adults and children weighing 35 to 45 kg (77 to 99 lb): 4 mg Serostim subcutaneously h.s.
Adults and children weighing less than 35 kg: 0.1 mg/kg Serostim subcutaneously daily h.s.
▶ **Long-term treatment of growth failure in children born small for gestational age who don't achieve catch-up growth by 2 years of age.** *Children:* 0.48 mg/kg Genotropin subcutaneously weekly, divided into five to seven doses.
▶ **Idiopathic short stature.** *Children:* Up to 0.37 mg/kg (Humatrope) subcutaneously weekly, divided into equal doses given 6 to 7 times per week.

Contraindications and cautions

• Contraindicated in patients with closed epiphyses or active underlying intracranial lesion.
• Don't reconstitute Humatrope with supplied diluent for patients with known sensitivity to either m-cresol or glycerin.
• Genotropin is contraindicated in patients with PWS who are severely obese or have severe respiratory impairment.
🜂 **Lifespan:** In pregnant and breast-feeding women, drug isn't indicated. In children with

hypothyroidism and in those whose GH deficiency is caused by an intracranial lesion, use cautiously; these children should be examined frequently for progression or recurrence of underlying disease.

Adverse reactions

CNS: headache, weakness.
CV: mild, transient edema.
Hematologic: *leukemia.*
Metabolic: mild hyperglycemia, hypothyroidism.
Musculoskeletal: localized muscle pain.
Other: injection site pain, *antibodies to GH.*

Interactions

Drug-drug. *Corticosteroids, corticotropin:* May inhibit growth response to GH with long-term use. Monitor patient.

Effects on lab test results

• May increase glucose, inorganic phosphorus, alkaline phosphatase, and parathyroid hormone levels.

Pharmacokinetics

Absorption: Unknown.
Distribution: Unknown.
Metabolism: About 90% metabolized in liver.
Excretion: About 0.1% excreted unchanged in urine. *Half-life:* 20 to 30 minutes.

Route	Onset	Peak	Duration
I.M, SubQ	Unknown	7½ hr	12–48 hr

Action

Chemical effect: Purified GH of recombinant DNA origin that stimulates linear, skeletal muscle, and organ growth.
Therapeutic effect: Stimulates growth.

Available forms

Genotropin injection: 1.5 mg (about 4.5 international units/vial), 5.8 mg (about 17.4 international units/vial), 13.8 mg (about 41.4 international units/vial)
Genotropin Miniquick injection: 0.2 mg/vial, 0.4 mg/vial, 0.6 mg/vial, 0.8 mg/vial, 1 mg/vial, 1.2 mg/vial, 1.4 mg/vial, 1.6 mg/vial, 1.8 mg/vial, 2 mg/vial
Humatrope injection: 2 mg (about 6 international units/vial), 5 mg (about 15 international units/vial), 6 mg (18 international units/car-

tridge), 12 mg (36 international units/cartridge), 24 mg (72 international units/cartridge)
Norditropin injection: 4 mg (about 12 international units/ml), 8 mg (about 24 international units/ml), 5 mg/1.5 ml cartridges, 10 mg/1.5 ml cartridges, 15 mg/1.5 ml cartridges
Nutropin injection: 5 mg (about 15 international units/vial), 10 mg (about 30 international units/vial)
Nutropin AQ injection: 10 mg (about 30 international units/vial)
Saizen injection: 5 mg (about 15 international units/vial)
Serostim injection: 4 mg (about 12 international units/vial), 5 mg (about 15 international units/vial), 6 mg (about 18 international units/vial)
Somatropin depot injection: 13.5 mg/vial, 18 mg/vial, 22.5 mg/vial

NURSING PROCESS

⚖ Assessment

• Assess child's growth before starting therapy, and regularly thereafter to monitor the drug's effectiveness.
• Ensure adults taking Saizen for GH replacement have GH deficiency alone or with multiple hormone deficiencies (result of pituitary or hypothalamic disease, surgery, radiation, or trauma) or had GH deficiency during childhood and confirmed deficiency as an adult.
• Be alert for adverse reactions.
• Toxicity in neonates may occur from exposure to benzyl alcohol used in drug as preservative.
• Conduct regular checkup with monitoring of height, blood, and radiologic studies.
• Observe patient for signs of glucose intolerance and hyperglycemia.
• Monitor patient's periodic thyroid function tests for hypothyroidism, which may require treatment with thyroid hormone.
• Assess patient's and family's knowledge of drug therapy.

🔲 Nursing diagnoses

• Delayed growth and development related to lack of adequate endogenous GH
• Ineffective health maintenance related to adverse metabolic reactions
• Deficient knowledge related to drug therapy

S

⟫ Planning and implementation

• To prepare solution, inject supplied diluent into vial containing drug by aiming stream of liquid against glass wall of vial. Then swirl vial with gentle rotary motion until contents are completely dissolved; don't shake vial.

• After reconstitution, solution should be clear. Don't inject solution if it's cloudy or contains particles.

• Store reconstituted drug in refrigerator; use within 14 days.

• If sensitivity to diluent develops, drugs may be reconstituted with sterile water for injection. When drug is reconstituted in this manner, use only one reconstituted dose per vial, refrigerate solution if it isn't used immediately after reconstitution, use reconstituted dose within 24 hours, and discard unused portion.

• If final height is achieved, or epiphyseal fusion occurs, do not continue therapy.

• Excessive glucocorticoid therapy inhibits growth-promoting effect of somatropin. In patient with corticotropin deficiency, adjust glucocorticoid-replacement dosage carefully to avoid growth inhibition.

ⓢ ALERT: Don't confuse somatropin with somatrem or sumatriptan.

Patient teaching

• Inform parents that child with endocrine disorders (including GH deficiency) may develop slipped capital epiphyses. Tell them to notify prescriber if child begins limping.

🗹 Evaluation

• Patient exhibits growth.

• Patient's thyroid function studies and glucose level are normal.

• Patient and family state understanding of drug therapy.

sotalol hydrochloride
(SOH-tuh-lol high-droh-KLOR-ighd)
Betapace, Betapace AF, Sotacor ◆ ◇

Pharmacologic class: beta blocker
Therapeutic class: antiarrhythmic, antihypertensive, antianginal
Pregnancy risk category: B

Indications and dosages

▶ **Documented, life-threatening ventricular arrhythmias.** *Adults:* Initially, 80 mg Betapace P.O. b.i.d. Dosage is increased q 2 to 3 days as needed and tolerated; most patients respond to 160 to 320 mg daily. A few patients with refractory arrhythmias have received as much as 640 mg daily.

☒ **Adjust-a-dose:** For patients with renal impairment, if creatinine clearance is 30 to 60 ml/minute, interval is increased to q 24 hours; if clearance is 10 to 30 ml/minute, give q 36 to 48 hours; if clearance is less than 10 ml/minute, individualize dosage.

▶ **To maintain normal sinus rhythm (delayed recurrence of atrial fibrillation or flutter) in patients with symptomatic atrial fibrillation or flutter who are currently in sinus rhythm.** *Adults:* Initially, 80 mg Betapace AF P.O. b.i.d. If initial dose doesn't reduce the frequency of relapses of atrial fibrillation or flutter and patient has a QTc interval of less than 520 msec, may increase to 120 mg P.O. b.i.d. after 3 days. Maximum, 160 mg P.O. b.i.d.

☒ **Adjust-a-dose:** For patients with renal impairment, if creatinine clearance is 40 to 60 ml/minute, give once daily.

Contraindications and cautions

• Contraindicated in patients hypersensitive to the drug or any of its components, and patients with severe sinus node dysfunction, sinus bradycardia, second- or third-degree AV block in absence of an artificial pacemaker, congenital or acquired long-QT interval syndrome, cardiogenic shock, uncontrolled heart failure, or bronchial asthma. Don't give to patients with a creatinine clearance less than 40 ml/minute.

• Use cautiously in patients with renal impairment, sick sinus syndrome, or diabetes mellitus.

⚘ **Lifespan:** In pregnant women, use cautiously. In breast-feeding women and in children, safety and effectiveness haven't been established.

Adverse reactions

CNS: asthenia, headache, dizziness, weakness, fatigue, sleep problems, light-headedness.
CV: *bradycardia, arrhythmias, heart failure, AV block, proarrhythmic events (ventricular tachycardia, PVCs, ventricular fibrillation),* edema, palpitations, chest pain, ECG abnormalities, hypotension.

GI: *nausea,* vomiting, diarrhea, dyspepsia.
Respiratory: dyspnea, ***bronchospasm.***

Interactions

Drug-drug. *Antiarrhythmics:* May have additive effects. Avoid using together.
Antihypertensives, catecholamine-depleting drugs (such as guanethidine, haloperidol, and reserpine): May enhance hypotensive effects. Monitor patient closely.
Calcium channel blockers: May enhance myocardial depression. Monitor patient carefully.
Clonidine: May enhance rebound effect seen after withdrawal of clonidine. May cause life-threatening or fatal increases in blood pressure. Stop sotalol several days before withdrawing clonidine.
General anesthetics: May cause additional myocardial depression. Monitor patient closely.
Insulin, oral antidiabetics: May cause hyperglycemia and mask its symptoms. Adjust dosage.
Prazosin: May increase the risk of orthostatic hypotension in the early phases of use together. Assist patient to stand slowly until effects are known.
Drug-food. *Any food:* May increase drug absorption. Give drug on an empty stomach.

Effects on lab test results

• May increase glucose level.

Pharmacokinetics

Absorption: Well absorbed, with bioavailability of 90% to 100%. Food may interfere with absorption.
Distribution: Unknown; doesn't bind to proteins and crosses blood-brain barrier poorly.
Metabolism: Not metabolized.
Excretion: Excreted primarily in urine in unchanged form. *Half-life:* 12 hours.

Route	Onset	Peak	Duration
P.O.	Unknown	2½–4 hr	Unknown

Action

Chemical effect: Depresses sinus heart rate, slows AV conduction, decreases cardiac output, and lowers systolic and diastolic blood pressure.
Therapeutic effect: Restores normal sinus rhythm, lowers blood pressure, and relieves angina.

Available forms

Tablets: 80 mg, 120 mg, 160 mg, 240 mg

NURSING PROCESS

Assessment

• Assess patient's condition before starting therapy, and regularly thereafter to monitor the drug's effectiveness.
• Monitor patient's electrolyte levels and ECG regularly, especially if patient is taking diuretics. Electrolyte imbalances, such as hypokalemia and hypomagnesemia, may enhance QT interval prolongation and increase risk of serious arrhythmias such as torsades de pointes.
• Be alert for adverse reactions and drug interactions.
• Assess patient's and family's knowledge of drug therapy.

Nursing diagnoses

• Ineffective health maintenance related to underlying condition
• Fatigue related to adverse reactions
• Deficient knowledge related to drug therapy

Planning and implementation

• Because proarrhythmic events may occur at start of therapy and during dose adjustments, patient should be hospitalized. Facilities and personnel should be available to monitor cardiac rhythm and interpret ECG.
• Although patient receiving I.V. lidocaine can start therapy with sotalol without ill effect, other antiarrhythmics should be stopped before starting therapy with sotalol. Therapy typically is delayed until two or three half-lives of withdrawn drug have elapsed. After withdrawal of amiodarone, sotalol shouldn't be given until QT interval normalizes.
• Adjust dose slowly, allowing 2 to 3 days between dose increases for adequate monitoring of QT intervals and for drug levels to reach steady-state level.
ALERT: The baseline QTc interval must be 450 msec or less in order to start a patient on Betapace AF. During initiation and adjustment, monitor QT interval 2 to 4 hours after each dose. If the QTc interval is 500 msec or longer, reduce dose or stop drug.
ALERT: Don't confuse sotalol with Stadol. Don't substitute Betapace AF for Betapace.

S

Patient teaching

• Explain importance of taking drug as prescribed, even when feeling well. Instruct patient not to stop drug suddenly.

• Tell patient to take drug 1 hour before or 2 hours after meals.

• Teach patient how to check his pulse rate.

☑ Evaluation

• Patient responds well to therapy.

• Patient states energy-conserving measures to combat fatigue.

• Patient and family state understanding of drug therapy.

spironolactone
(spih-ron-uh-LAK-tohn)
Aldactone, Novospiroton ♦ , Spiractin ◇

Pharmacologic class: mineralocorticoid receptor antagonist
Therapeutic class: potassium-sparing diuretic
Pregnancy risk category: NR

Indications and dosages

▶ **Edema.** *Adults:* 25 to 200 mg P.O. daily or in divided doses.
Children: 3.3 mg/kg P.O. daily or in divided doses.

▶ **Essential hypertension.** *Adults:* 50 to 100 mg P.O. daily or in divided doses.
Children: 1 to 2 mg/kg P.O. b.i.d.

▶ **Diuretic-induced hypokalemia.** *Adults:* 25 to 100 mg P.O. daily when P.O. potassium supplements are contraindicated.

▶ **Diagnosis of primary hyperaldosteronism.** *Adults:* 400 mg P.O. daily for 4 days (short test) or 3 to 4 weeks (long test). If hypokalemia and hypertension are corrected, presumptive diagnosis of primary hyperaldosteronism is made.

▶ **To manage primary hyperaldosteronism.** *Adults:* 100 to 400 mg P.O. daily. In patients unwilling or unable to undergo surgery, start with 400 mg daily and then maintain at lowest possible dose.

▶ **Hirsutism‡.** *Adults:* 50 to 200 mg P.O. daily.

▶ **Premenstrual syndrome‡.** *Adults:* 25 mg P.O. q.i.d. beginning on day 14 of menstrual cycle.

▶ **Heart failure in patients taking an ACE inhibitor and a loop diuretic with or without digoxin‡.** *Adults:* Initially, 12.5 to 25 mg P.O. daily.

▶ **To decrease risk of metrorrhagia‡.** *Adults:* 50 mg P.O. b.i.d. on days 4 through 21 of menstrual cycle.

▶ **Acne vulgaris‡.** *Adults:* 100 mg P.O. daily.

Contraindications and cautions

• Contraindicated in patients with anuria, acute or progressive renal insufficiency, rapidly deteriorating renal function, or hyperkalemia.

• Contraindicated in patients taking amiloride or triamterene concomitantly.

• Use cautiously in patients with fluid or electrolyte imbalances, impaired kidney function, or hepatic disease.

☀ **Lifespan:** In pregnant women, use cautiously. In breast-feeding women, safety and effectiveness haven't been established.

Adverse reactions

CNS: headache, drowsiness, lethargy, confusion, ataxia.
GI: diarrhea, gastric bleeding, ulceration, cramping, gastritis, vomiting.
GU: impotence, menstrual disturbances.
Hematologic: *agranulocytosis.*
Metabolic: *hyperkalemia,* hyponatremia, mild acidosis, dehydration.
Skin: urticaria, hirsutism, maculopapular eruptions, erythematous rash.
Other: drug fever, gynecomastia, breast soreness, *anaphylaxis, angioedema.*

Interactions

Drug-drug. *ACE inhibitors, indomethacin, other potassium-sparing diuretics, potassium supplements:* May increase risk of hyperkalemia. Don't use together, especially in patients with renal impairment.
Aspirin, other salicylates: May block diuretic effect of spironolactone. Antihypertensive effect of drug not affected. Monitor edema, ascites, fluid overload.
Digoxin: May alter digoxin clearance, increasing risk of digoxin toxicity. Monitor digoxin level.
Warfarin, other anticoagulants: May decrease effectiveness of anticoagulants. Monitor PT and INR, increase dosage as needed.

Drug-food. *Potassium-containing salt substitutes, potassium-rich foods (such as citrus fruits, tomatoes):* May increase risk of hyperkalemia. Tell patient to use low-potassium salt substitutes and to eat high-potassium foods cautiously.

Effects on lab test results

- May increase BUN, creatinine, and potassium levels. May decrease sodium level.
- May decrease granulocyte count.
- May falsely increase serum digoxin level.

Pharmacokinetics

Absorption: About 90%.
Distribution: More than 90% protein-bound.
Metabolism: Metabolized rapidly and extensively.
Excretion: Canrenone and other metabolites excreted primarily in urine, minimally in feces. *Half-life:* 1¼ to 2 hours.

Route	Onset	Peak	Duration
P.O.	Unknown	1–2 hr	Unknown

Action

Chemical effect: Antagonizes aldosterone in distal tubule.
Therapeutic effect: Promotes water and sodium excretion and hinders potassium excretion, lowers blood pressure, and helps to diagnose primary hyperaldosteronism.

Available forms

Tablets: 25 mg, 50 mg, 100 mg

NURSING PROCESS

Assessment

- Assess patient's condition before starting therapy, and regularly thereafter to monitor the drug's effectiveness. Maximum antihypertensive response may be delayed up to 2 weeks.
- Monitor electrolyte levels, fluid intake and output, weight, and blood pressure.
- Be alert for adverse reactions and drug interactions.
- Assess patient's and family's knowledge of drug therapy.

Nursing diagnoses

- Excess fluid volume related to presence of edema
- Impaired urinary elimination related to diuretic therapy
- Deficient knowledge related to drug therapy

Planning and implementation

- Give drug with meals to enhance absorption.
- Protect drug from light.
- Inform laboratory that patient is taking spironolactone because it may interfere with some laboratory tests that measure digoxin levels.

ALERT: Don't confuse Aldactone with Aldactazide.

Patient teaching

ALERT: To prevent serious hyperkalemia, warn patient not to eat large amounts of potassium-rich foods and not to use potassium-containing salt substitutes or potassium supplements.

- Tell patient to take drug with meals and, if possible, early in day to avoid interruption of sleep by nocturia.

Evaluation

- Patient shows no signs of edema.
- Patient demonstrates adjustment of lifestyle to deal with altered patterns of urinary elimination.
- Patient and family state understanding of drug therapy.

stavudine (2,3-didehydro-3-deoxythymidine, d4T)

(stay-VYOO-deen)
Zerit, Zerit XR

Pharmacologic class: nucleoside reverse transcriptase inhibitor
Therapeutic class: antiretroviral
Pregnancy risk category: C

Indications and dosages

▶ **Patients with advanced HIV infection who are intolerant of or unresponsive to other antivirals.** *Adults and children who weigh 60 kg (132 lb) or more:* 40 mg P.O. q 12 hours, or 100 mg P.O. extended-release daily.
Adults and children who weigh more than 30 kg (66 lb) but less than 60 kg: 30 mg P.O. q 12 hours, or 75 mg P.O. extended-release daily.

Children who weigh less than 30 kg: 1 mg/kg q 12 hours if at least 14 days old. If 13 days old or less, give 0.5 mg/kg q 12 hours.

N **Adjust-a-dose:** For patients with renal impairment adjust dosage as follows. If creatinine clearance 26 to 50 ml/min, give 20 mg q 12 hours if ≥ 60 kg or 15 mg q 12 hours if < 60 kg; if creatinine clearance is 10 to 25 ml/min, give 20 mg q 24 hours if ≥ 60 kg or 15 mg q 24 hours if < 60 kg. For adults undergoing hemodialysis, give 20 mg q 24 hours if ≥ 60 kg or 15 mg q 24 hours if < 60 kg. Give dose after hemodialysis.

Contraindications and cautions

• Contraindicated in patients hypersensitive to the drug or any of its components.
• Don't use Zerit XR in patients with creatinine clearance of 50 ml/minute or less.
• Use cautiously in patients with renal impairment or a history of peripheral neuropathy.
☀ **Lifespan:** In pregnant women, use cautiously. In breast-feeding women, safety and effectiveness haven't been established.

Adverse reactions

CNS: asthenia, peripheral neuropathy, headache, malaise, insomnia, anxiety, depression, nervousness, dizziness, fever.
CV: chest pain.
EENT: conjunctivitis.
GI: abdominal pain, diarrhea, nausea, vomiting, anorexia, dyspepsia, constipation, weight loss, *pancreatitis.*
Hematologic: *neutropenia, thrombocytopenia,* anemia, *leukopenia.*
Hepatic: *hepatotoxicity,* severe hepatomegaly with steatosis.
Metabolic: *lactic acidosis.*
Musculoskeletal: myalgia, *back pain, arthralgia.*
Respiratory: *dyspnea.*
Skin: rash, diaphoresis, pruritus, maculopapular rash.
Other: *chills,* breast enlargement, redistribution or accumulation of body fat.

Interactions

Drug-drug. *Didanosine, hydroxyurea:* May increase risk of lactic acidosis, hepatotoxicity, pancreatitis, peripheral neuropathy. Monitor patient closely.

Doxorubicin, ribavirin: May increase risk of toxicities. Use together cautiously.
Ketoconazole, ritonavir: May increase stavudine level. Monitor patient closely.
Methadone: May decrease stavudine absorption. Avoid using together.
Myelosuppressants: May cause additive myelosuppression. Avoid using together.
Zidovudine: May inhibit stavudine phosphorylation. Don't use together.

Effects on lab test results

• May increase liver enzyme levels. May decrease hemoglobin level and hematocrit.
• May decrease neutrophil and platelet counts.

Pharmacokinetics

Absorption: Rapid with mean absolute bioavailability of 86.4% for immediate release, slower and less bioavailability with extended release form.
Distribution: Equally between RBCs and plasma; binds poorly to proteins.
Metabolism: Not extensive.
Excretion: About 40% renal. *Half-life:* 1 to 2 hours.

Route	Onset	Peak	Duration
P.O.	Unknown	≤ 1 hr	8 hr
P.O. extended-release	Unknown	3 hr	24 hr

Action

Chemical effect: Prevents replication of HIV by interfering with enzyme reverse transcriptase.
Therapeutic effect: Inhibits HIV replication.

Available forms

Capsules: 15 mg, 20 mg, 30 mg, 40 mg
Capsules (extended-release): 37.5 mg, 50 mg, 75 mg, 100 mg.
Powder for oral solution: 1 mg/ml

NURSING PROCESS

⚗ **Assessment**
• Assess patient's condition before starting therapy, and regularly thereafter to monitor the drug's effectiveness.
• Periodically monitor CBC and levels of creatinine, AST, ALT, and alkaline phosphatase.

• Be alert for adverse reactions and drug interactions.

• Assess patient's and family's knowledge of drug therapy.

Nursing diagnoses

• Infection related to presence of HIV
• Disturbed sensory perception (peripheral) related to drug-induced peripheral neuropathy
• Deficient knowledge related to drug therapy

Planning and implementation

ALERT: Peripheral neuropathy appears to be major dose-limiting adverse effect. If it occurs, temporarily stop giving the drug; then resume at 50% of recommended dose.

• Dose is calculated based on patient's weight.

ALERT: Don't confuse drug with other antivirals that may use initials for identification.

• Motor weakness that mimics Guillain-Barré syndrome (including respiratory failure) may occur in HIV-positive patient taking this drug with other antiretrovirals, usually in those with lactic acidosis. Monitor patient for evidence of lactic acidosis, including generalized fatigue, GI problems, tachypnea, or dyspnea. Symptoms may continue or worsen when stopping drug. In patients with these symptoms, promptly stop antiretroviral therapy and perform a full medical workup immediately. Permanently stopping drug should be considered.

• Monitor patient for pancreatitis, especially when this drug is used with didanosine or hydroxyurea. Use caution when restarting drug after confirmed diagnosis of pancreatitis.

• If patient has trouble swallowing capsule, mix contents of the capsule in applesauce or yogurt. Instruct patient not to chew or crush the beads while swallowing.

Patient teaching

• Tell patient that drug may be taken with or without food.

• Advise patient that he can't take drug if he experienced peripheral neuropathy while taking other nucleoside analogues or if his treatment plan includes cytotoxic antineoplastics.

• Warn patient not to take any other drugs for HIV or AIDS (especially street drugs) unless prescriber has approved them.

• Teach patient signs and symptoms of peripheral neuropathy—pain, burning, aching, weakness, or pins and needles in limbs—and tell him to report these immediately.

• Tell patient to report symptoms of lactic acidosis, including fatigue, GI problems, dyspnea or tachypnea.

• Tell patient to report symptoms of pancreatitis, including abdominal pain, nausea, vomiting, weight loss or fatty stools.

Evaluation

• Patient's infection is controlled.
• Patient maintains normal peripheral neurologic function.
• Patient and family state understanding of drug therapy.

streptokinase
(strep-toh-KIGH-nayz)
Streptase

Pharmacologic class: plasminogen activator
Therapeutic class: thrombolytic enzyme
Pregnancy risk category: C

Indications and dosages

▶ **Arteriovenous cannula occlusion.** *Adults:* 250,000 international units in 2 ml I.V. solution by I.V. pump infusion into each occluded limb of cannula over 25 to 35 minutes. Clamp cannula for 2 hours. Then aspirate contents of cannula, flush with saline solution, and reconnect.

▶ **Venous thrombosis, pulmonary embolism, arterial thrombosis and embolism.** *Adults:* Loading dose is 250,000 international units by I.V. infusion over 30 minutes. Sustaining dose is 100,000 international units/hour by I.V. infusion for 72 hours for deep vein thrombosis and 100,000 international units/hour over 24 hours by I.V. infusion pump for pulmonary embolism.

▶ **Lysis of coronary artery thrombi after acute MI.** *Adults:* I.V. infusion preferred using 1,500,000 international units infused over 60 minutes. Or, if using intracoronary infusion, the total dose for intracoronary infusion is 140,000 international units. Loading dose is 15,000 to 20,000 international units by coronary catheter over 15 seconds to 2 minutes, followed by infusion of maintenance dose of 2,000 international units/minute for 60 minutes.

▼ I.V. administration

● Reconstitute each drug vial with 5 ml of normal saline solution for injection. Further dilute to 45 ml.
● Don't shake; roll gently to mix. Some precipitate may be present; discard if large amounts appear. Filter solution with 0.8-micron or larger filter. Use within 8 hours.
● Store powder at room temperature and refrigerate after reconstitution.
⊗ **Incompatibilities**
Dextrans, other I.V. drugs.

Contraindications and cautions

● Contraindicated in patients with ulcerative wounds, active internal bleeding, uncontrolled hypercoagulation, chronic pulmonary disease with cavitation, subacute bacterial endocarditis or rheumatic valvular disease, visceral or intracranial malignant neoplasms, ulcerative colitis, diverticulitis, severe hypertension, acute or chronic hepatic or renal insufficiency, recent stroke, recent trauma with possible internal injuries, or recent cerebral embolism, thrombosis, or hemorrhage.
● Also contraindicated within 10 days after intra-arterial diagnostic procedure or any surgery, including liver or kidney biopsy, lumbar puncture, thoracentesis, paracentesis, or extensive or multiple cutdowns.
● I.M. injections and other invasive procedures are contraindicated during streptokinase therapy.
● Use cautiously when treating arterial embolism that originates from left side of heart because of danger of cerebral infarction.
⚖ **Lifespan:** In pregnant women, use cautiously. In breast-feeding women and in children, safety and effectiveness haven't been established.

Adverse reactions

CNS: polyradiculoneuropathy, headache, fever.
CV: hypotension, vasculitis, *reperfusion arrhythmias,* flushing.
EENT: periorbital edema.
GI: nausea.
Hematologic: *bleeding.*
Musculoskeletal: musculoskeletal pain.
Respiratory: minor breathing difficulty, *bronchospasm, pulmonary edema.*
Skin: urticaria, pruritus.
Other: phlebitis at injection site, *hypersensitivity reactions (anaphylaxis), delayed hyper-*

sensitivity reactions (interstitial nephritis, vasculitis, serum-sickness–like reactions), *angioedema.*

Interactions

Drug-drug. *Anticoagulants:* May increase risk of bleeding. Monitor patient closely.
Antifibrinolytics, such as aminocaproic acid: May inhibit and reverse streptokinase activity. Use only when indicated during streptokinase therapy.
Aspirin, dipyridamole, drugs that affect platelet activity, indomethacin, phenylbutazone: May increase risk of bleeding. Monitor patient closely. Combined therapy with low-dose aspirin (162.5 mg) or dipyridamole has improved acute and long-term results.

Effects on lab test results

● May increase PT, PTT, and INR. May decrease hemoglobin level and hematocrit.

Pharmacokinetics

Absorption: Administered I.V.
Distribution: Unknown.
Metabolism: Insignificant.
Excretion: Removed from circulation by antibodies and reticuloendothelial system. *Half-life:* First phase, 18 minutes; second phase, 83 minutes.

Route	Onset	Peak	Duration
I.V.	Immediate	20 min–2 hr	4 hr

Action

Chemical effect: Activates plasminogen in two steps. Plasminogen and streptokinase form a complex that exposes plasminogen-activating site. Plasminogen is then converted to plasmin by cleavage of peptide bond.
Therapeutic effect: Dissolves blood clots.

Available forms

Injection: 250,000 international units, 750,000 international units, and 1.5 million international units in vials for reconstitution

NURSING PROCESS

℞ **Assessment**
● Assess patient's condition before starting therapy, and regularly thereafter to monitor the drug's effectiveness.

• Assess patient for increased risk of bleeding (such as from recent surgery, stroke, trauma, or hypertension) before starting therapy.
• Before starting therapy, draw blood to determine APTT and PT. Rate of I.V. infusion depends on thrombin time and streptokinase resistance. Then repeat studies often and keep laboratory flow sheet on patient's chart to monitor APTT, PT, hemoglobin level, and hematocrit.
• Monitor patient for excessive bleeding q 15 minutes for first hour, q 30 minutes for second through eighth hours, then once q shift.
• Monitor pulse rates, color, and sensation of limbs q hour.
• Be alert for adverse reactions and drug interactions.
• Assess patient's and family's knowledge of drug therapy.

⊕ **Nursing diagnoses**
• Ineffective cardiopulmonary tissue perfusion related to condition
• Risk for deficient fluid volume related to potential for bleeding
• Deficient knowledge related to drug therapy

▶ **Planning and implementation**
• Drug should be used only by prescriber with experience in thrombotic disease management and in a setting where close monitoring can be performed.
• Before using streptokinase to clear an occluded arteriovenous cannula, try flushing with heparinized saline solution.
Ⓢ **ALERT:** To check for hypersensitivity reactions, give 100 international units I.D.; wheal and flare response within 20 minutes means patient is probably allergic. Monitor vital signs frequently.
• If patient has had either recent streptococcal infection or recent treatment with streptokinase, higher loading dose may be needed.
• If bleeding occurs, stop therapy and notify prescriber. Pretreatment with heparin or drugs affecting platelets causes high risk of bleeding but may improve long-term results.
• Have aminocaproic acid available to treat bleeding and corticosteroids to treat allergic reactions.
• Have typed and crossmatched packed RBCs and whole blood ready to treat hemorrhage.

• Keep involved limb in straight alignment to prevent bleeding from infusion site.
• Avoid unnecessary handling of patient, and pad side rails. Bruising is more likely during therapy.
• Keep venipuncture sites to minimum; use pressure dressing on puncture sites for at least 15 minutes.
Ⓢ **ALERT:** Immediately notify prescriber if hypersensitivity occurs. Antihistamines or corticosteroids may be used to treat mild reactions. If severe reaction occurs, stop infusion and notify prescriber.
• Heparin by continuous infusion is usually started within 1 hour after stopping streptokinase. Use infusion pump to give heparin.
• In patient with acute MI, thrombolytic therapy may decrease infarct size, improve ventricular function, and decrease risk of heart failure. Drug must be given within 6 hours of onset of symptoms for optimal effect.
Patient teaching
• Tell patient to report oozing, bleeding, or signs of hypersensitivity immediately.

☑ **Evaluation**
• Patient responds well to therapy.
• Patient maintains adequate fluid balance.
• Patient and family state understanding of drug therapy.

streptomycin sulfate
(strep-toh-MIGH-sin SUL-fayt)

Pharmacologic class: aminoglycoside
Therapeutic class: antibiotic
Pregnancy risk category: D

Indications and dosages
▶ **Streptococcal endocarditis.** *Adults:* 1 g I.M. q 12 hours for 1 week, and then 500 mg q 12 hours for 1 week, given with penicillin. *Adults older than age 60:* 500 mg I.M. q 12 hours for 14 days.
▶ **Primary and adjunct treatment in tuberculosis.** *Adults:* 1 g or 15 mg/kg I.M. (up to 1 g) daily or 25 to 30 mg/kg (up to 1.5 g) two or three times weekly.
Children: 20 to 40 mg/kg (up to 1 g) I.M. daily in divided doses injected deep into large muscle mass or 25 to 30 mg/kg (up to 1 g) two or three

S

times weekly. Given with other antituberculars but not with capreomycin. Continue until sputum specimen becomes negative.

▶ **Enterococcal endocarditis.** *Adults:* 1 g I.M. q 12 hours for 2 weeks, and then 500 mg q 12 hours for 4 weeks, given with penicillin.

▶ **Tularemia.** *Adults:* 1 to 2 g I.M. daily in divided doses injected deep into upper outer quadrant of buttocks. Continue for 7 to 14 days until patient is afebrile for 5 to 7 days.

§ **Adjust-a-dose:** For patients with renal impairment, initial dose is the same as for normal renal function. Subsequent doses and frequency determined by renal function study results and blood levels. If creatinine clearance is 50 to 80 ml/minute, give 7.5 mg/kg q 24 hours; if 10 to 50 ml/minute, give 7.5 mg/kg q 24 to 72 hours; if less than 10 ml/minute, give 7.5 mg/kg q 72 to 96 hours.

Contraindications and cautions

• Contraindicated in patients hypersensitive to the drug or other aminoglycosides and patients with labyrinthine disease.
• Use cautiously in patients with impaired kidney function or neuromuscular disorders.
☀ **Lifespan:** In pregnant women, drug is contraindicated. In breast-feeding women and in the elderly, use cautiously.

Adverse reactions

CNS: *neuromuscular blockade.*
EENT: ototoxicity.
GI: vomiting, nausea.
GU: *nephrotoxicity.*
Hematologic: eosinophilia, *leukopenia, thrombocytopenia.*
Respiratory: *apnea.*
Skin: exfoliative dermatitis.
Other: hypersensitivity reactions, *angioedema, anaphylaxis.*

Interactions

Drug-drug. *Atracurium, doxacurium, mivacurium, pancuronium, rocuronium, tubocurarine, vecuronium:* May increase the effects of nondepolarizing muscle relaxant, including prolonged respiratory depression. Use together only when necessary. Dose of nondepolarizing muscle relaxant may need to be reduced.
Cephalosporins: May increase risk of nephrotoxicity. Use together cautiously.

Dimenhydrinate: May mask symptoms of streptomycin-induced ototoxicity. Use together cautiously.
I.V. loop diuretics (such as furosemide): May increase ototoxicity. Use together cautiously.
Other aminoglycosides, acyclovir, amphotericin B, cisplatin, methoxyflurane, vancomycin: May increase risk of nephrotoxicity. Monitor patient.

Effects on lab test results

• May increase BUN, creatinine, and nonprotein nitrogen levels. May decrease hemoglobin level and hematocrit.
• May increase eosinophil count. May decrease WBC and platelet counts.

Pharmacokinetics

Absorption: Unknown after I.M. administration.
Distribution: Wide distribution, although CSF penetration is low; 36% protein-bound.
Metabolism: None.
Excretion: Mainly in urine; less in bile. *Half-life:* 2 to 3 hours.

Route	Onset	Peak	Duration
I.M.	Unknown	1–2 hr	Unknown

Action

Chemical effect: Inhibits protein synthesis by binding directly to 30S ribosomal subunit.
Therapeutic effect: Kills bacteria.

Available forms

Injection: 400 mg/ml, 1 g/2.5-ml ampules

NURSING PROCESS

⚡ Assessment

• Assess patient's infection before starting therapy, and regularly thereafter to monitor the drug's effectiveness.
• Obtain specimen for culture and sensitivity tests before first dose except when treating tuberculosis. Start therapy pending test results.
⑤ **ALERT:** Obtain blood for peak streptomycin level 1 to 2 hours after I.M. injection; for trough levels, draw blood just before next dose. Don't use heparinized tube because heparin is incompatible with aminoglycosides.
• Evaluate patient's hearing before therapy, during therapy, and 6 months after therapy ends.

Reactions may be *common*, uncommon, *life-threatening*, or COMMON AND LIFE-THREATENING.

• Be alert for adverse reactions and drug interactions.

• Assess patient's and family's knowledge of drug therapy.

⊕ **Nursing diagnoses**

• Infection related to presence of susceptible bacteria

• Disturbed sensory perception (auditory) related to drug-induced adverse reactions

• Deficient knowledge related to drug therapy

▷ **Planning and implementation**

• Protect hands when preparing drug because drug is irritating.

• Inject drug deep into upper outer quadrant of buttocks. Rotate injection sites.

⊛ **ALERT:** Never give streptomycin I.V.

• Encourage adequate fluid intake. Patient should be well hydrated while taking drug to minimize chemical irritation of renal tubules.

• In primary treatment of tuberculosis, stop drug when sputum becomes negative.

Patient teaching

• Warn patient that injection may be painful.

• Emphasize the need to drink at least 2,000 ml daily (if not contraindicated) during therapy.

• Instruct patient to report hearing loss, roaring noises, or fullness in ears or dizziness immediately.

☑ **Evaluation**

• Patient is free from infection.

• Patient's auditory function remains normal.

• Patient and family state understanding of drug therapy.

succimer
(SUK-sih-mer)
Chemet

Pharmacologic class: heavy metal antagonist
Therapeutic class: chelate
Pregnancy risk category: C

Indications and dosages

▶ **Lead poisoning in children with blood lead levels above 45 mcg/dl.** *Children:* 10 mg/kg or 350 mg/m² q 8 hours for 5 days. Round dose to nearest 100 mg (see table). For next 2 weeks, decrease interval to q 12 hours.

Weight (kg)	Dose (mg)
8–15	100
16–23	200
24–34	300
35–44	400
≥ 45	500

Contraindications and cautions

• Contraindicated in patients hypersensitive to the drug or any of its components.

• Use cautiously in patients with compromised kidney function.

• Monitor patient for neutropenia. If absolute neutrophil count falls below 1,200/mm³, stop drug.

▒ **Lifespan:** None reported.

Adverse reactions

CNS: drowsiness, dizziness, sensory motor neuropathy, sleepiness, paresthesia, headache.
CV: *arrhythmias.*
EENT: plugged ears, cloudy film in eyes, otitis media, watery eyes, sore throat, rhinorrhea, nasal congestion.
GI: nausea, vomiting, diarrhea, loss of appetite, abdominal cramps, hemorrhoidal symptoms, metallic taste, loose stools, stomach pain.
GU: decreased urination, difficult urination, proteinuria, *flank pain.*
Hematologic: intermittent eosinophilia, *neutropenia.*
Musculoskeletal: leg, kneecap, back, or rib pain.
Respiratory: cough, head cold.
Skin: papular rash, herpetic rash, mucocutaneous eruptions, pruritus.
Other: *flulike syndrome,* candidiasis.

Interactions

None reported.

Effects on lab test results

• May increase AST, ALT, alkaline phosphatase, and cholesterol levels.

• May increase eosinophil and platelet counts.

• May cause false-positive results for ketones in urine using nitroprusside reagents (Ketostix) and falsely decreased levels of uric acid and CK.

S

Pharmacokinetics

Absorption: Rapid but variable.
Distribution: Unknown.
Metabolism: Rapid and extensive.
Excretion: 39% excreted in feces unchanged; remainder excreted mainly in urine. *Half-life:* 48 hours.

Route	Onset	Peak	Duration
P.O.	Unknown	1–2 hr	Unknown

Action

Chemical effect: Forms water-soluble complexes with lead and increases its excretion in urine.
Therapeutic effect: Relieves signs and symptoms of lead poisoning.

Available forms

Capsules: 100 mg

NURSING PROCESS

⚏ Assessment

• Assess child's condition before starting therapy, and regularly thereafter to monitor the drug's effectiveness.
• Measure severity by initial blood lead level and by rate and degree of rebound of blood lead level. Use severity as guide for more frequent blood lead monitoring.
• Monitor transaminase level and neutrophil count before starting therapy, and at least weekly during therapy. Transient, mild elevations of transaminase level may occur. Monitor patient with history of hepatic disease more closely.
• Monitor patient at least once weekly for rebound blood lead levels. Elevated blood lead levels and associated symptoms may return rapidly after drug is stopped because of redistribution of lead from bone to soft tissues and blood.
• Be alert for adverse reactions.
• If adverse GI reactions occur, monitor patient's hydration.
• Evaluate parents' knowledge of drug therapy.

⊞ Nursing diagnoses

• Ineffective health maintenance related to presence of lead poisoning
• Risk for deficient fluid volume related to drug-induced adverse GI reactions
• Deficient knowledge related to drug therapy

⊳ Planning and implementation

• Course of treatment lasts 19 days. Repeated courses may be needed if indicated by weekly monitoring of blood lead levels.
• A minimum of 2 weeks between courses is recommended unless high blood lead level indicates need for immediate therapy.
⊛ **ALERT:** Administration of succimer with other chelates isn't recommended. Patient who has received edetate calcium disodium with or without dimercaprol may use succimer as subsequent therapy after 4-week interval.
• Maintain adequate fluid intake.
Patient teaching
• Tell parents of child who can't swallow capsule to open it and sprinkle contents on small amount of soft food. Or, medicated beads from capsule may be poured on spoon and followed with flavored beverage such as a fruit drink.
• Help parents identify and remove sources of lead in child's environment. Chelation therapy isn't a substitute for preventing further exposure.
• Tell parents to consult prescriber if rash occurs. Consider possibility of allergic or other mucocutaneous reactions each time drug is used.

☑ Evaluation

• Patient responds well to therapy.
• Patient maintains adequate hydration.
• Parents state understanding of drug therapy.

succinylcholine chloride (suxamethonium chloride)
(SUK-seh-nil-KOH-leen KLOR-ighd)
Anectine, Anectine Flo-Pack, Quelicin, Scoline◇, Sucostrin

Pharmacologic class: depolarizing neuromuscular blocker
Therapeutic class: skeletal muscle relaxant
Pregnancy risk category: C

Indications and dosages

▶ **Adjunct to anesthesia to induce skeletal muscle relaxation; to facilitate intubation and assist with mechanical ventilation or orthopedic manipulations (drug of choice); to lessen muscle contractions in pharmacologically or electrically induced seizures.** *Adults:*

Dosage depends on anesthetic used, individual needs, and response. Give 0.6 mg/kg I.V. over 10 to 30 seconds; then give 2.5 mg/minute, p.r.n. Or, 2.5 to 4 mg/kg I.M. up to maximum of 150 mg I.M. in deltoid muscle. For short procedures, the optimum dose range is 0.3 to 1.1 mg/kg. The average dose is 0.6 mg/kg. Maximum paralysis occurs in 2 minutes. Recovery time is in 4 to 6 minutes. For long procedures, the average rate for adults is 2.5 to 4.3 mg/minutes For prolonged muscular relaxation, give intermittent I.V. injections of 0.3 to 1.1 mg/kg, then 0.04 to 0.07 mg/kg.
Children: 1 to 2 mg/kg I.V. or 2.5 to 4 mg/kg I.M. Maximum I.M. dose is 150 mg.

▼ I.V. administration

• Use immediately after reconstitution.
• Store injectable form in refrigerator. Store powder form at room temperature in tightly closed container.
• Solutions of 0.1% to 0.2% are common for I.V. infusions (1 to 2 mg/ml).
⊗ **Incompatibilities**
Barbiturates, nafcillin, sodium bicarbonate, solutions with pH above 4.5, thiopental sodium.

Contraindications and cautions

• Contraindicated in patients hypersensitive to the drug or any of its components and in patients with abnormally low pseudocholinesterase level, angle-closure glaucoma, personal or family history of malignant hyperthermia, or penetrating eye injury.
• Use cautiously in debilitated patients, those taking quinidine or digoxin therapy, and those with severe burns or trauma, electrolyte imbalances, hyperkalemia, paraplegia, spinal neuraxis injury, stroke, degenerative or dystrophic neuromuscular disease, myasthenia gravis, myasthenic syndrome of lung cancer, bronchogenic carcinoma, dehydration, thyroid disorders, collagen diseases, porphyria, fractures, muscle spasms, eye surgery, pheochromocytoma, respiratory depression, or hepatic, renal, or pulmonary impairment.
❦ **Lifespan:** In women undergoing cesarean section and in breast-feeding women, use large doses cautiously. In the elderly, use cautiously.

Adverse reactions

CV: *bradycardia,* tachycardia, hypertension, hypotension, *arrhythmias,* flushing, *cardiac arrest.*
EENT: increased intraocular pressure.
Musculoskeletal: muscle fasciculation, *postoperative muscle pain,* myoglobinemia.
Respiratory: *prolonged respiratory depression, apnea, bronchoconstriction.*
Other: *malignant hyperthermia,* excessive salivation, allergic or idiosyncratic hypersensitivity reactions *(anaphylaxis).*

Interactions

Drug-drug. *Aminoglycoside antibiotics, including amikacin, gentamicin, kanamycin, neomycin, and streptomycin; anticholinesterases, such as echothiophate, edrophonium, neostigmine, physostigmine, and pyridostigmine; general anesthetics, such as enflurane, halothane, and isoflurane; polymyxin antibiotics, such as colistin and polymyxin B sulfate:* May potentiate neuromuscular blockade, leading to increased skeletal muscle relaxation and potentiation of effect. Use cautiously during surgical and postoperative periods.
Cyclophosphamide, lithium, MAO inhibitors: May cause prolonged apnea. Avoid using together; monitor patient closely.
Digoxin: May cause arrhythmias. Use together cautiously.
Methotrimeprazine, opioid analgesics: May potentiate neuromuscular blockade, leading to increased skeletal muscle relaxation and, possibly, respiratory paralysis. Use cautiously.
Parenteral magnesium sulfate: May potentiate neuromuscular blockade, leading to increased skeletal muscle relaxation and, possibly, respiratory paralysis. Use cautiously, preferably with reduced doses.
Drug-herb. *Melatonin:* May potentiate blocking properties of succinylcholine. Discourage using together.

Effects on lab test results

• May increase myoglobin and potassium levels.

Pharmacokinetics

Absorption: Unknown.
Distribution: Distributed in extracellular fluid and rapidly reaches its site of action.

S

Rapid onset   *Liquid form contains alcohol.   ◆ Canada   ◇ Australia   †OTC   ✐ Photoguide   ‡ Off-label use

Metabolism: Occurs rapidly by plasma pseudocholinesterase.
Excretion: About 10% excreted unchanged in urine. *Half-life:* Unknown.

Route	Onset	Peak	Duration
I.V.	≤ 1 min	1–2 min	4–10 min
I.M.	2–3 min	Unknown	10–30 min

Action

Chemical effect: Prolongs depolarization of muscle end plate.
Therapeutic effect: Relaxes skeletal muscles.

Available forms

Injection: 20 mg/ml, 50 mg/ml, 100 mg/ml; 100-mg
Powder for infusion: 500-mg, and 1-g vials

NURSING PROCESS

Assessment

- Assess patient's condition before starting therapy and regularly thereafter to monitor the drug's effectiveness.
- Monitor baseline and ongoing electrolyte levels and vital signs (check respiratory rate q 5 to 10 minutes during infusion).
- Monitor respiratory rate and pulse oximetry closely until patient is fully recovered from neuromuscular blockade, as evidenced by tests of muscle strength (hand grip, head lift, and ability to cough).
- Be alert for adverse reactions and drug interactions.
- Assess patient's and family's knowledge of drug therapy.

Nursing diagnoses

- Ineffective health maintenance related to underlying condition
- Ineffective breathing pattern related to drug's effect on respiratory muscles
- Deficient knowledge related to drug therapy

Planning and implementation

ALERT: Only give drug if you are skilled in airway management.
- The drug of choice for procedures less than 3 minutes and for orthopedic manipulations—use caution in fractures or dislocations.
- Give sedatives or general anesthetics before neuromuscular blockers. Neuromuscular blockers don't induce unconsciousness or alter pain threshold.
- Keep airway clear. Have emergency respiratory support equipment immediately available.

ALERT: Careful drug calculation is essential. Always verify with another professional.
- To evaluate patient's ability to metabolize drug, give 10-mg I.M. or I.V. test dose after patient is anesthetized. No respiratory depression or transient depression for up to 5 minutes indicates drug may be given. Don't give subsequent doses if patient develops respiratory paralysis sufficient to permit endotracheal intubation. (Recovery within 30 to 60 minutes.)
- Give deep I.M., preferably high into deltoid muscle.
- Give analgesics.

ALERT: Don't use reversing drugs. Unlike with nondepolarizing drugs, giving neostigmine or edrophonium with this depolarizing drug may worsen neuromuscular blockade.
- Repeated or continuous infusions of succinylcholine aren't advised, because they may reduce response or prolong muscle relaxation and apnea.

Patient teaching
- Explain all events and happenings to patient because he can still hear.
- Reassure patient that he is being monitored at all times.
- Inform patient that postoperative stiffness is normal and will soon subside.

Evaluation

- Patient responds well to therapy.
- Patient maintains adequate respiratory patterns with mechanical assistance.
- Patient and family state understanding of drug therapy.

sucralfate

(SOO-krahl-fayt)
Carafate

Pharmacologic class: pepsin inhibitor
Therapeutic class: antiulcerative
Pregnancy risk category: B

Indications and dosages

▶ **Maintenance therapy for duodenal ulcer.** *Adults:* 1 g P.O. b.i.d., before meals.

▶ Therapy for up to 8 weeks for duodenal ulcer; gastric ulcer‡. *Adults:* 1 g P.O. q.i.d. 1 hour before meals and h.s.

Contraindications and cautions

• Use cautiously in patients with chronic renal impairment.

⚠ **Lifespan:** In pregnant women, use cautiously. In breast-feeding women, use cautiously; it's unknown if the drug appears in breast milk. In children, safety and effectiveness haven't been established.

Adverse reactions

CNS: dizziness, sleepiness, headache, vertigo.
GI: constipation, nausea, gastric discomfort, diarrhea, bezoar formation, vomiting, flatulence, dry mouth, indigestion.
Musculoskeletal: back pain.
Skin: rash, pruritus.

Interactions

Drug-drug. *Antacids:* May decrease binding of drug to gastroduodenal mucosa, impairing effectiveness. Don't give within 30 minutes of each other.
Cimetidine, digoxin, phenytoin, ranitidine, tetracycline, theophylline: May decrease absorption. Separate doses by at least 2 hours.
Ciprofloxacin, lomefloxacin, moxifloxacin, norfloxacin, ofloxacin: May decrease absorption of the quinolone, reducing anti-infective response. If use together can't be avoided, give at least 6 hours apart.

Effects on lab test results

None reported.

Pharmacokinetics

Absorption: About 3% to 5%. Acts locally.
Distribution: Distributed to GI tract and small amount to tissues.
Metabolism: None.
Excretion: About 90% excreted in feces; absorbed drug excreted unchanged in urine. *Half-life:* 6 to 20 hours.

Route	Onset	Peak	Duration
P.O.	Unknown	≤ 6 hr	Unknown

Action

Chemical effect: May adhere to and protect ulcer's surface by forming barrier.

Therapeutic effect: Aids in duodenal ulcer healing.

Available forms

Suspension: 500 mg/5 ml, 1 g/10 ml
Tablets: 1 g

NURSING PROCESS

⚕ **Assessment**
• Assess patient's GI symptoms before starting therapy, and regularly thereafter to monitor the drug's effectiveness.
• Be alert for adverse reactions and drug interactions.
• Monitor patient for severe, persistent constipation.
• Assess patient's and family's knowledge of drug therapy.

⊕ **Nursing diagnoses**
• Impaired tissue integrity related to presence of duodenal ulcer
• Constipation related to drug-induced adverse GI reactions
• Deficient knowledge related to drug therapy

▷ **Planning and implementation**
• Give drug on an empty stomach for best results.
Patient teaching
• Instruct patient to take drug 1 hour before each meal and bedtime.
• Tell patient to continue on prescribed regimen to ensure complete healing. Pain and ulcerative symptoms may subside within first few weeks of therapy.
• Urge patient to avoid cigarette smoking because it may increase gastric acid secretion and worsen disease. Also tell patient to avoid alcohol, chocolate, and spicy foods.
• Tell patient to sleep with head of bed elevated.
• Tell patient to avoid large meals within 2 hours of bedtime.

☑ **Evaluation**
• Patient's ulcer pain is gone.
• Patient maintains normal bowel elimination patterns.
• Patient and family state understanding of drug therapy.

S

sufentanil citrate
(soo-FEN-tih-nil SIGH-trayt)
Sufenta, Sufentanil Citrate Injection

Pharmacologic class: opioid agonist
Therapeutic class: analgesic, anesthetic
Pregnancy risk category: C
Controlled substance schedule: II

Indications and dosages

▶ **Adjunct to general anesthetic.** *Adults:* 1 to 2 mcg/kg I.V. with nitrous oxide and oxygen for 1- to 2-hour duration anesthesia in procedures lasting less than 8 hours. Maintain analgesia with 10 to 25 mcg/kg I.V. in increments for surgical stress or lightening of anesthesia. Or, 2 to 8 mcg/kg I.V. for more complicated procedures lasting longer than 8 hours; duration of anesthesia 2 to 8 hours. Maintain analgesia with 10 to 50 mcg/kg I.V. in increments for surgical stress or lightening of anesthesia. Adjust maintenance infusion rates based on the induction dose so that the total dose does not exceed 1 mcg/kg/hr of expected surgical time.
▶ **As primary anesthetic.** *Adults and children age 12 and older:* 8 to 30 mcg/kg I.V. with 100% oxygen and muscle relaxant. Maintain anesthesia with 0.5 to 10 mcg/kg for surgical stress; base the maintenance infusion rate on the induction dose so that the total dose for the procedure does not exceed 30 mcg/kg.
Children ages younger than age 12: For induction and maintenance of anesthesia during cardiovascular surgery, 10 to 25 mcg/kg I.V. with 100% oxygen. Maintenance doses of up to 25 to 50 mcg are recommended.
Adjust-a-dose: Reduce dosage in geriatric patients, debilitated patients, and neonates. Base dose on ideal body weight in obese patients whose body weight exceeds 20% of ideal body weight
▶ **Epidural analgesia during labor and vaginal delivery.** *Adults and children age 12 and older:* 10 to 15 mcg administered with 10 ml bupivacaine 0.125% with or without epinephrine. Mix drug and bupivacaine together before administration. Doses can be repeated twice (for a total of 3 doses) at 1 hour or longer intervals until delivery.

▼ I.V. administration

• Drug is analgesic at doses less than 8 mcg/kg and is anesthetic at doses equal to or greater than 8 mcg/kg.
• For obese patient weighing more than 20% above ideal body weight, base dosage calculations on lean body weight.
• Give drug by direct I.V. injection. May be given by intermittent I.V. infusion, but compatibility and stability in I.V. solutions aren't fully known.
• Don't exceed 1 mcg/kg/hour of expected surgical time.
⊗ **Incompatibilities**
Acidic solutions, diazepam, lorazepam, phenobarbital, phenytoin, thiopental.

Contraindications and cautions

• Contraindicated in patients hypersensitive to the drug or any of its components.
• Drug isn't recommended for prolonged use.
• Use cautiously in debilitated patients and in patients with head injury, decreased respiratory reserve, or pulmonary, hepatic, or renal disease.
⚠ **Lifespan:** In pregnant women, use only if benefits outweigh potential risks to the fetus. In breast-feeding women and in children, safety and effectiveness haven't been established. In the elderly, use cautiously and at a lower dose.

Adverse reactions

CNS: chills, somnolence.
CV: *hypotension,* hypertension, *bradycardia,* tachycardia, *arrhythmias,* increased cardiac index.
GI: nausea, vomiting.
Musculoskeletal: intraoperative muscle movement.
Respiratory: chest wall rigidity, *apnea, bronchospasm,* respiratory depression.
Skin: *pruritus,* erythema.

Interactions

Drug-drug. *Anesthetic agents:* May affect cardiovascular status. Monitor patient closely.
Beta blockers: May need lower doses of sufentanil. Assess patient.
CNS depressants: May have additive effects. Use together cautiously.
Drug-lifestyle. *Alcohol use:* May have additive effects. Discourage using together.

Effects on lab test results

None reported.

Reactions may be *common,* uncommon, *life-threatening,* or COMMON AND LIFE-THREATENING.

Pharmacokinetics

Absorption: Administered I.V.
Distribution: Highly protein-bound and redistributed rapidly.
Metabolism: Probably in liver and small intestine.
Excretion: Primarily in urine. *Half-life:* About 2½ hours.

Route	Onset	Peak	Duration
I.V.	1–2 min	1–2 min	¾–5 min

Action

Chemical effect: Binds with opioid receptors in CNS, altering perception of and emotional response to pain through unknown mechanism.
Therapeutic effect: Relieves pain and promotes loss of consciousness.

Available forms

Injection: 50 mcg/ml in 1-ml, 2-ml, and 5-ml ampules

NURSING PROCESS

Assessment
• Assess patient's condition before starting therapy, and regularly thereafter to monitor the drug's effectiveness.
• Because drug decreases rate and depth of respirations, monitor patient's arterial oxygen saturation to help assess respiratory depression.
• Monitor respiratory rate of neonates exposed to drug during labor.
• Monitor postoperative vital signs.
• Be alert for adverse reactions and drug interactions.
• Assess patient's and family's knowledge of drug therapy.

Nursing diagnoses
• Ineffective health maintenance related to underlying condition
• Ineffective breathing pattern related to respiratory depression
• Deficient knowledge related to drug therapy

Planning and implementation
• Only personnel specifically trained in use of I.V. anesthetics should give drug.
• When used at doses larger than 8 mcg/kg, postoperative mechanical ventilation and observation are essential because of prolonged respiratory depression.
• Keep opioid antagonist (naloxone) and resuscitation equipment available.
• If respiratory rate falls below 12 breaths/minute, notify prescriber.
• For epidural use, administer by slow injection. Closely monitor respiration following each administration of drug mixture.
ALERT: High doses can produce muscle rigidity reversible by neuromuscular blockers; however, patient must be artificially ventilated.
ALERT: Don't confuse sufentanil with alfentanil or fentanyl, or Sufenta with Survanta.
Patient teaching
• Inform patient and family that drug will be used as part of patient's anesthesia.

Evaluation
• Patient responds well to therapy.
• Patient maintains adequate ventilation with mechanical support, if needed.
• Patient and family state understanding of drug therapy.

sulfasalazine
(salazosulfapyridine, sulphasalazine)
(sul-fuh-SAL-uh-zeen)
Azulfidine, Azulfidine EN-Tabs, PMS-Sulfasalazine E.C.◆, Salazopyrin◆, Salazopyrin EN-Tabs◆◇, S.A.S.-500◆, S.A.S. Enteric-500◆

Pharmacologic class: sulfonamide
Therapeutic class: anti-inflammatory
Pregnancy risk category: B

Indications and dosages

▶ **Mild to moderate ulcerative colitis, adjunct therapy in severe ulcerative colitis.**
Adults: Initially, 3 to 4 g P.O. daily in evenly divided doses. May begin with a lower dose of 1 to 2 g/day to avoid GI intolerance; usual maintenance dosage is 1 to 2 g P.O. daily in divided doses q 6 hours. Dosage may be started with 1 to 2 g, with gradual increase to minimize adverse effects.
Children older than age 2: Initially, 40 to 60 mg/kg P.O. daily, divided into three to six

doses; then 30 mg/kg daily in four doses. If GI intolerance occurs, reduce dosage.
▶ **Rheumatoid arthritis in patients who have responded inadequately to salicylates or NSAIDs.** *Adults:* 2 g P.O. daily b.i.d. in evenly divided doses. Dosage may be started at 0.5 to 1 g daily and be gradually increased over 3 weeks to reduce GI intolerance.
▶ **Patients with polyarticular-course juvenile rheumatoid arthritis who have responded inadequately to salicylates or other NSAIDs.** *Children age 6 and older:* 30 to 50 mg/kg P.O. daily in two divided doses (as delayed-release tablet). Maximum dose is 2 g daily. To reduce GI intolerance, start with one-fourth to one-third of planned maintenance dose and increase weekly until maintenance dose is reached at 1 month.
▶ **Crohn's disease‡.** *Adults:* 3 to 6 g P.O. in divided doses.

Contraindications and cautions

• Contraindicated in patients hypersensitive to the drug or its metabolites, and patients with porphyria or intestinal or urinary obstruction.
• Use cautiously and in reduced dosages in patients with impaired liver or kidney function, severe allergy, bronchial asthma, or G6PD deficiency.
※ **Lifespan:** In pregnant women, use cautiously. In breast-feeding women, use cautiously; it's unknown if the drug appears in breast milk. In infants younger than age 2, drug is contraindicated.

Adverse reactions

CNS: headache, depression, *seizures,* hallucinations.
GI: *nausea, vomiting, diarrhea,* abdominal pain, anorexia, stomatitis.
GU: *toxic nephrosis with oliguria and anuria,* crystalluria, hematuria, oligospermia, infertility.
Hematologic: *agranulocytosis, aplastic anemia,* megaloblastic anemia, *thrombocytopenia, leukopenia,* hemolytic anemia.
Hepatic: jaundice, *hepatotoxicity.*
Skin: *erythema multiforme, Stevens-Johnson syndrome,* generalized skin eruption, *epidermal necrolysis,* exfoliative dermatitis, photosensitivity reactions, urticaria, pruritus.
Other: *hypersensitivity reactions* (serum sickness, drug fever, anaphylaxis).

Interactions

Drug-drug. *Antibiotics:* May alter action of sulfasalazine by altering internal flora. Monitor patient closely.
Digoxin: May reduce digoxin absorption. Monitor patient closely.
Folic acid: May decrease absorption. No intervention needed.
Hormonal contraceptives: May decrease contraceptive effectiveness and increases risk of breakthrough bleeding. Suggest nonhormonal contraceptive.
Iron: May lower sulfasalazine level by iron chelation. Monitor patient closely.
Oral anticoagulants: May increase anticoagulant effect. Monitor patient for bleeding.
Oral antidiabetics: May increase hypoglycemic effect. Monitor glucose level.
Drug-herb. *Dong quai, St. John's wort:* May increase risk of photosensitivity. Discourage using together.

Effects on lab test results

• May increase AST and ALT levels. May decrease hemoglobin level and hematocrit.
• May decrease granulocyte, platelet, RBC, and WBC counts.

Pharmacokinetics

Absorption: Poor; 70% to 90% transported to colon, where intestinal flora metabolize drug to its active ingredients, which exert their effects locally. One metabolite, sulfapyridine, is absorbed from colon, but only small portion of metabolite 5-aminosalicylic acid is absorbed.
Distribution: Distributed locally in colon. Distribution of absorbed metabolites is unknown.
Metabolism: Divided by intestinal flora in colon.
Excretion: Systemically absorbed sulfasalazine is excreted chiefly in urine. *Half-life:* 6 to 8 hours.

Route	Onset	Peak	Duration
P.O.			
parent drug	Unknown	1½–6 hr	Unknown
metabolites	Unknown	12–24 hr	Unknown

Action

Chemical effect: Unknown.
Therapeutic effect: Relieves inflammation in GI tract.

Reactions may be *common,* uncommon, *life-threatening,* or COMMON AND LIFE-THREATENING.

Available forms

Oral suspension: 250 mg/5 ml
Tablets (with or without enteric coating):
500 mg

NURSING PROCESS

🔍 Assessment
• Assess patient's condition before starting therapy, and regularly thereafter to monitor the
drug's effectiveness.
• Monitor CBC and liver function tests at baseline, every other week for first 3 months, monthly for next 3 months, then as needed.
• Be alert for adverse reactions and drug interactions.
• Monitor patient's hydration throughout drug
therapy.
• Assess patient's and family's knowledge of
drug therapy.

⊕ Nursing diagnoses
• Acute pain related to inflammation of GI tract
• Risk for deficient fluid volume related to
drug-induced adverse GI reactions
• Deficient knowledge related to drug therapy

▷ Planning and implementation
• Minimize adverse GI reaction by spacing dos-
es evenly and giving after food intake.
• Drug colors alkaline urine orange-yellow.
🟢 **ALERT:** If patient shows evidence of hypersen-
sitivity, stop immediately and notify prescriber.
🟢 **ALERT:** Don't confuse sulfasalazine with sulfisoxazole, salsalate, or sulfadiazine.
Patient teaching
• Instruct patient to take drug after meals and to
space doses evenly.
• Warn patient that drug may cause skin and
urine to turn orange-yellow and may permanently stain soft contact lenses yellow.
• Warn patient to avoid direct sunlight and ultraviolet light, to prevent photosensitivity reaction.
• Instruct patient to notify physician immediately with complaints of pallor, sore throat, purpura
or jaundice.

✔ Evaluation
• Patient is free from pain.
• Patient maintains adequate hydration.
• Patient and family state understanding of drug
therapy.

sulfinpyrazone
(sul-fin-PEER-uh-zohn)
Anturan ♦ , Anturane

Pharmacologic class: uricosuric
Therapeutic class: platelet aggregation inhibi-
tor, uricolytic
Pregnancy risk category: NR

Indications and dosages
▶ **Intermittent or chronic gouty arthritis.**
Adults: Initially, 100 mg to 200 mg P.O. b.i.d.
during the first week; then 200 mg to 400 mg
P.O. b.i.d. Maximum dosage is 800 mg daily.
After urate level is controlled, dosage can sometimes be reduced to 200 mg daily in divided
doses.
▶ **Prophylaxis of thromboembolic disorders,
including angina, MI, transient (cerebral)
ischemic attacks, and presence of prosthetic
heart valves‡.** *Adults:* 600 to 800 mg P.O. daily
in divided doses to decrease platelet aggregation.

Contraindications and cautions
• Contraindicated in patients hypersensitive to
pyrazole derivatives (including oxyphenbutazone and phenylbutazone) and patients with active peptic ulcer, symptoms of GI inflammation
or ulceration, or blood dyscrasias.
• Use cautiously in patients with healed peptic
ulcer.
⚡ **Lifespan:** In pregnant women, use cautiously. In breast-feeding women and in children,
safety and effectiveness haven't been established.

Adverse reactions
GI: *nausea, dyspepsia,* epigastric pain, reactivation of peptic ulcerations.
Hematologic: *blood dyscrasias,* anemia, *leukopenia, agranulocytosis, thrombocytopenia,
aplastic anemia.*
Respiratory: *bronchoconstriction* in patients
with aspirin-induced asthma.
Skin: rash.

Interactions
Drug-drug. *Aspirin, niacin, salicylates:* May
inhibit uricosuric effect of sulfinpyrazone. Don't
use together.

S

Cholestyramine: May bind and delay absorption of sulfinpyrazone. Give sulfinpyrazone at least 1 hour before or 4 to 6 hours after cholestyramine.

Oral anticoagulants: May increase anticoagulant effect and risk of bleeding. Use together cautiously.

Oral antidiabetics: May increase effects. Monitor glucose level closely.

Probenecid: May inhibit renal excretion of sulfinpyrazone. Use together cautiously.

Protein-bound drugs: May cause interaction. Monitor patient for toxicity.

Theophylline: May increase theophylline clearance. Monitor level.

Verapamil: May decrease verapamil effect. Monitor patient.

Drug-lifestyle. *Alcohol use:* May decrease drug effectiveness. Discourage using together.

Effects on lab test results

● May increase BUN and creatinine levels. May decrease hemoglobin level and hematocrit.
● May decrease RBC, WBC, granulocyte, and platelet counts.

Pharmacokinetics

Absorption: Complete.
Distribution: 98% to 99% protein-bound.
Metabolism: Rapid.
Excretion: Excreted in urine; about 50% excreted unchanged. *Half-life:* 3 hours.

Route	Onset	Peak	Duration
P.O.	Unknown	1–2 hr	4–6 hr

Action

Chemical effect: Blocks renal tubular reabsorption of uric acid, increasing excretion, and inhibits platelet aggregation.

Therapeutic effect: Relieves signs and symptoms of gouty arthritis.

Available forms

Capsules: 200 mg
Tablets: 100 mg

NURSING PROCESS

☒ Assessment

● Assess patient's condition before starting therapy, and regularly thereafter to monitor the drug's effectiveness.

● Monitor BUN level, CBC, and kidney function studies periodically during long-term use.
● Monitor fluid intake and output. Therapy may lead to renal colic and formation of uric acid stones until acid levels are normal (about 6 mg/dl).
● Be alert for adverse reactions and drug interactions.
● Assess patient's and family's knowledge of drug therapy.

✚ Nursing diagnoses

● Ineffective health maintenance related to presence of gouty arthritis
● Risk for injury related to drug-induced adverse CNS reactions
● Deficient knowledge related to drug therapy

▷ Planning and implementation

● Give drug with milk, food, or antacids to minimize GI disturbances.
● Encourage patient to drink fluids to maintain minimum daily output of 2 to 3 L. Alkalinize urine with sodium bicarbonate or other agent. Keep in mind that alkalinizers are used therapeutically to increase drug activity, preventing urolithiasis.
● Drug is recommended for patient unresponsive to probenecid. Suitable for long-term use; neither cumulative effects nor tolerance develops.
● Drug contains no analgesic or anti-inflammatory and is of no value during acute gout attacks.
● Drug may increase frequency, severity, and length of acute gout attacks during first 6 to 12 months of therapy. Give prophylactic colchicine or another anti-inflammatory during first 3 to 6 months.
● Lifelong therapy may be needed in patient with hyperuricemia.
● Drug decreases urinary excretion of aminohippuric acid, interfering with laboratory test results.
🛈 **ALERT:** Don't confuse Anturane with Artane or Antabuse.

Patient teaching
● Warn patient with gout not to take aspirin-containing drugs because they may precipitate gout. Acetaminophen may be used for pain.
● Tell patient to take drug with food, milk, or antacid. Also instruct him to drink plenty of water.

Reactions may be *common,* uncommon, *life-threatening*, or COMMON AND LIFE-THREATENING.

• Instruct patient with gout to avoid foods high in purine, such as anchovies, liver, sardines, kidneys, sweetbreads, peas, and lentils.
• Inform patient and family that drug must be taken regularly or gout attacks may result. Tell patient to see prescriber regularly so blood levels can be monitored and dosage adjusted if needed.

☑ **Evaluation**
• Patient regains and maintains normal uric acid level.
• Patient doesn't experience injury from adverse CNS reactions.
• Patient and family state understanding of drug therapy.

sulindac
(SUL-in-dak)
Aclin◇, Apo-Sulin◆, Clinoril, Novo-Sundac◆

Pharmacologic class: NSAID
Therapeutic class: analgesic, anti-inflammatory
Pregnancy risk category: B (D in third trimester)

Indications and dosages
▶ **Osteoarthritis, rheumatoid arthritis, ankylosing spondylitis.** *Adults:* Initially, 150 mg P.O. b.i.d.; increase to 200 mg b.i.d., p.r.n.
▶ **Acute subacromial bursitis or supraspinatus tendinitis, acute gouty arthritis.** *Adults:* 200 mg P.O. b.i.d. for 7 to 14 days. Reduce dose as symptoms subside.

Contraindications and cautions
• Contraindicated in patients hypersensitive to the drug or any of its components, and in patients for whom aspirin or NSAIDs precipitate asthma, rhinitis, urticaria, nasal polyps, angioedema, bronchospasm, or other allergic or anaphylactoid symptoms.
• Use cautiously in patients with history of ulcers and GI bleeding, renal dysfunction, hepatic dysfunction, compromised cardiac function or hypertension, or conditions predisposing to fluid retention.
⚕ **Lifespan:** In pregnant women, drug isn't recommended. In breast-feeding women and in children, safety and effectiveness haven't been established.

Adverse reactions
CNS: dizziness, headache, nervousness, psychosis.
CV: hypertension, *heart failure,* palpitations, edema.
EENT: tinnitus, transient visual disturbances.
GI: *epigastric distress,* peptic ulceration, *pancreatitis, GI bleeding,* occult blood loss, nausea, constipation, dyspepsia, flatulence, anorexia.
GU: interstitial nephritis, nephrotic syndrome, *renal failure.*
Hematologic: *aplastic anemia, thrombocytopenia, neutropenia, agranulocytosis,* hemolytic anemia.
Skin: *rash,* pruritus.
Other: drug fever, *anaphylaxis,* hypersensitivity syndrome, *angioedema.*

Interactions
Drug-drug. *ACE inhibitors:* May decrease antihypertensive effects of these drugs. Monitor blood pressure.
Anticoagulants: May increase risk of bleeding. Monitor PT closely.
Aspirin, NSAIDs: May decrease sulindac level and increase risk of adverse GI reactions. Avoid using together.
Cyclosporine: May increase nephrotoxicity of cyclosporine. Monitor renal function.
Diflunisal, dimethyl sulfoxide (DMSO): May decrease metabolism of sulindac to its active metabolite, reducing its effectiveness. Topical DMSO used with sulindac has caused severe peripheral neuropathy. Don't use together.
Diuretics: May increase effects of regular diuretics on blood pressure, but decrease effects of potassium-sparing diuretics. Monitor blood pressure and electrolytes.
Lithium: May decrease lithium levels. Monitor patient and blood levels carefully.
Methotrexate: May increase methotrexate toxicity. Avoid using together.
Probenecid: May increase levels of sulindac and its active metabolite. Monitor patient for toxicity.
Sulfonamides, sulfonylureas, other highly protein-bound drugs: May displace these drugs from protein-binding sites, leading to increased toxicity. Monitor patient closely for toxicity.

S

Effects on lab test results

• May increase BUN, creatinine, liver enzyme, and potassium levels. May decrease hemoglobin level and hematocrit.
• May increase bleeding time. May decrease platelet, neutrophil, and granulocyte counts.

Pharmacokinetics

Absorption: 90% absorbed.
Distribution: Highly protein-bound.
Metabolism: Drug is inactive and metabolized in liver to an active sulfide metabolite.
Excretion: Excreted in urine. *Half-life:* Parent drug, 8 hours; active metabolite, about 16 hours.

Route	Onset	Peak	Duration
P.O.	Unknown	2–4 hr	Unknown

Action

Chemical effect: Unknown; produces anti-inflammatory, analgesic, and antipyretic effects, possibly by inhibiting prostaglandin synthesis.
Therapeutic effect: Relieves pain and inflammation.

Available forms

Tablets: 100 mg ◇ , 150 mg, 200 mg

NURSING PROCESS

⏱ Assessment

• Assess patient's condition before starting therapy and regularly thereafter to monitor the drug's effectiveness.
• Periodically monitor liver and kidney function and CBC in patient taking long-term therapy.
• Be alert for adverse reactions and drug interactions.
• Assess patient's and family's knowledge of drug therapy.

⚏ Nursing diagnoses

• Acute pain related to presence of arthritis
• Impaired tissue integrity related to drug's adverse effect on GI mucosa
• Deficient knowledge related to drug therapy

⧉ Planning and implementation

• Notify prescriber of adverse reactions.
Patient teaching
• Tell patient to take drug with food, milk, or antacids to reduce adverse GI reactions.

• Advise patient to refrain from driving or performing other hazardous activities that require mental alertness until the drug's CNS effects are known.
• Teach patient signs and symptoms of GI bleeding, and tell him to contact prescriber immediately if they occur. Serious GI toxicity, including peptic ulceration and bleeding, can occur in patient taking NSAIDs despite absence of GI symptoms.
⑤ **ALERT:** Tell patient to notify prescriber immediately if easy bruising or prolonged bleeding occurs.
• Instruct patient to report any edema and to have his blood pressure checked monthly. Drug causes sodium retention but may not affect kidneys as much as other NSAIDs.
• Instruct patient not to take aspirin, aspirin-containing products, or other NSAIDs with sulindac.
• Tell patient to notify prescriber and undergo complete eye examination if visual disturbances occur.

☑ Evaluation

• Patient is free from pain.
• Patient doesn't experience adverse GI reactions.
• Patient and family state understanding of drug therapy.

sumatriptan succinate

(soo-muh-TRIP-ten SEK-seh-nayt)
Imitrex

Pharmacologic class: selective 5-hydroxytryptamine (5-HT$_1$) receptor agonist
Therapeutic class: antimigraine drug
Pregnancy risk category: C

Indications and dosages

▶ **Acute migraine attacks (with or without aura).** *Adults:* 6 mg subcutaneously. Maximum recommended dose is two 6-mg injections in 24 hours, separated by at least 1 hour. Or, 25 to 100 mg P.O. initially. If response isn't achieved in 2 hours, may give second dose of 25 to 100 mg. Additional doses may be used in at least 2-hour intervals. Maximum daily oral dose, 200 mg. Or, 5 mg, 10 mg, or 20 mg administered once in one nostril. May repeat once

after 2 hours for maximum daily inhalation dose of 40 mg. For 10-mg dose, give a single 5-mg dose in each nostril.
► **Acute treatment of cluster headache episodes.** *Adults:* 6 mg subcutaneously. Maximum recommended dose is two 6-mg injections in 24 hours, separated by at least 1 hour.
◙ **Adjust-a-dose:** For patients with hepatic impairment, don't exceed maximum single oral dose of 50 mg.

Contraindications and cautions

• Contraindicated in patients hypersensitive to the drug or any of its components, and in patients with history, symptoms, or signs of ischemic cardiac, cerebrovascular (stroke, transient ischemic attack), or peripheral vascular (ischemic bowel disease) syndromes, or MI.
• Contraindicated in patients with uncontrolled hypertension, severe hepatic impairment (oral form), and hemiplegic or basilar migraines.
• Contraindicated within 24 hours of another 5-HT agonist or ergotamine-containing drug and within 14 days of MAO inhibitor therapy (oral form only; decrease dosage of sumatriptan if given by injection while patient is on an MAO inhibitor).
• Don't give drug I.V.; it can cause coronary vasospasms.
• Use cautiously in patients who may have unrecognized coronary artery disease (CAD), such as postmenopausal women, men older than age 40, and patients with risk factors for CAD.
⚠ **Lifespan:** In pregnant women and women who intend to become pregnant, use cautiously. In breast-feeding women and in children, safety and effectiveness haven't been established.

Adverse reactions

CNS: *dizziness, vertigo,* drowsiness, headache, anxiety, malaise, fatigue.
CV: *atrial fibrillation, ventricular fibrillation, ventricular tachycardia, coronary artery vasospasm, transient myocardial ischemia, MI,* pressure or tightness in chest, hypertension.
EENT: discomfort of throat, nasal cavity or sinus, mouth, jaw, or tongue; altered vision.
GI: abdominal discomfort, dysphagia, diarrhea; nausea, vomiting, unusual or bad taste (nasal spray).
Musculoskeletal: myalgia, muscle cramps, neck pain.

Respiratory: upper respiratory inflammation and dyspnea (P.O.).
Skin: diaphoresis.
Other: *warm or hot sensation; burning sensation;* heaviness, pressure, or tightness; tight feeling in head; cold sensation; numbness; flushing, *tingling, injection site reaction* (subcutaneous).

Interactions

Drug-drug. *Ergot and ergot derivatives; other serotonin$_{1B/1D}$ agonists:* May prolong vasospastic effects. Don't use within 24 hours of sumatriptan therapy.
MAO inhibitors: May reduce sumatriptan clearance. Avoid using sumatriptan tablets or nasal spray within 2 weeks of stopping MAO inhibitor. Use injection cautiously in patients and decrease sumatriptan dose.
SSRIs: May cause weakness, hyperreflexia, and incoordination. Monitor patient closely if use together is warranted.
Drug-herb. *Horehound:* May enhance serotonergic effects. Discourage using together.

Effects on lab test results

None reported.

Pharmacokinetics

Absorption: Rapid after P.O. administration but with low absolute bioavailability (about 15%); absorbed well from injection site after subcutaneous administration.
Distribution: Drug has low protein-binding of about 14% to 21%.
Metabolism: About 80%, in liver.
Excretion: Excreted primarily in urine. *Half-life:* About 2 hours.

Route	Onset	Peak	Duration
P.O.	30 min	2–4 hr	Unknown
SubQ	10–20 min	1–2 hr	Unknown
Intranasal	Rapid	1–2 hr	Unknown

Action

Chemical effect: Unknown; thought to selectively activate vascular serotonin (5-HT) receptors. Stimulation of specific receptor subtype 5-HT$_1$, present on cranial arteries and the dura mater, causes vasoconstriction of cerebral vessels but has minimal effects on systemic vessels, tissue perfusion, and blood pressure.
Therapeutic effect: Relieves acute migraine pain.

Available forms

Injection: 6 mg/0.5 ml (12 mg/ml) in 0.5-ml prefilled syringes and vials
Nasal spray: 5 mg/spray; 20 mg/spray
Tablets: 25 mg, 50 mg, 100 mg (base) ◆

NURSING PROCESS

🏥 Assessment
• Assess patient's condition before starting therapy and regularly thereafter to monitor the drug's effectiveness.
• Be alert for adverse reactions and drug interactions.
• Assess patient's and family's knowledge of drug therapy.

⊞ Nursing diagnoses
• Acute pain related to presence of acute migraine attack
• Risk for injury related to drug-induced adverse reactions
• Deficient knowledge related to drug therapy

❯ Planning and implementation
• If patient has risk of unrecognized CAD, give first dose with prescriber present.
• Give single tablet whole with fluids as soon as patient complains of migraine symptoms. Give second tablet if symptoms come back, but no sooner than 2 hours after first tablet.
• Maximum recommended subcutaneous dosage in 24-hour period is two 6-mg injections separated by at least 1 hour. If patient doesn't experience relief, notify prescriber.
• Patient will most likely experience relief within 1 to 2 hours.
• Redness or pain at injection site should subside within 1 hour after injection.
⚠ **ALERT:** Serious adverse cardiac effects can follow administration of this drug, but such events are rare.
• If patient doesn't experience relief, notify prescriber.
⚠ **ALERT:** Don't confuse sumatriptan with somatropin.

Patient teaching
• Make sure patient understands that drug is intended only to treat migraine attack, not to prevent or reduce number of attacks.
• Tell patient that drug may be given at any time during migraine attack but should be given as soon as symptoms appear.

• Drug is available in spring-loaded injector system that makes it easy for the patient to give injection to himself. Review detailed information with patient. Make sure patient understands how to load injector, give injection, and dispose of used syringes.
• Instruct patient taking P.O. form when and how often to take drug. Warn patient not to take more than 200 mg within 24 hours.
• Instruct patient to use intranasal spray in one nostril. (If giving 10 mg, 1 spray into each nostril.) A second spray may be used if headache returns, but not before 2 hours has elapsed from the first use.
• Tell patient who experiences persistent or severe chest pain to call prescriber immediately. Patient who experiences pain or tightness in throat, wheezing, heart throbbing, rash, lumps, hives, or swollen eyelids, face, or lips should stop using drug and call prescriber.
• Tell woman who is pregnant or intends to become pregnant not to take this drug.

✅ Evaluation
• Patient is free from pain.
• Patient doesn't experience injury from adverse CV reactions.
• Patient and family state understanding of drug therapy.

tacrine hydrochloride
(TAK-reen high-droh-KLOR-ighd)
Cognex

Pharmacologic class: centrally acting reversible anticholinesterase
Therapeutic class: psychotherapeutic for Alzheimer's disease
Pregnancy risk category: C

Indications and dosages

▶ **Mild to moderate dementia of Alzheimer's type.** *Adults:* Initially, 10 mg P.O. q.i.d. After 4 weeks, if patient tolerates drug and transaminase levels aren't elevated, increase dosage to 20 mg q.i.d. After another 4 weeks, increase

---

Reactions may be *common*, uncommon, *life-threatening*, or COMMON AND LIFE-THREATENING.

dosage to 30 mg q.i.d. If still tolerated, increase to 40 mg q.i.d. after another 4 weeks.

⧄ Adjust-a-dose: For patients with ALT level three to five times the upper limit of normal (ULN) range, reduce dosage by 40 mg daily and monitor ALT level weekly until normal. If ALT is more than five times ULN, stop therapy and monitor patient for signs and symptoms of hepatitis. May rechallenge when ALT returns to normal. With rechallenge dosing: Monitor ALT weekly for 16 weeks, then monthly for 2 months, and every 3 months thereafter.

Contraindications and cautions

• Contraindicated in patients hypersensitive to the drug or acridine derivatives, and in those who have previously developed drug-related jaundice and been confirmed with elevated total bilirubin level of more than 3 mg/dl.

• Use cautiously in patients with sick sinus syndrome or bradycardia; those at risk for peptic ulceration (including patients taking NSAIDs or those with history of peptic ulcer); those with history of hepatic disease; and those with renal disease, asthma, prostatic hyperplasia, or other urinary outflow impairment.

⚖ Lifespan: In pregnant and breast-feeding women, drug isn't recommended. In children, drug isn't indicated.

Adverse reactions

CNS: agitation, ataxia, insomnia, abnormal thinking, somnolence, depression, anxiety, *headache,* fatigue, *dizziness,* confusion.
CV: chest pain, facial flushing.
EENT: rhinitis.
GI: *nausea, vomiting,* anorexia, *diarrhea,* dyspepsia, loose stools, changes in stool color, constipation.
Hepatic: jaundice.
Metabolic: weight loss.
Musculoskeletal: myalgia.
Respiratory: upper respiratory tract infection, cough.
Skin: rash.

Interactions

Drug-drug. *Anticholinergics:* May decrease effectiveness of anticholinergics. Monitor patient closely.
Anticholinesterases, cholinergics (such as bethanechol): May have additive effects. Monitor patient for toxicity.

Cimetidine: May increase tacrine levels. Monitor patient for toxicity.
Fluvoxamine: May increase tacrine levels. Monitor patient.
Succinylcholine: May enhance neuromuscular blockade and prolong duration of action. Monitor patient.
Theophylline: May increase theophylline level and prolong theophylline half-life. Carefully monitor theophylline level, and adjust dosage.
Drug-food. *Any food:* May decrease drug absorption. Tell patient to take drug on empty stomach.
Drug-lifestyle. *Smoking:* May decrease levels of drug. Monitor response.

Effects on lab test results

• May increase ALT and AST levels.

Pharmacokinetics

Absorption: Rapid with absolute bioavailability of about 17%. Food reduces bioavailability by 30% to 40%.
Distribution: About 55% bound to plasma proteins.
Metabolism: Undergoes first-pass metabolism, which is dose-dependent; extensively metabolized.
Excretion: Excreted in urine. *Half-life:* 2 to 4 hours.

Route	Onset	Peak	Duration
P.O.	Unknown	30 min–3 hr	Unknown

Action

Chemical effect: Reversibly inhibits enzyme cholinesterase in CNS, allowing buildup of acetylcholine.
Therapeutic effect: Improves thinking in patients with Alzheimer's disease.

Available forms

Capsules: 10 mg, 20 mg, 30 mg, 40 mg

NURSING PROCESS

⧉ Assessment
• Assess patient's cognitive ability before starting therapy and regularly thereafter to monitor the drug's effectiveness.
• Monitor ALT level every other week from at least week 4 to week 16 of therapy. If ALT is twice the ULN range, monitor weekly. If no

T

problems occur, decrease frequency of testing to every 3 months. Whenever dosage is increased, resume monitoring every other week.
• Assess patient's and family's knowledge of drug therapy.

⊕ **Nursing diagnoses**
• Disturbed thought processes related to Alzheimer's disease
• Diarrhea related to drug-induced adverse GI reactions
• Deficient knowledge related to drug therapy

❯ **Planning and implementation**
• Stop drug if patient has evidence of jaundice, increase in total serum bilirubin, or hypersensitivity. Don't resume therapy.
• If patient doesn't improve in 3 to 6 months, consider stopping the drug.
• Give drug between meals. If GI upset becomes a problem, give drug with meals, although level may drop by 30% to 40%.
• If drug is stopped for 4 weeks or more, restart at the basic dose and adjust according to the schedule, as if the patient were being started on drug for the first time.
• Obtain order for antidiarrheal, if indicated.
Patient teaching
• Inform patient and family that drug doesn't alter underlying degenerative disease. Instead, it may alleviate symptoms of Alzheimer's disease.
• Explain to patient and family that the effect of therapy depends on taking the drug at regular intervals.
Ⓢ**ALERT:** Instruct caregivers when to give drug. Explain that dosage adjustment is integral to safe use. Abruptly stopping or reducing daily dose by 80 mg or more may trigger behavioral disturbances and cognitive decline.
• Advise patient and caregivers to report immediately any significant adverse effects or changes in status.

☑ **Evaluation**
• Patient exhibits improved cognitive ability.
• Patient or caregiver states that drug-induced diarrhea hasn't occurred.
• Patient and family state understanding of drug therapy.

tacrolimus
(tek-roh-LYE-mus)
Prograf

Pharmacologic class: macrolide
Therapeutic class: immunosuppressant
Pregnancy risk category: C

Indications and dosages
❯ **Prophylaxis of organ rejection in allogenic liver transplantation.** *Adults:* 0.03 to 0.05 mg/kg I.V. daily as continuous infusion given at least 6 hours after transplantation. P.O. therapy should be substituted as soon as possible, with first dose given 8 to 12 hours after discontinuing I.V. infusion. Recommended initial P.O. dosage is 0.1 to 0.15 mg/kg daily in two divided doses q 12 hours. Adjust dosage according to response.
Children: Initially, 0.03 to 0.05 mg/kg I.V. daily, followed by 0.15 to 0.2 mg/kg P.O. daily on schedule similar to that for adults; adjust dosage, p.r.n.
❯ **Prophylaxis of organ rejection in allogenic kidney transplantation.** *Adults:* 0.03 to 0.05 mg/kg I.V. daily as continuous infusion given at least 6 hours after transplantation. P.O. therapy should be substituted as soon as possible. Recommended initial P.O. dosage is 0.2 mg/kg daily administered in two divided doses q 12 hours. Initial dose may be given within 24 hours of transplantation but must be delayed until creatinine equals or exceeds 4 mg/dl.
❯ **Crohn's disease‡.** 200 mcg/kg P.O. daily in 2 divided doses for 10 weeks.

▼ **I.V. administration**
• Dilute drug with normal saline solution injection or D_5W injection to 0.004 to 0.02 mg/ml before use.
• Each required daily dose of diluted drug is infused continuously over 24 hours.
• Monitor patient continuously during first 30 minutes of infusion; then check frequently for anaphylaxis.
• Keep epinephrine 1:1,000 available to treat anaphylaxis.
• Store diluted solution for no more than 24 hours in glass or polyethylene containers. Don't store drug in polyvinyl chloride container.

⊗ **Incompatibilities**
Solutions or I.V. drugs with a pH above 9, such as acyclovir and ganciclovir.

Contraindications and cautions

• Contraindicated in patients hypersensitive to the drug or any of its components. I.V. form contraindicated in patients hypersensitive to castor oil derivatives.
• Use cautiously in patients with renal or hepatic impairment.
⚠ **Lifespan:** In pregnant or breast-feeding women, drug isn't recommended.

Adverse reactions

CNS: asthenia, headache, tremor, insomnia, paresthesia, delirium, *coma,* pain, fever, *neurotoxicity.*
CV: hypertension, peripheral edema.
GI: ascites, diarrhea, nausea, constipation, anorexia, vomiting, abdominal pain.
GU: abnormal kidney function, UTI, oliguria, *nephrotoxicity.*
Hematologic: *anemia,* leukocytosis, THROMBOCYTOPENIA.
Metabolic: *hyperkalemia,* hypokalemia, hyperglycemia, *hypomagnesemia.*
Musculoskeletal: *back pain.*
Respiratory: pleural effusion, atelectasis, dyspnea.
Skin: photosensitivity reactions.
Other: *anaphylaxis.*

Interactions

Drug-drug. *Bromocriptine, cimetidine, clarithromycin, clotrimazole, cyclosporine, danazol, diltiazem, erythromycin, ethinyl estradiol, fluconazole, itraconazole, ketoconazole, methylprednisolone, metoclopramide, nefazodone, nicardipine, nifedipine, omeprazole, protease inhibitors, verapamil:* May increase tacrolimus level. Monitor patient for adverse effects.
Carbamazepine, phenobarbital, phenytoin, rifabutin, rifampin: May decrease tacrolimus level. Monitor effectiveness of tacrolimus.
Cyclosporine: May increase risk of excess nephrotoxicity. Don't give together.
Immunosuppressants (except adrenocorticosteroids): May over-suppress immune system. Monitor patient closely, especially during times of stress.

Inducers of CYP enzyme system: May increase tacrolimus metabolism and decrease plasma level. Dosage adjustment may be needed.
Inhibitors of CYP enzyme system: May decrease tacrolimus metabolism and increase plasma level. Dosage adjustment may be needed.
Nephrotoxic drugs (such as aminoglycosides, amphotericin B, cisplatin, cyclosporine): May cause additive or synergistic effects. Monitor patient closely.
Viral vaccines: May interfere with immune response to live-virus vaccines.
Drug-herb. *St. John's wort:* May decrease tacrolimus level. Monitor effectiveness of tacrolimus.
Drug-food. *Any food:* May inhibit drug absorption. Tell patient to take drug on an empty stomach.
Grapefruit juice: May increase drug level in liver transplant patients. Discourage use together.

Effects on lab test results

• May increase glucose, creatinine, and BUN levels. May decrease magnesium and hemoglobin levels and hematocrit. May increase or decrease potassium level.
• May increase liver function test values and WBC and platelet counts.

Pharmacokinetics

Absorption: Variable. Food reduces absorption and bioavailability of drug.
Distribution: Distribution between whole blood and plasma depends on several factors, such as hematocrit, temperature of separation of plasma, drug level, and protein level. Drug is 75% to 99% protein-bound.
Metabolism: Extensive.
Excretion: Primarily in bile. *Half-life:* 33 to 56 hours.

Route	Onset	Peak	Duration
P.O., I.V.	Unknown	1½–3½ hr	Unknown

Action

Chemical effect: Unknown; may inhibit T-lymphocyte activation, which results in immunosuppression.
Therapeutic effect: Prevents organ rejection.

Available forms

Capsules: 0.5 mg, 1 mg, 5 mg
Injection: 5 mg/ml

NURSING PROCESS

⏱ Assessment
• Obtain history of patient's organ transplant before starting therapy, and reassess regularly to monitor the drug's effectiveness.
• Monitor patient for signs of neurotoxicity and nephrotoxicity, especially in those receiving high dosage or those with renal dysfunction.
• Obtain potassium and glucose levels regularly. Monitor patient for hyperglycemia.
• Drug increases risk of infections, lymphomas, and other cancers.
• Be alert for adverse reactions and drug interactions.
• Assess patient's and family's knowledge of drug therapy.

⊕ Nursing diagnoses
• Risk for injury related to organ transplant rejection
• Ineffective protection related to drug-induced immunosuppression
• Deficient knowledge related to drug therapy

▶ Planning and implementation
• Child with normal kidney and liver function may need a higher dose than an adult.
• Patient with hepatic or renal dysfunction needs lowest possible dosage.
• Black renal transplant patients may require higher doses.
• Give adrenocorticosteroids with this drug.
• Give oral drug on empty stomach.
• Because of risk of anaphylaxis, use injection only in patient who can't take oral form.
• Don't use other immunosuppressants (except for adrenocorticosteroids) during therapy.
• Avoid potassium-sparing diuretics during therapy.
• Hepatic transplant trough levels are best maintained at 5 to 20 nanograms (ng)/ml 1 to 2 months post-transplant. Renal transplant trough levels are best maintained at 7 to 20 ng/ml between post-transplant months 1 to 3, and then 1 to 5 ng/ml for post-transplant months 4 to 12.
Patient teaching
• Instruct patient to take drug on empty stomach and not to take it with grapefruit juice.
• Explain need for repeated tests during therapy to monitor adverse reactions and drug effectiveness.

• Advise woman of childbearing age to notify prescriber if she becomes pregnant or plans to do so.
• Instruct patient to check with prescriber before taking other drugs.

✓ Evaluation
• Patient doesn't exhibit signs and symptoms of organ rejection.
• Patient doesn't develop serious complications as result of drug-induced adverse reactions.
• Patient and family state understanding of drug therapy.

tacrolimus (topical)
(tack-row-LYE-mus)
Protopic

Pharmacologic class: macrolide
Therapeutic class: immunosuppressant
Pregnancy risk category: C

Indication and dosages
▶ **Moderate to severe atopic dermatitis in patients unresponsive to other therapies or unable to use other therapies because of risks.** *Adults:* Apply thin layer of 0.03% or 0.1% strength to affected areas twice daily and rub in completely. Continue for 1 week after affected area clears.
Children ages 2 to 15 years: Apply thin layer of 0.03% strength to affected areas twice daily and rub in completely. Continue for 1 week after affected area clears.

Contraindications and cautions
• Contraindicated in patients hypersensitive to the drug or any of its components.
• Don't use in patients with Netherton's syndrome or generalized erythroderma.
⚠ **Lifespan:** In pregnant women, use only if benefits to the patient outweigh risks to the fetus. In breast-feeding women, the drug appears in breast milk; weigh benefits to the mother against risks to the infant. In children ages 2 to 15, use only 0.03% ointment.

Adverse reactions
CNS: *headache, fever,* hyperesthesia, asthenia, insomnia, pain.
CV: face edema, peripheral edema.

Reactions may be *common,* uncommon, *life-threatening*, or COMMON AND LIFE-THREATENING.

EENT: *otitis media, pharyngitis,* rhinitis, sinusitis, conjunctivitis.
GI: diarrhea, vomiting, nausea, abdominal pain, gastroenteritis, dyspepsia.
GU: dysmenorrhea.
Hematologic: lymphadenopathy.
Musculoskeletal: back pain, myalgia.
Respiratory: *increased cough, asthma,* pneumonia, bronchitis.
Skin: *skin burning, pruritus, skin erythema, skin infection,* eczema herpeticum, pustular rash, *folliculitis,* urticaria, maculopapular rash, rash, fungal dermatitis, acne, sunburn, tingling, benign skin neoplasm, skin disorder, vesiculobullous rash, dry skin, herpes zoster, eczema, exfoliative dermatitis, contact dermatitis.
Other: flulike symptoms, accidental injury, infection, lack of drug effect, alcohol intolerance, periodontal abscess, cyst, herpes simplex, allergic reaction.

Interactions

Drug-drug. *CYP 3A4 inhibitors (erythromycin, itraconazole, ketoconazole, fluconazole):* May interfere with effects of tacrolimus. Use together cautiously.
Drug-lifestyle. *Sun exposure:* May cause risk of phototoxicity. Tell patient to avoid or minimize exposure to artificial or natural sunlight.

Effects on lab test results

None reported.

Pharmacokinetics

Absorption: Immediate, with no systemic accumulation.
Distribution: Unknown.
Metabolism: Unknown.
Excretion: Unknown. *Half-life:* Unknown.

Route	Onset	Peak	Duration
Topical	Unknown	Unknown	Unknown

Action

Chemical effect: May inhibit T-lymphocyte activation in the skin, which causes immunosuppression. Also inhibits the release of mediators from mast cells and basophils in skin.
Therapeutic effect: Improves skin condition.

Available forms

Ointment: 0.03%, 0.1%

NURSING PROCESS

Assessment
• Assess patient's underlying condition before starting therapy, and reassess regularly to monitor the drug's effectiveness.
• Assess patient with infected atopic dermatitis; clear infections at treatment site before using drug.
• Assess patient's and family's knowledge of drug therapy.

Nursing diagnoses
• Impaired skin integrity related to underlying skin condition
• Acute pain related to drug-induced adverse effects
• Deficient knowledge related to tacrolimus therapy

Planning and implementation
• Drug is used only for short-term or intermittent therapy.
• Use only after other treatments have failed because of a possible risk of cancer with Protopic.
• **ALERT:** Don't use occlusive dressings over drug. This may promote systemic absorption.
• Drug may increase the risk of varicella zoster, herpes simplex virus, and eczema herpeticum.
• Assess all cases of lymphadenopathy to determine etiology. If a clear etiology is unknown or acute mononucleosis is diagnosed, consider stopping drug.
• Monitor all cases of lymphadenopathy until resolution.
• Local adverse effects are most common during the first few days of therapy.
Patient teaching
• Tell patient to wash hands before and after applying drug and to avoid applying drug to wet skin. Skin should be completely dry before applying drug.
• Instruct patient not to use bandages or other occlusive dressings.
• Tell patient not to bathe, shower, or swim immediately after application because doing so could wash the ointment off.
• Advise patient to avoid or minimize exposure to natural or artificial sunlight.
• Tell patient that, if he needs to be outdoors after applying drug, he should wear loose-fitting clothing that covers the treated area. Check with prescriber regarding sunscreen use.

T

- Tell patient not to use drug for any disorder other than that for which it was prescribed.
- Instruct patient to report adverse reactions.
- Tell patient to store the ointment at room temperature.

☑ Evaluation
- Patient has improved skin condition.
- Patient states that pain management techniques are effective.
- Patient and family state understanding of drug therapy.

tadalafil
(tah-DAH-lah-phil)
Cialis

Pharmacologic class: phosphodiesterase type 5 inhibitor
Therapeutic class: erectile dysfunction drug, vasodilating agent
Pregnancy risk category: B

Indications and dosages

▶ **Erectile dysfunction.** *Men:* 10 mg P.O. as a single dose, p.r.n., before sexual activity. Range is 5 to 20 mg based on effectiveness and tolerance. Maximum, one dose daily.
🖼 Adjust-a-dose: For patients with renal impairment, if creatinine clearance is 31 to 50 ml/ minute, starting dosage is 5 mg once daily and maximum dosage is 10 mg taken once q 48 hours; if 30 ml/minute or less, maximum dosage is 5 mg once daily. For patients with mild to moderate hepatic impairment (Child-Pugh class A or B), dosage shouldn't exceed 10 mg daily. For patients taking potent CYP 3A4 inhibitors (such as erythromycin, itraconazole, ketoconazole, ritonavir), don't exceed one 10-mg dose q 72 hours.

Contraindications and cautions

- Contraindicated in patients hypersensitive to the drug or any of its components, and in those taking nitrates or alpha blockers (other than tamsulosin 0.4 mg once daily). Drug isn't recommended for patients with severe hepatic impairment (Child-Pugh class C), MI within 90 days, New York Heart Association Class II or greater heart failure within 6 months, stroke within 6 months, uncontrolled arrhythmias,

blood pressure lower than 90/50 mm Hg or higher than 170/100 mm Hg, unstable angina, or angina that occurs during sexual intercourse. Drug also isn't recommended for patients whose cardiac status makes sexual activity inadvisable and for those with hereditary degenerative retinal disorders.
- Use cautiously in patients taking potent CYP 3A4 inhibitors and in patients with bleeding disorders, significant peptic ulceration, or renal or hepatic impairment. Use cautiously in patients with conditions that predispose them to priapism (such as sickle cell anemia, multiple myeloma, or leukemia), anatomical penis abnormalities, or left ventricular outflow obstruction.
🜲 **Lifespan:** Drug is for men only. In elderly men, consider a lower dose because they may be more sensitive to drug effects.

Adverse reactions

CNS: headache.
CV: flushing.
EENT: nasal congestion.
GI: dyspepsia.
Musculoskeletal: back pain, limb pain, myalgia.

Interactions

Drug-drug. *Alpha blockers (except tamsulosin 0.4 mg daily), nitrates:* May enhance hypotensive effects. Avoid using together.
Potent CYP 3A4 inhibitors (such as erythromycin, itraconazole, ketoconazole, ritonavir): May increase tadalafil level. Patient shouldn't exceed 10 mg q 72 hours.
Rifampin and other CYP 3A4 inducers: May decrease tadalafil level. Monitor patient closely.
Drug-food. *Grapefruit:* May increase drug level. Discourage use together. Monitor patient closely.
Drug-lifestyle. *Alcohol use:* May increase risk of headache, dizziness, orthostatic hypotension, and increased heart rate. Discourage use together.

Effects on lab test results

None reported.

Pharmacokinetics

Absorption: Median effect occurs in 2 hours.
Distribution: Distributed into tissues. 97% protein-bound.
Metabolism: Mainly through CYP 3A4 isoenzymes.

Excretion: In feces and urine. *Half-life:* 17½ hours.

Route	Onset	Peak	Duration
P.O.	Immediate	½–6 hr	Unknown

Action

Chemical effect: Prevents the breakdown of cyclic guanosine monophosphate (cGMP) by phosphodiesterase, thus increasing cGMP levels. **Therapeutic effect:** Prolongs smooth muscle relaxation and promotes blood flow into the corpus cavernosum.

Available forms

Tablets (film-coated): 5 mg, 10 mg, 20 mg

NURSING PROCESS

⚎ Assessment

Ⓢ **ALERT:** Sexual activity may increase cardiac risk. Assess patient's cardiac risk before he starts drug.
• Before patient starts drug, assess for underlying causes of erectile dysfunction.
• Assess patient's and family's knowledge of drug therapy.

⊞ Nursing diagnoses

• Sexual dysfunction related to patient's underlying condition
• Risk for injury related to potential for prolonged erections or priapism
• Deficient knowledge related to drug therapy

⊠ Planning and implementation

• Drug may cause transient decreases in supine blood pressure.
• Drug increases risk of prolonged erections and priapism.
Patient teaching
• Warn patient that taking drug with nitrates or alpha blockers could cause a serious drop in blood pressure, raising the risk of heart attack or stroke.
• Tell patient to seek immediate medical attention if he develops chest pain after taking the drug.
• Urge patient to seek emergency medical care if his erection lasts more than 4 hours.
• Tell patient to take drug about 60 minutes before anticipated sexual activity. Explain that drug has no effect without sexual stimulation.

• Warn patient not to change dose unless directed by prescriber.
• Caution patient against drinking large amounts of alcohol while taking drug.

☑ Evaluation

• Sexual activity improves with drug therapy.
• Patient doesn't experience injury from prolonged erection or priapism.
• Patient and family state understanding of drug therapy.

tamoxifen citrate

(teh-MOKS-uh-fen SIGH-trayt)
Apo-Tamox ◆ Nolvadex, Nolvadex-D ◆ ◇ , Novo-Tamoxifen ◆ , Soltamox, Tamofen ◆ , Tamone ◆

Pharmacologic class: nonsteroidal antiestrogen
Therapeutic class: antineoplastic
Pregnancy risk category: D

Indications and dosages

▶ **Advanced postmenopausal breast cancer.** *Women:* 20 to 40 mg P.O. b.i.d.
▶ **Adjunct treatment for breast cancer.** *Adults:* 10 mg P.O. b.i.d. to t.i.d. for no more than 5 years.
▶ **Reduction of breast cancer risk.** *High-risk women:* 20 mg P.O. daily for 5 years.
▶ **Ductal carcinoma in situ (DCIS).** *Adults:* 20 mg P.O. daily for 5 years.
▶ **Stimulation of ovulation‡.** *Women:* 5 to 40 mg P.O. b.i.d. for 4 days.
▶ **McCune–Albright syndrome and precocious puberty‡.** *Children ages 2 to 10:* 20 mg P.O. daily. Treat for up to 12 months.
▶ **Mastalgia‡.** *Women:* 10 mg P.O. daily for 10 months.

Contraindications and cautions

• Contraindicated in patients hypersensitive to the drug or any of its components, in women receiving coumarin-type anticoagulants, and in those with history of deep vein thrombosis or pulmonary emboli.
• Use cautiously in patients with leukopenia or thrombocytopenia.
⚹ **Lifespan:** In pregnant or breast-feeding women, drug isn't recommended. Patient should avoid pregnancy for at least 2 months after stop-

T

---

ping drug. In children, safety and effectiveness haven't been established.

Adverse reactions

CNS: confusion, weakness, headache, sleepiness, ***stroke.***
CV: hot flushes.
EENT: corneal changes, cataracts, retinopathy.
GI: nausea, vomiting, diarrhea.
GU: vaginal discharge and bleeding, irregular menses, amenorrhea, ***endometrial cancer, uterine sarcoma.***
Hematologic: ***leukopenia, thrombocytopenia.***
Hepatic: fatty liver, cholestasis, *hepatic necrosis.*
Metabolic: hypercalcemia, weight changes, fluid retention.
Musculoskeletal: brief exacerbation of pain from osseous metastases.
Respiratory: pulmonary embolism.
Skin: skin changes, rash.
Other: temporary bone or tumor pain.

Interactions

Drug-drug. *Antacids:* May affect absorption of enteric-coated tablet. Don't use within 2 hours of tamoxifen dose.
Bromocriptine: May elevate tamoxifen level. Monitor patient for toxicity.
Coumadin-type anticoagulants: May cause significant increase in anticoagulant effect. Monitor patient, PT, and INR closely.
Cytotoxic drugs (methotrexate, fluorouracil): May increase risk of thromboembolic events. Monitor patient, PT, and INR closely.

Effects on lab test results

- May increase BUN, creatinine, calcium, and liver enzyme levels.
- May decrease WBC and platelet counts.

Pharmacokinetics

Absorption: Appears to be well absorbed.
Distribution: Widely in total body water.
Metabolism: Extensive by the liver.
Excretion: Drug and metabolites excreted mainly in feces, mostly as metabolites. *Half-life:* More than 7 days.

Route	Onset	Peak	Duration
P.O.	4–10 wk	Unknown	Several wk

Action

Chemical effect: Exact antineoplastic action is unknown; acts as estrogen antagonist.
Therapeutic effect: Hinders function of breast cancer cells.

Available forms

Tablets: 10 mg, 20 mg
Tablets (enteric-coated): 10 mg, 20 mg
Oral solution: 10 mg/5 ml

NURSING PROCESS

Assessment

- Assess patient's breast cancer before starting therapy and regularly thereafter to monitor the drug's effectiveness.
- Monitor CBC closely in patient with leukopenia or thrombocytopenia.
- Monitor lipid levels during long-term therapy in patient with hyperlipidemia.
- Monitor calcium level in early stages of therapy; drug may compound hypercalcemia related to bone metastases.
- Be alert for adverse reactions.
- Monitor patient's hydration status if adverse GI reaction occurs.
- Assess patient's and family's knowledge of drug therapy.

Nursing diagnoses

- Ineffective health maintenance related to presence of breast cancer
- Risk for deficient fluid volume related to drug-induced adverse GI reactions
- Deficient knowledge related to drug therapy

Planning and implementation

- Make sure patient swallows enteric-coated tablets whole.

ALERT: Serious events (including uterine cancer, stroke, DVT, and pulmonary embolism) are linked to use in women at high risk for cancer and women with DCIS. Prescribers should discuss potential benefits and risks with women considering drug to reduce risk of developing breast cancer. The benefits outweigh risks in women already diagnosed with breast cancer.

Patient teaching

- Tell patient to use oral solution within 3 months of opening and not to freeze nor refrigerate.

• Instruct patient to report symptoms of pulmonary embolism (chest pain, difficulty breathing, rapid breathing, sweating or fainting).

• Tell patient to report symptoms of stroke (headache, vision changes, confusion, difficulty speaking or walking, and weakness of face, arm or leg, especially on one side of the body).

• Reassure patient that acute bone pain during drug therapy usually means that drug will produce good response. Tell her to take an analgesic for pain.

• Encourage patient who is taking or has taken drug to have regular gynecologic examinations because of increased risk of uterine cancer.

• If patient is taking drug to reduce risk of breast cancer, teach proper technique for breast self-examination.

• Tell patient that annual mammograms are important.

• Advise patient to use barrier form of contraception because short-term therapy induces ovulation in premenopausal women.

• Advise woman of childbearing age to avoid becoming pregnant during therapy and for at least 2 months following discontinuation of therapy. Tell her to consult with prescriber before becoming pregnant.

☑ **Evaluation**
• Patient responds well to drug.
• Patient maintains adequate hydration.
• Patient and family state understanding of drug therapy.

tamsulosin hydrochloride
(tam-soo-LOH-sin high-droh-KLOR-ighd)
Flomax

Pharmacologic class: alpha$_{1A}$ antagonist
Therapeutic class: benign prostatic hypertrophy agent
Pregnancy risk category: B

Indications and dosages

▶ **BPH.** *Men:* 0.4 mg P.O. once daily, given 30 minutes after same meal each day. If no response after 2 to 4 weeks, increase dosage to 0.8 mg P.O. once daily.

Contraindications and cautions

• Contraindicated in patients hypersensitive to the drug or any of its components.

• Use with caution in patients who have experienced hepatic or renal insufficiency, priapism, sulfa allergy, or orthostasis.

☲ **Lifespan:** Drug is indicated for men only.

Adverse reactions

CNS: asthenia, *dizziness, headache,* insomnia, somnolence, syncope, vertigo.
CV: chest pain, orthostatic hypotension.
EENT: amblyopia, pharyngitis, *rhinitis,* sinusitis.
GI: diarrhea, nausea.
GU: abnormal ejaculation.
Musculoskeletal: back pain.
Respiratory: cough, *rhinitis.*
Other: decreased libido, *infection,* tooth disorder.

Interactions

Drug-drug. *Alpha blockers:* May interact with tamsulosin. Avoid using together.
Cimetidine: May decrease tamsulosin clearance. Use cautiously.
Warfarin: Study results are inconclusive. Use together cautiously.

Effects on lab test results

None reported.

Pharmacokinetics

Absorption: More than 90%. Food increases bioavailability by 30%.
Distribution: Distributed into extracellular fluids. Extensively bound to protein (94% to 99%).
Metabolism: Primarily metabolized by CYP 450 enzymes in the liver.
Excretion: 76% of drug eliminated in urine; 21% in feces. *Half-life:* 9 to 13 hours.

Route	Onset	Peak	Duration
P.O.	Unknown	4–5 hr	9–15 hr

Action

Chemical effect: Selectively blocks alpha receptors in the prostate, leading to relaxation of smooth muscles in the bladder neck and prostate, which improves urine flow and reduces symptoms of BPH.
Therapeutic effect: Improves urine flow.

Available forms

Capsules: 0.4 mg

⚖ Assessment

• Assess patient for signs of prostatic hyperplasia, including frequency of urination, nocturnal urination, and urinary hesitancy.
• Monitor patient for decreases in blood pressure and notify prescriber.
• Assess patient's and family's knowledge of drug therapy.

⊕ Nursing diagnoses

• Risk for injury related to decreased blood pressure and resulting syncope
• Impaired urinary elimination related to underlying prostatic hyperplasia
• Deficient knowledge related to drug therapy

⊠ Planning and implementation

• Symptoms of BPH and cancer of the prostate are similar; cancer should be ruled out before therapy starts.
• If therapy is interrupted for several days or more, restart therapy at one capsule daily.
• Drug may cause a sudden drop in blood pressure, especially after the first dose or when changing doses.
• Patients having cataract surgery may develop intraoperative floppy iris syndrome; alert surgeon so he can modify his surgical technique as appropriate.
⑧ **ALERT:** Don't confuse Flomax with Fosamax.
Patient teaching
• Instruct patient not to crush, chew, or open capsules.
• Tell patient to get up slowly from chair or bed when therapy starts and to avoid situations where injury could occur because of syncope. Advise him that drug may cause a sudden drop in blood pressure, especially after the first dose or when changing doses.
• Instruct patient not to drive or perform hazardous tasks for 12 hours after the initial dose or a change in dose, until response can be monitored.
• Tell patient to take drug about 30 minutes after same meal each day.
• If patient needs cataract surgery, urge him to tell surgeon that he takes tamsulosin.

☑ Evaluation

• Patient doesn't experience sudden decreases in blood pressure.
• Patient experiences normal urinary elimination patterns.
• Patient and family state understanding of drug therapy.

tegaserod maleate
(teh-GAS-uh-rahd MALL-ee-ayt)
Zelnorm

Pharmacologic class: 5-HT$_4$ receptor partial agonist
Therapeutic class: irritable bowel drug
Pregnancy risk category: B

Indications and dosages

▶ **Short-term treatment for irritable bowel syndrome, when the primary bowel symptom is constipation.** *Women:* 6 mg P.O. b.i.d. before meals for 4 to 6 weeks. May add another 4- to 6-week course for patients who respond to therapy at 4 to 6 weeks.
▶ **Chronic idiopathic constipation.** *Adults younger than age 65:* 6 mg P.O. b.i.d. before meals.

Contraindications and cautions

• Contraindicated in patients hypersensitive to the drug or any of its components, and in those with severe renal impairment, moderate or severe hepatic impairment, a history of bowel obstruction, symptomatic gallbladder disease, suspected sphincter of Oddi dysfunction or abdominal adhesions, or frequent or current diarrhea.
⚕ **Lifespan:** In pregnant women, use drug only if clearly needed. In breast-feeding women, either stop breast-feeding or use a different drug, taking into account the importance of the drug to the mother. In children, safety and effectiveness haven't been established.

Adverse reactions

CNS: *headache,* dizziness, migraine.
GI: *abdominal pain,* diarrhea, nausea, flatulence, ischemic colitis.
Musculoskeletal: back pain, arthropathy, leg pain.
Other: accidental injury.

Interactions

Drug-drug. *Digoxin:* May reduce peak level and exposure of digoxin by 15%. Use cautiously.
Drug-food. *Food:* May reduce bioavailability of drug. Advise patient to take drug on an empty stomach.

Effects on lab test results

None reported.

Pharmacokinetics

Absorption: Food reduces bioavailability by 40% to 65%.
Distribution: About 98% protein-bound.
Metabolism: By two pathways. The first is hydrolysis, followed by oxidation and conjugation. The second is direct glucuronidation.
Excretion: Two-thirds of dose unchanged in feces, with the remaining one-third in the urine, primarily as the metabolite. *Half-life:* Unknown.

Route	Onset	Peak	Duration
P.O.	Unknown	1 hr	Unknown

Action

Chemical effect: Binds with high affinity to 5-HT$_4$ receptors and acts as an agonist. Activating 5-HT$_4$ receptors in the GI tract stimulates the peristaltic reflex and intestinal secretion and inhibits visceral sensitivity.
Therapeutic effect: Relieves constipation.

Available forms

Tablets: 2 mg, 6 mg

NURSING PROCESS

⚕ Assessment

• Assess patient's condition before starting therapy, and reassess regularly to monitor the drug's effectiveness.
• Monitor patient for diarrhea and abdominal pain.
• Assess patient's and family's knowledge of drug therapy.

⊞ Nursing diagnoses

• Constipation related to irritable bowel syndrome
• Diarrhea related to adverse effect of tegaserod maleate therapy
• Deficient knowledge related to drug therapy

⊠ Planning and implementation

• Give drug on an empty stomach before a meal.
• If patient experiences new or sudden worsening of abdominal pain, or rectal bleeding, stop drug.
• Patient may develop diarrhea during therapy; in most cases, diarrhea occurs within the first week of therapy and resolves with continued therapy.
• If serious cases of diarrhea with symptoms of hypovolemia, hypotension, and syncope occur, stop giving the drug. Don't use the drug in a patient who has frequent diarrhea.
• Discontinue drug in patients who develop ischemic colitis or other forms of intestinal ischemia characterized by rectal bleeding, bloody diarrhea, or abdominal pain. Don't resume treatment with tegaserod if ischemic colitis is discovered.

Patient teaching

• Tell patient to take drug on an empty stomach, before a meal.
• Inform patient she may have diarrhea during therapy. Tell her to report severe diarrhea or diarrhea accompanied by severe cramping, abdominal pain, or dizziness.
• Tell patient not to take drug if she now has or often has diarrhea.
• Tell patient to report new or worsening abdominal pain.
• Tell patient not to use drug during pregnancy or breast-feeding.

☑ Evaluation

• Patient expresses relief from constipation.
• Patient reports no diarrhea.
• Patient and family state understanding of drug therapy.

telithromycin
(tay-lith-roh-MY-seen)
Ketek

Pharmacologic classification: ketolide
Therapeutic classification: antibiotic
Pregnancy risk category: C

Indications and dosages

▶ **Acute bacterial exacerbation of chronic bronchitis caused by** *Streptococcus pneumo-*

niae, Haemophilus influenzae, or *Moraxella catarrhalis;* acute bacterial sinusitis caused by *S. pneumoniae, H. influenzae, M. catarrhalis,* or *Staphylococcus aureus. Adults:* 800 mg P.O. once daily for 5 days.

▶ Mild to moderate community-acquired pneumonia caused by *S. pneumoniae* (including multi–drug-resistant isolates), *H. influenzae, M. catarrhalis, Chlamydophila pneumoniae,* or *Mycoplasma pneumoniae. Adults:* 800 mg P.O. once daily for 7 to 10 days.

⊠ **Adjust-a-dose:** For patient with renal impairment and a creatinine clearances less than 30 ml/minute, including patients on dialysis, give 600 mg P.O. once daily. On dialysis days, give after session complete. For patient who also has hepatic impairment, give 400 mg once daily.

Contraindications and cautions

• Contraindicated in patients hypersensitive to telithromycin or any macrolide antibiotic. Don't give to patients with congenitally prolonged QTc interval, patients with ongoing proarrhythmic conditions (such as uncorrected hypokalemia or hypomagnesemia or significant bradycardia), or patients who are taking Class IA antiarrhythmics (such as quinidine, procainamide), Class III antiarrhythmics (such as dofetilide), cisapride, or pimozide.

• Not recommended for patients with myasthenia gravis; drug may worsen symptoms and increase the risk of acute respiratory failure.

• Use cautiously in patients with a history of hepatitis or jaundice caused by drug.

☀ **Lifespan:** In pregnant or breast-feeding women, use cautiously. In children, safety and effectiveness haven't been established.

Adverse reactions

CNS: dizziness, headache.
CV: prolonged QTc interval, *ventricular arrhythmias, torsade de pointes.*
Hepatic: hepatic dysfunction, *hepatitis, hepatotoxicity.*
EENT: blurred vision, diplopia, difficulty focusing.
GI: *diarrhea, pseudomembranous colitis,* loose stools, nausea, taste disturbance, vomiting.

Interactions

Drug-drug. *Atorvastatin, lovastatin, simvastatin:* May increase levels of these drugs, in-

creasing the risk of myopathy. Avoid use together.
Benzodiazepines (midazolam): May increase benzodiazepine level. Monitor patient closely, and consider adjusting benzodiazepine dosage.
Cisapride: May increase QTc level. Avoid concomitant use.
CYP 3A4 inducers (carbamazepine, phenobarbital, phenytoin): May decrease telithromycin level. Avoid use together.
CYP 3A4 inhibitors (itraconazole, ketoconazole): May increase telithromycin level. Monitor patient closely.
Digoxin: May increase digoxin level. Monitor digoxin levels.
Drugs metabolized by the CYP system (such as carbamazepine, cyclosporine, hexobarbital, phenytoin, sirolimus, tacrolimus): May increase serum levels of these drugs, increasing or prolonging their effects. Use together cautiously, and monitor patient closely.
Ergot alkaloid derivatives (such as ergotamine): May increase the risk of ergot toxicity, characterized by severe peripheral vasospasm and dysesthesia. Avoid use together.
Metoprolol: May increase metoprolol level. Use together cautiously.
Oral anticoagulants: May increase the effects of the anticoagulant. Monitor PT and INR during co-administration.
Pimozide: May increase pimozide level. Use together is contraindicated.
Rifampin: May decrease telithromycin level significantly. Avoid use together.
Sotalol: May decrease sotalol level. Monitor patient for lack of effect.
Theophylline: May increase theophylline level and cause nausea and vomiting. Separate telithromycin and theophylline doses by 1 hour.

Effects on lab test results

• May increase AST and ALT levels.
• May increase platelet count.

Pharmacokinetics

Absorption: Bioavailability is about 57%.
Distribution: Drug is 60% to 70% protein-bound.
Metabolism: About 50% is by CYP 3A4.
Elimination: 13% excreted unchanged in urine, and 7% excreted unchanged in feces. *Half-life:* 10 hours.

Route	Onset	Peak	Duration
P.O.	Unknown	1 hr	Unknown

Action

Chemical effect: Inhibits bacterial protein synthesis.
Therapeutic effect: Hinders or kills susceptible bacteria.

Available forms

Tablets: 300 mg, 400 mg

NURSING PROCESS

⏣ Assessment

• Assess patient's history of allergies, especially to macrolides, before starting therapy.
• Obtain patient's medical history before starting therapy, including a list of drugs he's taking.
• Obtain sample for culture and sensitivity tests prior to giving the first dose. Start therapy pending test results.
• Be alert for adverse reactions and drug interactions.
• Assess patient for diarrhea during therapy; patients with diarrhea may have pseudomembranous colitis.
• Assess patient's and family's knowledge of drug therapy.

⊕ Nursing diagnoses

• Ineffective health maintenance related to presence of susceptible bacteria
• Risk for deficient fluid volume related to potential for drug-induced adverse GI reactions
• Deficient knowledge related to drug therapy

⯈ Planning and implementation

• Monitor electrolyte levels before starting therapy and periodically thereafter. Electrolyte imbalances must be corrected before or during therapy to avoid proarrhythmic conditions.
• Obtain hematologic, renal and hepatic studies before starting therapy and during therapy.
• Drug may cause visual disturbances, particularly in women and patients younger than age 40. Adverse visual effects occur most often after the first or second dose, last several hours, and sometimes return with later doses. For some patients, the symptoms will resolve during treatment; for others, they'll continue until treatment is complete.

⊛ **ALERT:** Drug may prolong the QTc interval. Rarely, an irregular heartbeat may cause the patient to faint.
• Monitor patient for signs and symptoms of liver problems, such as jaundice, pale stools, darkened urine, weakness, and abdominal pain.

Patient teaching

• Urge patient to take this drug exactly as prescribed until all of the tablets are gone, even if he feels better before the prescription is finished.
• Tell patient that drug can be taken with or without food.
• Explain that this drug may cause vision disturbances, usually after the first or second dose and for up to a few hours at a time. Caution the patient to avoid hazardous activities.
• Tell patient to report diarrhea or any episodes of fainting that occur while taking this drug.
• Instruct patient to store tablets at room temperature.
• Tell patient to report new onset of weakness, abdominal pain, or other symptoms of liver problems.

☑ Evaluation

• Patient is free from infection.
• Patient maintains adequate hydration with therapy.
• Patient and family state understanding of drug therapy.

telmisartan
(tel-mih-SAR-tan)
Micardis

Pharmacologic class: angiotensin II receptor antagonist
Therapeutic class: antihypertensive
Pregnancy risk category: C (D in second and third trimesters)

Indications and dosages

▶ **Hypertension (used alone or with other antihypertensives).** *Adults:* 40 mg P.O. daily. Blood pressure response is dose-related between 20 and 80 mg daily.

Contraindications and cautions

• Contraindicated in patients hypersensitive to the drug or any of its components.

T

• Use cautiously in patients with renal and hepatic insufficiency and in those with an activated renin-angiotensin system, such as volume- or salt-depleted patients (those being treated with high doses of diuretics, for example).

⚞ **Lifespan:** In pregnant women, don't use. If pregnancy is suspected, notify prescriber because drug should be stopped. Breast-feeding women should stop breast-feeding or use another drug, taking into account importance of drug therapy. In children, safety and effectiveness haven't been established.

Adverse reactions

CNS: dizziness, pain, fatigue, headache.
CV: chest pain, hypertension, peripheral edema.
EENT: pharyngitis, sinusitis.
GI: abdominal pain, diarrhea, dyspepsia, nausea.
GU: UTI.
Musculoskeletal: back pain, myalgia.
Respiratory: cough, upper respiratory tract infection.
Other: flulike symptoms.

Interactions

Drug-drug. *Digoxin:* May increase digoxin level. Monitor digoxin level closely.
Warfarin: May slightly decrease warfarin level. Monitor INR.

Effects on lab test results

• May increase liver enzyme and creatinine levels. May decrease hemoglobin level and hematocrit.

Pharmacokinetics

Absorption: Readily absorbed.
Distribution: Highly protein-bound; volume of distribution is about 500 L.
Metabolism: Metabolized by conjugation to an inactive metabolite.
Excretion: Mainly excreted unchanged in feces.
Half-life: 24 hours.

Route	Onset	Peak	Duration
P.O.	Unknown	30 min–1 hr	24 hr

Action

Chemical effect: Blocks the vasoconstrictive and aldosterone-secreting effects of angiotensin II by selectively blocking the binding of angiotensin II to the AT_1 receptor in many tissues, such as vascular smooth muscle and the adrenal gland.
Therapeutic effect: Lowers blood pressure.

Available forms

Tablets: 40 mg, 80 mg

NURSING PROCESS

✍ Assessment

• In patient whose renal function may depend on the activity of the renin-angiotensin-aldosterone system, such as those with severe heart failure, use of ACE inhibitors and angiotensin-receptor antagonists may be related to oliguria or progressive azotemia and (rarely) to acute renal failure or death.
• In patient with biliary obstruction, drug level may elevate because of inability to excrete drug.
• Drug isn't removed by hemodialysis; orthostatic hypotension may develop in patient undergoing dialysis. Closely monitor blood pressure.
• Assess patient's and family's knowledge of drug therapy.

⊡ Nursing diagnoses

• Risk for injury related to presence of hypertension
• Ineffective cerebral and cardiopulmonary tissue perfusion related to drug-induced hypotension
• Deficient knowledge related to drug therapy

❯ Planning and implementation

• Most of the antihypertensive effect is present within 2 weeks. Maximal blood pressure reduction is generally attained after 4 weeks. If blood pressure isn't controlled by drug alone, a diuretic may be added.
• If hypotension occurs, place patient in supine position and give normal saline solution I.V. if needed.

Patient teaching
• Inform woman of childbearing age of consequences of second- and third-trimester exposure to drug. Instruct patient to immediately report suspected pregnancy to prescriber.
• Tell patient that transient hypotension may occur. Instruct him to lie down if feeling dizzy and to climb stairs slowly and rise slowly to standing position.
• Instruct patient with heart failure to notify prescriber about decreased urine output.

Reactions may be *common*, uncommon, *life-threatening*, or COMMON AND LIFE-THREATENING.

• Teach patient other means to reduce blood pressure, such as diet control, exercise, smoking cessation, and stress reduction.

• Inform patient that drug shouldn't be removed from blister-sealed packet until immediately before use.

☑ **Evaluation**

• Patient doesn't experience injury from underlying disease.

• Patient doesn't experience hypotension and maintains adequate tissue perfusion.

• Patient and family state understanding of drug therapy.

temazepam

(teh-MAZ-ih-pam)
Euhypnos◇, Normison◇, Restoril, Temaze◇

Pharmacologic class: benzodiazepine
Therapeutic class: sedative-hypnotic
Pregnancy risk category: X
Controlled substance schedule: IV

Indications and dosages

▶ **Short-term therapy for insomnia.** *Adults:* 15 to 30 mg P.O. 30 minutes before bedtime. 7.5 mg may be sufficient in some patients *Elderly or debilitated patients:* Initiate therapy with 7.5 mg P.O. h.s. until response is determined.

Contraindications and cautions

• Contraindicated in patients hypersensitive to benzodiazepines.

• Use cautiously in patients with chronic pulmonary insufficiency, impaired liver or kidney function, severe or latent depression, suicidal tendencies, or history of drug abuse.

▲ **Lifespan:** In pregnant women, drug is contraindicated. In breast-feeding women, drug isn't recommended. In children, safety and effectiveness haven't been established.

Adverse reactions

CNS: *drowsiness, dizziness, lethargy,* disturbed coordination, daytime sedation, confusion, nightmares, vertigo, euphoria, weakness, headache, fatigue, nervousness, anxiety, depression.
CV: hypotension, palpitations.

EENT: blurred vision.
GI: diarrhea, nausea, dry mouth.
Respiratory: dyspnea.
Other: physical or psychological dependence.

Interactions

Drug-drug. *CNS depressants, including opioid analgesics:* May increase CNS depression. Use together cautiously.
Drug-herb. *Calendula, catnip, hops, lady's slipper, lemon balm, passion flower, sassafras, skullcap, valerian, yerba maté:* May increase sedative effects. Monitor patient closely; discourage use together.
Kava: May cause excessive sedation. Discourage use together.
Drug-lifestyle. *Alcohol use:* May cause additive CNS effects. Strongly discourage use together.

Effects on lab test results

• May increase liver enzyme levels.

Pharmacokinetics

Absorption: Well absorbed.
Distribution: Distributed widely throughout body; 98% protein-bound.
Metabolism: Metabolized in liver to primarily inactive metabolites.
Excretion: Metabolites excreted in urine. *Half-life:* 10 to 17 hours.

Route	Onset	Peak	Duration
P.O.	Unknown	1–2 hr	Unknown

Action

Chemical effect: May act on limbic system, thalamus, and hypothalamus of CNS to produce hypnotic effects.
Therapeutic effect: Promotes sleep.

Available forms

Capsules: 7.5 mg, 15 mg, 20 mg◇, 30 mg

T

NURSING PROCESS

☑ **Assessment**

• Assess patient's sleeping disorder before starting therapy and regularly thereafter to monitor the drug's effectiveness.

• Assess mental status before starting therapy. An elderly patient is more sensitive to drug's adverse CNS effects.

• Be alert for adverse reactions and drug interactions.
• Assess patient's and family's knowledge of drug therapy.

[⊕] Nursing diagnoses
• Disturbed sleep pattern related to presence of insomnia
• Risk for injury related to drug-induced adverse CNS reactions
• Deficient knowledge related to drug therapy

Planning and implementation
• Before leaving the bedside, make sure patient who is depressed, suicidal, or drug-dependent, or who has history of drug abuse has swallowed the capsule to prevent hoarding.
• Use drug on an "as needed" basis.
• Supervise walking, and raise bed rails, particularly for geriatric patients.
ALERT: Don't confuse Restoril with Vistaril.
Patient teaching
• Warn patient to avoid activities that require mental alertness or physical coordination.

☑ Evaluation
• Patient states that drug induces sleep.
• Patient doesn't experience injury from adverse CNS reactions.
• Patient and family state understanding of drug therapy.

tenecteplase
(te-NEK-te-plase)
TNKase

Pharmacologic class: recombinant tissue plasminogen activator
Therapeutic class: thrombolytic
Pregnancy risk category: C

Indications and dosages
▶ **Reduction of mortality from acute MI.** *Adults who weigh less than 60 kg (132 lb):* 30 mg (6 ml) by I.V. bolus over 5 seconds.
Adults who weigh 60 to 69 kg (132 to 152 lb): 35 mg (7 ml) by I.V. bolus over 5 seconds.
Adults who weigh 70 to 79 kg (153 to 174 lb): 40 mg (8 ml) by I.V. bolus over 5 seconds.
Adults who weigh 80 to 89 kg (175 to 196 lb): 45 mg (9 ml) by I.V. bolus over 5 seconds.
Adults who weigh 90 kg (197 lb) or more: 50 mg (10 ml) by I.V. bolus over 5 seconds. Maximum dose is 50 mg.

I.V. administration
• Use syringe prefilled with sterile water for injection and inject entire contents into drug vial. Don't use bacteriostatic water for injection.
• Gently swirl solution once mixed. Don't shake. Make sure contents are completely dissolved.
• Draw up the appropriate dose needed from the reconstituted vial with the syringe and discard any unused portion.
• Give drug immediately once reconstituted, or refrigerate and use within 8 hours.
• Give drug in a designated line.
• Give heparin with tenecteplase, but not in the same I.V. line.
⊗ **Incompatibilities**
Solutions containing dextrose.

Contraindications and cautions
• Contraindicated in patients with active internal bleeding; history of stroke; intracranial or intraspinal surgery or trauma within the previous 2 months; intracranial neoplasm, aneurysm, or arteriovenous malformation; severe uncontrolled hypertension; or known bleeding diathesis.
• Use cautiously in patients who have had recent major surgery (such as coronary artery bypass graft), organ biopsy, or obstetrical delivery, or previous puncture of noncompressible vessels. Also use cautiously in patients with recent trauma, recent GI or GU bleeding, high risk of left ventricular thrombus, acute pericarditis, hypertension (systolic 180 mm Hg or above, diastolic 110 mm Hg or above), severe hepatic dysfunction, hemostatic defects, subacute bacterial endocarditis, septic thrombophlebitis, diabetic hemorrhagic retinopathy, or cerebrovascular disease.
Lifespan: In pregnant women, use cautiously. In breast-feeding women, use cautiously; it's unknown if the drug appears in breast milk. In children, safety and effectiveness haven't been established. In patients age 75 and older, give cautiously; weigh drug benefits against the risk of increased adverse effects.

Adverse reactions
CNS: ***stroke, intracranial hemorrhage,*** fever.

CV: *major hematoma, minor hematoma,* coronary reperfusion arrhythmias, *cholesterol embolism.*
EENT: pharyngeal bleeding, epistaxis.
GI: *GI bleeding,* nausea, vomiting.
GU: hematuria.
Hematologic: bleeding at puncture sites.

Interactions

Drug-drug. *Anticoagulants (heparin, vitamin K antagonists), drugs that alter platelet function (acetylsalicylic acid, dipyridamole, glycoprotein IIb/IIIa inhibitors):* May increase risk of bleeding when used before, during, or after therapy with tenecteplase. Use cautiously.

Effects on lab test results

• May increase PT, PTT, and INR.

Pharmacokinetics

Absorption: Administered I.V.
Distribution: Related to weight and is an approximation of plasma volume.
Metabolism: Primarily hepatic.
Excretion: Unknown. *Half-life:* 20 minutes to 2 hours.

Route	Onset	Peak	Duration
I.V.	Immediate	Immediate	20–24 min

Action

Chemical effect: Binds to fibrin and converts plasminogen to plasmin. Specificity to fibrin decreases systemic activation of plasminogen and the resulting breakdown of circulating fibrinogen.
Therapeutic effect: Dissolves blood clots.

Available forms

Injection: 50 mg

NURSING PROCESS

Assessment
• Assess underlying condition before starting therapy, and reassess regularly thereafter to monitor the drug's effectiveness.
• Monitor ECG for reperfusion arrhythmias.
• Assess pain before therapy and reassess regularly.
• Assess patient's and family's knowledge of drug therapy.

Nursing diagnoses
• Ineffective tissue perfusion, coronary, related to presence of blood clots
• Acute pain related to MI
• Deficient knowledge related to tenecteplase therapy

Planning and implementation
• Minimize arterial and venous punctures during therapy.
• Avoid noncompressible arterial punctures and internal jugular and subclavian venous punctures.
• Monitor patient for bleeding. If serious bleeding occurs, immediately stop giving heparin and antiplatelet drugs.
• Cholesterol embolism is rarely related to thrombolytic use, but may be lethal. Signs and symptoms may include livedo reticularis "purple toe" syndrome, acute renal failure, gangrenous digits, hypertension, pancreatitis, MI, cerebral infarction, spinal cord infarction, retinal artery occlusion, bowel infarction, and rhabdomyolysis.
Patient teaching
• Inform patient about proper dental care to avoid excessive gum bleeding.
• Advise patient to immediately report any adverse effects or excess bleeding.
• Explain use of drug to patient and family.

Evaluation
• Patient regains tissue perfusion with dissolution of blood clots.
• Patient is relieved of pain.
• Patient and family state understanding of drug therapy.

teniposide (VM-26)
(teh-NIP-uh-sighd)
Vumon

Pharmacologic class: podophyllotoxin
Therapeutic class: antineoplastic
Pregnancy risk category: D

Indications and dosages

▶ Refractory childhood acute lymphoblastic leukemia. *Children:* Optimum dosage hasn't been established. One protocol is 165 mg/m²

I.V. twice weekly for eight or nine doses, usually with other drugs.

🛇 **Adjust-a-dose:** Consider dosage adjustments in patients with renal and hepatic insufficiency. Patients with Down's syndrome may have increased sensitivity to the drug; begin therapy with a reduced dose, and monitor patient.

▼ I.V. administration

• Preparation and administration are linked to carcinogenic, mutagenic, and teratogenic risks for personnel. Follow institutional policy to reduce risks.
• Dilute drug in D_5W or normal saline solution injection to concentration of 0.1, 0.2, 0.4, or 1 mg/ml. Don't agitate vigorously; precipitation may form. Discard cloudy solutions.
• Don't give drug through membrane-type in-line filter because diluent may dissolve filter.
• Infuse over 45 to 90 minutes to prevent hypotension. If hypotension occurs, stop infusion.
• Ensure careful placement of catheter. Extravasation can cause local tissue necrosis or sloughing.
• Prepare and store in glass containers. Solutions containing 0.5 to 1 mg/ml teniposide are stable for 4 hours; those containing 0.1 to 0.2 mg/ml are stable for 6 hours at room temperature.
⊗ **Incompatibilities**
Heparin, idarubicin. Don't mix with other drugs or solutions.

Contraindications and cautions

• Contraindicated in patients hypersensitive to the drug or to polyoxyethylated castor oil (an injection vehicle).
• Use cautiously in patients with myelosuppression.
※ **Lifespan:** In pregnant and breast-feeding women, drug isn't recommended.

Adverse reactions

CV: hypotension from rapid infusion.
GI: nausea, vomiting, mucositis, diarrhea.
Hematologic: myelosuppression, *leukopenia, neutropenia, thrombocytopenia*, anemia.
Skin: alopecia; tissue necrosis, sloughing, or phlebitis at injection site.
Other: *hypersensitivity reactions* (chills, fever, urticaria, tachycardia, *bronchospasm*, dyspnea, hypotension, flushing).

Interactions

Drug-drug. *Methotrexate:* May increase clearance and intracellular levels of methotrexate. Monitor patient closely.
Sodium salicylate, sulfamethizole, tolbutamide: May displace teniposide from protein-binding sites and increase toxicity. Monitor patient closely.

Effects on lab test results

• May increase uric acid level. May decrease hemoglobin level and hematocrit.
• May decrease RBC, WBC, platelet, and neutrophil counts.

Pharmacokinetics

Absorption: Administered I.V.
Distribution: Distributed mainly in liver, kidneys, small intestine, and adrenals. Drug crosses blood-brain barrier to limited extent; highly bound to plasma proteins.
Metabolism: Metabolized extensively in liver.
Excretion: About 40% eliminated through kidneys as unchanged drug or metabolites. *Half-life:* 5 hours.

Route	Onset	Peak	Duration
I.V.	Unknown	Unknown	Unknown

Action

Chemical effect: Acts in late S or early G2 phase of cell cycle, thus preventing cells from entering mitosis.
Therapeutic effect: Prevents reproduction of leukemic cells.

Available forms

Injection: 50 mg/5 ml

🔍 Assessment

• Assess patient's condition before starting therapy and regularly thereafter to monitor the drug's effectiveness.
• Obtain baseline blood counts and kidney and liver function tests, then monitor periodically.
• Monitor blood pressure before therapy and at 30-minute intervals during infusion.
• Be alert for adverse reactions and drug interactions.
• Assess patient's and family's knowledge of drug therapy.

Nursing diagnoses
• Ineffective health maintenance related to presence of leukemia
• Ineffective protection related to drug-induced immunosuppression
• Deficient knowledge related to drug therapy

Planning and implementation
• Some prescribers may decide to use drug despite patient's history of hypersensitivity because therapeutic benefits may outweigh risks. Give antihistamines and corticosteroids to these patients before infusion begins, and monitor them closely during drug administration.
ALERT: Have diphenhydramine, hydrocortisone, epinephrine, and appropriate emergency equipment available to establish airway in case of anaphylaxis.
ALERT: Report systolic blood pressure below 90 mm Hg, and stop infusion.
Patient teaching
• Tell patient to immediately report discomfort at the I.V. site.
• Encourage adequate fluid intake to increase urine output and facilitate excretion of uric acid.
• Review infection-control and bleeding precautions to take during therapy.
• Reassure patient that hair should grow back after therapy stops.
• Instruct patient and parents to notify prescriber if adverse reactions occur.

Evaluation
• Patient responds well to drug.
• Patient doesn't develop serious complications from immunosuppression.
• Patient and family state understanding of drug therapy.

tenofovir disoproxil fumarate
(teh-NAH-fuh-veer diso-PRAHK-sul FOO-mah-rate)
Viread

Pharmacologic class: nucleotide reverse transcriptase inhibitor
Therapeutic class: antiretroviral
Pregnancy risk category: B

Indications and dosages
▶ **HIV-1 infection, with other antiretrovirals.**
Adults: 300 mg P.O. once daily without regard

to food. When given with didanosine, give 2 hours before or 1 hour after didanosine.
Adjust-a-dose: For creatinine clearance between 30 and 49 ml/minute, administer 300 mg every 48 hours. For creatinine clearance between 10 and 29 ml/minute, administer 300 mg twice a week.
For hemodialysis patients, administer 300 mg every 7 days or after a total of 12 hours of hemodialysis.

Contraindications and cautions
• Contraindicated in patients hypersensitive to the drug or any of its components.
• Use cautiously in patients with hepatic impairment or risk factors for liver disease, and in patients with renal impairment.
Lifespan: In pregnant women, use only if the benefits to the woman outweigh the risks to the fetus. Breast-feeding women should stop breast-feeding or use another drug. In children, safety and effectiveness haven't been established. In the elderly, use cautiously because they are more likely to have renal impairment and to be receiving other drug therapy.

Adverse reactions
CNS: asthenia, headache, depression, peripheral neuropathy, fever, insomnia.
CV: chest pain.
GI: abdominal pain, anorexia, diarrhea, flatulence, *nausea*, vomiting, dyspepsia.
GU: glycosuria, *renal toxicity.*
Hematologic: *neutropenia.*
Hepatic: *hepatomegaly with steatosis, hepatotoxicity.*
Metabolic: hyperglycemia, weight loss, *lactic acidosis.*
Musculoskeletal: decreased bone density, back pain, myalgias.
Skin: fat accumulation and redistribution, sweating, rash.

Interactions
Drug-drug. *Acyclovir, cidofovir, ganciclovir, valacyclovir, valganciclovir (drugs that reduce renal function or compete for renal tubular secretion):* May increase level of tenofovir or other renally eliminated drugs. Monitor patient for adverse effects.
Atazanavir: May decrease atazanavir levels, causing resistance. Give both drugs with ritonavir.

Rapid onset   *Liquid form contains alcohol.   ♦Canada   ◊Australia   †OTC   ⊘Photoguide   ‡Off-label use

Didanosine (buffered formulation): May increase didanosine bioavailability. Monitor patient for didanosine-related adverse effects, such as bone marrow suppression, GI distress, and peripheral neuropathy. Give tenofovir 2 hours before or 1 hour after didanosine.

Effects on lab test results

• May increase amylase, AST, ALT, creatinine kinase, serum and urine glucose, and triglyceride levels. May decrease HIV-1 RNA levels.
• May decrease neutrophil and CD4 cell counts.

Pharmacokinetics

Absorption: In fasting patients, tenofovir is poorly absorbed (bioavailability 25%) with peak level occurring in about 1 hour. A high-fat meal delays the peak by 1 hour but increases bioavailability to 40%.
Distribution: Tenofovir has low binding to plasma and proteins.
Metabolism: Neither tenofovir nor tenofovir disoproxil fumarate is metabolized by liver enzymes, including CYP enzymes.
Excretion: Renal, through glomerular filtration and active tubular secretion. *Half-life:* Unknown.

Route	Onset	Peak	Duration
P.O.	Unknown	1–2 hr	Unknown

Action

Chemical effect: Tenofovir disoproxil fumarate is hydrolyzed to produce tenofovir. Tenofovir undergoes sequential phosphorylations to yield tenofovir diphosphate. Tenofovir diphosphate is a competitive antagonist of HIV reverse transcriptase.
Therapeutic effect: Inhibits HIV replication.

Available forms

Tablets: 300 mg as the fumarate salt (equivalent to 245 mg of tenofovir disoproxil)

NURSING PROCESS

☼ Assessment
• Assess patient's viral infection before starting therapy and regularly thereafter to monitor the drug's effectiveness.
• Assess patient for risk of severe adverse reactions. Antiretrovirals, alone or combined, have been linked to lactic acidosis and severe (including fatal) hepatomegaly with steatosis. These effects may occur without elevated transaminase levels. Risk is increased for women, obese patients, and those exposed to antiretrovirals long-term. Monitor all patients for hepatotoxicity, including lactic acidosis and hepatomegaly with steatosis.
• Assess patient's and family's knowledge of drug therapy.

☼ Nursing diagnoses
• Noncompliance related to long-term therapy
• Risk for infection related to presence of HIV
• Deficient knowledge related to drug therapy

☼ Planning and implementation
• Antiretrovirals have been linked to the accumulation and redistribution of body fat, resulting in central obesity, peripheral wasting, and development of a buffalo hump. The long-term effects of these changes are unknown. Monitor patients for changes in body fat.
• Tenofovir may be linked to bone abnormalities (osteomalacia and decreased bone mineral density) and renal toxicity (increased creatinine and phosphaturia levels). Monitor patient carefully during long-term therapy.
• Drug may lead to decreased HIV-1 RNA levels and CD4 cell counts.
• The effects of tenofovir on the progression of HIV infection are unknown.
• Because of a high rate of early virologic resistance, triple antiretroviral therapy with abacavir, lamivudine, and tenofovir shouldn't be used as a new therapy regimen for untreated or pre-treated patients. Monitor patients currently controlled with this drug combination and those who use this combination in addition to other antiretroviral drugs, and consider modifying therapy.
• Because of a high rate of early virologic failure and emergence of resistance, therapy with tenofovir with didanosine and lamivudine isn't recommended as a new treatment regimen for therapy-naïve or experienced patients with HIV infection. Patients currently on this regimen should be considered for treatment modification.
Patient teaching
• Instruct patient to take tenofovir with a meal to enhance bioavailability.
• Tell patient to report adverse effects, including nausea, vomiting, diarrhea, flatulence, and headache.

☑ Evaluation
• Patient complies with therapy regimen.
• Patient has reduced signs and symptoms of infection.
• Patient and family state understanding of drug therapy.

terazosin hydrochloride
(ter-uh-ZOH-sin high-droh-KLOR-ighd)
Hytrin◊

Pharmacologic class: selective alpha$_1$ blocker
Therapeutic class: antihypertensive
Pregnancy risk category: C

Indications and dosages
► **Hypertension.** *Adults:* Initially, 1 mg P.O. h.s., increased gradually based on response. Usual dosage range is 1 to 5 mg daily. Maximum, 20 mg daily.
► **Symptomatic BPH.** *Adults:* Initially, 1 mg P.O. h.s. Dosage increased in stepwise manner to 2 mg, 5 mg, and 10 mg once daily to achieve optimal response. Most patients require 10 mg daily for optimal response.

Contraindications and cautions
• Contraindicated in patients hypersensitive to the drug or any of its components.
❀ **Lifespan:** In pregnant women, use cautiously. In breast-feeding women, use cautiously; it's unknown if the drug appears in breast milk. In children, safety and effectiveness haven't been established.

Adverse reactions
CNS: *asthenia, dizziness, headache,* nervousness, paresthesia, somnolence.
CV: palpitations, orthostatic hypotension, tachycardia, *peripheral edema,* atrial fibrillation.
EENT: nasal congestion, sinusitis, blurred vision.
GI: nausea.
GU: impotence, priapism.
Hematologic: *thrombocytopenia.*
Musculoskeletal: back pain, muscle pain.
Respiratory: dyspnea.
Other: decreased libido.

Interactions
Drug-drug. *Antihypertensives:* May cause excessive hypotension. Use together cautiously. *Clonidine:* May decrease antihypertensive effect of clonidine. Monitor patient.
Drug-herb. *Butcher's broom:* May cause diminished effect. Discourage using together.

Effects on lab test results
• May decrease total protein, albumin, and hemoglobin levels and hematocrit.
• May decrease platelet and WBC counts.

Pharmacokinetics
Absorption: Rapid with about 90% of dose being bioavailable.
Distribution: About 90% to 94% plasma protein–bound.
Metabolism: In liver.
Excretion: About 40% in urine, 60% in feces, mostly as metabolites. Up to 30% may be unchanged. *Half-life:* About 12 hours.

Route	Onset	Peak	Duration
P.O.	≤ 15 min	2–3 hr	24 hr

Action
Chemical effect: Decreases blood pressure by vasodilation produced in response to blockade of alpha$_1$-adrenergic receptors. Improves urine flow by blocking alpha$_1$ receptors in smooth muscle of bladder neck and prostate, thus relieving urethral pressure and reestablishing urine flow.
Therapeutic effect: Lowers blood pressure and relieves symptoms of BPH.

Available forms
Capsules: 1 mg, 2 mg, 5 mg, 10 mg

NURSING PROCESS

☜ Assessment
• Assess patient's condition before starting therapy and regularly thereafter to monitor the drug's effectiveness.
• Assess and monitor patient for prostate cancer, as it may resemble BPH.
• Monitor blood pressure frequently.
• Be alert for adverse reactions and drug interactions.
• Assess patient's and family's knowledge of drug therapy.

T

⊞ Nursing diagnoses
• Risk for injury related to presence of hypertension
• Sexual dysfunction related to drug-induced impotence
• Deficient knowledge related to drug therapy

⊠ Planning and implementation
• Use cautiously with initial dose, and monitor patient—especially elderly patient—for postural hypotension.
ⓈALERT: If drug is stopped for several days, begin again at the initial dose and adjust regimen.
Patient teaching
• Tell patient not to stop drug but to call prescriber if adverse reaction occurs.
• Tell patient to take the first dose at bedtime. If he must get up, he should do so slowly to prevent dizziness or blackouts.
• Warn patient to avoid activities that require mental alertness for 12 hours after first dose.
• Teach patient other means to reduce blood pressure, such as diet control, exercise, smoking cessation, and stress reduction.

☑ Evaluation
• Patient's blood pressure is normal.
• Patient develops and maintains positive attitude toward his sexuality despite impotence.
• Patient and family state understanding of drug therapy.

terbutaline sulfate
(ter-BYOO-tuh-leen SUL-fayt)
Brethine, Bricanyl

Pharmacologic class: beta$_2$ agonist
Therapeutic class: bronchodilator
Pregnancy risk category: B

Indications and dosages

▶ **Bronchospasm in patients with reversible obstructive airway disease.** *Adults and children older than age 15:* Initially, 2.5 mg P.O. t.i.d. or q.i.d. Increase to 5 mg P.O. t.i.d. at 6-hour intervals while awake. Maximum, 15 mg daily. Or, 0.25 mg subcutaneously. May repeat in 15 to 30 minutes. Maximum, 0.5 mg q 4 hours.
Children ages 12 to 15: 2.5 mg P.O. t.i.d. Maximum, 7.5 mg daily.

▶ **Premature labor‡.** *Adults:* Initially, 2.5 to 10 mcg/minute I.V.; increase dose gradually as tolerated in 10- to 20-minute intervals until desired effects are achieved. Maximum dosages range from 17.5 to 30 mcg/minute, although dosages of up to 80 mcg/minute have been used cautiously. Continue infusion for at least 12 hours after uterine contractions stop. Maintenance therapy, 2.5 to 10 mg P.O. q 4 to 6 hours.

▽ I.V. administration
• Protect injection from light. If discolored, don't use.
• Monitor uterine response, maternal blood pressure, and maternal and fetal heart rates. Also monitor patient for circulatory overload and pulmonary edema.
⊗ **Incompatibilities**
Bleomycin.

Contraindications and cautions
• Contraindicated in patients hypersensitive to the drug or any of its components, or to sympathomimetic amines.
• Use cautiously in patient with CV disorders, hyperthyroidism, diabetes, or seizure disorders.
≋ **Lifespan:** In pregnant women, use cautiously. In breast-feeding women, use cautiously; it's unknown if the drug appears in breast milk. In children age 11 and younger, safety and effectiveness haven't been established.

Adverse reactions
CNS: nervousness, tremor, headache, drowsiness, dizziness, weakness.
CV: *palpitations,* tachycardia, *arrhythmias,* flushing, hypertension, chest discomfort.
EENT: tinnitus.
GI: *vomiting,* nausea, heartburn.
Metabolic: hypokalemia.
Respiratory: *paradoxical bronchospasm,* dyspnea.
Skin: diaphoresis.

Interactions
Drug-drug. *CNS stimulants:* May increase CNS stimulation. Avoid use together.
Cyclopropane, digoxin, halogenated inhaled anesthetics, levodopa: May increase risk of arrhythmias. Monitor patient closely.
MAO inhibitors: May cause severe hypertension (hypertensive crisis). Don't use together.

Reactions may be *common,* uncommon, *life-threatening,* or COMMON AND LIFE-THREATENING.

Propranolol, other beta blockers: May block bronchodilating effects of terbutaline. Avoid use together.
Sympathomimetics: May cause additive cardiovascular effects. Avoid use together.
Theophylline derivatives: May increase risk of cardiotoxic effects. Avoid use together.

Effects on lab test results

• May increase liver enzyme levels. May decrease potassium level.

Pharmacokinetics

Absorption: 33% to 50% of P.O. dose; unknown for subcutaneous
Distribution: Widely distributed throughout body.
Metabolism: Partially metabolized in liver to inactive compounds.
Excretion: Excreted primarily in urine. *Half-life:* Unknown.

Route	Onset	Peak	Duration
P.O.	30 min	2–3 hr	4–8 hr
SubQ	≤ 15 min	30–60 min	1½–4 hr

Action

Chemical effect: Relaxes bronchial smooth muscle by acting on beta$_2$-adrenergic receptors.
Therapeutic effect: Improves breathing ability.

Available forms

Injection: 1 mg/ml
Tablets: 2.5 mg, 5 mg

NURSING PROCESS

🔖 Assessment

• Assess patient's condition before starting therapy and regularly thereafter to monitor the drug's effectiveness.
• Monitor patient closely for toxicity.
• Assess patient's and family's knowledge of drug therapy.

🔲 Nursing diagnoses

• Ineffective breathing pattern related to underlying respiratory condition
• Pain related to drug-induced headache
• Deficient knowledge related to drug therapy

🔳 Planning and implementation

• For subcutaneous administration, inject in lateral deltoid area.
• If bronchospasm develops during therapy, notify prescriber immediately.
• Mild analgesic may be used to treat drug-induced headache.
⑨ ALERT: Don't confuse terbutaline with tolbutamide or terbinafine.
Patient teaching
• Explain to patient and family why drug is needed.
• Instruct patient to report paradoxical bronchospasm, and tell him to stop drug if it happens.
• Warn patient that tolerance may develop with prolonged use.

🔳 Evaluation

• Patient's breathing is improved.
• Patient's headache is relieved with mild analgesic.
• Patient and family state understanding of drug therapy.

teriparatide (rDNA origin)
(tehr-ih-PAHR-uh-tyd)
Forteo

Pharmacologic class: recombinant human parathyroid hormone (PTH)
Therapeutic class: antiosteoporotic
Pregnancy risk category: C

Indications and dosages

▶ **Osteoporosis in postmenopausal women at high risk for fracture; to increase bone mass in men with primary or hypogonadal osteoporosis who are at high risk for fracture.**
Adults: 20 mcg subcutaneously in thigh or abdominal wall once daily.

Contraindications and cautions

• Contraindicated in patients hypersensitive to the drug or any of its components. Don't give to patients who have had radiation to the skeleton, those with Paget's disease or unexplained alkaline phosphatase elevations, or those at increased risk for osteosarcoma, such as children. Don't give drug to patients with bone metastases, a history of skeletal malignancies, or metabolic bone diseases other than osteoporosis. Avoid use in patients with hypercalcemia or primary hyperparathyroidism. Don't continue therapy beyond 2 years.

• Use cautiously in patients with active or recent urolithiasis and in patients with hepatic, renal, or cardiac disease.

⚝ **Lifespan:** In pregnant and breast-feeding women, drug isn't recommended. In children, safety and effectiveness haven't been established.

Adverse reactions

CNS: asthenia, depression, dizziness, headache, insomnia, syncope, vertigo, *pain.*
CV: angina pectoris, hypertension, orthostatic hypotension.
EENT: pharyngitis, rhinitis.
GI: constipation, diarrhea, dyspepsia, nausea, tooth disorder, vomiting.
Metabolic: hypercalcemia.
Musculoskeletal: *arthralgia,* leg cramps, neck pain.
Respiratory: dyspnea, cough, pneumonia.
Skin: rash, sweating.

Interactions

Drug-drug. *Calcium supplements:* May increase urinary calcium excretion. Dosage may need adjustment.
Digoxin: Hypercalcemia may predispose patient to digitalis toxicity. Use together cautiously.

Effects on lab test results

• May increase calcium and uric acid levels. May decrease phosphorus level.
• May increase urinary calcium and phosphorus excretion.

Pharmacokinetics

Absorption: Rapid and extensive, with level peaking after about 30 minutes. Availability is about 95%.
Distribution: Unknown.
Metabolism: Unknown for drug, but PTH is metabolized in the liver.
Excretion: Unknown for drug, but PTH is excreted by the kidneys. Elimination is rapid.
Half-life: 1 hour.

Route	Onset	Peak	Duration
SubQ	Rapid	30 min	3 hr

Action

Chemical effect: Regulates calcium and phosphorus metabolism in bones and kidneys, increases calcium, and decreases phosphorus levels.
Therapeutic effect: Decreases risk of fractures in patients with osteoporosis.

Available forms

Injection: 750 mcg/3 ml in a prefilled pen

NURSING PROCESS

⚎ Assessment

⚠ **ALERT:** Because of the risk of osteosarcoma, give drug only to patient for whom benefits outweigh risks.
• If patient could have urolithiasis or hypercalciuria, measure urinary calcium excretion before therapy.
• Assess patient's and family's knowledge of drug therapy.

⚎ Nursing diagnoses

• Risk for falls related to presence of osteoporosis
• Chronic pain related to adverse drug effects
• Deficient knowledge related to drug therapy

⚎ Planning and implementation

• Monitor patient for orthostatic hypotension, which may occur within 4 hours of dosing.
• Track calcium levels. If patient develops persistent hypercalcemia, stop drug and evaluate its possible cause.
• Safety and effectiveness haven't been established for use beyond 2 years.
Patient teaching
• Instruct patient on the proper use and disposal of the prefilled pen.
• Tell patient not to share pen with others.
• Advise patient to sit or lie down if drug causes a fast heart beat, light-headedness, or dizziness. Tell patient to report persistent or worsening symptoms.
• Instruct patient to report persistent symptoms of hypercalcemia (nausea, vomiting, constipation, lethargy, and muscle weakness).

⚎ Evaluation

• Patient doesn't fall.
• Patient reports no pain or states that pain is controlled by therapy.

Reactions may be *common,* uncommon, *life-threatening*, or COMMON AND LIFE-THREATENING.

• Patient and family state understanding of drug therapy.

testolactone
(tes-tuh-LAK-tohn)
Teslac

Pharmacologic class: aromatase inhibitor
Therapeutic class: antineoplastic
Pregnancy risk category: C
Controlled substance schedule: III

Indications and dosages

▶ **Advanced postmenopausal breast cancer.**
Women: 250 mg P.O. q.i.d. Some patients may benefit from 2 g per day. Therapy should continue for at least 3 months unless disease actively progresses.

Contraindications and cautions

• Contraindicated in patients hypersensitive to the drug or any of its components, and in men with breast cancer.
⚖ **Lifespan:** In pregnant women, use cautiously. In breast-feeding women, drug isn't recommended. In children, drug isn't indicated.

Adverse reactions

CNS: paresthesia, peripheral neuropathy.
CV: increased blood pressure, edema.
GI: nausea, vomiting, diarrhea, anorexia, glossitis.
Skin: erythema, nail changes, alopecia.
Other: hot flashes.

Interactions

Drug-drug. *Oral anticoagulants:* May increase pharmacologic effects. Monitor patient carefully.

Effects on lab test results

• May decrease estradiol levels. May increase plasma calcium levels.
• May increase 24-hour urinary excretion of creatine.

Pharmacokinetics

Absorption: Good.
Distribution: Widely distributed in total body water.
Metabolism: Extensively metabolized in liver.

Excretion: Testolactone and its metabolites excreted primarily in urine. *Half-life:* Unknown.

Route	Onset	Peak	Duration
P.O.	6–12 wk	Unknown	Unknown

Action

Chemical effect: Unknown; may change tumor's hormonal environment and alter neoplastic process.
Therapeutic effect: Hinders breast cancer cell activity.

Available forms

Tablets: 50 mg

NURSING PROCESS

⬚ Assessment
• Assess patient's breast cancer before starting therapy and regularly thereafter to monitor the drug's effectiveness.
• Monitor fluid and electrolyte levels, especially calcium level.
• Assess patient's and family's knowledge of drug therapy.

⬚ Nursing diagnoses
• Ineffective health maintenance related to presence of breast cancer
• Disturbed sensory perception (tactile) related to drug-induced paresthesia and peripheral neuropathy
• Deficient knowledge related to drug therapy

⬚ Planning and implementation
• Encourage patient to drink fluids to aid calcium excretion, and encourage exercise to prevent hypercalcemia. Immobilized patient is prone to hypercalcemia.
• Higher-than-recommended doses don't promote remission.
• Continue therapy for at least 3 months unless disease actively progresses.
Patient teaching
• Inform patient that therapeutic response isn't immediate; it may take up to 3 months for benefit to be noted.
• Encourage patient to exercise and drink plenty of fluids to help prevent hypercalcemia.
• Tell patient to report adverse effects.

T

☑ Evaluation
• Patient responds well to drug.
• Patient lists ways to protect against risk of injury caused by diminished tactile sensation.
• Patient and family state understanding of drug therapy.

testosterone
(tess-TOSS-teh-rohn)
Andronaq-50, Histerone-50, Histerone 100, Testamone 100, Testaqua, Testoject-50

testosterone cypionate
Andronate 100, Andronate 200, depAndro 100, depAndro 200, Depotest, Depo-Testosterone, Duratest-100, Duratest-200, T-Cypionate, Testred Cypionate 200, Virilon IM

testosterone enanthate
Andro L.A. 200, Andropository 200, Andryl 200, Delatest, Delatestryl, Durathate-200, Everone 200, Testrin-P.A.

testosterone propionate
Malogen in Oil◆, Testex

Pharmacologic class: androgen
Therapeutic class: hormone replacement, antineoplastic
Pregnancy risk category: X
Controlled substance schedule: III

Indications and dosages
▶ **Hypogonadism.** *Men:* 10 to 25 mg testosterone I.M. two to three times weekly. Or, 50 to 400 mg testosterone cypionate or testosterone enanthate I.M. q 2 to 4 weeks. Or, 10 to 25 mg testosterone propionate I.M. two to three times weekly. Another alternative is 75 to 150 mg of testosterone cypionate or enanthate I.M. every 7 to 10 days.
▶ **Delayed puberty.** *Boys:* 25 to 50 mg testosterone or testosterone propionate I.M. two or three times weekly for up to 6 months.
▶ **Metastatic breast cancer 1 to 5 years after menopause.** *Women:* 100 mg testosterone I.M. three times weekly. Or, 50 to 100 mg testosterone propionate I.M. three times weekly. Or, 200 to 400 mg testosterone cypionate or testosterone enanthate I.M. q 2 to 4 weeks.

▶ **Postpartum breast pain and engorgement.** *Adults:* 25 to 50 mg testosterone or testosterone propionate I.M. daily for 3 to 4 days.

Contraindications and cautions
• Contraindicated in men with breast or prostate cancer; patients with hypercalcemia; and those with cardiac, hepatic, or renal decompensation.
⚥ Lifespan: In pregnant and breast-feeding women, drug is contraindicated. In children, use cautiously because of risk of accelerated bone maturation leading to short stature. In the elderly, use cautiously.

Adverse reactions
CNS: headache, anxiety, depression, paresthesia, sleep apnea syndrome.
CV: edema.
GI: nausea.
GU: hypoestrogenic effects in women *(acne; edema; oily skin; hirsutism; hoarseness; weight gain;* clitoral enlargement; decreased or increased libido; flushing; diaphoresis; vaginitis, including itching, drying, and burning; vaginal bleeding; menstrual irregularities), excessive hormonal effects in boys and men (prepubertal: premature epiphyseal closure, *acne,* priapism, *growth of body and facial hair,* phallic enlargement; postpubertal: testicular atrophy, oligospermia, decreased ejaculatory volume, impotence, gynecomastia, epididymitis), bladder irritability.
Hematologic: polycythemia, suppression of clotting factors.
Hepatic: reversible jaundice, *cholestatic hepatitis.*
Metabolic: hypercalcemia.
Skin: local edema, hypersensitivity skin signs and symptoms.
Other: pain and induration at injection site.

Interactions
Drug-drug. *Hepatotoxic drugs:* May increase risk of hepatotoxicity. Monitor patient closely.
Insulin, oral antidiabetics: May alter dosage requirements. Monitor glucose level in diabetic patients.
Oral anticoagulants: May alter dosage requirements. Monitor PT and INR.

Effects on lab test results
• May increase sodium, potassium, phosphate, cholesterol, liver enzyme, calcium, and creati-

nine levels. May decrease thyroxine-binding globulin and total T_4 levels.
• May increase RBC count and resin uptake of T_3 and T_4.

Pharmacokinetics

Absorption: Unknown.
Distribution: 98% to 99% protein-bound, primarily to testosterone–estradiol-binding globulin.
Metabolism: In liver.
Excretion: In urine. *Half-life:* 10 to 100 minutes.

Route	Onset	Peak	Duration
I.M.	Unknown	Unknown	Unknown

Action

Chemical effect: Stimulates target tissues to develop normally in androgen-deficient men. Drug may have some antiestrogen properties, making it useful to treat certain estrogen-dependent breast cancers. Its action in postpartum breast engorgement isn't known because drug doesn't suppress lactation.
Therapeutic effect: Increases testosterone level, inhibits some estrogen activity, and relieves postpartum breast pain and engorgement.

Available forms

testosterone
Injection (aqueous suspension): 25 mg/ml, 50 mg/ml, 100 mg/ml
testosterone cypionate
Injection (in oil): 100 mg/ml, 200 mg/ml
testosterone enanthate
Injection (in oil): 200 mg/ml
testosterone propionate
Injection (in oil): 100 mg/ml

NURSING PROCESS

☷ Assessment

• Assess patient's condition before starting therapy and regularly thereafter to monitor the drug's effectiveness.
• Periodically monitor calcium level and liver function test results.
• Monitor hemoglobin and hematocrit for polycythemia.
• Monitor prepubertal boys by X-ray for rate of bone maturation.
• Be alert for adverse reactions and drug interactions.

• Assess patient's and family's knowledge of drug therapy.

☷ Nursing diagnoses

• Ineffective health maintenance related to underlying condition
• Disturbed body image related to drug-induced adverse androgenic reactions
• Deficient knowledge related to drug therapy

❯ Planning and implementation

• Give daily dose requirement in divided doses for best results.
• Store preparations at room temperature. If crystals appear, warm and shake bottle to disperse them.
• Inject deep into upper outer quadrant of gluteal muscle. Rotate sites to prevent muscle atrophy. Report soreness at site because of possibility of postinfection furunculosis.
• Unless contraindicated, use with diet high in calories and protein taken in small, frequent meals.
• Report signs of virilization in woman.
• Edema generally can be controlled with sodium restriction or diuretics.
Ⓢ **ALERT:** Therapeutic response in breast cancer usually appears within 3 months. If signs of disease progression appear, stop giving the drug. In metastatic breast cancer, hypercalcemia usually signals progression of bone metastases. Report signs of hypercalcemia.
• Androgens may alter results of laboratory studies during therapy and for 2 to 3 weeks after therapy ends.
Ⓢ **ALERT:** Testosterone and methyltestosterone aren't interchangeable. Don't confuse testosterone with testolactone.
Patient teaching
• Tell patient to use effective barrier-method contraception during therapy.
• Instruct man to report priapism, reduced ejaculatory volume, and gynecomastia. Drug may need to be stopped.
• Inform woman that virilization may occur. Tell her to report androgenic effects immediately. Stopping drug will prevent further androgenic changes but probably won't reverse those already present.
• Teach patient to recognize and report signs of hypoglycemia.
• Instruct patient to follow dietary measures to combat drug-induced adverse reactions.

✅ Evaluation
- Patient responds well to drug.
- Patient states acceptance of altered body image.
- Patient and family state understanding of drug therapy.

testosterone transdermal system
(tess-TOSS-teh-rohn tranz-DER-mal SIHS-tum)
Androderm, AndroGel, Testim, Testoderm, Testoderm TTS

Pharmacologic class: androgen
Therapeutic class: hormone replacement
Pregnancy risk category: X
Controlled substance schedule: III

Indications and dosages

▶ **Primary or hypogonadotropic hypogonadism.** *Men:* One 6-mg Testoderm patch applied to scrotal area daily. If scrotal area is too small for 6-mg patch, start with 4-mg patch. Patch worn for 22 to 24 hours daily. Or, 5 mg Androderm daily either as two 2.5-mg systems or one 5-mg system applied h.s. to clean, dry skin on back, abdomen, upper arms, or thighs. Or, one 5-mg Testoderm TTS patch applied to arm, back, or upper buttock daily. Or, 5 g, 7.5 g, or 10 g AndroGel applied to upper arms, shoulders, and abdomen daily. Or, 5 or 10 g Testim, applied to upper arms and shoulders daily.

Contraindications and cautions

- Contraindicated in patients hypersensitive to the drug or any of its components, and in patients with known or suspected breast or prostate cancer.
- Use cautiously in patients with renal, hepatic, or cardiac disease.
- ☀ **Lifespan:** In women, drug is contraindicated. In children, drug isn't indicated. In elderly men, use cautiously because they may be at greater risk for prostatic hyperplasia or prostate cancer.

Adverse reactions

CV: *stroke,* headache, depression.
GI: *GI bleeding.*
GU: prostatitis, prostate abnormalities, UTI.

Skin: acne, *pruritus,* irritation, *blister under system,* allergic contact dermatitis; burning, induration (at application site).
Other: gynecomastia, breast tenderness.

Interactions

Drug-drug. *Antidiabetics:* May alter antidiabetic dosage requirements. Monitor glucose level.
Oral anticoagulants: May alter anticoagulant dosage requirements. Monitor PT and INR.
Oxyphenbutazone: May elevate oxyphenbutazone levels. Monitor patient for adverse reactions.

Effects on lab test results

- May increase sodium, potassium, phosphate, cholesterol, liver enzyme, calcium, and creatinine levels.
- May increase RBC count.

Pharmacokinetics

Absorption: Absorbed from scrotal skin after application.
Distribution: Chiefly bound to sex–hormone-binding globulin.
Metabolism: Metabolized in liver.
Excretion: Excreted in urine. *Half-life:* 10 to 100 minutes.

Route	Onset	Peak	Duration
Transdermal	Unknown	2–4 hr	2 hr after removal

Action

Chemical effect: Stimulates target tissues to develop normally in androgen-deficient men.
Therapeutic effect: Increases testosterone in androgen-deficient men.

Available forms

Transdermal system: 2.5 mg/day, 4 mg/day, 5 mg/day, 6 mg/day
1% gel: 2.5 g and 5 g packets, 75 g nonaerosol metered pump, 5 g tube

NURSING PROCESS

📋 Assessment
- Assess patient's condition before starting therapy and regularly thereafter to monitor the drug's effectiveness.
- Because long-term use of systemic androgens is linked to polycythemia, monitor hematocrit

and hemoglobin values periodically in patient on long-term therapy.
• Periodically assess liver function tests, lipid profiles, and prostatic acid phosphatase and prostate-specific antigen levels.
• Be alert for adverse reactions and drug interactions.
• Assess patient's and family's knowledge of drug therapy.

⊞ Nursing diagnoses
• Sexual dysfunction related to androgen deficiency
• Risk for impaired skin integrity related to drug-induced irritation at application site
• Deficient knowledge related to drug therapy

⊠ Planning and implementation
• Apply Testoderm system on clean, dry scrotal skin. Dry shave scrotal hair (don't use chemical depilatories).
• Apply Androderm to clean, dry skin on back, abdomen, upper arms, or thighs.
• Apply Testoderm TTS to clean, dry skin on arm, back, or upper buttock.
🟀 **ALERT:** Don't confuse Testoderm with Estraderm.
• Apply gel by rubbing entire dose into skin, then don't allow patient to bathe for 2 to 6 hours.
Patient teaching
• Teach patient how to apply transdermal system.
• Tell patient to fully prime the AndroGel pump by depressing the pumping mechanism three times before first use and discarding that portion. For 5 g dose, he should pump 5 times, for 7.5 g, 6 times, and for 10 g, 8 times. The gel can be pumped into the palm of the hand then applied to application sites.
• Tell patient that topical testosterone preparations can cause virilization in women sexual partners. Advise these women to report acne or changes in body hair. Tell patient to wear a shirt during close physical contact or to wash site if applied within 2 to 6 hours of contact.
• Advise patient to report to prescriber persistent erections, nausea, vomiting, changes in skin color, or ankle edema.

🗹 Evaluation
• Patient states that he can resume normal sexual activity.

• Patient maintains normal skin integrity.
• Patient and family state understanding of drug therapy.

tetanus immune globulin, human
(TET-nuss ih-MYOON GLOH-byoo-lin)
BayTet

Pharmacologic class: immune serum
Therapeutic class: tetanus prophylaxis
Pregnancy risk category: C

Indications and dosages
▶ **Tetanus exposure.** *Adults and children age 7 and older:* 250 units I.M.
Children younger than age 7: 4 units/kg I.M.
▶ **Tetanus.** *Adults and children:* Single doses of 3,000 to 6,000 units I.M. Optimal dosage hasn't been established.

Contraindications and cautions
• In patients with thrombocytopenia or coagulation disorders, I.M. injection is contraindicated unless potential benefits outweigh risks.
🌣 **Lifespan:** In pregnant women, use cautiously. In breast-feeding women, use cautiously; it's unknown if the drug appears in breast milk.

Adverse reactions
GU: slight fever, nephrotic syndrome.
Other: hypersensitivity reactions; *anaphylaxis; angioedema;* pain, stiffness, erythema at injection site.

Interactions
Drug-drug. *Live-virus vaccines:* May interfere with response. Defer administration of live-virus vaccines for 3 months after administration of tetanus immune globulin.
Measles, mumps, rubella, and varicella vaccines: Tetanus antibodies may interfere with immune response. Separate vaccines by 3 months.

Effects on lab test results
None reported.

Pharmacokinetics
Absorption: Slow.
Distribution: Unknown.

T

Metabolism: Unknown.
Excretion: Unknown. *Half-life:* About 28 days.

Route	Onset	Peak	Duration
I.M.	Unknown	2–3 days	4 wk

Action

Chemical effect: Provides passive immunity to tetanus.
Therapeutic effect: Prevents tetanus.

Available forms

Injection: 250 units per vial or syringe

NURSING PROCESS

⚖ Assessment
• Obtain history of injury, tetanus immunizations, last tetanus toxoid injection, allergies, and reaction to immunizations.
• Antibodies remain at effective level for about 4 weeks (several times the duration of antitoxin-induced antibodies), which protects patient for incubation period of most tetanus cases.
• Be alert for adverse reactions and drug interactions.
• Assess patient's and family's knowledge of drug therapy.

⊕ Nursing diagnoses
• Risk for injury related to potential for tetanus to occur
• Deficient knowledge related to drug therapy

≥ Planning and implementation
⑤ **ALERT:** Have epinephrine 1:1,000 available to treat hypersensitivity reactions.
• Use drug if wound is more than 24 hours old or if patient has had fewer than two tetanus toxoid injections.
• Keep drug refrigerated.
• Thoroughly clean wound and remove all foreign matter.
• Inject drug into deltoid muscle for adult or child age 3 and older and into anterolateral aspect of thigh in neonate or child younger than age 3.
⑤ **ALERT:** Don't confuse drug with tetanus toxoid. Tetanus immune globulin isn't a substitute for tetanus toxoid, which should be given at same time to produce active immunization. Don't give at same site as toxoid.

Patient teaching
• Warn patient that pain and tenderness at injection site may occur. Suggest mild analgesic for pain relief.
• Tell patient to document date of tetanus immunization, and encourage him to keep immunization current.

☑ Evaluation
• Patient doesn't develop tetanus.
• Patient and family state understanding of drug therapy.

tetracycline hydrochloride
(tet-ruh-SIGH-kleen high-droh-KLOR-ighd)
Achromycin†, Apo-Tetra ◆, Novo-Tetra ◆, Nu-Tetra ◆, Sumycin, Tetrex ◇, Topicycline

Pharmacologic class: tetracycline
Therapeutic class: antibiotic
Pregnancy risk category: D

Indications and dosages

▶ **Infections caused by sensitive gram-negative and gram-positive organisms, including *Chlamydia, Mycoplasma, Rickettsia*, and organisms that cause trachoma.** *Adults:* 1 to 2 g P.O. divided into two to four doses for 10-14 days.
Children older than age 8: 25 to 50 mg/kg P.O. daily divided into four doses.
▶ **Uncomplicated urethral, endocervical, or rectal infection caused by *Chlamydia trachomatis*.** *Adults:* 500 mg P.O. q.i.d. for at least 7 days.
▶ **Brucellosis.** *Adults:* 500 mg P.O. q 6 hours for 3 weeks combined with 1 g of streptomycin I.M. q 12 hours first week and daily the second week.
▶ **Gonorrhea in patients sensitive to penicillin.** *Adults:* Initially, 1.5 g P.O.; then 500 mg q 6 hours for 4 days.
▶ **Syphilis in nonpregnant patients sensitive to penicillin.** *Adults:* 500 mg P.O. q.i.d. for 15 days.
▶ **Acne.** *Adults and adolescents:* Initially, 125 to 250 mg P.O. q 6 hours; then 125 to 500 mg daily or q other day. Or, apply 3% ointment or 2.2% solution to affected areas daily or b.i.d.

▶ **Lyme disease‡.** *Adults:* 250 to 500 mg P.O. q.i.d. for 10 to 30 days.
▶ **Adjunct therapy for acute transmitted epididymitis (children older than age 8); pelvic inflammatory disease; and infection with** *Helicobacter pylori‡. Adults:* 500 mg P.O. q.i.d. for 10 to 14 days.
▶ **Malaria.‡** *Adults:* 250 mg P.O. q.i.d. for 7 days with quinine sulfate.
Children older than age 8: 25 mg/kg daily in 4 divided doses for 7 days with quinine sulfate.

Contraindications and cautions

• Contraindicated in patients hypersensitive to tetracyclines.
• Use cautiously in patients with impaired kidney or liver function.
❧ **Lifespan:** In women in the last half of pregnancy and in children younger than age 8, use cautiously, if at all, because drug may cause permanent discoloration of teeth, enamel defects, and bone-growth retardation. In breast-feeding women, drug isn't recommended.

Adverse reactions

CNS: dizziness, headache, *intracranial hypertension (pseudotumor cerebri).*
CV: *pericarditis.*
EENT: sore throat, glossitis, dysphagia.
GI: anorexia, *epigastric distress, nausea,* vomiting, *diarrhea,* esophagitis, oral candidiasis, stomatitis, enterocolitis, inflammatory lesions in anogenital region.
Hematologic: *neutropenia, thrombocytopenia,* eosinophilia.
Musculoskeletal: retardation of bone growth if used in children younger than age 9.
Skin: *candidal superinfection,* maculopapular and erythematous rashes, urticaria, photosensitivity reactions, increased pigmentation.
Other: permanent discoloration of teeth, enamel defects, *hypersensitivity reactions.*

Interactions

Drug-drug. *Antacids (including sodium bicarbonate); antidiarrheals containing bismuth subsalicylate, kaolin, or pectin; laxatives containing aluminum, calcium, or magnesium:* May decrease antibiotic absorption. Give tetracyclines 1 hour before or 2 hours after these drugs.
Ferrous sulfate, other iron products, zinc: May decrease antibiotic absorption. Give tetracyclines 2 hours before or 3 hours after iron.

Hormonal contraceptives: May decrease contraceptive effectiveness and increase risk of breakthrough bleeding. Recommend nonhormonal form of birth control.
Lithium carbonate: May alter lithium level. Monitor patient.
Methoxyflurane: May cause severe nephrotoxicity with tetracyclines. Monitor patient carefully.
Oral anticoagulants: May potentiate anticoagulant effects. Monitor PT and adjust anticoagulant dosage.
Penicillins: May interfere with bactericidal action of penicillins. Avoid using together.
Drug-food. *Milk, dairy products, other foods:* May decrease drug absorption. Give drug 1 hour before or 2 hours after these products.
Drug-lifestyle. *Sun exposure:* May cause photosensitivity reactions. Urge patient to avoid prolonged or unprotected exposure to sunlight.

Effects on lab test results

• May increase BUN and liver enzyme levels.
• May increase eosinophil count. May decrease platelet and neutrophil counts.
• May cause false-negative reading with glucose enzymatic tests (Diastix).

Pharmacokinetics

Absorption: 75% to 80%. Food or milk products significantly reduces.
Distribution: Distributed widely in body tissues and fluids. CSF penetration is poor. Drug is 20% to 67% protein-bound.
Metabolism: None.
Excretion: Excreted primarily unchanged in urine. *Half-life:* 6 to 11 hours.

Route	Onset	Peak	Duration
P.O.	Unknown	2–4 hr	Unknown

Action

Chemical effect: Unknown; may act by binding to 30S ribosomal subunit of microorganisms, thus inhibiting protein synthesis.
Therapeutic effect: Hinders bacterial activity.

Available forms

Capsules: 250 mg, 500 mg
Ointment†: 3%
Oral suspension: 125 mg/5 ml
Topical solution: 2.2 mg/ml

T

NURSING PROCESS

⚙ Assessment
• Assess patient's infection before starting therapy and regularly thereafter to monitor the drug's effectiveness.
• Obtain specimen for culture and sensitivity tests before giving the first dose. Start therapy pending test results.
• If adverse GI reaction occurs, monitor hydration.
• Be alert for adverse reactions and drug interactions.
• Assess patient's and family's knowledge of drug therapy.

⚙ Nursing diagnoses
• Risk for infection related to presence of susceptible bacteria
• Risk for deficient fluid volume related to drug-induced adverse GI reactions
• Deficient knowledge related to drug therapy

⚙ Planning and implementation
ⓘ **ALERT:** Check expiration date. Outdated or deteriorated tetracyclines have been linked to reversible nephrotoxicity (Fanconi's syndrome).
• Give drug on empty stomach.
• Don't expose drug to light or heat.
Patient teaching
• Tell patient to take drug with full glass of water on empty stomach, at least 1 hour before or 2 hours after meals. Also, tell him to take drug at least 1 hour before bedtime to prevent esophagitis. Explain that effectiveness of drug is reduced when taken with milk or other dairy products, food, antacids, or iron products.
• Tell patient to take drug exactly as prescribed, even after he feels better, and to take entire amount prescribed.
• Warn patient to avoid direct sunlight and ultraviolet light. Recommend sunscreen to help prevent photosensitivity reactions. Tell him that photosensitivity persists after drug is stopped.
• Advise patient that topical forms of the drug may stain skin and clothing.
• Tell patient using topical preparation to wash, rinse, and thoroughly dry the affected area before applying the drug. Also, advise him to avoid getting it in his eyes, nose, mouth, or other mucous membranes.

☑ Evaluation
• Patient is free from infection.
• Patient maintains adequate hydration.
• Patient and family state understanding of drug therapy.

theophylline
(thee-OFF-ih-lin)
Immediate-release liquids
Accurbron*, Aquaphyllin, Asmalix*, Bronkodyl*, Elixomin*, Elixophyllin*, Lanophyllin*, Slo-Phyllin, Theolair

Immediate-release tablets and capsules
Bronkodyl, Elixophyllin, Nuelin◇, Slo-Phyllin

Timed-release capsules
Elixophyllin SR, Nuelin-SR◇, Slo-bid Gyrocaps, Slo-Phyllin, Theo-24, Theobid Duracaps, Theochron, Theospan-SR, Theovent Long-Acting

Timed-release tablets
Quibron-T/SR Dividose, Respbid, Sustaire, T-Phyl, Theochron, Theolair-SR, Theo-Sav, Theo-Time, Theo-X, Uniphyl

theophylline sodium glycinate

Pharmacologic class: xanthine derivative
Therapeutic class: bronchodilator
Pregnancy risk category: C

Indications and dosages

▶ **Oral theophylline for acute bronchospasm in patients not already receiving theophylline.** *Adults (nonsmokers):* Loading dose of 6 mg/kg P.O.; then 3 mg/kg q 6 hours for two doses. Maintenance dosage is 3 mg/kg q 8 hours.
Children ages 9 to 16 and young adult smokers: Loading dose of 6 mg/kg P.O.; then 3 mg/kg q 4 hours for three doses; then 3 mg/kg q 6 hours.
Children ages 6 months to 9 years: Loading dose of 6 mg/kg P.O.; then 4 mg/kg q 4 hours for three doses; then 4 mg/kg q 6 hours.
Older adults or those with cor pulmonale: Loading dose of 6 mg/kg P.O.; then 2 mg/kg q 6 hours for two doses; then 2 mg/kg q 8 hours.

Reactions may be *common*, uncommon, *life-threatening*, or COMMON AND LIFE-THREATENING.

§ **Adjust-a-dose:** For adults with heart failure or liver disease, give loading dose of 6 mg/kg P.O.; then 2 mg/kg q 8 hours for two doses; then 1 to 2 mg/kg q 12 hours.

▶ **Parenteral theophylline for patients not receiving theophylline.** *Adults (nonsmokers):* Loading dose of 4.7 mg/kg given slow I.V.; then maintenance infusion of 0.55 mg/kg/hour I.V. for 12 hours; then 0.39 mg/kg/hour.

Adults (otherwise healthy smokers): Loading dose of 4.7 mg/kg given slow I.V.; then maintenance infusion of 0.79 mg/kg/hour I.V. for 12 hours; then 0.63 mg/kg/hour.

Older adults or those with cor pulmonale: Loading dose of 4.7 mg/kg given slow I.V.; then maintenance infusion of 0.47 mg/kg/hour I.V. for 12 hours; then 0.24 mg/kg/hour.

Adults with heart failure or liver disease: Loading dose of 4.7 mg/kg given slow I.V.; then maintenance infusion of 0.39 mg/kg/hour I.V. for 12 hours; then 0.08 to 0.16 mg/kg/hour.

Children ages 9 to 16: Loading dose of 4.7 mg/kg given slow I.V.; then maintenance infusion of 0.79 mg/kg/hour I.V. for 12 hours; then 0.63 mg/kg/hour.

Children ages 6 months to 9 years: Loading dose of 4.7 mg/kg given slow I.V.; then maintenance infusion of 0.95 mg/kg/hour I.V. for 12 hours; then 0.79 mg/kg/hour.

▶ **Oral and parenteral theophylline for acute bronchospasm in patients receiving theophylline.** *Adults and children:* Each 0.5 mg/kg I.V. or P.O. (loading dose) increases plasma level by 1 mcg/ml. Ideally, dose is based on current theophylline level. In emergencies, some clinicians recommend 2.5 mg/kg P.O. dose of rapidly absorbed form if no obvious signs of theophylline toxicity are present.

▶ **Chronic bronchospasm.** *Adults and children:* 16 mg/kg or 400 mg P.O. daily (whichever is less) given in three or four divided doses at 6- to 8-hour intervals. Or, 12 mg/kg or 400 mg P.O. daily (whichever is less) using extended-release preparation given in two or three divided doses at 8- or 12-hour intervals. Dosage increased as tolerated at 2- to 3-day intervals to maximum dosage as follows:

Adults and children age 16 and older: 13 mg/kg or 900 mg P.O. daily (whichever is less) in divided doses.

Children ages 12 to 16: 18 mg/kg P.O. daily in divided doses.

Children ages 9 to 12: 20 mg/kg P.O. daily in divided doses.

Children ages 1 to 9: 24 mg/kg P.O. daily in divided doses.

Children younger than age 1 ‡*:* Loading dose is 1 mg/kg P.O. or I.V. for each 2-mcg/ml increase in theophylline level desired. Maintenance dosage for premature neonates up to 40 weeks postconception age is 1 mg/kg q 12 hours. Maintenance dosage for term neonates up to age 4 weeks is 1 to 2 mg/kg q 12 hours; 1 to 2 mg/kg q 8 hours in those age 4 to 8 weeks; and 1 to 3 mg/kg q 6 hours in those older than age 8 weeks.

▶ **Cystic fibrosis** ‡. *Infants:* 10 to 20 mg/kg I.V. daily.

▶ **Promotion of diuresis; Cheyne-Stokes respirations; paroxysmal nocturnal dyspnea** ‡. *Adults:* 200 to 400 mg I.V. bolus as a single dose.

▼ I.V. administration

● Use commercially available infusion solution, or mix drug in D_5W.
● Use infusion pump for continuous infusion.
⊗ **Incompatibilities**
Ascorbic acid, ceftriaxone, cimetidine, hetastarch, phenytoin.

Contraindications and cautions

● Contraindicated in patients with active peptic ulcer or seizure disorders and in those who are hypersensitive to xanthine compounds (caffeine, theobromine).
● Don't use extended-release forms for acute bronchospasm.
● Use cautiously in patients with COPD, cardiac failure, cor pulmonale, cardiac arrhythmias, renal or hepatic disease, peptic ulceration, hyperthyroidism, diabetes mellitus, glaucoma, severe hypoxemia, hypertension, compromised cardiac or circulatory function, angina, acute MI, or sulfite sensitivity.
❧ **Lifespan:** In pregnant women, use cautiously. In breast-feeding women, use is discouraged; infants of breast-feeding women may exhibit irritability, insomnia, or fretting. In young children, infants, neonates, and the elderly, use cautiously.

Adverse reactions

CNS: *restlessness, dizziness,* headache, *insomnia,* irritability, *seizures,* muscle twitching.

CV: palpitations, sinus tachycardia, extrasystoles, flushing, *marked hypotension, arrhythmias.*
GI: *nausea, vomiting,* diarrhea, epigastric pain.
Respiratory: increased respiratory rate, *respiratory arrest.*

Interactions

Drug-drug. *Adenosine:* May decrease antiarrhythmic effectiveness. Higher doses of adenosine may be needed.
Allopurinol, cimetidine, fluoroquinolones (such as ciprofloxacin), influenza virus vaccine, macrolide antibiotics (such as erythromycin), hormonal contraceptives: May decrease hepatic clearance of theophylline and elevate theophylline level. Monitor patient for toxicity.
Barbiturates, carbamazepine, phenytoin, rifampin: May enhance metabolism and decrease theophylline blood level. Monitor patient for decreased effect.
Carteolol, pindolol, propranolol, timolol: May act antagonistically, reducing the effects of one or both drugs. The elimination of theophylline may also be reduced. Monitor theophylline level and patient closely.
Nadolol: May antagonize drug; may cause bronchospasm in sensitive patients. Use together cautiously.
Drug-herb. *Cacao tree:* May inhibit drug metabolism. Discourage use together.
Cayenne: May increase drug absorption. Discourage use together.
St. John's wort: May decrease drug effectiveness. Discourage use together.
Drug-food. *Any food:* May accelerate absorption. Give drug on an empty stomach.
Caffeine: May decrease hepatic clearance of theophylline and elevate theophylline level. Monitor patient for toxicity.
Drug-lifestyle. *Smoking:* May increase drug elimination, increasing dosage requirements. Monitor drug response and level.

Effects on lab test results

• May increase free fatty acid level.

Pharmacokinetics

Absorption: Well absorbed. Food may further alter rate of absorption, especially of some extended-release preparations.
Distribution: Distributed throughout extracellular fluids; approximately 50% protein bound,

equilibrium between fluid and tissues occurs within 1 hour of I.V. loading dose.
Metabolism: In liver to inactive compounds.
Excretion: About 10% excreted unchanged in urine. *Half-life:* Adults, 7 to 9 hours; smokers, 4 to 5 hours; children, 3 to 5 hours; premature infants, 20 to 30 hours.

Route	Onset	Peak	Duration
P.O.			
regular	15–60 min	1–2 hr	Unknown
enteric-coated	15–60 min	1–2 hr	5 hr
extended-release	15–60 min	1–2 hr	4–7 hr
I.V.	15 min	15–30 min	Unknown

Action

Chemical effect: Inhibits phosphodiesterase, the enzyme that degrades cAMP, and relaxes smooth muscle of bronchial airways and pulmonary blood vessels.
Therapeutic effect: Improves breathing ability.

Available forms

theophylline
Capsules: 100 mg, 200 mg
Capsules (extended-release): 50 mg, 60 mg, 65 mg, 75 mg, 100 mg, 125 mg, 130 mg, 200 mg, 250 mg, 260 mg, 300 mg
D₅W injection: 200 mg in 50 ml or 100 ml; 400 mg in 100 ml, 250 ml, 500 ml, or 1,000 ml; 800 mg in 500 ml or 1,000 ml
Elixir: 27 mg/5 ml, 50 mg/5 ml*
Oral solution: 27 mg/5 ml, 50 mg/5 ml
Syrup: 27 mg/5 ml, 50 mg/5 ml
Tablets: 100 mg, 125 mg, 200 mg, 250 mg, 300 mg
Tablets (chewable): 100 mg
Tablets (extended-release): 100 mg, 200 mg, 250 mg, 300 mg, 400 mg, 500 mg, 600 mg
theophylline sodium glycinate
Elixir: 110 mg/5 ml (equivalent to 55 mg of anhydrous theophylline/5 ml)

NURSING PROCESS

✍ Assessment

• Assess patient's condition before starting therapy and regularly thereafter to monitor the drug's effectiveness.

• Monitor vital signs; measure fluid intake and output. Expect effects such as improvement in quality of pulse and respirations.

• Metabolism rate varies among individuals; dosage is determined by monitoring response, tolerance, pulmonary function, and drug level. Therapeutic level is 10 to 20 mcg/ml in adults and 5 to 15 mcg/ml in children.

• Be alert for adverse reactions and drug interactions.

⊛ **ALERT:** Monitor patient for signs and symptoms of toxicity, including tachycardia, anorexia, nausea, vomiting, diarrhea, restlessness, irritability, and headache. The presence of any of these signs or symptoms in a patient taking theophylline warrants checking theophylline level and adjusting dose as indicated.

• If adverse GI reaction occurs, monitor hydration.

• Assess patient's and family's knowledge of drug therapy.

🔠 **Nursing diagnoses**
• Impaired gas exchange related to presence of bronchospasm
• Risk for deficient fluid volume related to drug-induced adverse GI reactions
• Deficient knowledge related to drug therapy

▨ **Planning and implementation**
• Give oral drug around the clock, using sustained-release product at bedtime.

⊛ **ALERT:** Don't confuse sustained-release form with standard-release form.

• Dose may need to be increased in a cigarette smoker or a habitual marijuana smoker; smoking causes drug to be metabolized faster.

• Daily dose may need to be decreased in a patient with heart failure or hepatic disease, or in a geriatric patient, because metabolism and excretion may be decreased.

⊛ **ALERT:** Don't confuse Theolair with Thyrolar.

Patient teaching
• Instruct patient not to dissolve, crush, or chew sustained-release products. For child unable to swallow capsules, sprinkle contents of capsules over soft food and tell patient to swallow without chewing.

• Supply instructions for home care and dosage schedule.

• Tell patient to relieve GI symptoms by taking oral drug with full glass of water after meals, although food in stomach delays absorption.

• Instruct patient to take drug regularly, as directed.

• Inform geriatric patient that dizziness may occur at start of therapy.

• Have patient change position slowly and avoid hazardous activities.

• Tell patient to check with prescriber before taking other drugs, including OTC drugs. OTC drugs may contain ephedrine with theophylline salts; excessive CNS stimulation may result.

• If patient's dose is stabilized while he is smoking and he then quits smoking, tell him to notify his prescriber; the dose may need to be reduced.

☑ **Evaluation**
• Patient demonstrates improved gas exchange, exhibited in arterial blood gas values and respiratory status.
• Patient maintains adequate hydration.
• Patient and family state understanding of drug therapy.

thiamine hydrochloride (vitamin B₁)
(THIGH-eh-min high-droh-KLOR-ighd)
Betamin◇, Beta-Sol◇, Biamine, Thiamilate†

Pharmacologic class: water-soluble vitamin
Therapeutic class: nutritional supplement
Pregnancy risk category: A

Indications and dosages
▶ **RDA.** *Men age 19 and older:* 1.2 mg P.O. daily.
Boys ages 14 to 18: 1.2 mg P.O. daily.
Women age 19 and older: 1.1 mg P.O. daily.
Girls ages 14 to 18: 1 mg P.O. daily.
Pregnant women: 1.4 mg P.O. daily.
Breast-feeding women: 1.5 mg P.O. daily.
Children ages 9 to 13: 0.9 mg P.O. daily.
Children ages 4 to 8: 0.6 mg P.O. daily.
Children ages 1 to 3: 0.5 mg P.O. daily.
Infants age 6 months to 1 year: 0.3 mg P.O. daily.
Neonates and infants younger than age 6 months: 0.2 mg P.O. daily.
▶ **Beriberi.** *Adults:* Depending on severity, 10 to 20 mg I.M. t.i.d. for 2 weeks, followed by

T

dietary correction and multivitamin supplement containing 5 to 10 mg of thiamine daily for 1 month.
Children: Depending on severity, 10 to 50 mg I.M. daily for several weeks with adequate diet.
▶ **Wet beriberi with myocardial failure.**
Adults and children: 10 to 30 mg I.V. for emergency therapy.
▶ **Wernicke's encephalopathy.** *Adults:* Initially, 100 mg I.V.; then 50 to 100 mg I.V. or I.M. daily until patient is consuming regular balanced diet.

▼ I.V. administration

● Keep epinephrine available to treat anaphylaxis; give large I.V. doses cautiously.
● If patient has history of hypersensitivity reactions, apply skin test before starting therapy.
● Dilute drug before administration.
⊗ **Incompatibilities**
Alkali carbonates, barbiturates, citrates, erythromycin estolate, kanamycin, streptomycin, sulfites. Don't use with materials that yield alkaline solutions. Unstable in alkaline solutions.

Contraindications and cautions

● Contraindicated in patients hypersensitive to thiamine products.
⚞ **Lifespan:** In pregnant women, use cautiously if dose exceeds RDA.

Adverse reactions

CNS: restlessness, weakness.
CV: *CV collapse,* cyanosis.
EENT: tightness of throat.
GI: nausea, *hemorrhage.*
Respiratory: *pulmonary edema.*
Skin: feeling of warmth, pruritus, urticaria, diaphoresis.
Other: tenderness and induration after I.M. administration, *hypersensitivity reactions, anaphylactic shock.*

Interactions

None significant.

Effects on lab test results

None reported.

Pharmacokinetics

Absorption: Absorbed readily after small P.O. doses; after large P.O. dose, total amount absorbed is limited. In alcoholics and in patients

with cirrhosis or malabsorption, GI absorption is decreased. When given with meals, drug's GI rate of absorption decreases, but total absorption remains same. After I.M. dose, rapid and complete.
Distribution: Widely distributed. When intake exceeds minimal requirements, tissue stores become saturated.
Metabolism: In liver.
Excretion: In urine. *Half-life:* Unknown.

Route	Onset	Peak	Duration
P.O., I.V., I.M.	Unknown	Unknown	Unknown

Action

Chemical effect: Combines with adenosine triphosphate to form coenzyme needed for carbohydrate metabolism.
Therapeutic effect: Restores normal thiamine level.

Available forms

Elixir: 250 mcg/5 ml
Injection: 100 mg/ml, 200 mg/ml
Tablets: 5 mg†, 10 mg†, 25 mg†, 50 mg†, 100 mg†, 250 mg†, 500 mg†
Tablets (enteric-coated): 20 mg

NURSING PROCESS

⚕ Assessment

● Assess patient's condition before starting therapy and regularly thereafter to monitor the drug's effectiveness.
● Be alert for adverse reactions.
● Assess patient's and family's knowledge of drug therapy.

⚕ Nursing diagnoses

● Imbalanced nutrition: less than body requirements related to presence of thiamine deficiency
● Diarrhea related to drug-induced adverse GI reactions
● Deficient knowledge related to drug therapy

▶ Planning and implementation

● Use parenteral route only when P.O. route isn't feasible.
● For treating alcoholic patient, give thiamine before dextrose infusions to prevent encephalopathy.
● Drug malabsorption is most likely in a patient with alcoholism, cirrhosis, or GI disease.

• Significant deficiency can occur in about 3 weeks of thiamine-free diet. Thiamine deficiency usually requires simultaneous therapy for multiple deficiencies.

• If breast-fed infant develops beriberi, give drug to both mother and child.

⊛ **ALERT:** Don't confuse thiamine with Thorazine.

Patient teaching

• Stress proper nutritional habits to prevent recurrence of deficiency.

☑ Evaluation

• Patient regains normal thiamine level.

• Patient maintains normal bowel pattern.

• Patient and family state understanding of drug therapy.

thioridazine hydrochloride
(thigh-oh-RIGH-duh-zeen high-droh-KLOR-ighd)
Aldazine ◇, Apo-Thioridazine ♦, Mellaril*, Mellaril Concentrate, Novo-Ridazine ♦, PMS Thioridazine ♦

Pharmacologic class: phenothiazine (piperidine derivative)
Therapeutic class: antipsychotic
Pregnancy risk category: C

Indications and dosages

▶ **Schizophrenia in patients who don't respond to treatment with other antipsychotic drugs.** *Adults:* Initially, 50 to 100 mg P.O. t.i.d., with gradual, incremental increases up to 800 mg daily in divided doses, if needed. Dosage varies.
Children: Initially, 0.5 mg/kg P.O. daily in divided doses. Increase dose gradually to optimum therapeutic effect. Maximum dose is 3 mg/kg/day.

▶ **Short-term treatment of major depression in patients who also have varying degrees of anxiety.** *Adults:* 25 mg P.O. t.i.d. Maximum dose is 200 mg daily.

▶ **Agitation, anxiety, depressed mood, tension, sleep disturbances, and fears.** *Geriatric patients:* 25 mg P.O. t.i.d. Maximum dose is 200 mg daily.

Contraindications and cautions

• Contraindicated in patients hypersensitive to the drug or any of its components, and in those with CNS depression, severe hypertensive or hypotensive cardiac disease, coma, reduced levels of CYP 2D6 isoenzyme, congenital long-QT syndrome, or a history of cardiac arrhythmias.

• Don't give to patients taking fluvoxamine, propranolol, pindolol, fluoxetine, or drugs that inhibit the CYP 2D6 enzyme or that prolong the QT interval.

• Use cautiously in debilitated patients and in patients with hepatic disease, CV disease, respiratory disorder, hypocalcemia, seizure disorder, severe reactions to insulin or electroconvulsive therapy, and exposure to extreme heat or cold (including antipyretic therapy) or organophosphate insecticides.

⚹ **Lifespan:** In pregnant women, use cautiously. In breast-feeding women, use cautiously; it's unknown if the drug appears in breast milk. In the elderly, use cautiously.

Adverse reactions

CNS: extrapyramidal reactions, tardive dyskinesia, sedation, EEG changes, dizziness, *neuroleptic malignant syndrome.*
CV: *orthostatic hypotension,* tachycardia, ECG changes.
EENT: ocular changes, blurred vision, retinitis pigmentosa.
GI: dry mouth, constipation.
GU: *urine retention,* dark urine, menstrual irregularities, inhibited ejaculation.
Hematologic: transient leukopenia, *agranulocytosis,* hyperprolactinemia.
Hepatic: cholestatic jaundice.
Metabolic: weight gain, increased appetite.
Skin: mild photosensitivity reactions.
Other: gynecomastia, allergic reaction.

Interactions

Drug-drug. *Antacids:* May inhibit absorption of oral phenothiazines. Separate doses by at least 2 hours.
Barbiturates, lithium: May decrease phenothiazine effect. Monitor patient.
Centrally acting antihypertensives: May decrease antihypertensive effect. Monitor blood pressure.
Fluoxetine, fluvoxamine, pindolol, propranolol, drugs that inhibit the CYP 2D6 enzyme system, and drugs that prolong the QT interval: May in-

crease risk of serious or fatal cardiac arrhythmias. Don't use together.

Other CNS depressants: May increase CNS depression. Use together cautiously.

Drug-herb. *Dong quai, St. John's wort:* May increase photosensitivity reactions. Discourage use together.

Kava: May increase risk of dystonic reactions. Discourage use together.

Milk thistle: May decrease liver toxicity caused by phenothiazines. If drug and herb are used together, monitor liver enzyme levels.

Yohimbe: May increase risk for yohimbe toxicity. Discourage use together.

Drug-lifestyle. *Alcohol use:* May increase CNS depression, particularly psychomotor skills. Strongly discourage use.

Sun exposure: May increase photosensitivity reactions. Advise patient to avoid prolonged or unprotected exposure to sunlight.

Effects on lab test results

• May increase liver enzyme and prolactin levels.
• May decrease granulocyte and WBC counts.

Pharmacokinetics

Absorption: Erratic and variable, although P.O. concentrates and syrups are more predictable than tablets.

Distribution: Distributed widely in body; 91% to 99% protein-bound.

Metabolism: Metabolized extensively by liver by the CYP 2D6 enzyme system.

Excretion: Excreted mostly as metabolites in urine, some in feces. *Half-life:* 20 to 40 hours.

Route	Onset	Peak	Duration
P.O.	Varies	Unknown	Unknown

Action

Chemical effect: Unknown; probably blocks postsynaptic dopamine receptors in brain.

Therapeutic effect: Manages symptoms of schizophrenia.

Available forms

Oral concentrate: 30 mg/ml, 100 mg/ml* (3% to 4.2% alcohol)
Oral suspension: 25 mg/5 ml, 100 mg/5 ml
Tablets: 10 mg, 15 mg, 25 mg, 50 mg, 100 mg, 150 mg, 200 mg

NURSING PROCESS

Assessment

• Assess patient's condition before starting therapy and regularly thereafter to monitor the drug's effectiveness.
• Monitor patient for tardive dyskinesia. It may occur after prolonged use or months or years later. It may disappear spontaneously or persist for life, despite stopping the drug.
• Monitor therapy with weekly bilirubin tests during first month, periodic blood tests (CBC and liver function), and ophthalmologic tests (long-term therapy).
⚠ ALERT: Monitor patient for symptoms of neuroleptic malignant syndrome (extrapyramidal effects, hyperthermia, autonomic disturbance), which is rare but can be fatal. It may not relate to length of drug use or type of neuroleptic; however, more than 60% of patients are men.
• Before starting therapy, perform baseline ECG and measure potassium level. Don't give Mellaril to a patient with a QTc interval longer than 450 msec. Stop drug in patients with a QTc longer than 500 msec.
• Assess patient's and family's knowledge of drug therapy.

Nursing diagnoses

• Disturbed thought processes related to underlying condition
• Risk for injury related to drug-induced adverse CNS reactions
• Deficient knowledge related to drug therapy

Planning and implementation

⚠ ALERT: Different liquid formulations have different concentrations. Check dosage.
⚠ ALERT: Mellaril prolongs the QT interval in a dose-related manner.
• Prevent contact dermatitis by keeping drug away from skin and clothes. Wear gloves when preparing liquid forms.
• Dilute liquid concentrate with water or fruit juice just before giving.
• Shake suspension well before using.
• Don't abruptly stop giving the drug unless the patient experiences a severe adverse reaction. Abruptly stopping long-term therapy may cause gastritis, nausea, vomiting, dizziness, tremors, feeling of warmth or cold, diaphoresis, tachycardia, headache, or insomnia.

• Report jaundice, symptoms of blood dyscrasia (fever, sore throat, infection, cellulitis, weakness), or persistent extrapyramidal reactions (longer than a few hours), especially in pregnant women and in children, and withhold drug.
• Acute dystonic reactions may be treated with diphenhydramine.
ALERT: Don't confuse thioridazine with Thorazine; don't confuse Mellaril with Elavil.

Patient teaching

• Warn patient to avoid activities that require alertness until the drug's CNS effects are known. Drowsiness and dizziness usually subside after a few weeks.
• Tell patient to watch for orthostatic hypotension, especially with parenteral administration. Advise patient to change position slowly.
• Tell patient not to drink alcohol while taking drug.
• Instruct patient to report urine retention or constipation.
• Inform patient that drug may discolor urine.
• Tell patient to watch for and notify prescriber of blurred vision.
• Advise patient to relieve dry mouth with sugarless gum or hard candy.
• Tell patient to use sun block and to wear protective clothing to avoid photosensitivity reactions.

☑ Evaluation

• Patient's behavior and communication exhibit improved thought processes.
• Patient doesn't experience injury from adverse CNS reactions.
• Patient and family state understanding of drug therapy.

thiotepa

(thigh-oh-TEE-puh)
Thioplex

Pharmacologic class: alkylating drug
Therapeutic class: antineoplastic
Pregnancy risk category: D

Indications and dosages

▶ **Breast and ovarian cancers, lymphoma, Hodgkin's disease.** *Adults and children older than age 12:* 0.3 to 0.4 mg/kg I.V. q 1 to 4 weeks or 0.2 mg/kg for 4 to 5 days at intervals of 2 to 4 weeks.
▶ **Bladder tumor.** *Adults and children older than age 12:* 60 mg in 30 to 60 ml of normal saline solution instilled in bladder for 2 hours once weekly for 4 weeks.
▶ **Neoplastic effusions.** *Adults and children older than age 12:* 0.6 to 0.8 mg/kg intracavitarily or intratumor q 1 to 4 weeks.
▶ **Malignant meningeal neoplasm‡.** *Adults:* 1 to 10 mg/m^2 intrathecally, once to twice weekly.

I.V. administration

• Follow facility policy to minimize risks. Preparation and administration of parenteral form are linked to mutagenic, teratogenic, and carcinogenic risks to personnel.
• Reconstitute drug with 1.5 ml of sterile water for injection. Don't reconstitute with other solutions.
• Further dilute solution with normal saline solution injection, D_5W, dextrose 5% in normal saline solution for injection, Ringer's injection, or lactated Ringer's injection.
• Drug may be given by rapid I.V. administration in doses of 0.3 to 0.4 mg/kg at intervals of 1 to 4 weeks.
• If pain occurs at insertion site, dilute further or use local anesthetic. Make sure drug doesn't infiltrate.
• Refrigerate and protect dry powder from direct sunlight.
• Solutions are stable for up to 5 days if refrigerated. Solution should be clear to slightly opaque. Discard if solution appears very opaque or contains precipitate.

⊗ **Incompatibilities**
Cisplatin, filgrastim, minocycline, vinorelbine.

Contraindications and cautions

• Contraindicated in patients hypersensitive to the drug or any of its components and in those with severe bone marrow, hepatic, or renal dysfunction.
• Use cautiously in patients with mild bone marrow suppression or renal or hepatic dysfunction.
Lifespan: In pregnant and breast-feeding women, drug isn't recommended. In children age 12 and younger, safety and effectiveness haven't been established.

T

Adverse reactions

CNS: headache, dizziness, fatigue, weakness, fever.
EENT: blurred vision, *laryngeal edema*, conjunctivitis.
GI: *nausea, vomiting,* abdominal pain, anorexia, stomatitis.
GU: amenorrhea, decreased spermatogenesis, dysuria, urine retention, hemorrhagic cystitis.
Hematologic: *leukopenia, thrombocytopenia, neutropenia,* anemia.
Respiratory: *asthma.*
Skin: urticaria, rash, dermatitis, alopecia.
Other: hypersensitivity reactions, pain at injection site, *anaphylaxis.*

Interactions

Drug-drug. *Alkylating drugs, radiation therapy:* May intensify toxicity rather than enhance therapeutic response. Avoid using together.
Anticoagulants, aspirin: May increase bleeding risk. Avoid using together.
Neuromuscular blockers: May prolong muscular paralysis. Monitor patient closely.
Succinylcholine: May increase apnea. Monitor patient closely.

Effects on lab test results

● May increase uric acid level. May decrease pseudocholinesterase and hemoglobin levels and hematocrit.
● May decrease lymphocyte, platelet, WBC, RBC, and neutrophil counts.

Pharmacokinetics

Absorption: Absorption from bladder after instillation ranges from 10% to 100% of instilled dose; also variable after intracavitary administration. Increased by certain pathologic conditions.
Distribution: Crosses blood-brain barrier.
Metabolism: Metabolized extensively in liver.
Excretion: Drug and its metabolites excreted in urine. *Half-life:* 2¼ hours.

Route	Onset	Peak	Duration
I.V., bladder instillation, intracavitary	Unknown	Unknown	Unknown

Action

Chemical effect: Cross-links strands of cellular DNA and interferes with RNA transcription, causing growth imbalance that leads to cell death.
Therapeutic effect: Kills certain cancer cells.

Available forms

Injection: 15-mg vials

NURSING PROCESS

☲ Assessment
● Assess patient's condition before starting therapy and regularly thereafter to monitor the drug's effectiveness.
● Adverse GU reactions are reversible in 6 to 8 months.
● Monitor CBC weekly for at least 3 weeks after giving the last dose.
● Monitor uric acid level.
● Be alert for adverse reactions and drug interactions.
● Assess patient's and family's knowledge of drug therapy.

⊕ Nursing diagnoses
● Ineffective health maintenance related to presence of neoplastic disease
● Ineffective protection related to drug-induced immunosuppression
● Deficient knowledge related to drug therapy

▷ Planning and implementation
● Drug can be given by all parenteral routes, including direct injection into tumor.
● Dehydrate patient 8 to 10 hours before bladder instillation. Instill drug into bladder by catheter; ask patient to retain solution for 2 hours. If discomfort is too great with 60 ml, reduce volume to 30 ml. Reposition patient q 15 minutes for maximum area contact.
● When intracavitary use is needed, for neoplastic effusions, mix drug with 2% procaine hydrochloride or epinephrine hydrochloride 1:1,000.
● Report WBC count below 3,000/mm³ or platelet count below 150,000/mm³ and stop drug.
● To prevent hyperuricemia with resulting uric acid nephropathy, allopurinol may be used with adequate hydration.
Patient teaching
● Tell patient to watch for signs of infection (fever, sore throat, fatigue) and bleeding (easy bruising, nosebleeds, bleeding gums, melena).

Tell patient to take temperature daily and to report even mild infections.
• Instruct patient to avoid OTC products containing aspirin.
• Advise woman of childbearing age to avoid becoming pregnant during therapy and to consult with prescriber if pregnancy is suspected.

☑ **Evaluation**
• Patient responds well to drug.
• Patient doesn't develop serious complications from drug-induced immunosuppression.
• Patient and family state understanding of drug therapy.

thiothixene
(thigh-oh-THIKS-een)
Navane

thiothixene hydrochloride
Navane*

Pharmacologic class: thioxanthene
Therapeutic class: antipsychotic
Pregnancy risk category: C

Indications and dosages

▶ **Mild to moderate psychosis.** *Adults and children age 12 and older:* Initially, 2 mg P.O. t.i.d. Increase gradually to 15 mg daily.
▶ **Severe psychosis.** *Adults and children age 12 and older:* Initially, 5 mg P.O. b.i.d. Increase gradually to 20 to 30 mg daily. Maximum recommended dosage is 60 mg daily.

Contraindications and cautions

• Contraindicated in patients hypersensitive to the drug or any of its components and in those with circulatory collapse, coma, CNS depression, or blood dyscrasia.
• Use cautiously in patients with history of seizure disorder or during alcohol withdrawal. Also use cautiously in debilitated patients and in patients with CV disease (may cause sudden drop in blood pressure), glaucoma, prostatic hyperplasia, or exposure to extreme heat.
🔥 **Lifespan:** In pregnant women, use cautiously. In breast-feeding women, use cautiously; it's unknown if the drug appears in breast milk. In children younger than age 12, drug isn't recommended. In the elderly, use cautiously.

Adverse reactions

CNS: extrapyramidal reactions (pseudoparkinsonism, dystonias, akathisia), tardive dyskinesia, sedation, pseudoparkinsonism, EEG changes, dizziness, restlessness, agitation, insomnia, *neuroleptic malignant syndrome.*
CV: *orthostatic hypotension,* tachycardia, ECG changes.
EENT: ocular changes, *blurred vision,* nasal congestion.
GI: dry mouth, constipation.
GU: *urine retention,* menstrual irregularities, inhibited ejaculation.
Hematologic: transient leukopenia, leukocytosis, agranulocytosis.
Hepatic: jaundice.
Metabolic: weight gain.
Skin: mild photosensitivity reactions.
Other: gynecomastia, allergic reaction.

Interactions

Drug-drug. *Anticholinergics:* May potentiate anticholinergic effects. Use together cautiously
Antihypertensives: May potentiate antihypertensive effects. Use together cautiously.
Other CNS depressants: May increase CNS depression. Avoid using together.
Drug-herb. *Nutmeg:* May cause a loss of symptom control or interfere with therapy for psychiatric illnesses. Discourage using together.
Drug-lifestyle. *Alcohol use:* May increase CNS depression. Discourage using together.
Sun exposure: May increase photosensitivity reactions. Advise patient to avoid prolonged or unprotected exposure to sunlight.

Effects on lab test results

• May increase liver enzyme levels.
• May decrease granulocyte count. May increase or decrease WBC count.

Pharmacokinetics

Absorption: Rapid.
Distribution: Distributed widely in body; 91% to 99% protein-bound.
Metabolism: Minimal.
Excretion: Most of drug excreted as parent drug in feces. *Half-life:* 20 to 40 hours.

Route	Onset	Peak	Duration
P.O.	Several wk	Unknown	Unknown

T

Action
Chemical effect: Unknown; probably blocks postsynaptic dopamine receptors in brain.
Therapeutic effect: Relieves signs and symptoms of psychosis.

Available forms
thiothixene
Capsules: 1 mg, 2 mg, 5 mg, 10 mg, 20 mg
thiothixene hydrochloride
Oral concentrate: 5 mg/ml*

NURSING PROCESS

⚗ Assessment
● Assess patient's psychosis before starting therapy and regularly thereafter to monitor the drug's effectiveness.
● Watch for orthostatic hypotension; monitor blood pressure.
● Monitor patients, especially children, for tardive dyskinesia. It may occur after prolonged use or may not appear until months or years later. It may disappear spontaneously or persist for life, despite stopping the drug.
● Monitor therapy with weekly bilirubin tests during first month, periodic blood tests (CBC and liver function), and ophthalmologic tests for those in long-term therapy.
(§) **ALERT:** Monitor patient for symptoms of neuroleptic malignant syndrome (extrapyramidal effects, hyperthermia, autonomic disturbance), which is rare but can be fatal. It isn't necessarily related to length of drug use or type of neuroleptic; however, more than 60% of patients are men.
● Be alert for adverse reactions and drug interactions.
● Assess patient's and family's knowledge of drug therapy.

⊞ Nursing diagnoses
● Disturbed thought processes related to presence of psychosis
● Risk for injury related to drug-induced adverse CNS reactions
● Deficient knowledge related to drug therapy

❱ Planning and implementation
● Prevent contact dermatitis by keeping drug away from skin and clothes. Wear gloves when preparing liquid form.

● Dilute liquid concentrate with water or fruit juice just before giving.
● Slight yellowing of concentrate is common and doesn't affect potency. Discard markedly discolored solutions.
● Don't abruptly stop giving the drug unless warranted by a severe adverse reaction. Abruptly stopping long-term therapy may cause gastritis, nausea, vomiting, dizziness, tremors, feeling of warmth or cold, diaphoresis, tachycardia, headache, or insomnia.
● Report jaundice, symptoms of blood dyscrasia (fever, sore throat, infection, cellulitis, weakness), or persistent extrapyramidal reactions (longer than a few hours), especially in pregnant woman or in child, and withhold dose.
● Acute dystonic reactions may be treated with diphenhydramine.
(§) **ALERT:** Don't confuse Navane with Nubain or Norvasc.
Patient teaching
● Warn patient to avoid activities that require alertness until the drug's CNS effects are known. Drowsiness and dizziness usually subside after a few weeks.
● Tell patient not to drink alcohol while taking drug.
● If urine retention or constipation occurs, instruct patient to notify prescriber.
● Tell patient to relieve dry mouth with sugarless gum or hard candy.
● To avoid photosensitivity reactions, tell patient to use sun block and wear protective clothing.
● Tell patient to watch for orthostatic hypotension; advise patient to change position slowly.

✓ Evaluation
● Patient's behavior and communication exhibit improved thought processes.
● Patient doesn't experience injury from adverse CNS reactions.
● Patient and family state understanding of drug therapy.

thyroid
(THIGH-royd)
Armour Thyroid, Thyroid USP

Pharmacologic class: hormone
Therapeutic class: thyroid replacement
Pregnancy risk category: A

Reactions may be *common,* uncommon, *life-threatening*, or COMMON AND LIFE-THREATENING.

Indications and dosages

► **Hypothyroidism.** *Adults:* Initially, 30 mg P.O. daily; increase by 15 mg q 14 to 30 days, depending on disease severity, until desired response is achieved. Usual maintenance dosage is 60 to 180 mg P.O. daily as a single dose.
► **Congenital hypothyroidism.** *Children older than age 12:* May approach adult dosage (60 to 180 mg daily), depending on response.
Children ages 6 to 12: 60 to 90 mg P.O. daily.
Children ages 1 to 5: 45 to 60 mg P.O. daily.
Children ages 6 to 12 months: 30 to 45 mg P.O. daily.
Children younger than age 6 months: 15 to 30 mg P.O. daily.

Contraindications and cautions

• Contraindicated in patients hypersensitive to the drug or any of its components, and those with acute MI uncomplicated by hypothyroidism, untreated thyrotoxicosis, or uncorrected adrenal insufficiency.
• Use cautiously in patients with renal insufficiency, an ischemic state, or angina pectoris, hypertension, or other CV disorder. Also use cautiously in patients with myxedema, diabetes mellitus, or diabetes insipidus.
❄ **Lifespan:** In breast-feeding women, use cautiously. In the elderly, use cautiously.

Adverse reactions

CNS: *nervousness, insomnia,* tremor, headache.
CV: tachycardia, ***arrhythmias,*** angina pectoris, increased blood pressure, ***cardiac decompensation and collapse.***
GI: diarrhea, vomiting.
GU: menstrual irregularities.
Metabolic: weight loss, heat intolerance.
Musculoskeletal: accelerated rate of bone maturation in infants and children.
Skin: diaphoresis.
Other: allergic reactions.

Interactions

Drug-drug. *Antacids, calcium supplements:* May decrease effectiveness of thyroid hormone. Separate doses by at least 4 hours.
Cholestyramine: May impair thyroid absorption. Separate doses by 4 to 5 hours.
Digoxin: May decrease digoxin level in hyperthyroidism. Monitor level.
Growth hormone: May interfere with growth response. Monitor effects.

Insulin, oral antidiabetics: May alter glucose level. Monitor level, and adjust dosage, p.r.n.
I.V. phenytoin: May cause release of free thyroid. Monitor patient for tachycardia.
Oral anticoagulants: May increase PT. Monitor PT and INR; adjust dosage, p.r.n.
Sympathomimetics (such as epinephrine): May increase risk of coronary insufficiency. Monitor patient closely.
Theophylline: May decrease theophylline clearance. Monitor level.
Tricyclic antidepressants: May increase risk of toxicity for both drugs. Monitor levels.

Effects on lab test results

• May alter thyroid function test results.

Pharmacokinetics

Absorption: Absorbed from GI tract.
Distribution: Highly protein-bound.
Metabolism: Not fully understood.
Excretion: Not fully understood. *Half-life:* T$_4$, 7 days; T$_3$, 2 days.

Route	Onset	Peak	Duration
P.O.	Unknown	Unknown	Unknown

Action

Chemical effect: Not clearly defined; stimulates metabolism of body tissues by accelerating cellular oxidation.
Therapeutic effect: Raises thyroid hormone level.

Available forms

Tablets: 15 mg, 30 mg, 60 mg, 90 mg, 120 mg, 180 mg, 240 mg, 300 mg
Tablets (enteric-coated): 60 mg, 120 mg

NURSING PROCESS

Assessment
• Assess patient's thyroid condition before starting therapy and regularly thereafter to monitor the drug's effectiveness.
• Monitor pulse rate and blood pressure.
• In children, sleeping pulse rate and morning basal temperature guide therapy.
• In patient with coronary artery disease who must receive drug, watch for possible coronary insufficiency.
• Be alert for adverse reactions and drug interactions.

• Assess patient's and family's knowledge of drug therapy.

⊞ **Nursing diagnoses**
• Ineffective health maintenance related to presence of hypothyroidism
• Disturbed sleep pattern related to drug-induced insomnia
• Deficient knowledge related to drug therapy

▷ **Planning and implementation**
• Drug requirements are about 25% lower in patients older than age 60 than in young adults.
⊛ **ALERT:** Don't confuse Thyrolar with thyroid.
Patient teaching
• Tell patient to take drug at same time each day, preferably before breakfast, to maintain constant levels.
• Suggest that patient take drug in the morning to prevent insomnia.
• Advise patient who has achieved stable response not to change brands.
• Instruct patient (especially an elderly patient) to immediately notify the prescriber about dyspnea, tachycardia, or symptoms of overdose, such as chest pain, palpitations, sweating, and nervousness.
• Tell patient to report unusual bleeding and bruising.

☑ **Evaluation**
• Patient regains normal thyroid function.
• Patient expresses importance of taking thyroid in morning if insomnia occurs.
• Patient and family state understanding of drug therapy.

tiagabine hydrochloride
(tigh-AG-ah-been high-droh-KLOR-ighd)
Gabitril

Pharmacologic class: GABA uptake inhibitor
Therapeutic class: anticonvulsant
Pregnancy risk category: C

Indications and dosages

▶ **Adjunctive therapy in partial seizures.**
Adults: Initially, 4 mg P.O. once daily. Total daily dosage may be increased by 4 to 8 mg at weekly intervals until response is noted or up to 56 mg daily. Divide dose b.i.d. to q.i.d.

Children ages 12 to 18: Initially, 4 mg P.O. once daily. Total daily dosage may be increased by 4 mg at the beginning of week 2 and by 4 to 8 mg/week until response is noted or up to 32 mg daily. Divide dose b.i.d. to q.i.d.
⬓ **Adjust-a-dose:** Dosage may be decreased in patients with hepatic insufficiency.

Contraindications and cautions

• Contraindicated in patients hypersensitive to the drug or any of its components.
⚶ **Lifespan:** In pregnant women, use only if clearly needed. In breast-feeding women, use cautiously; it's unknown if drug appears in breast milk. In children younger than age 12, safety and effectiveness haven't been established.

Adverse reactions

CNS: generalized weakness, *dizziness, asthenia, somnolence, nervousness,* tremor, difficulty with concentration and attention, insomnia, ataxia, confusion, speech disorder, difficulty with memory, paresthesia, depression, emotional lability, abnormal gait, hostility, language problems, agitation, pain.
CV: vasodilation.
EENT: nystagmus, pharyngitis.
GI: abdominal pain, *nausea,* diarrhea, vomiting, increased appetite, mouth ulcerations.
Musculoskeletal: myasthenia.
Respiratory: increased cough.
Skin: rash, pruritus.

Interactions

Drug-drug. *Carbamazepine, phenobarbital, phenytoin:* May increase tiagabine clearance. Monitor patient for loss of therapeutic effect. May need to increase tiagabine dose.
CNS depressants: May increase CNS effects. Use cautiously.
Drug-lifestyle. *Alcohol use:* May increase CNS effects. Discourage using together.

Effects on lab test results

None reported.

Pharmacokinetics

Absorption: Rapid and more than 95%. Absolute bioavailability is 90%.
Distribution: About 96% bound to plasma protein.
Metabolism: Likely to be metabolized by CYP 3A isoenzymes.

Excretion: About 25% is excreted in urine; 63% in feces. *Half-life:* 7 to 9 hours.

Route	Onset	Peak	Duration
P.O.	Rapid	45 min	7–9 hr

Action

Chemical effect: Unknown; may enhance the activity of GABA, the major inhibitory neurotransmitter in the CNS. It binds to recognition sites related to the GABA uptake carrier and may thus permit more GABA to be available for binding to receptors on postsynaptic cells.
Therapeutic effect: Prevents partial seizures.

Available forms

Tablets: 2 mg, 4 mg, 12 mg, 16 mg

NURSING PROCESS

Assessment

- Assess patient's seizure disorder before starting therapy and regularly thereafter to monitor the drug's effectiveness.
- Assess patient's compliance with therapy at each follow-up visit.

ALERT: Monitor patient carefully for status epilepticus, because sudden death may occur in patient taking an anticonvulsant.

- Assess patient for adverse reactions and drug interactions.
- Assess patient's and family's knowledge of drug therapy.

Nursing diagnoses

- Risk for injury related to seizure disorder
- Impaired physical mobility related to drug-induced generalized weakness
- Deficient knowledge related to drug therapy

Planning and implementation

- In patient with impaired liver function, lower initial and maintenance doses or longer dosage intervals may be needed.

ALERT: Never abruptly stop giving the drug, because seizure frequency may increase. Stop giving the drug gradually unless safety concerns require a more rapid withdrawal.
ALERT: Drug may cause seizures and status epilepticus in patients without a history of epilepsy. Nonepileptic patients who develop seizures should stop drug and be evaluated for underlying seizure disorder. Prescribers are discouraged from using the drug for off-label indications.

- Patient who isn't receiving at least one enzyme-inducing antiepileptic when starting therapy may require lower dose or slower dose adjustments.
- Report breakthrough seizure activity to prescriber.

ALERT: Don't confuse tiagabine with tizanidine; both have 4-mg starting doses.

Patient teaching

- Advise patient to take drug only as prescribed.
- Advise patient to take drug with food.
- Warn patient that drug may cause dizziness, somnolence, and other symptoms and signs of CNS depression. Advise patient to avoid driving and other potentially hazardous activities that require mental alertness until the drug's CNS effects are known.
- Tell woman to notify prescriber if she becomes pregnant or plans to become pregnant during therapy.
- Tell woman to notify prescriber if planning to breast-feed because drug may appear in breast milk.

Evaluation

- Patient is free from seizure activity.
- Patient receives therapeutic dose and doesn't experience muscle weakness.
- Patient and family state understanding of drug therapy.

ticarcillin disodium

(tigh-kar-SIL-in digh-SOH-dee-um)
Ticar, Ticillin ◇

Pharmacologic class: extended-spectrum penicillin, alpha-carboxypenicillin
Therapeutic class: antibiotic
Pregnancy risk category: B

Indications and dosages

▶ **Severe systemic infections caused by susceptible strains of gram-positive and especially gram-negative organisms (including *Pseudomonas* and *Proteus*).** *Adults and children older than age 1 month:* 200 to 300 mg/kg I.V. daily in divided doses q 4 to 6 hours.

▶ **Uncomplicated UTI.** *Adults and children weighing 40 kg (88 lb) or more:* 1 g I.V. or I.M. q 6 hours.
Infants and children older than age 1 month and weighing less than 40 kg: 50 to 100 mg/kg I.V. or I.M. daily in divided doses q 6 to 8 hours.
▶ **Complicated UTI.** *Adults:* 150 to 200 mg/kg daily in divided doses every 4 or 6 hours.
◩ **Adjust-a-dose:** For patients with renal impairment, give the initial loading dose of 3 g I.V.; then base I.V. doses on creatinine clearance. If creatinine clearance is 30 to 60 ml/minute, dosage is 2 g I.V. q 4 hours; if clearance is 10 to 29 ml/minute, 2 g I.V. q 8 hours; if below 10 ml/minute, 2 g q 12 hours or 1 g I.M. q 6 hours; and if below 10 ml/minute with hepatic dysfunction, 2 g q 24 hours or 1 g I.M. q 12 hours.

▼ I.V. administration

• Reconstitute drug in vials using D_5W, normal saline solution injection, sterile water for injection, or other compatible solution.
• Reconstitute 3-g piggyback vials with a minimum of 30 ml compatible solution; if diluting with 50 ml diluent, dilute to 60 mg/ml. If diluting with 100 ml diluent, dilute to 30 mg/ml.
• Add 4 ml of diluent for each gram of drug to obtain 200 mg/ml. May dilute further, if desired.
• For direct injection, give slowly to avoid vein irritation. For intermittent infusion, give over 30 minutes to 2 hours. Infusing with a concentration of 50 mg/ml may reduce vein irritation.
• Continuous infusion may cause vein irritation. Change site q 48 hours.
⊗ **Incompatibilities**
Aminoglycosides, amphotericin B, ciprofloxacin, doxapram, fluconazole, gentamicin, methylprednisolone sodium succinate, vancomycin.

Contraindications and cautions

• Contraindicated in patients hypersensitive to penicillins.
• Use cautiously in patients with other drug allergies, especially to cephalosporins (possible cross-sensitivity), and those with impaired kidney function, hemorrhagic conditions, hypokalemia, or sodium restrictions (contains 5.2 to 6.5 mEq sodium/g).
⚜ **Lifespan:** In pregnant women and breastfeeding women, use cautiously.

Adverse reactions

CNS: *seizures,* neuromuscular excitability, lethargy, asterixis, stupor.
CV: vein irritation, phlebitis.
GI: nausea, diarrhea, vomiting.
Hematologic: *leukopenia, neutropenia,* eosinophilia, *thrombocytopenia,* granulocytopenia, hemolytic anemia.
Metabolic: hypokalemia.
Other: *hypersensitivity reactions, anaphylaxis,* overgrowth of nonsusceptible organisms, pain at injection site.

Interactions

Drug-drug. *Hormonal contraceptives:* May decrease effectiveness of hormonal contraceptives. Recommend an additional form of contraception during penicillin therapy.
Lithium: May alter renal elimination of lithium. Monitor lithium level closely.
Methotrexate: May decrease renal clearance of methotrexate. Monitor patient carefully.
Probenecid: May increase level of ticarcillin and other penicillins. Probenecid may be used for this purpose.

Effects on lab test results

• May increase ALT, AST, alkaline phosphatase, LDH, and sodium levels. May decrease potassium and hemoglobin levels and hematocrit.
• May increase eosinophil count. May decrease platelet, WBC, neutrophil, and granulocyte counts.

Pharmacokinetics

Absorption: Unknown after I.M. administration.
Distribution: Distributed widely. Penetrates minimally into CSF with non-inflamed meninges; 45% to 65% protein-bound.
Metabolism: About 13% metabolized by hydrolysis to inactive compounds.
Excretion: Excreted mostly in urine; also in bile. *Half-life:* About 1 hour.

Route	Onset	Peak	Duration
I.V.	Immediate	Immediate	Unknown
I.M.	Unknown	30–75 min	Unknown

Action

Chemical effect: Inhibits cell wall synthesis during microorganism multiplication; bacteria resist penicillins by producing penicillinase en-

zymes that convert penicillins to inactive penicilloic acid. Drug resists these enzymes.
Therapeutic effect: Kills bacteria.

Available forms

Injection: 1 g, 3 g
I.V. infusion: 3 g

NURSING PROCESS

Assessment
• Assess patient's infection before starting therapy and regularly thereafter to monitor the drug's effectiveness.
• Before giving drug, find out if patient is allergic to penicillin. Negative history of penicillin allergy is no guarantee against future allergic reaction.
• Obtain specimen for culture and sensitivity tests before giving the first dose. Start therapy pending test results.
• Monitor potassium level.
• Monitor CBC and platelet count.
• Monitor INR in patient taking warfarin therapy because drug may prolong PT.
• Be alert for adverse reactions and drug interactions.
• If adverse GI reaction occurs, monitor patient's hydration.
• Assess patient's and family's knowledge of drug therapy.

Nursing diagnoses
• Risk for infection related to presence of susceptible bacteria
• Risk for deficient fluid volume related to drug-induced adverse GI reactions
• Deficient knowledge related to drug therapy

Planning and implementation
• Lower the dose in a patient with renal impairment.
• Reconstitute drug for I.M. use in vials with sterile water for injection, normal saline solution injection, or lidocaine 1% (without epinephrine). Use 2 ml of diluent per gram of drug.
• Inject I.M. dose deep into large muscle. Don't exceed 2 g per injection.
• Give drug at least 1 hour before bacteriostatic antibiotics.
• Drug is typically used with another antibiotic, such as gentamicin.

ALERT: Institute seizure precautions. Patient with high drug level may develop seizures.
Patient teaching
• Instruct patient to report adverse reactions.

Evaluation
• Patient is free from infection.
• Patient maintains adequate hydration.
• Patient and family state understanding of drug therapy.

ticarcillin disodium and clavulanate potassium
(tigh-kar-SIL-in digh-SOH-dee-um and KLAV-yoo-lan-nayt poh-TAH-see-um)
Timentin

Pharmacologic class: extended-spectrum penicillin, beta-lactamase inhibitor
Therapeutic class: antibiotic
Pregnancy risk category: B

Indications and dosages

▶ **Systemic and urinary tract infections.**
Adults weighing 60 kg (132 lb) or more: 3.1 g (3 g ticarcillin and 100 mg clavulanic acid) I.V. q 4 to 6 hours.
▶ **Moderate gynecologic infections.** *Adults weighing 60 kg or more:* 200 mg of ticarcillin/kg daily I.V. in divided doses q 6 hours.
▶ **Severe gynecologic infections.** *Adults weighing 60 kg or more:* 300 mg of ticarcillin/kg daily I.V. in divided doses q 4 hours.
▶ **Systemic, urinary tract, and gynecologic infections.** *Adults weighing less than 60 kg:* 200 to 300 mg/kg I.V. daily (based on ticarcillin content) in divided doses q 4 to 6 hours.
Children age 3 months and older and weighing less than 60 kg: For mild to moderate infections, 200 mg of ticarcillin/kg I.V. daily in divided doses q 6 hours. For severe infections, 300 mg/kg daily in divided doses q 4 hours.
Children age 3 months and older weighing 60 kg or more: For mild to m oderate infections, 3.1 g (3 g ticarcillin and 100 mg clavulanic acid) I.V. q 6 hours; for severe infections, q 4 hours.
Adjust-a-dose: For patients with renal impairment, if creatinine clearance is greater than

T

60 ml/minute, give 3.1 g q 4 hours; if 30 to 60 ml/minute, give 2 g q 4 hours; if 10 to 30 ml/minute, give 2 g q 8 hours; if less than 10 ml/minute, give 2 g q 12 hours; and if less than 10 ml/minute and the patient has hepatic dysfunction, give 2 g q 24 hours. If the patient is on peritoneal dialysis, give 3.1 g q 12 hours and if the patient is on hemodialysis, give 2 g q 12 hours and 3.1 g after hemodialysis.

▼ I.V. administration

• Reconstitute drug with 13 ml of sterile water for injection or normal saline solution injection.
• Further dilute to maximum of 10 to 100 mg/ml (based on ticarcillin component). In fluid-restricted patient, dilute to maximum of 48 mg/ml if using D_5W, 43 mg/ml if using normal saline solution injection, or 86 mg/ml if using sterile water for injection.
• Infuse over 30 minutes.
⊗ **Incompatibilities**
Aminoglycosides, amphotericin B, cisatracurium, other anti-infectives, sodium bicarbonate, vancomycin.

Contraindications and cautions

• Contraindicated in patients hypersensitive to penicillins.
• Use cautiously in patients with other drug allergies, especially to cephalosporins (possible cross-sensitivity), and those with impaired kidney function, hemorrhagic condition, hypokalemia, or sodium restrictions (contains 4.5 mEq sodium/g).
⚖ **Lifespan:** In pregnant women, use cautiously. In breast-feeding women, use cautiously; it's unknown if the drug appears in breast milk.

Adverse reactions

CNS: *seizures,* neuromuscular excitability, headache, giddiness, lethargy, asterixis, stupor.
CV: vein irritation, phlebitis.
GI: nausea, diarrhea, stomatitis, vomiting, epigastric pain, flatulence, *pseudomembranous colitis,* taste and smell disturbances.
Hematologic: *leukopenia, neutropenia,* eosinophilia, *thrombocytopenia,* granulocytopenia, hemolytic anemia, anemia.
Metabolic: hypokalemia.
Other: *hypersensitivity reactions, anaphylaxis,* overgrowth of nonsusceptible organisms, pain at injection site.

Interactions

Drug-drug. *Hormonal contraceptives:* May decrease effectiveness of hormonal contraceptives. Recommend an additional form of contraception during ticarcillin therapy.
Lithium: May alter renal elimination of lithium. Monitor level closely.
Methotrexate: May decrease renal clearance of methotrexate. Monitor levels.
Probenecid: May increase blood level of ticarcillin. Probenecid may be used for this purpose.

Effects on lab test results

• May increase ALT, AST, alkaline phosphatase, LDH, and sodium levels. May decrease potassium and hemoglobin levels and hematocrit.
• May increase eosinophil count. May decrease platelet, WBC, neutrophil, and granulocyte counts.

Pharmacokinetics

Absorption: Administered I.V.
Distribution: Ticarcillin disodium distributed widely; penetrates minimally into CSF with noninflamed meninges. Clavulanic acid penetrates pleural fluid, lungs, and peritoneal fluid.
Metabolism: About 13% of ticarcillin dose metabolized by hydrolysis to inactive compounds; clavulanic acid is thought to undergo extensive metabolism but its fate is unknown.
Excretion: Ticarcillin excreted primarily in urine; also excreted in bile. Clavulanate's metabolites are excreted in urine. *Half-life:* About 1 hour.

Route	Onset	Peak	Duration
I.V.	Immediate	Immediate	Unknown

Action

Chemical effect: Inhibits cell wall synthesis during microorganism replication; clavulanic acid increases ticarcillin's effectiveness by inactivating beta lactamases, which destroy ticarcillin.
Therapeutic effect: Kills susceptible bacteria.

Available forms

Injection: 3 g ticarcillin and 100 mg clavulanic acid

Reactions may be *common,* uncommon, *life-threatening,* or COMMON AND LIFE-THREATENING.

NURSING PROCESS

☞ Assessment
• Assess patient's infection before starting therapy and regularly thereafter to monitor the drug's effectiveness.
• Before giving drug, find out if patient is allergic to penicillin. Negative history of penicillin allergy is no guarantee against future allergic reaction.
• Obtain specimen for culture and sensitivity tests before giving the first dose. Start therapy pending test results.
• Monitor CBC and platelet count.
• Be alert for adverse reactions and drug interactions.
• If adverse GI reactions occur, monitor patient's hydration.
• Assess patient's and family's knowledge of drug therapy.

⊞ Nursing diagnoses
• Risk for infection related to presence of susceptible bacteria
• Risk for deficient fluid volume related to drug-induced adverse GI reactions
• Deficient knowledge related to drug therapy

⧰ Planning and implementation
• Lower the dose in patient with renal impairment.
• Give drug at least 1 hour before bacteriostatic antibiotics.
Patient teaching
• Instruct patient to report adverse reactions immediately.

☑ Evaluation
• Patient is free from infection.
• Patient maintains adequate hydration.
• Patient and family state understanding of drug therapy.

ticlopidine hydrochloride
(tigh-KLOH-peh-deen high-droh-KLOR-ighd)
Ticlid

Pharmacologic class: platelet aggregation inhibitor
Therapeutic class: antithrombotic
Pregnancy risk category: B

Indications and dosages
▶ **To reduce risk of thrombotic stroke in patients with history of stroke or stroke precursors.** *Adults:* 250 mg P.O. b.i.d. with meals.
▶ **Prevention of coronary artery stent thrombosis.** *Adults:* 250 mg P.O. b.i.d. for 30 days. As an alternative, a loading dose of 500 mg may be given, followed by 250 mg b.i.d. for 10 to 14 days following successful stent placement.

Contraindications and cautions
• Contraindicated in patients hypersensitive to the drug or any of its components and in those with hematopoietic disorders (such as neutropenia, thrombocytopenia, or disorders of hemostasis), active pathologic bleeding (such as peptic ulceration or active intracranial bleeding), or severe hepatic impairment.
• Drug is reserved for patients intolerant to aspirin.
⚘ **Lifespan:** In pregnant women, use cautiously. In breast-feeding women, drug isn't recommended. In children, safety and effectiveness haven't been established.

Adverse reactions
CNS: dizziness, *intracerebral bleeding.*
CV: vasculitis.
EENT: epistaxis, conjunctival hemorrhage.
GI: *diarrhea,* nausea, dyspepsia, vomiting, flatulence, anorexia, *abdominal pain, bleeding.*
GU: hematuria, nephrotic syndrome, dark-colored urine.
Hematologic: *neutropenia, agranulocytosis, pancytopenia, immune thrombocytopenia.*
Hepatic: *hepatitis,* cholestatic jaundice.
Metabolic: hyponatremia.
Musculoskeletal: arthropathy, myositis.
Respiratory: allergic pneumonitis.
Skin: *rash,* purpura, pruritus, urticaria, *thrombocytopenic purpura,* ecchymoses.
Other: *hypersensitivity reactions, postoperative bleeding,* systemic lupus erythematosus, serum sickness.

Interactions
Drug-drug. *Antacids:* May decrease ticlopidine level. Separate administration times by at least 2 hours.
Aspirin: May potentiate aspirin effects on platelets. Don't use together.

T

Cimetidine: May decrease clearance of ticlopidine and increase risk of toxicity. Avoid using together.
Digoxin: May slightly decrease digoxin level. Monitor level.
Heparin, oral anticoagulants: Safety of combined use hasn't been established. Stop these drugs before starting ticlopidine.
Theophylline: May decrease theophylline clearance and risk of toxicity. Monitor patient closely, and adjust theophylline dosage.
Drug-herb. *Red clover:* May increase risk of bleeding. Caution against using together.

Effects on lab test results

• May increase ALT, AST, and alkaline phosphatase levels. May decrease sodium level.
• May decrease neutrophil, WBC, RBC, platelet, and granulocyte counts.

Pharmacokinetics

Absorption: Rapid and extensive; enhanced by food.
Distribution: 98% bound to proteins and lipoproteins.
Metabolism: Extensively metabolized by liver. More than 20 metabolites have been identified; unknown if parent drug or active metabolites are responsible for pharmacologic activity.
Excretion: 60% excreted in urine and 23% in feces. *Half-life:* 1½ hours after single dose; 4 to 5 days after multiple doses.

Route	Onset	Peak	Duration
P.O.	Unknown	2 hr	Unknown

Action

Chemical effect: Unknown; may block adenosine diphosphate-induced platelet-fibrinogen and platelet-platelet binding.
Therapeutic effect: Prevents blood clots from forming.

Available forms

Tablets: 250 mg

NURSING PROCESS

Assessment

• Assess patient's condition before starting therapy and regularly thereafter to monitor the drug's effectiveness.

• Obtain baseline liver function tests before starting therapy. Monitor test results closely, especially during first 4 months of therapy, and repeat when liver dysfunction is suspected.
• Determine baseline CBC and WBC differentials, repeat at second week of therapy and q 2 weeks until end of third month. If patient shows signs of declining neutrophil count, or if count falls 30% below baseline, test more frequently. After first 3 months, obtain CBC and WBC differential counts only in patient showing signs of infection.
• Be alert for adverse reactions and drug interactions.
• Assess patient's and family's knowledge of drug therapy.

Nursing diagnoses

• Impaired cerebral tissue perfusion related to stroke potential or history
• Ineffective protection related to drug-induced adverse hematologic reactions
• Deficient knowledge related to drug therapy

Planning and implementation

• Thrombocytopenia may occur rarely. Report platelet count of 80,000/mm³ or less, and stop giving the drug. Give 20 mg of methylprednisolone I.V. to normalize bleeding time within 2 hours. Platelet transfusions also may be used.
• When used preoperatively, drug may decrease risk of graft occlusion in patient receiving coronary artery bypass grafts and reduce severity of drop in platelet count in patient receiving extracorporeal hemoperfusion during open heart surgery.

Patient teaching

• Tell patient to take drug with meals; this substantially increases bioavailability and improves GI tolerance.
• Tell patient to avoid aspirin-containing products and to check with prescriber before taking OTC drugs.
• Explain that drug prolongs bleeding time, but that patient should report unusual or prolonged bleeding. Advise him to tell dentist and other health care providers that he is taking this drug.
• Stress importance of regular blood tests.
• Because neutropenia can increase risk of infection, tell patient to promptly report such signs as fever, chills, and sore throat.

• If drug is substituted for a fibrinolytic or anticoagulant, tell patient to stop those drugs before starting ticlopidine.

• Advise patient to stop drug 10 to 14 days before elective surgery.

• Tell patient to report yellow skin or sclera, severe or persistent diarrhea, rashes, subcutaneous bleeding, light-colored stools, and dark urine.

✓ Evaluation

• Patient maintains adequate cerebral perfusion.

• Patient doesn't develop serious complications.

• Patient and family state understanding of drug therapy.

tigecycline
(tie-geh-SIGH-kleen)
Tygacil

Pharmacologic class: glycylcycline antibacterial
Therapeutic class: antibiotic
Pregnancy risk category: D

Indications and dosages

▶ **Complicated skin and skin structure infections; complicated intra-abdominal infections.** *Adults:* Initially 100 mg I.V.; then 50 mg q 12 hours for 5 to 14 days. Infuse drug over 30 to 60 minutes.

☒ **Adjust-a-dose:** For patients with severe hepatic impairment, give initial dose of 100 mg I.V. and then 25 mg I.V. q 12 hours.

▽ I.V. administration

• Reconstitute powder with 5.3 ml of normal saline solution or D_5W to yield 10 mg/ml.

• Gently swirl the vial until the powder dissolves.

• Immediately withdraw the dose from the vial and add it to 100 ml of normal saline solution or D_5W. The maximum concentration is 1 mg/ml.

• Inspect the I.V. solution for particulates and discoloration (green or black) before giving it. Reconstituted solution should be yellow to orange.

• Immediately dilute reconstituted drug for I.V. infusion.

• Use a dedicated I.V. line or a Y-site, and flush the line with normal saline or D_5W before and after infusion.

• Infuse the drug over 30 to 60 minutes.

• Store unopened vials at room temperature in the original package. Store diluted solution at room temperature for up to 6 hours, or refrigerate for up to 24 hours.

⊗ **Incompatibilities**
Amphotericin B, chlorpromazine, methylprednisolone, voriconazole.

Contraindications and cautions

• Contraindicated in patients hypersensitive to tigecycline.

• Use cautiously in patients with severe hepatic impairment and in those hypersensitive to tetracycline antibiotics. Also use cautiously as monotherapy in patients with complicated intra-abdominal infections caused by intestinal perforation.

⚕ **Lifespan:** In pregnant women, use drug only if benefits to patient outweigh risks to fetus. In breast-feeding women, use cautiously; it isn't known if drug appears in breast milk. In children, safety and effectiveness haven't been established. Older adults may be more sensitive to drug's adverse effects.

Adverse reactions

CNS: *pseudotumor cerebri,* asthenia, dizziness, fever, headache, insomnia, pain.
CV: hypertension, hypotension, peripheral edema.
GI: abdominal pain, constipation, *diarrhea,* dyspepsia, *nausea, vomiting.*
Hematologic: anemia, leukocytosis, *thrombocytopenia.*
Metabolic: hyperglycemia, hypokalemia, hypoproteinemia.
Musculoskeletal: back pain.
Respiratory: cough, dyspnea.
Skin: local reaction, phlebitis, pruritus, rash, sweating.
Other: abnormal healing, abscess, allergic reaction, infection, *sepsis.*

Interactions

Drug-drug. *Hormonal contraceptives:* May decrease contraceptive effectiveness. Advise patient to use nonhormonal form of contraception during treatment.
Warfarin: May increase risk of bleeding. Monitor INR.

T

Effects on lab test results

• May increase alkaline phosphatase, amylase, bilirubin, BUN, creatinine, LDH, AST, and ALT levels. May decrease potassium, protein, calcium, sodium, and hemoglobin levels and hematocrit. May increase or decrease blood glucose levels.
• May increase INR, PT, APTT, and WBC count. May decrease platelet count.

Pharmacokinetics

Absorption: Administered I.V.
Distribution: Serum protein binding is about 70 to 90%. Extensively distributed in tissues.
Metabolism: Not extensively metabolized in the liver.
Excretion: Eliminated mainly through bile and feces as unchanged drug and metabolites. A lesser amount is eliminated via the kidneys.
Half life: 27 to 42 hours.

Route	Onset	Peak	Duration
I.V.	Unknown	Unknown	Unknown

Action

Chemical effect: Inhibits protein translation in bacteria by binding to the 30S ribosomal unit.
Therapeutic effect: Kills susceptible bacteria.

Available forms

Lyophilized powder: 50-mg vials

NURSING PROCESS

Assessment

• Assess patient for tetracycline allergy before giving drug.
• Obtain specimen for culture and sensitivity tests before giving first dose. Therapy may begin pending test results.
• If patient develops diarrhea, monitor him closely for pseudomembranous colitis.
• If patient has abdominal infection caused by intestinal perforation, monitor him for sepsis.
• Evaluate patient's and family's knowledge of drug therapy.

Nursing diagnoses

• Infection related to presence of susceptible bacteria
• Risk for deficient fluid volume related to drug-induced adverse GI reactions
• Deficient knowledge related to drug therapy

Planning and implementation

• Be alert for potentially dangerous toxicities of tetracyclines, such as photosensitivity, pseudotumor cerebri, pancreatitis and anti-anabolic action (increased BUN level, azotemia, acidosis, and hypophosphatemia).
• Excessive doses may increase the risk of nausea and vomiting. Drug isn't removed by hemodialysis.

Patient teaching
• Tell patient that drug is used to treat only bacterial infections, not viral infections.
• Explain that it's common to feel better after a few days of therapy. Stress that patient will need to finish the full course of treatment even if he feels better before it's finished.
• Tell patient to report burning or pain at the I.V. site.
• Tell women of childbearing age to avoid becoming pregnant during treatment. Urge those who use hormonal contraception to also use barrier contraception during treatment.
• Advise patient to notify a health care provider if pregnancy is suspected or confirmed.

Evaluation

• Patient is free from infection.
• Patient maintains adequate hydration.
• Patient and family state understanding of drug therapy.

tinidazole

(ty-NIH-duh-zohl)
Tindamax

Pharmacologic class: antiprotozoal
Therapeutic class: anti-infective
Pregnancy risk category: C (X in first trimester)

Indications and dosages

▶ **Trichomoniasis caused by** *Trichomonas vaginalis.* *Adults:* 2 g P.O. as a single dose taken with food. Sexual partners should be treated at the same time with the same dose.
▶ **Giardiasis caused by** *Giardia lamblia* (*G. duodenalis*). *Adults:* 2 g P.O. as a single dose taken with food.
Children older than age 3: 50 mg/kg (up to 2 g) as a single dose taken with food.

▶ **Intestinal amebiasis caused by** *Entamoeba*
histolytica. Adults: 2 g P.O. daily for 3 days,
taken with food.
Children older than age 3: 50 mg/kg (up to 2 g)
P.O. daily for 3 days, taken with food.
▶ **Amebic liver abscess (amebiasis).** *Adults:*
2 g P.O. daily for 3 to 5 days, taken with food.
Children older than age 3: 50 mg/kg (up to 2 g)
P.O. daily for 3 to 5 days, taken with food.
⧉ **Adjust-a-dose:** For patients on hemodialysis,
give an additional dose equal to one-half the recommended dose after the hemodialysis session.

Contraindications and cautions

• Contraindicated in patients hypersensitive to
the drug, its components, or other nitroimidazole derivatives.
• Use cautiously in patients with CNS disorders
and in those with blood dyscrasias or hepatic
dysfunction.
⧉ **Lifespan:** In pregnant women, drug is contraindicated during the first trimester; during the
second and third trimesters, use if benefits to the
patient outweigh risks to the fetus. Breast-feeding women should stop breast-feeding or use
another drug; they should wait 3 days after the
last dose before resuming breast-feeding. In
children age 3 and younger, safety and effectiveness haven't been established. In elderly patient, dose selection should reflect the possibility of decreased liver or kidney function and
other medical conditions or drug therapies.

Adverse reactions

CNS: dizziness, fatigue, headache, malaise, peripheral neuropathy, *seizures,* weakness.
GI: anorexia, constipation, cramps, dyspepsia,
metallic taste, nausea, vomiting.
Other: hypersensitivity reactions.

Interactions

Drug-drug. *Cholestyramine:* May decrease oral
bioavailability of tinidazole. Separate doses to
minimize this effect.
Cyclosporine, tacrolimus: May increase cyclosporine and tacrolimus levels. Monitor patient
closely for toxicity, including headache, nausea,
vomiting, nephrotoxicity, and electrolyte abnormalities.
Disulfiram: May increase abdominal cramping,
nausea, vomiting, headaches, and flushing. If

patient took disulfiram during previous 2 weeks,
don't give tinidazole.
*Drugs that induce CYP, such as fosphenytoin,
phenobarbital, phenytoin, and rifampin:* May
increase tinidazole elimination. Monitor patient.
*Drugs that inhibit CYP, such as cimetidine and
ketoconazole:* May prolong tinidazole half-life
and decrease clearance. Monitor patient.
Fluorouracil: May decrease fluorouracil clearance, increasing adverse effects without added
benefit. Monitor patient for rash, nausea, vomiting, stomatitis, and leukopenia.
Fosphenytoin, phenytoin: May prolong phenytoin half-life and decrease clearance of I.V.
drug. Monitor patient for toxicity.
Lithium: May increase lithium level. Monitor
patient and serum lithium and creatinine levels.
Oxytetracycline: May antagonize tinidazole. Assess patient for lack of effect.
Warfarin and other oral anticoagulants: May
increase anticoagulant effect. Anticoagulant
dosage may need adjustment and for up to
8 days after tinidazole therapy.
Drug-herb. *St. John's wort:* May increase or
decrease tinidazole levels. Discourage use together.
Drug-lifestyle. *Alcohol and alcohol-containing
products:* May increase abdominal cramping,
nausea, vomiting, headaches, and flushing. Discourage use together and for 3 days after stopping tinidazole.

Effects on lab test results

• May increase AST, ALT, glucose, LDH, and
triglyceride levels.
• May decrease WBC count.

Pharmacokinetics

Absorption: Rapid, complete, and unaffected
by food.
Distribution: Into body tissues, fluids, and
breast milk. Crosses the blood-brain and placen-
tal barriers. About 12% bound to plasma proteins.
Metabolism: Mainly by CYP 3A4 enzymes and
partially by oxidation, hydroxylation, and conjugation in the liver.
Excretion: By liver and kidneys, with 20% to
25% in the urine and 12% in the feces. *Half-
life:* About 12 to 14 hours.

Route	Onset	Peak	Duration
P.O.	Unknown	1½ hr	Unknown

Action

Chemical effect: Against *Trichomonas,* action may result from reduction of the compound's nitro group into a free nitro radical. Mechanism of action against *Giardia* and *Entamoeba* is unknown.

Therapeutic effect: Hinders growth of susceptible organisms.

Available forms

Tablets: 250 mg, 500 mg

NURSING PROCESS

✏ Assessment

• Assess patient's infection before starting therapy and regularly thereafter to monitor the drug's effectiveness.
• Children should be monitored closely if therapy exceeds 3 days.
• Be alert for adverse reactions and drug interactions.
⚠ **ALERT:** Stop giving the drug immediately if abnormal neurologic signs occur, such as seizures or numbness of the limbs.
• Assess patient's and family's knowledge of drug therapy.

🔢 Nursing diagnoses

• Risk for injury related to drug-induced adverse neurological reactions
• Risk for deficient fluid volume related to drug-induced adverse GI reactions
• Deficient knowledge related to drug therapy

▶ Planning and implementation

• For patients unable to swallow tablets, a suspension may be made by grinding 2 g of tinidazole into a powder and mixing with 10 ml of cherry syrup. Transfer to a graduated amber container with several rinses of cherry syrup to a final volume of 30 ml.
• Drug is stable for 7 days at room temperature. Shake well.
• Give drug with food to minimize adverse GI effects.
• If candidiasis develops during therapy, give an antifungal.
Patient teaching
• Tell patient to take drug with food.
• Warn patient not to drink alcohol or use alcohol-containing products while taking tinidazole and for 3 days afterward.

• Advise patient to immediately report pregnancy.
• If patient is being treated for a sexually transmitted disease, explain that sexual partners should be treated at the same time.

☑ Evaluation

• Patient does not experience adverse neurological effects.
• Patient maintains adequate hydration during drug therapy.
• Patient and family state understanding of drug therapy.

tinzaparin sodium
(TIN-zuh-pear-in SOE-dee-um)
Innohep

Pharmacologic class: low–molecular-weight heparin (LMWH)
Therapeutic class: anticoagulant
Pregnancy risk category: B

Indications and dosages

▶ **Adjunct treatment (with warfarin sodium) of symptomatic deep vein thrombosis with or without pulmonary embolism.**
Adults: 175 anti-factor Xa international units per kg of body weight subcutaneously once daily for at least 6 days and until the patient is adequately anticoagulated with warfarin (INR at least 2) for 2 consecutive days. Begin warfarin when appropriate, usually within 1 to 3 days after tinzaparin starts. The volume to be given may be calculated as follows:

$$\text{Patient weight in kg} \times 0.00875 \text{ ml/kg} = \text{volume to be given (in ml)}$$

▶ **Deep vein thrombosis prophylaxis‡.**
Adults: 3,500 anti-factor Xa international units or 50 anti-factor Xa international units/kg daily for patients at moderate to high risk, respectively. Start 1 to 2 hours before surgery, and continue for 5 to 10 days. For prophylaxis in orthopedic procedures: 75 anti-factor Xa international units/kg daily starting 12 to 24 hours postoperatively. Alternative: 4,500 anti-factor Xa international units 12 hours before orthopedic surgery followed by 4,500 anti-factor Xa international units daily.

Contraindications and cautions

• Contraindicated in patients hypersensitive to the drug or to heparin, sulfites, benzyl alcohol, or pork products. Also contraindicated in patients with active major bleeding and patients with current or previous heparin-induced thrombocytopenia.

• Use cautiously in patients with increased risk of hemorrhage, such as those with bacterial endocarditis, uncontrolled hypertension, diabetic retinopathy, or congenital or acquired bleeding disorders (such as hepatic failure, amyloidosis, GI ulceration, or hemorrhagic stroke). Also use cautiously in patients being treated with platelet inhibitors, in patients who have recently undergone brain, spinal, or ophthalmologic surgery, and in patients with renal insufficiency.

• Use cautiously in patients with neuraxial (spinal or epidural) anesthesia or spinal puncture because these patients have an increased risk of neurologic injury and epidural or spinal hematoma.

• Use cautiously in patients with severe renal impairment and creatinine clearance less than 30 ml/minute.

♨ **Lifespan:** In pregnant women, use cautiously and only when clearly needed. Vaginal bleeding has been reported in pregnant women receiving tinzaparin; use only if benefits outweigh risks. In breast-feeding women, use cautiously; it's unknown if the drug appears in breast milk. In children, safety and effectiveness haven't been established. In the elderly, use cautiously because they may have reduced elimination of drug.

Adverse reactions

CNS: headache, fever, dizziness, insomnia, confusion, *cerebral or intracranial bleeding,* pain.
CV: *arrhythmias,* chest pain, hypotension, hypertension, *MI, thromboembolism,* tachycardia, dependent edema, angina pectoris.
EENT: epistaxis, ocular hemorrhage.
GI: anorectal bleeding, constipation, flatulence, hematemesis, hemarthrosis, *GI hemorrhage,* melena, nausea, vomiting, dyspepsia, *retroperitoneal or intra-abdominal bleeding.*
GU: dysuria, hematuria, UTI, urine retention, *vaginal hemorrhage.*
Hematologic: granulocytopenia, *thrombocytopenia,* anemia, *agranulocytosis,* pancytopenia, *hemorrhage.*
Musculoskeletal: back pain.

Respiratory: pneumonia, respiratory disorder, *pulmonary embolism,* dyspnea.
Skin: bullous eruption, cellulitis, *injection site hematoma,* pruritus, purpura, rash, skin necrosis, wound hematoma.
Other: *hypersensitivity reactions,* spinal or *epidural hematoma,* infection, impaired healing, allergic reaction, congenital anomaly, *fetal death, fetal distress.*

Interactions

Drug-drug. *Oral anticoagulants, platelet inhibitors (such as dextran, dipyridamole, NSAIDs, salicylates, sulfinpyrazone), thrombolytics:* May increase the risk of bleeding. Use together cautiously, and monitor patient.

Effects on lab test results

• May increase AST and ALT levels. May decrease hemoglobin level and hematocrit.
• May increase granular leukocyte count. May decrease granulocyte, platelet, RBC, and WBC counts.

Pharmacokinetics

Absorption: Plasma levels peak in 4 to 5 hours.
Distribution: The volume of distribution is similar in magnitude to that of blood volume, which suggests that distribution is limited to the central compartment.
Metabolism: Drug is partially metabolized by desulfation and depolymerization, similar to that of other LMWHs.
Excretion: The primary route of elimination is renal. *Half-life:* 3 to 4 hours.

Route	Onset	Peak	Duration
SubQ	2–3 hr	4–5 hr	Unknown

Action

Chemical effect: Inhibits reactions that lead to blood clotting, including the formation of fibrin clots. The drug also acts as a potent co-inhibitor of several activated coagulation factors, especially factors Xa and IIa (thrombin). It also induces release of tissue factor pathway inhibitor, which may contribute to the antithrombotic effect.
Therapeutic effect: Reduces the ability of blood to clot.

T

Available forms

Injection: 20,000 anti-Xa international units per ml in 2-ml vials

NURSING PROCESS

⚖ Assessment

• Assess patient's condition before starting therapy and regularly thereafter to monitor the drug's effectiveness.
• Monitor platelet count during therapy. If platelet count falls below 100,000/mm³, stop drug.
• Periodically monitor CBC and stool tests for occult blood during therapy.
• Drug may affect PT and INR levels. Patients who also receive warfarin should have blood drawn for PT and INR tests just before the next scheduled dose of this drug.
• Drug contains sodium metabisulfite, which may cause allergic reactions in susceptible people.
• Weigh patient before starting therapy to calculate accurate dose.
• Assess patient's and family's knowledge of drug therapy.

⊞ Nursing diagnoses

• Ineffective protection related to increased risk of bleeding
• Ineffective tissue perfusion, peripheral, related to deep vein thrombosis
• Deficient knowledge related to tinzaparin sodium therapy

▷ Planning and implementation

• Dose is based on actual body weight.
• If patient develops serious bleeding or receives a large overdose, replace volume and hemostatic blood elements (such as RBCs, fresh frozen plasma, and platelets) p.r.n. If this treatment is ineffective, consider giving protamine sulfate.
• ⊛ **ALERT:** Don't give I.M. or I.V., and don't mix with other injections or infusions.
• ⊛ **ALERT:** Drug can't be interchanged (unit for unit) with heparin or other LMWHs.
• While giving the drug, have the patient lie or sit down. Give drug by deep subcutaneous injection into the abdominal wall. Insert the whole length of the needle into a skin fold held between your thumb and forefinger. Hold the skin fold throughout the injection. To minimize

bruising, don't rub the injection site after administration.
• Rotate injection sites between the right and left anterolateral and posterolateral abdominal wall.
• Use an appropriate calibrated syringe to ensure withdrawal of the correct volume of drug from vial.
• ⊛ **ALERT:** When neuraxial anesthesia (epidural or spinal anesthesia) or spinal puncture is used, the patient is at risk for spinal hematoma, which can result in long-term or permanent paralysis. Watch for evidence of neurologic impairment. Consider the risks and benefits of neuraxial intervention in patients being anticoagulated with LMWHs or heparinoids.
• Store drug at room temperature.

Patient teaching
• Inform patient that co-administration of warfarin will begin within 1 to 3 days of tinzaparin administration. Explain the importance of warfarin therapy.
• Stress the importance of laboratory monitoring to ensure effectiveness and safety of therapy.
• Instruct patient to take safety measures to prevent cuts and bruises (such as using a soft toothbrush and an electric razor).
• Review the warning signs of bleeding, and instruct the patient to report evidence of bleeding immediately.
• Gasping syndrome may occur in premature infants who receive large amounts of benzyl alcohol. Warn patient about the risks of becoming pregnant during therapy.

☑ Evaluation

• Patient states appropriate bleeding precautions to take.
• Patient's peripheral neurovascular status returns to baseline.
• Patient and family state understanding of tinzaparin sodium therapy.

tiotropium bromide
(tee-oh-TROPE-ee-um BROH-mighd)
Spiriva

Pharmacologic class: long-acting anticholinergic (antimuscarinic)
Therapeutic class: bronchodilator
Pregnancy risk category: C

Indications and dosages

▶ **Maintenance therapy for bronchospasm in COPD, including chronic bronchitis and emphysema.** *Adults:* One capsule (18 mcg) inhaled orally once daily using the HandiHaler inhalation device.

Contraindications and cautions

• Contraindicated in patients hypersensitive to atropine, its derivatives, ipratropium, or any component of the product.

• Use cautiously in patients with creatinine clearance of 50 ml/minute or less and patients with angle-closure glaucoma, prostatic hyperplasia, or bladder neck obstruction.

※ **Lifespan:** In pregnant women, use cautiously. In breast-feeding women, use cautiously; it's unknown if the drug appears in breast milk. In children, safety and effectiveness haven't been established.

Adverse reactions

CNS: depression, paresthesia.
CV: *angina pectoris,* chest pain, edema.
EENT: cataract, dysphonia, epistaxis, glaucoma, laryngitis, pharyngitis, rhinitis, *sinusitis.*
GI: abdominal pain, constipation, *dry mouth,* dyspepsia, gastroesophageal reflux, stomatitis, vomiting.
GU: UTI.
Metabolic: hypercholesterolemia, hyperglycemia.
Musculoskeletal: arthritis, leg pain, myalgia, skeletal pain.
Respiratory: *paradoxical bronchospasm,* cough, upper respiratory tract infection.
Skin: rash.
Other: *accidental injury, angioedema,* allergic reaction, candidiasis, flulike syndrome, herpes zoster, infections.

Interactions

Drug-drug. *Anticholinergics:* May increase the risk of adverse reactions. Avoid using together.

Effects on lab test results

• May increase cholesterol and glucose levels.

Pharmacokinetics

Absorption: Poorly absorbed from GI tract; absolute bioavailability is 19.5% after inhaling dry powder. Plasma levels peak 3 hours after inhalation.

Distribution: Extensively bound to tissues and 72% bound to plasma proteins.
Metabolism: Small amounts by CYP 2D6 and 3A4 pathways.
Excretion: About 14% in urine, the rest in feces. *Half-life:* 5 to 6 days.

Route	Onset	Peak	Duration
Inhalation	30 min	3 hr	> 24 hr

Action

Chemical effect: Competitive, reversible inhibition of muscarinic receptors leads to bronchodilation.
Therapeutic effect: Improves breathing.

Available forms

Capsules for inhalation: 18 mcg

NURSING PROCESS

▨ Assessment

• Obtain baseline assessment of patient's respiratory status before starting therapy, and assess frequently thereafter to monitor the drug's effectiveness.

• Be alert for adverse reactions; eye pain, blurred vision, visual halos, colored images, or red eyes may be signs of acute narrow-angle glaucoma.

③ **ALERT:** Watch for evidence of hypersensitivity (especially angioedema) and paradoxical bronchospasm.

• Assess patient's and family's knowledge of drug therapy.

▦ Nursing diagnoses

• Impaired gas exchange related to underlying respiratory condition

• Risk for activity intolerance related to underlying pulmonary condition

• Deficient knowledge related to drug therapy

▷ Planning and implementation

• Drug is for maintenance treatment of COPD, not for acute bronchospasm.

• Capsules aren't for oral ingestion. Give them only by oral inhalation and only with the HandiHaler device.

• Capsules may be stored at room temperature prior to use. Remove capsule for oral inhalation from blister card just before use. Capsules should not be stored in the HandiHaler device.

T

• To give the drug, place the capsule in the center chamber of the HandiHaler device. Close the mouthpiece until it clicks, but leave the dust cap open. Press the piercing button one time. Instruct the patient to breathe out completely, raise HandiHaler device to his mouth, and close his lips tightly around the mouthpiece. The patient should keep his head upright and inhale slowly and deeply at a rate sufficient to hear the capsule vibrate. After the patient has inhaled until his lungs are full, have him hold his breath for as long as is comfortable while simultaneously taking the HandiHaler device out of his mouth; he then resumes normal breathing. The patient shouldn't ever breathe into the mouthpiece. The patient should inhale again to ensure a full dose of the drug.

• After taking the daily dose, dispose of the capsule and close the HandiHaler mouthpiece and dust cap for storage.

• Signs of overdose include dry mouth, bilateral conjunctivitis, altered mental state, tremors, abdominal pain, and severe constipation. Alert prescriber if overdose is suspected, and provide supportive care.

Patient teaching
• Inform patient that drug is for maintenance treatment of COPD and not for immediate relief of breathing problems.

• Explain that capsules are for inhalation and shouldn't be swallowed.

• Provide full instructions for the HandiHaler device.

• Tell patient not to get the powder in his eyes.

• Review the signs and symptoms of hypersensitivity (especially angioedema) and paradoxical bronchospasm. Tell patient to stop the drug and contact the prescriber if they arise.

• Advise patient to report eye pain, blurred vision, visual halos, colored images, or red eyes immediately.

• Tell patient to keep capsules in sealed blisters and to remove each capsule just before use. Caution against storing capsules in the Handi-Haler device.

• Instruct patient to store capsules at 77° F (25° C) and not to expose them to extreme temperatures or moisture.

🅜 **Evaluation**
• Patient's respiratory signs and symptoms improve.
• Patient's activity intolerance improves.

• Patient and family state understanding of drug therapy.

tipranavir
(tih-PRAN-uh-veer)
Aptivus

Pharmacologic class: non-peptidic protease inhibitor
Therapeutic class: antiretroviral
Pregnancy risk category: C

Indications and dosages

▶ **HIV-1 in patients with viral replication who are highly treatment-experienced or have HIV-1 strains resistant to multiple protease inhibitors.** *Adults:* 500 mg P.O. twice daily with 200 mg of ritonavir. Give with food.

Contraindications and cautions

• Contraindicated in patients hypersensitive to any ingredients of the product, patients with moderate (Child-Pugh class B) and severe (Child-Pugh class C) hepatic insufficiency, and patients taking drugs that depend on CYP 3A for clearance, such as amiodarone, astemizole, bepridil, cisapride, dihydroergotamine, ergonovine, ergotamine, flecainide, methylergonovine, midazolam, pimozide, propafenone, quinidine, terfenadine, and triazolam.

• Use cautiously in patients with sulfonamide allergy, diabetes, liver disease, hepatitis B or C, or hemophilia A or B.

⚖ **Lifespan:** In pregnant women, use only if benefits to the patient outweigh risks to the fetus. If patient is pregnant or becomes pregnant and is exposed to drug, register her with the Antiretroviral Pregnancy Registry at 800-258-4263. Breast-feeding isn't recommended during treatment. Iin children, safety and effectiveness haven't been established. In elderly patients, use cautiously because these patients are more likely to have decreased organ function, multi-drug therapy, and multiple illnesses.

Adverse reactions

CNS: asthenia, depression, dizziness, fatigue, headache, insomnia, pyrexia, malaise, peripheral neuropathy, sleep disorder, somnolence.

GI: abdominal distention, abdominal pain, *diarrhea*, dyspepsia, flatulence, GERD, nausea, *pancreatitis*, vomiting.
GU: renal insufficiency.
Hematologic: anemia, *neutropenia, thrombocytopenia.*
Hepatic: *hepatic failure*, hepatitis.
Metabolic: anorexia, decreased appetite, dehydration, diabetes mellitus, facial wasting, hyperglycemia, weight loss.
Musculoskeletal: muscle cramps, myalgia.
Respiratory: bronchitis, cough, dyspnea.
Skin: acquired lipodystrophy, exanthem, lipoatrophy, lipohypertrophy, pruritus, *rash.*
Other: flulike illness, hypersensitivity, reactivation of herpes simplex and varicella zoster.

Interactions

Drug-drug. *Amiodarone, bepridil, flecainide, propafenone, quinidine:* May increase levels of these drugs and risk of serious or life-threatening arrhythmias. Avoid use together.
Astemizole, cisapride, pimozide, terfenadine: May cause serious or life-threatening arrhythmias. Avoid use together.
Atorvastatin: May increase levels of both drugs. Start with lowest dose of atorvastatin, and monitor patient closely or consider other drugs.
Clarithromycin: May increase levels of both drugs. If patient's creatinine clearance is 30 to 60 ml/minute, decrease clarithromycin dose by 50%. If creatinine clearance is less than 30 ml/minute, decrease clarithromycin dose by 75%.
Cyclosporine, sirolimus, tacrolimus: May cause unpredictable interaction. Monitor drug levels closely until they've stabilized.
Desipramine: May increase desipramine level. Decrease dose, and monitor desipramine level.
Dihydroergotamine, ergonovine, ergotamine, methylergonovine: May cause acute ergot toxicity, including peripheral vasospasm and ischemia of extremities. Avoid use together.
Diltiazem, felodipine, nicardipine, nisoldipine, verapamil: May cause unpredictable interaction. Use together cautiously, and monitor patient closely.
Disulfiram, metronidazole: May cause disulfiram reaction. Use together cautiously.
Estrogen-based hormone therapy: May decrease estrogen level, and rash may occur. Monitor patient carefully. Advise using nonhormonal contraception.

Fluoxetine, paroxetine, sertraline: May increase levels of these drugs. Adjust dosages as needed.
Glimepiride, glipizide, glyburide, pioglitazone, repaglinide, tolbutamide: May affect glucose levels. Monitor glucose level carefully.
Lovastatin, simvastatin: May increase risk of myopathy and rhabdomyolysis. Avoid use together.
Meperidine: May increase normeperidine metabolite. Avoid use together.
Methadone: May decrease methadone level by 50%. Consider increased methadone dose.
Midazolam, triazolam: May cause prolonged or increased sedation or respiratory depression. Avoid use together.
Rifampin: May lead to loss of virologic response and resistance to tipranavir and other protease inhibitors. Avoid use together.
Rifabutin: May increase rifabutin level. Decrease rifabutin dose by 75%.
Sildenafil, tadalafil, vardenafil: May increase levels of these drugs. Tell patient to use together cautiously. Tell him not to exceed 25 mg of sildenafil in 48 hours, 10 mg of tadalafil in 72 hours, or 2.5 mg of vardenafil in 72 hours.
Warfarin: May cause unpredictable reaction. Check INR often.
Drug-herb. *St. John's wort:* May lead to loss of virologic response and resistance to drug and class. Warn patient to avoid use together.

Effects on lab test results

• May increase total cholesterol, triglyceride, blood glucose, amylase, lipase, ALT, and AST levels.
• May decrease WBC count.

Pharmacokinetics

Absorption: Limited; bioavailability is increased when taken with a high-fat meal.
Distribution: 99.9% bound to plasma proteins.
Metabolism: Mediated by CYP; few plasma metabolites found.
Excretion: Mostly unchanged in feces; some in urine. *Half life:* 4.8 to 6 hours.

Route	Onset	Peak	Duration
P.O.	Unknown	3 hr	Unknown

Action

Chemical effect: Inhibits virus-specific processing of polyproteins in HIV-1 infected cells, thus preventing formation of mature virions.

T

Therapeutic effect: Produces immature, noninfectious virus.

Available forms

Capsules: 250 mg

NURSING PROCESS

⁂ Assessment
• Carefully obtain patient's drug history. Many drugs may interact with tipranavir.
• Obtain liver function tests at start of treatment and often during treatment.
• Obtain cholesterol and triglyceride levels at start of and periodically during therapy.
• If patient has diabetes, monitor blood glucose level closely. Hyperglycemia may occur.
• Monitor patient for evidence of hepatitis, such as fatigue, malaise, anorexia, nausea, jaundice, bilirubinemia, acholic stools, liver tenderness, and hepatomegaly.
• Monitor patient for cushingoid symptoms, such as central obesity, buffalo hump, peripheral wasting, facial wasting, and breast enlargement.
• Evaluate patient's and family's knowledge of drug therapy.

⁂ Nursing diagnoses
• Risk for injury related to potential for many drugs to interact with tipranavir
• Potential for ineffective protection related to drug-induced adverse hematologic reactions
• Deficient knowledge related to drug therapy

⧐ Planning and implementation
⊛ **ALERT:** Don't give this drug to treatment-naive patients.
• To be effective, drug must be given with 200 mg of ritonavir and other antiretrovirals.
⊛ **ALERT:** Patients who have chronic hepatitis B or C have an increased risk of hepatotoxicity.
• If patient has indicators of hepatitis, stop drug.
Patient teaching
• Explain that drug doesn't cure HIV infection and doesn't reduce the risk of transmitting the virus to others.
⊛ **ALERT:** Warn patient that many drugs may interfere with tipranavir. Urge patient to tell prescriber about all prescription drugs, OTC drugs, and herbal products he takes.
• Tell patient that drug is effective only when taken with ritonavir and other antiretroviral drugs.

• Instruct patient to take drug with food.
• Urge patient to stop drug and contact prescriber if he has evidence of hepatitis, such as fatigue, malaise, anorexia, nausea, jaundice, bilirubinemia, acholic stools, or liver tenderness.
• If patient uses hormonal contraceptives, advise additional or alternative contraception during treatment.
• Tell patient that redistribution or accumulation of body fat may occur.

☑ Evaluation
• Patient doesn't experience drug interactions.
• Patient doesn't experience any serious adverse hematologic effects.

tobramycin sulfate
(toh-bruh-MIGH-sin SUL-fayt)
Nebcin, Tobi

Pharmacologic class: aminoglycoside
Therapeutic class: antibiotic
Pregnancy risk category: D

Indications and dosages

▶ **Serious infections caused by sensitive strains of** *Citrobacter, Enterobacter, Escherichia coli, Klebsiella, Proteus, Providencia, Pseudomonas, Serratia,* **and** *Staphylococcus aureus. Adults and children with normal renal function:* 3 mg/kg I.M. or I.V. daily divided q 8 hours. Up to 5 mg/kg daily divided q 6 to 8 hours for life-threatening infections.
Neonates younger than age 1 week or premature infants: Up to 4 mg/kg I.V. or I.M. daily in two equal doses q 12 hours.
▶ **Bronchopulmonary** *Pseudomonas aeruginosa* **in cystic fibrosis patients.** *Adults and children 6 years and older:* 300 mg by oral inhalation every 12 hours. Intervals should never be less than 6 hours apart, and cycle should be for 28 days, followed by at least 28 days off.

▼ I.V. administration

• Dilute in 50 to 100 ml of normal saline solution or D_5W for adults and in less volume for children.
• Infuse over 20 to 60 minutes. After I.V. infusion, flush line with normal saline solution or D_5W.

⊗ **Incompatibilities**
Allopurinol; amphotericin B; beta lactam antibiotics; dextrose 5% in Isolyte E, M, or P; heparin sodium; hetastarch; indomethacin; I.V. solutions containing alcohol; other I.V. drugs; propofol; sargramostim.

Contraindications and cautions

• Contraindicated in patients hypersensitive to aminoglycosides.
• Use cautiously in patients with impaired kidney function or neuromuscular disorders.
⚶ **Lifespan:** In pregnant and breast-feeding women, drug isn't recommended. In the elderly, use cautiously.

Adverse reactions

CNS: headache, lethargy, confusion, disorientation.
EENT: ototoxicity.
GI: nausea, vomiting, diarrhea.
GU: *nephrotoxicity.*
Hematologic: anemia, eosinophilia, *leukopenia, thrombocytopenia, agranulocytosis.*
Other: hypersensitivity reactions, *anaphylaxis.*

Interactions

Drug-drug. *Acyclovir, amphotericin B, cephalothin, cisplatin, methoxyflurane, other aminoglycosides, vancomycin:* May increase nephrotoxicity. Use together cautiously.
Atracurium, doxacurium, mivacurium, pancuronium, rocuronium, tubocurarine, vecuronium: May increase the effects of nondepolarizing muscle relaxant, including prolonged respiratory depression. Use together only when necessary. Dose of nondepolarizing muscle relaxant may need to be reduced.
Dimenhydrinate: May mask symptoms of ototoxicity. Use cautiously.
General anesthetics: May potentiate neuromuscular blockade. Monitor patient closely.
I.V. loop diuretics (such as furosemide): May increase ototoxicity. Use together cautiously.
Parenteral penicillins (such as ticarcillin): May inactivate tobramycin. Don't mix.

Effects on lab test results

• May increase BUN, creatinine, and nonprotein nitrogen and nitrogenous compound levels. May decrease calcium, magnesium, potassium, and hemoglobin levels and hematocrit.

• May increase eosinophil count. May decrease WBC, platelet, and granulocyte counts.

Pharmacokinetics

Absorption: Unknown.
Distribution: Widely distributed, although CSF penetration is low, even in patients with inflamed meninges. Protein-binding is minimal.
Metabolism: None.
Excretion: Excreted primarily in urine; small amount may be excreted in bile. Oral inhalation form is excreted in sputum. *Half-life:* 2 to 3 hours.

Route	Onset	Peak	Duration
I.V.	Immediate	Immediate	8 hr
I.M.	Unknown	30–90 min	8 hr
Inhalation	Unknown	10 min	Unknown

Action

Chemical effect: Inhibits protein synthesis by binding directly to 30S ribosomal subunit.
Therapeutic effect: Kills susceptible bacteria.

Available forms

Injection: 40 mg/ml, 10 mg/ml (pediatric)
Powder for injection: 30 mg/ml after reconstitution
Premixed parenteral injection for I.V. infusion: 60 mg or 80 mg in normal saline solution
Solution for nebulization: 300 mg/5 ml.

NURSING PROCESS

Assessment
• Assess patient's infection before starting therapy and regularly thereafter to monitor the drug's effectiveness.
• Obtain specimen for culture and sensitivity tests before giving the first dose. Start therapy pending test results.
• Weigh patient and review baseline kidney function studies before starting therapy.
• Assess patient's hearing before starting therapy and during therapy. Report tinnitus, vertigo, or hearing loss.
• Monitor kidney function (output, specific gravity, urinalysis, BUN and creatinine levels, and creatinine clearance).
• Be alert for adverse reactions and drug interactions.
• Assess patient's and family's knowledge of drug therapy.

T

⊕ Nursing diagnoses
- Risk for infection related to susceptible bacteria
- Risk for injury related to potential for drug-induced nephrotoxicity
- Deficient knowledge related to drug therapy

▶ Planning and implementation
- Don't use commercially packaged products in normal saline solution for I.M. injection. For I.M. administration use tobramycin from multidose vial or prefilled syringes.
- Draw blood for peak tobramycin level 1 hour after I.M. injection and 30 minutes to 1 hour after infusion ends; draw blood for trough level just before next dose. Don't collect blood in heparinized tube because heparin is incompatible with drug.
- ⊛ **ALERT:** Peak levels higher than 12 mcg/ml and trough levels higher than 2 mcg/ml may be linked to increased risk of toxicity.
- Nebulizer treatment for inhaled tobramycin should last 15 minutes. Drug shouldn't be diluted or admixed with other drugs.
- Notify prescriber of signs of decreasing kidney function.
- Keep patient well hydrated during therapy to minimize chemical irritation of renal tubules.
- If no response occurs in 3 to 5 days, therapy may be stopped and new specimens obtained for culture and sensitivity testing.
- ⊛ **ALERT:** Don't confuse tobramycin with Trobicin.

Patient teaching
- Emphasize need to drink 2 L of fluid each day.
- Instruct patient to report adverse reactions.

☑ Evaluation
- Patient is free from infection.
- Patient maintains normal kidney function.
- Patient and family state understanding of drug therapy.

tolcapone
(TOHL-cah-pohn)
Tasmar

Pharmacologic class: COMT inhibitor
Therapeutic class: antiparkinsonian
Pregnancy risk category: C

Indications and dosages
▶ **Adjunct to levodopa and carbidopa for signs and symptoms of idiopathic Parkinson's disease.** *Adults:* Initially, 100 mg P.O. t.i.d. (with levodopa and carbidopa). Recommended daily dosage is 100 mg P.O. t.i.d., although 200 mg P.O. t.i.d. may be given if the anticipated benefit is justified. If starting therapy with 200 mg t.i.d. and dyskinesia occurs, reduce dosage of levodopa. Maximum, 600 mg daily.

Contraindications and cautions
- Contraindicated in patients hypersensitive to the drug or any of its components and in patients with liver disease, elevated ALT or AST values, or history of nontraumatic rhabdomyolysis, hyperpyrexia, or confusion possibly related to drug. Also contraindicated in patients withdrawn from drug because of evidence of drug-induced hepatocellular injury.
- Use cautiously in patients with severe renal impairment.
- ⚖ **Lifespan:** In pregnant women, use only if benefits to patient outweigh risks to fetus. In breast-feeding women, use cautiously.

Adverse reactions
CNS: *dyskinesia, sleep disorder, dystonia, excessive dreaming, somnolence, dizziness, confusion, headache, hallucinations,* hyperkinesia, hypertonia, fatigue, falling, syncope, balance loss, depression, tremor, speech disorder, paresthesia, agitation, irritability, mental deficiency, hyperactivity, hypokinesia, fever.
CV: *orthostatic complaints,* chest pain, chest discomfort, palpitations, hypotension.
EENT: pharyngitis, tinnitus, sinus congestion.
GI: *nausea, anorexia, diarrhea,* flatulence, *vomiting,* constipation, abdominal pain, dyspepsia, dry mouth.
GU: UTI, urine discoloration, hematuria, micturition disorder, urinary incontinence, impotence.
Hematologic: *bleeding.*
Hepatic: *hepatic failure.*
Musculoskeletal: *muscle cramps,* stiffness, arthritis, neck pain.
Respiratory: bronchitis, dyspnea, upper respiratory tract infection.
Skin: increased sweating, rash.
Other: burning, influenza.

Interactions

Drug-drug. *CNS depressants:* May enhance sedative effects. Use cautiously.
Nonselective MAO inhibitors (phenelzine, tranylcypromine): May increase risk of hypertensive crisis. Don't use together.

Effects on lab test results

• May increase liver function test values.

Pharmacokinetics

Absorption: Rapid. Absolute bioavailability is 65%.
Distribution: Not widely distributed into tissues; more than 99.9% is bound to plasma proteins.
Metabolism: Almost complete, mainly by glucuronidation.
Excretion: 60% excreted in urine and 40% in feces. *Half-life:* 2 to 3 hours.

Route	Onset	Peak	Duration
P.O.	Unknown	2 hr	Unknown

Action

Chemical effect: Unknown; may reversibly inhibit human erythrocyte COMT when given with levodopa and carbidopa, resulting in a decrease in levodopa clearance and a twofold increase in levodopa bioavailability. Decreased clearance of levodopa prolongs half-life of levodopa from 2 to 3½ hours.
Therapeutic effect: Improves physical mobility in patients with parkinsonism.

Available forms

Tablets: 100 mg, 200 mg

NURSING PROCESS

⚕ Assessment

• Assess patient's history of Parkinson's disease before starting therapy, and reassess during therapy to monitor the drug's effectiveness.
• Monitor liver enzyme levels before therapy, then q 2 to 4 weeks during first 6 months of therapy, then periodically thereafter because of risk of liver toxicity. Stop giving the drug if levels are elevated or if patient has signs or symptoms of liver dysfunction. If dose is increased to maximum, resume monistoring as described.
• Assess patient's risk for physical injury because of drug's adverse CNS effects.

• Monitor patient for orthostatic hypotension and syncope.
• Assess patient's and family's knowledge of drug therapy.

⊞ Nursing diagnoses

• Impaired physical mobility related to underlying Parkinson's disease
• Disturbed thought processes related to drug-induced CNS adverse reactions
• Deficient knowledge related to drug therapy

⊳ Planning and implementation

⑤ **ALERT:** Be sure patient has provided written informed consent before drug is used. Give drug only to patient taking levodopa and carbidopa who doesn't respond to, or who isn't an appropriate candidate for, other adjunctive therapies because of risk of liver toxicity.
• Give first dose of the day with first daily dose of levodopa and carbidopa.
• Patient with severe renal dysfunction may need a lower dose.
• Don't give the drug, and notify prescriber, if hepatic transaminases are elevated or if patient appears jaundiced or complains of nausea, upper right quadrant pain, fatigue, lethargy, anorexia, pruritus, or dark urine.
• Because of risk of liver toxicity, stop giving the drug if patient shows no benefit within 3 weeks.
• Because of highly protein-bound nature of drug, dialysis doesn't significantly remove drug.
• If severe diarrhea linked to therapy occurs, notify prescriber.
Patient teaching
• Advise patient to take drug exactly as prescribed.
• Teach patient signs of liver dysfunction (jaundice, fatigue, loss of appetite, persistent nausea, pruritus, dark urine, or right upper quadrant tenderness) and instruct him to report them immediately.
• Warn patient about risk of orthostatic hypotension; tell him to use caution when rising from a seated or lying position.
• Instruct patient to avoid hazardous activities until the drug's CNS effects are known.
• Tell patient nausea may occur at the start of therapy.
• Inform patient about risk of increased dyskinesia or dystonia.
• Tell patient to report planned, suspected, or known pregnancy during therapy.

T

• Instruct patient to report adverse effects to prescriber, including diarrhea and hallucinations.
• Inform patient that drug may be taken without regard to meals.

☑ Evaluation
• Patient exhibits improved mobility with reduction of muscular rigidity and tremor.
• Patient remains mentally alert.
• Patient and family state understanding of drug therapy.

tolterodine tartrate
(tohl-TER-oh-deen TAR-trate)
Detrol, Detrol LA

Pharmacologic class: muscarinic receptor antagonist
Therapeutic class: anticholinergic
Pregnancy risk category: C

Indications and dosages

▶ Overactive bladder in patients with symptoms of urinary frequency, urgency, or urge incontinence. *Adults:* 2 mg P.O. b.i.d. Dosage may be lowered to 1 mg P.O. b.i.d. based on patient response and tolerance. Or, 4 mg of extended-release capsule P.O. daily; may be decreased to 2 mg P.O. daily.
⧉ Adjust-a-dose: For patients with significantly reduced hepatic or renal function and patients taking drug that inhibits CYP 3A4 isoenzyme system, give 1 mg P.O. b.i.d. or 2 mg P.O. daily of extended-release capsules.

Contraindications and cautions

• Contraindicated in patients hypersensitive to the drug or any of its components and in those with uncontrolled angle-closure glaucoma or urine or gastric retention.
• Use cautiously in patients with significant bladder outflow obstruction, GI obstructive disorders (such as pyloric stenosis), controlled angle-closure glaucoma, or hepatic or renal impairment.
⚝ Lifespan: In preganant wimen, use only if benefits outweigh risks. Breast-feeding women should either stop breast-feeding or use another drug. In children, safety and effectiveness haven't been established.

Adverse reactions

CNS: fatigue, paresthesia, vertigo, dizziness, *headache,* nervousness, somnolence.
CV: hypertension, chest pain.
EENT: abnormal vision, xerophthalmia, pharyngitis, rhinitis, sinusitis.
GI: *dry mouth,* abdominal pain, constipation, diarrhea, dyspepsia, flatulence, nausea, vomiting.
GU: dysuria, micturition frequency, urine retention, UTI.
Metabolic: weight gain.
Musculoskeletal: arthralgia, back pain.
Respiratory: bronchitis, cough, upper respiratory tract infection.
Skin: pruritus, rash, erythema, dry skin.
Other: flulike syndrome, falls, fungal infection, infection.

Interactions

Drug-drug. *Antifungals (itraconazole, ketoconazole, miconazole), cyclosporine, CYP 3A4 inhibitors (such as macrolide antibiotics clarithromycin and erythromycin), vincristine:* May increase tolterodine concentration. Don't give tolterodine doses above 1 mg b.i.d. (2 mg daily of extended-release capsules) with these drugs.

Effects on lab test results

None reported.

Pharmacokinetics

Absorption: Well absorbed with about 77% bioavailability. Peak level occurs within 1 to 2 hours after administration. Food increases bioavailability by 53%.
Distribution: Volume of distribution is about 113 L, 96% protein-bound.
Metabolism: Primarily by oxidation by the CYP 2D6 pathway and forms an active 5-hydroxymethyl metabolite.
Excretion: Mostly recovered in urine, the rest in feces. Less than 1% of dose is recovered as unchanged drug, and 5% to 14% is recovered as the active metabolite. *Half-life:* 1¾ to 3½ hours.

Route	Onset	Peak	Duration
P.O.	Unknown	1–2 hr	Unknown

Action

Chemical effect: A competitive muscarinic receptor antagonist. Both urinary bladder contraction and salivation are mediated via cholinergic muscarinic receptors.

Therapeutic effect: Relieves symptoms of overactive bladder.

Available forms

Capsules (extended-release): 2 mg, 4 mg
Tablets: 1 mg, 2 mg

NURSING PROCESS

☑ Assessment
• Assess baseline bladder function before starting therapy, and reassess frequently to monitor the drug's effectiveness.
• Be alert for adverse reactions and drug interactions.
• Assess patient's and family's knowledge of drug therapy.

⊞ Nursing diagnoses
• Impaired urinary elimination related to underlying medical condition
• Urine retention related to drug-induced adverse effects
• Deficient knowledge related to drug therapy

▷ Planning and implementation
• Food increases the absorption of tolterodine, but no dose adjustment is needed.
• If patient has urine retention, notify prescriber and prepare for urinary catheterization.
• Dry mouth is the most common adverse reaction.
Patient teaching
• Tell patient that sugarless gum, hard candy, or saliva substitute may help relieve dry mouth.
• Advise patient to avoid driving or other potentially hazardous activities until visual effects of drug are known.
• Instruct patient to immediately report signs of infection, urine retention, or GI problems.

▨ Evaluation
• Patient experiences improved bladder function with drug therapy.
• Patient doesn't experience urine retention.
• Patient and family state understanding of drug therapy.

topiramate
(toh-PEER-uh-mayt)
Topamax

Pharmacologic class: sulfamate-substituted monosaccharide
Therapeutic class: antiepileptic
Pregnancy risk category: C

Indications and dosages

▶ **Adjunctive therapy for partial seizures, primary generalized tonic-clonic seizures, or Lennox-Gastaut syndrome.** *Adults:* For partial onset seizures, 200 to 400 mg P.O. daily in two divided doses. For primary generalized tonic-clonic seizures, 400 mg P.O. daily in two divided doses. Start at 25 to 50 mg daily, and adjust to an effective dose in increments of 25 to 50 mg weekly.
Children ages 2 to 16: 5 to 9 mg/kg P.O. daily in two divided doses. Begin dosage adjustment at 1 to 3 mg/kg nightly for 1 week. Then increase at 1- to 2-week intervals by 1 to 3 mg/kg daily to achieve optimal response.
▶ **Prevention of migraine headaches.** *Adults:* Week one, 25 mg P.O. q p.m. for 7 days. Week two, 25 mg P.O. b.i.d. for 7 days. Week three, 25 mg P.O. q a.m. and 50 mg P.O. q p.m. for 7 days. Maintenance dose 50 mg P.O. bid. If needed, may use longer intervals between dose adjustments.
▶ **Initial monotherapy in patients with partial onset or primary generalized tonic-clonic seizures.** *Adults and children age 10 or older:* The recommended daily dose is 400 mg P.O. divided b.i.d. (morning and evening). To achieve this dose, adjust as follows. The first week, give 25 mg P.O. b.i.d. The second week, give 50 mg P.O. b.i.d. The third week, give 75 mg P.O. b.i.d. The fourth week, give 100 mg P.O. b.i.d. The fifth week, give 150 mg P.O. b.i.d. The sixth week, give 200 mg P.O. b.i.d.
☒ **Adjust-a-dose:** For patients with creatinine clearance less than 70 ml/minute, reduce dosage by 50%. For patients on hemodialysis, may need to give supplemental doses to avoid rapid drops in drug level during prolonged dialysis treatment.

Contraindications and cautions

• Contraindicated in patients hypersensitive to the drug or any of its components.

T

1256 topiramate

• Use cautiously in patients with hepatic and renal impairment. Also use cautiously with other drugs that predispose patients to heat-related disorders, including other carbonic anhydrase inhibitors and anticholinergics.

⚄ **Lifespan:** In pregnant and breast-feeding women, use cautiously.

Adverse reactions

CNS: fever, *fatigue*, abnormal coordination, aggression, agitation, apathy, asthenia, *ataxia, confusion,* depression, depersonalization, *dizziness,* emotional lability, euphoria, **generalized tonic-clonic seizures,** hallucinations, hyperkinesia, hypertonia, hypesthesia, hypokinesia, insomnia, *nervousness, nystagmus, paresthesia,* personality disorder, *psychomotor slowing,* psychosis, *somnolence, speech disorders,* stupor, **suicide attempts,** *tremor,* vertigo, malaise, mood problems, difficulty with concentration, attention, language, or *memory.*
CV: chest pain, palpitations, edema, hot flushes.
EENT: *abnormal vision,* conjunctivitis, *diplopia,* eye pain, hearing problems, pharyngitis, sinusitis, tinnitus.
GI: taste perversion, abdominal pain, *anorexia,* constipation, diarrhea, dry mouth, dyspepsia, flatulence, gastroenteritis, gingivitis, *nausea,* vomiting.
GU: amenorrhea, dysuria, dysmenorrhea, hematuria, impotence, intermenstrual bleeding, menstrual disorder, menorrhagia, micturition frequency, renal calculi, urinary incontinence, UTI, vaginitis, leukorrhea.
Hematologic: anemia, epistaxis, *leukopenia.*
Metabolic: weight changes.
Musculoskeletal: arthralgia, back or leg pain, muscular weakness, myalgia, rigors.
Respiratory: bronchitis, cough, dyspnea, *upper respiratory tract infection.*
Skin: acne, alopecia, increased sweating, pruritus, rash.
Other: body odor, flulike syndrome, breast pain, decreased libido.

Interactions

Drug-drug. *Carbamazepine:* May decrease topiramate levels. Monitor patient.
Carbonic anhydrase inhibitors (acetazolamide, dichlorphenamide): May increase risk of renal calculus formation. Avoid use together.
CNS depressants: May increase risk of topiramate-induced CNS depression and other adverse cognitive and neuropsychiatric events. Use cautiously.
Hormonal contraceptives: May decrease effectiveness. Report changes in bleeding patterns; urge patient to use nonhormonal contraceptive.
Phenytoin: May decrease topiramate level and increase phenytoin level. Monitor levels.
Valproic acid: May decrease valproic acid and topiramate levels. Monitor patient.
Drug-lifestyle. *Alcohol use:* May increase risk of topiramate-induced CNS depression and other adverse cognitive and neuropsychiatric events. Discourage use together.

Effects on lab test results

• May increase liver enzyme levels. May decrease bicarbonate and hemoglobin levels and hematocrit.
• May decrease WBC count.

Pharmacokinetics

Absorption: Rapid.
Distribution: Up to 17% bound to plasma proteins.
Metabolism: Not extensive.
Excretion: Primarily eliminated unchanged in urine. *Half-life:* 21 hours.

Route	Onset	Peak	Duration
P.O.	Unknown	2 hr	Unknown

Action

Chemical effect: May block action potential, suggestive of a sodium channel blocking action. May also potentiate activity of GABA and antagonize ability of kainate to activate the amino acid (glutamate) receptor.
Therapeutic effect: Prevents partial-onset seizures.

Available forms

Capsules, sprinkle: 15 mg, 25 mg
Tablets: 25 mg, 50 mg, 100 mg, 200 mg

NURSING PROCESS

⚄ Assessment
• Assess patient's seizure disorder before starting therapy and regularly thereafter to monitor the drug's effectiveness.
• Carefully monitor patient taking topiramate with other antiepileptic drugs; dose adjustment may be needed to achieve optimal response.

Reactions may be *common,* uncommon, *life-threatening,* or COMMON AND LIFE-THREATENING.

• Oligohidrosis and hyperthermia have been infrequently reported, mainly in children. Monitor patient closely, especially in hot weather.

• Becasue Topamax inhibits carbonic anhydrase, it may cause hyperchloremic, non-anion gap metabolic acidosis from renal bicarbonate. Usually, this occurs early in treatment, although it may happen at any time. Assess patient for factors that may predispose him to acidosis, such as renal disease, severe respiratory disorders, status epilepticus, diarrhea, surgery, ketogenic diet, or drugs.

• Monitor patient for serious symptoms of acute and chronic metabolic acidosis, which include abnormal heart rhythms and stupor. Less severe complications include fatigue, anorexia, and hyperventilation. Left untreated, the acidosis can cause kidney damage, osteoporosis, or osteomalacia—also called rickets, in children.

• Assess patient's compliance with therapy at each follow-up visit.

• Assess patient's and family's knowledge of drug therapy.

⊕ **Nursing diagnoses**
• Risk for injury related to seizure disorder
• Acute pain related to increased risk of renal calculi formation
• Deficient knowledge related to drug therapy

▷ **Planning and implementation**
• Renal insufficiency requires a lower dose. For hemodialysis patients, supplemental doses may be needed to avoid rapid drops in drug levels during prolonged dialysis.

• Measure baseline and periodic serum bicarbonate levels during topiramate treatment. If metabolic acidosis develops and persists, consider reducing the dose or stopping the drug (using dose tapering). If patient continues on drug despite persistent acidosis, alkali treatment should be considered.

⑤ **ALERT:** If an ocular adverse event occurs, characterized by acute myopia and secondary angle-closure glaucoma, stop drug.

⑤ **ALERT:** Don't confuse Topamax with Toprol-XL, Tegretol, or Tegretol-XR.

Patient teaching
• Tell patient to maintain adequate fluid intake during therapy to minimize risk of forming renal calculi.

• Advise patient not to drive or operate hazardous machinery until the drug's CNS effects are known.

• Tell patient that drug may decrease effectiveness of hormonal contraceptives, and suggest barrier-method birth control.

• Tell patient to avoid crushing or breaking tablets because of bitter taste.

• Tell patient that drug can be taken without regard to food.

• Tell patient to notify prescriber immediately if he experiences changes in vision.

☑ **Evaluation**
• Patient is free from seizure activity.
• Patient maintains adequate hydration to prevent renal calculus formation.
• Patient and family state understanding of drug therapy.

topotecan hydrochloride
(toh-poh-TEE-ken high-droh-KLOR-ighd)
Hycamtin

Pharmacologic class: antitumor drug
Therapeutic class: antineoplastic
Pregnancy risk category: D

Indications and dosages

▶ **Metastatic carcinoma of ovary after failure of initial or subsequent chemotherapy; small-cell lung cancer after failure of first-line chemotherapy.** *Adults:* 1.5 mg/m^2 by I.V. infusion over 30 minutes, daily for 5 consecutive days, starting on day 1 of a 21-day cycle, for minimum of four cycles in absence of tumor progression.

⑤ **Adjust-a-dose:** For patients with renal impairment, if creatinine clearance is 20 to 39 ml/minute, decrease dosage to 0.75 mg/m^2. If severe neutropenia occurs, reduce dose by 0.25 mg/m^2 for subsequent courses. Or, in severe neutropenia, give granulocyte-colony stimulating factor (GSF) after subsequent course (before resorting to dose reduction) starting from day 6 of the course (24 hours after topotecan administration).

▽ **I.V. administration**
• Prepare drug under a vertical laminar flow hood while wearing gloves and protective cloth-

T

ing. If drug contacts skin, wash immediately and thoroughly with soap and water. If mucous membranes are affected, flush with water.

● Reconstitute drug in each 4-mg vial with 4 ml sterile water for injection.

● Dilute appropriate volume of reconstituted solution in normal saline solution or D₅W before use.

● Infuse over 30 minutes.

● Protect unopened vials of drug from light. Reconstituted vials stored at 68° to 77° F (20° to 25° C) and exposed to ambient lighting are stable for 24 hours.

⊗ **Incompatibilities**

Dexamethasone, mitomycin.

Contraindications and cautions

● Contraindicated in patients hypersensitive to the drug or any of its components and in patients with severe bone marrow depression.

🜲 **Lifespan:** In pregnant and breast-feeding women, drug is contraindicated.

Adverse reactions

CNS: fever, fatigue, asthenia, headache, paresthesia.

GI: nausea, vomiting, diarrhea, constipation, abdominal pain, stomatitis, anorexia.

Hematologic: *neutropenia, leukopenia, thrombocytopenia, anemia.*

Respiratory: *dyspnea.*

Skin: alopecia.

Other: *sepsis.*

Interactions

Drug-drug. *Cisplatin:* May increase severity of myelosuppression. Use both drugs very cautiously.

Filgrastim (6-GCSF): May prolong duration of neutropenia. Don't give GCSF until day 6 of regimen, 24 hours after completion of topotecan therapy.

Effects on lab test results

● May increase ALT, AST, and bilirubin levels. May decrease hemoglobin level and hematocrit.

● May decrease WBC, platelet, and neutrophil counts.

Pharmacokinetics

Absorption: Administered I.V.

Distribution: About 35% bound to plasma proteins.

Metabolism: Metabolized by liver.

Excretion: 30% excreted in urine. *Half-life:* 2 to 3 hours.

Route	Onset	Peak	Duration
I.V.	Unknown	Unknown	Unknown

Action

Chemical effect: Results from damage to DNA produced during DNA synthesis when replication enzymes interact with the complex formed.

Therapeutic effect: Kills certain cancer cells.

Available forms

Injection: 4-mg single-dose vial

NURSING PROCESS

🖉 **Assessment**

● Assess patient's and family's knowledge of drug therapy.

● Assess patient's underlying condition before and frequently during therapy.

● Monitor patient's CBC frequently during therapy.

● Be alert for adverse reactions and drug interactions.

⊞ **Nursing diagnoses**

● Ineffective health maintenance related to neoplastic disease

● Deficient knowledge related to drug therapy

⊠ **Planning and implementation**

⊛ **ALERT:** Patient must have a baseline neutrophil count greater than 1,500/mm³ and platelet count greater than 100,000/mm³ before therapy can start.

● Frequent monitoring of peripheral blood cell count is critical. Don't give repeated doses until neutrophil count is greater than 1,000/mm³, platelet count is greater than 100,000/mm³, and hemoglobin is greater than 9 mg/dl.

Patient teaching

● Instruct patient to promptly report sore throat, fever, chills, or unusual bleeding or bruising.

● Advise woman of childbearing age not to become pregnant, and not to breast-feed, during therapy.

● Tell patient and family about need for close monitoring of blood cell counts.

☑ Evaluation
- Patient shows positive response to drug.
- Patient and family state understanding of drug therapy.

torsemide
(TOR-seh-mighd)
Demadex

Pharmacologic class: loop diuretic
Therapeutic class: diuretic, antihypertensive
Pregnancy risk category: B

Indications and dosages

▶ **Diuresis in patients with heart failure.**
Adults: Initially, 10 to 20 mg P.O. or I.V. once daily. If response is inadequate, double dose until response is obtained. Maximum, 200 mg daily.
▶ **Diuresis in patients with chronic renal impairment.** *Adults:* Initially, 20 mg P.O. or I.V. once daily. If response is inadequate, double dose until response is obtained. Maximum, 200 mg daily.
▶ **Diuresis in patients with hepatic cirrhosis.** *Adults:* Initially, 5 to 10 mg P.O. or I.V. once daily with aldosterone antagonist or potassium-sparing diuretic. If response is inadequate, double dose until response is obtained. Maximum, 40 mg daily.
▶ **Hypertension.** *Adults:* Initially, 5 mg P.O. daily. Increase to 10 mg in 4 to 6 weeks if needed and tolerated. If response is still inadequate, add another antihypertensive.

▽ I.V. administration

- Drug may be given by direct injection over at least 2 minutes. Rapid injection may cause ototoxicity. Don't give more than 200 mg at a time.
- Switch to oral form as soon as possible.
⊗ **Incompatibilities**
None reported.

Contraindications and cautions

- Contraindicated in patients hypersensitive to the drug or other sulfonylurea derivatives and in those with anuria.
- Use cautiously in patients with hepatic disease, cirrhosis, or ascites; sudden changes in fluid and electrolyte balance may precipitate hepatic coma.

☳ **Lifespan:** In pregnant women, use cautiously. In breast-feeding women, use cautiously; it's unknown if the drug appears in breast milk. In children, safety and effectiveness haven't been established. In geriatric patients, use cautiously.

Adverse reactions

CNS: asthenia, dizziness, headache, nervousness, insomnia, syncope.
CV: *ventricular tachycardia,* ECG abnormalities, chest pain, edema, orthostatic hypotension.
EENT: rhinitis, sore throat.
GI: diarrhea, constipation, nausea, dyspepsia, *hemorrhage.*
GU: excessive urination, impotence.
Metabolic: *dehydration,* electrolyte imbalances, including *hypokalemia, hypomagnesemia,* hypocalcemia, hyperuricemia, hyperglycemia; *hypochloremic alkalosis.*
Musculoskeletal: arthralgia, myalgia.
Respiratory: cough.
Other: excessive thirst, gout.

Interactions

Drug-drug. *Chlorothiazide, chlorthalidone, hydrochlorothiazide, indapamide, metolazone:* May cause excessive diuretic response resulting in serious electrolyte abnormalities or dehydration. Adjust doses carefully and monitor patient for this effect.
Cholestyramine: May decrease absorption of torsemide. Separate administration times by at least 3 hours.
Indomethacin: May decrease diuretic effectiveness in sodium-restricted patients. Avoid use together.
Lithium, ototoxic drugs (such as aminoglycosides, ethacrynic acid): May increase toxicity of these drugs. Avoid use together.
NSAIDs: May potentiate nephrotoxicity of NSAIDs. Use together cautiously.
Probenecid: May decrease diuretic effectiveness. Avoid use together.
Salicylates: May decrease excretion, possibly leading to salicylate toxicity. Avoid use together.
Spironolactone: May decrease renal clearance of spironolactone. Dosage adjustments aren't needed.
Drug-herb. *Licorice:* May cause rapid potassium loss. Discourage use together.

T

Effects on lab test results

• May increase glucose, BUN, creatinine, cholesterol, and uric acid levels. May decrease calcium, potassium, and magnesium levels.

Pharmacokinetics

Absorption: Little first-pass metabolism.
Distribution: Extensively bound to plasma protein.
Metabolism: 80% hepatically metabolized.
Excretion: 22% to 34% excreted unchanged in urine. *Half-life:* 3½ hours.

Route	Onset	Peak	Duration
P.O.	1 hr	1–2 hr	6–8 hr
I.V.	≤ 10 min	≤ 1 hr	6–8 hr

Action

Chemical effect: Enhances excretion of sodium, chloride, and water by acting on ascending portion of loop of Henle.
Therapeutic effect: Promotes water and sodium excretion and lowers blood pressure.

Available forms

Injection: 10 mg/ml
Tablets: 5 mg, 10 mg, 20 mg, 100 mg

NURSING PROCESS

☑ Assessment
• Assess patient's condition before starting therapy and regularly thereafter to monitor the drug's effectiveness.
• Monitor an elderly patient, who is especially susceptible to excessive diuresis, with potential for circulatory collapse and thromboembolic complications.
• During rapid diuresis and routinely with long-term use, monitor fluid intake and output, electrolyte levels, blood pressure, weight, and pulse rate. Drug may cause profound diuresis and water and electrolyte depletion.
• Watch for signs of hypokalemia, such as muscle weakness and cramps.
• Be alert for adverse reactions and drug interactions.
• Assess patient's and family's knowledge of drug therapy.

☒ Nursing diagnoses
• Excess fluid volume related to presence of edema

• Risk for injury related to presence of hypertension
• Deficient knowledge related to drug therapy

▶ Planning and implementation
• Give oral drug in morning to prevent nocturia.
• Make sure patient is on a high-potassium diet; refer patient to a dietitian for guidance. Foods rich in potassium include citrus fruits, tomatoes, bananas, dates, and apricots.
⊗ **ALERT:** Don't confuse torsemide with furosemide.

Patient teaching
• Tell patient to take drug in the morning to prevent sleep interruption.
• Advise patient to change position slowly to prevent dizziness.
• Advise patient to immediately report ringing in ears because it may indicate toxicity.
• Tell patient to check with prescriber or pharmacist before taking OTC drugs.

☑ Evaluation
• Patient shows no signs of edema.
• Patient's blood pressure is normal.
• Patient and family state understanding of drug therapy.

tramadol hydrochloride
(TRAM-uh-dohl high-droh-KLOR-ighd)
Ultram

Pharmacologic class: opioid agonist
Therapeutic class: analgesic
Pregnancy risk category: C

Indications and dosages

▶ **Moderate to moderately severe pain.**
Adults: 50 to 100 mg P.O. q 4 to 6 hours, p.r.n. Maximum dosage is 400 mg daily.
☒ **Adjust-a-dose:** Maximum dosage in patients older than age 75 is 300 mg daily. For patients with cirrhosis, give 50 mg P.O. q 12 hours. For patients with renal impairment, if creatinine clearance is less than 30 ml/minute, give dose q 12 hours. Maximum, 200 mg daily. Hemodialysis patients can receive their regular dose on same day of dialysis.

Contraindications and cautions

- Contraindicated in patients hypersensitive to the drug or any of its components, and in those with acute intoxication from alcohol, hypnotics, centrally acting analgesics, opioids, or psychotropic drugs.
- Use cautiously in patients at risk for seizures or respiratory depression; patients with increased intracranial pressure or head injury, acute abdominal conditions, or renal or hepatic impairment; and patients physically dependent on opioids.

Lifespan: In pregnant women and in children, safety and effectiveness haven't been established. In breast-feeding women, drug isn't recommended.

Adverse reactions

CNS: *dizziness, vertigo, headache, somnolence, CNS stimulation, asthenia,* anxiety, confusion, coordination disturbance, malaise, euphoria, nervousness, sleep disorder, ***seizures.***
CV: vasodilation.
EENT: visual disturbances.
GI: *nausea, constipation, vomiting,* dyspepsia, dry mouth, diarrhea, abdominal pain, anorexia, flatulence.
GU: urine retention, urinary frequency, menopausal symptoms.
Musculoskeletal: hypertonia.
Respiratory: ***respiratory depression.***
Skin: *pruritus,* sweating, rash.

Interactions

Drug-drug. *Carbamazepine:* May increase tramadol metabolism. Patients receiving long-term carbamazepine therapy at dosage of up to 800 mg daily may require up to twice the recommended dose of tramadol.
CNS depressants: May have additive effects. Use together cautiously. Dosage of tramadol may need to be reduced.
MAO inhibitors, SSRIs: May increase risk of seizures. Monitor patient closely.
Drug-herb. *5-hydroxytryptophan (5-HTP), SAMe, St. John's wort:* May increase serotonin level. Discourage use together.

Effects on lab test results

- May increase liver enzyme level. May decrease hemoglobin level and hematocrit.

Pharmacokinetics

Absorption: Rapid and almost complete.
Distribution: About 20% bound to plasma proteins.
Metabolism: Extensively metabolized.
Excretion: 30% excreted in urine as unchanged drug and 60% as metabolites. *Half-life:* 6 to 7 hours.

Route	Onset	Peak	Duration
P.O.	Unknown	2 hr	Unknown

Action

Chemical effect: Unknown; centrally acting synthetic analgesic compound not chemically related to opioids that is thought to bind to opioid receptors and inhibit reuptake of norepinephrine and serotonin.
Therapeutic effect: Relieves pain.

Available forms

Tablets: 50 mg

NURSING PROCESS

Assessment

- Assess patient's pain before starting therapy and regularly thereafter to monitor the drug's effectiveness.
- Monitor CV and respiratory status.

ALERT: Closely monitor patient at risk for seizures; drug may reduce seizure threshold.

- Monitor patient for drug dependence. Tramadol can produce dependence similar to that of codeine or dextropropoxyphene and thus has potential to be abused.
- Be alert for adverse reactions and drug interactions.
- Assess patient's and family's knowledge of drug therapy.

Nursing diagnoses

- Acute pain related to underlying condition
- Risk for constipation related to drug-induced adverse GI reactions
- Deficient knowledge related to drug therapy

Planning and implementation

- For better analgesic effect, give drug before onset of intense pain.
- If respiratory rate decreases or falls below 12 breaths/minute, withhold dose and notify prescriber.

T

• Because constipation is a common adverse effect, anticipate need for laxative therapy.

⊛ **ALERT:** Don't confuse tramadol with trazodone or trandolapril.

Patient teaching

• Instruct patient to take drug only as prescribed and not to increase dosage or dosage interval unless instructed by prescriber.

• Tell ambulatory patient to be careful when getting out of bed and walking. Warn outpatient to refrain from driving and performing other potentially hazardous activities that require mental alertness until drug's CNS effects are known.

• Instruct patient to check with prescriber before taking OTC drugs; drug interactions can occur.

☑ **Evaluation**

• Patient is free from pain.

• Patient regains normal bowel pattern.

• Patient and family state understanding of drug therapy.

trandolapril

(tran-DOH-luh-pril)
Mavik

Pharmacologic class: ACE inhibitor
Therapeutic class: antihypertensive
Pregnancy risk category: C (D in second and third trimesters)

Indications and dosages

▶ **Hypertension.** *Adults:* For patient not receiving a diuretic, initially 1 mg for a nonblack patient and 2 mg for a black patient P.O. once daily. If response isn't adequate, dosage may be increased at intervals of at least 1 week. Maintenance dosage is 2 to 4 mg daily for most patients. Some patients receiving 4-mg once-daily doses may need b.i.d. doses. For patient also receiving diuretic, initial dose is 0.5 mg P.O. once daily. Subsequent dosages adjusted based on blood pressure response.

▶ **Heart failure or left ventricular dysfunction after acute MI.** *Adults:* Initiate therapy 3 to 5 days after MI with 1 mg P.O. daily. Adjust as tolerated to target dosage of 4 mg daily.

Contraindications and cautions

• Contraindicated in patients hypersensitive to the drug or any of its components and in pa-

tients with a history of angioedema with previous therapy with ACE inhibitor.

• Use cautiously in patients with impaired renal function, heart failure, or renal artery stenosis.

⚘ **Lifespan:** In pregnant women, drug is contraindicated. Breast-feeding women should stop breast-feeding or stop the drug. In children, safety and effectiveness haven't been established.

Adverse reactions

CNS: dizziness, headache, fatigue, drowsiness, insomnia, paresthesia, vertigo, anxiety.
CV: chest pain, first-degree AV block, *bradycardia,* edema, flushing, hypotension, palpitations.
EENT: epistaxis, throat irritation.
GI: diarrhea, dyspepsia, abdominal distention, abdominal pain or cramps, constipation, vomiting, *pancreatitis.*
GU: urinary frequency, impotence.
Hematologic: *neutropenia, leukopenia.*
Metabolic: *hyperkalemia,* hyponatremia.
Respiratory: dry, persistent, tickling, nonproductive cough; dyspnea; upper respiratory tract infection.
Skin: rash, pruritus, pemphigus.
Other: *anaphylaxis, angioedema,* decreased libido.

Interactions

Drug-drug. *Diuretics:* May increase risk of excessive hypotension. Monitor blood pressure closely.
Lithium: May increase lithium level and lithium toxicity. Avoid use together; monitor lithium level.
Potassium-sparing diuretics, potassium supplements: May increase risk of hyperkalemia. Monitor potassium level closely.
Drug-herb. *Licorice:* May increase sodium retention and blood pressure. Discourage use together.
Drug-food. *Salt substitutes containing potassium:* May increase risk of hyperkalemia. Monitor potassium level closely.

Effects on lab test results

• May increase BUN, creatinine, potassium, uric acid, and liver enzyme levels. May decrease sodium level.

• May decrease neutrophil and WBC counts.

Reactions may be *common,* uncommon, *life-threatening*, or COMMON AND LIFE-THREATENING.

Pharmacokinetics

Absorption: Food slows absorption.
Distribution: 80% protein-bound.
Metabolism: Metabolized in liver.
Excretion: In urine and feces. *Half-life:* 5 to 10 hours. Longer in patients with renal impairment.

Route	Onset	Peak	Duration
P.O.			
drug	Unknown	1 hr	Unknown
metabolite	4–10 hr	1 hr	Unknown

Action

Chemical effect: Inhibits circulating and tissue ACE activity, which reduces angiotensin II formation, decreases vasoconstriction and aldosterone secretion, and increases plasma renin.
Therapeutic effect: Lowers blood pressure.

Available forms

Tablets: 1 mg, 2 mg, 4 mg

NURSING PROCESS

❖ Assessment

• Monitor patient's blood pressure and potassium level before starting therapy and during therapy.
• Monitor patient for hypotension. If possible, stop diuretic therapy 2 to 3 days before starting drug.
• Monitor patient for jaundice, and immediately alert prescriber if it occurs.
• Monitor patient's compliance with therapy.
• Assess patient's and family's knowledge of drug therapy.

⊕ Nursing diagnoses

• Risk for injury related to hypertension
• Deficient knowledge related to drug therapy

▷ Planning and implementation

• Take steps to prevent or minimize orthostatic hypotension.
• Maintain patient's nondrug therapies, such as sodium restriction, stress management, smoking cessation, and exercise program.
• ⊛ ALERT: Angioedema that involves the tongue, glottis, or larynx may be fatal because of airway obstruction. Have resuscitation equipment readily available for maintaining a patent airway;

give appropriate therapy, including epinephrine 1:1,000 (0.3 to 0.5 ml) subcutaneously.
Patient teaching
• Advise patient to report infection and other adverse reactions.
• Tell patient to avoid salt substitutes.
• Tell patient to use caution in hot weather and during exercise.
• Tell woman to immediately report suspected pregnancy.
• Advise patient about to undergo surgery or anesthesia to inform prescriber of use of drug.

☑ Evaluation

• Patient's blood pressure is normal.
• Patient and family state understanding of drug therapy.

trastuzumab
(trahs-TOO-zuh-mab)
Herceptin

Pharmacologic class: monoclonal antibody
Therapeutic class: antineoplastic
Pregnancy risk category: B

Indications and dosages

▶ **Monotherapy for patients with metastatic breast cancer whose tumors overexpress the human epidermal growth factor receptor 2 (HER2) protein and who have received one or more chemotherapy regimens for their metastatic disease; or with paclitaxel for metastatic breast cancer in patients whose tumors overexpress the HER2 protein and who haven't received chemotherapy for their metastatic disease.** *Adults:* Initial loading dose of 4 mg/kg I.V. over 90 minutes. If the initial loading dose is well tolerated, maintenance dosage is 2 mg/kg I.V. weekly as a 30-minute I.V. infusion.

▼ I.V. administration

• Reconstitute drug in each vial with 20 ml of bacteriostatic water for injection, USP, 1.1% benzyl alcohol preserved, as supplied, to yield a multidose solution containing 21 mg/ml. Immediately after reconstitution, label vial for drug expiration 28 days from date of reconstitution.
• If patient is hypersensitive to benzyl alcohol, drug must be reconstituted with sterile water for

T

injection. Drug reconstituted with sterile water for injection must be used immediately; unused portion must be discarded. Avoid other reconstitution diluents.

• Determine dose (mg) of drug needed, based on loading dose of 4 mg/kg or maintenance dose of 2 mg/kg. Calculate volume of 21-mg/ml solution and withdraw amount from vial; add it to an infusion bag containing 250 ml of normal saline solution.

• Don't give as an I.V. push or bolus.

• Vials of drug are stable at 36° to 46° F (2° to 8° C) before reconstitution. Discard reconstituted solution after 28 days. Store drug solution diluted in normal saline solution for injection at 36° to 46° F before use; it's stable for up to 24 hours.

⊗ **Incompatibilities**
Other I.V. drugs or dextrose solutions.

Contraindications and cautions

• Use cautiously in patients with cardiac dysfunction. Watch closely for ventricular dysfunction and heart failure, and stop drug if signs of decreased left ventricular dysfunction develop.

• Use cautiously in patients hypersensitive to drug or its components. Severe hypersensitivity reactions, infusion reactions, and pulmonary events can develop. Hypersensitivity reaction typically occurs during or within 24 hours of administration.

≉ **Lifespan:** In pregnant women, use only if clearly needed. Breast-feeding women should stop breast-feeding during therapy and for 6 months after the last dose, or they should use another drug. In children, safety and effectiveness haven't been established. In the elderly, use cautiously.

Adverse reactions

CNS: *pain, fever, headache, asthenia, insomnia, dizziness,* paresthesia, depression, peripheral neuritis, neuropathy.
CV: tachycardia, *heart failure,* peripheral edema, edema, *left ventricular dysfunction.*
EENT: rhinitis, pharyngitis, sinusitis.
GI: nausea, diarrhea, vomiting, anorexia, abdominal pain.
GU: UTI.
Hematologic: anemia, *leukopenia.*
Musculoskeletal: bone pain, arthralgia, *back pain.*
Respiratory: cough, dyspnea.

Skin: *rash,* acne.
Other: chills, infection, flulike syndrome, allergic reaction, herpes simplex, *hypersensitivity reactions, anaphylaxis.*

Interactions

Drug-drug. *Anthracyclines, cyclophosphamide:* May increase risk of cardiotoxic effects. Monitor patient closely.
Paclitaxel: May decrease clearance of trastuzumab. Monitor patient closely.

Effects on lab test results

• May decrease hemoglobin level and hematocrit.
• May decrease WBC count.

Pharmacokinetics

Absorption: Administered I.V.
Distribution: Volume is 44 ml/kg.
Metabolism: Unknown.
Excretion: Unknown. *Half-life:* 1 to 32 days.

Route	Onset	Peak	Duration
I.V.	Unknown	Unknown	Unknown

Action

Chemical effect: Recombinant DNA-derived monoclonal antibody that selectively binds to HER2. Inhibits proliferation of human tumor cells that overexpress HER2.
Therapeutic effect: Hinders function of specific breast cancer tumor cells that overexpress HER2.

Available forms

Injection: lyophilized sterile powder containing 440 mg per vial

NURSING PROCESS

✐ **Assessment**
• Before beginning therapy, make sure patient has had a thorough baseline cardiac assessment, including history, physical examination, and evaluation, to see if he's at risk for developing cardiotoxicity.
• Use drug only in patients with metastatic breast cancer whose tumors have HER2 protein overexpression.
• Assess patient for chills and fever, especially during the first infusion.

Reactions may be *common,* uncommon, **life-threatening**, or COMMON AND LIFE-THREATENING.

• Monitor patient closely for signs and symptoms of cardiac dysfunction, especially if also receiving anthracyclines and cyclophosphamide.
• Monitor patient for dyspnea, increased cough, paroxysmal nocturnal dyspnea, peripheral edema, and S₃ gallop. Monitor patients also receiving chemotherapy closely for cardiac dysfunction or failure, anemia, leukopenia, diarrhea, and infection.
• Assess patient's and family's knowledge of drug therapy.

🔢 **Nursing diagnoses**
• Imbalanced nutrition: less than body requirements related to drug-induced GI adverse effects
• Decreased cardiac output related to drug-induced decreased left ventricular function
• Deficient knowledge related to drug therapy

▷ **Planning and implementation**
• Treat first-dose, infusion-related symptoms with acetaminophen, diphenhydramine, and meperidine (with or without reducing the rate of infusion).
• If patient experiences a significant decrease in cardiac function, notify prescriber.
Patient teaching
• Tell patient about possibility of first-dose, infusion-related adverse effects.
• Instruct patient to notify prescriber immediately if signs and symptoms of cardiac dysfunction develop, such as shortness of breath, increased cough, or peripheral edema.
• Instruct patient to report adverse effects to prescriber.

✔ **Evaluation**
• Patient doesn't experience adverse GI effects (nausea, vomiting, diarrhea).
• Patient doesn't exhibit dyspnea, increased cough, paroxysmal nocturnal dyspnea, peripheral edema, or S₃ gallop as result of drug-induced cardiac dysfunction.
• Patient and family state understanding of drug therapy.

travoprost
(TRA-voe-prost)
Travatan

Pharmacologic class: prostaglandin analogue
Therapeutic class: antiglaucoma drug, ocular antihypertensive
Pregnancy risk category: C

Indications and dosages

▶ **Reduction of elevated intraocular pressure (IOP) in patients with open-angle glaucoma or ocular hypertension who are intolerant of other IOP-lowering drugs, or in patients who have had insufficient responses to other IOP-lowering drugs.** *Adults:* 1 drop in conjunctival sac of affected eye once daily in evening.

Contraindications and cautions

• Contraindicated in patients hypersensitive to the drug, benzalkonium chloride, or other components.
• Use cautiously in patients with renal or hepatic impairment, active intraocular inflammation (iritis, uveitis), or risk factors for macular edema. Also use cautiously in aphakic patients and pseudophakic patients with a torn posterior lens capsule.
• Don't use in patients with angle-closure glaucoma or inflammatory or neovascular glaucoma.
⚠ **Lifespan:** In pregnant women and in women attempting to become pregnant, drug isn't recommended. In breast-feeding women, use cautiously; it's unknown if the drug appears in breast milk. In children, safety and effectiveness haven't been established.

Adverse reactions

CNS: anxiety, depression, headache, pain.
CV: angina pectoris, *bradycardia,* chest pain, hypertension, hypotension.
EENT: *ocular hyperemia, decreased visual acuity, eye discomfort, foreign body sensation, eye pain, eye pruritus,* conjunctival hyperemia, abnormal vision, blepharitis, blurred vision, cataracts, conjunctivitis, dry eyes, eye disorders, iris discoloration, keratitis, lid margin crusting, photophobia, subconjunctival hemorrhage, tearing, sinusitis.
GI: dyspepsia, GI disorder.

T

GU: prostate disorder, urinary incontinence, UTI.
Metabolic: hypercholesterolemia.
Musculoskeletal: arthritis, back pain.
Respiratory: bronchitis, sinusitis.
Other: accidental injury, cold syndrome, infection.

Interactions

Drug-herb. *Areca, jaborandi:* May cause additive effects. Discourage use together.

Effects on lab test results

• May increase cholesterol level.

Pharmacokinetics

Absorption: Absorbed through the cornea.
Distribution: Levels peak within 30 minutes.
Metabolism: Hydrolyzed by esterases in the cornea to its active free acid. The liver primarily metabolizes the active acid of drug reaching the systemic circulation.
Excretion: Within 1 hour. *Half-life:* 45 minutes.

Route	Onset	Peak	Duration
Ophthalmic	Unknown	30 min	Unknown

Action

Chemical effect: May increase uveoscleral outflow.
Therapeutic effect: Reduces IOP.

Available forms

Ophthalmic solution: 0.004%

NURSING PROCESS

Assessment
• Assess patient's condition before starting therapy and regularly thereafter to monitor the drug's effectiveness.
• If a pregnant woman or a woman attempting to become pregnant accidentally comes in contact with drug, immediately cleanse the exposed area thoroughly with soap and water.
• Assess patient's and family's knowledge of drug therapy.

Nursing diagnoses
• Acute pain related to adverse EENT effects of drug
• Risk for activity intolerance related to decreased visual acuity

• Deficient knowledge related to travoprost therapy

Planning and implementation
• Have patient remove contact lenses before you give the drug. Lenses may be reinserted 15 minutes afterward.
• If multiple ophthalmic drugs are being used, separate doses by at least 5 minutes.
• Temporary or permanent increased pigmentation of the iris and eyelid may occur as well as increased pigmentation and growth of the eyelashes.
Patient teaching
• Teach patient to instill drops, and advise him to wash hands before and after doing so. Warn him not to touch dropper or tip to eye or surrounding tissue.
• Advise patient to apply light pressure on lacrimal sac for 1 minute after instillation to minimize systemic absorption of drug.
• Tell patient to remove contact lenses before instilling solution and to leave them out for 15 minutes afterward.
• Advise patient that, if more than one ophthalmic drug is being used, the drugs should be given at least 5 minutes apart.
• Tell patient receiving treatment to only one eye about the potential for increased brown pigmentation of the iris, eyelid skin darkening, and increased length, thickness, pigmentation, or number of lashes in the treated eye.
• Tell patient that, if eye trauma or infection occurs or if eye surgery is needed, he should seek medical advice before continuing to use the multidose container.
• Advise patient to immediately report conjunctivitis or lid reactions.
• Stress importance of compliance with recommended therapy.
• Tell patient to discard container within 6 weeks of removing it from the sealed pouch.
• Tell pregnant woman or woman attempting to become pregnant that, if she accidentally comes in contact with drug, she should immediately cleanse the exposed area thoroughly with soap and water.

Evaluation
• Patient denies pain.
• Patient's activity level improves.
• Patient and family state understanding of travoprost therapy.

Reactions may be *common*, uncommon, *life-threatening*, or COMMON AND LIFE-THREATENING.

trazodone hydrochloride
(TRAYZ-oh-dohn high-droh-KLOR-ighd)
Desyrel, Desyrel Dividose

Pharmacologic class: triazolopyridine derivative
Therapeutic class: antidepressant
Pregnancy risk category: C

Indications and dosages

▶ **Depression.** *Adults:* Initially, 150 mg P.O. daily in divided doses. Increase by 50 mg daily q 3 to 4 days, p.r.n. Average daily dose ranges from 150 to 400 mg. Maximum, 600 mg daily for inpatients or 400 mg daily for outpatients.
▶ **Aggressive behavior‡.** *Adults:* 50 mg P.O. b.i.d.
▶ **Panic disorder‡.** *Adults:* 300 mg P.O. daily.

Contraindications and cautions

• Contraindicated in patients in initial recovery phase of MI and in patients hypersensitive to drug.
• Use cautiously in patients with cardiac disease and in those at risk for suicide.
🜲 **Lifespan:** In pregnant women, breast-feeding women, and children, safety and effectiveness haven't been established.

Adverse reactions

CNS: *suicidal thinking, drowsiness, dizziness,* nervousness, fatigue, confusion, tremor, weakness, hostility, syncope, anger, nightmares, vivid dreams, headache, insomnia.
CV: orthostatic hypotension, tachycardia, hypertension, shortness of breath.
EENT: blurred vision, tinnitus, nasal congestion.
GI: dry mouth, dysgeusia, constipation, nausea, vomiting, anorexia.
GU: urine retention, priapism, hematuria.
Hematologic: anemia.
Skin: rash, urticaria, diaphoresis.
Other: decreased libido.

Interactions

Drug-drug. *Antihypertensives:* May increase hypotensive effect of trazodone. Monitor blood pressure; antihypertensive dosage may have to be decreased.
Clonidine, CNS depressants: May increase CNS depression. Avoid use together.
CYP 3A4 inducers (carbamazepine): May reduce trazodone level. Monitor patient closely; he may need an increased dose of trazodone.
CYP 3A4 inhibitors (ketoconazole, ritonavir, and indinavir): May slow the clearance of trazodone and increase trazodone levels. May cause nausea, hypotension, and fainting. Consider decreasing trazodone dose.
Digoxin, phenytoin: May increase levels of these drugs. Monitor patient for toxicity.
MAO inhibitors: May cause an unknown interaction. Use together cautiously.
Phenothiazines: May increase trazodone level. Monitor toxic effects.
Venlafaxine, SSRIs: May cause serotonin syndrome. Don't use together.
Drug-herb. *St. John's wort:* May cause serotonin syndrome. Discourage use together.
Drug-lifestyle. *Alcohol use:* May increase CNS depression. Discourage use together.

Effects on lab test results

• May increase ALT and AST levels. May decrease hemoglobin level and hematocrit.

Pharmacokinetics

Absorption: Well absorbed from GI tract. Food delays absorption but increases amount of drug absorbed by 20%.
Distribution: Distributed widely in body; isn't concentrated in any particular tissue.
Metabolism: Metabolized by liver.
Excretion: About 75% excreted in urine; remainder excreted in feces. *Half-life:* First phase, 3 to 6 hours; second phase, 5 to 9 hours.

Route	Onset	Peak	Duration
P.O.	Unknown	1–2 hr	Unknown

Action

Chemical effect: Unknown, although it inhibits serotonin uptake in brain; not a tricyclic derivative.
Therapeutic effect: Relieves depression.

Available forms

Tablets (film coated): 50 mg, 100 mg
Tablets (scored): 150 mg, 300 mg

NURSING PROCESS

Assessment
- Assess patient's condition before starting therapy and regularly thereafter to monitor the drug's effectiveness.
- Be alert for adverse reactions and drug interactions.
- Assess patient's and family's knowledge of drug therapy.

Nursing diagnoses
- Disturbed thought processes related to presence of depression
- Risk for injury related to drug-induced adverse CNS reactions
- Deficient knowledge related to drug therapy

Planning and implementation
- Give after meal or light snack for optimal absorption and to decrease risk of dizziness.
- Don't abruptly stop giving the drug, but stop it at least 48 hours before surgery.
- If an adverse reaction occurs, notify prescriber.

ALERT: Don't confuse trazodone with tramadol.

Patient teaching
- Instruct patient to take drug after a meal or light snack.

ALERT: Advise patient to notify prescriber immediately if priapism (prolonged, painful erection unrelated to sexual stimulation) occurs; emergency interventions are needed within 6 hours to prevent permanent erectile dysfunction.
- Warn patient to avoid activities that require alertness and good psychomotor coordination until the drug's CNS effects are known; drowsiness and dizziness usually subside after first few weeks.
- Teach patient's family how to recognize signs of suicidal tendency or suicidal ideation.

Evaluation
- Patient's behavior and communication exhibit improved thought processes.
- Patient doesn't experience adverse CNS reactions.
- Patient and family state understanding of drug therapy.

treprostinil sodium
(treh-PROSS-ti-nil soh-dee-UHM)
Remodulin

Pharmacologic class: vasodilator
Therapeutic class: antihypertensive
Pregnancy risk category: B

Indications and dosages

▶ **New York Heart Association Class II to IV pulmonary arterial hypertension (PAH) to reduce symptoms caused by exercise.** *Adults:* Initially, 1.25 nanograms/kg/minute by continuous subcutaneous or I.V. infusion. If the initial dose can't be tolerated, reduce infusion rate to 0.625 nanograms/kg/minute. Increase by increments of no more than 1.25 nanograms/kg/minute each week for the first 4 weeks and then by no more than 2.5 nanograms/kg/minute each week for the duration of infusion. Maximum infusion rate is 40 nanograms/kg/minute. To determine the subcutaneous infusion rate in ml/hour, use this formula:

Infusion rate (ml/hr) =
[dosage (nanograms/kg/min)
× body weight (kg) × 0.00006]
÷ drug strength (mg/ml)

When using an appropriate infusion pump and reservoir, a predetermined intravenous infusion rate should first be selected to allow for a desired infusion period length of up to 48 hours between system changeovers. Typical intravenous infusion system reservoirs have volumes of 50 or 100 ml. With this selected intravenous infusion rate (ml/hr), the diluted intravenous Remodulin concentration (mg/ml) can be calculated using the following formula:

Diluted I.V. concentration (mg/ml) =
[dosage (nanograms/kg/min)
× weight (kg) × 0.00006]
÷ I.V. infusion rate (ml/minute)

The amount of Remodulin injection needed to make the required diluted intravenous Remodulin concentration for the given reservoir size can then be calculated using the following formula:

Amount of Remodulin injection (ml) =
[diluted I.V. concentration (mg/ml)
÷ vial strength (mg/ml)]
✕ total volume of diluted Remodulin
solution in reservoir (ml)

The calculated amount of Remodulin injection is then added to the reservoir along with the sufficient volume of diluent to achieve the desired total volume in the reservoir.
◨ **Adjust-a-dose:** In patients with mild or moderate hepatic insufficiency, initial dose is 0.625 nanograms/kg of ideal body weight per minute; increase cautiously.

▼ I.V. administration

• Remodulin must be diluted with either sterile water for injection or normal saline solution injection.
• Drug must be administered through a surgically placed, indwelling central venous catheter.
• Diluted Remodulin is stable at ambient temperature for up to 48 hours at concentrations as low as 0.004 mg/ml (4,000 nanograms/ml).
• Patient must have access to a backup infusion pump and infusion sets.
⊗ **Incompatibilities**
Other I.V. drugs.

Contraindications and cautions

• Contraindicated in patients hypersensitive to the drug or to structurally related compounds.
• Use cautiously in patients with hepatic or renal impairment.
⚠ **Lifespan:** In pregnant women, use only if clearly needed. In breast-feeding women, use cautiously; it's unknown if the drug appears in breast milk. In children, safety and effectiveness haven't been established; select dose cautiously. In the elderly, use cautiously.

Adverse reactions

CNS: dizziness, *headache,* fatigue.
CV: vasodilation, hypotension, edema, chest pain, *right ventricular heart failure.*
GI: diarrhea, nausea.
Respiratory: dyspnea.
Skin: *rash,* pruritus, pallor.
Other: *jaw pain, infusion site pain,* infusion site reaction.

Interactions

Drug-drug. *Anticoagulants:* May increase risk of bleeding. Monitor patient closely for bleeding.
Antihypertensives, diuretics, vasodilators: May worsen reduction in blood pressure. Monitor blood pressure.

Effects on lab test results

None reported.

Pharmacokinetics

Absorption: Rapid and complete. 100% bioavailable.
Distribution: 91% bound to plasma proteins.
Metabolism: By the liver. Five metabolites are known, but their activity isn't.
Excretion: In the urine, 4% as unchanged drug and 64% as metabolites. *Half-life:* 2 to 4 hours.

Route	Onset	Peak	Duration
I.V., SubQ	Unknown	Unknown	Unknown

Action

Chemical effect: Acts by direct vasodilation of pulmonary and systemic arterial vascular beds and inhibition of platelet aggregation.
Therapeutic effect: Reduces pulmonary artery pressure.

Available forms

Injection: 1 mg/ml, 2.5 mg/ml, 5 mg/ml, 10 mg/ml

NURSING PROCESS

⚕ Assessment

• Assess patient's condition before starting therapy and regularly thereafter to monitor the drug's effectiveness.
• Make sure adequate monitoring and emergency care are available when starting therapy.
• Assess patient's ability to accept, place, and care for subcutaneous catheter and to use infusion pump.
• Assess patient's ability to accept and care for I.V. catheter and to use the infusion pump.
• Be alert for adverse reactions and drug interactions.
• Assess patient's and family's knowledge of drug therapy.

T

🔛 Nursing diagnoses

- Activity intolerance related to presence of pulmonary hypertension
- Acute pain related to adverse drug effect of headache
- Deficient knowledge related to drug therapy

▷ Planning and implementation

- Drug should be used only by prescribers experienced in the diagnosis and treatment of PAH.
- Give by continuous subcutaneous infusion via a self-inserted subcutaneous catheter, using an infusion pump designed for subcutaneous drug delivery. Or give by continuous I.V. infusion through an indwelling central venous catheter.
- The infusion pump should be small and light-weight; be adjustable to approximately 0.002 ml/hour; have occlusion or no-delivery, low-battery, programming-error, and motor-malfunction alarms; have delivery accuracy of ± 6% or better; and be positive-pressure driven.
- The reservoir should be made of polyvinyl chloride, polypropylene, or glass.
- A single syringe can be given up to 72 hours at 99° F (37° C).
- Use a single vial no longer than 14 days after the initial introduction into the vial.
- Inspect for particulate matter and discoloration before giving.
- Unopened vials are stable until the date indicated when stored at 59° to 77° F (15° to 25° C).
- If patient doesn't improve or if symptoms worsen, increase dose. If patient has excessive effects or unacceptable infusion site symptoms, decrease dose.
- Don't abruptly stop giving the drug or reduce the dose by a large amount; symptoms of PAH may worsen.

Patient teaching

- Tell patient drug is infused continuously through subcutaneous or I.V. catheter, via an infusion pump.
- Inform patient that therapy will be needed for prolonged period, possibly years.
- Inform patient that many side effects may be related to the underlying disease (dyspnea, fatigue, chest pain, right ventricular failure, pallor).
- Tell patient that the most common local reactions are pain, erythema, induration, and rash at the infusion site.

☑ Evaluation

- Patient states activity intolerance is improving.
- Patient doesn't have headache.
- Patient and family state understanding of drug therapy.

triamcinolone
(trigh-am-SIN-oh-lohn)
Aristocort, Atolone, Kenacort

triamcinolone acetonide
Kenaject-40, Kenalog-10, Kenalog-40, Tac-3, Tac-40, Triam-A, Triamonide 40, Tri-Kort, Trilog

triamcinolone diacetate
Amcort, Aristocort Forte, Aristocort Intralesional, Clinacort, Triam Forte, Trilone, Tristoject

triamcinolone hexacetonide
Aristospan Intra-Articular, Aristospan Intralesional

Pharmacologic class: glucocorticoid
Therapeutic class: anti-inflammatory, immunosuppressant
Pregnancy risk category: C

Indications and dosages

▶ **Severe inflammation or immunosuppression.** *Adults:* 4 to 48 mg triamcinolone P.O. daily, in one to four divided doses. Or, initially, 2.5 to 60 mg triamcinolone acetonide I.M. Additional doses of 20 to 100 mg may be given, p.r.n., at 6-week intervals. Or, 2.5 to 15 mg intra-articularly, or up to 1 mg intralesionally, p.r.n. Or, 40 mg triamcinolone diacetate I.M. weekly; or 5 to 48 mg by intralesional or sublesional injections (at 1- to 2-week intervals); or 2 to 40 mg by intra-articular, intrasynovial, or soft tissue injection (may repeat at 1- to 8-week intervals). Or, with triamcinolone hexacetonide, use up to 0.5 mg per square inch of affected skin intralesionally, or 2 to 20 mg intra-articularly q 3 to 4 weeks, p.r.n.
Children: Base dosage on the the disease severity and the response instead of age and body weight or surface area. Taper to a stop as soon as possible

Contraindications and cautions

• Contraindicated in patients hypersensitive to the drug or any of its components, and in those with systemic fungal infections.

• Use cautiously in patients with GI ulcer, renal disease, hypertension, osteoporosis, diabetes mellitus, hypothyroidism, cirrhosis, diverticulitis, nonspecific ulcerative colitis, recent intestinal anastomoses, thromboembolic disorders, seizures, myasthenia gravis, heart failure, tuberculosis, ocular herpes simplex, emotional instability, or psychotic tendencies.

☀ **Lifespan:** In pregnant women, use cautiously. In breast-feeding women, use cautiously; it's unknown if the drug appears in breast milk.

Adverse reactions

CNS: *euphoria, insomnia,* psychotic behavior, *pseudotumor cerebri,* vertigo, headache, paresthesia, *seizures.*
CV: *heart failure,* hypertension, edema, *arrhythmias,* thrombophlebitis, *thromboembolism.*
EENT: cataracts, glaucoma.
GI: *peptic ulceration,* GI irritation, increased appetite, *pancreatitis,* nausea, vomiting.
GU: menstrual irregularities.
Metabolic: hypokalemia, hyperglycemia, carbohydrate intolerance.
Musculoskeletal: muscular weakness, osteoporosis, growth suppression in children.
Skin: delayed wound healing, acne, various skin eruptions, bruising, petechiae.
Other: *acute adrenal insufficiency* during times of increased stress; susceptibility to infections; hirsutism; cushingoid state (moonface, buffalo hump, central obesity).

Interactions

Drug-drug. *Aspirin, indomethacin, other NSAIDs:* May increase risk of GI distress and bleeding. Give together cautiously.
Barbiturates, phenytoin, rifampin: May decrease corticosteroid effect. Increase corticosteroid dosage.
Drugs that deplete potassium (such as thiazide diuretics): May increase potassium-wasting effects of triamcinolone. Monitor potassium level.
Oral anticoagulants: May alter dosage requirements. Monitor PT closely.
Skin-test antigens: Mat decrease response. Defer skin testing.

Toxoids, vaccines: May decrease antibody response and increase risk of neurologic complications. Avoid use together.

Effects on lab test results

• May increase glucose and cholesterol levels. May decrease potassium and calcium levels.

Pharmacokinetics

Absorption: Readily after P.O. administration. Variable after other routes of administration.
Distribution: To muscle, liver, skin, intestines, and kidneys. Extensively bound to plasma proteins. Only unbound portion is active.
Metabolism: In liver.
Excretion: In urine; insignificant quantities also excreted in feces. *Half-life:* 18 to 36 hours.

Route	Onset	Peak	Duration
P.O., I.M., intralesional, intra-articular, intrasynovial	Varies	Varies	Varies

Actions

Chemical effect: Not clearly defined; decreases inflammation, mainly by stabilizing leukocyte lysosomal membranes; suppresses immune response; stimulates bone marrow; and influences protein, fat, and carbohydrate metabolism.
Therapeutic effect: Relieves inflammation and suppresses immune system function.

Available forms

triamcinolone
Syrup: 4 mg/5 ml
Tablets: 4 mg, 8 mg
triamcinolone acetonide
Injection (suspension): 3 mg/ml, 10 mg/ml, 40 mg/ml
triamcinolone diacetate
Injection (suspension): 25 mg/ml, 40 mg/ml
triamcinolone hexacetonide
Injection (suspension): 5 mg/ml, 20 mg/ml

NURSING PROCESS

⚖ Assessment
• Assess patient before and after starting therapy; monitor weight, blood pressure, and electrolyte level.

T

• Watch for adverse reactions, drug interactions, depression, or psychotic episodes, especially with high doses.
• Assess patient's and family's knowledge of drug therapy.

⊞ Nursing diagnoses
• Ineffective health maintenance related to underlying condition
• Risk for injury related to drug-induced adverse reactions
• Deficient knowledge related to drug therapy

❯ Planning and implementation
• Drug isn't used for alternate-day therapy.
• Always adjust to lowest effective dose.
• For better results and less toxicity, give once-daily dose in morning.
• Give oral dose with food when possible to reduce GI irritation.
• For adults, give I.M. injection deep into gluteal muscle; rotate injection sites to prevent muscle atrophy.
• Don't use 10-mg/ml strength for I.M. administration.
• Assist prescriber with intralesional, intra-articular, or intrasynovial administration.
• Don't use 40-mg/ml strength for I.D. or intralesional administration.
• ⑨ ALERT: Parenteral form isn't for I.V. use; different salt formulations aren't interchangeable.
• Don't use diluents that contain preservatives; flocculation may occur.
• Unless contraindicated, give low-sodium diet high in potassium and protein. Give potassium supplements, p.r.n.
• Gradually reduce drug dose after long-term therapy. After abruptly stopping the drug, the patient may experience rebound inflammation, fatigue, weakness, arthralgia, fever, dizziness, lethargy, depression, fainting, orthostatic hypotension, dyspnea, anorexia, or hypoglycemia. After prolonged use, sudden withdrawal may be fatal.
• ⑨ ALERT: Don't confuse triamcinolone with Triaminicin, Triaminic, or Triaminicol.
Patient teaching
• Tell patient not to abruptly stop taking the drug without prescriber's consent.
• Instruct patient to take oral drug with food.
• Teach patient signs of early adrenal insufficiency (fatigue, muscle weakness, joint pain,

fever, anorexia, nausea, dyspnea, dizziness, and fainting).
• Instruct patient to wear or carry medical identification at all times.
• Warn patient receiving long-term therapy about cushingoid symptoms, and tell him to report sudden weight gain and swelling to prescriber.
• Tell patient to report slow healing.
• Advise patient receiving long-term therapy to consider exercise or physical therapy. Also tell patient to ask prescriber about vitamin D or calcium supplements.

☑ Evaluation
• Patient responds well to drug.
• Patient doesn't experience injury from adverse reactions.
• Patient and family state understanding of drug therapy.

---

triamcinolone acetonide
(trigh-am-SIN-oh-lohn as-EE-tuh-nighd)
Azmacort, Nasacort HFA

Pharmacologic class: glucocorticoid
Therapeutic class: anti-inflammatory, immunosuppressant
Pregnancy risk category: C

Indications and dosages
▶ **Corticosteroid-dependent asthma.** *Adults:* 2 inhalations t.i.d. to q.i.d. Maximum, 16 inhalations daily. In some patients, maintenance can be accomplished when total daily dose is given b.i.d.
Children ages 6 to 12: 1 or 2 inhalations t.i.d. to q.i.d. or 2 to 4 inhalations b.i.d. Maximum, 12 inhalations daily.
▶ **Treatment of nasal symptoms of seasonal and perennial allergic rhinitis.** *Adults and children age 12 years and older:* (Nasacort HFA) 2 sprays into each nostril once daily. May increase to 4 sprays into each nostril once daily. Adjust to minimum effective dosage.
Children age 12 years and older: (Nasacort HFA) 2 sprays into each nostril once daily. Adjust to minimum effective dosage.

Reactions may be *common*, uncommon, *life-threatening*, or COMMON AND LIFE-THREATENING.

Contraindications and cautions

• Contraindicated in patients hypersensitive to the drug or any of its components, and in those with status asthmaticus.

• Use cautiously, if at all, in patients with tuberculosis of respiratory tract; untreated fungal, bacterial, or systemic viral infections; or ocular herpes simplex. Also use cautiously in patients receiving systemic corticosteroids.

✹ **Lifespan:** In pregnant women, use cautiously. In breast-feeding women, drug isn't recommended.

Adverse reactions

CNS: *headache* (Nasacort HFA).
CV: facial edema.
EENT: dry or irritated nose or throat, hoarseness; *sneezing,* nasal irritation, rhinitis (Nasacort HFA).
GI: *oral candidiasis,* dry or irritated tongue or mouth.
Respiratory: cough, wheezing.
Other: *hypothalamic-pituitary-adrenal function suppression,* adrenal insufficiency.

Interactions

None significant.

Effects on lab test results

None reported.

Pharmacokinetics

Absorption: Slow.
Distribution: Without spacer, about 10% to 25% of dose goes to airways; remainder goes to mouth and throat and is swallowed. Spacer may help a greater percentage reach lungs.
Metabolism: Metabolized in liver. Some drug that reaches lungs may be metabolized locally.
Excretion: Excreted in urine and feces. *Half-life:* 18 to 36 hours; 5.4 hours (HFA)

Route	Onset	Peak	Duration
Inhalation	1–4 wk	Unknown	Unknown
Intranasal	Unknown	4 hr	Unknown

Action

Chemical effect: May decrease inflammation by stabilizing leukocyte lysosomal membranes.
Therapeutic effect: Improves breathing ability.

Available forms

Inhalation aerosol: 100 mcg/metered spray
Nasal aerosol: 55 mcg/actuation.

NURSING PROCESS

⚗ Assessment

• Assess patient's asthma or allergic rhinitis before starting therapy and regularly thereafter to monitor the drug's effectiveness.
• Be alert for adverse reactions.
• Assess patient's and family's knowledge of drug therapy.

⊕ Nursing diagnoses

• Ineffective breathing pattern related to presence of asthma
• Impaired tissue integrity related to drug's adverse effect on oral mucosa
• Deficient knowledge related to drug therapy

❯ Planning and implementation

• Patient who has recently been transferred to oral inhaled steroids from systemic administration of steroids may need to be placed back on systemic steroids during periods of stress or severe asthma attacks.
• Taper oral therapy slowly.
• If patient is also to receive bronchodilator by inhalation, give bronchodilator first, wait several minutes, and then give triamcinolone.
• If more than one inhalation is ordered for each dose, wait 1 minute between inhalations.
• Store drug between 36° and 86° F (2° and 30° C).
⊛ **ALERT:** Don't confuse triamcinolone with Triaminicin, Triaminic, or Triaminicol.
Patient teaching
• Inform patient that inhaled steroids don't provide relief for emergency asthma attacks.
• Instruct patient to use drug as prescribed, even when feeling well.
• Advise patient to ensure delivery of proper dose by gently warming canister to room temperature before using and by using the spacer. Patient can carry canister in his pocket to keep it warm.
• Instruct patient requiring bronchodilator to use it several minutes before triamcinolone. Tell him to wait 1 minute before repeat inhalations and to hold his breath for a few seconds to enhance drug action.

T

• Teach patient to check mucous membranes frequently for signs of fungal infection.
• Tell patient to prevent oral fungal infections by gargling or rinsing mouth with water after each use of inhaler but not to swallow water.
• Tell patient to keep inhaler clean and unobstructed by washing it with warm water and drying it thoroughly after use.
• Instruct patient to contact prescriber if response to therapy decreases; prescriber may need to adjust dosage. Tell patient not to exceed recommended dosage on his own.
• Instruct patient to wear or carry medical identification at all times.

☑ Evaluation
• Patient exhibits improved breathing ability.
• Patient maintains normal oral mucosa integrity.
• Patient and family state understanding of drug therapy.

triamterene
(trigh-AM-tuh-reen)
Dyrenium

Pharmacologic class: potassium-sparing diuretic
Therapeutic class: diuretic
Pregnancy risk category: B

Indications and dosages
▶ **Edema.** *Adults:* Initially, 100 mg P.O. b.i.d. after meals. Total daily dose shouldn't exceed 300 mg.

Contraindications and cautions
• Contraindicated in patients hypersensitive to the drug or any of its components, and in those with anuria, severe or progressive renal disease or dysfunction, severe hepatic disease, or hyperkalemia.
• Use cautiously in patients with impaired liver function or diabetes mellitus, and in debilitated patients.
❋ **Lifespan:** In pregnant women, use cautiously. In breast-feeding women, safety and effectiveness haven't been established. In children, safety and effectiveness haven't been established. In the elderly, use cautiously.

Adverse reactions
CNS: dizziness, weakness, fatigue, headache.
CV: hypotension.
GI: dry mouth, nausea, vomiting, diarrhea, stomatitis.
GU: azotemia, interstitial nephritis, nephrolithiasis.
Hematologic: megaloblastic anemia related to low folic acid levels, *thrombocytopenia, agranulocytosis.*
Hepatic: jaundice.
Metabolic: HYPERKALEMIA, *acidosis,* hypokalemia, hyponatremia, hyperglycemia.
Musculoskeletal: muscle cramps.
Skin: photosensitivity reactions, rash.
Other: *anaphylaxis.*

Interactions
Drug-drug. *ACE inhibitors, potassium supplements:* May increase risk of hyperkalemia. Don't use together.
Amantadine: May increase risk of amantadine toxicity. Don't use together.
Lithium: May decrease lithium clearance, increasing risk of lithium toxicity. Monitor lithium level.
NSAIDs (indomethacin): May increase risk of nephrotoxicity. Avoid use together.
Quinidine: May interfere with some laboratory tests that measure quinidine level. Inform laboratory that patient is taking triamterene.
Drug-food. *Potassium-containing salt substitutes, potassium-rich foods:* May increase risk of hyperkalemia. Discourage use together.
Drug-lifestyle. *Sun exposure:* May increase risk of photosensitivity reactions. Urge patient to avoid prolonged or unprotected exposure to sunlight.

Effects on lab test results
• May increase BUN, creatinine, glucose, and uric acid levels. May decrease sodium and hemoglobin levels and hematocrit. May increase or decrease potassium level.
• May increase liver function test values. May decrease RBC, granulocyte, and platelet counts.

Pharmacokinetics
Absorption: Rapid; extent varies.
Distribution: About 67% protein-bound.
Metabolism: By hydroxylation and sulfation.
Excretion: In urine. *Half-life:* 100 to 150 minutes.

Route	Onset	Peak	Duration
P.O.	2–4 hr	6–8 hr	7–9 hr

Action

Chemical effect: Inhibits sodium reabsorption and potassium and hydrogen excretion by direct action on distal tubule.
Therapeutic effect: Promotes water and sodium excretion.

Available forms

Capsules: 50 mg, 100 mg

NURSING PROCESS

Assessment

• Assess patient's edema before starting therapy and regularly thereafter. Full effect of triamterene is delayed 2 to 3 days when used alone.
• Monitor blood pressure, and BUN and electrolyte levels.
• Watch for blood dyscrasia.
• Be alert for adverse reactions and drug interactions.
• Assess patient's and family's knowledge of drug therapy.

Nursing diagnoses

• Excess fluid volume related to underlying condition
• Ineffective health maintenance related to drug-induced hyperkalemia
• Deficient knowledge related to drug therapy

Planning and implementation

• Give drug after meals, to minimize nausea.
• **ALERT:** Withdraw drug gradually to minimize excessive rebound potassium excretion.
• Drug is less potent than thiazides and loop diuretics and is useful as adjunct to other diuretic therapy. Triamterene is usually used with potassium-wasting diuretics.
• When used with other diuretics, lower initial dose of each drug and adjust to individual requirements.
• **ALERT:** Don't confuse triamterene with trimipramine.
Patient teaching
• Tell patient to take drug after meals.
• **ALERT:** Warn patient to avoid excessive ingestion of potassium-rich foods, potassium-containing salt substitutes, and potassium supplements to prevent serious hyperkalemia.

• Instruct patient to avoid direct sunlight, wear protective clothing, and use sunblock to prevent photosensitivity reactions.

Evaluation

• Patient exhibits no signs of edema.
• Patient's potassium level is normal.
• Patient and family state understanding of drug therapy.

triazolam

(trigh-AH-zoh-lam)
Alti-Triazolam ♦**, Apo-Triazo** ♦**, Halcion, Novo-Triolam** ♦

Pharmacologic class: benzodiazepine
Therapeutic class: sedative-hypnotic
Pregnancy risk category: X
Controlled substance schedule: IV

Indications and dosages

▶ **Insomnia.** *Adults:* 0.125 to 0.5 mg P.O. h.s. *Adults older than age 65:* 0.125 mg P.O. h.s.; increased, p.r.n., to 0.25 mg P.O. h.s.

Contraindications and cautions

• Contraindicated in patients hypersensitive to benzodiazepines.
• Use cautiously in patients with impaired liver or kidney function, chronic pulmonary insufficiency, sleep apnea, depression, suicidal tendencies, or history of drug abuse.
Lifespan: In pregnant women, drug is contraindicated. In breast-feeding women, drug isn't recommended. In children, safety and effectiveness haven't been established.

Adverse reactions

CNS: *drowsiness, dizziness, headache,* rebound insomnia, amnesia, light-headedness, lack of coordination, confusion, depression, nervousness, ataxia.
GI: nausea, vomiting, stomatitis.
Other: physical or psychological abuse.

Interactions

Drug-drug. *Cimetidine, erythromycin, hormonal contraceptives, isoniazid, ranitidine:* May cause prolonged triazolam blood level. Monitor patient for increased sedation.

Diltiazem: May increase CNS depression and prolong effects of triazolam. Use lower dose of triazolam.

Fluconazole, itraconazole, ketoconazole, miconazole: May increase and prolong drug levels, CNS depression, and psychomotor impairment. Don't use together.

Other CNS depressants, including opioid analgesics, other psychotropic drugs, anticonvulsants, antihistamines: May cause excessive CNS depression. Use together cautiously.

Other potent CYP 3A inhibitors, such as nefazodone: May decrease clearance of triazolam. Don't use together.

Drug-herb. *Calendula, catnip, hops, lady's slipper, lemon balm, passion flower, sassafras, skullcap, valerian, yerba maté:* May increase risk of sedative effects. Monitor patient closely if used together.

Kava: May cause excessive sedation. Discourage use together.

Drug-food. *Grapefruit juice:* May delay drug onset and increase effects. Advise patient to avoid use together.

Drug-lifestyle. *Alcohol use:* May cause additive CNS effects. Strongly discourage use together.

Effects on lab test results

• May increase liver function test values.

Pharmacokinetics

Absorption: Good.
Distribution: Widely distributed; 90% protein-bound.
Metabolism: In liver.
Excretion: In urine. *Half-life:* 1½ to 5½ hours.

Route	Onset	Peak	Duration
P.O.	Unknown	1–2 hr	Unknown

Action

Chemical effect: May act on limbic system, thalamus, and hypothalamus of CNS to produce hypnotic effects.
Therapeutic effect: Promotes sleep.

Available forms

Tablets: 0.125 mg, 0.25 mg

NURSING PROCESS

✒ Assessment

• Assess patient's condition before starting therapy and regularly thereafter to monitor the drug's effectiveness.
• Assess mental status and neurologic function before starting therapy. An elderly patient is more sensitive to the drug's CNS effects.
• Be alert for adverse reactions and drug interactions.
• Assess patient's and family's knowledge of drug therapy.

⊕ Nursing diagnoses

• Disturbed sleep pattern related to underlying disorder
• Risk for injury related to drug-induced adverse CNS reactions
• Deficient knowledge related to drug therapy

⟫ Planning and implementation

• Take precautions to prevent hoarding or intentional overdose by patient who is depressed, suicidal, or drug-dependent or who has a history of drug abuse.
• Store drug in cool, dry place away from light.
• Institute safety precautions once drug has been given.
• **ALERT:** Don't confuse Halcion with Haldol or halcinonide.

Patient teaching

• Warn patient not to take more than prescribed amount because overdose can occur at total daily dosage of 2 mg (four times the highest recommended amount).
• Warn patient about performing activities that require mental alertness or physical coordination. For inpatient, supervise walking and raise bed rails, particularly for geriatric patient.
• Inform patient that drug is very short-acting and therefore has less tendency to cause morning drowsiness.
• Tell patient that rebound insomnia may develop for 1 or 2 nights after stopping therapy.

✓ Evaluation

• Patient states that drug produces sleep.
• Patient doesn't experience injury from adverse CNS reactions.
• Patient and family state understanding of drug therapy.

Reactions may be *common*, uncommon, *life-threatening*, or COMMON AND LIFE-THREATENING.

trifluoperazine hydrochloride
(trigh-floo-oh-PER-eh-zeen high-droh-KLOR-ighd)
Apo-Trifluoperazine ♦ , Novo-Flurazine ♦

Pharmacologic class: phenothiazine (piperazine derivative)
Therapeutic class: antipsychotic, antiemetic
Pregnancy risk category: C

Indications and dosages

► **Anxiety.** *Adults:* 1 to 2 mg P.O. b.i.d. Maximum, 6 mg daily. Don't use for longer than 12 weeks.
► **Schizophrenia and other psychotic disorders.** *Adult outpatients:* 1 to 2 mg P.O. b.i.d., increased p.r.n. Or, 1 to 2 mg deep I.M. q 4 to 6 hours, p.r.n.
Adult inpatients: 2 to 5 mg P.O. b.i.d.; may increase gradually to 40 mg daily.
Children ages 6 to 12 (hospitalized or under close supervision): 1 mg P.O. daily or b.i.d.; may increase gradually to 15 mg daily, if needed.

Contraindications and cautions

• Contraindicated in patients hypersensitive to phenothiazines and in patients experiencing coma, CNS depression, bone marrow suppression, or liver damage.
• Use cautiously in debilitated patients and in patients with CV disease (may cause drop in blood pressure), seizure disorder, glaucoma, or prostatic hyperplasia. Also use cautiously in patients exposed to extreme heat.
⚠ **Lifespan:** In pregnant or breast-feeding women and in children younger than age 6, safety and effectiveness haven't been established. In the elderly, use cautiously.

Adverse reactions

CNS: *extrapyramidal reactions, tardive dyskinesia,* pseudoparkinsonism, dizziness, drowsiness, insomnia, fatigue, headache, *neuroleptic malignant syndrome.*
CV: *orthostatic hypotension,* tachycardia, ECG changes.
EENT: ocular changes, *blurred vision.*
GI: dry mouth, constipation, nausea.
GU: *urine retention,* menstrual irregularities.
Hematologic: *transient leukopenia, agranulocytosis.*

Hepatic: cholestatic jaundice.
Metabolic: weight gain.
Skin: *photosensitivity reactions,* sterile abscesses, rash.
Other: allergic reaction, pain at I.M. injection site, gynecomastia, inhibited lactation.

Interactions

Drug-drug. *Antacids:* May inhibit absorption of oral phenothiazines. Separate doses by at least 2 hours.
Barbiturates, lithium: May decrease phenothiazine effect. Monitor patient.
Centrally acting antihypertensives: May decrease antihypertensive effect. Monitor blood pressure.
CNS depressants: May increase CNS depression. Use together cautiously.
Propranolol: May increase levels of both propranolol and trifluoperazine. Monitor patient closely.
Warfarin: May decrease effect of oral anticoagulants. Monitor PT and INR.
Drug-herb. *Dong quai, St. John's wort:* May increase photosensitivity reactions. Discourage use together.
Ginkgo: May decrease adverse effects of thioridazine. Monitor patient.
Kava: May increase risk of dystonic reactions. Discourage use together.
Milk thistle: May decrease liver toxicity caused by phenothiazines. Discourage use together; monitor liver enzyme levels if used together.
Yohimbe: May increase risk of yohimbe toxicity. Discourage use together.
Drug-lifestyle. *Alcohol use:* May increase CNS depression, particularly psychomotor skills. Strongly discourage use together.
Sun exposure: May cause photosensitivity reactions. Urge patient to avoid prolonged or unprotected exposure to sunlight.

Effects on lab test results

• May increase liver enzyme levels.
• May decrease WBC and granulocyte counts.

Pharmacokinetics

Absorption: Variable with P.O. use; rapid after I.M. use.
Distribution: Widely distributed; 91% to 99% protein-bound.
Metabolism: Extensively by liver.

Excretion: Primarily in urine; some in feces.
Half-life: 20 to 40 hours.

Route	Onset	Peak	Duration
P.O., I.M.	Up to several wk	Unknown	Unknown

Action

Chemical effect: Unknown; probably blocks postsynaptic dopamine receptors in brain.
Therapeutic effect: Relieves anxiety and signs and symptoms of psychotic disorders.

Available forms

Injection: 2 mg/ml
Oral concentrate: 10 mg/ml
Tablets (regular and film-coated): 1 mg, 2 mg, 5 mg, 10 mg

NURSING PROCESS

⊞ Assessment

• Assess patient's condition before starting therapy and regularly thereafter to monitor the drug's effectiveness.
• Watch for orthostatic hypotension, especially with parenteral use.
• Monitor patient for tardive dyskinesia, which may occur after prolonged use. It may not appear until months or years later and may disappear spontaneously or persist for life, despite stopping the drug.
• Monitor therapy with weekly bilirubin tests during first month, periodic blood tests (CBC and liver function), and ophthalmologic tests (long-term use).
⊛ **ALERT:** Monitor patient for symptoms of neuroleptic malignant syndrome (extrapyramidal effects, hyperthermia, autonomic disturbance), which is rare but can be fatal. It isn't necessarily related to length of drug use or type of neuroleptic; however, more than 60% of patients are men.
• Assess patient's and family's knowledge of drug therapy.

⊞ Nursing diagnoses

• Anxiety related to underlying condition
• Disturbed thought processes related to underlying psychotic disorder
• Deficient knowledge related to drug therapy

⊠ Planning and implementation

• Although there is little likelihood of contact dermatitis, those sensitive to phenothiazine drugs should avoid direct contact. Wear gloves when preparing liquid forms.
• Dilute liquid concentrate with 60 ml of tomato or fruit juice, carbonated beverage, coffee, tea, milk, water, or semisolid food.
• Give deep I.M. only in upper outer quadrant of buttocks. Massage slowly afterward to prevent sterile abscess. Injection may sting.
• Protect solution or concentrate from light. Slight yellowing of drug is common; it doesn't affect potency. Discard markedly discolored solutions.
• Keep patient supine for 1 hour after drug administration, and advise him to change position slowly.
• Don't abruptly stop giving the drug unless a severe adverse reaction occurs. Abruptly stopping long-term therapy may cause gastritis, nausea, vomiting, dizziness, tremor, feeling of warmth or cold, diaphoresis, tachycardia, headache, insomnia, anorexia, muscle rigidity, altered mental status, or evidence of autonomic instability.
• Don't give the dose, and notify prescriber, if patient develops jaundice, symptoms of blood dyscrasia (fever, sore throat, infection, cellulitis, weakness), or extrapyramidal reactions longer than a few hours, especially in pregnant women and in children.
• Acute dystonic reactions may be treated with diphenhydramine.
⊛ **ALERT:** Don't confuse trifluoperazine with triflupromazine.

Patient teaching
• Teach patient or caregiver how to prepare oral form of drug.
• Warn patient to avoid activities that require alertness or good psychomotor coordination until drug's CNS effects are known; drowsiness and dizziness usually subside after a few weeks.
• Tell patient not to drink alcohol during therapy.
• Instruct patient to report urine retention or constipation.
• Tell patient to use sun block and wear protective clothing to avoid photosensitivity reactions.
• Tell patient to relieve dry mouth with sugarless gum or hard candy.

☑ Evaluation

• Patient's anxiety is reduced.
• Patient's behavior and communication exhibit improved thought processes.
• Patient and family state understanding of drug therapy.

trihexyphenidyl hydrochloride
(trigh-heks-eh-FEEN-ih-dil high-droh-KLOR-ighd)
Apo-Trihex ♦ , Artane ♦ , Trihexy-2, Trihexy-5

Pharmacologic class: anticholinergic
Therapeutic class: antiparkinsonian
Pregnancy risk category: C

Indications and dosages

▶ **All forms of parkinsonism and adjunct treatment with levodopa in management of parkinsonism.** *Adults:* 1 mg P.O. first day, then increased by 2 mg q 3 to 5 days until total of 6 to 10 mg is given daily. Usually given t.i.d. with meals. Sometimes given q.i.d. (last dose h.s.) Postencephalitic parkinsonism may require total daily dosage of 12 to 15 mg.
▶ **Drug-induced extrapyramidal reactions.** *Adults:* 5 to 15 mg P.O. daily. Initial dose of 1 mg may control some reactions.

Contraindications and cautions

• Contraindicated in patients hypersensitive to the drug or any of its components.
• Use cautiously in patients with glaucoma; cardiac, hepatic, or renal disorders; obstructive disease of the GI or GU tract; or prostatic hyperplasia.
≋ **Lifespan:** In pregnant women, safety and effectiveness haven't been established. In breast-feeding women, drug isn't recommended. In children, safety and effectiveness haven't been established. In the elderly, watch for mental confusion or disorientation.

Adverse reactions

CNS: nervousness, dizziness, headache, hallucinations, drowsiness, weakness.
CV: tachycardia.
EENT: blurred vision, mydriasis, increased intraocular pressure.
GI: *dry mouth,* constipation, *nausea,* vomiting.
GU: urinary hesitancy, urine retention.

Interactions

Drug-drug. *Amantadine:* May have additive anticholinergic reactions, such as confusion and hallucinations. Reduce dosage of trihexyphenidyl before giving.
Levodopa: May increase drug effect. May require lower doses of both drugs.
Drug-lifestyle. *Alcohol use:* May increase sedative effects. Discourage use together.

Effects on lab test results

None reported.

Pharmacokinetics

Absorption: Readily absorbed.
Distribution: Unknown; crosses blood-brain barrier.
Metabolism: Unknown.
Excretion: In urine. *Half-life:* 5½ to 10¾ hours.

Route	Onset	Peak	Duration
P.O.	1 hr	2–3 hr	6–12 hr

Action

Chemical effect: Unknown; blocks central cholinergic receptors, helping to balance cholinergic activity in basal ganglia.
Therapeutic effect: Improves physical mobility in patients with parkinsonism.

Available forms

Elixir: 2 mg/5 ml
Tablets: 2 mg, 5 mg

NURSING PROCESS

℞ Assessment

• Assess patient's condition before starting therapy and regularly thereafter to monitor the drug's effectiveness.
③ **ALERT:** Gonioscopic ocular evaluation and monitoring of intraocular pressure are needed, especially in a patient older than age 40.
• Be alert for adverse reactions and drug interactions. Adverse reactions are dose-related and usually transient.
• Assess patient's and family's knowledge of drug therapy.

⊕ Nursing diagnoses

• Impaired physical mobility related to presence of parkinsonism

T

• Risk for injury related to drug-induced adverse CNS reactions
• Deficient knowledge related to drug therapy

> **Planning and implementation**
• Dose may need to be increased gradually in a patient who develops drug tolerance.
• Give drug with meals.
Patient teaching
• Warn patient that drug may cause nausea if taken before meals.
• Tell patient to avoid activities that require alertness until the drug's CNS effects are known.
• Advise patient to report urinary hesitancy or urine retention.
• Tell patient to relieve dry mouth with cool drinks, ice chips, sugarless gum, or hard candy.

☑ **Evaluation**
• Patient exhibits improved physical mobility.
• Patient doesn't experience injury from adverse reactions.
• Patient and family state understanding of drug therapy.

trimethobenzamide hydrochloride
(trigh-meth-oh-BEN-zuh-mighd high-droh-KLOR-ighd)
Tebamide, T-Gen, Ticon, Tigan, Triban, Trimazide

Pharmacologic class: ethanolamine-related antihistamine
Therapeutic class: antiemetic
Pregnancy risk category: C

Indications and dosages

► **Nausea, vomiting.** *Adults:* 250 mg P.O. t.i.d. or q.i.d.; or 200 mg I.M. or P.R. t.i.d. or q.i.d.
► **Prevention of postoperative nausea and vomiting.** *Adults:* 200 mg I.M. or P.R. as single dose before or during surgery; if needed, repeat 3 hours after termination of anesthesia. Limit use to prolonged vomiting from known cause.
Children weighing 13 to 40 kg (28 to 88 lb): 100 to 200 mg P.O. or P.R. t.i.d. or q.i.d.
Children weighing less than 13 kg: 100 mg P.R. t.i.d. or q.i.d. Don't use in premature or newborn infants.

Contraindications and cautions

• Contraindicated in patients hypersensitive to the drug or any of its components. Suppositories are contraindicated in patients hypersensitive to benzocaine hydrochloride or similar local anesthetics.
⚖ **Lifespan:** In pregnant women, use cautiously. In breast-feeding women, safety and effectiveness haven't been established. In children, use cautiously. In children with viral illness, drug isn't recommended because it may contribute to development of Reye's syndrome.

Adverse reactions

CNS: *drowsiness,* dizziness, headache, disorientation, depression, Parkinsonian-like symptoms, *coma, seizures.*
CV: hypotension.
EENT: blurred vision.
GI: diarrhea.
Hepatic: jaundice.
Musculoskeletal: muscle cramps.
Skin: hypersensitivity reaction (pain, stinging, burning, redness, swelling at I.M. injection site).

Interactions

Drug-drug. *CNS depressants:* May cause additive CNS depression. Avoid use together.
Drug-lifestyle. *Alcohol use:* May cause additive CNS depression. Discourage use together.

Effects on lab test results

None reported.

Pharmacokinetics

Absorption: About 60% after P.O. use; unknown after P.R. or I.M. use.
Distribution: Unknown.
Metabolism: About 50% to 70%, probably in liver.
Excretion: In urine and feces. *Half-life:* 7 to 9 hours.

Route	Onset	Peak	Duration
P.O.	10–20 min	Unknown	3–4 hr
I.M.	15–30 min	Unknown	2–3 hr
P.R.	Unknown	Unknown	Unknown

Action

Chemical effect: Unknown; may act on chemoreceptor trigger zone to inhibit nausea and vomiting.

Reactions may be *common*, uncommon, *life-threatening*, or COMMON AND LIFE-THREATENING.

Therapeutic effect: Prevents or relieves nausea and vomiting.

Available forms

Capsules: 100 mg, 250 mg
Injection: 100 mg/ml
Suppositories: 100 mg, 200 mg

NURSING PROCESS

⏸ Assessment
• Assess patient's condition before starting therapy and regularly thereafter to monitor the drug's effectiveness.
• Be alert for adverse reactions and drug interactions.
• Assess patient's and family's knowledge of drug therapy.

⊞ Nursing diagnoses
• Risk for deficient fluid volume related to potential for or presence of nausea and vomiting
• Diarrhea related to drug-induced adverse GI reactions
• Deficient knowledge related to drug therapy

⧨ Planning and implementation
• Inject I.M. dose deep into upper outer quadrant of gluteal region to reduce pain and local irritation.
• Refrigerate suppositories.
• If skin hypersensitivity reaction occurs, don't give the drug.
⊛ ALERT: Don't confuse Tigan with Ticar.
Patient teaching
• Advise patient of possibility of drowsiness and dizziness, and caution against driving or performing other activities requiring alertness until the drug's CNS effects are known.
• Warn patient that giving the drug I.M. may be painful.
• If patient will be using suppositories, instruct him to remove foil and, if needed, moisten suppository with water for 10 to 30 seconds before inserting. Tell him to store suppositories in refrigerator.

☑ Evaluation
• Patient maintains adequate hydration with cessation of nausea and vomiting.
• Patient maintains normal bowel pattern.
• Patient and family state understanding of drug therapy.

trimethoprim
(trigh-METH-uh-prim)
Alprim◇, Primsol, Proloprim, Trimpex, Triprim◇

Pharmacologic class: synthetic folate antagonist
Therapeutic class: antibiotic
Pregnancy risk category: C

Indications and dosages

▶ **Acute otitis media caused by susceptible strains of *S. pneumoniae* and *H. influenzae.*** *Children age 6 months and older:* 10 mg/kg Primsol daily in divided doses q 12 hours for 10 days.
▶ **Uncomplicated UTIs caused by *E. coli, P. mirabilis, Klebsiella pneumoniae,* Enterobacter species, coagulase-negative *Staphylococcus* species (including *S. saprophyticus*).** *Adults:* 100 mg (10 ml) q 12 hours, or 200 mg (20 ml) daily for 10 days.
▶ **Prophylaxis of chronic and recurrent UTIs‡.** *Adults:* 100 mg P.O. h.s. for 6 weeks to 6 months.
▶ **Traveler's diarrhea‡.** *Adults:* 200 mg P.O. b.i.d. for 3 to 5 days.
▶ ***Pneumocystis jiroveci (carinii)* pneumonia‡.** *Adults:* 5 mg/kg P.O. t.i.d. with dapsone 100 mg daily for 21 days.
⧉ Adjust-a-dose: For patients with renal impairment, if creatinine clearance is 15 to 30 ml/minute, give half of the recommended dose q 12 hours; if less than 15 ml/minute, don't use drug.

Contraindications and cautions

• Contraindicated in patients hypersensitive to the drug or any of its components, and in those with documented megaloblastic anemia caused by folate deficiency.
• Use cautiously in patients with hepatic impairment.
⚘ Lifespan: In pregnant women, use cautiously. In breast-feeding women, drug isn't recommended. In children younger than age 12, safety and effectiveness (other than of Primsol) haven't been established.

Adverse reactions

CNS: fever.

T

GI: epigastric distress, nausea, vomiting, diarrhea, glossitis.
Hematologic: *thrombocytopenia, leukopenia,* megaloblastic anemia, *methemoglobinemia.*
Skin: *rash, pruritus,* exfoliative dermatitis.

Interactions

Drug-drug. *Phenytoin:* May decrease phenytoin metabolism and increase its level. Monitor patient for toxicity.

Effects on lab test results

• May increase BUN, creatinine, bilirubin, and aminotransferase levels. May decrease hemoglobin level and hematocrit.
• May decrease platelet and WBC counts.

Pharmacokinetics

Absorption: Quick and complete.
Distribution: Widely distributed. About 42% to 46% protein-bound.
Metabolism: Less than 20% in liver.
Excretion: Mostly in urine. *Half-life:* 8 to 11 hours.

Route	Onset	Peak	Duration
P.O.	Unknown	1–4 hr	Unknown

Action

Chemical effect: Interferes with action of dihydrofolate reductase, inhibiting bacterial synthesis of folic acid.
Therapeutic effect: Inhibits certain bacteria.

Available forms

Oral solution: 50 mg/5 ml
Tablets: 100 mg, 200 mg

NURSING PROCESS

Assessment
• Assess patient's infection before starting therapy and regularly thereafter to monitor the drug's effectiveness.
• Obtain urine specimen for culture and sensitivity tests before giving the first dose. Start therapy pending test results.
ALERT: Monitor CBC routinely. Signs and symptoms such as sore throat, fever, pallor, and purpura may be early indications of serious blood disorders. Prolonged use of trimethoprim at high doses may cause bone marrow suppression.

• Be alert for adverse reactions and drug interactions.
• If adverse GI reactions occur, monitor hydration.
• Assess patient's and family's knowledge of drug therapy.

Nursing diagnoses
• Infection related to presence of susceptible bacteria
• Risk for deficient fluid volume related to drug-induced adverse GI reactions
• Deficient knowledge related to drug therapy

Planning and implementation
• Because resistance to trimethoprim develops rapidly when given alone, it's usually given with other drugs.
ALERT: Trimethoprim is also used with sulfamethoxazole; don't confuse the two products.
Patient teaching
• Instruct patient to take drug as prescribed, even if he feels better.

Evaluation
• Patient is free from infection.
• Patient maintains adequate hydration.
• Patient and family state understanding of drug therapy.

triptorelin pamoate
(trip-TOE-reh-lin PAM-o-eight)
Trelstar Depot, Trelstar LA

Pharmacologic class: synthetic luteinizing hormone-releasing hormone (LHRH) analogue
Therapeutic class: antineoplastic
Pregnancy risk category: X

Indications and dosages

▶ **Palliative treatment of advanced prostate cancer.** *Men:* 3.75 mg Trelstar Depot I.M. given monthly as a single injection, or 11.25 mg Trelstar LA I.M. into either buttock q 12 weeks.

Contraindications and cautions

• Contraindicated in patients hypersensitive to the drug or any of its components, other LHRH agonists, or LHRH.
• Use cautiously in patients with metastatic vertebral lesions or upper or lower urinary tract

obstruction during the first few weeks of therapy.

• Use cautiously in patients with hepatic and renal impairment; they have a level of exposure to drug two to four times higher than normal.

⚄ **Lifespan:** Drug is used for men only. In boys, safety and effectiveness haven't been studied.

Adverse reactions

CNS: *spinal cord compression,* pain, headache, dizziness, fatigue, insomnia, emotional lability.
CV: hypertension.
GI: diarrhea, vomiting.
GU: urine retention, UTI, impotence.
Hematologic: anemia.
Musculoskeletal: *skeletal pain,* leg pain.
Skin: pruritus.
Other: *hot flushes,* pain at injection site.

Interactions

Drug-drug. *Hyperprolactinemic drugs:* May decrease pituitary gonadotropin-releasing hormone (GnRH) receptors. Don't use together.

Effects on lab test results

• May increase glucose, BUN, AST, ALT, and alkaline phosphatase. May transiently increase testosterone level. May decrease hemoglobin level and hematocrit.

Pharmacokinetics

Absorption: Maintains level over a period of a month.
Distribution: No evidence of protein-binding.
Metabolism: Unknown, but is unlikely to involve hepatic microsomal enzymes; no metabolites have been identified.
Excretion: By both liver and kidneys. *Half-life:* 2 to 3 hours.

Route	Onset	Peak	Duration
I.M.	Unknown	Unknown	1 mo

Action

Chemical effect: Is a potent inhibitor of gonadotropin secretion. In men, testosterone declines to a level typically seen in surgically castrated men. As a result, tissues and functions that depend on these hormones become inactive.
Therapeutic effect: Decreases effects of sex hormones on tumor growth in the prostate gland.

Available forms

Injection: 3.75 mg, 11.25 mg

NURSING PROCESS

⚄ Assessment

• Assess patient's condition before starting therapy and regularly thereafter to monitor the drug's effectiveness.
• Monitor testosterone and prostate-specific antigen levels.
• Assess patient's and family's knowledge of drug therapy.

⊞ Nursing diagnoses

• Ineffective health maintenance related to underlying condition
• Acute pain related to adverse drug effects
• Deficient knowledge related to drug therapy

⊳ Planning and implementation

• Give drug only under the supervision of an experienced prescriber.
ⓢ **ALERT:** Only sterile water may be used as a diluent.
• Dilute vial with 2 ml of sterile water for injection. Shake well until suspension appears milky. Use 20 G needle.
• Change the injection site periodically.
• Monitor patients with metastatic vertebral lesions or upper or lower urinary tract obstruction during the first few weeks of therapy.
• Initially, drug causes a transient increase in testosterone levels. As a result, signs and symptoms of prostate cancer may worsen during the first few weeks of therapy.
• Patients may experience worsening of symptoms or onset of new symptoms, including bone pain, neuropathy, hematuria, or urethral or bladder outlet obstruction.
ⓢ **ALERT:** Spinal cord compression, which can lead to paralysis and possibly death, may occur. If spinal cord compression or renal impairment develops, give standard treatment. In extreme cases, immediate orchiectomy is considered.
• If patient has an allergic reaction, immediately stop giving the drug, treat symptoms, and give supportive care.
• Diagnostic tests of pituitary-gonadal function conducted during and after therapy may be misleading.
• Reconstitute powder with 2 ml sterile water, using a 20-gauge needle.

T

Patient teaching
- Inform the patient about adverse reactions.
- Tell patient that symptoms (including bone pain, neuropathy, hematuria, or urethral or bladder outlet obstruction) may worsen during the first few weeks of therapy.
- Inform patient that a blood test will be used to monitor response to therapy.

☑ Evaluation
- Patient responds well to drug.
- Patient denies pain.
- Patient and family state understanding of drug therapy.

trospium chloride
(TROSE-pee-uhm KLOHR-ighd)
Sanctura

Pharmacologic class: anticholinergic
Therapeutic class: antispasmodic, antimuscarinic
Pregnancy risk category: C

Indications and dosages
▶ **Overactive bladder with symptoms of urinary urge incontinence, urgency, and frequency.** *Adults younger than age 75:* 20 mg P.O. b.i.d. taken on an empty stomach or at least 1 hour before a meal.
Adults age 75 and older: Based on patient tolerance, reduce dose to 20 mg once daily.
Ⓢ **Adjust-a-dose:** If patient's creatinine clearance is less than 30 ml/minute, give 20 mg P.O. once daily h.s.

Contraindications and cautions
- Contraindicated in patients hypersensitive to the drug or any of its components and in patients with or at risk for urine retention, gastric retention, or uncontrolled narrow-angle glaucoma.
- Use cautiously in patients with significant bladder outflow obstruction, obstructive GI disorders, ulcerative colitis, intestinal atony, myasthenia gravis, renal insufficiency, moderate or severe hepatic impairment, or controlled narrow-angle glaucoma.
- ♨ **Lifespan:** In pregnant women, use only if benefits to the patient outweigh risks to the fetus. In breast-feeding women, use cautiously;

it's unknown if the drug appears in breast milk. In children, safety and effectiveness haven't been established. In an elderly patient, use a lower dose because there may be an increased risk of anticholinergic effects.

Adverse reactions
CNS: fatigue, headache.
EENT: dry eyes.
GI: abdominal pain, *constipation, dry mouth,* dyspepsia, flatulence.
GU: urine retention.

Interactions
Drug-drug. *Anticholinergics:* May increase dry mouth, constipation, or other adverse effects. Monitor patient.
Digoxin, metformin, morphine, pancuronium, procainamide, tenofovir, vancomycin: May alter elimination of these drugs or trospium, increasing levels. Monitor patient closely.
Drug-food. *High-fat food:* May decrease absorption by up to 80%. Give trospium at least 1 hour before meals or on an empty stomach.
Drug-lifestyle. *Alcohol use:* May increase drowsiness. Discourage use together.

Effects on lab test results
None reported.

Pharmacokinetics
Absorption: Less than 10%. Taking drug after a high-fat meal significantly decreases absorption. It should be taken at least 1 hour before meals or on an empty stomach.
Distribution: Mostly in plasma. Protein-binding is 50% to 85%.
Metabolism: Not defined. Major pathway is most likely is the liver.
Excretion: About 85% appears in feces and about 6% in urine. *Half-life:* About 20 hours.

Route	Onset	Peak	Duration
P.O.	Unknown	5–6 hr	Unknown

Action
Chemical effect: Opposes the effect of acetylcholine on muscarinic receptors, reducing smooth muscle tone in the bladder and increasing maximum bladder capacity and volume at first contraction.
Therapeutic effect: Relieves symptoms of overactive bladder.

Available forms

Tablets: 20 mg

NURSING PROCESS

⚖ Assessment
• Assess patient before starting therapy to determine baseline bladder function, and reassess during therapy to monitor the drug's effectiveness.
• Monitor patient for decreased gastric motility and constipation.
• Assess patient's and family's knowledge of drug therapy.

⊕ Nursing diagnoses
• Impaired urinary elimination related to underlying medical condition
• Impaired oral mucous membrane related to drug-induced adverse effects
• Deficient knowledge related to drug therapy

▷ Planning and implementation
• If the patient has bladder-outflow obstruction, watch for evidence of urine retention.
• If the patient has urine retention, notify prescriber and prepare for urinary catheterization.
• Dry mouth and constipation are the most frequently reported adverse effects.
Patient teaching
• Tell patient to take drug on an empty stomach, at least 1 hour before meals.
• Discourage use of other drugs that may cause dry mouth, constipation, blurred vision, or urine retention.
• Tell patient that alcohol may increase drowsiness and fatigue. Urge him not to drink alcohol to excess while taking drug.
• Explain that drug may decrease sweating and increase the risk of heatstroke when used in hot environments or during strenuous activities.
• Urge patient to avoid activities that are hazardous or require mental alertness until the drug's CNS effects are known.

☑ Evaluation
• Patient experiences improved bladder function with drug therapy.
• Patient does not experience dry mouth or controls adverse effect with sugarless gum, hard candy, or saliva substitute.
• Patient and family state understanding of drug therapy.

unoprostone isopropyl
(yoo-noh-PROST-ohn igh-soh-PROH-pul)
Rescula

Pharmacologic class: docosanoid
Therapeutic class: antiglaucoma drug, ocular antihypertensive
Pregnancy risk category: C

Indications and dosages

▶ **Reduction of intraocular pressure (IOP) in patients with open-angle glaucoma or ocular hypertension who can't tolerate or who respond inadequately to other IOP-lowering drugs.** *Adults:* 1 drop in the affected eye b.i.d.

Contraindications and cautions

• Contraindicated in patients hypersensitive to drug, benzalkonium chloride, or any other component.
• Use cautiously in patients with active intraocular inflammation (uveitis) or with angle-closure, inflammatory, or neovascular glaucoma. Also use cautiously in patients with renal or hepatic impairment.
⚖ Lifespan: In pregnant women, use only if benefits to the patient outweigh risks to the fetus. In breast-feeding women, use cautiously; it's unknown if the drug appears in breast milk. In children, safety and effectiveness haven't been established.

Adverse reactions

CNS: dizziness, headache, insomnia, pain.
CV: hypertension.
EENT: abnormal vision, blepharitis, cataracts, conjunctivitis, corneal lesion, *dry eyes,* eye discharge, *eye burning or stinging,* eye discomfort, eye irritation, eye hemorrhage, decreased length of eyelashes, *increased length of eyelashes,* eyelid disorder, foreign body sensation, keratitis, lacrimal disorder, pharyngitis, photophobia, rhinitis, sinusitis, vitreous disorder, *eye itching, injection of eye.*
Metabolic: diabetes mellitus.
Musculoskeletal: back pain.

Respiratory: bronchitis, increased cough, pharyngitis, increased cough.
Other: accidental injury, allergic reaction, flu-like syndrome.

Interactions

None reported.

Effects on lab test results

None reported.

Pharmacokinetics

Absorption: Absorbed through the cornea and conjunctival epithelium. Systemic absorption is minimal.
Distribution: Unknown.
Metabolism: Hydrolyzed by esterases to form unoprostone free acid.
Excretion: Rapid. Metabolites are excreted mainly in urine. *Half-life:* 14 minutes.

Route	Onset	Peak	Duration
Ophthalmic	Unknown	Unknown	Unknown

Action

Chemical effect: Unknown. Thought to increase the outflow of aqueous humor.
Therapeutic effect: Reduces IOP.

Available forms

Ophthalmic solution: 0.15% (1.5 mg/ml)

NURSING PROCESS

Assessment
• Assess patient's condition before starting therapy and regularly thereafter to monitor the drug's effectiveness.
• Assess solution carefully before instilling. Serious eye damage and blindness may result from using contaminated solutions.
• Evaluate patient's and family's knowledge of drug therapy.

Nursing diagnoses
• Noncompliance related to long-term therapy
• Risk for injury related to adverse EENT effects of drug
• Deficient knowledge related to drug therapy

Planning and implementation
• Avoid touching the tip of the container to the eye because this may contaminate the applicator and cause infection.
• Have patient who wears contact lenses remove them before giving drug. Drug contains benzalkonium chloride, which may be absorbed by the lenses. He may reinsert them 15 minutes after drug use.
• When giving an additional ophthalmic drug, separate doses by 5 minutes.
• Store drug at room temperature.
Patient teaching
• Instruct patient to avoid touching the tip of the container to the eye because this could contaminate the tip and cause an eye infection.
• Instruct patient who wears contact lenses to remove lenses before using drug and to wait at least 15 minutes after using the drug before reinserting them.
• Tell patient that drug may permanently darken eye color. Change may be gradual, over months to years.
• Instruct patient to report adverse effects, especially conjunctivitis (pink eye) or eyelid reactions.
• If eye trauma or infection occur, or if ocular surgery is planned, tell patient to notify prescriber before continuing to use a multidose container.
• Tell patient that drug may be used with other ocular drugs, but that doses should be separated by 5 minutes.

Evaluation
• Patient is compliant with drug therapy.
• Patient sustains no injury.
• Patient and family state understanding of drug therapy.

urokinase
(yoo-roh-KIGH-nays)
Abbokinase

Pharmacologic class: enzyme
Therapeutic class: thrombolytic
Pregnancy risk category: B

Indications and dosages

▶ **Lysis of acute massive pulmonary emboli and pulmonary emboli accompanied by un-**

stable hemodynamics. *Adults:* For I.V. infusion only by constant infusion pump. Priming dose: 4,400 international units/kg over 10 minutes, followed with 4,400 international units/kg/hour for 12 hours. Flush any drug remaining in the I.V. tubing with a volume of compatible I.V. solution about equal to that of the tubing at 15 ml/hour.

▶ **Venous catheter occlusion‡.** *Adults:* Instill 5,000 international units into occluded line.

▽▼ I.V. administration

• Add 5 ml of sterile water for injection to vial. Don't use bacteriostatic water for injection to reconstitute; it contains preservatives. Use immediately after reconstitution.
• Dilute further with normal saline solution or D_5W solution before infusion.
• Solution may be filtered through a 0.45 micron or smaller filter before administration.
• Give by infusion pump. Total volume of fluid given shouldn't exceed 200 ml.
• Store powder at 36° to 46° F (2° to 8° C).
⊗ **Incompatibilities**
Other I.V. drugs.

Contraindications and cautions

• Contraindicated in patients with active internal bleeding; aneurysm; arteriovenous malformation; bleeding diathesis; visceral or intracranial cancer; ulcerative colitis; diverticulitis; severe hypertension; hemostatic defects, including those secondary to severe hepatic or renal insufficiency; uncontrolled hypocoagulation; subacute bacterial endocarditis or rheumatic valvular disease; history of stroke; recent trauma with possible internal injuries; or recent cerebral embolism, thrombosis, or hemorrhage.
• Also contraindicated within 10 days after intra-arterial diagnostic procedure or surgery (liver or kidney biopsy, lumbar puncture, thoracentesis, paracentesis, or extensive or multiple cutdowns); and within 2 months after intracranial or intraspinal surgery.
• I.M. injections and other invasive procedures are contraindicated during urokinase therapy.
⚕ **Lifespan:** In pregnant women, drug should be used only when clearly needed. Drug is contraindicated during the first 10 days postpartum. In children, safety and effectiveness haven't been established.

Adverse reactions

CNS: fever, *stroke,* hemiplegia.
CV: *reperfusion arrhythmias,* tachycardia, transient hypotension or hypertension.
GI: nausea, vomiting.
Hematologic: *bleeding.*
Respiratory: *bronchospasm,* minor breathing difficulties.
Skin: phlebitis, rash.
Other: *anaphylaxis,* chills.

Interactions

Drug-drug. *Anticoagulants:* May increase risk of bleeding. Monitor patient closely.
Aspirin, dipyridamole, indomethacin, phenylbutazone, other drugs affecting platelet activity: May increase risk of bleeding. Monitor patient closely.

Effects on lab test results

• May decrease hemoglobin level and hematocrit.
• May increase PT, PTT, and INR.

Pharmacokinetics

Absorption: Administered I.V.
Distribution: Rapidly cleared from circulation; most of drug accumulates in kidneys and liver.
Metabolism: Rapid, in liver.
Excretion: Small amount excreted in urine and bile. *Half-life:* 10 to 20 minutes.

Route	Onset	Peak	Duration
I.V.	Immediate	20 min–2 hr	4 hr

Action

Chemical effect: Activates plasminogen by directly cleaving peptide bonds at two sites.
Therapeutic effect: Dissolves blood clots in lungs, coronary arteries, and venous catheters.

Available forms

Injection: 250,000 international units/vial

U

NURSING PROCESS

⚕ **Assessment**
• Assess patient's condition before starting therapy and regularly thereafter to monitor the drug's effectiveness.
• Assess patient for contraindications to therapy.
• Monitor patient for excessive bleeding q 15 minutes for first hour, q 30 minutes for sec-

ond through eighth hours, then once every shift. Pretreatment with drugs affecting platelets places patient at high risk for bleeding.
• Monitor pulse rates and color and sensation of limbs every hour.
• Keep laboratory flow sheet on patient's chart to monitor PTT, PT, INR, hemoglobin level, and hematocrit.
• Be alert for adverse reactions and drug interactions.
• Assess patient's and family's knowledge of drug therapy.

⊞ **Nursing diagnoses**
• Ineffective tissue perfusion (cardiopulmonary, peripheral) related to presence of blood clot(s)
• Ineffective protection related to drug-induced bleeding
• Deficient knowledge related to drug therapy

⊠ **Planning and implementation**
• Have typed and crossmatched RBCs, whole blood, and aminocaproic acid available to treat bleeding, and keep corticosteroids available to treat allergic reactions.
• Keep venipuncture sites to a minimum; use pressure dressing on puncture sites for at least 15 minutes.
• Keep limb being treated in alignment to prevent bleeding from infusion site.
• Don't handle the patient unnecessarily; pad side rails. Bruising is more likely during therapy.
• To prevent recurrent thrombosis, start heparin by continuous infusion when patient's thrombin time has decreased to less than twice the normal control value after urokinase has been stopped.
Ⓢ **ALERT:** Rare reports of orolingual edema, urticaria, cholesterol embolization, and infusion reactions causing hypoxia, cyanosis, acidosis, and back pain have occurred in patients receiving this drug.
Patient teaching
• Instruct patient to report symptoms of bleeding and other adverse reactions.

🗹 **Evaluation**
• Patient regains normal tissue perfusion with dissolution of blood clots.
• Patient doesn't experience serious complications from drug-induced bleeding.
• Patient and family state understanding of drug therapy.

ursodiol
(ur-sih-DIGH-al)
Actigall

Pharmacologic class: bile acid
Therapeutic class: gallstone-dissolving drug
Pregnancy risk category: B

Indications and dosages
▶ **Dissolution of gallstones smaller than 20 mm in diameter in patients who are poor candidates for surgery or who refuse surgery.**
Adults: 8 to 10 mg/kg P.O. daily in two or three divided doses.
▶ **Prevention of gallstone formation in obese patients experiencing rapid weight loss.**
Adults: 300 mg P.O. b.i.d.

Contraindications and cautions
• Contraindicated in patients hypersensitive to the drug or other bile acids and in patients with chronic hepatic disease, unremitting acute cholecystitis, cholangitis, biliary obstruction, gallstone-induced pancreatitis, or biliary fistula.
⚖ **Lifespan:** In pregnant women, use cautiously. In breast-feeding women, use cautiously; it's unknown if the drug appears in breast milk. In children, safety and effectiveness haven't been established.

Adverse reactions
CNS: *headache,* fatigue, anxiety, depression, *dizziness,* sleep disorders.
EENT: rhinitis.
GI: *nausea, vomiting, dyspepsia,* metallic taste, *abdominal pain,* biliary pain, cholecystitis, *diarrhea, constipation,* stomatitis, flatulence.
GU: UTI.
Musculoskeletal: arthralgia, myalgia, back pain.
Respiratory: cough.
Skin: pruritus, rash, dry skin, urticaria, hair thinning, diaphoresis.

Interactions
Drug-drug. *Antacids that contain aluminum, cholestyramine, colestipol:* May bind ursodiol and prevent its absorption. Avoid use together.
Clofibrate, estrogens, hormonal contraceptives: May increase hepatic cholesterol secretion; may

counteract effects of ursodiol. Avoid use together.

Effects on lab test results

● May decrease liver enzyme levels in patients with liver disease.

Pharmacokinetics

Absorption: About 90%.
Distribution: Conjugated and then secreted into hepatic bile ducts. Drug in bile is concentrated in gallbladder and expelled into duodenum in gallbladder bile. A small amount appears in systemic circulation.
Metabolism: In liver. A small amount undergoes bacterial degradation with each cycle of enterohepatic circulation.
Excretion: Primarily in feces with very small amount in urine. *Half-life:* Unknown.

Route	Onset	Peak	Duration
P.O.	Unknown	1–3 hr	Unknown

Action

Chemical effect: Unknown; probably suppresses hepatic synthesis and secretion of cholesterol as well as intestinal cholesterol absorption. After long-term administration, ursodiol can solubilize cholesterol from gallstones.
Therapeutic effect: Dissolves cholesterol gallstones.

Available forms

Capsules: 300 mg

NURSING PROCESS

Assessment

● Assess patient's condition before starting therapy and regularly thereafter to monitor the drug's effectiveness.
● Usually, therapy is long-term and requires ultrasound images of gallbladder q 6 months. If partial stone dissolution doesn't occur within 12 months, it's unlikely that complete dissolution will. Safety of use for longer than 24 months hasn't been established.
● **ALERT:** Monitor liver function test results, including AST and ALT levels, at beginning of therapy, after 1 month, after 3 months, and then q 6 months during therapy. Abnormal test results may indicate worsening of disease. A he-

patotoxic metabolite of drug may form in some patients.
● Be alert for adverse reactions and drug interactions.
● If adverse GI reaction occurs, monitor patient's hydration.
● Assess patient's and family's knowledge of drug therapy.

Nursing diagnoses

● Risk for injury related to presence of gallstones
● Risk for deficient fluid volume related to drug-induced adverse GI reactions
● Deficient knowledge related to drug therapy

Planning and implementation

● Drug won't dissolve calcified cholesterol stones, radiolucent bile pigment stones, or radiopaque stones.
Patient teaching
● Tell patient about alternative therapies, including watchful waiting (with no intervention) and cholecystectomy because relapse rate after bile acid therapy may be as high as 50% after 5 years.

Evaluation

● Patient is free from gallstones.
● Patient maintains adequate hydration.
● Patient and family state understanding of drug therapy.

valacyclovir hydrochloride
(val-ay-SIGH-kloh-veer high-droh-KLOR-ighd)
Valtrex

Pharmacologic class: synthetic purine nucleoside
Therapeutic class: antiviral
Pregnancy risk category: B

Indications and dosages

▶ **Herpes zoster (shingles) in immunocompetent patients.** *Adults:* 1 g P.O. q 8 hours for 7 days.

⑤ Adjust-a-dose: For patient with renal impairment, if creatinine clearance is 30 to 49 ml/minute, give 1 g q 12 hours; if 10 to 29 ml/minute, give 1 g q 24 hours; if less than 10 ml/minute, give 500 mg q 24 hours.
▶ **Initial episodes of genital herpes in immunocompetent adults.** *Adults:* 1 g P.O. q 12 hours for 10 days.
⑤ Adjust-a-dose: For patients with renal impairment, if creatinine clearance is 10 to 29 ml/minute, give 1 g q 24 hours; if less than 10 ml/minute, give 500 mg q 24 hours.
▶ **Recurrent genital herpes in immunocompetent patients.** *Adults:* 500 mg P.O. q 12 hours for 3 days.
⑤ Adjust-a-dose: For patients with renal impairment, if creatinine clearance is 29 ml/minute or less, give 500 mg q 24 hours.
▶ **Chronic suppression of recurrent genital herpes.** *Adults:* 1 g P.O. once daily.
⑤ Adjust-a-dose: For patients with renal impairment, if creatinine clearance is 29 ml/minute or less, give 500 mg q 24 hours.
▶ **Chronic suppression of genital herpes in patients with a history of 9 or fewer recurrences per year.** *Adults:* 500 mg P.O. daily.
⑤ Adjust-a-dose: For patients with renal impairment, if creatinine clearance is 29 ml/minute or less, give 500 mg q 48 hours.
▶ **Chronic suppression of recurrent genital herpes in HIV-infected patients with CD4 count of 100/mm³ or more.** *Adults:* 500 mg P.O. twice daily. Safety and effectiveness of therapy beyond 6 months hasn't been established.
⑤ Adjust-a-dose: For patients with renal impairment, if creatinine clearance is 29 ml/minute or less, give 500 mg q 24 hours.
▶ **Cold sores (herpes labialis).** *Adults:* 2 g P.O. for two doses, taken about 12 hours apart.
⑤ Adjust-a-dose: For patient with renal impairment, if creatinine clearance is 30 to 49 ml/minute, give 1 g q 12 hours for two doses; if 10 to 29 ml/minute, give 500 mg q 12 hours for two doses; if less than 10 ml/minute, give 500 mg as a single dose.

Contraindications and cautions

• Contraindicated in patients hypersensitive to or intolerant of valacyclovir, acyclovir, or components of their formulations.
• Drug isn't recommended for immunocompromised patients. Thrombotic thrombocytopenic

purpura and hemolytic uremic syndrome have been fatal in some patients with advanced HIV disease and in bone marrow transplant and renal transplant recipients.
• Use cautiously in patients with renal impairment and in those receiving other nephrotoxic drugs.
⚘ **Lifespan:** In pregnant women, use only if benefits to the patient outweigh risks to the fetus. In breast-feeding women, use cautiously; it's unknown if the drug appears in breast milk. In children, safety and effectiveness haven't been established. In elderly patients, a lower dose may be needed, depending on underlying renal status.

Adverse reactions

CNS: *headache,* dizziness, depression.
GI: *nausea,* vomiting, diarrhea, abdominal pain.
GU: dysmenorrhea.
Musculoskeletal: arthralgia.

Interactions

Drug-drug. *Cimetidine, probenecid:* May reduce rate (but not extent) of conversion from valacyclovir to acyclovir and reduce renal clearance of acyclovir, thereby increasing acyclovir level. Monitor patient for possible toxicity.

Effects on lab test results

• May increase AST, ALT, alkaline phosphatase, and creatinine levels. May decrease hemoglobin level and hematocrit.
• May decrease WBC and platelet counts.

Pharmacokinetics

Absorption: Rapid; absolute bioavailability of about 54.5%.
Distribution: Protein-binding ranges from 13.5% to 17.9%.
Metabolism: Rapid; nearly completely converted to acyclovir and L-valine by first-pass intestinal or hepatic metabolism.
Excretion: In urine and feces. *Half-life:* Averages 2½ to 3¼ hours.

Route	Onset	Peak	Duration
P.O.	30 min	Unknown	Unknown

Action

Chemical effect: Rapidly converted to acyclovir, which becomes incorporated into viral

DNA and inhibits viral DNA polymerase, thereby inhibiting viral replication.
Therapeutic effect: Inhibits susceptible viral growth of herpes zoster.

Available forms

Caplets: 500 mg, 1,000 mg

NURSING PROCESS

Assessment
• Assess patient's infection before starting therapy.
• Assess patient's and family's knowledge of drug therapy.

Nursing diagnoses
• Risk for infection related to herpes zoster
• Deficient fluid volume related to adverse GI reactions
• Deficient knowledge related to drug therapy

Planning and implementation
• Although overdose hasn't been reported, precipitation of acyclovir in renal tubules may occur when solubility (2.5 mg/ml) is exceeded in the intratubular fluid. In the event of acute renal failure and anuria, the patient may benefit from hemodialysis until kidney function is restored.
ALERT: Don't confuse valacyclovir (Valtrex) with valganciclovir (Valcyte).
Patient teaching
• Inform patient that drug may be taken with or without food.
• Review signs and symptoms of herpes infection (rash, tingling, itching, and pain), and advise patient to notify prescriber immediately if they occur. Treatment should begin as soon as possible after symptoms appear, preferably within 48 hours.

Evaluation
• Patient is free from infection.
• Patient maintains adequate hydration.
• Patient and family state understanding of drug therapy.

valganciclovir
(val-gan-SYE-kloh-veer)
Valcyte

Pharmacologic class: synthetic nucleoside
Therapeutic class: antiviral
Pregnancy risk category: C

Indications and dosages

▶ **Active CMV retinitis in patients with AIDS.** *Adults:* Induction dose is 900 mg (two 450-mg tablets) P.O. b.i.d. with food for 21 days; maintenance dose is 900 mg P.O. once daily with food.
▶ **Inactive CMV retinitis.** *Adults:* 900 mg P.O. once daily with food.
▶ **Prevention of CMV in kidney, heart, and pancreas-kidney transplants.** *Adults:* 900 mg P.O. daily with food 10 days before through 100 days after transplant.
Adjust-a-dose: Patients with renal impairment need adjusted dose. For creatinine clearance of 40 to 59 ml/minute, 450 mg b.i.d. for induction followed by 450 mg daily for maintenance. For creatinine clearance of 25 to 39 ml/minute, 450 mg daily for induction followed by 450 mg every two days for maintenance. For creatinine clearance of 10 to 24 ml/minute, 450 mg every other day for induction followed by 450 mg twice weekly for maintenance.

Contraindications and cautions

• Contraindicated in patients hypersensitive to valganciclovir or ganciclovir or in liver transplant patients. Safety and effectiveness in the prevention of CMV disease in other solid-organ transplant patients, such as lung transplant patients, haven't been established.
• Don't use in patients receiving hemodialysis.
• Use cautiously in patients with cytopenias and in those who have received immunosuppressants or radiation.
Lifespan: In pregnant women, use only if benefits to the woman outweigh risks to the fetus. In breast-feeding women, use cautiously; it's unknown whether drug appears in breast milk. In children, safety and effectiveness haven't been established.

V

Adverse reactions

CNS: *pyrexia, headache, insomnia,* peripheral neuropathy, paresthesia, *seizures,* psychosis, hallucinations, confusion, agitation.
EENT: retinal detachment.
GI: *diarrhea, nausea, vomiting, abdominal pain.*
Hematologic: NEUTROPENIA, anemia, *thrombocytopenia, pancytopenia, bone marrow depression, aplastic anemia.*
Other: catheter-related infection, *sepsis,* local or systemic infections, *hypersensitivity reactions.*

Interactions

Drug-drug. *Didanosine:* May increase absorption of didanosine. Monitor patient closely for didanosine toxicity.
Immunosuppressants, zidovudine: May increase risk of neutropenia, anemia, thrombocytopenia, and bone marrow depression. Monitor CBC.
Mycophenolate mofetil: May increase levels of both drugs in renally impaired patients. Use together carefully.
Probenecid: May decrease renal clearance of ganciclovir. Monitor patient for ganciclovir toxicity.
Drug-food. *Any food:* May increase absorption of drug. Give drug with food.

Effects on lab test results

• May increase creatinine level. May decrease hemoglobin level and hematocrit.
• May decrease RBC, WBC, neutrophil, and platelet counts.

Pharmacokinetics

Absorption: Well absorbed from GI tract. Higher when taken with food.
Distribution: Minimal binding to proteins.
Metabolism: In intestinal wall and liver to ganciclovir.
Excretion: Eliminated renally. *Half-life:* 4 hours.

Route	Onset	Peak	Duration
P.O.	Unknown	1–3 hr	Unknown

Action

Chemical effect: Converted to ganciclovir, which inhibits replication of viral DNA synthesis of CMV.
Therapeutic effect: Inhibits CMV.

Available forms

Tablets: 450 mg

NURSING PROCESS

⚗ Assessment

• Assess patient's condition before starting therapy and regularly thereafter to monitor the drug's effectiveness.
• Obtain baseline laboratory studies before starting therapy and reassess regularly.
• Assess patient's and family's knowledge of drug therapy.

⊕ Nursing diagnoses

• Risk for imbalanced fluid volume related to adverse GI effects
• Ineffective protection related to adverse hematologic reactions
• Deficient knowledge related to valganciclovir therapy

❯ Planning and implementation

• Adhere to dosage guidelines for valganciclovir because ganciclovir and valganciclovir aren't interchangeable, and overdose may occur.
• Cytopenia may occur at any time during treatment and may increase with continued use. Cell counts usually recover 3 to 7 days after stopping the drug. Monitor patient's CBC closely and frequently throughout therapy.
• No drug interaction studies have been conducted; however, because drug is converted to ganciclovir, drug interactions probably are similar.
• Drug may cause temporary or permanent inhibition of spermatogenesis.
⚠ **ALERT:** Severe leukopenia, neutropenia, anemia, pancytopenia, bone marrow depression, aplastic anemia and thrombocytopenia may occur. If patient's absolute neutrophil count is less than 500/mm³, platelet count is less than 25,000/mm³, or hemoglobin level is less than 8 g/dl, don't use the drug.
• Overdose may cause severe or even fatal bone marrow depression and renal toxicity; if overdose occurs, maintain adequate hydration and consider hematopoietic growth factors. Dialysis may be used to reduce level.
⚠ **ALERT:** Don't confuse valganciclovir with valacyclovir.

Patient teaching

• Instruct women of childbearing age to use contraception during treatment. Instruct men to use barrier contraception during and for 90 days after treatment.
• Inform patient about infection control and bleeding precautions.
• Tell patient to take drug with food.

☑ Evaluation

• Patient remains well hydrated throughout therapy.
• Patient has no serious adverse hematologic reactions.
• Patient and family state understanding of drug therapy.

valproate sodium
(val-PROH-ayt SOH-dee-um)
Depacon, Depakene, Epilim◇, Valpro◇

valproic acid
Depakene

divalproex sodium
Depakote✔, Depakote ER, Depakote Sprinkle, Epival ◆

Pharmacologic class: carboxylic acid derivative
Therapeutic class: anticonvulsant
Pregnancy risk category: D

Indications and dosages

▶ **Simple and complex absence seizures, mixed seizure types (including absence seizures).** *Adults and children:* Initially, 15 mg/kg P.O. or I.V. daily; then increase by 5 to 10 mg/kg daily at weekly intervals up to maximum of 60 mg/kg daily. Don't use Depakote ER in children younger than age 10.
▶ **Mania.** *Adults:* Initially, 750 mg divalproex sodium (delayed-release) P.O. daily in divided doses. Adjust dosage based on patient's response; maximum dosage is 60 mg/kg daily.
▶ **Prevention of migraine headache.** *Adults:* Initially, 250 mg divalproex sodium (delayed-release) P.O. b.i.d. Some patients may need up to 1,000 mg daily. Or, 500 mg Depakote ER P.O. daily for 1 week; then 1,000 mg P.O. daily.

▶ **Complex partial seizures.** *Adults and children age 10 and older:* 10 to 15 mg/kg P.O. or I.V. daily; then increase by 5 to 10 mg/kg daily at weekly intervals, up to 60 mg/kg daily.
§ **Adjust-a-dose:** For elderly patients, use lower initial dose and adjust more slowly.

▼ I.V. administration

• Dilute with at least 50 ml of a compatible diluent (D_5W, saline solution, lactated Ringer's injection).
• Give I.V. over 1 hour. Don't exceed 20 mg/minute.
• Use of I.V. therapy for more than 14 days hasn't been studied.
⊗ **Incompatibilities**
None reported.

Contraindications and cautions

• Contraindicated in patients hypersensitive to the drug or any of its components and in patients with hepatic dysfunction or urea cycle disorder.
⚞ **Lifespan:** In pregnant and breast-feeding women, drug isn't recommended. In children younger than age 10, safety and effectiveness of Depakote ER haven't been established. In elderly patients, start at lower dose and adjust dose more slowly.

Adverse reactions

CNS: *sedation,* emotional upset, depression, psychosis, aggressiveness, hyperactivity, behavioral deterioration, muscle weakness, tremor, ataxia, headache, dizziness, incoordination.
EENT: nystagmus, diplopia.
GI: *nausea, vomiting, indigestion,* diarrhea, abdominal cramps, constipation, increased appetite and weight gain, anorexia, *pancreatitis.*
Hematologic: petechiae, bruising, eosinophilia, *hemorrhage, leukopenia, bone marrow suppression, thrombocytopenia.*
Hepatic: *toxic hepatitis, hepatotoxicity.*
Skin: rash, alopecia, pruritus, photosensitivity reactions, *erythema multiforme, Stevens-Johnson syndrome.*
Other: *flulike syndrome,* infection.

Interactions

Drug-drug. *Aspirin, chlorpromazine, cimetidine, felbamate:* May cause valproic acid toxicity. Use together cautiously and monitor levels.

V

Benzodiazepines, other CNS depressants: May cause excessive CNS depression. Avoid use together.

Carbamazepine: May result in carbamazepine CNS toxicity (acute psychotic reaction). Carefully monitor levels.

Cholestyramine: May decrease valproate level. Monitor patient for decreased effect.

Erythromycin: May increase valproate level. Monitor patient for toxicity.

Lamotrigine: May inhibit lamotrigine metabolism. Decrease lamotrigine dosage when valproic acid therapy starts.

Phenobarbital: May increase phenobarbital level. Monitor patient closely.

Phenytoin: May increase or decrease phenytoin level and increase metabolism of valproic acid. Monitor patient closely.

Rifampin: May decrease valproate level. Monitor level.

Warfarin: May displace warfarin from binding sites. Monitor PT and INR.

Drug-herb. *Glutamine:* May increase risk of seizures. Discourage use together.

White willow: May increase risk of adverse effects because herb contains substances similar to aspirin. Discourage use together.

Drug-lifestyle. *Alcohol use:* May cause excessive CNS depression. Discourage use together.

Effects on lab test results

• May increase ALT, AST, and bilirubin levels.
• May increase eosinophil count and bleeding time. May decrease platelet and WBC counts.
• May produce false-positive test results for ketones in urine.

Pharmacokinetics

Absorption: Valproate sodium and divalproex sodium quickly convert to valproic acid, which is then quickly and almost completely absorbed.
Distribution: Throughout body; 80% to 95% protein-bound.
Metabolism: In liver.
Excretion: Primarily in urine; some excreted in feces and exhaled in air. *Half-life:* 6 to 16 hours.

Route	Onset	Peak	Duration
P.O.	Unknown	1–4 hr	Unknown
I.V.	Unknown	Unknown	Unknown

Action

Chemical effect: Unknown; may increase brain levels of GABA, which transmits inhibitory nerve impulses in CNS.
Therapeutic effect: Prevents and treats certain types of seizure activity.

Available forms

valproate sodium
Injection: 100 mg/ml
Syrup: 250 mg/5 ml
valproic acid
Capsules: 250 mg
Syrup: 200 mg/5 ml ♦
Tablets (crushable): 100 mg ♦
Tablets (enteric-coated): 200 mg ♦, 500 mg ♦
divalproex sodium
Capsules (containing coated particles): 125 mg
Tablets (delayed-release): 125 mg, 250 mg, 500 mg
Tablets (extended-release): 500 mg

NURSING PROCESS

▨ Assessment
• Assess patient's condition before starting therapy and regularly thereafter to monitor the drug's effectiveness.
• Monitor drug level; therapeutic level is 50 to 100 mcg/ml.
• Before starting drug and periodically thereafter, monitor liver function studies, platelet counts, and PT.
• Be alert for adverse reactions and drug interactions.
• Assess patient's and family's knowledge of drug therapy.

▨ Nursing diagnoses
• Risk for trauma related to seizure activity
• Disturbed thought processes related to drug-induced adverse CNS reactions
• Deficient knowledge related to drug therapy

▷ Planning and implementation
• To switch adults and children ages 10 and older taking Depakote for seizures to Depakote ER, give dose of new drug that's 8% to 20% larger than previous drug dose.
• Don't give syrup to patient who needs sodium restriction. Check with prescriber.

• Give drug with food or milk to minimize adverse GI reaction.

• Suddenly stopping the drug may worsen seizures. If adverse reaction develops, call prescriber immediately.

⑧ **ALERT:** Serious or fatal hepatotoxicity may follow nonspecific symptoms, such as malaise, fever, and lethargy. If patient has suspected or apparently substantial hepatic dysfunction, notify prescriber immediately and stop giving the drug.

• Patients at high risk for developing hepatotoxicity include those with congenital metabolic disorders, mental retardation, or organic brain disease; those taking other anticonvulsants; and children younger than age 2.

• Divalproex sodium carries a lower risk of adverse GI effects than other drug forms.

• If tremors occur, notify prescriber. Dosage may need to be reduced.

⑧ **ALERT:** Fatal hyperammonemic encephalopathy may occur in patients with a urea cycle disorder, particularly ornithine transcarbamylase deficiency. Evaluate patients with risk factors for urea cycle disorders before starting therapy. If symptoms of unexplained hyperammonemic encephalopathy occur during therapy, stop drug; give prompt, appropriate treatment; and evaluate for underlying urea cycle disorder.

Patient teaching

• Tell patient that drug may be taken with food or milk to reduce adverse GI effects.

• Instruct patient not to chew capsules and not to crush or chew extended-release tablets.

• Tell patient and parents that syrup shouldn't be mixed with carbonated beverages.

• Tell patient and parents to keep drug out of children's reach.

• Warn patient and parents not to stop drug therapy abruptly.

• Advise patient to refrain from driving or performing other potentially hazardous activities that require mental alertness until drug's CNS effects are known.

🗹 **Evaluation**

• Patient is free from seizure activity.

• Patient maintains normal thought processes.

• Patient and family state understanding of drug therapy.

valsartan
(val-SAR-tin)
Diovan

Pharmacologic class: angiotensin II receptor blocker
Therapeutic class: antihypertensive
Pregnancy risk category: C (D in second and third trimesters)

Indications and dosages

▶ **Hypertension, used alone or with other antihypertensives.** *Adults:* Initially, 80 mg P.O. once daily. Expect a reduction in blood pressure in 2 to 4 weeks. If additional antihypertensive effect is needed, increase dosage to 160 or 320 mg daily, or add a diuretic. (Addition of a diuretic has a greater effect than dose increases above 80 mg.) Usual dosage range is 80 to 320 mg daily.

▶ **Heart failure (New York Heart Association classes II to IV).** *Adults:* Initially, 40 mg P.O. b.i.d. Increase as tolerated to 80 mg b.i.d. Maximum dosage is 160 mg b.i.d. Avoid using with ACE inhibitors or beta blockers.

▶ **To reduce cardiovascular death in stable post-MI patients with left ventricular failure or dysfunction.** *Adults:* 20 mg P.O. b.i.d. Initial dose may be given as soon as 12 hours following MI. Increase dose to 40 mg b.i.d. within 7 days. Increase subsequent doses as tolerated to target dose of 160 mg b.i.d.

Contraindications and cautions

• Contraindicated in patients hypersensitive to the drug or any of its components.

• Use cautiously in patients with severe renal or hepatic disease.

⚠ **Lifespan:** During second or third trimester of pregnancy or in breast-feeding women, don't give drug. In children, safety and effectiveness haven't been established.

Adverse reactions

CNS: fatigue, *dizziness,* headache, insomnia, vertigo.
CV: edema, hypotension, postural hypotension, syncope.
EENT: pharyngitis, rhinitis, sinusitis, blurred vision.

V

GI: abdominal pain, diarrhea, nausea, dyspepsia.
GU: renal impairment.
Hematologic: *neutropenia.*
Metabolic: *hyperkalemia.*
Musculoskeletal: arthralgia, back pain.
Respiratory: cough, upper respiratory tract infection.
Other: viral infection, *angioedema.*

Interactions

Drug-drug. *Other angiotensin II blockers, potassium sparing diuretics, potassium supplements:* May increase potassium level. Avoid use together.
Drug-food. *Salt substitutes containing potassium:* May increase potassium level. In heart failure patients, may also increase creatinine level. Discourage use together.

Effects on lab test results

• May increase potassium level.
• May decrease neutrophil count.

Pharmacokinetics

Absorption: Bioavailability about 25%; food decreases absorption.
Distribution: Not extensive; 95% bound to proteins.
Metabolism: In liver and kidneys.
Excretion: In urine and feces. *Half-life:* 6 hours.

Route	Onset	Peak	Duration
P.O.	< 2 hr	2–4 hr	24 hr

Action

Chemical effect: Blocks binding of angiotensin II to receptor sites in vascular smooth muscle and adrenal gland.
Therapeutic effect: Inhibits pressor effects of renin-angiotensin system.

Available forms

Tablets: 40 mg, 80 mg, 160 mg, 320 mg

NURSING PROCESS

Assessment

• Monitor patient for hypotension. Correct volume and sodium depletions before starting drug.
• Assess patient's and family's knowledge of drug therapy.

Nursing diagnoses

• Risk for injury related to presence of hypertension
• Deficient knowledge related to drug therapy

Planning and implementation

• Drug can be given with or without food.
Patient teaching
• Tell woman to notify prescriber if she becomes pregnant.
• Teach patient other means of reducing blood pressure, including proper diet, exercise, smoking cessation, and stress reduction.

Evaluation

• Patient's blood pressure becomes normal.
• Patient and family state understanding of drug therapy.

vancomycin hydrochloride
(van-koh-MIGH-sin high-droh-KLOR-ighd)
Vancocin, Vancoled

Pharmacologic class: glycopeptide
Therapeutic class: antibiotic
Pregnancy risk category: C

Indications and dosages

▶ **Severe staphylococcal infections when other antibiotics are ineffective or contraindicated.** *Adults:* 500 mg I.V. q 6 hours, or 1 g q 12 hours.
Children: 40 mg/kg I.V. daily in divided doses q 6 hours.
Neonates: Initially, 15 mg/kg; then 10 mg/kg I.V. daily, divided q 12 hours for first week after birth; then q 8 hours up to age 1 month.
▶ **Endocarditis prophylaxis for dental procedures.** *Adults:* 1 g I.V. slowly over 1 hour, starting 1 hour before procedure.
Children: 20 mg/kg I.V. over 1 hour, starting 1 hour before procedure.
Adjust-a-dose: For patients with renal impairment, adjust I.V. dosage.
▶ **Antibiotic-related pseudomembranous and staphylococcal enterocolitis.** *Adults:* 125 to 500 mg P.O. q 6 hours for 7 to 10 days. *Children:* 40 mg/kg P.O. daily in divided doses q 6 to 8 hours for 7 to 10 days. Maximum, 2 g daily.

Reactions may be *common*, uncommon, *life-threatening*, or COMMON AND LIFE-THREATENING.

▼ I.V. administration

• Dilute in 200 ml of saline solution injection or D_5W.
• Infuse over 60 minutes.
• Check site daily for phlebitis and irritation. Watch for irritation and infiltration; extravasation can cause tissue damage and necrosis.
• If red-man syndrome occurs because drug is infused too rapidly, stop infusion and report to prescriber.
• Refrigerate I.V. solution after reconstitution, and use within 96 hours.

⊗ **Incompatibilities**
Albumin, alkaline solutions, aminophylline, amobarbital, amphotericin B, aztreonam, cephalosporins, chloramphenicol, chlorothiazide, corticosteroids, dexamethasone sodium phosphate, foscarnet, heavy metals, heparin, hydrocortisone, idarubicin, methotrexate, nafcillin, penicillin G potassium, pentobarbital, phenobarbital, phenytoin, piperacillin, piperacillin sodium-tazobactam sodium, sargramostim, sodium bicarbonate, ticarcillin disodium, ticarcillin disodium and clavulanate potassium, vitamin B complex with C, warfarin.

Contraindications and cautions

• Contraindicated in patients hypersensitive to the drug or any of its components.
• Use cautiously in patients receiving other neurotoxic, nephrotoxic, or ototoxic drugs; patients older than age 60; and those with impaired liver or kidney function, hearing loss, or allergies to other antibiotics.
⚖ **Lifespan:** In pregnant women, use cautiously. In breast-feeding women, safety and effectiveness haven't been established.

Adverse reactions

CNS: fever, pain.
CV: hypotension.
EENT: tinnitus, ototoxicity.
GI: nausea.
GU: *nephrotoxicity, pseudomembranous colitis.*
Hematologic: eosinophilia, *leukopenia.*
Respiratory: wheezing, dyspnea.
Skin: red-man syndrome (maculopapular rash on face, neck, trunk, and limbs with rapid I.V. infusion; pruritus and hypotension with histamine release).
Other: chills, *anaphylaxis,* superinfection, thrombophlebitis at injection site.

Interactions

Drug-drug. *Aminoglycosides, amphotericin B, cisplatin, pentamidine:* May increase risk of nephrotoxicity and ototoxicity. Monitor patient closely.

Effects on lab test results

• May increase BUN and creatinine levels.
• May increase eosinophil counts. May decrease neutrophil and WBC counts.

Pharmacokinetics

Absorption: Minimal systemic absorption with P.O. administration. (Drug may accumulate in patients with colitis or renal failure.)
Distribution: In body fluids; achieves therapeutic level in CSF if meninges inflamed.
Metabolism: Unknown.
Excretion: In urine with parenteral administration; in feces with P.O. administration. *Half-life:* 6 hours.

Route	Onset	Peak	Duration
P.O.	Unknown	Unknown	Unknown
I.V.	Immediate	Immediate	Unknown

Action

Chemical effect: Hinders bacterial cell wall synthesis, damaging bacterial plasma membrane and making cell more vulnerable to osmotic pressure.
Therapeutic effect: Kills susceptible bacteria.

Available forms

Capsules: 125 mg, 250 mg
Powder for injection: 500-mg, 1-g vials
Powder for oral solution: 1-g, 10-g bottles

NURSING PROCESS

📋 **Assessment**
• Assess patient's infection before starting therapy and regularly thereafter to monitor the drug's effectiveness.
• Obtain urine specimen for culture and sensitivity tests before giving first dose. Start therapy pending test results.
• Obtain hearing evaluation and kidney function studies before starting therapy, and repeat during therapy.
• Check levels regularly, especially in geriatric patients, premature infants, and those with decreased renal function.

V

• Be alert for adverse reactions and drug interactions.
• Assess patient's and family's knowledge of drug therapy.

⊞ **Nursing diagnoses**
• Risk for infection related to presence of susceptible bacteria
• Risk for injury related to drug-induced adverse reactions
• Deficient knowledge related to drug therapy

▷ **Planning and implementation**
• In patient with renal dysfunction, use a lower dose.
⊛ **ALERT:** Oral administration is ineffective for systemic infections, and I.V. administration is ineffective for pseudomembranous (*Clostridium difficile*) diarrhea.
• Oral form is stable for 2 weeks when refrigerated.
• Don't give drug I.M.
• When using drug to treat staphylococcal endocarditis, give for at least 4 weeks.
Patient teaching
• Tell patient to take entire amount of drug exactly as directed, even after he feels better.
• Tell patient to stop taking the drug and immediately report any adverse reactions, especially fullness or ringing in ears.

✓ **Evaluation**
• Patient is free from infection.
• Patient doesn't experience injury from adverse reactions.
• Patient and family state understanding of drug therapy.

vardenafil hydrochloride
(var-DEN-ah-phill high-droh-KLOR-ighd)
Levitra✔

Pharmacologic class: selective inhibitor of cyclic guanosine monophosphate (cGMP)–specific phosphodiesterase type 5 (PDE5)
Therapeutic class: erectile dysfunction drug
Pregnancy risk category: B

Indications and dosages
▶ **Erectile dysfunction.** *Men:* 10 mg P.O. p.r.n., 1 hour before sexual activity. Dose range

is 5 to 20 mg based on effectiveness and tolerance. Maximum, 1 dose daily.
Men age 65 and older: Initial dose is 5 mg P.O. p.r.n., 1 hour before sexual activity. Maximum, 1 dose daily.
⧄ **Adjust-a-dose:** For patients with moderate hepatic impairment (Child-Pugh class B), initial dose is 5 mg daily, p.r.n., not to exceed 10 mg daily. Patients taking ritonavir shouldn't exceed 2.5 mg in a 72-hour period. Patients taking itraconazole 400 mg daily or ketoconazole 400 mg daily shouldn't exceed 2.5 mg daily. Patients taking erythromycin, itraconazole 200 mg daily, or ketoconazole 200 mg daily shouldn't exceed 5 mg daily.

Contraindications and cautions
• Contraindicated in patients hypersensitive to the drug or any of its components and in those taking nitrates or alpha blockers.
• Use cautiously in patients with unstable angina; hypotension (systolic pressure lower than 90 mm Hg); uncontrolled hypertension (blood pressure higher than 170/110 mm Hg); stroke, life-threatening arrhythmia, or MI within 6 months; severe cardiac failure; severe hepatic impairment (Child-Pugh class C); end-stage renal disease requiring dialysis; hereditary degenerative retinal disorders; hepatic or renal dysfunction; anatomical deformation of the penis; or prolonged QT interval. Also use cautiously in patients taking Class IA or Class III antiarrhythmics and in those with conditions that predispose them to priapism (sickle cell anemia, multiple myeloma, or leukemia).
⚖ **Lifespan:** Only indicated for men. Men age 65 and older have reduced drug clearance.

Adverse reactions
CNS: *headache,* dizziness.
CV: flushing.
EENT: rhinitis, sinusitis, visual changes.
GI: dyspepsia, nausea.
Musculoskeletal: back pain.
Other: flulike syndrome.

Interactions
Drug-drug. *Alpha blockers:* May increase hypotensive effects. Don't use together.
Erythromycin, itraconazole 200 mg daily, ketoconazole 200 mg daily: May increase vardenafil level. Don't exceed 5 mg daily.

Itraconazole 400 mg daily, ketoconazole 400 mg daily: May increase vardenafil level. Don't exceed 2.5 mg daily.
Nitrates: May increase hypotensive effects. Don't use together.
Ritonavir: May increase vardenafil level. Don't exceed 2.5 mg in a 72-hour period.
Drug-food. *High-fat meals:* May decrease peak level of drug. Advise patient to take on an empty stomach.

Effects on lab test results
• May increase CK level.

Pharmacokinetics
Absorption: Rapid. Absolute bioavailability is 15%.
Distribution: Both drug and its major active metabolite are 95% bound to proteins. Protein-binding is reversible and independent of drug level.
Metabolism: Primarily through CYP 3A4, along with CYP 3A5 and CYP 2C isoenzymes. N-demethylation converts drug into the major metabolite, which accounts for 7% of drug.
Excretion: Predominately in feces. *Half-life:* 4 to 5 hours.

Route	Onset	Peak	Duration
P.O.	Immediate	30–120 min	Unknown

Action
Chemical effect: Selectively inhibits cGMP-specific PDE5 and prevents the breakdown of cGMP by phosphodiesterase, leading to increased cGMP level and prolonged smooth muscle relaxation promoting the flow of blood into the corpus cavernosum.
Therapeutic effect: Stimulates penile erection.

Available forms
Tablets: 2.5 mg, 5 mg, 10 mg, 20 mg

NURSING PROCESS

🗒 Assessment
• Assess patient's erectile dysfunction before starting therapy and regularly thereafter to monitor the drug's effectiveness.
• Be alert for adverse reactions and drug interactions.
• Assess patient's and family's knowledge of drug therapy.

🗒 Nursing diagnoses
• Sexual dysfunction related to process of erectile dysfunction
• Chronic low self-esteem related to erectile dysfunction
• Deficient knowledge related to drug therapy

📑 Planning and implementation
⚕ ALERT: Because of cardiac risk during sexual activity, drug increases risk for patients with underlying CV disease.
Patient teaching
• Tell patient that drug doesn't protect against sexually transmitted diseases and that he should use protective measures to prevent infection.
• Advise patient that drug is most rapidly absorbed if taken on an empty stomach.
• Tell patient to notify prescriber of visual changes.
• Instruct patient to seek medical attention if erection persists for more than 4 hours because of risk of permanent erectile dysfunction.
• Tell patient to take drug 60 minutes before anticipated sexual activity. The drug will have no effect in the absence of sexual stimulation.
• Tell patient not to take drug more than once per day.

☑ Evaluation
• Patient states improvement in sexual functioning.
• Patient demonstrates increased self-esteem.
• Patient and family state understanding of drug therapy.

vasopressin (ADH)
(VAY-soh-preh-sin)
Pitressin

Pharmacologic class: posterior pituitary hormone
Therapeutic class: ADH, peristaltic stimulant
Pregnancy risk category: C

Indications and dosages
▶ **Neurogenic diabetes insipidus.** *Adults:* 5 to 10 units I.M. or subcutaneously b.i.d. to q.i.d., p.r.n. Range 5 to 60 units daily. Or, intranasally (aqueous solution used as spray or applied to cotton balls) in individualized doses, based on response.

V

Children: 2.5 to 10 units I.M. or subcutaneously b.i.d. to q.i.d., p.r.n. Or, intranasally (aqueous solution used as spray or applied to cotton balls) in individualized doses.

▶ **Postoperative abdominal distention.** *Adults:* Initially, 5 units (aqueous) I.M.; then q 3 to 4 hours, increasing dose to 10 units, if needed. Reduce dose proportionately for children.

▶ **To expel gas before abdominal X-ray.** *Adults:* 10 units subcutaneously 2 hours before X-ray; then again 30 minutes later.

▶ **Provocative testing for growth hormone and corticotropin release‡.** *Adults:* 10 units I.M.
Children: 0.3 units/kg I.M.

▶ **GI hemorrhage‡.** *Adults:* 0.2 to 0.4 units/minute I.V. Increase up to 0.9 units/minute p.r.n. Or, 0.1 to 0.5 units/minute intra-arterially.

▶ **Pulseless arrest (ventricular fibrillation, rapid ventricular tachycardia, asystole, pulseless electrical activity)‡.** *Adults:* 40 units I.V. as a single one-time dose.

▼ I.V. administration

• Drug is used I.V. for G.I. hemorrhage and pulseless arrest only.
• For GI hemorrhage, dilute with normal saline solution or D_5W to 0.1 to 1 unit/ml.
• For pulseless arrest, give as bolus during advanced cardiac life support (ACLS).
⊗ **Incompatibilities**
None reported.

Contraindications and cautions

• Contraindicated in patients with chronic nephritis accompanied by nitrogen retention.
• Use cautiously in preoperative and postoperative polyuric patients and those with seizure disorders, migraine headache, asthma, CV disease, heart failure, renal disease, goiter with cardiac complications, arteriosclerosis, or fluid overload.
⚖ **Lifespan:** In pregnant women, use cautiously. In breast-feeding women, use cautiously; it's unknown if the drug appears in breast milk. In children and the elderly, use cautiously.

Adverse reactions

CNS: tremor, vertigo, headache.
CV: angina in patients with vascular disease, vasoconstriction, *arrhythmias, pulseless arrest,*

myocardial ischemia, circumoral pallor, decreased cardiac output.
GI: abdominal cramps, nausea, vomiting, flatulence.
Skin: cutaneous gangrene, diaphoresis.
Other: water intoxication (drowsiness, listlessness, headache, confusion, weight gain, *seizures, coma),* hypersensitivity reactions (urticaria, *angioedema, bronchoconstriction, anaphylaxis).*

Interactions

Drug-drug. *Carbamazepine, chlorpropamide, clofibrate, fludrocortisone, tricyclic antidepressants:* May increase antidiuretic response. Use together cautiously.
Demeclocycline, heparin, lithium, norepinephrine: May decrease antidiuretic activity. Use together cautiously.
Drug-lifestyle. *Alcohol use:* May decrease antidiuretic activity. Discourage use together.

Effects on lab test results

None reported.

Pharmacokinetics

Absorption: Unknown.
Distribution: Throughout extracellular fluid without evidence of protein-binding.
Metabolism: Most of drug is destroyed rapidly in liver and kidneys.
Excretion: In urine. *Half-life:* 10 to 20 minutes.

Route	Onset	Peak	Duration
I.V	Unknown	Unknown	Unknown
I.M., SubQ, intranasal	Unknown	Unknown	2–8 hr

Action

Chemical effect: Increases permeability of renal tubular epithelium to adenosine monophosphate and water; epithelium promotes reabsorption of water and produces concentrated urine (ADH effect).
Therapeutic effect: Promotes water reabsorption and stimulates GI motility.

Available forms

Injection: 0.5-, 1-, and 10-ml ampules (20 units/ml)

NURSING PROCESS

▨ Assessment
• Assess patient's condition before starting therapy and regularly thereafter to monitor the drug's effectiveness.
• Monitor specific gravity of urine, and fluid intake and output, to aid evaluation of drug effectiveness.
• To prevent possible seizures, coma, and death, observe patient closely for early signs of water intoxication.
• Frequently monitor patient's blood pressure; watch for hypertension or lack of response to drug, which may be indicated by hypotension. Also monitor daily weight.
• Be alert for adverse reactions and drug interactions.
• Assess patient's and family's knowledge of drug therapy.

▨ Nursing diagnoses
• Risk for deficient fluid volume related to polyuria from diabetes insipidus
• Diarrhea related to drug-induced increased GI motility
• Deficient knowledge related to drug therapy

▷ Planning and implementation
• Drug may be used for transient polyuria resulting from ADH deficiency related to neurosurgery or head injury.
• To reduce adverse reactions, use minimum effective dose.
• Give drug with one to two glasses of water to reduce adverse reactions and improve therapeutic response.
• A rectal tube facilitates gas expulsion after vasopressin injection.
• In cardiac emergencies, use 2006 ACLS pulseless arrest protocol guide.
• ⚠ ALERT: Never inject during first stage of labor; doing so may cause uterus to rupture.
• Aqueous solution can be used as a nasal spray or applied to cotton balls. Follow manufacturer's guidelines for intranasal use.
• ⚠ ALERT: Don't confuse vasopressin with desmopressin.
Patient teaching
• Instruct patient how to give drug. Tell patient taking drug subcutaneously to rotate injection sites to prevent tissue damage.

• Stress importance of monitoring fluid intake and output.
• Tell patient to immediately notify prescriber if an adverse reaction occurs.

▨ Evaluation
• Patient maintains adequate hydration.
• Patient doesn't experience diarrhea.
• Patient and family state understanding of drug therapy.

vecuronium bromide
(veh-kyoo-ROH-nee-um BROH-mighd)

Pharmacologic class: nondepolarizing neuromuscular blocker
Therapeutic class: skeletal muscle relaxant
Pregnancy risk category: C

Indications and dosages
▶ **Adjunct to general anesthesia; to facilitate endotracheal intubation; to provide skeletal muscle relaxation during surgery or mechanical ventilation. Dosage depends on anesthetic used, individual needs, and response. Dosages are representative and must be adjusted.** *Adults and children age 10 and older:* Initially, 0.08 to 0.1 mg/kg I.V. bolus. During prolonged surgery, may give maintenance doses of 0.01 to 0.015 mg/kg within 25 to 40 minutes of initial dose. Maintenance doses may be given q 12 to 15 minutes in patients receiving balanced anesthesia. Or, drug may be given by continuous I.V. infusion of 1 mcg/kg/minute initially, then 0.8 to 1.2 mcg/kg/minute.
Children younger than age 10: May require slightly higher initial dose as well as supplementation slightly more often than adults.

▼ I.V. administration
• Give drug by rapid I.V. injection. Or, 10 to 20 mg may be added to 100 ml of compatible solution and given by I.V. infusion.
• Compatible solutions include D_5W, normal saline solution for injection, dextrose 5% in normal saline solution for injection, and lactated Ringer's injection.
• Store reconstituted solution in refrigerator. Discard after 24 hours.

V

⊗ **Incompatibilities**

Alkaline solutions, amphotericin B, diazepam, furosemide, thiopental.

Contraindications and cautions

• Contraindicated in patients hypersensitive to bromides.

• Use cautiously in patients with altered circulation caused by CV disease and edematous states and in patients with hepatic disease, severe obesity, bronchogenic carcinoma, electrolyte disturbances, or neuromuscular disease.

🌺 **Lifespan:** In pregnant woman, use cautiously. In breast-feeding women, use cautiously; it's unknown if the drug appears in breast milk. In the elderly, use cautiously.

Adverse reactions

Musculoskeletal: skeletal muscle weakness.
Respiratory: respiratory insufficiency, *apnea.*

Interactions

Drug-drug. *Amikacin, gentamicin, neomycin, streptomycin, tobramycin:* May increase the effects of nondepolarizing muscle relaxant, including prolonged respiratory depression. Use together only when necessary. May need to reduce dose of nondepolarizing muscle relaxant.
Bacitracin; clindamycin; general anesthetics, such as enflurane, halothane, isoflurane; kanamycin; other skeletal muscle relaxants; polymyxin antibiotics, such as colistin, polymyxin B sulfate; quinidine; tetracyclines: May potentiate neuromuscular blockade, leading to increased skeletal muscle relaxation and potentiation of effect. Use cautiously during surgical and postoperative periods.
Carbamazepine, phenytoin: May decrease the effects of vecuronium. May need to increase dose of the vecuronium.

Effects on lab test results

None reported.

Pharmacokinetics

Absorption: Administered I.V.
Distribution: In extracellular fluid; rapidly reaches its site of action (skeletal muscles); 60% to 90% protein-bound.
Metabolism: Hepatic; rapid and extensive.
Excretion: In feces and urine. *Half-life:* 20 minutes.

Route	Onset	Peak	Duration
I.V.	≤ 1 min	3–5 min	25–30 min

Action

Chemical effect: Prevents acetylcholine from binding to receptors on motor end plate, thus blocking depolarization.
Therapeutic effect: Relaxes skeletal muscle.

Available forms

Injection: 10 mg/vial, 20 mg/vial

NURSING PROCESS

🔅 **Assessment**

• Assess patient's condition before starting therapy and regularly thereafter to monitor the drug's effectiveness.

• Monitor respiratory rate closely until patient is fully recovered from neuromuscular blockade as evidenced by tests of muscle strength (hand grip, head lift, and ability to cough).

• Be alert for adverse reactions and drug interactions.

• Assess patient's and family's knowledge of drug therapy.

🔅 **Nursing diagnoses**

• Ineffective health maintenance related to underlying condition

• Ineffective breathing pattern related to drug's effect on respiratory muscles

• Deficient knowledge related to drug therapy

🔅 **Planning and implementation**

• Keep airway clear. Have emergency respiratory support equipment available immediately.

• Drug should be used only by personnel skilled in airway management.

• Previous administration of succinylcholine may enhance neuromuscular blocking effect and duration of action.

• Give sedatives or general anesthetics before neuromuscular blockers. Neuromuscular blockers don't obtund consciousness or alter pain threshold.

• Give analgesics for pain.

• Nerve stimulator and train-of-four monitoring are recommended to confirm antagonism of neuromuscular blockade and recovery of muscle strength. Before attempting pharmacologic reversal with neostigmine, some evidence of spontaneous recovery should be seen.

⊛ **ALERT:** Careful dose calculation is essential. Always verify with another health care professional.
• Don't give by I.M. injection.
Patient teaching
• Explain all events and happenings to patient because he can still hear.
• Reassure patient that he is being monitored at all times.

🗹 **Evaluation**
• Patient responds well to drug.
• Patient maintains effective breathing pattern with mechanical assistance.
• Patient and family state understanding of drug therapy.

venlafaxine hydrochloride
(ven-leh-FAKS-een high-droh-KLOR-ighd)
Effexor, Effexor XR⊘

Pharmacologic class: neuronal serotonin, norepinephrine, and dopamine reuptake inhibitor
Therapeutic class: antidepressant
Pregnancy risk category: C

Indications and dosages

▶ **Depression.** *Adults:* Initially, 75 mg P.O. daily in two or three divided doses, or 75 mg (extended-release) P.O. once daily with food. With both forms, increase dosage as tolerated and needed in increments of 75 mg daily at intervals of no less than 4 days. For moderately depressed outpatients, usual maximum dosage is 225 mg daily; in certain severely depressed patients, dosage may be as high as 350 mg daily.
▶ **Generalized or social anxiety disorder.** *Adults:* 75 mg extended-release capsules P.O. once daily. May increase p.r.n. in increments of 75 mg daily at intervals of no less than 4 days to maximum of 225 mg daily.
▶ **Prevention of major depressive disorder relapse‡.** *Adults:* 100 to 200 mg P.O. daily, or 75 to 225 mg (extended-release) P.O. daily.
▶ **Panic disorder.** *Adults:* Initially, 37.5 mg (extended-release) P.O. daily for 1 week. Then, increase dose to 75 mg daily. If no response, increase by up to 75 mg daily in no less than weekly intervals, p.r.n., to a maximum dosage of 225 mg daily.

🖎 **Adjust-a-dose:** For patients with hepatic impairment, reduce total daily dose by one-half. For patients with mild to moderate renal impairment (GFR of 10 to 70 ml/minute), reduce total daily dose by one-quarter to one-half. In patients undergoing hemodialysis, don't give the dose until dialysis session is completed; reduce daily dose by one-half.

Contraindications and cautions

• Contraindicated in patients hypersensitive to the drug or any of its components and in those who took an MAO inhibitor within 14 days.
• Use cautiously in patients with renal impairment or diseases, in those with conditions that could affect hemodynamic responses or metabolism, and in those with a history of mania or seizures.
≉ **Lifespan:** In pregnant women, use cautiously. In breast-feeding women, use cautiously; it's unknown if the drug appears in breast milk. In children, safety and effectiveness haven't been established.

Adverse reactions

CNS: *asthenia, headache, somnolence, dizziness, nervousness,* insomnia, anxiety, tremor, abnormal dreams, paresthesia, agitation.
CV: hypertension.
EENT: blurred vision.
GI: *nausea, constipation,* vomiting, *dry mouth, anorexia,* diarrhea, dyspepsia, flatulence.
GU: *abnormal ejaculation,* impotence, urinary frequency, impaired urination.
Metabolic: weight loss.
Skin: *diaphoresis,* rash.
Other: yawning, chills, infection.

Interactions

Drug-drug. *Haloperidol:* May increase haloperidol level. Use together cautiously.
Phenelzine, selegiline, tranylcypromine: May cause serotonin syndrome, which includes CNS irritability, shivering, and altered consciousness. Don't give together. Wait at least 2 weeks after stopping an MAO inhibitor before giving any SSRI.
Trazodone: May cause serotonin syndrome. Avoid use together.
Drug-herb. *St. John's wort:* May increase sedative-hypnotic effects. Discourage use together.

V

Yohimbe: May cause additive stimulation. Discourage use together.

Effects on lab test results

None reported.

Pharmacokinetics

Absorption: About 92%.
Distribution: About 25% to 29% protein-bound in plasma.
Metabolism: Extensively metabolized in liver.
Excretion: Excreted in urine. *Half-life:* 5 hours.

Route	Onset	Peak	Duration
P.O.	Unknown	Unknown	Unknown

Action

Chemical effect: Blocks reuptake of norepinephrine and serotonin into neurons in CNS.
Therapeutic effect: Relieves depression.

Available forms

Capsules (extended-release): 37.5 mg, 75 mg, 150 mg
Tablets: 25 mg, 37.5 mg, 50 mg, 75 mg, 100 mg

NURSING PROCESS

▨ Assessment

• Assess patient's depression before starting therapy and regularly thereafter to monitor the drug's effectiveness.
• Carefully monitor blood pressure. Venlafaxine therapy is linked to sustained, dose-dependent increases in blood pressure. Greatest increases (averaging about 7 mm Hg above baseline) occur in patients taking 375 mg daily.
• Be alert for adverse reactions and drug interactions.
• Assess patient's and family's knowledge of drug therapy.

⊞ Nursing diagnoses

• Disturbed thought processes related to presence of depression
• Risk for injury related to drug-induced adverse CNS reactions
• Deficient knowledge related to drug therapy

▷ Planning and implementation

• Give drug with food.

⊛ **ALERT:** If given for 6 weeks or more, don't abruptly stop giving the drug; taper dosage over a 2-week period.
• Closely monitor patients being treated for depression for signs and symptoms of worsening condition and suicidal ideation, especially when therapy starts or dosage is adjusted. Symptoms may include agitation, insomnia, anxiety, aggressiveness, and panic attacks.

Patient teaching
• Instruct patient to take drug with food.
• Warn patient to avoid hazardous activities until the drug's CNS effects are known.
• Caution patient not to become pregnant during treatment. Neonates exposed to drug late in the third trimester have developed complications requiring prolonged hospitalization, respiratory support, and tube feeding, possibly related to serotonin syndrome.
• Tell patient it may take several weeks before the full antidepressant effect is seen.
• Tell patient not to drink alcohol while taking drug and to notify prescriber before taking other medications, including OTC preparations, because of possible interactions.
• Instruct patient to notify prescriber if adverse reaction occurs.
• Urge family members to closely monitor the patient for signs of worsening condition and suicidal ideation.

▨ Evaluation

• Patient's behavior and communication exhibit improved thought processes.
• Patient doesn't experience injury from adverse CNS reactions.
• Patient and family state understanding of drug therapy.

verapamil hydrochloride
(veh-RAP-uh-mil high-droh-KLOR-ighd)
Anpec◇, Anpec SR◇, Apo-Verap♦, Calan✐, Calan SR, Cordilox◇, Cordilox SR◇, Covera-HS, Isoptin◇, Isoptin SR, Novo-Veramil♦, Nu-Verap♦, Veracaps SR◇, Verelan, Verelan PM

Pharmacologic class: calcium channel blocker
Therapeutic class: antianginal, antihypertensive, antiarrhythmic
Pregnancy risk category: C

Indications and dosages

▶ **Vasospastic angina; classic chronic, stable angina pectoris; unstable angina; chronic atrial fibrillation.** *Adults:* Starting dose is 80 mg P.O. q 6 to 8 hours. Increase at weekly intervals, p.r.n. Some patients may need up to 480 mg daily. Or, 180 mg Covera-HS P.O. h.s.; maximum, 480 mg P.O. daily h.s.

▶ **Supraventricular arrhythmias.** *Adults:* 0.075 to 0.15 mg/kg (5 to 10 mg) by I.V. push over 2 minutes with ECG and blood pressure monitoring. If no response occurs, give a second dose of 10 mg (0.15 mg/kg) 30 minutes after the initial dose.

Children ages 1 to 15: 0.1 to 0.3 mg/kg as I.V. bolus over 2 minutes. If no response, repeat in 30 minutes.

Children younger than age 1: 0.1 to 0.2 mg/kg as I.V. bolus over at least 2 minutes with continuous ECG monitoring. If no response, repeat in 30 minutes.

▶ **Prevention of recurrent paroxysmal supraventricular tachycardia.** *Adults:* 240 to 480 mg P.O. daily in three or four divided doses.

▶ **To control ventricular rate in digitalized patients with chronic atrial flutter or atrial fibrillation.** *Adults:* 240 to 320 mg P.O. in three or four divided doses.

▶ **Hypertension.** *Adults:* Start therapy with sustained-release capsules at 120 mg (240 mg for Verelan) P.O. daily in the morning. Adjust dosage based on effectiveness 24 hours after dose. Increase in increments of 120 mg daily to a maximum of 480 mg daily. Or, Covera-HS 180 mg P.O. daily h.s. or Verelan PM 200 mg P.O. h.s.

▼ I.V. administration

• Give drug by direct injection into vein or into tubing of free-flowing, compatible I.V. solution.
• Compatible solutions include D₅W, half-normal and normal saline solutions, and Ringer's and lactated Ringer's solutions.
• Give I.V. doses slowly over at least 2 minutes (3 minutes for geriatric patients) to minimize risk of adverse reactions.
• Perform continuous ECG and blood pressure monitoring during administration.

⊗ **Incompatibilities**
Albumin, aminophylline, amphotericin B, ampicillin sodium, co-trimoxazole, dobutamine, hydralazine, nafcillin, oxacillin, propofol, sodium bicarbonate, solutions with a pH greater than 6.

Contraindications and cautions

• Contraindicated in patients hypersensitive to the drug or any of its components and in those with severe left ventricular dysfunction; cardiogenic shock; second- or third-degree AV block or sick sinus syndrome, except in presence of functioning pacemaker; atrial flutter or fibrillation and accessory bypass tract syndrome; severe heart failure (unless secondary to verapamil therapy); or severe hypotension.
• I.V. verapamil is contraindicated in patients with ventricular tachycardia and in those receiving I.V. beta blockers.
• Use cautiously in patients with increased intracranial pressure or hepatic or renal disease.
⚠ **Lifespan:** In pregnant women, use cautiously. In breast-feeding women, avoid drug; it apears in breast milk. In the elderly, use cautiously.

Adverse reactions

CNS: dizziness, headache, asthenia.
CV: transient hypotension, *heart failure, bradycardia, AV block, ventricular asystole, ventricular fibrillation,* peripheral edema.
GI: constipation, nausea.
Respiratory: *pulmonary edema.*
Skin: rash.

Interactions

Drug-drug. *Acebutolol, atenolol, betaxolol, carteolol, esmolol, metoprolol, nadolol, penbutolol, pindolol, propranolol, timolol:* May increase the effects of both drugs. Monitor cardiac function closely, and decrease dosages, p.r.n.
Antihypertensives, quinidine: May cause hypotension. Monitor blood pressure.
Carbamazepine, digoxin: May increase levels of these drugs. Monitor patient for toxicity.
Cyclosporine: May increase cyclosporine level. Monitor cyclosporine level.
Disopyramide, flecainide, propranolol, other beta blockers: May cause heart failure. Use together cautiously.
Lithium: May decrease lithium level. Monitor patient closely.
Rifampin: May decrease oral bioavailability of verapamil. Monitor patient for lack of effect.
Drug-herb. *Black catechu:* May cause additive effects. Tell patient to use together cautiously.
Yerba maté: May decrease clearance of yerba maté methylxanthines and cause toxicity. Discourage concomitant use.

V

Drug-food. *Any food:* May increase drug absorption. Tell patient to take drug with food.
Drug-lifestyle. *Alcohol use:* May enhance effects of alcohol. Discourage use together.

Effects on lab test results

• May increase ALT, AST, alkaline phosphatase, and bilirubin levels.

Pharmacokinetics

Absorption: Rapid and complete from GI tract after P.O. administration; only about 20% to 35% reaches systemic circulation.
Distribution: About 90% of circulating drug is bound to proteins.
Metabolism: In liver.
Excretion: In urine as unchanged drug and active metabolites. *Half-life:* 6 to 12 hours.

Route	Onset	Peak	Duration
P.O.	1–2 hr	1–9 hr	8–24 hr
I.V.	Rapid	Immediate	1–6 hr

Action

Chemical effect: Not clearly defined; inhibits calcium ion influx across cardiac and smooth-muscle cells, thus decreasing myocardial contractility and oxygen demand. Drug also dilates coronary arteries and arterioles.
Therapeutic effect: Relieves angina, lowers blood pressure, and restores normal sinus rhythm.

Available forms

Capsules (extended-release): 120 mg, 180 mg, 240 mg
Capsules (sustained-release): 120 mg, 160 mg ◊, 80 mg, 200 mg, 240 mg, 360 mg
Injection: 2.5 mg/ml
Tablets: 40 mg, 80 mg, 120 mg, 160 mg ◊
Tablets (extended-release): 100 mg, 120 mg, 180 mg, 200 mg, 240 mg, 300 mg
Tablets (sustained-release): 120 mg, 180 mg, 240 mg

NURSING PROCESS

⧉ Assessment
• Assess patient's condition before starting therapy and regularly thereafter to monitor the drug's effectiveness.
• Monitor blood pressure at start of therapy and during dosage adjustments.

• Monitor liver function studies during long-term treatment.
• Be alert for adverse reactions and drug interactions.
• Assess patient's and family's knowledge of drug therapy.

⧉ Nursing diagnoses
• Acute pain related to presence of angina
• Decreased cardiac output related to presence of arrhythmia
• Deficient knowledge related to drug therapy

⧉ Planning and implementation
• Give lower doses to patient with severely compromised cardiac function or to a patient taking beta blockers.
• Give drug with food, but keep in mind that giving extended-release tablets with food may decrease rate and extent of absorption. It also produces smaller fluctuations of peak and trough levels.
• If drug is being used to terminate supraventricular tachycardia, prescriber may have patient perform vagal maneuvers after receiving drug.
• Assist patient with walking because dizziness may occur.
• If patient has signs of heart failure, such as swelling of hands and feet or shortness of breath, notify prescriber.
⧉ ALERT: Don't confuse Isoptin with Intropin; don't confuse Verelan with Vivarin, Voltaren, Ferralyn, or Virilon.
Patient teaching
• Instruct patient to take drug with food.
• If patient is kept on nitrate therapy during adjustment of oral verapamil dosage, urge continued compliance. S.L. nitroglycerin, especially, may be taken p.r.n. when angina is acute.
• Encourage patient to increase fluid and fiber intake to combat constipation. Give stool softener.
• Instruct patient to report adverse reactions, especially swelling of hands and feet and shortness of breath.

⧉ Evaluation
• Patient has reduced severity or frequency of angina.
• Patient regains normal cardiac output with restoration of normal sinus rhythm.
• Patient and family state understanding of drug therapy.

---

vinblastine sulfate (VLB)
(vin-BLAH-steen SUL-fayt)
Velban, Velbe ♦ ◇

Pharmacologic class: vinca alkaloid
Therapeutic class: antineoplastic
Pregnancy risk category: D

Indications and dosages

▶ **Breast or testicular cancer, Hodgkin's and non-Hodgkin's lymphoma, choriocarcinoma, lymphosarcoma, mycosis fungoides, Kaposi's sarcoma, histiocytosis.** *Adults:* 0.1 mg/kg or 3.7 mg/m² I.V. weekly or q 2 weeks. May be increased to maximum of 0.5 mg/kg or 18.5 mg/m² weekly according to response. If WBC count is less than 4,000/mm³, don't repeat dose.
▶ **Letterer-Siwe disease (histiocytosis X).** *Children:* 6.5 mg/m². Adjust dosage by hematologic response.
▶ **Hodgkin's disease.** *Children:* 6 mg/m² with other drugs. Adjust dosage by hematologic response.
▶ **Testicular germ cell carcinoma.** *Children:* 3 mg/m² with other drugs. Adjust dosage by hematologic response.
⧉ Adjust-a-dose: If bilirubin level is greater than 3 mg/dl, decrease dosage by half.

▼ I.V. administration

● Preparation and administration of parenteral form are linked to carcinogenic, mutagenic, and teratogenic risks. Follow facility policy to reduce risks.
● Reconstitute drug in 10-mg vial with 10 ml of saline solution injection or sterile water. This yields 1 mg/ml.
● Inject drug directly into vein or running I.V. line over 1 minute. Drug also may be given in 50 ml of D₅W or normal saline solution infused over 15 minutes.
● If extravasation occurs, stop infusion immediately and notify prescriber. Manufacturer recommends that moderate heat be applied to area of leakage. Local injection of hyaluronidase may help disperse drug. Some clinicians prefer to apply ice packs on and off q 2 hours for 24 hours, with local injection of hydrocortisone or normal saline solution.

● Refrigerate reconstituted solution. Discard after 30 days.
⊗ **Incompatibilities**
Cefepime, furosemide, heparin.

Contraindications and cautions

● Contraindicated in patients with severe leukopenia or bacterial infection.
● Use cautiously in patients with hepatic dysfunction.
⚖ **Lifespan:** In pregnant women, give only if clearly needed. In breast-feeding women, drug isn't recommended; it isn't known if drug appears in breast milk.

Adverse reactions

CNS: depression, paresthesia, peripheral neuropathy and neuritis, numbness, loss of deep tendon reflexes, *seizures, stroke,* headache.
CV: hypertension, *MI, phlebitis.*
EENT: pharyngitis.
GI: nausea, vomiting, ulcer, *bleeding,* constipation, ileus, anorexia, diarrhea, abdominal pain, stomatitis.
GU: oligospermia, aspermia, urine retention.
Hematologic: anemia, *leukopenia* (nadir on days 4 to 10; lasts another 7 to 14 days), *thrombocytopenia.*
Metabolic: hyperuricemia, *weight loss.*
Musculoskeletal: uric acid nephropathy, *muscle pain and weakness.*
Respiratory: *acute bronchospasm,* shortness of breath.
Skin: reversible alopecia, vesiculation, cellulitis, necrosis with extravasation.

Interactions

Drug-drug. *Erythromycin, other drugs that inhibit CYP pathway:* May increase toxicity of vinblastine. Monitor patient closely.
Mitomycin: May increase risk of bronchospasm and shortness of breath. Monitor patient closely.
Phenytoin: May decrease phenytoin level. Monitor patient closely.

Effects on lab test results

● May increase uric acid level. May decrease hemoglobin level and hematocrit.
● May decrease WBC and platelet counts.

Pharmacokinetics

Absorption: Administered I.V.

V

Distribution: Widely in body tissues; crosses blood-brain barrier but doesn't achieve therapeutic level in CSF.
Metabolism: Partially in liver to active metabolite.
Excretion: Primarily in bile as unchanged drug; smaller portion excreted in urine. *Half-life:* Alpha phase, 3 minutes; beta phase, 1½ hours; terminal phase, 25 hours.

Route	Onset	Peak	Duration
I.V.	Unknown	Unknown	Unknown

Action

Chemical effect: Arrests mitosis in metaphase, blocking cell division.
Therapeutic effect: Inhibits replication of certain cancer cells.

Available forms

Injection: 10-mg vials (lyophilized powder), 1 mg/ml in 10-ml vials

NURSING PROCESS

Assessment

- Assess patient's condition before starting therapy and regularly thereafter to monitor the drug's effectiveness.
- Before therapy and each dose, monitor CBC. Leukopenic effects reach lowest point in 4 to 10 days, with recovery in 7 to 14 days.

ALERT: After giving drug, monitor patient for development of life-threatening acute bronchospasm. Reaction is most likely if patient also receives mitomycin.

- Be alert for adverse reactions and drug interactions.
- Assess patient for numbness and tingling in hands and feet. Assess gait for early evidence of footdrop. Drug is less neurotoxic than vincristine.
- Assess patient's and family's knowledge of drug therapy.

Nursing diagnoses

- Ineffective health maintenance related to presence of neoplastic disease
- Ineffective protection related to drug-induced adverse hematologic reactions
- Deficient knowledge related to drug therapy

Planning and implementation

- Give antiemetic before giving drug.
- Don't give drug into limb with compromised circulation.

ALERT: Drug is fatal if given intrathecally; it's for I.V. use only.

- If acute bronchospasm occurs after administration, notify prescriber immediately.
- Make sure patient maintains adequate fluid intake to facilitate excretion of uric acid.
- If stomatitis occurs, stop giving the drug and notify prescriber.
- Don't repeat dose more frequently than q 7 days to prevent severe leukopenia.

ALERT: Don't confuse vinblastine with vincristine or vindesine.

Patient teaching

- Teach patient about infection control and bleeding precautions.
- Warn patient that alopecia may occur, but that it's usually reversible.
- Tell patient to report adverse reactions promptly.
- Encourage adequate fluid intake to increase urine output and facilitate excretion of uric acid.

Evaluation

- Patient responds well to drug.
- Patient doesn't develop serious complications from adverse hematologic reactions.
- Patient and family state understanding of drug therapy.

vincristine sulfate

(vin-KRIH-steen SUL-fayt)
Oncovin, Vincasar PFS

Pharmacologic class: vinca alkaloid
Therapeutic class: antineoplastic
Pregnancy risk category: D

Indications and dosages

► **Breast cancer‡, acute lymphoblastic and other leukemias, Hodgkin's disease, non-Hodgkin's lymphoma, neuroblastoma, rhabdomyosarcoma, Wilms' tumor.** *Adults:* 1.4 mg/m^2 I.V. weekly. Maximum, 2 mg weekly.
Children weighing more than 10 kg (22 lb): 1.5 to 2 mg/m^2 I.V. weekly. Maximum single dose is 2 mg.

Children weighing 10 kg or less: 0.05 mg/kg I.V. once weekly.

▼ I.V. administration

• Preparation and administration of parenteral form are linked to carcinogenic, mutagenic, and teratogenic risks. Follow facility policy to reduce risks.

• Inject drug directly into vein or running I.V. line slowly over 1 minute. Drug also may be given in 50 ml of D₅W or normal saline solution infused over 15 minutes.

• If drug extravasates, stop infusion immediately and notify prescriber. Apply heat on and off q 2 hours for 24 hours. Give 150 units of hyaluronidase to area of infiltrate.

• All vials (1-, 2-, and 5-mg) contain 1 mg/ml solution and should be refrigerated.

⊗ **Incompatibilities**
Cefepime, furosemide, idarubicin, sodium bicarbonate.

Contraindications and cautions

• Contraindicated in patients hypersensitive to the drug or any of its components and in those with demyelinating form of Charcot-Marie-Tooth syndrome. Don't give drug to patients who are receiving radiation therapy through sites that include the liver.

• Use cautiously in patients with hepatic dysfunction, neuromuscular disease, or infection.

❋ **Lifespan:** In pregnant or breast-feeding women, drug isn't recommended.

Adverse reactions

CNS: acute uric acid neuropathy, fever, peripheral neuropathy, sensory loss, loss of deep tendon reflexes, paresthesia, wristdrop and footdrop, headache, ataxia, cranial nerve palsies, jaw pain, hoarseness, vocal cord paralysis, *seizures, coma, permanent neurotoxicity.*
CV: hypotension, hypertension, *phlebitis.*
EENT: visual disturbances, diplopia, optic and extraocular neuropathy, ptosis.
GI: diarrhea, *constipation, cramps,* ileus that mimics surgical abdomen, *nausea, vomiting,* anorexia, dysphagia, *intestinal necrosis, stomatitis.*
GU: urine retention, dysuria, polyuria.
Hematologic: anemia, *leukopenia, thrombocytopenia.*
Metabolic: hyponatremia, hyperuricemia, weight loss.

Musculoskeletal: muscle weakness and cramps.
Respiratory: *acute bronchospasm.*
Skin: rash, *reversible alopecia,* cellulitis at injection site, severe local reaction with extravasation.
Other: SIADH.

Interactions

Drug-drug. *Asparaginase:* May decrease hepatic clearance of vincristine. Monitor patient closely for toxicity.
Calcium channel blockers: May increase vincristine accumulation. Monitor patient for toxicity.
Digoxin: May decrease digoxin effects. Monitor digoxin level.
Mitomycin: May increase frequency of bronchospasm and acute pulmonary reactions. Monitor patient closely.
Phenytoin: May decrease phenytoin level. Monitor patient closely.

Effects on lab test results

• May increase uric acid level. May decrease sodium and hemoglobin levels and hematocrit.
• May decrease WBC and platelet counts.

Pharmacokinetics

Absorption: Administered I.V.
Distribution: Wide. Bound to erythrocytes and platelets; crosses blood-brain barrier but doesn't achieve therapeutic level in CSF.
Metabolism: Extensively in liver.
Excretion: Primarily in bile; smaller portion excreted in urine. *Half-life:* First phase, 4 minutes; second phase, 2¼ hours; terminal phase, 85 hours.

Route	Onset	Peak	Duration
I.V.	Unknown	Unknown	Unknown

Action

Chemical effect: Arrests mitosis in metaphase, blocking cell division.
Therapeutic effect: Inhibits replication of certain cancer cells.

Available forms

Injection: 1 mg/ml in 1-, 2-, and 5-ml multiple-dose vials; 1 mg/ml in 1- and 2-ml preservative-free vials

V

NURSING PROCESS

🕮 Assessment
• Assess patient's condition before starting therapy and regularly thereafter to monitor the drug's effectiveness.
⚉ **ALERT:** After giving drug, monitor patient for development of life-threatening acute bronchospasm. Reaction is most likely to occur if patient also receives mitomycin.
• Monitor patient for hyperuricemia, especially if he has leukemia or lymphoma.
• Be alert for adverse reactions and drug interactions.
• Check for depression of Achilles tendon reflex, numbness, tingling, footdrop or wristdrop, difficulty in walking, ataxia, and slapping gait. Also check ability to walk on heels.
• Monitor bowel function. Constipation may be early sign of neurotoxicity.
• Assess patient's and family's knowledge of drug therapy.

⊞ Nursing diagnoses
• Ineffective health maintenance related to presence of neoplastic disease
• Ineffective protection related to drug-induced adverse hematologic reactions
• Deficient knowledge related to drug therapy

❱ Planning and implementation
• Give antiemetic before drug.
• Don't give drug to one patient as single dose. The 5-mg vials are for multiple-dose use.
⚉ **ALERT:** Drug is fatal if given intrathecally; it's for I.V. use only.
• Because of risk of neurotoxicity, don't give drug more than once a week. Children are more resistant to neurotoxicity than adults. Neurotoxicity is dose-related and usually reversible.
• If acute bronchospasm occurs after giving the drug, immediately notify the prescriber.
• Maintain good hydration and give allopurinol to prevent uric acid nephropathy.
• If SIADH develops, fluid restriction may be needed.
• Give stool softener, laxative, or water before each dose to help prevent constipation.
⚉ **ALERT:** Don't confuse vincristine with vinblastine or vindesine.

Patient teaching
• Instruct patient on infection control and bleeding precautions.

• Warn patient that alopecia may occur, but that it's usually reversible.
• Tell patient to report adverse reactions promptly.
• Encourage fluid intake to facilitate excretion of uric acid.
• Advise woman of childbearing age not to become pregnant during therapy. Also recommend that she consult with prescriber when planning a pregnancy.

🗹 Evaluation
• Patient responds well to drug.
• Patient doesn't develop serious complications from adverse hematologic reactions.
• Patient and family state understanding of drug therapy.

vinorelbine tartrate
(vin-oh-REL-been TAR-trayt)
Navelbine

Pharmacologic class: semisynthetic vinca alkaloid
Therapeutic class: antineoplastic
Pregnancy risk category: D

Indications and dosages

▶ **Alone or as adjunct therapy with cisplatin for first-line treatment of ambulatory patients with nonresectable advanced non–small-cell lung cancer; alone or with cisplatin in stage IV of non–small-cell lung cancer; with cisplatin in stage III of non–small-cell lung cancer.** *Adults:* 30 mg/m² I.V. weekly. In combination treatment, same dosage used along with 120 mg/m² of cisplatin, given on days 1 and 29, and then q 6 weeks.
▶ **Breast cancer ‡.** *Adults:* 20 to 30 mg/m² I.V. over 20 to 60 minutes weekly. Or, 30 mg/m² over 3 to 5 minutes. If used in combination therapy, give 25 or 30 mg/m² I.V. in periodic doses. If used with mitoxantrone and ifosfamide, give 12 mg/m² I.V. in periodic doses.
⧄ **Adjust-a-dose:** Dosage adjustments are made according to hematologic toxicity or hepatic insufficiency, whichever results in lower dosage. If patient's granulocyte count falls between 1,000/mm³ and 1,500/mm³, reduce dosage by half. If three consecutive doses are skipped because of granulocytopenia, stop drug.

▼ I.V. administration

• Drug must be diluted.
• Give drug I.V. over 6 to 10 minutes into side port of free-flowing I.V. line that is closest to I.V. bag.
• After the infusion, flush the line with 75 to 125 ml of D₅W or normal saline solution.

⊗ **Incompatibilities**
Acyclovir, allopurinol, aminophylline, amphotericin B, ampicillin sodium, cefazolin, cefoperazone, cefotetan, ceftriaxone, cefuroxime, fluorouracil, furosemide, ganciclovir, methylprednisolone, mitomycin, piperacillin, sodium bicarbonate, thiotepa, trimethoprim-sulfamethoxazole.

Contraindications and cautions

• Contraindicated in patients with pretreatment granulocyte counts below 1,000/mm³.
• Use cautiously in patients whose bone marrow may have been compromised by previous exposure to radiation therapy or chemotherapy or whose bone marrow is still recovering from previous chemotherapy. Also use cautiously in patients with hepatic impairment.
🜲 **Lifespan:** In pregnant and breast-feeding women, drug isn't recommended. In children, safety and effectiveness haven't been established.

Adverse reactions

CNS: peripheral neuropathy, asthenia, fatigue.
GI: nausea, vomiting, anorexia, diarrhea, constipation, stomatitis, paralytic ileus.
Hematologic: *bone marrow suppression, granulocytopenia,* LEUKOPENIA, *anemia.*
Hepatic: *bilirubinemia.*
Musculoskeletal: jaw pain, chest pain, myalgia, arthralgia, loss of deep tendon reflexes.
Respiratory: dyspnea, pneumonia, *ARDS.*
Skin: *alopecia,* rash.
Other: SIADH, injection site pain or reaction.

Interactions

Drug-drug. *Cisplatin:* May increase risk of bone marrow suppression when given with cisplatin. Monitor hematologic status closely.
Mitomycin: May cause pulmonary reactions. Monitor patient's respiratory status closely.

Effects on lab test results

• May increase bilirubin level. May decrease hemoglobin level and hematocrit.

• May decrease liver function test values and granulocyte, WBC, and platelet counts.

Pharmacokinetics

Absorption: Administered I.V.
Distribution: Widely in body tissues and bound to lymphocytes and platelets.
Metabolism: Extensively in liver.
Excretion: Primarily in bile; smaller portion excreted in urine. *Half-life:* 27¾ to 43½ hours.

Route	Onset	Peak	Duration
I.V.	Unknown	Unknown	Unknown

Action

Chemical effect: Arrests mitosis in metaphase, blocking cell division.
Therapeutic effect: Inhibits replication of selected cancer cells.

Available forms

Injection: 10 mg/ml, 50 mg/5 ml

NURSING PROCESS

📖 **Assessment**
• Assess patient's condition before starting therapy and regularly thereafter to monitor the drug's effectiveness.
• Monitor patient closely for hypersensitivity reactions.
• To determine dose before each treatment, monitor patient's peripheral blood count and bone marrow.
• Be alert for adverse reactions and drug interactions.
• Assess patient for numbness and tingling in hands and feet. Assess gait for early evidence of footdrop.
⑤ **ALERT:** Monitor patient's deep tendon reflexes; loss may indicate cumulative toxicity.
• Assess patient's and family's knowledge of drug therapy.

⊞ **Nursing diagnoses**
• Ineffective health maintenance related to presence of neoplastic disease
• Ineffective protection related to drug-induced adverse hematologic reactions
• Deficient knowledge related to drug therapy

▶ **Planning and implementation**
• Give antiemetic before giving drug.

V

• Check patient's granulocyte count before administration; it should be 1,000/mm³ or more. If it's less, don't give the dose, and notify the prescriber.

• Take care to avoid extravasation because drug can cause considerable irritation, localized tissue necrosis, and thrombophlebitis. If extravasation occurs, stop drug immediately and inject remaining portion of dose into a different vein.

⊛ ALERT: Drug is fatal if given intrathecally; it's for I.V. use only.

• Drug may be a contact irritant, and solution must be handled and given with care. Gloves are recommended. Avoid inhaling vapors and allowing drug to contact skin or mucous membranes, especially those of eyes. In case of contact, wash with copious amounts of water for at least 15 minutes.

Patient teaching

• Instruct patient on infection control and bleeding precautions.

• Warn patient that alopecia may occur, but that it's usually reversible.

• Instruct patient not to take other drugs, including OTC preparations, unless approved by prescriber.

• Instruct patient to tell prescriber about signs and symptoms of infection (fever, chills, malaise) because drug has immunosuppressant activity.

⛓ Evaluation

• Patient responds well to drug.

• Patient doesn't develop serious complications from adverse hematologic reactions.

• Patient and family state understanding of drug therapy.

vitamin A (retinol)
(VIGH-tuh-min ay)
Aquasol A, Palmitate-A 5000

Pharmacologic class: fat-soluble vitamin
Therapeutic class: vitamin
Pregnancy risk category: A (C at higher-than-recommended doses)

Indications and dosages

▶ **RDA.** RDAs are in retinol equivalents (RE). 1 RE has activity of 1 mcg of all-trans retinol, 6 mcg of beta carotene, or 12 mcg of carotenoid provitamins.
Men older than age 11: 1,000 mcg RE or 5,000 international units.
Pregnant women and women older than age 11: 800 mcg RE or 4,000 international units.
Breast-feeding women (first 6 months): 1,300 mcg RE or 6,500 international units.
Breast-feeding women (second 6 months): 1,200 mcg RE or 6,000 international units.
Children ages 7 to 10: 700 mcg RE or 3,500 international units.
Children ages 4 to 6: 500 mcg RE or 2,500 international units.
Children ages 1 to 3: 400 mcg RE or 2,000 international units.
Neonates and infants younger than age 1: 375 mcg RE or 1,875 international units.

▶ **Severe vitamin A deficiency.** *Adults and children older than age 8:* 100,000 international units I.M. or P.O. daily for 3 days, followed by 50,000 international units I.M. or P.O. daily for 2 weeks; then 10,000 to 20,000 international units P.O. daily for 2 months. Follow with adequate dietary nutrition and RE vitamin A supplements.
Children ages 1 to 8: 17,500 to 35,000 international units I.M. daily for 10 days.
Infants younger than age 1: 7,500 to 15,000 international units I.M. daily for 10 days.

▶ **Maintenance dosage to prevent recurrence of vitamin A deficiency.** *Children ages 1 to 8:* 5,000 to 10,000 international units P.O. daily for 2 months; then adequate dietary nutrition and RE vitamin A supplements.

Contraindications and cautions

• Contraindicated for oral administration in patients with malabsorption syndrome; if malabsorption is from inadequate bile secretion, oral route may be used with administration of bile salts (dehydrocholic acid). Also contraindicated in patients hypersensitive to other ingredients in product and in those with hypervitaminosis A.

• I.V. administration contraindicated except for special water-miscible forms intended for infusion with large parenteral volumes. I.V. push of vitamin A of any type is also contraindicated (anaphylaxis or anaphylactoid reactions and death have resulted).

☙ **Lifespan:** In pregnant women, use cautiously. In breast-feeding women, use cautiously, avoiding doses exceeding RE.

Adverse reactions

CNS: irritability, headache, *increased intracranial pressure,* fatigue, lethargy, malaise.
EENT: papilledema, exophthalmos.
GI: anorexia, epigastric pain, vomiting, polydipsia.
GU: hypomenorrhea, polyuria.
Hepatic: jaundice, hepatomegaly, *cirrhosis.*
Metabolic: slow growth, decalcification of bone, hypercalcemia, periostitis, premature closure of epiphyses, migratory arthralgia, cortical thickening over radius and tibia.
Skin: alopecia; dry, cracked, scaly skin; pruritus; lip fissures; erythema; inflamed tongue, lips, and gums; massive desquamation; increased pigmentation; night sweats.
Other: splenomegaly, *anaphylactic shock.*

Interactions

Drug-drug. *Cholestyramine resin, mineral oil:* May decrease GI absorption of fat-soluble vitamins. If needed, give mineral oil h.s.
Hormonal contraceptives: May increase vitamin A level. Monitor patient.
Isotretinoin, multivitamins containing vitamin A: May increase risk of toxicity. Avoid use together.
Neomycin (oral): May decrease vitamin A absorption. Avoid use together.
Warfarin: May increase risk of bleeding. Monitor PT and INR closely; monitor patient for bleeding.

Effects on lab test results

• May increase liver enzyme and calcium levels.

Pharmacokinetics

Absorption: Absorbed readily and completely if fat absorption is normal; larger doses or regular dose in patients with fat malabsorption, low protein intake, or hepatic or pancreatic disease may be absorbed incompletely. Because vitamin A is fat-soluble, absorption requires bile salts, pancreatic lipase, and dietary fat.
Distribution: Stored (primarily as palmitate) in liver. Normal adult liver stores are sufficient to provide vitamin A requirements for 2 years. Lesser amounts of retinyl palmitate are stored in kidneys, lungs, adrenal glands, retinas, and intraperitoneal fat. Vitamin A circulates bound to specific alpha-1 protein, retinol-binding protein.
Metabolism: In liver.

Excretion: Retinol (fat-soluble) combines with glucuronic acid and is metabolized to retinal and retinoic acid. Retinoic acid undergoes biliary excretion in feces. Retinal, retinoic acid, and other water-soluble metabolites are excreted in urine and feces. *Half-life:* Unknown.

Route	Onset	Peak	Duration
P.O., I.M.	Unknown	3–5 hr	Unknown

Action

Chemical effect: Stimulates retinal function, bone growth, reproduction, and integrity of epithelial and mucosal tissues.
Therapeutic effect: Raises vitamin A level in body.

Available forms

Capsules: 10,000 international units, 15,000 international units, 25,000 international units, 50,000 international units
Drops: 30 ml with dropper (50,000 international units/0.1 ml)
Injection: 2-ml vials (50,000 international units/ml with 0.5% chlorobutanol, polysorbate 80, butylated hydroxyanisole, and butylated hydroxytoluene)
Tablets: 5,000 international units, 10,000 international units

NURSING PROCESS

⅏ Assessment

• Assess patient's vitamin A intake from fortified foods, dietary supplements, self-administered drugs, and prescription drug sources before starting therapy, and reassess regularly thereafter to monitor the drug's effectiveness.
• If dose is high, watch for adverse reactions. Acute toxicity may result from a single dose of 25,000 international units/kg; 350,000 international units in infants and over 2 million international units in adults may also be acutely toxic. Doses that don't exceed RE are usually nontoxic.
• Chronic toxicity in infants (age 3 to 6 months) may result from doses of 18,500 international units daily for 1 to 3 months. In adults, chronic toxicity has resulted from doses of 50,000 international units daily for more than 18 months; 500,000 international units daily for 2 months,

V

and 1 million international units daily for 3 days.
• Be alert for drug interactions.
• Assess patient's and family's knowledge of drug therapy.

🖉 Nursing diagnoses
• Imbalanced nutrition: less than body requirements related to inadequate intake
• Ineffective health maintenance related to vitamin A toxicity caused by excessive intake
• Deficient knowledge related to drug therapy

⊠ Planning and implementation
• Adequate vitamin A absorption requires suitable protein, vitamin E, zinc intake, and bile secretion; give supplemental salts, if needed. Zinc supplements may be needed in patient receiving long-term total parenteral nutrition.
• Liquid preparations may be mixed with cereal or fruit juice to be given by NG tube.
• I.M. absorption is most rapid and complete with aqueous preparations, intermediate with emulsions, and slowest with oil suspensions.
⊛ ALERT: Give parenteral form by I.M. route or continuous I.V infusion in total parenteral nutrition. Never give as I.V. bolus.
• Protect drug from light.
Patient teaching
• Warn patient against taking megadoses of vitamins without specific indications. Also stress that he not share prescribed vitamins with others.
• Explain importance of avoiding prolonged use of mineral oil while taking this drug because it reduces vitamin A absorption.
• Review the signs and symptoms of vitamin A toxicity, and tell patient to report them immediately.
• Advise patient to consume adequate protein, vitamin E, and zinc, which, along with bile, are needed for vitamin A absorption.
• Instruct patient to store vitamin A in tight, light-resistant container.

🎞 Evaluation
• Patient regains normal vitamin A level.
• Patient doesn't exhibit signs and symptoms of vitamin A toxicity.
• Patient and family state understanding of drug therapy.

vitamin C (ascorbic acid)
(VIGH-tuh-min see)
Ascorbicap†, Cebid Timecelles†, Cecon†, Cenolate†, Cetane†, Cevalin†, Cevi-Bid, Ce-Vi-Sol*, Dull-C†, Flavorcee†, N'ice Vitamin C Drops†, Penta-vite ◇, Redoxon ♦, Vita-C†

Pharmacologic class: water-soluble vitamin
Therapeutic class: vitamin
Pregnancy risk category: A (C at higher-than-recommended doses)

Indications and dosages
▶ **RDA.** *Men:* 90 mg.
Women: 75 mg.
Pregnant women ages 14 to 18: 80 mg.
Pregnant women ages 19 to 50: 85 mg.
Breast-feeding women ages 14 to 18: 115 mg.
Breast-feeding women ages 19 to 50: 120 mg.
Boys ages 9 to 13: 45 mg.
Boys ages 14 to 18: 75 mg.
Girls ages 9 to 13: 45 mg.
Girls ages 14 to 18: 65 mg.
Children ages 4 to 8: 25 mg.
Children ages 1 to 3: 15 mg.
Infants ages 6 months to 1 year: 50 mg.
Neonates and infants younger than age 6 months: 40 mg.
▶ **Frank and subclinical scurvy.** *Adults:* Depending on severity, 300 mg to 1 g P.O., subcutaneously, I.M., or I.V. daily; then at least 50 mg daily for maintenance.
Children: Depending on severity, 100 to 300 mg P.O., subcutaneously, I.M., or I.V. daily; then at least 30 mg daily for maintenance.
Premature infants: 75 to 100 mg P.O., I.M., I.V., or subcutaneously daily.
▶ **Extensive burns, delayed fracture or wound healing, postoperative wound healing, severe febrile or chronic disease states.**
Adults: 300 to 500 mg P.O., subcutaneously, I.M., or I.V. daily for 7 to 10 days. For extensive burns, 1 to 2 g daily.
Children: 100 to 200 mg P.O., subcutaneously, I.M., or I.V. daily.
▶ **Prevention of vitamin C deficiency in patients with poor nutritional habits or increased requirements.** *Adults:* 70 to 150 mg P.O., subcutaneously, I.M., or I.V. daily.

Reactions may be *common*, uncommon, *life-threatening*, or COMMON AND LIFE-THREATENING.

Pregnant or breast-feeding women: 70 to 150 mg P.O., subcutaneously, I.M., or I.V. daily.
Children: at least 40 mg P.O., subcutaneously, I.M., or I.V. daily.
Infants: at least 35 mg P.O., subcutaneously, I.M., or I.V. daily.
▶ **Potentiation of methenamine in urine acidification.** *Adults:* 4 to 12 g P.O. daily in divided doses.

▽ I.V. administration

● Avoid rapid I.V. administration. It may cause faintness or dizziness.
● Give I.V. infusion cautiously in patients with renal insufficiency.
● Protect solution from light and refrigerate ampules.
⊗ **Incompatibilities**
Many drugs.

Contraindications and cautions

⚍ **Lifespan:** In pregnant women, give only if clearly needed. In breast-feeding women, use cautiously.

Adverse reactions

CNS: faintness, dizziness with rapid I.V. administration.
GI: diarrhea.
GU: acid urine, oxaluria, renal calculi.
Other: discomfort at injection site.

Interactions

Drug-drug. *Aspirin (high doses):* May increase risk of ascorbic acid deficiency. Monitor patient closely.
Estrogen, hormonal contraceptives: May increase level of estrogen. Monitor patient.
Oral iron supplements: May increase iron absorption. A beneficial drug interaction. Encourage use together.
Warfarin: May decrease anticoagulant effect. Monitor patient closely.
Drug-herb. *Bearberry:* May inactivate bearberry in urine. Discourage use together.

Effects on lab test results

None reported.

Pharmacokinetics

Absorption: After P.O. use, absorbed readily; may be reduced with very large doses or in pa-

tients with diarrhea or GI diseases. Unknown for I.M and subcutaneous use.
Distribution: Widely in body with high levels in liver, leukocytes, platelets, glandular tissues, and lens of eyes. Protein-binding is low.
Metabolism: In liver.
Excretion: In urine. Renal excretion is directly proportional to blood levels. *Half-life:* Unknown.

Route	Onset	Peak	Duration
P.O., I.V., I.M., SubQ	Unknown	Unknown	Unknown

Action

Chemical effect: Stimulates collagen formation and tissue repair; involved in oxidation-reduction reactions throughout body.
Therapeutic effect: Raises vitamin C level in body.

Available forms

Capsules (timed-release): 500 mg†
Crystals: 100 g (4 g/tsp)†, 500 g (4 g/tsp)†
Injection: 100 mg/ml, 250 mg/ml, 500 mg/ml
Lozenges: 60 mg†
Oral liquid: 50 ml (35 mg/0.6 ml)*†
Oral solution: 60 mg/ml†, 100 mg/ml†
Powder: 100 g (4 g/tsp)†, 500 g (4 g/tsp)†
Syrup: 20 mg/ml in 120 ml†, 480 ml†; 500 mg/ 5 ml in 5 ml†, 120 ml†, 480 ml†
Tablets: 25 mg†, 50 mg†, 100 mg†, 250 mg†, 500 mg†, 1,000 mg†
Tablets (chewable): 50 mg, 100 mg†, 250 mg†, 500 mg†, 1,000 mg†
Tablets (effervescent): 1,000 mg sugar-free†
Tablets (timed-release): 500 mg†, 1,000 mg†, 1,500 mg

NURSING PROCESS

⚕ Assessment
● Assess patient's condition before starting therapy and regularly thereafter to monitor the drug's effectiveness.
● When giving for urine acidification, check urine pH to ensure effectiveness.
● Be alert for adverse reactions and drug interactions.
● If adverse GI reactions occur, monitor patient's hydration.
● Assess patient's and family's knowledge of drug therapy.

V

Rapid onset   *Liquid form contains alcohol.   ◆ Canada   ◇ Australia   †OTC   ⌀ Photoguide   ‡ Off-label use

🖳 Nursing diagnoses
● Imbalanced nutrition: less than body requirements related to inadequate intake
● Risk for deficient fluid volume related to drug-induced adverse GI reactions
● Deficient knowledge related to drug therapy

▷ Planning and implementation
● Give P.O. solution directly into mouth, or mix with food.
● Dissolve effervescent tablets in glass of water immediately before giving.
● Utilization of vitamin may be better with I.M. route, the preferred parenteral route.

Patient teaching
● Stress proper nutritional habits to prevent recurrence of deficiency.
● Advise patient with vitamin C deficiency to decrease or stop smoking.

☑ Evaluation
● Patient regains normal vitamin C level.
● Patient maintains adequate hydration.
● Patient and family state understanding of drug therapy.

vitamin D

cholecalciferol (vitamin D₃)
(koh-lih-kal-SIF-eh-rol)
Delta-D, Vitamin D₃

ergocalciferol (vitamin D₂)
(er-goh-kal-SIF-er-ohl)
Calciferol, Drisdol, Radiostol Forte ◆

Pharmacologic class: fat-soluble vitamin
Therapeutic class: vitamin
Pregnancy risk category: A, C with doses over the RDA

Indications and dosages

▶ **RDA for cholecalciferol.** *Adults older than age 70:* 600 international units.
Adults ages 51 to 70: 400 international units.
Adults age 50 and younger and children: 200 international units.
Pregnant or breast-feeding women: 400 international units.
▶ **Rickets and other vitamin D deficiency diseases.** *Adults:* Initially, 12,000 international units P.O. or I.M. daily; increase by response up to 500,000 international units daily. After correcting deficiency, patient should have adequate diet and take supplements.
▶ **Hypoparathyroidism.** *Adults and children:* 50,000 to 200,000 international units P.O. or I.M. daily with calcium supplement.
▶ **Familial hypophosphatemia.** *Adults:* 10,000 to 80,000 international units P.O. or I.M. daily with phosphorus supplement.

Contraindications and cautions

● Contraindicated in patients with hypercalcemia, hypervitaminosis A, or renal osteodystrophy with hyperphosphatemia.
● Use cautiously in cardiac patients, especially those receiving digoxin, and in patients with increased sensitivity to these drugs.
● Give ergocalciferol cautiously to patients with impaired kidney function, heart disease, renal calculi, or arteriosclerosis.
※ **Lifespan:** In pregnant women, use cautiously. In breast-feeding women, use cautiously.

Adverse reactions

Adverse reactions listed are usually seen only in vitamin D toxicity.
CNS: headache, weakness, somnolence, overt psychosis, irritability.
CV: calcifications of soft tissues including heart, *arrhythmias,* hypertension.
EENT: rhinorrhea, conjunctivitis (calcific), photophobia.
GI: anorexia, nausea, vomiting, constipation, dry mouth, metallic taste, polydipsia.
GU: polyuria, albuminuria, hypercalciuria, nocturia, impaired kidney function, reversible azotemia.
Metabolic: hypercalcemia, hyperthermia, weight loss.
Musculoskeletal: bone and muscle pain, bone demineralization.
Skin: pruritus.
Other: decreased libido.

Interactions

Drug-drug. *Cholestyramine resin, mineral oil:* May inhibit GI absorption of oral vitamin D. Space doses. Use together cautiously.
Corticosteroids: May antagonize effect of vitamin D. Monitor vitamin D level closely.
Digoxin: May increase risk of arrhythmias. Monitor calcium level.

Phenobarbital, phenytoin: May increase vitamin D metabolism, which decreases half-life as well as drug's effectiveness. Monitor patient closely.
Thiazide diuretics: May cause hypercalcemia in patients with hypoparathyroidism. Monitor patient closely.
Verapamil: May increase risk of atrial fibrillation because of increased calcium. Monitor patient closely.

Effects on lab test results

• May increase BUN, creatinine, AST, ALT, urine urea, albumin, calcium, and cholesterol levels.

Pharmacokinetics

Absorption: From small intestine with P.O. administration; unknown for I.M. administration.
Distribution: Throughout body; bound to proteins stored in liver.
Metabolism: In liver and kidneys.
Excretion: Primarily in bile; small amount excreted in urine. *Half-life:* 24 hours.

Route	Onset	Peak	Duration
P.O., I.M.	2–24 hr	3–12 hr	Varies

Action

Chemical effect: Promotes absorption and utilization of calcium and phosphate, helping to regulate calcium homeostasis.
Therapeutic effect: Helps to maintain normal calcium and phosphate levels in body.

Available forms

Capsules: 1.25 mg (50,000 international units)
Injection: 12.5 mg (500,000 international units)/ml
Oral liquid: 8,000 international units/ml in 60-ml dropper bottle
Tablets: 400 international units, 1,000 international units

NURSING PROCESS

⚚ Assessment
• Assess patient's condition before starting therapy and regularly thereafter to monitor the drug's effectiveness.
• **ALERT:** Monitor patient's eating and bowel habits; dry mouth, nausea, vomiting, metallic taste, and constipation may be early evidence of toxicity.

• Monitor serum and urine calcium, potassium, and urea levels when high doses are used.
• Be alert for adverse reactions and drug interactions.
• Assess patient's and family's knowledge of drug therapy.

⊞ Nursing diagnoses
• Imbalanced nutrition: less than body requirements related to inadequate intake
• Ineffective health maintenance related to vitamin D toxicity
• Deficient knowledge related to drug therapy

⊳ Planning and implementation
• Use I.M. injection of vitamin D dispersed in oil for patient unable to absorb P.O. form.
• Doses of 60,000 international units a day can cause hypercalcemia.
• Malabsorption from inadequate bile or hepatic dysfunction may require addition of exogenous bile salts with oral form.
• Patient with hyperphosphatemia requires dietary phosphate restrictions and binding agents to avoid metastatic calcifications and renal calculus formation.
Patient teaching
• Warn patient of dangers of increasing dose without consulting prescriber. Vitamin D is fat-soluble.
• Tell patient taking vitamin D to restrict his intake of magnesium-containing antacids.

☑ Evaluation
• Patient regains normal vitamin D level.
• Patient doesn't develop vitamin D toxicity.
• Patient and family state understanding of drug therapy.

vitamin E (tocopherol)

(VIGH-tuh-min EE)
Amino-Opti-E†, Aquasol E Drops†, E-Complex-600†, E-200 I.U. Softgels†, E-400 I.U. Softgels†, E-Vitamin Succinate†, Mixed E 400 Softgels, Mixed E 1000 Softgels, Vitamin E with Mixed Tocopherols, Vita-Plus E Softgels†

Pharmacologic class: fat-soluble vitamin
Therapeutic class: vitamin
Pregnancy risk category: A

V

Indications and dosages

► **RDA.** RDAs are in α-tocopherol equivalents (α-TE). One α-TE equals 1 mg of D-α tocopherol or 1.49 international units.
Adults, pregnant women: 15 α-TE.
Breast-feeding women: 19 α-TE.
Children ages 14 to 18: 15 α-TE.
Children ages 9 to 13: 11 α-TE.
Children ages 4 to 8: 7 α-TE.
Children ages 1 to 3: 6 α-TE.
Infants ages 7 to 12 months: 5 α-TE.
Infants age 6 months and younger: 4 α-TE.
► **Vitamin E deficiency in adults and in children with malabsorption syndrome.** *Adults:* Depending on severity, 60 to 75 international units P.O. daily.
Children: 1 international unit/kg P.O. daily.

Contraindications and cautions

None reported.
🜲 **Lifespan:** In pregnant women, use cautiously. In breast-feeding women, use cautiously.

Adverse reactions

None reported.

Interactions

Drug-drug. *Cholestyramine resin, mineral oil:* May inhibit GI absorption of oral vitamin E. Space doses. Use together cautiously.
Iron: May catalyze oxidation and increase daily requirements. Give separately.
Oral anticoagulants: May increase hypoprothrombinemic effects, possibly causing bleeding. Monitor patient closely.
Vitamin K: May antagonize effects of vitamin K with large doses of vitamin E. Avoid use together.

Effects on lab test results

None reported.

Pharmacokinetics

Absorption: GI absorption depends on presence of bile. Only 20% to 60% of vitamin obtained from dietary sources is absorbed. As dosage increases, fraction of vitamin E absorbed decreases.
Distribution: To all tissues and stored in adipose tissues.
Metabolism: In liver.
Excretion: Primarily in bile; small amount excreted in urine. *Half-life:* Unknown.

Route	Onset	Peak	Duration
P.O.	Unknown	Unknown	Unknown

Action

Chemical effect: May act as an antioxidant and protect RBC membranes against hemolysis.
Therapeutic effect: Raises vitamin E level in body.

Available forms

Capsules: 100 international units, 200 international units†, 400 international units†, 600 international units†, 1,000 international units†
Drops: 15 international units/0.3 ml
Liquid: 15 international units/30 ml
Oral solution: 50 international units/ml
Tablets (chewable): 100 international units, 200 international units†, 400 international units†, 500 international units, 600 international units, 800 international units, 1,000 international units

NURSING PROCESS

⚖ **Assessment**
● Assess patient's condition before starting therapy and regularly thereafter to monitor the drug's effectiveness.
● Monitor patient with liver or gallbladder disease for response to therapy. Adequate bile is essential for vitamin E absorption.
● Be alert for drug interactions.
● Assess patient's and family's knowledge of drug therapy.

⚙ **Nursing diagnoses**
● Imbalanced nutrition: less than body requirements related to inadequate intake
● Deficient knowledge related to drug therapy

❭ **Planning and implementation**
● Requirements increase with rise in dietary polyunsaturated acids.
● Make sure patient swallows tablets or capsules whole.
● Store drug in tightly closed, light-resistant container.
● If patient has malabsorption caused by lack of bile, give vitamin E with bile salts.
● Hypervitaminosis E symptoms include fatigue, weakness, nausea, headache, blurred vision, flatulence, diarrhea.

Reactions may be *common*, uncommon, *life-threatening*, or COMMON AND LIFE-THREATENING.

Patient teaching

• Tell patient not to crush tablets or open capsules. An oral solution and chewable tablets are commercially available.

• Discourage patient from taking megadoses, which can cause thrombophlebitis. Vitamin E is fat-soluble.

✓ Evaluation

• Patient regains normal vitamin E level.

• Patient and family state understanding of drug therapy.

voriconazole

(vhor-i-KHAN-a-zawl)

Vfend

Pharmacologic class: synthetic triazole
Therapeutic class: antifungal
Pregnancy risk category: D

Indications and dosages

▶ **Invasive aspergillosis; serious infections caused by *Fusarium* species and *Scedosporium apiospermum* in patients intolerant of or refractory to other therapy.** *Adults:* Initially, 6 mg/kg I.V. q 12 hours for two doses; then 4 mg/kg I.V. q 12 hours for maintenance. Switch to P.O. form as tolerated, using the following maintenance dosages:
Adults weighing 40 kg (88 lb) or more: Maintenance dosage, 200 mg P.O. q 12 hours. May increase to 300 mg P.O. q 12 hours, if needed.
Adults weighing less than 40 kg: Maintenance dosage, 100 mg P.O. q 12 hours. May increase to 150 mg P.O. q 12 hours, if needed.

▶ **Candidemia in non-neutropenic patients; candida infections of the kidney, abdomen, bladder wall, wounds, and skin (disseminated).** *Adults:* Initially, 6 mg/kg I.V. q 12 hours for two doses; then 4 mg/kg I.V. q 12 hours for maintenance. If patient unable to tolerate maintenance dose, decrease to 3 mg/kg. Switch to P.O. form as tolerated, using the maintenance dosages shown here.
Adults who weigh 40 kg (88 lb) or more: 200 mg P.O. q 12 hours. May increase to 300 mg P.O. q 12 hours, if needed.
Adults who weigh less than 40 kg: 100 mg P.O. q 12 hours. May increase to 150 mg P.O. q 12 hours, if needed.

Adjust-a-dose: In patients with mild to moderate hepatic cirrhosis, decrease the maintenance dosage by one-half.

▶ **Esophageal candidiasis.** *Adults weighing 40 kg or more:* 200 mg P.O. q 12 hours. Treat for a minimum of 14 days and for at least 7 days following resolution of symptoms.
Adults weighing less than 40 kg: 100 mg P.O. q 12 hours. Treat for a minimum of 14 days and for at least 7 days following resolution of symptoms.

I.V. administration

• Reconstitute powder with 19 ml of sterile water for injection to obtain a volume of 20 ml of clear concentrate containing 10 mg/ml of drug. If a vacuum doesn't pull the diluent into the vial, discard the vial. Shake vial until all the powder is dissolved.

• Further dilute the 10-mg/ml solution to a concentration of 5 mg/ml or less. Follow the manufacturer's instructions for diluting.

• Infuse over 1 to 2 hours, at a concentration of 5 mg/ml or less and a maximum of 3 mg/kg hourly.

• Infusion reactions, including flushing, fever, sweating, tachycardia, chest tightness, dyspnea, faintness, nausea, pruritus, and rash, may occur as soon as infusion starts. If reaction occurs, notify prescriber. Infusion may need to be stopped.

• Monitor creatinine level in patient with moderate to severe renal dysfunction (creatinine clearance less than 50 ml/minute). If creatinine level increases, consider changing to P.O. form.

• Store unreconstituted vials at controlled room temperature (59° to 86° F [15° to 30° C]). Use reconstituted solution immediately.

⊗ Incompatibilities

Blood products, electrolyte supplements, 4.2% sodium bicarbonate infusion.

Contraindications and cautions

• Contraindicated in patients hypersensitive to the drug or any of its components and in those with rare hereditary problems of galactose intolerance, Lapp lactase deficiency, or glucose-galactose malabsorption. Also contraindicated in patients taking rifampin, carbamazepine, long-acting barbiturates, sirolimus, rifabutin, ergot alkaloids, pimozide, quinidine, efavirenz, or ritonavir.

V

• Use cautiously in patients hypersensitive to other azoles. Use I.V. form cautiously in patients with creatinine clearance less than 50 ml/minute.
⚖ **Lifespan:** In pregnant women, don't use; drug can harm fetus. In breast-feeding women, use cautiously; it's unknown whether drug appears in breast milk. In children younger than age 12, safety and effectiveness haven't been established.

Adverse reactions

CNS: fever, headache, hallucinations, dizziness.
CV: tachycardia, hypertension, hypotension, peripheral edema, vasodilation, *prolonged QT interval.*
EENT: *abnormal vision,* photophobia, chromatopsia, dry mouth.
GI: abdominal pain, nausea, vomiting, diarrhea.
GU: *acute renal failure.*
Hepatic: cholestatic jaundice.
Metabolic: hypokalemia, hypomagnesemia.
Skin: rash, pruritus.
Other: chills.

Interactions

Drug-drug. *Benzodiazepines, calcium channel blockers, lovastatin, omeprazole, sulfonylureas, vinca alkaloids:* May increase levels of these drugs. Adjust dosages of these drugs, and monitor patient for adverse effects.
Carbamazepine, long-acting barbiturates, rifabutin, rifampin: May decrease voriconazole level. Avoid use together.
Coumarin anticoagulants, warfarin: May significantly increase PT. Monitor PT or other appropriate anticoagulant test results.
Cyclosporine, tacrolimus: May increase levels of these drugs. Reduce dosages of these drugs, and monitor levels. Adjust doses and monitor levels of these drugs when voriconazole is stopped.
Efavirenz: May significantly decrease voriconazole level and significantly increase efavirenz level. Avoid use together.
Ergot alkaloids (such as ergotamine), sirolimus: May increase levels of these drugs. Avoid use together.
HIV protease inhibitors (amprenavir, nelfinavir, saquinavir), nonnucleoside reverse transcriptase inhibitors (delavirdine): May increase levels of both drugs. Monitor patient for adverse effects.

Phenytoin: May decrease voriconazole level and increase phenytoin level. Increase voriconazole maintenance dose, and monitor phenytoin level.
Pimozide, quinidine: May increase levels of these drugs, possibly leading to QT prolongation and torsades de pointes. Avoid use together.
Ritonavir: May significantly decrease voriconazole level. Avoid use together.
Drug-lifestyle. *Sun exposure:* May cause photosensitivity reaction. Tell patient to avoid excessive or unprotected sun exposure.

Effects on lab test results

• May increase AST, ALT, bilirubin, alkaline phosphatase, and creatinine levels. May decrease potassium, magnesium, and hemoglobin levels and hematocrit.
• May decrease platelet, WBC, and RBC counts.

Pharmacokinetics

Absorption: Oral bioavailability is about 96%.
Distribution: Extensive. Protein-binding is 58%.
Metabolism: By the CYP 2C19, 2C9, and 3A4.
Excretion: Via hepatic metabolism, with less than 2% excreted unchanged in the urine. *Half-life:* Depends on dose.

Route	Onset	Peak	Duration
P.O., I.V.	Immediate	1–2 hr	12 hr

Action

Chemical effect: Inhibits an essential step in fungal ergosterol biosynthesis.
Therapeutic effect: Kills susceptible fungi.

Available forms

Injection: 200 mg
Powder for oral suspension: 45 g (40 mg/ml after reconstitution)
Tablets: 50 mg, 200 mg

NURSING PROCESS

▨ **Assessment**
• Assess patient's condition before starting therapy and regularly thereafter to monitor the drug's effectiveness.
• Monitor liver function test results throughout therapy. Monitor patient who develops abnormal liver function test results for more severe hepatic dysfunction.

- Monitor renal function during treatment.
- If treatment lasts more than 28 days, monitor visual acuity, visual fields, and color perception.
- Assess patient's and family's knowledge of drug therapy.

⊞ Nursing diagnoses
- Risk for infection related to presence of fungus
- Risk for injury related to adverse CNS effects of drug
- Deficient knowledge related to drug therapy

▷ Planning and implementation
- Use oral form in patient with moderate to severe renal impairment unless benefits of I.V. use outweigh risks.
- Reconstitute powder for oral suspension with 46 ml of water. Shake the bottle vigorously for about 1 minute. Remove cap, push bottle adaptor into neck of the bottle, and replace cap. The reconstituted suspension should be shaken for about 10 seconds before each use. Administer using the supplied oral dispenser.
- The reconstituted oral suspension should not be mixed with any other medication or flavoring agent and should not be further diluted. Reconstituted suspension can be stored at a controlled room temperature (59° to 86° F [15 to 30° C]) for 14 days.
- If patient develops signs and symptoms of liver disease that may be caused by therapy, stop drug.

Patient teaching
- Tell patient to take oral drug at least 1 hour before or 1 hour after a meal.
- Advise patient to avoid driving or operating machinery while taking drug, especially at night, because vision changes, including blurring and photophobia, may occur.
- Tell patient to avoid strong, direct sunlight during therapy.
- Tell woman of childbearing potential to use effective contraception during treatment.

✔ Evaluation
- Infection is successfully treated.
- Patient doesn't sustain any injury.
- Patient and family state understanding of drug therapy.

WXY

warfarin sodium
(WAR-feh-rin SOH-dee-um)
Coumadin◊, Jantoven, Warfilone ◆

Pharmacologic class: coumarin derivative
Therapeutic class: anticoagulant
Pregnancy risk category: X

Indications and dosages

▶**Pulmonary embolism related to deep vein thrombosis, MI, rheumatic heart disease with heart valve damage, prosthetic heart valves, chronic atrial fibrillation.** *Adults:* Initially, 2 to 5 mg P.O. or I.V daily for 2 to 4 days. Use PT and INR determinations to establish optimal dose. Usual maintenance dosage, 2 to 10 mg daily.

▼I.V. administration

- Reconstitute by adding 2.7 ml of sterile water for injection to vial of 5 mg of warfarin. Resulting solution contains 2 mg/ml.
- Inject dose slowly over 1 to 2 minutes.
⊗ **Incompatibilities**
None reported.

Contraindications and cautions

- Contraindicated in patients with bleeding or hemorrhagic tendencies, GI ulcerations, severe hepatic or renal disease, severe uncontrolled hypertension, subacute bacterial endocarditis, polycythemia vera, or vitamin K deficiency. Also contraindicated in patients who have had recent eye, brain, or spinal cord surgery.
- Use cautiously in patients with diverticulitis, colitis, mild or moderate hypertension, mild or moderate hepatic or renal disease, drainage tubes in any orifice, or regional or lumbar block anesthesia. Also use cautiously if patient has any condition that increases the risk of hemorrhage.
⚠ **Lifespan:** In pregnant women, drug is contraindicated. In breast-feeding women, use cautiously; it's unknown if the drug appears in breast milk. Infants, especially neonates, may be more susceptible to anticoagulants because of vitamin K deficiency. In elderly patients, use a

W

lower dose because they have an increased risk of bleeding.

Adverse reactions

CNS: headache, *fever.*
GI: anorexia, nausea, vomiting, cramps, *diarrhea,* mouth ulcerations, sore mouth, melena.
GU: hematuria, excessive menstrual bleeding.
Hematologic: *hemorrhage.*
Hepatic: *hepatitis,* jaundice.
Skin: dermatitis, urticaria, necrosis, gangrene, alopecia, *rash.*

Interactions

Drug-drug. *Acetaminophen:* May increase bleeding with more than 2 weeks of acetaminophen therapy at dosages of more than 2 g/day. Monitor patient carefully.
Allopurinol, amiodarone, anabolic steroids, cephalosporins, chloramphenicol, cimetidine, clofibrate, danazol, diazoxide, diflunisal, disulfiram, erythromycin, ethacrynic acid, fluoroquinolones, glucagon, heparin, influenza virus vaccine, isoniazid, lovastatin, meclofenamate, methimazole, methylthiouracil, metronidazole, miconazole, nalidixic acid, neomycin (oral), pentoxifylline, propafenone, propoxyphene, quinidine, sulfonamides, tamoxifen, tetracyclines, thiazides, thrombolytics, thyroid drugs, tricyclic antidepressants, vitamin E: May increase PT. Monitor patient for bleeding. Reduce anticoagulant dosage.
Anticonvulsants: May increase levels of phenytoin and phenobarbital. Monitor patient for toxicity.
Barbiturates, carbamazepine, corticosteroids, corticotropin, hormonal contraceptives containing estrogen, mercaptopurine, methaqualone, nafcillin, rifampin, spironolactone, sucralfate, trazodone: May decrease PT with reduced anticoagulant effect. Monitor patient carefully.
Chloral hydrate, glutethimide, propylthiouracil, sulfinpyrazone: May increase or decrease PT. Avoid use, if possible. Monitor patient carefully.
Cholestyramine: May decrease response when given too close together. Give 6 hours after oral anticoagulants.
NSAIDs, salicylates: May increase PT and ulcerogenic effects. Don't use together.
Sulfonylureas (oral antidiabetics): May increase hypoglycemic response. Monitor glucose level.
Drug-herb. *Angelica:* May significantly prolong PT when used together. Discourage use together.

Arnica, ginkgo biloba, ginseng, motherwort, pau d'arco, red clover: May increase risk of bleeding. Discourage use together.
Drug-food. *Foods or enteral products containing vitamin K:* May impair anticoagulation. Tell patient to maintain consistent daily intake of leafy green vegetables.
Drug-lifestyle. *Alcohol use:* May increase anticoagulant effects. Discourage alcohol intake; however, one or two drinks daily are unlikely to affect warfarin response.

Effects on lab test results

• May increase ALT and AST levels.
• May increase INR, PT, and PTT.

Pharmacokinetics

Absorption: Rapid and complete.
Distribution: Highly bound to proteins, especially albumin.
Metabolism: In liver.
Excretion: Metabolites reabsorbed from bile and excreted in urine. *Half-life:* 1 to 3 days.

Route	Onset	Peak	Duration
P.O.	½–3 days	Unknown	2–5 days
I.V.	Unknown	Unknown	2–5 days

Action

Chemical effect: Inhibits vitamin K–dependent activation of clotting factors II, VII, IX, and X, formed in liver.
Therapeutic effect: Reduces ability of blood to clot.

Available forms

Powder for injection: 5 mg
Tablets: 1 mg, 2 mg, 2.5 mg, 3 mg, 4 mg, 5 mg, 6 mg, 7.5 mg, 10 mg

NURSING PROCESS

⚕ Assessment

• Assess patient's condition before starting therapy and regularly thereafter to monitor the drug's effectiveness.
• Draw blood to establish baseline coagulation parameters before starting therapy.
⊛ ALERT: INR determinations are essential for proper control. Clinicians typically try to maintain INR at two to three times normal; risk of bleeding is high when INR exceeds six times normal.

Reactions may be *common,* uncommon, *life-threatening,* or COMMON AND LIFE-THREATENING.

• Be alert for adverse reactions and drug interactions. An elderly patient or a patient with renal or hepatic failure is especially sensitive to warfarin effect.
• Regularly inspect patient for bleeding gums, bruises on arms or legs, petechiae, nosebleed, melena, tarry stools, hematuria, and hematemesis.
• Observe the breast-fed infant of a mother taking the drug for unexpected bleeding.
• Assess patient's and family's knowledge of drug therapy.

Nursing diagnoses
• Risk for injury related to potential for blood clot formation from underlying condition
• Ineffective protection related to increased risk of bleeding
• Deficient knowledge related to drug therapy

Planning and implementation
• Give drug at same time each day.
• I.V. form may be obtained from manufacturer for rare patient who can't have oral therapy. Follow guidelines carefully to prepare and give the drug.
• Because onset of action is delayed, heparin sodium is commonly given during first few days of treatment. When heparin is given simultaneously, blood for PT shouldn't be drawn within 5 hours of intermittent I.V. heparin administration. Blood for PT may be drawn at any time during continuous heparin infusion.
ALERT: If patient has a fever and rash, notify the prescriber immediately and don't give the dose; these symptoms may signal severe adverse reactions.
• The drug's anticoagulant effect can be neutralized by vitamin K injections.
• Drug is best oral anticoagulant for patient taking antacids or phenytoin.

Patient teaching
• Stress importance of compliance with prescribed dosage and follow-up appointments. Patient should wear or carry medical identification that indicates his increased risk of bleeding.
• Instruct patient and family to watch for signs of bleeding and to immediately notify the prescriber if they occur.
• Warn patient to avoid OTC products containing aspirin, other salicylates, or drugs that may interact with warfarin.
• Tell patient to notify prescriber if menses are heavier than usual; dosage adjustment may be needed.
• Tell patient to use an electric razor when shaving, to avoid scratching skin, and to use soft toothbrush.
• Instruct patient to read food labels. Food and enteral feedings that contain vitamin K may impair anticoagulation.
• Tell patient to daily eat a consistent amount of leafy green vegetables that contain vitamin K. Eating varying amounts may alter anticoagulant effects.

Evaluation
• Patient doesn't develop blood clots.
• Patient states appropriate bleeding precautions to take.
• Patient and family state understanding of drug therapy.

Z

zafirlukast
(zay-FEER-loo-kast)
Accolate

Pharmacologic class: synthetic, selective peptide leukotriene receptor antagonist
Therapeutic class: anti-inflammatory, bronchodilator
Pregnancy risk category: B

Indications and dosages
▶ **Prevention and long-term treatment of chronic asthma.** *Adults and children age 12 and older:* 20 mg P.O. b.i.d. taken 1 hour before or 2 hours after meals.
Children ages 5 to 11: 10 mg P.O. b.i.d. taken 1 hour before or 2 hours after meals.
▶ **Prevention of seasonal allergic rhinitis** ‡. *Adults:* 20 to 40 mg P.O. as a single dose before exposure to allergen.

Contraindications and cautions
• Contraindicated in patients hypersensitive to the drug or any of its components.

• Use cautiously in patients with hepatic impairment.

⚜ **Lifespan:** In pregnant women, drug should be used only if clearly needed. In breast-feeding women, drug shouldn't be given because it appears in breast milk. In children younger than age 5, safety and effectiveness haven't been established. In the elderly, use cautiously.

Adverse reactions

CNS: *headache,* asthenia, dizziness, pain, fever.
GI: nausea, diarrhea, abdominal pain, vomiting, dyspepsia.
Musculoskeletal: myalgia, back pain.
Other: infection, accidental injury.

Interactions

Drug-drug. *Aspirin:* May increase zafirlukast level. Monitor patient.
Erythromycin, theophylline: May decrease zafirlukast level. Monitor patient.
Warfarin: May increase PT. Monitor PT and INR levels, and adjust dosage of anticoagulant.
Drug-food. *Any food:* May reduce rate and extent of drug absorption. Give drug 1 hour before or 2 hours after meals.

Effects on lab test results

• May increase liver enzyme levels.

Pharmacokinetics

Absorption: Rapid.
Distribution: Unknown.
Metabolism: Extensive.
Excretion: Mainly in feces; 10% in urine. *Half-life:* 10 hours.

Route	Onset	Peak	Duration
P.O.	Unknown	3 hr	Unknown

Action

Chemical effect: Selectively competes for leukotriene receptor sites. Blocks inflammatory action and inhibits bronchoconstriction.
Therapeutic effect: Improves breathing.

Available forms

Tablets: 10 mg, 20 mg

NURSING PROCESS

⚗ Assessment
• Assess patient's and family's understanding of drug therapy.

⊞ Nursing diagnoses
• Impaired gas exchange related to bronchospasm
• Deficient knowledge related to drug therapy

⟩ Planning and implementation
⟳ **ALERT:** Don't use drug for reversing bronchospasm in acute asthma attack.
⟳ **ALERT:** Reducing dose may rarely cause eosinophilia, vasculitic rash, worsening pulmonary symptoms, cardiac complications, or neuropathy, such as Churg-Strauss syndrome.
Patient teaching
• Tell patient to keep taking drug even if symptoms disappear.
• Advise patient to continue taking other antiasthmatics.
• Instruct patient to take drug 1 hour before or 2 hours after meals.

☑ Evaluation
• Patient demonstrates improved gas exchange.
• Patient and family state understanding of drug therapy.

---

zalcitabine (ddC, dideoxycytidine)
(zal-SIGH-tuh-been)
Hivid

Pharmacologic class: nucleoside analogue
Therapeutic class: antiretroviral
Pregnancy risk category: C

Indications and dosages

▶ **Advanced HIV infection (CD4+ T-cell count below 300/mm³) in patients with significant deterioration.** *Adults and adolescents age 13 and older weighing at least 30 kg (66 lb):* 0.75 mg P.O. q 8 hours given with other antiretrovirals.

Contraindications and cautions

• Contraindicated in patients hypersensitive to the drug or any of its components.

• Use cautiously in patients with peripheral neuropathy, baseline cardiomyopathy, or history of heart failure. Use cautiously in patients with creatinine clearance less than 55 ml/minute because they may be at increased risk for toxicity. Use cautiously in patients with hepatic failure; drug regimen (zalcitabine and zidovudine) may worsen hepatic dysfunction in patients with hepatic impairment. Use cautiously in patients with history of pancreatitis; rarely, pancreatitis is fatal in patients receiving zalcitabine.
⚠ **Lifespan:** In pregnant women and in children younger than age 13, safety and effectiveness haven't been established. Advise breast-feeding women to feed their infants another way, to reduce risk of transmitting HIV.

Adverse reactions

CNS: *peripheral neuropathy, headache, fatigue,* dizziness, confusion, *seizures,* impaired concentration, amnesia, insomnia, depression, tremor, hypertonia, asthenia, agitation, abnormal thinking, anxiety, *fever.*
CV: *cardiomyopathy, heart failure,* chest pain.
EENT: pharyngitis, ocular pain, abnormal vision, ototoxicity, nasal discharge.
GI: nausea, vomiting, diarrhea, abdominal pain, anorexia, constipation, stomatitis, esophageal ulcer, glossitis, *pancreatitis.*
Hematologic: anemia, *neutropenia, leukopenia, thrombocytopenia.*
Hepatic: hepatomegaly, *hepatic toxicity.*
Respiratory: cough.
Metabolic: *lactic acidosis.*
Musculoskeletal: myalgia, arthralgia.
Skin: pruritus; night sweats; *erythematous, maculopapular, or follicular rash;* urticaria.

Interactions

Drug-drug. *Aminoglycosides, amphotericin B, foscarnet, other drugs that may impair kidney function:* May increase risk of nephrotoxicity. Avoid use together.
Antacids containing aluminum or magnesium: May decrease absorption of zalcitabine. Separate administration times.
Chloramphenicol, cisplatin, dapsone, disulfiram, ethionamide, glutethimide, gold salts, hydralazine, iodoquinol, isoniazid, metronidazole, nitrofurantoin, phenytoin, ribavirin, vincristine, and other drugs that can cause peripheral neuropathy: May increase risk of peripheral neuropathy. Avoid use together.

Cimetidine, probenecid: May increase zalcitabine level. Monitor patient carefully.
Pentamidine: May increase risk of pancreatitis. Avoid use together.
Drug-food. *Any food:* May decrease rate of drug absorption. Give drug on empty stomach.

Effects on lab test results

• May increase alkaline phosphatase, ALT, and AST levels. May decrease hemoglobin level and hematocrit. May alter glucose level.
• May decrease neutrophil, WBC, and platelet counts.

Pharmacokinetics

Absorption: Mean absolute bioavailability is above 80%. Administering drug with food decreases rate and extent of absorption.
Distribution: Enters CNS.
Metabolism: Probably insignificant in liver; phosphorylation to active form occurs within cells.
Excretion: Primarily in urine. *Half-life:* 2 hours.

Route	Onset	Peak	Duration
P.O.	Unknown	1–2 hr	Unknown

Action

Chemical effect: Inhibits replication of HIV by blocking viral DNA synthesis.
Therapeutic effect: Reduces symptoms linked to advanced HIV infection.

Available forms

Tablets: 0.375 mg, 0.75 mg

NURSING PROCESS

Assessment
• Assess patient's condition before starting therapy and regularly thereafter to monitor the drug's effectiveness.
• Assess patient for signs of peripheral neuropathy, characterized by numbness and burning in limbs.
• Be alert for adverse reactions and drug interactions.
• Assess patient's and family's knowledge of drug therapy.

Nursing diagnoses
• Risk for infection related to presence of HIV

Z

• Disturbed sensory perceptions (tactile) related to drug-induced peripheral neuropathy
• Deficient knowledge related to drug therapy

▷ **Planning and implementation**
• Adjust dosage in patient with moderate to severe renal failure.
• Don't give drug with food because it decreases rate and extent of absorption.
• If signs and symptoms of peripheral neuropathy occur, notify prescriber. If symptoms are on both sides and persist beyond 72 hours, withhold the drug. If symptoms persist or worsen beyond 1 week, stop drug permanently. If peripheral neuropathy resolves to minor symptoms, reintroduce at 0.375 mg P.O. q 8 hours. If drug isn't withdrawn, peripheral neuropathy may be irreversible and may progress to sharp, shooting pain or severe continuous burning pain requiring opioid analgesics.
• If this drug is stopped because of toxicity, resume recommended dose for zidovudine (100 mg q 4 hours).
⊛ **ALERT:** Don't confuse drug with other antivirals that use initials for identification.
Patient teaching
• Inform patient that drug doesn't cure HIV infection and that opportunistic infections may occur despite continued use. Review safe sex practices with patient.
• Inform patient that peripheral neuropathy is the major adverse reaction and that pancreatitis is the major life-threatening adverse reaction. Review signs and symptoms of these adverse reactions, and instruct patient to call prescriber immediately if they appear.
• Instruct woman of childbearing age to use effective contraceptive during drug therapy.

☑ **Evaluation**
• Patient responds well to drug.
• Patient doesn't develop peripheral neuropathy.
• Patient and family state understanding of drug therapy.

zaleplon
(ZAL-eh-plon)
Sonata

Pharmacologic class: pyrazolopyrimidine
Therapeutic class: hypnotic

Pregnancy risk category: C
Controlled substance schedule: IV

Indications and dosages

▶ **Short-term treatment of insomnia.** *Adults:* 10 mg P.O. h.s.; may increase dose to 20 mg if needed. Low-weight adults may respond to 5-mg dose.
Elderly and debilitated patients: Initially, 5 mg P.O. h.s.; doses over 10 mg aren't recommended.
⟦ **Adjust-a-dose:** For patients with mild to moderate hepatic impairment and those taking cimetidine, give 5 mg P.O. daily.

Contraindications and cautions

• Don't use in patients with severe hepatic impairment.
• Use cautiously in debilitated patients, in those with compromised respiratory function, and in those with signs and symptoms of depression.
⚘ **Lifespan:** In pregnant and breast-feeding women, drug isn't recommended. In children, safety and effectiveness haven't been established. In elderly patients, use cautiously.

Adverse reactions

CNS: *headache,* amnesia, dizziness, somnolence, depression, hypertonia, nervousness, depersonalization, hallucinations, vertigo, difficulty concentrating, anxiety, paresthesia, hypesthesia, tremor, asthenia, migraine, malaise, fever.
CV: chest pain, peripheral edema.
EENT: abnormal vision, conjunctivitis, eye pain, ear pain, hyperacusis, epistaxis, parosmia.
GI: constipation, dry mouth, anorexia, dyspepsia, nausea, abdominal pain, colitis.
GU: dysmenorrhea.
Musculoskeletal: arthritis, myalgia, back pain.
Respiratory: bronchitis.
Skin: pruritus, rash, photosensitivity reactions.

Interactions

Drug-drug. *Carbamazepine, phenobarbital, phenytoin, rifampin, other drugs that induce CYP 3A4:* May reduce effectiveness of zaleplon. Consider a different hypnotic.
Cimetidine: May cause pharmacokinetic interaction. For patient taking cimetidine, use an initial zaleplon dose of 5 mg.
CNS depressants (imipramine, thioridazine): May produce additive CNS effects. Use cautiously together.

Reactions may be *common,* uncommon, *life-threatening*, or COMMON AND LIFE-THREATENING.

Drug-food. *High-fat foods, heavy meals:* May prolong absorption, delaying peak zaleplon level by about 2 hours; sleep onset may be delayed. Separate drug from meals.
Drug-lifestyle. *Alcohol use:* May increase CNS effects. Discourage use together.

Effects on lab test results

None reported.

Pharmacokinetics

Absorption: Rapid and almost complete. Levels peak within 1 hour. Taking drug after a high-fat or heavy meal delays peak levels by about 2 hours.
Distribution: Substantially into extravascular tissues. Protein-binding is about 60%.
Metabolism: Extensive, primarily by aldehyde oxidase and, to a lesser extent, CYP 3A4 to inactive metabolites. Less than 1% of dose is excreted unchanged in urine.
Excretion: Rapid. *Half-life:* 1 hour.

Route	Onset	Peak	Duration
P.O.	1 hr	1 hr	3–4 hr

Action

Chemical effect: Has a chemical structure unrelated to benzodiazepines but interacts with the GABA and benzodiazepine receptor complex in the CNS. Modulation of this complex is hypothesized to be responsible for sedative, anxiolytic, muscle relaxant, and anticonvulsant effects of benzodiazepines.
Therapeutic effect: Promotes sleep.

Available forms

Capsules: 5 mg, 10 mg

NURSING PROCESS

Assessment
- Carefully assess patient because sleep disturbances may be a symptom of an underlying physical or psychiatric disorder.
- Closely monitor elderly or debilitated patient, or patient with compromised respiratory function because of illness.
- Monitor patient for drug abuse and dependence.
- Assess patient's and family's knowledge of drug therapy.

Nursing diagnoses
- Disturbed sleep pattern related to presence of insomnia
- Risk for injury related to drug-induced adverse CNS reactions
- Deficient knowledge related to drug therapy

Planning and implementation
- Don't give drug with or following a high-fat or heavy meal.
- Because drug works rapidly, give only immediately before bedtime or after patient has been unable to sleep.
- Adverse reactions are usually dose-related. Give lowest effective dose.
- Limit hypnotic use to 7 to 10 days. If hypnotics will be taken for more than 3 weeks, prescriber should reevaluate patient.
- The potential for drug abuse and dependence exists. Drug shouldn't be given as more than a 1-month supply.
Patient teaching
- Advise patient that drug works rapidly and should be taken immediately before bedtime or after trying unsuccessfully to sleep.
- Advise patient to take drug only if he can sleep undisturbed for at least 4 hours.
- Warn patient that drowsiness, dizziness, lightheadedness, and difficulty with coordination occur most often within 1 hour after taking drug.
- Advise patient to avoid performing activities that require mental alertness until the drug's CNS effects are known.
- Advise patient not to drink alcohol while taking drug and to notify prescriber before taking any prescription or OTC drugs.
- Tell patient not to take drug after a high-fat or heavy meal.
- Advise patient to report any continued sleep problems despite use of drug.
- Inform patient that dependence can occur, and that drug is recommended for short-term use only.
- Warn patient not to abruptly stop drug because withdrawal symptoms, including unpleasant feelings, stomach and muscle cramps, vomiting, sweating, shakiness, and seizures, may occur.
- Tell patient that insomnia may recur for a few nights after stopping drug, but should resolve on its own.
- Advise patient that zaleplon may cause changes in behavior and thinking, including out-

Z

going or aggressive behavior, loss of personal identity, confusion, strange behavior, agitation, hallucinations, worsening of depression, or suicidal thoughts. Tell patient to notify prescriber immediately if any of these problems occur.

☑ **Evaluation**

• Patient states that drug effectively promotes sleep.
• Patient doesn't experience injury as a result of drug-induced adverse CNS reactions.
• Patient and family state understanding of drug therapy.

zanamivir
(zah-NAM-ah-veer)
Relenza

Pharmacologic class: neuraminidase inhibitor
Therapeutic class: antiviral
Pregnancy risk category: C

Indications and dosages

▶ **Uncomplicated acute illness caused by influenza A and B virus in patients who have been symptomatic for no more than 2 days.**
Adults and children age 7 and older: 2 oral inhalations (one 5-mg blister per inhalation for a total dose of 10 mg) b.i.d. using the Diskhaler inhalation device for 5 days. Give two doses on the first day of treatment with at least 2 hours between doses. Subsequent doses should be about 12 hours apart (in the morning and evening) at about the same time each day.

Contraindications and cautions

• Contraindicated in patients hypersensitive to the drug or any of its components.
• Use cautiously in patients with severe or decompensated COPD, asthma, or other underlying respiratory disease.
⚠ **Lifespan:** In pregnant women, use only if benefits outweigh risks. In breast-feeding women, use cautiously; it's unknown if the drug appears in breast milk. In children younger than age 7, safety and effectiveness haven't been established.

Adverse reactions

CNS: headache, dizziness.

EENT: nasal signs and symptoms; sinusitis; ear, nose, and throat infections.
GI: diarrhea, nausea, vomiting.
hemaologic: lymphopenia, *neutropenia.*
Respiratory: *bronchospasm,* bronchitis, cough.

Interactions

None reported.

Effects on lab test results

• May increase ALT, AST, and CK.
• May decrease lymphocyte and neutrophil counts.

Pharmacokinetics

Absorption: About 4% to 17%, with peak levels occurring 1 to 2 hours following a 10-mg dose.
Distribution: Less than 10% protein binding.
Metabolism: Not metabolized.
Excretion: Excreted unchanged in the urine within 24 hours. Unabsorbed drug is excreted in feces. *Half-life:* 2½ to 5¼ hours.

Route	Onset	Peak	Duration
Inhalation	Unknown	1–2 hr	Unknown

Action

Chemical effect: Probably inhibits the enzyme neuraminidase on the surface of the influenza virus, possibly altering virus particle aggregation and release. When neuraminidase is inhibited, the virus can't escape from its host cell to attack others, thereby inhibiting the process of viral proliferation.
Therapeutic effect: Lessens the symptoms of influenza.

Available forms

Powder for inhalation: 5 mg per blister

NURSING PROCESS

🔲 **Assessment**

• Obtain accurate patient medical history before starting therapy.
• Lymphopenia, neutropenia, and a rise in liver enzyme and CK levels may occur during treatment. Monitor patient appropriately.
• Monitor patient for bronchospasm and decline in lung function. If they occur, stop giving the drug.
• Assess patient's and family's knowledge of drug therapy.

Reactions may be *common,* uncommon, *life-threatening,* or COMMON AND LIFE-THREATENING.

⊞ Nursing diagnoses
• Risk for infection related to influenza virus
• Imbalanced nutrition: less than body requirements related to drug's adverse GI effects
• Deficient knowledge related to drug therapy

⧉ Planning and implementation
• Have patient exhale fully before inserting the mouthpiece. Then, keeping the Diskhaler level, have patient close his lips around the mouthpiece, and have him breathe in steadily and deeply. Instruct patient to hold his breath for a few seconds after inhaling to help keep the drug in his lungs.
• If patient is scheduled to use an inhaled bronchodilator for asthma, have him use his bronchodilator before starting therapy. In patient with underlying respiratory disease, have a fast-acting bronchodilator available in case of wheezing.
• Safety and effectiveness of drug haven't been established for influenza prevention. Use of drug shouldn't affect annual influenza vaccination.
• No data exist to suggest that drug is effective when started more than 48 hours after symptoms start.
Patient teaching
• Teach patient how to properly use the drug with the Diskhaler inhalation device, and tell him to carefully read the instructions.
• Advise patient to keep the Diskhaler level when loading and inhaling drug. Tell patient to check inside the mouthpiece of the Diskhaler before each use to make sure it's free of foreign objects.
• Instruct patient with respiratory disease who has an impending scheduled dose of inhaled bronchodilator to take it before taking zanamivir. Tell patient with asthma to have a fast-acting bronchodilator available in case of wheezing during therapy.
• Tell patient to finish the entire 5-day course even if he feels better and symptoms improve before the fifth day.
• Inform patient that zanamivir hasn't been shown to reduce the risk of transmitting influenza virus to others.

☑ Evaluation
• Patient recovers from influenza.
• Patient doesn't experience adverse GI effects.
• Patient and family state understanding of drug therapy.

zidovudine (azidothymidine, AZT)
(zigh-DOH-vyoo-deen)
Apo-Zidovudine ♦ , Novo-AZT ♦ , Retrovir

Pharmacologic class: thymidine analogue
Therapeutic class: antiretroviral
Pregnancy risk category: C

Indications and dosages
▶ **HIV infection.** *Adults:* 600 mg P.O. daily in divided doses given with other antiretrovirals. Or, for patients who can't take the oral form, 1 mg/kg I.V. over 1 hour, q 4 hours around the clock until oral therapy can be used.
Children ages 6 weeks to 12 years: 160 mg/m^2 P.O. q 8 hours. Maximum, 200 mg q 8 hours. Give with other antiretrovirals.
▷ **Adjust-a-dose:** Patients with end-stage renal disease (creatinine clearance less than 15 ml/minute) maintained on dialysis should receive 1 mg/kg I.V. q 6 to 8 hours.
▶ **To prevent maternal-fetal HIV transmission.** *Pregnant women past 14 weeks' gestation:* 100 mg P.O. five times daily until the start of labor. Then, 2 mg/kg I.V. over 1 hour followed by a continuous I.V. infusion of 1 mg/kg/hour until the umbilical cord is clamped.
Neonates: 2 mg/kg P.O. q 6 hours starting within 12 hours after birth and continuing until age 6 weeks. Or, give 1.5 mg/kg via I.V. infusion over 30 minutes q 6 hours.
▷ **Adjust-a-dose:** For patients on hemodialysis or peritoneal dialysis, give 100 mg P.O. q 6 to 8 hours. For patients with mild to moderate hepatic dysfunction or liver cirrhosis, reduce daily dose.
▶ **Prophylaxis after occupational exposure to HIV‡.** *Adults:* 600 mg P.O. daily in two or three divided doses for 4 weeks given with other antiretrovirals.

▼ I.V. administration
• Dilute drug before use. Remove calculated dose from vial; add to D$_5$W to yield no more than 4 mg/ml.
• Adding solution to biological or colloidal fluids (such as blood products and protein solutions) isn't recommended.
• Infuse drug over 1 hour at constant rate; give q 4 hours around the clock. Avoid rapid infusion or bolus injection.

Z

Rapid onset   *Liquid form contains alcohol.   ♦ Canada   ◇ Australia   †OTC   ⌀Photoguide   ‡Off-label use

• Solution is physically and chemically stable for 24 hours at room temperature and for 48 hours if refrigerated at 36° to 46° F (2° to 8° C). Store undiluted vials at 59° to 77° F (15° to 25° C) and protect them from light.

⊗ **Incompatibilities**
Biological or colloidal solutions, such as blood products or protein-containing solutions; meropenem.

Contraindications and cautions

• Contraindicated in patients hypersensitive to the drug or any of its components.
• Use cautiously and with close monitoring in patients with advanced symptomatic HIV infection and in those with severe bone marrow depression. Also use cautiously in patients with hepatomegaly, hepatitis, or other known risk factors for hepatic disease.
⚠ **Lifespan:** In breast-feeding women, drug shouldn't be used. In an elderly patient, use cautiously.

Adverse reactions

CNS: asthenia, headache, *seizures,* paresthesia, malaise, insomnia, dizziness, somnolence, fever.
GI: nausea, anorexia, abdominal pain, vomiting, constipation, diarrhea, dyspepsia, taste perversion.
Hematologic: *bone marrow suppression, agranulocytosis, thrombocytopenia.*
Metabolic: *lactic acidosis.*
Musculoskeletal: myalgia.
Skin: *rash,* diaphoresis.

Interactions

Drug-drug. *Atovaquone, fluconazole, methadone, probenecid, valproic acid:* May increase levels of zidovudine. Adjust dosage if needed.
Doxorubicin, ribavirin, stavudine: May antagonize zidovudine. Avoid use together.
Ganciclovir, interferon alfa, other bone marrow suppressants or cytotoxic drugs: May increase hematologic toxicity of zidovudine. Use cautiously as with other reverse transcriptase inhibitors.
Nelfinavir, rifampin, ritonavir: May decrease bioavailability of zidovudine. Dosage adjustment isn't needed.
Phenytoin: May alter phenytoin level and decrease zidovudine clearance by 30%. Monitor patient closely.

Effects on lab test results

• May increase ALT, AST, alkaline phosphatase, and LDH levels. May decrease hemoglobin level and hematocrit.
• May decrease granulocyte and platelet counts.

Pharmacokinetics

Absorption: Rapid.
Distribution: Preliminary data reveal good CSF penetration; about 36% protein-bound.
Metabolism: Rapid, to inactive compound.
Excretion: In urine. *Half-life:* 1 hour.

Route	Onset	Peak	Duration
P.O.	Unknown	30–90 min	Unknown
I.V.	Immediate	30–90 min	Unknown

Action

Chemical effect: Prevents replication of HIV by inhibiting the enzyme reverse transcriptase.
Therapeutic effect: Reduces symptoms of HIV infection.

Available forms

Capsules: 100 mg
Injection: 10 mg/ml
Syrup: 50 mg/5 ml
Tablets: 300 mg

NURSING PROCESS

🔎 **Assessment**
• Assess patient's condition before starting therapy and regularly thereafter to monitor the drug's effectiveness.
• Monitor CBC with differential and platelet counts q 2 weeks to detect anemia or agranulocytosis.
• Be alert for adverse reactions and drug interactions.
• Assess patient's and family's knowledge of drug therapy.

🔧 **Nursing diagnoses**
• Infection related to presence of HIV
• Ineffective protection related to drug-induced adverse hematologic reactions
• Deficient knowledge related to drug therapy

▶ **Planning and implementation**
• Drug temporarily decreases illness and risk of death in certain patients with AIDS or AIDS-related complex.

Reactions may be *common,* uncommon, *life-threatening,* or COMMON AND LIFE-THREATENING.

• Optimum duration of treatment and optimum dosage for effectiveness with minimum toxicity aren't yet known.
⑤ **ALERT:** Notify prescriber of abnormal hematologic study results. Significant anemia (hemoglobin level of less than 7.5 g/dl or reduction of more than 25% of baseline) or significant neutropenia (granulocyte count of less than 750/mm³ or reduction of more than 50% from baseline) may warrant interrupting therapy until marrow begins to recover.

Patient teaching
• Advise patient that blood transfusions may be needed during treatment. Drug often causes low RBC count.
• Stress importance of compliance with every-4-hour dosing. Suggest ways to avoid missing doses, perhaps by using an alarm clock.
• Warn patient not to take other drugs for AIDS (especially street drugs) unless approved by prescriber. Some supposed AIDS cures may interfere with drug's effectiveness.
• Advise pregnant HIV-infected women that drug therapy only reduces risk of HIV transmission to neonates. Long-term risks to infants are unknown.
• Advise health care worker considering drug as prophylaxis after occupational exposure (such as after needle-stick injury) that its safety and effectiveness haven't been proven.

✔ Evaluation
• Patient exhibits reduced severity and frequency of symptoms linked to HIV infection.
• Patient doesn't develop complications from therapy.
• Patient and family state understanding of drug therapy.

ziprasidone
(zi-PRAY-si-done)
Geodon

Pharmacologic class: atypical antipsychotic
Therapeutic class: psychotropic
Pregnancy risk category: C

Indications and dosages

▶ **Symptomatic schizophrenia.** *Adults:* Initially, 20 mg P.O. b.i.d. with food. Dosages are highly individualized. Dosage adjustments should occur no sooner than q 2 days, but to allow for lowest possible doses, the interval should be several weeks. Effective dosage range is usually 20 to 80 mg b.i.d. Maximum recommended dosage is 100 mg b.i.d.
▶ **Rapid control of acute agitation in schizophrenic patients.** *Adults:* 10 to 20 mg I.M. as a single dose. Doses of 10 mg may be given q 2 hours; doses of 20 mg may be given q 4 hours. Maximum cumulative dose is 40 mg daily.
▶ **Acute bipolar mania, including manic and mixed episodes, with or without psychotic features.** *Adults:* 40 mg P.O. b.i.d. on day 1. Increase to 60 or 80 mg P.O. b.i.d. on day 2 with subsequent adjustments based on patient response within the range of 40 to 80 mg b.i.d. Give with food.

Contraindications and cautions

• Contraindicated in patients hypersensitive to the drug or any of its components. Also contraindicated in patients taking drugs that prolong QT interval and in those who have a QTc interval longer than 500 msec. Contraindicated in patients with a history of QT-interval prolongation, congenital QT-interval syndrome, recent MI, and uncompensated heart failure.
• Use cautiously in patients with acute diarrhea and in patients with a history of bradycardia, hypokalemia, seizures, aspiration pneumonia, or hypomagnesemia.
• Give I.M. ziprasidone with caution to patients with impaired renal function.
⚖ **Lifespan:** In pregnant women, use only if benefits outweigh risks. Breast-feeding women should stop breast-feeding or shouldn't use the drug. In children, safety and effectiveness haven't been established. In the elderly, safety and effectiveness of I.M. use haven't been established.

Adverse reactions

P.O. use
CNS: dystonia.
CV: tachycardia.
EENT: abnormal vision.
Musculoskeletal: myalgia.
Respiratory: cough.
Skin: rash.
I.M. use
CNS: speech disorders.
CV: vasodilation.
GU: priapism.
Musculoskeletal: back pain.

Z

Skin: sweating.
Other: flulike syndrome, tooth disorder.
Both routes
CNS: *neuroleptic malignant syndrome, somno-lence,* akathisia, dizziness, extrapyramidal symptoms, hypertonia, asthenia; *headache, dizziness,* anxiety, insomnia, agitation, cog-wheel rigidity, paresthesia, personality disorder, psychosis, *suicide attempt.*
CV: orthostatic hypotension; hypertension, *bradycardia.*
EENT: rhinitis.
GI: *nausea,* constipation, dyspepsia, diarrhea, dry mouth, anorexia, abdominal pain, *rectal hemorrhage,* vomiting, dyspepsia.
GU: dysmenorrhea.
Metabolic: hyperglycemia.
Skin: injection site pain, furunculosis.

Interactions

Drug-drug. *Antihypertensives:* May enhance hypotensive effects. Monitor blood pressure.
Carbamazepine: May decrease levels of ziprasi-done. Higher doses of ziprasidone may be need-ed to achieve desired effect.
Drugs that increase dopamine level, such as lev-odopa and dopamine agonists: May have antag-onistic effect on ziprasidone. Use together cau-tiously.
Drugs that lower potassium and magnesium lev-els, such as diuretics: May increase risk of ar-rhythmias. If giving together, monitor potassium and magnesium levels.
Drugs that prolong QT interval, including ar-senic trioxide, chlorpromazine, dofetilide, dolasetron mesylate, droperidol, gatifloxacin, halofantrine, levomethadyl acetate, mefloquine, mesoridazine, moxifloxacin, pentamidine, pi-mozide, probucol, quinidine, sotalol, sparflox-acin, tacrolimus, thioridazine, or other class IA and III antiarrhythmics: May increase risk of ar-rhythmias when used together. Don't give to-gether.
Itraconazole, ketoconazole: May increase ziprasidone level. Lower doses of ziprasidone may be needed to achieve desired effect.

Effects on lab test results

● May increase glucose level.

Pharmacokinetics

Absorption: Doubled when taken with food, which is recommended. Level peaks in about 6 to 8 hours.
Distribution: Highly protein-bound.
Metabolism: Hepatic metabolism; no active metabolites. Less than one-third of the drug is metabolized through the CYP system, mainly via CYP 3A4 and partly via CYP 1A2.
Excretion: Unknown. *Half-life:* 2¼ to 7 hours.

Route	Onset	Peak	Duration
P.O.	1–3 days	6–8 hr	12 hr
I.M.	Unknown	1 hr	Unknown

Action

Chemical effect: May work by antagonizing dopamine and serotonin, the neurotransmitters usually targeted for treatment of positive and negative symptoms of schizophrenia. Blocking these neurotransmitters allows symptomatic im-provement with minimal adverse effects in the extrapyramidal system.
Therapeutic effect: Relieves psychotic signs and symptoms of schizophrenia.

Available forms

Capsules: 20 mg, 40 mg, 60 mg, 80 mg
Injection: 20-mg/ml single-dose vials (after re-constitution)

NURSING PROCESS

℞ Assessment

● Assess patient's condition before starting ther-apy and regularly thereafter to monitor the drug's effectiveness.
● Assess and monitor patient who experiences dizziness, palpitations, or syncope.
● Drug may prolong QT interval. Other antipsy-chotics should be considered in patient with a history of QT-interval prolongation, acute MI, congenital QT-interval syndrome, and other conditions that place the patient at risk for life-threatening arrhythmias. Don't give other drugs that prolong the QT interval with ziprasidone.
● Patient taking antipsychotics is at risk for de-veloping neuroleptic malignant syndrome or tar-dive dyskinesia.
● Electrolyte disturbances, such as hypokalemia or hypomagnesemia, increase the risk of ar-rhythmias. Before starting therapy, monitor

potassium and magnesium levels and correct imbalances.
• Assess patient's and family's knowledge of drug therapy.

⊞ **Nursing diagnoses**
• Disturbed thought processes related to underlying condition
• Risk for fall related to adverse CNS effects of drug
• Deficient knowledge related to ziprasidone therapy

▶ **Planning and implementation**
• Don't adjust dosage sooner than q 2 days. Longer intervals may be needed because symptoms may take 4 to 6 weeks to respond.
• Monitor patient for prolonged QT interval during therapy. Further monitor patient with symptoms of arrhythmias. If QTc interval is greater than 500 msec, stop drug.
⊛ **ALERT:** Hyperglycemia may occur in patient taking drug. Regularly monitor patient with diabetes. Patient with risk factors for diabetes should undergo fasting blood glucose testing at baseline and periodically during therapy. Monitor every patient for symptoms of hyperglycemia including polydipsia, polyuria, polyphagia, and weakness; if symptoms develop, perform fasting blood glucose testing. Hyperglycemia may be reversible when antipsychotic is stopped.
• Immediately treat patient with symptoms of neuroleptic malignant syndrome, which can be life-threatening.
• Monitor patient for tardive dyskinesia.
• If long-term ziprasidone therapy is needed, switch to P.O. route as soon as possible. Effect of I.M. administration for more than 3 consecutive days isn't known.
• Don't give drug I.M. to schizophrenic patient already taking ziprasidone P.O.
• Give oral drug with food, which increases the effect.
• For I.M. use, add 1.2 ml of sterile water for injection to vial and shake vigorously until entire drug is dissolved.
• Don't mix I.M. injection with any other product besides sterile water for injection.
• Inspect for particulate matter and discoloration before administration, whenever solution and container permit.

• Store dry form at room temperature. Store reconstituted form for up to 24 hours at room temperature or up to 7 days refrigerated (36° to 46° F [2° to 8° C]). Protect from light.
Patient teaching
• Tell patient to take drug with food.
• Tell patient to immediately report to prescriber symptoms of dizziness, fainting, irregular heart beat, or relevant cardiac problems.
• Advise patient to report to prescriber any recent episodes of diarrhea.
• Advise patient to report to prescriber abnormal movements.
• Tell patient to report to prescriber sudden fever, muscle rigidity, or change in mental status.

⊠ **Evaluation**
• Patient demonstrates reduced psychotic symptoms with drug therapy.
• Patient doesn't fall.
• Patient and family state understanding of drug therapy.

zoledronic acid
(zoe-LEH-druh-nick ASS-id)
Zometa

Pharmacologic class: bisphosphonate
Therapeutic class: antihypercalcemic
Pregnancy risk category: D

Indications and dosages
▶ **Hypercalcemia related to malignancy.**
Adults: 4 mg by I.V. infusion over at least 15 minutes. If albumin-corrected calcium level doesn't return to normal, consider retreatment with 4 mg. Allow at least 7 days to pass before retreatment to allow a full response to the initial dose.
▶ **Multiple myeloma and bone metastases of solid tumors (given with standard antineoplastic therapy). Prostate cancer should have progressed after treatment with at least one hormonal therapy.** *Adults:* 4 mg infused over at least 15 minutes q 3 to 4 weeks. Duration of treatment in studies was 15 months for prostate cancer, 12 months for breast cancer and multiple myeloma, and 9 months for other solid tumors.

Z

⊠ **Adjust-a-dose:** For patients with creatinine clearance of 50 to 60 ml/minute, give 3.5 mg. If clearance is 40 to 49 ml/minute, give 3.3 mg. If clearance is 30 to 39 ml/minute, give 3 mg.

For patients with normal baseline creatinine level but an increase of 0.5 mg/dl during therapy, and in those with abnormal baseline creatinine level who have an increase of 1 mg/dl, withhold drug. Resume treatment only when creatinine level has returned to within 10% of baseline value.

▼ I.V. administration

• Reconstitute by adding 5 ml of sterile water to each vial. Powder must be completely dissolved.
• Withdraw 5 ml for 4 mg of drug and mix in 100 ml of normal saline solution or D₅W.
• To withdraw the appropriate dose for a patient with creatinine clearance 60 ml/minute or less: withdraw 4.4 ml for the 3.5 mg dose, 4.1 ml for the 3.3 mg dose, and 3.8 ml for the 3 mg dose.
• Inspect solution for particulate matter and discoloration before giving it.
• The drug must be given as an I.V. infusion over at least 15 minutes. Give drug as a single I.V. solution in a line separate from all other drugs.
• If not used immediately after reconstitution, solution must be refrigerated and given within 24 hours.

⊗ **Incompatibilities**
Other I.V. drugs; solutions that contain calcium, such as lactated Ringer's solution.

Contraindications and cautions

• Contraindicated in patients with clinically significant hypersensitivity to drug, other bisphosphonates, or ingredients in formulation.
• Not recommended in patients with hypercalcemia of malignancy with creatinine greater than 4.5 mg/dl. Not recommended in patients with bone metastases with creatinine greater than 3.0 mg/dl.
• Use cautiously in patients with aspirin-sensitive asthma because other bisphosphonates may cause bronchoconstriction in these patients.
⚕ **Lifespan:** In pregnant women, don't use. Women of childbearing age should avoid becoming pregnant. In breast-feeding women, use cautiously; it's unknown if the drug appears in breast milk. In children, safety and effectiveness

haven't been established. In elderly patients, monitor renal function.

Adverse reactions

Hypercalcemia
CNS: *headache,* somnolence, anxiety, confusion, agitation, *insomnia, depression, dizziness,* fever.
CV: hypotension.
GI: nausea, constipation, diarrhea, abdominal pain, vomiting, anorexia, dysphagia.
GU: *renal failure,* UTI, candidiasis.
Hematologic: anemia, *granulocytopenia, thrombocytopenia, pancytopenia.*
Metabolic: dehydration.
Musculoskeletal: *skeletal pain,* arthralgia, osteonecrosis of the jaw.
Respiratory: *dyspnea, cough,* pleural effusion.
Other: PROGRESSION OF CANCER, infection.
Bone metastases
CNS: *headache, anxiety, insomnia, depression, paresthesia, hypoesthesia,* fatigue, weakness, *dizziness,* fever.
CV: hypotension, leg edema.
GI: *nausea, constipation, diarrhea, abdominal pain, vomiting, anorexia, increased appetite.*
GU: *UTI, renal failure.*
Hematologic: anemia, *neutropenia.*
Metabolic: dehydration, weight loss.
Musculoskeletal: *skeletal pain, arthralgia, myalgia, back pain,* osteonecrosis of the jaw.
Respiratory: *dyspnea, cough.*
Skin: alopecia, dermatitis.
Other: PROGRESSION OF CANCER, rigors, infection.

Interactions

Drug-drug. *Aminoglycosides, loop diuretics:* May have additive effects to lower calcium level. Give together cautiously, and monitor calcium level.
Thalidomide: May increase risk of renal dysfunction in multiple myeloma patients. Use together cautiously.

Effects on lab test results

• May increase creatinine level. May decrease calcium, phosphorus, magnesium, potassium, and hemoglobin levels and hematocrit.
• May decrease RBC, WBC, and platelet counts.

Pharmacokinetics

Absorption: Administered I.V.
Distribution: Protein-binding of about 22%.
Postinfusion decline of level is consistent with a triphasic process: Low level observed up to 28 days after a dose.
Metabolism: Doesn't inhibit CYP enzymes or undergo biotransformation in vivo.
Excretion: Primarily via the kidneys. *Half-life:* Alpha is 0.23 hours; beta is 1.75 hours for early distribution. *Terminal half-life:* 167 hours.

Route	Onset	Peak	Duration
I.V.	Unknown	Unknown	7–28 days

Action

Chemical effect: Inhibits bone resorption, probably by inhibiting osteoclast activity and osteoclastic resorption of mineralized bone and cartilage, decreasing calcium release induced by the stimulatory factors produced by tumors.
Therapeutic effect: Lowers calcium level in malignant disease.

Available forms

Injection: 4 mg zoledronic acid, 220 mg mannitol, and 24 mg sodium citrate

NURSING PROCESS

▧ Assessment

• Assess patient's condition before starting therapy and regularly thereafter to monitor the drug's effectiveness.
• Assess kidney function before and during therapy because drug is excreted mainly via the kidneys. The risk of adverse reactions may be greater in a patient with renal impairment. If patient has renal impairment, give drug only if benefits outweigh risks, and at a lower dose.
• Measure creatinine level before each dose.
• Make sure patient is adequately hydrated before giving drug; urine output should be about 2 L daily.
• Assess patient's dental health before starting therapy. Make sure patient has had a dental exam with appropriate preventive dentistry before being treated with bisphosphonates, especially patients with cancer, those receiving chemotherapy or corticosteroids, and those with poor oral hygiene.
• Assess patient's and family's knowledge of drug therapy.

▧ Nursing diagnoses

• Ineffective protection related to adverse hematologic effects
• Ineffective health maintenance related to underlying condition
• Deficient knowledge related to drug therapy

▷ Planning and implementation

ⓈALERT: A significant decline in renal function could progress to renal failure; single doses shouldn't exceed 4 mg, and infusion should last at least 15 minutes.
ⓈALERT: After giving drug, carefully monitor renal function and calcium, phosphate, magnesium, and creatinine levels.
• Other bisphosphonates have been linked to bronchoconstriction in patients with asthma and aspirin sensitivity.
• Give patient an oral calcium supplement of 500 mg and a multiple vitamin containing 400 international units of vitamin D daily.
Patient teaching
• Review the use and administration of drug with patient and family.
• Instruct patient to report adverse effects promptly.
• Explain the importance of periodic laboratory tests to monitor therapy and renal function.
• Advise patient to notify prescriber if she is pregnant.

▧ Evaluation

• Patient has no adverse hematologic reactions.
• Patient shows improvement in condition.
• Patient and family state understanding of drug therapy.

zolmitriptan
(zohl-muh-TRIP-tan)
Zomig, Zomig-ZMT

Pharmacologic class: selective 5-hydroxytryptamine (5-HT$_1$) receptor agonist
Therapeutic class: antimigraine drug
Pregnancy risk category: C

Indications and dosages

▶ **Acute migraine headache.** *Adults:* Initially, 2.5 mg or less P.O. increased to 5 mg per dose, p.r.n. If headache returns after initial dose, second dose may be given after 2 hours. Maxi-

Z

mum dose is 10 mg in 24-hour period. Or, give 2.5 mg P.O. of orally disintegrating tablets; don't break tablets in half. Or, 5 mg (one nasal spray) into one nostril. If headache returns after initial dose, a second dose may be given after 2 hours. Maximum dose is 10 mg in 24-hour period.

◪ **Adjust-a-dose:** For patients with liver disease, use doses lower than 2.5 mg. Also, don't use orally disintegrating tablets; they shouldn't be split. Avoid use of nasal spray because doses lower than 5 mg can't be given.

Contraindications and cautions

• Contraindicated in patients hypersensitive to the drug or any of its components, in those with uncontrolled hypertension, and in those with symptoms or findings consistent with ischemic heart disease (angina pectoris, history of MI or documented silent ischemia), coronary artery vasospasm (including Prinzmetal's variant angina), or other significant heart disease.
• Avoid use within 24 hours of other 5-HT$_1$ agonists or drugs containing ergot, or within 2 weeks of stopping MAO inhibitor therapy. Also avoid use in patients with hemiplegic or basilar migraine.
• Use cautiously in patients with liver disease and in patients who may be at risk for coronary artery disease, such as postmenopausal women, men older than age 40, or patients with hypertension, hypercholesterolemia, obesity, diabetes, smoking, or family history of coronary artery disease.

⚜ **Lifespan:** In pregnant women, use cautiously. In breast-feeding women, use cautiously; it's unknown if the drug appears in breast milk. In children, safety and effectiveness haven't been established.

Adverse reactions

CNS: somnolence, vertigo, *dizziness,* hypesthesia, paresthesia, asthenia, pain.
CV: palpitations, *coronary artery vasospasm, transient myocardial ischemia, MI, ventricular tachycardia, ventricular fibrillation;* pain, tightness, pressure, or heaviness in chest.
EENT: pain, tightness, or pressure in the neck, throat, or jaw.
GI: dry mouth, dyspepsia, dysphagia, nausea.
Musculoskeletal: myalgia, myasthenia.
Skin: sweating.
Other: warm or cold sensations.

Interactions

Drug-drug. *Cimetidine:* May double half-life of zolmitriptan. Monitor patient closely.
Ergot-containing drugs, serotonin$_{1B/1D}$ agonists: May cause additive effects. Avoid use within 24 hours of almotriptan.
Hormonal contraceptives: May increase levels of zolmitriptan. Monitor patient closely.
MAO inhibitors: May increase levels of zolmitriptan. Avoid use of drug within 2 weeks of stopping MAO inhibitor therapy.
SSRIs: May cause additive serotonin effects, resulting in weakness, hyperreflexia, or incoordination. If given together, monitor patient closely.

Effects on lab test results

• May increase glucose level.

Pharmacokinetics

Absorption: Well absorbed following P.O. administration, with an absolute bioavailability of 40%.
Distribution: 25% bound to protein.
Metabolism: Converted to active N-desmethyl metabolite.
Excretion: About 65% of dose is recovered in urine (8% unchanged) and 30% in feces. *Half-life:* 3 hours.

Route	Onset	Peak	Duration
P.O.	Unknown	2 hr	3 hr
P.O. orally disintegrating	Unknown	2 hr	Unknown
Nasal spray	5 min	3 hr	Unknown

Action

Chemical effect: Selective serotonin receptor agonist causes constriction of cranial blood vessels and inhibits proinflammatory neuropeptide release.
Therapeutic effect: Relieves migraine headache pain.

Available forms

Nasal spray: 5 mg
Tablets: 2.5 mg, 5 mg
Tablets (orally disintegrating): 2.5 mg, 5 mg

NURSING PROCESS

⚕ Assessment
• Assess patient's history of migraine headaches before starting therapy and regularly thereafter to monitor the drug's effectiveness.
• Assess patient for history of coronary artery disease, hypertension, arrhythmias, or presence of risk factors for coronary artery disease.
• Monitor liver function test results before starting drug therapy, and report abnormalities.
• Use drug only when a clear diagnosis of migraine has been established.
• Assess patient's and family's knowledge of drug therapy.

⚙ Nursing diagnoses
• Acute pain related to presence of migraine headache
• Impaired cardiopulmonary tissue perfusion related to drug-induced adverse cardiac events
• Deficient knowledge related to drug therapy

❯ Planning and implementation
• Use a lower dose in a patient with moderate to severe hepatic impairment; don't give orally disintegrating tablets because they can't be split.
• Don't give drug to prevent migraine headaches or to treat hemiplegic migraines, basilar migraines, or cluster headaches.
• ⏺ ALERT: Don't give drug within 24 hours of ergot-containing drugs or within 2 weeks of MAO inhibitor.
Patient teaching
• Tell patient that drug is intended to relieve the symptoms of migraines, not to prevent them.
• Advise patient to take drug as prescribed. Caution against taking a second dose unless instructed by prescriber. Tell patient that if a second dose is indicated and permitted, he should take it at least 2 hours after initial dose.
• Advise patient to immediately report pain or tightness in chest or throat, heart throbbing, rash, skin lumps, or swelling of face, lips, or eyelids.
• Tell woman not to take drug if she's planning or suspects a pregnancy.
• Instruct patient to remove the orally disintegrating tablet from the blister pack just before use and to let it dissolve on the tongue.
• Advise patient not to break the orally disintegrating tablets in half.

☑ Evaluation
• Patient has relief from migraine headache.
• Patient doesn't experience pain or tightness in the chest or throat, arrhythmias, increases in blood pressure, or MI.
• Patient and family state understanding of drug therapy.

zolpidem tartrate
(ZOHL-peh-dim TAR-trayt)
Ambien✍, Ambien CR

Pharmacologic class: imidazopyridine
Therapeutic class: hypnotic
Pregnancy risk category: B
Controlled substance schedule: IV

Indications and dosages
❯ **Short-term management of insomnia.**
Adults: 10 mg P.O. (immediate release) or 12.5 mg P.O. (extended release) immediately before h.s.
⬡ **Adjust-a-dose:** *Elderly patients:* 5 mg P.O. (immediate release) or 6.25 mg (extended release) immediately before h.s. Maximum daily dose is 10 mg (immediate release) or 6.25 mg (extended release).
Debilitated patients and those with hepatic insufficiency: 5 mg P.O. immediately before h.s. Maximum daily dose is 10 mg. If using the extended release tablet, maximum daily dose is 6.25 mg.

Contraindications and cautions
• Use cautiously in patients with conditions that could affect metabolism or hemodynamic responses and in those with compromised respiratory status, because hypnotics may depress respiratory drive. Also use cautiously in patients with depression or history of alcohol or drug abuse.
• ⚘ Lifespan: In pregnant women, use cautiously. In breast-feeding women, drug isn't recommended. In children, safety and effectiveness haven't been established.

Adverse reactions
CNS: daytime drowsiness, light-headedness, abnormal dreams, amnesia, dizziness, *headache,* hangover effect, sleep disorder, lethargy, depression.

Z

CV: palpitations.
EENT: sinusitis, pharyngitis.
GI: nausea, vomiting, diarrhea, dyspepsia, constipation, abdominal pain, dry mouth.
Musculoskeletal: back or chest pain, myalgia, arthralgia.
Skin: rash.
Other: flulike syndrome, hypersensitivity reactions.

Interactions

Drug-drug. *CNS depressants:* May increase CNS depression. Use together cautiously.
Drug-food. *Any food:* May decrease rate and extent of absorption. Tell patient to take drug on an empty stomach.
Drug-lifestyle. *Alcohol use:* May cause excessive CNS depression. Discourage use together.

Effects on lab test results

None reported.

Pharmacokinetics

Absorption: Rapid. Food delays drug absorption.
Distribution: Protein-binding is about 92.5%.
Metabolism: In liver.
Excretion: Primarily in urine. *Half-life:* 2½ hours.

Route	Onset	Peak	Duration
P.O.	Rapid	30 min–2 hr	Unknown

Action

Chemical effect: Interacts with one of three identified GABA and benzodiazepine receptor complexes but isn't a benzodiazepine. Exhibits hypnotic activity but has no muscle relaxant or anticonvulsant properties.
Therapeutic effect: Promotes sleep.

Available forms

Tablets: 5 mg, 10 mg
Extended-release tablets: 6.25 mg, 12.5 mg

NURSING PROCESS

Assessment

- Assess patient's condition before starting therapy and regularly thereafter to monitor the drug's effectiveness.
- Be alert for adverse reactions and drug interactions.
- Assess patient's and family's knowledge of drug therapy.

Nursing diagnoses

- Disturbed sleep pattern related to presence of insomnia
- Risk for injury related to drug-induced adverse CNS reactions
- Deficient knowledge related to drug therapy

Planning and implementation

- Drug has a rapid onset of action; give when patient is ready to sleep.
- Use hypnotics only for short-term management of insomnia, usually 7 to 10 days. Persistent insomnia may indicate primary psychiatric or medical disorder.
- Because most adverse reactions are dose-related, use smallest effective dose in all patients, especially those who are elderly or debilitated.
- Give drug at least 1 hour before meals or 2 hours after meals.

ALERT: Don't confuse Ambien with Amen.

Patient teaching

- Tell patient to take drug immediately before going to bed.
- For faster onset, instruct patient not to take drug with or immediately after a meal. Food decreases drug's absorption.

ALERT: Tell patient not to crush, chew, or divide the extended-release tablets.

- Warn patient about performing activities that require mental alertness or physical coordination. For inpatient, supervise walking and raise bed rails, particularly for geriatric patient.

Evaluation

- Patient states that drug effectively promotes sleep.
- Patient doesn't experience injury from adverse CNS reactions.
- Patient and family state understanding of drug therapy.

Herbal
Medicines

aloe

Reported uses

• Externally as a topical gel for minor burns, sunburn, cuts, frostbite, skin irritation, and other wounds and abrasions
• Amenorrhea, asthma, colds, seizures, bleeding, and ulcers. Preparations also used to treat acne, AIDS, arthritis, blindness, bursitis, cancer, colitis, depression, diabetes, glaucoma, hemorrhoids, multiple sclerosis, peptic ulcers, and varicose veins

Cautions

• External preparations shouldn't be used by people hypersensitive to herb or those with a history of allergic reactions to plants in the Liliaceae family (such as garlic, onions, and tulips).
• Aloe shouldn't be taken orally by people with cardiac or kidney disease (because of risk of hypokalemia and disturbance of cardiac rhythm), by those with intestinal obstruction, and by those with Crohn's disease or ulcerative colitis.
⚘ Lifespan: Pregnant women, breast-feeding women, and children shouldn't use.

Adverse reactions

CV: *arrhythmias.*
GI: painful intestinal spasms, damage to intestinal mucosa, harmless brown discoloration of intestinal mucous membranes, *severe hemorrhagic diarrhea.*
GU: *kidney damage,* red discoloration of urine, *reflex stimulation of uterine musculature causing miscarriage or premature birth.*
Metabolic: fluid and electrolyte loss, hypokalemia.
Musculoskeletal: muscle weakness, accelerated bone deterioration.
Skin: contact dermatitis, delayed healing of deep wounds.

Interactions

Herb-drug. *Antiarrhythmics, digoxin:* Oral form may lead to toxic reaction. Monitor patient closely.
Corticosteroids, diuretics: Increases potassium loss. Monitor patient for signs of hypokalemia.

Disulfiram: Tincture contains alcohol and could precipitate a disulfiram reaction. Discourage use together.
Herb-herb. *Licorice:* Increases risk of potassium deficiency. Discourage use together.

angelica

Reported uses

• Gynecologic disorders, postmenopausal symptoms, menstrual discomfort, anemia, and mild peptic discomfort, such as GI spasms, flatulence, bloating, colic, and loss of appetite; to strengthen the heart; to improve circulation in the limbs; and to relieve osteoporosis, hay fever, cough, asthma, bronchitis, acne, and eczema

Cautions

• People with diabetes should use caution because various species of this plant contain polysaccharides that may disrupt glucose control.
⚘ Lifespan: Pregnant or breast-feeding women shouldn't use angelica because it may have stimulant effects on the uterus.

Adverse reactions

CV: hypotension.
Skin: photodermatitis, phototoxicity.

Interactions

Herb-drug. *Antacids, H_2-receptor antagonists, proton pump inhibitors, sucralfate:* Herb may increase acid production in the stomach and may interfere with absorption of these drugs. Discourage use together.
Anticoagulants: Excessive amounts of herb may potentiate anticoagulant effects. Monitor patient for bleeding.
Herb-lifestyle. *Sun exposure:* Photosensitivity reaction may occur. Advise a person taking angelica to avoid unprotected or prolonged exposure to sunlight.

bilberry

Reported uses

• Visual and circulatory problems, glaucoma, cataracts, diabetic retinopathy, macular degeneration, varicose veins, and hemorrhoids
• To improve night vision

Cautions

• Urge caution in those taking anticoagulants. Herb may be unsuitable for those with a bleeding disorder.
≋ Lifespan: Pregnant and breast-feeding women should avoid herb.

Adverse reactions

Other: *toxic reaction.*

Interactions

Herb-drug. *Anticoagulants, antiplatelets:* Inhibits platelet aggregation, possibly increasing the risk of bleeding. Monitor patient.
Disulfiram: May cause disulfiram reaction if herbal preparation contains alcohol. Advise patient to avoid use together.

capsicum

Reported uses

• Bowel disorders, chronic laryngitis, and peripheral vascular disease
• Counterirritants and external analgesics
• Topical preparation FDA-approved for temporary relief of pain from rheumatoid arthritis, osteoarthritis, postherpetic neuralgia (shingles), and diabetic neuropathy.
• FDA-tested for psoriasis, intractable pruritus, vitiligo, phantom limb pain, mastectomy pain, Guillain-Barré syndrome, neurogenic bladder, vulvar vestibulitis, apocrine chromhidrosis, and reflex sympathetic dystrophy
• In personal defense sprays and for refractory pruritus and pruritus caused by renal failure

Cautions

• People hypersensitive to herb or chili pepper products should avoid capsicum. Those with irritable bowel syndrome should avoid it because capsicum has irritant and peristaltic effects.
• Those with asthma who use capsicum may experience more bronchospasms.
≋ Lifespan: Pregnant women should avoid capsicum because of possible uterine stimulant effects.

Adverse reactions

EENT: blepharospasm, extreme burning pain, lacrimation, conjunctival edema, hyperemia, burning pain in nose, sneezing, serous discharge.
GI: oral burning, diarrhea, gingival irritation, bleeding gums.
Respiratory: *bronchospasm,* cough, retrosternal discomfort.
Skin: transient skin irritation, itching, stinging, erythema without vesicular eruption, contact dermatitis.

Interactions

Herb-drug. *ACE inhibitors:* Increases risk of cough when applied topically. Monitor patient closely.
Anticoagulants: May alter anticoagulant effects. Monitor PT and INR closely; tell patient to avoid use together.
Antiplatelets, heparin and low–molecular-weight heparin, warfarin: Increases risk of bleeding. Advise patient to avoid use together. If used together, monitor patient for bleeding.
Aspirin, salicylic acid compounds: Reduces bioavailability of these drugs. Discourage use together.
MAO inhibitors: Herb increases catecholamine secretion and increases risk of hypertensive crisis. Discourage use together.
Theophylline: Herb increases theophylline absorption. Discourage use together.
Herb-herb. *Feverfew, garlic, ginger, ginkgo, ginseng:* Increases anticoagulant effects of capsicum, and increases risk of bleeding. Discourage use together. Anyone who uses them together should be monitored closely for bleeding.

cat's claw

Reported uses

• GI problems, including inflammatory bowel disease (Crohn's disease or ulcerative colitis) diverticulitis, gastritis, dysentery, ulcerations and hemorrhoids, and to enhance immunity
• Systemic inflammatory diseases such as arthritis and rheumatism
• By cancer patients for its antimutagenic effects
• With zidovudine to stimulate the immune system by patients with HIV infection
• As a contraceptive

Cautions

• Those who have had transplant surgery, and those who have an autoimmune disease, multiple sclerosis, or tuberculosis should avoid use. Anyone who has a coagulation disorder or takes an anticoagulant should also avoid use.
• People with a history of peptic ulcer disease or gallstones should use caution when taking this herb because it stimulates stomach acid secretion.
⚠ **Lifespan:** Women who are pregnant or breast-feeding shouldn't use this herb.

Adverse reactions

CV: hypotension.

Interactions

Herb-drug. *Antihypertensives:* May potentiate hypotensive effects. Discourage use together.
Immunosuppressants: May counteract therapeutic effects because herb has immunostimulant properties. Discourage use together.
Herb-food. *Food:* May enhance absorption of herb.

chamomile

Reported uses

• Sedation or relaxation (main use)
• Stomach disorders, such as GI spasms and other GI inflammatory conditions
• Insomnia

• Menstrual disorders, migraine, epidermolysis bullosa, eczema, eye irritation, throat discomfort, and hemorrhoids
• As a topical bacteriostat and mouthwash

Cautions

• Probably an abortifacient, and some of its components may have teratogenic effects.
• Urge caution in those hypersensitive to components of volatile oils and in those at risk for contact dermatitis.
• Safety in people with liver or kidney disorders hasn't been established, and they should avoid use.
⚠ **Lifespan:** Discourage use by pregnant or breast-feeding women. Herb shouldn't be given to babies or children younger than age 2.

Adverse reactions

EENT: conjunctivitis, eyelid angioedema.
GI: nausea, vomiting.
Skin: eczema, contact dermatitis.
Other: *anaphylaxis.*

Interactions

Herb-drug. *Anticoagulants:* May potentiate effects. Discourage use together.
Other drugs: Potential for decreased absorption of drugs because of antispasmodic activity of herb in the GI tract. Discourage use together.

echinacea

Reported uses

• As a wound-healing agent for abscesses, burns, eczema, varicose ulcers of the leg, and other skin wounds
• As a nonspecific immunostimulant for the supportive treatment of upper respiratory tract infections, the common cold, and UTIs

Cautions

• Shouldn't be used by anyone with severe illness, such as HIV infection, collagen disease, leukosis, multiple sclerosis, tuberculosis, or autoimmune disease.
⚠ **Lifespan:** Discourage use by pregnant or breast-feeding women because effects of herb are unknown.

*Liquid may contain alcohol.

Adverse reactions

CNS: fever.
GI: nausea, vomiting, unpleasant taste, minor GI symptoms.
GU: diuresis.
Other: tachyphylaxis, allergic reaction in patients allergic to plants belonging to the daisy family.

Interactions

Herb-drug. *Disulfiram, metronidazole:* Herbal products that contain alcohol may cause a disulfiram reaction. Discourage use together.
Immunosuppressants such as cyclosporine: Decreases effectiveness of these drugs. Discourage use together.
Herb-lifestyle. *Alcohol use:* Echinacea preparations containing alcohol may enhance CNS depression. Discourage use together.

eucalyptus

Reported uses

• Internally and externally as an expectorant and for infections and fevers
• Topically to treat sore muscles and rheumatism

Cautions

• People who have had an allergic reaction to eucalyptus or its vapors should avoid use.
• Those who have liver disease or intestinal tract inflammation shouldn't use.
• Essential oil preparations shouldn't be applied to an infant's or child's face because of risk of severe bronchial spasm.
⚠ **Lifespan:** Pregnant and breast-feeding women shouldn't use.

Adverse reactions

CNS: delirium, dizziness, *seizures.*
EENT: miosis.
GI: epigastric burning, nausea, vomiting.
Musculoskeletal: muscular weakness.
Respiratory: *asthma-like attacks.*

Interactions

Herb-drug. *Antidiabetics:* Enhances effects. Discourage use together.

Other drugs: Eucalyptus oil induces detoxication enzyme systems in the liver and may affect any drug metabolized in liver. Watch for intended drug effects and toxic reactions.
Herb-herb. *Other herbs that cause hypoglycemia (basil, glucomannan, Queen Anne's lace):* Decreases glucose level. Advise caution.

fennel

Reported uses

• To increase milk secretion, promote menses, facilitate birth, and increase libido
• As an expectorant to manage cough and bronchitis
• Mild spastic disorders of the GI tract, feelings of fullness, and flatulence
• Upper respiratory tract infections in children (syrup)

Cautions

• Should be used cutiously by people allergic to other members of the Umbelliferae family, such as celery, carrots, or mugwort.
• Discourage use in those with a history of seizures.
⚠ **Lifespan:** In pregnant women, discourage use.

Adverse reactions

CNS: *seizures,* hallucinations.
GI: nausea, vomiting.
Respiratory: *pulmonary edema.*
Skin: photodermatitis, contact dermatitis.
Other: allergic reaction.

Interactions

Herb-drug. *Anticonvulsants, drugs that lower the seizure threshold:* Increases risk of seizure. Monitor patient very closely.
Herb-lifestyle. *Sun exposure:* Increases risk of photosensitivity reactions. Person taking fennel should wear protective clothing and sunscreen and should limit exposure to direct sunlight.

Bold italic type indicates that reaction may be life-threatening.

feverfew

Reported uses

- As an antipyretic
- Psoriasis, toothache, insect bites, rheumatism, asthma, stomachache, and menstrual problems
- Migraine prophylaxis

Cautions

- Shouldn't be taken internally by anyone allergic to members of the daisy, or Asteraceae, family—including yarrow, southernwood, wormwood, chamomile, marigold, goldenrod, coltsfoot, and dandelion—or anyone who has had previous reaction to herb.
- Those taking anticoagulants such as warfarin and heparin should use herb cautiously.
- ☀ **Lifespan:** Pregnant women shouldn't use because of herb's potential abortifacient properties. Breast-feeding women shouldn't use. Children shouldn't use.

Adverse reactions

CNS: dizziness.
CV: tachycardia.
GI: GI upset, mouth ulcerations.
Skin: contact dermatitis.

Interactions

Herb-drug. *Anticoagulants, antiplatelet drugs including aspirin and thrombolytics:* Herb inhibits prostaglandin synthesis and platelet aggregation. Monitor patient for increased bleeding.

flax

Reported uses

- Constipation, functional disorders of the colon resulting from laxative abuse, irritable bowel syndrome, and diverticulitis
- As a supplement to decrease the risk of hypercholesterolemia and atherosclerosis
- As a poultice for areas of local inflammation

Cautions

- People with an ileus or esophageal stricture, and those experiencing an acute inflammatory illness of the GI tract, should avoid use.
- ☀ **Lifespan:** Pregnant and breast-feeding women, and those planning to become pregnant shouldn't use.

Adverse reactions

GI: diarrhea, flatulence, nausea.

Interactions

Herb-drug. *Laxatives, stool softeners:* Possible increase in laxative actions of herb. Discourage use together.
Oral drugs: Because of herb's fibrous content and binding potential, drug absorption may be altered or prevented. Advise patient to avoid taking herb within 2 hours of a drug.

garlic

Reported uses

- To decrease total cholesterol level, decrease triglyceride level, and increase HDL level
- To help prevent atherosclerosis because of its effect on blood pressure and platelet aggregation
- To decrease the risk of cancer, especially cancer of the GI tract; of stroke; and of MI
- Cough, colds, fevers, and sore throats
- Asthma, diabetes, inflammation, heavy metal poisoning, constipation, and athlete's foot
- As an antimicrobial and to reduce symptoms in patients with AIDS

Cautions

- Shouldn't be used by anyone sensitive to garlic or other members of the Liliaceae family or by those with GI disorders, such as peptic ulcer or reflux disease.
- ☀ **Lifespan:** Herb shouldn't be used by pregnant women because it has oxytocic effects.

Adverse reactions

CNS: dizziness.
GI: halitosis; irritation of mouth, esophagus, and stomach; nausea; vomiting.

Hematologic: decreased hemoglobin production and lysis of RBCs (with long-term use or excessive amounts).
Skin: contact dermatitis, diaphoresis.
Other: allergic reaction, *anaphylaxis,* garlic odor.

Interactions

Herb-drug. *Anticoagulants, NSAIDs, prostacyclin:* May increase bleeding time. Discourage use together.
Antidiabetics: Glucose level may be decreased further. Advise caution if using together, and tell patient to monitor glucose level closely.
Drugs metabolized by the enzyme CYP 2E1 (such as acetaminophen): Decreases metabolism of these drugs. Monitor patient for therapeutic effects and toxic reaction.
Herb-herb. *Herbs with anticoagulant effects:* Increases bleeding time. Discourage use together.
Herbs with antihyperglycemic effects: Glucose level may be further decreased. Advise caution and close monitoring of glucose level.

ginger

Reported uses

● As an antiemetic, GI protectant, anti-inflammatory for arthritis treatment, CV stimulant, antitumor agent, antioxidant, and as therapy for microbial and parasitic infestations
● Seasickness, morning or motion sickness, and postoperative nausea and vomiting, and to provide relief from pain and swelling caused by rheumatoid arthritis, osteoarthritis, or muscular discomfort

Cautions

● People with gallstones or with an allergy to herb should avoid use.
● Those with bleeding disorders should avoid using large amounts of herb.
● Anyone taking a CNS depressant or an antiarrhythmic should use ginger cautiously.

⚘ **Lifespan:** Pregnant women should avoid using large amounts of herb.

Adverse reactions

CNS: CNS depression.
CV: *arrhythmias,* increased bleeding time.
GI: heartburn.

Interactions

Herb-drug. *Anticoagulants and other drugs that can increase bleeding time:* May further increase bleeding time. Discourage use together.
Herb-herb. *Herbs that may increase bleeding time:* May further increase bleeding time. Discourage use together.

ginkgo

Reported uses

● Primarily to manage cerebral insufficiency, dementia, and circulatory disorders such as intermittent claudication
● Headaches, asthma, colitis, impotence, depression, altitude sickness, tinnitus, cochlear deafness, vertigo, premenstrual syndrome, macular degeneration, diabetic retinopathy, and allergies
● As an adjunctive treatment for pancreatic cancer and schizophrenia
● In addition to physical therapy for Fontaine stage IIIB peripheral arterial disease to decrease pain during ambulation with a minimum of 6 weeks of treatment

Cautions

● People with a history of an allergic reaction to ginkgo or any of its components and those with increased risk of intracranial hemorrhage (hypertension, diabetes) should avoid use.
● Anyone taking an antiplatelet or an anticoagulant should avoid use because of the increased risk of bleeding.
● Herb should be avoided before surgery.
⚘ **Lifespan:** Pregnant women shouldn't use.

Adverse reactions

CNS: headache, *seizures, subarachnoid hemorrhage.*
GI: diarrhea, flatulence, nausea, vomiting.

Bold italic type indicates that reaction may be life-threatening.

Skin: contact hypersensitivity reaction, dermatitis.

Interactions

Herb-drug. *Anticoagulants, antiplatelets, high-dose vitamin E:* May increase the risk of bleeding. Discourage use together.
MAO inhibitors: Theoretically, herb can potentiate the activity of these drugs. Advise patient to stop taking herb.
SSRIs: Herb extracts may reverse the sexual dysfunction caused by these drugs. Urge patient to consult prescriber before using together.
Warfarin: Possibly increases INR when taken together. Monitor INR.
Herb-herb. *Garlic and other herbs that increase bleeding time:* Potentiates anticoagulant effects. Advise caution.

ginseng

Reported uses

• To minimize or reduce the activity of the thymus gland
• As a sedative, demulcent (soothes irritated or inflamed internal tissues or organs), aphrodisiac, antidepressant, sleep aid, and diuretic
• To improve stamina, concentration, healing, stress resistance, vigilance, and work efficiency and to improve well-being in elderly people with debilitated or degenerative conditions
• To decrease fasting glucose and hemoglobin A1c levels and for hyperlipidemia, hepatic dysfunction, and impaired cognitive function

Cautions

• Should be used cautiously by anyone with CV disease, hypertension, hypotension, or diabetes, and by those receiving steroid therapy.
☙ Lifespan: In pregnant or breast-feeding women, discourage use; effects are unknown.

Adverse reactions

CNS: headache, insomnia, nervousness.
CV: chest pain, palpitations, hypertension.
EENT: epistaxis.
GI: diarrhea, nausea, vomiting.
GU: impotence, vaginal bleeding.

Skin: pruritus, skin eruptions (with ginseng abuse).
Other: breast pain.

Interactions

Herb-drug. *Anticoagulants, antiplatelet drugs:* May decrease the effects of these drugs. Monitor PT and INR.
Antidiabetics, insulin: Increases hypoglycemic effects. Monitor glucose level.
Drugs metabolized by CYP 3A4: Herb may inhibit this enzyme system. Monitor patient for clinical effects and toxicity.
Phenelzine, other MAO inhibitors: May cause headache, irritability, visual hallucinations, and other interactions. Discourage use together.
Warfarin: Herb may decrease drug effect. Discourage using herb.

goldenseal

Reported uses

• GI disorders, gastritis, peptic ulceration, anorexia, postpartum hemorrhage, dysmenorrhea, eczema, pruritus, tuberculosis, cancer, mouth ulcerations, otorrhea, tinnitus, and conjunctivitis
• As a wound antiseptic, diuretic, laxative, and anti-inflammatory agent
• To shorten the duration of acute *Vibrio cholera* diarrhea and diarrhea caused by some species of *Giardia, Salmonella, Shigella,* and some Enterobacteriaceae
• To improve biliary secretion and function in hepatic cirrhosis

Cautions

• People with hypertension, heart failure, or arrhythmias, or severe renal or hepatic disease should avoid use.
☙ Lifespan: Pregnant or breast-feeding women shouldn't use. Infants shouldn't use.

Adverse reactions

CNS: sedation, reduced mental alertness, hallucinations, delirium, paresthesia, paralysis.
CV: hypotension, hypertension, *asystole, heart block.*
GI: nausea, vomiting, diarrhea, GI cramping, mouth ulcerations.

*Liquid may contain alcohol.

Hematologic: megaloblastic anemia from decreased vitamin B absorption, *leukopenia.*
Respiratory: *respiratory depression.*
Skin: contact dermatitis.

Interactions

Herb-drug. *Anticoagulants:* May reduce anticoagulant effect. Discourage use together.
Antidiabetics, insulin: Increases hypoglycemic effects. Discourage use together; advise patient to monitor glucose levels closely.
Antihypertensives: May reduce or enhance hypotensive effect. Discourage use together.
Beta blockers, calcium channel blockers, digoxin: May interfere with or enhance cardiac effects. Discourage use together.
Cephalosporins, disulfiram, metronidazole: May cause disulfiram-like reaction when taken with liquid herbal preparations. Discourage use together.
CNS depressants, such as benzodiazepines: May enhance sedative effects. Discourage use together.
Herb-lifestyle. *Alcohol use:* May enhance sedative effects. Discourage use together.

grapeseed, pinebark

Reported uses

• As an antioxidant for circulatory disorders (hypoxia from atherosclerosis, inflammation, and cardiac or cerebral infarction)
• Pain, limb heaviness, and swelling from peripheral circulatory disorders and to treat inflammatory conditions, varicose veins, and cancer

Cautions

• People with liver dysfunction should use cautiously.
🕭 **Lifespan:** No considerations reported.

Adverse reactions

Hepatic: *hepatotoxicity.*

Interactions

None reported.

kava

Reported uses

• Nervous anxiety, stress, and restlessness
• Orally as a sedative, to promote wound healing, and for headaches, seizure disorders, the common cold, respiratory tract infection, tuberculosis, and rheumatism
• Urogenital infections, including chronic cystitis, venereal disease, uterine inflammation, menstrual problems, and vaginal prolapse
• As an aphrodisiac
• As juice, for skin diseases, including leprosy
• As a poultice, for intestinal problems, otitis, and abscesses

Cautions

• People hypersensitive to herb or any of its components should avoid it. Depressed people should avoid herb because of possible sedative activity; those with endogenous depression should avoid it because of increased risk of suicide.
• People with renal disease, thrombocytopenia, or neutropenia should use cautiously.
🕭 **Lifespan:** Pregnant women shouldn't use this herb because of possible loss of uterine tone. Breast-feeding women shouldn't use. Children shouldn't use.

Adverse reactions

CNS: mild euphoric changes characterized by feelings of happiness, fluent and lively speech, and increased sensitivity to sounds; morning fatigue, sedation, *suicidal thoughts.*
EENT: visual accommodation disorders, pupil dilation, disorders of oculomotor equilibrium.
GI: mild GI disturbances, mouth numbness.
GU: hematuria.
Hematologic: increased RBC count, decreased platelets and lymphocytes.
Metabolic: reduced levels of albumin, total protein, bilirubin, and urea; increased HDL cholesterol.
Respiratory: *pulmonary hypertension.*
Skin: scaly rash.

Interactions

Herb-drug. *Antiplatelet drugs, type B MAO inhibitors:* Possible additive effects. Monitor patient closely.

Bold italic type indicates that reaction may be life-threatening.

Barbiturates, benzodiazepines: Kava lactones potentiate the effects of CNS depressants, leading to toxicity. Discourage use together.
Levodopa: Possible reduced effectiveness of levodopa therapy in patients with Parkinson's disease, apparently because of dopamine antagonism. Advise patient to use cautiously.
Herb-herb. *Calamus, calendula, California poppy, capsicum, catnip, celery, couch grass, elecampane, German chamomile, goldenseal, gotu kola, hops, Jamaican dogwood, lemon balm, sage, sassafras, shepherd's purse, Siberian ginseng, skullcap, stinging nettle, St. John's wort, valerian, wild lettuce, yerba maté:* Additive sedative effects may occur. Advise great caution.
Herb-lifestyle. *Alcohol use:* Increases risk of CNS depression and liver damage. Discourage use together.

milk thistle

Reported uses
● Dyspepsia, liver damage from chemicals, Amanita mushroom poisoning, support in inflammatory liver disease and cirrhosis, loss of appetite, and gallbladder and spleen disorders
● As a liver protectant

Cautions
● Herb shouldn't be used by people hypersensitive to it or to plants in the Asteraceae family. Use in decompensated cirrhosis isn't recommended.
🐾 **Lifespan:** Pregnant and breast-feeding women shouldn't use.

Adverse reactions
GI: nausea, vomiting, diarrhea.

Interactions
Herb-drug. *Aspirin:* May improve aspirin metabolism in people with liver cirrhosis. Advise person to consult prescriber before use.
Cisplatin: May prevent kidney damage by cisplatin. Advise patient to consult prescriber before use.
Disulfiram: Herbal products that contain alcohol may cause a disulfiram-like reaction. Discourage use together.

Hepatotoxic drugs: May prevent liver damage from butyrophenones, phenothiazines, phenytoin, acetaminophen, and halothane. Advise patient to consult prescriber before use.
Tacrine: Silymarin reduces adverse cholinergic effects when given together. Advise patient to consult prescriber before use.

nettle

Reported uses
● Allergic rhinitis, osteoarthritis, rheumatoid arthritis, kidney stones, asthma, and BPH
● As a diuretic, an expectorant, a general health tonic, a blood builder and purifier, a pain reliever and anti-inflammatory, and a lung tonic for ex-smokers
● Eczema, hives, bursitis, tendinitis, laryngitis, sciatica, and premenstrual syndrome
● Possibly hay fever and irrigation of the urinary tract

Cautions
🐾 **Lifespan:** Herb shouldn't be used by women who are pregnant or breast-feeding because of its diuretic and uterine stimulation properties. Children shouldn't use.

Adverse reactions
CV: edema.
GI: gastric irritation, gingivostomatitis.
GU: decreased urine formation; *oliguria;* increased diuresis in patients with arthritic conditions and those with myocardial or chronic venous insufficiency.
Skin: topical irritation, burning sensation.

Interactions
Herb-drug. *Disulfiram:* Possible disulfiram reaction if taken with liquid extract or tincture. Discourage use together.
Herb-lifestyle. *Alcohol use:* Possible additive effect from liquid extract and tincture. Discourage alcohol use.

*Liquid may contain alcohol.

passion flower

Reported uses

- As a sedative, a hypnotic, and an antispasmodic for treating muscle spasms
- As an analgesic for menstrual cramping, pain, or migraines
- For neuralgia, generalized seizures, hysteria, nervous agitation, and insomnia
- Crushed leaves and flowers topically for cuts and bruises

Cautions

- Excessive amounts may cause sedation and may potentiate MAO inhibitor therapy.
- Those with liver disease or a history of alcoholism should avoid products that contain alcohol.
- ❧ **Lifespan:** Women who are pregnant or breast-feeding shouldn't use.

Adverse reactions

CNS: drowsiness, headache, flushing, agitation, confusion, psychosis.
CV: *shock,* tachycardia, hypotension, *ventricular arrhythmias.*
GI: nausea, vomiting.
Respiratory: *asthma.*
Other: allergic reaction.

Interactions

Herb-drug. *Disulfiram, metronidazole:* Herbal products that contain alcohol may cause a disulfiram-like reaction. Discourage use together.
Hexobarbital: Increases sleeping time; other barbiturate effects may be potentiated. Monitor patient's level of consciousness carefully.
MAO inhibitors: Actions can be potentiated by herb. Discourage use together.

primrose, evening

Reported uses

- Infusion for sedative and astringent properties
- Asthmatic coughs, GI disorders, whooping cough, psoriasis, multiple sclerosis, asthma, Raynaud's disease, and Sjögren's syndrome

- Poultices made from oil to speed wound healing
- Pruritic symptoms of atopic dermatitis and eczema, breast pain and tenderness from premenstrual syndrome, benign breast disease, and diabetic neuropathy
- In rheumatoid arthritis, to improve symptoms and reduce the need for pain medication; also used to lower serum cholesterol, improve hypertension, and decrease platelet aggregation
- To calm hyperactive children
- To reduce mammary tumors from baseline size

Cautions

- Urge caution or discourage use in people with schizophrenia and in those taking antiseizure drugs.
- ❧ **Lifespan:** In pregnant women, discourage use; effects are unknown.

Adverse reactions

CNS: headache, *temporal lobe epilepsy.*
CV: *thrombosis.*
GI: nausea.
Skin: rash.
Other: inflammation, *immunosuppression.*

Interactions

Herb-drug. *Phenothiazines:* May increase risk of seizures. Discourage use together.

Saint John's wort

Reported uses

- Depression, bronchial inflammation, burns, cancer, enuresis, gastritis, hemorrhoids, hypothyroidism, insect bites and stings, insomnia, kidney disorders, and scabies, and as a wound-healing agent
- HIV infection
- Topically for phototherapy of skin diseases, including psoriasis, cutaneous T-cell lymphoma, warts, and Kaposi's sarcoma

Cautions

- Transplant patients maintained on cyclosporine therapy should avoid this herb because of the risk of organ rejection.

Bold italic type indicates that reaction may be life-threatening.

❧ **Lifespan:** Pregnant women and both men and women planning pregnancy shoudn't use this herb because of mutagenic risk to sperm cells and oocytes and adverse effects on reproductive cells.

Adverse reactions

CNS: fatigue, neuropathy, restlessness, headache.
GI: digestive complaints, fullness sensation, constipation, diarrhea, nausea, abdominal pain, dry mouth.
Skin: photosensitivity reactions, pruritus.
Other: delayed hypersensitivity.

Interactions

Herb-drug. *Amitriptyline, chemotherapeutics, cyclosporine, digoxin, drugs metabolized by the CYP enzyme system, hormonal contraceptives, protease inhibitors, theophylline, and warfarin:* Decreases effectiveness of these drugs. May require drug dosage adjustment. Monitor patient closely; discourage use together.
Barbiturates: Decreases sedative effects. Monitor patient closely.
Indinavir: Substantially reduces drug level, causing loss of therapeutic effects. Discourage use together.
MAO inhibitors, including phenelzine and tranylcypromine: May increase effects and cause toxicity and hypertensive crisis. Discourage use together.
Opioids: Increases sedative effects. Discourage use together.
Reserpine: Antagonizes effects of reserpine. Discourage use together.
SSRIs, such as citalopram, fluoxetine, paroxetine, sertraline: Increases risk of serotonin syndrome. Discourage use together.
Herb-herb. *Herbs with sedative effects, such as calamus, calendula, California poppy, capsicum, catnip, celery, couch grass, elecampane, German chamomile, goldenseal, gotu kola, Jamaican dogwood, kava, lemon balm, sage, sassafras, shepherd's purse, Siberian ginseng, skullcap, stinging nettle, valerian, wild carrot, and wild lettuce:* May enhance effects of herbs. Discourage use together.
Herb-food. *Tyramine-containing foods such as beer, cheese, dried meats, fava beans, liver, wine, and yeast:* May cause hypertensive crisis when used together. Advise person to separate food from herb.

Herb-lifestyle. *Alcohol use:* May increase sedative effects. Discourage use together.
Sun exposure: Increases risk of photosensitivity reaction. Advise person to avoid unprotected or prolonged exposure to sunlight.

saw palmetto

Reported uses

• As a mild diuretic
• GU problems such as BPH and to increase sperm production, breast size, and sexual vigor

Cautions

• Those with breast cancer or hormone-dependent illnesses other than BPH should avoid this herb.
❧ **Lifespan:** Women of childbearing potential and women who are pregnant or breast-feeding shouldn't use this herb.

Adverse reactions

CNS: headache.
CV: hypertension.
GI: abdominal pain, constipation, diarrhea, nausea.
GU: dysuria, impotence, urine retention.
Musculoskeletal: back pain.
Other: decreased libido.

Interactions

Herb-drug. *Adrenergics, hormones, hormone-like drugs:* May cause estrogen, androgen, and alpha-blocking effects. Drug dosages may need adjustment if patient takes this herb. Monitor patient closely.

valerian

Reported uses

• Menstrual cramps, restlessness and sleep disorders from nervous conditions, and other symptoms of psychological stress, such as anxiety, nervous headaches, and gastric spasms
• Topically as a bath additive for restlessness and sleep disorders

*Liquid may contain alcohol.

Cautions

• People with hepatic impairment shouldn't use this herb because of the risk of hepatotoxicity.
• People with acute or major skin injuries, fever, infectious diseases, cardiac insufficiency, or hypertonia shouldn't bathe with valerian products.

≋ **Lifespan:** Women who are pregnant or breast-feeding shouldn't use this herb; it's effects are unknown.

Adverse reactions

CNS: excitability, headache, insomnia.
CV: cardiac disturbance.
EENT: blurred vision.
GI: nausea.
Other: hypersensitivity reaction.

Interactions

Herb-drug. *Barbiturates, benzodiazepines:* May have additive effects. Monitor patient closely.
CNS depressants: May have additive effects. Discourage use together.
Disulfiram: Disulfiram reaction may occur if herbal extract or tincture contains alcohol. Discourage use together.
Herb-herb. *Herbs with sedative effects, such as catnip, hops, kava, passion flower, skullcap:* May increase sedative effects. Advise caution.
Herb-lifestyle. *Alcohol use:* May increase sedative effects. Discourage using together.

Bold italic type indicates that reaction may be life-threatening.

Appendices
and Index

Glossary

Agranulocytosis: an abnormal blood condition characterized by a severe reduction in the number of granulocytes, basophils, eosinophils, and neutrophils that results in high fever, exhaustion, and bleeding ulcers of the throat, mucous membranes, and GI tract; an acute disease that may be an adverse reaction to drug or radiation therapy.

Allergic reaction: a local or general reaction after exposure to an allergen to which the patient has already been exposed and sensitized; may range from localized dermatitis to anaphylaxis.

Alopecia: absence or loss of hair.

Angioedema: a potentially life-threatening condition characterized by sudden swelling of tissue in the face, neck, lips, tongue, throat, hands, feet, genitals, or intestine.

Aplastic anemia: a deficiency of all of the formed elements of the blood related to bone marrow failure; caused by neoplastic bone marrow disease or by destruction of the bone marrow by exposure to toxic chemicals, radiation, or certain drugs; also known as *pancytopenia.*

Arthralgia: any pain that affects a joint.

Azotemia: a toxic condition caused by renal insufficiency and subsequent retention of urea in the blood; also called *uremia.*

Cushing's syndrome: a metabolic disorder caused by increased production of adrenocorticotropic hormone from a tumor of the adrenal cortex or of the anterior lobe of the pituitary gland, or by excessive intake of glucocorticoids; characterized by central obesity, "moon face," glucose intolerance, growth suppression in children, and weakening of the muscles.

Disseminated intravascular coagulation (DIC): a life-threatening coagulopathy resulting from overstimulation of the body's clotting and anticlotting processes in response to disease, septicemia, neoplasms, obstetric emergencies,

severe trauma, prolonged surgery, and hemorrhage.

Eosinophilia: an increase in the number of eosinophils in the blood accompanying many inflammatory conditions; substantial increases are considered a reflection of an allergic response.

Erythema: redness of the skin caused by dilation and congestion of the superficial capillaries, often a sign of inflammation or infection.

Gray baby syndrome: a life-threatening condition that can occur in newborns (especially premature one) who are given chloramphenicol for a bacterial infection such as meningitis; symptoms, usually appearing 2 to 9 days after therapy has begun, include vomiting, loose green stools, refusal to suck, hypotension, cyanosis, low body temperature, and CV collapse; the baby becomes limp and has a gray coloring.

Hemolytic anemia: a disorder characterized by the premature destruction of RBCs; anemia may be minimal or absent, reflecting the ability of the bone marrow to increase production of RBCs.

Hepatitis: inflammation of the liver, usually from a viral infection but sometimes from toxic agents.

Hirsutism: excessive growth of dark, coarse body hair in a characteristically male pattern.

Hypercalcemia: greater-than-normal amounts of calcium in the blood; signs and symptoms include confusion, anorexia, abdominal pain, muscle pain, and weakness.

Hyperglycemia: greater-than-normal amounts of glucose in the blood; signs and symptoms include excessive hunger, thirst, frequent urination, fatigue, weight loss, blurred vision, and poor wound healing.

Hyperkalemia: greater-than-normal amounts of potassium in the blood; signs and symptoms include nausea, fatigue, weakness, and palpitations or irregular pulse.

Hypermagnesemia: greater-than-normal amounts of magnesium in the blood; toxic levels may cause cardiac arrhythmias and may depress deep tendon reflexes and respiration.

Hypernatremia: greater-than-normal amounts of sodium in the blood; signs and symptoms include confusion, seizures, coma, dysrhythmic muscle twitching, lethargy, tachycardia, and irritability.

Hyperplasia: an increase in the number of cells.

Hypersensitivity reaction: an abnormal and undesirable reaction in response to a foreign agent; classified by the mechanism involved and the time it takes to occur and assigned a rating of 1 through 4 (Types I, II, III, IV).

Hypocalcemia: less-than-normal amounts of calcium in the blood; signs and symptoms of severe hypocalcemia include cardiac arrhythmias and muscle cramping and twitching as well as numbness and tingling of the hands, feet, lips, and tongue.

Hypoglycemia: less-than-normal amounts of glucose in the blood; signs and symptoms include weakness, drowsiness, confusion, hunger, dizziness, pallor, irritability, tremor, sweating, headache, a cold and clammy feeling, rapid heart beat, and if left untreated, delirium, coma, and death.

Hypokalemia: less-than-normal amounts of potassium in the blood; signs and symptoms include palpitations, muscle weakness or cramping, paresthesias, frequent urination, delirium, depression, and GI complaints such as constipation, nausea, vomiting, and abdominal cramping.

Hypomagnesemia: less-than-normal amounts of magnesium in the blood; signs and symptoms include nausea, vomiting, muscle weakness, tremors, tetany, and lethargy.

Hyponatremia: less-than-normal amounts of sodium in the blood; signs and symptoms may range from mild anorexia, headache, or muscle cramps to obtundation, coma, or seizures.

Leukocytosis: an abnormal increase in the number of circulating WBCs; types are basophilia, eosinophilia, and neutrophilia.

Leukopenia: an abnormal decrease in the number of WBCs to fewer than 5,000/mm^3.

Myalgia: diffuse muscle pain, usually occurring with malaise.

Nephrotic syndrome: an abnormal kidney condition characterized by marked proteinuria, hypoalbuminemia, and edema.

Neuroleptic malignant syndrome: the rarest and most serious of the neuroleptic-induced movement disorders, a neurologic emergency in most cases; signs and symptoms include fever, rigidity, tremor, drowsiness, and confusion progressing to stupor and coma, seizures, and cardiac arrhythmias.

Neutropenia: an abnormal decrease in the number of circulating neutrophils in the blood.

Pancytopenia: a deficiency of all of the formed elements of the blood related to bone marrow failure caused by neoplastic bone marrow disease or by destruction of the bone marrow after exposure to toxic chemicals, radiation, or certain drugs; also known as *aplastic anemia.*

Pharmacodynamics: the study of drug action in the body at the tissue site; includes uptake, movement, binding, and interactions.

Pharmacokinetics: the study of the action of drugs within the body, including the routes and mechanisms of absorption and excretion, the rate at which a drug's action begins, the duration of effect, the biotransformation of the substance in the body, and the effects and routes of metabolite excretion.

Pseudomembranous colitis: a complication of antibiotic therapy that causes severe local tissue inflammation of the colon; signs and symptoms include watery diarrhea, abdominal pain or cramping, and low-grade fever.

Pseudotumor cerebri: benign intracranial hypertension, most common in women ages 20 to 50, caused by increased pressure within the brain; symptoms include headache, dizziness, nausea, vomiting, and ringing or rushing sound in the ears.

Pruritus: itching.

Psoriasis: a common skin disorder characterized by the eruption of red, silvery-scaled maculopapules, predominantly on the elbows, knees, scalp, and trunk.

Reye's syndrome: an encephalopathy that affects children; linked to the use of aspirin and other salicylate-containing drug, as well as other causes; the syndrome may follow an upper respiratory infection or chicken pox; its onset is rapid, usually starting with irritable, combative behavior and vomiting, progressing to semiconsciousness, seizures, coma, and possibly death.

Serotonin syndrome: a typically mild, yet potentially serious drug-related condition most often reported in patients taking two or more drugs that increase CNS serotonin levels; the most common combinations involve MAO inhibitors, SSRIs, and tricyclic antidepressants; signs and symptoms include confusion, agitation, restlessness, rapid heart rate, muscle rigidity or twitching, tremors, and nausea.

Serum sickness: an immune complex disease appearing 1 or 2 weeks after infection of a foreign serum or serum protein, with local and systemic reactions, such as urticaria, fever, general lymphadenopathy, edema, arthritis, and occasionally albuminuria or severe nephritis.

Syncope: a brief loss of consciousness caused by oxygen deficiency to the brain, often preceded by a feeling of dizziness; have the patient lie down or place his head between his knees to prevent it.

Thrombocytopenia: an abnormal decrease in the number of platelets in the blood, predisposing the patient to bleeding disorders.

Thrombocytopenic purpura: a bleeding disorder characterized by a marked decrease in the number of platelets, causing multiple bruises, petechiae, and hemorrhage into the tissues.

Tinnitus: sound in one or both ears, such as buzzing, ringing, or whistling, occurring without external stimuli; it may be from an ear infection, the use of certain drugs, a blocked auditory tube or canal, or head trauma.

Urticaria: an itchy skin condition characterized by pale wheals with well-defined red edges; this may be the result of an allergic response to insect bites, food, or drugs.

Avoiding dangerous abbreviations

The Joint Commission on Accreditation of Healthcare Organizations (JCAHO) requires every health care facility to specify which abbreviations are approved for staff use and which shouldn't be used. To help guide this process, JCAHO also has created a list of abbreviations, acronyms, and symbols that are dangerous because they increase the risk of medication errors, especially when hand-written. This core do-not-use list includes the following items.

Do not use	Potential problem	Use instead
U (unit)	Mistaken for "0" (zero), the number "4" (four), or "cc"	Write "unit."
IU (international unit)	Mistaken for IV (intravenous) or the number "10" (ten)	Write "international unit."
q.d. (daily) q.o.d. (every other day)	Mistaken for each other. The period after the "q" mistaken for "i" and the "o" mistaken for "i"	Write "daily" or "every other day."
Trailing zero (X.0 mg) Lack of leading zero (.X mg)	Decimal point is missed	Write "X mg" or "0.X mg."
MS, MSO₄, MgSO₄	Can mean morphine sulfate or magnesium sulfate Confused for one another	Write "morphine sulfate" or "magnesium sulfate."

Pregnancy risk categories

The FDA has assigned a pregnancy risk category to each drug based on available clinical and preclinical information. The five categories (A, B, C, D, X) reflect a drug's potential to cause birth defects. Although drugs should ideally be avoided during pregnancy, sometimes they're needed; this rating system permits rapid assessment of the risk-benefit ratio. Drugs in category A are generally considered safe to use in pregnancy; drugs in category X are generally contraindicated.

• A: Adequate studies in pregnant women haven't shown a risk to fetus.
• B: Animal studies haven't shown a risk to fetus, but controlled studies haven't been conducted in pregnant women; or animal studies have shown an adverse effect on fetus, but adequate studies in pregnant women haven't shown a risk to fetus.
• C: Animal studies have shown an adverse effect on fetus, but adequate studies haven't been conducted in pregnant women. The benefits from use in pregnant women may be acceptable despite risks.

• D: The drug may cause risk to fetus, but the potential benefits of use in pregnant women may be acceptable despite the risks (such as in a life-threatening situation or a serious disease for which safer drugs can't be used or are ineffective).
• X: Studies in animals or humans show fetal abnormalities, or adverse-reaction reports indicate evidence of fetal risk. The risks involved clearly outweigh potential benefits.
• NR: Not rated.

Controlled substance schedules

Drugs regulated under the jurisdiction of the Controlled Substances Act of 1970 are divided into the following groups or schedules:

• Schedule I (C-I): High abuse potential and no accepted medical use. Examples include heroin, cocaine, and LSD.
• Schedule II (C-II): High abuse potential with severe dependence liability. Examples include opioids, amphetamines, and some barbiturates.
• Schedule III (C-III): Less abuse potential than schedule II drugs and moderate dependence liability. Examples include nonbarbiturate sedatives, nonamphetamine stimulants, anabolic steroids, dronabinol, and limited amounts of certain opioids.
• Schedule IV (C-IV): Less abuse potential than schedule III drugs and limited dependence liability. Examples include some sedatives, anxiolytics, and non-opioid analgesics.

• Schedule V (C-V): Limited abuse potential. This category includes mainly small amounts of opioids, such as codeine, used as antitussives or antidiarrheals. Under federal law, limited quantities of certain C-V drugs may be purchased without a prescription directly from a pharmacist if allowed under specific state laws. The purchaser must be at least age 18 and must furnish suitable identification. All such transactions must be recorded by the dispensing pharmacist.

Toxic drug–drug interactions

Interaction	Drugs	Interacting drugs
Decreased corticosteroid effects	*corticosteroids* (betamethasone, cortisone, dexamethasone, fludrocortisone, hydrocortisone, methylprednisolone, prednisolone, prednisone, triamcinolone)	*rifamycins* (rifabutin, rifampin, rifapentine)
Digoxin toxicity and arrhythmias	*digoxin* (Lanoxin)	*tetracyclines* (demeclocycline, doxycycline, minocycline, tetracycline) *thiazide diuretics* (chlorothiazide, hydrochlorothiazide, indapamide, methyclothiazide, metolazone, polythiazide, trichlormethiazide) *verapamil* (Calan)
Hearing loss	*aminoglycosides* (amikacin, gentamicin, kanamycin, neomycin, netilmicin, streptomycin, tobramycin)	*loop diuretics* (bumetanide, ethacrynic acid, furosemide, torsemide)
Increased bleeding	*warfarin* (Coumadin)	*alteplase* (Activase, tPA) *androgens* [17-alkyl] (danazol, fluoxymesterone, methyltestosterone, oxandrolone) *cimetidine* (Tagamet) *fibric acids* (clofibrate, fenofibrate, gemfibrozil) *cranberry juice* *salicylates* (aspirin, methylsalicylate)
		amiodarone (Cordarone, Pacerone) *azole antifungals* (fluconazole, itraconazole, ketoconazole, miconazole, voriconazole) *macrolide antibiotics* (azithromycin, clarithromycin, erythromycin) *metronidazole* (Flagyl) *quinine derivatives* (quinidine, quinine) *quinolones* (ciprofloxacin, levofloxacin, moxifloxacin, norfloxacin, ofloxacin) *sulfinpyrazone* (Anturane) *sulfonamides* (sulfasalazine, sulfisoxazole trimethoprim-sulfamethoxazole) *thyroid hormones* (levothyroxine, liothyronine, liotrix, thyroid) *vitamin E*
Increased potassium level	*potassium-sparing diuretics* (amiloride, spironolactone, triamterene)	*angiotensin-converting enzyme (ACE) inhibitors* (benazepril, captopril, enalapril, fosinopril, lisinopril, moexipril, perindopril, quinapril, ramipril, trandolapril) *angiotensin II receptor antagonists* (candesartan, eprosartan, irbesartan, losartan, olmesartan, telmisartan, valsartan) *potassium preparations* (potassium acetate, potassium phosphate, potassium bicarbonate, potassium chloride, potassium citrate, potassium gluconate, potassium iodide, potassium phosphate)

Nursing considerations

- Avoid use together, if possible.
- Effects may persist for 2 to 3 weeks after stopping therapy.

- Use together cautiously.
- Monitor serum digoxin levels. The therapeutic range for digoxin is 0.8 to 2 nanograms/ml.
- Effects of tetracyclines on digoxin may persist for several months after the antibiotic is stopped.
- Monitor serum potassium and magnesium levels if patient is taking both thiazide diuretics and digoxin.
- Monitor patient for evidence of digoxin toxicity, including arrhythmias (such as bradycardia, atrioventricular [AV] block, ventricular ectopy), lethargy, drowsiness, confusion, hallucinations, headache, syncope, vision disturbance, nausea, anorexia, vomiting, or diarrhea.

- Use together cautiously.
- Patients with renal insufficiency are at greater risk.
- Irreversible hearing loss is more likely with this combination than when either drug is used alone.

- Avoid use together, if possible.
- If drugs must be used together, monitor coagulation values carefully; the dosage requirements for warfarin will be decreased.
- Suggest taking a different histamine$_2$ antagonist.
- Aspirin doses of 500 mg or more daily cause a greater risk.

- Use together cautiously.
- Monitor prothrombin time and international normalized ratio closely when starting or stopping any of these drugs.
- Bleeding effects may persist after interacting drug is stopped.
- Typically, the warfarin dose needs to be reduced.
- Vitamin E doses of less than 400 mg daily may not have this effect.

- Use together cautiously.
- High-risk patients include those with renal impairment, type 2 diabetes, decreased renal perfusion, and those who are elderly.
- Don't use potassium preparations and potassium-sparing diuretics unless the patient has severe hypokalemia that isn't responding to either drug class alone.
- Monitor the patient's potassium level; also monitor patient for palpitations, chest pain, nausea and vomiting, paresthesias, and muscle weakness.

(continued)

Interaction	Drugs	Interacting drugs
Increased risk of pregnancy, breakthrough bleeding	*barbiturates* (amobarbital, butabarbital, pentobarbital, phenobarbital, primidone, secobarbital)	*hormonal contraceptives* (Ortho-Evra, Yasmin-28)
Life-threatening hypertension	*clonidine* (Catapres)	*beta blockers* (acebutolol, atenolol, betaxolol, carteolol, esmolol, metoprolol, nadolol, penbutolol, pindolol, propranolol, timolol)
		tricyclic antidepressants (amitriptyline, amoxapine, clomipramine, desipramine, doxepin, imipramine, nortriptyline, protriptyline, trimipramine)
	monoamine oxidase (MAO) inhibitors (isocarboxazid, phenelzine, tranylcypromine)	*anorexiants* (amphetamine, benzphetamine, dextroamphetamine, methamphetamine, phentermine)
		methylphenidate (dexmethylphenidate, Concerta)
Methotrexate toxicity	*methotrexate* (Rheumatrex, Trexall)	*nonsteroidal anti-inflammatory drugs (NSAIDs)* (diclofenac, etodolac, fenoprofen, flurbiprofen, ibuprofen, indomethacin, ketoprofen, ketorolac, meclofenamate, nabumetone, naproxen, oxaprozin, piroxicam, sulindac, tolmetin) *penicillins* (amoxicillin, ampicillin, carbenicillin, cloxacillin, dicloxacillin, nafcillin, oxacillin, penicillin G, penicillin V, piperacillin, ticarcillin)
Reduced penicillin effectiveness	*penicillins* (amoxicillin, ampicillin, carbenicillin, cloxacillin, dicloxacillin, nafcillin, oxacillin, Penicillin G, Penicillin V, piperacillin, ticarcillin)	*tetracyclines* (demeclocycline, doxycycline, minocycline, tetracycline)
Rhabdomyolysis and myopathy	*HMG-CoA reductase inhibitors* (atorvastatin, fluvastatin, lovastatin, pravastatin, rosuvastatin, simvastatin)	*cyclosporine* (Neoral) *gemfibrozil* (Lopid) *protease inhibitors* (amprenavir, atazanavir, indinavir, lopinavir with ritonavir, nelfinavir, ritonavir, saquinavir)
		macrolide antibiotics (azithromycin, clarithromycin, erythromycin)
Serious cardiac events	*quinidine*	*verapamil* (Calan)
Serotonin syndrome	*selective serotonin reuptake inhibitors (SSRIs)* (fluoxetine, paroxetine, sertraline)	*risperidone* (Risperdal)

Nursing considerations

- Use together cautiously.
- Suggest use of an alternative barrier form of contraception during therapy with both drugs.

- Use together cautiously.
- Monitor blood pressure closely when starting and stopping clonidine and beta blockers simultaneously; stop the beta blocker first.
- Use together is contraindicated.

- Avoid using these drugs together, if possible.
- Several deaths have occurred as a result of hypertensive crisis leading to cerebral hemorrhage.
- Monitor patient for hypertension, hyperpyrexia, and seizures.
- Hypertensive reaction may occur for several weeks after stopping an MAO inhibitor.

- Use together is contraindicated.

- Use together cautiously.
- Monitor patient for mouth sores, hematemesis, diarrhea with melena, nausea and weakness, and bone marrow suppression.
- Methotrexate toxicity is less likely to occur with weekly low-dose methotrexate regimens for rheumatoid arthritis and other inflammatory diseases.
- Longer leucovorin rescue should be considered when giving NSAIDs and methotrexate at antineoplastic doses.
- Obtain methotrexate levels twice weekly for the first 2 weeks of concurrent penicillin and methotrexate therapy.

- Avoid use together, if possible.

- Use of nelfinavir with simvastatin is contraindicated.
- Avoid use together, if possible.
- Monitor patient taking an HMG-CoA reductase inhibitor and gemfibrozil for signs of acute renal failure, including decreased urine output, elevated blood urea nitrogen and creatinine levels, edema, dyspnea, tachycardia, distended neck veins, nausea, vomiting, weakness, fatigue, confusion, and agitation.
- Monitor patient for fatigue, muscle aches and weakness, joint pain, unintentional weight gain, seizures, dramatically increased serum creatine kinase level, and dark, red, or cola-colored urine.

- Use together cautiously.
- Monitor patient for rhabdomyolysis, especially 5 to 21 days after starting the macrolide antibiotic.

- Use together only when there are no other alternatives.
- Monitor patient for hypotension, bradycardia, ventricular tachycardia, and AV block.
- Tell patient to report diaphoresis, dizziness, or blurred vision as well as palpitations, shortness of breath, dizziness or fainting, and chest pain.
- Complications of this interaction may be noticed after as little as 1 day or as long as 5 months of combined therapy.

- Monitor patient carefully if an SSRI is started or stopped or if dosage is changed during risperidone therapy. Risperidone levels may increase.
- Assess patient for central nervous system (CNS) irritability, increased muscle tone, muscle twitching or jerking, and changes in level of consciousness (LOC).
- Although average doses of fluoxetine and paroxetine may cause this interaction, higher doses of sertraline (greater than 100 mg daily) are needed.

(continued)

Interaction	Drugs	Interacting drugs
Serotonin syndrome (continued)	SSRIs (citalopram, fluoxetine, fluvoxamine, nefazodone, paroxetine, sertraline, venlafaxine)	selective 5-HT$_1$ receptor agonists (almotriptan, eletriptan, frovatriptan, naratriptan, rizatriptan, sumatriptan, zolmitriptan)
	serotonin reuptake inhibitors (citalopram, escitalopram, fluoxetine, fluvoxamine, nefazodone, paroxetine, sertraline, venlafaxine)	MAO inhibitors (isocarboxazid, phenelzine, selegiline, tranylcypromine)
		sibutramine (Meridia) sympathomimetics (amphetamine, dextroamphetamine, methamphetamine, phentermine)
Severe arrhythmias	dofetilide (Tikosyn)	thiazide diuretics (chlorothiazide, hydrochlorothiazide, indapamide, methyclothiazide, metolazone, polythiazide, trichlormethiazide) verapamil (Calan)
	pimozide (Orap)	SSRIs (citalopram, sertraline)
	quinolones (gatifloxacin, levofloxacin, moxifloxacin)	antiarrhythmics (amiodarone, bretylium, disopyramide, procainamide, quinidine, sotalol) erythromycin (E-mycin, Eryc) phenothiazines (chlorpromazine, fluphenazine, mesoridazine, perphenazine, prochlorperazine, promethazine, thioridazine) tricyclic antidepressants (amitriptyline, amoxapine, clomipra-mine, desipramine, doxepin, imipramine, nortriptyline, trimipramine)
		ziprasidone (Geodon)
	thioridazine (Mellaril)	fluoxetine (Prozac)
Severe hypotension	nitrates (amyl nitrite, isosorbide dinitrate, isosorbide mononitrate, nitroglycerin)	sildenafil (Viagra) tadalafil (Cialis) vardenafil (Levitra)
	protease inhibitors (amprenavir, indinavir, nelfinavir, ritonavir, saquinavir)	sildenafil (Viagra) tadalafil (Cialis) vardenafil (Levitra)
Severe muscular depression	cholinesterase inhibitors (ambenonium, edrophonium, neostigmine, pyridostigmine)	Corticosteroids (betamethasone, corticotrophin, cortisone, cosyntropin, dexamethasone, fludrocortisone, hydrocortisone, methylprednisolone, prednisolone, prednisone, triamcinolone)

Nursing considerations

- Avoid combining these drugs if possible.
- If concurrent use can't be avoided, start with the lowest dosages possible, and observe the patient closely.
- Stop the selective 5-HT$_1$ receptor agonist at the first sign of interaction. Begin an antiserotonergic drug such as cyproheptadine (Periactin).
- Some patients may note increased frequency of migraine and reduced effectiveness of antimigraine drugs if a serotonin reuptake inhibitor is begun.
- Monitor patient for evidence of serotonin syndrome, including CNS irritability, motor weakness, shivering, muscle twitching, and altered LOC.

- Don't use these drugs together.
- Allow 1 week after stopping nefazodone or venlafaxine before giving an MAO inhibitor.
- Allow 2 weeks after stopping citalopram, escitalopram, fluvoxamine, paroxetine, or sertraline before giving an MAO inhibitor.
- Allow 5 weeks after stopping fluoxetine before giving an MAO inhibitor.
- Allow 2 weeks after stopping an MAO inhibitor before giving any serotonin reuptake inhibitor.
- Serotonin syndrome effects include CNS irritability, motor weakness, shivering, myoclonus, and altered LOC.
- The selective MAO type-B inhibitor selegiline has been given with fluoxetine, paroxetine, or sertraline to patients with Parkinson disease without negative effects.

- Don't use these drugs together, if possible.
- If this combination must be used, carefully monitor the patent for adverse effects, which require immediate medical attention.
- Monitor the patient closely for increased CNS effects, such as anxiety, jitteriness, agitation and restlessness, plus dizziness, nausea, vomiting, motor weakness, shivering, myoclonus, and altered LOC.

- Use together is contraindicated.
- In the event of inadvertent use together, monitor electrocardiogram for excessive prolongation of the QTc interval or the development of ventricular arrhythmias.
- Use of a thiazide diuretic increases potassium excretion.
- Monitor renal function and QTc interval every 3 months during dofetilide and verapamil therapy.

- Use together is contraindicated.
- Life-threatening risk is from prolongation of the QTc interval.

- Use of class IA or III antiarrhythmics, erythromycin, phenothiazines, or tricyclic antidepressants with levofloxacin should be avoided.
- Gatifloxacin and moxifloxacin may be used with caution and increased monitoring with phenothiazines and tricyclic antidepressants but should be avoided with antiarrhythmics and erythromycin.

- Use together is contraindicated.

- Use together is contraindicated.
- Risk increases proportional to increased dose of thioridazine.

- Use together is contraindicated.
- Before giving a nitrate, find out if a patient with chest pain has taken a drug for erectile dysfunction during the previous 24 to 48 hours.

- Use together is contraindicated.
- Tell patient to take sildenafil exactly as prescribed. Dosage may be reduced to 25 mg and an interval of at least 48 hours between drugs may be needed.

- If given together in a patient with myasthenia gravis, watch for severe muscle deterioration unresponsive to cholinesterase inhibitor therapy.
- Be prepared to provide respiratory support and mechanical ventilation, as needed.
- Corticosteroid therapy may have long-term benefits in patients with myasthenia gravis.

Combination drug products

Accuretic

Generic components
Tablets
10 mg quinapril and 12.5 mg hydrochlorothiazide
20 mg quinapril and 12.5 mg hydrochlorothiazide
20 mg quinapril and 25 mg hydrochlorothiazide

Dosages
Adults: 1 tablet P.O. per day in the morning. Adjust drug using the individual products; then switch to appropriate dosage of the combination product.

Activella
femHRT

Generic components
Tablets
2.5 mcg ethinyl estradiol and 0.5 mg norethindrone acetate (femHRT)
5 mcg ethinyl estradiol and 1 mg norethindrone acetate (femHRT)
1 mg ethinyl estradiol and 0.5 mg norethindrone acetate (Activella)

Dosages
Signs and symptoms of menopause and prevention of osteoporosis
Women with intact uterus: 1 tablet P.O. daily.

Adderall
Adderall XL
Controlled Substance Schedule (CSS) II

Generic components
Tablets
5 mg: 1.25 mg dextroamphetamine sulfate, 1.25 mg dextroamphetamine saccharate, and 1.25 mg amphetamine aspartate, 1.25 mg amphetamine sulfate
7.5 mg: 1.875 mg dextroamphetamine sulfate, 1.875 mg dextroamphetamine saccharate,
1.875 mg amphetamine aspartate, and 1.875 mg amphetamine sulfate
10 mg: 2.5 mg dextroamphetamine sulfate, 2.5 mg dextroamphetamine saccharate, 2.5 mg amphetamine aspartate, and 2.5 mg amphetamine sulfate
12.5 mg: 3.125 mg dextroamphetamine sulfate, 3.125 mg dextroamphetamine saccharate, 3.125 mg amphetamine aspartate, and 3.125 mg amphetamine sulfate
15 mg: 3.75 mg dextroamphetamine sulfate, 3.75 mg dextroamphetamine saccharate, 3.75 mg amphetamine aspartate, and 3.75 mg amphetamine sulfate
20 mg: 5 mg dextroamphetamine sulfate, 5 mg dextroamphetamine saccharate, 5 mg amphetamine aspartate, and 5 mg amphetamine sulfate
30 mg: 7.5 mg dextroamphetamine sulfate, 7.5 mg dextroamphetamine saccharate, 7.5 mg amphetamine aspartate, and 7.5 mg amphetamine sulfate
Capsules (extended-release)
5 mg: 1.25 mg dextroamphetamine sulfate, 1.25 mg dextroamphetamine saccharate, 1.25 mg amphetamine aspartate, and 1.25 mg amphetamine sulfate
10 mg: 2.5 mg dextroamphetamine sulfate, 2.5 mg dextroamphetamine saccharate, 2.5 mg amphetamine aspartate, and 2.5 mg amphetamine sulfate
15 mg: 3.75 mg dextroamphetamine sulfate, 3.75 mg dextroamphetamine saccharate, 3.75 mg amphetamine aspartate, and 3.75 mg amphetamine sulfate
20 mg: 5 mg dextroamphetamine sulfate, 5 mg dextroamphetamine saccharate, 5 mg amphetamine aspartate, and 5 mg amphetamine sulfate
25 mg: 6.25 mg dextroamphetamine sulfate, 6.25 mg dextroamphetamine saccharate, 6.25 mg amphetamine aspartate, and 6.25 mg amphetamine sulfate
30 mg: 7.5 mg dextroamphetamine sulfate, 7.5 mg dextroamphetamine saccharate, 7.5 mg amphetamine aspartate, and 7.5 mg amphetamine sulfate

Dosages
Narcolepsy
Adults and children age 12 and older: Initially, 10 mg immediate-release tablet daily. Increase by 10 mg weekly to maximum dose of

60 mg in two or three divided doses q 4 to
6 hours.
Children ages 6 to 12: Initially, 5 mg immediate-release tablet P.O. daily. Increase by 5 mg at
weekly intervals to maximum of 60 mg in divided doses.
Attention deficit hyperactivity disorder
Adults: 20 mg extended-release capsules P.O.
daily.
Adolescents ages 13 to 17: Initially, 10 mg extended-release capsule P.O. daily. Increase after
1 week to 20 mg daily if needed.
Children age 6 and older: Initially, 5 mg immediate-release tablet P.O. daily or b.i.d. Increase by 5 mg at weekly intervals until expected response. Dosage should rarely exceed
40 mg.
Children ages 6 to 12: 10 mg extended-release
capsule P.O. daily in a.m. Increase by 5 to
10 mg in weekly intervals to a maximum dose
of 30 mg.
Children ages 3 to 5: Initially 2.5 mg immediate-release tablet P.O. daily. Increase by 2.5 mg
at weekly intervals until optimal response. Divide total daily amount into two or three doses
and give 4 to 6 hours apart.

Advicor

Generic components
Tablets
20 mg lovastatin and 500 mg niacin
20 mg lovastatin and 1,000 mg niacin

Dosages
Adults: 1 tablet daily P.O. at night.

Aggrenox

Generic components
Capsules
25 mg aspirin and 200 mg dipyridamole

Dosages
Adults: To decrease risk of stroke, 1 capsule
P.O. b.i.d. in the morning and evening. Swallow
capsule whole; may be taken with or without
food.

Aldactazide

Generic components
Tablets
25 mg spironolactone and 25 mg hydrochlorothiazide
50 mg spironolactone and 50 mg hydrochlorothiazide

Dosages
Adults: One to eight 25 mg spironolactone and
25 mg hydrochlorothiazide tablets daily. Or, one
to four 50 mg spironolactone and 50 mg hydrochlorothiazide tablets daily.

Aldoclor

Generic components
Tablets
250 mg methyldopa and 150 mg chlorothiazide
250 mg methyldopa and 250 mg chlorothiazide

Dosages
Adults: 1 tablet P.O. per day taken in the morning. Adjust dosage using the individual products; then switch to the combination product
when patient's adjustment schedule is stable.

Aldoril
Aldoril D

Generic components
Tablets
250 mg methyldopa and 15 mg hydrochlorothiazide
250 mg methyldopa and 25 mg hydrochlorothiazide
500 mg methyldopa and 30 mg hydrochlorothiazide
500 mg methyldopa and 50 mg hydrochlorothiazide

Dosages
Adults: 1 tablet P.O. daily, in the morning. Adjust dosage using the individual products; then
switch to the combination product when patient's adjustment schedule is stable.

Alor 5/500
Azdone
Damason-P
Lortab ASA
Panasal 5/500
CSS III

Generic components
Tablets
500 mg aspirin and 5 mg hydrocodone bitartrate

Dosages
Moderate to moderately severe pain
Adults: 1 or 2 tablets q 4 hours. Maximum dosage, 8 tablets in 24 hours.

Anexsia 5/325
Norco 5/325
CSS III

Generic components
Tablets
325 mg acetaminophen and 5 mg hydrocodone bitartrate

Dosages
Moderate to moderately severe pain
Adults: 1 to 2 tablets q 4 to 6 hours. Maximum dosage, 12 tablets in 24 hours.

Anexsia 5/500
Co-Gesic
Lorcet HD
Lortab 5/500
Panacet 5/500
Vicodin
CSS III

Generic components
Tablets
500 mg acetaminophen and 5 mg hydrocodone bitartrate

Dosages
Moderate to moderately severe pain
Adults: 1 to 2 tablets q 4 to 6 hours. Maximum dosage, 8 tablets in 24 hours.

Anexsia 7.5/325
Norco 7.5/325
CSS III

Generic components
Tablets
325 mg acetaminophen and 7.5 mg hydrocodone bitartrate

Dosages
Moderate to moderately severe pain
Adults: 1 to 2 tablets q 4 to 6 hours. Maximum dosage, 12 tablets in 24 hours.

Anexsia 7.5/650
Lorcet Plus
CSS III

Generic components
Tablets
650 mg acetaminophen and 7.5 mg hydrocodone bitartrate

Dosages
Arthralgia, bone pain, dental pain, headache, migraine, moderate pain
Adults: 1 to 2 tablets q 4 hours. Maximum dosage, 6 tablets in 24 hours.

Anexsia 10/660
Vicodin HP
CSS III

Generic components
Tablets
660 mg acetaminophen and 10 mg hydrocodone bitartrate

Dosages
Arthralgia, bone pain, dental pain, headache, migraine, moderate pain
Adults: 1 tablet q 4 to 6 hours. Maximum dosage, 6 tablets in 24 hours.

Atacand HCT

Generic components
Tablets
16 mg candesartan and 12.5 mg hydrochlorothiazide
32 mg candesartan and 12.5 mg hydrochlorothiazide

Dosages
Adults: 1 tablet P.O. daily in the morning. Adjust dosage using the individual products; then switch to appropriate dosage.

Avalide

Generic components
Tablets
150 mg irbesartan and 12.5 mg hydrochlorothiazide
300 mg irbesartan and 12.5 mg hydrochlorothiazide
300 mg irbesartan and 25 mg hydrochlorothiazide

Dosages
Adults: 1 tablet P.O. daily. Adjust dosage with individual products; then switch to combination product when patient's condition is stabilized. Maximum daily dose, 300 mg irbesartan and 25 mg hydrochlorothiazide.

Benicar HCT

Generic components
Tablets
20 mg olmesartan and 12.5 mg hydrochlorothiazide
40 mg olmesartan and 12.5 mg hydrochlorothiazide
40 mg olmesartan and 25 mg hydrochlorothiazide

Dosages
Adults: 1 tablet P.O. per day in the morning. Adjust dosage using the individual products; then switch to the combination product when patient's adjustment schedule is stable.

BiDil

Generic components
Tablets
20 mg isosorbide dinitrate and 37.5 mg hydralazine

Dosages
Adults: 1 to 2 tablets P.O. t.i.d.

Capital with Codeine
Tylenol with Codeine Elixir
CSS V

Generic components
Elixir
120 mg acetaminophen and 12 mg codeine phosphate/5 ml

Dosages
Mild to moderate pain
Adults: 15 ml q 4 hours.

Capozide

Generic components
Tablets
25 mg captopril and 15 mg hydrochlorothiazide
50 mg captopril and 15 mg hydrochlorothiazide
25 mg captopril and 25 mg hydrochlorothiazide
50 mg captopril and 25 mg hydrochlorothiazide

Dosages
Adults: 1 to 2 tablets P.O. daily, in the morning. Adjust dosage using the individual products; then switch to the combination product when patient's adjustment schedule is stable.

Clorpres
Combipres

Generic components
Tablets
15 mg chlorthalidone and 0.1 mg clonidine hydrochloride
15 mg chlorthalidone and 0.2 mg clonidine hydrochloride

15 mg chlorthalidone and 0.3 mg clonidine hydrochloride

Dosages
Adults: 1 to 2 tablets per day P.O. in the morning. Adjust dosage using the individual products; then switch to the combination product when patient's adjustment schedule is stable

CombiPatch

Generic components
Transdermal patch
0.05 mg/day estradiol and 0.14 mg/day norethindrone
0.05 mg/day estradiol and 0.25 mg/day norethindrone

Dosages
To relieve menopause symptoms
Women: Change patch twice a week.

Combivent

Generic components
Metered-dose inhaler
18 mcg ipratropium bromide and 90 mcg albuterol

Dosages
Bronchospasm with COPD in patients who require more than a single bronchodilator
Adults: Two inhalations q.i.d. Not for use during acute attack. Use caution with known sensitivity to atropine, soy, or peanuts.

Corzide

Generic components
Tablets
40 mg nadolol and 5 mg bendroflumethiazide
80 mg nadolol and 5 mg bendroflumethiazide

Dosages
Adults: 1 tablet P.O. per day in the morning. Adjust dosage using the individual products; then switch to the combination product when patient's adjustment schedule is stable.

Darvocet-A500
CSS IV

Generic components
Tablets
500 mg acetaminophen and 100 mg propoxyphene napsylate

Dosages
Mild to moderate pain
Adults: 1 tablet q 4 hours. Maximum dosage, 8 tablets in 24 hours.

Darvocet-N50
CSS IV

Generic components
Tablets
325 mg acetaminophen and 50 mg propoxyphene napsylate

Dosages
Mild to moderate pain
Adults: 2 tablets q 4 hours. Maximum dosage, 12 tablets in 24 hours.

Darvocet-N100
CSS IV

Generic components
Tablets
650 mg acetaminophen and 100 mg propoxyphene napsylate

Dosages
Mild to moderate pain
Adults: 1 tablet q 4 hours. Maximum dosage, 6 tablets in 24 hours.

Diovan HCT

Generic components
Tablets
80 mg valsartan and 12.5 mg hydrochlorothiazide
160 mg valsartan and 12.5 mg hydrochlorothiazide
160 mg valsartan and 25 mg hydrochlorothiazide

Dosages
Adults: 1 tablet per day P.O. Not for initial therapy; start using each component first.

Dyazide

Generic components
Capsules
37.5 mg triamterene and 25 mg hydrochlorothiazide

Dosages
Adults: 1 to 2 capsules daily.

Empirin with Codeine No. 3
CSS III

Generic components
Tablets
325 mg aspirin and 30 mg codeine phosphate

Dosages
Fever and mild to moderate pain
Adults: 1to 2 tablets q 4 hours. Maximum dosage, 12 tablets in 24 hours.

Empirin with Codeine No. 4
CSS III

Generic components
Tablets
325 mg aspirin and 60 mg codeine phosphate

Dosages
Fever and mild to moderate pain
Adults: 1 tablet q 4 hours. Maximum dosage, 6 tablets in 24 hours.

Endocet 5/325
Percocet 5/325
Roxicet
CSS II

Generic components
Tablets
325 mg acetaminophen and 5 mg oxycodone hydrochloride

Dosages
Moderate to moderately severe pain
Adults: 1 tablet q 6 hours. Maximum dosage, 12 tablets in 24 hours.

Endocet 7.5/325
Percocet 7.5/325
CSS II

Generic components
Tablets
325 mg acetaminophen and 7.5 mg oxycodone hydrochloride

Dosages
Moderate to moderately severe pain
Adults: 1 tablet q 6 hours. Maximum dosage, 8 tablets in 24 hours.

Endocet 7.5/500
Percocet 7.5/500
CSS II

Generic components
Tablets
500 mg acetaminophen and 7.5 mg oxycodone hydrochloride

Dosages
Moderate to moderately severe pain
Adults: 1 to 2 tablets q 4 to 6 hours. Maximum dosage, 8 tablets in 24 hours.

Endocet 10/325
Percocet 10/325
CSS II

Generic components
Tablets
325 mg acetaminophen and 10 mg oxycodone hydrochloride

Dosages
Moderate to moderately severe pain
Adults: 1 tablet q 6 hours. Maximum dosage, 6 tablets in 24 hours.

Endodan
Percodan
CSS II

Generic components
Tablets
325 mg aspirin, 4.5 mg oxycodone hydrochloride, and 0.38 mg oxycodone terephthalate

Dosages
Moderate to moderately severe pain
Adults: 1 tablet q 6 hours. Maximum dosage, 12 tablets in 24 hours.

Epzicom

Generic components
Tablets
600 mg abacavir with 300 mg lamivudine

Dosages
Adults: 1 tablet daily, taken without regard to food and with other antiretrovirals.

Eryzole
Pediazole

Generic components
Granules for oral suspension
Erythromycin ethylsuccinate (equivalent of 200 mg erythromycin activity) and 600 mg sulfisoxazole per 5 ml when reconstituted according to manufacturer's directions

Dosages
Acute otitis media
Children: 50 mg/kg/day erythromycin and 150 mg/kg/day sulfisoxazole in divided doses q.i.d. for 10 days. Give without regard to meals. Refrigerate after reconstitution; use within 14 days.

Fiorinal with Codeine
Fioricet with Codeine
CSS III

Generic components
Capsules
325 mg acetaminophen, 50 mg butalbital, 40 mg caffeine, and 30 mg codeine phosphate

Dosages
Headache, mild to moderate pain
Adults: 1 to 2 capsules q 4 hours. Maximum dosage, 6 capsules in 24 hours.

Hyzaar

Generic components
Tablets
50 mg losartan and 12.5 mg hydrochlorothiazide
100 mg losartan and 25 mg hydrochlorothiazide

Dosages
Adults: 1 tablet per day P.O. in the morning. Not for initial therapy; start using each component and if desired effects are obtained, Hyzaar may be used.

Inderide

Generic components
Tablets
40 mg propranolol hydrochloride and 25 mg hydrochlorothiazide
80 mg propranolol hydrochloride and 25 mg hydrochlorothiazide

Dosages
Adults: 1 tablet P.O. b.i.d. Adjust dosage using the individual products; then switch to the combination product when patient's adjustment schedule is stable. Maximum total daily dose shouldn't exceed 160 mg propranolol and 50 mg hydrochlorothiazide.

Lexxel

Generic components
Extended-release tablets
5 mg enalapril maleate and 2.5 mg felodipine
5 mg enalapril maleate and 5 mg felodipine

Dosages
Adults: 1 tablet per day P.O. Adjust dosage using the individual products; then switch to the combination product when patient's adjustment schedule is stable. Make sure that patient swallows tablet whole. Don't cut, crush, or allow him to chew.

Limbitrol
Limbitrol DS

Generic components
Tablets
5 mg chlordiazepoxide and 12.5 mg amitriptyline
10 mg chlordiazepoxide and 25 mg amitriptyline

Dosages
Adults: 10 mg chlordiazepoxide with 25 mg amitriptyline 3 to 4 times per day up to 6 times daily. For patients who don't tolerate the higher doses, 5 mg chlordiazepoxide with 12.5 mg amitriptyline 3 to 4 times per day. Reduce dosage after initial response.

Lopressor HCT

Generic components
Tablets
50 mg metoprolol and 25 mg hydrochlorothiazide
100 mg metoprolol and 25 mg hydrochlorothiazide
100 mg metoprolol and 50 mg hydrochlorothiazide

Dosages
Adults: 1 tablet P.O. per day. Adjust dosage using the individual products; then switch to the combination product when patient's adjustment schedule is stable..

Lorcet 10/650
CSS III

Generic components
Tablets
650 mg acetaminophen and 10 mg hydrocodone bitartrate

Dosages
Moderate to moderately severe pain
Adults: 1 tablet q 4 to 6 hours. Maximum dosage, 6 tablets in 24 hours.

Lortab 2.5/500
CSS III

Generic components
Tablets
500 mg acetaminophen and 2.5 mg hydrocodone bitartrate

Dosages
Moderate to moderately severe pain
Adults: 1 to 2 tablets q 4 to 6 hours. Maximum dosage, 8 tablets in 24 hours.

Lortab 7.5/500
CSS III

Generic components
Tablets
500 mg acetaminophen and 7.5 mg hydrocodone bitartrate

Dosages
Moderate to moderately severe pain
Adults: 1 tablet q 4 to 6 hours. Maximum dosage, 8 tablets in 24 hours.

Lortab 10/500
CSS III

Generic components
Tablets
500 mg acetaminophen and 10 mg hydrocodone bitartrate

Dosages
Moderate to moderately severe pain
Adults: 1 tablet q 4 to 6 hours. Maximum dosage, 6 tablets in 24 hours.

Lortab Elixir
CSS III

Generic components
Elixir
167 mg acetaminophen and 2.5 mg/5 ml hydrocodone bitartrate

Dosages
Moderately severe pain
Adults: 15 ml q 4 to 6 hours. Maximum dosage, 90 ml/day.

Lotensin HCT

Generic components
Tablets
5 mg benazepril and 6.25 mg hydrochlorothiazide
10 mg benazepril and 12.5 mg hydrochlorothiazide
20 mg benazepril and 12.5 mg hydrochlorothiazide
20 mg benazepril and 25 mg hydrochlorothiazide

Dosages
Adults: 1 tablet per day P.O. in the morning. Adjust dosage using the individual products; then switch to the combination product when patient's adjustment schedule is stable.

Lotrel

Generic components
Capsules
2.5 mg amlodipine and 10 mg benazepril
5 mg amlodipine and 10 mg benazepril
5 mg amlodipine and 20 mg benazepril
10 mg amlodipine and 20 mg benazepril

Dosages
Adults: 1 tablet P.O. daily in the morning. Monitor patient for hypertension and adverse effects closely over first 2 weeks and regularly thereafter.

Maxzide

Generic components
Tablets
75 mg triamterene and 50 mg hydrochlorothiazide

Dosages
Adults: 1 tablet daily.

Micardis HCT

Generic components
Tablets
40 mg telmisartan and 12.5 mg hydrochlorothiazide
80 mg telmisartan and 12.5 mg hydrochlorothiazide
80 mg telmisartan and 25 mg hydrochlorothiazide

Dosages
Adults: 1 tablet P.O. per day; may be adjusted up to 160 mg telmisartan and 25 mg hydrochlorothiazide, based on patient's response.

Minizide

Generic components
Tablets
1 mg prazosin and 0.5 mg polythiazide
2 mg prazosin and 0.5 mg polythiazide
5 mg prazosin and 0.5 mg polythiazide

Dosages
Adults: 1 capsule P.O. b.i.d. or t.i.d. Adjust drug using the individual products; then switch to appropriate dosage of the combination product.

Moduretic

Generic components
Tablets
5 mg amiloride and 50 mg hydrochlorothiazide

Dosages
Adults: 1 to 2 tablets per day with meals.

Monopril-HCT

Generic components
Tablets
10 mg fosinopril and 12.5 mg hydrochlorothiazide
20 mg fosinopril and 12.5 mg hydrochlorothiazide

Dosages
Adults: 1 tablet P.O. per day in the morning. Adjust dosage using the individual products, then switch to appropriate dosage of the combination product.

Norco 325/10
CSS III

Generic components
Tablets
325 mg acetaminophen and 10 mg hydrocodone bitartrate

Dosages
Moderate to moderately severe pain
Adults: 1 tablet q 4 to 6 hours. Maximum dosage, 6 tablets in 24 hours.

Percocet 2.5/325
CSS II

Generic components
Tablets
325 mg acetaminophen and 2.5 mg oxycodone hydrochloride

Dosages
Moderate to moderately severe pain
Adults: 1 to 2 tablets q 4 to 6 hours. Maximum dosage, 12 tablets in 24 hours.

Percocet 10/650
CSS II

Generic components
Tablets
650 mg acetaminophen and 10 mg oxycodone hydrochloride

Dosages
Moderate to moderately severe pain
Adults: 1 tablet q 4 hours. Maximum dosage, 6 tablets in 24 hours.

Prefest

Generic components
Tablets
1 mg estradiol and 0.09 mg norgestimate

Dosages
Moderate to severe symptoms of menopause; to prevent osteoporosis
Women with intact uterus: 1 tablet/day P.O. (3 days of pink tablets: estradiol alone; followed by 3 days of white tablets: estradiol and norgestimate combination; continue cycle uninterrupted).

Premphase

Generic components
Tablets
0.625 mg conjugated estrogens; 0.625 mg conjugated estrogens with 5 mg medroxyprogesterone

Dosages
Moderate to severe symptoms of menopause and prevention of osteoporosis
Women with intact uterus: 1 tablet per day P.O. Use estrogen alone on days 1 to 14 and estrogen-medroxyprogesterone tablet on days 15 to 28.

Prempro

Generic components
Tablets
0.3 mg conjugated estrogen and 1.5 mg medroxyprogesterone
0.45 mg conjugated estrogen and 1.5 mg medroxyprogesterone
0.625 mg estrogen and 2.5 mg medroxyprogesterone
0.625 mg conjugated estrogen and 5 mg medroxyprogesterone

Dosages
To relieve symptoms of menopause; to prevent osteoporosis
Women with intact uterus: 1 tablet per day P.O.

Prinzide
Zestoretic

Generic components
Tablets
10 mg lisinopril and 12.5 mg hydrochlorothiazide
20 mg lisinopril and 12.5 mg hydrochlorothiazide
20 mg lisinopril and 25 mg hydrochlorothiazide

Dosages
Adults: 1 tablet per day P.O. taken in the morning. Adjust dosage using the individual products; then switch to the combination product when patient's adjustment schedule is stable.

Roxicet 5/500
Roxilox
Tylox
CSS II

Generic components
Tablets
500 mg acetaminophen and 5 mg oxycodone hydrochloride

Dosages
Moderate to moderately severe pain
Adults: 1 tablet q 6 hours.

Roxicet Oral Solution
CSS II

Generic components
Solution
325 mg acetaminophen and 5 mg/5 ml oxycodone hydrochloride

Dosages
Moderate to moderately severe pain
Adults: 5 ml q 6 hours. Maximum dosage, 60 ml in 24 hours.

Symbyax

Generic components
Capsules
6 mg olanzapine and 25 mg fluoxetine
6 mg olanzapine and 50 mg fluoxetine
12 mg olanzapine and 25 mg fluoxetine
12 mg olanzapine and 50 mg fluoxetine

Dosages
Adults: 1 capsule daily in the evening. Begin with 6 mg/25 mg capsule and adjust according to efficacy and tolerability.

Talacen
CSS IV

Generic components
Tablets
650 mg acetaminophen and 25 mg pentazocine hydrochloride

Dosages
Mild to moderate pain
Adults: 1 tablet q 4 hours. Maximum dosage, 6 tablets in 24 hours.

Talwin Compound
CSS IV

Generic components
Tablets
325 mg aspirin and 12.5 mg pentazocine hydrochloride

Dosages
Moderate pain
Adults: 2 tablets q 6 to 8 hours. Maximum dosage, 8 tablets in 24 hours.

Talwin NX
CSS IV

Generic components
Tablets
0.5 mg naloxone and 50 mg pentazocine hydrochloride

Dosages
Moderate to severe pain
Adults: 1 to 2 tablets q 3 to 4 hours. Maximum dosage, 12 tablets daily.

Tarka

Generic components
Tablets
1 mg trandolapril and 240 mg verapamil
2 mg trandolapril and 180 mg verapamil
2 mg trandolapril and 240 mg verapamil
4 mg trandolapril and 240 mg verapamil

Dosages
Adults: 1 tablet P.O. per day, taken with food. Adjust dosage using the individual products; then switch to the combination product when patient's adjustment schedule is stable. Make sure that patient swallows tablet whole. Don't cut, crush, or allow him to chew.

Teczem

Generic components
Extended-release tablets
5 mg enalapril maleate and 180 mg diltiazem hydrochloride

Dosages
Adults: 1 to 2 tablets per day P.O. in the morning. Adjust dosage using the individual products; then switch to the combination product when patient's adjustment schedule is stable. Make sure that patient swallows tablet whole. Don't cut, crush, or allow him to chew.

Tenoretic

Generic components
Tablets
50 mg atenolol and 25 mg chlorthalidone
100 mg atenolol and 25 mg chlorthalidone

Dosages
Adults: 1 tablet P.O. daily in the morning. Adjust dosage using the individual products; then switch to appropriate dosage.

Teveten HCT

Generic components
Tablets
600 mg eprosartan and 12.5 mg hydrochlorothiazide
600 mg eprosartan and 25 mg hydrochlorothiazide

Dosages
Adults: 1 tablet P.O. each day. Establish dosage with each component alone before using the combination product; if blood pressure isn't controlled on 600 mg/25 mg tablet, 300 mg eprosartan may be added each evening.

Trizivir

Generic components
Tablets
300 mg abacavir, 300 mg zidovudine, and 150 mg lamivudine

Dosages
Adults: 1 tablet P.O. b.i.d. Carefully monitor patient for hypersensitivity reactions.

Truvada

Generic components
Tablets
200 mg emtricitabine with 300 mg tenofovir

Dosages
Adults and adolescents weighing more than 40 kg (88 lb): 1 tablet daily, taken without regard to food and with other antiretrovirals.

Tylenol with Codeine No. 2
CSS III

Generic components
Tablets
300 mg acetaminophen and 15 mg codeine phosphate

Dosages
Fever, mild to moderate pain
Adults: 1 to 2 tablets q 4 hours. Maximum dosage, 12 tablets in 24 hours.

Tylenol with Codeine No. 3
CSS III

Generic components
Tablets
300 mg acetaminophen and 30 mg codeine phosphate

Dosages
Fever, mild to moderate pain
Adults: 1 to 2 tablets q 4 hours. Maximum dosage, 12 tablets in 24 hours.

Tylenol with Codeine No. 4
CSS III

Generic components
Tablets
300 mg acetaminophen and 60 mg codeine phosphate

Dosages
Fever, mild to moderate pain
Adults: 1 tablet q 4 hours. Maximum dosage, 12 tablets in 24 hours.

Tylox 5/500
CSS II

Generic components
Tablets
500 mg acetaminophen and 5 mg oxycodone hydrochloride

Dosages
Moderate to moderately severe pain
Adults: 1 capsule q 6 hours. Maximum dosage, 8 capsules in 24 hours.

Uniretic

Generic components
Tablets
7.5 mg moexipril and 12.5 mg hydrochlorothiazide
15 mg moexipril and 25 mg hydrochlorothiazide

Dosages
Adults: 0.5 to 2 tablets per day. Not for initial therapy. Adjust dose to maintain appropriate blood pressure.

Vaseretic

Generic components
Tablets
5 mg enalapril maleate and 12.5 mg hydrochlorothiazide
10 mg enalapril maleate and 25 mg hydrochlorothiazide

Dosages
Adults: 1 to 2 tablets per day P.O. in the morning. Adjust dosage using the individual products; then switch to the combination product when patient's adjustment schedule is stable. Make sure that patient swallows tablet whole. Don't cut, crush, or allow him to chew.

Vicodin ES
CSS III

Generic components
Tablets
750 mg acetaminophen and 7.5 mg hydrocodone bitartrate

Dosages
Moderate to moderately severe pain
Adults: 1 tablet q 4 to 6 hours. Maximum dosage, 5 tablets in 24 hours.

Vytorin

Generic components
Tablets
10 mg ezetimibe with 10, 20, 40, or 80 mg simvastatin

Dosages
Adults: 1 tablet daily, taken in the evening with a cholesterol-lowering diet and exercise. Dosage of simvastatin in the combination may be adjusted based on patient response. If given with a bile sequestrant, must be given at least 2 hours before or 4 hours after the bile sequestrant.

Wygesic
CSS IV

Generic components
Tablets
650 mg acetaminophen and 65 mg propoxyphene napsylate

Dosages
Mild to moderate pain
Adults: 1 tablet q 4 hours. Maximum dosage, 6 tablets in 24 hours.

Ziac

Generic components
Tablets
2.5 mg bisoprolol and 6.25 mg hydrochlorothiazide
5 mg bisoprolol and 6.25 mg hydrochlorothiazide
10 mg bisoprolol and 6.25 mg hydrochlorothiazide

Dosages
Adults: 1 tablet daily P.O. in morning. Initial dose is 2.5/6.25 mg tablet P.O. daily.
Adjust dosage within 1 week; optimum antihypertensive effect may require 2 to 3 weeks.

Zydone 5/400
CSS III

Generic components
Tablets
400 mg acetaminophen and 5 mg hydrocodone bitartrate

Dosages
Moderate to moderately severe pain
Adults: 1 to 2 tablets q 4 to 6 hours. Maximum dosage, 8 tablets in 24 hours.

Zydone 7.5/400
CSS III

Generic components
Tablets
400 mg acetaminophen and 7.5 mg hydrocodone bitartrate

Dosages
Moderate to moderately severe pain
Adults: 1 tablet q 4 to 6 hours. Maximum dosage, 6 tablets in 24 hours.

Zydone 10/400
CSS III

Generic components
Tablets
400 mg acetaminophen and 10 mg hydrocodone bitartrate

Dosages
Moderate to moderately severe pain
Adults: 1 tablet q 4 to 6 hours. Maximum dosage, 6 tablets in 24 hours.

Dialyzable drugs

The amount of a drug removed by dialysis differs among patients and depends on several factors, including the patient's condition, the drug's properties, length of dialysis and dialysate used, rate of blood flow or dwell time, and purpose of dialysis. This table indicates the effect of conventional hemodialysis on selected drugs.

Drug	Level reduced by hemodialysis?	Drug	Level reduced by hemodialysis?
acebutolol	Yes	carmustine	No
acetaminophen	Yes (may not influence toxicity)	cefaclor	Yes
		cefadroxil	Yes
acetazolamide	No	cefazolin	Yes
acyclovir	Yes	cefepime	Yes
allopurinol	Yes	cefoperazone	Yes
alprazolam	No	cefotaxime	Yes
amikacin	Yes	cefotetan	Yes (only by 20%)
amiodarone	No	cefoxitin	Yes
amitriptyline	No	cefpodoxime	Yes
amlodipine	No	ceftazidime	Yes
amoxicillin	Yes	ceftibuten	Yes
amoxicillin and clavulanate potassium	Yes	ceftizoxime	Yes
		ceftriaxone	No
amphotericin B	No	cefuroxime	Yes
ampicillin	Yes	cephalexin	Yes
ampicillin and sulbactam sodium	Yes	cephalothin	Yes
aprepitant	No	cephradine	Yes
ascorbic acid	Yes	chloral hydrate	Yes
aspirin	Yes	chlorambucil	No
atenolol	Yes	chloramphenicol	Yes (very small amount)
azathioprine	Yes	chlordiazepoxide	No
aztreonam	Yes	chloroquine	No
bivalirudin	Yes	chlorpheniramine	Yes
bretylium	No	chlorpromazine	No
busulfan	Yes	chlorthalidone	No
captopril	Yes	cilastatin	Yes
carbamazepine	No	cimetidine	Yes
carbenicillin	Yes	ciprofloxacin	Yes (only by 10%)
carboplatin	Yes	cisplatin	No
carisoprodol	Yes	clavulanic acid	Yes

Drug	Level reduced by hemodialysis	Drug	Level reduced by hemodialysis
clindamycin	No	fluconazole	Yes
clofibrate	No	flucytosine	Yes
clonazepam	No	fluorouracil	No
clonidine	No	fluoxetine	No
clorazepate	No	flurazepam	No
cloxacillin	No	foscarnet	Yes
codeine	No	fosinopril	No
colchicine	No	furosemide	No
cortisone	No	gabapentin	Yes
co-trimoxazole	Yes	ganciclovir	Yes
cyclophosphamide	Yes	gemcitabine	Yes
diazepam	No	gemfibrozil	No
diazoxide	Yes	gemifloxacin	Yes
diclofenac	No	gentamicin	Yes
dicloxacillin	No	glipizide	No
didanosine	Yes	glyburide	No
digoxin	No	guanfacine	No
diltiazem	No	haloperidol	No
diphenhydramine	No	heparin	No
dipyridamole	No	hydralazine	No
disopyramide	Yes	hydrochlorothiazide	No
doxazosin	No	hydroxyzine	No
doxepin	No	ibuprofen	No
doxorubicin	No	ifosfamide	Yes
doxycycline	No	imipenem and cilastatin	Yes
emtricitabine	Yes	imipramine	No
enalapril	Yes	indapamide	No
ertapenem	Yes	indomethacin	No
erythromycin	Yes (only by 20%)	insulin	No
ethacrynic acid	No	irbesartan	No
ethambutol	Yes (only by 20%)	iron dextran	No
ethosuximide	Yes	isoniazid	Yes
famciclovir	Yes	isosorbide	Yes
famotidine	No	isradipine	No
fenoprofen	No	kanamycin	Yes
flecainide	No		(continued)

Drug	Level reduced by hemodialysis	Drug	Level reduced by hemodialysis
ketoconazole	No	morphine	No
ketoprofen	Yes	nabumetone	No
labetalol	No	nadolol	Yes
levetiracetam	Yes	nafcillin	No
levofloxacin	No	naproxen	No
lidocaine	No	nelfinavir	No
linezolid	Yes	nifedipine	No
lisinopril	Yes	nimodipine	No
lithium	Yes	nitazoxanide	No
lomefloxacin	No	nitrofurantoin	Yes
lomustine	No	nitroglycerin	No
loracarbef	Yes	nitroprusside	Yes
loratadine	No	nizatidine	No
lorazepam	No	norfloxacin	No
mechlorethamine	No	nortriptyline	No
mefenamic acid	No	octreotide	Yes
meperidine	No	ofloxacin	Yes
meprobamate	Yes	olanzapine	No
mercaptopurine	Yes	omeprazole	No
meropenem	Yes	oxacillin	No
mesalamine	Yes	oxazepam	No
metformin	Yes	paroxetine	No
methadone	No	penicillin G	Yes
methotrexate	Yes	pentamidine	No
methyldopa	Yes	pentazocine	Yes
methylprednisolone	Yes	perindopril	Yes
metoclopramide	No	phenobarbital	Yes
metolazone	No	phenylbutazone	No
metoprolol	Yes	phenytoin	No
metronidazole	Yes	piperacillin	Yes
mexiletine	Yes	piperacillin and tazobactam	Yes
miconazole	No	piroxicam	No
midazolam	No	prazosin	No
minocycline	No	prednisone	No
minoxidil	Yes	pregabalin	Yes
misoprostol	No	primidone	Yes

Drug	Level reduced by hemodialysis	Drug	Level reduced by hemodialysis
procainamide	Yes	triazolam	No
promethazine	No	trimethoprim	Yes
propoxyphene	No	valacyclovir	Yes
propranolol	No	valganciclovir	Yes
protriptyline	No	valproic acid	No
pyrazinamide	Yes	valsartan	No
pyridoxine	Yes	vancomycin	Yes
quinapril	No	verapamil	No
quinidine	Yes	vigabatrin	Yes
quinine	Yes	warfarin	No
ranitidine	Yes	zolpidem	No
rifampin	No		
ritodrine	Yes		
salsalate	Yes		
sertraline	No		
sotalol	Yes		
stavudine	Yes		
streptomycin	Yes		
sucralfate	No		
sulbactam	Yes		
sulfamethoxazole	Yes		
sulindac	No		
tazobactam	Yes		
temazepam	No		
theophylline	Yes		
ticarcillin	Yes		
ticarcillin and clavulanate	Yes		
timolol	No		
tirofiban	Yes		
tobramycin	Yes		
tocainide	Yes		
tolbutamide	No		
topiramate	Yes		
topotecan	Yes		
trandolapril	Yes		
trazodone	No		

Herb–drug interactions

Herb	Drug	Possible effects
aloe (dried juice from leaf [latex])	antiarrhythmics, digoxin	May lead to hypokalemia, which may potentiate digoxin and antiarrhythmics.
	thiazide diuretics, other potassium-wasting drugs, such as corticosteroids	May cause additive effect of potassium wasting.
	oral drugs	May decrease drug absorption because of more rapid GI transit time.
	stimulant laxatives	May increase risk of potassium loss.
bilberry	anticoagulants, antiplatelets	Decreases platelet aggregation.
	hypoglycemics, insulin	May increase insulin level, causing hypoglycemia; additive effect with antidiabetics.
capsicum	ACE inhibitors	May cause cough.
	anticoagulants, antiplatelets	Decreases platelet aggregation and increases fibrinolytic activity, prolonging bleeding time.
	antihypertensives	May interfere with antihypertensives by increasing cate-cholamine secretion.
	aspirin, NSAIDs	Stimulates GI secretions to help protect against NSAID-induced GI irritation.
	CNS depressants, such as barbiturates, benzodiazepines, opioids	Increases sedative effect.
	cocaine	May increase effects of drug and risk of adverse reactions, including death. Use together includes exposure to capsicum in pepper spray.
	H_2 blockers, proton-pump inhibitors	Decreases effects of the increased catecholamine secretion by herb.
	hepatically metabolized drugs	May increase hepatic metabolism of drugs by increasing G6PD and adipose lipase activity.
	MAO inhibitors	May decrease efficacy because of increased acid secretion by capsicum.
	theophylline	Increases absorption of theophylline, possibly leading to higher drug level or toxicity.
chamomile	anticoagulants	Warfarin constituents in herb may enhance drug therapy and prolong bleeding time.
	drugs requiring GI absorption	May delay drug absorption.

Herb	Drug	Possible effects
chamomile *(continued)*	drugs with sedative properties, such as benzodiazepines	May cause additive effects and adverse reactions.
	iron	Tannic acid content in herb may reduce iron absorption.
echinacea	hepatotoxic drugs	Hepatotoxicity may increase with drugs known to elevate liver enzyme levels.
	immunosuppressants	Herb may counteract drugs.
	warfarin	Increases bleeding time without increased INR.
evening primrose oil	anticonvulsants	Lowers seizure threshold.
	antiplatelets, anticoagulants	Increases risk of bleeding and bruising.
feverfew	anticoagulants, antiplatelets	May decrease platelet aggregation and increase fibrinolytic activity.
	methysergide	May potentiate drug.
garlic	anticoagulants, antiplatelets	Enhances platelet inhibition, leading to increased anticoagulation.
	antihyperlipidemics	May have additive lipid-lowering properties.
	antihypertensives	May cause additive hypotension.
	cyclosporine	May decrease efficacy of drug. May induce metabolism and decrease drug level to subtherapeutic; may cause rejection.
	hormonal contraceptives	May decrease efficacy of drugs.
	insulin, other drugs causing hypoglycemia	May increase insulin level, causing hypoglycemia, an additive effect with these drugs.
	nonnucleotide reverse transcriptase inhibitors (NNRTIs)	May affect metabolism of these drugs.
	saquinavir	Decreases drug level, causing therapeutic failure and increased viral resistance.
ginger	anticoagulants, antiplatelets	Inhibits platelet aggregation by antagonizing thromboxane synthetase and enhancing prostacyclin, leading to prolonged bleeding time.
	antidiabetics	May interfere with diabetes therapy because of hypoglycemic effects.
	antihypertensives	May antagonize drug effects.
	barbiturates	May enhance drug effects.

(continued)

Herb	Drug	Possible effects
ginger *(continued)*	calcium channel blockers	May increase calcium uptake by myocardium, leading to altered drug effects.
	chemotherapy	May reduce nausea caused by chemotherapy.
	H_2 blockers, proton-pump inhibitors	May decrease efficacy because of increased acid secretion by herb.
ginkgo	anticoagulants, antiplatelets	May enhance platelet inhibition, leading to increased anticoagulation.
	anticonvulsants	May decrease effectiveness of drugs.
	drugs known to lower seizure threshold	May further reduce seizure threshold.
	insulin	Ginkgo leaf extract can alter insulin secretion and metabolism, affecting glucose level.
	thiazide diuretics	Ginkgo leaf may increase blood pressure.
ginseng	alcohol	Increases alcohol clearance, possibly by increasing activity of alcohol dehydrogenase.
	anabolic steroids, hormones	May potentiate effects of drugs. Estrogenic effects of herb may cause vaginal bleeding and breast nodules.
	antibiotics	Herb may enhance effects of some antibiotics.
	anticoagulants, antiplatelets	Decreases platelet adhesiveness.
	antidiabetics	May enhance glucose-lowering effects.
	antipsychotics	Because of CNS stimulant activity, avoid use with these drugs.
	digoxin	May falsely elevate drug level.
	furosemide	May decrease diuretic effect with this drug.
	immunosuppressants	May interfere with drug therapy.
	MAO inhibitors	Potentiates action of MAO inhibitors. May cause insomnia, headache, tremors, and hypomania.
	stimulants	May potentiate drug effects.
	warfarin	Causes antagonism of warfarin, resulting in a decreased INR.

Herb	Drug	Possible effects
goldenseal	antihypertensives	Large amounts of herb may interfere with blood pressure control.
	CNS depressants, such as barbiturates, benzodiazepines, opioids	Increases sedative effect.
	diuretics	Causes additive drug effect.
	general anesthetics	May potentiate hypotensive action of drugs.
	heparin	May counteract anticoagulant effect of drug.
	H_2 blockers, proton-pump inhibitors	May decrease efficacy because of increased acid secretion by herb.
grapeseed	warfarin	Increases effects and INR because of tocopherol content of herb.
green tea	acetaminophen, aspirin	May increase efficacy of these drugs by as much as 40%.
	adenosine	May inhibit hemodynamic effects of drug.
	albuterol, isoproterenol, metaproterenol, terbutaline	May increase the cardiac inotropic effect of these drugs.
	clozapine	May cause acute worsening of psychotic symptoms.
	disulfiram	Increases risk of adverse effects of caffeine; decreases clearance and increases half-life of caffeine.
	ephedrine	Increases risk of agitation, tremors, and insomnia.
	hormonal contraceptives	Decreases clearance by 40% to 65%. Increases effects and adverse effects.
	lithium	Abrupt caffeine withdrawal increases drug level; may cause lithium tremor.
	MAO inhibitors	Large amounts of herb may precipitate hypertensive crisis.
	mexiletine	Decreases caffeine elimination by 50%. Increases effects and adverse effects.
	verapamil	Increases caffeine level by 25%; increases effects and adverse effects.
	warfarin	Causes antagonism resulting from vitamin content of herb.
hawthorn berry	cardiovascular drugs	May potentiate or interfere with conventional therapies used for congestive heart failure, hypertension, angina, and arrhythmias.
	CNS depressants	Causes additive effects.

(continued)

Herb	Drug	Possible effects
hawthorn berry (continued)	coronary vasodilators	Causes additive vasodilator effects when used with theophylline, caffeine, papaverine, sodium nitrate, adenosine, and epinephrine.
	digoxin	Causes additive positive inotropic effect, with potential for drug toxicity.
kava	alcohol	Potentiates depressant effect of alcohol and other CNS depressants.
	benzodiazepines	Use with these drugs may result in comalike states.
	CNS depressants or stimulants	May hinder therapy with CNS stimulants.
	hepatotoxic drugs	May increase risk of liver damage.
	levodopa	Decreases efficacy because of dopamine antagonism by herb.
licorice	antihypertensives	Decreases effect of drug therapy. Large amounts of herb cause sodium and water retention and hypertension.
	aspirin	May provide protection against aspirin-induced damage to GI mucosa.
	corticosteroids	Causes additive and enhanced effects of drugs.
	digoxin	Herb causes hypokalemia, which predisposes to drug toxicity.
	hormonal contraceptives	Increases fluid retention and potential for increased blood pressure resulting from fluid overload.
	hormones	Interferes with estrogen or antiestrogen therapy.
	insulin	Causes hypokalemia and sodium retention.
	spironolactone	Decreases effects of drug.
ma huang (ephedra)	amitriptyline	May decrease hypertensive effects of herb.
	caffeine	Increases risk of stimulatory adverse effects of ephedra and caffeine and risk of hypertension, myocardial infarction, stroke, and death.
	caffeine, CNS stimulants, theophylline	Causes additive CNS stimulation.
	dexamethasone	Increases clearance and decreases efficacy of drug.
	digoxin	Increases risk of arrhythmias.
	hypoglycemics	Decreases drug effect because of hyperglycemia caused by herb.

Herb	Drug	Possible effects
ma huang (ephedra) (continued)	MAO inhibitors	Potentiates drugs.
	oxytocin	May cause hypertension.
	theophylline	May increase risk of stimulatory adverse effects.
melatonin	CNS depressants, such as barbiturates, benzodiazepines, opioids	Increases sedative effect.
	fluoxetine	Improves sleep in some patients with major depressive disorder.
	fluvoxamine	May significantly increase melatonin level; may decrease melatonin metabolism.
	immunosuppressants	May stimulate immune function and interfere with drug therapy.
	isoniazid	May enhance effects of drug against some *Mycobacterium* species.
	nifedipine	May decrease efficacy of drug; increases heart rate.
	verapamil	Increases melatonin excretion.
milk thistle	drugs causing diarrhea	Increases bile secretion and often causes loose stools. May increase effect of other drugs commonly causing diarrhea.
	hepatotoxic drugs, such as acetaminophen, butyrophenones, ethanol, phenothiazines, phenytoin	May have liver membrane-stabilization and antioxidant effects, leading to protection from liver damage.
	indinavir	May decrease trough level of drug, reducing virologic response.
nettle	anticonvulsants	May increase sedative adverse effects; may increase risk of seizure.
	anxiolytics, hypnotics, opioids	May increase sedative adverse effects.
	iron	Tannic acid content of herb may reduce iron absorption.
	warfarin	Antagonism resulting from vitamin K content of aerial parts of herb.
passion flower	CNS depressants, such as barbiturates, benzodiazepines, opioids	Increases sedative effect.
St. John's wort	5-hydroxytriptamine$_1$ (5-HT$_1$) agonists (triptans)	Increases risk of serotonin syndrome.
	alcohol, opioids	Enhances the sedative effect of these drugs.
	anesthetics	May prolong effect of drugs.

(continued)

Herb	Drug	Possible effects
St. John's wort (continued)	barbiturates	Decreases drug-induced sleep time.
	cyclosporine	Decreases drug level below therapeutic levels, threatening transplanted organ rejection.
	digoxin	May reduce drug level, which decreases therapeutic effects.
	human immunodeficiency virus (HIV) protease inhibitors, indinavir, NNRTIs	Induces cytochrome P-450 metabolic pathway, which may decrease therapeutic effects of drugs using this pathway for metabolism. Avoid use together because of the potential for subtherapeutic antiretroviral level and insufficient virologic response that could lead to resistance or class cross-resistance.
	hormonal contraceptives	Increases breakthrough bleeding; decreases level and efficacy of drugs.
	irinotecan	Decreases drug level by 50%.
	iron	Tannic acid content of herb may reduce iron absorption.
	MAO inhibitors, nefazodone, SSRIs, trazodone	Causes additive effects with MAO inhibitors, SSRIs, and other antidepressants, potentially leading to serotonin syndrome, especially when combined with SSRIs.
	photosensitizing drugs	Increases photosensitivity.
	reserpine	Antagonizes effects of drug.
	sympathomimetic amines, such as pseudoephedrine	Causes additive effects.
	theophylline	May decrease drug level, making the drug less effective.
	warfarin	May alter INR. Reduces efficacy of anticoagulant, requiring increased dosage of drug.
valerian	alcohol	May be risk of increased sedation.
	CNS depressants, sedative hypnotics	Enhances effects of these drugs.
	iron	Tannic acid content of herb may reduce iron absorption.

Table of equivalents and conversions

Metric system equivalents

Metric weight

1 kilogram (kg or Kg)	=	1,000 grams (g or gm)
1 gram	=	1,000 milligrams (mg)
1 milligram	=	1,000 micrograms (mcg)
0.6 g	=	600 mg
0.3 g	=	300 mg
0.1 g	=	100 mg
0.06 g	=	60 mg
0.03 g	=	30 mg
0.015 g	=	15 mg
0.001 g	=	1 mg

Metric volume

1 liter (l or L)	=	1,000 milliliters (ml)*
1 milliliter	=	1,000 microliters (mcl)

Household		Metric
1 teaspoon (tsp)	=	5 ml
1 tablespoon (T or tbs)	=	15 ml
2 tablespoons	=	30 ml
8 ounces	=	240 ml
1 pint (pt)	=	473 ml
1 quart (qt)	=	946 ml
1 gallon (gal)	=	3,785 ml

Weight conversions

1 oz = 30 g   1 lb = 453.6 g   2.2 lb = 1 kg

Temperature conversions

Centigrade degrees	Fahrenheit degrees	Centigrade degrees	Fahrenheit degrees	Centigrade degrees	Fahrenheit degrees
41.1	106.0	38.1	100.6	35.1	95.2
41.0	105.8	38.0	100.4	35.0	95.0
40.9	105.6	37.9	100.2	34.9	94.8
40.8	105.4	37.8	100.0	34.8	94.6
40.7	105.2	37.7	99.8	34.7	94.4
40.6	105.0	37.6	99.6	34.6	94.2
40.4	104.8	37.4	99.4	34.4	94.0
40.3	104.6	37.3	99.2	34.3	93.8
40.2	104.4	37.2	99.0	34.2	93.6
40.1	104.2	37.1	98.8	34.1	93.4
40.0	104.0	37.0	98.6	34.0	93.2
39.9	103.8	36.9	98.4	33.9	93.0
39.8	103.6	36.8	98.2	33.8	92.8
39.7	103.4	36.7	98.0	33.7	92.6
39.6	103.2	36.5	97.8	33.6	92.4
39.4	103.0	36.4	97.6	33.4	92.2
39.3	102.8	36.3	97.4	33.3	92.0
39.2	102.6	36.2	97.2	33.2	91.8
39.1	102.4	36.1	97.0	33.1	91.6
39.0	102.2	36.0	96.8	33.0	91.4
38.9	102.0	35.9	96.6	32.9	91.2
38.8	101.8	35.8	96.4	32.8	91.0
38.7	101.6	35.7	96.2	32.7	90.8
38.6	101.4	35.6	96.0	32.6	90.6
38.4	101.2	35.4	95.8	32.4	90.4
38.3	101.0	35.3	95.6	32.3	90.2
38.2	100.8	35.2	95.4	32.2	90.0

*1 ml = 1 cubic centimeter (cc); however, ml is the preferred measurement term.

Adverse reactions misinterpreted as age-related changes

In elderly patients, adverse drug reactions can easily be misinterpreted as the typical signs and symptoms of aging. The table below, which shows possible adverse reactions for common drug classifications, can help you avoid such misinterpretations.

Drug Classifications	Agitation	Anxiety	Arrhythmias	Ataxia	Changes in appetite	Confusion	Constipation	Depression
ACE inhibitors						●	●	●
Alpha₁ adrenergic blockers		●					●	●
Antianginals	●	●	●			●		
Antiarrhythmics			●				●	
Anticholinergics	●	●	●			●	●	
Anticonvulsants	●		●	●	●	●	●	●
Antidepressants, tricyclic	●	●	●	●	●	●	●	
Antidiabetics, oral								
Antihistamines						●	●	●
Antilipemics							●	
Antiparkinsonians	●	●		●	●	●	●	●
Antipsychotics	●	●	●	●	●	●	●	●
Barbiturates	●	●	●			●		
Benzodiazepines	●			●		●	●	●
Beta blockers		●	●					●
Calcium channel blockers		●	●				●	
Corticosteroids	●					●		●
Diuretics						●		
NSAIDs		●				●	●	●
Opioids	●	●				●	●	●
Skeletal muscle relaxants	●	●		●		●		●
Thyroid hormones			●		●			

Difficulty breathing	Disorientation	Dizziness	Drowsiness	Edema	Fatigue	Hypotension	Insomnia	Memory loss	Muscle weakness	Restlessness	Sexual dysfunction	Tremors	Urinary dysfunction	Visual changes
		●			●	●	●				●			●
		●	●	●	●	●	●				●		●	●
		●	●	●	●	●	●			●	●		●	●
●		●			●	●								
	●	●	●		●			●	●				●	●
●		●	●	●	●	●	●					●	●	●
●	●	●	●		●	●	●			●		●	●	●
		●			●									
	●	●	●		●							●	●	●
		●			●			●		●	●		●	●
	●	●	●		●	●			●			●	●	●
		●	●		●	●	●			●		●	●	●
●	●		●		●	●			●					
●	●	●	●		●			●	●	●		●	●	●
●	●	●			●	●					●		●	●
●		●		●	●	●					●		●	●
				●	●		●		●					●
		●			●	●	●					●		
		●	●		●		●		●					●
●	●	●	●		●	●	●	●		●			●	●
		●	●		●	●	●					●		
							●					●		

Drugs that shouldn't be crushed

Slow-release, enteric-coated, encapsulated-bead, wax-matrix, sublingual, and buccal drug forms are made to release their active ingredients over a certain period of time or at preset points after administration. Crushing these drug forms can dramatically affect their absorption rate and increase the risk of adverse reactions.

Other reasons not to crush some drug forms include taste, tissue irritation, and unusual formulation—for example, a capsule within a capsule, a liquid within a capsule, or a multiple-compressed tablet. Some drugs shouldn't be crushed because they're teratogenic. Avoid crushing the following brand-name drugs, for the reasons noted beside them.

Accutane (irritant)
Aciphex (delayed release)
Actifed 12-Hour (sustained release)
Adalat CC (sustained release)
Advicor (extended release)
Aggrenox (extended release)
Allegra D (extended release)
Allerest 12 Hour (sustained release)
Altocor (extended release)
Ambien CR (extended release)
Amnesteem (irritant)
Ansaid (taste)
Arthrotec (delayed release)
Asacol (delayed release)
Aspirin (enteric coated)
Atrohist LA (long acting)
Augmentin XR (extended release)
Avinza (extended release)
Azulfidine EN-tabs (enteric coated)
Biaxin XL (extended release)
Biohist LA (long acting)
Bisacodyl (enteric coated)
Bontril Slow-Release (slow release)
Bromfed (slow release)
Bromfed-PD (slow release)
Bronkodyl SR (slow release)
Calan SR (sustained release)
Carbatrol (extended release)
Cardizem CD, LA, SR (slow release)
Cartia XT (extended release)
Ceclor CD (slow release)
Ceftin (strong, persistent taste)
Cellcept (teratogenic)
Chloral Hydrate (liquid within a capsule, taste)

Chlor-Trimeton Allergy 8-hour and 12-hour (slow release)
Choledyl SA (slow release)
Cipro XR (extended release)
Claritin-D 12-hour (slow release)
Claritin-D 24-hour (slow release)
Cleocin (taste)
Colace (liquid within a capsule)
Colazal (granules within capsules must reach colon intact)
Colestid (protective coating)
Compazine Spansules (slow release)
Concerta (extended release)
Contac 12 Hour, Maximum Strength 12 Hour (slow release)
Cotazym-S (enteric coated)
Covera-HS (extended release)
Creon (enteric coated)
Cytovene (irritant)
Cytoxan (toxic)
Dallergy, Dallergy-Jr (slow release)
Deconamine SR (slow release)
Depakene (slow release, mucous membrane irritant)
Depakote (enteric coated)
Depakote ER (extended release)
Desyrel (taste)
Dexedrine Spansule (slow release)
Diamox Sequels (slow release)
Dilacor XR (extended release)
Dilatrate-SR (slow release)
Diltia XT (extended release)
Dimetane Extentabs (extended release)
Dimetapp Extentabs (slow release)
Ditropan XL (slow release)

Dolobid (irritant)
Donnatel Extentabs (extended release)
Doxidan Liquigels (liquid within capsule)
Drisdol (liquid filled)
Dristan (protective coating)
Drixoral (slow release)
Dulcolax (enteric coated)
Dynabac (slow release)
DynaCirc CR (slow release)
Easprin (enteric coated)
Ecotrin (enteric coated)
Ecotrin Maximum Strength (enteric coated)
E.E.S. 400 Filmtab (enteric coated)
Effexor XR (extended release)
Emend (hard gelatin capsule)
E-Mycin (enteric coated)
Entex LA (slow release)
Entex PSE (slow release)
Equanil (extended release)
Ergostat (sublingual)
Eryc (enteric coated)
Ery-Tab (enteric coated)
Erythrocin Stearate (enteric coated)
Erythromycin Base (enteric coated)
Eskalith CR (slow release)
Extendryl JR, SR (slow release)
Feldene (mucous membrane irritant)
Feosol (enteric coated)
Feratab (enteric coated)
Fergon (slow release)
Fero-Folic 500 (slow release)
Fero-Grad-500 (slow release)
Ferro-Sequel (slow release)

Feverall Children's Capsules, Sprinkle (taste)

Flomax (slow release)

Fumatinic (slow release)

Geocillin (taste)

Glucophage XR (extended release)

Glucotrol XL (slow release)

Glumetza (extended release)

Guaifed (slow release)

Guaifed-PD (slow release)

Guaifenex LA (slow release)

Guaifenex PPA (slow release)

Guaifenex PSE (slow release)

Guaimax-D (slow release)

Hydergine LC (sublingual)

Hytakerol (liquid filled)

Iberet (slow release)

ICAPS Plus (slow release)

ICAPS Time Release (slow release)

Ilotycin (enteric coated)

Imdur (slow release)

Inderal LA (slow release)

Indocin SR (slow release)

InnoPran XL (extended release)

Ionamin (slow release)

Isoptin SR (sustained release)

Isordil Sublingual (sublingual)

Isordil Tembids (slow release)

Isosorbide Dinitrate Sublingual (sublingual)

Kaletra (extended release)

Kaon-Cl (slow release)

K-Dur (slow release)

Klor-Con (slow release)

Klotrix (slow release)

K-Tab (slow release)

Levbid (slow release)

Levsinex Timecaps (slow release)

Lithobid (slow release)

Macrobid (slow release)

Mestinon Timespans (slow release)

Metadate CD, ER (extended release)

Methylin ER (extended release)

Micro-K Extencaps (slow release)

Modane (enteric coated)

Motrin (taste)

MS Contin (slow release)

Mucinex (extended release)

Naprelan (slow release)

Nexium (sustained release)

Niaspan (extended release)

Nicotinic acid (slow release)

Nitroglyn (slow release)

Nitrostat (sublingual)

Noctec (liquid within capsule)

Norflex (slow release)

Norpace CR (slow release)

Oramorph SR (slow release)

Oruvail (extended release)

OxyContin (slow release)

Pancrease (enteric coated)

Pancrease MT (enteric coated)

Paxil CR (controlled-release)

PCE (slow release)

Pentasa (controlled release)

Phazyme (slow release)

Phazyme 95 (slow release)

Phenytek (extended release)

Plendil (slow release)

Prelu-2 (slow release)

Prevacid, Prevacid SoluTab (delayed release)

Prilosec (slow release)

Prilosec OTC (delayed-release)

Pro-Banthine (taste)

Procanbid (slow release)

Procardia (delayed absorption)

Procardia XL (slow release)

Propecia (adverse effects when handled by pregnant women)

Proscar (adverse effects when handled by pregnant women)

Protonix (delayed release)

Proventil Repetabs (slow release)

Prozac Weekly (slow release)

Quibron-T/SR (slow release)

Quinaglute Duratabs (extended release)

Quinidex Extentabs (slow release)

Respaire SR (slow release)

Respbid (extended release)

Risperdal M-Tab (delayed-release)

Ritalin-LA, -SR (slow release)

Rondec-TR (slow release)

Roxanol SR (sustained release)

Sinemet CR (slow release)

Slo-bid Gyrocaps (slow release)

Slo-Niacin (slow release)

Slo-Phyllin GG, Gyrocaps (slow release)

Slow FE (slow release)

Slow-K (slow release)

Slow-Mag (slow release)

Sorbitrate (sublingual)

Sotret (irritant)

Sudafed 12 Hour (slow release)

Sular (extended release)

Surfac Liquigels (liquid within capsule)

Tegretol-XR (extended release)

Ten-K (slow release)

Tenuate Dospan (slow release)

Tessalon Perles (slow release)

Theochron (slow release)

Theoclear LA (slow release)

Theo-24 (slow release)

TheoDur (extended release)

Thorazine Spansules (slow release)

Tiazac (sustained release)

Topamax (taste)

Toprol XL (extended release)

Trental (slow release)

Tylenol Extended Relief (slow release)

Uniphyl (slow release)

Vantin (taste)

Verelan, Verelan PM (slow release)

Volmax (slow release)

Voltaren (enteric coated)

Voltaren-XR (extended release)

Wellbutrin SR (sustained release)

Xanax XR (extended release)

Zerit XR (extended release)

Zomig-ZMT (delayed-release)

ZORprin (slow release)

Zyban (slow release)

Zyrtec-D 12 hour (extended release)

Normal laboratory test values

Normal values may differ from laboratory to laboratory. Standard International units are abbreviated SI.

Hematology

Bleeding time
Template: 3–6 min (SI, 3–6 m)
Ivy: 3–6 min (SI, 3–6 m)
Duke: 1–3 min (SI, 1–3 m)

Fibrinogen, plasma
200–400 mg/dl (SI, 2–4 g/L)

Hematocrit
Men: 42%–52% (SI, 0.42–0.52)
Women: 36%–48% (SI, 0.36–0.48)

Hemoglobin, total
Men: 14–17.4 g/dl (SI, 140–174 g/L)
Women: 12–16 g/dl (SI, 120–160 g/L)

Partial thromboplastin time, activated
21–35 sec (SI, 21–35 sec)

Platelet aggregation
3–5 min (SI, 3–5 min)

Platelet count
140,000–400,000/mm^3 (SI, 140–400 × 10^9/L)

Prothrombin time
10–14 sec (SI, 10–14 sec); INR for patients not receiving warfarin, 1.12–1.46; INR for patients receiving warfarin, 2–3 (SI, 2–3) (those with prosthetic heart valve, 2.5–3.5 [SI, 2.5–3.5])

Red blood cell count
Men: 4.5–5.5 million/mm^3 (SI, 4.5–5.5 × 10^{12}/L) venous blood
Women: 4–5 million/mm^3 (SI, 4–5 × 10^{12}/L) venous blood

Red blood cell indices
Mean corpuscular volume: 82–98 femtoliters
Mean corpuscular hemoglobin: 26–34 picograms/cell
Mean corpuscular hemoglobin concentration: 31–37 g/dl

Reticulocyte count
0.5%–1.5% (SI, 0.005–0.025) of total RBC count

White blood cell count
4,500–10,500 cells/mm^3

White blood cell differential, blood
Neutrophils: 54%–75% (SI, 0.54–0.75)
Lymphocytes: 25%–40% (SI, 0.25–0.4)
Monocytes: 2%–8% (SI, 0.02–0.08)
Eosinophils: up to 4% (SI, up to 0.04)
Basophils: up to 1% (SI, up to 0.01)

Blood chemistry

Alanine aminotransferase
Adults: 10–35 units/L (SI, 0.17–0.6 µkat/L)
Newborns: 13–45 units/L (SI, 0.22–0.77 µkat/L)

Amylase, serum
Adults ≥ age 18: 30–175 units/L (SI, 0.5–2.83 µkat/L)

Arterial blood gases
pH: 7.35–7.45 (SI, 7.35–7.45)
Paco$_2$: 35–45 mm Hg (SI, 4.7–5.3 kPa)
Pao$_2$: 80–100 mm Hg (SI, 10.6–13.3 kPa)
HCO$_3^-$: 22–26 mEq/L (SI, 22–25 mmol/L)
Sao$_2$: 94%–100% (SI, 0.94–1.00)

Aspartate aminotransferase
Men: 14–20 units/L (SI, 0.23–0.33 µkat/L)
Women: 7–34 units/L (SI, 0.12–0.58 µkat/L)

Bilirubin, serum
Adults, total: 0.2–1 mg/dl (SI, 3.5–17 µmol/L)
Neonates, total: 1–10 mg/dl (SI, 17–170 µmol/L)
Neonates, unconjugated indirect: 0–10 mg/dl (SI, 0–170 µmol/L)

Blood urea nitrogen
8–20 mg/dl (SI, 2.9–7.5 mmol/L)

Calcium, serum
Adults: 8.2–10.2 mg/dl (SI, 2.05–2.54 mmol/L)
Children: 8.6–11.2 mg/dl (SI, 2.15–2.79 mmol/L)

Carbon dioxide, total blood
22–26 mEq/L (SI, 22–26 mmol/L)

Cholesterol, total serum
Men: < 205 mg/dl (SI, < 5.30 mmol/L) (desirable)
Women: < 190 mg/dl (SI, < 4.90 mmol/L) (desirable)

Creatine kinase, isoenzymes
CK–BB: none
CK–MB: 0–7%
CK–MM: 96–100%

Creatinine, serum
Adults: 0.6–1.3 mg/dl (SI, 53–115 μmol/L)

Glucose, plasma, fasting
70–110 mg/dl (SI, 3.9–6.1 mmol/L)

Glucose, plasma, 2-hour postprandial
< 145 mg/dl (SI, < 8 mmol/L)

Lactate dehydrogenase
Total: 71–207 units/L in adults (SI, 1.2–3.52 μkat/L)
LD1: 14%–26% (SI, 0.14–0.26)
LD2: 29%–39% (SI, 0.29–0.39)
LD3: 20%–26% (SI, 0.20–0.26)
LD4: 8%–16% (SI, 0.08–0.16)
LD5: 6%–16% (SI, 0.06–0.16)

Lipase
< 160 units/L (SI, < 2.72 μkat/L)

Magnesium, serum
1.8–2.6 mg/dl (SI, 0.74–1.07 mmol/L)

Phosphates, serum
2.7–4.5 mg/dl (SI, 0.87–1.45 mmol/L)

Potassium, serum
3.8–5 mEq/L (SI, 3.5–5 mmol/L)

Protein, serum
Total: 6.3–8.3 g/dl (SI, 64–83 g/L)
Albumin fraction: 3.5–5 g/dl (SI, 35–50 g/L)

Sodium, serum
135–145 mEq/L (SI, 135–145 mmol/L)

Triglycerides, serum
Men > age 20: 40–180 mg/dl (SI, 0.11–2.01 mmol/L)
Women > age 20: 10–190 mg/dl (SI, 0.11–2.21 mmol/L)

Uric acid, serum
Men: 3.4–7 mg/dl (SI, 202–416 μmol/L)
Women: 2.3–6 mg/dl (SI, 143–357 μmol/L)

English-to-Spanish drug phrase translator

Medication history

Do you take any medications?
– Prescription?
– Over-the-counter?
– Other?

¿Toma usted medicamentos?
– ¿Bajo receta?
¿De venta libre?
– ¿Otro?

Which prescription medications do you take routinely?
Which over-the-counter medications do you take routinely?
– How often do you take them?
– Once daily?
– Twice daily?
– Three times daily?
– Four times daily?
– More often?

¿Qué medicamentos bajo receta toma como rutina?
¿Qué medicamentos de venta libre toma como rutina?
– ¿Con qué frecuencia los toma?
– ¿Una vez al día?
– ¿Dos veces al día?
– ¿Tres veces al día?
– ¿Cuátro veces al día?
– ¿Con más frecuencia?

Why do you take these medications?

¿Por qué toma estos medicamentos?

What is the dosage for each medication?

¿Cuál es la dosis para cada medicamento?

Are you allergic to any medications?

¿Es usted alérgico(a) a algún medicamento?

Medication teaching

Purpose of the medication
This medication will:
– elevate your blood pressure.
– improve circulation to your _____.
– lower your blood pressure.
– lower your blood sugar.
– make your heart rhythm more even.
– raise your blood sugar.
– reduce or prevent the formation of blood clots.
– remove fluid from your body.
– remove fluid from your feet, ankles, or legs.

– remove fluid from your lungs so that they work better.
– remove fluid from your pancreas so that it works better.
– kill the bacteria in your _____.
– slow down your heart rate.
– soften your bowel movements.
– speed up your heart rate.
– help your body to use insulin more efficiently.

Este medicamento:
– elevará su presión sanguínea.
– mejorará la circulación a su _____.
– reducirá su presión sanguínea.
– reducirá el nivel de azúcar en su sangre.
– hará que su ritmo cardiaco sea más uniforme.
– elevará el nivel de azúcar en su sangre.
– reducirá o evitará la formación de coágulos.
– eliminará el liquido de su cuerpo.
– eliminará el liquido de sus pies, tobillos o piernas.
– eliminará el liquido de sus pulmones para que funcionen mejor.
– eliminará el liquido de su páncreas para que funcione mejor.
– matará las bacterias en su _____.
– hará más lento su ritmo cardiaco.
– ablandará sus evacuaciones intestinales.
– acelerará su ritmo cardiaco.
– ayudará a su cuerpo a usar la insulina de manera más eficaz.

This medication will help you to:
- breathe better.
- fight infections.
- relax.
- sleep.
- think more clearly.

Este medicamento le ayudará a:
- respirar mejor.
- combatir infecciones.
- relajarse.
- dormir.
- pensar con mayor claridad.

This medication will relieve or reduce:
- the acid production in your stomach.
- anxiety.
- bladder spasms.
- burning in your stomach or chest.
- burning when you urinate.
- diarrhea.
- muscle cramps.
- nausea.
- pain in your ____.

Este medicamento le aliviará o reducirá:
- la producción de ácido en su estómago.
- la ansiedad.
- los espasmos en la vejiga.
- el ardor en su estómago o pecho.
- el ardor al orinar.
- la diarrea.
- los calambres musculares.
- las nauseas.
- el dolor en su ____.

Medication administration

I would like to give you:
- an injection.
- an I.V. medication.
- a liquid medication.
- a medicated cream or powder.
- a medication through your epidural catheter.

- a medication through your rectum.
- a medication through your ____ tube.
- a medication under your tongue.
- some pill(s).
- a suppository.

Quisiera darle:
- una inyección.
- un medicamento por vía intravenosa.
- un medicamento en forma líquida.
- un medicamento en pomada o polvo.
- un medicamento a través de su catéter epidural.
- un medicamento por vía rectal.
- un medicamento a través de su tubo de ____.
- un medicamento debajo de la lengua.
- algunas píldoras.
- un supositorio.

This is how you take this medication.

Así se toma este medicamento.

If you can't swallow this pill, I can get it in another form.

Si usted no logra tragar esta píldora, puede obtenerla en otra forma.

If you can't swallow a pill, you can crush it and mix it in soft food.

Si usted no logra tragar una píldora, puede molerla y mezclarla con alimentos blandos.

I need to mix this medication in juice or water.

Necesito mezclar este medicamento en jugo o agua.

I need to give you this injection in your:
- abdomen.
- buttocks.
- hip.
- outer arm.
- thigh.

Necesito ponerle esta inyección en:
- el abdomen.
- las nalgas.
- la cadera.
- la parte externa el brazo.
- el muslo.

Some medications are coated with a special substance to protect your stomach from getting upset.

Algunos medicamentos están revestidos con una sustancia especial para protegerlo(a) contra malestar estomacal.

Do not chew:
– enteric-coated pills.
– long-acting pills.
– capsules.
– sublingual medication.

No masque:
– píldoras con recubrimiento entérico.
– píldoras de efecto prolongado.
– cápsulas.
– medicamentos sublinguales.

Ask your doctor or pharmacist whether you can:
– mix your medication with food or fluids.

– take your medication with or without food.

Pregunte a su médico o farmacéutico si usted puede:
– mezclar su medicamento con alimentos o líquidos.
– tomar su medicamento con o sin alimentos.

You need to take your medication:
– after meals.
– before meals.
– on an empty stomach.
– with meals or food.

Usted debe tomar su medicamento:
– después de las comidas.
– antes de las comidas.
– con el estómago vacío.
– con comidas o alimentos.

Skipping doses
If you skip or miss a dose:
– Take it as soon as you remember it.
– Wait until the next dose.
– Call the doctor if you are not sure.
– Do not take an extra dose.

Si usted se salta u omite una dosis:
– Tómela apenas se acuerde.
– Espere hasta la próxima dosis.
– Llame a su médico si no está seguro(a).
– No tome una dosis adicional.

Adverse effects
Some common adverse effects of _____ are:

Algunos afectos adversos comunes de _____ son:

– constipation
– diarrhea
– difficulty sleeping
– dry mouth
– fatigue
– headache
– itching
– light-headedness
– nausea
– poor appetite
– rash
– upset stomach
– weight loss or gain
– frequent urination.

– constipación
– diarrea
– dificultad para dormir
– boca seca
– fatiga
– dolor de cabeza
– picazón (comezón)
– mareos
– náuseas
– disminución del apetito
– erupción
– malestar estomacal
– aumento o pérdida de peso
– orinar con frecuencia.

These adverse effects:
– will go away after your body gets used to the medication.
– may persist as long as you take the medication.

Estos efectos adversos:
– desaparecerán cuanao su cuerpo se acostumbre al medicamento.
– podrán persistir mientras usted tome el medicamento.

If you have an adverse reaction to your medication, call your doctor right away.

Si usted tiene una reacción adversa a su medicamento, llame a su médico de inmediato.

Other concerns

Tell your doctor if you are pregnant or breast-feeding.

Dígale a su médico si usted está embarazada o amamantando.

While you are taking this medication, ask your doctor if:
– you can safely take other over-the-counter medications.
– you can drink alcoholic beverages.
– your medications interact with each other.

Mientras tome este medicamento, pregúntele a su médico si:
– usted puede tomar otros medicamentos de venta libre sin peligro.
– usted puede tomar bebidas alcohólicas.
– sus medicamentos tienen interacción entre si.

Storing medication

You should keep your medication:
– in a cool, dry place.
– in the refrigerator.
– at room temperature.
– out of direct sunlight.
– away from heat.
– away from children.

Usted debe guardar sus medicamentos:
– en un lugar fresco y seco.
– en el refrigerador.
– al temperatura ambiente.
– fuera de la luz directa del sol.
– lejos del calor.
– lejos del alcance de los niños.

Subcutaneous injection

To give yourself an injection, follow these steps:
– Draw up the medication.
– Replace the cap carefully.
– Decide where you are going to give the injection.
– Clean the skin area with alcohol.
– Gently pinch up a little skin over the area.

– Using a dartlike motion, stab the needle into your skin.
– Gently pull back on the plunger to see if there is any blood in the syringe.
– Steadily push the medication into your skin.

– Pull the needle out.
– Apply gentle pressure with the alcohol wipe.

– Dispose of the needle in a proper receptacle.

Para ponerse una inyección, haga lo siguiente:
– Extraiga el medicamento.
– Vuelva a colocar la tapa con cuidado.
– Decida dónde colocará la inyección.
– Limpie el área de la piel con alcohol.
– Suavemente, pellizque un poco de la piel sobre el área.

– Con un movimiento como si estuviera arrojando un dardo, penetre la piel con la aguja.
– Tire suavemente del émbolo para ver si hay sangre en la jeringa.
– Coloque el medicamento en la piel de manera uniforme.
– Retire la aguja.
– Aplique presión suave con un paño con alcohol.

– Deseche la aguja en un recipiente apropiado.

Insulin preparation and administration

The doctor has ordered insulin for you.

El médico le ha recetado insulina.

To draw up insulin, follow these steps:

– Wipe the rubber top of the insulin bottle with alcohol.

Para extraer la insulina, siga los siguientes pasos:
– Limpie la tapa de goma del frasco de insulina con alcohol.

– Remove the needle cap.
– Pull out the plunger until the end of the plunger in the barrel aligns with the number of units of insulin that you need.
– Push the needle through the rubber top of the insulin bottle.
– Inject the air into the bottle.
– Without removing the needle from the bottle, turn it upside down.
– Withdraw the plunger until the end of the plunger aligns with the number of units you need.
– Gently pull the needle out of the bottle.

– Retire la tapa de la aguja.
– Tire del émbolo hasta que la extremidad del émbolo en la barril esté al nivel de la cantidad de unidades de insulina que usted necesita.
– Empuje la aguja a través de la tapa de goma del frasco de insulina.
– Inyecte el aire dentro del frasco.
– Sin retirar la aguja del frasco, gírelo boca abajo.
– Retire el émbolo hasta que la extremidad del émbolo esté al nivel de la cantidad de unidades que necesita.
– Suavemente, retire la aguja del frasco.

To mix insulin, follow these steps:

– Wipe the rubber tops of the insulin bottles with alcohol.
– Gently roll the cloudy insulin between your palms.
– Remove the needle cap.
– Pull out the plunger until the end of the plunger in the barrel aligns with the number of units of NPH or Lente insulin that you need.
– Push the needle through the rubber top of the cloudy insulin bottle.
– Inject the air into the bottle.
– Remove the needle.
– Pull out the plunger until the end of the plunger in the barrel aligns with the number of units of clear regular insulin that you need.
– Push the needle through the rubber top of the clear insulin bottle.
– Inject the air into the bottle.
– Without removing the needle, turn the bottle upside down.
– Withdraw the plunger until it aligns with the number of units of clear regular insulin that you need.
– Gently pull the needle out of the bottle.
– Push the needle into the cloudy (NPH or Lente) insulin without injecting it into the bottle.
– Withdraw the plunger until you reach your total dosage of insulin in units (regular combined with NPH or Lente).
– We will practice again.

Para mezclar la insulina siga los siguientes pasos:

– Limpie las tapas de goma de los frascos de insulina con alcohol.
– Suavemente, gire el frasco de insulina turbia entre las palmas de la mano.
– Retire la tapa de la aguja.
– Tire del émbolo hasta que la extremidad del émbolo en el barril esté alineado con la cantidad de unidades de NPH o Lente que usted necesita.
– Empuje la aguja a través de la tapa de goma del frasco de insulina clara.
– Inyecte el aire en el frasco.
– Sin retirar la aguja, gire el frasco boca abajo.
– Tire del émbolo hasta que este al nivel de la cantidad de unidades de insulina común clara que usted necesita.
– Empuje la aguja a través de la tapa de goma del frasco de insulina clara.
– Inyecte el aire en el frasco.
– Sin retirar la aguja, gire el frasco boca abajo.

– Tire del émbolo hasta que al nive de la cantidad de unidades de insulina común clara que usted necesita.
– Suavemente, retire la aguja del frasco.
– Empuje la aguja hacia dentro de la insulina turbia (NPH o Lente) sin inyectarla en el frasco.
– Tire del émbolo hasta llegar ala dosis total de insulina en unidades (común combinada con NPH o Lente).
– Practicaremos nuevamente.

Home care phrases

Wash your hands before touching medications.	Lávese las manos antes de tocar medicamentos.
Check the medication bottle for name, dose, and frequency (how often it's supposed to be taken).	Verifique el nombre, dosis y frecuencia (cada cuanto lo debe tomar) en al frasco del medicamento.
Check the expiration date on all medications.	Verifique la fecha de vencimiento de todos los medicamentos.
Store medications according to pharmacy instructions.	Almacene los medicamentos de acuerdo con las instrucciones de la farmacia.
Under adequate lighting, read medication labels carefully before taking doses.	Con luz adecuada, lea las etiquetas de los medicamentos con mucho cuidado antes de tomar las dosis.
Don't crush medication without first asking the doctor or pharmacist.	No machaque el medicamento sin preguntar al médico o al farmacéutico.
Contact your doctor if a new or unexpected symptom or another problem appears.	Contacte a su médico si aparece u síntoma nuevo o imprevisto u otro problema.
Don't stop taking medication unless instructed by your doctor.	No deje de tomar el medicamento sin indicación médica.
Discard outdated medications.	Deseche los medicamentos vencidos.
Never take someone else's medications.	Nunca tome los medicamentos de otra persona.
Keep a record of your current medications.	Mantenga un registro de sus medicamentos actuales.

General drug therapy phrases

Drug classes

Analgesic	Analgésico
Anesthetic	Anestético
Antacid	Antiácido
Antianginal agent	Agente antianginal
Antianxiety agent	Agente ansiolítico
Antiarrhythmic agent	Agente antiarrítmico
Antibiotic	Antibiótico
Anticancer agent	Agente anticarcinógeno
Anticoagulant	Anticoagulante
Anticonvulsant	Anticonvulsivante
Antidepressant	Antidepresivo
Antidiarrheal	Antidiarreico
Antifungal agent	Agente antifúngico
Antigout agent	Agente antigota

Antihistamine	Antihistamínico
Antihyperlipemic agent	Agente hiperlipémico
Antihypertensive agent	Agente antihipertenso
Anti-inflammatory agent	Agente antiinflamatorio
Antimalarial agent	Agente antimalárico
Antiparkinsonian agent	Agente antiparkinsoniano
Antipsychotic agent	Agente antipsicótico
Antipyretic	Antipirético
Antiseptic	Antiséptico
Antispasmodic	Antiespasmódico
Antithyroid agent	Agente antitiroideo
Antituberculosis agent	Agente antituberculoso
Antitussive agent	Agente antitusígeno
Antiviral agent	Agente antiviral
Appetite stimulant	Estimulante para el apetito
Appetite suppressant	Supresor de apetito
Bronchodilator	Broncodilatador
Decongestant	Descongestivo
Digestant	Digestivo (agente que estimula la digestión)
Diuretic	Diurético
Emetic	Emético
Fertility agent	Agente para la fertilidad
Hypnotic	Hipnótico
Insulin	Insulina
Laxative	Laxante
Muscle relaxant	Relajante de músculos
Oral contraceptive	Anticonceptivo oral
Oral hypoglycemic agent	Agente hipoglucémico oral
Sedative	Sedante
Steroid	Esteroide
Thyroid hormone	Hormona de la glándula tiroides
Vaccine	Vacuna
Vasodilator	Vasodilatador
Vitamin	Vitamina

Preparations

Capsule	Cápsula
Cream	Pomada
Drops	Gotas
Elixir	Elixir
Inhaler	Inhalador

Injection	Inyección
Lotion	Loción
Lozenge	Pastilla
Powder	Polvo
Spray	Atomizador
Suppository	Supositorio
Suspension	Suspensión
Syrup	Jarabe
Tablet	Tableta

Frequency

Once daily	Una vez al día
Twice daily	Dos veces al día
Three times daily	Tres veces al día
Four times daily	Cuatro veces al día
In the morning	Por la mañana
With meals	Con las comidas
Before meals	Antes de las comidas
After meals	Después de las comidas
Before bedtime	Antes de acostarse
When you have____	Cuando Ud. tome____
Only when you need it	Sólo cuando lo necesite
Every four hours	Cada cuatro horas
Every six hours	Cada seis horas
Every eight hours	Cada ocho horas

Acknowledgments

We would like to thank the following companies for granting us permission to include their drugs in the full-color photoguide.

Abbott Laboratories
Depakote®
Hytrin®
Kaletra®

AstraZeneca LP
Arimidex®
Crestor®
Prilosec®
Tenormin®
Toprol-XL®

Aventis Pharmaceuticals
DiaBeta®
Lasix®

Bayer Corporation
Cipro®
Levitra®

Biovail Pharmaceuticals, Inc.
Cardizem®
Cardizem CD®
Cardizem LA®
Vasotec®

Bristol-Myers Squibb Company
Capoten®
Coumadin®
Monopril®
Pravachol®

Elan Pharmaceuticals, Inc.
Frova®

Forest Pharmaceuticals, Inc.
Campral®
Celexa®
Lexapro®

GlaxoSmithKline
Reproduced with permission of GlaxoSmithKline.
Avandia®
Combavir®
Imitrex®
Lanoxin®
Lotronex®
Retrovir®
Wellbutrin®
Wellbutrin SR®
Zyban®

Janssen Pharmaceutica, Inc.
Risperdal®
Risperdal® M-Tab™

King Pharmaceuticals, Inc.
Levoxyl®

Eli Lilly and Company
Copyright Eli Lilly and Company. Used with Permission.
Cymbalta®
Prozac®

Mallinckrodt, Inc.
Pamelor®

Merck & Co., Inc.
Used with permission.
Cozaar®
Crixivan®
Fosamax®
Mevacor®
Pepcid®
Prinivil®
Sinemet®
Sinemat CR®
Singulair®
Zocor®

Merck/Schering-Plough
Used with permission.
Zetia™

Merck Santé
An associate of Merck KGaA, Darmstadt, Germany
Glucophage®
Glucophage XR®

Novartis Pharmaceuticals, Inc.
Enablex®
Ritalin®

Ortho-McNeil Pharmaceutical
Levaquin®

Otsuka Pharmaceutical Company, Ltd.
Abilify®

Pfizer, Inc.
Photographed with pemission of Pfizer Inc. All rights reserved.
Accupril®
Bextra®
Calan®
Cardura®
Celebrex®
Demulen®
Detrol®
Diflucan®
Dilantin® Kapseals®
Glucotrol®
Glucotrol XL®
Lipitor®
Lopid®
Midrol®
Micronase
Neurontin®
Nitrostat®
Norvasc®

Pletal®
Procardia®
Procardia XL®
Provera®
Relpax®
Viagra®
Zithromax®
Zoloft®
Zyrtec®

**Pharmacia Corporation, a
Pfizer, Inc. corporation**
Registered Trademarks of
Pharmacia Corporation, a
Pfizer Inc. corporation. All
rights reserved. Courtesy of
Pfizer Inc.
Calan®
Micronase®
Provera®
Xanax®

Presutti Laboratories, LLC
Tindamax®

**Procter & Gamble
Pharmaceuticals, Inc.**
Actonel®

Purdue Pharma L.P.
OxyContin®

Roche Laboratories, Inc.
Valium®

Salix Pharmaceuticals, Inc.
Xifaxan®

Sanofi-Synthelabo, Inc.
Ambien®

**Schering Corporation and
Key Pharmaceuticals, Inc.**
Clarinex®
K-Dur®

Sepracor, Inc.
Lunesta®

Tap Pharmaceuticals, Inc.
Prevacid®

**Warner Chilcott Laborato-
ries, Inc.**
Duricef®
Eryc®
Estrace®

Wyeth Pharmaceuticals
The appearance of these
tablets and capsules is a trade-
mark of Wyeth Pharmaceuticals, Philadelphia, Pa.
Effexor XR®
Phenergan®

Index

t refers to a table; **boldface** refers to the drug's monograph; ***boldface italic*** refers to a full-color photograph.

Alzheimer's disease
(continued)
rivastigmine for, 1119
tacrine for, 1190
amantadine hydrochloride, 58,
60, **133–135**
Amaryl, 637
ambenonium, drug interactions
with, 1364t–1365t
Ambien, 1337, *C16*
Ambien CR, 1337
AmBisome, 155
Amcort, 1270
Amebiasis
chloroquine for, 314
erythromycin for, 511
metronidazole for, 850
minocycline for, 861
tinidazole for, 1242
Amen, 807
Amenorrhea
bromocriptine for, 235
medroxyprogesterone ac-
etate for, 807
norethindrone for, 926
Amerge, 899
Americium contamination, pen-
tetate calcium trisodium
for, 1005
A-MethaPred, 841
amethopterin, **834–837**
Amevive, 116
amikacin sulfate, 39, **135–137**
drug interactions with,
1360t–1361t
Amikin, 135
amiloride, 1374
drug interactions with,
1360t–1361t
Aminoglycosides, 39–40
drug interactions with,
1360t–1361t
Amino-Opti-E, 1317
aminophylline, 86, **137–139**
Aminoxin, 1078
amiodarone hydrochloride, 44,
139–142
Amitone, 257
amitriptyline hydrochloride, 50,
142–143, 1373
amitriptyline pamoate, 50
amlodipine besylate, 42, 55,
63, **144–145**, 1374
amlodipine besylate and atorvastatin calcium, **145–146**
Amniocentesis, Rho(D) im-
mune globulin, human, for,
1102
amobarbital sodium, 61
drug interactions with,
1362t–1363t

amoxapine, 50
amoxicillin and clavulanate
potassium, 78, **147–149**
amoxicillin trihydrate, 78,
149–151
drug interactions with,
1362t–1363t
Amoxil, 149
amoxycillin trihydrate, **149–151**
amphetamine aspartate, 1366
amphetamine sulfate, 1366
Amphocin, 151
Amphojel, 132
amphotericin B desoxycholate,
151–153
amphotericin B lipid complex,
153–155
amphotericin B liposomal,
155–157
ampicillin, 78, **157–159**
drug interactions with,
1362t–1363t
ampicillin sodium, **157–159**
ampicillin sodium and sulbactam sodium, 78, **159–161**
ampicillin trihydrate, 78,
157–159
Ampicin ◆, 157
Ampicyn Injection ◇, 157
Ampicyn Oral ◇, 157
Amprace ◇, 483
amprenavir, 60, **161–163**
drug interactions with,
1364t–1365t
Amylase, serum, 1396t
amyl nitrate, drug interactions
with, 1364t–1365t
Amyotrophic lateral sclerosis,
riluzole for, 1111
Anacin, 99
Anacin Maximum Strength As-
pirin Free, 99
Anacobin ◆, 366
Anafranil, 346
Ana-Guard, 495
anakinra, **164–165**
Analgesia. *See* Pain
Anaphylaxis, epinephrine for,
495
Anaprox, 897
Anaprox DS, 897
anastrozole, **165–166**
Anatensol ◇, 589
Ancasal ◆, 178
Ancef, 278
Ancobon, 579
Ancolan ◇, 806
Ancotil ◇, 579
Androderm, 1218
AndroGel, 1218
Andro L.A. 200, 1216

Andronaq-50, 1216
Andronate 100, 1216
Andronate 200, 1216
Andropository 200, 1216
Andryl 200, 1216
Anectine, 1178
Anectine Flo-Pack, 1178
Anemia
azacitidine for, 195
chlorambucil for, 309
cyanocobalamin for, 366
darbepoetin alfa for, 387
epoetin alfa for, 501–502
folic acid for, 602–603
iron dextran for, 720
iron sucrose for, 722
leucovorin for, 755
lymphocyte immune globulin
for, 795
pyridoxine for, 1078
sodium ferric gluconate
complex for, 1158
Anergan 50, 1064
Anesthesia
atracurium for, 192
butorphanol for, 249
epinephrine to prolong effect
of, 495
fentanyl for, 566
meperidine for, 818
midazolam for, 856
mivacurium for, 869
nalbuphine for, 893
pancuronium for, 974
phenylephrine for,
1018–1019
rocuronium for, 1122
succinylcholine for, 1178
sufentanil for, 1182
vecuronium for, 1301
Anexsia 5/325, 1368
Anexsia 5/500, 1368
Anexsia 7.5/325, 1368
Anexsia 7.5/650, 1368
Anexsia 10/660, 1368
angelica, **1341**
Angina
abciximab for, 93
acebutolol for, 97
amiodarone for, 139
amlodipine and atorvastatin
for, 145
amlodipine for, 144
aspirin for, 178
atenolol for, 184
atorvastatin to reduce risk
of, 1878
bivalirudin for, 226
clopidogrel for, 351
dalteparin for, 382
diltiazem for, 429

---

t refers to a table; **boldface** refers to the drug's monograph; ***boldface italic*** refers to a full-color photograph.

---

t refers to a table; **boldface** refers to the drug's monograph; ***boldface italic*** refers to a full-color photograph.

B

baclofen, 81, **204–206**
Bacteremia. *See also* Septicemia
cefoperazone for, 285
cefotaxime for, 287
cefoxitin for, 288
ceftazidime for, 283
ceftizoxime for, 296
ceftriaxone for, 298
chloramphenicol for, 311
linezolid for, 775
Bacterial infection
amikacin for, 135
amoxicillin and clavulanate
potassium for, 147
amoxicillin for, 149
ampicillin for, 157–158
ampicillin sodium and sulbactam sodium for,
159–160
azithromycin for, 200–201
aztreonam for, 202
cefaclor for, 275–276
cefadroxil for, 277
cefazolin for, 278
cefdinir for, 280
cefditoren for, 281
cefixime for, 283
cefoperazone for, 285
cefotaxime for, 287
cefoxitin for, 288
cefpodoxime for, 290
cefprozil for, 292
ceftazidime for, 283
ceftibuten for, 295
ceftizoxime for, 296
ceftriaxone for, 298
cefuroxime for, 300
cephalexin for, 305
chloramphenicol for, 311
ciprofloxacin for, 330
clarithromycin for, 336–337
clindamycin for, 339
co-trimoxazole for, 364
daptomycin for, 385
doxycycline for, 465
ertapenem for, 508–509
erythromycin for, 511–512
gatifloxacin for, 627
gatifloxacin ophthalmic solution for, 629
gemifloxacin for, 631
gentamicin for, 635
imipenem and cilastatin
sodium for, 684
levofloxacin for, 768–769
linezolid for, 775
loracarbef for, 787
meropenem for, 821
metronidazole for, 850–851

Bacterial infection *(continued)*
minocycline for, 861
moxifloxacin for, 882
moxifloxacin hydrochloride
ophthalmic solution for,
884
nafcillin for, 891
neomycin for, 906
nitrofurantoin for, 917
norfloxacin for, 928
ofloxacin for, 934
penicillin G benzathine for,
992
penicillin G potassium for,
994
penicillin G procaine for, 996
penicillin G sodium for, 998
penicillin V for, 1000
piperacillin sodium and
tazobactam sodium for,
1030
quinupristin and dalfopristin
for, 1088
streptomycin for, 1175
telithromycin for, 1201
tetracycline for, 1220
ticarcillin and clavulanate
potassium for, 1237
ticarcillin for, 1235
tigecycline for, 1241
tobramycin for, 1250
trimethoprim for, 1281
vancomycin for, 1296
Bacterial vaginosis
clindamycin for, 339
metronidazole for, 851
Bactrim, 364
Bactrim DS, 364
Bactrim I.V., 364
BAL in Oil, 431
Balminil DMI, 412
balsalazide disodium, **206–207**
Balziva, 540
Banophen, 432
Banophen Caplets, 432
Baraclude, 490
Barbiturates, 61–62
adverse reactions misinterpreted as age-related
changes, 1392t–1393t
drug interactions with,
1362t–1363t
Baridium, 1014
Barium examination, lactulose
to induce bowel evacuation after, 744
Bartter's syndrome, indomethacin for, 694
Basal cell carcinoma, fluorouracil for, 585
basiliximab, **207–209**

Bayer Aspirin, 178
BayHep B, 657
BayRab, 1091
BayRho-D Full Dose, 1102
BayRho-D Mini-Dose, 1102
BayTet, 1219
BCNU, **270–271**
beclomethasone dipropionate,
209–210
beclomethasone dipropionate
monohydrate, **210–211**
Beconase AQ, 210
Bedoz ♦, 366
Beepen-VK, 1000
Beesix, 1078
Behavior disorders, haloperidol
for, 652
Bejel, penicillin G benzathine
for, 992
Beldin, 432
Bell/ans, 1155
Bemote, 419
Benadryl, 432
Benadryl 25, 432
Benadryl Kapseals, 432
benazepril hydrochloride, 40,
54, **212–213**, 1374
bendroflumethiazide, 1370
Benicar, 939
Benicar HCT, 1369
Benign prostatic hyperplasia
alfuzosin for, 120
doxazosin for, 456
dutasteride for, 473
finasteride for, 574
tamsulosin for, 1199
terazosin for, 1211
Bentyl, 419
Bentylol ♦, 419
Benuryl ◊, 1056
Benylin Adult, 412
Benylin Cough, 432
Benylin Pediatric, 412
Benzodiazepine reversal,
flumazenil for, 583
Benzodiazepines, adverse reactions misinterpreted as
age-related changes,
1392t–1393t
benztropine mesylate, 46, 58,
213–215
benzylpenicillin benzathine,
992–994
benzylpenicillin potassium,
994–996
benzylpenicillin procaine,
996–998
benzylpenicillin sodium,
998–1000
Beriberi, thiamine for,
1225–1226

---

t refers to a table; **boldface** refers to the drug's monograph; ***boldface italic*** refers to a full-color photograph.

---

t refers to a table; **boldface** refers to the drug's monograph; *boldface italic* refers to a full-color photograph.

---

t refers to a table; **boldface** refers to the drug's monograph; ***boldface italic*** refers to a full-color photograph.

Fero-Gradumet, 569
Ferretts, 569
Ferrlecit, 1158
ferrous fumarate, 72, **569–571**
ferrous gluconate, 72, **569–571**
ferrous sulfate, 72, **569–571**
ferrous sulfate, dried, **569–571**
Fertinic◆, 569
Fetal distress, oxytocin, synthetic injection, for assessment of, 963
Fever
acetaminophen for, 99
aspirin for, 178
ibuprofen for, 674
ketoprofen for, 737
FeverAll Children's, 99
FeverAll Infants, 99
FeverAll Junior Strength, 99
feverfew, **1345**
drug interactions with, 1385t
fexofenadine hydrochloride,
53, **571–572**
Fibrinogen, plasma, 1396t
Fibrositis, cyclobenzaprine for,
368
filgrastim, **572–574**
finasteride, **574–575**
Fioricet with Codeine, 1372
Flagyl, 850
Flagyl 375, 850
Flagyl ER, 850
Flagyl I.V. RTU, 850
Flatulence, activated charcoal
for, 105
Flavorcee, 1314
flax, **1345**
flecainide acetate, 44,
575–577
Fleet Bisacodyl, 222
Fleet Enema, 1160
Fleet Laxative, 222
Fleet Pediatric Enema, 1160
Fleet Phospho-soda, 1160
Fleet Prep Kit, 222
Flexeril, 368
Flomax, 1199
Flonase, 593
Florical, 254
Florinef, 582
Flovent Diskus◆, 593
Flovent HFA, 593
Flovent Inhalation Aerosol, 593
Flow rates, calculation of, 10
Floxin, 934
Floxin Otic, 934
fluconazole, **577–579**
flucytosine, **579–580**
Fludara, 580
fludarabine phosphate, 57,
580–582

fludrocortisone acetate, 67,
582–583
drug interactions with,
1360t–1361t
flumazenil, **583–585**
FluMist, 698
5-fluorocytosine, **579–580**
Fluoroplex, 585
fluorouracil, 57, **585–587**
5-fluorouracil, **585–587**
fluoxetine hydrochloride,
587–589, 1376
drug interactions with,
1362t–1365t
fluphenazine, 80
fluphenazine decanoate,
589–591
fluphenazine hydrochloride,
589–591
flurazepam hydrochloride,
591–592
Flushing, octreotide for, 933
flutamide, **592–593**
fluticasone propionate,
593–596
fluticasone propionate and salmeterol inhalation powder,
596–599
fluvastatin sodium, 56,
599–600
drug interactions with,
1362t–1363t
fluvoxamine maleate, **601–602**
drug interactions with,
1364t–1365t
Focalin, 405
Focalin XR, 405
folic acid, **602–604**
Folic acid antagonist overdose,
leucovorin for, 755
Folic acid deficiency, folic acid
for, 602, 603
folinic acid, **755–756**
Follicular lymphoma
chlorambucil for, 309
interferon alfa for, 712
Folvite, 602
fondaparinux sodium, 47,
604–606
Foradil Aerolizer, 606
formoterol fumarate inhalation
powder, **606–608**
Formulex◆, 419
Fortamet, 827
Fortaz, 293
Forteo, 1213
Fosamax, 119
Fosamax Plus D, 119
fosamprenavir calcium, 60,
608–610
foscarnet sodium, 60, **610–612**

Foscavir, 610
fosinopril sodium, 40, 54,
612–613, 1375
fosphenytoin sodium, 48,
613–615
Fraction method for dosage
calculation, 5–6
Fracture healing, vitamin C for,
1314
Fragmin, 382
Frilone, 1270
Frova, 615, **C8**
frovatriptan succinate,
615–617
frusemide, **618–620**
5-FU, **585–587**
fulvestrant, **617–618**
Fumasorb, 569
Fumerin, 569
Fungal infection
amphotericin B desoxy-
cholate for, 151
amphotericin B lipid complex
for, 153
amphotericin B liposomal
for, 155
caspofungin for, 274
fluconazole for, 577
flucytosine for, 579
itraconazole for, 732
ketoconazole for, 735
micafungin for, 854
nystatin for, 931
sertaconazole for, 1141
voriconazole for, 1319
Fungizone, 151
Furadantin, 917
Furalan, 917
furosemide, 68, **618–620**
Furoside◆, 618
Fusarium infection, voriconazole for, 1319
Fuzeon, 485

G

gabapentin, 48, **620–622**
Gabitril, 1234
Galactorrhea, bromocriptine
for, 235
galantamine hydrobromide,
622–624
Gallstones, ursodiol for, 1288
gamma globulin, **688–690**
ganciclovir, 60, **624–626**
ganirelix acetate, **626–627**
Garamycin, 635
garlic, **1345–1346**
drug interactions with, 1385t
Gastric cancer
doxorubicin for, 460
fluorouracil for, 585

Orthopedic manipulations,
succinylcholine for, 1178
Orthopedic surgery
dalteparin for, 382
enoxaparin for, 487
fondaparinux for, 604
Orthostatic hypotension, flu-
drocortisone for, 582
Ortho Tri-Cyclen, 540
Ortho Tri-Cyclen Lo, 540
Orthovisc, 658
Or-Tyl, 419
Orudis, 737
Orudis-E ♦, 737
Orudis KT, 737
Orudis SR ♦ ◊, 737
Oruvail, 737
Os-Cal, 254
Os-Cal 500 ♦, 254
Os-Cal Chewable ♦, 254
oseltamivir phosphate, 60,
949–950
Osmitrol, 801
Osteitis deformans. *See*
Paget's disease of bone
Osteoarthritis
acetaminophen for, 99
celecoxib for, 302
diclofenac for, 417
diflunisal for, 423
etodolac for, 553
high–molecular-weight
hyaluronan for, 658
ibuprofen for, 673
indomethacin for, 693
ketoprofen for, 737
meloxicam for, 811
nabumetone for, 889
naproxen for, 897
oxaprozin for, 953
sulindac for, 1187
Osteogenesis imperfecta, calcitonin (salmon) for, 251
Osteolytic bone lesions,
pamidronate for, 972
Osteomyelitis, nafcillin for, 891
Osteopetrosis, interferon gam-
ma-1b for, 716
Osteoporosis
alendronate for, 119
calcitonin (salmon) for, 251
ibandronate for, 672
raloxifene for, 1092
risedronate for, 1112
teriparatide (rDNA origin) for,
1213
Osteoporosis prevention
alendronate for, 119
estradiol and norgestimate
for, 524

Osteoporosis prevention
(continued)
estradiol for, 521
estrogens, conjugated, for,
527
estrogens, esterified, for,
529
estropipate for, 531
Osteosarcoma
cisplatin for, 333
methotrexate for, 834
Otic drug administration,
28–29
Otitis externa, ofloxacin for,
935
Otitis media
amoxicillin and clavulanate
potassium for, 147
azithromycin for, 201
cefaclor for, 275
cefdinir for, 280
cefixime for, 283
cefpodoxime for, 290
cefprozil for, 292
ceftibuten for, 295
ceftriaxone for, 298
cefuroxime for, 300
cephalexin for, 305
clarithromycin for, 337
co-trimoxazole for, 364
loracarbef for, 787
ofloxacin for, 935
trimethoprim for, 1281
Ovarian cancer
carboplatin for, 267
chlorambucil for, 309
cisplatin for, 333
cyclophosphamide for, 369
doxorubicin for, 460
doxorubicin hydrochloride liposomal for, 463
ifosfamide for, 678
melphalan for, 813
paclitaxel for, 964
thiotepa for, 1229
topotecan for, 1257
Ovarian failure
estradiol for, 521
estrogens, conjugated, for,
527
estrogens, esterified, for,
529
estropipate for, 531
Ovarian hyperstimulation, inhibition of luteinizing hormone surges during,
ganirelix for, 626
Ovcon-35, 540
Ovcon-50, 540

Overactive bladder
darifenacin for, 389
oxybutynin for, 958
solifenacin for, 1164
tolterodine for, 1254
trospium for, 1284
Ovral, 540
Ovulation stimulation
clomiphene for, 344
tamoxifen for, 1197
oxacillin sodium, 78
drug interactions with,
1362t–1363t
oxaliplatin, **951–953**
oxaprozin potassium, 75,
953–954
oxazepam, **954–956**
oxcarbazepine, 48, **956–958**
oxybutynin chloride, **958–959**
oxycodone hydrochloride, 76,
960–961
in combination drug prod-
ucts, 1371–1372, 1375,
1376, 1378
oxycodone pectinate, **960–961**
oxycodone terephthalate, 1372
OxyContin, 960, *C12*
Oxydess II, 410
Oxydose, 960
OxyFAST, 960
OxyIR, 960
oxymorphone hydrochloride,
961–962
OxyNorm ◊, 960
oxytetracycline hydrochloride,
83
oxytocin, synthetic injection,
962–964
Oxytocin challenge test, oxytocin, synthetic injection,
for, 963
Oxytrol, 958
Oysco, 254
Oysco 500 Chewable, 254
Oyst-Cal 500, 254
Oystercal 500, 254
Oyster Shell Calcium-500, 254

P
Pacerone, 139
paclitaxel, **964–966**
paclitaxel protein-bound particles, **966–968**
Paget's disease of bone
alendronate for, 119
calcitonin (salmon) for, 251
pamidronate for, 972
risedronate for, 1112
Pain
acetaminophen for, 99
amitriptyline for, 142

---

t refers to a table; **boldface** refers to the drug's monograph; *boldface italic* refers to a full-color photograph.

---

t refers to a table; **boldface** refers to the drug's monograph; ***boldface italic*** refers to a full-color photograph.

---

t refers to a table; **boldface** refers to the drug's monograph; *boldface italic* refers to a full-color photograph.
